Immunologic Disorders in Infants & Children

Immunologic Disorders in Infants & Children

4th Edition

E. Richard Stiehm, MD
Chief, Division of Immunology/Allergy
UCLA Department of Pediatrics
Professor of Pediatrics
University of California School of Medicine
Los Angeles, California

W.B. SAUNDERS COMPANY
A Division of Harcourt Brace & Company
Philadelphia • London • Toronto • Montreal • Sydney • Tokyo

W.B. SAUNDERS COMPANY
A Division of Harcourt Brace & Company

The Curtis Center
Independence Square West
Philadelphia, Pennsylvania 19106

Library of Congress Cataloging-in-Publication Data

Immunologic disorders in infants and children/[edited by] E. Richard
Stiehm.—4th ed.

p.   cm.

Includes bibliographical references and index.

ISBN 0–7216–4948–3

1. Immunologic diseases in children.   2. Developmental
immunology.   I. Stiehm, E. Richard   [DNLM: 1. Immunologic
Diseases—in infancy & childhood.   WD 300 I324 1996]

RJ385.I46 1996

618.92'97—dc20

DNLM/DLC   95–8333

Immunologic Disorders in Infants and Children, Fourth Edition   ISBN 0–7216–4948–3

Printed in the United States of America.

Last digit is the print number: 9   8   7   6   5   4   3   2   1

Dedication of the 4th Edition

To my University of Wisconsin mentors,
Harold F. Deutsch
and
Robert F. Schilling,
and colleagues
Arthur J. Ammann
and
Richard Hong.

Dedication of the First Edition

To
Marie D. Stiehm,
Judith H. Stiehm,
and Jamie, Carrie, and Meredith
and to
John and Rose Fulginiti,
Shirley L. Fulginiti,
and John, Jeff, Laura, and Paul.

Preface to the First Edition

Twenty-five years ago, the thymus was a mystery organ that was irradiated for respiratory stridor, organ transplantation was science fiction, a gamma globulin determination was a sophisticated research effort, the function of the lymphocyte was not known, and the immunodeficiencies were not yet discovered. Since then a bountiful harvest of immunologic information has been gathered by the combined efforts of physicians, biochemists, microbiologists, pathologists, and other scientists. A significant portion has relevance to human health and disease and has been collected under the heading of clinical immunology. This book is concerned with the clinical immunology of infancy and childhood.

Like other specialty fields, clinical pediatric immunology is primarily concerned with a specific group of related illnesses necessitating special investigative procedures—the primary immunodeficiency diseases. Unlike most other specialties, pediatric immunology widens its horizons to include such related areas as collagen diseases, infectious diseases, allergies, transplantation, and immunization procedures. Further, the field encompasses many aspects of endocrine, hematologic, renal, neurologic, gastrointestinal, and malignant diseases, and thus it is especially attractive to the physician who enjoys the entire scope of pediatric medicine. In sum, pediatric immunology has some relevance and contribution to the whole of pediatrics.

This book has been written by men and women from 18 universities in North America and Europe whose own careers have been devoted to some aspect of clinical immunology. Writing with both the specialist and the generalist in mind, the contributors have combined the basic knowledge of the immunologic system with clinical descriptions of immunologic disorders.

The book begins with the development and biology of the immune response and the components of the immunologic system (Part One), continues with a detailed exposition of the immunodeficiencies (Part Two), and concludes with a group of chapters detailing the immunologic aspects of various pediatric disorders (Part Three). Included in Part One is a review by Dr. Robert Good of the major experiments in nature which have served as the impetus for the advances in clinical immunology.

The terminology employed for the immunoglobulin classes, complement components, and immunodeficiencies is that recommended by the World Health Organization. The terminology for the primary immunodeficiencies has only recently been codified, and since many eponyms are well established in the literature (e.g., Wiskott-Aldrich syndrome), we have added these to avoid ambiguity. Except in the section on immunodeficiences (Part Two), no attempt has been made to present complete bibliographies. In the other sections, key references to summary and review articles are often used.

A suitable subtitle for a primarily American work on pediatric immunology might be "A Tale of Two Cities." The cities are not London and Paris in the 1780's but Minneapolis and Boston in the 1960's. The pediatric departments of the University of Minnesota and Harvard, under the leadership of Good, Janeway, and Gitlin, have provided much of the information in this volume and served as the training grounds for many of the contributors. Others, including the editors, have indirectly benefited from the stimulation from these centers. In 1859 Dickens stated about the 1780's that "It was the best of times, it was the worst of times." In 1973, it is the best of times for physicians concerned with the exciting and challenging aspects of immunologic disorders; for most patients, it is still the worst of times, because, with rare exceptions, therapy is unrewarding. The outlook should be bright; one large cloud is the diminution of support for the further exposition of this subject.

The skilled secretarial assistance of Mrs. Paulette Stroehnisch and Mrs. Donna Keller is acknowledged. The editorial guidance of Mr. Albert Meier and Mr. Michael Jackson of the W. B. Saunders Company is greatly appreciated.

E. Richard Stiehm
Vincent A. Fulginiti

Preface to the 4th Edition

This volume, first published in 1973 and now appearing as Edition 4, might be subtitled "The 7-Year Itch." In the first 3 years between editions, the itch is in remission; in the next 3 years, the itch intensifies; and in the final year, it is all-consuming—but suddenly relieved by publication! Despite the itch, the personal advantage of editing a text in a fast-moving field is the knowledge gained by reading and reviewing each sentence of each chapter. Indeed, I believe this is the only medical text I have read cover to cover since medical school.

Editing is a unique way to learn; it is more intense than reading, more specific than listening, more efficient than lecturing, and more encompassing than writing. During this process, I was amazed at how much I learned and how much I did not at first understand. In the latter situation, the authors were cajoled into shortening, clarifying, or simplifying. The aim was to make the book understandable to the practicing pediatrician, to pediatric residents and fellows, and to medical students with a minimal background in immunology.

As in previous editions, the book is subdivided into three parts: Development and Function of the Immune System (Chapters 1 to 8), Immunodeficiency Disorders (Chapters 9 to 19), and Immunologic Aspects of Pediatric Illnesses (Chapters 20 to 32). Within each part, new authors (32), new topics (many), and new chapters (2) have been added. Appendices on leukocyte CD (cluster designation) antigens and cytokines have also been added.

In Chapters 2, 3, and 4, the interaction of the cells of the immune system is outlined in considerably more detail and complexity than in previous editions, mostly because of new knowledge of cell surface antigens, recently discovered cytokines, and the identification of adhesion molecules. New material on the molecular biology of antibody synthesis has been added to Chapter 3, and a new section on dendritic cells has been added to Chapter 6. Much information on the secretory immune system, including breast milk and the enteromammary circulation, has been added to Chapter 8.

The most extensive changes are present in Part II. The functional defects of the immature immune system are outlined in detail in Chapter 10. Chapters 11 through 19 describe 47 primary and 35 secondary immunodeficiencies as listed in the World Health Organization Classification. The genes for several of these diseases have recently been identified (e.g., X-linked agammaglobulinemia, the hyper-IgM syndrome), and the texts on pathogenesis reflect these findings. Other syndromes have been subdivided into distinct clinical entities (e.g., severe combined immunodeficiency and chronic granulomatous disease), which are explained. New treatments such as gene therapy, cytokine administration, and transplantation are discussed. A new chapter (Chapter 18) devoted to pediatric HIV infection, including its virology, immunology, clinical manifestations, and treatment, has been included.

Part III includes a new chapter (Chapter 21) on dermatologic disorders and expanded coverage of hematologic disorders, including malignancy in immunodeficiency states. New therapies, such as methotrexate for arthritis, intravenous immunoglobulin for Kawasaki disease, and oral tolerance for multiple sclerosis, are discussed. The information on pediatric transplantation (Chapter 32) is completely updated and includes a worldwide survey of bone marrow transplantation for primary immunodeficiencies.

I wish to acknowledge the assistance of several colleagues who made important contributions to the success of the first three editions of this book but are not represented in Edition 4. These include Arthur Ammann of the University of California, San Francisco, now scientific director of The Pediatric AIDS Foundation; Alfred Michael of the University of Minnesota; Leslie Weiner of the University of Southern California; and the late Michael Miller of the University of California, Davis.

I also wish to acknowledge several authors who are long-term "survivors" (i.e., contributors) of all four editions. These include Per Brandtzaeg, Rebecca Buckley, Max Cooper, Alfred Fish, Lars Hanson, Richard Hong, Alexander Lawton, David Pearlman, Paul Quie, and Jane Schaller. Their early contributions were so valuable that I have asked them over and over to rewrite their respective chapters. Among these, Richard Hong bears special thanks; he has authored or coauthored nine chapters in four editions, including the very complex and detailed chapters on T-cell immunodeficiencies.

Finally, the support of W.B. Saunders, and particularly Judith Fletcher, Medical Editor, and Carol Robins, Senior Copy Editor, is acknowledged. I also want to thank my assistants Deborah Kutnik and Jennifer Kwon for devoted help. Their patience and hard work contributed greatly to this effort and helped to alleviate the "7-year itch."

E. RICHARD STIEHM

Contributors

Jon S. Abramson, M.D.
Professor and Vice-Chairman, Department of Pediatrics, Bowman Gray School of Medicine of Wake Forest University. Attending Staff, North Carolina Baptist Hospital, Winston-Salem, North Carolina.
The Polymorphonuclear Leukocyte System

Melvin Berger, M.D., Ph.D.
Professor of Pediatrics, Case Western Reserve University. Chief, Immunology/Allergy Division, Department of Pediatrics, Rainbow Babies and Children's Hospital and University Hospitals of Cleveland, Cleveland, Ohio.
The Serum Complement System

C. Warren Bierman, M.D.
Clinical Professor of Pediatrics, University of Washington School of Medicine. Co-director of Allergy Training Program. Chief, Division of Allergy, Children's Hospital Medical Center, Seattle, Washington.
Allergic Disorders

Athos Bousvaros, M.D.
Instructor, Department of Pediatrics, Harvard Medical School, and Division of Gastroenterology, Children's Hospital, Boston, Massachusetts.
Gastroenterologic and Liver Disorders

Per Brandtzaeg, Ph.D.
Professor of Pathology, The Medical Faculty, University of Oslo. Chief, Laboratory for Immunohistochemistry and Immunopathology (LIIPAT), The National Hospital of Norway, Rikshospitalet, Oslo, Norway.
The Mucosal Defense System

Jonathan Braun, M.D., Ph.D.
Associate Professor, Department of Pathology and Laboratory Medicine, UCLA School of Medicine, Los Angeles, California.
The B-Lymphocyte System

Rebecca H. Buckley, M.D.
J. Buren Sidbury Professor of Pediatrics and Immunology, Duke University School of Medicine. Chief, Division of Allergy and Immunology, Department of Pediatrics, Duke University Medical Center, Durham, North Carolina.
Disorders of the IgE System; Transplantation

James D. Cherry, M.D., M.Sc.
Professor of Pediatrics and Chief, Division of Pediatric Infectious Diseases, University of California School of Medicine. Attending Physician, UCLA Medical Center, Los Angeles, California.
Infection in the Compromised Host

Loran T. Clement, M.D.
Professor of Pediatrics, University of California School of Medicine, Los Angeles, California.
Cellular Interactions in the Human Immune Response; Disorders of the T-Cell System

Mary Ellen Conley, M.D.
Professor of Pediatrics (Federal Express Professor of Pediatrics), University of Tennessee College of Medicine. Director, Program in Genetic Immunodeficiencies, St. Jude Children's Research Hospital, Memphis, Tennessee.
Immunodeficiency Disorders: General Considerations

Max D. Cooper, M.D.
Professor of Medicine, Pediatrics, and Microbiology, University of Alabama at Birmingham. Investigator, Howard Hughes Medical Institute, Birmingham, Alabama.
Ontogeny of Immunity

Charlotte Cunningham-Rundles, M.D., Ph.D.
Professor of Pediatrics, Medicine, and Biochemistry, Mount Sinai Medical Center, New York, New York.
Disorders of the IgA System

Steven D. Douglas, M.D.
Professor of Pediatrics and Microbiology, University of Pennsylvania School of Medicine. Section Chief for Immunology and Director, Clinical Immunology Laboratory, The Children's Hospital of Philadelphia, Philadelphia, Pennnsylvania.
The Mononuclear Phagocyte and Dendritic Cell Systems; Disorders of the Mononuclear Phagocytic System

Ralph D. Feigin, M.D.
J. S. Abercrombie Professor of Pediatrics and Chairman of the Department of Pediatrics, Baylor College of Medicine. Physician-in-Chief, Texas Children's Hospital, and Pediatrics Service, Harris County Hospital District, and Chief, Pediatric Service, The Methodist Hospital, Houston, Texas.
Infection in the Compromised Host

Alexandra H. Filipovich, M.D.
Professor of Pediatrics, University of Minnesota
Medical School. Director of Pediatric Immunology,
University of Minnesota Hospitals and Clinics,
Minneapolis, Minnesota.
*Immune-Mediated Hematologic and Oncologic Disorders,
Including Epstein-Barr Virus Infection*

Terri H. Finkel, M.D., Ph.D.
Associate Professor, University of Colorado Medical
School. Associate Member, National Jewish Center
for Immunology and Respiratory Medicine, Denver,
Colorado.
The T-Lymphocyte System

Alfred J. Fish, M.D.
Professor of Pediatrics, University of Minnesota,
Department of Pediatrics, Division of Nephrology,
Minneapolis, Minnesota.
Renal Disorders

John O. Fleming, M.D.
Professor, Department of Neurology and
Department of Medical Microbiology and
Immunology, University of Wisconsin. Director,
Multiple Sclerosis Clinic, University of Wisconsin
Hospital and Clinics, Madison, Wisconsin.
Immunologic Diseases of the Nervous System

Michael M. Frank, M.D.
Professor and Chairman, Department of Pediatrics,
Duke University. Staff, Duke Children's Hospital,
Duke University Medical Center, Durham, North
Carolina.
The Serum Complement System

Richard A. Gatti, M.D.
Professor, University of California School of
Medicine, Los Angeles, California.
Disorders of the T-Cell System

Erwin W. Gelfand, M.D.
Professor of Pediatrics and Microbiology/
Immunology, University of Colorado Medical
School. Chairman, Pediatrics, National Jewish
Center for Immunology and Respiratory Medicine,
Denver, Colorado.
The T-Lymphocyte System

Janis V. Giorgi, Ph.D.
Professor of Medicine, University of California
School of Medicine, Los Angeles, California.
*Appendix 1: Cluster Designation Nomenclature for
Human Leukocyte Differentiation Antigens*

Randall M. Goldblum, M.D.
Professor, Departments of Pediatrics and Human
Biological Chemistry and Genetics, University of
Texas Medical Branch, University of Texas Medical
School at Galveston, Galveston, Texas.
The Mucosal Defense System

Thomas Gross, M.D., Ph.D.
Assistant Professor of Pediatrics and Pathology and
Microbiology, University of Nebraska Medical
School. Staff, University of Nebraska Medical
Center, Omaha, Nebraska.
*Immune-Mediated Hematologic and Oncologic Disorders,
Including Epstein-Barr Virus Infection*

Jon M. Hanifin, M.D.
Professor of Dermatology, Oregon Health Sciences
University, Portland, Oregon.
Dermatologic Disorders

Lars Å. Hanson, M.D., Ph.D.
Professor and Chairman, Department of Clinical
Immunology, University of Göteborg. Physician-in-
Chief, Clinical Immunology Laboratory, Sahlgren's
Hospital, Göteborg, Sweden.
The Mucosal Defense System

Richard Hong, M.D.
Professor of Pediatrics, University of Vermont
College of Medicine. Attending Physician, Fletcher-
Allen Health Care, Burlington, Vermont.
Disorders of the T-Cell System

Richard B. Johnston, Jr., M.D.
Adjunct Professor and Chief, Section of
Immunology, Department of Pediatrics, Yale
University School of Medicine, New Haven,
Connecticut. Medical Director, March of Dimes
Birth Defects Foundation, White Plains, New York.
Disorders of the Complement System

Harumi Jyonouchi, M.D.
Assistant Professor of Pediatrics, University of
Minnesota Medical School. Staff, University of
Minnesota Hospital and Clinics, Minneapolis,
Minnesota.
*Immune-Mediated Hematologic and Oncologic Disorders,
Including Epstein-Barr Virus Infection*

Naynesh R. Kamani, M.D.
Director, Division of Clinical Immunology, and
Associate Director, Bone Marrow Transplant
Program, Miami Children's Hospital, Miami,
Florida.
Disorders of the Mononuclear Phagocytic System

Gerald T. Keusch, M.D.
Professor of Medicine, Tufts University School of
Medicine. Chief, Division of Geographic Medicine
and Infectious Diseases, New England Medical
Center, Boston, Massachusetts.
Immunologic Mechanisms in Infectious Diseases

Charles H. Kirkpatrick, M.D.
Professor of Medicine and Immunology, Division of
Allergy and Clinical Immunology, University of
Colorado School of Medicine. Director of Research,
Innovative Therapeutics, Inc., Denver, Colorado.
Disorders of the T-Cell System

Mark W. Kline, M.D.
Associate Professor of Pediatrics, Baylor College of Medicine. Attending Physician, Texas Children's Hospital, Houston, Texas.
The Secondary Immunodeficiencies; Active and Passive Immunization in the Prevention of Infectious Diseases

Alexander R. Lawton, M.D.
Edward C. Stahlman Professor of Pediatric Physiology and Cell Metabolism and Professor of Microbiology and Immunology, Vanderbilt University School of Medicine, Nashville, Tennessee.
Ontogeny of Immunity

David B. Lewis, M.D.
Associate Professor of Pediatrics, University of Washington. Attending Staff, Children's Hospital and Medical Center, Seattle, Washington.
The Physiologic Immunodeficiency of Immaturity

Noel K. MacLaren, M.D.
Professor and Chairman, Department of Pathology, and Professor of Pediatrics, University of Florida College of Medicine. Chief, Department of Pathology and Laboratory Medicine, Shands Teaching Hospital, Gainesville, Florida.
Autoimmune Endocrinopathies

Laurie C. Miller, M.D.
Assistant Professor of Pediatrics, Tufts University School of Medicine. Attending Pediatric Rheumatologist, The Floating Hospital for Children at New England Medical Center, Boston, Massachusetts.
Rheumatic Disorders

Elaine L. Mills, M.D.
Associate Professor, Departments of Pediatrics and Microbiology and Immunology, McGill University. Director, Division of Infectious Diseases, Montreal Children's Hospital, Montreal, Quebec, Canada.
Disorders of the Polymorphonuclear Phagocytic System

Lynne Morrison, M.D.
Assistant Professor of Dermatology, Oregon Health Sciences University, Portland, Oregon.
Dermatologic Disorders

Francisco J. D. Noya, M.D.
Assistant Professor of Pediatrics, McGill University. Pediatrician, Montreal Children's Hospital, Montreal, Quebec, Canada.
Disorders of the Polymorphonuclear Phagocytic System

Hans D. Ochs, M.D.
Professor of Pediatrics, University of Washington. Chief, Immunology Clinic, Children's Hospital and Medical Center, Seattle, Washington.
Disorders of the B-Cell System

David S. Pearlman, M.D.
Clinical Professor of Pediatrics, University of Colorado Medical School. Associate, Colorado Allergy and Asthma Clinic, PC, Denver, Colorado.
Allergic Disorders

Laurie A. Penix, M.D.
Assistant Professor of Pediatrics, Yale University School of Medicine, New Haven, Connecticut.
The Physiologic Immunodeficiency of Immaturity

John K. Pfaff, M.D.
Staff Pulmonologist, Naval Medical Center, Department of Pediatrics, Portsmouth, Virginia.
Pulmonary Disorders

Philip A. Pizzo, M.D.
Professor of Pediatrics, Uniformed Services University of the Health Sciences, F. Edward Hébert School of Medicine. Chief of Pediatrics and Head, Infectious Disease Section, National Cancer Institute, National Institutes of Health, Bethesda, Maryland.
Pediatric Human Immunodeficiency Virus Infection

Susan F. Plaeger, Ph.D.
Associate Professor of Pediatrics, University of California School of Medicine. Associate Director, Clinical Immunology Research Laboratory, UCLA Medical Center, Los Angeles, California.
Appendix 2: Principal Human Cytokines

Paul G. Quie, M.D.
Regent's Professor of Pediatrics, University of Minnesota School of Medicine. Attending Physician, University of Minnesota Hospital, Minneapolis, Minnesota.
The Polymorphonuclear Leukocyte System; Disorders of the Polymorphonuclear Phagocytic System

Robert L. Roberts, M.D., Ph.D.
Assistant Professor of Pediatrics, University of California School of Medicine, Los Angeles, California.
Disorders of the Polymorphonuclear Phagocytic System

Robert S. Rust, M.D.
Assistant Professor of Neurology and Pediatrics, University of Wisconsin. Director of Child Neurology, University of Wisconsin Hospitals and Clinics, Madison, Wisconsin.
Immunologic Diseases of the Nervous System

Eric T. Sandberg, M.D.
Formerly, Assistant Professor, Department of Pediatrics, Baylor College of Medicine. Physician, Kelsey-Seybold Clinic. Staff, Texas Children's Hospital, Houston, Texas.
The Secondary Immunodeficiencies

Jane G. Schaller, M.D.
Professor and Chairman, Department of Pediatrics, Tufts University School of Medicine. Pediatrician-in-Chief, The Floating Hospital for Children at New England Medical Center, Boston, Massachusetts.
Rheumatic Disorders

Ralph S. Shapiro, M.D.
Assistant Professor of Pediatrics, University of Minnesota Medical School. Staff, University of Minnesota Hospital and Clinics, Minneapolis, Minnesota.
Immune-Mediated Hematologic and Oncologic Disorders, Including Epstein-Barr Virus Infection

William T. Shearer, M.D., Ph.D.
Professor of Pediatrics and Microbiology and Immunology, Baylor College of Medicine. Chief, Allergy and Immunology Service, Texas Children's Hospital, Houston, Texas.
The Secondary Immunodeficiencies; Active and Passive Immunization in the Prevention of Infectious Diseases

E. Richard Stiehm, M.D.
Professor of Pediatrics, and Chief, Division of Immunology/Allergy, University of California School of Medicine. Attending Pediatrician, UCLA Medical Center, Los Angeles, California.
The B-Lymphocyte System; Immunodeficiency Disorders: General Considerations

Lynn M. Taussig, M.D.
Professor of Pediatrics, University of Colorado School of Medicine. President and CEO, National Jewish Center for Immunology and Respiratory Medicine, Denver, Colorado.
Pulmonary Disorders

Lori B. Tucker, M.D.
Assistant Professor of Pediatrics, Tufts University School of Medicine. Pediatric Rheumatologist, The Floating Hospital for Children at New England Medical Center, Boston, Massachusetts.
Rheumatic Disorders

Gareth Tudor-Williams, M.R.C.P.
Visiting Scientist, Pediatric Branch, National Cancer Institute, National Institutes of Health, Bethesda, Maryland.
Pediatric Human Immunodeficiency Virus Infection

Beth A. Vogt, M.D.
Assistant Professor of Pediatrics, Case Western Reserve University School of Medicine. Attending Physician, Rainbow Babies and Children's Hospital, Division of Pediatric Nephrology, Cleveland, Ohio.
Renal Disorders

W. Allan Walker, M.D.
Conrad Taff Professor of Nutrition and Pediatrics, Harvard Medical School. Professor of Nutrition, Harvard School of Public Health. Chief, Combined Program in Pediatric Gastroenterology and Nutrition, Children's Hospital and Massachusetts General Hospital, Boston, Massachusetts.
Gastroenterologic and Liver Disorders

J. Gary Wheeler, M.D.
Associate Professor of Pediatrics, Divisions of Infectious Diseases, Allergy, and Clinical Immunology, University of Arkansas for Medical Sciences. Attending Staff, Arkansas Children's Hospital, Little Rock, Arkansas.
The Polymorphonuclear Leukocyte System

Christopher B. Wilson, M.D.
Professor of Pediatrics and Immunology, University of Washington. Head, Division of Infectious Diseases, Immunology, and Rheumatology, Children's Hospital Medical Center, Seattle, Washington.
The Physiologic Immunodeficiency of Immaturity

Jerry Winkelstein, M.D.
Professor of Pediatrics and Molecular Microbiology and Immunology, Johns Hopkins University. Director, Division of Allergy and Immunology, Johns Hopkins Hospital, Baltimore, Maryland.
Disorders of the B-Cell System

William Ernest Winter, M.D.
Associate Professor, Department of Pathology and Laboratory Medicine, University of Florida, Gainesville, Florida.
Autoimmune Endocrinopathies

Mervin C. Yoder, M.D.
Associate Professor of Pediatrics and Biochemistry and Molecular Biology, Indiana University School of Medicine. Attending Neonatologist, James Whitcomb Riley Hospital for Children, Indiana University Medical Center, Indianapolis, Indiana.
The Mononuclear Phagocyte and Dendritic Cell Systems

Contents

PART I

DEVELOPMENT AND FUNCTION OF THE IMMUNE SYSTEM

Chapter 1

Ontogeny of Immunity

Alexander R. Lawton and Max D. Cooper

The cells of the immune system are derived from a relatively small pool of pluripotential hematopoietic stem cells (HSCs) present in the fetal liver, omentum, and ultimately the bone marrow. In response to inductive signals from specialized microenvironments, HSCs enter one of two major differentiation pathways. One generates several lineages of specialized effector cells, which constitute the innate immune system. These include the professional phagocytes (polymorphonuclear leukocytes, monocytes, and macrophages), specialized antigen-presenting cells (dendritic cells of germinal centers, Langerhans' cells of skin), and purveyors of the mediators of inflammation (mast cells, basophils, and eosinophils). The second pathway generates the two major classes of lymphocytes, T cells and B cells, which form the adaptive immune system.

Collectively, the lymphocytes of the adaptive immune system have the capacity to recognize specifically an almost limitless number of antigens; individually, each cell expresses one receptor (in the case of T cells, perhaps two receptors [Padovan et al., 1993]). In addition to having unique receptors, mature lymphoid cells have distinct effector functions ranging from the secretion of antibodies to the direct killing of other cells.

Lymphocytes express a variety of membrane molecules that determine their migration patterns and communicate signals to and from other lymphocytes. They also secrete soluble cytokines that regulate the functions of the cells of the innate immune system and of other lymphocytes. The result is a network of interacting cells that resembles the central nervous system in its organizational complexity and capacity for learning.

Each step in the developmental process that generates the lymphoid system is genetically controlled. The number of structural and regulatory genes involved is quite large; therefore, the potential for genetic defects resulting in abnormal function of the immune system is great. Just as the elucidation of enzymatic defects responsible for inborn errors of metabolism depends on the identification of each step in a metabolic pathway, understanding lymphoid differentiation defects requires appreciation of the sequence and regulation of normal lymphoid development. The study of the ontogeny of lymphocytes offers the great advantage of isolating some of the early events of their differentiation from the complex regulatory interactions occurring in mature animals.

In this chapter we describe the major steps in the

development of T and B lymphocytes. We briefly discuss the maturation of the integrated functions of these cells and the characteristics that distinguish the immune responses of the fetus and newborn from those of older children or adults.

T- AND B-CELL SYSTEMS

Lymphoid development occurs along two distinct pathways, leading to populations of cells that have different functions and phenotypic markers. The thymus is the induction site for T cells, which are responsible for those effector functions termed *cell-mediated immunity*. B cells, which are collectively responsible for the synthesis and secretion of humoral antibodies, constitute the second major limb of the lymphoid system. The name is derived from their primary developmental sites, the bursa of Fabricius in birds and bone marrow in mammals.

Surface Markers

Hematopoietic cells, including T and B cells, are identified and characterized in blood and tissues by labeled monoclonal antibodies that recognize some unique component of the cell membrane. An international committee assigns *cluster of differentiation* (CD) numbers to markers recognized by several different monoclonal antibodies that have uniform physical characteristics and cellular distribution. The number of CD molecules is increasing rapidly, as is knowledge of their structure and function. A list of CD designations and descriptions of the proteins they represent is included in Appendix 1 at the end of this book.

B lymphocytes are classically distinguished by the presence of surface immunoglobulin (Ig), predominantly of the IgM and IgD isotypes, and the B cell–specific glycoproteins CD19 and CD20. A number of membrane proteins recognized by widely available monoclonal antibodies are used to identify T cells. The predominant T-cell receptor (TCR) consists of a heterodimeric antigen recognition unit of α and β chains linked to a multichain signaling complex recognized by CD3 monoclonal antibodies. Included in this complex are coreceptor molecules CD4 and CD8 and the tyrosine phosphatase CD45. The last is found on all hematopoietic cells, but it is of particular importance because the expression of different isoforms distinguishes naive from memory T cells (Janeway, 1992). A much smaller T-cell population has an antigen recognition unit consisting of γ and δ chains and generally lacks CD4 and CD8.

A third class of lymphoid cells can be defined by the use of monoclonal antibodies. These are variously called null cells, natural killer (NK) cells, or large granular lymphocytes. These cells are nonphagocytic and lack the antigen-specific receptors of T or B cells, but they share both markers and some functions with macrophages and T cells. The ability to efficiently lyse antibody-coated target cells (antibody-dependent cellular cytotoxicity) and the capacity to kill certain target cells without prior sensitization (NK activity) are the important functions of these cells. Insight into the specificity of NK cells is now beginning to emerge (Moretta et al., 1992).

B and T cells are developmentally independent, have distinctive cell membrane characteristics, occupy different areas in lymphoid tissues, have different patterns of recirculation, and can be grouped into effectors of humoral and cellular immunity, respectively. This distinctiveness should not obscure the fact that these two systems use related gene families and common mechanisms for the generation of diverse receptors and are remarkably interrelated in terms of their functions. A discussion of the extent and mechanisms of these interactions is beyond the scope of this chapter. Nevertheless, we briefly outline some of the phenomena that are relevant to an understanding of the ontogeny of immunity.

T-Cell Subsets

T cells with αβ receptors are divided into two non-overlapping classes distinguished by expression of either CD4 or CD8 on the cell membrane. CD4 binds to conserved sites on class II proteins of the major histocompatibility complex (MHC); CD8 binds to class I MHC molecules. The receptors of CD4$^+$ T cells recognize foreign peptides derived from extracellular antigens that have been ingested and processed by professional antigen-presenting cells and are presented bound to MHC II molecules. CD8$^+$ T cells recognize peptides bound to MHC I molecules; these peptides are usually derived from proteins synthesized by the presenting cell. CD4$^+$ T cells perform as helpers for the differentiation of B cells and cytotoxic T cells and as activators of various cells of the innate immune system, such as macrophages and eosinophils. CD8$^+$ cells function as cytotoxic effectors. Because MHC I molecules are expressed by all nucleated cells and are associated on the cell surface with endogenously synthesized peptides, CD8$^+$ cells are particularly suited to recognize and destroy virus-infected cells and perhaps tumor cells.

CD4$^+$ cells are divisible into functional sets based on the patterns of cytokines they produce. Cells designated helper T1 (T$_H$1) produce interleukin (IL-2) and interferon (IFN-γ) as predominant cytokines and mediate delayed-type hypersensitivity reactions. Helper T2 (T$_H$2) cells produce mostly IL-4 and IL-5 and serve as helpers for B-cell differentiation. The development of T$_H$1 and T$_H$2 cells is a post-thymic, antigen-driven differentiation process. The type of T cell emerging from an encounter appears to be determined by properties of the antigen, the antigen-presenting cells, the cytokine environment, and the genetic background of the host (Mossman and Coffman, 1989; Sher and Coffman, 1992).

B- and T-Cell Cooperation

With few exceptions, the production of specific antibodies requires an interactive collaboration among antigen-presenting cells, T cells, and B cells. Professional antigen-presenting cells (phagocytic macrophages, follicular dendritic cells in the germinal centers of lymph nodes, and Langerhans' cells in the skin) ingest protein antigens and digest them into peptides. Relevant peptides are bound intracellularly to nascent class II MHC proteins and exported to the cell membrane. B lymphocytes are able to process soluble protein antigens and are extremely efficient in presenting the antigens recognized by their receptors (Lanzavecchia, 1990).

T cells become activated when their receptors bind to peptides residing in the groove of MHC molecules. Full activation of CD4[+] T cells requires a co-stimulatory signal delivered when the T-cell molecule CD28 reacts with members of a family of B7 molecules expressed by antigen-presenting cells and excited B cells (Freeman et al., 1993; Linsley and Ledbetter, 1993). Activated CD4[+] T cells transiently express a surface glycoprotein called CD40 ligand (CD40L), which binds to CD40 on B cells. The ligation of CD40 transmits a signal to B cells that makes them competent to proliferate, undergo isotype switching, and differentiate to antibody-secreting plasma cells (Noelle et al., 1992; Purkerson and Isakson, 1992). These last steps are driven by various cytokines, and it is these cytokines that determine which isotypes will be produced. For example, IL-4 directs switching to IgG1 and IgE, and IL-10 is needed for IgA synthesis (Defrance et al., 1992; Purkerson and Isakson, 1992).

T-cell regulation of the antibody response is also exerted in a negative sense. Mechanisms for T-cell suppression have eluded molecular definition, although the phenomenon is reproducible. The recognition that T cells differentiate into distinct subsets secreting groups of cytokines with opposing immunoregulatory effects is providing new ways of investigating this problem (Bloom et al., 1992).

B cells and their products, the antibody molecules, also serve both immunoregulatory and effector functions. A landmark in immunologic thought occurred with the publication in 1974 of Jerne's network theory of immune regulation. The network consists of idiotypes—unique antigenic determinants associated with the combining site of antibody molecules—and successive generations of auto–anti-idiotypic antibodies that they may provoke. The idea that immunization results in the production not only of antibodies but also of autologous anti-idiotypic antibodies and T cells has been verified in several species (Paul and Bona, 1982), including humans (Geha, 1983; Colley, 1990). Idiotypic regulation may be responsible for the amplification or the suppression of immune responses and is clearly one of the mechanisms by which T-cell immunity and B-cell immunity are linked. The expression of anti-idiotypic antibodies occurs in certain autoimmune diseases. For example, antibodies to the acetylcholine receptor found in patients with myasthenia gravis seem regularly to stimulate an anti-idiotypic response (Dwyer et al., 1983).

The importance of understanding these humoral and cellular interactions is potentially immense. There is much evidence that immunoregulatory abnormalities occur in immunodeficiency diseases, and autoimmunity is such a disorder by definition. Unraveling the mechanisms by which T-cell and B-cell interactions are responsible for the induction and maintenance of tolerance should eventually lead to ways of inducing specific tolerance to cellular antigens in humans; such an accomplishment would be an unparalleled advance in the field of organ transplantation. How some of these relationships play a role in the maturation of the immunologic capacity of the human fetus and newborn is discussed at the end of this chapter.

Stem Cell Compartment

All cells of the immune system are derived from pleuripotential hematopoietic stem cells, which are first found within the blood islands of the yolk sac. During embryogenesis, they migrate to other sites of hematopoiesis: the liver, spleen, and bone marrow. The bone marrow is the major repository of HSCs during adult life.

During the last decade, techniques have been developed for the isolation of both human and mouse HSCs and for their propagation in vitro (Golde, 1991). The more than 1000-fold enrichment of marrow stem cells has been accomplished by the combination of negative selection to remove lineage-committed cells and positive selection with monoclonal antibodies to stem-cell membrane proteins (Ikuta et al., 1992). Human progenitors express the CD34 glycoprotein. The long-term cultivation of stem cells is dependent on a combination of soluble growth factors and contact with a marrow-derived population of stromal cells (Dorshkind, 1990).

HSCs from the same highly enriched population can generate both T-cell and B-cell lineages following migration to the thymus or bone marrow, respectively. It remains to be established whether there is a committed lymphoid stem cell incapable of myeloid differentiation and whether independent precursors for T- and B-cell development exist (Ikuta et al., 1992).

T-CELL DEVELOPMENT

T-Cell Receptor (TCR) Diversity

The role of central lymphoid organs is the generation and education of large numbers of T and B cells having an immensely diverse repertoire of receptors for antigens. This process occurs throughout life but is the defining element of the ontogeny of immunity. The mechanisms for the generation of receptor diversity are described briefly here and in greater detail in Chapters 2 and 4.

T-cell and B-cell receptors for antigen are the products of related but distinct clusters of genes belonging to the large immunoglobulin gene superfamily. Receptor diversity is generated from relatively small sets of germline genes by DNA rearrangement. The same recombinase enzyme creates functional TCR and Ig receptor genes by a *looping out mechanism,* whereby the DNA separating two segments to be joined is deleted as a circle (Schatz et al., 1992). Seven extended loci of similarly organized genes arranged in tandem are involved in this recombinational process.

TCRs are of two types, $\alpha\beta$ and $\gamma\delta$. The $\alpha\beta$ types are expressed on the great majority of T cells. T cells with $\gamma\delta$ receptors are the first to appear in the thymus and may serve specialized functions. With regard to organization of their constituent genes, the α and δ chains are similar to immunoglobulin light chains, and the β and γ chains resemble heavy chains. The genes for the 90-kd TCR polypeptides are formed by recombination of gene segments called variable (V), diversity (D), joining (J), and constant (C). The β gene family consists of approximately 20 V_β genes, a set of D_β genes, and two sets of several J_β genes each associated with a C_β gene. The last are called $C_\beta 1$ and $C_\beta 2$. The α and δ gene families lack D genes but are otherwise similarly organized. The γ and δ families contain many fewer V genes than do the α and β families. Functional genes are generated by sequential rearrangements. To form a β gene, for example, a D_β gene is translocated and joined to one of the J_β genes. A second recombination links a V_β gene to that D-J segment and generates a functional transcriptional unit. Depending upon the J gene used, the chain will be of either the $\beta 1$ or $\beta 2$ type. A single V-J joining event creates functional α and δ genes.

Receptor diversity is created at several levels of this process, which is common to the TCR and immunoglobulin gene families. The V, D, and J genes inherited in the germline all contribute to the structure of the antigen-binding site, so that each possible combination of these units may produce a different specificity. The splice sites of D-J and V-D-J joints are imprecise and are also subject to the addition of random nucleotides by the enzyme terminal deoxynucleotidyltransferase (TdT). This mechanism, called *N diversity*, makes a particularly large contribution to the generation of diverse TCRs of the $\alpha\beta$ type. Finally, different combinations of α with β or of γ with δ chains produce distinct receptor specificities. The $\gamma\delta$ TCRs have a restricted repertoire because there are relatively few germline V genes in these families and because they do not use the N diversity mechanism (discussed in the next section).

These mechanisms create an immensely diverse repertoire of receptor specificities from relatively few inherited genes. Imprecise splicing of gene segments and the random addition of untemplated nucleotides produce diversity at the cost of generating a high proportion of defective genes resulting from changes in reading frames or from the introduction of stop codons. This cost is easily met by the production of an excess of lymphocytes in the thymus and bone marrow. Another certain consequence of these random processes is the production of receptors with specificity for antigenic determinants of self. The clones of lymphocytes bearing such receptors are subject to censorship in their sites of origin but are also regulated in peripheral lymphoid tissues. The occasional development of serious autoimmune disease may be counted as an unavoidable cost of having an immune system sufficiently diverse to recognize virtually any foreign antigen. Finally, these mechanisms suggest that selective pressures during

evolution have acted primarily to increase diversity rather than preserve particular useful receptor specificities. This idea is supported by the many different strategies that are successfully used to create antibody and TCR diversity in different species (McCormack et al., 1991).

Thymus Development

The thymus is derived from elements of three primitive germ layers: the endoderm of the third pharyngeal pouch; the ectoderm of the third brachial cleft; and mesenchymal elements, at least a portion of which are of neural crest origin (Bockman and Kirby, 1984). These tissue elements migrate caudally to their eventual location in the anterior mediastinum. Beginning in about the seventh week of gestation in humans, blood-borne stem cells enter the thymus and are induced to begin lymphoid differentiation.

In birds (Jotereau and Le Douarin, 1982) and mice (Ikuta et al., 1992), the thymus initially becomes receptive to the immigration of circulating HSCs in cyclic periods that last a few days and are separated by somewhat longer periods during which it is refractory. This pattern appears to be due to chemotactic activity generated by the thymus epithelium. In birds, a soluble form of β_2-microglobulin has been identified as a stem cell chemotactic factor (Dunon et al., 1990).

The earliest waves of HSCs to populate the mouse thymus express distinct developmental programs. T cells generated at 14 to 17 days of gestation have a homogeneous TCR consisting of $V\gamma3$ and $V\delta1$ polypeptides. These cells are precursors of dendritic epidermal cells of the skin (Havran and Allison, 1990; Ikuta et al., 1992). The next wave of T cells expresses $V\gamma4$ and $V\delta1$ and migrates to mucosal epithelia. T cells expressing $V\gamma2$ and $V\gamma5$ as well as those with an $\alpha\beta$ TCR develop subsequently. Only fetal HSCs have the capacity to express $V\gamma3$ TCR, and they do so only in the fetal thymus environment. An additional developmentally determined characteristic of the TCR is the junctional diversity at the V-J and V-D-J joints. The fetal $V\gamma3$ and $V\gamma4$ lack inserted nucleotides at these joints, whereas abundant N nucleotides are an important source of diversity in adult TCRs. It is speculated that a similar developmental clock of stem cells may regulate the switch from fetal to adult globin in erythroid development and programmed expression of TCRs in T-cell development (Ikuta et al., 1992).

Early development of the human thymus is described in elegant studies by Haynes and colleagues (Lobach et al., 1985; Haynes et al., 1988a and b) and by Campana and coworkers (1989). Figure 1–1 summarizes the main steps in this developmental pathway. CD7, a marker present on mature T cells, is expressed by hematopoietic cells before the beginning of thymic lymphopoiesis. CD7+ cells, which also contain cytoplasmic CD3, accumulate in prethymic mesenchyme from 7 to 8 weeks of gestation. These investigators postulated that because the epithelial thymus is poorly vascularized at this time, the CD7+ cells migrate directly into the epithelial rudiment. CD7+ cells from thorax or

THYMOCYTE DIFFERENTIATION

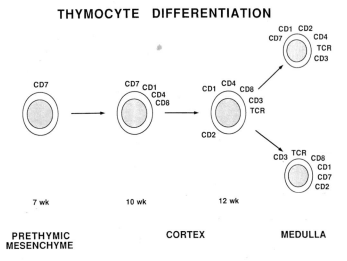

Figure 1–1. T-cell development within the thymus. The locations and Cluster of Differentiation (CD) markers for the major steps in thymocyte differentiation are indicated. Both positive and negative selection occur at the double positive CD4$^+$CD8$^+$ stage (see text). (From Lawton AR. Ontogeny of immunity. In Coulam C, Faulk WP, McIntyre JH, eds. Immunological Obstetrics. New York, Norton Medical Books, 1992, p. 29.)

liver cultured with IL-2 and other cytokines generated progeny with markers of mature thymocytes: CD2, CD3, CD4, CD8, and αβ TCRs. The same population cultured under different conditions could give rise to myeloid colonies, indicating their pluripotential nature. In a subsequent study, a population of CD7$^+$CD3$^-$CD4$^-$CD8$^-$ cells isolated from postnatal thymus generated γδ TCR and CD8$^+$ cells on culture (Denning et al., 1989). This suggests that in humans as well as mice, αβ TCR and γδ TCR populations originate from distinct stem cells.

Campana and colleagues (1989) have delineated several stages of T-cell differentiation in the fetal thymus. The least mature proliferating cell population is marked by membrane CD7 and cytoplasmic CD3. Before 18 weeks of gestation, these cells are TdT negative; after this time, they are TdT positive. These cells subsequently express cytoplasmic TCR β chain, CD4, CD8, and CD1. The next stage is marked by membrane expression of CD3 and αβ TCR and by loss of TdT. Finally, the mature medulary cells lose CD4 or CD8 and are no longer in cycle. Cells expressing the γδ TCR are infrequent at all stages of development.

Transgenic Mouse Studies

Studies using TCR transgenic mice have provided a remarkably detailed view of the major functional events of intrathymic T-cell development. The genes encoding TCR α and β chains from a T cell of known specificity and MHC-restriction, including the regulatory elements that ensure the expression of this TCR by most or all developing thymocytes, are introduced into the germline to create these animals. Selective breeding is then used to manipulate the environment in which these cells develop. These studies have been performed by several groups, but the most important results are particularly well illustrated by the elegant experiments of von Boehmer and colleagues (reviewed by von Boehmer, 1990). The TCR used in these studies recognized the HY antigen, expressed by male but not female mice of the same strain, in association with the class I H-2D^b MHC antigen. Transgenic mice were

backcrossed to alter the MHC background, or alternatively backcrossed to *SCID* mice to silence the expression of any endogenous TCR.*

The αβ transgenic mice had accelerated development of thymocytes bearing CD3, CD4, and CD8, indicating that expression of these coreceptors is dependent on TCR expression. When introduced into mice, the αβ transgene restored normal production of thymocytes. Transfer of only the β transgene raised thymocyte numbers moderately and permitted expression of CD4 and CD8. Rearrangement and expression of the complete αβ TCR are thus necessary for the generation of an expanded population of CD4$^+$CD8$^+$ thymocytes.

The H-2D^b restricted transgenes were derived from a CD8$^+$ T-cell clone. In female transgenic mice of this MHC haplotype, there was an expanded population of CD4$^-$CD8$^+$ thymocytes and a corresponding reduction of mature CD4$^+$CD8$^-$ cells. The latter population expressed endogenous α chain in combination with the transgenic β chain, whereas the former expressed the transgenic αβ TCR. In transgenic females of the D^d haplotype, there was no such selection for CD8$^+$ T cells; both CD8$^+$ and CD4$^+$ mature cells expressed endogenous α genes with the β transgene. Thus T cells having a receptor with the proper fit for a self-MHC molecule (in this case, T cells with the complete αβ transgene) are positively selected in the thymus. The MHC molecule determines whether the CD4$^+$CD8$^+$ T cell will retain CD8 (for class I MHC) or CD4 (for class II MHC).

The fate of T cells bearing the transgenic TCR in male mice of D^b haplotype was quite different. Their thymuses contained 10-fold fewer cells than those of females, and virtually all expressed the transgenic TCR but neither CD4 nor CD8. In control D^d mice, the thymuses of male and female mice were indistinguishable. These results indicate that T cells having receptors that bind avidly to self-antigens are eliminated in the

---

*The *SCID* (severe combined immunodeficiency) mouse has a defective recombinase enzyme that cannot make the gene rearrangements needed to create either T-cell or Ig receptors. Generation of both T and B cells is severely compromised.

thymus. Deletion by apoptosis occurs in immature CD4$^+$CD8$^+$ cells and therefore affects both CD4$^+$ and CD8$^+$ mature subsets.*

Experiments with radiation chimeras have demonstrated that positive selection is dependent on thymus epithelium, whereas expression of the restricting MHC molecule on bone marrow–derived cells is sufficient for negative selection to occur.

Determinants of Thymic Development

During the last two decades there have been many attempts to characterize soluble factors important in the development and function of the thymus. The identification of the defective gene in X-linked severe combined immunodeficiency has led to a breakthrough in this area. The defective gene encoded a protein then known only as the γ chain of the IL-2 receptor (Noguchi et al., 1993b). The investigators who made the discovery immediately suspected additional functions for this protein because inability to produce IL-2 caused a form of severe combined immunodeficiency in which T cells were present in normal numbers (Weinberg and Parkman, 1990). Additional experiments have demonstrated that this polypeptide, renamed common γ chain, is a component of the receptors for IL-4, IL-7, and perhaps other cytokines (Noguchi et al., 1993a; Russell et al., 1993). It is thus likely that the factors that drive thymocyte proliferation and differentiation include multiple polyfunctional cytokines acting in concert.

Ontogeny of Peripheral T Cells

CD7$^+$ cells with cytoplasmic expression of CD3 appear in fetal liver and perithymic mesenchyme at 7 to 10 weeks of gestation. T cells with membrane αβ TCR and CD3 begin to accumulate in fetal liver at about 10 weeks of gestation and are subsequently found in other lymphoid tissues. Cells with γδ TCR have not been found in human fetal liver and are rare in thymus (Campana et al., 1989). Specific responses to histocompatibility antigens are demonstrable in the thymus by 12 weeks and in the spleen by 15 weeks (Asantila et al., 1974a and b). The ability of infants born at 24 weeks of gestation to survive in the hostile environment of the intensive care nursery is good evidence that a heterogeneous population of functional T cells is present by this time. Since maturation of T-cell functions such as development of T$_H$1 and T$_H$2 cells is antigen driven, it is unlikely that qualitative changes take place between midgestation and birth in the sheltered intrauterine environment. The capabilities of neonatal T cells, which are discussed in detail in Chapter 10 (Wilson et al., 1991), are probably identical to those of fetal cells from midgestation to birth.

---

*Apoptosis is a term used to describe genetically programmed cell death.

B-CELL DEVELOPMENT

Stages of B-Cell Development

As is the case for T cells, the development of B cells occurs in discontinuous steps. The first stage involves the generation of a large and diverse repertoire of clones of B cells expressing unique receptors for antigen from a relatively small number of stem cell precursors. The generation of clonal diversity of B cells is analogous to intrathymic T-cell development, except that it is localized sequentially in different tissues rather than occurring in a single organ. This process is genetically programmed and regulated by soluble and cell-associated signals of the inductive microenvironments.

Several steps in early B-cell generation can be identified. Progenitor B cells (pro-B) are dividing and have begun the process of rearrangement of immunoglobulin heavy-chain genes. Production of μ heavy chain in the cell cytoplasm signals successful rearrangement and marks the transition from pro-B and pre-B cell. Rearrangement of light-chain genes usually (but not always) occurs after heavy-chain rearrangement. Synthesis of intact light chain permits efficient assembly and transfer of monomeric IgM molecules to the cell surface. The expression of cell surface Ig receptor marks the transition from pre-B to immature B cells (Fig. 1–2).

The second stage of B-cell differentiation is initiated by the binding of antigen and is usually dependent on the receipt of signals from activated T cells. Appropriately stimulated B cells proliferate and differentiate to form memory cells or antibody-secreting plasma cells. Only a small fraction of the B cells generated during the first stage survive to encounter antigens and complete their differentiation; the remainder are believed to undergo programmed cell death. The primary B-cell population is continuously renewed throughout life.

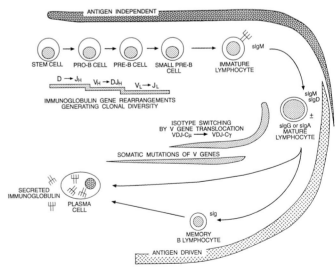

Figure 1–2. Developmental stages of B cells. The discontinuity of antigen-independent and antigen-driven events is indicated. (From Lawton AR, B Cell development. In Polin RA, Fox WW, eds. Fetal and Neonatal Physiology. Philadelphia, WB Saunders, 1992, pp 1432–1438.)

The major steps in B-cell development are diagrammed in Figure 1–2 and are detailed in Chapter 3.

Sites of B-Cell Generation

Primary development of B cells in birds occurs in an organ called the bursa of Fabricius. Experiments demonstrating the contrasting effects of bursectomy and thymectomy on immune functions of chickens were seminal in recognition of distinct T- and B-cell lineages (Cooper et al., 1966). The parallels between bursa and thymus are striking.

The bursa originates as a dorsal evagination of the hindgut, forming a hollow epithelial organ with a lumen continuous with the cloaca. Beginning at about the seventh day of embryogenesis in the chicken, blood-borne stem cells enter the bursal mesenchyme, where some develop into granulocytes. Others migrate into the epithelium and begin lymphoid differentiation. These lymphoepithelial buds develop into the large follicles of the mature bursa. As is the case for the thymus, the influx of stem cells seems to be controlled by a property of the epithelial bursa that maintains its attractiveness for stem cells from developmental day 7 to 11 (Le Douarin et al., 1975). The first recognizable event of B-cell development in the bursa is the onset of IgM synthesis by a few cells in the primordial follicles at 12 days. Thereafter, the number of B lymphocytes spawned within the bursa rises geometrically, with a mean doubling time of approximately 10 hours. Emigration of lymphocytes from the bursa begins before hatching.

The successive sites of B-cell development in humans and other mammals are the omentum and liver in early fetal life and the bone marrow as it becomes the hematopoietic organ (Kamps and Cooper, 1982; Bofill et al., 1985). The omentum may be the primary site for development of a distinct subset of B cells bearing the CD5 marker, which may be involved in autoimmunity (Solvason and Kearney, 1992).

B-Cell Receptor Diversity

Immunoglobulin genes are organized in three families that encode heavy chains, κ light chains, and λ light chains. Each family contains tandem arrays of V and J genes (light chains) or V, D, and J genes (heavy chains) upstream from the genes of the constant region. The heavy-chain family is located on chromosome 14; κ light chains are on chromosome 2, and λ light chains are on chromosome 22. The immunoglobulin gene loci are organized in a manner similar to that already described for TCR genes. The heavy-chain cluster contains several hundred V_H genes, a number of D_H genes, six J_H genes, and nine functional C_H genes (μ, δ, γ3, γ1, α1, γ2, γ4, ε, α2). The κ locus has a single $C_κ$ gene downstream from several $J_κ$ genes, and the λ locus has several $J_λ C_λ$ pairs. V(D) and J genes encode the antibody-combining site; C genes determine the antibody class and light-chain type.

Functional immunoglobulin genes are formed by sequential DNA rearrangements mediated by a highly specialized recombinase enzyme that recognizes conserved signal sequences that flank the coding segments to be joined (Schatz et al., 1992). The recombinase mediates formation of a loop or hairpin structure, clips the DNA at the signal sequences, and reanneals the opened DNA to form a coding joint and a signal joint. The signal joint forms a circle of DNA containing the sequence that originally separated the two coding segments; this DNA is subsequently degraded. The coding joint splices, for example, a D gene to a J gene.

The precise location of splice junctions in coding joints is variable. Additional nucleotides may be added through the action of TdT to generate N diversity, as described earlier for the TCR. The imprecision in the formation of coding joints increases diversity in the antigen-binding site but also results in many ineffectual rearrangements. That evolution has favored diversity is indicated by the fact that the signal joints forming the discarded circular DNA are precise and lack random nucleotide insertions.

Rearrangements occur in order, beginning with D-J gene splicing in the heavy-chain locus (Alt et al., 1992). A functional D-J rearrangement is followed by translocation of a V_H gene. If translocation is successful, the cell makes the transition from pro-B to pre-B by initiating synthesis of μ chain (Cooper and Burrows, 1990). Nascent μ chains combine in the endoplasmic reticulum with a surrogate light chain (ψLC), the product of two pre-B cell–specific genes called λ5 (mouse) or 14.1 (human) and V_{pre-B}. The complex of μ and ψLC may be transported to the cell surface (Tsubata and Reth, 1990). Although ψLC is produced in pro-B as well as pre-B cells, it is expressed on the surface of only the most mature pre-B cells (Lassoued et al., 1993).

Light-chain rearrangement usually follows productive heavy-chain rearrangement but may occur independently (Kubagawa et al., 1989). κ chains are generally rearranged before λ chains. Sequential rearrangements of a particular $V_κ$ to different $J_κ$ genes may occur within a single clone (Caton, 1990). For the most part, however, a functional rearrangement at a particular locus inhibits further rearrangements at that locus, resulting in the characteristic allelic exclusion of the polypeptides of lymphocyte receptors. Whether this series of gene rearrangements is precisely regulated or entirely stochastic remains controversial. The end result is clear: each newly generated B cell expresses a single unique receptor, but the population of B cells contains many different receptor specificities.

Mice with disruptions of λ5 genes have greatly reduced production of B cells (Kitamura et al., 1992), indicating that the ψLC must play an important role in the differentiation of these cells (Ehlich et al., 1993; Lassoued et al., 1993). The daily production of B cells in the bone marrow is far greater than the numbers of cells entering the peripheral lymphoid pool (Osmond 1991), suggesting that a large number of progenitors are destined for programmed cell death. It may be that expression of μ-ψLC complex on the cell surface prevents apoptosis.

Ontogeny of V-Gene Expression

The fetal repertoire of expressed V genes is both restricted and conserved. Most of the fetal V_H genes of mice map close to the D locus, which suggests a location-dependent mechanism for V_H readout (Perlmutter et al., 1985). The human fetal repertoire is similarly restricted, but the expressed genes are scattered throughout the locus, making the positional hypothesis less likely (Schroeder et al., 1987; Schroeder and Wang, 1990; Adderson et al., 1992; Willems van Dijk et al., 1992). There is less junctional diversity at V-D-J splice sites in fetal heavy chains than in neonatal heavy chains, apparently reflecting developmental delay in expression of TdT (Raaphorts et al., 1992). Because these splice junctions are located in CDR3, a region of antigen contact, diversity is further restricted. The neonatal repertoire is substantially more diverse than that of the fetus, containing a broader spectrum of V, D, and J genes, somatic mutations, and longer CDR3 regions owing to greater N-region diversity (Mortari et al., 1993).

Experimental evidence in inbred mice strongly implies ordered expression of particular antibody specificities during ontogeny (Sigal et al., 1977; Cancro et al., 1979). Restricted V gene use might contribute to this developmental program, but it is not likely the major factor. This is so because somatic junctional diversity and mutations play such a large role in the determination of antibody specificity. Another mechanism is suggested by the discovery that the murine fetal B-cell population is dominated by clones that secrete polyspecific antibodies and are connected through idiotypic interactions (Vakil and Kearney, 1986; Vakil et al., 1986). B cells producing idiotypes associated with polyspecific autoantibodies are prominent in fetal spleen (Kipps et al., 1990).

B cells that bear CD5 are associated with the production of polyreactive autoantibodies (Casali and Notkins, 1989) and are present in relatively high proportions during fetal life. The fetal omentum is the site of genesis of this subset of B cells (Solvason and Kearney, 1992). It is tempting to speculate that V_H restriction, a uniquely connected repertoire, and the ontogenetic prominence of CD5$^+$ B cells are related and might explain the programmed expression of particular specificities. In fetal mice, however, both conventional and CD5$^+$ cells use restricted (but different) sets of V genes (Jeong and Teale, 1990).

Immature B Cells and Tolerance to Self

An inevitable consequence of the processes involved in generation of diversity is the production of some clones with receptors for self-antigens. Newly emerging B cells are susceptible to negative selection should they encounter their antigen in the proper context. This phenomenon is called *clonal abortion.* Experiments with transgenic mice have elucidated several levels of B-cell tolerance that depend on the affinity of the autoreactive antibody, the concentration of antigen, and whether the antigen is anchored in cell membranes.

Goodnow (1992) has bred lysozyme-transgenic mice to mice that are transgenic for a high-affinity antibody to lysozyme, creating a model in which nearly all emerging B cells are self-reactive. When the lysozyme gene is engineered so as to be expressed on cell membranes, mature B cells do not appear in spleen or lymph nodes, but the bone marrow contains a normal complement of B cells bearing membrane IgM. If lysozyme is secreted instead of membrane bound, the consequences depend on the relative concentrations of the antigen. Relatively high concentrations induce a state of *clonal anergy,* in which B cells that recognize the autoantigen are present but unresponsive. When the concentration of lysozyme is low, B-cell development is unimpeded and function is normal. This state is called *clonal ignorance* (Goodnow, 1992).

Susceptibility to clonal deletion is a property of immature B cells. Treatment of neonatal mice with anti-μ antibodies blocks B-cell development; delay of the start of treatment until the mice are 1 week old changes this outcome (Lawton and Cooper, 1974). In vitro parallels include the irreversible receptor modulation that follows treatment of B cells from infant mice with antibodies to μ chains (Raff et al., 1975), induction of tolerance to immunogenic forms of antigen (Metcalf and Klinman, 1976), and distinctly different signal transduction pathways following cross-linking of the IgM receptor (Yellen et al., 1991).

Goodnow's observation (1992) that the population of immature B cells in the marrow is not diminished in the transgenic clonal deletion model may indicate that cell death requires time and may occur after the cells have exited the bone marrow.

Development of Isotype Diversity

B cells expressing any other isotype originate from precursors that express membrane IgM (mIgM) by a process called *isotype switching.* This concept originated with biologic observations and experiments (Nossal et al., 1964; Cooper et al., 1971; Lawton and Cooper, 1974) but now has an easily appreciated molecular explanation. IgM is necessarily expressed first because the C_μ gene is proximate to the J genes and the intron between J6 and C_μ contains important transcriptional enhancers. Two mechanisms are recognized for expression of isotypes whose genes are downstream of Cμ. Differential *splicing* of a transcript including V-D-J-C_μ-C_δ may generate independent messenger RNAs (mRNAs), V-D-J-C_μ and V-D-J-C_δ, which are translated to μ and δ chains having identical V regions (Tucker, 1985). This mechanism accounts for the large number of B cells that co-express mIgM and mIgD receptors with identical specifity. The second mechanism, called *switch recombination,* involves translocation of a V-D-J gene from its location upstream of C_μ to a new *switch site* in the 5' flanking region of another C_H gene, for example $C_\alpha1$ (Honjo, 1983). Switch recombination is generally antigen driven, T-cell dependent, and directed by the cytokine environment in which it occurs (Purkerson and Isakson, 1992). For example, IL-4 promotes switching of precursors bearing mIgM and mIgD to IgE production while differentiating into plasma cells.

Expression of multiple isotypes by individual B cells occurs consistently at particular times during fetal life. B lymphocytes can first be detected in human fetal liver at approximately 9 weeks of gestation. These cells have IgM on their surface but lack other immunoglobulin classes (Gathings et al., 1977; Bofill et al., 1985). Most also fail to bind aggregated IgG (Fc receptor). Lymphocytes expressing other immunoglobulin classes begin to appear in low frequency at 10 to 12 weeks of gestation (Fig. 1–3). IgG-positive cells have been found by 10 weeks, and cells bearing IgD and IgA appear to develop slightly later. The number of B lymphocytes in liver and in other developing organs increases rapidly at 12 to 15 weeks of gestation. By 15 weeks of gestation, the proportion of immunoglobulin-bearing cells in blood, spleen, and lymph nodes is the same as that found in adults. Moreover, the distribution of B lymphocytes bearing different immunoglobulin classes is also similar to that in adults (Lawton et al., 1972; Hayward and Ezer, 1974; Gupta et al., 1976; Gathings et al., 1977).

B-cell isotype expression on fetal and neonatal cells differs from that on adult cells: expression of mIgA or mIgG occurs exclusively on cells that also express mIgM with or without mIgD (Gathings et al., 1977; Gandini et al., 1981), whereas adult B cells expressing mIgG or mIgA have only the single isotype. The mechanism for multiple isotype expression by single B cells is not known, but RNA processing seems most plausible (reviewed by Lawton, 1986). The importance of this observation is that it marks relatively immature B cells. Cells bearing mIgA in patients with selective IgA deficiency and mIgG B cells in patients with common variable immunodeficiency have the same phenotype (Conley and Cooper, 1982; Fiorilli et al., 1986).

B cells diffusely distributed in lymph nodes at 16 to 17 weeks of gestation express CD21 (complement receptor 2 and the Epstein-Barr virus receptor) and are largely IgD positive. The organization of primary follicles around follicular dendritic cells from 17 weeks on is associated with the expression of CD5. The development of splenic follicles follows the same pattern but occurs a few weeks later (Bofill et al., 1985).

MATURATION OF THE IMMUNE SYSTEM

It has long been recognized that, in comparison with the older child or adult, the fetus and newborn have a sluggish immune response, most clearly defined as a reduced capacity to produce antibodies of the IgG or IgA classes to protein antigens or antibodies of any class to carbohydrate antigens. One of the goals of the study of ontogeny has been to understand, and perhaps learn to circumvent, these impediments to effective immunization against serious infectious diseases of infancy.

The first problem became particularly interesting with the discovery of the long gap between the development of B lymphocytes bearing IgG or IgA isotypes on their membranes late in the first trimester and the expression of adult concentrations of these isotypes in serum in middle to late childhood (Stiehm and Fudenberg, 1966; Buckley et al., 1968). The inability of newborn B lymphocytes able to synthesize and express these isotypes on their membranes to differentiate into secretory plasma cells became a focus of ontogenetic investigation. The later observation that fetal B cells share an immature phenotype with B cells from patients with common variable immunodeficiency and isolated IgA deficiency (Conley and Cooper, 1982; Fiorilli et al., 1986) made this problem even more interesting. Functional studies comparing in vitro responses of neonatal B and T cells with those of adult cells implicated both T and B cells in the impaired capacity to produce IgG and IgA. In addition to providing poor helper function, neonatal T cells were active suppressors (Hayward and Lawton, 1977). The inability of

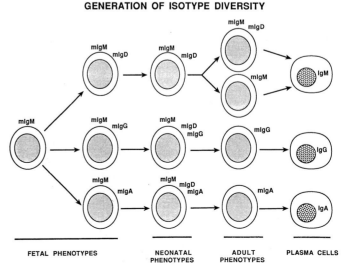

GENERATION OF ISOTYPE DIVERSITY

Figure 1–3. Development of intraclonal isotype diversity. The expression of multiple cell surface isotypes (other than IgM and IgD) is characteristic of immature B cells. (From Lawton, AR. B Cell development. In Polin RA, Fox WW, eds. Fetal and Neonatal Physiology. Philadelphia, WB Saunders, 1992, pp 1432–1438.)

FETAL PHENOTYPES   NEONATAL PHENOTYPES   ADULT PHENOTYPES   PLASMA CELLS

neonatal B cells to efficiently produce IgG or IgA isotypes was confirmed through the use of polyclonal stimulants that were completely (pokeweed mitogen), partially (*Nocardia* water-soluble mitogen), or not (Epstein-Barr virus) T-cell dependent (Tosato et al., 1980; Andersson, et al., 1981; Miyawaki, et al., 1981).

All of these studies are technically flawed because the stimulants used address only a small fraction of the total B-cell population: preactivated cells, which are unlikely to be present in neonatal blood (Anderson et al., 1988, and references therein). Investigations that have used an efficient culture system in which B-cell differentiation is initiated by direct contact with anti–CD3-activated T cells (capable of inducing plasma cell differentiation in 50% to 90% of peripheral blood B cells) have nevertheless confirmed the earlier results (Splawski et al., 1991). Along with adult cells, neonatal lymphocytes of both T and B lineages were induced to proliferate, and the T cells produced as much IL-2 as do adult cells; however, little or no immunoglobulin was produced. Neonatal T cells could initiate proliferation of adult B cells, but little immunoglobulin was produced. Adult T cells provided help for IgM production, but not IgG or IgA production, by neonatal B cells.

The functional deficits of neonatal cells can be overcome by the addition of exogenous IL-2 and either IL-4 or IL-6. The effect of IL-2 is critical, because antibodies to the IL-2 receptor eliminate immunoglobulin production in the presence of any of these lymphokines. No cytokine-specific patterns of isotype secretion were observed in these experiments (Splawski and Lipsky, 1991). These results indicate that neonatal B cells require both a competence signal provided by direct contact with activated T cells and higher concentrations of IL-2 and IL-4 or IL-6 than do adult B cells to undergo differentiation into plasma cells. Neonatal T cells produce sufficient IL-2 to drive T-cell proliferation, but they do not provide the additional cytokines required to support optimal B-cell differentiation.

Differential expression of isoforms of the tyrosine phosphatase CD45 distinguish adult $CD4^+$ T cells with helper activity (CD45RO) from those with suppressor/inducer function (CD45RA). CD45RO cells, which constitute 50% of adult but only 5% of neonatal $CD4^+$ cells, appear to represent a memory population derived from virgin CD45RA cells. These CD45RA cells account for 90% of neonatal $CD4^+$ cells (Clement et al., 1988, 1990; Janeway, 1992). The small number of $CD45RO^+CD4^+$ cells present in neonatal blood has helper activity equivalent to the same population of adult cells, whether stimulated by pokeweed mitogen or anti-CD3. The reciprocal $CD45RA^+$ neonatal T-cell population actively suppresses the helper function of CD45RO cells. This radiation-sensitive suppressor activity is absent from adult $CD45RA^+$ cells. Neonatal $CD45RA^+$ cells stimulated by mitogen and cultured for long periods with IL-2 lose suppressor activity, become $CD45RA^-$ and acquire helper function (Clement et al., 1988, 1990).

Neonatal T cells produce quantities of IL-2 and tumor necrosis factor α and β similar to those made by adult cells, but they make little or no IFN-γ, IL-3, IL-4, IL-5, IL-6, or granulocyte-macrophage colony-stimulating factor (Ehlers and Smith, 1991; Lewis et al., 1991; Wilson et al., 1991). The differences in cytokine secretion are due to reduced numbers of cells making a given cytokine. For example, IFN-γ was produced by 40% of adult but only 3% of neonatal T cells analyzed by in situ hybridization (Lewis et al., 1991). The synthesis of diverse cytokines by T cells is linked to their activation. For example, the frequency of adult $CD4^+$ cells containing mRNA for IFN-γ or for IL-4 was highest in the CD45RO fraction, intermediate in unfractionated cells, and extremely low in CD45RA cells (Wilson et al., 1991). Neonatal cells stimulated by anti-CD3 and cultured with IL-2 for 7 to 10 days produced an adult pattern of cytokine expression (Ehlers and Smith, 1991). This requirement for post-thymic differentiation, almost certainly an antigen-driven process in vivo, must contribute to, if not completely account for, the deficiencies in neonatal helper function.

Discovery of the gene defect in X-linked immunodeficiency with hyper-IgM has provided a new model for the functional immaturity of neonatal B cells. Data from several studies indicated that B cells from hyper IgM patients could not produce IgG or IgA when co-cultivated with normal T cells stimulated by pokeweed mitogen, whereas patients' T cells provided help for secretion of these isotypes by normal B cells (Geha et al., 1979; Levitt et al., 1983). One study had concordant results for normal T cells but described a leukemic T cell that could induce hyper-IgM B cells to produce both isotypes (Mayer et al., 1986). The hyper-IgM gene encodes gp39, the CD40 ligand, which is not expressed on activated T cells in most affected males. B cells from these patients activated by cross-linking of CD40 with antibody or cells constitutively expressing the CD40 ligand are able to switch to synthesis of diverse isotypes (Allen et al., 1993; Aruffo, et al., 1993). Together, these data suggest that either prolonged or repeated signaling through CD40 is required to bring B cells to a state of full differentiation competence. The lack of such stimulation is a logical explanation for the functional immaturity of neonatal B cells.

The inability of newborn animals and humans to respond to carbohydrate antigens (reviewed by Davie, 1985) remains an enigma. Might the characteristic restrictions in expression of V_H genes constrain diversity to the extent that important epitopes of carbohydrate antigens are not recognized?

The developmental period during which the murine B-cell repertoire exhibits restricted diversity occupies approximately 1 prenatal and 2 postnatal weeks; even very young mice exhibit considerable clonal diversity (Cancro et al., 1979). Based on the histologic appearance of lymphoid tissues and the relative numbers of peripheral T and B cells, the immune system of the newborn mouse is at a developmental stage equivalent to that of the human newborn at 12 to 16 weeks. Given the mechanisms for the generation of diversity and the long gestational period in humans, it is unlikely that diversity is a limiting factor. This theoretical view is supported by the excellent responses of young infants to protein-carbohydrate conjugate vaccines (Adderson et al., 1992).

SUMMARY

The generation of clonal diversity of T and B cells begins early in gestation and proceeds at a rapid rate by parallel mechanisms. The lack of precision of the V-D-J recombinase enzyme in making coding joints for immunoglobulin and TCR genes, and the creation of untemplated nucleotides at joints through the action of TdT, stand in striking contrast to the fidelity of other enzymes involved in DNA replication and repair, emphasizing the evolutionary advantage of diversity in the immune system. Efficient mechanisms for the elimination of inevitable autoreactive clones of both T and B cells have been developed.

The long-recognized immaturities of neonatal T and B cells are beginning to achieve molecular definition. The new findings emphasize the importance of maturation events occurring in the peripheral rather than central lymphoid organs, and further study may lead to new strategies for immunization of the very young infant.

References

Adderson EE, Johnston MJ, Shackelford PG, Carroll WL. Development of the human antibody repertoire. Pediatr Res 32:257–263, 1992.

Allen RC, Armitage RJ, Conley ME, Rosenblatt H, Jenkins A, Copeland NG, Bedell MA, Edelhoff S, Disteche CM, Simoneaux DK, Fanslow WC, Belmont J, Spriggs MK. CD40 ligand gene defects responsible for X-linked hyper-IgM syndrome. Science 259:990–993, 1993.

Alt FW, Oltz EM, Young F, Groman J, Taccioli G, Chen J. VDJ recombination. Immunol Today 13:306–314, 1992.

Anderson SJ, Hummell DS, Lawton AR. Differentiation of human B lymphocyte subpopulations induced by an alloreactive helper T cell clone. J Clin Immunol 8:275–284, 1988.

Andersson U, Bird AG, Britton S, Palacios R. Humoral and cellular immunity in humans studied at the cell level from birth to two years of age. Immunol Rev 57:5–38, 1981.

Aruffo A, Farrington M, Hollenbaugh D, Li X, Milatovich A, Nonoyama S, Bajorath J, Grosmaire LS, Stenkamp R, Neubauer M, Roberts RL, Noelle RJ, Ledbetter JA, Francke U, Ochs HD. The CD40 ligand gp39 is defective in activated T cells from patients with X-linked hyper-IgM syndrome. Cell 72:291–300, 1993.

Asantila T, Vahala J, Toivanen P. Generation of functional diversity of T cell receptors. Immunogenetics 1:407–415, 1974a.

Asantila T, Vahala J, Toivanen P. Response of human fetal lymphocytes in xenogeneic mixed leukocyte culture: phylogenetic and ontogenetic aspects. Immunogenetics 1:272–290, 1974b.

Bloom BR, Modlen RL, Salgame P. Stigma variations: observations on suppressor T cells and leprosy. Annu Rev Immunol 10:453–488, 1992.

Bockman DE, Kirby ML. Dependence of thymus development on derivatives of neural crest. Science 223:498–500, 1984.

Bofill M, Janossy G, Janossa M, Burford GD, Seymour GJ, Wernet P, Kelemen E. Human B cell development. II. Subpopulations in the human fetus. J Immunol 134:1531–1538, 1985.

Buckley RH, Dees SC, O'Fallon WM. Serum immunoglobulins: I. Levels in normal children and in uncomplicated childhood allergy. Pediatrics 41:600–611, 1968.

Campana D, Janossy G, Coustan-Smith E, Amlot PL, Tian WT, Ip S, Wong L. The expression of T cell receptor–associated proteins during T cell ontogeny in man. J Immunol 142:57–66, 1989.

Cancro MP, Wylie DE, Gerhard W, Klinman NR. Patterned acquisition of gene antibody repertoire: diversity of the hemagglutinin-specific B cell repertoire in neonatal BALB/c mice. Proc Natl Acad Sci U S A 76:6577–6581, 1979.

Casali P, Notkins AL. Probing the human B cell repertoire with EBV: polyreactive antibodies and CD5+ B lymphocytes. Annu Rev Immunol 7:513–535, 1989.

Caton AJ. A single pre-B cell can give rise to antigen-specific B cells that utilize distinct immunoglobulin gene rearrangements. J Exp Med 172:815–825, 1990.

Clement LT, Yamashita N, Martin AM. The functionally distinct subpopulations of human helper/inducer T lymphocytes defined by anti CD45R antibodies derive sequentially from a differentiation pathway that is regulated by activation-dependent post-thymic differentiation. J Immunol 141:1464–1470, 1988.

Clement LT, Vink PE, Bradley GE. Novel immunoregulatory functions of phenotypically distinct subpopulations of CD4+ cells in the human neonate. J Immunol 145:102–108, 1990.

Colley DG. Occurrence, roles, and uses of idiotypes and anti-idiotypes in parasitic diseases. In Cerny J, Hiernaux J, eds. Idiotypic Networks and Diseases. Washington DC, American Society for Microbiology, 1990, pp 71–105.

Conley ME, Cooper MD. Immature IgA B cells in IgA deficient patients. N Engl J Med 305:495–497, 1982.

Cooper MD, Burrows PD. B cell differentiation. In Honjo T, Alt FW, Rabbits TH, eds. Immunoglobulin Genes. San Diego, Academic Press, 1990, pp 1–21.

Cooper MD, Kincade PW, Lawton AR. Thymus and bursal function in immunologic development. A new theoretical model of plasma cell differentiation. In Kagan BM, Stiehm ER, eds. Immunologic Incompetence. Chicago Year Book, 1971, pp 81–104.

Cooper MD, Peterson RDA, South MA, Good RA. The functions of the thymus system and bursa system in the chicken. J Exp Med 123:75–102, 1966.

Davie JM. Antipolysaccharide immunity in man and animals. In Sell SH, Wright PF, eds. Hemophilus Influenzae: Epidemiology, Immunology, and Prevention of Disease. New York. Elsevier Biomedical, 1985, pp 129–134.

Defrance T, Vanbervliet F, Brière F, Durand I, Rousset F, Banchereau J. Interleukin 10 and transforming growth factor β cooperate to induce anti–CD40-activated naive human B cells to secrete immunoglobulin A. J Exp Med 175:671–682, 1992.

Denning SM, Kurtzberg J, Leslie DS, Haynes BF. Human post-natal CD4−CD8−CD3− thymic T cell precursors differentiate in vitro into T cell receptor γδ-bearing cells. J Immunol 142:2988–2997, 1989.

Dorshkind K. Regulation of hematopoiesis by bone marrow stromal cells. Annu Rev Immunol 8:111–138, 1990.

Dunon D, Kaufman J, Salomonsen J, Skjoldt K, Vainio O, Thiery JP, Imhof BA. T cell precursor migration towards beta 2-microglobulin is involved in thymus colonization of chicken embryos. EMBO J 9:3315–3322, 1990.

Dwyer DS, Bradley RJ, Urquhart CK, Kearney JF. Naturally occurring antibodies in myasthenia gravis patients. Nature 301:611–614, 1983.

Ehlers S, Smith KA. Differentiation of T cell lymphokine gene expression: the in vitro acquisition of T cell memory. J Exp Med 173:25–36, 1991.

Ehlich A, Schaal S, Gu H, Kitamura D, Müller W, Rajewsky K. Immunoglobulin heavy and light chain genes rearrange independently at early stages of B cell development. Cell 72:695–704, 1993.

Fiorilli M, Crescenzi M, Carbonari M, Tedesco L, Russo G, Gaetano C, Aiuti F. Phenotypically immature IgG-bearing B cells in patients with hypogammaglobulinemia. J Clin Immunol 6:21–25, 1986.

Freeman GJ, Gribben JG, Boussiotis VA, Ng JW, Restivo VA Jr, Lombard LA, Gray GS, Nadler LM. Cloning of B7-2: a CTLA-4 counter-receptor that costimulates human T cell proliferation. Science 262:909–911, 1993.

Gandini M, Kubagawa H, Gathings WE, Lawton AR. Expression of three immunoglobulin isotypes by individual B cells during development: implications for heavy chain switching. Am J Reprod Immunol 1:161–163, 1981.

Gathings WE, Lawton AR, Cooper MD. Immunofluorescent studies on the development of pre-B cells, B lymphocytes, and immunoglobulin isotype diversity. Eur J Immunol 7:804–810, 1977.

Geha RS. Presence of circulating anti–idiotype-bearing cells after booster immunizations with tetanus toxoid (TT) and inhibition of anti TT antibody synthesis by auto–anti-idiotypic antibody. J Immunol 130:1634–1639, 1983.

Geha RS, Hyslop N, Alami S, Farah F, Schneeberger EE, Rosen FS. Hyper IgM immunodeficiency (dysgammaglobulinemia). J Clin Invest 64:385–391, 1979.

Golde DW. The stem cell. Sci Am 265:86–93, Dec. 1991.

Goodnow CC. Transgenic mice and analysis of B-cell tolerance. Annu Rev Immunol 10:489–518, 1992.

Gupta S, Pahwa R, O'Reilly RO, Good RA, Siegal FP. Ontogeny of lymphocyte subpopulations in human fetal liver. Proc Natl Acad Sci U S A 73:919–922, 1976.

Havran WL, Allison JP. Origin of thy-1$^+$ dendritic epidermal cells from fetal thymic precursors. Nature 344:68–70, 1990.

Haynes BF, Martin ME, Kay HH, Kurtzberg J. Early events in human T cell ontogeny. Phenotypic characterization and immunohistologic localization of T cell precursors in early human fetal tissues. J Exp Med 168:1061–1080, 1988a.

Haynes BF, Singer KH, Denning SM, Martin ME. Analysis of expression of CD2, CD3, and T cell antigen receptor molecules during early fetal thymic development. J Immunol 141:3776–3784, 1988b.

Hayward AR, Ezer G. Development of lymphocyte populations in human thymus and spleen. Clin Exp Immunol 17:169–178, 1974.

Hayward AR, Lawton AR. Induction of plasma cell differentiation of human fetal lymphocytes: evidence for functional immaturity of T and B cells. J Immunol 119:1213–1217, 1977.

Honjo T. Immunoglobulin genes. Annu Rev Immunol 1:499–528, 1983.

Ikuta K, Uchida N, Friedman J, Weissman IL. Lymphocyte development from stem cells. Annu Rev Immunol 10:759–783, 1992.

Janeway CA Jr. The T cell receptor as a multicomponent signalling machine: CD4/CD8 coreceptors and CD45 in T cell activation. Annu Rev Immunol 10:645–674, 1992.

Jeong HD, Teale JM. Contribution of the CD5$^+$ B cell to D-proximal V$_H$ family expression early in ontogeny. J Immunol 145:2725–2729, 1990.

Jerne NK. Towards a network theory of the immune system. Ann Immunol 125C:373–389, 1974.

Jotereau FV, Le Douarin NM. Demonstration of a cyclic renewal of the lymphocyte precursor cells in the quail thymus during embryonic and perinatal life. J Immunol 129:1869–1877, 1982.

Kamps WA, Cooper MD. Microenvironmental studies of pre B and B cell development in human and mouse fetuses. J Immunol 129:526–531, 1982.

Kipps TJ, Robbins BA, Carson DA. Uniform high frequency expression of autoantibody-associated crossreactive idiotypes in the primary B cell follicles of human fetal spleen. J Exp Med 171:189–196, 1990.

Kitamura D, Kudo A, Schaal S, Müeller W, Melchers R, Rajewsky K. A critical role of λ5 protein in B cell development. Cell 69:823–831, 1992.

Kubagawa H, Cooper MD, Carroll AJ, Burrows PD. Light-chain gene expression before heavy-chain rearrangement in pre-B cells transformed by Epstein-Barr virus. Proc Natl Acad Sci U S A 86:2356–2360, 1989.

Lanzavecchia A. Receptor-mediated antigen uptake and its effect on antigen presentation to class II–restricted T lymphocytes. Annu Rev Immunol 6:773–793, 1992.

Lassoued K, Nuñez CA, Billips L, Kubagawa H, Monteiro RC, LeBien T, Cooper MD. Expression of surrogate light chain receptors is restricted to a late stage in pre–B cell differentiation. Cell 73:73–86, 1993.

Lawton AR. Ontogeny of B cells: relations to immunodeficiency diseases. Clin Immunol Immunopathol 40:5–12, 1986.

Lawton AR, Asofsky R, Hylton MD, Cooper MD. Suppression of immunoglobulin class synthesis in mice: I. Effects of treatment with antibody to μ chain. J Exp Med 135:277–297, 1972.

Lawton AR, Cooper MD. Modification of B lymphocyte differentiation by anti-immunoglobulins. In Cooper MD, Warner NL, eds. Contemporary Topics in Immunobiology, Vol. 3. New York. Plenum Publishing 1974, pp 193–225.

Le Douarin NM, Houssaint E, Jotereau FV, Belo M. Origin of haemopoietic stem cells in the embryonic bursa of Fabricius and bone marrow studied through interspecies chimaeras. Proc Natl Acad Sci U S A 72:2701–2705, 1975.

Levitt D, Haber P, Rich K, Cooper MD. Hyper IgM immunodeficiency. J Clin Invest 72:1650–1657, 1983.

Lewis DB, Yu CC, Meyer J, English BK, Kahn SJ, Wilson CB. Cellular and molecular mechanisms for reduced interleukin 4 and interferon-gamma production by neonatal T cells. J Clin Invest 87:194–202, 1991.

Linsley PS, Ledbetter JA. The role of the CD28 receptor during T cell responses to antigen. Annu Rev Immunol 11:191–212, 1993.

Lobach DF, Hensley LL, Ho W, Haynes BF. Human T cell antigen expression during the early stages of fetal thymic maturation. J Immunol 135:1752–1759, 1985.

Mayer L, Kwan SP, Thompson C, Ko HS, Chiorazzi N, Waldmann T, Rosen F. Evidence for a defect in "switch" T cells in patients with immunodeficiency and hyperimmunoglobulinemia M. N Engl J Med 314:409–413, 1986.

McCormack WT, Tjoelker LW, Thompson CB. Avian B cell development: generation of an immunoglobulin repertoire by gene conversion. Annu Rev Immunol 9:219–241, 1991.

Metcalf ES, Klinman NR. *In vitro* tolerance induction of neonatal murine B cells. J Exp Med 143:1327–1340, 1976.

Miyawaki T, Moriya N, Nagaoki T, Taniguchi N. Maturation of B cell differentiation ability and T cell regulatory function in infancy and childhood. Immunol Rev 57:61–87, 1981.

Moretta L, Ciccone E, Moretta A, Höglund P, Öhlén C, Kärre K. Allorecognition by NK cells: nonself or no self. Immunol Today 13:300–306, 1992.

Mortari F, Wang JY, Schroeder HW Jr. Human cord blood antibody repertoire: mixed population of V$_H$ gene segments and CDR 3 distribution in the expressed Cα and Cγ repertoires. J Immunol 150:1348–1357, 1993.

Mossman TR, Coffman RL. T$_H$1 and T$_H$2 cells: different patterns of lymphokine secretion lead to different functional properties. Annu Rev Immunol 7:145–173, 1989.

Noelle RJ, Roy M, Shepherd DM, Stamenkovic I, Ledbetter JA, Aruffo A. A 39-kDa protein on activated helper T cells binds CD40 and transducts a signal for cognate activation of B cells. Proc Natl Acad Sci U S A 89:6550–6554, 1992.

Noguchi M, Nakamura Y, Russell SM, Ziegler SF, Tsang M, Cao X, Leonard WJ. Interleukin-2 receptor γ chain: a functional component of the interleukin-7 receptor. Science 262:1877–1880, 1993a.

Noguchi M, Yi H, Rosenblatt HM, Filipovich AH, Adelstein S, Modi WS, McBride OW, Leonard WJ. Interleukin-2 receptor γ chain mutation results in X-linked severe combined immunodeficiency in humans. Cell 73:147–157, 1993b.

Nossal GJV, Szenberg A, Ada GL, Austin CM. Single cell studies on 19S antibody production. J Exp Med 119:485–502, 1964.

Osmond DG. Proliferation kinetics and the lifespan of B cells in central and peripheral lymphoid organs. Curr Opin Immunol 3:179–185, 1991.

Padovan E, Casorati G, Dellabona P, Meyer S, Brockhaus M, Lanzavecchia A. Expression of two T cell receptor α chains: dual receptor T cells. Science 262:422–424, 1993.

Paul WE, Bona C. Regulatory idiotypes and immune networks: a hypothesis. Immunol Today 3:230–234, 1982.

Perlmutter RM, Kearney JF, Chang SP, Hood LE. Developmentally controlled expression of immunoglobulin V$_H$ genes. Science 227:1597–1601, 1985.

Purkerson J, Isakson P. A two-signal model for regulation of immunoglobulin isotype switching. FASEB J 6:3245–3252, 1992.

Raaphorts FM, Timmers E, Keuter MJH. Restricted utilization of germ line V$_H$3 genes and short diverse third complementarity-determining regions (CDR3) in human fetal B lymphocyte immunoglobulin heavy chain gene rearrangements. Eur J Immunol 22:247–251, 1992.

Raff MC, Owen JJT, Cooper MD, Lawton AR, Megson M, Gathings WE. Differences in susceptibility of mature and immature mouse B lymphocytes to anti–immunoglobulin-induced immunoglobulin suppression in vitro: possible implications for B cell tolerance to self. J Exp Med 142:1052–1064, 1975.

Russell SM, Keegan AD, Harada N, Nakamura Y, Noguchi M, Leland P, Friedmann MC, Miyajima A, Puri RK, Paul WE, Leonard WJ. Interleukin-2 receptor γ chain: a functional component of the interleukin-4 receptor. Science 262:1881–1883, 1993.

Schatz DG, Oettinger MA, Schlissel MS. V(D)J recombination: molecular biology and regulation. Annu Rev Immunol 10:359–384, 1992.

Schroeder HW Jr, Hillson JL, Perlmutter RM. Early restriction of the human antibody repertoire. Science 238:791–793, 1987.

Schroeder HW Jr, Wang JY. Preferential utilization of conserved immunoglobulin heavy chain variable gene segments during human fetal life. Proc Natl Acad Sci U S A 87:6146–6150, 1990.

Sher A, Coffman RL. Regulation of immunity to parasites by T cells and T cell–derived cytokines. Annu Rev Immunol 10:385–409, 1992.

Sigal NH, Pickard AR, Metcalf ES, Gearhart PJ, Klinman NR. Expression of phosphorylcholine specific B cells during murine development. J Exp Med 146:933–948, 1977.

Solvason N, Kearney JF. The human fetal omentum: a site of B cell generation. J Exp Med 175:397–404, 1992.

Splawski JB, Jelinek DF, Lipsky PE. Delineation of the functional capacity of human neonatal lymphocytes. J Clin Invest 87:545–553, 1991.

Splawski JB, Lipsky PE. Cytokine regulation of immunoglobulin secretion by neonatal lymphocytes. J Clin Invest 88:967–977, 1991.

Stiehm ER, Fudenberg HH. Serum levels of immunoglobulins in health and disease: a survey. Pediatrics 37:715–727, 1966.

Tosato G, Magrath IT, Koski IR, Dooley NJ, Blaese RM. B cell differentiation and immunoregulatory T cell function in human cord blood lymphocytes. J Clin Invest 66:383–388, 1980.

Tsubata T, Reth M. The products of the pre-B cell specific genes ($\lambda 5$ and VpreB) and the immunoglobulin μ chain form a complex that is transported to the cell surface. J Exp Med 172:973–976, 1990.

Tucker PW. Transcriptional regulation of IgM and IgD. Immunol Today 6:181–182, 1985.

Vakil M, Kearney J. Functional characterization of monoclonal auto–anti-idiotype antibodies isolated from the early B cell repertoire of BALB/c mice. Eur J Immunol 16:1151–1158, 1986.

Vakil M, Sauter H, Paige C, Kearney, J. *In vivo* suppression of perinatal multispecific B cells results in a distortion of the adult B cell repertoire. Eur J Immunol 16:1159–1165, 1986.

von Boehmer H. Developmental biology of T cells in T cell–receptor transgenic mice. Annu Rev Immunol 6:531–556, 1990.

Weinberg K, Parkman R. Severe combined immunodeficiency due to a specific defect in the production of interleukin-2. N Engl J Med 322:1718–1723, 1990.

Willems van Dijk K, Milner LA, Sasso EH, Millner ECB. Chromosomal organization of the heavy chain variable region gene segments comprising the human fetal antibody repertoire. Proc Natl Acad Sci U S A 89:10403–10434, 1992.

Wilson CB, Lewis DB, English KB. T cell development in the fetus and neonate. Adv Exp Med Biol 310:17–29, 1991.

Yellen AJ, Glenn W, Sukhatme VP, Cao X, Monroe JG. Signaling through surface IgM in tolerance-susceptible immature murine B lymphocytes: developmentally regulated differences in transmembrane signaling in splenic B cells from adult and neonatal mice. J Immunol 146:1446–1454, 1991.

Chapter 2

The T-Lymphocyte System

Erwin W. Gelfand and Terri H. Finkel

Thymus-dependent, or T, lymphocytes are responsible for cell-mediated immunity and are essential for the development of antigen-specific antibody responses. The central role of the thymus was first recognized in mice and rabbits who were subjected to thymectomy (Archer and Pierce, 1961; Miller and Osoba, 1967). Studies in athymic, or nude, mice provided more direct evidence for the role of the thymus in T-cell differentiation (Sato et al., 1976). An endocrine function for the thymus was suggested by experiments using thymic tissue enclosed in cell-impermeable diffusion chambers and cell-free thymus extracts to restore immune competence in neonatally thymectomized animals (Miller and Osoba, 1967). Indeed, a number of thymic humoral factors have been suggested to contribute to T-cell differentiation within the thymus and in the peripheral lymphoid tissues. The immunologic role of these factors has been investigated in different bioassays (Bach and Carnaud, 1976; Trainin et al., 1980), and a number of clinical trials were initiated in the therapy of primary and secondary disorders of T-cell function. In the last several years, there has been little enthusiasm for studying their role as immune modulators.

A number of different experimental approaches have contributed to an understanding of the functional development of human T cells. A major source of continuing information has derived from the careful analysis of a number of immunodeficiency disorders. As these disorders often manifest as examples of the arrest of T-cell maturation, they provide a clearer understanding of the role of different enzymes and growth factors in

T-cell differentiation than can be achieved by studying in vitro systems. The recent genetic and biochemical characterization of different types of severe combined immunodeficiency disorders (SCIDs) and antibody deficiency disorders has revealed a critical role for different kinases, growth factors, and growth factor receptors in the development of the T-lymphocyte system. These studies in humans have been complemented by genetic manipulation of mice, in so-called knock-out experiments, in which gene targeting has been used to examine the role of specific proteins in T-cell development and function.

A second important source of information on T-cell development is the monitoring of T-cell function following immune or hematologic reconstitution. Following reconstitution there is recapitulation of T-cell ontogeny. During normal lymphocyte maturation, many of the stages in T-cell development are highly dynamic, and at any given time, each of these stages may exist only transiently and in small numbers of cells. Lymphoblasts from patients with T-cell leukemia may serve as examples of cells "frozen," or arrested, at distinct stages of differentiation. Finally, the ability to identify distinct T-cell subsets with monoclonal antibodies has significantly advanced our understanding of the T-lymphocyte system in man.

DEVELOPMENT

Anatomy and Embryology of the Thymus

The thymus gland arises from the ventral portions of the third and fourth pharyngeal pouches. It appears that during morphogenesis of the human thymus gland, the fibrous capsule, stroma, and vessels are derived from mesodermal or mesoectodermal (mesenchymal) tissue. The cortical epithelial component of the thymic microenvironment is thought to be derived from the ectodermal bronchial cleft; the medullary epithelium is derived from the third pharyngeal pouch endoderm. Until 7 to 8 weeks gestational age, the thymic epithelial rudiments are virtually devoid of lymphoid cells. By 9 weeks, thymocytes are detectable. Between 7 to 10 weeks' gestation, the thymus gland descends from the neck into the upper and anterior mediastinum.

In relation to total body size, the thymus is largest at birth. With increasing age, there is progressive involution with infiltration of fatty tissue. The gland is highly organized, consisting of numerous lobules and a well-demarcated outer cortex and inner medulla. The cortex contains densely packed small lymphocytes, whereas lymphocytes are more dispersed in the medulla. Prominent in the medulla are the reticuloepithelial cells that form Hassall's bodies (Fig. 2–1).

As discussed later, the anatomic compartmentalization of the thymus is paralleled by a phenotypic compartmentalization of thymocytes. In the cortex, the cells express the immature T-cell marker CD1 and may be double-negative or double-positive for CD4 and CD8. As the cells mature, they acquire increased expression of CD3 and in the medulla become single-positive for CD4 or CD8. Within the thymus, it is the thymic stromal cells that nurture differentiation, development, and even positive and negative selection. Different stromal subsets likely play different functional roles in their interactions with developing intrathymic lymphocytes. These different thymic stromal cells express an array of surface molecules (homing, adhesion, major histocompatibility complex) and form a precise architecture essential for thymic lymphocyte maturation.

Acquisition of Immune Competence in the Fetal Thymus

The high degree of organization within the thymus is attained by 10 to 12 weeks' gestation. At this age, fetal thymocytes can respond to the T-cell mitogen phytohemagglutinin and to allogeneic cells in a mixed leukocyte response (August et al., 1971). Transplantation of 10- to 12-week-old fetal thymocytes into immunodeficient recipients has resulted in graft-versus-host disease. This early acquisition of immune competence likely explains the ability of premature infants to actively reject a transplant or to demonstrate normal responses in in vitro tests of T-lymphocyte function. In contrast to mice, this early fetal T-cell immunocompetence in humans accounts for the overall lack of sequelae to neonatal thymectomy.

Intrathymic T-Cell Maturation

It is generally accepted that cells in hematopoietic tissues of embryos (yolk sac, fetal liver, bone marrow) migrate or are attracted to the thymus, where the processes of T-cell differentiation are initiated. In a series of studies of chick-quail hybrids, LeDourain and Jotereau (1975) have defined the contributions of endodermal epithelium, thymic mesenchyma, and blood-borne extrinsic elements to the histogenesis of the thymus.

The first detectable lymphoid elements of the embryonic thymus are blood-borne cells with a large nucleus and basophilic cytoplasm. Subsequent pathways of T-cell differentiation within the thymus have been inferred, based on in vivo studies of T-cell maturation, in vitro studies of human T-cell maturation using thymus epithelial cell cultures and culture-derived supernatant fluid, or by phenotypic compartmentalization of cells within the thymus (Gelfand and Dosch, 1982).

ORGANIZATION

Lymphocyte Compartmentalization, Recirculation, and Homing

The lymphoid system is functionally compartmentalized in vivo into defined primary, secondary, and tertiary lymphoid organs. Primary lymphoid tissues, the bone marrow and thymus, contribute by producing mature but antigen-naive lymphocytes. The secondary

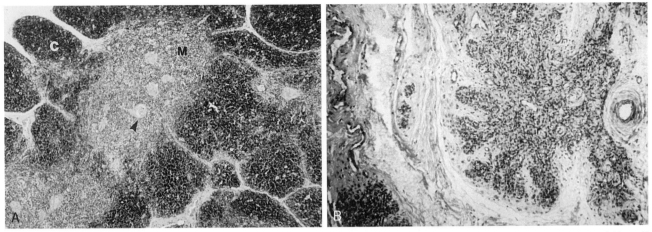

Figure 2–1. *A,* Normal thymus illustrating lobular structure of cortex (c) and medulla (m), corticomedullary differentiation and Hassall's corpuscles *(arrow)* in the medulla. *B,* Typical hypoplastic thymus from x-linked severe combined immunodeficiency disease illustrating lack of lobular structure and absence of corticomedullary demarcation and Hassall's corpuscles.

lymphoid tissues include lymph nodes, the spleen, and gut-associated lymphoid tissues and are specialized for the accumulation and presentation of antigen to both naive and memory lymphocyte subsets. The remaining, or tertiary, lymphoid tissues contain few lymphoid elements but can be induced to recruit lymphocytes when challenged—for example, in the setting of inflammation. Within each tissue, discrete microenvironments, characterized by different lymphocyte subsets and stromal elements, exist.

Lymphocyte homing encompasses the physiologic processes by which lymphocytes seek out or localize to particular tissues and their specific microenvironments. In these processes, adhesive interactions involved in lymphocyte-endothelial cell recognition play major roles. Thus, lymphocyte homing/recirculation is largely determined by the differential regulation of adhesion and de-adhesion. Adhesion to tissue components also plays a critical role in determining the tendency of a given lymphocyte to recirculate by regulating the ability of that cell type to pass through a particular tissue, appear in the lymph, and return to the circulation. Some lymphocyte subsets, such as intraepithelial T cells, remain firmly attached to their microenvironments, recirculating very little. Others, such as small, resting T cells, constantly recirculate over 12 to 24

cycles. One adhesive interaction central to the regulation of lymphocyte homing is that between blood-borne lymphocytes and postcapillary venular endothelium. The regulation of expression of lymphocyte receptors and their vascular ligands control to a large degree the overall functioning of the immune system.

Increasingly, lymphocyte and endothelial cell adhesion molecules are being identified (reviewed in Picker and Butcher, 1992; Mackay, 1992, Weissman, 1994). These molecules form several distinct families, including (Table 2–1):

1. The selectin family of leukocyte and endothelial cell c-type lectins.
2. Oligosaccharide ligands for the selectins.
3. Heterodimeric, activation-dependent integrins of the β1 and β2 classes, as well as novel βp-β7 integrins.
4. Members of the immunoglobulin family of cell adhesion molecules.
5. CD44, a proteoglycan-like molecule.

Primary Lymphoid Organs—Bone Marrow and Thymus

The production of T cells is initiated from hematopoietic stem cells in the marrow, but little T-cell differenti-

Table 2–1. Surface Molecules Involved in Lymphocyte-Endothelial Cell Interactions and Lymphocyte Homing

Lymphocyte Molecule	Structure	Endothelial Ligand	Function
L-selectin (LAM-1)	Selectin	MECA-79 PNAd	Lymphocyte homing to lymph nodes
α4β1 (VLA-4)	Integrin	VCAM-1/Fibronectin	Lymphocyte homing to inflammatory sites
α4β7 (LPAM-2)	Integrin	MAdCAM-1	Lymphocyte homing to gut
α5β1 (VLA-5)	Integrin	Fibronectin	
α6β1 (VLA-6)	Integrin	Laminin	Homing of pre-T cells to thymus
LFA-1	Integrin	ICAM-1/ICAM-2	Secondary adhesion molecule
CD31 (PECAM)	Immunoglobulin-related	CD31	Homing of naive T cells to lymph node
CLA (sialyl-Lewis X) cutaneous lymphocyte antigen	Sugar	ELAM-1	Recruitment to skin inflammatory sites
CD44 (Pgp-1, HCAM)	Cartilage link protein	Hyaluronate	General adhesion molecule

ation occurs there. Further differentiation occurs for the majority of T-cell precursors in the thymic microenvironment, which requires an obligatory bloodborne homing stage. Little is known about bone marrow–to–thymus migration, but this translocation in humans involves T lineage–committed precursors with the phenotype CD7[+], CD2[+], cytoplasmic CD3[+] and preservation of the progenitor cell antigen, CD34. About 1% of thymocytes constitute this population of cells. CD34 is rapidly lost when T cells become CD4/CD8 double-positive.

Among the receptors that may control migration of pre-T cells to mouse thymus is CD44 (Pgp-1) (Reichart et al., 1986). This adhesion receptor is expressed on bone marrow prothymocytes and the most immature thymocyte subset. LECAM-1 is also expressed at high levels on the most immature human and mouse thymocytes (Reichart et al., 1986; Picker et al., 1990). These receptors, which also participate in lymphocyte-postcapillary high endothelial venule (HEV) interactions, may be involved in pre–T-cell localization to the thymus. Within the thymus, the complex processes of positive and negative selection critical to shaping of the T-cell repertoire occur (see following).

These processes generate αβ T-cell receptors expressing T lymphocytes capable of responding to appropriately presented foreign antigens, which then emigrate from the thymus. By this time, they express the homing receptors required for their accumulation in secondary lymphoid tissues and for localizing within T-cell microenvironments.

An exception to this pattern involves the unique subsets of γδ-bearing T cells that are associated with discrete epithelial sites. Some of these subsets pass through the thymus, whereas others, such as intestinal intraepithelial T cells, may be independent of the thymus and migrate directly from bone marrow to gut, where they undergo terminal differentiation.

Secondary Lymphoid Organs—Lymph Node, Spleen, Peyer's Patches

These sites are the principal sites of homing of naive T cells. In these sites are specialized areas of antigen accumulation that contain subpopulations of immune accessory cells that are efficient in antigen processing and presentation. Lymph nodes are the termination point of lymphatic vessels that drain lymph from most tissues of the body and carry antigens to these nodes. The spleen filters the blood and accumulates bloodborne antigens for lymphocytes in the white pulp. The Peyer's patches of the gastrointestinal mucosa and similar lymphoid accumulations in the respiratory tract are specialized in passing antigen across the epithelial barrier for presentation to the organized lymphoid tissues. Lymph nodes and Peyer's patches have distinct postcapillary venules for recruiting lymphocytes, the HEVs.

Lymphocytes that encounter specific antigen within a secondary lymphoid organ become activated. As a result, lymphocyte surface integrin expression is upregulated, including LFA-1 and β1 integrins (VLA-pro-

teins), which mediate strong transient adhesion to cellular and extracellular matrix at the site of stimulation (Springer, 1990; Dustin and Springer, 1991). A second consequence of antigenic stimulation is the clonal expansion and differentiation of lymphocytes into effector and memory cells. These populations differ in their migratory properties from naive lymphocytes. Memory/effector cells migrate efficiently into tertiary organs and become selective in their ability to access peripheral lymph nodes rather than mucosal lymphoid tissues.

Homing to lymph nodes is targeted by binding of the lymphocyte (selectin) homing receptor LECAM-1 to the tissue-selective vascular adhesion molecule, the peripheral lymph node vascular addressin (PNAd). In contrast to naive T cells (which all express LECAM-1), memory T cells are subdivided into LECAM-1[+] and LECAM-1[−] (Picker et al., 1990). The activation-dependent leukocyte integrin, LFA-1, has also been shown to participate in lymphocyte interactions with lymph node HEVs to some degree through the endothelial cell ligand ICAM-1. In Peyer's patches, the α4 integrins are involved in lymphocyte interactions with HEV via VCAM-1 or fibronectin (Elices et al, 1990). Peyer's patch HEVs are also rich in a mucosal addressin called MAdCAM-1 that binds mucosa-homing lymphoid subsets through interaction with α4, β7 integrin (Berlin et al., 1993).

Tertiary Lymphoid Tissues

The best studied tertiary lymphoid tissues are associated with epithelial surfaces such as the gastrointestinal tract, the respiratory tract, the skin, and the reproductive tract. At these sites, the lymphocytes are primarily in intraepithelial locations. Recirculation through these tertiary tissues preferentially involves activated memory T cells expressing LFA-1, ICAM-1, α4 integrins, LFA-3 and CD44 (Sanders et al., 1988; Picker et al., 1990). The majority of the cells are also CD45RO[+] memory T cells (in contrast to the CD45RA[+] naive T cells). The attraction of memory T cells may also reflect involvement of memory lymphocyte-selective chemoattractants such as RANTES (Schall, 1991). After prolonged stimulation, the tertiary tissues take on appearances similar to that of a lymph node or Peyer's patch. With this transformation—for example, in skin—the infiltrating T cells are predominantly CLA[+](sialyl-Lewis X) with the superficial dermal venules expressing the vascular counter-receptor for CLA, ELAM-1 (Picker et al., 1991).

Adhesion Molecule Defects

The important role of these adhesion molecules and adhesive interactions is underscored by the defects that accompany congenital deficiency of some of these molecules. An inherited defect in the synthesis of CD18, the common β chain of β2 integrins, causes a syndrome called *leukocyte adhesion defect type 1* (Bowen et al., 1982; Anderson and Springer, 1987). Affected patients suffer from severe recurrent bacterial infections, characteristically without pus formation, despite markedly elevated systemic leukocyte counts. The defect leads to abnormal leukocyte adhesion that is mediated by CD11/CD18 on the neutrophil surface and by other molecules, including ICAM-1, on endothelial cells (see Chapter 15).

A second defect affects the first adhesive step, the rolling phenomenon that is mediated by selectins that specifically recognize structures containing sialyl-Lewis X. This form of leukocyte adhesion defect (LAD-type 2) was ascribed to a congenital defect of endogenous fucose metabolism resulting in the failure to synthesize fucosylated carbohydrate molecules, including sialyl-Lewis X. This defect also results in severe recurrent pyogenic infections and defective neutrophil mobility (Etzioni et al., 1992).

FUNCTIONAL DIFFERENTIATION

Shaping the T-Cell Repertoire

T lymphocytes are involved in multiple arms of the immune response, including the regulation of immunoglobulin production, the mediation of delayed hypersensitivity and graft rejection, and defense against a variety of pathogenic viruses, fungi, or facultative intracellular parasites. The different regulatory and effector functions mediated by T cells represent the work of populations of T cells that can be distinguished by the expression of different cell surface proteins. In order for these specific functions to occur, the T cell must first recognize an antigen that initiates the T-cell immune response.

T-cell antigen recognition is a complicated process that is considerably different in many ways from antigen recognition by B cells, although they share some principles in common. T cells recognize antigens bound to self–major histocompatibility complex (MHC) gene products in humans (Benacerraf and McDevitt, 1972; Zinkernagel and Doherty, 1975; Bjorkmann et al., 1987), the class I molecules (HLA-A, -B, -C), and class II molecules (HLA-DR, -DQ, and -DP) expressed on antigen presenting cells (APC). In general, CD4$^+$ T cells recognize endocytosed antigenic peptides bound to class II molecules and CD8$^+$ T cells recognize endogenous peptides bound to class I molecules (Biddison et al., 1982; Meuer et al., 1982; Brodsky and Guagliardi, 1991).

T-Cell Receptor

Recognition of foreign antigens is through the T-cell receptor for antigen (TCR) (Fig. 2–2). TCRs expressed on the surface of T cells are composed of either the heterodimeric proteins alpha (α) and beta (β) or gamma (γ) and delta (δ). Each of these protein chains has a variable (V), joining (J), and constant region (C), encoded by noncontiguous gene segments (Williams and Barclay, 1988). The genetic organization of the TCR genes is similar to the organization of the immunoglobulin genes. It is the mixing and matching of individual V, J, and C regions by a process of sequential gene rearrangement that generates the diversity of TCR antigen recognition patterns necessary for discernment of the thousands of known antigens. Although the TCR is required for recognition and binding of foreign antigen, the CD3 complex is required for expression and function of the TCR (see later). The CD3 complex

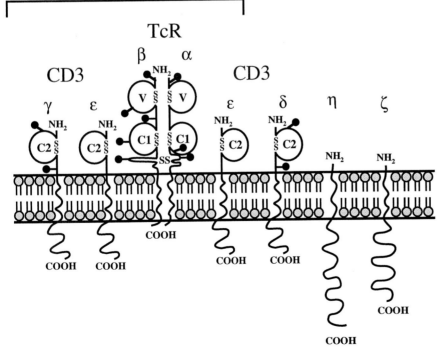

Figure 2–2. The TCR:CD3 complex. Shown are the α and β chains, required for recognition and binding of foreign antigen, and the CD3 complex (γ, ε, δ) and ζ and η chains, required for expression and function of the T-cell receptor. The circles in the figure represent domains, predicted from primary sequences; V and C domains show homology with the V and C domains of immunoglobulin molecules. Presumed N-linked carbohydrate sites are shown by the symbol.

is composed of at least five proteins that are noncovalently associated with the αβ or γδ TCR molecules: gamma (CD3-γ), delta (CD3-δ), and epsilon (CD3-ε), encoded on human chromosome 11, and zeta (ζ) or a ζ-family member, encoded on human chromosome 1 (Weissman et al., 1988).

As discussed previously, the TCR recognizes antigen bound in the groove of an MHC molecule (Fig. 2–3). This interaction involves the variable regions of both the α and β chains and any individual antigen activates only approximately 0.01% of the T-cell repertoire. In contrast, proteins encoded by microorganisms that activate between 5% and 30% of the T-cell repertoire because they require interaction with only the β-chain of the TCR have recently been identified (Herman et al., 1991). These proteins have therefore been named "superantigens" and likely play a critical role in shaping the T-cell repertoire and in many aspects of health and disease.

Clonal Selection

Positive Selection

Based on studies in mice, specificity for self is acquired by most αβ+ T cells in the thymus, where precursor T cells learn to recognize antigens expressed by cells within the thymus (Zinkernagel and Doherty, 1979). As discussed earlier, T lineage–committed precursors bearing CD34 but without CD4 or CD8 migrate from the bone marrow to the cortical region of the thymus (Fig. 2–4). In ontogeny, a small population of T cells expressing the γδ TCR appear first and exit the thymus in waves to populate the tertiary lymphoid organs (Fowlkes and Pardoll, 1989). The majority of immature thymocytes, appearing slightly later in thymus development, transit to the thymic medulla and sequentially express CD4 and CD8. It is at this stage that αβ gene rearrangement occurs, first for the β-chain and then for the α-chain (Raulet et al, 1985).

Although a particular T cell can express only a single β-chain as a result of a process called *allelic exclusion*, the α-chain is not similarly regulated, a fact that may have interesting consequences for positive selection (see later). The α- and β-chain pair in association with the CD3 molecules are expressed on the surface of the T cell at about one tenth of the level found on mature T cells.

At this immature stage of development, the sampling (or repertoire) of TCRs is random, determined solely by the genetics of the individual and by the rules of αβ gene rearrangement. However, the majority of these T cells will never leave the thymus but will be eliminated by the dual processes of positive and negative selection. In order for T cells that can appropriately respond to foreign antigen bound to self-MHC to mature, immature thymocytes must go through an educational process called *positive selection.*

Although the biochemical events leading to positive selection are not understood, studies using mice transgenic for a single TCR of known specificity (so-called monoclonal mice) have shown that during thy-

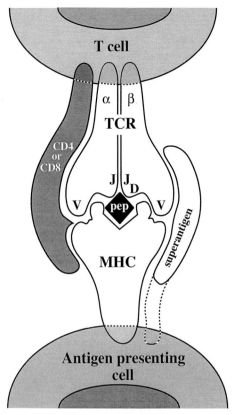

Figure 2–3. Interactions involved in T-cell recognition of conventional antigens and superantigens. Peptide fragments (pep) of protein antigens are bound in a groove in major histocompatibility complex (MHC) molecules expressed on antigen-presenting cells (APCs). During an interaction between a T cell and an APC, MHC-bound peptides come into contact with the hypervariable regions of the T-cell receptor. This region is formed by the variable (V), diversity (D), and joining (J) gene segments, which rearrange during T-cell development. Superantigens, which can be soluble or cell-bound, facilitate the interaction between a T cell and an APC by binding to the sides of MHC and TCR molecules. These regions of MHC and TCR are relatively invariant. Therefore, superantigens activate a very high proportion of T cells. For recognition of both conventional antigens and superantigens, the interaction between the T cell and APC is strengthened by binding and signaling of CD4 or CD8.

mic development, only those T cells bearing TCRs specific for self-MHC are allowed to survive (von Boehmer, 1990). As predicted, all of the mature T cells in these mice bear the CD4 coreceptor if the TCR is specific for class II MHC and the CD8 coreceptor if the TCR is specific for class I MHC. If an immature thymocyte has the "wrong" specificity, recent data suggest that it may have a second chance at survival by rearranging and expressing a second α-chain to pair with its first β-chain. Only after positive selection are the gene products responsible for gene rearrangement (the recombinase-activating genes) down-regulated, thus limiting TCR expression for that particular cell (Turka et al., 1991).

Negative Selection

A second selective gauntlet that the immature thymocyte must survive is "negative selection." Negative

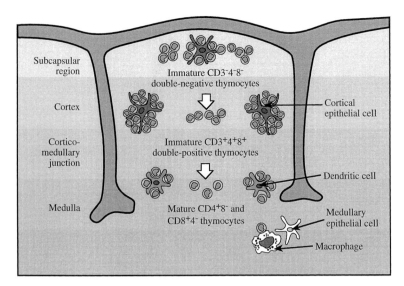

Figure 2–4. Changes in cell surface molecules during T-cell development in the thymus. The CD4, CD8, and T-cell receptor (TCR) molecules are the most important cell surface molecules in identifying thymocyte subpopulations. The most immature cell population in the thymus is found in the subcapsular region of the cortex and does not express any of these molecules. Since these cells do not express CD4 or CD8, they are called "double-negative" thymocytes. After migrating deeper into the thymic cortex, αβ T cells mature through a stage where both CD4 and CD8, as well as low levels of the TCR, are expressed by the same cell. These cells are known as "double-positive" thymocytes. If these cells bind self-MHC, they lose expression of either CD4 or CD8 and increase the level of expression of the TCR. These cells are the mature, "single-positive" thymocytes found in the medulla, and they are exported from the thymus to the peripheral lymphoid organs.

selection, or clonal deletion, ensures that the TCR does not induce autoimmunity by responding to self-MHC molecules in the absence of foreign antigen. Elegant studies using TCR-transgenic mice or mice with endogenous or exogenous superantigens have shown that cells bearing autoreactive TCRs are deleted by apoptosis (programmed cell death) before release from the thymus (see Fig. 2–2) (Kappler et al., 1987; Murphy et al., 1990).

Thymocytes that successfully pass the tests of positive and negative selection mature to medullary thymocytes bearing CD4 *or* CD8 and high levels of antigen receptor. Medullary thymocytes are largely phenotypically and functionally mature and by poorly understood processes, exit the thymus to populate the secondary and tertiary lymphoid organs.

A critical question of T-cell development for which answers are still rudimentary is how can a T cell with a single antigen receptor be both positively and negatively selected using that same antigen receptor? Hypotheses that have been advanced include the following:

1. Peptides that positively and negatively select have different affinities for the TCR.
2. Thymocytes at different developmental stages are susceptible to positive or negative selection.
3. The ligand (APC or peptide) responsible for positive selection is different from the ligand responsible for negative selection. Whereas the role that the latter two mechanisms play in signaling for positive versus negative selection is controversial, recent data suggest that the same antigenic peptide can lead to positive *or* negative selection, the outcome being determined by the affinity and density of the peptide ligand (Fig. 2–5) (Marrack and Parker, 1994).

Role of Soluble Factors

The discussion has thus far focused on the critical role of direct interactions between developing thymocytes and the stromal cells of the thymus in shaping T-

cell development. Although less well studied, "thymic humoral factors" and other lymphokines known to be secreted in the thymus are also likely to play an important role in thymocyte differentiation. (Lymphokines and other cytokines are discussed below and in Chapter 4).

Interestingly, recent studies of mutant mice lacking specific cytokines (cytokine "knock-out" mice) have not revealed marked effects of the missing cytokine on T-cell development. However, rather than arguing for the nonessential nature of an individual cytokine, these findings point to the characteristic redundancy of cytokines; that is, each cytokine has multiple functions, and any one function is generally mediated by more than one cytokine (Paul, 1989).

Table 2–2 summarizes the effects of cytokines on intrathymic T-cell development. IL-1 is produced by thymic epithelial cells and pre-T cells. Although IL-1 does not act as a growth factor by itself, it can cooperate with other intrathymic cytokines (such as IL-2) to induce proliferation of human thymic T-cell precursors (He and Kabelitz, 1994). Although IL-2 messenger ribonucleic acid (mRNA) is absent in human postnatal thymocytes and stromal cells, IL-2 has effects on these cells and could enter the thymus through the bloodstream. An IL-2–dependent autocrine pathway of growth stimulation has been described in human thy-

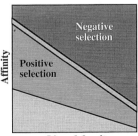

Figure 2–5. The affinity and density of the peptide ligand may determine the fate of developing T cells in the thymus. (After M. Bevan.)

Table 2–2. Summary of Cytokine Effects on Intrathymic T-Cell Development

Interleukin	Growth-Promoting Effect on							Induction of Expression of	
	pro-T	pre-T	TN	DN	DP	CD4+SP	CD8+SP	TCRαβ	TCRγδ
IL-1*	?	−	−	+	−	±	±	?	?
IL-2	+ +	+ +	+ +	+	−	+	+	+ +	+
IL-4	+ +	+ +	+ +	+	±	±	+ +	+	+ +
IL-6*	−	−	−	−	−	+	+	?	?
IL-7	+ + +	+ + +	+ + +	+ + +	−	+	+ +	−	+ + +

*Costimulatory activity.

Key: ? = Not clear; − = no effect; ± = weak effect; + = moderate effect; + + = strong effect; + + + = very strong effect.

Abbreviations: TN = triple negative (CD3⁻, CD4⁻, CD8⁻); DN = double negative (CD3⁺, CD4⁻, CD8⁻); DP = double positive (CD3⁺, CD4⁺, CD8⁺); CD4⁺SP = CD4⁺ single positive; CD8⁺SP = CD8⁺ single positive; TCR = T-cell receptor.

mic T-cell precursors, in which an IL-2/IL-2Rβ interaction induces the expression of IL-2Rα, leading to high affinity IL-2R expression and cellular proliferation (Toribio et al., 1989). In addition to its growth-promoting effects, IL-2 may influence thymocyte differentiation by promoting maturation of αβ T cells (Barcena et al., 1991).

IL-4 is a cytokine produced by activated T cells of the T_H2 phenotype. Its pleiotropic effects on cells of the immune system are summarized later in Table 2–4. IL-4 acts as a growth and differentiation factor for human thymic T cell precursors and in vitro preferentially induces maturation of γδ T cells. IL-6, like IL-1, appears to function primarily as a costimulator of thymocyte proliferation. IL-7 has growth-promoting effects, particularly on the earliest T-cell precursors (see Table 2–4) and may be an inductive factor for γδ, but not αβ, T-cell maturation (Watanabe et al., 1991).

Along with these cytokines, additional cytokines (Table 2–4) have been shown to be constitutively produced by thymocytes or thymic stromal cells. These include IL-3, GM-CSF, leukemia inhibitory factor, stem cell factor, IL-1 receptor antagonist 2, TNF-α, lymphotoxin (TNF-β), and interferon gamma (IFN-γ), although the effects of these cytokines on T-cell development remain to be clarified. Clearly, more research is needed, particularly into the effects of these growth factors on thymic selection and shaping of the T-cell repertoire.

Finally, although the thymus plays a predominant role in T-cell education, some of the T-cell repertoire (notably γδ⁺ T cells but also, for example, αβ⁺ intestinal epithelial lymphocytes) is shaped in extrathymic locations. In addition, the T cell is not immutable even after selection, since surface receptor and cytokine expression may be altered by activation, by the acquisition of immunologic memory, by infection, and by malignancy, thus impacting T-cell function.

T-CELL ACTIVATION

T-Cell Signaling

Mature antigen-specific T lymphocytes are generally in a resting or quiescent state, requiring antigen stimulation to exit from the G₀ stage of the cell cycle. As discussed, it is through the T-cell receptor (TCR) that antigens, pathogens, or foreign substances are recognized and through it that a series of signal transduction events are initiated. These signals are not only fundamental for the initiation of T-cell responses but as previously discussed, are involved in developmental decisions as well. The signal transduction events triggered through the antigen (T-cell) receptor are slowly being unraveled. TCRs recognize short peptide antigens that have been proteolytically processed and bound to (antigen presentation) self–major histocompatibility complex (MHC) molecules on the surface of the antigen presenting cell (APC).

In addition to the TCR itself, other surface molecules, coreceptors or accessory (costimulatory) molecules contribute to T-cell activation. Coreceptors, such as CD4 or CD8, are important in antigen-receptor signal transduction since they contribute to the initiation of signals and amplify the interaction between the antigen complex and antigen receptor. Costimulatory molecules, such as CD2 and CD28, interact with ligands on the APC and induce independent signal transduction events that influence the cellular response.

T-Cell Receptor Interactions with Protein Tyrosine Kinases

In all cell types, protein tyrosine phosphorylation is important in the initiation of cellular responses. The TCR has no intrinsic protein tyrosine kinase (PTK) activity but activates a number of cytoplasmic PTKs. There are two distinct classes of PTKs involved in T-cell activation, members of the Src family, including Lck and Fyn and the non-Src kinases, ZAP-70 and Syk. These PTKs interact with the TCR and with each other (Fig. 2–6). One tyrosine phosphatase (PTPase), CD45, is also important in regulating TCR-induced signal transduction.

The TCRs have separate antigen-binding and signal-transduction units, and they form a complex at the plasma membrane. The antigen-binding subunit consists of the α- and β-chains and is noncovalently associated with the CD3-δ, CD3-ε, and CD3-γ chains and a ζ-chain–containing dimer. The cytoplasmic domains of these associated invariant chains are responsible for coupling the TCR to the intracellular signaling machin-

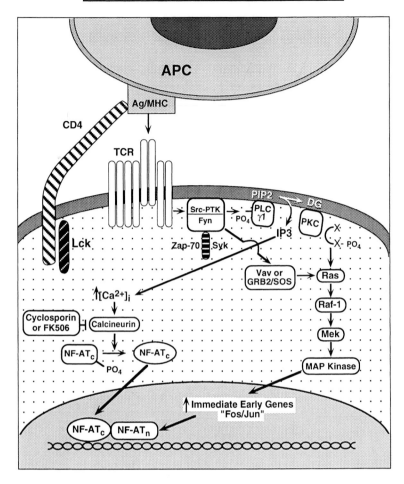

Consequences of Antigen Receptor Induced Tyrosine Phosphorylation

Figure 2–6. Signaling pathways are induced following antigen-presenting cell/T-cell receptor interaction. APC = antigen-presenting cell; Ag-MHC = antigen/major histocompatibility complex class II interaction; Src-PTK = Src family protein tyrosine kinases; PIP2 = phosphatidylinositol bisphosphate; DG = diacylglycerol; PKC = protein kinase C; PLC-γ1 = phospholipase C-γ 1; IP3 = inositol trisphosphate; NF-AT = nuclear factor of activated T cells; n = nuclear; c = cytosolic.

ery (Weiss, 1991). Common cytoplasmic domain sequence motifs couple these proteins to intracellular PTKs. These motifs consist of paired tyrosines and leucines and are called *antigen recognition activation motifs* (ARAM) or *tyrosine-based activation motifs* (TAM) (Samelson and Klausner, 1992).

Because the TCR has neither intrinsic PTK or PTPase function, the ARAM sequences appear to be both necessary and sufficient for the induction of protein tyrosine phosphorylation in T cells, likely by direct interaction with cytoplasmic PTKs. Currently, the clearest role for a Src family member in T-cell signal transduction is Lck. This PTK interacts with the cytoplasmic domains of the co-receptors CD4 and CD8 (Rudd, 1990; Veillette et al., 1991). Lck also interacts with the ARAMs in the ζ chain and the CD3-ε chain. Phosphorylation of the ARAMs then leads to recruitment of other molecules involved in signal transduction, such as ZAP-70.

Biochemical studies also implicate a role for Fyn in T-cell signal transduction, demonstrating a functional interaction with the TCR complex. As with overexpression of Lck, overexpression of Fyn increases the sensitivity to TCR stimulation (Davidson et al., 1992). ZAP-70 is a PTK expressed exclusively in T cells and NK

cells (Chan et al., 1992), whereas Syk is expressed preferentially in B cells, myeloid cells, and thymocytes (Taniguchi et al., 1991). Although not associated with the TCR in the basal state, ZAP-70 is rapidly recruited to the phosphorylated ζ and CD3-ε chains following TCR stimulation (Chan et al., 1991). In thymocytes, Syk may substitute to some extent for ZAP-70, but not completely, as demonstrated in ZAP-70 deficient patients, who positively select CD4[+] cells (but not CD8[+] T cells), although these cells remain nonfunctional (Gelfand et al., 1995) (see Chapter 12). The results suggest that the TCR interacts with two PTKs sequentially. One of these, likely a Src family member, first phosphorylates the ARAM, leading to the recruitment of ZAP-70. The coreceptor binding of both CD4 and CD8 to Lck further amplifies effective signal transduction at low antigen concentrations (Weiss and Littman, 1994).

Studies of T-cell lines deficient in CD45 expression demonstrate that CD45 is required for TCR signal transduction, including PTK activation (Koretzky et al., 1990, 1991). The target of the CD45 phosphatase is the negative regulatory site of tyrosine phosphorylation in Lck (or Fyn). In opposition to CD45, these negative regulatory sites of Src PTKs are phosphorylated by Csk, a widely expressed PTK (Okada et al., 1991).

T-Cell Receptor–Induced Tyrosine Phosphorylation

As a result of stimulation of the TCR, a number of cytoplasmic and membrane proteins become phosphorylated. In many cases, the identity and particularly the function of these phosphoproteins are not known.

Ras Activation in T Cells

Stimulation of the TCR induces a marked and rapid activation of Ras, a GTP-binding protein (Downward et al., 1992; Patel et al., 1994). Receptor tyrosine kinases regulate Ras activity through interactions with the guanine nucleotide exchange proteins, Sos and Vav (Polakis and McCormick, 1993; Schlessinger, 1993). The downstream effectors of Ras function have been identified in T cells (see Fig. 2–6) (Franklin et al., 1994). Ras interacts directly with the serine/threonine kinase Raf-1, which in turn regulates the activity of the kinase cascade that includes MEK (MAP kinase kinase) and MAP kinase. This complex of kinases has been implicated in the regulation of nuclear events involved in cell growth and differentiation. Activation of Ras has also been correlated with the transcriptional activation of the IL-2 gene.

Activation of Ca²⁺ Influx and the Phosphatidylinositol Second Messenger Systems

Stimulation of the TCR also leads to rapid increases in free cytosolic Ca^{2+} concentrations ($[Ca^{2+}]_i$) and the generation of the second messengers inositol 1,4,5-trisphosphate (IP_3) and diacylglycerol (DG) (Gelfand, 1990). The second messengers are liberated as a consequence of the activation of phospholipase C-γ1 (PLC-γ1), resulting in the hydrolysis of phosphatidylinositol 4,5-bisphosphate (see Fig. 2–6). Accumulated data indicate that stimulation of the TCR induces tyrosine phosphorylation and activation of PLC-γ1. Release of IP_3 is responsible for the TCR-induced rapid increases in ($[Ca^{2+}]_i$) resulting from the release of Ca^{2+} from sequestered stores in the cytoplasm. IP_3 may also regulate the influx of Ca^{2+} across the plasma membrane, although the mechanisms regulating the transport of Ca^{2+} through non–voltage-gated channels in the plasma membranes of stimulated T cells is not entirely clear (Berridge, 1993). Release of DG activates protein kinase C. Increases in $[Ca^{2+}]_i$, especially secondary to transmembrane influx, appear necessary for IL-2 gene transcription.

Inhibitors of PTK prevent TCR-induced changes in $[Ca^{2+}]_i$, IP_3 production, activation of PKC and IL-2 production. Activation of a major transcriptional enhancer of the IL-2 gene, nuclear factor of activated T cells (NF-AT), appears dependent on these increases in $[Ca^{2+}]_i$. Calcineurin, a calcium-calmodulin–dependent phosphatase, required for dephosphorylation of the cyto-

plasmic component of NF-AT, is the target of the immunosuppressive drugs cyclosporine and FK506 (see Fig. 2–6) (Schrieber and Crabtree, 1992).

Tyrosine Kinases in T-Cell Development

The signals generated as a consequence of the activation of some PTKs are also fundamental in developmental pathways. Mice deficient in Lck have an arrest early in thymocyte development from the CD4/CD8 double-negative to the CD4/CD8 double-positive stage, and the few peripheral T cells that do develop have decreased responses to TCR stimulation (Molina et al., 1992; Levin et al., 1993). In contrast, in mice in which the Fyn gene has been disrupted, no gross T-cell developmental abnormalities were observed, implying that the events associated with TCR-mediated positive and negative selection are independent of Fyn (Appleby et al., 1992; Stein et al., 1992). Thymocytes from such mice show a TCR-signaling defect that appears most pronounced in a mature thymocyte subset but less so in peripheral T cells. These findings indicate that Fyn may play an important role in TCR signal transduction in a developmentally restricted T-cell compartment. The phenotype of mice in which the CD45 gene has been disrupted is also altered. T-cell development is impaired at the CD4/CD8 double-positive stage, and a reduced number of T cells are detected in the periphery (Kishihara et al., 1993).

Recently, a form of severe combined immunodeficiency disease (SCID) with decreased CD8⁺ cells has been associated with *ZAP-70 deficiency* (Arpaia et al., 1994; Chan et al., 1994; Elder et al., 1994) (see Chapter 12). In these cases, the thymus appears normal with apparently normal numbers of CD4/CD8 double-positive cells, although in the periphery only CD4⁺ cells are detected. These CD4⁺ cells do not signal through the TCR, although the thymocytes appear to signal normally (Gelfand et al., 1995). It thus appears that ZAP-70 may not be required for the positive selection of CD4⁺ cells but is essential for CD8⁺ T-cell selection. In peripheral CD4⁺ T cells, ZAP-70 appears essential for TCR-induced signaling.

Signaling Through the Interleukin-2 Complex

Interleukin-2 (IL-2) is produced by T cells in response to activation and stimulates T cells through specific surface receptors (IL-2 receptors, IL-2R). IL-2 has additional biological effects including induction of B-cell proliferation and differentiation, proliferation and maturation of oligodendroglial cells, activation of lymphokine-activated killer (LAK) cells and activation of natural killer cell function. The human IL-2 gene is localized on chromosome 4q.

The IL-2R is a heterotrimeric complex consisting of single α, β, and γ subunits. The failure to express a normal IL-2R γ-chain has been associated with X-linked SCID (Noguchi et al., 1993; Puck et al., 1993) (see Chapter 12). Association of all three chains forms the high-affinity receptor complex. Interaction of IL-2 with its receptor initiates a series of responses, some of which are shared with TCR-induced activation of T cells, but others are different (reviewed by Terada et al., 1994a). Activation of T cells through the IL-2R is not associated with hydrolysis of phosphatidylinositol 4,5-bisphosphate, release of IP_3 or DG, activation of PKC, or increases in $[Ca^{2+}]_i$. Triggering of the IL-2R results in the tyrosine phosphorylation of a number of proteins, implicating certain PTKs. Activation of Lck and a novel PTK called Emt follows IL-2/IL-2R interaction, as does activation of phosphatidylinositol-3 kinase (PI-3 kinase).

It also appears that the downstream cascade of Ras/Raf-1/MEK/MAP kinase activation results from T-cell activation through the IL-2R. Within minutes of addition of IL-2, the serine threonine kinase, p70 S6 kinase (p70^{S6K}), is activated. p70^{S6K} is responsible for *in vivo* phosphorylation of ribosomal S6 protein, which regulates messenger RNA transcription. p70^{S6K} may be the target for the immunosuppressive agent rapamycin, and addition of this drug inhibits IL-2–dependent T-cell proliferation (Terada et al., 1994b). This contrasts with cyclosporin A and FK506, which inhibit IL-2 production but do not interfere with IL-2–dependent T-cell proliferation.

Costimulatory and Accessory Molecules

A growing number of surface molecules other than growth factor receptors have been identified in T-cell activation. Some of these receptors are expressed on both resting and activated T cells, whereas others are more restricted, suggesting involvement at certain phases of the cell cycle. These may act in different ways, some by transmitting a signal independent of the TCR, others by increasing intercellular adhesion, and others by augmenting or sustaining signals delivered through the TCR. Among the major costimulatory surface proteins are the following:

CD4/CD8. CD4 and CD8 function in MHC-restricted antigen presentation by binding to invariant regions of the MHC molecules on the antigen-presenting cell, thereby enhancing antigen recognition and signaling by the TCR. The ligands for CD4 and CD8 are the invariant regions of class II and class I MHC molecules, respectively (Konig et al., 1992). The cytosolic PTK, Lck, is present in T cells, in part associated with CD4 and CD8 (Veillette et al., 1991). Although not linked directly to the TCR complex in resting cells, CD4 and CD8 become associated with the TCR when engaged by the complex of antigen and MHC on the surface of the antigen-presenting cell (see Fig. 2–6). This association between CD4 and Lck is essential for antigen-specific signal transduction (Glaichenhaus et al., 1991). Cross-linking of either CD4 or CD8 induces the autophosphorylation and activation of Lck.

CD2. CD2 is an adhesion receptor expressed on T cells and NK cells. The ligand for CD2 is CD58 (LFA-3). CD2 is able to release intracellular Ca^{2+}, stimulate transmembrane influx of Ca^{2+}, and activate phospholipase C in T cells. It is unlikely that CD2 can function independently of the TCR, and it may play its major role through adhesion rather than cell signaling.

CD28. Increasing evidence supports the important role of the CD28 adhesion receptor and the costimulatory signal it provides. CD28 is a 44-kd glycoprotein expressed on the surface of most peripheral blood T cells and thymocytes (June et al., 1990). It is a member of a receptor family that includes CTLA-4, a molecule expressed on activated T cells. The ligand for CD28 is the B7 or BB-1 receptor, a 45-kd antigen expressed on activated B cells and monocytes. B7 interacts with both CD28 and CTLA-4 and markedly augments T-cell activation and proliferation. The biochemical pathway used by CD28 is not well delineated. Ligation of CD28 does not lead to calcium mobilization, and it triggers a pattern of tyrosine phosphorylation that differs from TCR-induced tyrosine phosphorylation.

Other Molecules. Other molecules may augment T cell responses, including LFA-1 following addition of its ligand ICAM-1 (see Table 2–1). The integrins VLA-4, VLA-5, and VLA-6 are also able to provide costimulatory effects to T cells.

Purine Enzymes in Lymphocyte Ontogeny

A number of enzymes important in nucleotide/nucleoside metabolism have a restricted distribution in different lymphocyte subpopulations (Martin and Gelfand, 1981). Enzymatic activity may be used to identify distinct stages of lymphocyte maturation and to provide some understanding of the pathogenesis of a number of the immunodeficiency diseases associated with abnormalities of these pathways.

Terminal Deoxynucleotidyl Transferase (TdT). TdT adds deoxymononucleotides to segments of DNA and is restricted in distribution to immature lymphocytes. Many TdT-positive bone marrow cells are prethymic precursor T cells. Confirmation of these observations is the increase in TdT activity in athymic animals treated with thymic hormone. A majority of thymocytes also contain a high level of TdT, whereas peripheral T cells contain little.

Adenosine Deaminase (ADA). ADA activity is highest in thymocytes with decreasing levels in secondary lymphoid organs (spleen, lymph nodes) and in circulating T cells. In rats, levels in cortical thymocytes are three- to tenfold higher than in medullary thymocytes or peripheral T cells.

Purine Nucleoside Phosphorylase (PNP). Levels of PNP appear inversely correlated with ADA levels in T cells at various stages of differentiation. As a result, PNP activity increases as T cells mature, highest levels occurring in circulating T cells and in secondary lymphoid organs.

Deoxycytidine Kinase. Deoxycytidine kinase is a central enzyme in the phosphorylation of nucleosides and deoxynucleosides. Highest levels of activity of this enzyme have been demonstrated in thymocytes, and lower activity is found in peripheral blood T lymphocytes.

Ecto-5′-Nucleotidase. Ecto-5′-nucleotidase, CD73, is a purine salvage enzyme attached to the external plasma membrane of human lymphocytes by a glycosyl phosphatidylinositol linkage. CD73 functions by catalyzing the dephosphorylation of purine and pyrimidine ribonucleosides and deoxynucleosides to the corresponding nucleosides. Approximately one third of adult peripheral T cells express CD73, and enzyme activity in thymocytes is lower than in circulating T cells. Patients with a variety of immunodeficiency disorders, including SCID, Wiskott-Aldrich syndrome, hypogammaglobulinemia, acquired immunodeficiency syndrome (AIDS), and Omenn syndrome have reduced or virtually absent levels of CD73 expression or low to absent levels of enzymatic activity.

HETEROGENEITY OF T-CELL FUNCTION

Antigen-specific cell-mediated immune responses are carried out by T lymphocytes; generally, specific responses are mediated by distinct subsets of T cells. With advances in detecting subpopulations of T cells as a result of identification of new surface molecules, increasingly complex interactions between subsets of cells are being defined. The major responses mediated by T cells are the support/regulation of immunoglobulin production, cytotoxicity, and delayed hypersensitivity. A major mechanism whereby T cells control the extent or magnitude of these responses is through their secretion or response to soluble factors produced by activated cells of the immune system. In some cases, a particular T cell responds to its own secreted product in an autocrine response (e.g., the response to IL-2). In other circumstances, the T cell responds to the secreted product of another cell in a paracrine response (e.g., the response of T cells to IL-1 secreted by macrophages). Some of the cellular interactions in the immune system and the soluble factors involved are described in Chapter 4 and Tables 2–3 and 2–4.

gp39/CD40 Interaction and Immunoglobulin Production

CD40 is a molecule expressed on the surface of many cell types, including B lymphocytes, and is a member of the tumor necrosis factor receptor family (Spriggs et al., 1993). Knowledge about the function of this receptor on B cells derived initially from studies using monoclonal antibodies to CD40. A diverse array of biologic activities results from signaling through CD40. These include B-cell proliferation; enhanced production of IgG, IgM, and IgE; and rescue from programmed cell death (apoptosis). In most instances, the response to CD40 signaling is dependent on various cytokines; in concert with IL-4, CD40 signaling triggers marked increases in IgE production.

The human ligand for CD40 (CD40L) is a 39-kD membrane glycoprotein, gp39, expressed primarily on the surface of activated T cells. Genetic studies localized the gene for gp39 to the q26 region of the human X chromosome. Soon after, studies performed in a number of laboratories identified gp39 gene defects as the cause of X-linked hyper-IgM syndrome, a syndrome

characterized by normal to elevated levels of serum IgM but little or no IgG, IgA, or IgE (see Chapter 11). To date, nucleotide sequencing of gp39 mRNA from different kindreds has identified point mutations within the extracellular domain, deletions and point mutations in the transmembrane domain, and defects in translational regulation.

Based on the studies in affected individuals and in vitro and in vivo data, it is clear that gp39 is absolutely essential for B-cell isotype switching. It appears that T cells, or perhaps certain T-cell subsets, become activated in response to antigen and up-regulate the expression of many surface molecules. One of these, gp39, interacts with its cognate receptor on B cells and, in the presence of cytokines (especially IL-4), triggers the B cells to proliferate and produce the more mature immunoglobulin isotypes.

The T$_H$1/T$_H$2 Paradigm

The provision of helper cell function by CD4$^+$ T cells for immunoglobulin production by B cells and enhancement of the microbicidal activity of macrophages suggested that although both were induced by T cells, the factors, or cytokines, mediating these interactions were quite distinct. Studies of long-term clones of murine CD4$^+$ T cells demonstrated two patterns of cytokine production: one type produced IL-2, IFN-γ, and TNF-β and was designated T$_H$1; the other type secreted IL-4, IL-5, IL-6, and IL-10, and was designated T$_H$2. Both types generally produce IL-3, IL-13, and GM-CSF as well. The T$_H$1 clones enhance cellular immunity and macrophage activity, whereas the T$_H$2 clones support differentiation of B cells into antibody-producing cells.

The phenotypic distinction between T$_H$1 and T$_H$2 cells has best been established in long-term clones in which the cytokine-producing profile rarely changes. In vivo and in short-term clones, overlap in the cytokines produced may be observed. The development of precursor, or T$_H$0, cells (which secrete both IL-4 and IFN-γ) into T$_H$1 or T$_H$2 cells appears to be controlled by specific cytokines (Fig. 2–7) (Swain et al, 1991). Thus, IL-4

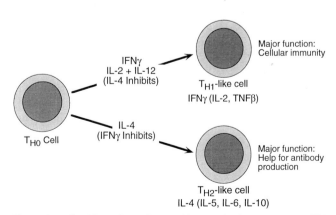

Figure 2–7. Cytokines determine cytokine-producing phenotype. IFN = interferon; IL: = interleukin.

Table 2–3. Cytokine Receptor Gene Families

Family	Distinguishing Features	Ligands of Member Receptors
Hematopoietin (cytokine receptor)	4-cysteines in extracellular domain; a conserved Trp-Ser-x-Trp-Ser motif	
Multichain		IL-2, IL-3, IL-5, IL-6, GM-CSF, Epo
Single chain		IL-4, IL-7, EPO, G-CSF
TNF family		TNF, CD27, CD30, CD40
IL-3 family	Common β subunit	IL-3, IL-5, GM-CSF
IL-6 family	Common β subunit	IL-6, IL-11, LIF
IL-8 family		IL-8, RANTES, PF-4
Tyrosine kinase family	Intrinsic tyrosine kinase activity in cytoplasmic domain	M-CSF, SCF
TGF-β family		TGF-β
Interferon family		IFN-α, IFN-β, IFN-ω, IFN-γ, IL-10
Immunoglobulin superfamily	Ig-like extracellular domain	IL-1, IL-6, M-CSF, G-CSF, SCF

Modified from Oppenheim JJ, Ruscetti FW, Faltyneke C. Cytokines. In Stites DP, Terr AI, Parslow TG, eds. Basic and Clinical Immunology, 8th ed. East Norwalk, Conn, Appleton and Lange, 1994, pp. 105–123.

supports differentiation into T_H2 cells, and IFN-γ directs differentiation into T_H1 cells. The former can be inhibited by IFN-γ, and the latter may be inhibited by IL-4.

The selective expansion of T_H2 cells is thought to play a critical role in allergic diseases. T_H2 cells are essential for inducing IgE synthesis because of the selective ability of IL-4 to induce immunoglobulin gene switching to the epsilon locus. In addition, they enhance allergic responses, since IL-4 and IL-3 are mast cell growth factors and IL-5 induces the proliferation and differentiation of eosinophils. Allergen-specific $CD4^+$ T-cell clones established from atopic patients also have a T_H2-lymphokine profile, whereas helper–T cell clones from the same patients to nonallergenic proteins have a T_H1-like profile. Antigens expressed on parasites also appear to evoke a T_H2 response.

T-CELL CYTOKINES

Cytokines are the regulatory proteins of the immune system that influence the growth, differentiation, repair, expansion, and activation of cells involved in specific immunity and inflammation. More than 100 protein and peptides fit this description; most are small, 20 to 60 kd proteins made principally by T lymphocytes (lymphokines) or monocyte-macrophages (monokines) but also by endothelial cells, stromal cells, other leukocytes, and somatic cells. With a few exceptions—erythropoietin (EPO), granulocyte colony–stimulating factor (G-CSF), granulocyte-macrophage colony–stimulating factor (GM-CSF)—they are not normally present in the blood stream to exert their effect on a distant site (endocrine function) but instead exert their action on cells in the immediate vicinity of the synthesizing cell (paracrine function) or on themselves (autocrine function). In certain illnesses (e.g., septic shock, acute infection, or inflammation), cytokines are released into the blood stream or tissue compartment (e.g., cerebrospinal fluid, joint capsule), but because of their rapid clearance, detectable levels are not maintained for any appreciable length of time.

The stimulus for production of cytokines is cell activation, either specifically by antigens (plus costimulatory signals), monoclonal antibodies, or nonspecifically by mitogens, superantigens, other cytokines, or endotoxins. Their striking activity at low concentrations derives from the presence on target cells of high-affinity receptors, many of which have been isolated and cloned. Several of these receptors structurally resemble each other and can be grouped into one of nine cytokine-receptor families (Table 2–3).

The cytokine system is extremely complex because:

1. Multiple cells secrete the same cytokine.
2. Multiple cells respond to the same cytokine.
3. Multiple cytokines have similar actions on particular cells.
4. A stimulus to one cytokine may stimulate production of other cytokines.
5. Some cytokines stimulate or inhibit the synthesis of other cytokines.
6. The cytokines often work together to produce synergistic or sometimes opposing effects.

Thus, the terms *pleotropic* and *redundant* are appropriately applied to the cytokines and the cytokine network.

Cytokines affecting T cells can be grouped for functional purposes into four groups:

1. Those regulating lymphocyte growth and differentiation.
2. Those activating other effector cells.
3. Those mediating natural immunity and inflammation.
4. Those regulating hematopoiesis.

Table 2–4 details the principal cytokines produced or influenced by T cells. Several excellent reviews are available (Howard et al., 1993; Oppenheim et al., 1994; Lederer and Abbas, 1995).

Cytokines Regulating Lymphocyte Growth and Development (IL-2, IL-4, IL-7, IL-10, TGF-β)

Interleukin-2. Among the cytokines affecting lymphocyte growth and development, interleukin-2 (IL-2) is the predominant cytokine. It is the major autocrine and paracrine T-cell growth factor; it is produced by activated T cells and essential for T cell clonal proliferation. It is a 133–amino acid, 15.4-kD protein encoded

Table 2–4. Cytokines Produced by or Influencing T Lymphocytes

Cytokine	Other Nomenclature	Principal Cell Source	Principal Actions
1. Regulators of Lymphocyte Growth			
IL-2*	T-cell growth factor	T_H1, NK	Stimulates T prolif., Tc, NK, B; induces IL-2R on T and B cells
IL-4*	B-cell growth factor I	T_H2, mast	Stimulates B proliferation, IgE synthesis, T_H2 responses; inhibits T_H1 responses
IL-7*		Epi, S	Stimulates T and B growth, thymocytes
IL-10*	Cytokine synthesis inhibiting factor	T_H2	Inhibits T_H1 responses, cytokine synthesis; stimulates B and Ig synthesis
TGF-β*	Transforming growth factor beta	T, MΦ, B, placental cells, bone, kidney	Inhibits T, NK, cytokine synthesis
2. Activators of Effector Cells			
IL-5*	B-cell growth factor II, T replacing factor	T_H2, mast	Stimulates Eo growth, differentiation, and activation
IL-12	NK cell stimulating factor	B, MΦ	Stimulates NK, Tc, IFN-γ, T_H1 responses; inhibits T_H2 responses
IFN-γ*	Macrophage activating factor, immune IFN, Type III IFN	T_H1, NK	Activates MΦ, NK, PMN, inhibits T_H2 responses, induces MHC Class I and II IL-I–like effects, tumor necrosis
TNF-β	Lymphotoxin	T_H1	IL-1–like effects; tumor necrosis
3. Modulators of Natural Immunity			
IL-1α and β	Lymphocyte activating factor, B-cell activating factor	MΦ	Stimulates proliferation of act T, stimulates B proliferation, Ig synthesis, stimulates inflammation, acute-phase reactants
IL-6*	B-cell stimulating factor, IFN-β₂	T_H2, B, MΦ, Endo, Epi, F	Stimulates T, B, Ig synthesis, acute-phase reactants
IL-8	Neutrophil activating factor	MΦ, PMN, NK	Chemoattractant for PMN, T, Baso
TNF-α	Cachectin	MΦ, other	IL-1–like effects, tumor necrosis
IFN-α	Leukocyte IFN, type I IFN	MΦ, PMN, T, other	Antiviral; activates MΦ, NK, Tc
IFN-β	Fibroblast IFN, type II IFN	F, MΦ, Epi	Antiviral; activates MΦ, NK, Tc
4. Hematopoietic Factors			
IL-3*	Multicolony-stimulating factor	T	Stimulates MΦ, PMN, Eo, Meg
IL-11		S	Stimulates hematopoiesis, thrombopoiesis
SCF	Stem cell factor	Hepatocytes, endo, epi, S	Stimulates multiple cell types
G-CSF	Granulocyte colony-stimulating factor	Mo, F	Stimulates PMN
GM-CSF	Granulocyte-monocyte colony-stimulating factor	T, Mo, Endo	Stimulates PMN, Eo, Meg
M-CSF	Monocyte colony-stimulating factor	T, Mo, Endo, Epi	Stimulates Mo, placental cells
EPO	Erythropoietin	Kidney cells	Stimulates erythropoiesis

*Mainly secreted by T cells.

Abbreviations: B = B cells; Baso = basophils; CSF = colony-stimulating factor; Endo = endothelial cells; Eo = eosinophils; Epi = epithelial cells; EPO = erythropoietin; F = fibroblasts; IFN = interferon; Ig = immunoglobulin; IL = interleukin; Meg = megakaryocytes; Mo = monocytes; MΦ = macrophages; NK = natural killer cells; S = stromal cells; T = T cells; Tc = cytotoxic T cells; T_H = T helper cells; TNF = tumor necrosis factor.

by a single gene on human chromosome 14. It was discovered in 1976 in the supernatant of mitogen-activated lymphocytes as a substance that stimulated the growth of T cells (Morgan et al., 1976). It resembles IL-4 and GM-CSF in its three-dimensional structure.

Resting T cells synthesize no IL-2, but on antigen activation in the presence of costimulatory factors, or following mitogen or anti-CD3 activation, CD4 cells and to a lesser extent CD8 and NK cells begin to produce IL-2 within 2 or 3 hours of activation, reaching maximal production within 6 to 12 hours and unless restimulation occurs, ceasing by 24 hours.

Activation of T cells initiates transcription of the IL-2 gene to IL-2 mRNA. This process involves both ubiquitous nuclear factors (e.g., NF-κB) and lymphoid specific factors (e.g., NF-AT and NF–IL-2A); the former is inhibited by cyclosporin and FK-506. Cells that are functionally anergic may also have blocked IL-2 transcription. Secreted IL-2 has a very short half-life in the circulation and acts primarily on the cell that secreted it or on an adjacent cell.

IL-2 stimulates the expansion of the CD4 T-helper cells that have recognized the antigen–MHC complex and to a lesser extent, CD8 cytotoxic T lymphocytes that recognize class I MHC–associated endogenously synthesized peptide antigens. There is some activation of adjacent T cells but in the absence of high-affinity IL-2 receptors on unstimulated T cells, this stimulation is not as vigorous as that for activated cells that express the high-affinity IL-2 receptor. IL-2 also stimulates T_H1

cells to secrete IFN-γ, TNF-β, and TGF-β, and perhaps other cytokines. Thus, IL-2 has a predominant effect on T$_H$1 responses.

IL-2 also enhances proliferation and antibody secretion by B cells, either when antigen-activated or following B-cell polyclonal activators. IL-2 also induces immunoglobulin class switching, which favors IgG2 subclass antibody synthesis. IL-2 enhances the proliferation and cytotoxic activity of NK cells, acting synergistically with IL-12. NK cells, if cultured for 2 to 5 days with a high concentration of IL-2, differentiate into lymphokine-activated killer cells (LAK), which are highly cytotoxic and show a wider spectrum of target cell activity than do NK cells. Such cells grown in vitro and autotransfused are used in tumor cytotherapy.

IL-2 is also a weak activator of monocytes and macrophages, promoting their secretion of H_2O_2, TNF-α, and IL-6. IL-2 may also activate polymorphonuclear neutrophils (PMNs) and eosinophils.

Interleukin-2 Receptors. In order for a cell to respond to IL-2, it needs an IL-2 receptor, expressed either constitutively or following activation. There are high-, medium-, and low-affinity IL-2 receptors.

The high-affinity IL-2 receptor complex (IL-2R) consists of an α chain (IL-2Rα), 35 kD; a β chain (IL2Rβ), 75 kD; and a γ chain (IL-2Rγ), 64 kD. The latter contains the signaling component of IL-2R (and also of IL-4R and IL-7R). The intermediate affinity receptor is the IL-2Rβ/IL-2Rγ complex on resting T cells and NK cells. The low-affinity IL-2 receptor is the IL-2Rβ alone, expressed on some T cells, fibroblasts, and other cells.

As noted, the high-affinity IL-2R is not present on resting T cells but is expressed within 1 to 2 days of activation when the IL-2Rα chain becomes expressed. The IL-2Rα chain, identified by the anti-Tac monoclonal antibody CD25, a crucial component of the high-affinity IL-2 receptor, has a very short cytoplasmic tail, too short to transduce signals by itself. CD25 is often used to assess the presence of activated T cells. IL-2R is only transiently expressed on activated T cells, disappearing within 4 to 7 days. T cells transformed with human T-cell leukemia virus (HTLV-1), the agent responsible for adult T-cell leukemia, constitutively express IL-2R. Since the IL-2R complex (α, β, and γ chains) binds IL-2 with a high affinity, it will initiate intracellular signaling on exposure to low levels of IL-2.

Most resting T cells expressing the intermediate-affinity receptor respond only to high concentrations of IL-2. NK cells also express the intermediate-affinity IL-2R and thus also respond to high levels of IL-2.

Monoclonal antibodies to CD25 (anti IL-2Rα, anti-Tac) attached to toxins may be of value in treatment of adult T-cell leukemia or graft-versus-host disease, illnesses with high levels of circulating or tissue-activated T cells.

Interleukin-4 and Interleukin-4R. IL-4 is a 20 kD glycoprotein with a chemical structure similar to GM-CSF and IL-2, encoded on chromosome 5. It is secreted by activated CD4 T$_H$2 cells on antigen recognition. It was initially identified as a B-cell growth or stimulatory factor because it causes expansion of activated B cells and induces MHC class II expression on B cells. It also promotes a switch to IgE production and increased expression of Fc receptor εI (FcεRI) on eosinophils.

IL-4 suppresses the induction and function of T$_H$1 cells, thus inhibiting cellular immunity and stimulating a T$_H$2 antibody response with eosinophilia and IgE production. IL-4 also activates macrophages and increases MHC class II expression while inhibiting the production of the inflammatory cytokines IL-1, IL-6, IL-8 and TNF-α. IL-13, a T$_H$2 product, shares properties with IL-4. IFN-γ and IL-4 have almost directly opposing actions. IL-4 production is also inhibited by cyclosporine and FK506.

IL-4R are present on lymphocytes, monocyte/macrophages, and endothelial cells. IL-4R belongs to the single-chain cytokine receptor family, along with the receptors for IL-7, G-CSF and EPO (Table 2–3). Soluble IL-4R in the serum may inhibit IL-4–mediated responses.

IL-7. IL-7 is a 25 kD glycoprotein secreted by bone marrow stromal cells. It is a growth factor for pre-B, B, thymocyte and T cells. It may also stimulate T-cell receptor rearrangement in fetal thymocytes. It induces LAK-cell activity but to a lesser extent than does IL-2. It may also activate macrophages and stimulate proinflammatory monokines.

IL-10. IL-10 is a heterodimer of 18 kD encoded on chromosome 1. It is produced by T$_H$2 cells, CD8 T cells, monocytes, activated B cells and keratinocytes. IL-10 inhibits the production of IL-2 and IFN-γ by T$_H$1 cells, and other cytokine production by NK cells and macrophages; it thus has been called *cytokine synthesis–inhibiting factor*. It also inhibits antigen presentation by macrophages. The net effect of IL-10 is to favor antibody synthesis and to inhibit cellular immune responses. The IL-10 gene shares homology with that of the Epstein-Barr virus (EBV); indeed, productive EBV infection may increase IL-10 and shut down antiviral defenses.

Transforming Growth Factor–Beta (TGF-β). TGF-β was initially identified as a fibroblast growth factor implicated in normal healing. However, it has pronounced antiproliferative and anti-inflammatory effects on macrophages, endothelial cells, T, B, and NK cells, and inhibits the secretion of proinflammatory cytokines. It is produced by a variety of cells, including T and B cells; activated macrophages; and cells of the placenta, bone, and kidney. It may also promote switching to IgA synthesis following oral antigen stimulation and may help to mediate oral tolerance.

Cytokines Activating Other Cells (IL-5, IL-12, IFN-γ, TNF-β)

IL-5. IL-5 is a 20 kD glycoprotein encoded on chromosome 5 and produced by T$_H$2 cells. First described as a growth factor for murine B cells, it has minimal effects on human B cells but has as its major effect the stimulation of eosinophil growth, differentiation, and activation.

IL-5 is made by the same T$_H$2 subset as IL-4, and by upregulating the expression of FcεRs on eosinophils, works synergistically with IL-4. IL-5–activated eosinophils recognize IgE on parasites and degranulate to release major basic proteins of eosinophils and other toxic granule proteins. IL-5 also activates basophils to release allergic mediators such as histamine.

The IL-5 receptor is a 60 kD molecule of the type I cytokine family. High levels of IL-5R are present on eosinophils.

IL-12. IL-12 is produced by B cells and macrophages and shares many biologic activities with IL-2, notably augmentation of NK cell and T-cell cytotoxicity. It often works synergistically with IL-2. IL-12 is a 35 kD protein structurally similar to IL-6 and GM-CSF.

IL-12 activates NK cells to a greater degree than does IL-2 and stimulates IFN-γ synthesis by NK cells. It also enhances the production and function of LAK cells and cytotoxic T cells. IL-12 promotes T_H1 responses and suppresses T_H2 responses by inhibiting IL-4, IL-10, and IgE synthesis.

IFN-γ. IFN-γ (type III, or immune interferon) is an 18 kD protein that shares some antiviral activity with IFN-α and IFN-β, but in many respects it is quite different from them. It is primarily secreted by activated CD4 T_H1 cells and to some degree by NK cells. Nearly all cells have IFN-γ receptors and respond to IFN-γ by upregulating expression of MHC classes I and II. This latter action promotes antigen presentation by CD4 lymphocytes. IFN-γ is a strong activator of macrophages (thus deriving its alternative name of macrophage activity factor), enhancing their microbicidal, cytotoxic, and secretory functions, notably IL-1, IL-6, IL-8, and IFN-α secretion. IFN-γ also stimulates NK and phagocytic cells. Thus IFN-γ enhances T_H1 activity and inhibits T_H2 responses. It also inhibits IL-4 activation of IgE synthesis by B cells.

Tumor Necrosis Factor–β. TNF-β, also called *lymphotoxin,* is synthesized by activated T_H1 cells. It causes many of the same effects as TNF-α on other cells, including vascular thrombosis and tumor necrosis.

Cytokines Modulating Natural Immunity (IL-1, IL-6, IL-8; TNF-α; IFN-α, β)

IL-1α, IL-1β. The inflammatory cytokines, most of which are not produced by T cells, nevertheless have major effects on T-cell growth and activation. IL-1, also known as *lymphocyte-activating factor,* is primarily produced by macrophages but also by many other cell types. A major function is the activation of T_H1 cells following antigen presentation, and thus it serves as an important T-cell costimulatory signal. The two distinct forms, IL-1α and IL-1β are produced by different cells and are only 45% homologous but have very similar biologic activities. IL-1 stimulates B cell growth, activates acute phase reactants, induces fever, stimulates thymocyte and hematopoietic stem cell growth, and activates PMN and monocytic phagocytosis. IL-1 shares many of the stimulatory properties of TNF-α and TNF-β.

One remarkable feature of IL-1 is the presence of a natural receptor antagonist IL-RA, produced by many of the same cells that synthesize IL-1. Pharmacologic inhibition of IL-1 by corticosteroids or other drugs results in a strong anti-inflammatory response.

IL-6. IL-6 is a 22–30 kD glycoprotein encoded on chromosome 7 and produced primarily by T_H2 and B cells but also by endothelial and epithelial cells and fibroblasts. IL-6, along with IL-1, TNF-α, and TNF-β, stimulates T-cell immune responses, B-cell synthesis, and hepatic acute-phase reactants; it increases glucocorticoid production and bone resorption. IL-6 was initially called IFN-$\beta2$, but it has only weak antiviral activity.

A high-affinity IL-6 receptor is present on macrophages, hepatocytes, T cells, B cells, and plasma cells. The beta subunit of the IL-6 receptor (gp130) is shared by IL-11, leukocyte-inhibiting factor (LIF), and oncostatin M.

IL-8. IL-8 is one of the chemokines (others include platelet factor 4 and RANTES) made by monocytes, neutrophils, T cells, and somatic cells that chemoattract other cells, including neutrophils, T cells, and basophils. Thus, IL-8 is a major factor in the acute inflammatory response.

TNF-α. Tumor necrosis factor-α (TNF-α, or cachectin) is produced primarily by monocyte/macrophages but also by other somatic cells. It has a variety of properties similar to IL-1 and TNF-β and serves as a costimulatory signal for activation and proliferation of T and B cells. It stimulates IL-2 and IFN-γ receptors, inflammation, fever, and acute-phase reactants, and activates phagocytic cells. Two high-affinity TNF receptors have been identified. Inhibitors of TNF-α (and IL-1) are being explored as anti-inflammatory agents. Corticosteroids and TGF-β inhibit TNF-α.

Interferon-α and β. Interferon-α (leukocyte-IFN) and interferon-β (fibroblast-IFN) are produced by a variety of cells following infection with viruses, bacteria, or protozoa or contact with other stimuli (certain cytokines, double-stranded RNA). They induce a temporary antiviral state in a variety of cells, including T cells. They also upregulate MHC class I molecules and activate cytotoxicity in T cells and NK cells. There are 14 forms of IFN-α, all of which have the common antiviral property of inducing enzymes that degrade viral RNA and inhibit protein synthesis.

Hematopoietic Cytokines (IL-3, IL-11, SCF, CSFs, EPO)

The final group of T cell cytokines are the hematopoietic growth factors (see Table 2–4). Most do not influence T cells and only IL-3, GM-CSF, and M-CSF are synthesized by T cells. They serve to stimulate the formation and release of various blood cells in the bone marrow. Many of the hematopoietic factor receptors are structurally similar to the other cytokines. Unlike most cytokines, SCF, M-CSF, and EPO are present in low quantities in the circulation. GM-CSF, G-CSF, and EPO are available for therapeutic use.

Contributed by E. Richard Stiehm

EVALUATION OF T-LYMPHOCYTE FUNCTION

T-Cell Subset Enumeration

A screening evaluation begins with enumeration of the crucial cell populations. The initial evaluation includes a blood count and calculation of absolute numbers of lymphocytes. Since T cells constitute 70% or more of the peripheral blood lymphocytes, lymphopenia ($<$ 1000 to 1500 lymphocytes/mm^3) usually represents a depletion of T cells. Marked differences in T-cell numbers occur at various ages, so that age-matched controls must be used (see Chapter 9).

Among the primary immunodeficiencies, lymphopenia is observed in some forms of severe combined immunodeficiency (SCID), particularly in association with a deficiency of adenosine deaminase, in purine nucleoside phosphorylase deficiency, and in cartilage-hair hypoplasia. T-cell lymphopenia can also be secondary to viral infections (e.g., AIDS), malnutrition, autoimmune diseases, hematopoietic malignancy, or loss, as in intestinal lymphangiectasia.

With the increased availability of monoclonal antibodies to cell surface proteins, major and minor populations of T cells can be identified and enumerated by immunofluorescence. In normals, a general "rule of thumb" is that the number of CD2$^+$ T cells equals CD3$^+$ T cells equals CD4$^+$ + CD8$^+$ T cells. Discrepancies may indicate an increased number of NK (CD16$^+$) cells or an increase in the number of $\gamma\delta$ T cells.

Delayed Hypersensitivity Skin Tests

The most direct way for assessing cell-mediated immunity is by performing delayed-type hypersensitivity skin testing. In vitro tests of T-cell function include stimulation of T cells by mitogens, antigens or allogeneic cells.

Delayed cutaneous hypersensitivity (DCH) is a localized immunologic skin response: the prototype is the tuberculin skin test. Because DCH is dependent on functional thymus-derived lymphocytes (T lymphocytes), it is used in screening for T-cell mediated immunity (CMI). Antigens generally used are mumps, *Trichophyton,* purified protein derivative (PPD), *Candida (Monilia),* tetanus, and diphtheria toxoid. To adequately assess CMI responses, several antigens should be used. All skin tests are done by intradermal injection of 0.1 ml of antigen and should be read after 48 to 72 hours for the maximal diameter of induration, which indicates intact cell-mediated immunity. Erythema is not an indication of DCH. A negative test often is not informative in infants younger than 2 years. Negative test findings may also result from insufficient material injected in an appropriate fashion or outdated solutions of test materials.

Lymphocyte Proliferation

Lymphocytes can be activated in vitro by the following:

1. Mitogens, such as phytohemagglutinin (PHA), pokeweed mitogen (PWM), or concanavalin A (Con A).
2. Antigens (such as PPD, *Candida,* streptokinase, tetanus, or diphtheria) if the patient has had prior encounter with the antigen or with superantigens, such as toxic shock syndrome toxin (TSST).

3. Allogeneic cells (mixed leukocyte reaction).
4. Monoclonal antibodies to T-cell surface molecules involved in signal transduction—for example, antibodies to CD3, CD2, CD28, and CD43.

T-lymphocyte activation can be assessed directly by the following methods:

- Measuring blastogenesis and/or proliferation of cells
- Expression of activation antigens
- Release of mediators

The proliferative response is assayed after 3 to 7 days by ^{3}H- or ^{14}C-labeled thymidine incorporation into DNA for 3 to 6 hours, followed by DNA extraction techniques or cell precipitation on filter paper and subsequent liquid scintillation counting.

Control values of unstimulated cultures vary from person to person and from day to day. Data on unstimulated and stimulated cultures should always be given. Soluble PHA and Con A require the presence of monocytes for stimulation of T cells; under certain conditions, however, such as when bound to particulate matter, they may also stimulate B cells. Pokeweed mitogen stimulates a response in both T and B cells, although T cells must be present for the B cells to be stimulated. The mixed leukocyte reaction (MLR) results from T-cell reactivity to MHC antigens displayed on allogeneic B cells and monocytes. It should be noted that when normal irradiated or mitomycin C–treated lymphocytes are the stimulators of an MLR, the normal T cells in the culture may secrete factors that induce blastogenesis in the patient's lymphocytes. Therefore, it is preferable to use B-cell lines or T-cell depleted normal cells as the stimulators.

Activated T cells express IL-2Rα (CD25), transferrin receptors (CD71), and MHC class II molecules (DR) not present or present in low numbers on resting T cells. T-cell populations to be assessed for their capacity to express these receptors are stimulated with a soluble lectin such as PHA and examined 24 to 48 hours following stimulation by direct or indirect immunofluorescence, using monoclonal antibodies to interleukin-2 (CD25), transferrin (CD71) receptors, or MHC class II molecules.

Activated T cells and monocytes synthesize and secrete interleukins-2, -4, -5 and -6; interferon-γ; and other cytokines. The supernatants of peripheral blood mononuclear cells stimulated by mitogens or the combination of a phorbol ester and calcium ionophore can be assessed for IL-2 by an enzyme-linked immunosorbent assay (ELISA) technique or by determining their capacity to stimulate ^{3}H-thymidine uptake in mouse IL-2–dependent cultured T-cell lines (e.g., the CTLL-2 cell line). The bioassay should be confirmed with blocking antibodies to IL-2. Specific in vitro systems or ELISAs exist to assess this and other cytokines.

Transplant Rejection

Cell-mediated immunity is responsible for the rejection of foreign tissue. The immune response to foreign transplantation antigens or alloantigens is characterized by the generation of cytotoxic T cells specifically directed against the sensitizing alloantigens. In the classic rejection reaction, generation of cytotoxic effector cells occurs among the CD8$^+$ cells. CD4$^+$ cells may play a major role by secreting IL-2, leading to the full expansion of the pool of cytotoxic CD8$^+$ effector T cells.

Evaluation of a transplant rejection response can be easily achieved by transplanting allogeneic skin. Rejection of a skin graft normally occurs within 14 to 28 days.

Graft-versus-host disease (GVHD) occurs when histoincompatible T cells attack tissues of a recipient who is unable to reject foreign cells. The requirements for such a reaction are histocompatibility differences between donor and recipient, immunocompetent T cells in the graft, and an immunodeficient host. This type of CMI response is similar to the rejection of a transplant but in reverse. A graft-versus-host reaction may result from the infusion of any blood product containing viable, immunocompetent T cells or following transplantation of fetal thymus, fetal liver, or bone marrow. The major target organs are the skin, liver, and gastrointestinal tract, and the patient presents with a maculopapular skin rash, hepatomegaly and jaundice, and diarrhea (Kruger et al., 1971).

Lymph Node or Thymus Biopsy

Because of the location of T and B cells in discrete areas of the lymph node, a biopsy of an antigenically stimulated node may aid in the evaluation of a patient. The biopsies may also prove helpful in difficult cases of T-cell deficiency in infants. Although a thymus biopsy can provide invaluable information, it should be performed only when the diagnosis is unclear and biopsy material will be used to further understand the pathogenesis of the T-cell deficiency.

Regulation of Immunoglobulin Production

Terminal differentiation of surface immunoglobulin-positive B lymphocytes into immunoglobulin-secreting plasma cells is regulated by different T-cell subpopulations. The CD4$^+$ population contains cells capable of promoting the terminal differentiation of B cells to an antibody secreting stage, whereas some cells among the CD8$^+$ subset inhibit this step. Although the different subsets may act directly on the B cells themselves, there are also complex T cell–T cell interactions described.

Cytotoxic Effector Cell Functions

Cytotoxic effector T-cell activity toward a variety of target cells can be induced by several different mechanisms. T lymphocytes, sensitized in vivo or in vitro against alloantigens, tumor antigens, or viral antigens are able to react specifically in vitro with target cells expressing the appropriate sensitizing antigen. The

generation of cytotoxic T lymphocytes predominantly resides in the CD8$^+$ population.

Another population of lymphocytes, the large granular lymphocytes that express CD8 but not CD3, are capable of lysing a variety of tumor targets without prior sensitization. Such natural killer cells also express surface antigens (CD16 and CD56) with selectivity for this group of cells. Although the T-cell antigen receptor is thought to be involved in the effector function of the cytotoxic T cell, the recognition structure on NK cells remains to be defined.

Cytokine Assays

Assays for cytokines are sometimes of value in defining an immune deficiency (see Chapter 9). The assays most commonly used are IL-1, IL-2, IFN-γ, and TNF-α, either by ELISA, immunoassays, or bioassays. Cytokines are rarely found in the circulation except following acute stress, injury, or therapeutic administration. Their assessment in the supernatant of cultured stimulated leukocytes may be of value in assessment of certain syndromes (e.g., IL-2 deficiency, Griscelli syndrome) or defining the T$_H$1/T$_H$2 cytokine profile in certain conditions.

Soluble cytokine receptor assays (e.g., IL-2R, IL-4R) are also available and may define states of immune activation or hypersensitivity.

ALTERATIONS OF CELL-MEDIATED IMMUNITY

Primary Immunodeficiency

Congenital, often genetic, isolated deficiencies of T-cell immunity are rare and are discussed in Chapter 12. Examples include congenital thymic aplasia (DiGeorge anomaly), cartilage-hair hypoplasia, and the T-cell deficiency associated with purine nucleoside phosphorylase deficiency. Deficiencies of cell-mediated immunity are manifested primarily by infection with fungal, viral, or protozoal (e.g., *Pneumocystis carinii*) organisms.

More commonly, primary disorders of cell-mediated immunity are accompanied by abnormalities of humoral immunity. Such disorders may be found in the heterogeneous group of patients with combined immunodeficiency disease, including those with deficiency of adenosine deaminase, cellular immunodeficiency with abnormal immunoglobulin production (Nezelof syndrome), ataxia-telangiectasia, and Wiskott-Aldrich syndrome. Most of these disorders manifest early in infancy with infections caused by a wide variety of microbial organisms.

Secondary Immunodeficiency

Secondary, or acquired, abnormalities of cell-mediated immunity are common (see Chapter 19). Cellular immunity is often transiently depressed by illness, particularly viral infection. Measles, rubella, rubeola, *Mycoplasma,* and a number of other viruses may result in lymphopenia and a depression of in vivo and in vitro lymphocyte function. Indeed, inoculation with live virus may transiently depress T-cell immunity. Malnutritional states are often accompanied by an impairment of cell-mediated immunity. Protein-calorie malnutrition and iron deficiency can lead to reduced cell-mediated immunity. Particularly impressive is the T-cell dysfunction associated with zinc or pyridoxine deficiency. Patients with malignancy or renal failure also demonstrate abnormalities of T-cell function. Patients receiving chemotherapy for malignancy or immunosuppressive drugs are at risk of developing infection as a result of the drug effects on the T-cell system. Antibodies to T cells (e.g., anti-CD3) or anti-lymphocyte globulin for the control of allograft rejection have a primary effect on the T-lymphocyte compartment of the immune response.

Many of the autoimmune disorders are accompanied by abnormalities of T-cell function. In addition to a decrease in numbers and function of the suppressor T-cell pool, diseases such as systemic lupus erythematosus may manifest marked abnormalities of T-cell function in vitro and in vivo. The process of aging is associated with progressive decline in T-cell function.

AIDS is a good example of the effect of lymphotropic retroviruses on T-cell immunity (see Chapter 18). Infection with the human immunodeficiency virus (HIV) has a profound impact on T-cell immunity. Such patients are lymphopenic; they are susceptible to a variety of fungal, viral, and protozoal organisms and Kaposi's sarcoma, and they lack delayed cutaneous hypersensitivity. In the laboratory, T-cell function in these patients is markely impaired, highlighted by a reduction in CD4$^+$ cells.

RESTORATION OF T-CELL FUNCTION

There have been many attempts to augment cell-mediated immunity through the use of immune potentiators or immune-modulating agents. These include drugs (e.g., levamisole, isoprinosine); bacille Calmette-Guérin (BCG); thymus factors; and T cell–derived factors, such as transfer factor, interleukins, and interferons. None of these attempts has reliably or reproducibly brought about an improvement of T-cell function or enhancement of immune function. In contrast, transplantation of bone marrow in patients with severe combined immunodeficiency disease and Wiskott-Aldrich syndrome has provided long-lasting reconstitution of the immune system (see Chapter 32).

Enzyme replacement therapy, adenosine deaminase in deficient individuals, may also provide varying degrees of immune reconstitution. Exciting new developments are emerging in the area of gene therapy. In certain rare cases, fetal thymus transplantation or transplantation of cultured thymus epithelium has resulted in reconstitution of T-cell immunity (see Chapter 12).

References

Anderson DC, Springer TA. Leukocyte adhesion deficiency: an inherited defect in the MAC-1, LFA-1, and p150,95 glycoproteins. Ann Rev Med 38:175–194, 1987.

Appleby MW, Gross JA, Cooke MP, Levin SD, Qian X, Perlmutter RM. Defective T cell receptor signaling in mice lacking the thymic isoform of p59^{fyn}. Cell 70:751–763, 1992.

Archer OK, Pierce JC. Role of the thymus in the development of the immune response. Fed Proc 20:26–36, 1961.

Arpaia E, Shahar M, Dadi H, Cohen A, Roifman CM. Defective T cell receptor signaling and CD8$^+$ thymic selection in humans lacking ZAP-70 kinase. Cell 76:947–958, 1994.

August CS, Berkel AI, Driscoll S, Merler E. Onset of lymphocyte function in the developing human fetus. Pediatr Res 5:539–545, 1971.

Bach JF, Carnaud C. Thymic factors. Progr Allergy 21:342–408, 1976.

Barcena A, Toribio ML, Gutierrez-Ramos JC, Kroemer G, Martinez AC. Interplay between IL-2 and IL-4 in human thymocyte differentiation: antagonism or agonism. Int Immunol 3:419–425, 1991.

Benacerraf B, McDevitt HO. Histocompatibility-linked immune response genes. Science 175:273–279, 1972.

Berlin C, Berg EL, Briskin MJ, Andrew DP, Kilshaw PJ, Holzmann B, Weissman IL, Hamann A, Butcher EC. α4β7 integrin mediates lymphocyte binding to the mucosal vascular addressin MAdCAM-1. Cell 74:185–195, 1993.

Berridge MJ. Inositol trisphosphate and calcium signalling. Nature 361:315–325, 1993.

Biddison WE, Rao PE, Talle MA, Goldstein G, Shaw S. Possible involvement of the OKT4 molecule in T cell recognition of class II HLA antigens: evidence from studies of cytotoxic T lymphocytes specific for SB antigens. J Exp Med 156:1065–1076, 1982.

Bjorkmann PJ, Saper MA, Samraoui B, Bennett WS, Strominger JL, Wiley DC. The foreign antigen binding site and T cell recognition region of class I histocompatibility antigens. Nature 329:512–518, 1987.

Bowen TJ, Ochs HD, Altman LC, Price TH, van Epps DE, Brantigan DL, Rosin RE, Perkins WD, Babior BM, Klebanoff SJ, Wedgwood RJ. Severe recurrent bacterial infections associated with defective adherence and chemotaxis in two patients with neutrophils deficient in a cell-associated glycoprotein. J Pediatr 101:932–940, 1982.

Brodsky FM, Guagliardi LE. The cell biology of antigen processing and presentation. Ann Rev Immunol 9:707–744, 1991.

Chan AC, Irving BA, Fraser JD, Weiss A. The ζ-chain is associated with a tyrosine kinase and upon T cell antigen receptor stimulation associates with ZAP-70, a 70-kilodalton tyrosine phosphoprotein. Proc Natl Acad Sci U S A 88:9166–9170, 1991.

Chan AC, Iwashima M, Turck CW, Weiss A. ZAP-70: a 70-kd protein-tyrosine kinase that associates with the TCR ζ chain. Cell 71:649–662, 1992.

Chan AC, Kadlecek TA, Elde ME, Filipovich AH, Kuo WL, Iwashima M, Parslow TG, Weiss A. ZAP-70 deficiency in an autosomal recessive form of severe combined immunodeficiency. Science 264:1599–1601, 1994.

Davidson D, Chow LML, Fournel M, Veillette A: Differential regulation of T cell antigen responsiveness by isoforms of the src-related tyrosine protein kinase p59^{fyn}. J Exp Med 175:1483–1492, 1992.

Downward J, Graves J, Cantrell D. The regulation and function of p21ras in T cells. Immunol Today 13:89–92, 1992.

Dustin ML, Springer TA. Role of lymphocyte adhesion receptors in transient interactions and cell locomotion. Ann Rev Immunol 9:27–66, 1991.

Elder ME, Liu D, Clever J, Chan AC, Hope TJ, Weiss A, Parslow TG. Human severe combined immunodeficiency due to a defect in ZAP-70, a T cell tyrosine kinase. Science 264:1596–1599, 1994.

Elices MJ, Osborn L, Takada Y, Crouse C, Luhowsky S, Hemler ME, Lobb RR. VCAM-1 on activated endothelium interacts with the leukocyte integrin VLA-4 at a site distinct from the VLA-4/fibronectin binding site. Cell 60:577–584, 1990.

Etzioni A, Frydman M, Pollack S, Avidor I, Phillips ML, Paulson JC, Gershoni-Baroch S. Severe recurrent infections due to a novel adhesion molecule defect. New Engl J Med 327:1789–1792, 1992.

Fowlkes BJ, Pardoll DM. Molecular and cellular events of T cell development. Adv Immunol 44:207–264, 1989.

Frank MM, Austen KF, Claman HN, Unancie ER. Boston, Little, Brown, 1995, pp 129–142.

Franklin RA, Tordai A, Patel H, Gardner AM, Johnson GL, Gelfand EW. Ligation of the T-cell receptor complex results in activation of the Ras/Raf-1/MEK/MAPK cascade in human T lymphocytes. J Clin Invest 93:2134–2140, 1994.

Gelfand EW. Ion movement, activation and signalling of T and B lymphocytes. In Cambier J, ed. Ligands, Receptors and Signal Transduction in Regulation of Lymphocyte Function. American Society for Microbiology, Washington, D.C., 1990, pp. 359–386.

Gelfand EW, Dosch HM. Differentiation of precursor T lymphocytes in man and delineation of the selective abnormalities in severe combined immune deficiency disease. Clin Immunol Immunopathol 25:303–315, 1982.

Gelfand EW, Weinberg K, Mazer B, Kadlecek T, Weiss A. Absence of ZAP-70 prevents signaling through the antigen receptor on peripheral blood T cells but not thymocytes. J Exp Med (in press), 1995.

Glaichenhaus N, Shastri N, Littman DR, Turner JM. Requirement for association of p56lck with CD4 in antigen specific signal transduction in T cells. Cell 64:511-520, 1991.

He W, Kabelitz D. Cytokines involved in intrathymic T cell development. Int Arch Allergy Immunol 105:203–210, 1994.

Herman A, Kappler JW, Marrack P, Pullen AM. Superantigens: mechanism of T-cell stimulation and role in immune responses. Ann Rev Immunol 9:745–772, 1991.

Howard MC, Miyajima A, Coffman R, In Paul WE, ed. T Cell Derived Cytokines and Their Receptors in Fundamental Immunology, 3rd ed. Raven Press, New York, 1993, pp. 763–800.

June CH, Ledbetter JA, Linsley PS, Thompson CB. Role of the CD28 receptor in T cell activation. Immunol Today 11:211–216, 1990.

Kappler JW, Roehm N, Marrack P. T cell tolerance by clonal elimination in the thymus. Cell 49:273–280, 1987.

Kishihara K, Penninger J, Wallace VA, Kündig TM, Kawai K, Wakeham A, Timms E, Pfeffer K, Ohashi PS, Thomas ML, Furlonger C, Paige CJ, Mak TW. Normal B lymphocyte development but impaired T cell maturation in CD45-exon 6 protein tyrosine phosphatase-deficient mice. Cell 74:143–156, 1993.

Konig R, Huang L-Y, Germain RN. MHC class II interaction with CD4 mediated by a region analogous to the MHC class I binding site for CD8. Nature 356:796–798, 1992.

Koretzky GA, Picus J, Thomas ML, Weiss A. Tyrosine phosphatase CD45 is essential for coupling T cell antigen receptor to the phosphatidylinositol pathway. Nature 346:66–68, 1990.

Koretzky G, Picus J, Schultz T, Weiss A. Tyrosine phosphatase CD45 is required for both T cell antigen receptor- and CD2-mediated activation of a protein-tyrosine kinase and interleukin-2 production. Proc Natl Acad Sci U S A 88:2037–2041, 1991.

Kruger GRF, Bernard CW, Delellis RA, Graw RG, Yankee RA, Leventhal BG, Rogentine CN, Herzig GP, Haltman RH, Henderson ES. Graft-versus-host disease. Am J Pathol 63:179–197, 1971.

Lederer JA, Abbas AK. Cytokines in specific immune responses. In Frank MM, Austein KF, Claman HN, Unanue ER, eds. Samter's Immunologic Diseases, 5th ed. Boston, Little Brown, 1995, pp. 129–142.

LeDourain NM, Jotereau FV. Tracing of cells of the avian thymus through embryonic life in interspecies chimeras. J Exp Med 142:17–31, 1975.

Levin SD, Anderson SJ, Forbush KA, Perlmutter RM. A dominant negative transgene defines a role for p56lck in thymopoiesis. EMBO J, 12:1671–1680, 1993.

Mackay CR. Migration pathways and immunologic memory among T lymphocytes. Semin Immunol 4:51–58, 1992.

Marrack P, Parker DC. A little of what you fancy. Nature 368:397, 1994.

Martin DW Jr, Gelfand EW. Biochemistry of diseases of immunodevelopment. Am Rev Biochem 50:845–877, 1981.

Meuer SC, Schlossman RF, Reinherz EL. Clonal analysis of human cytotoxic T lymphocytes: T4+ and T8+ effector T cells recognize products of different major histocompatibility complex regions. Proc Natl Acad Sci U S A 79:4395–4399, 1982.

Miller JFAP, Osoba D. Current concepts of the immunological function of the thymus. Physiol Rev 47:437–520, 1967.

Molina TJ, Kishihara K, Siderovski DP, van Ewijk W, Narendran A, Timms E, Wakeham A, Paige CJ, Harmann K-U, Veillette A, Davidson D, Mak TW. Profound block in thymocyte development in mice lacking p56lck. Nature 357:161–164, 1992.

Morgan DA, Ruscetti FW, Gallo RC. Selective *in vitro* growth of T lymphocytes from normal bone marrow. Science 193:1007–1110, 1976.

Murphy KM, Heimberger AB, Loh DH. Induction by antigen of intrathymic apoptosis of CD4+CD8+ TCRlo thymocytes *in vivo*. Science 250:1720–1723, 1990.

Noguchi M, Yi H, Rosenblatt HM, Filipovich AH, Adelstein S, Modi WS, McBride OW, Leonard WJ. Interleukin-2 receptor γ chain mutation results in X-linked severe combined immunodeficiency in humans. Cell 73:147–157, 1993.

Okada M, Nada S, Yamanashi NY, Yamamoto T, Nakagawa H. CSK: a protein-tyrosine involved in regulation of Src family kinases. J Biol Chem 266:24249–24252, 1991.

Oppenheim JJ, Ruscetti FW, Faltynek C. Cytokines. In Stites DP, Terr AI, Parslow TG, eds. Cytokines in Basic and Clinical Immunology, 8th ed. East Norwalk, Conn. Appleton and Lange, 1994, pp. 105–123.

Patel HR, Renz H, Terada N, Gelfand EW. Differential activation of p21ras in CD45RA+ and CD45RO+ human T lymphocytes. J Immunol 152:2830–2836, 1994.

Paul WE. Pleiotropy and redundancy: T cell–derived lymphokines in the immune response. Cell 57:521–524, 1989.

Picker LJ, Butcher EC. Physiological and molecular mechanisms of lymphocyte homing. Ann Rev Immunol 10:561–591, 1992.

Picker LJ, Kishimoto TK, Smith CW, Warnock RA, Butcher EC. ELAM-1 is an adhesion molecule for skin-homing T cells. Nature 349: 796–799, 1991.

Picker LJ, Terstappen LWMM, Rott LS, Streeter PR, Stein H, Butcher EC. Differential expression of homing-associated adhesion molecules by T-cell subsets in man. J Immunol 145:3247–3255, 1990.

Polakis P, McCormick F. Structural requirements for the interaction of p21ras with GAP, exchange factors, and its biological effector target. J Biol Chem 268:9157–9160, 1993.

Puck JM, Deschenes SM, Porter JC, Dutra AS, Brown CJ, Wallard HF, Heirthorn PS. The interleukin-2 receptor gamma chain maps to Xq 13.1 and is mutated in X-linked severe combined immunodeficiency, SCID XI. Mol Genet 2:1099–1104, 1993.

Raulet DH, Garman RD, Saito H, Tonegawa S. Developmental regulation of T-cell receptor gene expression. Nature 314:103–107, 1985.

Reichart RA, Weissman IL, Butcher EC. Phenotypic analysis of thymocytes that express homing receptors for peripheral lymph nodes. J Immunol 136:3521–3528, 1986.

Rudd CE. CD4, CD8 and the TCR-CD3 complex: a novel class of protein-tyrosine kinase receptor. Immunol Today, 11:400–406, 1990.

Samelson LE, Klausner RD. Tyrosine kinases and tyrosine-based activation motifs. Current research on activation via the T cell antigen receptor. J Biol Chem 267:24913–24916, 1992.

Sanders ME, Makgoba MW, Sharrow SO, Stephany D, Springer TA, Young HA, Shaw S. Human memory T lymphocytes express increased levels of three cell adhesion molecules (LFA-3, CD2, and LFA-1) and three other molecules (UCHL1, CDw29, and Pgp-1) and have enhanced IFN-γ production. J Immunol 140:1401–1407, 1988.

Sato VL, Waksal SD, Herzenberg LA. Identification and separation of pre-T-cells from nu/nu mice: differentiation by preculture with thymic reticuloepithelial cells. Cell Immunol 24:173–184, 1976.

Schall TJ. Biology of the RANTES/SIS cytokine family. Cytokine 3:1–18, 1991.

Schlessinger J. How receptor tyrosine kinases activate Ras. TIBS, 18:273–275, 1993.

Schreiber SL, Crabtree GR. The mechanism of action of cyclosporin A and FK506. Immunol Today 13:136–142, 1992.

Spriggs MK, Fanslow WC, Armitage RJ, Belmont J. The biology of the human ligand for CD40. J Clin Immunol 13:373–380, 1993.

Springer TA. Adhesion receptors of the immune system. Nature 346:426–433, 1990.

Stein PL, Lee H-M, Rich S, Soriano P. pp59fyn mutant mice display differential signaling in thymocytes and peripheral T cells. Cell 70:741–750, 1992.

Swain SL, Bradley LM, Croft M, Tonkonogy S, Atkins G, Weinberg AD, Duncan DD, Hedrick SM, Dutton RW, Huston G. Helper T-cell subsets: phenotype, function, and the role of lymphokines in regulating their development. Immunol Rev 123:115–144, 1991.

Taniguchi T, Kobayashi T, Kondo J, Takahashi K, Nakamura H, Suzuki J, Nagai K, Yamada T, Nakamura S, Yamamura H. Molecular cloning of a porcine gene syk that encodes a 72-kda protein-tyrosine kinase showing high susceptibility to proteolysis. J Biol Chem 266:15790–15796, 1991.

Terada N, Franklin RA, Lucas JJ, Gelfand, EW. T-cell signaling and activation through the IL-2 receptor complex. In Growth Factors and Signal Transduction in Development, pp. 75–95, 1994a.

Terada N, Patel HR, Takase K, Domenico J, Kohno K, Nairn AC, Lucas JJ, Gelfand EW. Rapamycin selectively inhibits translation of mRNAs encoding elongation factors and ribosomal proteins. Proc Natl Acad Sci U S A 91:11477–11481, 1994b.

Toribio ML, Gutierrez-Ramos JC, Pezzi L, Marcos MAR, Martinez AC. Interleukin-2–dependent autocrine proliferation in T-cell development. Nature 342:82–85, 1989.

Trainin N, Zaisov R, Yakir Y, Rotter V. Thymic hormones: characterization and perspectives. In Doria G, Eshkol A, eds. Proc. Serono Symposia, Vol. 27, The Immune System: Functions and Therapy of Dysfunction. London, Academic Press, 1980, pp. 159–169.

Turka LA, Schatz DG, Oettinger MA, Chun JJ, Gorka C, Lee K, McCormack WT, Thompson CB. Thymocyte expression of RAG-1 and RAG-2: termination by T cell receptor cross-linking. Science 253:778–781, 1991.

Veillette A, Abraham N, Caron L, Davidson D. The lymphocyte-specific tyrosine kinase p56[lck]. Semin Immunol 3:143–152, 1991.

von Boehmer H. Developmental biology of T cells in T cell receptor transgenic mice. Ann Rev Immunol 8:531–556, 1990.

Watanabe Y, Sudo J, Minato N, Ohnishi A, Katsura Y. Interleukin 7 preferentially supports the growth of $\gamma\delta$ T cell receptor–bearing T cells from fetal thymocytes in vitro. Int Immunol 3:1067–1075, 1991.

Weiss A. Molecular and genetic insights into T cell antigen receptor structure and function. Ann Rev Genet 25:487–510, 1991.

Weiss A, Littman DR. Signal transduction by lymphocyte antigen receptors. Cell 76:263–274, 1994.

Weissman AM, Hou D, Orloff DG, Madi WS, Seuanez H, O'Brien SU, Klausner RD. Molecular cloning and chromosomal localization of the human T-cell receptor ζ chain: distinction from the molecular CD3 complex. Proc Natl Acad Sci U S A 85:9709–9713,1988.

Weissman IL. Developmental switches in the immune system. Cell 76:207–218, 1994.

Williams AF, Barclay, AN. The immunoglobulin superfamily—domains for cell surface recognition. Ann Rev Immunol 6:381–405, 1988.

Zinkernagel RM, Doherty PC. H-2 compatibility requirement for T cell–mediated lysis of target cells infected with lymphocyte choriomeningitis virus: different cytotoxic T-cell specificities are associated with structures coded for in H-2K or H-2D. J Exp Med 141:1427–1436, 1975.

Zinkernagel RM, Doherty PC. MHC-restricted cytotoxic T-cells: studies on the biological role of polymorphic major transplantation antigens determining T-cell restriction-specificity, function, and responsiveness. Adv Immunol 27:51–177, 1979.

Chapter 3

The B-Lymphocyte System

Jonathan Braun and E. Richard Stiehm

THE IMMUNOGLOBULIN SYSTEM

The B-lymphocyte (B-cell) system comprises the cells capable of immunoglobulin synthesis (B cells and plasma cells), the precursors of these cells (pro-B cells and pre-B cells), and the products of these cells, the immunoglobulins. The entire system is directed toward one result, the production of a vast array of immunoglobulin molecules with different specificities (antibodies) that constitute the humoral immune system. Although different types (classes and subclasses) of immunoglobulins exist, they make up a single effector system that arises from a spectrum of B cells. This is in contrast to the T-cell system (see Chapter 2), which develops into several divergent and distinct effector systems. The immunoglobulins, the effector molecules of the B-lymphocyte system, are considered first; this includes a discussion of immunoglobulin receptors on various cells. The B cells that produce these immunoglobulins, the molecular events that give rise to immunoglobulin diversity, and the maturation of the B-cell system are then considered. Finally, clinical aspects of immunoglobulins and B cells are discussed.

The immunoglobulins (also termed immune serum globulins, or γ globulins) are proteins endowed with known antibody activity. Certain proteins related to them by chemical and antigenic structure are clearly immunoglobulins, but antibody activity has simply not been demonstrated for them—for example, myeloma proteins, Bence Jones proteins, and naturally occurring subunits of the immunoglobulins such as γ-chain fragments in γ-chain disease (World Health Organization [WHO], 1964). As discussed in detail later, immunoglobulins are proteins made solely by cells of B lineage that are capable of reacting specifically with antigens. The similarities of the various immunoglobulins in terms of molecular origin, structure, biologic activity, and cells of origin permit their consideration as a single system.

Immunoglobulin Structure

The immunoglobulins, as mediators of humoral, or antibody-dependent, immunity, are present as free molecules in the blood stream, tissues, and exocrine secretions. Immunoglobulins also exist as integral membrane proteins on B-cell surfaces and thereby serve the additional function of antigen recognition for the B cell–immunoglobulin system. The functions of free immunoglobulin are (1) to combine with antigen (e.g., show specific antibody activity) and (2) to participate in adjunctive biologic functions such as opsonization, neutralization, complement fixation, transport into secretions, and immune complex formation. Dif-

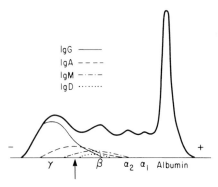

Figure 3–1. Electrophoretic distribution of the immunoglobulins. There is an approximate correlation between the gamma globulin on electrophoresis and the total of the immunoglobulins measured immunochemically. Immunoglobulin E (IgE) is present in such small concentrations that it contributes insignificantly to the γ globulin on electrophoresis.

ferent portions of the antibody molecule are involved in each; antigen binding is a property of the Fab, or *variable* (V), region of the molecule, and adjunctive biologic functions are properties of the Fc, or *crystallizable* region.

Immunoglobulin Heterogeneity

Sixty years ago, the plasma proteins were separated by salt fractionation into albumin and globulins. In 1937, Tiselius introduced electrophoresis, which separates proteins on the basis of electrical charge. This technique permitted resolution of the globulins into four fractions: γ, β, α2, and α1. At a pH of 8.6, the γ fraction migrates most slowly and α1 migrates most rapidly, next to albumin. Immunoglobulins from serum are primarily located in the γ fraction, but some are also present in the β and the α2 fractions. The distribution of different immunoglobulin classes in serum is illustrated in Figure 3–1.

Subsequently, extensive chemical, serologic, and molecular studies have indicated that antibodies (immunoglobulins) possess considerable heterogeneity and make up a group of related proteins. Immunoelectrophoresis has been especially valuable in delineating this heterogeneity (Fig. 3–2). Immunoelectrophoresis combines the migration of a protein solution (such as serum) in an electrical field (electrophoresis), followed

by immune precipitation in agar by an antiserum to the protein. The antiserum is placed in a trough parallel with the path of the electrophoretic migration to which the serum was subjected. The antiserum then diffuses toward the electrophoretically separated serum components. When a protein that reacts with the antiserum is encountered, a distinct arc of precipitation is formed.

Immunoelectrophoresis of normal human serum discloses 25 or more separate proteins; three of these—IgG, IgM, and IgA—have antibody activity and are missing in the serum of patients with agammaglobulinemia (see Fig. 3–2). In addition to these three antigenically distinct immunoglobulin classes, two other immunoglobulins—IgD and IgE—are present in normal serum but are below the level of detection of immunoelectrophoresis.

Other techniques are used to further define immunoglobulin heterogeneity and structure. Starch gel and acrylamide gel electrophoresis, which separate similarly charged proteins on the basis of size by their different rates of migration through the gels, have been used to separate immunoglobulins and their subunits into multiple fractions. The molecular weight (MW) of immunoglobulins can be estimated, using ultracentrifugation or filtration through dextran gels, such as Sephadex, which separates large-molecular-weight immunoglobulins (i.e., IgM) from other immunoglobulins.

Immunoglobulin structure can be visualized by use of the electron microscope. X-ray diffraction studies have been used to define the three-dimensional structure of immunoglobulin molecules (Nisonoff et al., 1975a). For this technique, however, pure crystallizable proteins or subunits, which are only occasionally available, are required.

Techniques to determine the exact amino acid sequence of proteins and peptides (sequence analysis) have been utilized to arrive at the primary structure of several myeloma proteins (Nisonoff et al., 1975b). Most recently, the ability to clone the deoxyribonucleic acid (DNA) sequences for the various constant region heavy and light genes has allowed the exact determination of the C-region composition (both DNA sequence and thereby the amino acid sequence) for all the immunoglobulins.

Nomenclature

The nomenclature of the immunoglobulin classes and their structural units, codified by the World Health

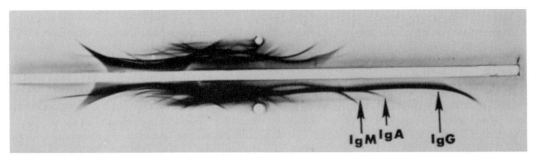

Figure 3–2. Immunoelectrophoretic analysis of an agammaglobulinemic serum *(top)* and a normal serum *(bottom)*. The trough contains a rabbit antiserum to normal human serum. Each of the precipitin arcs that is formed represents a unique protein. The normal serum demonstrates the three immunoglobulins (IgG, IgM, and IgA) that are missing from the serum of the agammaglobulinemic individual.

Table 3–1. Chain Structures of the Human Immunoglobulin Classes

Immunoglobulin Class	Heavy Chain	Light Chain	Other Chain(s)	Chain Formula
IgG	γ	κ		$\gamma_2\kappa_2$
		λ		$\gamma_2\lambda_2$
IgM	μ	κ	J	$(\mu_2\kappa_2)_5$-J
		λ	J	$(\mu_2\lambda_2)_5$-J
IgD	δ	κ		$\delta_2\kappa_2$
		λ	J	$\delta_2\lambda_2$
IgE	ϵ	κ		$\epsilon_2\kappa_2$
		λ	J	$\epsilon_2\lambda_2$
IgA	α	κ		$\alpha_2\kappa_2$
		λ	J	$\alpha_2\lambda_2$
Secretory IgA	α	κ	J, SC	$(\alpha_2\kappa_2)_2$-SC-J
		λ	J, SC	$(\alpha_2\lambda_2)_2$-SC-J

Abbreviations: J = joining; SC = secretory component.

Organization (WHO, 1964, 1970), is presented in Table 3–1. All immunoglobulins are designated Ig. The five classes are designated IgG, IgM, IgA, IgD, and IgE, all of which are present in normal adult serum (WHO, 1964, 1970). The class of immunoglobulin is determined by the heavy chain (μ, δ, γ, ϵ, or α) for IgM, IgD, IgG, IgE, and IgA, respectively. Each immunoglobulin molecule is composed of two pairs of polypeptide chains: one pair of identical heavy chains and one pair of identical light chains (Fig. 3–3).

There are two types of light chains, termed kappa (κ) and lambda (λ). Immunoglobulin molecules have either two κ chains or two λ chains, never one of each. These two light-chain types are common to all immunoglobulin classes; the heavy-chain pair is different in each immunoglobulin class. These are held together, in general, by sets of disulfide bridges between the heavy chains and between the light and heavy chains. In normal serum, molecules of each class are paired with sets of both κ and λ chains. Thus a complete immunoglobulin molecule is composed of at least four polypeptide chains; indeed, immunoglobulins were the first proteins that were clearly shown to be composed of the products of more than one gene.

IgM primarily exists as a pentamer of five monomeric units of paired light and heavy chains, with an additional single-polypeptide molecule, the joining (J) chain (Fig. 3–4). The J chain is common to all polymeric immunoglobulins (IgM and some IgA molecules). Secretory IgA present in exocrine gland secretions also is a polymeric molecule containing two and occasionally three IgA molecules, a J chain, and a secretory component (Tomasi, 1972) (see Fig. 3–4).

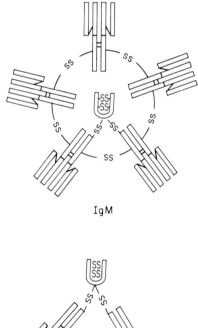

IgM

SECRETORY IgA

Figure 3–4. Structural models of polymeric serum IgM and secretory IgA. The U-shaped chain is the J (joining) chain, common to all polymeric immunoglobulins. SC is the secretory component of the secretory IgA molecule. The disulfide bonds (—S—S—) of the monomeric units are indicated by lines between the chains.

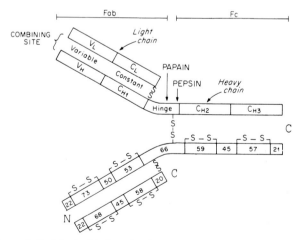

Figure 3–3. A typical IgG molecule. N indicates the amino terminal end and C the carboxyl terminal end. The intrachain and interchain disulfide bonds are indicated by —S—S—. Papain splits the molecule at the hinge region, so that two Fab fragments and one Fc fragment result. Pepsin splits the molecule at the hinge region, so that an F(ab')₂ fragment results.

Based on the chain structure of the immunoglobulin, the molecular composition of each of the immunoglobulin classes can be formulated (see Table 3–1).

Isotypes, Allotypes, and Idiotypes

Immunoglobulin molecules can be divided into three subdivisions, based on antigen differences within their structural subunits.

Isotypes are all present in normal individuals and include:

1. The five major immunoglobulin classes, based on major antigenic (and physicochemical) differences in their heavy chains (see Table 3–1).
2. The four IgG and two IgA subclasses, based on subtle antigenic variability within the heavy chains of IgG and IgA, respectively (Fig. 3–5).
3. The two light-chain types κ and λ.
4. Several λ chain subtypes. The last are dependent on the presence or absence of certain nonexclusive antigenic determinants termed Oz, Mz, Kern, and Mcg, initially identified on λ chain Bence Jones proteins (Solomon, 1976). Other λ subtypes may also exist (Schanfield and Van Loghem, 1986).

The *allotypes* are genetic markers present on certain heavy- and light-chain isotypes that are inherited in typical mendelian fashion. Thus only certain individuals carry these antigenic determinants. The allotypes associated with the γ heavy chain are designated Gm (γ marker); the allotypes associated with α and ε heavy chains are designated Am and Em respectively, and those associated with κ light chains are designated Km. No allotypes of IgM or λ light chains have been identified.

Idiotypes are unique antigenic determinants present in the V region of the immunoglobulin molecule. Idiotypes may be either *public* or *private* (Rajewsky and Takemori, 1983). A public idiotype represents a peptide sequence in one or more closely related V genes. It is thus detected commonly among different individuals and is genetically distributed in classic mendelian fashion (Stewart and Schwartz, 1994). The level of an idiotype in serum or membrane Ig depends on developmental and antigenic factors controlling the activity of the idiotype-positive B cells. For example, the most common public idiotype is 16/6 (encoded by the $V_H 26$ V gene). It is present in most individuals and is typically expressed at high levels (~10% of blood B cells and a similar fraction of serum IgM).

In contrast, a private idiotype is present in a unique clonal antibody, typically encoded by the peptide sequence of somatically mutated hypervariable regions. Such idiotypes thus intimately involve the antigen-binding site. Consequently, anti-idiotypic antibodies against these sites often block antigen binding. In addition, these anti-idiotypic antibodies can serve as mimics for antigen and elicit a humoral immune response similar to that produced by the authentic antigen. Use of this "internal image" strategy has been a productive research tool to define ligand-receptor interactions and also a novel immunization strategy (Bruck et al., 1986; Garcia et al., 1992). Private idiotypes have often been defined for M components: serum antibodies produced by pathologically activated (often malignant) B-cell clones. More broadly, idiotypes can be defined for any clonal immunoglobulin. From a practical standpoint, public and private idiotypes are defined by polyclonal or monoclonal anti-idiotypic antibodies, and these have been widely used in research on the antibody repertoire. Some anti-idiotypic reagents are now available commercially (Bahler et al., 1991).

In the course of a normal immune response, idiotype production is followed by an endogenous anti-idiotypic response, at both the cellular and the antibody levels (Kearney, 1993). Jerne's network theory (Jerne, 1974) states that such idiotype–anti-idiotype interactions form a dynamic idiotypic network that is essential for the development and control of the normal antibody response. The extent to which this interaction contributes to the normal immune regulation remains unresolved. However, it has proved both a disadvantage and an advantage in exogenous antibody therapy. Monoclonal antibodies have been administered for a variety of therapeutic purposes, but their efficacy is reduced by anti-idiotypic antibody responses, which shorten the agent's serum half-life and elicit other immune complex–related adverse reactions. This has driven the development of new recombinant antibody technologies to reduce antibody immunogenicity. Conversely, large doses of intravenous immunoglobulin are used therapeutically to suppress pathogenic auto-antibodies, and this effect has been attributed to the

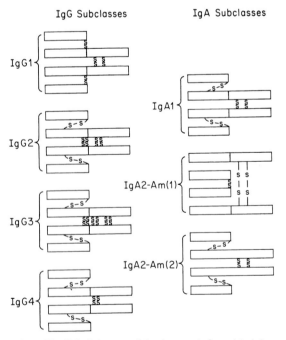

Figure 3–5. Disulfide linkages of the human IgG and IgA immunoglobulin subclasses. The heavy-chain cysteine residue of IgG1 forming the heavy-light disulfide bond is considerably closer to the C-terminal end than in the other IgG subclasses. The IgA2Am(1) molecule lacks the heavy-light disulfide bonds, which are linked by covalent bonds.

multiple anti-idiotypes present in these preparations (Dwyer, 1992).

Gm, Am, and Km Factors

Further variation in the immunoglobulins is based on the presence or absence of genetic differences in immunoglobulin amino acid sequences. These were first described by Grubb in 1956. These inherited markers—Gm, Am, and Km—are termed *allotypes* (genetic alternatives within the same species controlled by allelic genes) and are present in only certain individuals as determined by mendelian genetics.

Nomenclature

The nomenclature and a list of genetic immunoglobulin factors are presented in Table 3–2. The recommended nomenclature (WHO, 1965, 1970) labels the allotypes first by class and subclass (e.g., G1m) and then by allele (in parentheses). These factors are inherited in accordance with typical mendelian genetics (Natvig and Kunkel, 1973). At least 23 genetic factors are recognized (Schanfield and Van Loghem, 1986).

Three groups of genetic factors are recognized:

- Gm factors, present on the γ heavy chain of IgG and thus limited to IgG classes
- Am factors, present on the α2 heavy chain of IgA
- Km factors, present on the κ light chain and thus represented in all classes of immunoglobulins

In addition, allotypy has been described for IgE (Em) by Van Loghem and others (1984), using a monoclonal antibody.

Table 3–2. Genetic Factors of Human Immunoglobulins

Genetic Factor	Subclass or Chain Location
Factors at the Gm Locus	
G1m(1)	IgG1
G1m(2)	IgG1
G1m(3)	IgG1
G1m(17)	IgG1
G2m(23)	IgG2
G3m(5)	IgG3
G3m(6)	IgG3
G3m(10)	IgG3
G3m(11)	IgG3
G3m(13)	IgG3
G3m(14)	IgG3
G3m(15)	IgG3
G3m(16)	IgG3
G3m(21)	IgG3
G3m(24)	IgG3
G3m(26)	IgG3
G3m(27)	IgG3
G3m(28)	IgG3
Factors at the Am Locus	
A2m(1)	IgA2
A2m(2)	IgA2
Factors at the Km Locus	
Km(1)	κ
Km(2)	κ
Km(3)	κ

Methods of Detection

The usual method of detection of Ig allotypy is presented in Figure 3–6. Human O Rh-positive (D) erythrocytes are exposed to an incomplete Rh antibody (an IgG immunoglobulin), which coats but does not agglutinate them. This antibody is generally obtained from an Rh-negative multiparous woman sensitized by an Rh-positive fetus. The coated red blood cells are agglutinated by human sera with *rheumatoid factor* (an IgM antibody that reacts with an IgG immunoglobulin) when the rheumatoid factor is directed toward the immunoglobulin allotype of the coat. This agglutination reaction between the rheumatoid factor (agglutinator) and the IgG-coated erythrocyte can be inhibited by a serum whose IgG globulin has the same genetic determinant to which the rheumatoid factor is directed. If the added serum does not have the genetic determinant, no inhibition occurs and the rheumatoid factor agglutinates the coated erythrocyte. Thus, serum from an individual of G1m(1) type inhibits the agglutination of an anti-G1m(1) rheumatoid factor with a G1m(1)-coated erythrocyte.

The sera of frequently transfused individuals may also contain antibodies to immunoglobulin allotypes (because of exposure to allotypes of immunoglobulin that the individual lacks) and can be used as agglutinators instead of rheumatoid factors. These sera are generally preferable, since they have a higher degree of specificity (e.g., a narrower spectrum). The latter type of agglutinator is often called a *SNagg* (serum normal agglutinin) and is usually an IgG globulin; a rheumatoid factor is often called a *Ragg* (rheumatoid agglutinin) and is usually an IgM globulin (Fudenberg, 1963).

Instead of incomplete Rh antibodies, isolated myeloma proteins can be used as the coat. They are coupled to human O erythrocytes by means of bisdiazotized benzidine or chromium chloride. This may reduce the problem of multispecificity of the coat.

The inhibition of the agglutination system so described necessitates a pair of human serum reagents: a

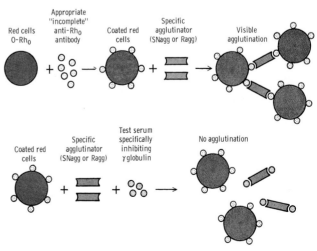

Figure 3–6. Method for typing genetic γ globulin factors. (From Engle RL Jr, Wallis LA. Immunoglobulinopathies. Springfield, Ill., Charles C Thomas, 1969.)

coat consisting of an incomplete Rh antibody, or myeloma protein, and a specific antibody (the SNagg and Ragg agglutinator) reactive to it for each factor to be tested. The procurement of reagents is cumbersome at best; indeed, the supply of the reagents for Km(2) and Km(3) typing is exceedingly scarce. Monoclonal antibodies to G1m(3) and a few G3m allotypes have been produced (Zelaschi et al, 1983; Nelson et al, 1994).

Gm Factors

The Gm groups are the most widely studied (see Table 3–2) (Nisonoff et al., 1975c). They are localized to the constant region of the γ heavy chain, and each is located on one of the IgG subclasses. Many of the Gm factors are inherited together; for example, G1m(1) and G1m(3) are either both present or both absent in any individual. Others seem to be allelic, including G1m(3) and G1m(4), and G3m(5) and G3m(12) (Steinberg, 1969). In many instances, the exact amino acid substitution is known; for example, G3m(21) and nG3m(21) differ as a result of a single amino acid substitution at position 296 of the C_H3 region; G3m(21) has tyrosine and nG3m(21) has phenylalanine at this position.

Although Gm factors are present on the heavy chain, G1m(3) and G1m(17) require the presence of light chains for their expression, probably because of conformational change when the light chain is separated from the heavy chain.

Isoallotypes and Allogroups

Isoallotypes are Gm determinants that are allotypic variants in one subclass of IgG but are present in all molecules of at least one other subclass. These isoallotypes, or nonmarkers, are designated by the letter *n* or a minus sign before the allelic factor notation. The notation indicates the allotype present when other subclasses are absent. Thus nG1m(1) is an allele on IgG1 molecules but is also present on all IgG2 and IgG3 molecules. Another isoallotype is nG3m(21), an allele for IgG3 but present on all IgG2 molecules (Nisonoff et al., 1975a).

Several markers are inherited together in a closely linked cluster termed an *allogroup*, or a haplotype. An example is G1m(1,17), nG2m(23), and G3m(21).

Biologic Levels of Significance of Gm Allotypes

Levels of specific IgG subclasses, IgD, and possibly the antibody response to certain antigens may be related to the Gm or Km type (Kunkel and Kindt, 1975). For example, normal subjects with IgG allotype G3m(5) have twice the IgG3 level of those having G3m(21). The antibody response to the polysaccharide capsule of *Haemophilus influenzae* of children with the Km(1) allotype is fivefold to 10-fold greater than in those children who lack this determinant (Granoff et al., 1984).

Gene deletions governing the Gm alleles may occur and may result in low levels of an IgG subclass; for example, when G3m(21) and G3m(5) are deleted, low levels of IgG1 result. In one symptomatic patient with hypogammaglobulinemia, heterozygous gene deletions

of IgG1 from one parent and of IgG3 from the other were present, resulting in extremely low levels of both IgG1 and IgG3 (Yount et al., 1970).

Certain populations have a high incidence of specific Gm factors that are absent or low in other populations, thus making Gm typing useful in anthropologic studies (Steinberg, 1969). For example, G1m(3) is present in 90% of whites but rare in blacks; G3m(6) is present in 25 to 50% of blacks but rare (< 1%) in whites. These observations can be used to determine the degree of racial admixture (e.g., there is approximately 30% white admixture among American blacks) as well as tribal migration patterns. Antibodies of certain genetic types may offer superior protection to microorganisms indigenous to various regions, thus explaining the marked variability of the Gm types from population to population.

Am Factors

A2m(1), one of the two allotypes of the IgA2 subclass, is unique among the immunoglobulins, inasmuch as the heavy and light chains are not joined by disulfide bonds; indeed, the two light chains are linked by disulfide bonds (see Fig. 3–5). The other allele of the IgA2 subclass, A2m(2), has the usual disulfide bond arrangement. The A2m(1) factor is present in 98% of whites and 51% of blacks. No relation between the Am type and the Gm or Km type exists (Vyas and Fudenberg, 1969).

Km Factors

Three allelic markers on the κ light chain—Km(1), Km(2), and Km(3)—have been described. Individuals who express Km(2) activity always express Km(1) activity. The amino acid substitutions responsible for this allotypy are shown in Table 3–3 (Solomon, 1976).

Anti-allotypic Antibodies

Anti-Gm antibodies may appear after multiple blood or γ globulin administrations (Allen and Kunkel, 1966) and under normal circumstances, in some newborns transiently exposed to maternal IgG different from their own (Steinberg and Wilson, 1963). Also, in one instance, an anti-Gm factor developed in a pregnant mother as a result of exposure to her infant's paternally derived Gm factor (Fudenberg and Fudenberg, 1964); this is analogous to sensitization of an Rh-negative mother by an Rh-positive infant. Anti-Gm antibodies are not a source of transfusion reactions. Maternal anti-Gm antibodies do not inhibit the synthesis of IgG by

Table 3–3. Relation Between the Km Allotypes and the Amino Acid Sequence of the Constant Region of the Kappa Light Chain

	Amino Acid Residue	
Allotype	Position 153	Position 191
Km (1)	Valine	Leucine
Km (1, 2)	Alanine	Leucine
Km (3)	Alanine	Valine

the fetus even when they are IgG antibodies and cross the placenta (Nathenson et al., 1971).

Physical and Chemical Properties of Immunoglobulins

The immunoglobulins are the plasma proteins with the slowest electrophoretic mobility at pH 8.6 and with isoelectric points near pH 7.3. Early characterization of immunoglobulin size was by ultracentrifugation constants, Svedberg units (S), hence the terms 7S γ globulin for IgG and 19S for IgM. Electron microscopic studies indicate that the monomeric Ig molecule is T-shaped, with the arms making a slight angle, so that the actual shape is between that of a T and a Y. The horizontal length is 120 Å, the vertical height 80 Å, and the width 35 Å (Labaw and Davies, 1971).

As noted, each immunoglobulin molecule is made up of two pairs of identical chains—two heavy and two light chains; these are held together by disulfide bonds and weak noncovalent forces. There are two antibody-combining sites, consisting of a portion of the heavy and light chains in the two amino terminal sections of the molecule—the Fab regions (see Figure 3–3). The single C-terminal end of the molecule contains the C, or constant, regions (Fc), which relate to the nonantigen-binding biologic properties of a given immunoglobulin.

The chemical and physical properties of the immunoglobulin classes are presented in Table 3–4. IgG has the broadest mobility but is principally located in the γ globulin region; in general, the other immunoglobulins have faster mobilities.

Serum IgM generally is a polymer (see Fig. 3–4) of five monomers, has a molecular weight of 900,000, and is held together by disulfide bonds. A single J chain is also linked to this complex by disulfide bridges. A J chain is made by the same B cells (plasma cells) that make the immunoglobulin. The MW of a J chain is 15,000; it serves to stabilize the multimeric complex.

Polymeric IgM may also be synthesized by B cells as a hexamer (six monomers) without a J chain. This minor form is much more efficient than pentameric IgM in complement fixation and accounts for most of this biologic activity of polymeric IgM (Randall et al., 1990).

Serum IgA often exists as a polymer of two or three monomers. When these immunoglobulins are in their polymeric form, a J chain is attached to stabilize the complex and protect it from degradation. Secretory IgA (see Fig. 3–4) is composed of two IgA monomers, a J chain, and another protein of 60,000 daltons—secretory component. In contrast to J chain, secretory component is synthesized by epithelial cells. It is actually a proteolytic fragment of the polyimmunoglobulin receptor used by these cells for cellular translocation of IgA from the basal to the apical cell surface. Proteolysis releases the complex (with the secretory component segment still attached) for luminal delivery (Tomasi, 1972; Aroeti et al., 1992) (see Chapter 8, The Mucosal Defense System).

Structural Subunits

A key source of knowledge of the structure of the immunoglobulin molecule has been its enzymatic breakdown by the proteolytic enzymes papain and pepsin and the subsequent characterization of the resulting fragments. Reducing agents and extremes of pH have also been used to obtain immunoglobulin fragments for structural studies. In more recent years, recombinant DNA technology has also been much used to produce synthetic antibodies engineered for conventional or novel antibody functions.

Papain Fragments

Porter (1959) studied digestion of a rabbit IgG antibody (to egg albumin) with papain in the presence of cysteine. The MW was reduced from 150,000 to 50,000; the fragmented antibody could no longer precipitate with egg albumin but could combine with it,

Table 3–4. Chemical and Physical Properties of the Immunoglobulin Classes

Characteristic	Immunoglobulin Class				
	IgG	*IgM*	*IgA*	*IgD*	*IgE*
Chains					
Heavy	γ	μ	α	δ	ε
Light	κ, λ	κ, λ	κ, λ	κ, λ	κ, λ
Monomer units	1	5	1–3	1	1
Electrophoretic mobility	γ_2–α_2	γ_1–α_1	γ_1–α_1	γ_1–β	γ_1–β
Principal mobility	γ_2	γ_1	β	γ	β
Sedimentation coefficient (Svedberg units)	6.7	19	7–15	7	8
Molecular weight	150,000	900,000	160–500,000	180,000	200,000
Percent carbohydrate	3	12	7.5–11	12–18	12
Serum concentration					
Adult mean (mg/dl)	1,200	120	200	3	0.01
Percent of total	70–80	5–10	10–15	<1	<0.01
Solubility	Euglobulin	Euglobulin	Pseudoglobulin	Pseudoglobulin	Pseudoglobulin
Sensitivity to mercaptans	0	+	+	?	?
Heat lability	±	+ +	+	+ + + +	+ + +
Number of subclasses	4	2	2	0	0
Genetic factors	Gm, Km	Km	Am, Km	Km	Km

as shown by its ability to inhibit combination of the antigen with intact antiserum. Porter fractionated the digested product and noted two types of subunits, one that combined with antigen (the Fab portion) and another that had most of the antigenic properties of the molecule and was crystallizable (the Fc portion). This important finding indicated that the intact molecule could be reduced to fragments that retain distinct biologic activities.

Human IgG immunoglobulin can also be digested with papain and results in the same important biologic fractions—a pair of Fab subunits that are antigen binding and a single Fc fragment that retains the characteristic biologic and antigenic properties of IgG (see Fig. 3–3). These fragments can be separated chromatographically or electrophoretically for chemical and biologic studies. The Fc fragment has a molecular weight of 48,000; the Fab fragment has a molecular weight of 52,000.

Pepsin Fragments

Pepsin can also be used to digest immunoglobulin (Nisonoff et al., 1960). Digestion of the 7S IgG molecule with pepsin results in a 5S fragment of 100,000 MW. This fragment, designated $F(ab')_2$, consists of the two linked Fab subunits; it retains bivalent antibody activity and can precipitate with antigen. It can be split into two identical single Fab units by reduction of disulfide bonds linking the two Fab fragments (see Fig. 3–3). The Fc portion is completely digested into multiple small fragments by pepsin.

Heavy and Light Chains

Edelman and Poulik (1961), using reduction with thiols in the presence of urea, cleaved IgG into smaller fragments, which were separated by gel filtration into heavy chains (MW 53,000) and light chains (MW 22,000) (see Fig. 3–3). Subsequent studies indicated that the Fab fraction resulting from papain or pepsin digestion is composed of the light chain and a portion of the heavy chain, whereas the Fc fraction is a portion of the heavy chain. This has led to the currently accepted model of the two-paired polypeptide chain structure joined by disulfide bonds (see Fig. 3–3).

Half-Molecules

Palmer and Nisonoff (1963) reduced the disulfide bonding between the two heavy chains of IgG to produce two half-molecules, each consisting of a single light chain and a single heavy chain. These half-molecules can be readily recombined; by using two half-molecules from different antibodies, a hybrid antibody with two specificities can be created (Fudenberg et al., 1963).

Properties of Subunits

The isolated fragments and chains have distinct properties. The distinct antigenic features of the classes and subclasses reside in the heavy chain; the distinct antigenic features of the types and subtypes reside in the light chain. The IgG Gm genetic factors are located on the γ heavy chains of IgG; the Am factors are located on the α2 heavy chain of IgA, and the Km factors are located on κ light chains.

The marked electrophoretic heterogeneity of the intact immunoglobulin molecules demonstrable by starch gel or acrylamide gel electrophoresis is largely a function of the heavy chain. The electrophoretic mobility of the intact molecule resembles that of the heavy chain, indicating that the electrical charge is primarily a heavy-chain characteristic.

The heavy chains are also the site of carbohydrate attachment in the molecule, primarily within the Fc fragment. Carbohydrate is important for proper folding and packing of the Fc region, and absent or aberrant glycosylation can result in intracellular degradation; production of a denatured, poorly functional protein; or unusual serum half-life and tissue sequestration (Jefferis, 1993). As stated earlier, the Fc fragment of the various heavy chains contains the determinants that enable the intact molecule to carry out its various effector functions other than antigen binding, such as complement fixation (for IgG and IgM), transport across the placenta (IgG), and binding to various cellular Fc receptors. Although most of these functions depend on interaction with Fc regions defined by peptide structure, other functions depend on recognition of the Fc carbohydrate, as in Fc receptor binding of IgA and IgM by certain lectins and glycosyltransferases (Tomana et al., 1993). Some V regions also display potential or demonstrated glycosylation sites, and the functional role of these glycans is an area of active investigation (Wright and Morrison, 1993).

Subclasses

The four IgG subclasses were initially defined by antigenic differences among the heavy chains of IgG myeloma proteins (Grey and Kunkel, 1964; Terry and Fahey, 1964). These antigenic differences among subclasses are less profound than among classes, so that rabbit antisera to IgG cannot distinguish between them. Mouse monoclonal antibodies from animals immunized with isolated myeloma proteins produce the best antisera for distinguishing between the IgG subclasses.

In addition to their antigenic differences, IgG subclasses differ in their structural, chemical, and biologic properties (Table 3–5). Of particular interest are the location and number of disulfide bonds, represented in Figure 3–5. This results in marked differences in susceptibility to papain cleavage. IgG3 is the most susceptible, IgG1 and IgG4 are intermediate, and IgG2 is relatively resistant to cleavage into the Fab and Fc fragments (Gergely et al., 1970). This susceptibility to proteolytic cleavage has been used to type isolated IgG molecules (Turner et al., 1970).

Two subclasses of IgA—IgA1 and IgA2—have been recognized. Normal serum IgA has 93% IgA1 and 7% IgA2 (Vaerman et al., 1968). Only IgA2 has the A2m(1) and A2m(2) genetic markers. The A2m(1) allotype lacks the disulfide bond linking the heavy and light chains but instead consists of disulfide-bonded light chains joined noncovalently to a pair of disulfide-bonded heavy chains (Grey et al., 1968) (see Fig. 3–5).

Table 3–5. Metabolic and Chemical Properties of the Human IgG Subclasses

Property	IgG1	IgG2	IgG3	IgG4
Molecular weight	146,000	146,000	165,000	146,000
Mean adult serum level (mg/dl)	840	240	80	40
Percentage of total IgG	70	20	7	3
Biologic half-life (days)	23	23	9	23
Gm markers	1, 2, 3, 17	23	5, 6, 10, 11, 13, 14, 15, 16, 21, 24, 26, 27, 28	
Susceptibility to proteolytic digestion	+ +	±	+ + + +	+ +

There is a considerably increased amount of IgA2 in the secretions (e.g., ~60% IgA2 and ~40% IgA1) as contrasted to the 9:1 ratio of IgA1 to IgA2 in the serum; this may confer resistance to secretory IgA–splitting enzymes known to be produced by bacteria in the gastrointestinal tract (Plaut et al., 1974).

Structure of the Heavy and Light Chains

Studies by numerous investigators, including 1973 Nobel prize winners R. R. Porter and G. M. Edelman, established the basic primary structure of light- and heavy-polypeptide chains of the immunoglobulin molecule (Edelman and Gall, 1969). All the chains are composed of similar (but clearly nonidentical), repeating homologous segments, called *domains*, of about 110 amino acid residues. Each domain contains a 60–amino acid loop stabilized by an intrachain disulfide bond.

Light chains are made up of two domains and vary in length between 211 and 217 amino acid residues. α, γ, and δ Heavy chains have 450 residues in four domains; μ and ε heavy chains have five domains, totaling 550 residues (Fig. 3–7). It is the N, or amino, terminal domain in both the light and heavy chains that makes up the Fab, or antigen-binding, section. Thus a typical complete IgG molecule has 1320 amino acid residues, whereas a dissociated IgM member has 1430 amino acids.

Constant and Variable Regions

The immunoglobulin chains consist of two distinct regions—the V, or *variable regions*, so designated because of the diversity of amino acid sequences found therein, and the C, or *constant regions*, so designated because of marked similarities of amino acid sequences among molecules of the same class and type.

The V region makes up the amino terminal domain (one half) of the light chain and constitutes one fourth or one fifth of the heavy chain. The V regions contain the antibody-combining site; the diversity of their amino acid sequences accounts for the large number of antibody specificities needed to react with all the antigens encountered by the body. This variability of sequence is not located equally throughout the V region of a given chain but is concentrated in three regions termed the *hypervariable regions (complementarity-determining regions* [CDRs]). Not surprisingly, these hypervariable regions fold in such a way as to constitute the critical portion of the antigen-binding cleft.

The C, or constant, regions include the carboxyl terminal domain (one half) of the light chains and the carboxyl terminal constituting three or four domains of the heavy chains. The C region accounts for the properties common to all immunoglobulins of a particular class; differences in their amino acid sequence result in isotypic or allotypic variants.

Light Chain

The amino terminal half of the κ light chain, the variable (V_κ) segment, is composed of 107 amino acids (see Fig. 3–7). There are four families of V_κ segments (V_κI–V_κIV), based on amino acid sequence similarity. There is much diversity within each family, since each family is composed of one to several nonidentical V_κ genes, and the V region of each individual antibody bears additional unique combinational and somatic mutations. The other half of the κ light chain is the constant (C_κ) segment, which is common to all κ light chains. Variants of the C_κ segment at two positions (see Table 3–3) make up the three Km allotypes.

The λ light chain is similarly constructed, with an amino terminal V region segment, V_λ, combined with a constant lambda segment, C_λ. There are nine V_λ families (V_λI–V_λIX), and each V_λ family is itself diverse as a result of multiple family gene members and somatic mutation. The constant segment of the λ light chain is

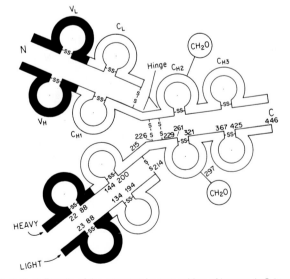

Figure 3–7. Details of the structural composition of human IgG immunoglobulin. The shaded areas of the chains are the variable (V) regions, and the unshaded areas are the constant (C) regions. Within each region are 60 amino acid loops stabilized by disulfide bonds (—S—S—), termed *domains*. The numbers refer to the amino acid positions of the cysteine residues that form disulfide bonds or are the attachment sites of carbohydrate.

formed from one of four different C_λ segments ($C_\lambda 1$, $C_\lambda 2$, $C_\lambda 3$, $C_\lambda 7$). These were originally designated as serologic isotypes (respectively: Mcg, Ke⁻Oz⁻, Ke⁻Oz⁺, Ke⁺Oz⁻) and show only modest sequence divergence (Vasicek and Leder, 1990).

Surrogate Light Chain

A novel surrogate light chain (ψL) with an interesting structure has also been identified (Melchers et al.,

1994) (Fig. 3–8). The protein consists of two noncovalently bound subunits, one V-like, the other C_λ-like. In humans, there is one V-like (Vpre-B) and four alternate C_λ-like proteins (14.1, 16.1, 16.2, and $C_\lambda 1$) (Evans and Hollis, 1991). Together, they constitute a light-chain structure that forms a conventional disulfide-linked monomer with the membrane form of μ heavy chain. ψL is almost exclusively limited in its localization to an intracellular compartment of pre-B cells and does

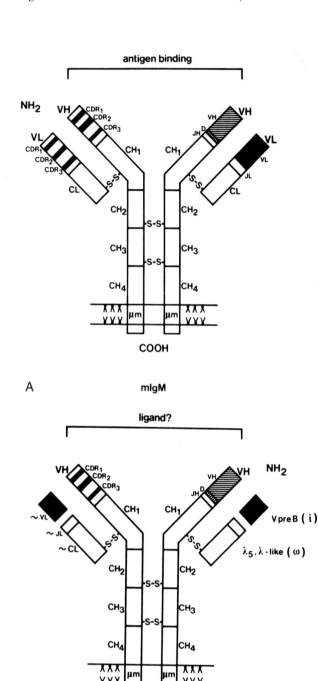

Figure 3–8. Diagram of the variable receptors found on mature or pre-B cells. *A,* Disulfide-linked heavy (H) and light (L) chains form a membrane IgM molecule with two identical antigen-binding sites. Within the μ-H chain, intracellular, transmembrane (μm), four constant ($C_H 1$–$C_H 4$), and three complementary-determining regions (CDR1–CDR3) are indicated relative to the V, D, and J segments. *B,* In pre-B cells, the variable μm chains are associated with ψL (covalently with the $\lambda 5$ subunit and noncovalently with the V pre-B subunit); $\lambda 5$ and V pre-B are alternately designated ω and ι, respectively. (From van Noesel CJM, van Lier RAW. Architecture of the human B-cell antigen receptors. Blood 82:363–373, 1993.)

not occur in secreted or serum immunoglobulin (see Cells of the B-Lymphocyte System). Since acute lymphocytic leukemia is commonly drawn from B cells of this stage, ψL represents a distinctive and useful marker for this disease.

Heavy Chain

The first 121 or so amino terminal residues of the heavy chain make up the variable V_H region. Three V_H subgroups, or "clans" (V_HI, V_HII, V_HIII), have been defined by amino acid similarity and are more commonly divided into seven families (V_H1–V_H7) that have been defined by nucleotide homology (Stewart and Schwartz, 1994). Heavy-chain V regions differ somewhat in size because of different lengths of the three hypervariable region segments. Heterogeneity in the first two hypervariable regions is usually encoded by the V_H gene, whereas the third hypervariable region differs as the result of the combinational and mutational processes that form this region.

The remaining amino acid residues form the constant (C_H) region. For immunoglobulins IgG, IgA, and IgD, this region is composed of three homologous C, or constant, region domains (C_H1, C_H2, and C_H3), counting from the amino terminal end (see Fig. 3–7). Isotype-specific sequences and function occur in each domain. For this reason, the domains are typically designated with their isotype as well (e.g., C_α1, C_α2, C_α3 for IgA; C_γ1, C_γ2, C_γ3 for IgG). In IgM and IgE, there is a fourth domain (C_μ4 and C_ϵ4, respectively). Any V_H region can be combined with a C region from any class of heavy chains. For this reason, antibodies of identical antigenic specificity occur that bear different heavy-chain isotypes. The molecular basis of alternate C_H use, termed switch recombination, is detailed below.

Hinge Region

The hinge region is a stretch of 20 to 100 amino acids between the C_H1 and the C_H2 segments of IgG, IgA, and IgD. This region permits mobility of the Fab portions for antigen combination and other biologic functions. It is not homologous with other parts of the light or heavy chains and shows distinct variability between classes and subclasses, which results in many distinct biologic and chemical properties. It also contains the cysteine residues that make up the heavy-heavy interchain disulfide bonds. IgM and IgE do not have recognizable hinge regions, but this function is subserved by an additional C region.

Antigen-Combining Site

The antigen-combining site of the Fab fragment is made up of portions of the V segments of the heavy and light chains (Nisonoff et al., 1975c). Within these segments are the hypervariable regions that are located near the residues forming the interchain disulfide bridge of the V, or variable, domains. The combining site is an invagination formed by the folding together of some 20 amino acid residues from the hypervariable regions. This results in a depression of 10 Å with an area of 500 Å, occupying 1% of the immunoglobulin surface. It can react with a peptide chain of four to six amino acid residues or an oligosaccharide chain of six glucose residues.

Cleavage of the heavy and light chains of the antigen-combining site abolishes its ability to combine with antigen. Antibody activity can be restored by recombining specific heavy and light chains that preferentially join together (Edelman et al., 1963). When other light chains (not specific for that antigen) are substituted and combined with specific heavy chains, recombination results in considerably less antibody activity (Kotynek and Franek, 1965). However, no activity results when specific light chains are combined with antigen-nonspecific heavy chains. Thus, both heavy and light chains are required for optimal steric configuration and activity of the combining site, but the heavy chain appears to make the more important contribution.

Summary of Immunoglobulin Chain Structures and Variants

Immunoglobulin structural heterogeneity is summarized in Table 3–6. There are nine heavy chains (four IgG subclasses, two IgA subclasses, plus IgM, IgD, and IgE). There are five conventional light chains (one κ and four λ), and four surrogate light chains (restricted to use in pre-B cell receptors). Genetic heterogeneity results in some diversity of these proteins among individuals (allotypes). V-region families are numerous for most immunoglobulin chains, and as discussed later, are highly diversified by somatic mechanisms.

Fc Receptors

Fc receptors (FcRs) are immunoglobulin-binding molecules on the surface of multiple cells and tissues that enable antibodies to undertake biologic functions independently of the antigenic binding site; they allow immunoglobulin molecules to serve as a ligand between the antigen and the Fc-bearing cell. Fc receptors have been identified (Table 3–7) for all the immuno-

Table 3–6. Summary of Immunoglobulin Chain Structures and Variants

---

Classes: IgG, IgM, IgA, IgD, IgE

Chains: Heavy, light

Heavy Chain:
　　Classes and subclasses: γ1, γ2, γ3, γ4, α1, α2, μ, δ, ϵ
　　Variable region families: V_H1, V_H2, V_H3, V_H4, V_H5, V_H6, V_H7
　　Allotypes of γ chains: Gm (18 types)
　　Allotypes of α chains: Am (2 types)
　　Allotypes of ϵ chains: Em (2 types)

Light Chain:
　　Types: κ, λ
　　Constant regions: C_κ, C_λ1, C_λ2, C_λ3, C_λ7
　　Variable regions: V_κI–V_κIV; V_λI–V_λ IX
　　Allotypes of κ chains: Km (3 types)

Surrogate light chain (ψL):
　　Constant regions: 14.1, 16.1, 16.2, C_λ1
　　Variable region: V pre-B

Table 3–7. Characteristics of Human Fc Receptors

Receptor	FcR Type	Ligand	CD	Molecular Weight (kd)	Cell Distribution
FcγRI	IgG high affinity	Monomeric IgG	CD64	72	Monocytes and macrophages Activated neutrophils and eosinophils
FcγRII	IgG low affinity	Complexed IgG	CD32	40	Monocytes and macrophages Neutrophils, basophils, eosinophils, B cells, T-cell subset Langerhans' cells Placental and endothelial cells
FcγRIII	IgG low affinity	Complexed IgG	CD16	50–70	K/NK cells Neutrophils Activated monocytes and macrophages T-cell subset Placental trophoblast Mesangial cells
FcεRI	IgE high affinity	IgE	—	50/32/7	Mast cells and basophils
FcεRII	IgE low affinity	IgE	CD23	45	Monocytes and macrophages Eosinophils B-cell subset Platelets
FcαR	IgA	IgA	—	50–70	Monocytes and macrophages Neutrophils T-cell subset B-cell subset NK cells Erythrocytes
FcμR	IgM	IgM	—	90	B cells Glandular epithelium Hepatocytes

Abbreviations: CD = cluster of differentiation; FcR = Fc receptor; kd = kilodalton; K = killer cell; NK = natural killer.

globulin classes except IgD (van de Winkel and Capel, 1993).

Most Fc receptors belong to the immunoglobulin supergene family (exception: FcεRII) and thus show structural homology with each other and their immunoglobulin ligands (Fig. 3–9). Fc receptors serve a crucial function in triggering cytotoxicity, secreting media-

tors, permitting phagocytosis, initiating the oxidative burst, and regulating antibody production (Table 3–8).

Several types and subtypes of Fc receptors can be defined, depending on their immunoglobulin ligand and their physicochemical, immunologic, and antigenic properties (see Table 3–8). Most are characterized by an extracellular region, a transmembrane region, and

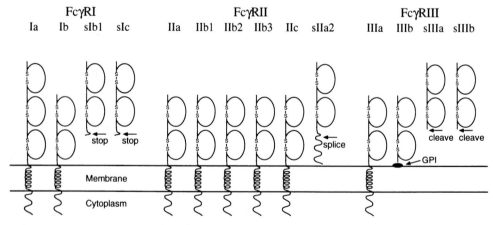

Figure 3–9. Schematic representation of the human IgG Fc γ receptor (FcγR) family. All of these receptors belong to the immunoglobulin supergene family with their extracellular regions composed of disulfide-bonded domains. Most have a transmembrane portion and a cytoplasmic tail. All classes of FcγR have members that are not anchored to the membrane. These soluble receptors (indicated by an s before the subunit name) are generated by three distinct mechanisms: (1) by stop codons in their extracellular domain (sFcγRIb1 and sFcγRIc), (2) by alternate RNA splicing (sFcγRIIa2), and (3) by proteolytic cleavage (sFcγRIIIa and sFcγRIIIb). The FcγRIIIb found on neutrophils is anchored by a glycosyl-phosphatidyl inositol (GPI) moiety without a transmembrane or cytoplasmic domain. (Redrawn from van de Winkel JGJ, Capel PJA. Human IgG Fc receptor heterogeneity: molecular aspects and clinical implications. Immunol Today 14:215–220, 1993.)

Table 3–8. Biologic Functions Triggered by FcγR
Engagement

Phagocytosis
Superoxide generation
Antibody-dependent cellular cytotoxicity (ADCC)
Cytokine release
Enhanced antigen presentation
Regulation of immunoglobulin production
Placental transport of IgG
Clearance of immune complexes

a cytoplasmic tail (see Fig. 3–9). Soluble forms of the Fc receptors also exist; they lack the transmembrane and cytoplasmic tail. These may be shed from activated leukocytes or synthesized *de novo*. These soluble receptors may have important immunoregulatory roles, such as control of immunoglobulin synthesis. The extracellular regions consist of two or three disulfide-bonded domains similar to those present in immunoglobulin.

Multiple genes control their synthesis; they are located on the long arm of chromosome 21. Separate genes control each of the Fc receptors (Ravetch and Kinet, 1991).

Molecules similar or identical to Fc receptors may be present on certain parasites and bacteria (notably staphylococcal protein A, and virus-infected cells), so that immunoglobulin binds to them nonspecifically.

Fc Receptors for IgG

Three types of Fc receptors for IgG (FcγR) exist (see Table 3–7). FcγRI (CD64) is distinguished primarily by its high affinity for monomeric IgG and is expressed constitutively only on monocytes and macrophages. It is also expressed on interferon γ-activated neutrophils and eosinophils. This receptor binds strongly with IgG1 and IgG3, slightly with IgG4, and not at all with IgG2.

Four isoforms of FcγRI exist: FcγRIa, sFcγRIb1, FcγRIb2, and FcγRIc. The sFcγRIb2 is the soluble receptor.

FcγRII (CD32) is a family of molecules encoded by three genes with six isoforms (FcγRIIa1, sFcγRIIa2, FcγRIIb1, FcγRIIb2, FcγRIIb3, and FcγRIIc) and binds primarily to complexed or aggregated IgG. It is expressed on multiple cells and is a low affinity receptor.

Genetic polymorphism exists for FcγRIIa. One allotype, FcγRIIa1, is present on monocytes and reacts with a mouse IgG1 mitogenic monoclonal antibody (41H16). Individuals with a proliferative response to this antibody are designated high responders (HRs), and individuals who do not react are designated low responders (LRs) (Gosselin et al., 1990). At least two other nonallelic polymorphisms exist for the FcRII isoforms.

FcRIII is a low affinity FcR, binding to complexed IgG and identified as the CD16 antigen. Two forms of FcγRIII exist; one is present on monocytes/macrophages, natural killer cells, and some T cells (FcγRIIIa), and a second form is present on neutrophils (FcγRIIIb). The latter is distinct, inasmuch as instead of a transmembrane anchoring domain, there is a phosphatidyl-inositol linkage to the neutrophil. FcγRIIIb does not mediate antibody-dependent cellular cytotoxicity (ADCC), probably because signal transduction does not occur. FcγRIIIa is the main FcR involved in ADCC of antibody-coated platelets in immune thrombocytopenic purpura.

Genes on chromosome 1 control FcγRIII synthesis; several polymorphic variants have been identified for both FcγRIIIa and FcγRIIIb. The latter include the allelic neutrophil antigens NA1 and NA2, sometimes involved in immune neutropenias.

Clinical Aspects of FcRγ

One mode of action of interferon-γ, used in the therapy of chronic granulomatous disease, may be to induce Fcγ receptors on neutrophils and eosinophils and enhance their expression on monocytes, thus increasing their antimicrobial activity.

The LR form of FcγRII may work synergistically with IgG2 antibodies to certain organisms, and individuals lacking this FcγRII (i.e., those with the HR phenotype) may be more susceptible to certain encapsulated bacteria, such as *Haemophilus influenzae* and pneumococci (van de Winkel and Capel, 1993).

Neutrophils from patients with paroxysmal nocturnal hemoglobinuria lack FcγRIIIb on their neutrophils but have FcγRIIIa on their natural killer cells (Selvaraj et al., 1988).

FcRγ function may require interaction with other receptors. For example, leukocyte adhesion defect-1 (LAD) patients lacking CD11b/CD18 may fail to trigger FcR-mediated phagocytosis and oxidative burst. Individuals totally lacking FcRγI have been reported, and they are apparently healthy (Ceuppens et al., 1988).

Fc Receptors for IgM, IgA, and IgE (FcµR, FcαR, and FcεR)

There are a number of proteins with FcαR activity. A highly glycosylated ~60-kd receptor is observed on a variety of leukocytes as well as on erythrocytes. This FcαR can induce reactive oxygen intermediates (Shen and Collins, 1989) and bacterial phagocytosis of neutrophils (Weisbart et al., 1988). Other classes of proteins with FcαR activity are distinguished by cell-type distribution and mode of Fcα recognition: galactosyltransferases (diverse cell types), asialoglycoprotein receptor (hepatocytes), and the polyimmunoglobulin receptor/secretory component (epithelium) (Tomana et al., 1993). These latter proteins also bind IgM.

A distinct FcµR is present on activated B cells and a possibly related structure occurs on T cells (Ohno et al., 1991; Nakamura et al., 1993). Little is known about the function of these receptors.

The high affinity FcεRI is expressed on mast cells and circulating basophils (Metzger et al., 1986). When bound IgE molecules are cross-linked by antigen, allergic mediators are released from mast cells and basophils to initiate the allergic response.

The low affinity FcεRII (CD23) is expressed on a broad range of cells and serves to regulate IgE responses. It is a 45-kd type II protein of the C-type lectin family and is thus quite different in structure from the other major Fc receptor proteins (Kikutani et al., 1986). A distinct second ligand for this receptor is CD21. It is often released as a soluble receptor and acts as a cytokine for B cells through it avidity for its alternate ligand, CD23 (Aubry et al., 1992).

Immunoglobulin Synthesis and Metabolism

Sites of Synthesis

Plasma cells and, to a much smaller extent, the less differentiated cells of the B-lymphocyte lineage synthesize immunoglobulins. These immunoglobulin-synthesizing cells are scattered throughout the body but are most abundant in the bone marrow and in the lamina propria of the respiratory and gastrointestinal tracts. Other significant sites include the spleen, lymph nodes, liver, and exocrine epithelia. Each cell synthesizes only one class or subclass of heavy chain and one type of light chain. The number of cells producing each class or subclass of immunoglobulin is proportional to the percentage of each immunoglobulin class within the body. Essentially all of the circulating immunoglobulin is derived from plasma cells.

IgM-producing plasma cells are morphologically distinct from immunoglobulin-producing cells of other classes. These cells have scant cytoplasm and a poorly developed endoplasmic reticulum; because they resemble a large lymphocyte, they often are termed *lymphocytoid plasma cells*. This morphologic difference permits a distinction between Waldenström's macroglobulinemia and multiple myeloma. There are no morphologic differences between plasma cells producing the other classes of immunoglobulins; multiple myelomas of the IgA, IgG, IgD, and IgE varieties are not distinguishable morphologically.

IgA production mainly occurs in mucosal sites as a result of homing properties of the B- and T-cell subsets committed to the immunoregulatory process required for IgA expression (Platts-Mills, 1979; Berlin et al., 1994) and other favorable factors in the mucosal milieu. Local mucosal plasma cells are the source of IgA used by mucosal epithelium for complexing with secretory component and for luminal transport. These cells are also the predominant source of serum IgA. Similarly, IgE-producing plasma cells are located mainly in the lymphoid tissue associated with the respiratory mucosa and the gastrointestinal tract.

Immunoglobulin is synthesized on the ribosomes within the plasma cell by the endoplasmic reticulum (Askonas and Williamson, 1966). Newly synthesized immunoglobulin is localized between the membranes of the endoplasmic reticulum (Fig. 3–10A) and may accumulate in inclusions called *Russell bodies* (Fig. 3–10B). Heavy and light chains are synthesized separately and combined before release, carbohydrate being added last. Polymeric IgM and IgA also follow this pattern; shortly before secretion, the J chain is added. The entire process takes only 30 minutes. There is not an exact balance between heavy-chain and light-chain synthesis. Normally, a slight excess of light chains is

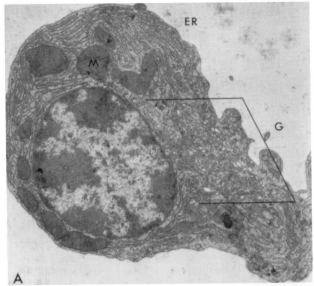

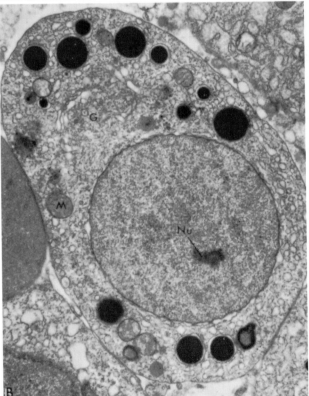

Figure 3–10. Ultrastructure of the plasma cell. *A,* An electron micrograph shows the extensive development of the rough-surfaced endoplasmic reticulum (ER) and the large area occupied by the Golgi zone *(bracket).* A material of homogeneous density is seen in the tubules of the ER, presumably representing γ globulin (× 13,000). *B,* An electron micrograph shows Russell bodies of varying sizes. M = mitochondria; G = Golgi zone; Nu = nucleolar mass with irregular outline (× 15,600). *(A and B from Zucker-Franklin D. Multiple myeloma. Semin Hematol 1:165–198, 1964.)*

synthesized, resulting in the presence of small numbers of free light chains.

It is estimated that each immunoglobulin-producing cell can synthesize 2000 molecules of immunoglobulin per second and 1.7×10^8 molecules per day. Based on an IgG synthesis rate of 35 mg/kg/day, there are 9.4×10^{18} immunoglobulin molecules produced per day by 5.5×10^{10} cells. The volume of this number of cells is only 10 ml (Engle and Wallis, 1969).

Distribution and Destruction

Although immunoglobulin can theoretically be stored in the plasma cells after synthesis, kinetic studies have shown that it is rapidly secreted from the cell. Because plasma cells release their immunoglobulins into the circulatory system, it is unnecessary for them to be concentrated in any particular region of the body. However, the production of IgA along the gastrointestinal tract and the synthesis of IgE adjacent to the respiratory mucosa are two examples of regional immunoglobulin synthesis that can thereby bring about an increased local concentration. Indeed, there is selective secretion of IgA into the gut and respiratory fluids, whereas IgE is concentrated in the nasal washings.

Immunoglobulin destruction occurs within granulocytes (after phagocytosis of immunoglobulin-coated bacteria and particles), in the cells of the reticuloendothelial system (particularly in the liver), and in the gastrointestinal tract. As much as 40% of the immunoglobulin may be broken down within the intestinal lumen. Small quantities of immunoglobulin are also lost through the kidneys.

Immunoglobulin Metabolism

Studies of immunoglobulin metabolism have been facilitated by techniques to isolate and purify the immunoglobulin classes and trace-label them, usually with radioactive iodine (^{131}I or ^{125}I) (Waldmann and Strober, 1969). Because of the difficulty in isolating normal IgM, IgA, IgD, and IgE in an undenatured state, most metabolic studies have been done with purified M-components. Even under optimal isolation conditions, some denaturation may occur, resulting in a spuriously rapid turnover.

By measuring the dilution of a known quantity of trace-labeled immunoglobulin, its rate of disappearance from the serum, and its rate of excretion in the urine and stools, one can calculate the half-life in the circulation and also the intravascular and extravascular distribution, the total body pool, the synthetic rate, and the amount of the total body pool synthesized per day (fractional catabolic rate) (Waldmann and Strober, 1969). These data are presented in Table 3–9.

Immunoglobulin metabolism has also been studied by the turnover of in vivo–labeled immunoglobulin (obtained by administering radioactive precursor compounds, such as ^{14}C amino acids), or by the disappearance rate of passively administered immunoglobulin or antibody. These studies have confirmed the findings obtained by the in vitro–labeling isotopic studies.

IgG

The rate of synthesis of IgG is 35 mg/kg/day under normal conditions, equivalent to synthesis of 2 g of IgG per day by a 70-kg adult. The mean half-life of IgG as

Table 3–9. Metabolic Properties of the Immunoglobulin Classes

	IgG	IgM	IgA	IgD	IgE
Mean adult serum concentration (mg/dl)	1200	120	200	3	0.01
Percentage of total immunoglobulin	70–80	5–10	10–15	<1	<0.01
Biologic half-life (days)	23	5	7	2.8	2.3
Distribution (percentage intravascular)	45	80	45	75	50
Total body pool (mg/kg)	1150	49	230	1.5	0.04
Synthetic rate (mg/kg/day)	35	7	25	0.4	0.02
Placental transfer	+	–	–	–	–
Fractional catabolic rate (percent of body content catabolized/day)	3	14	12	35	89

a class is about 23 days, the longest of any plasma protein. There is no difference in catabolic rate between autologous and homologous IgG. The half-life of IgG3 subclass is considerably shorter (i.e., 9 days) than the other IgG subclasses (see Table 3–5). The metabolic studies of normal IgG reflect a mean of all four subclasses.

IgG metabolism is regulated by the serum level of IgG, so that there is an increase in the fractional catabolic rate at higher IgG levels and a decrease at low levels. Thus, the IgG half-life in patients with agammaglobulinemia is prolonged to between 35 and 40 days; by contrast, the IgG half-life is shortened in multiple myeloma and other hypergammaglobulinemic states. High levels of other immunoglobulins or albumin do not influence IgG turnover.

IgA

The IgA half-life of 7 days is significantly shorter than that of IgG, despite similar molecular size and distribution (see Table 3–7). The lower serum level (mean, 200 mg/dl in adults) compared with IgG and its rapid catabolism results in a rate of synthesis of 25 mg/kg/day, nearly equivalent to that of IgG. Additional IgA, synthesized as secretory IgA in tears, saliva, gastrointestinal fluid, and so forth, makes IgA the immunoglobulin with the largest total synthesis. The catabolic rate of IgA (and of IgE and IgM) is independent of the level of IgA, IgE, or IgM.

IgM, IgD, and IgE

IgM is found primarily (75%) in the intravascular compartment. This feature, combined with its early appearance after antigenic stimulation and its opsonic and complement-fixing properties, suggests that IgM is a first line of defense against organisms entering the blood stream. The rate of synthesis of IgM (7 mg/kg/day) is considerably less than that of IgG or IgA, whereas its half-life is similar to that of IgA (7 days).

Both IgD and IgE have short serum half-lives (2.8 and 2.3 days, respectively) and correspondingly large fractional catabolic rates. As pointed out earlier, there is evidence for local synthesis of IgE at the mucosal surfaces, particularly of the upper respiratory tract. Although IgE has a measurable serum half-life, there are two pools of IgE—IgE in the circulation and IgE attached to mast cells or basophils. Such cytophilic IgE has a half-life of 2 to 3 weeks.

Placental Transfer

Placental transfer from mother to infant occurs for IgG alone. The Fc portion of the γ heavy chain has a special determinant that permits active transfer. The rate of maternal-fetal transfer is a function of maternal and fetal IgG levels and of age of the placenta (Gitlin, 1971). At low levels of maternal IgG, there is little IgG transfer; at higher levels of maternal IgG, transfer occurs in proportion to the maternal IgG level. Because of an immature placenta, premature infants at birth have low serum levels of IgG in inverse proportion to the gestational age (Hyvarinen et al., 1973).

The other immunoglobulins (IgM, IgA, IgD, and IgE) are not transferred across the placenta, with the result that certain antibodies present in the maternal circulation are absent in the infant. This is disadvantageous in some instances because most antibodies to gram-negative organisms are IgM globulins. On the other hand, maternal IgM isoagglutinins, which can cause ABO hemolytic disease of the newborn, and maternal IgE antibodies, which may cause allergic reactions, do not have access to the infant's circulation.

Clinical Implications

Commercial γ globulin preparations, although they contain immunoglobulins of all classes, are essentially all IgG from the point of view of therapeutic benefit. The biologic half-life of both the intravenous and intramuscular forms of IgG is somewhat less than 23 days in normal individuals because of some denaturation during processing. However, because of the feedback on IgG catabolism by the serum level of IgG, the actual half-life in patients with hypogammaglobulinemia is generally prolonged beyond 23 days. The difficulty in isolating IgM and IgA and their short half-lives make IgM and IgA preparations impractical for therapeutic use, despite theoretical advantages for individuals who lack IgM or IgA. Plasma can be used to supply IgM and IgA; however, the IgM and IgA content is relatively low, and therapeutic levels are not sustained for a significant period.

Several disorders of immunoglobulin metabolism are known. These include the *Wiskott-Aldrich syndrome*, in which there is hypercatabolism of IgG, and *myotonic dystrophy*. In addition, increased loss can occur through the gastrointestinal tract (e.g., in *protein-losing enteropathy*) and through the genitourinary tract (e.g., in *nephrotic syndrome*).

Biologic Properties of the Immunoglobulin Classes

IgG and IgG Subclasses

A summary of the biologic properties of the immunoglobulin classes is given in Table 3–10. IgG, normally representing about 80% of the serum immunoglobulin, is the chief component of the body's serologic defenses and contains most of the antibacterial, antiviral, anti-

Table 3–10. Biologic Properties of the Immunoglobulin Classes and IgG Subclasses

Property	IgG1	IgG2	IgG3	IgG4	IgM	IgA	IgD	IgE	Secretory IgA
First detectable antibody	−	−	−	−	+	−	−	−	−
Major part of secondary response	+	+	+	+	−	−	−	−	−
Placental transport	+ +	+	+ +	+ +	−	−	−	−	−
Complement activation via									
Classical pathway	+ +	+	+ +	−	−	−	−	−	−
Alternate pathway	−	−	−	−*	−	+ +	±	+	+
Reacts with *Staphylococcus aureus*									
Protein A	+ +	+ +	−	+ +	−	−	−	−	−
Agglutination	+	+	+	+	+ +	+ +	−	−	−
Opsonization	+	+	+	+	+ +	−	−	−	−
Virus neutralization	+	+	+	+	+	−	−	−	+
Hemolysis	+	+	+	+	+ +	−	−	−	−
Anaphylactic activity	−	−	−	−	−	−	−	+ +	−
Present in exocrine secretions	+	+	+	+	+	+	−	+	+ +
Cytophilic for									
Macrophages	+ +	±	+ +	±	−	−	−	+	−
Lymphocytes	+	±	+	±	−	−	−	−	−
Neutrophils	+	+	+	+	+	+	±	±	−
Platelets	+	+	+	+	−	−	−	−	−
Mast cells	−	−	−	−	−	−	−	+	−
Binding to Fc Receptors									
FcγRI	+ +	±	+ +	+	−	−	−	−	−
FcγRII	+ +	+	+ +	±	−	−	−	−	−
FcγRIII	+ +	±	+ +	±	−	−	−	−	−
FcαR	−	−	−	−	−	+	−	−	+
FcμR	−	−	−	−	+	−	−	−	−
FcεRI and FcεRII	−	−	−	−	−	−	−	+	−

Abbreviations: + + = Very strong; + = strong; ± = equivocal; − = absent.
*Aggregated IgG4 may activate alternate pathway.

protozoal, and antitoxic activity of the serum. Although IgG probably does little if any direct killing, IgG can activate the complement system, promote opsonization, and participate in antibody-dependent cytolytic reactions. The distribution of IgG within the tissues, because of its small molecular size, makes IgG the primary immunoglobulin participating in extravascular immune reactions. IgG can be thought of as guarding the tissues (including the alveoli) from bacterial infection. Passage across the placenta provides the term newborn with passive immunity for about 6 months.

An IgG antibody response after initial antigenic challenge is associated with the development of immunologic memory; on subsequent challenge, the anamnestic response is predominantly an IgG response. Most of the antibody following repetitive antigenic challenge is IgG. The long half-life of IgG and its association with the anamnestic response make it the ideal immunoglobulin for durable host immunity.

IgG antibodies are potent inhibitors and competitors of other immune responses. The inhibition of Rh sensitization by passive administration of IgG anti-Rh antibodies is used clinically in the prevention of Rh hemolytic disease of the newborn. Successful allergy desensitization in part results when highly avid blocking antibodies are developed that can prevent an allergen from reacting with an IgE-coated mast cell. This is particularly true of the blocking antibodies protective against systemic reactions such as that seen with stinging insects. Blocking antibodies are predominantly but not exclusively IgG antibodies.

All subclasses of IgG can fix complement except for IgG4. It alone is unable to bind to C1q and initiate the complement cascade. IgG1, IgG2, and IgG3 can promote phagocytosis, initiate chemotaxis, release anaphylatoxin, and lyse target cells.

IgG immunoglobulins have strong cytophilic properties and can interact with macrophages, neutrophils, lymphocytes, and platelets through Fc receptors on these cells (see Table 3–10). This interaction occurs via specific receptors for the Fc portion of the IgG subclasses found on these various cellular elements. The presence of specific IgG on target cells (tumor cells, heterologous erythrocytes, allogeneic lymphocytes) may permit antibody-dependent cytotoxicity by lymphocytes, neutrophils, and macrophages with Fc receptors.

IgG antibodies participate in various immunopathophysiologic reactions. IgG may rarely be involved in *anaphylactoid reactions* (type I), in which large amounts of IgG antibody may bind antigen in the circulation and activate anaphylatoxins from the complement cascade, as in transfusion reactions to IgA. More commonly, IgG is involved in *cytotoxic reactions* (type II), such as hemolytic anemia, or *immune complex reactions* (type III), such as serum sickness. Some investigators have attempted to ascribe reaginic properties (IgE-like) to IgG4, but the weight of evidence is that IgG4 subclass antibodies contain protective antibodies against immediate hypersensitivity reactions rather than being their instrument (Urbanek, 1988).

Antibody activity differs among the IgG subclasses.

Most treponemal antibodies are IgG1. Rh antibodies are usually of the IgG1 and IgG3 subclasses, occasionally of IgG4, but never of the IgG2 subclass (Frame et al., 1970). Coagulation factor VIII (antihemophiliac globulin) antibodies are limited to the IgG4 subclass (Anderson and Terry, 1968). Antibodies to polysaccharide antigens, such as antidextran and antilevan, generally belong to the IgG2 subclass. The ability of IgG to combine with staphylococcal protein A, a property of the Fc portion of the molecule, is present in IgG1, IgG2, and IgG4 subclasses but is lacking in IgG3 (Kronvall and Williams, 1969).

Patients with low levels of one or more IgG subclasses may demonstrate increased susceptibility to infection. Terry (1968) described a 3-month-old infant with low levels of IgG3 and increased susceptibility to infection. Schur and associates (1970) described three older patients who had lifelong susceptibility to pyogenic infection and selective subclass deficiencies. In one patient, levels of IgG1, IgG2, and IgG4 were low; in a second, IgG1, IgG2, and IgG3 were low; and in a third, IgG1 and IgG2 were low. All patients showed defective antibody responses and were benefited by γ globulin injections. Yount and colleagues (1970) described a patient with selective IgG3 deficiency. Beck and Heiner (1981) have suggested that patients with selective depression in IgG4 levels show an increased risk for recurrent pulmonary infection. Oxelius and colleagues (1981) have noted IgG2 deficiency in about one third of patients with selective IgA deficiency. Despite these cases, most patients with subclass imbalance show slightly decreased total IgG levels and poor antibody responses, thus fitting into other categories of antibody deficiency (see Chapter 11).

Therapeutic human immunoglobulin, mostly IgG, given in large doses has important biologic effects that provide therapeutic benefit in inflammatory and immunologic disorders (e.g., immune thrombocytopenic purpura, Kawasaki syndrome) (Dwyer, 1992; Ballow, 1994). These include:

1. Fc receptor blockade (mostly FcγRIII) with inhibition of uptake and lysis of antibody-coated cells (i.e., antibody dependent–cellular cytotoxicity).
2. Inhibition of pathogenic antibodies by anti-idiotypic activity or B-cell inhibition.
3. Down-regulation of T-cell activation.
4. Neutralization of microbial antigens or superantigens that may cause viral reactivation, T-cell activation, or endotoxin-stimulated cytokine release.
5. Modulation of complement-dependent immune damage to tissue and cells.

IgM

IgM antibodies are the earliest antibodies identified in phylogeny and in the developing fetus; they also are the first antibody class formed after antigenic stimulation. IgM antibodies appear within 4 days but do not persist; durable immunity is associated with IgG antibody. Indeed, if only an IgM response occurs, immunologic memory is not acquired. Presence of IgM antibodies to an infectious agent can often be used as an indicator of recent infection. The presence of IgM antibodies in a newborn infant indicates congenital or perinatal infection, since such antibodies cannot be acquired from the mother because of lack of transplacental passage.

IgM antibodies are excellent agglutinating antibodies, are unusually avid because of their multimeric nature and are complement fixing. The preponderance of IgM (80%) is localized within the intravascular system. IgM thus primarily assists the reticuloendothelial system in clearing the blood stream of bacteria and particles by opsonization and agglutination. The aggregating action is enhanced by the 10 combining sites on each polymeric IgM molecule. IgM is a strong activator of the classical pathway of complement by means of its interaction with C1; the 19S IgM molecule has 15 times the complement-activating activity of monomeric IgM or IgG1. The predominant intravascular localization, the ability to fix complement and act as an efficient opsonin, and the early appearance after antigenic challenge enable IgM to serve as the first serologic line of defense to bacterial infection. Individuals who lack IgM are susceptible to rapid, overwhelming sepsis.

Certain antigens do stimulate a persistent IgM antibody response, resulting in serum antibodies that are of the IgM class. These include: (1) antibodies to polysaccharide antigens (e.g., anti-A and anti-B isoagglutinins); (2) the Wassermann and heterophile antibodies; (3) typhoid O antibodies; and (4) antibodies to endotoxins of gram-negative organisms. Rheumatoid factors, cold agglutinins, and certain other autoantibodies also are predominantly IgM. These IgM antibodies do not depend (or depend little) on T-cell effects for their expression and therefore are often called *T-independent responses*.

IgM antibodies participate in cytotoxic hypersensitivity (type II) reactions, such as autoimmune hemolytic anemia. However, the clinical manifestations may differ from those seen with IgG antibodies and are often accentuated by the enhanced ability of IgM to activate complement. Likewise, IgM antibodies participate in immune complex (type III) formation and disease states.

IgM Monomers

Monomeric IgM appears on the surface of most of the B cells, where it functions as the central component of the B-cell antigen receptor. Naturally occurring 7S IgM monomers may also be present in normal serum and in cord serum (Bush et al., 1969). High concentration of monomeric IgM occurs in hypergammaglobulinemic states such as lupus erythematosus, rheumatoid arthritis, and Waldenström's macroglobulinemia. Monomeric IgM has also been noted in certain immunodeficiencies, notably ataxia-telangiectasia, and in dysgammaglobulinemia (Metzger, 1970). The IgM monomers may have antibody activity against blood group substances and cell nuclei. The IgM monomers are synthesized *de novo* and are not a result of the breakdown of polymeric IgM (Solomon and McLaughlin, 1970).

IgM monomers are the predominant form of IgM that is present on the surface of or within B cells. The attachment of the J chain and resulting polymerization may be defective in states in which serum monomeric IgM is present in excessive amounts.

IgA

Serum IgA globulin contains several varieties of antibodies, including isoagglutinins, and antibrucella, antidiphtheria, anti-insulin, and antipoliomyelitis antibodies. Serum IgA antibodies provide no known unique defense mechanism; indeed, most individuals who lack IgA are not unusually susceptible to systemic infections. Isolated IgA deficiency is a common abnormality, occurring in one of 700 normal subjects (see Chapter 14). Although IgA antibodies are found both in the circulation and in the tissues, their primary defense role is at mucosal surfaces after transport into local secretions.

Engagement of the Fcα receptor for IgA on neutrophils and monocytes and other cells by IgA-coated bacteria may initiate phagocytosis or superoxide generation (Golde et al., 1990).

IgA antibodies do not activate the classical pathway of complement but can activate the alternate pathway. This may aid in phagocytosis and killing of certain organisms. IgA has some bactericidal activity, particularly when combined with lysozyme and complement. IgA molecules may serve to combine with tissue antigens (from damaged organs) or exogenous protein antigens (coming primarily from the gastrointestinal tract) and prevent them from stimulating an immune response. By so doing, IgA antibodies prevent such antigens from provoking an antibody or a cell-mediated response that may be harmful. In individuals who lack IgA, there is a high incidence of autoantibodies to antigens such as thyroglobulin, adrenal tissue, DNA, and bovine milk proteins and also an increased risk of autoimmune disorders.

The serum monomeric IgA (MW 160,000) is structurally different from the dimeric secretory IgA (MW 500,000) found in exocrine secretions, and the latter contains a secretory piece and a J chain. The bulk of serum IgA (90%) is IgA1; most of secretory IgA (60%) is IgA2, but this ratio varies from secretion to secretion. IgA2, but not IgA1, is resistant to bacterial IgA protease. This resistance to proteolytic digestion makes IgA2 particularly suited for defense of mucosal surfaces.

Serum IgA is not specifically transported from the serum to the exocrine glands (Tomasi, 1972). However, a large portion of the serum IgA is produced in the plasma cells of the exocrine glands, where instead of being excreted as a secretory IgA, it diffuses into the circulation. Thus the serum IgA has the antibody specificities of the secretory IgA molecules, the chief antibody providing antiviral and antibacterial activity on mucous surfaces. Individuals who lack secretory IgA generally lack serum IgA. Such persons may experience increased infections involving primarily the upper respiratory system and sinuses. The structure and role of secretory IgA are further detailed in Chapter 8, The Mucosal Defense System.

IgD

IgD was discovered by the finding of a new myeloma protein unrelated to IgG, IgA, or IgM (Rowe and Fahey, 1965). It had the clinical and structural characteristics of an immunoglobulin, and with the use of monospecific antisera to this protein, it was possible to demonstrate small quantities of IgD in all normal adult serum (mean, 3 mg/dl). Although IgD has some antibody activity (to benzylpenicilloyl acid, diphtheria toxoid, bovine γ globulin, and cell nuclei) (Heiner and Rose, 1970), its primary biologic function is not, as for the other Ig classes, as a soluble effector molecule. This is highlighted by its low concentration in serum or secretions and by its inability to fix complement, cross the placenta, or interact with neutrophils or mast cells.

An important clue to the biologic role of IgD was the observation that IgD made up a disproportionately high percentage (up to 10%) of immunoglobulin bound to the membrane of B cells from newborns (Rowe et al., 1973). This is in marked contrast to the low levels of IgD in serum, including cord serum. Subsequent studies have identified IgD as being present on the majority of normal B lymphocytes, usually with surface IgM. This led to the proposal that IgD and IgM serve as antigen receptors on the lymphocyte surface, particularly during immune development. Further evidence for this has come from experiments showing that interaction with antibody to the IgD on B cells can dramatically alter the ability of those cells to develop a normal antibody response. Thus IgD appears to function primarily as an antigen receptor (along with membrane IgM on B cells) involved in regulation of B-cell development.

A few individuals have been identified with polyclonal hyperimmunoglobulinemia D. These patients have periodic fevers and lymphadenopathy (van der Meer et al., 1984; Hiemstra et al., 1989; Drenth et al., 1994) (see Chapter 11).

IgE

IgE, the anaphylactic, or reaginic, antibody, was the last immunoglobulin discovered (Ishizaka et al., 1966) and is the one present in the smallest concentration. Its elucidation was greatly facilitated by finding two patients with IgE myeloma, which permitted its isolation, structural analysis, and measurement by immunoassay. Like IgM and unlike IgG, IgD, or IgA, it has one extra heavy-chain segment and lacks a hinge region. Its MW is 200,000.

Reaginic Activity

IgE functions primarily as a trigger for immediate hypersensitivity (type I) reactions (Ishizaka et al., 1966). This occurs because IgE binds to basophils and mast cells located in the lungs, skin, peripheral blood, tonsils, and gastrointestinal tract. IgE binds to the high affinity Fcε receptor on such cells. Allergens (antigens) combine with IgE to initiate cell activation, leading to release of chemical mediators, such as histamine and leukotrienes. For this to occur, cross-linking of the IgE bound to the cell surface must occur. Such a reaction requires a bivalent antibody (isolated Fab fragments of IgE do not work) and a multivalent antigen (Ishizaka, 1974). Anti-IgE antisera can also be used to initiate the reaction, since it will bridge two bound IgE molecules.

IgE has a strong affinity for basophils and mast cells scattered throughout the body and persists for weeks on such cells. Triggering of the bound antigen-specific IgE results in varied hypersensitivity reactions, such as anaphylactic shock, bronchoconstriction, nasal mucosal rhinorrhea, urticaria, and gastrointestinal disturbances, depending on the site and degree of the reaction. Complement is not involved in these reactions, although aggregated IgE in vitro can activate the alternate complement system.

IgE is synthesized in the central lymphoid tissue (lymph nodes, spleen, bone marrow), the tonsils, and the exocrine glands. Most IgE-containing plasma cells are found in lymphoid tissue associated with the respiratory or gastrointestinal tract. IgE antibodies are not specifically secreted in exocrine fluids because they do not contain secretory component. Although IgE is found in higher than expected levels in fluids, such as nasal washings, this circumstance primarily results from increased local production and diffusion (Platts-Mills, 1979).

IgE Regulation

Several authors have dissected the stimulus for IgE production by B cells (Leung, 1993). The first signal is T cell–secreted interleukin-4 (IL-4), which switches immunoglobulin gene synthesis to the ε locus. The second signal, delivered by IL-4 along with contact with antigen-activated T cells, triggers messenger ribonucleic acid (mRNA) and IgE synthesis. T-cell contact in vivo can be replaced in vitro by Epstein-Barr virus, hydrocortisone, or a monoclonal antibody to CD40, a differentiation receptor on T cells. Certain cytokines (IL-4, IL-5, IL-6) amplify IgE synthesis, whereas others (IFN-α, IFN-γ, TGF-β) suppress IL-4–stimulated IgE synthesis. One type of T-helper cells (T_H1 cells) secrete IL-2 and IFN-γ, which inhibit IgE synthesis, whereas another type (T_H2 cells) secrete IL-4, IL-5, and IL-6, which promote IgE synthesis. T_H1 cells facilitate delayed hypersensitivity reactions, and T_H2 cells facilitate antibody responses. IL-4 also promotes the expression of low affinity FcεRII (CD23) on B cells and monocytes of patients with hyper-IgE states such as eczema and hyper-IgE syndrome (Vercelli and Geha, 1993).

IgE antibody responses are regulated by T lymphocytes to a greater degree than are those of other Ig classes (Hamaoka et al., 1973). Patients with profound antibody and cellular immunodeficiencies lack serum IgE, but several partial cellular immunodeficiencies syndromes are characterized by elevated levels of IgE, including the DiGeorge anomaly, Wiskott-Aldrich syndrome, and Hodgkin's disease. In experimental animals, IgE levels increase following thymectomy, whole-body irradiation, or the administration of antithymocyte serum or other immunosuppressive drugs. Similarly, following bone marrow transplantation, IgE levels may rise precipitously, particularly in the presence of graft-versus-host disease.

Beneficial Effects of IgE

A protective biologic role for IgE antibodies has been sought, since it is unlikely that a totally harmful immunoglobulin would persist in evolution. The high incidence of allergy in the general population suggests some survival advantage.

A possible clue to a beneficial biologic role of IgE is the repeated observation of marked elevation of serum IgE levels in the presence of intestinal parasitism. Experimental work in the rat infected with the intestinal parasite *Nippostrongylus brasiliensis* suggests one beneficial role (Bloch, 1972). When worms enter the gastrointestinal tract, IgE antiworm antibodies are formed. These may damage the worm and result in the release of more worm antigen and stimulation of more IgE antibody. Worm antigen reacts with IgE antibodies on the mast cell or eosinophil to release pharmacologic mediators; these in turn cause enlargement of the villi, edema of the intestinal wall, leakage of serum proteins into the gastrointestinal tract (including other immunoglobulins and complement), and worm expulsion. Treatment with antihistamines inhibits worm expulsion.

IgE may thus serve as a mechanism for defending against parasitism by inhibiting the attachment and entry of the invading organism by binding to the parasite, by IgE-mediated mast cell release, causing a flushing effect on the mucosal surface, and by increased local delivery of other defense effectors such as IgG, complement, macrophages, lymphocytes, and, particularly, eosinophils.

Another beneficial effect of IgE has been shown with experimental schistosomiasis in the rat. The schistosomes that penetrate the skin and migrate through the blood vessels are attacked by macrophages, which interact with the parasite in the presence of IgE antibodies. The macrophage FcεRII then binds to the parasite and brings about its destruction (Capron et al., 1975).

A third beneficial effect of IgE antibody may be the potentiation of an IgG antitoxic reaction. At the site of an allergic skin reaction induced by IgE antibody and antigen, considerably more diphtheria toxin is neutralized by serum antitoxin than at a nonsensitized site (Steinberg et al., 1974). The mechanism appears to be increased cutaneous permeability, permitting more serum antitoxin to diffuse into the reaginic area and to neutralize more toxin.

It has been noted that in developing countries the incidence of allergy in children seemingly is low, despite high levels of IgE. Although it was thought that the high levels of IgE caused by parasitism might compete for all the IgE sites on mast cells and in so doing inhibit other allergic reactions, this is not the case. Indeed, when such individuals are exposed to a more urban environment, the incidence of allergy approaches that of the more developed countries. The absence of detectable IgE (<1 ng/ml) does not appear to be associated with an enhanced susceptibility to infection, at least in more industrialized countries.

Recombinantly Engineered Antibodies

DNA recombinant technology has provided a flexible system for the production of antibodies and the creation of antibody structures with novel effector domains. This is a burgeoning area in immunology and biotechnology beyond the scope of the current volume and is outlined only briefly here. For more detailed reviews, the reader may consult a number of monographs (e.g., Winter and Milstein, 1991; Wright et al., 1992).

In this approach, the genes for the desired light- and heavy-chain V regions are cloned either from defined monoclonal antibody cell sources, or by use of enrichment and screening procedures to isolate the desired antibody specificity from V-region gene libraries (Hoogenboom et al., 1992; Sarvetnick et al., 1993). The use of polymerase chain reaction (PCR) amplification of V, or variable region, genes can make such cloning feasible within days or weeks in an experienced laboratory.

For screening of antibodies of a desired antigen-binding specificity, an important advance has been in an area termed phage display. In this approach, bacteriophages are used for the double purpose of carrying the cloned immunoglobulin V-region genes and inserting the surface expression of the V regions. Hence, such phages can be directly selected for the desired antigen-binding specificity (Fig. 3–11). Innovative methods are used to generate highly diverse synthetic gene libraries with the goal of creating a universal library from which any desired antibody specificity can be selected.

Compared with hybridoma-based technology, this approach presents several advantages and is likely to replace hybridomas for the isolation of antigen-specific monoclonal antibodies. The ability to create novel ligand-binding sites has prompted the use of these antibodies in applications far beyond the usual biomedical sphere, notably in chemical engineering antibody-mediated catalysis (Janda et al., 1993).

The functionality of the constant (C) region may also be modified in interesting ways. As noted earlier, "bare" Fab molecules, including a soluble form, can be produced directly by these expression systems. Such reagents are useful for analytic purposes, such as diagnostic laboratory tests for in vitro research purposes (e.g., for blood group antigens [Marks et al., 1993; Siegel and Silberstein, 1994]). Recombinant methods allow a particular Fab (technically, Fv) to be produced that duplicates any heavy-chain C region, including its specific biologic activity.

Monoclonal antibodies already have been employed for a variety of therapeutic purposes in vitro, either directly or as chemical conjugates with agents, such as immunotoxins (Bahler et al., 1991; Uckun et al., 1992; Amlot et al., 1993). An exciting research direction is the creation of synthetic C regions with novel functional activities. Thus heavy-chain C regions are re-

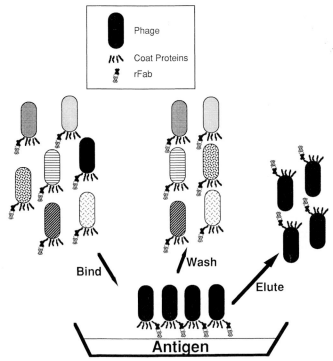

Figure 3–11. Strategy for selection of phage-expressing recombinant antibodies (rFab) on microwells coated with antigen. The heavy-chain variable region segment and C_H1 domain are recombinantly fused to the tip of the phage cIII coat protein. A conventional light chain is also expressed. Heavy- and light-chain segments pair and bond with disulfide in the conventional manner, creating a typical Fab, displayed as part of the phage coat protein. Diverse Fab libraries (>10^7 independent clones) can be readily prepared in this phage system, and antigen-specific members can be selected by serial adsorption, elution, and regrowth. (Adapted with permission from Braun J, et al. On the pathogenesis trail: what marker B-cell clones tell us about inflammatory bowel disease. In Sutherland LR, et al [eds.]. Inflammatory Bowel Disease. Amsterdam: Kluwer Academic Publishers, 1994, pp. 96–103.)

placed with enzymes, toxins, cell surface or barrier receptors, and cytokines. The immunoglobulin-cytokine fusion proteins are particularly notable, since they are the basis for a technologically distinct immuniza-tion strategy for malignant or autoimmune diseases (Tao and Levy, 1993).

CELLS OF THE B-LYMPHOCYTE SYSTEM

Pro-B and Pre-B Cells

The current view of the early stages of B-cell differ-entiation has emerged from flow cytometric studies of bone marrow populations in normal individuals (mouse and human) and transgenic mice manipulated for critical steps in the differentiative process (Melchers et al., 1994; van Noesel and van Lier, 1993) (Fig. 3–12). The earliest recognizable cell of the B-cell lineage is termed a pro-B cell: an early hemopoietic cell (CD45R$^+$, CD43$^+$), which is distinguished by the sur-face expression of the pan–B cell marker CD19 and a membrane complex composed of surrogate light chain (ψL) and one or more novel proteins of uncertain identity (the presumed surrogate heavy chain, ψH).

The next and more prevalent precursor of the B-cell population is the pre-B cell, distinguished from the pro-B stage as a CD43$^-$, CD19$^+$ cell bearing cyto-plasmic μ in the form of a novel ψL,μ complex (see Fig. 3–8). Pre-B cells are not found in the circulation but make up a small percentage (less than 5%) of bone marrow cells. These cells are present by the eighth week of gestation.

B Cells

The B lymphocyte is characterized by a variety of differentiation markers, and the presence of conven-tional immunoglobulin complex in the form of a sur-face-exposed integral membrane receptor (membrane immunoglobulin [Ig]). The B lymphocyte is a small, mobile, nonphagocytic cell present in the blood, bone marrow, lymph, lymphoid organs, and connective tis-sue. It is most commonly distinguished from other lymphoid cells by immunohistochemistry or flow cy-

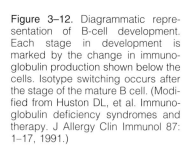

Figure 3–12. Diagrammatic repre-sentation of B-cell development. Each stage in development is marked by the change in immuno-globulin production shown below the cells. Isotype switching occurs after the stage of the mature B cell. (Modi-fied from Huston DL, et al. Immuno-globulin deficiency syndromes and therapy. J Allergy Clin Immunol 87: 1–17, 1991.)

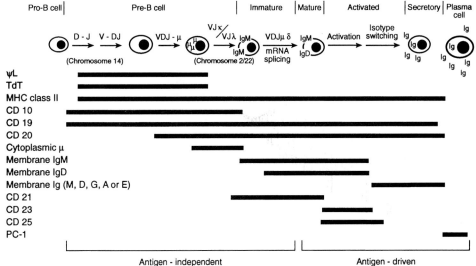

tometry detection of pan-B differentiation markers such as CD19 or CD20 and for membrane IgM or IgD. B cells can be identified in the circulation by the 11th week in utero.

B cells make up 10% to 20% of peripheral blood and thoracic duct lymphocytes; 20% to 30% of the lymphocytes of lymph nodes, spleen, and mucosal lamina propria; and most of the lymphocytes of the bone marrow, palatine tonsil, and intestinal Peyer's patches and appendix. They are rare in the thymus. Microanatomically, they are localized in the follicles, germinal centers, and medullary cords of lymph nodes; the follicles, germinal centers, marginal zone, and red pulp of spleen; and the central follicles of Peyer's patches. These microanatomic sites are the *B-cell areas*.

Membrane Ig of B cells serves as the antigen recognition unit, and signaling via this receptor is critical for many aspects of further B-cell activation and differentiation. Receptors for antigens in the form of immune complexes are specific for Fc (FcγRII [CD32] and in some B-cell subsets, FcμR and FcαR), C3b, C3d, and iC3b complement components; and complement receptors (CR1 [CD35], CR2 [CD21], and in some cases CR3 [CD11b/18]). CD21 also serves as the target for infection by Epstein-Barr virus. These receptors are commonly detected by using commercially available monoclonal antibodies. In addition, they may be detected functionally by rosetting with erythrocytes coated with antibody (EA) for Fc receptors or with antibody and complement (EAC) for complement, receptors. Unlike T cells, B cells lack the receptor for sheep erythrocytes (CD2); sheep erythrocyte rosetting is thus a common method for depleting T cells from B-cell preparations.

A fundamental gene required for the successful differentiation of B cells is *btk*, encoding one of an unusual family of tyrosine kinases. Serious mutations of this gene are the structural basis for Bruton's agammaglobulinemia and indicate that this gene is critical for successfully traversing the pre-B stage of development (Tsukada et al., 1993). More minor *btk* mutations are associated with several deficits at this and latter stages of B-cell function and humoral immunity (Rawlings et al., 1993). Curiously, *btk* is also expressed by nonlymphoid hemopoietic cells, but mutations in the gene have not been associated with functional disturbances in these cell types. This intracellular signaling pathway is thus of critical and specific importance throughout B-cell development. *Btk* and other components of this pathway are likely to emerge as the basis of other genetic disorders of humoral immunity and may be useful as therapeutic targets for immunologic and neoplastic B-cell disorders.

The B-Cell Antigen Receptor Complex

The immunoglobulin on the B-cell surface (~ 100,000 molecules per B cell) is generally not limited to one heavy-chain class. Most resting B cells express both membrane IgM and IgD (Vitetta and Uhr, 1975). Thus the class and subclass distribution of cell surface immunglobulin is considerably different from

that of serum (Fig. 3–13). This is because serum immunoglobulin does not originate from the abundant resting B-cell population but instead from the small population of end-differentiated, highly secretory plasma cells. The occasional B cells bearing membrane IgG and other "mature" isotypes represent cells that have further differentiated as a result of recent or remote antigenic experience (see later).

Membrane Ig is structurally distinct from secreted immunoglobulin because of a distinct C-region hydrophobic tail that anchors the Ig monomer in the plasma membrane as an integral membrane protein. The Ig monomer is disulfide-linked with two accessory proteins, Ig-α and Ig-β (Fig. 3–14) (Cambier et al., 1994). These proteins are in some cases critical for the proper intracellular translocation of typical membrane Ig isotypes to the cell surface. More importantly, they are central to the protein phosphorylation cascade that carries out the signaling activity of membrane Ig as an antigen receptor. Both Ig-α and Ig-β bear tyrosine-rich cytoplasmic peptide segments, designated TAM or ARH1 motifs. On antigen-mediated cross-linking of the antigen receptor complex, these motifs are phosphorylated. A number of protein kinases are physically associated with the B-cell antigen receptor (BCR), and

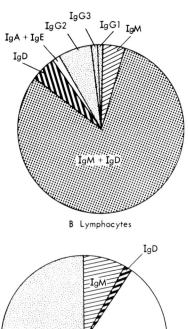

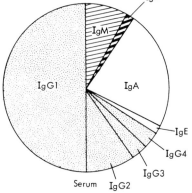

Figure 3–13. Class and subclass distribution of immunoglobulin on the B lymphocytes of the peripheral blood compared with the distribution of serum immunoglobulin. (From Hobart MJ, McConnell I. The Immune System: A Course on the Molecular and Cellular Basis of Immunity. London, Blackwell Scientific, 1975, p. 111.)

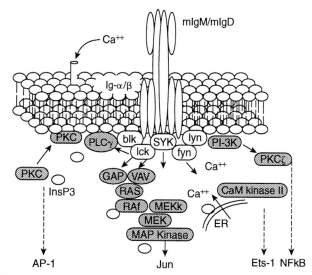

Figure 3–14. Model of intermediary events in B-cell antigen receptor–mediated signal transduction. (Redrawn from Cambier JC, Pleiman CM, Clark MR. Signal transduction by the B-cell antigen receptor and its coreceptors. Annu Rev Immunol 12:457–486, 1994. © 1994, by Annual Reviews, Inc.)

among these, *fyn* and *lyn* are thought to carry out this reaction. In turn, the phosphorylated sites bind and activate a second-level kinase, *syk* (see Fig. 3–14).

The activation of *syk* and other intermediary enzymes of the *Src* protein kinase family delivers the receptor signal to diverse intracellular targets. Some important substrates are key components of the processes controlling intracellular calcium levels, G proteins and their regulators, and cell cycle and transcriptional control genes. Although gaps remain in this scenario, this cascade is central to programming functionally defined B-cell activation and differentiation (see below). It is likely, therefore, that these signaling processes will be useful pharmacologic targets in the therapeutic control of B-cell dysfunction and malignancy. This structural and functional organization of the BCR is highly analogous to that of the T-cell antigen receptor complex (TCR).

Other B-Cell Antigen Receptors

B cells may also react with antigen indirectly through recognition of Fc and C3 structures decorating antigen within immune complexes. Although this mode of antigen interaction is nonspecific and indirect, it serves as an important component of the feedback system for B-cell differentiation. Ligand binding by the predominant FcγR on B cells, FcγRIIb (CD32), inactivates B-cell responsiveness to signaling via the BCR. FcγRIIb generates a unique phosphorylation cascade that interferes with the BCR-induced cascade. One likely kinase substrate affected by this interference is the γ2 isoform of phospholipase C, which is critical for the generation of the Ca^{2+} influx in BCR-induced B-cell activation.

Conversely, ligand binding by the predominant B-cell complement receptor (CR2) synergizes with the BCR in antigen-induced B-cell activation (Matsumoto et al., 1993). CR2 is a large protein complex, consisting

of CD21, CD19, Leu-13, and TAPA-1. Receptor signaling predominantly involves a kinase cascade, apparently with a pattern identical or complementary to that produced by the BCR. As a consequence, B-cell responsiveness to antigen is enhanced about 100-fold when compared with BCR activation alone. As noted previously, CD23 is an alternate ligand for CD21. Hence, soluble CD23 secreted by activated B cells further amplifies B-cell antigen responsiveness.

These points lead to the concept that initial antigenic response of B cells involves positive signaling by the BCR, and amplification by immune complexes of the initial wave of complement-fixing IgM. Subsequently, negative feedback occurs when a mature response with IgG production becomes predominant.

Activated B Cells

When activated by antigen and the appropriate T-cell and stromal signals (see The Antibody Response later), the mature resting B cell develops into an activated B cell. These activated B cells are morphologically distinguished by a larger size than that of resting B cells, having an increased cytoplasm, more open chromatin, and, often, prominent nucleoli. Most "histiocytes" in lymphoid tissues correspond to such B cells. Whereas most resting B cells are found in mantle zones, activated B cells are found in specialized microanatomic sites, such as germinal centers. Expression of certain differentiation antigens is selectively increased or decreased in activated B cells, although the particular pattern varies with the exact mode of activation (Table 3–11).

Membrane Ig levels are reduced in activated B cells for two reasons. First, the expression of membrane forms of immunoglobulin mRNA and its translation efficiency are reduced in these cells (see Membrane versus Secreted Immunoglobulins later in this chapter). In addition, antigens and other ligands of membrane Ig elicit a sequence of receptor redistribution and endocytosis. This process, "capping," is an active contractile and cytoskeletal mechanism that initially moves bound receptors from their uniform surface distribution to multiple small patches, coalescing rapidly into a cap at one cell pole, and interiorization (Taylor et al., 1971; Braun and Unanue, 1983).

One important consequence of this efficient receptor interiorization is the delivery of bound antigens for proteolytic processing and delivery to major histocompatibility complex (MHC) class II proteins for antigen processing in subsequent T cell–B cell interaction (Lanzavecchia, 1990). From a practical standpoint, this leaves the cell surface temporarily denuded until fresh immunoglobulin is resynthesized and thus prevents identification of activated B cells on the basis of membrane Ig.

Activated B cells generally produce higher relative and absolute levels of secreted antibody and often have switched heavy-chain classes to mature immunoglobulin isotypes. In fact, this B-cell population includes the precursors for cells undergoing plasma cell differentiation. Although such B cells are rarely found in normal

Table 3–11. Stage-Specific Membrane Proteins of Postantigenic B-Cell Development*

Receptor	Comments	Stage	Ligand
Class II MHC	HLA-D	Activated	TCR
CD5		Activated	CD72
CD23	FcεRII	Activated	CD21, IgE
CD25	IL-2 receptor	Activated	IL-2
CD22		Activated	
CD40		Activated	CD40L (gp39)
CD48	Blast-1	Activated	CD2
CD54	ICAM-1	Activated	CD11a/18
CD58	LFA-3	Activated	CD2
CD69		Activated	
CD71	Transferrin receptor	Activated	Transferrin
CD80	B7	Activated	CD28
Membrane IgD		Activated (reduced)	Antigen
CD44		Activated (reduced)	Hyaluronate
CD62L	L-selectin	Activated (reduced)	Endothelial glycoconjugate
PNA-binding glycoconjugates	Decreased α2,3-sialyltransferase	Activated (germinal center)	Stromal galactose-binding protein
CD10	Neutral endopeptidase	Activated (germinal center)	
CD38	ADP ribosyl cyclase	Activated (germinal center)	
CD49d	VLA-4	Activated (germinal center)	VCAM-1 of FDC
CDw75		Activated (germinal center)	
CD77	Globotriasyl ceramide	Activated (germinal center)	
PC-1	Alkaline phosphodiesterase	Plasma cell	

*Surface expression of these proteins is increased at the listed stage of development. In the case of membrane IgD, CD44, and CD62L, levels are selectively reduced in activated B cells. Many activation markers are elevated in the germinal center stage; those selectively expressed or of particular biologic significance in this stage are denoted.

blood, they are significantly elevated in conditions associated with activation of humoral immunity such as vaccination, systemic lupus erythematosus, or acquired immunodeficiency syndrome (AIDS).

Plasma Cells

The plasma cell is the most differentiated cell of the B-cell lineage (see Fig. 3–10). These cells have a characteristic morphology, featuring an eccentric nucleus with clumped chromatin around its periphery, and a deep-blue cytoplasm on Wright's stain. Plasma cells are easily recognizable in routine histologic specimens and are found (in decreasing order of abundance) in mucosal lamina propria, perivascular sinuses of bone marrow, splenic red pulp, and lymph node medulla. The infrequency of plasma cells in lymph nodes is actually a useful diagnostic criterion, since their abundance in this site is part of the distinguishing histopathology of various chronic inflammatory diseases and B-cell neoplasms of this stage (Waldenström's macroglobulinemia and plasma cell leukemia).

At this mature stage of B-cell development, the plasma cell has shifted to an exceptionally high relative and absolute level of secreted (versus membrane) Ig mRNA. Consequently, membrane Ig expression is minimal and usually undetectable, but it may devote as much as 30% of its protein synthesis to secretory antibody production. Unlike other B-cell states, plasma cells do not proceed to other differentiative stages but instead terminate after 1 to 2 weeks with cell death.

MOLECULAR GENERATION OF ANTIBODY DIVERSITY

One major question that has intrigued immunologists for decades centers on how the great diversity of antibody molecules might be generated. Despite an innumerable array of different antigens in the environment, the immune system is capable of producing a unique antibody to each novel antigen. The solution of this question has not only yielded information about how the immune system functions but also has provided initial insight into the organization and dynamic structure of the genetic material in higher organisms.

V-D-J Recombination

As discussed earlier, the variable (V) region of the immunoglobulin molecule constitutes its antigen-binding region. However, it was not known whether there were millions of such V-region genes (germline theory), whether there were a small number of such genes that underwent frequent mutation (somatic mutation theory), or whether these latter genes were able to recombine with each other (combinatorial theory). Beginning with the pioneering work of Tonegawa and colleagues in 1975, a comprehensive understanding has emerged (Tonegawa, 1983). The formation of a complete antibody molecule involves the combinatorial joining of a large number of V, or variable, region segments (V_L) and J_L (joining) for light-chain V regions and V_H, D_H (diversity) and J_H for heavy-chain V regions. These molecular junctions are routinely diversified by somatic mutation, and a further mutational process acts on the entire rearranged V-region segment in activated B cells. Thus, elements of all three theories have contributed to the current understanding of immunoglobulin gene recombination (Fig. 3–15).

The genetic information encoding both the V and constant (C) regions for the heavy chains in humans is found in chromosome 14 (Malcolm et al., 1982; Berman et al., 1988; Matsuda et al., 1993); that for κ and

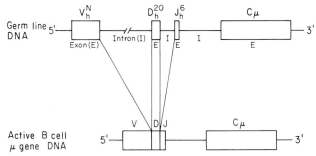

Figure 3–15. DNA splicing in the assembly of an active B-cell μ gene DNA. The future coding regions are the exons (E); the intervening sequences are the introns (I). To assemble an active μ gene, a V_H, D_H, and J_H exon are spliced together and the interposed introns deleted. With the formation of this continuous V-D-J region, the μ gene becomes active. The V-D-J region, which codes for the Fab region of the μ chain, is separated by a long intron from the μ constant region exons. There are numerous V_H regions, at least 20 D_H regions, and six J_H elements.

λ light chains is in chromosomes 2 and 22, respectively (Malcolm et al., 1982; Zachau, 1993; Vasicek and Leder, 1990). These loci each include approximately 100 functional V-region segments and five J segments. For heavy chain, there are about 30 D_H region elements. A major challenge has been to determine the mechanism that permits an orderly recombination of these segments at each locus, so that a single active immunoglobulin gene is formed for subsequent immunologic processes of the cell and its clonal progeny.

Many features of this mechanism are understood. In order to assemble segments in an orderly fashion, each is flanked by regulatory elements, called *recombination signal sequences* (RSSs). The RSS consists of a seven-nucleotide *(heptamer)* and a nine-nucleotide *(nonamer)* sequence, separated by either a ~12- or 23-nucleotide *spacer*. The heptamer-nonamer pair of the short-spacer RSS is complementary in sequence to the pair associated with the long spacer. DNA hybridization between these two RSS classes facilitates the assortment of proper segments and their ends and proper alignment for cutting and religation. Through a process of DNA excision and joining, the often vast segments of intervening DNA are removed, and an individual set of V_H, D_H, and J_H segments are brought into juxtaposition (Early et al., 1980; Gauss and Lieber, 1992). Such recombinations can readily be detected by Southern blot hybridization analysis, and uniquely sized V-D-J segments detected in this way are commonly used to identify and follow clonal populations in clinical illnesses such as B-cell leukemias and lymphomas.

At least some of the enzymes responsible for this process have been identified by biochemical, genetic, or molecular approaches. Among these, the central proteins are RAG-1 and RAG-2, which are critical for orchestrating the overall activity of the recombination system (Oettinger et al., 1990; van Noesel and van Lier, 1993). The specific components of this system are expressed only in pre-B cells and are turned off on completion of the recombination process, thus assuring that the antigen receptor of the B-cell clone remains constant over the lifetime of the cell and its progeny.

It is for this reason that some of these components (terminal transferase, RAG genes) are used as markers of the pre-B stage.

A number of genetic disorders have been identified in which the V-D-J recombination mechanism is impaired (Gauss and Lieber, 1992). In the human, the best example is ataxia-telangiectasia, which is associated with often aberrant immunoglobulin (and TCR) recombination products (Russo et al., 1989). However, the identity and function of the gene in this disease are still unknown. It should be noted that mutations of some specific V-D-J recombination pathway genes (such as RAG-1 and RAG-2) are lethal for fetal or neonatal development. This may account for the difficulty in identifying such mutants in immunogenetic disorders and may indicate that these genes have important but thus far uncharacterized roles in the development of other nonhemopoietic cell lineages.

The recombination process is critical for creating much of the diversity of the antigen-binding site. The V_H region element codes for the first two hypervariable regions that make up the antibody combining site, and these are defined by the particular V_H and V_L gene recombined by the B-cell clone. Some V genes are much more favored for recombination than others, and some of the predominant ones in the early fetus (e. g., $V_H 5$ and $V_H 6$) differ from those of postnatal life. As a result, only a portion (~10%) of the available genomically encoded V gene repertoire is commonly used (Huang and Stollar, 1993; Stewart and Schwartz, 1994).

A number of mechanisms are probably involved in the selective rearrangement of V genes: optimal RSS motifs, physical closeness to the downstream Ig locus (J cluster and C region), and flagging of favored V genes by special flanking "accessibility" regulatory segments. Presumably, these favored genes have been evolutionarily selected because of their importance in recognition of prevalent pathogens. For example, the $V_H 26$ gene is one such favored gene, and it has been shown to encode for a predominant protective antibody (anticapsular type B *H. influenzae* polysaccharide) in the response to *H. influenzae* infection (Adderson et al., 1993).

Finally, an emerging area is the existence of microbial B-cell superantigens (Goodglick and Braun, 1994). Such antigens interact with framework-defined V-region domains, and thus interact with a striking abundance (~1 to 10%) of B cells and serum Ig–sharing members of the same V_H gene family. Two of the B-cell superantigens currently known (protein A of *Staphylococcus aureus* and gp120 of HIV-1 [human immunodeficiency virus]) are virulence factors that co-opt antibodies ($V_H 3$ family) to facilitate the life cycle of the organism. It is thus possible that this may be a commonly used mechanism in microbial pathogenesis and a possible target for immunotherapy.

The third hypervariable region is created by the D_H segment and its junctions with V_H and J_H forms. In the human, several D segments may be fused in forward or reverse orientation to create a tandem D gene mosaic. Finally, somatic mutation occurs in the joined V_H-D_H-

The B-Lymphocyte System

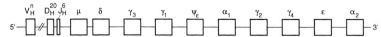

Figure 3–16. The linear array of the heavy-chain constant region coding sequences (exons) on the 14th chromosome. The μ gene is 5' (closest to the centromere); the $\alpha 2$ region is 3' and farthest away from the V_H elements. In actuality, each heavy-chain constant region is composed of three (γ, δ, and α) or four (μ and ϵ) separate exons with associated introns, each exon representing a domain of the heavy-chain constant region.

J_H elements, as a result of deletions of the elements at their ends, and insertion of nontemplated sequence by the enzyme terminal transferase. As a result, enormous diversity is observed in this hypervariable region. Because of the absence of D segments in the light-chain loci, third hypervariable regions are much more diverse in the heavy chain. Accordingly, structural studies of antibody-antigen interaction show that this region is particularly important for the avidity and selectivity of antigen binding.

Ontogenic factors are important in determining the repertoire of antibodies produced by an individual (Hardy and Hayakawa, 1991). As noted above, distinct V genes are favored in the fetus compared with the adult, and the same is true for D and J segments. Moreover, pre-B cells in the fetus differ in their enzymatic profile from those in the adult by the absence of terminal transferase and other enzymes that promote deletions and insertions of V-D-J junctions. As a result, the third hypervariable region in the fetus is shorter and much less diverse than in the adult. By the neonatal period, an adult pattern of antibody gene rearrangement has commenced, and these clones increasingly predominate in the first few years of life (Mortari et al., 1993). The ontogenic shift is thus likely to account for aspects of the qualitative deficit in humoral immune responses in the first years of life.

Heavy-Chain Class and Subclass Expression

As discussed earlier, there are five major classes of heavy chains plus four subclasses of IgG and two subclasses of IgA. All of the genetic material for these chains is found in a linear array of exons and introns downstream from the heavy-chain V_H region elements on chromosome 14. The order is as follows: μ, δ, $\gamma 3$, γ, $\Psi\epsilon$, $\alpha 1$, $\gamma 2$, $\gamma 4$, ϵ, and $\alpha 2$ (Fig. 3–16) (Honjo, 1983). The DNA for each heavy-chain constant region is composed of a cluster of exons, each representing a sample domain with introns between. The C, or constant, region domains are spliced together in the production of messenger RNA. The clusters of V_H, D_H, and J_H genes are located immediately upstream in the heavy-chain locus, and the rearranged V-D-J is recombined with any of the heavy-chain coding elements downstream. This permits the preservation of antigen specificity and idiotypy during class switching.

As with essentially all eukaryotic genes, functional immunoglobulin genes consist of series of exons, introns, and flanking DNA elements (Fig. 3–17). The seven or eight DNA segments that encode the actual protein sequence and are spliced together to form the

mature immunoglobulin RNA are called *exons*. These exons are separated by noncoding DNA segments, *introns*, which range in size from 50 to 10,000 nucleotides. Together, they form an immunoglobulin transcription unit, since they consist of the span synthesized by RNA polymerase into the primary RNA transcript. Regulation of transcription is encoded by DNA elements within some of the introns and certain segments of *flanking DNA elements*. The molecular and biochemical mechanisms involved in this regulatory system are not a focus of the present chapter but have been detailed in excellent reviews (e.g., Staudt and Leonardo, 1992).

An elegant feature of V-D-J recombination is that it brings together the different types of regulatory elements associated with the different immunoglobulin gene segments. As a result, recombination creates a functional transcription unit. From this unit, a large primary RNA transcript is produced, that in the case of heavy chain, includes the V_H-D_H-J_H and μ exons as well as the many intervening sequences. This primary RNA transcript then undergoes RNA splicing, a process by which the exons coding for the complete μ chain are brought into final continuous linear array (see Fig. 3–17).

A similar mechanism is also involved for IgD production. Since the μ and δ exon groups are so close together, a cell may make a long RNA transcript that includes both the μ and δ exon regions with the upstream V_H-D_H-J_H. The cell thus has RNA splicing alter-

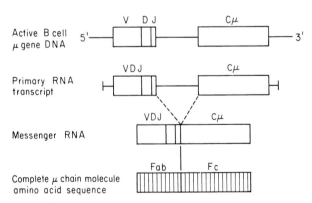

Figure 3–17. Steps in the production of an immunoglobulin molecule from an active immunoglobulin gene. A primary RNA transcript is made; this is an exact reflection of the active B-cell DNA. Messenger RNA is derived by splicing out the intervening RNA between the V-D-J regions and the heavy-chain constant region (in this case Cμ). Thus the messenger RNA now has the original coding sequences in a simple linear array. This is then read off by the polyribosomes on the endoplasmic reticulum, and a complete set of amino acids for a μ chain is assembled—the V-D-J region having coded for the Fab region and Cμ being represented by the constant region.

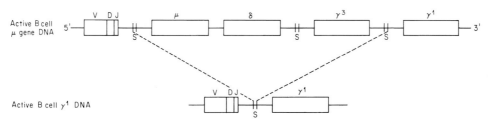

Figure 3–18. B-cell isotype switching at the level of immunoglobulin DNA. The assembled V-D-J region is moved downstream (3') and placed just 5' to the new isotype to be produced, in this case γ1. The joining occurs at specialized regions designated switch regions; these regions are represented by an *S* in the figure. Just as for the active μ gene, the V-D-J region is not brought exactly next to the γ1 DNA in the active B-cell DNA. All the DNA between the V-D-J region and the γ1 region (the μ, δ, and γ3 sequences) is deleted from the cell during the switch shown.

natives to make either μ or δ chain mRNA and can therefore make both μ and δ mRNA and both IgM and IgD protein (Moore et al., 1981). The relative levels of IgM and IgD are largely determined by preference of the splicing machinery for μ versus δ, although the mechanism for this alternate splicing selectivity is not yet resolved.

Expression of other heavy-chain isotypes requires a unique recombination event, *switch recombination*, which juxtaposes the V_H-D_H-J_H region to a different C-region exon group (Fig. 3–18). There are specialized regions of DNA, called *switch regions*, located in the upstream flank of each isotype cluster, which consists of numerous, tandemly arrayed, shorter and longer sequences. The homology of these sequences presumably facilitates hybridization for alignment of different isotype clusters during switch recombination (Dunnick and Stavnezer, 1990).

Activation of switch recombination involves additional regulatory elements in the switch regions that are isotype-specific. The current concept is that putative isotype-specific switch proteins selectively bind these elements, thereby promoting accessibility of the switch regions for the general recombination machinery. In support of this idea, cytokines known to selectively induce expression of certain isotypes (e. g., IL-4 for IgE; transforming growth factor–α (TGF-α) for IgA) promote accessibility of the corresponding isotype segments by transcriptional criteria (Harriman et al., 1993). Biologically, this process is normally induced by the antigenic and cognate T-cell interactions involved in differentiation of B cells to the germinal cell stage; cells expressing this activity are most abundant in this microanatomic site. B cells may recurrently recombine at switch regions, and this accounts for the occurrence of identical clones (by V-D-J recombination) with different heavy-chain normal or neoplastic B-cell populations.

Light-Chain Diversity

The situation for the two light chains is somewhat different from that for heavy chains, in that each light chain is encoded on a separate chromosome and has its own set of $V_L J_L$ segments (Fig. 3–19). The κ system is represented by only one C-region locus with five J_L-region segments. Thus, rearrangement of the κ V_L-J_L uses only the one κ constant (C) gene. The situation for the λ system is more complex. Here there are four sets of functional λ C-region exons; however, each C_L exon cluster is preceded by its own J_L region. Limited sequence information indicates that these make use of a single set of V_L region elements. There is no evidence for switching of λ subtypes.

Membrane versus Secreted Immunoglobulins

Immunoglobulin molecules exist in two major forms: secreted molecules free in body fluids and transmembrane proteins on cells of the B-cell lineage. The different roles of these immunoglobulin forms have been discussed previously. The generation of these distinct forms of immunoglobulin molecules can now also be understood at a molecular level. Just downstream from each heavy-chain exon cluster are two small exons.

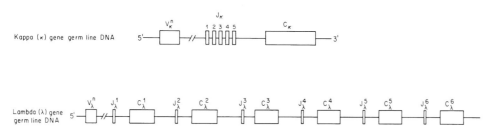

Figure 3–19. Molecular arrangement of the light-chain gene DNAs. κ Gene DNA is similar to that of the heavy chains—there is a cluster of $V_κ$ regions upstream of a group of five $J_κ$ elements. A single $V_κ$ combines with a $J_κ$ to make an active κ gene. There is only one $C_κ$ element, so there is nothing analogous to isotype switching. λ Gene DNA has a cluster of $V_λ$ regions, but there is a group of $C_λ$ elements, of which each element has a single J region associated with it. To create an active λ gene, the $V_λ$ is joined to one of the $J_λ$ regions. No λ subtype switching occurs, because there is no mechanism to separate and move a V region from a J region to another J and its associated $C_λ$.

One encodes a short, 20–amino acid hydrophilic tail found in secreted immunoglobulins, and the other encodes a longer tail (41 for μ and δ, ~60 for other heavy-chain isotypes), including a hydrophobic sequence and flanking positively charged cytoplasmic margin typical of regions that permit membrane anchoring of type 1 membrane proteins (Rogers et al., 1980). This membrane segment has also gained attention because of a potentially amphipathic central α-helix region and other sequence features involved in proper association with the BCR complex and in efficient biosynthesis and intracellular trafficking of the receptor (Cherayil et al., 1993).

Both the secreted and membrane exons are transcribed into the primary RNA transcript. Thus, for any heavy-chain class or subclass, the B cell can form by alternately splicing the mRNAs to produce membrane or secreted immunoglobulin or both. For example, plasma cells are distinguished from resting B cells not only by their high level of immunoglobulin transcription but also by their remarkable increase in the efficiency of secreted exon splicing (i.e., the ratio of secreted versus membrane exon formation in plasma cells is about 100-fold that of resting B cells).

V Gene Hypermutation

A unique mechanism of diversification in antibodies is V gene hypermutation. This process involves the accumulation of mutations specifically into the rearranged V-D-J_H and V-J_L gene segments and a short span of flanking DNA (Rothenfluh et al., 1993; Giusti and Manser, 1993). Studies by Weigert and colleagues first underscored the remarkably elevated rate of somatic region in this gene segment, which may exceed the background mutation rate by five to six orders of magnitude (Shlomchik et al., 1987). The mutations typically involve single nucleotides that are randomly distributed throughout the rearranged V(D)J segment. However, at the amino acid level, mutations are greatly favored in the first and second hypervariable regions. Analytically, this is judged by the ratio of replacement to silent mutations *(R:S ratio)* exceeding ~3, which is the ratio under neutral selection (reflecting the likelihood that a random mutation of a codon nucleotide will change the amino acid encoded). Conversely, the R:S ratio is substantially less than 3 in framework regions.

This selectivity does not reflect the hypermutation process itself but the action of antigenic selection on the population of cells with an initially neutral distribution of mutation. Thus, mutations involving the antigen-binding domain that improve binding activity are positively selected, and clones with such mutations progressively predominate. Overall, 10% to 20% of the V region–coding segment can accumulate mutations through V gene hypermutation, thereby introducing a burst of diversification in the clonal progeny of cells passing through this process and contributing the affinity maturation so important to the enhanced quality of the memory humoral immune response.

Biologically, this process occurs in the germinal center stage, and is thus a relatively late event in B-cell development involving antigenic and T cell–B cell (T-B) interaction, and overlapping in its expression with heavy-chain switch recombination (Jacob et al., 1993). One consequence is that the prevalence of such mutations in clones expressing IgM (versus other heavy-chain isotypes) is infrequent. Moreover, neoplastic B cells representative of the germinal center stage (follicular-type non-Hodgkin's lymphoma) show evidence of progressive V gene hypermutation, whereas it is absent or quiescent in those neoplasms representative of other stages (e.g., multiple myeloma, chronic lymphocytic leukemia, and acute leukemias of the pre-B type) (Wagner et al., 1994). In fact, V gene hypermutation has proved to be an obstacle to the therapeutic use of reagents directed against the tumor-specific immunoglobulin V regions in follicular lymphomas (Zelenetz et al., 1992).

THE ANTIBODY RESPONSE

Primary and Secondary Responses

When an individual is challenged with a previously unencountered antigen, there is a lag period of 10 to 14 days before the appearance of serum antibody. When antibody appears, it is predominantly of the IgM class, followed in a few days by IgG antibody. This is the *primary response.* Upon reintroduction of antigen, IgG reappears within 4 days and in quantities far greater than was present in the primary response. This rapid recall of antibody is the *memory, anamnestic,* or *secondary, response,* which may occur years after the primary response, may persist for a prolonged period of time, and may lead to high levels of antibody (Uhr, 1964). Similar events occur if there is protracted initial exposure to antigen as in an ongoing bacterial infection. The memory cells responsible for the secondary response are long-lived B lymphocytes that bear membrane Ig specific for the corresponding antigen as their surface antigen receptor.

Postantigenic B-Cell Development and Cellular Control of the Antibody Response

Successful postantigenic differentiation of B cells ultimately includes the selective clonal expansion and long-lived state of cells specific for relevant antigens. Typically, class switching to heavy-chain isotypes with the most suitable heavy-chain isotype and respective effector functions also occurs. Such differentiation involves stimulatory signals from antigen by the BCR, and cell-cell interaction with helper T cells, follicular dendritic cells of the germinal center, and their cell surface and secreted (cytokine) products. In order to consider these cellular interactions involved in antibody production, one can classify them according to three phases:

- Afferent, or inductive, phase
- Central, or proliferative, phase
- Efferent, or productive, phase

Afferent (Inductive) Phase

The afferent phase comprises the events between antigenic entry and contact with lymphocyte receptors. Antigen is first captured by nonlymphoid hematopoietic cells (monocyte/macrophage lineage and dendritic cells; the so-called reticuloendothelial system) of the spleen and lymph nodes.

In a process known as *antigen presentation*, the antigen is proteolyzed to small peptides in lysosomes and other intracellular compartments and is then complexed with class II *major histocompatibility complex proteins* (the *HLA-D* family in the human) through the action of a specialized peptide processing and delivery system (Germain and Margulies, 1993). Peptide-loaded HLA-D traffics to the macrophage surface and constitutes the form of antigen recognized by the T cell–antigen receptor as part of initial antigen-specific T-cell activation.

These cell types also express a variety of cell-cell interaction molecules at their cell surface and by local secretions that are critical cosignals required for T-cell activation. Quiescent B cells lack expression of several components of this interaction system and thus induce only abortive T-cell stimulation. In fact, the functional consequence of T cell–B cell interaction at this point is an anergic state for both cell types (Matzinger, 1994). Overall, this phase typically occurs in the first 2 to 3 days of an immune response and results in a population of activated T helper cells suitable for B-cell stimulation.

Central (Proliferative) Phase

Antigen in lymphoid tissue serves as a ligand for antigen-specific B cells through their membrane immunoglobulin (Ig) and stimulates an initial phase of B-cell activation through intracellular signals generated by the BCR, as described previously. Such activated cells move from G_0 to G_1 growth phase and elevate their expression of surface receptors relevant for T-B interaction: HLA-D, CD80 (B7), CD40, LFA-3, ICAM-1, and various cytokine receptors (for IL-2, IL-4, and IL-6). To further proceed in their differentiation, B cells require the signals generated by ligation of these receptors through the relevant counter-receptors and cytokines (Melchers et al., 1982; Teranishi et al., 1984; Clark and Ledbetter, 1994). Accordingly, the activated T helper cell is specialized for the expression of this very panel of ligands. For example, mutation of the CD40 ligand expressed by such T cells is responsible for the impaired B-cell development in hyper-IgM syndrome (Aruffo et al., 1993).

The interaction with activated T cells is intimate, since it generally requires antigen presentation by B cells. As a consequence, B-cell activation in vivo is usually restricted to antigen-specific B and T cells. This selectivity is important, since it assures that T helper cells can act as both a stimulus and gatekeeper for B-cell activation, and failure of this selectivity system is a major factor in the pathogenesis of autoimmunity.

The outcome of these antigenic and T-cell interactions is proliferating clones of B cells; the result is an expanded population of antigen-specific cells, some of which are programmed for plasma cell differentiation, others for a quiescent, long-lived memory state (MacLennan, 1994). Microanatomically, this central phase initially occurs (during the first 4 to 7 days) in foci at the borders of T-cell (interfollicular) and B-cell (follicular mantle zone) sites. However, many of these activated B cells rapidly migrate to germinal centers of B-cell follicles to undergo further proliferation, heavy-chain class switching, and somatic mutation.

Two key cell types involved in the germinal center microenvironment are *follicular dendritic cells* and *T helper cells*. The follicular dendritic cells are specialized for the capture of immune complexes and long-term retention and surface display of nonproteolyzed antigen. This role as a native antigen depot and perhaps other cell-cell interactions promote further antigen-driven B-cell stimulation (MacLennan, 1994).

The minor population of germinal center T helper cells is distinguished by a novel marker (CD57) and is thought to provide further positive selection through T cell/B cell interaction. Clonal expansion in the germinal center is largely controlled by the persistence of antigen and may continue for weeks in the wake of a typical microbial infection. However, individual B cells reside in the germinal center for only 1 to 2 days and then emigrate to local or distant sites. Germinal center emigrants give rise to the long-lived *memory cells*, a quiescent population representative of the antigenically selected B cells programmed for highly efficient reactivation on specific antigenic challenge (Gray, 1993).

Germinal center B cells that fail to compete successfully for these interactions undergo apoptotic (programmed cell) death, a fate of about 90% of the initial germinal center immigrants. This is reflected by both phenotypic and microanatomic distinctions of the germinal center B-cell population and the prominence of tingible-body macrophages laden with B-cell debris. Cells successfully stimulated during this period are distinguished by their expression of *bcl2*, which has a key role in rescuing germinal center B cells from apoptosis (MacLennan, 1994).

This point is relevant to the pathogenesis of follicular non-Hodgkin's lymphoma. Such cells are molecularly characterized by a tumor-specific mutation, in which the bcl-2 gene is aberrantly transposed to an active immunoglobulin gene, resulting in its constitutive expression (Bakhshi et al., 1985). As a consequence, such cells are at a proliferative advantage in the germinal center stage, since they do not require competition for the cell-cell interactions, which normally induce *bcl-2* expression. This pathogenic mechanism has been validated by model experiments in the mouse (Nunez et al., 1989) and provides an elegant biologic explanation for molecular oncogenesis in this neoplasm.

CD5+ B Cells—the B1 Population

A small population of B cells initially distinguished by their expression of the surface glycoprotein CD5+ (in humans) exists. CD5+ B cells (alternatively called *B1 cells*) possess properties distinct from conventional

B cells, including a unique ontogeny, phenotype, and adult tissue distribution (Kipps, 1989). Ontologically, B1 cells are representative of the initial, fetal wave of B-cell lymphopoiesis (Hardy and Hayakawa, 1991). B1 cells arise during development before conventional B cells and exist as the predominant B cell throughout early neonatal life. B1 cells are derived from hematopoietic stem cells in the fetal liver and omentum (Solvason and Kearney, 1992). In the adult, B1 cells are most abundant in the blood and follicular mantle zones of the spleen and in the small B-cell population in the thymus (Punnonen and de Vries, 1993).

The antibody repertoire of B1 cells is also unique. The B1-cell population uses a small set of V-region immunoglobulin genes; most, if not all, of these V genes encode reactivity against autoantigens, or idiotypes, or both. Based on this production of autoreactive antibodies, the increase in B1 cells in autoimmune-prone mice, and the increase in B1 cells in some human autoimmune diseases, B1 cells may play a key role in some types of autoimmune disease. A restricted V-gene usage is also seen in mouse and human B1 cell–derived malignancies. For example, there is a striking prevalence of certain V genes (V_H5, V_H421, V_H1051, and $V_\kappa325$) in human chronic lymphocytic leukemia and Waldenström's macroglobulinemia; thus it is postulated that surface immunoglobulin may play a role in the malignant clonal expansion of B1 cells (Kipps and Carson, 1993).

Efferent (Productive) Phase

The productive, or effector, phase of antibody production involves synthesis and secretion of immunoglobulin by plasma cells. Activated B cells emigrate from germinal centers to perivascular sites in bone marrow sinuses, mucosal lamina propria, or splenic red pulp. These sites support terminal differentiation of these cells to the plasma cell stage, a process independent of further antigen stimulation.

Also, some B-cell responses are elicited by antigens with limited, if any, T-cell interaction. Such *T-independent antigens* are typically hydrolase-resistant polysaccharides with dense epitope arrays and are efficiently captured by macrophages found in the splenic marginal zones (MacLennan, 1994). These structures provide poorly understood costimulatory signals that functionally substitute for those produced during T cell–B cell interaction. The consequence is proliferation and secretory IgM expression in a process independent of the germinal center and largely devoid of heavy-chain class switching or somatic mutation. The most common natural sources of such antigens are components of bacterial-cell walls, and this mode of plasma cell differentiation is favored in the spleen over other lymphoid sites. Consequently, T cell–independent responses are likely to serve a particularly important role in the protective response to bacteremic gram-positive bacterial infection.

Noncellular Factors Affecting Antibody Synthesis

Numerous factors influence the type and extent of the antibody response, including *exogenous* (antigenic) and *host-related* factors.

Exogenous Factors

Antigenic factors influencing the antibody response are:

- The chemical nature of the antigen
- The route of antigen entry
- The dose of antigen
- The presence of other antigens (antigenic competition)
- The presence of adjuvants

Chemical properties of the antigen that favor a strong antibody response include a large molecular weight, multiple similar antigenic groups, foreignness of the antigen, the presence of lipid and sugars, and a replicating (live) source of the antigen. A poor antibody response is associated with small molecular weight, an inability to metabolize the antigen, and a structural similarity of the antigen to the body's own tissues. Subcutaneous and intramuscular administration of antigen favors antibody production, whereas the intravenous route is less effective. Oral administration of antigen preferentially activates IgA responses; exposure to minute quantities of antigen, particularly through mucosal surfaces, favors the production of IgE antibodies.

Large antigen doses and the presence of an adjuvant favor antibody production. Very large or very small antigen doses are associated with poor antibody production or with the development of immunologic tolerance. The simultaneous administration of several antigens results in inhibition of antibody responses to secondary, or less immunogenic, antigens.

Host Factors

Host factors that influence antibody formation include age, size, genetic background, presence of pre-existing antibody, and general health of the host. At both extremes of age, unusual or deficient antibody responses occur, particularly in the newborn period (see Chapter 10, The Physiologic Immunodeficiency of Immaturity). Females are superior formers of antibody, both for pathogens and for autoantigens; the result is both increased resistance to infection and increased susceptibility to autoimmunity (Kenny and Gray, 1971).

The most physiologic regulator of antibody synthesis is the presence of antibody. Pre-existing antibody not only intercepts new antigen but also has a central inhibitory effect on the antibody-synthesizing cell (Weigle, 1973). In the primary response, the IgG antibody inhibits further IgM response. Transplacental antibody also inhibits the IgG response of the fetus.

CLINICAL ASPECTS OF B CELLS AND IMMUNOGLOBULINS

Enumeration and Analysis of B Cells

Estimation of peripheral blood B-, T-, and other lymphocyte subpopulations is of value in many clinical situations, particularly immunodeficiency. Generally, this is done by flow cytometry by means of monoclonal antibody–stained cells. Manual immunofluorescence techniques can also be used to enumerate the stained cells, but this method is laborious and imprecise. As indicated in Figure 3–12 and Table 3–11, a variety of membrane antigens that are useful for delineation of B cells have been defined.

In general, CD19 or CD20 is used to measure total B cells. These are B-cell markers that react with all B cells (pan-B markers) and with no other types of cells. Other B-cell markers react with some T cells (e.g., CD10) or with B cells at a limited developmental stage (CD21) and thus are less valuable for B-cell enumeration. Normal values for peripheral blood B cells at various ages are given in Chapter 9, Table 9–9.

B cells can also be identified by detecting immunoglobulin on the lymphocyte membrane by immunofluorescent techniques (WHO/IARC, 1974). With antisera directed against light chains or heavy-chain determinants, 10% to 20% of the peripheral blood lymphocytes show an immunofluorescent pattern indicating the presence of surface membrane immunoglobulin (sIg). When monovalent antisera specific for one or another immunoglobulin class or subclass are used, the relative percentages of B-cell subtypes can be estimated.

B cells have receptors for the Fc portion (Fc receptor) of immunoglobulin and the third component of complement, C3, and can thus form rosettes with sheep erythrocytes coated with IgG antibody (EA rosettes) or with antibody and complement (EAC rosettes). Because monocytes and certain lymphocytes lacking sIg (non–B cells) have Fc and C3 receptors, this method for B-cell enumeration is not generally employed.

Enumeration of B cells is indicated in evaluation of immunodeficiency and lymphoproliferative disorders. However, B-cell quantitation in immunodeficiency is rarely indicated if immunoglobulin levels are normal. In autoimmune disorders and other immunologic disorders in which B-cell dysfunction is suspected, B-cell quantitation may occasionally be of value. B cells likewise can be quantitated in tissue sections of lymph nodes, spleen, and other tissues.

Pre–B cells are evaluated by staining bone marrow cells for cytoplasmic μ chains in the absence of light-chain staining. This is generally done only in the evaluation of certain humoral immunodeficiencies and lymphoid malignancy. Although plasma cells may be quantitated by immunohistologic techniques, they are generally measured by routine histologic staining.

DNA analysis by Southern blot hybridization is widely used to determine the nature of the immunoglobulin rearrangements in lymphoid populations. This establishes whether the cells are of B-cell origin and, if so, whether they represent a monoclonal (malignant) or polyclonal (reactive) proliferation. For a monoclonal (lymphoproliferative) disorder, this type of analysis also reveals the stage of maturation of the B cells. This has been particularly revealing in acute lymphoblastic and chronic myelogenous leukemias in blast crisis, both of which represent B-cell neoplasms (Korsmeyer et al., 1983). This methodology has also been applied

to genomic Epstein-Barr virus, since the fingerprint integration site is an alternate to immunoglobulin rearrangements for identification of clonal B-cell populations (Shibata et al., 1993).

Polymerase chain reaction (PCR) offers convenient strategies to ascertain relative use of V genes and their extent of hypermutation (Huang and Stollar, 1993). This has been effective in characterizing the pace of B–cell repertoire reconstitution after bone marrow transplantation and the presence of clonal deficits in some immunodeficiencies, such as Wiskott-Aldrich syndrome and common variable immunodeficiency. PCR can also be used to characterize some types of genomic rearrangements, such as in the clinical detection of *bcl-2* translocation in follicular lymphoma.

Levels of B cells are decreased in some but not all antibody deficiency disorders. Particularly, in hypogammaglobulinemia with thymoma, the number of both pre-B cells and B cells is diminished; in X-linked agammaglobulinemia, B cells are very low but pre-B cells are present in normal numbers; and in common variable immunodeficiency, both B cells and pre-B cells are normal in number. High percentages and absolute levels of B cells are found in B-cell neoplasms (lymphoid malignancies). Monoclonality is suggested by the overabundance of a light-chain or heavy-chain isotype.

The numbers of T cells, B cells, natural killer (NK) cells, monocytes, or Ig-secreting plasma cells in body fluids (e.g., cerebrospinal or synovial fluid) or tissues (e.g., synovium or kidney) may help to define the immunologic mechanisms occurring in specific diseases. This has been applied particularly to the mononuclear cells derived from the lungs by bronchoalveolar lavage, a technique by which new insights into the immunopathophysiology of hypersensitivity pneumonitis and sarcoidosis have been gained.

Measurement of immunoglobulin synthesis by isolated B cells and assay of the effect on the immunoglobulin synthetic rate by other cells (suppressor and T helper cells) or serum factors are of value in certain immunodeficiency disorders (see Chapter 11, Disorders of the B-Cell System).

Immunoglobulin Assessment

Immunoglobulin levels and antibody function are assessed in many illnesses. Synthetic deficiencies of the immunoglobulins must initially be differentiated from loss of serum proteins. When the latter occurs, the total serum protein and other serum proteins (such as albumin and transferrin) are usually simultaneously reduced, and lymphopenia may be present. However, as a result of its low fractional catabolic rate, IgG may be decreased out of proportion to other serum proteins under conditions of extracorporeal loss.

Electrophoresis

Serum electrophoresis, either on paper, gel, or cellulose acetate, is sometimes used for detecting abnormalities of the serum proteins. There is some correlation between the electrophoretic γ globulin level and the sum of the individually measured immunoglobulins. This correlation is not absolute, since most IgM and IgA and some IgG molecules migrate in the β and α-2 regions of the electrophoretic field. Nevertheless, it is unusual to find hypogammaglobulinemia if the γ globulin level is normal by serum electrophoresis and if results of screening tests for antibody function are normal. However, isolated deficiency of IgA and IgM cannot be detected by electrophoresis.

Serum electrophoresis is also of value in hypergammaglobulinemic states. A broad increase in the γ globulin fraction is the usual finding, which indicates an increase in several immunoglobulin classes and subclasses. This polyclonal hypergammaglobulinemia is a nonspecific finding seen in chronic infection, inflammatory disorders, and liver diseases. In contrast to this pattern, a sharp (monoclonal) spike in the γ globulin region (or occasionally in the α and β globulins) denotes an increase of a single clone of immunoglobulin, an M-component. Monoclonal hypergammaglobulinemia is characteristically present in multiple myeloma or Waldenström's macroglobulinemia (Fig. 3–20).

Immunoelectrophoresis

Immunoelectrophoresis is a qualitative test for individual serum proteins that can be used to demonstrate the presence or absence of IgG, IgM, or IgA immunoglobulins. It also is useful for identifying the presence and class of M-components. Immunoelectrophoresis is not an especially sensitive technique, so that proteins present in low concentrations (less than 10 to 20 mg/dl) may not be detected. In pediatric diagnosis, immunoelectrophoresis is generally an unnecessary intermediate procedure because it must be followed by quantitative immunoglobulin determinations.

Immunoglobulin Quantitation

Quantitative immunoglobulin determinations to measure levels of IgG, IgM, IgA, IgE, and IgD (the last is not usually performed routinely) are available for evaluation of patients with frequent infections, allergy, and related disorders. Quantitative immunoglobulin determinations are often done by the radial diffusion technique, but this has now been replaced in large centers by laser nephelometry, radioimmunoassays (RIA), or enzyme-linked immunosorbent assays (ELISA). Since levels of immunoglobulins change with age, especially in the first year, the results must be compared with those of normal age-matched controls. Levels of IgG, IgM, IgA, and IgD immunoglobulins are generally reported in mg/dl, although mg/ml and g/L are also used. The use of International Units (except for IgE) is not yet widely accepted. Normal levels of immunoglobulin are given in Chapter 9, Table 9–12.

Immunoglobulin Subclasses and Genetic Factors

Although antisera for determination of some IgG subclasses and allotypes are commercially available, re-

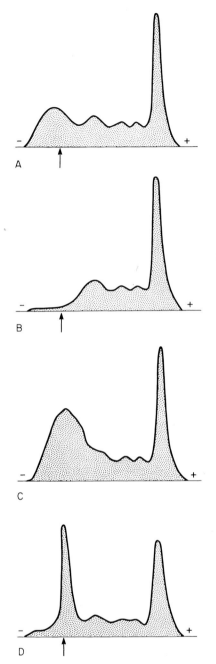

Figure 3–20. *A*, Electrophoretic pattern of normal serum. *B*, Agammaglobulinemic serum. *C*, Diffuse hypergammaglobulinemic serum. *D*, M-component hypergammaglobulinemic serum. The arrow indicates the point of application of the serum.

liable determinations must be done in research or reference laboratories performing these on a regular basis. Normal levels of IgG subclasses are given in Chapter 9, Table 9–16.

Immunoglobulins in Secretions and Fluids

The immunoglobulin content of the spinal fluid, joint fluid, urine, and exocrine gland secretions is often of clinical interest. Since these fluids are more dilute than serum, they often must be concentrated before analysis with radial diffusion techniques. However, the immunoassay in current use for immunoglobulin levels is capable of measuring these levels directly in most of the specimens. We have used tears to measure the immunoglobulins of external secretions; others have used saliva, nasal fluid, or gastric juice. Levels of IgG in cerebrospinal fluid are of considerable diagnostic value in multiple sclerosis.

Other Procedures

Other laboratory procedures available to evaluate immunoglobulins include:

- Erythrocyte sedimentation rate (ESR)
- Bence Jones urinary protein
- Euglobulin (Sia water test)
- Cryoglobulin

Sedimentation Rate

The ESR is elevated in active inflammation or tissue necrosis and is associated primarily with an increase in fibrinogen and secondarily with elevated γ globulin levels. The ESR may be low in the presence of agammaglobulinemia despite the presence of infection.

Bence Jones Protein

Monoclonal free light chains are excreted in the urine of some patients with multiple myeloma or Waldenström's macroglobulinemia. Urinary light chains from some patients precipitate when the urine is heated to 56°C, redissolved at higher temperatures, and reprecipitated with cooling. Light chains having these characteristics are called Bence Jones proteins. Because not all urinary monoclonal light chain proteins have these characteristics, a more reliable method for their detection in a concentrated (100×) sample of urine is the demonstration of a monoclonal spike on electrophoresis or a light-chain paraprotein arc on immunoelectrophoresis. The urinary protein reacts with antiserum to either κ or λ light chains but not to both.

Euglobulin

The Sia water test is a bedside test for high concentrations of euglobulin (a globulin insoluble at low ionic strength) and is characteristically positive in Waldenström's macroglobulinemia. A drop of serum is added to a cylinder of distilled water, and a flocculent precipitate or dense coagulum is noted immediately. Although characteristic of M-components, test results are occasionally positive in polyclonal hypergammaglobulinemias associated with chronic infection. This test is primarily of historical interest.

Cryoglobulin

Cryoglobulins are serum immunoglobulins that precipitate in the cold and redissolve at room temperature. Three general forms of cryoglobulins occur:

1. Monoclonal proteins (M-components), usually of the IgG or IgM classes.
2. Mixed cryoglobulins, composed of an array of normal immunoglobulins.
3. Cryoglobulins composed of a single clone of cold-reactive immunoglobulin but without a monoclonal gammopathy.

Generally, the latter two forms of cryoglobulins are associated with high levels of anti-immunoglobulin (rheumatoid factor) activity. When cryoglobulins are present in high concentrations, Raynaud's disease, cold urticaria, microthromboses, and peripheral gangrene may result.

Immunoglobulin Alterations in Health and Disease

Immunoglobulin Alterations with Age

Marked alterations in the levels of immunoglobulins occur during intrauterine life and the neonatal period (Fig. 3–21). The term newborn synthesizes little immunoglobulin at the time of birth but receives an adult level of IgG as a result of active transplacental transport from the mother (Stiehm and Fudenberg, 1966). Placental IgG transport begins at about 3 months' gestation. By term (40 weeks) the IgG level in the infant is slightly greater (110%) than the IgG level in the mother (Kohler and Farr, 1966). The cord blood level of IgG can be used to estimate the gestational age of the fetus (Yeung and Hobbs, 1968).

After birth, the IgG level in the infant decreases as a result of the normal catabolism of maternal IgG and the delay in the infant's own IgG synthesis. During this physiologic hypogammaglobulinemia, the IgG level generally falls to 300 to 500 mg/dl by 4 months. After 4 months, IgG synthesis increases slowly, and 60% of the adult IgG level of 1200 mg/dl is attained by 1 year. Adult levels are reached by age 10 years.

The physiologic dip in IgG levels to hypogammaglobulinemic levels (by adult standards) from the age of 2 to 6 months is a period that coincides with the peak

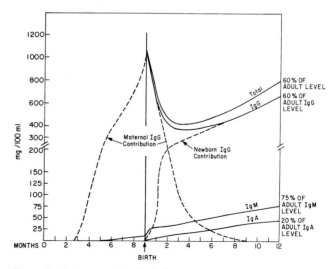

Figure 3–21. Immunoglobulin (IgG, IgM, and IgA) levels in the fetus and infant in the first year of life. The IgG of the fetus and newborn infant is solely of maternal origin. The maternal IgG disappears by the age of 9 months, by which time endogenous synthesis of IgG by the infant is well established. The IgM and IgA of the neonate are entirely endogenously synthesized, for maternal IgM and IgA do not cross the placenta.

incidence of many serious infections, such as *H. influenzae* meningitis, and of sudden, unexplained death in infancy. Because of their lower cord IgG levels, premature infants have a more prolonged and severe physiologic hypogammaglobulinemia and are more susceptible to neonatal infections.

Levels of IgG are slightly higher in postmature infants than in term infants. Further, IgA is occasionally elevated in postmature infants (above 5 mg/dl in 25% of the cases described by Ackerman et al., 1969). In infants with Down syndrome, IgG levels are decreased at birth, averaging 80% of the maternal concentrations (Miller et al., 1969).

IgM does not cross the placenta, but because of some in utero synthesis, it is present in infants with a mean level of 10 mg/dl (adult mean, 120 mg/dl). Within a week of birth, IgM synthesis accelerates, with the result that IgM is the chief immunoglobulin synthesized by the newborn infant. The stimulus for the accelerated IgM synthesis is probably the bacterial flora of the recently colonized gastrointestinal tract; thus premature infants, regardless of gestational age, demonstrate a similarly accelerated IgM synthesis immediately after birth. IgM levels reach 50% of adult values by age 6 months and 80% by 1 year.

Because most antibodies to gram-negative bacteria are IgM globulins, infants are not passively protected by transplacental antibodies to these organisms (Gitlin et al., 1963). Conversely, maternal IgG antibodies pass the placenta readily; thus the infant acquires passive protection to many bacterial and viral diseases for the first 6 months of life. In some circumstances, active immunization (e.g., to measles) is inhibited by this passive maternal IgG antibody, so that certain immunizations should be delayed until after the child is 15 months of age.

IgA, IgD, and IgE neither cross the placenta nor are synthesized in significant quantities by the newborn. Cord levels of these immunoglobulins are extremely low and rise slowly in the first year (Figs. 3–21 and 3–22), achieving levels of 10% to 25% of adult levels by 12 months of age. Adult levels are achieved by about age 15. Levels for each age are given in Chapter 9, Table 9–13).

Immunoglobulins in Congenital Infection

In congenital infection, cord blood IgM levels are increased, usually to levels exceeding 20 mg/dl (Stiehm et al., 1966). In about 1% to 3% of all infants, cord IgM is elevated. Although it is not always possible to identify an infection in these infants, they should be regarded as a high-risk group and watched carefully for infection. In infants with congenital rubella, toxoplasmosis, cytomegalic inclusion disease, and syphilis, IgM levels are usually, but not invariably, elevated; in infants with cytomegalovirus, IgA levels may also be elevated.

Elevated levels of IgM in cord blood may also occur as a result of leakage of blood from mother to fetus, resulting in a false-positive IgM test for congenital infection. Maternal to fetal leakage is responsible for

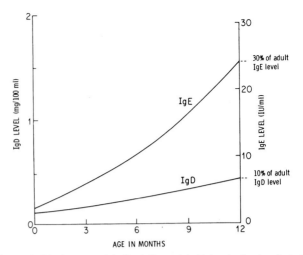

Figure 3–22. Immunoglobulin IgD and IgE levels in the first 12 months of life. Neither IgD nor IgE crosses the placenta, so these immunoglobulins are synthesized solely by the newborn. Note the different scales for IgD (mg/dl) and IgE (IU/ml) (1 IU = 2.4 ng).

about 5% to 10% of instances of elevated IgM and can be suspected if the cord IgA exceeds the cord IgM (since maternal IgA is higher than maternal IgM). It can be confirmed by a repeat assay of infant IgM and IgA levels; maternally derived IgM and IgA decrease after 3 or 4 days because of their rapid half-lives. By contrast, levels of IgM and IgA synthesized by the infant increase or are maintained.

Immunoglobulins in Antibody Immunodeficiencies

Several chapters of this text are devoted to the antibody deficiency disorders; most of these are associated with deficiency of one or more of the immunoglobulins. There are unusual instances in which immunoglobulin levels are normal but the immunoglobulins function poorly as antibodies. Thus tests for antibody function should be included in the evaluation of a patient with suspected immunodeficiency (see Chapters 9 and 11).

In most patients with antibody immunodeficiency, synthesis of immunoglobulins is defective. However, in certain disorders, hypogammaglobulinemia (total immunoglobulin levels < 400 mg/dl or an IgG globulin < 200 mg/dl) is due to excessive loss as a result of extracorporeal loss, e.g., nephrotic syndrome, protein-losing enteropathy, or hypercatabolism. In these disorders, levels of many serum proteins, not only serum immunoglobulins, are decreased. The IgG globulin survival is markedly shortened, in contrast to the normal or prolonged IgG survival in most antibody immunodeficiencies. Replacement of IgG is generally not indicated, since it will be rapidly lost. Furthermore, patients with these conditions usually do not experience the same degree of serious infection seen in conditions of defective immunoglobulin synthesis.

M-Components and Paraproteins

Considerable information about immunoglobulin structure has been derived from the study of individuals with excess amounts of a single serum or urinary immunoglobulin, termed an M-component or paraprotein. These proteins are characteristically found in patients with multiple myeloma or Waldenström's macroglobulinemia. An M-component is a homogeneous immunoglobulin present in large quantities, produced by a single clone of neoplastic cells. This monoclonal protein results in a single sharp spike on electrophoresis (see Fig. 3–20). This single peak, in contrast to the relatively broad peak of normal immunoglobulins, occurs as a result of the electrophoretic homogeneity of the component. Monoclonal antibodies produced by hybridoma techniques are laboratory-derived M-components limited to a single antigenic specificity.

The presence of large quantities of single M-components permits their isolation and characterization and has led to many important observations about the immunoglobulins. For example, recognition of the IgD and IgE immunoglobulin classes resulted from the study of individuals with previously undefined M-components. The entire amino acid sequence of a number of myeloma proteins has been established (Nisonoff et al., 1975a, 1975b).

M-component disorders are mostly of theoretical interest to the pediatrician, since multiple myeloma and macroglobulinemia have not been described in children. The incidence of M-components increases with age; in older individuals, low levels of M-component may occur without associated illness, and their serum concentration remains relatively stable for years. This disorder has been termed benign monoclonal gammopathy. M-components have been noted in some pediatric patients with combined immunodeficiency (Geha et al., 1974; DeFazio et al., 1975) and transiently in some patients following immunologic reconstitution by bone marrow transplantation (Rádl et al., 1971).

Myeloma or Macroglobulinemia M-Components

An M-component can belong to any immunoglobulin class. Multiple myeloma is associated with IgG, IgA, IgD, or IgE M-component; Waldenström's macroglobulinemia is associated with an IgM M-component. A myeloma M-component contains either κ or λ light chains, not both. If it is an IgG or IgA myeloma, it contains a heavy chain belonging to only one of the respective subclasses. Some myeloma cells produce κ or λ light chains only and therefore have light-chain M-components. M-components have limited allotypic determinants and idiotypic antigenic characteristics, indicating molecular homogeneity. Bence Jones protein is an M-component found in the urine (rarely in the serum) of patients with multiple myeloma or macroglobulinemia. Often there is an associated serum M-component. The Bence Jones proteins are dimers of either two κ or two λ light chains (40,000 daltons). The light-chain type is the same as the light-chain type of the corresponding serum M-component, since the Bence Jones protein simply results from excess synthesis of light chains not incorporated into intact immunoglobulin molecules.

The frequency of M-components among the classes of immunoglobulins reflects their relative serum concentration. IgG myeloma proteins are the most common, followed by IgA myeloma and IgM macroglobulinemia. IgD myelomas are extremely rare, and IgE myelomas have been found in only eight patients.

Heavy-Chain M-Components

The M-components of heavy-chain disease are homogeneous proteins completely lacking light chains (Franklin and Frangione, 1975; Franklin, 1976). Three types of heavy-chain disease involving the γ, μ, or α heavy chain have been identified; these are called γ, μ, and α heavy-chain disease. Clinically, the disorder resembles a lymphoreticular neoplasm. α Heavy-chain disease affects elderly individuals, who manifest lymphadenopathy (particularly that of Waldeyer's ring) and hepatosplenomegaly. α Heavy-chain disease occurs in younger individuals in areas around the Mediterranean Sea. It is generally associated with Mediterranean lymphoma, a malignant infiltration of the gastrointestinal tract that gives rise to diarrhea, malabsorption, and steatorrhea. μ Heavy-chain disease generally occurs with chronic lymphocytic leukemia; prominent features include vacuolated plasma cells and marked visceral involvement.

In all of these patients, there is an M-protein in the serum and occasionally in the urine that reacts with heavy-chain antisera. There is no associated light chain seen in γ or α heavy-chain disease. Structural studies on these proteins indicate that all the molecules have, in addition to absence of light chains, internal deletions of variable size, including deletions of the V region, the C region, and the hinge region. The heavy-chain fragments are the product of synthesis of protein from aberrant DNA rearrangements in the abnormal B cells rather than the product of degradation of normal heavy chains.

Amyloid

Amyloidosis, an extravascular deposition of homogeneous eosinophilic protein throughout the body, is a common complication of multiple myeloma, or it may exist as a primary disorder. Analysis of the amyloid protein in myeloma patients indicates that it is made up of homogeneous light chains related to Bence Jones protein. These light chains have the ability to fold into the characteristic β-pleated sheets of *amyloid L* (AL). In other patients, the amyloid protein is not a portion of the immunoglobulin molecule but is caused by the deposition of a reactive serum protein, *amyloid A* (AA).

Hypergammaglobulinemic Disorders

An immunoglobulin level greater than two standard deviations above the mean for age-matched controls is considered abnormally elevated. Some causes of selective immunoglobulin elevations are noted in Table 3–12. In certain immunodeficiencies, elevated levels of one or more immunoglobulins are noted, especially

Table 3–12. Some Nonmalignant Causes of
Immunoglobulin Elevations in Children

High levels of one or two immunoglobulins

Immunodeficiency diseases
Hyper-IgM immunodeficiency (↑ IgM)
Wiskott-Aldrich syndrome (↑ IgA, ↑ IgE)
Job's syndrome (↑ IgE)
Buckley's syndrome (↑ IgE)

Infections
Congenital infection (↑ IgM)
Infectious mononucleosis (↑ IgM)
Trypanosomiasis (↑ IgM)
Malaria (↑ IgM)
Kala-azar (↑ IgM)

Miscellaneous
Anaphylactoid purpura (↑ IgA)
Extrinsic allergy (↑ IgE)
Eczema (↑ IgE)
Kawasaki syndrome (↑ IgE)
Periarteritis nodosa (↑ IgE)
Cold agglutinin disease (↑ IgM)

High levels of all immunoglobulins

Immunodeficiencies
Chronic granulomatous disease
Acquired immunodeficiency syndrome

Infections
Intestinal parasitism (↑ ↑ IgE)
Visceral larva migrans
Chronic bacterial infections (osteomyelitis, endocarditis,
    abscesses, tuberculosis)

Collagen vascular diseases
Rheumatic fever
Rheumatoid arthritis
Lupus erythematosus
Ulcerative colitis
Regional enteritis

Liver diseases
Acute hepatitis
Chronic active hepatitis
Cirrhosis

Miscellaneous
Down syndrome
Hyperglobulinemic purpura
Pulmonary hypersensitivity diseases
Illicit intravenous drug use
Cystic fibrosis
Sarcoidosis

in immunodeficiency with hyper-IgM and in Wiskott-Aldrich syndrome (high IgA and IgE). Patients with AIDS often have elevated IgG and IgA levels with normal IgM even before multiple opportunistic infections. All pediatric patients with a total immunoglobulin level over 2000 mg/dl should be screened for HIV infection. Other chronic infections are associated with high levels of IgG and other immunoglobulins. By contrast, infectious mononucleosis, kala-azar, and trypanosomiasis are associated with selected elevation of IgM globulin.

In many collagen diseases, diffuse hypergammaglobulinemia is present. The degree of hypergammaglobulinemia reflects the duration and severity of the illness and often is correlated with the degree of elevation of the ESR. Certain families may have hypergammaglobulinemia and a high incidence of collagen disease. In liver diseases, high immunoglobulin levels are also observed; in chronic active hepatitis, the total immunoglobulin may exceed 4000 mg/dl. Patients with Down syndrome, especially institutionalized patients, have high levels of immunoglobulins, particularly of the IgG and IgA classes (Stiehm and Fudenberg, 1966). Chronic exposure to exogenous antigenic stimulation, as in hypersensitivity pneumonitis (such as pigeon breeder's lung), may also give rise to hypergammaglobulinemia. The finding of elevated levels of immunoglobulins, of itself, is not associated with unusual ability to fight infection.

References

Ackerman BD, Taylor WF, O'Loughlin BJ. Serum immunoglobulin levels in postmature infants. Pediatrics 43:956–962, 1969.

Adderson EE, Shackelford PG, Quinn A, Wilson PM, Cunningham MW, Insel RA, Carroll WL. Restricted immunoglobulin V$_H$ usage and VDJ combinations in the human response to *Haemophilus influenzae* type b capsular polysaccharide. Nucleotide sequences of monospecific anti-*Haemophilus* antibodies and polyspecific antibodies cross-reacting with self antigens. J Clin Invest 91:2734–2743, 1993.

Allen JC, Kunkel HG. Antibodies against gamma-globulin after repeated blood transfusions in man. J Clin Invest 45:29–39, 1966.

Amlot PL, Stone MJ, Cunningham D, Fay J, Newman J, Collins R, May R, McCarthy M, Richardson J, Ghetie V, Ramilo O, Thorpe PE, Uhr JW, Vitetta ES. A phage I study of anti–CD22-deglycosylated ricin A chain immunotoxin in the treatment of B-cell lymphomas resistant to conventional therapy. Blood 82:2624–2633, 1993.

Anderson BR, Terry WD. Gamma G4–globulin antibody causing inhibition of clotting factor VIII. Nature 217:174–175, 1968.

Aroeti B, Casanova J, Okamoto C, Cardone M, Pollack A, Tang K, Mostov K. Polymeric immunoglobulin receptor. Int Rev Cytol 137B:157–168, 1992.

Aruffo A, Farrington M, Hollenbaugh D, Li X, Milatovich A, Nonoyama S, Bajorath J, Grosmaire LS, Stenkamp R, Neubauer M, Roberts RL, Noelle RJ, Ledbetter JA, Francke U, Ochs HD. The CD40 ligand, gp39, is defective in activated T cells from patients with X-linked hyper-IgM syndrome. Cell 72:291–300, 1993.

Askonas BA, Williamson AR. Biosynthesis of immunoglobulins on polyribosomes and assembly of the IgG molecule. Proc Soc Lond [Biol] 166:232–243, 1966.

Aubry J-P, Pochon S, Graber P, Jansen KU, Bonnefoy J-Y. CD21 is a ligand for CD23 and regulates IgE production. Nature 358:505–507, 1992.

Bahler DW, Campbell MJ, Hart S, Miller RA, Levy S, Levy R. Ig V$_H$ gene expression among human follicular lymphomas. Blood 78:1561–1568, 1991.

Bakhshi A, Jensen JP, Goldman P, Wright JJ, McBride OW, Epstein AL, Korsmeyer SJ. Cloning the chromosomal breakpoint of t(14;18) human lymphomas clustering around J$_H$ on chromosome 14 and near a transcriptional unit on 18. Cell 41:899–906, 1985.

Ballow M. Mechanisms of action of intravenous immune serum globulin therapy. Pediatr Infect Dis J 13:806–811, 1994.

Beck CS, Heiner DC. Selective immunoglobulin G4 deficiency and recurrent infections of the respiratory tract. Am Rev Respir Dis 124:94–96, 1981.

Berlin C, Berg EL, Briskin MJ, Andrew DP, Kilshaw PJ, Holzmann B, Weissman IL, Hamann A, Butcher EC. α4β7 integrin mediates lymphocyte binding to the mucosal vascular addressin MAdCAM-1. Cell 74:185–194, 1994.

Berman JE, Mellis SJ, Pollock R, Smith CL, Suh H, Heinke B, Kowal C, Surti U, Chess L, Cantor CR, Alt FW. Content and organization of the human Ig VH locus: definition of three new VH families and linkage to the Ig CH locus. EMBO J 7:727–738, 1988.

Bloch KJ. The IgE system and parasitism: role of mast-cells, IgE, and other antibodies in host response to primary infection with *Nippostrongylus brasiliensis*. In Ishizaka K, Dayton DE Jr, eds. The Biological Role of the Immunoglobulin E System. Bethesda, Md.: Department of Health, Education, and Welfare, 1972, pp. 119–139.

Braun J, Unanue ER. The lymphocyte cytoskeleton and its control of surface receptor functions. Semin Hematol 20:322–326, 1983.

Braun J, Valles-Ayoub Y, Berberian L, Eggena M, Gordon LK, Targan SR. On the pathogenesis trail: what marker B cell clones tell us about inflammatory bowel disease. In Sutherland LR, Collins SM, Martin F, et al, eds: Inflammatory Bowel Disease: Basic Research, Clinical Implications, and Trends in Therapy. Dordrecht, The Netherlands, Kluwer Academic Publishing, 1994, pp. 96–103.

Bruck C, Co MS, Slaoui M, Gaulton GN, Smith T, Fields BN, Mullins JI, Greene MI. Nucleic acid sequence of an internal image-bearing monoclonal anti-idiotype and its comparison to the sequence of the external antigen. Proc Natl Acad Sci U S A 83:6578–6582, 1986.

Bush ST, Swedlund HA, Gleich GJ. Low molecular weight IgM in human sera. J Lab Clin Med 73:194–201, 1969.

Cambier JC, Pleiman CM, Clark MR. Signal transduction by the B cell antigen receptor and its coreceptors. Annu Rev Immunol 12:457–486, 1994.

Capron A, Dessaint JP, Capron M, Bazin H. Specific IgE antibodies in immune adherence of normal macrophages to *Schistosoma mansoni* schistosomules. Nature 253:474–475, 1975.

Ceuppens JL, Baroja ML, Van Vaeck F, Anderson CL. A defect in the membrane expression of high affinity 72 kD Fc receptors on phagocytic cells in four healthy subjects. J Clin Invest 82:572–578, 1988.

Cherayil BJ, MacDonald K, Waneck GL, Pillai S. Surface transport and internalization of the membrane IgM H chain in the absence of the Mb-1 and B29 proteins. J Immunol 151:11–20, 1993.

Clark EA, Ledbetter JA. How B and T cells talk to each other. Nature 367:425–428, 1994.

DeFazio SR, Criswell BS, Kimzey SL, South MA, Montgomery JR. A paraprotein in severe combined immunodeficiency disease detected by immunoelectrophoretic analysis of plasma. Clin Exp Immunol 19:563–570, 1975.

Drenth JPH, Haagsma CJ, van der Meer JWM, and International Hyper-IgD Study Group. Hyperimmunoglobulinemia D and periodic fever syndrome: The clinical spectrum in a series of 50 patients. Medicine 73:133–144, 1994.

Dunnick W, Stavnezer J. Copy choice mechanism of immunoglobulin heavy-chain switch recombination. Mol Cell Biol 10:397–400, 1990.

Dwyer JM. Manipulating the immune system with immune globulin. N Engl J Med 326:107–116, 1992.

Early P, Huang H, Davis M, Calame C, Hood L. An immunoglobulin heavy chain variable gene is generalized from three segments of DNA: V_H, D_H, and J_H. Cell 19:981–984, 1980.

Edelman GM, Gall WE. The antibody problem. Annu Rev Biochem 38:415–466, 1969.

Edelman GM, Olins DE, Gally JA, Zinder ND. Reconstitution of immunologic activity by interaction of polypeptide chains of antibodies. Proc Natl Acad Sci U S A 50:753–761, 1963.

Edelman GM, Poulik MD. Studies on structural units of the gamma globulins. J Exp Med 113:861–864, 1961.

Engle RL Jr, Wallis LA. Immunoglobulinopathies. Springfield, Ill., Charles C Thomas, 1969.

Evans RJ, Hollis GF. Genomic structure of the human Ig lambda 1 gene suggests that it may be expressed as an Ig lambda 14.1–like protein or as a canonical B-cell Ig lambda light chain: implications for Ig lambda gene evolution. J Exp Med 173:305–311, 1991.

Frame M, Mollison PL, Terry WD. Anti-Rh activity of human gamma G4 proteins. Nature 225:641–643, 1970.

Franklin EC. Some impacts of clinical investigation on immunology: surface IgD, IgE, and heavy-chain variants. N Engl J Med 294:531–537, 1976.

Franklin EC, Frangione B. Structural variants of human and murine immunoglobulins. In Inman FP, ed. Contemporary Topics in Molecular Immunology, Vol. 4. New York, Plenum Publishing, 1975, pp. 89–126.

Fudenberg HH. Hereditary human gamma globulin (Gm) groups: interpretations and extensions. Prog Allergy 7:1–31, 1963.

Fudenberg HH, Drews G, Nisonoff A. Serologic demonstration of dual specificity of rabbit bivalent hybrid antibody. J Exp Med 119:151–164, 1963.

Fudenberg HH, Fudenberg BR. Antibody to hereditary human gamma-globulin (Gm) factor resulting from maternal-fetal incompatibility. Science 145:170, 1964.

Garcia KC, Desiderio SV, Ronco PM, Verroust PJ, Amzel LM. Recognition of angiotensin II: antibodies at different levels of an idiotypic network are superimposable. Science 257:528–531, 1992.

Gauss GH, Lieber MR. The basis for the mechanistic bias for deletional over inversional V(D)J recombination. Genes Dev 6:1553–1561, 1992.

Geha RS, Schneeberger E, Gatien J, Rosen FS, Merler E. Synthesis of an M component by circulating B lymphocytes in severe combined immunodeficiency. N Engl J Med 290:726–728, 1974.

Gergely J, Fudenberg HH, Van Loghem E. The papain susceptibility of IgG myeloma proteins of different heavy chain subclasses. Immunochemistry 7:1–6, 1970.

Germain RN, Margulies DH. The biochemistry and cell biology of antigen processing and presentation. Annu Rev Immunol 11:403–450, 1993.

Gitlin D. Development and metabolism of the immune globulins. In Kagan BM, Stiehm ER, eds. Immunologic Incompetence. Chicago, Year Book, 1971, pp. 3–13.

Gitlin D, Rosen FS, Michael JG. Transient 19S gamma-1-globulin deficiency in the newborn infant and its significance. Pediatrics 3:197–208, 1963.

Giusti AM, Manser T. Hypermutation is observed only in antibody H chain region transcripts that have been recombined with endogenous Ig H DNA. Implications for the location of *cis*-acting elements required for somatic mutation. J Exp Med 177:797–809, 1993.

Golde DW, Baldwin GC, Weisbart RH. Responses of neutrophils to myeloid growth factors. CIBA Found Symp 148:62–71, 1990.

Goodglick L, Braun J. Revenge of the microbes: superantigens of the T and B cell lineage. Am J Pathol 144:623–636, 1994.

Gosselin EJ, Brown MF, Anderson CL, Zipf TF, Guyre PM. The monoclonal antibody 41H16 detects the leu 4 responder form of human FcγRII. J Immunol 144:1817–1822, 1990.

Granoff DM, Pandey JP, Boies E, Squires J, Munson RS Jr, Suarez B. Response to immunization with *Haemophilus influenzae* type b polysaccharide-pertussis vaccine and risk of *Haemophilus* meningitis in children with the Km(1) immunoglobulin allotype. J Clin Invest 74:1708–1714, 1984.

Gray D. Immunological memory. Annu Rev Immunol 11:49–77, 1993.

Grey HM, Abel CA, Yount WJ, Kunkel HG. A subclass of human gamma A globulins (IgA2) which lacks the disulfide bonds linking heavy and light chains. J Exp Med 128:1223–1236, 1968.

Grey HM, Kunkel HG. H chain subgroups of myeloma proteins and normal 7S gamma-globulins. J Exp Med 120:253–266, 1964.

Grubb R. Agglutination of erythrocytes coated with ''incomplete'' anti-Rh by certain rheumatoid arthritic sera and some other sera. Acta Pathol Microbiol Scand 35:195–197, 1956.

Hamaoka T, Katz DH, Benacerraf B. Hapten-specific IgE antibody responses in mice: II. Cooperative interaction between adoptively transferred T and B lymphocytes in the development of IgE response. J Exp Med 138:338–556, 1973.

Hardy RR, Hayakawa K. A developmental switch in B lymphopoiesis. Proc Natl Acad Sci U S A 88:11550–11554, 1991.

Harriman W, Volk H, Defranoux N, Wabl M. Immunoglobulin class switch recombination. Annu Rev Immunol 11:361–386, 1993.

Heiner DC, Rose B. A study of antibody responses by radioimmunodiffusion with demonstration of gamma-D antigen-binding activity in four sera. J Immunol 104:691–697, 1970.

Hiemstra I, Vossen JM, van der Meer JWM, Weemaes CMR, Out TA, Zegers BJM. Clinical and immunological studies in patients with an increased serum IgD level. J Clin Immunol 9:393–400, 1989.

Honjo T. Immunoglobulin genes. Annu Rev Immunol 1:499–536, 1983.

Hoogenboom HR, Winter G. By-passing immunisation. Human antibodies from synthetic repertoires of germline V_H gene segments rearranged in vitro. J Mol Biol 227:381–388, 1992.

Huang C, Stollar BD. A majority of Ig H chain cDNA of normal human adult blood lymphocytes resembles cDNA for fetal Ig and natural autoantibodies. J Immunol 151:5290–5300, 1993.

Hyvarinen M, Zeltzer P, Oh W, Stiehm ER. Influence of gestational age on serum levels of alpha-1-fetoprotein, IgG globulin and albumin in newborn infants. J Pediatr 82:430–437, 1973.

Ishizaka K. Immunoglobulin E and reaginic hypersensitivity. Johns Hopkins Med J 135:67–90, 1974.

Ishizaka K, Ishizaka R, Hornbrook MH. Physicochemical properties of human reaginic antibody. IV. Presence of a unique immunoglobulin as a carrier of reaginic antibody. J Immunol 97:75–85, 1966.

Jacob J, Przylepa J, Miller C, Kelsoe G. In situ studies of the primary immune response to (4-hydroxy-3-nitrophenyl) acetyl: III. The kinetics of V region mutation and selection in germinal center B cells. J Exp Med 178:1293–1307, 1993.

Janda KD, Shevlin CG, Lerner RA. Antibody catalysis of a disfavored chemical transformation. Science 259:490–493, 1993.

Jefferis R. The glycosylation of antibody molecules: functional significance. Glycoconjugate J 10:358–361, 1993.

Jerne NK. Toward a network theory of the immune system. Ann d'Immunol Inst Pasteur (Paris) 125C:373–389, 1974.

Kearney JF. Idiotypic networks. In Paul W, ed. Fundamental Immunology, 3rd ed. New York, Raven Press, 1993, pp. 887–902.

Kenny JF, Gray JA. Sex differences in immunologic response: studies of antibody production by individual cells after stimulus with *Escherichia coli* antigen. Pediatr Res 5:246–255, 1971.

Kikutani H, Inui S, Sato R, Barsumanian EL, Owaki H, Yamasaki L, Kaisho T, Uchibayashi N, Tsunasawa S, Sakiyama F, Suemura M, Kishimoto T. Molecular structure of human lymphocyte receptor for immunoglobulin E. Cell 47:657–665, 1986.

Kipps TJ. The CD5 B cell. Adv Immunol 47:117–185, 1989.

Kipps TJ, Carson DA. Autoantibodies in chronic lymphocytic leukemia and related systemic autoimmune diseases. Blood 81:2475–2487, 1993.

Kirsh IR, Morton CC, Nakahara K, Leder P. Human immunoglobulin heavy chain genes map to a region of translocations in malignant B lymphocytes. Science 216:301–303, 1982.

Kohler PF, Farr RS. Elevation of cord over maternal IgG immunoglobulin: evidence for an active placental IgG transport. Nature 210:1070–1071, 1966.

Korsmeyer SJ, Arnold A, Bakhski A, Ravetch JV, Siebenlist U, Haiter PA, Sharrow SO, Lekein TW, Kersey JH, Poplack DG, Leder P, Waldmann TA. Immunoglobulin gene rearrangement and cell surface antigen expression in acute lymphocytic leukemias of T cell and B cell precursor origin. J Clin Invest 71:301–313, 1983.

Kotynek O, Franek F. Unequal importance of different polypeptide chains for the determination of antibody specificity in bovine antidinitrophenyl antibodies: Collection of Czechoslovak. Chem Commun 30:3153–3163, 1965.

Kronvall G, Williams RC Jr. Differences in antiprotein A activity among IgG subgroups. J Immunol 103:828–833, 1969.

Kunkel HG, Kindt T. Allotypes and idiotypes. In Benacerraf B, ed. Immunogenetics and Immunodeficiency. Baltimore, University Park Press, 1975, pp 55–80.

Labaw LW, Davies DR. An electron microscopic study of human gamma-G1 immunoglobulin crystals. J Biol Chem 246:3760–3762, 1971.

Lanzavecchia A. Receptor-mediated antigen uptake and its effect on antigen presentation to class-II–restricted T lymphocytes. Annu Rev Immunol 8:773–794, 1990.

Leung DYM. Mechanisms controlling the human IgE response: new directions in the therapy of allergic diseases. Pediatr Res 33 (Suppl. 1):S56–S62, 1993.

Lin PS, Cooper AG, Wortis HH. Scanning electron microscopy of human T-cell and B-cell rosettes. N Engl J Med 289:548–551, 1973.

MacLennan ICM. Germinal centers. Annu Rev Immunol 12:117–139, 1994.

Malcolm S, Barton P, Murphy C, Ferguson-Smith MA, Bentley DL, Rabbitts TH. Localization of human immunoglobulin K light-chain variable region genes to the short arm of chromosome 2 by in situ hybridization. Proc Natl Acad Sci U S A 79:4957–4961, 1982.

Marks JD, Ouwehand WH, Bye JM, Finnern R, Gorick BD, Voak D, Thorpe SJ, Hughes-Jones NC, Winter G. Human antibody fragments specific for human blood group antigens from a phage display library. Biotechniques 11:1145–1149, 1993.

Matsuda F, Shin EK, Nagaoka H, Matsumura R, Haino M, Fukita Y, Takaishi S, Imai T, Riley JH, Anand R, Soeda E, Honjo T. Structure and physical map of 64 variable segments in the 3′ 0.8-megabase region of the human immunoglobulin heavy-chain locus. Nature Genet 3:88–94, 1993.

Matsumoto AK, Martin DR, Carter RH, Klickstein LB, Ahearn JM, Fearon DT. Functional dissection of the CD21/CD19/TAPA-1/Leu-13 complex of B lymphocytes. J Exp Med 178:1407–1417, 1993.

Matzinger P. Tolerance, danger, and the extended family. Annu Rev Immunol 12:991–1045, 1994.

McConnell I. T and B lymphocytes. In Hobart MJ, McConnell I, eds. The Immune System: A Course on the Molecular and Cellular Basis of Immunity. Oxford, Blackwell Scientific, 1975, pp. 98–119.

Melchers F, Anderson J, Curbel C, Leptin M, Lehnhardt W, Gerhard W, Zeathen J. Regulation of B lymphocyte replication and maturation. J Cell Biochem 19:315–321, 1982.

Melchers F, Haasner D, Grawunder U, Kalberer C, Karasuyama H, Winkler T, Rolink AG. Roles of Ig H and L chains and of surrogate H and L chains in the development of cells of the B lymphocyte lineage. Annu Rev Immunol 12:209–225, 1994.

Metzger H. Structure and function of gamma M macroglobulins. Adv Immunol 12:57–116, 1970.

Metzger H, Alcarez G, Hohman R, Kunet JP, Pribluda B, Quarto R. The receptor with high affinity for immunoglobulin E. Annu Rev Immunol 4:419–470, 1986.

Miller ME, Mellman MJ, Cohen MM, Kohn G, Dietz WH Jr. Depressed immunoglobulin G in newborn infants with Down's syndrome. J Pediatr 75:996–1000, 1969.

Moore KW, Rogers J, Hunkapiller I, Early P, Nottenberg C, Weissman I, Bazin H, Wall R, Hood L. Expression of IgD may use both DNA rearrangement and RNA splicing mechanisms. Proc Natl Acad Sci U S A 78:1800–1804, 1981.

Mortari F, Wang J-Y, Schroeder HW Jr. Human cord blood antibody repertoire: mixed population of V$_H$ gene segments and CDR3 distribution in the expressed C-alpha and C-gamma repertoires. J Immunol 150:1348–1357, 1993.

Nakamura T, Kubagawa H, Ohno T, Cooper MD. Characterization of an IgM Fc-binding receptor on human T cells. J Immunol 151:6933–6941, 1993.

Nathenson G, Schorr JB, Litwin D. Gm factor fetomaternal gammaglobulin incompatibility. Pediatr Res 4:2–9, 1971.

Natvig JB, Kunkel HG. Human immunoglobulins, classes, subclasses, genetic variants, and idiotypes. Adv Immunol 16:1–59, 1973.

Nelson PN, Goodall M, Jefferis R. Characterization of putative monoclonal anti-G3m(μ) and anti-G3m(γ) reagents and their antigenic determinants. Immunol Invest 23:39–43, 1994.

Nisonoff A, Hopper JE, Spring SB. The three-dimensional structure of immunoglobulins. In The Antibody Molecule. New York, Academic Press, 1975a, pp. 209–237.

Nisonoff A, Hopper JE, Spring SB. Amino acid sequences in human immunoglobulins and in mouse light chains. In The Antibody Molecule. New York, Academic Press, 1975b, pp. 138–208.

Nisonoff A, Hopper JE, Spring SB. Allotypes of rabbit, human, and mouse immunoglobulins. In The Antibody Molecule. New York, Academic Press, 1975c, pp. 346–406.

Nisonoff A, Wissler FC, Lipman LN. Properties of the major component of a peptic digest of rabbit antibody. Science 132:1770–1771, 1960.

Nunez G, Seto M, Seremetis S, Ferrero D, Grignani F, Korsmeyer SJ, Dalla-Favera R. Growth- and tumor-promoting effects of deregulated BCL2 in human B-lymphoblastoid cells. Proc Natl Acad Sci U S A 86:4589–4593, 1989.

Oettinger MA, Schatz DG, Gorka C, Baltimore D. RAG-1 and RAG-2, adjacent genes that synergistically activate V(D)J recombination. Science 248:1517–1523, 1990.

Ohno T, Kubagawa H, Sanders SK, Cooper MD. Biochemical nature of the Fcμ receptor on human B-lineage cells. J Exp Med 172:1165–1172, 1991.

Okudaira H, Ishizaka K. Reaginic antibody formation in the mouse. II. Participation of long-lived antibody-forming cells in persistent antibody formation. Cell Immunol 50:188, 1981.

Oxelius V-A, Laurell A-B, Lindquist B, Golebiowska H, Axelsson U, Bjorkander J, Hanson LA. IgG subclasses in selective IgA deficiency: importance of IgG2-IgA deficiency. N Engl J Med 304:1476–1477, 1981.

Palmer JL, Nisonoff A. Reduction and reoxidation of a critical disulfide bond in the rabbit antibody molecule. J Biol Chem 238:2393–2398, 1963.

Platts-Mills TAE. Local production of IgG, IgA, and IgE antibodies in grass pollen hay fever. J Immunol 123:2218–2225, 1979.

Plaut AG, Genco RJ, Tomasi TB Jr. Isolation of an enzyme from

Streptococcus sanguis, which specifically cleaves IgA. J Immunol 113:289–291, 1974.

Porter RR. Hydrolysis of rabbit gamma-globulin and antibodies with crystalline papain. Biochem J 73:119–126, 1959.

Punnonen J, de Vries JE. Characterization of a novel CD2$^+$ human thymic B cell subset. J Immunol 151:100–110, 1993.

Rádl J, Dooren LJ, Eijsvoogel VP, Van Went JJ, Hijmans W. An immunological study during posttransplantation follow-up of a case of severe combined immunodeficiency. Clin Exp Immunol 10:367–382, 1971.

Rajewsky K, Takemori T. Genetics, expression, and functions of idiotypes. Annu Rev Immunol 1:609–641, 1983.

Randall TD, King LB, Corley RB. The biological effects of IgM hexamer formation. Eur J Immunol 20:1971–1979, 1990.

Ravetch JV, Kinet JP. Fc receptors. Annu Rev Immunol 9:457–492, 1991.

Rawlings DJ, Saffran DC, Tsukada S, Largaespada DA, Grimaldi JC, Cohen L, Mohr RN, Bazan JF, Howard M, Copeland NG, Jenkins NA, Witte ON. Mutation of unique region of Bruton's tyrosine kinase in immunodeficient XID mice. Science 261:358–361, 1993.

Rogers J, Early P, Carter C, Calame C, Bond M, Hood L, Wall R. Two mRNAs with different 3′ ends encode membrane bound and secreted forms of immunoglobulin mu chain. Cell 20:303–308, 1980.

Rothenfluh HS, Taylor L, Bothwell ALM, Both GW, Steele EJ. Somatic hypermutation in 5′ flanking regions of heavy-chain antibody variable regions. Eur J Immunol 23:2152–2159, 1993.

Rowe DS, Fahey JL. A new class of human immunoglobulins. I. Unique myeloma protein. J Exp Med 121:171–184, 1965.

Rowe DS, Hug K, Forni L, Pernis B. Immunoglobulin D as a lymphocyte receptor. J Exp Med 138:965–972, 1973.

Russo G, Isobe M, Gatti R, Finan J, Batuman O, Huebner K, Nowell PC, Croce CM. Molecular analysis of a t(14;14) translocation in leukemic T-cells of an ataxia-telangiectasia patient. Proc Natl Acad Sci U S A 86:602–606, 1989.

Sarvetnick N, Gurushanthaiah D, Han N, Prudent J, Schultz P, Lerner R. Increasing the chemical potential of the germline antibody repertoire. Proc Natl Acad Sci U S A 90:4008–4011, 1993.

Schanfield MS, van Loghem EV. Human immunoglobulin allotypes. In Weir DM, ed. Handbook of Experimental Immunology. Vol 3, Genetics and Molecular Immunology, 4th ed. Oxford, Blackwell Publishing, 1986, pp. 94:1–17.

Schur PH, Borel H, Gelfand EW, Alper CA, Rosen F. Selective gamma-G globulin deficiencies in patients with recurrent pyogenic infections. N Engl J Med 283:631–634, 1970.

Selvaraj P, Rosse WF, Silber R, Springer TA. The major Fc receptor in blood has a phosphatidylinositol anchor and is deficient in paroxysmal nocturnal haemoglobinuria. Nature 333:565–567, 1988.

Shen L, Collins J. Monocyte superoxide secretion triggered by human IgA. Immunology 68:491–496, 1989.

Shibata D, Weiss LM, Hernandez AM, Nathwani BN, Bernstein L, Levine AM. Epstein-Barr virus–associated non-Hodgkin's lymphoma in patients infected with the human immunodeficiency virus. Blood 81:2102–2109, 1993.

Shlomchik MJ, Marshak-Rothstein A, Wolfowicz CB, Rothstein TL, Weigert MG. The role of clonal selection and somatic mutation in autoimmunity. Nature 328:805–811, 1987.

Siegel DL, Silberstein LE. Expression and characterization of recombinant anti-Rh(D) antibodies on filamentous phage: a model system for isolating human red blood cell antibodies by repertoire cloning. Blood 83:2334–2344, 1994.

Solomon A. Bence-Jones proteins and light chains of immunoglobulins. N Engl J Med 294:17–23, 91–98, 1976.

Solomon A, McLaughlin CL. Biosynthesis of low molecular weight (7S) and high molecular weight (19S) IgM. J Clin Invest 49:150–160, 1970.

Solvason N, Kearney JF. The human fetal omentum: a site of B cell generation. J Exp Med 175:397–404, 1992.

Staudt LM, Leonardo MJ. Transcriptional control of immunoglobulin genes. Annu Rev Immunol 9:373–398, 1992.

Steinberg AG. Globulin polymorphisms in man. Annu Rev Genet 3:25–52, 1969.

Steinberg AG, Wilson JA. Hereditary globulin factors and immune tolerance in man. Science 140:303–304, 1963.

Steinberg P, Ishizaka K, Norman PS. Possible role of IgE-mediated reaction in immunity. J Allergy Clin Immunol 54:359–366, 1974.

Stewart AK, Schwartz RS. Immunoglobulin V regions and the B cell. Blood 83:1717–1730, 1994.

Stiehm ER, Ammann AJ, Cherry JD. Elevated cord macroglobulins in the diagnosis of intrauterine infections. N. Engl J Med 275:971–977, 1966.

Stiehm ER, Fudenberg HH. Serum levels of immune globulins in health and disease: a survey. Pediatrics 37:715–727, 1966.

Tao M-H, Levy R. Idiotype/granulocyte-macrophage colony–stimulating factor fusion protein as a vaccine for B-cell lymphoma. Nature 362:755–758, 1993.

Taylor RB, Duffus PH, Ruff MC, De Petris S. Redistribution and pinocytosis of lymphocyte surface immunoglobulin molecules induced by anti-immunoglobulin antibody. Nature New Biol 233:225–229, 1971.

Teranishi T, Hirano T, Lin BH, Onoue K. Demonstration of the involvement of interleukin-2 in the differentiation of *Staphylococcus aureus* Cowan I–stimulated B-cells. J Immunol 133:3062–3067, 1984.

Terry WD. Variations in the subclasses of IgG. In Good RA, Bergsma D, eds. Immunologic Deficiency Diseases in Man. New York, National Foundation Press, 1968, pp. 357–361.

Terry WD, Fahey JL. Subclasses of human gamma-2-globulin based on differences in the heavy polypeptide chains. Science 146:400–401, 1964.

Tomana M, Zikan J, Moldoveanu Z, Kulhavy R, Bennett JC, Mestecky J. Interactions of cell-surface galactosyltransferase with immunoglobulins. Mol Immunol 30:265–275, 1993.

Tomasi TB Jr. Secretory immunoglobulins. N Engl J Med 287:500–506, 1972.

Tonegawa S. Somatic generation of antibody diversity. Nature 302:575–581, 1983.

Tsukada S, Saffran DC, Rawlings DJ, Parolini O, Cutler AR, Klisak I, Sparkes RS, Kubagawa H, Mohandas T, Quan S, Belmont JW, Cooper MD, Conley ME, Witte ON. Deficient expression of a B cell cytoplasmic tyrosine kinase in human X-linked agammaglobulinemia. Cell 72:279–290, 1993.

Turner MW, Bennich HH, Natvig JB. Simple method of subtyping human G-myeloma proteins based on sensitivity to pepsin digestion. Nature 225:853–855, 1970.

Uckun FM, Haissig S, Ledbetter JA, Fidler P, Myers DE, Kuebelbeck V, Weisdorf D, Gajl-Peczalska K, Kersey JH, Ramsay NKC. Developmental hierarchy during early human B-cell ontogeny after autologous bone marrow transplantation using autografts depleted of CD19$^+$ B-cell precursors by an anti-CD19 pan–B-cell immunotoxin containing pokeweed antiviral protein. Blood 79:3369–3379, 1992.

Uhr JW. Heterogeneity of the immune response. Science 145:457–464, 1964.

Urbanek R. IgG subclasses and subclass distribution in allergic disorders. In Skavaril F, Morrell A, Perret B, eds. Clinical Aspects of IgG Subclasses and Therapeutic implications. Monogr Allergy 16:33–40, 1988.

Vaerman JP, Heremans JF, Laurell CB. Distribution of alpha-chain subclasses in normal and pathological IgA-globulins. Immunology 14:425–432, 1968.

van der Meer JWM, Rádl J, Meyer CJL, Vossen JM, van Nieuwkoop JA, Lobatto S, van Furth R. Hyperimmunoglobulinaemia D and periodic fever: a new syndrome. Lancet 1:1087–1090, 1984.

van de Winkel JGJ, Capel PJA. Human IgG Fc receptor heterogeneity: molecular aspects and clinical implications. Immunol Today 14:215–220, 1993.

Van Loghem E, Aalberse RC, Matsumoto HA. A genetic marker of human IgE heavy chains, Em(1). Vox Sang 46:195–206, 1984.

van Noesel CJM, van Lier RAW. Architecture of the human B-cell antigen receptors. Blood 82:363–373, 1993.

Vasicek TJ, Leder P. Structure and expression of the human immunoglobulin lambda genes. J Exp Med 172:609–621, 1990.

Vercelli D, Geha RS. Control of IgE synthesis. In Middleton E Jr, et al., eds. Allergy: Principles and Practice, 4th ed. St. Louis, Mosby–Year Book, 1993, pp. 93–104.

Vitetta ES, Uhr JW. Immunoglobulin-receptors revisited. Science 189:964–969, 1975.

Vyas GN, Fudenberg HH. Am(1), the first genetic marker of human immunoglobulin A. Proc Natl Acad Sci U S A 64:1211–1216, 1969.

Wagner SD, Martinelli V, Luzzatto L. Similar patterns of V$_K$ gene usage but different degrees of somatic mutation in hairy cell leukemia, prolymphocytic leukemia, Waldenström's macroglobulinemia, and myeloma. Blood 83:3647–3653, 1994.

Waldmann TA, Strober N. Metabolism of immunoglobulins. Prog Allergy 13:1–110, 1969.

Weigle WO. Immunological unresponsiveness. Adv Immunol 16:61–122, 1973.

Weisbart RH, Kacena A, Schuh A, Golde DW. GM-CSF induces human neutrophil IgA-mediated phagocytosis by an IgA–Fc receptor activation mechanism. Nature 332:647–648, 1988.

WHO/IARC Technical Report: Identification, enumeration, and isolation of B- and T-lymphocytes from human peripheral blood. Scand J Immunol 3:521–532, 1974.

Winter G, Milstein C. Man-made antibodies. Nature 349:293–299, 1991.

World Health Organization (WHO). Nomenclature for human immunoglobulins. Bull WHO 30:447–450, 1964.

World Health Organization (WHO). Notation for genetic factors of human immunoglobulins. Bull WHO 33:721–724, 1965.

World Health Organization (WHO). Notation for human immunoglobulin subclasses. Bull WHO 35:953, 1966.

World Health Organization (WHO). An extension of the nomenclature for immunoglobulins. Immunochemistry 7:497–500, 1970.

Wright A, Morrison SL. Antibody variable region glycosylation: biochemical and clinical effects. Springer Semin Immunopathol 15:1–15, 1993.

Wright A, Shin S-U, Morrison SL. Genetically engineered antibodies: progress and prospects. CRC Crit Rev Immunol 12:125–168, 1992.

Yeung CY, Hobbs JR. Serum-gamma-G-globulin levels in normal, premature, post-mature, and ''small-for-dates'' newborn babies. Lancet 1:1167–1170, 1968.

Yount WJ, Hong R, Seligmann M, Good RA, Kunkel HC. Imbalances of gamma globulin subgroups and gene defects in patients with primary hypogammaglobulinemia. J Clin Invest 49:1957–1966, 1970.

Zachau HG. The immunoglobulin kappa locus—or what has been learned from looking closely at one-tenth of a percent of the human genome. Gene 135:167–173, 1993.

Zelaschi D, Newby C, Parsons M, Van West B, Cavalli-Sforza LL, Herzenberg LA. Human Ig allotypes: previously unrecognized determinants and alleles defined by monoclonal antibodies. Proc Natl Acad Sci U S A 80:3762–3766, 1983.

Zelenetz AD, Chen TT, Levy R. Clonal expansion in follicular lymphoma occurs subsequent to antigenic selection. J Exp Med 176:1137–1148, 1992.

Chapter 4

Cellular Interactions in the Human Immune Response

Loran T. Clement

For individuals interested in growth and development, the concept of cellular interactions occurring in an immune response should be familiar. In multicellular organisms, it is well accepted that orderly interactions among different cell types must occur for normal embryogenesis and for physiologic homeostasis thereafter. Furthermore, it is clear that abnormalities of these interactions may result in defects of serious consequence. Because the immune system must continually include cells capable of specific responses against new antigens, ongoing production of lymphoid cells is essential; thus, the cells and tissues that constitute the immune system never finish the process of growth and differentiation. Furthermore, immune cells must expand and mount vigorous memory responses upon re-exposure to previously encountered antigens. Thus, the two principal distinguishing features of the immune system, *antigen specificity* and *immunologic memory*, depend on intricate interactions among the different types of cells that make up the immune system.

In many respects, our understanding of the cellular interactions that occur during an immune response is more developed than is our knowledge of these events in other tissues. In large part, this is true because the basic functions of the immune system are performed by individual lymphocytes. Those studying the immune response have thus been able to isolate and grow individual cells in vitro in defined tissue culture media and to examine the structure and function of these cells (and their secreted products) in great detail. This discovery process has been nurtured by recent advances in monoclonal antibody technology and molecular biology. Lymphocytes with different effector functions or immunoregulatory capabilities can now be identified on the basis of their expression of different membrane proteins or their pattern of cytokine production. The ability to identify the cells involved in an immune response and to characterize the mechanisms by which these cells interact has also led to a markedly improved understanding of how defects or abnormalities of these interactions result in immune deficiencies or in the immune dysfunction found in an increasing number of diseases.

There are two principal mechanisms by which the cells that constitute the immune system interact. First, signaling may result from the physical interactions of the membrane proteins expressed by different cell types. In addition, lymphocytes and other cells involved in host defense mechanisms produce a large array of soluble factors, or cytokines, which mediate many of the intercellular communications between cells within the immune system. These soluble factors may act in an autocrine fashion, or they may influence cells found elsewhere in the body. In this chapter, the cells of the immune system, their cellular interactions, and the molecules mediating some of these interactions are introduced.

CELLS OF THE IMMUNE SYSTEM

Origin and Composition of the Immune System

The recognition of and reaction to foreign antigens by the immune system involves several different cell types (Kincade and Phillips, 1984; Paul, 1984). The primary effector cells of the immune system are lymphocytes. All lymphocytes are derived from pluripotent *stem cells* (Fig. 4–1), which originate in the embryonic yolk sac. During fetal development, these stem cells migrate, first to the fetal liver and, ultimately, to the bone marrow. Lymphocytes can be divided into three major classes:

1. *Thymus-derived lymphocytes,* or *T cells,* whose development is dependent on the thymus gland.
2. *B lymphocytes,* which develop in the liver during fetal life and in the bone marrow during adult life.
3. *Natural killer (NK) cells,* a population of large granular lymphocytes with cytotoxic functions.

Although it is clear that NK cells, which share certain features of myeloid cells and T lymphocytes, derive from bone marrow stem cells, the differentiation pathway by which these lymphoid cells are generated is currently poorly understood.

To perform the varied functions of the immune sys-

tem, lymphocytes (particularly T cells) must interact productively with another heterogeneous group of cells, which have been termed *accessory cells.* The majority (though not all) of the cells that perform these vital accessory cell functions are of monocyte/macrophage or B-lymphocyte lineage; thus, accessory cells derive from the same pluripotent stem cells that give rise to lymphoid cells.

The immune system is not localized to one anatomic site within the body. Rather, lymphoid tissues are found throughout the body. In addition to the primary (generative) lymphoid organs (thymus, bone marrow), lymphocytes and various accessory cell populations are organized in secondary lymphoid tissues throughout the body, such as in the spleen, lymph nodes, tonsils and adenoids, Peyer's patches, and lamina propria of various mucosal surfaces. Furthermore, large numbers of lymphocytes and monocytes circulate throughout the body, moving from the blood to tissues and recirculating back to the blood.

B Lymphocytes

The major contributions of B cells to the immune response are directly related to their ability to produce antibody molecules capable of binding to specific determinants (termed *epitopes*) of antigens. The first immunoglobulins produced by B cells consist of *membrane immunoglobulin* (Ig) molecules (Froland et al., 1971). These molecules are integral B-cell membrane proteins composed of two light chains (κ or λ), which are linked by disulfide bonds to two disulfide-linked heavy chains. The organization of the genetic elements that combine to produce immunoglobulin molecules is discussed in detail in Chapter 3, The B-Lymphocyte System.

Early in their ontogeny, B cells express *secretory IgM* and *secretory IgD* membrane immunoglobulins. These molecules are anchored to the cell membrane via the heavy-chain constant region; the variable regions of these molecules (which form the antigen-binding sites) are farthest from the membrane. Later in B-cell ontogeny, membrane IgG, IgA, or IgE molecules may be expressed. These integral membrane molecules are distinct from *cytophilic antibodies,* which bind to specific cell surface Fc receptors found on numerous cell types (e.g., NK cells) (Lobo et al., 1975).

The differentiation of B cells into antibody-secreting *plasma cells* is initiated when specific antigens bind to B-cell surface immunoglobulin receptor molecules. The resulting cross-linkage of these receptor molecules triggers a complex series of intracellular reactions, which are collectively referred to as *B-cell activation* (Figure 4–2). These activated B cells proliferate and mature into plasma cells, which secrete large amounts of antibody molecules that neutralize the noxious properties of certain antigens or serve as opsonins to promote antigen removal by phagocytosis. As discussed in Chapter 2, this maturational process is largely dependent on the actions of helper T cells. The immunoglobulin molecules produced by these plasma cells have the same antigen specificity (i.e., the same variable region sequences) as those expressed on their surfaces (Toneg-

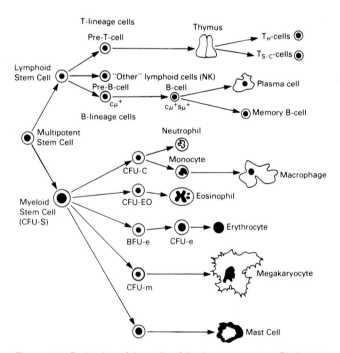

Figure 4–1. Derivation of the cells of the immune system. Pluripotent stem cells are derived from the yolk sac and ultimately reside in the bone marrow. Lymphocytes are derived from a lymphoid stem cell, whereas monocytes and macrophages are derived from myeloid stem cells. Lymphocytes can be divided into B-lineage cells and T-lineage cells. The differentiation pathway of natural killer (NK) lymphocytes is poorly defined. T_H = helper T; $T_{s/c}$ = suppressor/cytotoxic; $c\mu^+$ = cytoplasmic unit; $s\mu^+$ = surface unit; CFU = colony-forming unit; S = spleen; C = culture; EO = eosinophil; BFU-e = burst-forming unit–erythrocytic; CFU-e = colony-forming unit–erythrocytic; CFU-m = colony-forming unit–megakaryocytic.

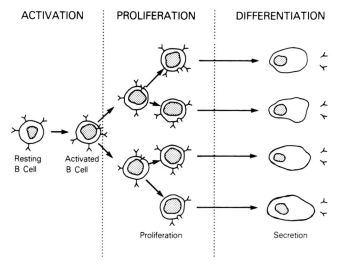

ACTIVATION   PROLIFERATION   DIFFERENTIATION

Resting B Cell   Activated B Cell   Proliferation   Secretion

Figure 4–2. Model for B-cell growth and differentiation. B lymphocytes are initially activated by antigen-mediated cross-linkage of their membrane surface immunoglobulin receptors. Signals generated by helper T cells then induce these activated B cells to undergo clonal proliferation. This may be followed by the terminal differentiation of these B cells into plasma cells that secrete antibody molecules.

awa, 1985). For the production of secretory IgM, messenger RNA (mRNA) sequences that encode for the transmembrane portion of the molecule are removed (Rogers et al., 1980), thereby yielding an immunoglobulin that cannot be anchored to the membrane. In other instances, there may be a "switch" of the constant region heavy-chain genes used during B-cell activation. This process, called *isotype switching*, results in the production of IgG, IgA, and IgE antibodies.

T Lymphocytes

In contrast to the limited functional repertoire of B cells, the functions of thymus-derived T cells are heterogeneous (see Chapter 2). These may be broadly categorized in the following fashion: (1) *delayed-type hypersensitivity* functions (many of which are mediated by myelomonocytic cells under the influence of T cell–derived cytokines), (2) *cytotoxic* host-defense functions, and (3) *immunoregulatory functions* (i.e., helper or suppressor functions that govern the magnitude and duration of other immune events).

Advances in understanding the cellular basis for the functional heterogeneity of T cells have come from several avenues. First, the ability to isolate and grow clones of T cells has provided the opportunity to study the attributes of single T cells and their progeny. Studies using T cells from patients with various immunodeficiency diseases and from patients with monoclonal T-cell neoplasms have also helped define the functional capacity of various human T-cell populations (Waldmann et al., 1974; Broder et al., 1976, 1978).

Finally, methods and reagents have been produced that enable identification of phenotypically and functionally distinct subpopulations of T lymphocytes. Early attempts to identify T-lymphocyte subpopulations employed heteroantisera (Evans et al., 1978), autoanti-

bodies (Morimoto et al., 1981), or analyses of the expression of Fc receptors for either IgG or IgM (Moretta et al., 1976; Shaw et al., 1979). The application of *monoclonal antibody* technology (Kohler and Milstein, 1975) and *flow cytometry* techniques has eclipsed these early approaches and revolutionized our understanding of the functional diversity of T cells and the complexity of the cellular interactions that regulate immune responses.

Because large numbers of monoclonal antibodies to human T cells (or subsets thereof) have been produced, workshops have been held to assign and codify the antigens recognized by various monoclonal antibodies using a *cluster of differentiation* (CD) nomenclature (Bernard et al., 1984). Some of the T-cell membrane proteins that have been identified by monoclonal antibodies are present on all T cells. Among the most prominent of these *pan–T-cell antigens* are CD3 and CD2 molecules.

CD3 Molecules. Expression of CD3 antigens is now generally regarded as the definitive marker for cells of T-lymphocyte lineage (Reinherz et al., 1979b). Membrane molecules expressing the CD3 antigen are first expressed during the intrathymic maturation of T cells (Reinherz et al., 1980a), and the density of antigen expression correlates with thymocyte maturation. The membrane molecules recognized by anti-CD3 antibodies are part of a CD3 molecular complex that contains as many as five different invariant proteins; three distinct, but structurally similar 20- to 25-kilodalton (kd) glycoprotein subunits (γ, δ, and ϵ chains) are complexed with a disulfide-linked dimer containing ζ or η chains (Borst et al., 1984; van den Elsen et al., 1984, 1985; Clevers et al., 1988). The heterodimeric *T-cell antigen receptor* (TCR) is also associated with this molecular complex. Thus, the membrane proteins recognized by anti-CD3 antibodies are critical components of the complex that triggers T-cell activation and function following exposure to exogenous antigen.

CD2 Molecules. The CD2 molecule is a glycoprotein 50 kd that is expressed by all human T cells, as well as by a subset of NK lymphocytes. The primary physiologic role of CD2 molecules appears to involve promoting the adhesion of T cells to other cell types (Bierer et al., 1989); in this regard, it has been shown that CD2 molecules mediate the curious ability of human T cells to bind to sheep erythrocytes (Froland, 1972; Kamoun et al., 1981; Verbi et al., 1982). This ability enables T cells to form rosettes with sheep erythrocytes and is the origin of the archaic synonym *erythrocyte rosette-forming cells*.

The ligand for CD2 molecules is the CD58 (leukocyte function–associated [LFA]–3) antigen, which is expressed by certain lymphocytes, monocytes, endothelial cells, and a variety of other cell types. The cellular interactions mediated by T-cell CD2 molecules appear to be of functional significance because antibodies to either the CD2 molecule or its ligand inhibit a number of T-cell functions (Sanchez-Madrid et al., 1982). Because certain anti-CD2 monoclonal antibodies are able to activate T cells, it has been proposed that

CD2 molecules may be a component of an alternative pathway of T-cell activation (Meuer et al., 1984).

In addition to these pan–T-cell molecules, numerous other T-cell membrane antigens have been identified with monoclonal antibodies. Many of these molecules mediate T-cell functions and may serve as markers for functionally distinct T-cell subpopulations. For example, the CD4 and CD8 antigens identify reciprocal subsets of T cells with distinct effector and immunoregulatory functions (Evans et al., 1981; Reinherz et al., 1980a). The functions of these molecules and the characteristics of the T-cell subsets they define are discussed later in the context of the functions they perform.

Accessory Cells

Although lymphocytes are the main effector cells of the immune system, the initiation of an immune response is dependent on the actions of other cell types, collectively referred to as accessory cells. The most prominent functions of these accessory cells involve the processing (degrading) of exogenous antigen and the subsequent presentation of antigenic peptides to T lymphocytes; this interactive process is discussed in detail later in this chapter. Most of these *antigen-presenting cells* (APCs) are of monocyte/macrophage lineage. They include blood monocytes, tissue macrophages, *Langerhans' cells* in skin, interdigitating *dendritic cells* in nodes and spleen, and microglial cells in neural tissues. In addition, it is clear that *B cells* may also act as APCs, particularly if they have been activated by the cross-linking of their antigen receptors; indeed, under some conditions, B cells may serve as the primary APCs (Ron and Sprent, 1987).

Finally, certain specialized epithelial or endothelial cells are also capable of processing and presenting antigens in a form that can be recognized by T cells, particularly after their exposure to cytokines that induce class II major histocompatibility complex (MHC) antigen expression, such as interferon-α (IFN-γ).

CELLULAR INTERACTIONS: HISTORICAL PERSPECTIVES

A new era in immunology began with the discovery that the thymus gland played a major role in the immune response (Miller, 1961; Archer et al., 1962). One of the first indications that several cell types might be interacting in the antibody response to foreign antigens was provided by the discovery that both thymus-derived T lymphocytes and bone marrow–derived B lymphocytes were necessary for murine antibody responses to occur (Claman et al., 1966). The T cells involved in this response were called *helper T cells* because they provided assistance necessary for antibody production by the B cells (Miller and Mitchell, 1969; Davies, 1969). These findings were followed closely by the observation of Mosier (1967) that adherent cells (monocytes/macrophages) as well as nonadherent lymphocytes were required for antibody responses. Thus, it appeared that at least three cell types were necessary

for murine antibody responses: helper T cells, bone marrow–derived B cells, and adherent accessory cells.

It was later shown that murine T cells could be subdivided into two populations differing in their expression of certain alloantigens (Cantor and Asofsky, 1972). The existence of T cells capable of actively suppressing antibody responses (suppressor T cells) was also discovered (Gershon and Kondo, 1970). T cells were also shown to have the capacity of disrupting the membrane integrity of other cells by a process termed *cytotoxicity* (Cerottini et al., 1970). Thus, it was clear that lymphocytes showed considerable heterogeneity in terms of their functional capabilities.

These observations set the stage for the discovery that T cells from one strain of inbred mice would not cooperate with B cells from a genetically different strain of inbred mice for an antibody response in vivo (Katz et al., 1973). Thus, there appeared to be genetically determined restrictions on the interaction of T cells and B cells. Similarly, it was shown that antigen-induced memory T cells would proliferate if presented with an appropriate antigen on the surface of macrophages, and that there were genetic restrictions in this interaction between T cells and accessory APCs (Rosenthal and Shevach, 1973). Subsequently, Zinkernagel and Doherty (1974) and Shearer and colleagues (1975) demonstrated that genetic restrictions also govern interactions between cytotoxic T cells and antigen-bearing target cells. In each case, these genetic restrictions were mapped to a set of MHC genes. These studies provided the foundation for much of our knowledge of the cellular interactions and the restrictions on these interactions occurring in the human immune response.

Most studies of the human immune response have been performed in vitro using mononuclear cells isolated from blood by density-gradient centrifugation by means of Ficoll-Hypaque gradients (Boyum, 1968). The ability to isolate human T cells by rosette formation with sheep erythrocytes (Chess et al., 1974) enabled analyses of the cellular interactions involved. In addition, certain patients with immune defects ("experiments of nature") provided important insights (Good, 1975; Waldmann et al., 1974). Most early studies of human cells examined the proliferative response of T cells activated in vitro by polyclonal mitogens, such as phytohemagglutinin (PHA), concanavalin A (Con A), and pokeweed mitogen (PWM). Comparable techniques using polyclonal T-cell activators were developed to assess B-cell immunoglobulin production (Wu et al., 1973), T-helper cell activity for immunoglobulin synthesis (Broder et al., 1976), T-suppressor cell activity for immunoglobulin synthesis (Waldmann et al., 1974), and cytotoxic T-cell function (Nelson et al., 1976).

The first in vitro studies of antigen-specific immune responses relied on the activation of cells by allogeneic stimulator cells in the mixed leukocyte reaction (MLR). These cultures were used to assess the proliferative responses of T cells (Bain et al., 1964) and the generation of alloantigen-specific cytotoxic T cells (Stejskal et al., 1974), which were then analyzed in short-term radioisotope-release cytotoxicity assays (Nelson, 1981).

Subsequently, antigen-specific methods for assessing T-cell proliferation or cytotoxic function have emerged (Bergholtz and Thorsby, 1978; Biddison et al., 1979; Yarchoan et al., 1982). The remainder of this chapter focuses primarily on the cell surface molecules and cellular interactions involved in these immune responses.

MEMBRANE MOLECULES MEDIATING CELLULAR INTERACTIONS

The basic framework of cell membranes is a double layer of lipid molecules (Bretscher, 1985). Residing within this lipid membrane are membrane proteins, which are of two general types: (1) globular proteins and glycoproteins (sugar-modified proteins) residing largely within the hydrophobic membrane, and (2) proteins and glycoproteins residing largely outside the cell membrane (Fig. 4–3). This second type of membrane protein typically has a hydrophobic string of amino acids (the transmembrane region) that spans the lipid bilayer, and a short, hydrophilic, intracellular tail that extends into the cytoplasm. The membrane proteins that play a role in the cell-cell communications within the immune system are largely of this variety. In addition, many of these membrane glycoproteins share sequence homology with immunoglobulin molecules and thus belong to what is termed the *immunoglobulin supergene family*. It has been speculated that the genes encoding for these molecules may have derived from a single gene that encodes a primordial integral cell surface glycoprotein involved in cell-cell recognition (Hood et al., 1985; Matsunaga, 1985).

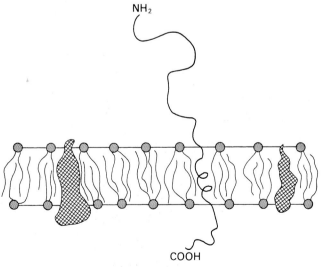

Figure 4–3. The basic components of cell membranes. Cell membranes consist of double layers of lipid molecules with hydrophilic heads (stippled) and hydrophobic tails that align themselves to form water-impermeable membranes. Incorporated in this lipid bilayer are glycoproteins; these may be either globular proteins (crosshatched), which reside largely within the membrane, or integral proteins, which are largely extracellular. A typical integral protein of this nature consists of a large extracellular domain (containing the NH$_2$-terminal amino acid), a transmembrane domain, and an intracytoplasmic tail (containing the carboxyl-terminal amino acid).

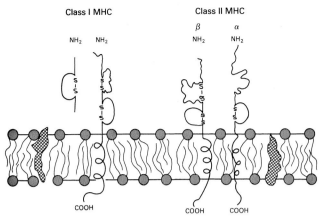

Figure 4–4. Schematic depiction of class I and class II major histocompatibility complex (MHC) antigens. Intrachain disulfide bonds are depicted by S—S. Those portions of the molecules that are polymorphic, and thus vary from individual to individual, are shown as irregular lines; those portions of the molecules that are largely invariant (constant) are shown as smooth lines.

The Major Histocompatibility Complex

The discovery of genes that are located in what is now termed the major histocompatibility gene complex (MHC) originated from studies examining the transplantation of different tissues between members of a species. Regardless of the species examined, a consistent finding of these studies was that tissues transplanted from one individual to an unrelated individual of the same species *(allografts)* did not survive. This barrier resulted from an immunologic attack against the tissue allografts, a process termed *rejection*. The molecules expressed by transplanted tissues that were responsible for this rejection phenomenon were called histocompatibility antigens (Sachs, 1984; Kindt and Robinson, 1984). It was subsequently found that the histocompatibility antigens that provoked the strongest, most rapid rejection of tissue allografts were encoded for by a set of closely linked genetic loci in a region referred to as the MHC.

Because an organism rarely encounters allogeneic cells from unrelated members of its species, it is not surprising that these cell surface molecules have functions other than providing a barrier against tissue transplantation. As mentioned previously, a seminal discovery for understanding the interactions of cells that constitute the immune system was the finding that the cell surface molecules that restrict the interactions among different cell types were encoded by genes that map to the MHC. In addition, these highly polymorphic MHC molecules govern intrathymic selection of T cells. Thus, MHC molecules provide the basis for discriminating *self* from *non-self* that lies at the heart of the remarkable specificity of the immune system.

The genetic locus of the human MHC is on chromosome 6. The MHC genes are inherited in haplotypic fashion from each parent and are codominantly expressed. The MHC has been subdivided into three major regions based on the molecules that these loci encode. The class I and class II MHC genes encode for two distinct groups of molecules that exhibit considerable intraclass structural similarities (Fig. 4–4). These molecules, which serve as restriction elements for T-cell antigen recognition, are discussed next. (In contrast, class III MHC gene products, a heterogeneous group of more than 20 proteins that includes a number of complement components, are not directly involved in cell interactions.)

Class I Major Histocompatibility Complex Antigens

The membrane molecules encoded for by class I MHC genes consist of a single integral membrane glycoprotein (molecular mass ~45 kd). These molecules have a large extracellular segment (consisting of three domains), a small transmembrane region, and a small intracytoplasmic tail. The extracellular portion of these molecules is associated noncovalently with a smaller glycoprotein (~12 kd) termed β_2-microglobulin, which in humans is encoded by a gene found on chromosome 15. This protein is necessary for the membrane expression of all class I molecules (Zylstra et al., 1990).

Class I MHC gene products are highly polymorphic (i.e., they differ among individuals of the same species) and represent, in humans, the cell surface human leukocyte antigens (HLAs) HLA-A, HLA-B, and HLA-C. There are approximately 20 different allelic forms of the HLA-A antigen, 50 forms of the HLA-B antigen, and 11 forms of the HLA-C antigen. In contrast, β_2-microglobulin exhibits no polymorphism. The HLA class I proteins and β_2-microglobulin both share considerable amino acid sequence homology with immunoglobulin constant region domains. Class I antigens are expressed on virtually all nucleated cells of humans; they are not expressed on erythrocytes.

Studies of the structure of class I MHC antigens have provided a model for the basis by which these molecules function as restriction elements for T-cell recognition of antigen (Sette et al., 1989; Shimojo et al., 1990). According to this model, a peptide-binding groove bordered by two of the extracellular domains of the class I α chain is formed in the tertiary conformation of these molecules. Prior to membrane expression of class I molecules, this groove must bind to endogenously generated peptides. If these peptides are non-self (as would be the case if they were generated by viral genes, for example), these molecules will be recognized as foreign by specific TCR molecules. The peptide-binding region of class I MHC molecules is distinct from the alloantigenic epitopes identified by serologic tissue-typing techniques. However, much of the sequence polymorphism of these molecules is located in areas that lie in the vicinity of this groove (Shimojo et al., 1990). Thus, polymorphism of class I antigens, as reflected in the three-dimensional structure of this groove, is a determinant of which peptides will bind to a particular class I molecule and the nature of the TCR that recognizes this complex.

Class II Major Histocompatibility Complex Antigens

Class II MHC products are heterodimers consisting of two noncovalently associated glycoproteins (see Fig. 4–4). The class II MHC antigens of humans are termed HLA-DR, HLA-DQ, and HLA-DP antigens. The two protein chains of class II MHC antigens are encoded by 12 to 15 distinct structural genes located within the HLA-D region of the MHC; many of these genes show considerable allelic polymorphism. The larger α chain has a molecular mass of approximately 33 kd, whereas the lighter β chain has a mass of approximately 28 kd. Because of the allelic polymorphism of the HLA-DB loci, the β chains of different class II molecules are generally more polymorphic than are the α chains, although sequence heterogeneity of the α chains of human HLA-DQ and HLA-DP is also seen. In contrast to class I antigens, class II MHC antigens are constitutively expressed only by B lymphocytes, monocytes, and certain other specialized cell types, such as Langerhans' cells (Dezutter-Dambuyant et al., 1984) and the large intrathymic *nurse cells* that engulf thymocytes (Ritter et al., 1981). However, expression of class II MHC molecules can be induced on certain other cell types, including activated T cells (Ko et al., 1979) and a variety of endothelial and epithelial populations, especially after exposure to IFN-γ. This finding has implications for current theories concerning the pathogenesis of autoimmune disorders (see Chapters 24 and 26).

The transcription of class II MHC structural genes is coordinately regulated by two or more *trans*-acting genes that are not linked to the MHC (Salter et al., 1985). These regulatory genes produce DNA-binding proteins that bind to conserved *cis*-active upstream promoter elements (termed the *X* and *Y* boxes) and thus initiate gene transcription. This process may also involve accessory proteins that organize class II promoters into a configuration accessible to binding proteins or otherwise enhance the association of DNA-binding proteins with promoter sequences (Kara and Glimcher, 1993).

The principal function identified for class II MHC antigens involves their pivotal role in the presentation of antigen to T cells. As described earlier for class I MHC molecules, it is believed that the three-dimensional conformation of these molecules forms a peptide-binding groove that binds fragments of processed exogenous antigen. When this complex is expressed on the surface of APCs, it is recognized as non-self by specific TCR molecules of T cells. Class II MHC antigens may also transduce activation signals during this interaction.

The initial characterization of the different class II MHC molecules expressed by human cells was achieved by serologic methods using defined alloantisera or monoclonal antibodies. In addition, class II MHC antigen expression can be assessed in the MLR. Although these typing techniques are still widely used for tissue transplantation, molecular methods for *oligotyping* class II genes are emerging (Tiercy et al., 1991) and promise to be important tools for future studies of the structure and function of class II MHC antigens and their possible role in the pathogenesis of disease.

T-Cell Antigen Receptor

The human T-cell antigen receptor (TCR) is a 90-kd disulfide-linked heterodimer (Acuto and Reinherz,

1985). The polypeptide chains that make up TCRs are encoded by distinct genes on separate chromosomes (see Chapter 2). Both chains are integral membrane glycoproteins with large extracellular domains, a transmembrane domain, and an intracytoplasmic tail. Two forms of this receptor have been identified. The TCR-2 receptor, which is expressed by 90% of T cells, consists of an α chain (51-kd) and a β chain (43-kd). The remaining 10% of T cells express the TCR-1 receptor, which is composed of disulfide-linked γ and δ chains. T cells expressing TCR-1 molecules may differentiate in extrathymic sites and appear to have a more limited repertoire than do T cells expressing TCR-2 molecules. As for B-cell immunoglobulin receptors, both TCR chains have variable and constant domains. However, the nature of the antigenic determinants recognized by TCR molecules (i.e., linear amino acid sequences of small peptide fragments) differs significantly from those bound by B-cell immunoglobulin receptors (i.e., conformational epitopes determined by the tertiary structure of intact antigen molecules).

As noted previously, TCR molecules are complexed with the CD3 subunits to form the CD3/TCR complex. Immunoprecipitation of the CD3 complex from cell surfaces coprecipitates TCR molecules (Borst et al., 1983), and modulation of CD3 molecules from the cell surface simultaneously removes TCR molecules (Meuer et al., 1983). Signals transduced by this complex are critical for initiating T-cell activation, and monoclonal antibodies reactive with either CD3 or TCR molecules are mitogenic for T cells (Van Wauwe et al., 1980). Similarly, in higher concentrations, these antibodies share the ability to inhibit numerous T-cell functions (Chang et al., 1981; Reinherz et al., 1981; Platsoucas and Good, 1981).

Accessory Molecules

It has become clear that the interaction of the CD3/TCR complex with foreign antigen in the context of self-MHC molecules is not sufficient to induce T-cell activation. In addition to this pivotal event, interactions between other membrane molecules and their ligands are also necessary for effective functioning of the immune system (Springer, 1990). These interactions serve two purposes; they increase the avidity or otherwise stabilize cellular interactions and transduce signals to the interior of the cells. Some of the membrane molecules that play important roles in these cell-cell interactions are shown in Table 4–1. Among these are the CD4 and CD8 antigens.

As discussed later, the extracellular domain of these molecules can bind to nonpolymorphic determinants of MHC antigens; CD4 molecules bind to class II MHC antigens, whereas CD8 molecules bind to class I MHC antigens (Bierer et al., 1989). If these interactions fail to occur, T-cell functions are adversely affected. For example, anti-CD4 antibodies inhibit CD4+ T-cell proliferation and cytotoxic responses induced by class II MHC molecules (Engleman et al., 1981; Biddison et al., 1982). In analogous fashion, anti-CD8 antibodies inhibit proliferative and cytotoxic responses of CD8+

Table 4–1. Membrane Molecules Mediating Cellular Interactions

Membrane Molecule	Ligand
CD4	Class II MHC antigens
CD8	Class I MHC antigens
CD2	CD58 (LFA-3)
CD5	CD72
CD40	CD40 ligand (gp39)
CD28	B7-1 (CD80) and B7-2
CD43	CD54
CD11a/CD18	CD54

cells to class I MHC antigens (Evans et al., 1981; Reinherz et al., 1981; Biddison et al., 1982). This antibody-mediated inhibition of the binding of CD4 and CD8 molecules to nonpolymorphic parts of class II and class I MHC antigens, respectively, interrupts the generation of signals required for activating the p56lck protein-tyrosine kinase associated with the intracytoplasmic tails of CD4 and CD8 molecules.

Another class of molecules that appears to be meaningfully involved in the cellular interactions of the immune system is the β2 integrin family. These heterodimeric proteins contain two chains: an α chain from the CD11 group, which distinguishes the different members of this family, and a β-subunit, termed CD18, which is common to all members of the subfamily. The expression of many members of this family is upregulated when cells are activated. Members of the β2 integrin family include the LFA-1 (CD11a/CD18) antigen; this molecule comprises a CD11a α chain (170–180 kd) that is noncovalently linked to the CD18 β chain (95 kd). Other members of this integrin family include the CR3 (CD11b/CD18) and CR4 (CD11c/CD18) complement receptors (Beller et al., 1982). The LFA-1 antigen is widely expressed on virtually all peripheral lymphocytes, thymocytes, granulocytes, monocytes, and one third of bone marrow cells (Krensky et al., 1984). The ligands for this integrin, called *intercellular adhesion molecule* (ICAM)–1 (CD54) and ICAM-2 (CD102), are also found on a variety of hematopoietic, lymphoid, and endothelial cell types. In view of the ubiquitous expression of these molecules, it is not surprising that these molecules mediate a variety of cellular interactions pertinent to the functions of the immune system. Thus, antibodies reactive with LFA-1 inhibit numerous immune functions, including the induction of T-cell proliferation by APCs and the priming and effector functions of cytotoxic cell populations (Sanchez-Madrid et al., 1982; Hildreth et al., 1983). In addition to mediating intercellular interactions, these integrins also help to regulate cell migration throughout the body.

As noted, the CD2 pan–T-cell antigen and its ligand, the CD58 (LFA-3) antigen, also mediate important interactions between T cells and other cell types. The CD58 molecule is expressed on 40 to 60% of peripheral T cells and B cells and on virtually all monocytes, platelets, endothelial cells, and fibroblasts. Both anti-CD2 and anti-CD58 antibodies inhibit T-cell proliferative responses to mitogens and antigens (Sanchez-

Madrid et al., 1982). Furthermore, both types of antibodies block T cell–mediated cytolytic function; the anti-CD2 antibodies block the binding of molecules expressed by the cytotoxic effector T cells, whereas the anti-CD58 antibodies impede the binding function of target cell molecules. Finally, as described later, interactions of the CD28 and CTLA-4 molecules expressed by T cells and their ligands, the B7 (CD80) and B7-2 molecules on APCs, provide a second signal during antigen presentation that is essential for T-cell activation; in the absence of this signal, T cells become unresponsive, resulting in *clonal anergy*, or tolerance.

ANTIGEN PROCESSING AND PRESENTATION

Generation of Antigenic Fragments

The initial event in the cascade of cellular interactions that leads to an immune response by T cells is the processing and subsequent presentation of antigen in a form that can be recognized by the TCR complex (Germain, 1993). Because less than 1% of an exogenous antigen load is processed in this immunologically relevant fashion, antigen processing and presentation appear to be rate-limiting steps in the immune response. As noted previously, APCs include monocytes, *tissue macrophages, Langerhans' cells* in skin, *interdigitating dendritic cells* in nodes and spleen, *microglial cells*, and *B lymphocytes* (Knight and Stagg, 1993). These cells appear to differ somewhat in their ability to serve as APCs for a particular immune response. For example, B cells appear to be particularly important as APCs for the T cell/B cell interactions involved in memory humoral responses (Finkelman et al., 1992). In contrast, monocyte-lineage cells and interdigitating dendritic cells appear to be the primary APCs for cell-mediated immune responses (Knight and Stagg, 1993).

The cellular organization of lymphoid tissues promotes the interaction of APCs with T cells. For example, interdigitating dendritic cells have numerous long processes that extend throughout the paracortical regions of lymph nodes. The proximity of these APCs to a large number of monospecific T cells thus enhances the likelihood that antigen presentation and immune response will ensue (Steinman, 1991).

Exogenous antigen is internalized by APCs via *phagocytosis, pinocytosis*, or receptor-mediated *endocytosis* in vesicles, which fuse with enzyme-rich lysosomes to form phagolysosomes (Lanzavecchia, 1990). The antigen is then degraded by limited proteolysis, producing multiple peptides. These linear peptide fragments may then complex with class II MHC antigens within these endosomes, or they may be delivered by transporter proteins to the rough endoplasmic reticulum, where they can associate with newly synthesized class I MHC molecules (Schwartz, 1990a.). As noted previously, it is believed that these antigen fragments bind to a peptide-binding groove formed by the three-dimensional conformation of MHC molecules. These assembled complexes are then re-expressed on the surface of

APCs in a form that can be recognized as non-self by specific TCR molecules of T cells.

The MHC molecules expressed by APCs influence antigen presentation both quantitatively and qualitatively. For example, the density of the membrane class II MHC antigens expressed by APCs directly affects the efficiency of antigen presentation; up-regulation (or de novo induction) of class II MHC expression enhances a cell's capability to present foreign antigen. In addition, because fragments of processed antigen must bind in the peptide-binding groove of MHC molecules, the ability of a particular fragment to bind to a particular MHC antigen depends on the structural characteristics of the groove; this, in turn, is determined by the amino acid sequence of the MHC molecule. Because much of the polymorphism of these molecules is located in areas that lie in the vicinity of the peptide-binding groove, MHC antigens differ in their ability to bind the various peptide fragments generated. Thus, the structural characteristics of MHC molecules affect the formation of these specific complexes that are recognized by specific T cells.

Although recognition of the antigen-MHC molecular complex on the surface of APCs by T-cell antigen receptor molecules provides a critical T-cell activation signal, the interaction of these cells is not mediated solely by these molecules. As noted previously, auxiliary interactions also occur between CD4 or CD8 molecules and the nonpolymorphic region of class II or class I MHC molecules. Ligand-receptor interactions between LFA-1 (CD11a/CD18) molecules and CD54 (ICAM-1) molecules and between CD2 molecules and CD58 (LFA-3) molecules also appear to be essential. These accessory interactions not only stabilize the cell-cell binding but also provide signals to each cell type that heighten their functions. Furthermore, there is considerable evidence that a second signal is also needed for T-cell activation and IL-2 production. Considerable attention has been focused on the CD28 and CTLA-4 T-cell membrane molecules and on the B7-1 (CD80) and B7-2 molecules expressed by B cells and other types of APCs as mediators of this second signal (Linsley et al., 1991; Gimmi et al., 1991; Freeman et al., 1993). There is evidence that a signal generated by the binding of these T-cell molecules to their APC ligands during antigen presentation is essential for T-cell activation. In the absence of this costimulatory signal, TCR-mediated signals may actually inactivate T cells such that they are unable to respond on re-exposure to antigen; this antigen-induced unresponsiveness is termed *clonal anergy* (Schwartz, 1990b; Harding et al., 1992).

Fruitful interactions of the many molecular ligands expressed by APCs and T cells generate a complex series of signals that collectively trigger T-cell activation (see Chapter 2). As discussed later, these activated T cells then produce and secrete a variety of cytokines that mediate the clonal expansion and functional differentiation of T and B cells and promote the delayed-type hypersensitivity functions of cells of monocyte/macrophage lineage (Fraser et al., 1993; Stout, 1993).

Superantigens

Superantigens are proteins produced by certain microorganisms that directly activate certain T cells; most are produced by bacteria, although some are virally produced (Kotzin et al., 1993). These substances have attracted considerable attention as a result of their ability to induce T-cell activation by a novel mechanism that involves the same molecules used by APCs and T cells for classical antigen recognition but independent of antigen processing or presentation.

Molecules that can act as superantigens have two binding elements. The first binds to a nonpolymorphic region of class II MHC molecules that is distinct from the peptide-binding groove; the other specifically binds to a site on the β TCR subunits that is encoded for by specific variable β ($V_β$) genes. The linkage of these molecules by superantigen proteins induces T-cell activation; all T cells expressing the $V_β$ gene product recognized by a given superantigen may be activated, regardless of their antigen recognition specificity. This process can influence the T-cell repertoire during intrathymic generation. Superantigens may produce tolerance and/or anergy of certain T-cell populations. In addition to their involvement in certain diseases, such as those caused by staphylococcal enterotoxins or the toxic shock syndrome toxin, superantigens may have a role in the pathogenesis of autoimmune disorders (Kotzin et al., 1993).

SOLUBLE FACTORS (CYTOKINES)

Many of the major advances in our understanding of the mechanisms by which lymphoid cells regulate the magnitude and duration of an immune response have been achieved as a result of the identification, characterization, and standardization of soluble factors produced by cells that constitute the immune system. It is now clear that cytokines regulate or influence virtually every aspect of immune cell growth, differentiation, and function. These factors, generally small, single-chain peptides, are produced by virtually all cell types in the immune system (particularly by T cells and monocytes). Although some cytokines are constitutively produced, most are synthesized and secreted as a consequence of activation signals that lead to cytokine gene expression. These soluble factors then produce their biologic effects by interacting with specific membrane receptors expressed by various cell types.

Although most of the cytokines that are produced by or act on cells of the immune system have unique attributes, certain noteworthy characteristics are commonly shared by these disparate factors:

1. The effects mediated by cytokines are typically pleiotropic, i.e., each cytokine has many effects, typically affecting multiple cell types.
2. There is functional redundancy, i.e., several different cytokines may perform a similar, or even identical, function.
3. Cytokines are often functionally linked with one another. This linking may be manifest as true synergy (in which two cytokines act together to produce a biologic effect much greater than the aggregate of their individual effects) or the cytokines may be components of a sequential *cascade* or network in which the action of one cytokine influences—positively or negatively—the production, function, or receptor expression of another cytokine.
4. One cytokine may be produced by many cell types.

Attempts to unravel the complexity of cytokine effects and interactions have benefited from a number of technical advances. Because the genes for most of these factors have been cloned, many of the factors can be synthesized by recombinant DNA technology, thereby providing significant amounts of highly purified material for studies investigating cytokine function and cytokine receptors and for the production of neutralizing antibodies. In addition, gene transfection techniques and the breeding of transgenic mice have provided important information. Finally, the use of site-directed mutagenesis to produce mutant cell lines and "knockout" mice in which a single cytokine gene is rendered inactive have provided insight into which essential functions are mediated by a given cytokine alone.

Most cytokines were initially named according to their ability to produce a particular biologic effect. As the ability to characterize biochemically and quantify these factors improved, it became clear that many of these nominal factors were structurally identical. This discovery has led to the adoption of a standardized interleukin nomenclature system for cytokines that have been suitably characterized (see Appendix 2). Although a detailed discussion of all soluble factors that can affect the human immune response is beyond the scope of this chapter, the characteristics of those factors that are particularly relevant to immune cell interactions are introduced next. A comprehensive list of cytokines is presented in Appendix 2.

Interleukin-1 (IL-1). The IL-1 family in humans is made up of two molecules: IL-α, a 33-kd molecule, and IL-1β, a 17-kd molecule. These molecules are produced by separate genes (Auron et al., 1984; March et al., 1985). Although they have only 24% homology, the two molecules use the same receptors. This cytokine is produced by a wide variety of cell types, but cells of monocyte origin appear to be particularly important sources. Because most cells in the body express receptors for IL-1, it is not surprising that this cytokine has extremely diverse biologic activities. Its effects on T cells, B cells, NK cells, monocytes, neutrophils, fibroblasts, hepatocytes, muscle cells, and numerous other tissues have been described (Dinarello, 1985; Akira et al., 1990). A prominent effect is to provide costimulatory signals that enhance T- and B-cell activation. IL-1 increases cytokine production by these (and other) cell types, up-regulates expression of cytokine receptors for IL-2, or both. IL-1 also has an important role as a mediator of tissue inflammation, enhancing prostaglandin synthesis, inducing enzyme production (especially collagenase), increasing the expression of adhesion molecules, and acting on the central nervous system to cause fever. Interestingly, the effects of IL-1 are counteracted by an IL-1 receptor antagonist. This 18-kd molecule binds to receptors for IL-1, thereby blocking their access to IL-1, but it provides no agonist signals.

Interleukin-2 (IL-2). Initially isolated and characterized as a T-cell growth factor (Morgan et al., 1976), IL-2 is a single protein of lymphocyte origin with relatively restricted biologic activities (Cantrell and Smith, 1984). This molecule (~15 kd) is encoded for by a single gene (Taniguchi et al., 1983). IL-2 is produced by T cells and, to a lesser extent, NK cells. Although CD4$^+$ T cells are the principal source, certain activated CD8$^+$ T cells can also produce this cytokine. In mice, most activated CD4$^+$ T cells can produce IL-2, although this ability is lacking or lost in type 2 helper T (T$_H$2) cells (discussed later). Studies of human T cells have shown that *naive* T cells produce more IL-2 than do memory cells; this is true for both the CD4$^+$ and CD8$^+$ subpopulations.

The primary functions of IL-2 are related to its ability to support lymphocyte proliferation and differentiation. This cytokine supports the clonal expansion of activated T cells, and it increases their production of other cytokines, such as IFN-γ. IL-2 also promotes T-cell differentiation; it is essential for the differentiation of activated cytotoxic T-lymphocyte (CTL) precursor cells into cytotoxic effector cells, and it is an important component for the post-thymic generation of memory T cells. Similarly, IL-2 is active as a growth factor for activated B cells and for NK cells, a property that is exploited for generating *lymphokine-activated killer (LAK) cells*. Finally, IL-2 may also activate macrophages.

The effects of IL-2 are mediated through specific cell surface receptors (Uchiyama et al., 1981; Leonard et al., 1983). The human IL-2 receptor is formed by three peptides and can exist in three forms. The β chain, a 75-kd molecule that is expressed at low levels by most resting lymphocytes, has intermediate affinity for IL-2. This chain is associated with a 64-kd γ chain, which is thought to endow the β chain with the ability to bind IL-2. In contrast, the low-affinity, 55-kd α-chain receptor (termed Tac or CD25) (Leonard et al., 1984; Nikaido et al., 1984), is expressed only following lymphocyte activation. The α chain complexes with the β chain to form the high-affinity IL-2 receptor. All IL-2 receptor components are up-regulated by the action of IL-2; this is also effected by IL-1 and IL-6. Soluble forms of the CD25 α-chain receptor are released by activated T cells and B cells (Rubin et al., 1985; Nelson et al., 1986) and are present in the serum in many disorders in which immune activity is high. Because this receptor binds IL-2, it may play an immunoregulatory role in the human immune response.

Interleukin-4 (IL-4). This cytokine, a 15-kd molecule initially described as a B-cell growth factor, has a number of important functions affecting humoral immune responses. IL-4, which is produced by activated T cells, mast cells, and basophils, is involved in early stages of B-cell activation, up-regulating the expression of B-cell class II MHC antigens and CD23

(an IgE receptor) antigens (Ambrus et al., 1985; Mehta et al., 1985). In addition, IL-4, which is perhaps the archetypic lymphokine produced by the T$_H$2 cell subset, induces isotype switching necessary for the production of IgG1 and IgE antibodies (Gascan et al., 1991). IL-4 also counteracts many of the effects of IFN-γ and thus inhibits the functions of type 1 helper T (T$_H$1) cells. IL-4 is able to induce T-cell differentiation in the thymus, and it acts as a growth factor (typically in an IL-2–independent fashion) for mature T cells. Finally, IL-4 is a potent mast-cell growth factor.

Interleukin-5 (IL-5). This cytokine was also first described as a B-cell growth factor. It is produced primarily by activated T cells (particularly T$_H$2 cells). In addition to its effects on B-cell proliferation and differentiation, IL-5 is a major factor inducing eosinophil differentiation and eosinophilia. A role for IL-5 in CTL differentiation has also been described.

Interleukin-6 (IL-6). In many respects, IL-6 is the epitome of a multifunctional cytokine (Akira et al., 1990). Although this 20-kd molecule is produced by many cell types (T and B cells, endothelial and epithelial cells, fibroblasts), cells of monocyte lineage are the main producers of IL-6 (Hirano et al., 1985). Its production is enhanced by IL-1 and tumor necrosis factor. IL-6 induces or augments the activation of many cell types. For T cells, IL-6 provides costimulatory signals, enhancing the responses of T cells to IL-2. For B-lineage cells, IL-6 appears to act primarily as a differentiation factor that increases the production of antibody by normally activated B cells. It also acts as a growth factor for myeloma/plasmacytoma cells. Among the other effects of IL-6 that are particularly well documented are its ability to increase platelet production and its ability to induce acute phase protein production by liver cells. Increased levels of IL-6 have been reported in a number of different autoimmune and immunodeficiency diseases.

The receptor for IL-6 is composed of two chains: an 80-kd molecule that has IL-6–binding properties, and a 130-kd molecule that acts as a signal transducer. The association of these subunits is triggered by the binding of IL-6 to the 80-kd receptor.

Interleukin-7 (IL-7). IL-7 is produced by stromal cells in the bone marrow and thymus. This cytokine was first described as a growth factor for pre-B cells in the bone marrow (Goodwin et al., 1989). However, there is evolving evidence that IL-7 can also promote the growth and differentiation of thymocytes and provide costimulatory signals for the activation of T cells (Welch et al., 1989). This cytokine also augments cytotoxic T-cell generation and lymphokine-activated killer activity (Alderson et al., 1990).

Interleukin-10 (IL-10). IL-10 was first described as a *cytokine synthesis inhibitory factor* (Moore et al., 1993). Interestingly, this cytokine has sequence homology and functional similarities to a factor produced by the *BCRF1* gene of the Epstein-Barr virus (De Waal Malefyt et al., 1991b). Among murine T cells, IL-10 is produced only by T$_H$2 cells; it may, however, be produced by both T$_H$1- and T$_H$2-like cells in humans (Del Prete et al., 1993). This cytokine is also produced by a number of other cell types, including B cells, macrophages, and mast cells. A major action of IL-10 is to inhibit the production of cytokines, especially IFN-γ, by T_H1 cells (Fiorentino et al., 1989). Thus, this action may indirectly enhance IgE production. IL-10 also exerts powerful inhibitory effects on cells of monocyte/macrophage lineage: (1) IL-10 inhibits production of IL-1, IL-6, and tumor necrosis factor–α (TNF-α) (De Waal Malefyt et al., 1991a; Ralph et al., 1992); (2) IL-10 has inhibitory effects on antigen presentation (De Waal Malefyt et al., 1991b), which is of particular importance for delayed-type hypersensitivity (i.e., T_H1-like) functions; and (3) IL-10 inhibits expression of the B7-1 (CD80) antigen, the ligand for the T-cell CD28 molecule that provides a second signal for T-cell activation (Ding et al., 1993). IL-10 may play a role in determining the nature of the inflammatory response in certain bacterial and parasitic infections. Finally, IL-10 may have a role in mast cell functions.

Interleukin-12 (IL-12). This relatively new cytokine was initially identified as an NK stimulatory factor. A 75-kd heterodimer composed of disulfide-linked 35- and 40-kd subunits, IL-12 is produced by B cells, monocyte/macrophage–lineage cells, and perhaps other types of accessory cells. The most notable effects identified for IL-12 to date involve T and NK cells. This factor acts as a costimulatory factor for T-cell activation and proliferation (particularly T_H1-like cells), and it enhances the cytotoxic activity of NK cells and MHC-unrestricted CTLs (Gately, 1993). Because IL-12 appears to be a major factor in the development of cell-mediated immunity, it has been hypothesized that this cytokine is an important mediator for the generation of T_H1-type cells (Trinchieri, 1993). Several lines of evidence support this view: (1) IL-12 is a potent stimulator of IFN-γ production (Germann et al., 1993); (2) IL-12 appears to counteract or inhibit T_H2-like functions (i.e., IgE production); and (3) the production of IL-12 is inhibited by IL-10, which is produced by T_H2-type cells.

Interferons. The interferons, a family of glycoprotein mediators, are synthesized by various cell types in response to viral infections or immune stimulation (Toy, 1983). Three major types of interferons (termed α, β, and γ) have been identified. Of these, IFN-γ is most prominent as a mediator of immune cell interactions. The gene for this molecule, which consists of a 40- to 50-kd dimer, has been cloned (Gray and Goeddel, 1982). IFN-γ is produced by activated CD4$^+$ and CD8$^+$ T cells and NK cells. Among murine CD4$^+$ cells, IFN-γ is produced exclusively by T_H1 cells. In humans, CD4$^+$ T cells with phenotypic properties of memory cells are the principal sources (Sanders et al., 1988).

IFN-γ has several prominent effects. First, it is the primary macrophage activation factor. This cytokine enhances the metabolic activity of monocyte/macrophage cells, increasing their capacity to produce reactive oxygen molecules, nitric oxide, and monokines such as IL-1 and IL-6. IFN-γ also increases membrane receptors for IgG (Itoh et al., 1980). Second, IFN-γ enhances expression of class I and class II MHC molecules on a variety of tissues, including epithelial cells and monocytes (Fellous et al., 1979; Koeffler et al., 1984); thus, these cells may either acquire or develop a heightened ability to present antigen after exposure to this cytokine. Third, IFN-γ has a number of important immunoregulatory properties. In murine systems, this cytokine enhances the production of certain IgG subclasses while inhibiting IgE and IgG1 production; IFN-γ may also modulate human IgG production (Harfast et al., 1981; Muraguchi et al., 1984), although its role in this regard is poorly defined. Fourth, IFN-γ induces cytotoxic cell function. A role in MHC-restricted CTL generation has been reported. In addition, IFN-γ significantly increases the cytotoxic activity of NK and killer cells (Trinchieri et al., 1978; Ortaldo et al., 1980) and of macrophages (Jett et al., 1980).

IMMUNOREGULATORY T-CELL SUBPOPULATIONS

Our understanding of the cellular basis for the functional heterogeneity of T lymphocytes has been greatly enhanced by the identification of membrane markers that distinguish functionally distinct subpopulations of human T cells. Among the first human T-cell subset markers to be identified were the *CD4* and *CD8 antigens* (Evans et al., 1978; Kung et al., 1979). Although the CD4 and CD8 molecules are co-expressed on a significant fraction of relatively immature thymocytes, most of the mature CD3$^+$ T cells that emigrate from the thymus are members of reciprocal subsets that express either the CD4 or CD8 antigen (Evans et al., 1978; Reinherz et al., 1980a). Studies of the effector and immunoregulatory functions of the cells constituting these broad T-cell subpopulations have provided major insights into the cellular interactions of the human immune response.

CD4$^+$ T-Cell Subset

Approximately 60% of peripheral T cells express the CD4 antigen, a membrane molecule with a molecular mass of 62 kd (Maddon et al., 1985). The extracellular portion of this molecule is capable of binding to nonpolymorphic determinants on class II MHC molecules, and the intracellular portion of the CD4 molecule is associated with the p56^{lck} protein-tyrosine kinase (Bierer et al., 1989).

Because CD4$^+$ T cells play a central role in the induction and regulation of most aspects of an immune response, this T-cell subpopulation is frequently referred to as the *helper/inducer subset*. When appropriately activated, CD4$^+$ T cells provide help essential for immunoglobulin biosynthesis by human B cells (Reinherz et al., 1979a and 1979b; Yarchoan et al., 1982). In addition, CD4$^+$ lymphocytes provide help for the efficient generation of CD8$^+$ cytotoxic effector cells (Reinherz et al., 1979c; Biddison et al., 1981). The CD4$^+$ T-cell subset contains the memory T cells that proliferate and secrete a broad array of cytokines in response to soluble recall antigens.

Finally, CD4$^+$ T cells are involved in the suppression

of immune responses, either by their direct action (Moore and Nesbitt, 1986) or via the induction of suppressor functions by CD8$^+$ T cells (Broder et al., 1978; Thomas et al., 1980; Gatenby et al., 1982; Morimoto et al., 1985b).

CD4$^+$ Subpopulations Defined by CD45 Isoform Expression

In view of the functional heterogeneity of CD4$^+$ T cells, efforts have been made to find phenotypic markers that identify functionally distinct subpopulations of human CD4$^+$ lymphocytes. Studies of the expression of two isoforms of the CD45 common leukocyte antigen family, the CD45RA and CD45RO membrane antigens, have proved to be particularly rewarding (Clement, 1992). The CD45 common leukocyte antigen family consists of a group of related membrane glycoproteins (or isoforms) that are variably expressed by cells of lymphoid or myeloid origin. The proteins that constitute this family, which range in molecular mass from 220 to 180 kd, appear to be involved in the regulation of transmembrane signals mediating T-, B-, and NK-lymphocyte activation (Pingel and Thomas, 1989; Schraven et al., 1989). The different isoforms are produced by alternative splicing of the mRNA produced by a single gene (Streuli et al., 1987). All isoforms share a common, large intracellular domain. This domain has protein-tyrosine-phosphatase activity, which may enzymatically activate T-cell protein-tyrosine kinases such as p56^{lck} (Tonks et al., 1988; Ledbetter et al., 1988). The differential use of three exons during mRNA splicing is responsible for creating the antigenic variability of the extracellular domains that distinguish different CD45 isoforms (Pulido and Sanchez-Madrid, 1989). It is unknown whether the differences in the extracellular portion of these isoforms have direct physiologic consequences for the functions of T cells.

The T-cell subsets defined by the CD45RA and CD45RO antigens are largely reciprocal; i.e., cells expressing one isoform generally do not express the other. The CD45RA antigen is first expressed by T-lineage cells relatively late during their intrathymic maturation and continues to be expressed by the vast majority of the "virgin" or naive T cells present in the immunologically naive neonate (Tedder et al., 1985a). With increasing age and antigenic exposure, however, CD45RA$^-$/RO$^+$ cells become more prevalent in the circulation and constitute the majority of cells in tissues and secondary lymphoid organs (Tedder et al., 1985a; Paoli et al., 1988; Janossy et al., 1989). The preferential homing and/or retention of CD45RO$^+$ T cells in tissues may be related to their increased expression of a variety of different adhesion molecules, including the LFA-1 (CD18/CD11a), LFA-3 (CD58), CD2, CD29, and ICAM-1 (CD54) molecules (Sanders et al., 1988; Mackay, 1991).

Functional Differences

Several key differences in the functional capabilities of the subsets of CD4$^+$ T cells defined by CD45RA and CD45RO expression have been described. Whereas CD4$^+$CD45RA$^+$ and CD4$^-$CD45RA$^-$-cells share the ability to proliferate in response to most mitogens or following stimulation with allogeneic cells in the MLR, the ability to proliferate in response to soluble memory recall antigens is unique to CD4$^+$CD45RA$^-$/RO$^+$ cells (Morimoto et al., 1985b; Tedder et al., 1985b; Smith et al., 1986). Similarly, the ability to provide help for antibody production is uniquely performed by the CD4$^+$CD45RA$^-$/RO$^+$ subset. This interaction requires the cognate interaction (i.e., direct cell-cell contact) of B cells with the CD4$^+$CD45RA$^-$/CD45RO$^+$ T cells (Sleasman et al., 1990). Although CD4$^+$CD45RA$^-$ memory cells are uniquely able to provide help for B-cell differentiation, this subpopulation does not perform all of the helper/inducer functions mediated by human CD4$^+$ cells. For example, CD4$^+$CD45RA$^+$ and CD4$^+$CD45RA$^-$ cells both have the ability to provide help for the generation of alloantigen-specific CD8$^+$ CTLs in the MLR (Yamashita et al., 1990).

In contrast, the major immunoregulatory functions described for CD4$^+$CD45RA$^+$ cells involve *suppression* of immune responses. First, CD4$^+$CD45RA$^+$ T cells can directly suppress immune responses (Moore and Nesbitt, 1986; Hirohata and Lipsky, 1989). This function is particularly prominent in the immunologically naive human neonate, in whom the dominant immunoregulatory function of cord blood CD4$^+$ cells is suppression mediated by CD4$^+$CD45RA$^+$ cells (Clement et al., 1990). In addition, CD4$^+$CD45RA$^+$ cells can induce suppressor activity by CD8$^+$ cells (Morimoto et al., 1985a). As a result of this property, cells with the CD4$^+$CD45RA$^+$ phenotype have been termed *suppressor/inducer* cells. Whether this subset is unique among CD4$^+$ T cells in its ability to perform suppressor/inducer functions is controversial (Damle et al., 1987).

Although the differential production of lymphokines has been used to characterize the functional heterogeneity of the murine T$_H$1 and T$_H$2 subsets (discussed next), there is little evidence suggesting that the subsets of human T cells identified by the expression of different CD45 isoforms are analogous to these subsets of murine helper T cells. Whereas CD45RA$^-$/RO$^+$ cells preferentially produce certain lymphokines, especially IFN-γ (Dohlsten et al., 1988; Sanders et al., 1988), CD45RA$^+$ cells appear to be more proficient in producing IL-2 (Akbar et al., 1991).

Differentiation Models

Two general models of differentiation have been proposed to describe the lineal relationship of the T-cell subsets defined by CD45RA and CD45RO antigen expression. Although these subsets could represent mature, phenotypically and functionally stable progeny arising from separate differentiation pathways, there is considerable experimental support for the hypothesis that CD45RA$^-$/RO$^+$ cells are memory cells that derive from naive or virgin CD45RA$^+$/RO$^-$ precursors via an activation-dependent post-thymic differentiation pathway (Tedder et al., 1985b; Serra et al., 1988; Akbar et al., 1988). During this maturational process, these cells acquire the ability to provide help for B-cell differentiation (Clement et al., 1988a). The permanence or unidirectional nature of this phenotypic and functional conversion remains controversial (Clement, 1992).

Altered frequencies of CD45RA$^+$ and CD45RO$^+$ T cells have been observed in a variety of different clinical conditions, particularly diseases manifesting altered immune function (Clement, 1992). A decline in the frequency of circulating CD4$^+$CD45RA$^+$ cells, with a corresponding increase in the frequency of CD4$^+$CD45RO$^+$ cells, has been described in a variety of inflammatory and autoimmune diseases. Alterations of the frequency of CD45RA$^+$ and CD45RO$^+$ T cells have also been reported in a variety of immune deficiency disorders (Clement et al., 1988b; LeBranchu et al., 1990) and following bone marrow transplantation. These findings may provide clues to the pathogenetic processes associated with certain diseases.

T$_H$1 and T$_H$2 Subsets

Two functionally distinct subsets of helper T cells (which have been termed T$_H$1 and T$_H$2) have been described and extensively characterized in the mouse (Street and Mosmann, 1991). Although a detailed discussion of these subsets is beyond the scope of this chapter, some of the concepts that have emerged from murine studies appear to be applicable to our understanding of human immune regulation, and evidence for the existence of T$_H$1 and T$_H$2 cells in humans is rapidly accumulating (Romagnani, 1991).

The T$_H$1 and T$_H$2 subsets are distinguished by functional rather than phenotypic criteria (Mosmann et al., 1986). These functional differences derive from the differential production of certain cytokines. Thus, T$_H$1 cells produce IL-2 and IFN-γ. These helper cells are most readily activated by antigen presented by monocyte-lineage cells. An important function of these cytokines is the regulation of delayed-type hypersensitivity responses mediated by T cells and monocytes; these include granuloma formation (which is associated with macrophage activation by IFN-γ), the killing of intracellular pathogens, and other aspects of tissue inflammation and reorganization. In contrast, T$_H$2 cells are more involved with regulating *humoral immunity*. The T$_H$2 subset of helper cells responds best to antigen presented by B cells. These cells preferentially produce the cytokines IL-4, IL-5, and IL-10. In addition to promoting IgG1 and IgE antibody responses, IL-4 and IL-10 both inhibit the production of IFN-γ and monokines, thereby inhibiting delayed-type hypersensitivity. Conversely, the proliferation of T$_H$2 cells and their ability to stimulate IgE production are inhibited or counteracted by IFN-γ.

Although early efforts to identify these subsets in humans were unrewarding, evidence supporting the existence of this helper-cell dichotomy in humans has been reported (Romagnani, 1991). It appears that the distinction of T$_H$1 and T$_H$2 in humans may be less rigorous than that described for mice. For example, virtually all human T cells can produce IL-2, although their capacity to do so may vary. In addition, it has been reported that IL-10, which is produced only by T$_H$2 cells in mice, is produced by both subsets in humans (Del Prete et al., 1993). In view of the striking functional dichotomy of these cells in mice (Street and Mosmann, 1991), clearer definition and characterization of these subsets in humans offers an attractive area for future study.

CD8$^+$ T-Cell Subset

The second major T-cell subpopulation, which contains 20 to 40% of circulating T cells, expresses CD8 molecules, which exist as multimeric complexes of disulfide-linked 34-kd glycoprotein subunits (Snow and Terhorst, 1983). The extracellular portion of CD8 molecules can bind to nonpolymorphic determinants on class I MHC molecules (Bierer et al., 1989). As with CD4 molecules, the intracellular portion of the CD8 molecule is associated with p56^{lck} protein-tyrosine kinase molecules. The CD8$^+$ subset contains the precursors of class I MHC–restricted virus-specific cytotoxic T cells (Biddison et al., 1981) as well as the cytotoxic effector cells responsible for most allogeneic cytotoxic reactions (Reinherz et al., 1979b). In addition, CD8$^+$ cells suppress a number of different immune responses, including B-cell immunoglobulin biosynthesis (Thomas et al., 1980; Reinherz et al., 1980b). As discussed later, this suppression requires interaction with the CD4$^+$ cells known as suppressor/inducer cells (Broder et al., 1978; Thomas et al., 1980; Gatenby et al., 1982; Morimoto et al., 1985a). Thus, the CD8$^+$ T-cell subset is frequently referred to as the *cytotoxic/suppressor subpopulation*.

Although many of the functions of CD4$^+$ and CD8$^+$ cells appear to be distinct, there are notable exceptions. For example, in contrast to alloreactive cytotoxic T cells directed against class I MHC alloantigens, which are CD8$^+$ T cells, the cytotoxic T cells that recognize and lyse allogeneic class II MHC–bearing target cell antigens or exogenous antigens (i.e., influenza virus) in the context of autologous class II MHC antigens (Biddison et al., 1982) have the CD4$^+$ phenotype. Similarly, certain CD4$^+$ cells can act as potent suppressor cells (Moore and Nesbitt, 1986). Thus, it is believed that the functional segregation of CD4$^+$ and CD8$^+$ T cells is most closely correlated with the ability of these two T-cell subsets to recognize antigen in association with class II and class I molecules, respectively.

CELLULAR INTERACTIONS NECESSARY FOR ANTIBODY PRODUCTION

The cellular interactions between helper T cells and B cells that result in antibody production involve both cognate interactions (i.e., mediated by cell-cell contact) and cytokine-mediated events (Parker, 1993). The initial stage of this bidirectional process is no different from that of CD4$^+$ T cells and other types of APCs. The cross-linkage of membrane immunoglobulin receptors by exogenous antigen provides an activation signal to the B cells, which express heightened amounts of class

II MHC antigens, other membrane molecules (i.e., CD23 and CD80 molecules), and receptors for IL-2 and various other cytokines. In addition, B cells process internalized antigen and re-express antigen fragments in the context of self-MHC antigens, thereby acquiring the potential to present antigen and activate CD4$^+$ T cells (particularly primed or memory T cells).

During the cognate interaction of B cells and CD4$^+$ T cells, the TCR molecules of T cells and the class II MHC molecules of B cells become polarized, migrating toward the junctional area of the respective lymphocytes. The resulting proximity of the TCR molecules and class II MHC molecules enhances the efficiency of antigen presentation and T-cell activation. Several important events accompany this process. First, there is up-regulation of the expression of numerous membrane molecules, such as integrins and other adhesion molecules, that are necessary for efficient T cell–B cell cognate interactions. In addition, the ligand for B-cell CD40 molecules appears on activated T cells (Castle et al., 1993). Interactions between CD40 and its 39-kd T-cell ligand appear to be essential for normal humoral immunity (Noelle et al., 1992); as noted in Chapter 11 (Disorders of the B-Cell System), mutations of the gene encoding for the T-cell ligand for CD40 are responsible for *X-linked hyper-IgM syndrome*. Activated T cells also produce cytokines (such as IL-2 and IL-4) that provide signals promoting B-cell proliferation (thereby leading to clonal expansion and memory B-cell production). Cytokines that promote the terminal differentiation of B cells into immunoglobulin-secreting plasma cells are also produced. Thus, this interaction of T and B cells generates effector populations that mediate both humoral and cell-mediated immune responses (Finkelman et al., 1992).

CELLULAR INTERACTIONS NECESSARY FOR CYTOTOXIC T-CELL GENERATION

The initial event in the generation of CTLs is the recognition of foreign antigen in the context of self-MHC molecules by T cells. For CD8$^+$ lymphocytes, which are the predominant cells responsible for this effector function, antigen is recognized in association with class I MHC molecules. In some instances, these antigenic fragments may be generated by the degradation of a foreign antigen (i.e., virally encoded proteins); in other cases, the peptides normally produced intracellularly by allogeneic cells may be seen as foreign. The binding of the TCR of the CD8$^+$ T cell to the complex of antigen bound to class I MHC molecules, in conjunction with accessory interactions between the T cell and the target cell that are mediated by CD8, LFA-1, CD28, and CD2 molecules, leads to T-cell activation. As noted later, these activated CD8$^+$ T cells then undergo cytokine-mediated differentiation into cytotoxic effector cells.

The generation of CD8$^+$ cytotoxic effector cells is considerably enhanced by CD4$^+$ helper T cells. In contrast to the cognate interactions of CD4$^+$ T cells with B cells that are essential for the induction of antibody production, the helper functions of CD4$^+$ T cells for CTL generation appear to be mediated exclusively by cytokines. The pivotal cytokine mediating the helper function of CD4$^+$ T cells for CTL differentiation is IL-2 (Gillis et al., 1981; Bass et al., 1992). Although a number of other T cell–derived cytokines (i.e., IL-4, IL-5, IL-6, IFN-γ) may influence this process, their actions appear to be costimulatory and to require the presence of IL-2.

The ability of different CD4$^+$ T cells to provide helper functions for CTL generation is closely associated with their ability to produce IL-2. For human CD4$^+$ T cells, this is in part determined by the nature of the activation stimulus. For example, CD4$^+$CD45RA$^+$ cells and CD4$^+$CD45RO$^+$ T cells both produce IL-2 when stimulated with allogeneic cells. Thus, in contrast to help for antibody production, which is mediated only by CD4$^+$CD45RA$^-$/RO$^+$ cells, both the CD4$^+$CD45RA$^+$ and CD4$^+$CD45RO$^+$ T-cell subsets are capable of providing help for the maturation of CD8$^+$ precursor cells into mature alloreactive cytotoxic effector cells (Yamashita et al., 1990).

Although CD4$^+$ T cells clearly can enhance CTL generation, it has become apparent that helper T cell–independent CTL generation in humans can also occur (Wee et al., 1982; Kung et al., 1991). This process, which is often suboptimal, appears to be related to the ability of certain CD8$^+$ precursor cells to produce IL-2. For the subsets of human CD8$^+$ T cells defined by CD45 isoforms, both the CD8$^+$CD45RA$^+$ and CD8$^+$CD45RA$^-$ subsets contain precursor cells capable of developing into alloreactive CTLs in the presence of activated CD4$^+$ T cells (Yamashita et al., 1989). In the absence of CD4$^+$ T cells, however, only CD8$^+$CD45RA$^+$ precursor cells can develop into CTLs (Bass et al., 1992). This restricted ability of human CD8$^+$ cells to undergo helper cell–independent differentiation into cytotoxic effector cells occurs as a result of the enhanced ability of the CD8$^+$CD45RA$^+$ subset to produce and use IL-2 in an autocrine fashion (Bass et al., 1992).

CELLULAR INTERACTIONS RESULTING IN IMMUNOSUPPRESSION

A number of early studies investigating the regulation of immunity demonstrated that immune responses were subject to down-regulation. These observations stimulated considerable interest in determining the cellular basis for this immunosuppression. Although various cell types (including monocytes, NK cells, and certain CD4$^+$ T cells) were found to suppress immune responses (particularly in vitro), CD8$^+$ T cells appeared to be particularly effective as suppressors of cellular and humoral immune responses, both in vitro and in vivo. Activated CD8$^+$ T cells were also shown to be responsible for mediating certain states of tolerance. In addition, it was found that CD8$^+$ suppressor cells often required the actions of a subset of CD4$^+$ T cells (termed *suppressor/inducer cells*) to mediate their functions (Broder et al., 1978; Thomas et al., 1980; Gatenby et al., 1982).

These early findings suggesting that the cells mediating immunosuppression might be functionally compartmentalized stimulated considerable efforts to determine whether a distinct subpopulation of CD8[+] T cells performed suppressor functions. Although early studies reported that distinct subpopulations of murine T cells identifiable by membrane markers such as I-J antigens or *idiotype/anti-idiotypic determinants* constituted an intricate suppressor-cell network, the initial burst of enthusiasm for this hypothesis dimmed after it was found that the postulated I-J region of the murine equivalent of the MHC did not exist.

There have been several reports that human CD8[+] suppressor T cells have unique phenotypic characteristics. Of particular interest has been a subset of CD8[+] T cells that express CR3 (CD11b/CD18) β_2-integrin molecules and the CD57 antigen but lack membrane CD28 molecules (Damle et al., 1983; Landay et al., 1983). These cells, which exert potent suppressor functions, have a number of functional and structural characteristics that differ from the reciprocal CD28[+]/CD11b[−] subset of CD8[+] cells (Clement et al., 1984). However, because these cells may also mediate cytotoxic functions (McFarland et al., 1992), they do not appear to represent a functionally distinct subpopulation of CD8[+] cells exclusively devoted to immunosuppression. Conversely, it is possible, or even likely, that other CD8[+] T-cell subsets can similarly suppress immune responses under certain conditions. Thus, whereas there is considerable evidence that CD8[+] T cells may suppress immune responses, the properties of the CD8[+] cells that may mediate these functions are poorly defined at present.

As noted previously, CD8[+] T cells do not appear to independently mediate immunosuppression; rather, the suppressor functions of CD8[+] T cells must be activated or induced by CD4[+] T cells. Because CD4[+] T cells provide helper functions necessary for numerous immune effector mechanisms (helper/inducer functions) and also stimulate suppressor activity by CD8[+] T cells (suppressor/inducer function), studies have been performed to determine whether these two dissimilar functions are performed by different subsets of CD4[+] T cells. As previously noted, studies of the nonoverlapping subsets of CD4[+] T cells defined by expression of CD45RA or CD45RO isoforms have shown that the cells that provide help for B-cell differentiation express the CD45RA[−]/CD45RO[+] phenotype. In contrast, it has been reported that the CD4[+] T cells that perform suppressor/inducer functions belong to the reciprocal CD4[+]CD45RA[+]/CD45RO[−] subset (Morimoto et al., 1985a, 1985b). Interestingly, these CD4[+]CD45RA[+] cells can also directly suppress immune responses (Moore and Nesbitt, 1986; Hirohata and Lipsky, 1989; Clement et al., 1990). Although it remains controversial whether these suppressor/inducer functions are uniquely performed by CD45RA[+]/CD45RO[−] cells (Damle et al., 1987), this conceptual model of immunoregulatory compartmentalization remains an attractive theory.

Although the mechanisms by which CD8[+] (or CD4[+]) T cells suppress immune responses are unknown, a number of diverse mechanisms may result in immunosuppression (Bloom et al., 1992). It may be mediated by the production of cytokines, such as IL-10 or *transforming growth factors* (TGF-β), which directly suppress various immune responses. The mutually antagonistic actions of IL-4 and IFN-γ for T_H1 and T_H2 cells, respectively, provides an alternative model for cytokine-mediated suppression of specific immune functions. Suppressor cells may also act to maintain states of tolerance, as has been described for T_H2 cells and transplantation tolerance (Lowry et al., 1993). This maintenance of tolerance could be accomplished by modulating the differential antigen presentation capabilities of different types of APCs or otherwise interrupting certain cell activation signals, thus resulting in clonal anergy, as is found in T cells that do not receive a requisite second signal during TCR-mediated activation. Definition of the cellular interactions and mechanisms by which immune functions may be suppressed offers an important challenge for the future.

References

Acuto O, Reinherz EL. The human T-cell receptor: Structure and function. N Engl J Med 312:1100–1111, 1985.

Akbar AN, Salmon M, Janossy G. The synergy between naive and memory T cells during activation. Immunol Today 12:184–188, 1991.

Akbar AN, Terry L, Timms A, Beverley PCL, Janossy G. Loss of CD45R and gain of UCHL1 reactivity is a feature of primed T cells. J Immunol 140:2171–2176, 1988.

Akira S, Hirano T, Kishimoto T. Biology of multifunctional cytokines: IL 6 and related molecules (IL 1 and TNF). FASEB J 4:2860–2867, 1990.

Alderson MR, Sassenfeld HM, Widmer MB. Interleukin-7 enhances cytolytic T lymphocyte generation and induces lymphokine-activated killer cells from human peripheral blood. J Exp Med 172:577–587, 1990.

Ambrus JL, Jurgensen CH, Brown EJ, Fauci AS. Purification to homogeneity of a high molecular weight human B-cell growth factor: demonstration of specific binding to activated B cells; and development of a monoclonal antibody to the factor. J Exp Med 162:1319–1335, 1985.

Archer OK, Pierce JC, Papermaster BW, Good RA. Reduced antibody response in thymectomized rabbits. Nature 195:191–193, 1962.

Auron PE, Webb AC, Rosenwasser LJ, Mucci SR, Rich A, Wolff SM, Dinarello CA. Nucleotide sequence of human monocyte interleukin-1 precursor cDNA. Proc Natl Acad Sci U S A 81:7907–7911, 1984.

Bain B, Vas MR, Lowenstein L. The development of large immature mononuclear cells in mixed lymphocyte cultures. Blood 23:108–116, 1964.

Bass H, Yamashita N, Clement LT. Heterogeneous mechanisms of human cytotoxic T lymphocyte generation. I. Differential helper cell requirement for the generation of cytotoxic effector cells from CD8[+] precursor subpopulations. J Immunol 149:2489–2495, 1992.

Beller EI, Springer TA, Schreiber RD. Anti–Mac-1 selectively inhibits the mouse and human type three complement receptor. J Exp Med 156:1000–1009, 1982.

Bergholtz BO, Thorsby E. HLA-D restriction of the macrophage-dependent response of immune human T lymphocytes to PPD in vitro: inhibition by anti–HLA-DR antisera. Scand J Immunol 8:63–73, 1978.

Bernard A, Boumsell L, Hill C. In Bernard A, Boumsell L, Dausett J, Milstein C, Schlossman SF, eds. Joint Report of the First International Workshop on Human Leukocyte Differentiation Antigens by the Investigators of the Participating Laboratories in Leukocyte Typing. New York, Springer-Verlag, 1984, pp 9–143.

Biddison WE, Shaw S, Nelson DL. Virus specificity of human influenza virus–immune cytotoxic T cells. J Immunol 122:660–664, 1979.

Biddison WE, Sharrow SO, Shearer GM. T cell subpopulations required for the human cytotoxic T lymphocyte response to influenza virus: evidence for T cell help. J Immunol 127:487–491, 1981.

Biddison WE, Rao PE, Talle MA, Goldstein G, Shaw S. Possible involvement of the OKT4 molecule in T cell recognition of class II HLA antigens: evidence from studies of cytotoxic T lymphocytes specific for SB antigens. J Exp Med 156:1065–1076, 1982.

Bierer BE, Sleckman BP, Ratnofsky SE, Burakoff SJ. The biological roles of CD2, CD4, and CD8 in T cell activation. Annu Rev Immunol 7:579–608, 1989.

Bloom BR, Salgame P, Diamond B. Revisiting and revising suppressor T cells. Immunol Today 13:131–136, 1992.

Borst J, Alexander S, Elder J, Terhorst C. The T3 complex on human T lymphocytes involves four structurally distinct glycoproteins. J Biol Chem 258:5135–5141, 1983.

Borst J, Coligan JE, Oettgen H, Pessano S, Malin R, Terhorst C. The delta and epsilon chains of the human T3/T-cell receptor complex are distinct polypeptides. Nature 312:455–458, 1984.

Boyum A. Separation of leukocytes from blood and bone marrow. Scand J Clin Lab Invest 21 (Suppl. 97):9–29, 1968.

Bretscher MS. The molecules of the cell membrane. Sci Am 253:100–110, 1985.

Broder S, Edelson RL, Lutzner MA, Nelson DL, MacDermott RP, Durm ME, Goldman CK, Mead BD, Waldmann TA. The Sezary syndrome: a malignant proliferation of helper T cells. J Clin Invest 58:1297–1306, 1976.

Broder S, Poplack D, Whang-Peng J, Durm M, Goldman C, Muul L, Waldmann TA. Characterization of a suppressor-cell leukemia. Evidence for the requirement of an interaction of two T cells in the development of human suppressor effect or cells. N Engl J Med 298:66–72, 1978.

Cantor H, Asofsky R. Synergy among lymphoid cells mediating the graft-versus-host response. III. Evidence for interaction between two types of thymus derived cells. J Exp Med 135:764–779, 1972.

Cantrell DA, Smith KA. The interleukin-2 T-cell system: a new cell growth model. Science 224:1312–1316, 1984.

Castle BE, Kishimoto K, Stearns C, Brown ML, Kehry MR. Regulation of expression of the ligand for CD40 on T helper lymphocytes. J Immunol 151:1777–1788, 1993.

Cerottini JS, Nordin AA, Brunner KT. In vitro cytotoxic activity of thymus cells sensitized to alloantigens. Nature 227:72–73, 1970.

Chang TW, Kung PC, Gingras SP, Goldstein G. Does OKT3 monoclonal antibody react with an antigen-recognition structure on human T cells? Proc Natl Acad Sci U S A 78:1805–1808, 1981.

Chess L, MacDermott RP, Schlossman SF. Immunologic functions of isolated human lymphocyte subpopulations: I. Quantitative isolation of human T and B cells and response to mitogens. J Immunol 113:1113–1121, 1974.

Claman HN, Chaperon EA, Triplett RF. Thymus-marrow cell combinations. Synergism in antibody production. Proc Soc Exp Biol Med 122:1167–1171, 1966.

Clement LT. Isoforms of the CD45 common leukocyte antigen family: markers for human T cell differentiation. J Clin Immunol 12:1–10, 1992.

Clement LT, Giorgi JV, Plaeger-Marshall S, Haas A, Stiehm ER, Martin AM. Abnormal differentiation of immunoregulatory T lymphocyte subpopulations in the major histocompatibility complex (MHC) class II antigen deficiency syndrome. J Clin Immunol 8:503–512, 1988a.

Clement LT, Grossi CE, Gartland GL. Morphological and phenotypic features of the subpopulation of Leu-2$^+$ cells that suppresses B cell differentiation. J Immunol 133:2461–2468, 1984.

Clement LT, Vink PE, Bradley GB. Novel immunoregulatory functions of phenotypically distinct subpopulations of CD4$^+$ cells in the human neonate. J Immunol 145:102–108, 1990.

Clement LT, Yamashita N, Martin AM. The functionally distinct subpopulations of human helper/inducer T lymphocytes defined by anti-CD45R antibodies derive sequentially from a differentiation pathway that is regulated by activation-dependent post-thymic differentiation. J Immunol 141:1464–1470, 1988b.

Clevers H, Alarcon B, Wileman T, Terhorst C. The T-cell receptor/CD3 complex: a dynamic protein ensemble. Annu Rev Immunol 6:629–662, 1988.

Damle NK, Childs AL, Doyle LV. Immunoregulatory T lymphocytes in man: soluble antigen-specific suppressor-inducer T lymphocytes are derived from the CD4$^+$CD45R$^-$p80$^+$ subpopulation. J Immunol 139:1501–1508, 1987.

Damle NK, Mohagheghpour N, Hansen JA, Engleman EG. Alloantigen-specific cytotoxic and suppressor T lymphocytes are derived from phenotypically distinct precursors. J Immunol 131:2296–2306, 1983.

Davies AJS. The thymus and the cellular basis of immunity. Transplant Rev 1:43–91, 1969.

De Waal Malefyt R, Abrams J, Bennett B, Figdor CG, de Vries JE. Interleukin-10 (IL-10) inhibits cytokine synthesis by human monocytes: an autoregulatory role of IL-10 produced by monocytes. J Exp Med 174:1209–1220, 1991a.

De Waal Malefyt R, Haanen J, Spits J, Roncarlo MG, te Velde A, Figdor CG, de Vries JE. Interleukin-10 (IL-10) and viral IL-10 strongly reduce antigen-specific human T cell proliferation by diminishing the antigen-presenting capacity of monocytes via down regulation of class II major histocompatibility complex expression. J Exp Med 174:915–924, 1991b.

Del Prete G, De Carli M, Almerigogna F, Giudizi MG, Biagiotti R, Romagnani S. Human IL-10 is produced by both type I helper (T_H1) and type 2 helper (T_H2) T cell clones and inhibits their antigen-specific proliferation and cytokine production. J Immunol 150:353–360, 1993.

Dezutter-Dambuyant C, Cordier G, Schmitt D, Faure M, Laquoi C, Thivolet J. Quantitative evaluation of two distinct cell populations expressing HLA-DR antigens in normal human epidermis. Br J Dermatol 111:1–11, 1984.

Dinarello CA. An update on human interleukin-1: from molecular biology to clinical relevance. J Clin Immunol 5:287–297, 1985.

Ding L, Linsley PS, Huang LY, Germain RN, Shevach EM. IL-10 inhibits macrophage costimulatory activity by selectively inhibiting the up-regulation of B7 expression. J Immunol 151:1224–1234, 1993.

Dohlsten M, Hedlund G, Sjogren H-O, Carlsson R. Two subsets of human CD4$^+$ T helper cells differing in kinetics and capacities to produce interleukin 2 and interferon-γ can be defined by the Leu-18 and UCHL1 monoclonal antibodies. Eur J Immunol 18:1173–1178, 1988.

Engleman EG, Benike CJ, Glickman E, Evans RL. Antibodies to membrane structures that distinguish suppressor/cytotoxic and helper T lymphocyte subpopulations block the mixed leukocyte reaction in man. J Exp Med 153:193–198, 1981.

Evans RL, Lazarus H, Penta AC, Schlossman SF. Two functionally distinct subpopulations of human T cells that collaborate in the generation of cytotoxic cells responsible for cell-mediated lympholysis. J Immunol 120:1423–1428, 1978.

Evans RL, Wall DW, Platsoucas CD, Siegal FP, Fikrig SH, Testa CM, Good RA. Thymus-dependent membrane antigens in man: inhibition of cell-mediated lympholysis by monoclonal antibodies to the TH2 antigen. Proc Natl Acad Sci U S A 78:544–551, 1981.

Fellous M, Kamaon M, Gresser I, Bono R. Enhanced expression of HLA antigens and β_2-microglobulin on interferon treated human lymphoblastoid cells. Eur J Immunol 9:446–449, 1979.

Finkelman FD, Lees A, Morris SC. Antigen presentation by B lymphocytes to CD4$^+$ T lymphocytes in vivo: importance for B lymphocyte and T lymphocyte activation. Semin Immunol 4:247–255, 1992.

Fiorentino DF, Bond MW, Mosmann TR. Two types of mouse helper T cells. IV. T_H2 clones secrete a factor that inhibits cytokine production by T_H1 clones. J Exp Med 170:2081–2095, 1989.

Fraser JD, Straus D, Weiss A. Signal transduction events leading to T cell lymphokine gene expression. Immunol Today 14:357–362, 1993.

Freeman GJ, Gribben JG, Boussiotis VA, Ng JW, Restivo VA, Lombard LA, Gray GS, Nadler LM. Cloning of B7-2: a CTLA-4 counterreceptor that costimulates human T cell proliferation. Science 262:909–911, 1993.

Froland SS. Binding of sheep erythrocytes to human lymphocytes. A probable marker of T lymphocytes. Scand J Immunol 3:269–280, 1972.

Froland SS, Natvig JB, Berdal P. Surface bound immunoglobulin as a marker of B lymphocytes in man. Nature (New Biol) 234:251–252, 1971.

Gascan H, Gauchat J-F, Roncarlo M-G, Yssel H, Spits H, de Vries JE. Human B cell clones can be induced to proliferate and to switch to IgE and IgG4 synthesis by interleukin-4 and a signal provided by activated CD4$^+$ T cell clones. J Exp Med 173:747–759, 1991.

Gately MK. Interleukin-12: a recently discovered cytokine with potential for enhancing cell-mediated immune responses to tumors. Cancer Invest 11:500–506, 1993.

Gatenby PA, Kansas GS, Xian CY, Evans RL, Engleman EG. Dissection of immunoregulatory subpopulations of T lymphocytes within the helper and suppressor sublineages in man. J Immunol 129:1997–2000, 1982.

Germain R. The biochemistry and cell biology of antigen processing and presentation. Annu Rev Immunol 11:403–450, 1993.

Germann T, Gately MK, Schoenhart DS, Lohoff M, Mattner F, Fischer S, Jim SC, Schmitt E, Rude E. Interleukin 12/T cell stimulatory factor, a cytokine with multiple effects on T$_H$1 but not T$_H$2 cells. Eur J Immunol 23:1762–1770, 1993.

Gershon RK, Kondo K. Cell interactions in the induction of tolerance: the role of thymic lymphocytes. Immunology 18:723–737, 1970.

Gillis S, Gillis AE, Henney CS. Monoclonal antibody directed against interleukin 2: 1. Inhibition of T lymphocyte mitogenesis and the in vitro differentiation of alloreactive cytotoxic T cells. J Exp Med 154:983–997, 1981.

Gimmi CD, Freeman J, Gribben JG, Sugita K, Freedman AS, Morimoto C, Nadler LM. B cell surface antigen B7 provides a costimulatory signal that induces T cells to proliferate and secrete interleukin-2. Proc Natl Acad Sci U S A 88:6575–6580, 1991.

Good RA. Immunodeficiencies of man and the new immunobiology. Birth Defects 11:xiii–xx, 1975.

Goodwin RG, Lupton S, Schmeirer A, Hjerrild KH, Jrzy R, Clevenger W, Gillis S, Cosman D, Namen AE. Human interleukin-7: molecular cloning and growth factor activity on human and murine B lineage cells. Proc Natl Acad Sci U S A 86:302–306, 1989.

Gray PW, Goeddel DV. Structure of the human immune interferon gene. Nature 298:859–863, 1982.

Harding FA, McArthur JG, Gross JA, Raulet DH, Allison JP. CD28-mediated signaling co-stimulates murine T cells and prevents induction of anergy in T cell clones. Nature 356:607–611, 1992.

Harfast B, Huddlestone JR, Casali P, Merigan TC, Oldstone MBA. Interferon acts directly on human B lymphocytes to modulate immunoglobulin synthesis. J Immunol 127:2146–2150, 1981.

Hildreth JEK, Gotch FM, Hildreth PDK, McMichael AJ. A human lymphocyte-associated antigen involved in cell-mediated lympholysis. Eur J Immunol 13:202–208, 1983.

Hirano T, Taga T, Nakano N, Yasukawa K, Kashiwamura S, Shimizu K, Nakajima K, Pyun KH, Kishimoto T. Purification to homogeneity and characterization of human B-cell differentiation factor (BCDF or BSFp-2). Proc Natl Acad Sci U S A 82:5490–5494, 1985.

Hirohata S, Lipsky PE. T cell regulation of human B cell proliferation and differentiation. Regulatory influences of CD45R$^+$ and CD45R$^-$ T4 cell subsets. J Immunol 142:2597–2604, 1989.

Hood L, Kronenberg M, Hunkapiller T. T cell antigen receptors and the immunoglobulin supergene family. Cell 40:225–229, 1985.

Itoh K, Inoue M, Kataoka S, Kumagai K. Differential effect of interferon expression of IgG- and IgM-Fc receptors on human lymphocytes. J Immunol 124:2589–2595, 1980.

Janossy G, Bofill M, Rowe D, Muir J, Beverley PCL. The tissue distribution of T lymphocytes expressing different CD45 polypeptides. Immunology 66:517–525, 1989.

Jett JR, Mantovani A, Herberman RB. Augmentation of human monocyte-mediated cytolysis by interferon. Cell Immunol 54:425–434, 1980.

Kamoun M, Martin PJ, Hansen JA, Brown MA, Siadak AW, Nowinski RC. Identification of a human T lymphocyte surface protein associated with the E-rosette receptor. J Exp Med 153:207–212, 1981.

Kara CJ, Glimcher L. Promoter accessibility within the environment of the MHC is affected in class II–deficient combined immunodeficiency. EMBO J 12:187–193, 1993.

Katz DH, Hamaoka T, Benacerraf B. Cell interactions between histocompatible T and B lymphocytes from allogeneic donor strains in humoral response to hapten-protein conjugates. J Exp Med 137:1405–1418, 1973.

Kincade PW, Phillips RA. B lymphocyte development. Fed Proc 44:2874–2881, 1984.

Kindt TJ, Robinson MA. Major histocompatibility complex antigens.

In Paul WE, ed. Fundamental Immunology, 2nd ed. New York, Raven Press, 1984, pp. 347–377.

Knight SC, Stagg AJ. Antigen-presenting cell types. Curr Opin Immunol 5:374–382, 1993.

Ko HS, Fu SM, Winchester RJ, Yu DT, Kunkel HG. Ia determinants on stimulated human T lymphocytes. Occurrence on mitogen- and antigen-activated T cells. J Exp Med 150:246–255, 1979.

Koeffler HP, Ranyard J, Yelton L, Billing R, Bohman R. Gamma-interferon induces expression of the HLA-D antigens on normal and leukemic human myeloid cells. Proc Natl Acad Sci U S A 81:4080–4084, 1984.

Kohler G, Milstein C. Continuous cultures of fused cells secreting antibody of predefined specificity. Nature 256:495–497, 1975.

Kotzin BL, Leung DY, Kappler J, Marrack P. Superantigens and their potential role in autoimmune disease. Adv Immunol 54:99–166, 1993.

Krensky AM, Sanchez-Madrid F, Springer TA, Burakoff SJ. Human lymphocyte function–associated antigens. Surv Immunol Res 3:39–44, 1984.

Kung JT, Castillo M, Heard P, Kerbacher K, Thomas CA. Subpopulations of CD8$^+$ cytotoxic T cell precursors collaborate in the absence of conventional CD4$^+$ helper T cells. J Immunol 146:1783–1792, 1991.

Kung PC, Goldstein G, Reinherz E, Schlossman SF. Monoclonal antibodies defining distinctive human T cell surface antigens. Science 206:347–350, 1979.

Landay A, Gartland GL, Clement LT. Characterization of a phenotypically distinct subpopulation of Leu 2$^+$ cells which suppresses T cell proliferative responses. J Immunol 131:2757–2761, 1983.

Lanzavecchia A. Receptor-mediated antigen uptake and its effect on antigen presentation to class II–restricted T lymphocytes. Annu Rev Immunol 8:773–793, 1990.

LeBranchu Y, Thibault G, Degenne D, Bardos P. Deficiency of CD4$^+$CD45R$^+$ T lymphocytes in common variable immunodeficiency. New Engl J Med 323:276–277, 1990.

Leonard WJ, Depper JM, Crabtree GR, Rudikoff SJ, Pumphrey J, Robb RJ, Kronke M, Svetlik PB, Peffer NJ, Waldmann TA, Greene WC. Molecular cloning and expression of cDNAs for the human interleukin-2 receptor. Nature 311:626–629, 1984.

Leonard WJ, Depper JM, Robb RJ, Waldmann TA, Greene WC. Characterization of the human receptor for T cell growth factor. Proc Natl Acad Sci U S A 80:6957–6960, 1983.

Linsley PS, Brady W, Grosmaire L, Aruffo A, Damle NK, Ledbetter JA. Binding of the B cell activation antigen B7 to CD28 costimulates T cell proliferation and interleukin-2 mRNA accumulation. J Exp Med 173:721–733, 1991.

Lobo RI, Westervelt FB, Horwitz DA. Identification of two populations of immunoglobulin-bearing lymphocytes in man. J Immunol 114:116–119, 1975.

Lowry RP, Takenuchi T, Cremisi H, Konieczeny B. T$_H$2-like effectors may function as antigen-specific suppressor cells in states of transplantation tolerance. Transplant Proc 25:324–326, 1993.

Mackay CR. T-cell memory: the connection between function, phenotype, and migration pathways. Immunol Today 12:189–193, 1991.

Maddon PJ, Littman DR, Godfrey M, Maddon DE, Chess L, Axel R. The isolation and nucleotide sequence of cDNA encoding the T cell surface protein T4: a new member of the immunoglobulin gene family. Cell 42:93–104, 1985.

March CJ, Mosley B, Arsen A, Cerretti DP, Braedt G, Price V, Gillis S, Henney CS, Kronheim SR, Grabstein K, Colon PJ, Hopp TP, Cosman D. Cloning, sequence, and expression of two distinct human interleukin-1 complementary DNAs. Nature 315:641–646, 1985.

Matsunaga T. Evolution of the immunoglobulin superfamily by duplication of complementarity. Immunol Today 6:260–263, 1985.

McFarland HI, Nahill SR, Maciaszek JW, Welsh RM. CD11b (Mac-1): a marker for CD8$^+$ cytotoxic T cell activation and memory in virus infection. J Immunol 149:1326–1333, 1992.

Mehta SR, Conrad D, Sandler R, Morgan J, Montagna R, Maizel AL. Purification of human B cell growth factor. J Immunol 135:3298–3302, 1985.

Meuer SC, Fitzgerald DA, Hussey RE, Hodgdon JC, Schlossman SF, Reinherz EL. Clonotypic structures involved in antigen-specific human T cell function: relationship to the T3 molecular complex. J Exp Med 157:705–719, 1983.

Meuer SC, Hussey RE, Fabbi M, Fox D, Acuto O, Fitzgerald KA, Hodgdon JC, Protentis JP, Schlossman SF, Reinherz EL. An alternative pathway of T-cell activation: a functional role for the 50 Kd T11 sheep erythrocyte receptor protein. Cell 36:897–906, 1984.

Miller JFAP. Immunologic function of the thymus. Lancet 2:748–749, 1961.

Miller JFAP, Mitchell GF. Thymus and antigen reactive cells. Transplant Rev 1:3–42, 1969.

Moore K, Nesbitt AM. Identification and isolation of OKT4+ suppressor cells with the monoclonal antibody WR16. Immunology 58:659–667, 1986.

Moore KW, O'Garra A, de Waal Malefyt R, Vieira P, Mosmann TR. Interleukin-10. Annu Rev Immunol 11:165–190, 1993.

Moretta L, Ferrarini M, Mingari MC, Moretta A, Webb SR. Subpopulations of human T cells identified by receptors for immunoglobulins and mitogen responsiveness. J Immunol 117:2171–2174, 1976.

Morgan DA, Ruscetti FW, Gallo R. Selective in vitro growth of T lymphocytes from normal human bone marrow. Science 193:1007–1008, 1976.

Morimoto C, Reinherz EL, Borel Y, Mantzouranis E, Steinberg AD, Schlossman SF. Autoantibody to an immunoregulatory inducer population in patients with juvenile rheumatoid arthritis. J Clin Invest 67:753–761, 1981.

Morimoto C, Letvin NL, Boyd AW, Hagan M, Brown HM, Kornacki MM, Schlossman SF. The isolation and characterization of the human helper inducer T cell subset. J Immunol 134:3762–3769, 1985a.

Morimoto C, Letvin NL, Distaso JA, Aldrich WR, Schlossman SF. The isolation and characterization of the human suppressor inducer T cell subset. J Immunol 134:1508–1515, 1985b.

Mosier DE. A requirement for two cell types for antibody formation in vitro. Science 158:1573–1575, 1967.

Mosmann TR, Cherwinski HM, Bond MW, Giedlin MA, Coffman RL. Two types of murine helper T cell clones. I. Definition according to profiles of lymphokine activity and secreted proteins. J Immunol 136:2348–2357, 1986.

Muraguchi A, Kerhl JH, Butler JL, Fauci AS. Regulation of human B-cell activation, proliferation, and differentiation by soluble factors. J Clin Immunol 4:337–347, 1984.

Nelson DL. Cell-mediated cytotoxicity. In Oppenheim JJ, Rosenstreich DL, Potter M, eds. Cellular Functions and Immunity and Inflammation. New York: Elsevier/North-Holland, 1981, pp. 187–205.

Nelson DL, Bundy BM, Pitchon HE, Blaese RM, Strober W. The effector cells in human peripheral blood mediating mitogen-induced cellular cytotoxicity and antibody-dependent cellular cytotoxicity. J Immunol 117:1472–1481, 1976.

Nelson DL, Rubin LA, Kurman CC, Fritz ME, Boutin B. An analysis of the cellular requirements for the production of soluble interleukin-2 receptors in vitro. J Clin Immunol 6:1–7, 1986.

Nikaido T, Shimuzu A, Ishida N, Sabe H, Teshigawara K, Maeda M, Uchiyama T, Yodoi J, Honjo T. Molecular cloning of cDNA encoding human interleukin-2 receptor. Nature 311:631–634, 1984.

Noelle RJ, Ledbetter JA, Aruffo A. CD40 and its ligand, an essential ligand-receptor pair for thymus-dependent B cell activation. Immunol Today 13:431–434, 1992.

Ortaldo JR, Pestka S, Slease RB, Rubenstein M, Herberman RB. Augmentation of human K-cell activity. Scand J Immunol 12:365–369, 1980.

Paoli PD, Battistin S, Santini GF. Age-related changes in human lymphocyte subsets: progressive reduction of the CD4 CD45R (suppressor inducer) population. Clin Immunol Immunopathol 48:290–296, 1988.

Parker DC. T cell-dependent B cell activation. Annu Rev Immunol 11:331–376, 1993.

Paul WE. The immune system: an introduction. In Paul WE, ed. Fundamental Immunology, 2nd ed. New York, Raven Press, 1984, pp. 3–21.

Pingel JT, Thomas ML. Evidence that the leukocyte-common antigen is required for antigen-induced T lymphocyte proliferation. Cell 58:1055–1065, 1989.

Platsoucas CD, Good RA. Inhibition of specific cell mediated cytotoxicity by monoclonal antibodies to human T-cell antigens. Proc Natl Acad Sci U S A 78:4500–4504, 1981.

Pulido R, Sanchez-Madrid F. Biochemical nature and topographic localization of epitopes defining four distinct CD45 antigen specificities. Conventional CD45, CD45R, 180 kDa(UCHL1) and 220/205/190 kDa. J Immunol 143:1930–1936, 1989.

Ralph P, Nakoinz I, Sampson-Johannes A, Fong S, Lowe D, Min H-Y, Lin L. IL-10, T lymphocyte inhibitor of human blood cell production of IL-1 and tumor necrosis factor. J Immunol 148:808–814, 1992.

Reinherz EL, Hussey RE, Fitzgerald K, Snow P, Terhorst C, Schlossman SF. Antibody directed at a surface structure inhibits cytolytic but not suppressor function of human T lymphocytes. Nature 294:168–170, 1981.

Reinherz EL, Kung PC, Goldstein G, Levey RH, Schlossman SF. Discrete stages of human intrathymic differentiation: analysis of normal thymocytes and leukemic lymphoblasts of T cell lineage. Proc Natl Acad Sci U S A 77:1588–1592, 1980a.

Reinherz EL, Kung PC, Goldstein G, Schlossman SF. Further characterization of the human inducer T cell subset defined by monoclonal antibody. J Immunol 123:2894–2896, 1979a.

Reinherz EL, Kung PC, Goldstein G, Schlossman SF. A monoclonal antibody with selective reactivity with functionally mature human thymocytes and all peripheral human T cells. J Immunol 134:1312–1317, 1979b.

Reinherz EL, Kung PC, Goldstein G, Schlossman SF. Separation of functional subsets of human T cells by a monoclonal antibody. Proc Natl Acad Sci U S A 76:4061–4065, 1979c.

Reinherz EL, Morimoto C, Penta AC, Schlossman SF. Regulation of B cell immunoglobulin secretion by functional subsets of T lymphocytes in man. Eur J Immunol 10:570–572, 1980b.

Ritter MA, Sauvage CA, Cotmore SF. The human thymus microenvironment: in vivo identification of thymic nurse cells and other antigenically-distinct subpopulations of epithelial cells. Immunology 44:439–446, 1981.

Rogers J, Early P, Carter C, Calame K, Bond M, Hood L, Wall R. Two mRNAs with different 3′ ends encode membrane-bound and secreted forms of immunoglobulin mu chain. Cell 20:303–312, 1980.

Romagnani S. Human T_H1 and T_H2 subsets: doubt no more. Immunol Today 12:256–257, 1991.

Ron Y, Sprent J. T cell priming in vivo: a major role for B cells in presenting antigen to T cells in lymph nodes. J Immunol 138:2848–2856, 1987.

Rosenthal AS, Shevach EM. Function of macrophages in antigen recognition by guinea pig T lymphocytes. I. Requirement for histocompatible macrophages and lymphocytes. J Exp Med 138:1194–1212, 1973.

Rubin LA, Kurman CC, Fritz ME, Biddison WE, Boutin B, Yarchoan R, Nelson DL. Soluble interleukin 2 receptors are released from activated lymphoid cells in vitro. J Immunol 135:3172–3177, 1985.

Sachs DH. The major histocompatibility complex. In Paul WE, ed. Fundamental Immunology, 2nd ed.New York, Raven Press, 1984, pp. 303–346.

Salter RD, Alexander J, Levine F, Pious D, Cresswell P. Evidence for two trans-acting genes regulating HLA class II antigen expression. J Immunol 135:4235–4238, 1985.

Sanchez-Madrid F, Krensky AM, Ware CF, Robbins E, Strominger JL, Burakoff SJ, Springer TA. Three distinct antigens associated with human T-lymphocyte–mediated cytolysis: LFA-1, LFA-2, and LFA-3. Proc Natl Acad Sci U S A 79:7489–7493, 1982.

Sanders ME, Makgoba MW, Sharrow SO, Stephany D, Springer TA, Young HA, Shaw S. Human memory lymphocytes express increased levels of three cell adhesion molecules (LFA-3, CD2, and LFA-1) and three other molecules (UCHL1, CDw29, and Pgp-1) and have enhanced IFN-γ production. J Immunol 140:1401–1408, 1988.

Schraven B, Roux M, Hutmacher B, Meuer SC. Triggering of the alternative pathway of human T cell activation involves members of the T200 family of glycoproteins. Eur J Immunol 19:397–403, 1989.

Schwartz AL. Cell biology of intracellular protein trafficking. Annu Rev Immunol 8:195–226, 1990a.

Schwartz RH. A cell culture model for T lymphocyte clonal anergy. Science 248:1349–1354, 1990b.

Serra HM, Krowka JF, Ledbetter JA, Pilarski LM. Loss of CD45R (Lp220) represents a post-thymic T cell differentiation event. J Immunol 140:1441–1445, 1988.

Sette A, Buus S, Appella E, Smith JA, Chesnut R, Miles C, Colon SM, Grey HM. Prediction of major histocompatibility complex binding regions of protein antigens by sequence pattern analysis. Proc Natl Acad Sci U S A 86:3296–3300, 1989.

Shaw S, Pichler WJ, Nelson DL. Fc receptors on human T lymphocytes. III. Characterization of subpopulations involved in cell-mediated lympholysis and antibody-dependent cellular cytotoxicity. J Immunol 122:599–604, 1979.

Shearer GM, Rhen TG, Garbarino CA. Cell mediated lympholysis of trinitrophenyl-modified cell surface components controlled by the H-2K and H-2D serological regions of the murine major histocompatibility complex. J Exp Med 141:1348–1364, 1975.

Shimojo N, Anderson RW, Mattson DH, Turner RV, Coligan JE, Biddison WE. The kinetics of peptide binding to HLA-A2 and the conformation of the peptide-A2 complex can be determined by amino acid side chains on the floor of the peptide binding groove. Internat Immunol 2:193–200, 1990.

Sleasman JW, Morimoto C, Schlossman S, Tedder TF. The role of functionally distinct helper T lymphocyte subpopulations in the induction of human B cell differentiation. Eur J Immunol 20:1357–1366, 1990.

Smith SH, Brown MH, Rowe D, Callard RE, Beverley PCL. Functional subsets of human helper-inducer cells defined by a new monoclonal antibody, UCHL1. Immunology 58:63–70, 1986.

Snow PM, Terhorst C. The T8 antigen is a multimeric complex of two distinct subunits on human thymocytes but consists of homomultimeric forms on peripheral blood T lymphocytes. J Biol Chem 258:14675–14681, 1983.

Springer TA. Adhesion receptors of the immune system. Nature 346:425–432, 1990.

Steinman RM. The dendritic cell system and its role in immunogenicity. Annu Rev Immunol 9:271–306, 1991.

Stejskal V, Harfast B, Holm G, Perlmann P. Cytotoxicity of human lymphocytes induced by pokeweed mitogen or in mixed lymphocyte culture. Specificity and nature of effector cells. Eur J Immunol 4:126–130, 1974.

Stout RD. Macrophage activation by T cells: cognate and noncognate signals. Curr Opin Immunol 5:398–403, 1993.

Street NE, Mosmann TR. Functional diversity of T lymphocytes due to secretion of different cytokine patterns. FASEB J 5:171–177, 1991.

Streuli M, Hall LR, Saga Y, Schlossman SF, Saito H. Differential usage of three exons generates at least five different mRNAs encoding human leukocyte common antigens. J Exp Med 166:1548–1566, 1987.

Taniguchi T, Matsui H, Fujita T, Takaoka C, Kashima N, Yoshimoto R, Hamuro J. Structure and expression of a cloned cDNA for human interleukin-2. Nature 302:305–310, 1983.

Tedder TF, Clement LT, Cooper MD. Human lymphocyte differentiation antigens HB-10 and HB-11. I. Ontogeny of antigen expression. J Immunol 134:2983–2988, 1985a.

Tedder TF, Cooper MD, Clement LT. Human lymphocyte differentiation antigens HB-10 and HB-11. II. Differential production of B cell growth and differentiation factors by distinct helper T cell subpopulations. J Immunol 134:2989–2994, 1985b.

Thomas Y, Sosman J, Irigoyen O, Friedman SM, Kung PC, Goldstein G, Chess L. Functional analysis of human T cell subsets defined by monoclonal antibodies. I. Collaborative T-T interactions in the immunoregulation of B cell differentiation. J Immunol 125:2402–2408, 1980.

Tiercy J-M, Jeannet M, Mach B. A new approach for the analysis of HLA class II polymorphism: HLA oligotyping. Blood Rev 7:9–15, 1991.

Tonegawa S. The molecules of the immune system. Sci Am 253:122–131, 1985.

Tonks NK, Charbonneau H, Diltz CD, Fischer EH, Walsh KA. Demonstration that the leukocyte common antigen CD45 is a protein tyrosine phosphatase. Biochemistry 27:8695–8704, 1988.

Toy JL. The interferons. Clin Exp Immunol 54:1–13, 1983.

Trinchieri G. IL-12 and its role in the generation of T_H1 cells. Immunol Today 14:335–338, 1993.

Trinchieri G, Santoli D, Koprowski H. Spontaneous cell mediated cytotoxicity in humans: role of interferon and immunoglobulins. J Immunol 120:1849–1855, 1978.

Uchiyama T, Nelson DL, Fleisher TA, Waldmann TA. A monoclonal antibody (anti-Tac) reactive with activated and functionally mature human T cells. II. Expression of Tac antigen on activated cytotoxic killer T cells, suppressor cells, and on one of two types of helper T cells. J Immunol 126:1398–1403, 1981.

van den Elsen P, Shepley B-A, Borst J, Coligan JE, Markham AF, Orkin S, Terhorst C. Isolation of cDNA clones encoding the 20K T3 glycoprotein of human T-cell receptor complex. Nature 312:413–418, 1984.

van den Elsen P, Shepley B-A, Cho M, Terhorst C. Isolation and characterization of a cDNA clone encoding the murine homologue of the human 20K T3/T-cell receptor glycoprotein. Nature 314:542–544, 1985.

Van Wauwe JP, De Mey JR, Goossens JG. OKT3: a monoclonal anti–human T lymphocyte antibody with potent mitogenic properties. J Immunol 124:2708–2713, 1980.

Verbi W, Greaves MF, Schneider C, Koubek K, Janossy G, Stein H, Kung P, Goldstein G. Monoclonal antibodies OKT11 and OKT11A have pan-T reactivity and black sheep erythrocyte receptors. Eur J Immunol 12:81–86, 1982.

Waldmann TA, Durm M, Broder S, Blackman M, Blaese M, Strober W. Role of suppressor T cells in pathogenesis of common variable hypogammaglobulinemia. Lancet 2:609–613, 1974.

Wee SL, Chen LK, Strassmann G, Bach FH. Helper cell independent cytotoxic clones in man. J Exp Med 156:1854–1858, 1982.

Welch PA, Namen AE, Goodwin RG, Armitage R, Cooper MD. Human interleukin-7: a novel T cell growth factor. J Immunol 143:3562–3567, 1989.

Wu LYF, Lawton AR, Cooper MD. Differentiation capacity of cultured B lymphocytes from immunodeficient patients. J Clin Invest 52:3180–3189, 1973.

Yamashita N, Clement LT. Phenotypic characterization of the postthymic differentiation of human alloantigen-specific $CD8^+$ cytotoxic T lymphocytes. J Immunol 143:1518–1523, 1989.

Yamashita N, Bullington R, Clement LT. Equivalent helper functions of human "naive" and "memory" $CD4^+$ T cells for the generation of alloreactive cytotoxic T lymphocytes. J Clin Immunol 10:237–246, 1990.

Yarchoan R, Biddison WE, Schneider HS, Nelson DL. Human T-cell subset requirements for the production of specific anti influenza virus antibody in vitro. J Clin Immunol 2:118–125, 1982.

Zinkernagel RM, Doherty PC. Restriction of in vitro T cell–mediated cytotoxicity in lymphocytic choriomeningitis within a syngeneic or semiallogeneic system. Nature 248:701–702, 1974.

Zylstra M, Bix M, Sinister NE, Loring JM, Raulet DH, Jaenisch R. Beta-2-microglobulin deficient mice lack $CD4^- 8^+$ cytolytic T cells. Nature 334:742–746, 1990.

Chapter 5

The Polymorphonuclear Leukocyte System

Jon S. Abramson, J. Gary Wheeler,
and Paul G. Quie

Polymorphonuclear leukocytes include neutrophils, eosinophils, and basophils. The *neutrophil* is a highly specialized cell whose primary function is to kill microbes. This chapter concentrates on the neutrophil, since most research has focused on this cell. A brief review of the structure and function of eosinophils and basophils is also included.

The major *end-stage events* occurring after neutrophil activation include chemotactic, phagocytic, secretory, and oxidative responses. Each response helps regulate the others, although certain stimuli induce one response without initiating the others (Weissmann et al., 1981). Activation steps that occur prior to end-stage functions include ligand-receptor binding, receptor-G protein interaction, generation or changes of second messengers (e.g., ionic fluxes, cyclic nucleotide levels, arachidonic acid metabolites), and protein kinase-induced phosphorylation and phosphatase-induced dephosphorylation of proteins. Different activation pathways lead to different end-stage functions.

Until the last decade, the neutrophil was thought to be a terminally differentiated cell whose main function was to kill bacterial pathogens by oxidative and secretory capabilities. The neutrophil was thought incapable of protein synthesis or cytokine production and therefore did not participate in the immune response to nonbacterial infections. However, we now know that neutrophils play a major role in the overall immune response to a variety of pathogens both by their traditional role of phagocytosis and microbial killing, and by the production of a number of *cytokines*, for example, interleukins (IL-1 to IL-6) and tumor necrosis factor-α (TNF) (Boxer and Todd, 1993).

This chapter reviews the current status of:

1. Neutrophil maturation.
2. Neutrophil activation pathways that regulate chemotactic, phagocytic, secretory, and oxidative activities.

3. The role of the neutrophil in the overall immune response.
4. The adverse consequences of neutrophil activation.

NEUTROPHILS

Neutrophil Maturation

Neutrophil maturation occurs within two frameworks: (1) the ontogeny of single cells and (2) the marrow response to a microbial challenge.

Granulocyte Differentiation

Single-cell development has been delineated through morphologic observations of normal and pathologic marrow and the development of tissue culture methods (Bainton et al., 1971; Quesenberry and Levitt, 1979; Wright, 1982; Golde, 1983).

Neutrophils arise from bone marrow *stem cells*. Stem cells proceed through several differentiation steps in which they lose their pluripotency and commit to granulocytic differentiation. The nomenclature for these cells is derived from the types of colony-forming units these cells propagate:

- CFU-GEMM (colony-forming unit–granulocyte, –erythroid, –monocyte, –megakaryocyte)
- CFU-GM (colony-forming unit–granulocyte, –macrophage)
- CFU-G (colony-forming unit–granulocyte)

The last of the progenitor pool (CFU-G) differentiate into committed myeloid cells of the neutrophil proliferative pools (NPP): myeloblasts, promyelocytes, and myelocytes.

Table 5–1. Contents of Granules in Neutrophils

Primary Granules (Azurophilic)	Secondary Granules (Specific)	Tertiary Granules
Myeloperoxidase	Lactoferrin	Gelatinase
Lysozyme	Lysosome	Cytochrome b
Acid hydrolases	B_{12}-binding protein	Ubiquinone
Neutral proteases (e.g., elastase)	Phospholipase A_2	CD11b, CD11c, CD18
Cationic antibacterial proteins	Collagenase Plasminogen activator	
Sialidase	Cytochrome b Sialidase	

Granule Development

The first differentiation step is the development of the early *promyelocyte*, also referred to as the *eogranulocyte* (Brederoo et al., 1983). During this stage, the earliest granule forms—nucleated granules—have been identified (Scott and Horn, 1970; Breton-Gorius et al., 1978; Wright, 1982; DeWald et al., 1982).

The late promyelocyte develops next and is characterized by primary or azurophilic cytoplasmic granules containing hydrolases, proteases, lysosome, and myeloperoxidase (Table 5–1). With further differentiation (*myelocytic* stage), there is a loss of the deep-blue appearance of the granules with Wright-Giemsa stain and a neutrophilic character is acquired. This is caused by an increase in secondary or specific granules. The staining characteristics of the granules can now distinguish neutrophils from basophils and eosinophils. Specific granules of the neutrophil myelocyte contain lactoferrin and vitamin B_{12}-binding protein; in the mature cell, they outnumber the azurophilic granules about twofold. The neutrophil granules are generated in the Golgi complex and bud off from the endoplasmic reticulum.

Abnormalities of budding occur in *Chédiak-Higashi syndrome* with the formation of giant coalesced granules (see Chapter 15).

Early stages of neutrophil development are characterized by the presence of mitochondria; later stages are marked by a proliferation of glycogen with few mitochondria. This change represents a shift from aerobic metabolism to glycolysis as the major source of cell energy (Beck, 1958; Scott and Horn, 1970).

Development of Membrane Receptors

The ontogeny of neutrophil surface receptors has become clarified primarily because of monoclonal antibody technology. The appearance of membrane adherence proteins, complement receptors, immunoglobulin receptors, and other cellular differentiation markers has been identified at different stages of neutrophil proliferation and differentiation.

Early myeloid differentiation can be characterized by the loss of CD34 (a stem cell marker), the transient appearance and disappearance of HLA-DR (on CFU-GEMM, CFU-GM, and CFU-G), the appearance of CD13 (aminopeptidase N) and CD38 (NAD glycohydrolase) in the myeloblast (Kanwar and Cairo, 1993). As shown in Figure 5–1, promyelocytes lack complement (CR3) and Fcγ (Fc gamma) receptors until they begin to differentiate. Fc gamma receptors (FcγR) are not present until the metamyelocyte stage (Fleit et al., 1984; Kanwar and Cairo, 1993). Membrane adherence proteins (e.g., CR3) and the Fc receptors are critical for *chemotaxis* and *phagocytosis*, and their acquisition parallels development of these functions.

Other factors play a role in these functions. For example, chemotaxis is reduced in early band forms compared to segmented forms (Boner et al., 1982). Immature neutrophils are more rigid, probably because of altered actin polymerization, and have delayed microbial ingestion, compared with mature cells (Lichtman and Weed, 1972; Altman and Stossel, 1974). Other surface receptors include erythrocyte and human granulocyte antigens (HGA). The granulocyte-specific antigens display considerable polymorphism and are responsible for immune neutropenias (particularly NA1 and NA2 antigens) and febrile transfusion reactions (Billett and Caren, 1985). Surface glycosylation patterns also change with maturation, and this affects

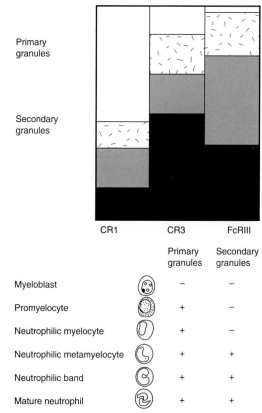

Figure 5–1. The increase in granules and surface proteins on neutrophils as they mature from myeloblasts *(top)* to mature neutrophils *(bottom)*. CR1, CR3, and FcRIII are initially absent from myeloblasts *(top portion of bars)* but begin to be expressed on the surface at different stages of myelopoiesis. Slight expression is depicted by the speckled pattern, moderate expression by the gray pattern, and strong expression by the black pattern. Primary granules appear at the promyelocyte stage and secondary granules appear at metamyelocyte stage. (From Kanwar VS, Cairo MS. Neonatal neutrophil maturation, kinetics, and function. In Abramson JS, Wheeler JG, eds. The Neutrophil. Oxford, England, Oxford University Press, 1993, pp. 1–16).

certain cell functions. Excessive N-acetyl neuraminic acid on immature cells has been associated with a high negative surface charge with inhibition of adhesion and cell-cell interactions (Lichtman and Weed, 1972). The loss of these sugars may make them more susceptible to phagocytosis by the reticuloendothelial system after programmed cell death *(apoptosis)*.

Granulocyte Kinetics During Infection

Myelopoiesis is now understood to be a cytokine orchestrated event. Most of the permissive myelopoietic cytokines have been cloned and their functions established using in vitro culture systems. Granulocyte colony-stimulating-factor (G-CSF), granulocyte-macrophage colony-stimulating factor (GM-CSF), IL-3 and IL-6, and stem cell factor (SCF) are glycoproteins (14,000 to 26,000 kD) that stimulate progenitor cells to differentiate. Most are derived from T lymphocytes, but monocytes, fibroblasts, endothelial cells, other reticuloendothelial cells, and even granulocytes synthesize cytokines to some degree (Boxer and Todd, 1993). See Appendix 2.

Interaction of various cytokines regulates the differentiation and interaction of neutrophil precursors. Several of these cytokines used alone in pharmacologic doses have dramatic effects on granulopoiesis (Vadhan-Raj et al., 1987; Nemunaitis et al., 1991). Cellular stromal interactions are also important in granulocyte differentiation. Other factors also affect proliferation and differentiation, both positively and negatively (chalones). The normal turnover of the neutrophil pool is negatively affected by drugs (e.g., lithium and antibiotics; the latter is reversible with recombinant G-CSF), illnesses (particularly viral), microbial products (e.g., endotoxin), and cellular products (e.g., lactoferrin and prostaglandin E). Finally, the ultimate egress of cells from marrow into the circulation is affected by IL-1, complement factors C3e and C3d,g, and intravenous immunoglobulin (IVIG) (Shigeoka, et al., 1988).

The blood neutrophil pool is partitioned into marginated and circulating components roughly equal in size. Neutrophils shift from the marginated to the circulating pool with stress (e.g., exercise, infection, labor) and in response to beta-agonists and IL-6. In adults the proliferative and storage pools may exceed circulating neutrophils by a factor of 5 to 10. According to rat models, the rate of production can be increased threefold (Kanwar and Cairo, 1993).

Under physiologic conditions, 9 to 11 days are required for neutrophil maturation and release into the circulation, based on generation times of 18 to 24 hours for myeloblasts and promyelocytes, 52 hours for myelocytes, and 96 to 144 hours for their appearance in the circulation (Fliedner et al., 1964a, 1964b; Cronkite and Vincent, 1970). With stress or infection, their turnover is accelerated; for example, in the neonate, reconstitution of the depleted marrow has occurred in less than 24 hours (Christensen et al., 1982; Wheeler et al., 1984b). Once the granulocyte leaves the marrow, its half-life in the circulation is 6 to 10 hours (Mauer et al., 1960). However, neutrophils remain fully func-

tional in whole blood up to 28 hours when stored in citrate-phosphate-dextrose anticoagulant at 4°C (McCullough et al., 1969; Wheeler et al., 1984a).

Granulocyte Kinetics and Function in the Fetus and Neonate

During fetal development, leukocytes are first produced in the liver at about 2 months' gestation. At about 5 months' gestation, the bone marrow replaces the liver as the primary hematopoietic center (Playfair et al., 1963). The bone marrow neutrophil storage pool of premature and term animals is considerably smaller than that of adults. Bacterial infection in human neonates leads to rapid exhaustion of the neutrophil storage pool and may result in *neutropenia* (Christensen et al., 1982; Erdman et al., 1982).

It is uncertain at what age the infant storage pool achieves normal adult size and whether attrition occurs with aging. The recent recognition of neutrophil programmed cell death (apoptosis) may be a mechanism by which cells remove themselves from the circulation.

In addition to the smaller neutrophil pool, neonatal neutrophils function poorly compared to those of older children and adults (Hill, 1987). This increases the neonate's risk for infection. Most studies of neonatal granulocyte function have been done on cord blood, which contains both immature neutrophils (released under the stress of birth) and mature neutrophils exposed to cytokines associated with delivery, placental separation, acidosis, and progesterone. Drugs used in delivery, such as anesthetics and antibiotics, may also alter the function of neonatal neutrophils (Frazier et al., 1982; Cotton et al., 1983; Lippa et al., 1983; White et al., 1983; Krumholz et al., 1993; Wheeler and Abramson, 1993).

Although controversy exists over which newborn neutrophil functions are truly abnormal, there is agreement that chemotaxis and adherence related functions are decreased. Neutrophil chemotaxis and serum chemotactic activity are abnormal, and chemotactic function does not reach adult levels until after 5 years of age (Miller, 1979; Mohandes et al., 1982; Sacchi et al., 1982; Anderson et al., 1983; Klein et al., 1977; Krause and Lew, 1987). Other neonatal abnormalities in diapedesis-related functions include decreased expression of adherence proteins (Smith JB, 1990; Bruce et al., 1987), and abnormal deformability, adherence, aggregation, and actin polymerization (Fontan et al., 1981; Mease et al., 1981; Krause et al., 1982; Olson et al., 1983; Hilmo and Howard, 1987).

Other abnormalities of neonatal granulocyte function are controversial. Frazier and associates (1982) found that cord blood neutrophils from elective non-labor cesarean sections have normal quantitative nitroblue tetrazolium reduction, oxygen consumption, and hexose monophosphate shunt activity. By contrast, *chemiluminescence* (another measure of oxidative metabolism) was found to be depressed 12 to 36 hours after birth (Mills et al., 1979).

Unlike neutrophils from normal newborns, neutrophils from stressed or premature neonates have decreased oxidative responses and microbial killing activity when compared with adult cells (Anderson et al., 1974; Wright et al., 1975; Mills et al., 1979; Shigeoka et al., 1979; Driscoll et al., 1990). This may explain the increased number of immature forms that accompany the neonate's response to stress. Phagocytosis is normal or supernormal (Mills et al., 1979; Harris et al., 1983), whereas degranulation has been less fully investigated. Ambruso and Johnston (1981) found that neutrophil lactoferrin levels are reduced in neonates, and Christensen and Rothstein (1985) found that a high turnover of neonatal neutrophils led to decreased primary granule (myeloperoxidase-containing) content. The calcium responses to some stimuli are abnormal in neonatal cells (Anderson et al., 1981), but studies of the signal transduction pathway, including G protein function, second messengers, and protein kinases, have not yet been accomplished.

Granulocyte Kinetics and Function in Older Adults

Less attention has focused on neutrophil function with aging. Oxidative-metabolic activities are consistently depressed in the neutrophils of geriatric adults, whereas chemotaxis is both normal and abnormal (Saltzmann and Peterson, 1987). Suzuki and colleagues (1983) demonstrated that degranulation decreases after age 50. Nagel et al. (1986) have shown abnormalities of phagocytosis of beads with aging. The production of some phosphoinositides and their subsequent second messengers may be compromised in neutrophils from geriatric patients, and this may alter their capacity to respond to infections (Lipschitz et al., 1991).

The effect of aging on neutrophil apoptosis is not known. Further studies should address the effects of aging on both neutrophil maturation and function.

Activation and Transmembrane Signaling

The neutrophil signal pathway is a complex series of events that eventually elicit one or more of the end-stage functions of the cell. During the past decade, data have accumulated that indicate different or divergent pathways for the various end-stage functions. The advantage in having different pathways available for neutrophil activation allows the cell to exhibit only the activity that is needed at the time; that is, the cell can move to the site of infection before activating its microbicidal functions.

Other mechanisms are available to control the type of end-stage response that is elicited. A process termed *deactivation* (down-regulation) can occur where low concentrations of a stimulus cause chemotaxis, but higher concentrations decrease chemotaxis and stimulate the respiratory burst. This is thought to be due to decreased membrane receptor numbers and/or affinity (Gallin, 1982; Cassimeris and Zigmond, 1990).

In contrast to down-regulation, *priming* (enhancement) of the respiratory burst occurs when the neutrophils are incubated with certain agents and then exposed to a different stimulus (Van Epps and Garcia,

1980; Yuo et al., 1991); these priming agents may themselves be unable to activate end-stage functions (e.g., GM-CSF) or do not induce end-stage functions at the low concentrations used for priming. As an example, at low concentrations N-formyl-methionyl-leucyl-phenylalanine (FMLP) causes priming; at higher concentrations, it induces chemotaxis and at still greater amounts produces respiratory burst activity. The exact mechanism for priming remains to be elucidated and probably varies for different agents. For example, GM-CSF priming is associated with up-regulation of a trimeric G protein (G_i2) (Durstin et al., 1993); priming with 1-oleoyl-2-acetylglycerol (OAG) is not thought to involve trimeric G proteins.

The neutrophil's regulatory mechanisms for controlling the type and extent of a given end-stage function are described in the text on end-stage functions. The following text reviews the neutrophil's signal activation pathways. For a more detailed discussion, see McPhail and Harvath (1993).

Ligand-Receptor Interaction

The first step of neutrophil activation is the binding of a *ligand* to a *receptor*. Neutrophils have receptors for several different ligands, including N-formyl peptides (e.g., FMLP), which are derived from cell wall products of invading microbes, and components generated by the host, including complement components (C5a and C3b), cytokines (interleukin 8 [IL-8], leukotriene B_4 [LTB_4], platelet activating factor [PAF]) and immunoglobulins (Lambeth, 1988; Harvath, 1991; McPhail et al., 1992b; Rosales and Brown, 1993). Many of these receptors are present on the neutrophil outer plasma membrane, even in the resting state, and are up-regulated from the lysosomal compartment upon stimulation (Table 5–2). Upon attachment of these ligands to their receptor, a complex series of events is started that initiates one or more end-stage functions, usually within 1 minute. Most, but not all ligands, can elicit all of the end-stage responses if there is a high enough concentration of the ligand. As a general rule, how-

Table 5–2. Neutrophil Surface Proteins

Class	Name	Synonym
Adhesion molecules	CD11a/CD18	LFA-1
	CD11b/CD18	CR3
	CD11c/CD18	gp150, 95
	L-selectin (CD62L)	
	sLe^x (CD15s)	LECAM-1, LAM-1
	VLA-6	
	LRI (leukocyte response integrin)	ECM binding protein
Antibody receptors	FCγRII	CD32
	FCγRIII	CD16
Complement receptors	CR1 (CD35)	C3b receptor
	CR2 (CD21)	C3d receptor
	CR3 (CD11b/CD18)	iC3b receptor Mac-1, Mo-1
	CR4 (CD11c/CD18)	C3b receptor gp150, 95

ever, ligands that are potent chemoattractants are less effective at eliciting the respiratory burst and vice versa. For example, IL-8 is a potent chemoattractant but elicits only a weak respiratory burst. This regulatory discrepancy is beneficial because it allows the neutrophil to arrive at the site of infection prior to eliciting a strong oxidative response.

G Protein Activity

G proteins are guanine nucleotide binding proteins that couple extracellular receptors to intracellular second messenger systems. Two classes of G proteins exist in cells. *Heterotrimeric* G proteins, consisting of alpha, beta, and gamma subunits, function as intermediaries linking the receptor to enzymes that generate second messengers (Bokoch, 1990). Association of receptors with heterotrimeric G proteins increases receptor binding affinity (Sklar, 1986). There are also small *monomeric* G proteins that function downstream in the activation cascade to help regulate end-stage functions (Quinn et al., 1989; Bokoch et al., 1991; Philips et al., 1991).

G proteins undergo guanine nucleotide exchange and guanosine triphosphate (GTP) hydrolysis. For trimeric G proteins, guanine nucleotide exchange occurs at the α-subunit. When GDP is bound to the α-subunit, the protein is inactive. Upon binding of the ligand to the receptor, the GDP is released and replaced with GTP. A conformational change occurs that allows the α-subunit to disassociate from the β/gamma complex, attach to the effector enzyme, and generate a second messenger. At least for some stimuli, the β-subunit may also interact with effector enzymes (Kleus et al., 1992). GTP hydrolysis then allows the G protein to go back to its inactive state (Fig. 5–2). GDP release is the most important rate-limiting step, and this is controlled by guanine nucleotide release proteins (GNRPs). For monomeric G proteins, the rate of release of GDP is also regulated by guanine nucleotide dissociation inhibitors (GDIs). For trimeric G proteins, the rate of GTP hydrolysis is not regulated by a protein; for monomeric G proteins, however, the rate of GTP hydrolysis is regulated by proteins termed *GTPase-activating proteins* (GAPs). The intracellular concentration of magnesium may also influence G protein activation (Freissmuth et al., 1989).

A variety of trimeric and monomeric G proteins are found in different cells. There are four known trimeric G proteins: G_s, G_q, G_i2, and G_i3. Some of the G proteins are altered by adenosine diphosphate (ADP)–ribosylating bacterial toxins, including pertussis, cholera, and botulism C_3 toxin; indeed these toxins are used to determine the role of G proteins in neutrophil function.

G_s couples adrenergic and other receptors to adenylate cyclase.

G_i proteins link N-formyl peptide receptors and probably other chemoattractant receptors to an effector enzyme. For instance, G_i2, a pertussis toxin–sensitive G protein, links FMLP receptors to phospholipase C). Al-

though G_i3 may be involved with chemoattractant receptors, less is known about this and G_q proteins.

Monomeric neutrophil G proteins include rap1A and rac, and these may be involved in regulating end-stage functions, including oxidative and secretory responses (Quinn et al., 1989; Dexter et al., 1990; Bokoch et al., 1991; Philips et al., 1991).

Generation and Role of Second Messengers

Concentrations of neutrophil second messengers increase dramatically upon cell stimulation. These include:

- Inositol triphosphate (IP_3)
- Ca^{2+}
- Diacylglycerol (DAG)
- Phosphatidic acid (PA)
- Arachidonic acid (AA)
- Cyclic nucleotides

Because different pathways are activated by various stimuli, not all second messengers are increased by a particular stimulus. For chemoattractant stimuli, the second messengers are generated either directly or indirectly in response to G protein activation of phospholipases (A_2, C and D) in the cell. For example, the activation of phospholipase C causes hydrolysis of

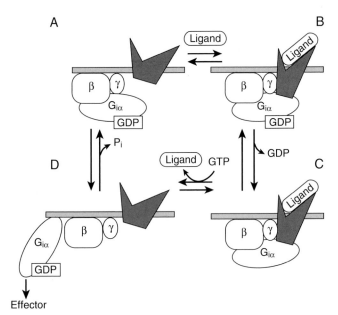

Figure 5–2. A simplified scheme of potential chemoattractant receptor and heterotrimeric G protein interactions. Receptor (black structure) dissociation from the G protein (*A* and *D*) results in a low receptor-binding affinity for the ligand, whereas receptor association with the G protein (*B* and *C*) confers a high binding affinity for the ligand. GTP binding to the α-subunit results in dissociation of the complex and GTPase activity. GTPase activity occurs only when GTP is bound to the α-subunit (*D*) and is absent in conditions represented in *A*, *B*, and *C*. During guanine nucleotide exchange, the complex may exist in a nucleotide-empty state (*B* and *C*). Several other receptor states (not shown) have been proposed. (From McPhail LC, Harvath L. Signal transduction in neutrophil oxidative metabolism and chemotaxis. In Abramson JS, Wheeler JG, eds. The Neutrophil. Oxford, England, Oxford University Press, 1993, pp. 63–107.)

phosphatidylinositol-4,5-biphosphate to DAG and IP_3, which in turn activates protein kinase C and increases the level of intracellular Ca^{2+}. In contrast, phorbol ester stimuli, which induce oxidative and secretory but not chemotactic activities, can directly activate protein kinase C without increasing intracellular Ca^{2+} (Sha'afi et al., 1983). Second messengers of the neutrophil have been reviewed (DiVirgilio et al., 1990; Reibman et al., 1990; Traynor-Kaplan, 1990; McPhail and Harvath, 1993).

The exact role of these second messengers in activating the functional responses of the neutrophil varies, depending on the end-stage function. In general, elevated levels of cyclic adenosine monophosphate (cAMP) have an inhibiting effect but increased levels of cyclic guanosine monophosphate (cGMP) and Ca^{2+} enhance neutrophil functions (Zurier et al., 1974; McPhail and Harvath, 1993). These messengers have a role in activating some cellular protein kinases, enzymes that cause phosphorylation of various proteins within the neutrophil (DiVirgilio et al., 1990; Reibman et al., 1990). Additionally, subcellular regional increases in intracellular Ca^{2+} occur during cell activation (Sawyer et al., 1985; Marks and Maxfield, 1990), which may regulate cytoskeletal changes influencing chemotactic activity. The intracellular site of action for the lipid mediators is not well defined, but the mediators may interact with phospholipases, protein kinases, and the reduced nicotinamide-adenine dinucleotide phosphate (NADPH) oxidase system (Agwu et al., 1991; McPhail et al., 1992a).

Protein Kinases and Phosphatases

Neutrophils have a number of kinases that can phosphorylate proteins at a serine, threonine, or tyrosine amino acid site (similarly, some phosphatases can dephosphorylate proteins). Many of these kinases are the target of secondary messengers and once activated cause phosphorylation of intracellular and some extracellular proteins. Inhibitors of protein kinases depress one or more end-stage cellular functions (Harvath et al., 1987; Tauber et al., 1990).

An example of neutrophil kinases are the cAMP- and cGMP-dependent kinases, which cause phosphorylation of the cytoskeletal proteins actin and vimentin, respectively. Whether phosphorylation is important in regulating the function of these cytoskeleton proteins is not clearly established. Neutrophil protein kinases and their substrates are reviewed by Huang (1989).

END-STAGE FUNCTIONS

Within 1 minute of ligand-receptor binding, a transmembrane signal is generated and the end-stage chemotactic, phagocytic, secretory, and/or oxidative activities are initiated. These activities allow the neutrophil to arrive at the site of microbial invasion, initiate killing and digestion, and control the infection. This process is usually efficient and completed without the benefit of antimicrobial drugs. However, patients with neutrophil abnormalities or neutropenia have an increased risk

for serious bacterial, fungal, and even viral diseases (see Chapter 15, Disorders of the Polymorphonuclear Phagocytic System). The following text reviews the biophysical events that allow these end-stage functions to occur.

Granulocyte Movement

Types of Cell Movement

Rapid movement of neutrophils to a site of microbial invasion is crucial for localizing and eliminating infection. The types of cell movement include:

- Nondirected (random) migration
- Stimulated nondirected migration (i.e., chemokinesis)
- Directed migration (i.e., chemotaxis)

There may be defects in the machinery needed for cell movement, an inability to increase the rate of migration, or a defect of directed migration (Gallin et al., 1980, Singer and Kupfer, 1986). The type of structural or biochemical defect determines which migration responses will be impaired. Abnormalities of membrane glycoprotein receptors, cytoskeletal assembly, lysosomal granules, and cyclic nucleotide levels all have been implicated in defective chemotaxis (see Chapter 15).

Chemoattractants and Receptor Binding

The initial event that initiates a chemotactic response is the generation of chemotactic stimuli. These stimuli include:

1. C5a, a complement fragment generated by activation of the complement cascade.
2. Secretion products from other cells (e.g., the cytokines IL-8 and PAF).
3. Arachidonic acid metabolites from the oxidation of neutrophil lipids (e.g., LTB_4).
4. Proteins of the coagulation pathway.
5. Microbial components, which activate complement and have chemotactic activity themselves; small-molecular-weight peptides, such as FMLP, are similar to bacterial chemoattractants and are used to study the chemotactic response.

Once chemotactic stimuli are generated, they attach to receptors on the cell's plasma membrane; this is termed *receptor-ligand interaction*. Chemoattractant receptors exist in interconvertible high and low affinity states, and association of a receptor with a G protein increases receptor binding affinity (Sklar, 1986). For the FMLP receptor, there are three affinity states:

1. The high affinity state consists of the reversibly bound ligand-receptor-G protein.
2. The low-affinity state consists of a reversibly bound ligand-receptor.
3. In the inactive state, the ligand is irreversibly bound to the receptor.

The association rate of the ligand to the receptor is

equivalent for the high and low affinity states; however, the dissociation rate differs by twofold and thus a critical difference between high and low receptor affinity states (Sklar et al., 1989; Fay et al., 1991).

Chemotactic factors attach to a specific receptor for that factor (Fletcher and Gallin, 1983; Sklar, 1986; Sklar and Omenn, 1990). Prior to ligand-receptor binding, neutrophils move in a random fashion; once the chemoattractant attaches to the plasma membrane, chemokinesis and chemotaxis proceed. The neutrophil can sense a 1% chemoattractant gradient from the front to the back of the cell and moves in the direction of the higher concentration (Zigmond, 1977). Fewer than 50% of neutrophils migrate in response to chemoattractants (Harvath et al., 1980). The cells that migrate to one chemoattractant are the same as those that migrate to other chemoattractants. The structural or biochemical difference between migrating and nonmigrating cells is not known, but it is not due to differences in ligand-receptor binding (Harvath and Leonard, 1982).

Chemotactic Activation Pathway

The activation pathways that elicit end-stage responses share the signal transduction machinery with other cells and include: (1) activation of phospholipases, (2) generation of second messengers, and (3) activation of protein kinases and phosphatases. However, some differences in these pathways for different end-stage functions exist.

Certain stimuli elicit only one type of response; for instance, phorbol myristate acetate invokes oxidative and secretory, but not chemotactic, activities. Furthermore, even among stimuli that cause chemotaxis, different pathways exist. For example, certain inhibitors of protein kinase (isoquinoline sulfonamides) decrease chemotaxis in response to FMLP, but not to LTB_4 (Harvath et al., 1987, 1991). These protein kinase inhibitors decrease chemotaxis but have no effect on oxidative activities in response to FMLP (Harvath et al., 1987).

Similarly, agents that disrupt the polymerization of actin during cytoskeleton assembly completely shut down chemotaxis, yet enhance secretion and the respiratory burst (McPhail and Snyderman, 1983; Norgauer et al., 1988). Thus, cytoskeleton assembly is unnecessary for completion of these later two responses. Oxidized derivatives of FMLP that bind to the receptor with lower affinity than the nonoxidized FMLP elicit an oxidative response but do not induce chemotaxis (Harvath and Aksamit, 1984). This suggests that binding affinity determines which activation pathway is elicited. Much remains to be learned about activation pathways, but it is clear that this diversity allows the neutrophil to select a specific end-stage function. This allows for a more focused attack against microbial invaders.

Within 10 seconds of chemoattractant-receptor binding, G proteins and their effector enzymes are activated; this results in generation of second messengers. For chemotactic activity, much research on second messengers has focused on the role of Ca^{2+}. Depletion of intracellular and extracellular calcium partially inhibits cell movement (Meshulam et al., 1986). Elevated intracellular calcium promotes the assembly of cytoskeleton F-actin and modifies actin-binding cytoskeleton proteins via calcium-mediated phosphorylation (Eberle et al., 1990). Neutrophils undergoing chemotaxis show localized increases in intracellular Ca^{2+}; this suggests that pseudopod formation is regulated by such changes. Although extracellular Ca^{2+} is not required for initiation of chemotaxis, it is important for sustained cell movement. The role of other intermediary messengers in chemotaxis is less clear (McPhail and Harvath, 1993).

Role of the Cytoskeleton in Cell Movement

Prior to chemotaxis, the cell shape changes from spherical to bipolar. A wide, undulating *pseudopod,* which forms thin anterior-extending lamellepodia containing large amounts of microfilament proteins, is at the leading edge of the cell. At the back of the cell are the nucleus and contractile *uropod* with long-extending retraction fibers by which the cell adheres to surfaces. The *centriole,* an organizing center for the *microtubule system,* is found between the nucleus and the leading edge (Malech et al., 1977; Gallin et al., 1980). The cell migrates by repetitive events, during which the *lamellepodia* is extended in the direction of the gradient and the uropod is retracted toward the body of the cell.

The neutrophil cytoskeleton is composed of microfilaments (containing actin), actin-binding proteins, intermediate filaments, and microtubules. These provide the components for contractile forces and cell movement. The polymerization of *globular actin (G-actin)* monomers into actin filaments (F-actin) occurs within seconds after chemoattractant-receptor binding, and it is actin that provides the force for cell movement (Singer and Kupfer, 1986; Omann et al., 1987).

Actin has two linear polymers of a globular protein wrapped in a helix shape, and *myosin* is composed of large molecules that are asymmetric. One end of the myosin molecule has a globular shape, which binds to actin and has an enzymatic site that hydrolyses adenosine triphosphate (ATP) (Adelstein, 1983). Contractile activity depends on the rate of hydrolysis of ATP, which is controlled by a calcium-calmodulin–dependent enzyme, myosin light-chain kinase. *Calmodulin* is a protein with four calcium binding sites; it binds to myosin light-chain kinase and causes the phosphorylation of myosin. This increases the rate of ATP hydrolysis and contractile activity of the microfilament proteins in the cell.

Other actin-binding proteins are involved in the reversible gelation and solation of the three-dimensional dynamically changing actin network. Microtubules that radiate from the centriole provide stability to the cytoskeleton and allow movement of lysosomal granules and locomotion. Agents that interfere with proteins involved with cytoskeleton function inhibit chemotaxis (Zigmond and Hirsch, 1972; Norgauer et al., 1988). Additionally, patients with congenital abnormalities of cytoskeleton function exhibit decreased chemotaxis (Coates et al., 1991; Southwick et al., 1988).

Role of Degranulation in Cell Movement

Lysosomal granules also regulate neutrophil chemotactic activity. Lysosomal granules are secreted into phagosomes, onto the plasma membrane and into extracellular spaces. Although discharge of granules into phagosomes is critical for microbicidal activity, specific granules also contribute to the chemotactic response. Exocytosis of lactoferrin may increase neutrophil surface charges and adherence to endothelial cells (Oseas et al., 1981; Boxer et al., 1982b). Indeed, a patient with absence of specific granules has exhibited markedly impaired adherence and chemotaxis, which was able to be restored by the addition of lactoferrin to the patient's cells in vitro (Boxer et al., 1982a). Other secretory products may also affect neutrophil adherence and chemotaxis (Gordon et al., 1979; Bockenstedt and Goetzl, 1980).

Secretion of neutrophil contents contributes significantly to inflammation at a local site. Certain lysosomal enzymes cleave complement components (Wright and Gallin, 1975, 1977) and induce formation of C5a by activating complement (Wright and Gallin, 1975, 1977; Wright and Klock, 1979). Other proteases can inactivate chemotactic factors, including C5a (Venge and Olsson, 1975; Wright and Gallin, 1977). Therefore, neutrophil secretion can both generate or inactivate chemotactic stimuli and thereby regulate cell movement.

Another mechanism by which the neutrophil localizes to a site of infection is by deactivation with downregulation of cell movement. Neutrophils possess an intracellular pool of chemoattractant receptors many times greater than the number of surface receptors. These intracellular receptors are translocated to the surface when the cells are stimulated (Gallin and Seligmann, 1984). Cells that vigorously degranulate (i.e., release of more than 30% of lysosomal enzymes) undergo deactivation with decreased numbers of chemotactic receptors and immigration of neutrophils from the circulation. Additional adherence molecules on neutrophils and endothelial cells may also be involved with diapedesis (Springer, 1990). A diagram for these interactions is presented in Figure 5–3 (Rosales and Brown, 1993).

Phagocytosis

Phagocytosis involves both attachment to receptors and subsequent engulfment of microbes. Neutrophils are usually activated by the attachment of opsonized microbes to specific receptors on the plasma membrane. The presence of complement and antibody on the bacteria reduces their hydrophilic forces and allows greater interaction of microbe and neutrophil. Thermodynamic particle-surface relationships may contribute to bacterial pathogenicity by inhibiting neutrophil attachment and phagocytosis. Nonpathogenic bacteria tend to be hydrophobic, and attachment to neutrophil

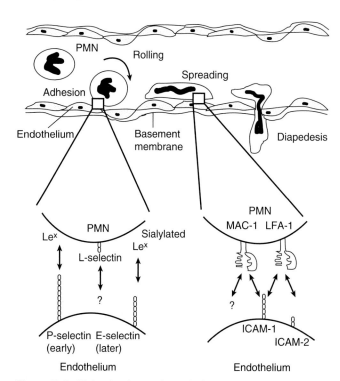

Figure 5–3. Molecular interactions during neutrophil adhesion to endothelium at sites of inflammation. The bottom half of the figure is an exploded view of the neutrophil–endothelial cell interface within the rectangle. (From Rosales C, Brown EJ. Neutrophil receptors and modulation of the immune response. In Abramson JS, Wheeler JG, eds. The Neutrophil. Oxford, England, Oxford University Press, 1993, pp. 23–62.)

receptors occurs readily even without *opsonization* (Van Oss et al., 1975; Kreutzer et al., 1979; Verhoef and Visser, 1993).

The receptor-ligand interaction causes alterations in cytoskeletal proteins (actin, myosin and actin-binding proteins), which are necessary for phagocytosis to occur. The actin microfilaments undergo polymerization in the region of the cell where receptor-ligand interaction has occurred. The polymerization allows the formation of pseudopodia (finger-like extensions of the plasma membrane) to occur. The plasma membrane surrounds the microbe, forming a phagocytic vacuole *(phagosome)*. Simultaneously, granules in the cytoplasm fuse with the phagosome and a new phagolysosome is produced (Verhoef and Visser, 1993). Phagocytosis of particles does not require activation of pertussis toxin-sensitive trimeric G proteins, phosphoinositide turnover, liberation of arachidonic acid, or increases in intracellular calcium (Rossi et al., 1989). Patients with neutrophils that have a defect only in phagocytosis have not been described.

Degranulation

Controlled degranulation can have a number of nonmicrobicidal effects, such as enhancement of chemotaxis due to the release of intracellular receptors and changes in plasma membrane surface charge. However, the main purpose of degranulation and lysosome-phagosome fusion is to kill pathogens.

Types of Granules

Table 5–1 lists the different granules, classified by differential centrifugation and by contents. *Primary granules* appear first during myelopoiesis and consist of two distinct populations with different densities. *Secondary* (specific) *granules* develop later; they have a uniform density (Wright, 1982) and give the cell its characteristic color on histologic staining. A third type, the *tertiary granule,* is defined by its major constituent gelatinase (DeWald et al., 1982; Verhoef and Visser, 1993).

Events Contributing to Degranulation

After receptor occupancy, two activation events initiate degranulation. The first stimulus is phagocytosis of opsonized particles and creation of an internalized pathogen in a phagosome. Through a series of events dependent on changes in cytoskeletal structures, localized fluctuation in intracellular electrolytes and specialized proteins *(annexins),* the membranes of phagosomes and granules fuse and degranulation occurs. The second stimulus is the direct stimulation of activation pathways, but without phagocytosis. This can be demonstrated in vitro by the use of agents such as calcium ionophore. These perturb the membrane, cause a shift in intracellular ions, and trigger degranulation of secondary (specific) granules. In general, specific granule contents are released extracellularly and primary granule contents are released intraphagosomally (Wright, 1988).

The in vitro data suggest that the release of specific, primary, and tertiary granules is under separate regulation. Whether this selected release of granules occurs in vivo is not yet established. The in vitro experiments suggest that the characteristics of bacteria, such as their glycosylation state, may dictate the type of granule release (Steadman et al., 1988).

In vitro FMLP stimulates the release of primary, secondary, and tertiary granules; at relatively low concentrations, FMLP stimulates the release of granules containing only FMLP receptors. Phorbol myristate acetate releases specific and tertiary granules but not primary granule (Goldstein et al., 1975a; Weissmann et al., 1981; Steadman et al., 1988). Other degranulation stimulants include receptor-dependent agents (e.g., leukotriene B_4, C3bi, FcRγ) and physical stimuli (e.g., hyperosmolality or hypo-osmolality).

Calcium Flux

During phagocytosis and activation, alterations in transmembrane potential (Korchak and Weissmann, 1978; Seligmann and Gallin, 1980) are followed by shifts in intracellular calcium and other ions. An increase of intracellular calcium is associated with degranulation (Korchak and Weissmann, 1980; Seligmann and Gallin, 1980; Weissmann et al., 1981). Intracellular calcium antagonists inhibit secretory responses (Weissmann et al., 1978).

Extracellular calcium enhances enzyme degranulation, but degranulation can occur in the absence of extracellular calcium (Smolen et al., 1980). Calcium may be necessary for degranulation to chemoattractants, such as FMLP and LTB$_4$, but intracellular calcium fluxes alone cannot activate degranulation (Rossi et al., 1988). Intracellular organelles that store calcium (Krause and Lew, 1987) allow for localized increases of calcium within the cell; these shifts in intracellular calcium occur in regions of the cell that are undergoing stimulation (Hoffstein, 1979; Weissmann et al., 1978; Wick and Hepler, 1982).

Certain stimuli, such as phorbol myristate acetate, can induce neutrophil degranulation without shifts in calcium distribution, indicating alternative pathways of transmembrane signaling (Sha'afi et al., 1983). Other cations may also contribute to transmembrane signaling (Kitagawa and Johnston, 1985). Anions can alkalinize the intralysosomal pH and decrease degranulation by inhibiting the fusion of lysosomal granules with phagocytic vacuoles (Korchak et al., 1980; Klempner and Styrt, 1983).

cAMP and Prostaglandins

A role for cyclic nucleotides and prostaglandins in degranulation has been suggested. Agents that elevate intracellular cAMP decrease lysosomal secretion, whereas agents that elevate intracellular cGMP augment degranulation (Zurier et al, 1974). Neutrophils can generate factors such as (1) arachidonic acid–derived prostaglandins of the E and F series, (2) thromboxane A$_2$ via the cyclooxygenase pathway and (3) hydroxyeicosatetraenoic acid, hydroperoxyeicosatetraenoic acid, and leukotrienes by the lipoxygenase pathway (Smolen et al., 1982), which may influence degranulation. Although certain prostaglandins, when added to neutrophils, produce sustained elevations of cAMP and inhibit degranulation (Weissmann et al., 1981), a direct role for prostaglandins in degranulation is unproven.

Cytoskeletal Changes

Cytoskeletal alterations occur during intracellular calcium shifts. Calcium binding and releasing proteins trigger a cascade of events involving microtubules, microfilaments, and other calcium-dependent proteins that lead to a change in the sol/gel status of the cytoplasm. Lysosomes and phagosomes drift toward each other as a leading wave of sol formation and result in lysosome-phagosome fusion. The molecular basis for this fusion involves fusion proteins termed *annexins* (Ernst, 1991).

The cytoskeleton is also involved in transport of lysosomal granules to the plasma membrane. Membrane perturbation is associated with assembly of microtubules (Goldstein et al., 1975a, 1975b; Hoffstein et al., 1976; Oliver, 1978). Agents that disrupt microtubule function alter the release of lysosomal enzymes (Zurier et al., 1974; Hoffstein et al., 1977).

One patient with recurrent infections had neutrophils that had abnormal microtubule assembly and diminished secretion of lysosomal granules in response to various stimuli (Gallin et al., 1978a).

Nonoxidative Killing of Microorganisms

Neutrophil killing of pathogens occurs by both oxidative and nonoxidative processes. The earliest evidence for nonoxidative killing arose from patients with chronic granulomatous disease who lack an oxidative burst. These patients exhibit defective killing of certain microbes but normal killing of others, implying the existence of alternative microbicidal mechanisms.

There are several methods of nonoxidative killing. The simplest is phagocytosis, during which some microbes (e.g., *Streptococcus pneumoniae*) are captured in the phagocytic vacuole and are killed by their own microbial waste. The second mechanism is killing by granule contents. When granules (see Table 5–1) are disrupted after lysosome-phagosome fusion, their enzymes digest the pathogens.

Several different enzymes exist. Granules contain cationic proteins that perturb the bacterial cell wall. One compound (50 to 60 kd) has been termed *bacterial/ permeability increasing protein* (BPI) (Weiss et al., 1982; Elsbach and Weiss, 1983). Two other *cationic antibacterial proteins* (CAP 37, CAP 57) have also been identified. Both BPI and CAP can kill certain gram-negative bacteria (Shafer et al., 1986; Weiss et al., 1978).

Another group of enzymes found in azurophil granules are the *defensins,* low-molecular-weight, antibiotic-like molecules. The two major defensins, NP-1 and NP-2, have antibacterial, fungal and viral activity that are time- and temperature-dependent. Defensins may be developmentally regulated, since fewer defensins are noted in infant cells (Ganz et al., 1985).

Lactoferrin, a major component of specific granules, kills by three possible mechanisms:

1. It interacts with the H_2O_2/halide/myeloperoxidase system (Ambruso and Johnston, 1981).
2. It scavenges iron from iron-dependent bacteria (Baggiolini et al., 1970; Green et al., 1971).
3. It is directly toxic to certain microbes (Kalmar and Arnold, 1988).

Neutrophil lactoferrin production may be decreased in certain illnesses, such as acute viral infections (Baynes et al., 1988).

Another nonoxidative killing mechanism is acidification of phagosomes. This process can activate certain acid enzymes that are involved in microbial killing (Goldstein, 1976; Mandell, 1970; Jensen and Bainton, 1973).

Once a pathogen is killed, digestive enzymes are available to degrade it within the phagosome, including *lysosome, elastase, collagenase,* and neutral *proteases* (Olsson et al., 1978; Elsbach and Weiss, 1981).

Oxidative Responses

Neutrophils possess several oxidant-dependent microbicidal mechanisms that kill a broad spectrum of microbiologic agents. Phagocytosis of microorganisms was first linked to oxygen consumption in 1933 (Baldridge and Gerard, 1933), but the crucial role of *oxygen radicals* in microbial killing was not truly appreciated until 1967, when patients with chronic granulomatous disease (CGD) were found to have defective oxidative metabolic responses (see Chapter 15). Since then, much study has been directed toward the mechanisms by which oxygen metabolites kill microorganisms. Any component of the neutrophil armamentarium leads to suboptimal cellular defenses, but certain defects (e.g., the oxidase deficiency of CGD, has more severe consequences than other defects (e.g., myeloperoxidase deficiency).

When neutrophils respond to chemotactic stimuli, a receptor-ligand interaction occurs, resulting in chemotactic activity. The same stimuli in higher concentrations can inhibit cell movement and activate the oxidative and *hexose monophosphate shunt pathways.* Nonchemotactic stimuli can also induce oxidative activity. Depending on the nature of the stimulant, preactivation state, and maturity of the cell, the *oxidative response* is preceded by pinocytosis, phagocytosis, and/or degranulation (Weisdorf et al., 1982; Karnovsky and Badwey, 1983; Verhoef and Visser, 1993). The signal transduction pathway leading to the oxidative response (Fig. 5–4) and the mechanisms of oxidative killing are discussed next.

The Respiratory Burst

The NADPH oxidase enzyme is responsible for the oxidative burst. It is inactive until an activation signal is generated by ligand-receptor binding (Segal, 1989; Clark, 1990; Smith and Curnutte, 1991; McPhail and Harvath, 1993). An electron cascade is necessary for reduction of O_2 to O_2^- (superoxide) by the oxidase. The hexose monophosphate shunt provides electrons for the cascade and the cytochrome component of the oxidase participates in electron transport (Karnovsky and Badwey, 1983; Borregaard et al., 1983, 1984).

The development of a cell-free system for NADPH oxidase activation has allowed identification of the components necessary for the respiratory burst (McPhail and Harvath, 1993). The oxidase is composed of a multicomponent system, including the membrane-associated heterodimeric cytochrome b_{558} (made up of a 91,000-kd glycoprotein and a 22,000-kd protein subunit) and two cytosolic components (47,000-kd and 67,000-kd proteins), which translocate to the cytochrome b on activation of the cell. The cytochrome b is the terminal component of the electron transport chain and transfers electrons directly to oxygen. Both cytosolic proteins are phosphorylated upon cell activation, but it is not known whether phosphorylation is a prerequisite for oxidase activity. All components of the oxidase system are required for normal respiratory burst activity. A defect in any of these components leads to the chronic granulomatous disease syndrome (see Chapter 15).

Studies utilizing the cell-free system have identified other components required for the respiratory burst. Monomeric G-proteins, such as rap1A, which copurifies with the cytochrome b_{558}, appears to be required because anti-rap1A antibodies inhibit the respiratory burst (Eukland et al., 1991). Lipids are required as

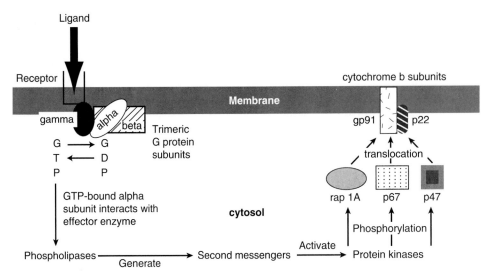

Figure 5–4. Potential scheme for oxygen radical generation resulting from membrane stimulation. For some stimuli (e.g., FMLP), receptor interaction at the neutrophil plasma membrane leads to changes in trimeric G protein conformation; for other stimuli (e.g., phorbol myristate acetate), trimeric G proteins may not be involved. Second messengers are then generated, followed by activation of protein kinases and phosphatases. The active NADPH oxidase enzyme is assembled at the membrane, and this requires the translocation of at least two cytosolic proteins (p47-phox and p67-phox) to the membrane. Monomeric G proteins appear to participate in the assembly of the oxidase (rap 1A interacts with cytochrome b_{558}). This leads to enhanced oxygen consumption, hexose monophosphate shunt activity, and generation of various oxygen species.

second messengers, but their role is unclear (Agwu et al., 1991). One tentative model of the activation of the oxidase system is shown in Figure 5–4.

Oxidative Killing

Once the oxidase is activated, oxygen is converted to superoxide. Metabolism of superoxide, either by superoxide dismutase (SOD) or by spontaneous dismutation (see Equation 1), results in other oxygen metabolites, including hydrogen peroxide, singlet oxygen, hydroxyl ions, and oxyhalides. These are often termed *reactive oxygen intermediates*.

$$\underset{\text{(superoxide)}}{O_2^- + O_2^-} + 2 H^+ \xrightarrow[\text{dismutase}]{\text{superoxide}}$$

$$\underset{\substack{\text{(hydrogen} \\ \text{peroxide)}}}{H_2O_2} + O_2 + \underset{\substack{\text{(singlet} \\ \text{oxygen)}}}{O_2^-} \quad [1]$$

$$H_2O_2 \xrightarrow{\text{catalase}} H_2O + O_2 \quad [2]$$

$$O_2^- + H_2O_2 \xrightarrow{\text{lactoferrin}}$$

$$\underset{\substack{\text{(hydroxyl} \\ \text{radical)}}}{OH\cdot} + \underset{\substack{\text{(hydroxyl} \\ \text{ion)}}}{OH^-} + O_2 + O_2^- \quad [3]$$

$$Cl^-(I^-) + H_2O_2 \xrightarrow{\text{myeloperoxidase}} \underset{\text{(oxyhalide)}}{HOCl^-(HOI^-)} + H_2O \quad [4]$$

Although 90% of neutrophil oxygen consumption leads to H_2O_2 production (Reiss and Roos, 1978), unstable intermediaries, such as the hydroxyl radical (OH·),

are important in microbial killing. Lactoferrin, a specific granule component, has an important role in OH· generation and helps to catalyze the reaction in Equation 3. Myeloperoxidase (MPO), an azurophilic granule component, modulates the generation of O_2^- (Stendahl et al., 1984) and catalyzes the generation of oxyhalide radicals (Equation 4). Thus, degranulation is intimately involved in regulating the respiratory burst.

Neutrophil microbicidal assays performed in anaerobic conditions suggest that oxidative mechanisms are important for killing of many bacteria. Certain organisms (e.g., *Staphylococcus aureus*) are killed poorly under anaerobic conditions (Mandell, 1974). Bacteria with high intrinsic levels of superoxide dismutase and catalase activity are less effectively killed by oxygen metabolites (Johnston et al., 1975; Mandell, 1975). Scavengers of H_2O_2, and hydroxyl radicals [OH^-, OH·, and singlet oxygen (O_2^-)], depress bacterial killing (Johnston et al., 1975; Mandell, 1975; Repine et al., 1981).

Oxygen radicals may be released into extracellular fluid or into phagosomes by neutrophils, but monocytes secrete oxygen metabolites only into the phagosomes (Babior, 1984). Extracellular release occurs mainly at points of microbial contact (Ohno et al., 1982), an important observation for nonphagocytizable microorganisms, such as fungi. If oxygen radicals leak into the cytoplasm, catalase, superoxide dismutase, and the glutathione reductase system usually prevent autolysis and neutrophil-induced tissue injury.

Role of Neutrophils in the Immune Response

Previously, the neutrophil was thought to be incapable of protein synthesis because of the relatively low amount of ribosomes and endoplasmic reticulum in mature cells. However, it is now known that neutrophils can synthesize messenger RNA (mRNA) and proteins, including neutrophil constituents (e.g., actin, CR1, CR3, FcR) and cytokines (e.g., IL-1, IL-6, IL-8), TNF, and each of the colony-stimulating factors [macrophage, granulocyte-macrophage and granulocyte]). The neutrophil's ability to produce and react to these proteins permits the neutrophil to interact with lymphocytes and macrophages (Ishibashi and Yamashita, 1987; Prior et al., 1992). A review of the neutrophil's role in the immune response is available (Lloyd and Oppenheim, 1992).

The neutrophil also participates in the killing of many fungi and certain viruses (Root and Cohen, 1981; Yamamoto et al., 1991; Klebanoff and Coombs, 1992). Clinically, patients with neutrophil-specific defects may have increased susceptibility to nonbacterial pathogens, including *Candida, Aspergillus,* and herpes simplex virus (Mills and Noya, 1993).

Microbial Survival Mechanisms

Certain microbes have mechanisms that allow them to survive within the phagocytic cell. These organisms evade phagocytosis and killing either by altering their own characteristics or by inducing cell dysfunction (Verhoef and Visser, 1993; Wheeler and Abramson, 1993). For example, *Salmonella typhimurium* exposed to sublethal concentrations of H_2O_2 induces antioxidant enzymes, competent DNA repair, and other stress proteins that permit survival to high concentrations of peroxide (Moran et al., 1986). *Mycobacterium tuberculosis, Histoplasma capsulatum, Toxoplasma gondii, Neisseria gonorrhoeae, Legionella,* and *Chlamydia* species inhibit lysosome-phagosome fusion by secreting fusion-inhibiting factors (Dumont and Robert, 1970; Jones and Hirsch, 1972; Goren et al., 1976; Densen and Mandell, 1978; Wyrick and Brownridge, 1978; Wilson et al., 1980).

Lysosome-phagosome fusion is inhibited by acidic sulfatides that accumulate in the granules following its secretion by *M. tuberculosis* (Goren et al., 1976). *S. typhimurium* and *Mycobacterium lepraemurium* replicate within phagocytic cells despite lysosome-phagosome fusion, since they are resistant to the antimicrobial factors of lysosomal granules (Hart et al., 1972; Carrol et al., 1979). Neutrophils incubated with certain strains of influenza A virus exhibit decreased secretion of lysosomal enzymes into phagosomal vacuoles that contain *S. aureus* (Abramson et al., 1982, 1984). Inhibition of degranulation by influenza virus correlates with decreased bactericidal capacity. Other mechanisms by which microbes alter the bactericidal capacity of neutrophils are noted in Table 5–3.

Neutrophil-Induced Tissue Injury

Neutrophils may cause tissue injury in several diseases, including adult respiratory distress syndrome, arthritis, asthma, atherosclerosis, cystic fibrosis, inflammatory bowel disease, ischemia-reperfusion injury,

Table 5–3. Microbial-Induced Perturbations of Important Neutrophil Functions in Microbicidal Activity*

Inhibition of Chemotactic-Related Responses†
Bacteria: *Bacteroides* spp, *Bordetella pertussis,*‡ *Capnocytophaga, Clostridium perfringens,*‡ *Escherichia coli,*† *Mycobacterium tuberculosis, Pseudomonas* spp,‡ *Staphylococcus aureus,*‡ *Vibrio cholerae* ‡
Fungi: *Aspergillus* spp
Viruses: CMV, enteroviruses, hepatitis B, HIV-1, herpes simplex, influenza A, rotavirus, RSV, rubeola

Inhibition of Killing
Bacteria: *B. pertussis†, Neisseria gonorrhoeae*
Fungi: *Aspergillus* spp
Viruses: CMV, EBV, enteroviruses, hepatitis B, HIV-1, influenza A, RSV

Inhibition of Phagocytosis
Bacteria: *Streptococcus pneumoniae, Staphylococcus aureus*
Viruses: CMV, hepatitis B, HIV-1, herpes simplex, mumps

Inhibition of Oxidative Metabolism
Bacteria: *B. pertussis,*‡ *C. perfringens,*‡ *Legionella pneumophila,*‡ *Listeria monocytogenes, Pasteurella haemolytica,*‡ *Pseudomonas* spp, *Salmonella typhi*
Fungi: *Candida albicans*
Viruses: CMV, EBV, enteroviruses, hepatitis B, herpes simplex, influenza A, RSV

Inhibition of Secretion
Bacteria: *B. pertussis,*‡§ *Chlamydia psittaci,*§ *M. tuberculosis,*§ *N. gonorrhoeae,*§ *S. pneumoniae, Staphylococcus pyogenes* ‡
Fungi: *C. albicans, Histoplasma capsulatum* §
Parasites: *Toxoplasma gondii*§
Viruses: CMV, enteroviruses, hepatitis B, HIV-1, herpes simplex, influenza A,§ rotavirus, RSV, rubeola

Resistance to Lysosomal Enzymes
Bacteria: *Mycobacterium lepraemurium, Salmonella typhimurium*
Parasites: *Leishmania mexicania*

*For a more detailed review, see Abramson & Wheeler, The Neutrophil. New York, Oxford University Press, 1993, pp. 139–181.

†Chemotactic-related functions include those involved in adherence and cell movement.

‡Alteration is due, at least in part, to a toxin produced by the bacteria.

§Notes microbes which can inhibit the fusion of lysosomes with phagosomes.

Abbreviations: CMV = cytomegalovirus; EBV = Epstein-Barr virus; HIV-1 = human immunodeficiency virus, type 1; RSV = respiratory syncytial virus; spp = species.

neutrophilic dermatoses, and psoriasis. Involvement of neutrophils is suggested by their high concentrations at the site of disease at the onset or during the active phase of the disease. In addition, neutrophil depletion in experimental models abrogates the severity of tissue damage. The neutrophil's role in adult respiratory distress syndrome and other illnesses is reviewed elsewhere (Leff and Repine, 1993).

Neutrophil tissue damage is brought about by the same mechanisms that kill microbes (i.e., oxygen radicals and granular contents). Tissue injury occurs when neutrophil products are secreted extracellularly and the normal physiologic systems that scavenge them, such as proteinase inhibitors (alpha$_1$-antitrypsin [alpha$_1$-antiproteinase], alpha$_2$-macroglobulin, and secretory leukoproteinase inhibitor) and antioxidants (glutathione and superoxide dismutase), are compromised. Another mechanism of tissue injury is the release of toxic products from neutrophils undergoing programmed death-apoptosis. Because neutrophils die at a rapid rate in the circulation, a reticuloendothelial scavenging system must remove them and their toxic contents. Interference with this system may induce tissue damage (Savill et al., 1993).

EOSINOPHILS

Normal Physiology

The eosinophil is the same size as the neutrophil, but it usually has a bilobed nucleus. The function and biology of eosinophils are reviewed elsewhere (Weller, 1991; McEwen, 1992). Their most distinctive feature is their large cytoplasmic specific granules, which contain basic proteins that stain with eosin and other acidic dyes. These proteins (i.e., major basic protein, eosinophilic peroxidase, eosinophil cationic protein, and eosinophil-derived neurotoxin/eosinophil protein X) are not found in neutrophils. "Small granules" are also found in the eosinophil and contain enzymes, such as arylsulfatase B and acid phosphatase. The protein that forms Charcot-Leyden crystals in tissue and sputum has lysophospholipase activity and is derived from either the primary granule or the plasma membrane. Important surface proteins on eosinophils include LFA-1 (CD11a/CD18), Mac-1 (CD11b/CD18), L-selectin, CD4 (in small amounts), and IgE and Fc receptors.

The regulation of eosinophil production has now been defined. Initial differentiation of the eosinophil is driven by IL-3, and both GM-CSF and IL-5 promote eosinophil proliferation. The T_H2 subset of CD4 lymphocytes is the source of IL-4 and IL-5, and these cells are increased in allergic (atopic) disorders. IL-5 regulation is complex, and the stimulus for a T_H2 cell response is not known. GM-CSF also increases human leukocyte antigen DR (HLA-DR) on eosinophils, allowing them to act as antigen-presenting cells (APCs) (Weller, 1992).

Eosinophil migration into tissues occurs in the late phase of immediate hypersensitivity and is initiated by eosinophil chemotactic factors. These include C5a, PAF, IL-2, IL-3, IL-5, IL-8, GM-CSF, RANTES (a gene encoding a novel T-cell specific molecule) and *lymphocyte chemotactic factor,* which binds to CD4 receptors. Eosinophils emigrate from the circulation by diapedesis across the endothelium using intracellular adhesion molecule (ICAM-1), E-selectin and vascular cell adhesion molecule (VCAM-1) as tethering molecules. The increased expression of VCAM-1 induced by IL-4 and the increased responsiveness of eosinophils to IL-4 may account for tissue eosinophilia (Resnick and Weller, 1993).

Degranulation occurs after cross-linking of immunoglobulin receptors, particularly by secretory IgA. Degranulation is enhanced by several cytokines, including IL-5, G-CSF, and GM-CSF (Abu-Ghazaleh et al., 1992). In certain diseases, eosinophils may appear partially degranulated (hypodense) and may be primed for greater activity (Fukuda and Gleich, 1989). The en-

gagement of certain eosinophil receptors can lead to a patterned release of specific granule components. For example, binding of IgE-allergen complexes to eosinophils causes the release of eosinophil peroxidase but not eosinophil cationic proteins (Capron et al., 1989).

Stimulated eosinophils and neutrophils metabolize arachidonic acid via the 5-lipoxygenase pathway; however, eosinophils elaborate leukotriene C4 (LTC_4) as the predominant metabolite but neutrophils release mostly LTB_4 (Weller, 1984). Eosinophils, like neutrophils, can generate toxic oxygen metabolites for microbicidal functions and tissue damage (see the next topic).

Eosinophils in Disease

The two known functions of the eosinophil are as an effector cell for killing helminths and as a modulator of immediate hypersensitivity reactions. The eosinophilic killing of parasites is suggested by the finding that many helminthic infections are associated with eosinophilia. In vitro studies show that eosinophils kill certain parasites (e.g., *Trichinella*) after direct contact with the helminth and release of their granules (Galli and Dvorak, 1979; Butterworth and David, 1981). Eosinophils also kill protozoa, but most protozoal infections do not elicit eosinophilia.

A role for eosinophils in regulating IgE-mediated *mast cell reactions* is suggested by the finding that certain eosinophil granules can degrade (Henderson et al., 1982) or inhibit the release of mast cell products (Hubscher, 1975).

The eosinophil, even more than the neutrophil, is associated with tissue damage in certain diseases, including:

- Allergic conditions (e.g., asthma, atopic dermatitis, allergic bronchopulmonary aspergillosis), immune deficiencies (e.g., Omenn syndrome)
- Skin disorders (e.g., allergic angiitis)
- Neoplastic disease (e.g., Hodgkin's disease and acute lymphocytic leukemia)
- Drug or toxin reactions (eosinophilia-myalgia syndrome)
- The hypereosinophilic syndrome, in which eosinophils infiltrate various organ systems (Weller, 1984)

The association of eosinophils with these diseases has been known for some time, but the role of the recruitment and priming of eosinophils by cytokines and the specific proteins released, such as major basic protein, has emerged (Bruijnzeel et al., 1992; Corrigan and Kay, 1992; Kapp, 1993). This has led to a better understanding of the effects of older medications (corticosteroids) and consideration of new therapies.

BASOPHILS

Normal Physiology

Basophils and mast cells are discussed together because of their similar cellular contents and assumed complicity in atopic disease. It has long been thought that basophils circulate in the blood and differentiate to mast cells in tissues. However, basophils are distinct cells with a separate marrow lineage and differ from tissue mast cells in morphology, response to corticosteroids, affinity for IgE, response to and production of mediators, and life span (Huntley, 1992; Valent and Bettelheim, 1992).

Hematopoietic factors that affect basophil differentiation and activation include IL-3, GM-CSF, and IL-5 (Hirai et al., 1992). Basophils contain metachromatic granules that stain with basic dyes and have larger granules than mast cells. Both cells have IgE surface receptors and contain most of the body's store of histamine and histamine decarboxylase (the enzyme involved in histamine synthesis). Other substances generated by these cells include leukotriene C_4, D_4, and E_4 (SRS-A); eosinophil chemotactic factor A; prostaglandin D_2; PAF; and enzymes that activate the Hageman factor–dependent inflammatory pathway. Basophils also contain a major basic protein and the Charcot-Leyden protein (Marone et al., 1989).

In contrast to mast cells, basophils are more sensitive to anti-IgE and non-IgE stimuli. Release of histamine and other granules contents is associated with cytoskeletal repolymerization, calcium flux, and arachidonic acid release. Agents that facilitate granule release, in addition to cross-linked IgE, include neuropeptides, IL-1, IL-3, IL-8, GM-CSF, FMLP and its analogs, anaphylatoxins (C3a, C4a, C5a), calcium ionophore, phorbol esters, and PAF (Hook et al., 1976; Glovsky et al., 1979; MacGlashan et al., 1983; Marone et al., 1989; Huntley, 1992; Lichtenstein and Bochner, 1991). Basophils are subject to immune modulation; when basophils are exposed to suboptimal concentrations of an antigen followed by optimal concentrations of the same antigen, there is a decreased release of granule contents (Baxter and Adamik, 1975; Dembo et al., 1979).

Basophils in Disease

The role of the mast cell in atopic diseases is well established, and a similar role for basophils has also been established. Basophils are less responsive to allergen challenge, although in vitro they can be used to diagnose allergic disease by assessing histamine release after antigenic challenge. Basophils are few, compared with tissue mast cells, but their progenitors are increased in the blood and secretions of atopic persons (Denburg et al., 1985; Lichtenstein and Bochner, 1991). The increased histamine content of asthmatic tissues during the late phase reaction is due to a basophilic infiltration. If the asthmatic person is pretreated with corticosteroids, the acute inflammatory response is unchanged, but the late phase response is abolished without basophilia or eosinophilia (Lichtenstein and Bochner, 1991).

Basophil histamine releasibility varies in different diseases and may be increased in atopic patients and decreased in children (Marone et al., 1986). Atopic individuals also have a greater sensitivity to cross-linking IgE signals than normal people (Lichtenstein and MacGlashan, 1986). Askenase et al. (1978) suggested that these basophils present antigen in delayed hypersensitivity reactions. Basophils may also present antigen during an anaphylactic reaction to an intravenously administered drug.

Acknowledgment: Supported by Grant AI-20506 from the National Institute of Health.

References

Abramson JS, Lewis JC, Lyles DS, Heller KA, Mills EL, Bass DA. Inhibition of neutrophil lysosome-phagosome fusion associated with influenza virus infection in vitro: role in depressed bactericidal activity. J Clin Invest 69:1393–1397, 1982.

Abramson JS, Parce JW, Lewis JC, Lyles DS, Mills EL, Nelson RD, Bass DA. Characterization of the effect of influenza virus on polymorphonuclear leukocyte membrane responses. Blood 64:131–138, 1984.

Abu-Ghazaleh RI, Kita H, Gleich GJ. Eosinophil activation and function in health and disease. Immunol Ser 57:137–167, 1992.

Adelstein RS. Regulation of contractile proteins by phosphorylation. J Clin Invest 72:1863–1866, 1983.

Agwu DE, McPhail LC, Sozani S, Bass DA, McCall CE. Phosphatidic acid as a second messenger in human polymorphonuclear leukocytes: Effects on activation of NADPH oxidase. J Clin Invest 88:531–539, 1991.

Altman AJ, Stossel TP. Functional immaturity of bone marrow bands and polymorphonuclear granulocytes. Br J Haematol 27:241–245, 1974.

Ambruso DR, Johnston RB. Lactoferrin enhances hydroxyl radical production by human neutrophils, neutrophil particulate fractions, and an enzymatic generating system. J Clin Invest 67:352–360, 1981.

Anderson DC, Pickering LK, Feigen RD. Leukocyte function in normal infected neonates. J Pediatr 85:420–425, 1974.

Anderson DC, Hughes BJ, Edwards MD, Buffone GJ, Baker CJ. Impaired chemotaxigenesis by type III group B streptococci in neonatal sera: relationship to diminished concentration of specific anticapsular antibody and abnormalities of serum complement. Pediatr Res 17:496–502, 1983.

Anderson DC, Hughes BJ, Smith CW. Abnormal mobility of neonatal polymorphonuclear leukocytes: relationship to impaired redistribution of surface adhesion sites by chemotactic factor or colchicine. J Clin Invest 68:863–874, 1981.

Arnaout MA. Leukocyte adhesion molecule deficiency: its structural basis, pathophysiology, and implications for modulating the inflammatory response. Immunol Rev 114:145–180, 1990.

Askenase FW, Debernardo R, Tauben D, Kashgarian M. Cutaneous basophil anaphylaxis. Immunology 35:741–755, 1978.

Babior BM. Oxidants from phagocytes: agents of defense and destruction. Blood 64:959–966, 1984.

Baggiolini M, DeDuve C, Masson PL, Heremans JF. Association of lactoferrin with specific granules in rabbit neutrophil leukocytes. J Exp Med 131:559–570, 1970.

Bainton DF, Ullyot JL, Farquhar MG. The development of neutrophilic polymorphonuclear leukocytes in human bone marrow. J Exp Med 134:907–934, 1971.

Baldridge CW, Gerard RW. The extra respiration of phagocytosis. Am J Physiol 133:235–236, 1933.

Baxter JH, Adamik R. Control of histamine release: effects of various conditions on rate of release and rate of cell desensitization. J Immunol 114:1034–1041, 1975.

Baynes RD, Bezwoda WR, Mansoor N. Neutrophil lactoferrin content in viral infections. Am J Clin Pathol 89:225–228, 1988.

Beck WS. The control of leukocyte glycolysis. J Biol Chem 232:251–270, 1958.

Billett JN, Caren LD. Human granulocyte antigens: current status and biological significance. Proc Soc Exp Biol Med 178:12–23, 1985.

Bockenstedt LK, Goetzl EJ. Constitutents of human neutrophils that mediate enhanced adherence to surfaces. J Clin Invest 65:1372–1381, 1980.

Bokoch GM. Signal transduction by GTP binding proteins during leukocyte activation: phagocytic cells. Curr Top Membr Transport 35:65–101, 1990.

Bokoch GM, Quilliam LA, Bohl BP, Jesaitis AJ, Quinn MT. Inhibition of rap1A binding to cytochrome b$_{558}$ of NADPH oxidase by phosphorylation of rap1A. Science 254:1794–1796, 1991.

Boner A, Zeligs BJ, Bellanti JA. Chemotactic responses of various differentiational stages of neutrophils from human cord and adult blood. Infect Immun 35:921–928, 1982.

Borregaard N, Heiple JM, Simons ER, Clark RA. Subcellular localization of the b-cytochrome component of the human neutrophil microbicidal oxidase: translocation during activation. J Cell Biol 97:52–61, 1983.

Borregaard N, Schwartz JH, Tauber AI. Protein secretion by stimulated neutrophils. J Clin Invest 74:455–459, 1984.

Boxer LA, Coates TD, Haak RA, Wolach JB, Hoffstein S, Baehner RL. Lactoferrin deficiency associated with altered granulocyte function. N Engl J Med 307:404–410, 1982a.

Boxer LA, Haak RA, Yang HH, Wolach JB, Whitcomb JA, Butterick CJ, Bahner RL. Membrane-bound lactoferrin alters the surface properties of polymorphonuclear leukocytes. J Clin Invest 70:1049–1057, 1982b.

Boxer LA, Todd RF. Therapeutic modulation of neutrophil number and function. In Abramson JS, Wheeler JG, eds. The Neutrophil. Oxford, England, Oxford University Press, 1993, pp. 263–302.

Brederoo P, van der Meulen J, Mommaas-Kienhuis AM. Development of the granule population in neutrophil granulocytes from bone marrow. Cell Tissue Res 234:469–496, 1983.

Breton-Gorius J, Coquin Y, Guichard J. Cytochemical distinction between azurophils and catalase-containing granules in leukocytes. Lab Invest 38:21–31, 1978.

Bruce MC, Baley JE, Medvik KA, Berger M. Impaired surface membrane expression of C3bi but not C3b receptros on neonatal neutrophils. Pediatr Res 21:306–311, 1987.

Bruijnzeel PL, Rihs S, Virchow JC Jr, Warringa RA, Moser R, Walker C. Early activation or ''priming'' of eosinophils in asthma. Schweiz Med Wochenschri 122:298–301, 1992.

Butterworth AE, David JR. Eosinophil function. N Engl J Med 304:154–156, 1981.

Capron M, Tomassini M, Torpier G, Kusnierz JP, MacDonald S, Capron A. Selectivity of mediators released by eosinophils. Int Arch Allergy Appl Immunol 88:54–58, 1989.

Carrol ME, Jackett PS, Aber VR, Lowrie DB. Phagolysosome formation, cyclic adenosine 3′,5′-monophosphate and the fate of *Salmonella typhimurium* within mouse peritoneal macrophages. J Gen Microbiol 110:421–429, 1979.

Cassimeris L, Zigmond SH. Chemoattractant stimulation of polymorphonuclear leukocyte locomotion. Semin Cell Biol 1:125–134, 1990.

Christensen RD, Rothstein G. Neutrophil myeloperoxidase concentration: changes with development and during bacterial infection. Pediatr Res 19:1278–1282, 1985.

Christensen RD, Rothstein G, Anstall HB, Bybee B. Granulocyte transfusions in neonates with bacterial infection, neutropenia and depletion of mature marrow neutrophils. Pediatrics 70:1–6, 1982.

Clark RA. The human neutrophil respiratory burst oxidase. J Infect Dis 161:1140–1147, 1990.

Coates TD, Torkildson JC, Torres M, Church JA, Howard TH. An inherited defect of neutrophil motility and microfilamentous cytoskeleton associated with abnormalities in 47-kd and 89-kd proteins. Blood 78:1338–1346, 1991.

Corrigan CJ, Kay AB. T cells and eosinophils in the pathogenesis of asthma. Immunol Today 13:501–507, 1992.

Cotton DJ, Seligmann B, O'Brien WF, Gallin JI. Selection defect in human neutrophil superoxide anion generation elicited by the chemoattractant N-formyl-methionyl-leucyl-phenylalanine in pregnancy. J Infect Dis 148:194–199, 1983.

Cronkite EP, Vincent PV. Granulocytopoiesis in hemopoietic cellular proliferation. In Strohlman F, ed. Hematopoietic Cellular Proliferation. New York, Grune & Stratton, 1970, pp. 211–228.

Dembo M, Goldstein B, Sobotka AK, Lichtenstein LM. Degranulation of human basophils: quantitative analysis of histamine release and desensitization due to a bivalent penicilloyl hapten. J Immunol 123:1864–1872, 1979.

Denburg JA, Telizyn S, Belda A, Dolovich J, Bienenstock J. Increased numbers of circulating basophil progenitors in atopic patients. J Allergy Clin Immunol 76:466–472, 1985.

Densen P, Mandell GL. Gonococcal interactions with polymorphonuclear neutrophils: importance of the phagosome for bactericidal activity. J Clin Invest 62:1161–1171, 1978.

DeWald B, Bretz U, Baggiolini M. Release of gelatinase from a novel secretory compartment of human neutrophils. J Clin Invest 70:518–525, 1982.

Dexter D, Rubins JB, Manning EC, Khachatrian L, Dickey BF. Compartmentalization of low molecular mass GTP-binding proteins among neutrophil secretory granules. J Immunol 145:1845–1850, 1990.

DiVirgilio F, Stendahl O, Pittet D, Lew PD, Pozzan T. Cytoplasmic calcium in phagocyte activation. Curr Top Membr Transport 35:180–205, 1990.

Driscoll MS, Thomas VL, Ramamurthy RS, Casto DT. Longitudinal evaluation of polymorphonuclear leukocyte chemiluminescence in premature infants. J Pediatr 116:429–434, 1990.

Dumont A, Robert A. Electron microscopic study of phagocytosis of *Histoplasma capsulatum* by hamster peritoneal macrophages. Lab Invest 23:278–286, 1970.

Durstin M, McColl SR, Gomez-Cambronero J, Naccache PH, Sha'afi R. Up-regulation of the amount of G$_i$2 associated with the plasma membrane in human neutrophils by granulocyte-macrophage colony stimulating factor. Biochem J 292:183–187, 1993.

Eberle M, Traynor-Kaplan AE, Sklar LA, Norgauer J. Is there a relationship between phosphatidylinositol triphosphate and F-actin polymerization in human neutrophils? J Biol Chem 265:16725–16728, 1990.

Elsbach P, Weiss J. A reevaluation of the roles of the oxygen-dependent and oxygen-independent microbicidal systems of phagocytes. Rev Infect Dis 5:843–853, 1983.

Elsbach P, Weiss J. Oxygen-independent bactericidal systems of polymorphonuclear leukocytes. Adv Inflammation Res 2:95–113, 1981.

Erdman SH, Christensen RD, Bradley PP, Rothstein G. Supply and release of storage neutrophils. Biol Neonate 41:132–137, 1982.

Ernst JD. Annexin III translocates to the periphagosomal region when neutrophils ingest opsonized yeast. J Immunol 146:3110–3114, 1991.

Eukland EA, Marshall M, Gibbs JB, Crean CD, Gabig TG. Resolution of a low molecular weight G protein in neutrophil cytosol required for NADPH oxidase activation and reconstitution by recombinant Krev-1 protein. J Biol Chem 266:13964–13970, 1991.

Fay SP, Posner RG, Swann WN, Sklar LA. Real-time analysis of the assembly of ligand, receptor, and G protein by quantitative fluorescence flow cytometry. Biochemistry 30:5066–5075, 1991.

Fleit HB, Wright SD, Durie CJ, Valinsky JE, Unkeless JC. Ontogeny of Fc receptors and complement receptor (CR3) during human myeloid differentiation. J Clin Invest 73:516–525, 1984.

Fletcher MP, Gallin JI. Human neutrophils contain an intracellular pool of putative receptors for the chemoattractant N-formyl-methionyl-leucyl-phenylalanine. Blood 62:792–799, 1983.

Fliedner TM, Cronkite EP, Killmann SA, Bond VP. Granulopoiesis: II. Emergence and pattern of labeling of neutrophilic granulocytes in humans. Blood 24:683–700, 1964a.

Fliedner TM, Cronkite EP, Robertson JS. Granulopoiesis: I. Senescence and random loss of neutrophil granulocytes in human beings. Blood 24:402–414, 1964b.

Fontan G, Lorente F, Garcia Rodriguez MC, Ojeda JA. *In vitro* human neutrophil movement in umbilical cord blood. Clin Immunol Immunopathol 20:224–230, 1981.

Frazier JP, Cleary TG, Pickering LK, Kohl S, Ross PJ. Leukocyte function in healthy neonates following vaginal and cesarean section deliveries. J Pediatr 101:269–272, 1982.

Freissmuth M, Casey PJ, Gilman AG. G-proteins control diverse pathways of transmembrane signaling. FASEB J 3:2125–2131, 1989.

Fukuda T, Gleich GJ. Heterogeneity of human eosinophils. J Allergy Clin Immunol 83:369–373, 1989.

Furie MB, Tancinco MCA, Smith CW. Monoclonal antibodies to leukocyte integrins CD11a/CD18 and CD11b/CD18 or intercellular adhesion molecule-1 inhibit chemoattractant-stimulated neutrophil transendothelial migration in vitro. Blood 78:2089–2097, 1991.

Galli ST, Dvorak HF. Basophils and mast cells: structure, function and role in hypersensitivity. In Gupta S, Good RA, eds. Cellular, Molecular and Clinical Aspects of Allergic Disorders. New York, Plenum Press, 1979, pp. 1–53.

Gallin JI. Role of neutrophil lysosomal granules in the evolution of the inflammatory response. In Karnovsky ML, Bolis L, eds. Phagocytosis—Past and Future. New York, Academic Press, 1982, pp. 519–541.

Gallin JI, Malech HL, Wright DG, Whisnant JK, Kirkpatrick CH. Recurrent severe infections in a child with abnormal leukocyte function: possible relationship to increased microtubule assembly. Blood 51:919–933, 1978a.

Gallin JI, Seligmann BE. Mobilization and adaption of human neutrophil chemoattract f-Met-Leu-Phe receptors. Fed Proc 43:2732–2736, 1984.

Gallin JI, Wright DG, Malech HL, Davis JM, Klempner MS, Kirkpatrick CH. Disorders of phagocyte chemotaxis. Ann Intern Med 92:520–538, 1980.

Gallin JI, Wright DG, Schiffmann E. Role of secretory events in modulating human neutrophil chemotaxis. J Clin Invest 62:1364–1374, 1978b.

Ganz T, Selsted ME, Szklarek D, Harwig SSL, Daherk E, Bainton DF, Lehrer RI: Defensins: natural peptide antibiotics of human neutrophils. J Clin Invest 76:27–35, 1985.

Glovsky MM, Hugli TE, Ishizaka T, Lichtenstein LM, Erickson BW. Anaphylatoxin-induced histamine release with human leukocytes: studies of C3a leukocyte binding and histamine release. J Clin Invest 64:804–811, 1979.

Golde DW. Production, distribution and fate of neutrophils. In Williams WJ, Beutler E, Erslev AJ, Lichtman MA, eds. Hematology, 3rd ed. New York, McGraw-Hill, 1983, pp. 759–765.

Goldstein IM. Polymorphonuclear leukocyte lysosomes and immune tissue injury. Prog Allergy 20:301–340, 1976.

Goldstein IM, Hoffstein ST, Weissman G. Mechanisms of lysosomal enzyme release from human polymorphonuclear leukocytes: effects of phorbol myristate acetate. J Cell Biol 66:647–652, 1975a.

Goldstein IM, Roos D, Weissman G, Kaplan H. Complement and immunoglobulin stimulate superoxide production by human leukocytes independently of phagocytosis. J Clin Invest 56:1155–1163, 1975b.

Gordon LI, Douglas SD, Kay NE, Yamada O, Osserman EF, Jacob HS. Modulation of neutrophil function by lysozyme. J Clin Invest 64:226–232, 1979.

Goren MB, D'Arcy Hart P, Young MR, Armstrong JA. Prevention of phagosome lysosome fusion in cultured macrophages by sulfatides of *Mycobacterium tuberculosis*. Proc Natl Acad Sci USA 73:2510–2514, 1976.

Green I, Kirkpatrick CH, Dale DC. Lactoferrin-specific localization in the nuclei of human polymorphonuclear neutrophilic leukocytes. Proc Soc Exp Biol Med 137:1311–1317, 1971.

Harris MC, Stroobant J, Cody CS, Douglas SD, Polin RA. Phagocytosis of group B streptococcus by neutrophils from newborn infants. Pediatr Res 17:358–361, 1983.

Hart PD, Armstrong JA, Brown CA, Draper P. Ultrastructural study of the behavior of macrophages toward parasitic mycobacteria. Infect Immun 5:803–807, 1972.

Harvath L. Neutrophil chemotactic factors. In Goldberg ID, ed. Cell Motility Factors. Basel, Birkhauser Verlag, 1991, pp. 35–52.

Harvath L, Aksamit RR. Oxidized N-formylmethionyl-leucylphenylalanine: effect on the activation of human monocyte and neutrophil chemotaxis and superoxide production. J Immunol 133:1471–1476, 1984.

Harvath L, Falk W, Leonard EJ. Rapid quantitation of neutrophil chemotaxis: use of a polyvinyl-pyrrolidone-free polycarbonate membrane in a multiwell assembly. J Immunol Methods 37:39–45, 1980.

Harvath L, Leonard EJ. Two neutrophil populations in human blood with different chemotactic activities: separation and chemoattractant binding. Infect Immun 36:443–449, 1982.

Harvath L, McCall CE, Bass DA, McPhail LC. Inhibition of human neutrophil chemotaxis by the protein kinase inhibitor, 1-(5-isoquinolinesulfonyl) piperazine. J Immunol 139:3055–3061, 1987.

Harvath L, Robbins JD, Russell AA, Seamon KB. Cyclic AMP and human neutrophil chemotaxis: elevation of cyclic AMP differentially affects chemotatic responsiveness. J Immunol 146:224–232, 1991.

Henderson WR, Jorg A, Klebanoff SJ. Eosinophil peroxidase-mediated inactivation of leukotrienes B$_4$, C$_4$ and D$_4$. J Immunol 128:2609–2613, 1982.

Hill HR. Biochemical, structural, and functional abnormalities of polymorphonuclear leukocytes in the neonate. Pediatr Res 22:375–382, 1987.

Hilmo A, Howard TH. F-actin content of neonate and adult neutrophils. Blood 69:945–949, 1987.

Hirai K, Morita Y, Miyamoto T. Hemopoietic growth factors regulate basophil function and lability. Immunol Ser 57:587–600, 1992.

Hoffstein S, Goldstein IM, Weissman G. Role of microtubule assembly in lysosomal enzyme secretion from human polymorphonuclear leukocytes. J Cell Biol 73:242–256, 1977.

Hoffstein S, Soberman R, Goldstein I, Weissman G. Concanavalin A induces microtubule assembly and specific granule discharge in human polymorphonuclear leukocytes. J Cell Biol 68:781–787, 1976.

Hoffstein ST. Ultrastructural demonstration of calcium loss from local regions of the plasma membrane of surface-stimulated human granulocytes. J Immunol 123:1395–1402, 1979.

Hook WA, Schiffmann E, Aswanikumar S, Siraganian RP. Histamine release by chemotactic, formyl methionine-containing peptides. J Immunol 117:594–596, 1976.

Huang CK. Protein kinases in neutrophils: a review. Membr Biochem 8:61–79, 1989.

Hubscher T. Role of the eosinophil in the allergic reactions: II. Release of prostaglandins from human eosinophilic leukocytes. J Immunol 114:1389–1396, 1975.

Huntley JF. Mast cells and basophils: a review of their heterogeneity and function. J Comp Pathol 107:349–372, 1992.

Ishibashi Y, Yamashita T. Effects of a phagocytosis-stimulating factor derived from polymorphonuclear neutrophils on the functions of macrophages. Infect Immun 55:1762–1766, 1987.

Jensen MS, Bainton DF. Temporal changes in pH within the phagocytic vacuole of the polymorphonuclear neutrophilic leukocyte. J Cell Biol 56:379–388, 1973.

Johnston RB Jr, Keele BB, Jr, Misra HP, Lehmeyer JE, Webb LS, Baehner RL, Rajagopalan KV. The role of superoxide anion generation in the phagocytic bactericidal activity: studies with normal and chronic granulomatous disease leukocytes. J Clin Invest 55:1357–1372, 1975.

Jones TC, Hirsch JG. The interaction between *Toxoplasma gondii* and mammalian cells. J Exp Med 136:1173–1194, 1972.

Kalmar JR, Arnold RR. Killing of *Actinobacillus actinomycetemcomitans* by human lactoferrin. Infect Immun 56:2552–2557, 1988.

Kanwar VS, Cairo MS. Neonatal neutrophil maturation, kinetics, and function. In Abramson JS, Wheeler JG, eds. The Neutrophil. Oxford, England, Oxford University Press, 1993, pp. 1–21.

Kapp A. The role of eosinophils in the pathogenesis of atopic dermatitis—eosinophilic granule proteins as markers of disease activity. Allergy 48:1–5, 1993.

Karnovsky ML, Badwey JA. Determinants of the production of active oxygen species by granulocytes and macrophages. J Clin Chem Clin Biochem 21:545–553, 1983.

Kitagawa S, Johnston RB Jr. Relationship between membrane potential changes and superoxide-releasing capacity in resident and activated mouse peritoneal macrophages. J Immunol 135:3417–3423, 1985.

Klebanoff SJ, Coombs RW. Viricidal effect of polymorphonuclear leukocytes on human immunodeficiency virus-1: role of the myeloperoxidase system. J Clin Invest 89:2014–2017, 1992.

Klein RB, Fischer TJ, Gard SE, Biberstein M, Rich KC, Stiehm ER. Decreased mononuclear and polymorphonuclear chemotaxis in human newborns, infants and young children. Pediatrics 60:467–472, 1977.

Klempner MS, Styrt B. Alkalinizing the intralysosomal pH inhibits degranulation of human neutrophils. J Clin Invest 72:1793–1800, 1983.

Kleus C, Scherubl H, Hescheler J, Schultz G, Wittig B. Different β-subunits determine G protein interaction with transmembrane receptors. Nature 358:424–426, 1992.

Korchak HM, Weissmann G. Changes in membrane potential of human granulocytes antecede the metabolic responses to surface stimulation. Proc Natl Acad Sci (U S A) 75:3818–3822, 1978.

Korchak HM, Weissmann G. Stimulus-response coupling in the human neutrophil: Transmembrane potential and the role of extracellular Na+. Biochim Biophys Acta 601:180–194, 1980.

Korchak HM, Eisenstat BA, Hoffstein ST, Dunham PB, Weissmann

G. Anion channel blockers inhibit lysosomal enzyme secretion from human neutrophils without affecting generation of superoxide anion. Proc Natl Acad Sci U S A 77:2721–2725, 1980.

Krause KH, Lew DP. Subcellular distribution of Ca^{2+} pumping sites in human neutrophils. J Clin Invest 80:107–116, 1987.

Krause PJ, Maderazo EG, Scroggs M. Abnormalities of neutrophil adherence in newborns. Pediatrics 69:184–187, 1982.

Kreutzer DL, Dreyfus LA, Robertson DC. Interaction of polymorphonuclear leukocytes with smooth and rough stains of *Brucella abortus*. Infect Immun 23:737–742, 1979.

Krumholz W, Demel C, Jung S, Meuthen G, Hempelmann G. The influence of intravenous anaesthetics on polymorponuclear leukocyte function. Can J Anaesth 40:770–774, 1993.

Lambeth JD. Activation of the respiratory burst in neutrophils: on the role of membrane-derived second messengers, Ca^{++}, and protein kinase C J Bioenerg Biomembr 20:709–733, 1988.

Leff JA, Repine JE. Neutrophil-mediated tissue injury. In Abramson JS, Wheeler JG, eds. The Neutrophil. Oxford, England, Oxford University Press, 1993, pp. 229–262.

Lichtenstein LM, Bochner BS. The role of basophils in asthma. Ann N Y Acad Sci 629:48–61, 1991.

Lichtenstein LM, MacGlashan DW Jr. The concept of basophil releasability. J Allerg Clin Immunol 77:291–293, 1986.

Lichtman MA, Weed RI. Alteration of the cell periphery during granulocyte maturation: relationship to cell function. Blood 39:301–316, 1972.

Lippa S, DeSole P, Meucci E, Littarru GP, DeFrancisci G, Magalini SI. Effect of general anesthetics on human granulocyte chemiluminescence. Experientia 39:1386–1387, 1983.

Lipschitz DA, Udupa SR, Indelicato SR, Das M. Effect of age on second messenger generation in neutrophils. Blood 78:1347–1354, 1991.

Lloyd AR, Oppenheim JJ. Poly's lament: the neglected role of the polymorphonuclear neutrophil in the afferent limb of the immune response. Immunol Today 13:169–172, 1992.

MacGlashan DW, Schleimer RP, Peters SP, Schulman ES, Adams K, Sobotka AK, Newball HH, Lichtenstein LM. Comparative studies of human basophils and mast cells. Fed Proc 42:2504–2509, 1983.

Malech HL, Root KR, Gallin JI. Structural analysis of human neutrophil migration: centriole, microtubule and microfilament orientation and function during chemotaxis. J Cell Biol 75:666–693, 1977.

Mandell GL. Intraphagosomal pH of human polymorphonuclear neutrophils. Proc Soc Exp Biol Med 134:447–449, 1970.

Mandell GL. Bactericidal activity of aerobic and anaerobic polymorphonuclear neutrophils. Infect Immun 9:337–341, 1974.

Mandell GL. Catalase, superoxide dismutase, and virulence of *Staphylococcus aureus*. J Clin Invest 55:561–566, 1975.

Marks PW, Maxfield FR. Local and global changes in cytosolic free calcium in neutrophils during chemotaxis and phagocytosis. Cell Calcium 11:181–190, 1990.

Marone G, Casolaro V, Cirillo R, Stellato C, Genovese A. Pathophysiology of human basophils and mast cells in allergic disorders. Clin Immunol Immunopathol 50:S24–S40, 1989.

Marone G, Poto S, diMartino L, Condorelli M. Human basophil releasability: I. Age-related changes in basophil releasability. J Allergy Clin Immunol 77:377–383, 1986.

Mauer AM, Athens JW, Ashenbrucker H, Cartwright GE, Wintrobe MM. Leukokinetic studies: II. A method for labeling granulocytes *in vitro* with radioactive di-isopropylfluorophosphate (DFP32). J Clin Invest 39:1482–1486, 1960.

McCullough J, Yunis EJ, Benson SJ, Quie PG. Effect of blood-bank storage on leukocyte function. Lancet 2:1333–1337, 1969.

McEwen BJ. Eosinophils: a review. Vet Res Commun 16:11–44, 1992.

McPhail LC, Ellenburg MD, Leone PA, Agwu DE, McCall CE, Qualliotine-Mann D, Strum SL. Molecular mechanism of activation of leukocyte superoxide production. In Jesaitis AJ, Dratz EA, eds. The Molecular Basis of Oxidative Damage by Leukocytes. Boca Raton, Fla., CRC Press, 1992a, pp. 11–24.

McPhail LC, Harvath L. Signal transduction in neutrophil oxidative metabolism and chemotaxis. In Abramson JS, Wheeler JG, eds. The Neutrophil. Oxford, England, Oxford University Press, 1993, pp. 63–107.

McPhail LC, Snyderman R. Activation of the respiratory burst enzyme in human polymorphonuclear leukocytes by chemoattractants and other soluble stimuli. J Clin Invest 72:192–200, 1983.

McPhail LC, Strum SL, Leone PA, Sozzani S. The neutrophil respiratory burst mechanism. In Coffey R, ed. Granulocyte Responses to Cytokines: Basic and Clinical Research. New York, Marcel Dekker, 1992b, pp. 47–76.

Mease AD, Burgess DP, Thomas PJ. Irreversible neutrophil aggregation: a mechanism of decreased newborn neutrophil chemotactic response. Am J Pathol 104:98–102, 1981.

Meshulam T, Proto P, Diamond RD, Melnick DA. Calcium modulation and chemotactic response divergent stimulation of neutrophil chemotaxis and cytosolic calcium response by the chemotactic peptide receptor. J Immunol 137:1954–1960, 1986.

Miller ME. Phagocyte function in the neonate: selected aspects. Pediatrics 64(Suppl):709–712, 1979.

Mills EL, Noya JD. Congenital neutrophil deficiencies. In Abramson JS, Wheeler JG, eds. The Neutrophil. Oxford, England, Oxford University Press, 1993, pp. 183–227.

Mills EL, Thompson T, Bjorksten B, Filipovich D, Quie PG. The chemiluminescence response and bactericidal activity of polymorphonuclear neutrophils from newborns and their mothers. Pediatrics 63:429–434, 1979.

Mohandes AE, Touranine JL, Osman M, Salle B. Neutrophil chemotaxis in infants of diabetic mothers and in preterms at birth. J Clin Lab Immunol 8:117–120, 1982.

Moran RW, Christman MF, Jacobson FS, Storz G, Ames BN. Hydrogen peroxide-inducible proteins in *Salmonella typhimurium* overlap with heat shock and other stress proteins. Proc Natl Acad Sci U S A 83:8059–8063, 1986.

Nagel JE, Hand K, Coon PJ, Adler WH, Bender BS. Age differences in phagocytes by polymorphonuclear leukocytes measured by flow cytometry. J Leukoc Biol 39:399–407, 1986.

Nemunaitis J, Rabinowe SN, Singer JW, Bierman PJ, Vose JM, Freedman AS, Onetto N, Gillis S, Oette D, Gold M, Buckner CD, Hansen JA, Ritz J, Applebaum FR, Armitage JO, Nadler LM. Recombinant granulocyte-macrophage colony-stimulating factor after autologous bone marrow transplantation for lymphoid cancer. N Engl J Med 324:1773–1778, 1991.

Norgauer J, Kownatzki E, Aktories K. Botulism C2 toxin aADP-ribosylates actin and enhances O_2^- production and secretion but inhibits migration of activated human neutrophils. J Clin Invest 82:1376–1382, 1988.

Ohno Y, Hirai K, Knaoh T, Uchino H, Ogawa K. Subcellular localization of H_2O_2 production in human neutrophils stimulated with particles and an effect of cytochalasin-B on the cells. Blood 60:253–260, 1982.

Oliver JM. Cell biology of leukocyte abnormalities: membrane and cytoskeletal function in normal and defective cells. Am J Pathol 93:221–270, 1978.

Olson TA, Ruymann FB, Cook BA, Burgess DP, Henson SA, Thomas PJ. Newborn polymorphonuclear leukocyte aggregation: a study of physical properties and ultrastructure using chemotactic peptides. Pediatr Res 17:993–997, 1983.

Olsson I, Odeberg H, Weiss J, Elsbach P. Bactericidal cationic proteins of human granulocytes. In Havemann K, Janoff A, eds. Neutral Proteases of Human Polymorphonuclear Leukocytes: Biochemistry, Physiology and Clinical Significance. Baltimore, Urban and Schwarzenberg, 1978, pp. 18–32.

Omann GM, Allen RA, Bokoch GM, Painter RG, Traynor AE, Sklar LA. Signal transduction and cytoskeletal activation in the neutrophil. Physiol Rev 67:285–322, 1987.

Oseas R, Yang HH, Baehner RL, Boxer LA. Lactoferrin: a promoter of polymorphonuclear leukocyte adhesiveness. Blood 57:939–945, 1981.

Philips MR, Abramson SB, Kolasinski SL, Haines KA, Weissman G, Rosenfield MG. Low molecular weight GTP-binding proteins in human neutrophil granule membranes. J Biol Chem 266:1289–1298, 1991.

Playfair JHL, Wolfendale MR, Kay HEM. The leukocytes of peripheral blood in the human foetus. Br J Haematol 9:336–344, 1963.

Prior C, Townsend PJ, Hughes DA, Haslam PL. Induction of lymphocyte proliferation by antigen-pulsed human neutrophils. Clin Exp Immunol 87:485–492, 1992.

Quesenberry P, Levitt L. Hematopoietic stem cells. N Engl J Med 301:755–760, 819–822, 868–872, 1979.

Quinn MT, Parkos CA, Walker L, Orkin SH, Dinauer MC, Jesaitis AJ. Association of ras-related protein with cytochrome b of human neutrophils. Nature 342:198–200, 1989.

Reibman J, Haines K, Weissmann G. Alterations in cyclic nucleotides and the activation of neutrophils. Curr Top Membr Transport 35:399–424, 1990.

Reiss M, Roos D. Differences in oxygen metabolism of phagocytosing monocytes and neutrophils. J Clin Invest 61:480–488, 1978.

Repine JE, Fox RB, Berger EM. Dimethyl sulfoxide inhibits killing of Staphylococcus aureus by polymorphonuclear leukocytes. Infect Immun 31:510–513, 1981.

Resnick MB, Weller PF. Mechanisms of eosinophil recruitment. Am J Respir Cell Molec Biol 8:349–355, 1993.

Root RK, Cohen MS. The microbicidal mechanisms of human neutrophils and eosinophils. Rev Infect Dis 3:565–597, 1981.

Rosales C, Brown EJ. Neutrophil receptors and modulation of the immune response. In Abramson JS, Wheeler JG, eds. The Neutrophil. Oxford, England, Oxford University Press, 1993, pp. 23–62.

Rossi AG, McMillan RM, MacIntyre DE. Agonist-induced calcium flux, phosphoinositide metabolism, aggregation and enzyme secretion in human neutrophils. Agent Action 24:272–281, 1988.

Rossi F, Bianca VD, Grzeskowiak M, Bazzoni F. Studies on molecular regulation of phagocytosis in neutrophils: Con A-mediated ingestion and associated respiratory burst independent of phosphoinositide turnover, rise in $[CA^{2+}]i$, and arachidonic acid release. J Immunol 142:1652–1660, 1989.

Sacchi F, Rondini G, Mingrat G, Stronati M, Gancia GP, Marseglia GL, Siccardi AG. Different maturation of neutrophil chemotaxis in term and preterm newborn infants. J Pediatr 101:273–274, 1982.

Savill J, Fadok V, Henson P, Haslett C. Phagocyte recognition of cells undergoing apoptosis. Immunol Today 14:131–136, 1993.

Saltzmann RL, Peterson PK. Immunodeficiency of the elderly. Rev Infect Dis 9:1127–1139, 1987.

Sawyer DW, Sullivan JA, Mandell GL. Intracellular free calcium location in neutrophils during phagocytosis. Science 230:663–666, 1985.

Scott RE, Horn RG. Ultrastructural aspects of neutrophil granulocyte development in humans. Lab Invest 23:202–215, 1970.

Segal AW. The electron transport chain of the microbicidal oxidase of phagocytic cells and the involvement in the molecular pathology of chronic granulomatous disease. J Clin Invest 83:1785–1793, 1989.

Seligmann BE, Gallin JI. Use of lipophilic probes of membrane potential to assess human neutrophil activation. J Clin Invest 66:493–503, 1980.

Sha'afi RI, White JR, Molski TF, Shefcyk J, Volpi M, Naccache PH, Feinstein MB. Phorbol 12-myristate 13-acetate activates rabbit neutrophils without an apparent rise in the level of intracellular free calcium. Biochem Biophys Res Commun 114:638–645, 1983.

Shafer WM, Martin LE, Spitznagel JK. Late intraphagosomal hydrogen ion concentration favors the in vitro antimicrobial capacity of a 37-kilodalton cationic granule protein of human neutrophil granulocytes. Infect Immun 53:651–655, 1986.

Shigeoka AO, Gobel R, Janatova J, Hill H. Neutrophil mobilization induced by complement fragments during experimental group B streptococcal (GBS) infection. Am J Pathol 133:623–629, 1988.

Shigeoka AO, Santos JI, Hill HR. Functional analysis of neutrophil granulocytes from healthy, infected, and stressed neonates. J Pediatr 95:454–460, 1979.

Singer SJ, Kupfer A. The directed migration of eukaryotic cells. Ann Rev Cell Biol 2:337–365, 1986.

Sklar LA. Ligand-receptor dynamics and signal amplification in the neutrophil. Adv Immunol 39:95–143, 1986.

Sklar LA, Mueller H, Omenn G, Oades Z. Three states for the formyl peptide receptor on intact cells. J Biol Chem 264:8483–8486, 1989.

Sklar LA, Omenn GM. Kinetics and amplification in neutrophil activation and adaption. Semin Cell Biol 1:115–123, 1990.

Smith CW, Kishimoto TK, Abbass O, Hughes B, Rothlein R, McIntyre LV, Butcher E, Anderson DC. Chemotactic factors regulate lectin adhesion molecule 1(LECAM-1)-dependent neutrophil adhesion to cytokine-stimulated endothelial cells in vitro. J Clin Invest 87:609–618, 1991.

Smith JB, Campbell DE, Ludomirsky A, Polin RA, Douglas SD, Gartz BZ, Harris MC. Expression of the complement receptors CR1 and CR3 and the Type III Fc$_\gamma$ receptor on neutrophils from newborn infants and from fetuses with Rh disease. Pediatr Res 28:120–126, 1990.

Smith RM, Curnutte JT. Molecular basis of chronic granulomatous disease. Blood 77:673–686, 1991.

Smolen JE, Korchak HM, Weissmann G. Increased levels of cyclic adenosine-3',5'-monophosphate in human polymorphonuclear leukocytes after surface stimulation. J Clin Invest 65:1077–1085, 1980.

Smolen JE, Korchak HM, Weissmann G. Stimulus-response coupling in neutrophils. Trends Pharmacol Sci 3:483–487, 1982.

Southwick FS, Dabiri GA, Stossel TP. Neutrophil actin dysfunction is a genetic disorder associated with partial impairment of neutrophil actin assembly in three family members. J Clin Invest 82:1525–1531, 1988.

Springer TA. Adhesion receptors of the immune system. Nature 346:425–434, 1990.

Steadman R, Topley N, Jenner DE, Davies M, Williams JD. Type 1 fimbriate E. coli stimulates a unique pattern of degranulation by human polymorphonuclear leukocytes. Infect Immun 56:815–822, 1988.

Stendahl O, Coble BI, Dahlgren C, Hed J, Molin L. Myeloperoxidase modulates the phagocytic activity of polymorphonuclear leukocytes: studies with cells from a myeloperoxidase deficient patient. J Clin Invest 73:366–373, 1984.

Suzuki K, Swenson C, Sasagawa S, Sakatani T, Watanabe M, Kobayashi M, Fujikura T. Age-related decline in lysosomal enzyme release from polymorphonuclear leukocytes after N-formyl-methionyl-leucyl-phenylalanine stimulation. Exp Hematol 11:1005–1013, 1983.

Tauber AI, Kanard AB, Ginis I. The role of phosphorylation in phagocyte activation. Curr Top Membr Transport 35:469–494, 1990.

Traynor-Kaplan AE. Phosphoinositide metabolism during phagocytic cell activation. Curr Top Membr Transport 35:303–332, 1990.

Vadhan-Raj S, Keating M, LeMaistre A, Hittelman WN, McCredie K, Trujillo JM, Broxmeyer HE, Henney C, Gutterman JU. Effects of recombinant human granulocyte-macrophage colony-stimulating factor in patients with myelodysplastic syndromes. N Engl J Med 317:1445–1452, 1987.

Valent P, Bettelheim P. Cell surface structures on human basophils and mast cells: biochemical and functional characterization. Adv Immunol 52:333–423, 1992.

Van Epps DE, Garcia ML. Enhancement of neutrophil function as a result of prior exposure to chemotactic factor. J Clin Invest 66:167–175, 1980.

Van Oss CJ, Gillman CF, Neuman AW. Phagocytic engulfment and cell adhesiveness as cellular surface phenomena. In Isenberg HD, ed. Microorganisms and Infectious Diseases, Vol. 2. New York, Marcel Dekker, 1975, pp. 1–16.

Venge P, Olsson I. Cationic proteins of human granulocytes: VI. Effects on the complement system and mediation of chemotactic activity. J Immunol 115:1505–1508, 1975.

Verhoef J, Visser MR. Neutrophil phagocytosis and killing: normal function and microbial evasion. In Abramson JS, Wheeler JG, eds. The Neutrophil, Oxford, England, Oxford University Press, 1993, pp. 109–137.

Weisdorf DJ, Craddock PR, Jacob HS. Glycogenolysis versus glucose transport in human granulocytes: differential activation in phagocytosis and chemotaxis. Blood 60:888–893, 1982.

Weiss J, Elsbach P, Olsson I, Odeberg H. Purification and characterization of a potent bactericidal and membrane active protein from the granules of human polymorphonuclear leukocytes. J Biol Chem 253:2664–2672, 1978.

Weiss J, Victor M, Stendhal O, Elsbach P. Killing of gram-negative bacteria by polymorphonuclear leukocytes. J Clin Invest 69:959–970, 1982.

Weissmann G, Hoffstein S, Korchak H, Smolen JE. The earliest membrane responses to phagocytosis: membrane potential changes and Ca^{++} loss in human granulocytes. Trans Assoc Am Physicians 91:90–103, 1978.

Weissmann G, Smolen J, Korchak H, Hoffstein S. The secretory code of the neutrophil. In Dingle JT, Gordon JL, eds. Cellular Interactions. New York, Elsevier, North-Holland, 1981, pp. 15–31.

Weller PF. Eosinophilia. J Allergy Clin Immunol 73:1–10, 1984.

Weller PF. The immunobiology of eosinophils. N Engl J Med 324:1110–1118, 1991.

Weller PF. Cytokine regulation of eosinophil function. Clin Immunol Immunopathol 62:S55–S59, 1992.

Wheeler JG, Abramson JS. Microbial and pharmacological induction of neutrophil dysfunction. In Abramson JS, Wheeler JG, eds. The

Neutrophil. Oxford, England, Oxford University Press, 1993, pp. 139–181.

Wheeler JG, Abramson JS, Ekstrand K. Function of irradiated polymorphonuclear leukocytes obtained by buffy-coated centrifugation. Transfusion 24:238–239, 1984a.

Wheeler JG, Chauvenet AR, Johnson CA, Dillard R, Block SM, Boyle R, Abramson JS. Neutrophil storage pool depletion in septic, neutropenic neonates. Pediatr Infect Dis 3:407–409, 1984b.

White IWC, Gelb AW, Wexler HR, Stiller CR, Keown PA. The effects of intravenous anaesthetic agents on human neutrophil chemiluminescence. Can Anesth Soc J 30:506–511, 1983.

Wick SM, Hepler PK. Selective localization of intracellular Ca^{2+} with potassium antimonate. J Histochem Cytochem 30:1190–1204, 1982.

Wilson CB, Tsai V, Remington JS. Failure to trigger the oxidative metabolic burst by normal macrophages: possible mechanism for survival of intracellular pathogens. J Exp Med 151:328–346, 1980.

Wright DG. The neutrophil as a secretory organ of host defense. In Gallin JI, Fauci AS, eds. Advances in Host Defense Mechanisms, Vol 1. New York, Raven Press, 1982, pp. 75–110.

Wright DG. Human neutrophil degranulation. Methods Enzymol 162:538–551, 1988.

Wright DG, Gallin JI. A functional differentiation of human neutrophil granules: generation of C5a by a specific (secondary) granule product and inactivation of C5a by azurophil (primary) granule products. J Immunol 119:1068–1076, 1977.

Wright DG, Gallin JI. Modulation of the inflammatory response by products released from human polymorphonuclear leukocytes during phagocytosis: generation and inactivation of the chemotactic factor C5a. Inflammation 1:23–39, 1975.

Wright DG, Klock JC. Functional changes in neutrophils collected by filtration leukapheresis and their relationship to cellular events that occur during adherence of neutrophils to nylon fibers. Exp Hematol 7(Suppl 4):11–23, 1979.

Wright WC, Ank BJ, Herbert J, Stiehm ER. Decreased bactericidal activity of leukocytes of stressed newborn infants. Pediatrics 56:579–584, 1975.

Wyrick PB, Brownridge EA. Growth of *Chlamydia psittaci* in macrophages. Infect Immun 19:1054–1060, 1978.

Yamamoto K, Miyoshi-Koshio T, Utsuki Y, Mizuno S, Suzuki K. Virucidal activity and viral modification by myeloperoxidase: a candidate for defense factor of human polymorphonuclear leukocytes against influenza virus. J Infect Dis 164:8–14, 1991.

Yuo A, Kitagawa S, Kasahara T, Matsushima K, Saito M, Takaku F. Stimulation and priming of human neutrophils by interleukin-8: cooperation with tumor necrosis factor and colony-stimulating factor. Blood 78:2708–2714, 1991.

Zigmond SH. Ability of polymorphonuclear leukocytes to orient in gradients of chemotactic factors. J Cell Biol 75:606–616, 1977.

Zigmond SH, Hirsch JG. Effects of cytochalsin B on polymorphonuclear leukocytes locomotion, phagocytosis and glycolysis. Exp Cell Res 73:383–393, 1972.

Zurier RB, Weissmann G, Hoffstein S, Kammerman SK, Tai HH. Mechanisms of lysosomal enzyme release from human leukocytes. J Clin Invest 53:297–309, 1974.

Chapter 6

The Mononuclear Phagocyte and Dendritic Cell Systems

Steven D. Douglas and Mervin C. Yoder

THE MONONUCLEAR PHAGOCYTE SYSTEM

Since the modern study of mammalian phagocytes began with Metchnikoff in the nineteenth century, classification of these cells with respect to structure-function relationships has been controversial. Studies of the ontogeny, kinetics, and function of phagocytic cells in animals have led to the concept of the mononuclear phagocyte system (MPS) (Van Furth et al., 1975); this is the most useful conceptual framework for these cells. The MPS, as presently defined, consists of bone marrow *promonocytes*, circulating blood *monocytes*, and both mobile and fixed tissue *macrophages* (Table 6–1). Vascular endothelium, reticulum cells, and dendritic cells of lymphoid germinal centers are not included, although terms used in the past, such as the *reticuloendothelial system*, denoted these cells and mononuclear phagocytes (MNPs) collectively. The justification for

the present classification of cells of the MPS includes numerous lines of investigation (Ackerman and Douglas, 1980), notably the following:

1. Most tissue macrophages, as identified morphologically in tissue sections, appear to have several important functional characteristics in common—particularly, pronounced phagocytic ability in vivo and in vitro and adhesiveness to glass or plastic surfaces in vitro.

2. Kinetic studies identify a bone marrow cell as precursor to the monocyte and the circulating monocyte as the precursor of most, although not all, tissue macrophages.

The functions of MNPs include the following:

1. Phagocytosis and digestion of microorganisms and tissue debris

2. Secretion of inflammatory mediators and regulators

Table 6–1. Cells Belonging to the Mononuclear Phagocyte System

Bone Marrow	Tissues	Body Cavities
Monoblasts	Macrophages occurring in	Pleural macrophages
Promonocytes	Connective tissue (histiocytes)	Peritoneal macrophages
Monocytes	Skin (histiocytes; Langerhans cells?)	
	Liver (Kupffer cells)	**Inflammation**
Blood	Spleen (red pulp macrophages)	Exudate macrophages
Monocytes	Lymph nodes (free and fixed macrophages; interdigitating cells?)	Epithelioid cells
	Thymus	Multinucleated giant cells
	Bone marrow (resident macrophages)	
	Bone (osteoclasts)	
	Synovia (Type A cell)	
	Lung (alveolar and tissue macrophages)	
	Mucosa-associated lymphoid tissues	
	Gastrointestinal tract	
	Genitourinary tract	
	Endocrine organs	
	Central nervous system (macrophages, [reactive] microglia, CSF macrophages)	

From Van Furth R. Development and distribution of mononuclear phagocytes in the normal steady state and inflammation. In Gallin JI, Goldstein IM, Snyderman R, eds. Inflammation: Basic Principles and Clinical Correlates. New York, Raven Press, 1988, p. 291.
Abbreviation: CSF = cerebrospinal fluid.

3. Interaction with antigen and lymphocytes in the generation of the immune response

4. Extracellular killing, as of some tumor cells

5. Other functions specific for macrophages of particular organs or tissues

Most investigations of MNP function have used tissue macrophages, both for technical reasons and also in the belief that these are the most important functional element in the MPS. Studies in humans, however, are more difficult, and the circulating blood monocyte is the most readily available MNP. After in vitro culture for 5 to 7 days, the monocyte develops macrophage-like properties (Zuckerman et al., 1979). The in vitro study of human MNP biology has been a useful model for examining macrophage physiology and function (Ackerman et al., 1981).

Origin and Development

All lymphohematopoietic cells arise from lineage-committed hematopoietic progenitor cells and, ultimately, from a pool of self-renewing pluripotent stem cells. During embryogenesis, primitive macrophages are the first hematopoietic cells to appear in the yolk sac. Later in gestation, when the fetal liver is the predominant site of hematopoiesis, first macrophages and then monocytes are produced (Kelemen et al., 1979). After birth and throughout childhood and adult life, hematopoiesis occurs in the bone marrow. In marrow, the *monoblast*, the MNP bone marrow precursor cell, differentiates to the promonocyte, and subsequently to the mature circulating monocyte (Douglas and Musson, 1986). The monoblast is a small, round cell that actively incorporates thymidine, is esterase- and peroxidase-negative, contains lysozyme, and has complement and IgG receptors. The promonocyte contains specific monocyte enzymes, has complement and IgG receptors, and is capable of phagocytosing particles. The promonocyte is also an actively dividing cell that undergoes several intramarrow mitoses before differentiating into the monocyte, at which time it moves into the intravascular compartment. Blood monocytes circulate for 1 to 4 days, then migrate into tissues. Some of the circulating blood monocytes bind to blood vessel walls, and this marginating pool represents approximately 75% of the total intravascular monocyte pool (Van Furth, 1980).

The resident tissue macrophages are replaced from the blood monocyte pool with defined turnover and exist as both fixed and free macrophages. Free macrophages are found in pleural, synovial, peritoneal, and alveolar spaces and in inflammatory sites. The generally less motile fixed tissue macrophages are present in splenic sinusoids, in the liver as Kupffer cells, in reticulum cells of the bone marrow, in the lamina propria of the gastrointestinal tract, in specific sites in lymph nodes, in bone as osteoclasts, and as microglia in the central nervous system (Van Furth, 1980). We have developed methods for isolation of purified populations of human peripheral blood monocytes and study of their in vitro differentiation (Zuckerman et al., 1979;

Hassan et al., 1986). In pathologic sites, tissue macrophages may undergo cell fusion and form multinucleated giant cells, which are the source of epithelioid cells in chronic granulomata (Adams, 1976).

Kinetics

The kinetics of human monocytes have been actively studied, both by use of in vivo pulse labeling with tritiated thymidine and by autotransfusion of monocytes labeled with ^{3}H-diisopropyfluorophosphate (Meuret et al., 1971, 1974, 1975; Whitlaw, 1972; Meuret and Hoffman, 1973). The total blood monocyte pool is made up of both a circulating monocyte pool and a marginal monocyte pool, the latter existing in normal individuals in a circulating monocyte pool–to–marginal monocyte pool ratio of approximately 1:3.5. The circulating monocyte pool is made up predominantly of cells in a G_1 state, which are released into the circulation following a maturation time in the bone marrow of between 50 and 60 hours. Under normal conditions, the bone marrow promonocyte pool produces approximately 7×10^6 monocytes/kg/hour. The half-disappearance time of labeled monocytes from the blood is considerably longer than for granulocytes (monocytes, approximately 70 hours; granulocytes, approximately 7 hours) (Meuret et al., 1974a, 1974b; Whitlaw, 1972; Athens et al., 1961). The mean absolute monocyte count in peripheral blood ranges from 1100/mm^3 during the first 2 weeks of life (when there is a relative monocytosis) to between 350/mm^3 and 700/mm^3 during the remainder of childhood (Yoder et al., 1992). The blood monocyte counts in normal subjects oscillate in a cycle that varies between 3 and 6 days in length. This is shorter than the cycle for polymorphonuclear leukocytes, platelets, and reticulocytes. In addition to this normal cyclical variation, perturbations in the monocyte count can occur following the injection of a number of different materials as well as in response to inflammation and disease (see Chapter 16, Disorders of the Mononuclear Phagocytic System). Usually, monocytopenia develops during endotoxin or steroid administration.

The tissue macrophage does not usually undergo division. It has a life span that has been estimated to range from 60 days to many years; however, an extremely small proportion (less than 5%) of tissue macrophages were found to synthesize deoxyribonucleic acid (DNA) and divide locally in the tissues (Van Furth et al., 1985). The macrophage does not return to the peripheral circulation; however, its ultimate fate is not precisely known.

Characterization

Morphology

The morphology of the MNP has been investigated by light microscopy, including histologic and cytochemical stains and phase-contrast, Nomarski, and reflection-contrast optics (Ploem, 1975; Zuckerman and Douglas, 1979). Scanning and transmission electron microscopy and freeze-fracture and freeze-etch procedures have also been used (Douglas, 1978; Ackerman and Douglas, 1980, 1983).

Light Microscopy

Monoblasts and promonocytes are the precursors of monocytes and bear finely dispersed nuclear chromatin and nucleoli when observed in stained films of the blood or bone marrow. Monoblasts lack distinctive features and are indistinguishable by light microscopy from the neutrophilic precursor, the myeloblast. Promonocytes are 12 to 18 μm in diameter and have characteristic deeply indented, irregularly shaped nuclei with condensed chromatin and numerous cytoplasmic microfilaments (Nichols et al., 1971; Nichols and Bainton, 1973).

Monocytes are found both in the blood and in tissues and body cavities, in which they exhibit morphologic variation. In the stained blood film, the diameter is 12 to 15 μm. The nucleus occupies about half the area of the cell in a film and is usually eccentrically placed. The nucleus is most often reniform but may be round or irregular. It contains a characteristic chromatin net with fine strands bridging small chromatin clumps. Chromatin aggregates are arranged along the internal aspect of the nuclear membrane. The nuclear chromatin pattern has been called "raked" because of its fine-stranded appearance. The cytoplasm is spread out, turns grayish-blue with Wright's stain, and contains a variable number of fine, pink-purple granules that at times are sufficiently numerous to give the entire cytoplasm a pink hue. Clear cytoplasmic vacuoles and a variable number of larger azurophilic granulations are often encountered in these cells.

Macrophages are heterogeneous in size and shape, ranging from 25 to 70 μm in diameter and appearing as oval, stellate, or spindle-shaped cells. The nucleus is eccentrically placed and contains finely dispersed chromatin and prominent nucleoli. Cytoplasmic granules and lysosomes are abundant and are indicative of the phagocytic nature of these cells. Numerous vacuoles characteristic of pinocytic cells are present near the cell periphery (Zuckerman et al., 1979).

Phase Microscopy

Under the phase-contrast microscope (Fig. 6–1), the monocyte nucleus shows a distinct chromatin pattern on a somewhat cloudy background. The cytoplasm is clear and gray. Mitochondria are extremely fine and on occasion form a small, juxtanuclear rosette surrounding the centrosome. The phase-dense cytoplasmic granules, varying in number, are generally at the limit of resolution of light microscopy and appear as fine intracytoplasmic dust. Monocytes contain several types of cytoplasmic vacuoles.

The monocyte generally assumes a triangular shape as it moves, with one point trailing behind and the other two points advancing before the cell. It adheres to and spreads on glass surfaces (Bessis, 1955; Fedorko and Hirsch, 1970; North, 1970). The extent of spreading is increased in the presence of antigen-antibody complexes, certain divalent metals, and proteolytic en-

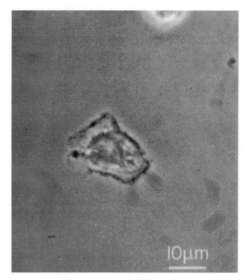

Figure 6–1. Human blood monocyte after in vitro culture for 1 hour. Note phase-dense thickening at the peripheral region of the cell signifying ruffling of the membrane. (Phase-contrast micrograph, original magnification ×400.) (From Ackerman SK, Douglas SD. In Carr I, Daems WT, eds. Reticuloendothelial System: Morphology. New York, Plenum Press, 1980, pp. 297–327.)

zymes (Rabinovitch and DeStefano, 1973; Rabinovitch et al., 1975; Douglas, 1976). The spread form of the monocyte is characteristic, with the nucleus and granulations located centrally and the abundant hyaloplasm about the periphery of the cell, terminating in a fringed border that displays characteristic undulating movement. The small monocyte may be difficult to distinguish from the large lymphocyte when examined by phase-contrast microscopy, although the two cells can be differentiated by the ability of small monocytes to adhere to glass surfaces.

Scanning Electron Microscopy

Figure 6–2 shows a scanning micrograph of a human monocyte following isolation and 1 hour in vitro culture (Ackerman and Douglas, 1978; Zuckerman et al., 1979). Prominent ruffles and small surface blebs are apparent. Extensive ruffling of the monocyte plasma membrane is of functional significance (Bumol and Douglas, 1977). The monocyte is both motile and phagocytic, and for these functions to be accomplished, there must be physical contact with fibers or cell surfaces. Reduction in the radius of curvature of the cell surface by formation of ruffles or microvilli may decrease repulsive forces when surface negative–charge groups on the cell approach and contact a negatively charged substratum or cell (Van Oss et al., 1975). Also, redundancy of the cell membrane may provide reserve membrane required for locomotion and for phagocytosis.

Transmission Electron Microscopy

The nucleus of the monocyte contains one or two small nucleoli surrounded by nucleolar-associated chromatin (DePetris et al., 1962; Sutton and Weiss, 1966; Cohn, 1968). The cytoplasm contains a relatively

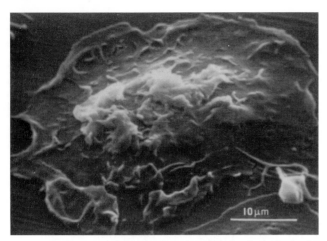

Figure 6–2. Blood monocyte cultured 1 hour in vitro. The cell is flattened against the substratum and possesses prominent surface ruffles. (Scanning electron micrograph, ×2750.) (From Ackerman SK, Douglas SD. In Carr I, Daems WT, eds. Reticuloendothelial System: Morphology. New York, Plenum Press, 1980, pp. 297–327.)

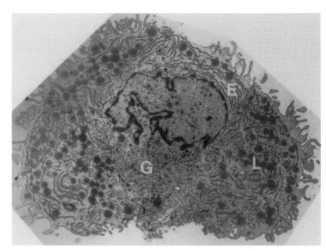

Figure 6–3. Monocyte-derived macrophage cultured 17 days in vitro. Note the presence of a Golgi zone (G) with scattered endoplasmic reticulum (E) and lipid vacuoles (L). (Transmission electron micrograph, ×6000.)

small quantity of endoplasmic reticulum and a variable quantity of ribosomes and polysomes. The mitochondria are usually numerous, small, and elongated. The Golgi complex is well developed. Centrioles and filamentous centriolar satellites can often be visualized. Microtubules and microfibrils are numerous (DePetris et al., 1962).

In cultures of macrophages, collections of microfilaments are present underneath the plasma membrane near sites of cell attachment either to a substratum or to ingestable particles (Reaven and Axline, 1973). Microfilaments are the main structural component of the contractile apparatus (Hartwig and Stossel, 1985). The cell surface is characterized by numerous microvilli and vesicles of micropinocytosis.

The cytoplasmic granules resemble the small granules found in the granulocytic series, measuring approximately 0.05 to 0.2 μm. They are dense and homogeneous and are surrounded by a limiting membrane. These granules, as with the lysosomal granules of other leukocytes, are packaged by the Golgi apparatus after their enzymatic content has been produced by the ribosomal complex of the cell (Cohn and Benson, 1966; Cohn, 1968; Wetzel et al., 1967; Nichols et al., 1971; Nichols and Bainton, 1973). These cytoplasmic granules contain acid phosphatase and arylsulfatase and are therefore primary lysosomes (Axline, 1970). After endocytosis, lysosomes fuse with the phagosome, forming secondary lysosomes (North, 1970). Monocyte granules may give a positive reaction for peroxidase, although in a large proportion of monocytes this reaction is negative (Breton-Gorius and Cuichard, 1969; Nichols et al., 1971; Nichols and Bainton, 1973). The monocyte-derived macrophage maintained in culture is characterized by many lysosomes, a well-developed Golgi zone, an extensive endoplasmic reticulum, and lipid vacuoles (Fig. 6–3).

Freeze-Fracture Microscopy

In the technique known as freeze-fracture microscopy, a cell suspension is first frozen and then placed

in a high-vacuum chamber and struck with a blunt edge. A fracture is propagated through the frozen specimen. The utility of the procedure comes from the remarkable finding that when the fracture encounters a cell, it tends to propagate along the interior of the plasma membrane and thus splits the lipid bilayer in half. After fracture, the specimen is coated with platinum, which is electron-dense, and viewed with transmission electron microscopy.

All cell types examined thus far by the freeze-fracture technique have shown intramembrane particles as the predominant feature of the topography of the interior of the bilayer (Figs. 6–4 and 6–5). In the erythrocyte, some particles contain intercalated membrane proteins (IMPs) (Weinstein et al., 1978), and this has been assumed to be the case with nucleated cells as well. The distribution of IMPs is dramatically altered in a number of cell systems by physiologic stimuli, e.g., hormonal stimulation. Profound changes in the distri-

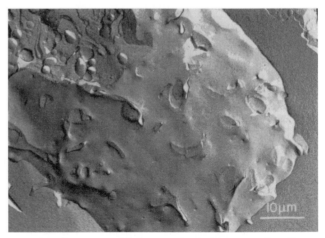

Figure 6–4. Human blood monocyte, freeze-fracture replica. (Survey view, ×18,000.) (From Ackerman SK, Douglas SD. In Carr I, Daems WT, eds. Reticuloendothelial System: Morphology. New York, Plenum Press, 1980, pp. 297–327.)

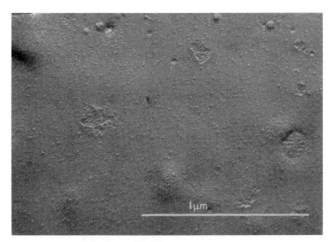

Figure 6–5. Human blood monocyte, freeze-fracture detail. Note the many small particles, normal distribution of which is random. These consist, at least in part, of intercalated membrane proteins (×67,500). (From Ackerman SK, Douglas SD. In Carr I, Daems WT, eds. Reticuloendothelial System: Morphology. New York, Plenum Press, 1980, pp. 297–327.)

bution of intramembrane particles on MNPs occur following binding of antibody-coated erythrocytes (Douglas, 1978). Since redistribution also occurs in some nonphagocytic Fc receptor–bearing cells (Douglas, 1978) and after exposure to aggregated IgG (Douglas et al., 1980), this alteration in intramembrane particles presumably reflects interaction with the Fc receptor.

Histochemistry

Macrophages contain a wide variety of hydrolytic enzymes that are synthesized in the rough endoplasmic reticulum and are packaged in units of membrane-bound vesicles known as lysosomes. Lysozyme, β-glucuronidase, acid phosphatase, cathepsins, hydrolases, and esteroproteases have all been described in macrophages (Axline and Cohn, 1970; Solotorovsky and Soderberg, 1972). These enzymes play an important role in intracellular digestion of phagocytized material and in the development and maintenance of inflammatory reactions. They also may be involved in microbial killing.

Nonspecific esterase is an enzyme on the external side of the plasma membrane (ectoenzyme) on alveolar macrophages (Jaubert et al., 1978) and blood monocytes (Bozdech and Bainton, 1981). Nonspecific esterase (Wachstein and Wolfe, 1958; Braunsteiner and Schmalzl, 1968, 1970; Li et al., 1973) is frequently used as a marker for monocytes, and the recent isolation and cloning of MNP esterase complementary deoxyribonucleic acid (cDNA) will facilitate the use of this enzyme as a MNP marker (Yourno, 1986; Zschunke et al., 1991; Scott et al., 1992). Monocyte esterases are inhibited by sodium fluoride, whereas the esterases of the granulocytic series are not. The nonspecific esterase reaction is positive in promyelocytes and myelocytes, and therefore analysis of fluoride inhibition is necessary to distinguish marrow monocytes from early myelocytes (Braunsteiner and Schmalzl, 1968).

Monocytes, neutrophils, and lymphocytes differ in hydrolytic enzyme content (Wachstein and Wolfe, 1958; Braunsteiner and Schmalzl, 1968, 1970; Li et al., 1973). Monocyte granules, although heterogeneous in size (0.3 to 0.6 μm), are not separable into populations by routine electron microscopic criteria, except in the rat (Van der Rhee et al., 1977). Identification of monocyte granule populations has depended on subcellular localization of monocyte enzymes by electron microscopic cytochemistry (Nichols et al., 1971).

Human marrow promonocytes and blood monocytes contain granules that make up two functionally distinct populations (Nichols et al., 1971; Nichols and Bainton, 1973). One population contains the enzymes acid phosphatase, arylsulfatase, and—in the human but not in the rabbit—peroxidase; these granules are therefore modified primary lysosomes and are analogous to the azurophil granules of the neutrophil. The monocyte azurophil granule population is heterogeneous with respect to cytochemical reactivity for peroxidase, acid phosphatase, and arylsulfatase (Nichols and Bainton, 1975; Bodel et al., 1977). Moreover, primary granules that are morphologically identical with other vesicles may be identified cytochemically as lysosomes. The content of the other population of monocyte granules is unknown; however, they lack alkaline phosphatase (Nichols and Bainton, 1975) and hence are not strictly analogous to the specific granules of neutrophils. The function of the lysosomal granule is presumably digestive; the purpose of the second population is not known.

About 10% of granules in normal human blood monocytes stain with reagents that identify complex acid carbohydrates, or *acid mucosubstances* (Parmley et al., 1978). These substances are found in leukemic monocyte granules as well as in granules of normal neutrophils (Horn and Spicer, 1964), and their function is unknown. Monocytes also have a weak but positive periodic acid–Schiff (PAS) reaction (for polysaccharides) and Sudan black B reaction (for lipids).

Cell Surface Antigenic Determinants

The MNP cell surface is rich in antigenic markers that have been studied with a variety of monoclonal antibodies. Studies of the expression of these antigens on human MNPs have led to better understanding of the origin, differentiation, and functions of MNPs (Todd and Schlossman, 1982; Dimitriu-Bona et al., 1983; Andreesen et al., 1986; Auger and Ross, 1992; Ho et al., 1992). Table 6–2 lists most of the antigenic determinants of MNP cells that are recognized as *clusters of differentiation* (CD) by the International Workshop on Human Leukocyte Differentiation Antigens (Barclay et al., 1993). These cell surface antigens function as cell recognition or adhesion molecules, enzymes, or receptors for growth factors, hormones, lipids, extracellular matrix molecules, or lectins (Gordon et al., 1988); some antigens are not well enough characterized to be assigned a specific cellular function. Most of these antigens are not expressed exclusively by MNP; however, unique patterns of antigen expression have been

Table 6–2. CD Antigens on Mononuclear Phagocyte Cells

CD Group	Molecule	Distribution on Hematopoietic Cells
4	T₄	Thymocytes, T cells, monocytes, macrophages
11b	CR3, OKM-1, Mac-1	Neutrophils, monocytes, platelets
11c	p150, 95	Monocytes, neutrophils, natural killer (NK) cells
w12	p150–160	Monocytes, neutrophils, platelets
13	gp150	Monocytes, neutrophils, some macrophages
14	LPS receptor	Monocytes, macrophages, dendritic cells, some neutrophils
15	Lewis X (Leˣ)	Neutrophils, eosinophils, monocytes, myeloid leukemia cells
16	FcγRIII	NK cells, macrophages, some monocytes
w17	Lactosylceramide	Neutrophils, monocytes, platelets
18	Integrin β2	Most leukocytes
23	FcεRII	B cells, activated macrophages, monocytes, platelets
25	IL-2 receptor	T and B cells, monocytes
31	PECAM-1	Monocytes, platelets, neutrophils
w32	FcγRII	Monocytes, neutrophils, B cells
33	p67	Monocytes, progenitor cells, myeloid leukemia cells
34	p105–120	Progenitor cells, myeloid and lymphoid leukemia cells
35	CR1	Erythrocytes, monocytes, macrophages, neutrophils
36	Platelet glycoprotein IV	Monocytes
43	Leukosialin	T cells, monocytes, macrophages, platelets
44	Phagocytic glycoprotein-1	T and B cells, monocytes, thymocytes, erythrocytes
45	B220, T200, Ly-5	All leukocytes
46	Membrane cofactor protein	T and B cells, NK cells, monocytes, platelets
48	gp41	Most leukocytes
49	Integrin α¹⁻⁶ chains	Most leukocytes
w50	p148/108	T and B cells, monocytes
53	gp21–28	Thymocytes, T and B cells, monocytes, osteoclasts
54	ICAM-1	Activated B and T cells, monocytes
58	LFA-3	Macrophages, B cells, thymocytes
61	Integrin β₃	Macrophages, osteoclasts, platelets
63	gp53	Platelets, monocytes, macrophages, B and T cells
64	FcγRI	Monocytes, macrophages, activated neutrophils
w65	Ceramide dodecasaccharide 4c	Monocytes, activated neutrophills
68	p110	Macrophages, monocytes, neutrophils
71	Transferrin receptor	Activated monocytes, neutrophils, B and T cells
74	MHC II-associated invariant chain	B cells, monocytes
w78	Leu 21	B cells, macrophages

Abbreviations: CD = cluster of differentiation; CR = complement receptor; ICAM = intercellular adhesion molecule; IL = interleukin; LFA = leukocyte function antigen; Mac = macrophage; MHC = major histocompatibility complex; PECAM = platelet endothelial cell adhesion molecule; T₄ = thyroxine; p = protein; gp = glycoprotein; LPS = lipopolysaccharides.

useful in defining developmentally regulated or tissue-specific MNP phenotypes (Todd and Schlossman, 1984; Andreesen et al., 1988, 1990; Terstappen et al., 1990; Buckley, 1991; Ho et al., 1992).

Metabolism

The metabolic activities of MNPs vary, depending on their degree of development, site of origin, and state of activation or stimulation (Cline, 1965; Bennett and Cohn, 1966; Cohn, 1968; Nelson, 1969; Karnovsky et al., 1973). The monocyte uses active aerobic glycolysis as a source of energy, whereas mature macrophages derive their energy from both glycolytic and aerobic pathways (Cline and Lehrer, 1968; Cohn, 1968). The degree to which macrophages depend on either aerobic or anaerobic processes appears to differ with their site of origin. Pulmonary macrophages manifest a high degree of oxygen consumption, gaining energy through oxidative phosphorylation (Hocking and Golde, 1979; Rossman and Douglas, 1988). Macrophages from other sites utilize anaerobic glycolysis as their main energy source.

These different characteristics appear to represent distinct functional advantages for the macrophages at each particular anatomic site. For example, it has been suggested that the capacity of nonalveolar macrophages to be metabolically active under anaerobic conditions is crucial to their ability to function optimally at sites of inflammation, where oxygen tension may be low. The dependence of the alveolar macrophage on aerobic sources of energy may represent a logical anatomic adaptation. However, this may be a disadvantage in situations of compromised pulmonary function because it has been shown that these cells have significantly reduced phagocyte capacity under conditions of low oxygen tension (Cline, 1970).

Biochemistry

Respiratory Burst

Stimulation of with soluble chemoattractants or through cell surface receptor–ligand interactions is associated with a dramatic increase in MNP oxygen consumption. This respiratory burst is not required for energy production but is necessary for superoxide anion, hydrogen peroxide, and hydroxyl radical production. A plasma membrane–bound enzyme complex

(NADPH oxidase) along with several cytosolic proteins converts molecular oxygen to superoxide anion. The reactive oxygen intermediates produced are further metabolized to free radicals and hypohalous acid and are used to kill ingested bacterial and fungal pathogens (Nathan, 1982, 1983). Respiratory burst activity diminishes as monocytes differentiate into macrophages, and tissue macrophages may rely more on oxygen-independent means to kill pathogens.

Lysosomes

Lysosomes are intracellular granular compartments composed of numerous enzymes and proteases. The primary function of these granules appears to be degradation of ingested materials. Acid hydrolases, lipases, ribonucleases, phosphatases, sulfatases, and neutral proteases are some of the constituents of lysosomes. Many of these proteins are not restricted to lysosomes and are secreted by MNPs on cytokine or complement stimulation, engagement of IgG-opsonized material through Fc receptors, or exposure to bacteria (Pantalone and Page, 1975; Lasser, 1983).

Biosynthesis and Secretion of Growth Factors and Cytokines

One of the mechanisms used by MNPs to influence local and systemic immune responses is the biosynthesis and secretion of numerous cytokines and growth factors (Table 6–3; Fig. 6–6). These regulatory molecules have pleiotropic effects that affect nearly all cell types, allowing for cell-to-cell communication among immune and nonimmune cells. Systemic as well as local events may be influenced by MNP cytokine secretion. Thus, normal homeostatic mechanisms such as core body temperature maintenance may be overridden in times of acute inflammation by the secretion of macrophage pyrogens interleukin-1 (IL-1), tumor necrosis factor (TNF-α), and IL-6 (see Table 6–3). These same cytokines alter liver metabolism and protein biosynthesis, resulting in liver secretion of acute-phase reactant proteins (Heinrich, 1990). B and T lymphocytes are activated to proliferate and differentiate in response to MNP secretion of IL-1 and IL-6 and the hematopoietic colony-stimulating factors CSF-1, GM-CSF, and G-CSF. The T lymphocyte–derived cytokines IL-6, G-CSF, and GM-CSF feed back to further stimu-

Table 6–3. Cytokines Secreted by Macrophages

Cytokine	Stimuli for Production	Biological Action
IFN-α	Viruses, bacteria	Antiviral; antimitotic; MHC Class II ($\uparrow$), NK activity ($\uparrow$); decreased c-*myc* expression
M-CSF	LPS, IL-1	Macrophage colonies; antiviral, induces PGE_2, plasminogen activator, IL-1, IFN-γ, TNF-α
GM-CSF	LPS, IL-1, TNF, retroviral infection	Granulocyte, eosinophil, macrophage colonies, radioprotection, protection from bacterial and parasitic infections; enhances neutrophil and eosinophil functions, PGE_2, IL-1, TNF, and O_2 induction
G-CSF	LPS, IL-1	Granulocyte colonies; terminal differentiation of myeloid cells; enhancement of neutrophil function
TNF-α	LPS and other microbial products, IL-2, GM-CSF, IL-1	Necrosis of tumors; endotoxic shock-like syndrome; cachexia; fever; IL-1; acute-phase protein response; antiparasitic; in vitro induction of ICAM-1, IL-1, GM-CSF, IL-6; up-regulation of MHC I and II expression
IL-1	Microbial products, TNF, GM-CSF, IL-2, antigen presentation	Immunoregulation (induction of IL-2, IL-4, IL-6, TNF); fever; acute-phase protein response; hypotension; slow wave sleep; induction of collagenase and PGE_2, bone and cartilage resorption in culture
IL-6	IL-1, TNF, PDGF	Proliferation of myeloma cell lines, hemopoietic cells (GM-CSF and IL-3-like action); induces IL-2R in T-cells; induces Ig production in B cells; induces acute-phase protein production by hepatocytes; fever
TGF-β		Inhibition of IL-2 effects; role in fibrosis and wound healing in vivo; anti-proliferative effects on hepatocytes, epithelial cells, T and B cells; influences integrin expression and differentiation; inhibits proliferative actions of EGF, PDGF, IL-2, and FGF
Basic FGF		Endothelial cell chemotaxis and growth; IFN-γ, IFN-β, PGE_2, LDL-receptor, c-myc, c-fos, amino acid transport; neutrophil activation; intracellular actin reorganization; augments synthesis of collagen; chemotaxis and proliferation of mesenchymal cells
EGF		Proliferation and differentiation of basal layer in epithelia; angiogenic; wound healing

Abbreviations: CSF = colony-stimulating factor; EGF = epidermal growth factor; FGF = fibroblast growth factor; G = granulocyte; ICAM = intracellular adhesion molecule; IFN = interferon; Ig = immunoglobulin; IL = interleukin; LDL = low-density lipoprotein; LPS = lipopolysaccharide; M = macrophage; PDGF = platelet-derived growth factor; TGF = transforming growth factor; TNF = tumor necrosis factor.
Adapted from Auger MJ, Ross JA. The biology of the macrophage. In Lewis CE, McGee JO, eds. The Macrophage. Oxford, England, IRL Press, 1992, pp. 1–74. By permission of Oxford University Press.

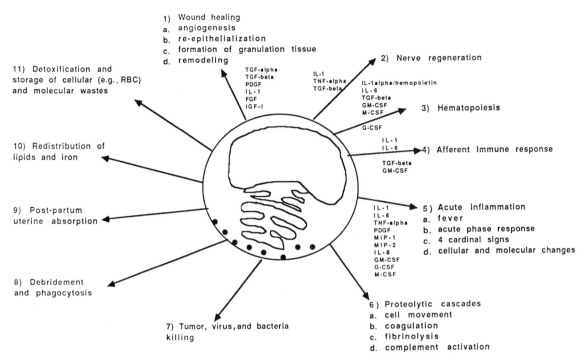

Figure 6–6. Growth factors produced by mononuclear phagocytes correlated with specific macrophage functions. (From Rappolee DA, Werb Z. Macrophage-derived growth factors. Curr Top Microbiol Immunol 181:87–140, 1992.)

late MNP secretion of growth factors and regulatory molecules and to increase bone marrow production of immature MNPs and granulocytes (Metcalf, 1987).

Other MNP-derived growth factors such as basic fibroblast growth factor, platelet-derived growth factor, and epidermal growth factor promote mesenchymal and epithelial cell growth and differentiation, whereas MNP secretion of transforming growth factor-β (TGF-β) has immunosuppressive and antiproliferative effects on a variety of immune and nonimmune cells (Lobb et al., 1986; Carpenter, 1987; Massague, 1987; Ross, 1987; Rappolee and Werb, 1992). Several anticytokine molecules have been identified in human MNPs. IL-1 receptor antagonist (IL-1ra) and TNF-soluble receptor-binding protein are secreted by MNP and serve to inhibit the effects of IL-1 and TNF, respectively, during acute and chronic inflammatory states (Seckinger et al., 1987, 1988; Arend et al., 1989).

Many techniques have been developed to assay for the biosynthesis and secretion of growth factors and cytokines by human MNPs. In most cases, growth factor and cytokine assays have been performed on isolated peripheral blood monocytes or monocyte-derived macrophages cultured and stimulated in vitro. Hamilton (1993) has indicated that some of the reported observations of cytokine secretion by stimulated human MNPs are contradictory. Comparisons between reports of cytokine secretion from MNPs must consider (1) method and site of MNP isolation, (2) purity of the isolated population, (3) state of differentiation of the isolated cells, (4) whether the cells were studied in suspension or adherent to tissue culture plates, (5) sensitivity and specificity of the assays, (6) whether

messenger ribonucleic acid (mRNA) or protein is measured, (7) quantification of secreted or cell-associated protein, (8) whether recombinant or native cytokines were used for stimulation of MNP secretion of additional cytokines, and (9) the medium and serum concentration used in the assay.

Other Secretory Products

More than 100 MNP secretory products have been studied (Nathan, 1987). Certain products are released on a constitutive basis and are little influenced by the tissue of origin or state of activation of the MNP (Davies, 1981). Other products are dependent on the activity of the cell in vitro or the site of origin in vivo (Rappolee and Werb, 1989). Table 6–4 lists some of the classes of MNP secretory products. Although some of these products are unique to the MNP, many are produced by other secretory cells (Nathan, 1987).

Selected Functions

Motility

An effective macrophage response to infection is predicated upon the ability to migrate and accumulate at an infection site. Macrophages, like neutrophils, are capable of both *random* and *directed* movement. Random migration is nondirected movement that occurs in the absence of attracting substances. Directed movement, or *chemotaxis*, refers to macrophage migration that occurs in response to identifiable chemotactic factors or stimuli and that is mediated by different types

Table 6–4. Secretory Products of Mononuclear
Phagocytes

Polypeptide hormones
Complement (C) components
Coagulation factors
Other enzymes
Inhibitors of enzymes and cytokines
Protease inhibitors
Proteins of extracellular matrix or cell adhesion
Other binding proteins
Bioactive oligopeptides
Bioactive lipids
Sterol hormones
Purine and pyrimidine products
Reactive oxygen intermediates
Reactive nitrogen intermediates

Modified from Nathan CF. Secretory products of macrophages, Journal of Clinical Investigation, 1987, vol. 79, pp. 319–326 by Copyright permission of the American Society for Clinical Investigation.

of receptors on phagocyte cell surfaces (Snyderman and Pike, 1989). A number of different methods have been used to study macrophage movement both in vivo (Rebuck and Crowley, 1955) and in vitro (Boyden, 1962).

Chemotaxis plays a major role in macrophage accumulation at the site of an infection. This process of cellular attraction is mediated by a number of chemotactic substances that either are produced as a result of activation of the complement pathway and the fibrinolytic and kinin-generating systems or are secreted by leukocytes (Gallin and Wolff, 1976). The complement pathway and the fibrinolytic and kinin-generating systems can be activated by a variety of substances, including antigen-antibody complexes, endotoxin, and even enzymes from macrophages and neutrophils released during the phagocytic process. C3a and C5a are the complement components that manifest chemotactic activity.

Plasminogen activator and kallikrein are chemotactic factors produced by the fibrinolytic and kinin-generating systems, respectively (Gallin and Kaplan, 1974). During the acute inflammatory response, leukotriene B4, platelet-activating factor, and neutrophil-derived chemotactic factor, produced by activated neutrophils, and platelet factor 4, platelet-derived growth factor, and TGF-β, produced by activated platelets, are potent chemotactic factors for human monocytes (Verghese and Snyderman, 1989). In addition, lymphocytes exposed to antigenic stimulation also produce substances that are capable of attracting MNPs (Ward et al., 1970). These lymphokines include lymphocyte-derived chemotactic factor (Altman et al., 1973), TNF-α and -β, and GM-CSF (Verghese and Snyderman, 1989). Certain compounds produced as a result of bacterial growth in vitro (Ward, 1968) also possess chemotactic activity for mononuclear phagocytes.

In addition to substances that stimulate macrophage motility, a number of biologically active inhibitors of mononuclear cell movement and inactivators of chemotactic factors have been described (Gallin and Wolff, 1976). Inhibition of MNP motility appears to play a significant role in accumulation of MNPs at sites of infection and inflammation. An important mediator of this phenomenon may be migration inhibition factor, a lymphokine released by antigen-stimulated lymphocytes that inhibits macrophage migration in vitro (David, 1973).

Migration of MNPs into areas of inflammation in tissues requires multiple receptor-ligand interactions between the MNP and capillary endothelial cells. In the systemic circulation, monocyte extravasation from postcapillary venules occurs in three stages (Butcher, 1991). Initially, monocytes rolling along the vascular endothelium make transient focal contact with the endothelial cells through a family of adhesion molecules called *selectins* (Fig. 6–7)(Lasky, 1992). *L-selectin* is constitutively expressed on the cell surface of monocytes and recognizes several types of carbohydrate molecules present on endothelial cell surface glycoproteins. *E-selectin* and *P-selectin* are adhesion molecules that are expressed only by activated endothelial cells (Carlos et al., 1991; Hakkert et al., 1991, Sanders et al., 1992). These selectins recognize several types of carbohydrate molecules expressed on monocyte cell surface glycoproteins.

The second phase of monocyte extravasation results in inhibition of monocyte rolling, with firm attachment of the monocyte to the activated endothelial cell (Carlos and Harlan, 1990). Adherence to endothelium is associated with overall activation of the monocyte and requires interaction of adhesion molecules of the integrin family on the monocyte with members of the immunoglobulin family on the endothelial cell (see Fig. 6–7). Specifically, heterodimeric monocyte cell surface CD11a/CD18, CD11b/CD18, and CD11c/CD18 mole-

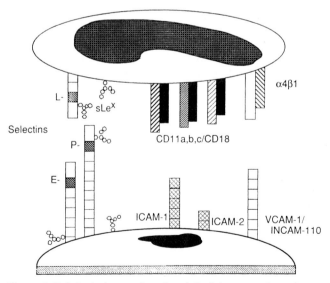

Figure 6–7. Selected examples of endothelial-mononuclear phagocyte adhesion molecules. Mononuclear phagocytes express cell surface carbohydrate and integrin (CD11a,b,c/CD18 and α4β1) molecules that can interact with ligand counter receptors on endothelial cells. Thus, adhesion of mononuclear phagocytes to endothelial cells is mediated by carbohydrate-selectin, integrin-ICAM, and integrin-VCAM-1/INCAM-110 interactions. (Reproduced with permission from Bevilacqua MP. Endothelial-leukocyte adhesion molecules. Annual Review of Immunology, Vol. 11, pp. 767–804, © 1993 by Annual Reviews Inc.)

cules bind to endothelial cell surface intercellular cell adhesion molecule-1 (ICAM-1) or -2 (ICAM-2) (Makgoba et al., 1988; Staunton et al., 1989; Arnaout, 1990; Springer, 1990). Monocytes also express another heterodimeric integrin family member composed of α4 and β1 chains that interacts with endothelial cell surface vascular cell adhesion molecule-1 (VCAM-1) and is associated with monocyte-endothelial adhesion on endothelial cell activation (Rice et al., 1990, 1991; Wellicome et al., 1990). The final step in monocyte extravasation involves chemotactic factor– or cytokine-directed transendothelial monocyte migration and emigration into the tissue toward the nidus of inflammation.

Several studies on the mechanisms that control pseudopod formation during macrophage movement have been performed. Actin is an abundant cytoplasmic protein that organizes into a three-dimensional network in the macrophage cortical cytoplasm (Hartwig and Stossel, 1985). Actin filaments attach to specific cell surface receptors (e.g., fibronectin receptors) that induce a change in cytoplasmic actin assemblies on binding to fibronectin. *Myosin* filaments that are present in macrophage cytoplasm control the contractility of the cells. Other proteins have been described, including gelsolin (Yin et al., 1981) and acumentin (Southwick and Hartwig, 1982), which serve to regulate actin filament assembly and macrophage mobility (Stossel, 1989). The observation that there is defective mononuclear phagocytic chemotaxis in a number of disease states (see Chapter 16) emphasizes the importance of an intact mononuclear phagocytic migratory response in host defense against infection and perhaps malignancy.

Endocytosis

The ability of macrophages to ingest a wide variety of materials is crucial to their immunologic function. Endocytosis is important in antigen processing, antimicrobial resistance, antineoplastic activity, removal of senescent cells and other "debris," and a number of other monocyte and macrophage functions. Two forms of endocytosis occur: *pinocytosis* and *phagocytosis*. The distinction between these two processes is related to the difference in the size and type of particles being ingested; the basic mechanisms are believed to be similar. Pinocytosis refers to the ingestion of microscopic fluid droplets. Phagocytosis describes the ingestion of larger particulate matter. Both processes involve interiorizing the respective materials in the cytoplasm. The actual interiorization phenomenon has been described in detail (Cohn, 1968; Gordon and Cohn, 1973). The ingested material becomes progressively surrounded by the plasma membrane through either invagination or engulfment by membrane extensions or microvilli. In this way, the particle comes to lie within a vesicle that is formed by the exterior plasma membrane of the cell. This vesicle becomes detached from the cell membrane and moves, apparently propelled by the undulating motion of the plasma membrane and cytoplasm, in a centripetal fashion toward the peri-Golgi region of the

cell. En route, these vesicles often fuse to form phagocytic vacuoles, or *phagosomes*. Phagosomes, in turn, fuse with the hydrolytic enzyme containing primary lysosomes and form *phagolysosomes*, in which the ultimate digestion process takes place.

Particulate material is not ingested without first becoming attached to the MNP cell surface membrane. Microorganisms that have been opsonized by complement, immunoglobulin (Ig), or both are more readily sequestered by the MNP cell surface membrane and ingested through cell surface receptors for complement component C3 products (C3b and C3bi) and the Fc portion of immunoglobulin (Horwitz, 1982; Ross et al., 1989). MNP receptors for the Fc domain of IgG (FcγR) belong to the immunoglobulin superfamily and are grouped in three primary classes; at least 12 isoforms of these molecules may be synthesized in humans (van de Winkel and Capel, 1993).

The receptor expressed by monocytes and macrophages that recognizes monomeric IgG is FcγRI (CD64). This high affinity receptor allows the MNP to bind and ingest bacteria with low concentrations of IgG that may not be recognized by neutrophils. A second receptor, FcγRII (CD32), is expressed by many leukocytes, including MNPs, and this receptor binds aggregated or complexed IgG. Neutrophils utilize FcγRII as the primary receptor in ingesting IgG-opsonized microorganisms. A third receptor, FcγRIII (CD16), is not expressed on circulating monocytes but is utilized by macrophages in the clearance of IgG-coated platelets and erythrocytes in vivo (Unkeless, 1989).

Several receptors expressed by MNPs bind fragments of complement (Law, 1988). Complement receptor 1 (CR1; CD35) expressed by monocytes and macrophages binds C3b, C4b, and iC3b. CR3 (CD11b/CD18) binds iC3b and is the primary MNP receptor used in binding serum-opsonized particles (Wright and Detmers, 1988). Neither CR1 or CR3 receptors on MNP can mediate phagocytosis of opsonized particles unless the MNP has been previously stimulated with phorbol esters or fibronectin (Wright and Griffin, 1985; Brown, 1986). The role of CR4 (CD11c/CD18) in mediating complement-opsonized material by MNPs remains unclear.

Monocytes and macrophages also express cell surface receptors that recognize specific carbohydrate moieties on the surface of microorganisms. Human macrophages express a receptor that recognizes proteins conjugated with *mannose* (Ezekowitz et al., 1990). This receptor is not expressed by monocytes but appears during monocyte-macrophage differentiation (Mokoena and Gordon, 1985; Lennartz et al., 1989). Since L-*fucose*–terminated proteins are bound by the mannose receptor, this receptor is often called the *mannose/fucose receptor* (Shepherd et al., 1982). Macrophages utilize the mannose receptor to directly recognize, bind, and ingest a variety of microorganisms, including *Candida albicans* and *Pneumocystis carinii* (Ezekowitz et al., 1990; Ezekowitz, 1992). Macrophage mannose receptor expression and function is down-regulated by interferon-γ (IFN-γ) exposure but is increased in dexamethasone- or vitamin D–pretreated cells (Mokoena and Gordon,

1985; Stahl, 1990). Additional lectin-like receptors expressed by MNPs include a β-glucan receptor on human monocytes (Czop and Austen, 1985) and a receptor on monocytes and macrophages that recognize advanced glycosylation end products (Vlassara et al., 1988, 1989).

Microbicidal Activity

Several different antimicrobial mechanisms have been identified in MNPs. These are generally divided into *oxygen-independent* and *oxygen-dependent* mechanisms. Several antimicrobial proteins and enzymes are present within the lysosomes of MNPs. Cathepsin G, azurocidin, proteinase 3, elastase, collagenase, arginase, ribonuclease deoxyribonuclease, defensins, and lysozyme are constituents of lysosomes that may account for the bacteriolytic activity of these intracellular organelles (Thorne et al., 1976; Selsted et al., 1985). Most of these proteins are active at neutral pH. The initial rise in pH to 7.0 to 8.0 in phagocytic vacuoles may create an optimal working environment for these antimicrobial proteins, and as the pH in the phagosome becomes acidic, these proteins become generally ineffective and acid hydrolases predominate (Thorne et al., 1976).

Oxygen-dependent mechanisms have been studied more extensively. These mechanisms also are important in tissue damage to a wide variety of cells and are linked to secretory responses and to other intracellular events. Reactive *oxygen* and *nitrogen intermediates* have a direct role in the killing of certain microorganisms. Microbicidal activity for certain organisms is decreased under conditions of anaerobiosis (Cline, 1970; Miller, 1971), emphasizing the role of oxygen-dependent killing.

Both hydrogen peroxide (H_2O_2) and myeloperoxidase play a major role in the microbicidal killing by MNPs (Baehner and Johnston, 1972; Klebanoff and Hamon, 1973). Monocytes from patients with chronic granulomatous disease have defective generation of H_2O_2 and manifest decreased microbicidal activity for catalase-forming bacteria (Davis et al., 1968; Nathan et al., 1969; Klebanoff, 1988; Dinauer and Orkin, 1992). Although myeloperoxidase is present in maturing monocytes, it cannot be found in fully mature macrophages (Van Furth and Cohn, 1968). The demonstration that monocytes from myeloperoxidase-deficient individuals are impaired in microbial killing compared with their mature macrophages is consistent with this observation.

Another oxygen-dependent antimicrobial system functioning in MNPs is derived from the oxidation of L-*arginine* to nitrate with the formation of reactive nitrogen intermediates (Nathan and Gabay, 1992). Nitric oxide, nitrogen dioxide, and nitrosamines are the bioactive antimicrobial molecules produced by this pathway when MNPs are appropriately stimulated (Nathan, 1991). Reactive nitrogen intermediate synthesis, as with synthesis of reactive oxygen intermediates, is highly regulated, being induced and inhibited by numerous cytokines (Ding et al., 1988; Lioy et al., 1993).

Normal macrophages require both a priming signal, such as IFN-γ or IFN-β, and an activating signal, such as lipopolysaccharide, muramyl dipeptide, or TNF-α, to fully induce production of reactive nitrogen intermediate from the L-arginine pathway (Hibbs et al., 1992).

Cytotoxic Activity

Macrophages are involved in the host defense against malignancy (Levy and Wheelock, 1974; Evans and Alexander, 1976; Hibbs, 1976). Macrophages can be activated to function as effector cells that are capable of inhibiting tumor growth. Chronic infection with a variety of organisms or injection of a number of inducing substances, such as endotoxin, lipid A, double-stranded ribonucleic acid (RNA), complete Freund's adjuvant, and pyran copolymer, will produce tumoricidal macrophages (Alexander, 1976). These nonspecifically cytotoxic macrophages exhibit selectivity in that they express cytotoxicity against transformed but not normal cells (Hibbs et al., 1972; Hibbs, 1973). However, in vitro studies have shown that destruction of tumor cells by macrophages is accomplished by two different mechanisms (Adams and Hamilton, 1984): macrophage-mediated tumor cytotoxicity is selective for neoplastic targets but is slow and independent of antibody; cell-mediated tumor cytotoxicity is rapid, specific, and dependent on antibody (Adams and Nathan, 1983).

Lymphocytes may play a cooperative role in the induction of tumoricidal macrophages. Lymphokines produced by nonspecific stimulation of lymphocytes in vitro can induce macrophages to become cytotoxic for syngeneic tumor cells (Piessens et al., 1975). In addition, the prolonged maintenance of nonspecific cytotoxic potential in an in vitro culture system requires a factor produced by an interaction between inducing antigen and sensitized lymphocytes (Hibbs, 1974). Under different experimental conditions, lymphocytes produce a *specific macrophage arming factor*, which renders macrophages specifically cytotoxic to the tumor to which the lymphocytes were originally sensitized (Evans and Alexander, 1971).

Several macrophage mediators, including TNF-α (Urban et al., 1986), IFN-γ (Adams and Hamilton, 1987), cytolytic proteases (Adams et al., 1980), oxygen radicals such as H_2O_2 (Nathan, 1982), and reactive nitrogen intermediates such as nitric oxide (Stuehr and Nathan, 1989; Higuchi et al., 1990; Keller et al., 1990), have also been implicated in macrophage tumor lysis and killing. Finally, macrophages may indirectly aid in tumor destruction by the production of substances such as *lymphocyte activation factor*, which enhance the antitumor response of lymphocytes.

Antigen Processing and Presentation

Studies in several laboratories have shown that there is a complex interaction between lymphocytes and macrophages during a primary immune response (Fig. 6–8). After uptake by macrophages, a part of the protein molecule escapes proteolysis and is recognized as antigen. Immunoregulatory molecules, including IFN-

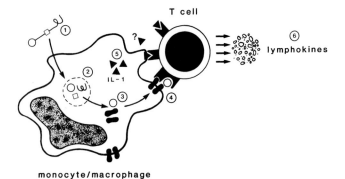

monocyte/macrophage

Figure 6–8. Events involved in macrophage processing and presentation of antigen to T lymphocytes. Most protein antigens (1) require internalization and phagolysosomal processing (2) and physical association with newly synthesized major histocompatibility antigen class II molecules (3) before presentation to T cells at the cell surface of the mononuclear phagocyte. Interleukin-1 (5) production in conjunction with antigen presentation (4) activates the T cell to release numerous lymphokines (6) that further activate macrophages, B cells, and T cells. (From Yoder MC, Hassan NF, Douglas SD. Mononuclear phagocyte system. In Polin RA, Fox WW, eds. Fetal and Neonatal Physiology, Vol. 2. Philadelphia, WB Saunders, 1992, pp. 1438–1461.)

γ and IL-1, modulate the interactions between lymphocytes and macrophages (Unanue and Allen, 1987a). Cells serving in antigen presentation have been shown to process antigen, express human leukocyte antigen (HLA) class II glycoprotein (Ia) on their surfaces, and secrete IL-1.

The exact mechanisms involved in intracellular antigen processing and degradation have yet to be determined (Unanue and Allen, 1987b). Initially, proteins enter the antigen-presenting cell (APC) following their interaction with plasma membrane. Degradation of the proteins occurs in acid vesicles to enable the generation of an immunogenic fragment complexed with the major histocompatibility determinant. Following protein degradation, some fragments proceed to the lysosome vesicles, while others complex directly with HLA class II molecules and appear on the cell surface (Geuze et al., 1983). Expression of HLA class II on different populations of macrophages correlates with their ability to present antigen to T cells (Beller, 1984).

Several lymphokines regulate HLA class II expression on the macrophage surface. IFN-γ increases HLA class II expression (Basham and Merigan, 1983); prostaglandins of the E class (Snyder et al., 1982), alpha-fetoprotein (Lu et al., 1984), and glucocorticoids (Snyder and Unanue, 1982) inhibit HLA class II expression. Similarly, IL-1 plays an important role in macrophage antigen presentation (Chu et al., 1984). IL-1 is secreted by macrophages after the T cell interacts with macrophage cell surface HLA class II antigens. The binding of IL-1 to its receptor on T-cell surfaces induces T-cell proliferation and secretion of IL-2. Recent investigation has identified a membrane-bound form of IL-1 required for antigen presentation by macrophages (Kurt-Jones et al., 1985). This membrane IL-1 is an integral membrane protein, distinct from the soluble IL-1 nonspecifically bound or fixed to the macrophage membrane.

Tissue Remodeling and Wound Healing

Macrophages are necessary for injured tissues and organs to heal properly (Leibovich and Ross, 1975; Riches, 1988). During the earliest phases of wound repair, monocytes are recruited to the injury site and, along with the resident tissue macrophages, participate in the débridement of the damaged tissue. Although macrophages secrete enzymes competent to degrade connective tissue matrices in vitro (Werb et al., 1980; Banda et al., 1985), endocytosis of matrix fragments leading to activation of the macrophages and IL-1 secretion may have a more widespread effect on damaged matrix dismantling by increasing collagenase synthesis and secretion by fibroblasts (Postlethwaite et al., 1983; Huybrechts-Godin et al., 1985). Macrophages further contribute in three general ways to heal the débrided wound and remodel the site to a preinjured state. Macrophages secrete numerous potent growth factors (see Fig. 6–6) for fibroblasts and mesenchymal cells. These are necessary for the production of the loose connective tissue and new blood capillaries that constitute granulation tissue, the provisional matrix utilized by fibroblasts to deposit structural matrix molecules (Polverini et al., 1977; Greenburg and Hunt, 1978). A direct role in provisional extracellular matrix synthesis has been demonstrated in macrophages by Brown et al. (1993); wound macrophages synthesized embryonic isoforms of fibronectin before fibroblast synthesis of these important elements of granulation tissue. Later in the wound-healing process, macrophages secrete factors that modulate fibroblast collagen production and, in cutaneous wounds, re-epithelialization (Rappolee and Werb, 1992; Schultz et al., 1987). Macrophages may also participate in the exaggerated deposition of fibroblast-derived matrix materials leading to tissue fibrosis (Wong and Wahl, 1989).

Activation

Macrophages obtained from animals that have become immune following sublethal infection manifest an impressive morphologic, metabolic, and functional metamorphosis and are said to be "activated." These cells are larger, have an increased tendency to spread (North, 1978), adhere more avidly to glass, and have more lysosomes, a more elaborate Golgi apparatus, and more ribosomes. Such activated macrophages also have increased metabolic and mitotic rates and are capable of increased pinocytosis and phagocytic activity (Cohn, 1978; Karnovsky and Lazdins, 1978). One of the more important functional correlates of these metabolic changes is the observation that activated macrophages are capable of enhanced microbicidal activity. Mackaness (1962) observed that following sublethal Listeria challenge mice were temporarily resistant to subsequent rechallenge with a much larger number of Listeria organisms. This increased resistance was in large part due to the fact that the macrophages from such animals had become "activated" and consequently were much more efficient in the killing of Listeria. However, macrophage activation is a nonspecific phenomenon, in that macrophages activated by infection with one intracellular organism express increased microbicidal activity toward antigenically different organisms. For example, animals infected with *Brucella abortus* become resistant to infection with *Listeria* (Blaese, 1975).

Numerous agents are known to nonspecifically activate macrophages via "nonimmune" mechanisms. For example, a common experimental technique used to elicit the production of large numbers of peritoneal macrophages in laboratory animals involves injection of a variety of irritant substances (such as peptone, casein, and mineral oil) into their peritoneal cavities. Macrophages elicited in this manner show morphologic and functional changes similar to macrophages activated through immune mechanisms (e.g., *Listeria* infection), although the degree of activation achieved by such nonimmune mechanisms does not appear to be as great (Karnovsky et al., 1973).

In addition to enhanced microbicidal activity, a number of other macrophage functions are stimulated by the activation process. For example, activated macrophages are known to have increased tumoricidal capacity (Alexander, 1973), accelerated movement (Poplack et al., 1976), the ability to produce a number of important biologically active substances (Wahl et al., 1975), and an enhanced ability to collaborate with immunocompetent cells in the production of specific antibody (Blaese, 1975). Thus, the activation process itself, although invoked in the macrophage response to infection, is important in a wide variety of macrophage functions.

Activation of the macrophage may not always lead to increases in tumoricidal or antimicrobial activity. The term *activation* is used to describe the effects of any stimulus on MNP morphology, physiology, or function. Thus, activation may refer to a change in the level of expression of one specific cell surface membrane receptor or to a change in the size of the cell without invoking any change in a complex function such as tumor cell killing or phagocytosis and killing of microbes. Adams and Hamilton (1988) have proposed that the term *macrophage activation* refer to macrophage acquisition of competence to complete some complex cell function. Scrutiny of the molecular events underlying and regulating macrophage activation has begun, and the most current concepts have been reviewed by Adams and Hamilton (1992).

THE DENDRITIC CELL SYSTEM

Dendritic cells are a distinct lineage of migratory leukocytes that primarily serve as accessory cells in initiation of primary immune responses. Members of this family share certain morphologic, kinetic, and functional characteristics and can be identified in discrete locations in lymphoid and nonlymphoid organs (Steinman and Cohn, 1973; Inaba et al., 1983; Tew et al., 1982). Although dendritic cells express certain cell surface antigenic features that resemble those of MNPs, they demonstrate poor phagocytic activity and weak or no adhesion to tissue culture surfaces and generally lack nonspecific esterase activity—three universal characteristics of mononuclear phagocytes (Tew et al., 1982). Nevertheless, there is compelling evidence for a common hematopoietic progenitor for cells of the dendritic cell system and the MNP system. The following text reviews the origin, kinetics, characterization, and tissue distribution of dendritic cells along with several well-recognized functions of these potent APCs.

Origin and Kinetics

In adult subjects, dendritic cells are derived from bone marrow hematopoietic progenitor cells (Katz et al., 1979; Volk-Platzer et al., 1984; Reid et al., 1990). During embryologic development, dendritic cells and macrophages have been identified as early as week 6 in the yolk sac (Janossy et al., 1986). By 12 weeks of gestation, dendritic cells are present in thymus, lymph nodes, spleen, and many nonlymphoid organs. In these tissues, dendritic cells occupy distinct sites that differ from the location of macrophages (Hofman et al., 1984; Janossy et al., 1986).

In the full-term newborn infant, dendritic cells can be cultured in vitro from cord blood hematopoietic progenitor cells if the cells are incubated with GM-CSF and TNF-α (Santiago-Schwarz et al., 1992; Caux et al., 1992). A common precursor for MNPs and dendritic cells was suggested by the presence of colony-forming unit–like clusters containing both macrophages and dendritic cells and a single peak of thymidine incorporation in the macrophage-dendritic cultures (Santiago-Schwarz et al., 1992).

A probable common bone marrow and peripheral blood hematopoietic precursor of MNPs and dendritic cells has been identified in adult human subjects (Reid et al., 1990; Thomas et al., 1993). In methylcellulose colony assays, pure colonies of dendritic-appearing cells and mixed colonies containing dendritic cells and macrophages were cultured from human adult bone marrow and peripheral blood mononuclear cells. The dendritic cells strongly expressed major histocompatibility complex (MHC) class II antigens, lacked nonspecific esterase, expressed some cell surface markers of skin Langerhans cells, and stimulated allogeneic mixed leukocyte reactions—all characteristic features of freshly isolated dendritic cells (Reid et al., 1990; Thomas et al., 1993). Although these findings strongly suggest a common myeloid origin for MNPs and dendritic cells, conclusive evidence using genetic markers is lacking.

The kinetics of dendritic cell production are not well delineated in humans, but mice and rat dendritic cells have a short life span. Murine splenic dendritic cells live an estimated 8 to 11 days, with similar turnover times for lymph node dendritic cells in rats. Some rat dendritic cells in nonlymphoid tissues live 2 to 4 weeks, and in one experiment human skin dendritic cells lived more than 9 weeks after transplantation to immunodeficient mice (Fossum, 1989). Some investigators propose heterogeneity in dendritic cell turnover, with rapidly and slowly dividing populations of cells in spleen and skin (Steinman, 1991; Chen et al., 1986). The ultimate fate of dendritic cells in lymphoid and non-lymphoid tissues is not known; most dendritic cells do not leave the organs they enter and are presumed to die in situ (Steinman, 1991; Fossum, 1989).

Characterization

Morphology

Dendritic cells from human peripheral blood have an irregular cell surface outline with an eccentrically placed, elongated, and often lobulated nucleus. These peripheral blood cells are of a size similar to circulating monocytes and have a nuclear-cytoplasmic ratio between 1:2 and 1:4 (Kamperdijk et al., 1989). Circulating dendritic cells have few cytoplasmic vacuoles, but those vacuoles present are located near the cell surface.

Tissue dendritic cells vary greatly in morphology, reflecting site-specific morphologic features (Fossum, 1989). In general, circulating dendritic cells may display a "veiled," extensively folded plasma membrane that becomes partitioned into numerous blunt pseudopodia that extend for varying lengths from the body of the cell (Fig. 6–9); these dendritic processes give rise to the name for this family of leukocytes (Tew et al., 1982). Ultrastructurally, the nuclear material is euchromatic; the cytoplasm contains mitochondria and strands of rough and smooth endoplasmic reticulum. Few granules are evident, and phagolysosomes are not present (Kamperdijk et al., 1989). Epidermal Langerhans cells contain unique organelles, called *Birbeck granules*, that are lost with in vitro culture (Austyn, 1987).

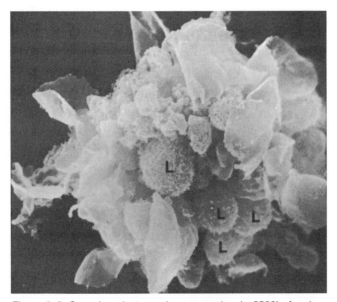

Figure 6–9. Scanning electron microscope view (×2500) of a dendritic cell clustering with several lymphocytes (L). The numerous dendritic cell surface membrane and cytoplasmic projections in the shape of sheets, pseudopods, and dendrites are characteristic of these cells. (From Steinman RM, et al. Dendritic cells. In Zucker-Franklin D, Greaves MF, Grossi CE, Marmont AM, eds. Atlas of Blood Cells: Function and Pathology, 2nd ed. Philadephia, Lea & Febiger, 1988, p. 360.)

Histochemistry

Nonspecific esterase activity is weak or nonexistent in dendritic cells. Dendritic cells, such as Langerhans cells, express acid phosphatase, adenosine triphosphatase (ATPase), 5'-nucleotidase, and aminopeptidase N (Stachura, 1989). These cells also express S100 protein, a product that is found in Schwann cells and melanocytes (Romani et al., 1991). Dipeptidyl aminopeptidase I and cathepsin B activity are low in human peripheral blood dendritic cells (Thomas et al., 1993).

Cell Surface Antigenic Determinants

No unique cell surface antigenic determinants have been identified that can be utilized to isolate and characterize human dendritic cells (Steinman, 1991). All human dendritic cells express 30–100 fold more HLA class II antigens (DP, DQ, DR) than the level expressed by resting MNPs (Steinman, 1991). Human dendritic cell precursors strongly express MHC class I and II molecules; moderately express CD11a,b,c/CD18, CD40, CD44, CD54, CD64, CD32, CD33, and CD34; and weakly express CD14 (Thomas et al., 1993). These purported precursors do not express CD16, CD19, CD3, or CD1 (Thomas et al., 1993). Mature dendritic cells express both MHC class I and class II molecules, as well as CD1, CD4, CD8, CD11a,b,c/CD18, CD25, CD40, CD54, and CD58, and weakly express CD23 and 32 (Steinman, 1991).

Tissue Distribution

Steinman (1991) has suggested that the dendritic cell system can be categorized in three groups by location:

- Nonlymphoid organ cells (Langerhans and interstitial dendritic cells)
- Circulating cells (afferent lymph veiled and blood dendritic cells)
- Lymphoid organ cells (dendritic and interdigitating cells)

Nonlymphoid Cells. Langerhans cells are the best studied nonlymphoid dendritic cells. These cells, which are probably derived from blood dendritic precursors, are capable of leaving the dermis and migrating through afferent lymph fluid to local lymph nodes (Silberberg-Sinakin et al., 1976; Hoefsmit et al., 1982). Dendritic cells are present in the interstitium of nearly all organs except the brain (Hart and McKenzie, 1990). In the lung, dendritic cells are present in the alveolar septa and just beneath the tracheobronchial epithelial cells, where the capture of aerosolized particulates is facilitated (Toews, 1991).

Circulating Cells. Afferent but not efferent lymph contains dendritic cells that can capture antigens throughout the body and carry the material to lymphoid tissues (Bujdoso et al., 1989). Dendritic cells in blood are a minor population (<0.1%) that may be difficult to identify morphologically from peripheral blood monocytes by light microscopy. If viewed by video microscopy, blood dendritic cells are unique in repeatedly protruding and retracting lamellipodia, or "veils" (Steinman, 1991). The role of the blood dendritic cells is unclear. These cells may be en route from bone marrow to nonlymphoid organs or may have left nonlymphoid organs to migrate to the spleen (Thomas et al., 1993).

Lymphoid Cells. In lymphoid tissues, dendritic cells are positioned so as to have maximal interaction with the T lymphocytes. Interdigitating dendritic cells are found clustered with T cells in lymph nodes. In the spleen, dendritic cells reside as interdigitating cells in the periarterial sheaths and are present in the periphery of T-cell areas, interrupting the marginal zone of macrophages (Fossum, 1989). Because T cells and antigenic material must traverse the marginal zone on leaving the arterial system, dendritic cells present a cellular barrier through which the T cells and antigens pass; thus, cell-to-cell communication between dendritic cells, T cells, and antigen is anatomically intimate (Steinman, 1991).

Selected Functions

Antigen Capture and Presentation

Whereas macrophages, B cells, and dendritic cells can serve as APCs, dendritic cells are the primary presenters of antigen to antigen-specific T cells after antigen administration (Bujdoso et al., 1989; Crowley et al., 1990). Dendritic cells need not express large amounts of the antigen to stimulate effective T-cell responses; only 250 molecules of antigen induces mitogenesis of primary T cells (Demotz et al., 1990). Dendritic cells demonstrate a highly efficient capacity to ingest material by endocytosis, move the material into acidic lysosomal compartments, combine newly synthesized MHC class II invariant chain with the liberated antigenic peptides, and present the MHC class II peptide material on the cell surface to the appropriate antigen-specific T cell (Steinman, 1991). Macrophage antigen processing and presentation is characterized by degradation of large quantities of material into antigenic peptides, rapid loss of antigen-presenting activity after pulsing with antigen, and a requirement for additional adjuvants to prime T cells in situ after antigen priming (Steinman, 1991). Dendritic cells are nearly 100 times more potent at antigen presentation and T-cell activation than macrophages (Romani et al., 1989). The prolonged (1 to 2 days) capacity to present antigen after pulsing and the ability to directly activate T cells in situ after antigen pulsing are unique features of dendritic cells (Inaba et al., 1990).

Transport of Captured Antigen

Dendritic cells are uniquely capable of transporting immunogenic material to lymphoid tissues. Some examples of in situ antigen capture and transport include T-cell stimulation by dendritic cells isolated from afferent lymph after intradermal administration of antigen (Bujdoso et al, 1989), T-cell activation by lymph node

dendritic cells after application of a contact allergen (Macatonia et al., 1987), and in situ activation of CD4$^+$ T cells in the draining lymph nodes of mice injected in the foot pads with splenic dendritic cells exposed to antigenic material in vitro (Inaba et al., 1990).

Activation of T-Lymphocyte Growth and Effector Function

Dendritic cells in lymph and blood preferentially "home" to T-cell areas of lymphoid organs. The mechanisms of homing are poorly understood, but dendritic cells express several cell surface molecules that have been implicated in leukocyte homing (Steinman, 1991; Thomas et al., 1993). Dendritic cells are also capable of tightly clustering with resting T cells in initiation of primary immune responses; macrophages and B cells are unable to do so (Inaba and Steinman, 1985; 1986). In some cases, dendritic cells bind T cells in an antigen-independent fashion that may facilitate subsequent antigen-specific interactions between antigen-presenting cells and clustered T cells (Inaba and Steinman, 1986). The mechanisms used and signals provided to T cells by dendritic cells that result in T-cell activation remain to be elucidated.

References

Ackerman SK, Douglas SD. Purification of human monocytes on microexudate-coated surfaces. J Immunol 120:1372–1374, 1978.

Ackerman SK, Douglas SD. Monocytes. In Carr I, ed. The Reticuloendothelial System, Vol. 1. New York, Plenum Press, 1980, pp. 297–328.

Ackerman SK, Douglas SD. Morphology of monocytes and macrophages. In Williams WJ, Beutler E, Erslev A, Rundles W, eds. Haematology, 3rd ed. New York, McGraw-Hill, 1983, pp. 837–847.

Ackerman SK, Zuckerman SH, Douglas SD. Isolation and culture of human blood monocytes. In Douglas SD, Quie PG, eds. Practical Methods in Clinical Immunology: Investigation of Phagocytes in Disease. London, Churchill Livingstone, 1981, pp. 66–75.

Adams DO. The granulomatous inflammatory response. Am J Pathol 84:164–191, 1976.

Adams DO, Hamilton TA. The cell biology of macrophage activation. Annu Rev Immunol 2:283–318, 1984.

Adams DO, Hamilton TA. Molecular transductional mechanisms by which IFN-α and other signals regulate macrophage development. Immunol Rev 97:5–27, 1987.

Adams DO, Hamilton TA. Phagocytic cells: cytotoxic activities of macrophages. In Gallin JI, Goldstein IM, Snyderman R, eds. Inflammation: Basic Principles and Clinical Correlates. New York, Raven Press, 1988, pp. 471–492.

Adams DO, Hamilton TA. Molecular basis of macrophage activation: diversity and its origins. In Lewis CE, McGee JO, eds. The Macrophage. Oxford, Oxford University Press, 1992, pp. 75–114.

Adams DO, Nathan CF. Molecular mechanisms in tumor-cell killing by activated macrophages. Immunol Today 4:166–170, 1983.

Adams DO, Kao KJ, Farb R, Pizzo SV. Effector mechanisms of cytolytically activated macrophages. J Immunol 124:292–300, 1980.

Alexander P. Activated macrophages and the anti-tumor action of BCG. Natl Cancer Inst Monograph 39:127–133, 1973.

Alexander P. The functions of the macrophage in malignant disease. Annu Rev Med 27:207–224, 1976.

Altman LC, Snyderman R, Oppenheim JJ, Mergenhagen SE. A human mononuclear leukocyte chemotactic factor: characterization, specificity, and kinetics of production by homologous leukocytes. J Immunol 110:801–810, 1973.

Andreesen R, Bross KJ, Osterholz J, Emmrich F. Human macrophage maturation and heterogeneity: analysis with a newly generated set of monoclonal antibodies to differentiation antigens. Blood 67:1257–1264, 1986.

Andreesen R, Brugger W, Scheibenbogen C, Kreutz M, Leser H, Rebin A, Lohr GW. Surface phenotype analysis of human monocyte to macrophage differentiation. J Leuk Biol 47:490–497, 1990.

Andreesen R, Gadd S, Costabel U, Leser HG, Speth V, Cesnik B, Atkins RC. Human macrophage maturation and heterogeneity: restricted expression of late differentiation antigens in situ. Cell Tissue Res 253:271–279, 1988.

Arend WP, Joslin FG, Thompson RC, Hannum CH. An interleukin-1 inhibitor from human monocytes: production and characterization of biological properties. J Immunol 143:1851–1858, 1989.

Arnaout MA. Structure and function of the leukocyte adhesion molecules CD11/CD18. Blood 75:1037–1050, 1990.

Athens JW, Haab OP, Raab SO, Mauer AM, Aslenbrucker H, Cartwright GE, Wintrobe MM. Leukokinetic studies. III. The total blood, circulating and marginal granulocyte pools, and the granulocyte turnover rate in normal subjects. J Clin Invest 40:989–995, 1961.

Auger MJ, Ross JA. The biology of the macrophage. In Lewis CE, McGee JO, eds. The Macrophage. Oxford, Oxford University Press, 1992, pp. 1–74.

Austyn JM. Lymphoid dendritic cells. Immunol 62:161–170, 1987.

Axline SG. Functional biochemistry of the macrophage. Semin Hematol 7:142–160, 1970.

Axline SG, Cohn ZA. In vitro induction of lysosomal enzymes by phagocytosis. J Exp Med 131:1239–1260, 1970.

Baehner RL, Johnston RB. Monocyte function in children with neutropenia and chronic infection. Blood 40:31–41, 1972.

Banda MJ, Clark EJ, Werb Z. Macrophage elastase: regulatory consequences of the proteolysis of non-elastin substrates. In Van Furth R, ed. Mononuclear Phagocytes. Dordrecht, Netherlands, Martinus Nijhoff, 1985, pp. 295–300.

Barclay NA, Birkeland ML, Brown MH, Beyers AD, Davis SJ, Somoza C, Williams AF. The Leukocyte Antigen Facts Book. Orlando, Fla., Harcourt Brace Jovanovich, 1993, pp. 1–269.

Basham TY, Merigan TC. Recombinant interferon-gamma increases HLA-DR synthesis and expression. J Immunol 130:1492–1494, 1983.

Beller DI. Functional significance of the regulation of macrophage Ia expression. Eur J Immunol 14:138–143, 1984.

Bennett WE, Cohn ZA. The isolation and selected properties of blood monocytes. J Exp Med 123:145–149, 1966.

Bessis M. Cytologic aspects of immunohematology: a study with phase contrast cinematography. Ann NY Acad Sci 59:986–995, 1955.

Blaese RM. Macrophages and the development of immunocompetence. In Bellanti JA, Dayton DA, eds. The Phagocytic Cell in Host Resistance. New York, Raven Press, 1975, pp. 309–320.

Bodel PT, Nichols BA, Bainton DF. Appearance of peroxidase reactivity within the rough ER of blood monocytes after surface adherence. J Exp Med 145:264–274, 1977.

Boyden S. The chemotactic effect of mixtures of antibody and antigen on polymorphonuclear leukocytes. J Exp Med 115:453–466, 1962.

Bozdech MJ, Bainton DF. Identification of α-naphthyl butyrate esterase as a plasma membrane ectoenzyme of monocytes and as a discrete intracellular membrane–bounded organelle in lymphocytes. J Exp Med 153:182–185, 1981.

Braunsteiner H, Schmalzl F. Étude cytochemique des monocytes: mise en evidence d'une esterase caracteristique. Nouv Rev Fr Hematol 9:678–687, 1968.

Braunsteiner H, Schmalzl F. Cytochemistry of monocytes and macrophages. In Van Furth R, ed. Mononuclear Phagocytes. Oxford, Blackwell Scientific Publications, 1970, pp. 62–81.

Breton-Gorius J, Cuichard J. Étude au microscopé electronique de la localisation des peroxydases dans les cellules de la moelle asseuse humaine. Nouv Rev Fr Hematol 9:678–687, 1969.

Brown EJ. The role of extracellular matrix protein in the control of phagocytosis. J Leuk Biol 39:579–591, 1986.

Brown LF, Dubin D, Lavikgne L, Logan B, Dvorak HF, Van de Water L. Macrophages and fibroblasts express embryonic fibronectins during cutaneous wound healing. Am J Pathol 142:793–801, 1993.

Buckley PJ. Phenotypic subpopulations of macrophages and dendritic cells in human spleen. Scan Electron Microsc 5:147–158, 1991.

Bujdoso R, Hopkins J, Dutra BM, Young P, McConnell I. Characterization of sheep afferent lymph dendritic cells and their role in antigen carriage. J Exp Med 170:1285–1302, 1989.

Bumol TF, Douglas SD. Human monocyte cytoplasmic spreading in vitro: early kinetics and scanning electron microscopy. Cell Immunol 34:70–78, 1977.

Butcher EC. Leukocyte-endothelial cell recognition: three (or more) steps to specificity and diversity. Cell 67:1033–37, 1991.

Carlos TM, Harlan JM. Membrane proteins involved in phagocyte adherence to endothelium. Immunol Rev 114:5–28, 1990.

Carlos T, Kovach N, Schwartz B, Rosa M, Newman B, Wayner E, Benjamin C, Osborn L, Labb R, Harlan J. Human monocytes bind to two cytokine-induced adhesive ligands on cultured human endothelial cells: endothelial-leukocyte adhesion molecule-1 and vascular cell adhesion molecule-1. Blood 77:2261–2271, 1991.

Carpenter G. Receptors for epidermal growth factor and other polypeptide mitogens. Annu Rev Biochem 56:881–914, 1987.

Caux C, Dezutter-Dambuyant C, Schmitt D, Bancherau J. GM-CSF and TNF-α cooperate in the generation of dendritic Langerhans cells. Nature 360:258–261, 1992.

Chen H-D, Ma C, Yuan J-T, Wang Y-K, Silvers WK. Occurrence of donor Langerhans cells in mouse and rat chimeras and their replacement in skin grafts. J Invest Dermatol 86:630–633, 1986.

Chu E, Rosenwasser LJ, Dinarello CA, Lareau M, Geha RS. Role of interleukin-1 in antigen-specific T cell proliferation. J Immunol 132:1311–1316, 1984.

Cline MJ. Metabolism of the circulating leukocyte. Physiol Rev 45:674–720, 1965.

Cline MJ. Bactericidal activity of human macrophages: analysis of factors influencing the killing of listeria monocytogenes. Infect Immun 2:156–161, 1970.

Cline MJ, Lehrer RI. Phagocytosis by human monocytes. Blood 32:423–435, 1968.

Cohn ZA. The structure and function of monocytes and macrophages. Adv Immunol 9:163–214, 1968.

Cohn ZA. The activation of mononuclear phagocytes: fact, fancy, and future. J Immunol 121:813–816, 1978.

Cohn ZA, Benson B. The differentiation of mononuclear phagocytes: morphology, cytochemistry, and biochemistry. J Exp Med 121:153–170, 1965.

Crowley M, Inaba K, Steinman RM. Dendritic cells are the principal cells in mouse spleen bearing immunogenic fragments of foreign proteins. J Exp Med 172:383–386, 1990.

Czop JK, Austen KF. A glucan-inhibitable receptor on human monocytes: its identity with the phagocytic receptor for particulate activators of the alternative complement pathway. J Immunol 134:2588–2593, 1985.

David JR. Lymphocyte mediators and cellular hypersensitivity. N Engl J Med 288:143–149, 1973.

Davies P. Secretory functions of mononuclear phagocytes: overview and methods for preparing conditioned supernatants. In Adams DO, Edelson PJ, Koren H, eds. Methods for Studying Mononuclear Phagocytes. New York, Academic Press, 1981, pp. 549–560.

Davis WC, Huber H, Douglas SD, Fudenberg HH. A defect in circulating mononuclear phagocytes in chronic granulomatous disease of childhood. J Immunol 101:1093–1095, 1968.

Demotz S, Grey HM, Sette A. The minimal number of class II MHC–antigen complexes needed for T cell activation. Science 249:1029–1030, 1990.

DePetris S, Karlsbad G, Pernis B. Filamentous structures in the cytoplasm of normal mononuclear phagocytes. J Ultrastruct Res 7:39–55, 1962.

Dimitriu-Bona A, Burmester GR, Waters SJ, Winchester RJ. Human mononuclear phagocyte differentiation antigens. I. Patterns of antigenic expression on the surface of human monocytes and macrophages defined by monoclonal antibodies. J Immunol 130:145–152, 1983.

Dinauer MC, Orkin SH. Chronic granulomatous disease. Annu Rev Med 43:117–124, 1992.

Ding A, Nathan CF, Stuehr DJ. Release of reactive nitrogen intermediates and reactive oxygen intermediates from mouse peritoneal macrophages: comparison of activating cytokines and evidence for independent production. J Immunol 141:2407–2412, 1988.

Douglas SD. Human monocyte spreading in vitro: inducers and effects on Fc and C3 receptors. Cell Immunol 21:344–349, 1976.

Douglas SD. Alterations in intramembrane particle distribution during interaction of erythrocyte-bound ligands with immunoprotein receptors. J Immunol 120:131–157, 1978.

Douglas SD, Musson RA. Phagocytic defects: monocytes/macrophages. Clin Immunol Immunopathol 40:62–68, 1986.

Douglas SD, Zuckerman SH, Cody CS. Alterations in intramembrane particle distribution during interaction of erythrocyte-bound ligands with immunoprotein receptors. Effect of the membrane mobility agent A_2C on immunologic and nonimmunologic ligand binding. J Reticuloendothel Soc 28:91–102, 1980.

Evans R, Alexander P. Rendering macrophages specifically cytotoxic by a factor released from immune lymphoid cells. Transplantation 12:227–229, 1971.

Evans R, Alexander P. Mechanisms of extracellular killing of nucleated mammalian cells by macrophages. In Nelson DS, ed. Immunobiology of the Macrophage. New York, Academic Press, 1976, pp. 536–576.

Ezekowitz RAB. The mannose receptor and phagocytosis. In Van Furth R, ed. Mononuclear Phagocytes. Dordrecht, Netherlands, Kluwer Academic Publishers, 1992, pp. 208–213.

Ezekowitz RAB, Sostry K, Bailly P, Warner A. Molecular characterization of the human macrophage receptor: demonstration of multiple carbohydrate recognition-like domains and phagocytosis of yeasts in Cos-1 cells. J Exp Med 172:1785–1794, 1990.

Fedorko M, Hirsch JG. Structure of monocytes and macrophages. Semin Hematol 7:109–124, 1970.

Fossum S. The life history of dendritic leukocytes (DL). Curr Topics Pathol 79:101–124, 1989.

Gallin JI, Kaplan AP. Mononuclear cell chemotactic activity of kallikrein and plasminogen activator and its inhibition by C1 inhibitor and $\alpha2$ macroglobulin. J Immunol 113:1928–1934, 1974.

Gallin JI, Wolff SM. Leucocyte chemotaxis: physiological considerations and abnormalities. Clin Haematol 4:567–607, 1976.

Geuze HJ, Slot JW, Strous GJAM, Lodish HF, Schwartz AL. Intracellular site of asialoglycoprotein receptor–ligand uncoupling: double-label immunoelectron microscopy during receptor-mediated endocytosis. Cell 323:277–287, 1983.

Gordon S, Cohn SA. The macrophage. Int Rev Cytol 36:171–214, 1973.

Gordon S, Perry VH, Rabinowitz S, Chung L, Rosen H. Plasma membrane receptors of the mononuclear phagocyte system. J Cell Sci (Suppl 9):1–26, 1988.

Greenburg GB, Hunt TK. The proliferation response in vitro of vascular endothelial and smooth muscle cells exposed to wound fluid and macrophages. J Cell Physiol 97:353–360, 1978.

Hakkert BC, Kuijpers TW, Leewenberg JFM, Van Mourik JA, Ross D. Neutrophil and monocyte adherence to and migration across monolayers of cytokine-activated endothelial cells: the contribution of CD18, ELAM-1, VLA-4. Blood 78:2721–2726, 1991.

Hamilton JA. Colony-stimulating factors, cytokines, and monocyte-macrophages: some controversies. Immunol Today 14:18–24, 1993.

Hart DNJ, McKenzie JL. Interstitial dendritic cells. Int Rev Immunol 6:128–149, 1990.

Hartwig JH, Stossel TP. Macrophage movement. In Van Furth R, ed. Mononuclear Phagocytes: Characteristics, Physiology and Function. Dordrecht, Netherlands, Martinus Nijhoff Publishers, 1985, pp. 329–335.

Hassan NF, Campbell DE, Douglas SD. Purification of human monocytes on gelatin-coated surfaces. J Immunol Methods 95:273–276, 1986.

Heinrich PC. Interleukin-6 and the acute phase protein response. Biochem J 265:621–636, 1990.

Hibbs JB. Macrophage nonimmunologic recognition of target cell factors related to contact inhibition. Science 180:868–870, 1973.

Hibbs JB. Heterocytolysis by macrophages activated by bacillus Calmette-Guerin: lysosome exocytosis into tumor cells. Science 184:471, 1974.

Hibbs JB. Role of activated macrophages in nonspecific resistance to neoplasia. J Reticuloendothel Soc 20:223–231, 1976.

Hibbs JB, Granger DL, Krahenbuhl JL, Adams LB. Synthesis of nitric oxide from L arginine: a cytokine-inducible pathway with antimicrobial activity. In Van Furth R, ed. Mononuclear Phagocytes. Dordrecht, Netherlands, Kluwer Academic Publishers, 1992, pp. 279–292.

Hibbs JB, Lambert LH, Remington JS. In vitro nonimmunologic destruction of cells with abnormal growth characteristics by adjuvant-activated macrophages. Proc Soc Exp Biol Med 139:1049–1052, 1972.

Higuchi M, Higachi N, Taki H, Osawa T. Cytolytic mechanisms of activated macrophages. Tumor necrosis factor and L-arginine-dependent mechanisms act synergistically as the major cytolytic mechanisms of activated macrophages. J Immunol 144:1425–1431, 1990.

Ho W-Z, Lioy J, Song L, Cutilli JR, Polin RA, Douglas SD. Infection of cord blood monocyte–derived macrophages with human immunodeficiency virus type 1. J Virol 66:573–579, 1992.

Hocking WG, Golde DW. The pulmonary-alveolar macrophage. N Engl J Med 301:580–587, 1979.

Hoefsmit ECM, Duijverstyn AM, Kamperdijk WA. Relation between Langerhans cells, veiled cells, and interdigitating cells. Immunobiology 161:255–265, 1982.

Hofman FM, Danilous JA, Taylor CR. HLA-DR (Ia)–positive dendritic-like cells in human fetal nonlymphoid tissues. Transplantation 37:590–594, 1984.

Horn RG, Spicer SS. Sulfated mucopolysaccharide and basic protein in certain granules of rabbit leukocytes. Lab Invest 13:1–15, 1964.

Horwitz MA. Phagocytosis of microorganisms. Rev Infect Dis 4:104–123, 1982.

Huybrechts-Godin G, Peeters-Joris C, Voes G. Partial characterization of the macrophage factor that stimulates fibroblasts to produce collagenase and to degrade collagen. Biochim Biophys Acta 846:51–54, 1985.

Inaba K, Metlay JP, Crowley MT, Steinman RM. Dendritic cells pulsed with protein antigens in vitro can prime antigen-specific MHC-restricted T cells in situ. J Exp Med 172:631–640, 1990.

Inaba K, Steinman RM. Accessory cell–T lymphocyte interactions: antigen-dependent and independent clustering. J Exp Med 163:247–261, 1986.

Inaba K, Steinman RM. Protein-specific helper T lymphocyte formation initiated by dendritic cells. Science 229:475–479, 1985.

Inaba K, Steinman RA, van Voorhis WC, Muramatsu S. Dendritic cells are critical accessory cells for thymus-dependent antibody responses in mouse and man. Proc Natl Acad Sci U S A 80:6041–6049, 1983.

Janossy G, Bofiel M, Pouler LW, Rawlings E, Burford GD, Navarette C, Ziegler A, Keleman E. Separate ontogeny of two macrophage-like accessory cell populations in the human fetus. J Immunol 136:4354–4360, 1986.

Jaubert F, Monnel JP, Danel C, Cretien J, Nezelof C. The location of nonspecific esterase in human lung macrophages. Histochemistry 59:141–147, 1978.

Kamperdijk EWA, Bos HJ, Bellen RHJ, Hoefsmit ECM. Morphology and ultrastructure of dendritic cells. In Zembala M, Asherson GL, eds. Human Monocytes. London, Academic Press, 1989, pp. 17–25.

Karnovsky ML, Lazdins JK. Biochemical criteria for activated macrophages. J Immunol 121:809–813, 1978.

Karnovsky ML, Lazdins J, Simmons SR. Metabolism of activated mononuclear phagocytes at rest and during phagocytosis. In Van Furth R, ed. Mononuclear Phagocytes in Immunity, Infection and Pathology. Oxford, Blackwell Scientific Publications, 1973, pp. 423–439.

Katz SI, Tamaki K, Salles D. Epidermal Langerhans cells are derived from cells originating in bone marrow. Nature 282:324–327, 1979.

Kelemen E, Calvo W, Fleidner TM. Atlas of Human Hematopoietic Development. New York, Springer-Verlag, 1979, pp. 1–261.

Keller R. Susceptibility of normal and transformed cell lines to cytostatic and cytocidal effects exerted by activated macrophages. J Natl Cancer Inst 56:369–374, 1976.

Keller R, Geiges M, Keist R. L-Arginine–dependent reactive nitrogen intermediates as mediators of tumor cell killing by activated macrophages. Cancer Res 50:1421–1425, 1990.

Klebanoff SJ. Phagocytic cells: products of oxygen metabolism. In Gallin JI, Goldstein IM, Snyderman R, eds. Inflammation: Basic Principles and Clinical Correlates. New York, Raven Press, 1988, pp. 391–444.

Klebanoff SJ, Hamon CB. Antimicrobial systems of mononuclear phagocytes. In Van Furth R, ed. Mononuclear Phagocytes in Immunity, Infection and Pathology. Oxford, Blackwell Scientific Publications, 1973, pp. 507–531.

Kurt-Jones EA, Beller DI, Mizel SB, Unanue ER. Identification of a membrane-associated interleukin 1 in macrophages. Proc Natl Acad Sci USA 82:1204–1208, 1985.

Lasky LA. Selectins: interpreters of cell-specific carbohydrate information during inflammation. Science 258:964–969, 1992.

Lasser A. The mononuclear phagocyte system: a review. Hum Pathol 14:108–126, 1983.

Law SKA. C3 receptors on macrophages. J Cell Sci (Suppl. 9):67–97, 1988.

Leibovich SJ, Ross R. The role of the macrophage in wound repair. A study with hydrocortisone and antimacrophage serum. Am J Pathol 78:71–100, 1975.

Lennartz MR, Cole FS, Stahl P. Biosynthesis and processing of the mannose receptor in human macrophages. J Biol Chem 264:2385–2390, 1989.

Levy MH, Wheelock EF. The role of macrophages in defense against neoplastic disease. Adv Cancer Res 20:131–163, 1974.

Li CY, Lam KW, Yam LT. Esterases in human leukocytes. J Histochem Cytochem 21:1–12, 1973.

Lioy J, Ho W-Z, Cutilli JR, Polin RA, Douglas SD. Thiol suppression of human immunodeficiency virus type 1 replication in primary cord blood monocyte–derived macrophages in vitro. J Clin Invest 91:495–498, 1993.

Lobb RR, Harper JW, Fett JW. Purification of heparin-binding growth factors. Ann Biochem 154:1–14, 1986.

Lu CY, Changelian PS, Unanue ER. Alpha-Fetoprotein inhibits macrophage expression of Ia antigen. J Immunol 132:1722–1727, 1984.

Macatonia SE, Knight SC, Edwards AJ, Griffiths S, Fryer P. Localization of antigen on lymph node dendritic cells after exposure to the contact sensitizer fluorescein isothiocyanate. J Exp Med 166:1654–1667, 1987.

Mackaness GB. Cellular resistance to infection. J Epidemiol Med 116:381–406, 1962.

Makgoba MW, Sanders ME, Luce G, Dustin ML, Springer TA, Clark EA, Mannoni P, Shaw S. ICAM-1a ligand for LFA-1–dependent adhesion of B, T, and myeloid cells. Nature 331:86–88, 1988.

Massague J. The TGF-beta family of growth and differentiation factors. Cell 49:437–438, 1987.

Metcalf D. The molecular control of normal and leukemic granulocytes and macrophages. Proc R Soc Lond (Biol) 230:389–423, 1987.

Meuret G, Hoffman G. Monocyte kinetic studies in normal and disease states. Br J Haematol 24:275–285, 1973.

Meuret G, Bammert J, Hoffman G. Kinetics of human monocytopoiesis. Blood 44:801–816, 1974a.

Meuret G, Bremer C, Bammert J, Ewen J. Oscillation of blood monocyte counts in healthy individuals. Cell Tissue Kinet 7:223–230, 1974b.

Meuret G, Detel V, Kilz HP, Senn HJ, Van Lessen H. Human monocytopoiesis in acute and chronic inflammation. Acta Haemat 54:328–335, 1975.

Meuret G, Djawari D, Berlet R, Hoffmann G. Kinetics, cytochemistry, and DNA synthesis of blood monocytes in man. In DiLuzio NR, Flemming K, eds. The Reticulo-endothelial System and Immune Phenomena. New York, Plenum Press, 1971, pp. 33–46.

Miller TE. Metabolic events involved in the bactericidal activity of normal mouse macrophages. Infect Immun 3:390–397, 1971.

Mokoena T, Gordon S. Human macrophage activation modulation of mannosyl, fucosyl receptor in vitro by lymphokines, gamma and alpha interferons, and dexamethasone. J Clin Invest 75:624–635, 1985.

Nathan CF. Mechanisms and modulation of macrophage activation. Behring Inst Mitt 888:200–207, 1991.

Nathan CF. Secretory products of macrophages. J Clin Invest 79:319–326, 1987.

Nathan CF. Mechanisms of macrophage antimicrobial activity. Trans R Soc Trop Med Hyg 77:620–630, 1983.

Nathan CF. Secretion of oxygen intermediates: role in effector functions of activated macrophages. Fed Proc 41:2206–2211, 1982.

Nathan CF, Gabay J. Antimicrobial mechanisms of macrophages. In Van Furth R, ed. Mononuclear Phagocytes. Dordrecht, Netherlands, Kluwer Academic Publishers, 1992, pp. 259–267.

Nathan Dg, Baehner RL, Weaver DK. Failure of nitroblue tetrazolium reduction in the phagocytic vacuoles of leukocytes in chronic granulomatous disease. J Clin Invest 48:1895–1904, 1969.

Nelson DS. Macrophages and Immunity. Amsterdam, North-Holland Publishing, 1969.

Nichols BA, Bainton DF. Differentiation of human monocytes in bone marrow and blood: sequential formation of two granule populations. Lab Invest 29:27–40, 1973.

Nichols BA, Bainton DF. Ultrastructure and cytochemistry of mononuclear phagocytes. In Van Furth R, ed. Mononuclear Phagocytes in Immunity, Infection and Pathology. Oxford, Blackwell Scientific Publications, 1973, pp. 17–55.

Nichols BA, Bainton DF, Farquhar MG. Differentiation of monocytes: origin, nature and fate of their azurophil granules. J Cell Biol 50:498–515, 1971.

North RJ. The concept of the activated macrophage. J Immunol 121:806–808, 1978.

North RJ. Endocytosis. Semin Hematol 7:161–171, 1970.

Pantalone RM, Page RC. Lymphokine-induced production and release of lysosomal enzymes by macrophages. Proc Natl Acad Sci U S A 72:2091–2094, 1975.

Parmley RT, Spicer SS, O'Dell RF. Ultrastructural identification of acid complex carbohydrate in cytoplasmic granules of normal and leukaemic human monocytes. Br J Haematol 39:33–39, 1978.

Piessens WF, Churchill WH, David JR. Macrophages activated in vitro with lymphocyte mediators kill neoplastic but not normal cells. J Immunol 114:293–299, 1975.

Ploem JS. Reflection contrast microscopy as a tool in investigation of the attachment of living cells to glass surface. In Van Furth R, ed. Mononuclear Phagocytes in Immunity, Infection and Pathology. London, Blackwell Scientific Publications, 1973, pp. 405–422.

Polverini PJ, Cotran RS, Gimbrone MA, Unanue ER. Activated macrophages induce vascular proliferation. Nature 269:804–806, 1977.

Poplack DG, Sher NA, Chaparas SD, Blaese RM. The effect of mycobacterium bovis (bacillus Calmette-Gúerin) on macrophage random migration, chemotaxis, and pinocytosis. Cancer Res 36:1233–1237, 1976.

Postlethwaite AE, Lachman LB, Mainardi CL, Kang AH. Interleukin 2 stimulation of collagenase production by cultured fibroblasts. J Exp Med 157:801–806, 1983, pp. 49–86.

Rabinovitch M, DeStefano MJ. Macrophages spreading in vitro. I. Inducers of spreading. Exp Cell Res 77:323–334, 1973.

Rabinovitch M, Manejias RE, Nussenzweig V. Selective phagocytic paralysis induced by immobilized immune complexes. J Exp Med 142:827–838, 1975.

Rappolee DA, Werb Z. Macrophage secretions: a functional perspective. Bull Inst Pasteur 87:361–394, 1989.

Rappolee DA, Werb Z. Macrophage-derived growth factors. Curr Top Microbiol Immunol 181:87–140, 1992.

Reaven EP, Axline SG. Subplasmalemmal microfilaments and microtubules in resting and phagocytizing cultivated macrophages. J Cell Biol 59:12–27, 1973.

Rebuck JW, Crowley JH. A method of studying leukocytic functions in vivo. Ann N Y Acad Sci 59:757–805, 1955.

Reid CDL, Fryer PR, Clifford C, Kirk A, Tikerpae J, Knight SC. Identification of hematopoietic progenitors of macrophages and dendritic Langerhans cells (DL-CFU) in human bone marrow and peripheral blood. Blood 76:1139–1149, 1990.

Rice GE, Munro JM, Bevilacqua MP. Inducible cell adhesion molecule 110 (INCAM-110) is an endothelial receptor for lymphocytes. A CD11/CD18–independent adhesion mechanism. J Exp Med 171:1369–1374, 1990.

Rice GE, Munro JM, Corless C, Bevilacqua MP. Vascular and nonvascular expression of INCAM-110. A target for mononuclear leukocyte adhesion in normal and inflamed human tissues. Am J Pathol 138:385–393, 1991.

Riches DWH. The multiple roles of macrophages in wound healing. In Clark RAF, Henson PM, eds. The Molecular and Cellular Biology of Wound Repair. New York, Plenum Press, 1988, pp. 213–239.

Romani N, Fritsch P, Schuler G. Identification and phenotype of Langerhans cells. In Schuler G, ed. Epidermal Langerhans Cells. Boca Raton, Fla., CRC Press, 1991.

Romani N, Korde S, Crowley M, Witmer-Pack M, Livingstone AM, Fathman CG, Inaba K, Steinman RM. Presentation of exogenous protein antigens by dendritic cells to T cell clones: intact protein is presented best by immature epidermal Langerhans cells. J Exp Med 169:1169–1178, 1989.

Ross GD, Walport MJ, Hogg N. Receptors for IgG Fc and fixed C3.

In Zembala M, Asherson GL, eds. Human Monocytes. London, Academic Press, 1989, pp. 123–140.

Ross R. Platelet-derived growth factor. Annu Rev Med 38:71–79, 1987.

Rossman MD, Douglas SD. The alveolar macrophage-receptors and effector cells function. In Daniele RP, ed. Pulmonary Immunology and Immunologic Diseases of the Lung. London, Blackwell Scientific Publications, 1988, pp. 168–183.

Sanders WE, Wilson RW, Ballantyne CM, Beaudet AL. Molecular cloning and analysis of in vivo expression of murine P-selectin. Blood 80:795–800, 1992.

Santiago-Schwarz F, Belilos E, Diamond B, Carson SE. TNF in combination with GM-CSF enhances the differentiation of neonatal cord blood stem cells into dendritic cells and macrophages. J Leukoc Biol 52:274–281, 1992.

Schultz GS, White M, Mitchell R, Brown G, Lynch J, Twardzik DR, Todaro GJ. Epithelial wound healing enhanced by transforming growth factor-α and vaccinia growth factor. Science 235:350–3542, 1987.

Scott CS, Patel D, Keen JN. Purification of human monocyte-specific esterase (MSE): molecular and kinetic characteristics. Br J Haematol 81:470–479, 1992.

Seckinger P, Isaaz S, Dayer JM. A human inhibitor of tumor necrosis factor-α. J Exp Med 167:1511–1516, 1988.

Seckinger P, Williamson K, Balavione J-F, Mach B, Mazzi G, Shaw A, Dayer JM. A urine inhibitor of interleukin-1 activity affects both interleukin-1α and 1β but not tumor necrosis factor α. J Immunol 139:1541–1545, 1987.

Selsted ME, Szklarek D, Ganz T, Lehrer RI. Activity of rabbit leukocyte peptides against Candida albicans. Infect Immun 49:202–207, 1985.

Shepherd V, Campbell E, Senior R, Stahl P. Characterization of the mannose/fucose receptor on human mononuclear phagocytes. J Reticuloendothel Soc 32:423–431, 1982.

Silberberg-Sinakin I, Thorbecke G, Baer RL, Rosenthal SA, Berezowsky V. Antigen-bearing Langerhans cells in skin, dermal lymphatics and in lymph nodes. Cell Immunol 25:137–151, 1976.

Snyder DD, Unaue ER. Corticosteroids inhibit murine macrophage Ia expression and interleukin-1 production. J Immunol 129:1803–1805, 1982.

Snyder DS, Beller DI, Unanue ER. Prostaglandins modulate macrophage Ia expression. Nature 229:163–165, 1982.

Snyderman R, Pike MC. Structure and function of monocytes and macrophages. In McCarty DJ, ed. Arthritis and Allied Conditions. Philadelphia, Lea & Febiger, 1989, pp. 306–335.

Solotorovsky M, Soderberg L. Host-parasite interactions with macrophages in culture. In Laskin AI, Lechavalier H, eds. Macrophages and Cellular Immunity. Cleveland, CRC Press, 1972, pp. 77–123.

Southwick FS, Hartwig JH. Acumentin, a protein in macrophages which caps the pointed ends of actin filaments. Nature 297:303, 1982.

Springer TA. Adhesion receptors of the immune system. Nature 346:425–434, 1990.

Stachura J. Cytochemistry of monocytes and macrophages. In Zembala M, Asherson GL, eds. Human Monocytes. London, Academic Press, 1989, pp. 27–36.

Stahl P. The macrophage mannose receptor: current status. Am J Respir Cell Mol Biol 2:317–318, 1990.

Staunton DE, Dustin ML, Springer TA. Functional cloning of ICAM-2, a cell adhesion ligand for LFA-1 homologous to ICAM-1. Nature 339:61–64, 1989.

Steinman RM. The dendritic cell system and its role in immunogenicity. Annu Rev Immunol 9:271–296, 1991.

Steinman RM, Cohn ZA. Identification of a novel cell type in peripheral lymphoid organs of mice. J Exp Med, 137:1142–1147, 1973.

Stossel TP. From signal to pseudopod: how cells control cytoplasmic actin assembly. J Biol Chem 264:18261–18264, 1989.

Stuehr DJ, Nathan CF. Nitric oxide: a macrophage product responsible for cytostasis and respiratory inhibition in tumor target cells. J Exp Med 169:1543–1545, 1989.

Sutton JS, Weiss L. Transformation of monocytes in tissue culture into macrophages, epitheliod cells, and multinucleated giant cells. J Cell Biol 28:303–332, 1966.

Terstappen LWMM, Hollander Z, Meiners H, Loken MR. Quantitative comparison of myeloid antigens on five lineages of mature peripheral blood cells. J Leuk Biol 48:138–148, 1990.

Tew JG, Thorbecke J, Steinman RM. Dendritic cells in the immune response. Characteristics and recommended nomenclature. J Reticuloendothel Soc 31:371–380, 1982.

Thomas R, Davis LS, Lipshy PE. Isolation and characterization of human peripheral blood dendritic cells. J Immunol 150:821–834, 1993.

Thorne KJI, Oliver RC, Barnet AJ. Lysis and killing of bacteria by lysosomal proteinases. Infect Immun 14:555–563, 1976.

Todd RF III, Schlossman SF. Analysis of antigenic determinants on human monocytes and macrophages. Blood 59:775–786, 1982.

Todd RF III, Schlossman SF. Utilization of monoclonal antibodies in the characterization of monocyte-macrophage differentiation antigens. In Bellanti JA, Herscowitz HB, eds. The Reticuloendothelial System. New York, Plenum Publishing, 1984, pp. 87–112.

Toews GB. Pulmonary dendritic cells: sentinels of lung-associated lymphoid tissues. Am J Resp Cell Mol Biol 4:204–205, 1991.

Unanue ER, Allen PM. The basis for the immunoregulatory role of macrophages and other accessory cells. Science 236:551–557, 1987a.

Unanue ER, Allen PM. The immunoregulatory role of the macrophage. Hosp Pract 22:63–80, 1987b.

Unkeless JC. Function and heterogeneity of human Fc receptors for immunoglobulin G. J Clin Invest 83:355–361, 1989.

Urban JL, Shepard HM, Rothstein JL, Sugarman BJ, Schreiber H. Tumor necrosis factor: a potent effector molecule for tumor cell killing by activated macrophages. Proc Natl Acad Sci U S A 83:5233–5237, 1986.

Van de Winkel JGJ, Capel PJA. Human IgG Fc receptor heterogeneity: molecular aspects and clinical implications. Immunol Today 14:215–221, 1993.

Van der Rhee HJ, de Winter CPM, Daems WT. Fine structure and peroxidatic activity of rat blood monocytes. Cell Tissue Res 185:1–16, 1977.

Van Furth R. Cells of the mononuclear phagocyte system: nomenclature in terms of sites and conditions. In Van Furth R, ed. Mononuclear Phagocytes—Functional Aspects. Dordrecht, Netherlands, Martinus Nijhoff Publishers, 1980, pp. 1–40.

Van Furth R, Cohn ZA. The origin and kinetics of mononuclear phagocytes. J Exp Med 128:415–435, 1968.

Van Furth R, Diesselhoff den Dulk MMC, Sluiter W, Van Dissel JT. New perspective on the kinetics of mononuclear phagocytes. In Van Furth R, ed. Mononuclear Phagocytes: Characteristics, Physiology and Function. Dordrecht, Netherlands, Martinus Nijhoff Publishers, 1985, pp. 201–209.

Van Furth R, Langevoort HL, Schaberg A. Mononuclear phagocytes in human pathology—proposal for an approach to improved classification. In Van Furth R, ed. Mononuclear Phagocytes in Immunity, Infection and Pathology. London, Blackwell Scientific Publications, 1975, pp. 1–16.

Van Oss CJ, Gillman CF, Neuman AW. Phagocytic Engulfment and Adhesiveness as Cellular Surface Phenomena. New York, Marcel Dekker, 1975, pp. 1–153.

Verghese MW, Snyderman R. Chemotaxis and chemotactic factors. In Zembala M, Asherson GL, eds. Human Monocytes. Oxford, Oxford University Press, 1989, pp. 167–176.

Vlassara H, Brownlee IM, Manogue KR, Dinarillo CA, Pasagian A. Cachectin/TNF and IL-1 induced by glucose-modified proteins: role in normal tissue remodeling. Science 240:1546–1548, 1988.

Vlassara H, Moldawer L, Chan B. Macrophage/monocyte receptor for nonenzymatically glycosylated proteins is upregulated by cachectin/tumor necrosis factor. J Clin Invest 84:1813–1820, 1989.

Volk-Platzer B, Stingl G, Wolff K, Hinterberg W, Schnedl W. Cytogenetic identification of allogeneic epidermal Langerhans cells in a bone marrow-graft recipient. N Engl J Med 310:1123–1127, 1984.

Wachstein M, Wolfe G. The histochemical demonstration of esterase activity in human blood and bone marrow smears. J Histochem Cytochem 6:457, 1958.

Wahl LM, Wahl SM, Mergenhagen SE, Martin GR. Collagenase production by lymphokine-activated macrophages. Science 187:261–263, 1975.

Ward PA. Chemotaxis of mononuclear cells. J Exp Med 128:1201–1221, 1968.

Ward PA, Remold HG, David JR. The production by antigen-stimulated lymphocytes of a leukotactic factor distinct from migratory inhibitory factor. Cell Immunol 1:162–174, 1970.

Weinstein RS, Khoudadad JK, Steck TL. Ultrastructural characterization of proteins at the natural surfaces of the red cell membrane. In Brewer GJ, ed. The Red Cell. New York, Alan R Liss, 1978, pp. 413–427.

Wellicome SM, Thornhill MH, Pitzalis C, Thomas DS, Lanchburg JSS, Panayi GS, Haskard DO. A monoclonal antibody that detects a novel antigen on endothelial cells that is induced by tumor necrosis factor, IL-1, or lipopolysaccharide. J Immunol 144:2558–2565, 1990.

Werb Z, Banda MJ, Jones PA. Degradation of connective tissue matrices by macrophages. I. Proteolysis of elastin, glycoproteins, and collagen by proteinases isolated from macrophages. J Exp Med 152:1340–1357, 1980.

Wetzel BK, Spicer SS, Horn RG. Fine structural localization of acid and alkaline phosphatases in cells of rabbit blood and bone marrow. J Histochem Cytochem 15:311–334, 1967.

Whitlaw DW. Observations on human monocyte kinetics after pulse labeling. Cell Tissue Kinet 5:3111–3117, 1972.

Wong HL, Walh SM. Tissue repair and fibrosis. In Zembala M, Asherson GL, eds. Human Monocytes. London, Academic Press, 1989, pp. 383–394.

Wright SD, Detmer PA. Adhesion-promoting receptors on phagocytes. J Cell Sci 9(Suppl):99–120, 1988.

Wright SD, Griffin FM. Activation of phagocytic cells' C3 receptors for phagocytosis. J Leuk Biol 38:327–339, 1985.

Yin HL, Hartwig JH, Maruyama K, Stossel TP. Ca^{2+} control of actin filament length. Effect of macrophage gelsolin on actin polymerization. J Biol Chem 256:9693–9697, 1981.

Yoder MC, Hassan SF, Douglas SD. Mononuclear phagocyte system. In Polin RA, Fox WW, eds. Fetal and Neonatal Physiology. Philadelphia, WB Saunders, 1992, pp. 1438–1461.

Yourno J. Monocyte nonspecific esterase: purification and subunit structure. Blood 68:479–487, 1986.

Zschunke F, Salmassi A, Kreipe H, Buck H, Parwaresch MR, Radzun HJ. cDNA cloning and characterization of human monocyte/macrophage serine esterase-1. Blood 78:506–512, 1991.

Zuckerman SH, Douglas SD. Mononuclear phagocytes: plasma membrane receptors and dynamics. Annu Rev Microbiol 33:267–307, 1979.

Zuckerman SH, Ackerman SK, Douglas SD. Long-term peripheral blood monocyte cultures: establishment and morphology of primary human monocyte-macrophage cell culture. Immunology 38:401–411, 1979.

Chapter 7

The Serum Complement System

Melvin Berger and Michael M. Frank

As originally described at the end of the nineteenth century, complement referred to the heat-labile, nonspecific principles in serum required to lyse bacteria that had been sensitized with the heat-stable, specific component now recognized as antibody. Early in this century, it became apparent that this bactericidal activity required the sequential activation of multiple factors or components. With sensitized erythrocytes used as a model, the lytic process has been studied in detail and characterized mathematically (Mayer, 1961; Borsos and Rapp, 1970). With modern biochemical technology, the individual proteins of this classical, antibody-dependent pathway of activation have been isolated and characterized, and the basis of complement activity is now understood on a molecular level.

In the 1950s another pathway of complement activation was described by Pillemer and colleagues (1954). Initially, this was termed the *properdin system,* but it is now referred to as the *alternative pathway* because it is activated by an alternative series of proteins that bypass the early components of the classical pathway. The alternative pathway does not require specific antibody but is activated by certain types of surfaces, including the surface of many microbes as well as a particle of yeast cell walls often used as a model, called *zymosan.* The proteins that constitute this pathway have also been isolated and characterized, and their relationships to the classical pathway components have been defined (Müller-Eberhard and Schreiber, 1980).

The components of the classical and alternative pathways, together with their important regulatory factors, thus comprise more than 19 unique serum proteins, plus additional membrane proteins. The properties of all of these proteins are summarized in Table 7–1. The originally described activity of the complement system, lysis of bacteria or erythrocytes, is still its most commonly recognized function. However, many other functions have subsequently been attributed to this complex system of proteins. These include the generation of peptide fragments that serve as potent mediators of inflammation and attractants for phagocytic cells and the formation of opsonins that have essential functions in the host defense against infection. Complement also plays critical roles in solubilization and clearance

133

Table 7–1. Physicochemical Properties of Complement Components and Inhibitor Proteins

Component	Molecular Weight	Serum Concentration, μg/ml	Chain Structure
Classical Pathway			
C1q	390,000	190	6 each α, β, γ
C1r	95,000	100	1 chain
C1s	85,000	80	1 chain
C4 (β_{1E})	209,000	430	α, β, γ
C2	117,000	30	1 chain
C3 (β_{1C})	190,000	1400	α, β
C5	206,000	75	α, β
C6	95,000	60	1 chain
C7	120,000	55	1 chain
C8	163,000	80	α, β, γ
C9	79,000	160	1 chain
Alternative Pathway			
P (properdin)	223,000	25	4 identical chains
D (C3 proactivator convertase)	25,000	1–5	1 chain
B (C3 proactivator, glycine rich β-glycoprotein)	100,000	200	1 chain
Control Proteins			
C1 esterase inhibitor (C1EI, C1 INH)	105,000	180	1 chain
	570,000	?	8 identical chains
C4 binding protein	100,000	50	α, β
I (C3b/C4b inactivator, C3 INA)	150,000	520	1 chain
H (β_{1H} globulin)	80,000	600	1 chain
S Protein (vitronectin)			
*Membrane bound control proteins**		*CD Designation*	
Decay accelerating factor (DAF)	70–80,000	CD55	1 chain
Membrane cofactor protein (MCP)	48–68,000	CD46	1 chain
Complement receptor type 1 (CR1)	190–220,000	CD35	1 chain
Protectin, membrane inhibitor of reactive lysis (MIRL)	18–25,000	CD59	1 chain
Homologous restriction factor (HRF), C8 binding protein	65,000	Not assigned	1 chain

*Absent in serum; present on multiple cells identified by monoclonal antibodies to specific surface antigens.
Abbreviation: CD = cluster of differentiation.

of immune complexes by the reticuloendothelial system and in immunologic homeostasis, such as initiating antibody responses, modulating lymphocyte activation, and establishing immunologic memory. Thus, understanding the mechanisms of complement activation, its biologic effects, and its regulation has become a major endeavor of modern immunologic research.

More detailed discussions of the complement system are available in a collection of selected reviews by Müller-Eberhard (1983/1984), a comprehensive textbook by Rother and Till (1988), and a set of reviews of current concepts of complement physiology (Lachmann, 1994).

NOMENCLATURE

A uniform set of symbols for the components and intermediates involved in complement activation has been adopted by the World Health Organization and is now in general use (Austen et al., 1968; Alper et al., 1981). The classical pathway components were assigned numbers in the order of their discovery and are thus designated C1 through C9. They also act in numeric sequence except for C4, which is the second

protein in the cascade. The alternative pathway components or factors are referred to by the letters B, D, and P, which correspond to the previously used names (listed in Table 7–1). The two soluble control proteins that regulate activation of this pathway have also been assigned letters: H for β_{1H} and I for the C3b/C4b inactivator. The proteins that control the earliest steps of the classical pathway activation retain their original names, C1 esterase inhibitor and C4 binding protein. C1 is composed of three distinct and separate subunits denoted by C1q, C1r, and C1s. None of the other components have distinct subunits, but for those that contain more than one peptide chain, the first three letters of the Greek alphabet are used to designate the separate chains: α denoting the largest, β the next, and γ the smallest.

Most laboratory studies of the function of complement components employ hemolytic assays using sheep erythrocytes as the particle to be lysed. The target erythrocyte is denoted by E and the specific antibody by A. As complement components bind to the surface, their number is added (i.e., EAC1 or EAC142). Many of the steps in the activation of both pathways involve limited proteolytic cleavages, and the cleavage products are usually denoted by lower case letters (e.g.,

C3a and C3b). The actual polypeptide chains cleaved are designated with a prime mark, so that upon cleavage, the α chain of native C3 becomes the α' chain of C3b. Enzymatically active intermediates or complexes are denoted by a bar over the fragments involved, as in $\overline{\text{C3bBb}}$, the alternative pathway C3 convertase. Proteins that have lost their ability to act as convertases are given the lower case letter i, as in iC3b (formerly, the i came after the component, as in C3bi). This designation is important because even though iC3b is not active in convertases, it still plays an important role in opsonization by binding to its specific receptor, CR3 (see later discussion).

COMPLEMENT ACTIVATION

The Classical Pathway

C142 Activation

The classical pathway is initiated when C1 binds to an antigen-antibody complex and becomes activated. C1 normally circulates in the blood as a macromolecular complex held together in the presence of calcium. C1q itself has a molecular weight of 400,000 and is composed of 18 polypeptide chains of three types (six each of α, β, and γ). These are bound together to form six triple-helical collagen-like strands with a globular structure at the end of each one, giving the appearance under an electron microscope of a bunch of tulips (Porter and Reid, 1978). The strand-like domains of C1q are rich in glycine, hydroxylysine, and hydroxyproline and can be digested by collagenase. The globular domains contain the sites that bind to antibody molecules. Although monomeric immunoglobulin (IgG) can interact weakly with C1q, activation requires binding of more than one of the globular domains of a single C1q molecule to individual Fc portions of the immunoglobulin.

IgM is an efficient activator of C1, presumably because the five Fc portions of this molecule are all linked together. A single IgM molecule is thus sufficient to activate the classical pathway, although studies suggest that more than one of the antigen-binding sites of the IgM molecule must be engaged in order for activation to occur.

Activation by IgG requires two or more molecules to be brought into close proximity, as in an antigen-antibody complex or on a cell surface. In hemolytic systems or with particulate activators in general, this requirement for a doublet of IgG means that many thousands of IgG molecules must be deposited on an erythrocyte or bacterium for two of them to be close enough to bind with and activate a single C1 molecule. Human IgG subclasses 1, 2, and 3 can activate C1, but IgG4, IgA, IgD, and IgE cannot. The C1q interacts noncovalently with the CH_2 domain of the immunoglobulin molecule, but it is not clear whether a conformational change is induced in this domain when the immunoglobulin binds antigen, which then promotes C1q binding, or whether antigen binding is required just to bring the Fc fragments into appropriate proximity to form a C1 fixing site.

Macromolecular C1 contains two molecules each of C1r and C1s in addition to the C1q. Each C1r is a single polypeptide chain with a molecular weight of 85,000 daltons, and each C1s is a single chain of similar molecular weight (Reid and Porter, 1981; Ziccardi, 1981; Cooper, 1983). These subunits are also globular and associated with the stalk region on the C1q molecule. C1r and C1s are activated when the globular ends of the C1q bind to antibody molecules, probably by conformational changes that occur when multiple sites interact with the immunoglobulins. During activation, each of the C1r chains is cleaved into a larger fragment of approximately 56,000 daltons and a smaller fragment of 27,000 daltons, which contains an active site serine and has protease activity. These active proteases then carry out similar cleavages on $\overline{\text{C1s}}$ that form the active $\overline{\text{C1s}}$ molecules (Sim, 1981). The $\overline{\text{C1s}}$ then acts as the protease that cleaves and activates C4 and C2, but it can also cleave synthetic esters. Hence, it is sometimes referred to as C1 esterase because this activity is more easily studied in the laboratory.

After binding and activation of C1, the C1s subunit can cleave and activate the next protein in the sequence, C4 (Fig. 7–1). This component is made up of three chains; α, with a molecular weight of 93,000, β, with a molecular weight of 78,000, and γ, with a molecular weight of 34,000. Activation is accomplished by cleavage at a single site on the α chain giving rise to C4a, a small fragment (molecular weight, 9000) that diffuses away, and C4b, the remainder of the molecule, which can continue the activation cascade. C4 activation is biochemically similar to C3 activation (discussed later), and the major fragment, C4b, is transiently able

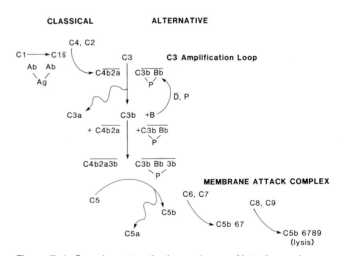

Figure 7–1. Complement activation pathways. Note the analogous function of $\overline{\text{C4b2a}}$, the classical pathway C3 convertase, and $\overline{\text{C3bBb}}$, the alternative pathway C3 convertase. Addition of another molecule of C3b to each of these leads to formation of the respective C5 convertases. The alternative pathway convertases are shown here in their properdin stabilized forms. Note that only the active fragments, C3a and C5a, are indicated; inactive cleavage fragments are not shown. (Modified from Berger M, Frank MM. Complement. In Wedgwood RJ, Davis SD, Ray CG, Kelley VC, eds. Infections in Children. Philadelphia, JB Lippincott, 1982, pp. 86–108.)

to bind covalently to the cell surface or immune complex. A single active C$\overline{1}$ complex can cleave multiple C4 molecules so that many C4b molecules may cluster around a single original C1 fixing site, providing the first amplification step of the complement cascade.

The bound C4b molecules have no enzymatic activity *per se*, but provide binding sites for C2, the next protein in the sequence (Fig. 7–1). C2 bound to C4b is a substrate for C$\overline{1s}$, which again cleaves at a single site, uncovering the enzymatic activity that is carried on the larger fragment, C2a. The interaction of C2a with C4b is stabilized by C2b (Nagasawa and Stroud, 1977). This complex then functions as the C3 convertase, with C4b providing the binding site for native C3 and C$\overline{2a}$, the proteolytic active site, which is serine-dependent. The C$\overline{4b2a}$ complex is held together by weak, noncovalent interactions and decays spontaneously with loss of the C2a. Each C4b can promote cleavage of multiple C2 molecules by C$\overline{1s}$. Activation is thus more efficient on a surface where the C1 complex and C4b remain bound in close proximity. In the fluid phase, diffusion makes it difficult to sustain the multiple protein-protein interactions necessary for C$\overline{1s}$ to cleave C2.

C3 Activation

Activation of C3 by the classical pathway C3 convertase C$\overline{4b2a}$ also involves a single specific proteolytic cleavage (see Fig. 7–1). C3 is present at the highest serum concentration of any of the complement components, 1.0 to 1.5 mg/ml, and it plays central roles in both the classical and alternative pathways of activation. It also has important biologic activity in opsonization and immune complex clearance and is thus the focal point of much complement research. Native C3 is a glycoprotein (molecular weight, 190,000) that is composed of an α chain (molecular weight, 115,000) linked by disulfide bonds to a β chain (molecular weight, 75,000) (Fig. 7–2). Activation by C$\overline{4b2a}$ by the alternative pathway C3 convertase or nonspecific activation by other serine proteases appears to be identical, with release of C3a, a 77 amino acid fragment from the NH_2 terminal of the α chain. This small fragment has anaphylatoxin activity (discussed later). The remaining large fragment, C3b, undergoes a complex conformational change exposing an internal thioester in the C3d region of the α' chain, remote from the initial cleavage site (see Fig. 7–2). Studies by Tack and colleagues led to the discovery of this unusually reactive chemical structure, which is shared by C4 and α$_2$-macroglobulin and accounts for the ability of these proteins to bind covalently to their targets (Tack et al., 1980; Harrison et al., 1981; Thomas et al., 1982.)

The peptide chain that contains this bond has the following sequence:

—Gly—Cys*—Gly—Glu—Glu*—Asn—Met—

The asterisks indicate the cysteine residue that provides the thiol and the glutamate residue that provides the acyl moiety of the thioester. This group is usually protected in a hydrophobic pocket in the native molecule. Upon exposure, however, it is subject to nucleophilic

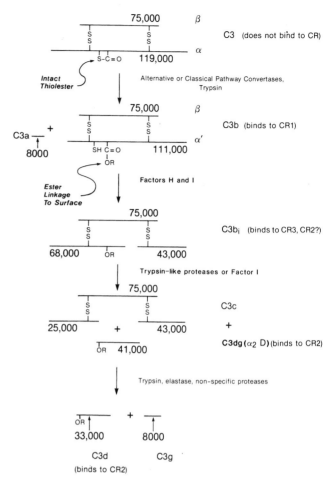

Figure 7–2. Schematic polypeptide chain structure of C3 and its cleavage fragments. Note that the site of cleavage by the convertases is toward the NH_2-terminal of the α chain, remote from the thioester site. This activation step may be accompanied by a transesterification reaction, resulting in surface-bound C3b (shown), or the thioester may react with H_2O, in which case the carboxyl moiety would be COOH, resulting in fluid phase C3b. A conformational change accompanies this process and allows C3b to bind to CR1. Further cleavage by factor I in the presence of factor H or CR1 leads to production of C3bi, which binds to CR3, then to release of C3c, which is actually a three-chain molecule with a molecular weight of 145,000. Cleavage by factor I stops at this point, leaving α$_2$D in serum or C3dg bound. Additional cleavage by nonspecific proteases releases a small fragment (C3g), leaving C3d bound. (Adapted from Harrison RA, Lachmann PJ. The physiological breakdown of the third component of complement. Mol Immunol 17:9–20, 1980. With kind permission from Elsevier Science Ltd, Kidlington, United Kingdom; and Ross GD, et al. J Exp Med 158:334–352, 1983. Copyright permission of The Rockefeller University Press, New York.)

attack and thus becomes highly reactive. This unique structure can then participate in transesterification reactions in which the acyl moiety is transferred from the thiol to another electron-rich acceptor, forming a new covalent bond (Sim et al., 1981; Hostetter et al., 1982).

Acceptors can include the oxygen atoms of hydroxyl groups on cell surface carbohydrates, glycoprotein side chains, or amino acids. Binding of C3b to one of these groups occurs by ester linkages that are resistant to detergents but can be released by high pH or hydroxylamine (Law et al., 1979). The thioester may also react with amino groups, forming amide linkages resistant to hydrolysis except under the most rigorous laboratory conditions. If the thioester does not react with a suitable acceptor within a very brief half-life, the oxygen atom of water will provide the necessary pair of electrons, resulting in fluid phase C3b. Because the thioester remains available for a matter of only milliseconds before reacting with water, the newly cleaved C3b is referred to as *nascent* and the thioester as the *labile* binding site (because its ability to bind to biologic targets is only transient).

Once the thioester has reacted with water, the fluid phase C3b is no longer capable of strong interactions with targets. Biologic acceptors for C4b and C3b binding include cell surface carbohydrates of red cells and bacteria as well as antibody molecules (Goers and Porter, 1978; Campbell et al., 1980; Brown et al., 1983). Chemicals that can disrupt the hydrophobic pocket of native C3 and C4 or low-molecular-weight nucleophiles that can diffuse in and react directly with the thioester will inactivate these molecules, thus explaining the sensitivity of the complement system to inactivation by thiocyanate, ammonia, and hydrazine.

During complement activation, many C3 molecules are cleaved. Some are hydrolyzed and remain in free solution, but many are deposited on the cell surface. Some of these are too far from their activation site to participate in furthering the activation sequence. These molecules may, nevertheless, have important biologic activity in opsonization, one of the major functions of the complement system, as well as in activating the alternative pathway (discussed later).

C5 to C9 Activation

Those C3b molecules that do bind in close proximity to C4b2a serve as binding sites for C5 and thus transform the C3 convertase function of C4b2a into the C5 convertase, C4b2a3b, with C2a again providing the proteolytic active site. The cleavage of C5 is analogous to that of C4 and C3 in that an NH_2-terminal fragment of the α chain is released. Designated C5a, it has a molecular weight of 11,000 and potent anaphylatoxin activity. In addition, it is a chemoattractant and activator of neutrophils. In contrast to C4 and C3, with which it shares several common molecular characteristics, C5 does not contain an internal thiol ester and does not bind covalently to cells.

C5b is unstable and rapidly loses activity in the reaction sequence unless it binds to C6. This forms an active complex that can bind to membranes and/or interact with C7. On interaction with C6 and C7, the hydrophobic properties of C5b increase, and the complex is capable of inserting into membrane lipid bilayers in much the same way that detergents interact with lipids. Similar to C6 and C7, the remaining components, C8 and C9, are activated in numeric sequence without requiring proteolytic cleavage and form the *membrane attack complex* that can lyse biologic membranes (see Cytolysis and the Membrane Attack Complex).

Control of Classical Pathway Activation

Since activation of the complement cascade leads not only to cell lysis but also to the release of cleavage fragments such as C3a and C5a, which can have local and systemic toxic effects, the body could not tolerate unchecked activation of this system. Of course, the degree of activation depends on the amounts of the native precursor proteins present in serum as well as on the amount and type of antigen-antibody complexes initiating the cascade. An inherent limit on activation is imposed by the requirement for the proteins to act in sequence and the limited stability of the intermediates before they spontaneously lose activity or dissociate from the multimolecular assemblies in which they act. Because complement is a self-amplification system, there is a critical dependence on the density of active intermediates at a given site and time. These considerations may partly explain why complement activation is much more efficient on the surface of a cell or a large immune complex than in free solution.

Additional regulation of complement activation is provided by specific inhibitor proteins. The first of these is C1 esterase inhibitor, a single-chain protein with a molecular weight of 105,000 and an extraordinarily large sugar content (35% to 40%). This protein reacts with exposed sites on C1r and C1s, eliminating their activity, dissociating them from C1q, and forming a large, extremely stable complex (Ziccardi and Cooper, 1979). This protein is a member of the family of serine protease inhibitors termed *serpins*; these can inhibit several other plasma proteases involved in the contact and clotting cascades (Patston et al., 1991). Its absence or reduced activity results in the condition known as hereditary angioedema (see Chapter 17, Disorders of the Complement System).

C4b and the classical pathway C3 convertase are also regulated by a specific protein, C4 binding protein. Binding of this protein to C4b promotes dissociation of C2a from the enzyme and facilitates the further cleavage of C4b by C4b/C3b inactivator, also known as factor I. Action of factor I on the α′ chain of C4b results in the loss of the ability to act in the convertase and, after multiple cleavages, the release of most of the C4b molecule, leaving only the C4d fragment bound to the surface or immune complex, in a manner similar to that shown for C3b in Figure 7–2 (Fujita et al., 1978).

The Alternative Pathway

The alternative pathway of complement activation also involves the formation of convertases analogous to those previously described (Müller-Eberhard and Schreiber, 1980). The major difference is that specific antibody is not required to initiate the process. This pathway appears to be phylogenetically older than the classical pathway and can provide natural resistance in the early stages of infection, before the immune system has had time to respond by synthesizing specific antibody. Bacterial and other polysaccharides, endotoxins, yeast cell wall particles, and aggregated immunoglobulins, including IgA and IgE, are all capable of activating the alternative pathway. The chemical nature of the surface that initiates activation partly determines this capability (discussed in Role of the Surface).

The first component of the alternative pathway is C3b, which may be produced by classical pathway activation or by nonspecific proteolytic attack. The alternative pathway can also be activated by a form of C3 that has not been activated by proteolytic cleavage but resembles C3b because its thioester has been hydrolyzed by water (Pangburn and Müller-Eberhard, 1980). This process probably goes on continuously at a slow rate and accounts for the previously observed fluid phase C3 "tickover," providing a basal level of activity that can be rapidly amplified in the presence of a suitable surface without the need for additional recognition or initiating factors. Thus, C3b plays a role analogous to that of the C4b in the classical pathway and serves as a binding site for factor B, which is biochemically and functionally homologous to C2.

When factor B is bound to C3b, it becomes susceptible to activation by a single specific proteolytic cleavage carried out by factor D. Factor D is a low-molecular-weight (25,000) serine protease that apparently circulates in its active form in plasma at all times but at very low concentration, 1 to 5 μg/ml. D can cleave B only when it is bound to C3b and has no other known natural substrates. After cleavage, a small fragment (Ba) diffuses away and the large fragment (Bb) remains associated with C3b to form the alternative pathway C3 convertase ($\overline{C3bBb}$). In this enzyme, the C3b continues to function like C4b by providing a binding site for additional C3 molecules and Bb functions like C2a in providing the proteolytically active site.

Once again, the nascent C3b molecules can have a number of different fates. A few will bind very closely to the $\overline{C3bBb}$ enzyme and will complex with it, providing a binding site for C5. This transforms the C3 convertase to a C5 convertase just as in the classical pathway, and Bb is thus able to cleave the C5. After activation of C5 by this enzyme, the later components continue to act in sequence exactly as in classical pathway activation resulting in the formation of the membrane attack complex and leading to cell lysis.

C3 Control Proteins and the C3 Amplification Loop

Soluble Proteins

The soluble proteins are summarized in Table 7–1. Just as formation of the initial C3 convertase of the alternative pathway has many features similar to the corresponding classical pathway enzyme, its regulation also has some analogous features. First, the $\overline{C3bBb}$ complex has only a limited half-life and decays spontaneously by losing Bb. The protein properdin (P), for which the alternative pathway was originally named, can bind to the alternative pathway C3 and C5 convertases and stabilize them against the loss of Bb, thus prolonging their activity. On the other hand, the protein β_{1H} or factor H can act analogously to C4-binding protein and promote dissociation of Bb by binding to

C3b. If the complex decays spontaneously, the C3b can continue to serve as a binding site for additional factor B molecules, and activation will continue. When factor H binds, however, it promotes the cleavage of C3b by the same enzyme that cleaves C4b, factor I or the C4b/C3b inactivator. The iC3b that remains after cleavage by factor I still has opsonic activity, but it no longer promotes activation of B. This action of factors H and I is also important in limiting the rate of the spontaneous C3 tickover in the fluid phase. Patients who are deficient in either of these proteins have continuous activation of the alternative pathway, resulting in conversion of C3 to circulating C3b.

Membrane Proteins

In addition to the soluble proteins that regulate complement activation at the convertase level, a family of structurally related integral cell membrane proteins has similar regulatory activities (Table 7–2). These proteins play an important role in protecting body cells against activation of autologous complement on their surfaces, which may occur in autoimmune diseases or when extrinsic antigens are passively adsorbed onto their surfaces. Like the soluble proteins, these membrane proteins inhibit complement activation by binding to one component of a convertase (i.e., C4b or C3b) and displacing another (i.e., $\overline{C2a}$ or Bb), thus inactivating the convertase. Because the convertase activity would decay spontaneously when its noncovalently bound components dissociated naturally, this function of the regulatory molecules is referred to as *accelerating decay of the convertase*. In addition to accelerating decay, some of these regulatory molecules serve as cofactors that enable factor I to cleave and inactivate the C3b or C4b to which they have bound. This prevents the C3b or C4b from participating in the formation of any new convertase complexes. As reviewed in Table 7–2, different members of this family are capable of either or both of these regulatory functions.

Complement receptor type 1, or CR1, has both of these activities; the 70,000-dalton protein known as *decay accelerating factor* (DAF) promotes dissociation of the classical and alternative pathway convertases but does not serve as a cofactor for cleavage by factor I. The clinical importance of DAF is suggested by its absence in paroxysmal nocturnal hemoglobinuria (see Paroxysmal Nocturnal Hemoglobinuria) and by the observation that tumor cells that express high levels of DAF are resistant to immunologic attack and complement-mediated lysis (Cheung et al, 1988).

In contrast to DAF, the 48,000- to 68,000-dalton protein termed *membrane cofactor protein* (MCP) facilitates cleavage of C4b and C3b by factor I but by itself does not affect binding of Bb or C2a, the enzymatically active subunits of the convertases.

Structural Homology of C3b and C4b Regulatory Proteins: Regulators of Complement Activation Gene Family

All of these proteins, including factor H and C4bp, share a high degree of structural homology. This is not unexpected because they all bind to C3b and/or C4b,

Table 7–2. Protein Regulators of Complement Activation

Protein	Abbreviation	Molecular Weight	Number of Short Concensus Repeats (SCRs)	Dissociation of C3 and C5 Convertases		Factor I Cofactor Activity for	
				Alternative	Classical	C3b	C4b
Factor H, β_{1H} (p)*	H	150,000	20	+	−	+	−
C4 binding protein (p)	C4bp	570,000 (Octomer)	8	−	+	−	+
Decay accelerating factor (CD55)	DAF	70,000–80,000	4	+	+	−	−
Membrane cofactor protein (CD46)	MCP	45,000–70,000	4	−	−	+	+
Complement receptor type 1 C3b/C4b receptor (CD35)	CR1	205,000–250,000	30	+	+	+	+
Complement receptor type 2 C3d receptor (CD21)	CR2	145,000	15/16	−	−	−	−

*p indicates plasma proteins; membrane proteins are indicated by CD number.

Adapted from Ahearn JM, Fearon DT. Structure and function of the complement receptors, CR1 (CD35) and CR2 (CD21). Adv Immunol 46:183–219, 1989; Weisman HF, Bartow T, Leppo MK, et al. Soluble human complement receptor type 1: in vivo inhibitor of complement suppressing post-ischemic myocardial inflammation and necrosis. Science 249:146–151, 1990.

which are themselves highly homologous. The type 2 complement receptor, which binds C3d, also shares structural homology with these regulatory proteins, even though it does not apparently share their activity. The genes for all of these proteins are clustered together in band q32 on human chromosome 1 in what have been termed the *regulators of complement activation*, or RCA gene cluster (Carroll et al., 1988, Bora et al., 1989).

The basic structural unit of these proteins is a highly conserved 60- to 65-amino acid short consensus repeat (SCR), which contains two disulfide bonds that give it a double-looped structure. The individual proteins contain different numbers of these SCRs (see Table 7–2) grouped into long homologous repeats that form the C3b or C4b binding sites. It seems likely that they have all evolved from a common primordial gene corresponding to the SCR. For this reason, the proteins themselves are considered to constitute a distinct family, although other membrane receptors not related to the complement system (e.g., the interleukin-2 [IL-2] receptor) also contain structures highly homologous with the complement regulatory protein SCRs.

Role of the Surface

As noted previously, the chemical nature of the surface on which the initial C3b is deposited also plays an important role in determining the extent of alternative pathway activation. This occurs because the surface exerts an important influence on the competition between factors H and B for binding to the C3b. As shown in Figure 7–3, surfaces that favor alternative pathway activation are those that allow or promote binding of B. On these surfaces, the C3b is in a protected site where it is not cleaved by factor I; thus, alternative pathway activation continues. Because the newly generated C3b molecules also deposit on this activating surface and can form new convertases, a positive feedback loop is begun and marked amplification can occur. Surfaces that favor binding of factor H

promote cleavage and inactivation of C3b by factor I, and alternative pathway activation does not occur.

Role of Sialic Acid

An important determinant of whether a surface will be an activator is its sialic acid content. Although most human cells contain a considerable amount of surface sialic acid, many bacterial polysaccharides, endotoxins, and cell walls are devoid of this sugar; hence, the deposition of a small amount of C3b on most bacteria leads to the rapid and continued activation of this C3b amplification loop in the presence of alternative pathway components B and D and additional C3. This results in heavy opsonization with C3b and/or activation of the later components and cell lysis, limiting the pathogenicity of organisms that activate the alternative pathway.

Laboratory studies show that removal of the surface sialic acid from sheep erythrocytes transforms them into good activators of the alternative pathway and have confirmed that this activation is accompanied by a 10- to 20-fold drop in the affinity with which factor H binds to the C3b on these cells (Fearon, 1978; Kazatchkine et al., 1979). Because of the ability of factor H to recognize surfaces that have characteristics in common with normal human cells and inhibit activation, the alternative pathway provides a primitive mechanism for distinguishing non-self from self without requiring specific antibody. Interestingly, the strains of *Escherichia coli* and group B streptococcus that are such dangerous pathogens for the neonate contain sialic acid in their capsular polysaccharides and are poor activators of the alternative pathway (Edwards et al., 1982; Stevens et al., 1978).

Role of Antibody

As noted above, antibodies other than IgG and IgM can activate the alternative pathway. F(ab')$_2$ fragments can also activate the alternative pathway, even on sur-

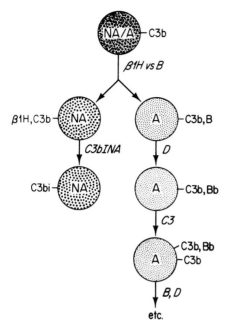

Figure 7–3. Control of alternative pathway activation by competition between B and H (β1H) for binding to membrane-associated C3b. C3b binds to both nonactivating (NA) and activating (A) cell surfaces, and discrimination between these surfaces by the alternative pathway occurs after this step. On a nonactivating cell, certain membrane constituents, such as sialic acid, promote the binding of β_{1H} (factor H), which facilitates conversion of C3b to C3bi by factor I, the C3b inactivator (C3bINA). On an activating cell, these membrane constituents are diminished or absent, and binding of B leads to formation of C3bB, which catalyzes deposition of more C3b, allowing activation of the C3 amplification loop. (Reprinted by permission, from Fearon DT, Austen KF. The alternative pathway of complement: a system for host resistance to microbial infection. The New England Journal of Medicine, 303:259–263, 1980.)

faces that would otherwise be nonactivating (Winkelstein and Shin, 1974; Moore et al., 1981). Because antibodies are known to provide good acceptor sites for nascent C3b, it is not surprising that antibody-bound C3b might be protected from the action of factors H and I, and studies with fluid phase complexes confirm this (Fries et al., 1984). Another likely effect of antibody is to cover up some of the sites that would favor factor H binding. This has been suggested for antibody against the capsule of group B streptococcus, which may mask the sialic acid moieties of the polysaccharide (Edwards et al., 1980).

Nonimmunologic Complement Activation

Nonimmunologic activation of complement can occur when plasma comes into contact with certain materials or when certain substances are injected into the blood stream. C1 can be activated directly by complexes of heparin with protamine, certain bacterial lipopolysaccharides, and other repeating-charge polymers. In addition, many serine proteases have overlapping specificity so that plasmin or trypsin is capable of directly activating C1s and C3. Plasmin activation may be important when the fibrinolytic system is activated in vivo, and trypsin activation has been an important tool for in vitro studies.

An excellent example of nonimmunologic activation of the alternative pathway occurs when blood is passed through cellulose membranes during hemodialysis or in certain pump oxygenators. This commonly results in transient leukopenia and pulmonary dysfunction and has been shown to be caused by activation of the alternative pathway by the cellulose, leading to the interaction of complement fragments (particularly C5a) with circulating neutrophils (Craddock et al., 1977; Jacob et al., 1980; Chenowith et al., 1981). These leukocytes then aggregate and plug pulmonary capillaries, and additional vasoactive substances may be released. Although the symptoms are usually mild, severe hypoxia and cardiovascular decompensation may occur in patients with preexisting cardiovascular or pulmonary impairment. Similar mechanisms probably contribute to the severe pulmonary dysfunction that occurs in the adult respiratory distress syndrome (Hammerschmidt et al., 1980).

Another condition in which nonimmunologic activation of the alternative pathway may have pathologic consequences is in the rare disease porphyria cutanea tarda, in which ultraviolet irradiation apparently causes photoactivation of abnormal circulating porphyrins. These porphyrins then react with skin proteins, transforming them into activators of the alternative pathway. This leads to local complement activation, which generates anaphylatoxins and causes inflammatory damage to the involved skin (Lim et al., 1984). Burns and ischemia also may lead to structural changes in tissue proteins and exposure of intracellular structures. Activation of the alternative pathway, C1, or both may occur in those situations, leading to formation of membrane attack complexes, attraction of neutrophils, and enhanced tissue damage.

Iodinated radiographic contrast media are commonly infused intravenously and are associated with adverse allergic-type reactions in as many as 5% of patients. These reactions do not appear to be IgE-mediated, and their mechanism remains unknown. One possibility is suggested by the capability of these low-molecular-weight compounds to bind directly to a variety of serum proteins and by the observation that they may nonspecifically activate proteolytic enzymes. There have been reports of depression of clotting factors and consumption of complement components by adding these media to normal serum (Arroyave and Tan, 1977; Kolb et al., 1978). The alternative pathway may be activated under these conditions, or direct proteolytic attack on C3 or C5 may occur, resulting, in either case, in the generation of C3a, C5a, or both. These anaphylatoxins could lead to histamine release from mast cells and to the activation of other mediator systems, resulting in a full-blown allergic reaction even though true IgE-mediated hypersensitivity is not demonstrable.

BIOLOGIC EFFECTS OF COMPLEMENT ACTIVATION

Anaphylatoxins and Chemoattractants

As discussed previously, activation of C4, C3, and C5 is accompanied by release of C4a, C3a, and C5a, which are peptides of 74 to 77 amino acid residues from the NH_2 end of the α chain of each molecule. These small peptides do not participate in further reactions of the activation sequence but remain in the fluid phase. C4a has a molecular weight of 8650, is nonglycosylated, and has only weak biologic activity (Gorski et al., 1979). C3a is a 9000-dalton peptide released when C3 is cleaved by the convertase of either the classical or alternative pathway. C5a is a similar peptide with a molecular weight of 11,000; it is released by corresponding cleavage of C5. These fragments have similar amino acid sequences and contain a helical portion as well as several disulfide bonds that form a rigid, complex loop in the peptide chain (Hugli, 1984). The higher molecular weight of C5a is due to the presence of a large carbohydrate moiety that accounts for 25 to 30% of this fragment's weight. These peptides are highly basic and possess great stability with respect to temperature and pH.

The anaphylatoxin activity of C3a is about 100 times greater than that of C4a when measured by the wheal-and-flare response of normal human skin. This response is caused by histamine and other mediators released when the anaphylatoxins bind to specific receptors on the surface of mast cells and basophils and cause these cells to degranulate. This degranulation is independent of IgE and is noncytotoxic. Although many of the responses to the anaphylatoxins are secondary effects of the mast cell–derived mediators, it is believed that some smooth muscle contraction is induced as a direct effect of C3a binding (Hugli and Müller-Eberhard, 1978). In addition, Marom and colleagues (1985) have shown that C3a induces mucus secretion by human lung explants that is not histamine dependent.

The anaphylatoxin activity of C5a is approximately 100- to 200-fold that of C3a in human skin. Besides its anaphylatoxin activity, C5a is an important chemoattractant for neutrophils and monocytes. C3a is apparently devoid of this activity, and C5a is now believed to be the major chemotactic factor formed during activation of the complement system. Previous reports of a chemotactic complex of C5, C6, and C7 may have resulted from slow dissociation of C5a from this larger complex. C5a has a number of other effects on neutrophils, including aggregation, increased adherence to endothelial surfaces, increased oxidase activity, and increased enzyme secretion. There have also been descriptions of C5a "helper" factors as well as inhibitors, but the exact nature and biologic importance of these proteins remains uncertain (Goldstein and Perez, 1980).

All of these anaphylatoxins are rapidly inactivated by serum carboxypeptidase-N (formerly called carboxypeptidase-B or serum anaphylatoxin inactivator), which cleaves an essential carboxyl terminal arginine from each of these peptides. Although these des-Arg forms lose most of their anaphylatoxin activity, C5a des-Arg retains considerable chemoattractant and neutrophil-activating activity for which the carbohydrate moiety is important (Gerard and Hugli, 1981).

Radioimmunoassays for these anaphylatoxins are used as sensitive monitors of complement activation. The presence of circulating C3a des-Arg most reliably reflects in vivo anaphylatoxin generation because the affinity of C5a for cell surface receptors is so high that this peptide does not persist in the circulation a long time (Chenowith and Hugli, 1980). Because release of these highly active factors allows complement activation to mimic classical IgE-mediated anaphylaxis, use of these assays should lead to a marked improvement in understanding a variety of apparently non–IgE-mediated anaphylactoid reactions.

Opsonization, Immune Complex Clearance, and C3 Receptors

An important biologic function of the complement system is its participation in phagocytosis of microorganisms and facilitation of the clearance of immune complexes by the reticuloendothelial system (RES). Arguably, these are the most important physiologic roles of complement in vivo, and breakdown in these functions is critically involved in most immune complex diseases (Schifferli et al., 1986, Fearon, 1988). These effects are mediated primarily by the interaction of C3 fragments bound to the surface of the organism or to antigen-antibody complexes with specific receptors on the plasma membranes of phagocytic cells. Four distinct receptors for different fragments of C3 have been identified and are designated CR1 (CD35), CR2 (CD21), CR3 (CD11b/CD18), and CR4 (CD11c/CD18) (Berger et al., 1982; Fearon and Wong, 1983; Arnaout and Colten, 1984). In addition, a receptor for C1q has also been described; it may have a role in phagocytic host defenses (Goodman and Tenner, 1992).

CR1 (CD35)

Native C3 does not effectively interact with any of these receptors, but upon cleavage, conformational changes take place that result in a more than 1000-fold increase in the affinity for C3b binding to CR1 (Berger et al., 1981). C4b can also bind to CR1, a single-chain glycoprotein with a molecular weight of approximately 220,000 that, when extracted from membranes with detergent, associates to form a 1.2×10^6 dalton molecule (Fearon, 1979, 1980). Studies with antibodies against CR1 indicate that CR1 is the C3b receptor on human erythrocytes, polymorphonuclear leukocytes, B lymphocytes, and monocytes (Fearon, 1980). CR1 is also found on the podocytes of glomerular epithelial cells (Gelfand et al., 1975). CR1 is a traditional transmembrane molecule with a short cytoplasmic tail and a single long extracellular region. This region consists of 28 or more (in different allotypes) repeats of a highly homologous, or *consensus* sequence of 60 to 65 amino acids each of which contains two internal disulfide-bonded loops. Similar short consensus repeats are found in the other regulators of complement activation that bind C3b and C4b and in other proteins that do not interact with the complement system. In CR1 and other regulators of complement activation, the SCRs are further organized in groups of seven into long homologous repeats that actually form the C3b and C4b binding sites (Fearon, 1988; Wilson et al., 1987).

The study of complement receptors and their role in host defense began with the observation by Nelson (1953) of a phenomenon he called *immune adherence.* This refers to the observation that bacteria coated with antibody and complement adhered to erythrocytes, which increased their phagocytosis by neutrophils. Studies in monkeys (Cornacoff et al., 1983) have demonstrated that preformed immune complexes rapidly fix complement upon injection into the blood stream and are then carried by the *immune adherence receptors* (i.e., CR1) on the erythrocytes. This facilitates their rapid removal from the circulation by hepatic macrophages, apparently by an analogous mechanism.

In most experimental systems, the interaction of particle-bound C3b with plasma membrane C3b receptors facilitates adherence, but this is insufficient to induce phagocytosis. Cell activation and ingestion requires a second signal, which can be provided by the interaction of a few particle-bound IgG molecules with Fc receptors on the phagocyte (Griffin et al., 1975; Ehlenberger and Nussenzweig, 1977). Although this is true for sheep erythrocytes and some bacteria, other bacteria and zymosan can be ingested when coated with C3b alone. Studies by Pommier and coworkers (1983) indicated that bound fibronectin may also provide a second signal to induce phagocytosis of C3b-coated particles.

Unlike IgG, IgM does not provide a second signal because phagocytes do not have receptors for the Fc portion of IgM. In vivo studies of the clearance of erythrocytes sensitized with IgM and C3b but not IgG are consistent with these results; these erythrocytes are not effectively removed from the circulation by RES macrophages (Frank et al., 1977). Although resting macrophages do not phagocytose erythrocytes opsonized with C3b, thioglycolate-stimulated macrophages or macrophages activated in vitro by phorbol esters are capable of phagocytosing C3b-coated erythrocytes without additional stimuli (Bianco et al., 1975; Wright and Silverstein, 1982).

These findings are analogous to the in vivo situation in animals injected with bacille Calmette-Guérin (BCG), which activates their macrophages. C3b-coated erythrocytes are then cleared from the circulation and phagocytosed much more effectively (Frank et al., 1977). Griffin and colleagues have shown that a T-cell–derived lymphokine alters the function of macrophage-complement receptors so that additional activating signals are no longer required to initiate phagocytosis (Griffin and Griffin, 1979; Griffin and Mullinax, 1981). Interaction of C3b with its receptor has also been reported to induce other effects, including histaminase release from neutrophils, secretion of factor I from lymphocytes, and production of prostaglandins by monocytes.

CR2 (CD21)

CR2 is a distinct receptor for C3d. This is a single-chain glycoprotein recognized by monoclonal antibod-ies B2 and HB5 (Iida et al., 1983; Weis et al., 1984) that has now been designated CD21. CR2 shares overall structural homology with CR1 and maps to the same gene locus as CR1 on chromosome 1 band q32, but the arrangement of the smaller number of short consensus repeats into long homologous regions differs (Weis et al., 1988; Ahearn and Fearon, 1989).

CR2 is most prominently expressed on B lymphocytes and probably plays an important role in stimulating and modulating the activity of these cells. CR2 is also found on follicular dendritic cells, where it likely plays a role in retention of antigen-antibody complexes and stimulation of antibody responses, and on some T lymphocytes and epithelial cells. Although CR2 can facilitate the cleavage of iC3b to C3d by factor I, it is not established that CR2 has any role in phagocytosis or immune complex clearance. Interestingly, CR2 has been determined to be the receptor for the Epstein-Barr virus (EBV) apparently because the gp350/220 of the virus shares homology with C3d (Ahearn and Fearon, 1989; Nemerow, et al., 1989) (see later, Molecular Mimicry of Complement Proteins by Infectious Agents).

CR3 (CD11b/CD18)

Following cleavage of bound C3b by factors H and I, the resulting iC3b is inactive in both classical and alternative pathway convertases and has a greatly reduced affinity for CR1 (see Fig. 7–2). However, this form of the molecule still has important opsonic activity (Stossel et al., 1975) and binds to a distinct receptor termed CR3. As with CR1, binding of some particles to CR3 may be followed by phagocytosis, although the details of this process and the requirements for additional signals are still being defined. This receptor, found on phagocytic cells, has been identified with the use of monoclonal antibodies. CR3 is a dimer with an α chain of 155,000 daltons and a β chain of 95,000 daltons (CD11b). It belongs to a family of cell surface proteins, termed *integrins,* that share common β chains but have different α chains that determine their binding activity (Sanchez-Madrid et al., 1983). The monoclonal antibodies that bind to this protein include OKM1, Mac-1, Leu-15, and Mol. Most of these antibodies block the binding of iC3b coated erythrocytes to human neutrophils and monocytes, and inhibit other activities of these cells (Beller et al., 1982; Arnaout et al., 1983; Wright et al., 1983). Other members of the leukocyte β integrin family include LFA-1 (CD11a/CD18) and P150/95 (CD11c/CD18) which is also considered CR4. LFA-1 is a major adhesion molecule on lymphocytes, as is CR3 (also termed Mac-1) on neutrophils and monocytes. These molecules play important roles in the binding of circulating cells to endothelial cells and thus help regulate their trafficking throughout the body.

CR4 (CD11c/CD18)

P150/95 (CD11c/CD18) is also referred to as CR4 and apparently has weak affinity for iC3b, C3dg, or both. This is the most prominently expressed member of the leukocyte β-integrin family on tissue macrophages (Myones et al., 1988.) Although some workers have proposed that it helps to promote phagocytosis, neither its exact binding specificity nor its role in promoting phagocytosis has been clearly defined.

Leukocyte Adhesion Defect Type 1

The three different α chains of the leukocyte integrin family (CD11a, 11b, and 11c) are all dependent on the common β chain (CD18) for proper insertion into the cell membrane. Deficiency of CD18 thus causes an inability to express any of these proteins and results in the syndrome of leukocyte adhesion defect type 1. Clinical features include delayed separation of the umbilical cord, persistent leukocytosis, and recurrent infections (Crowley et al., 1980; Arnaout et al., 1982; Bowen et al., 1982). Other immunologic abnormalities are also present. There are severe and moderate forms caused by different mutations. Neutrophils from these patients have diminished ability to bind and ingest iC3b-coated particles and have decreased adherence and chemotaxis in vitro because the same molecule (CD11b/CD18) serves as CR3 and as the major adherence protein. Interestingly, normal newborns are also partially deficient in this protein, which may contribute to their increased susceptibility to infection (Bruce et al., 1987; Abughali et al., 1994).

Role of Adhesion Molecules

The interactions between circulating leukocytes and endothelial cells have been the subject of intense investigation. Dynamic changes in adherence interactions are of major importance not only in directing neutrophils to sites of infection but also in regulating the trafficking of lymphocytes and all types of inflammatory responses.

In addition to the integrins, another class of adhesion molecules, called *selectins,* is also involved. Under normal conditions, circulating neutrophils have weak interactions with endothelial cells that cause them to roll along the vessel wall, pushed forward by the flow but not adhering tightly. This weak or rolling adherence is caused by the interaction of L-selectin on the neutrophil surface with a sialylated ligand on the endothelial cells (Hogg, 1992; Cronstein and Weissmann, 1993).

When endothelial cells are activated (i.e., by endotoxin, IL-1 and/or tumor necrosis factor [TNF]), they first increase expression of P-selectin and E-selectin, which bind to L-selectin and other sialylated ligands on the polymorphonuclear neutrophil leukocyte, respectively, slowing it down and increasing its chances of being activated by chemoattractants or other cytokines, such as IL-8. These, in turn, cause shedding of the weak adhesion molecule L-selectin from the neutrophil and also cause increases in both the number and affinity of β-integrin molecules (CD11b/CD18) on the neutrophil surface. The major endothelial ligand for CD11b/CD18 is an intracellular adhesion molecule (ICAM-1), whose expression is also induced by IL-1 and TNF, for example. The interaction between

ICAM-1 and β integrins is quite strong; it holds the neutrophil in place despite the shear forces of capillary flow, allowing the neutrophil to begin migrating across the endothelial wall. ICAM-1 also serves as a ligand for CD11a/CD18 (LFA-1); thus, its expression leads to adherence of lymphocytes, monocytes, and eosinophils.

Lymphocytes, monocytes, and eosinophils have an additional type of integrin called VLA-4, which binds to an endothelial cell ligand called vascular cell adhesive molecule (VCAM) (Hemler, 1990). Because VLA-4 is not prominently expressed on neutrophils, the relative expression of ICAM versus VCAM can determine the nature of the local inflammatory response. ICAM and VCAM are members of the immunoglobulin superfamily; the selectins all contain the types of structural motifs found in CR1 and the other RCA proteins. Blocking of any of the three types of adhesion molecules—integrins, selectins, or ICAM/VCAMs—by monoclonal antibodies can be used to modify immune and inflammatory responses in animal models and will surely lead to new forms of therapy for a wide variety of diseases in the near future.

Modulation of CR Expression

There are relatively few C3b or iC3b receptors on the surface of resting neutrophils in peripheral blood; on exposure to chemoattractants, however, these proteins are rapidly brought to the surface by translocation from an intracellular pool. Thus, each activated cell may express 40,000 to 50,000 CR1 molecules and 80,000 to 100,000 CR3 molecules (Fearon and Collins, 1983; Berger et al., 1984). Enhanced expression of CR1 and CR3 is important in increasing the adherence and phagocytic activity of cells at inflammatory sites (Kay et al., 1979). CR1 and CR3 are also found on large granular lymphocytes and can enhance antibody-dependent cellular cytotoxicity in a manner analogous to their role in enhancing phagocytosis (Perlmann et al., 1981).

As noted earlier, the neutrophils of newborn babies are partially deficient in CR3 and do not increase expression of this molecule normally when they are activated, although they do increase CR1 expression equally to the neutrophils of adults (Bruce et al., 1987; Abughali et al., 1994). This deficient CR3 expression contributes to decreased adherence, chemotaxis, and phagocytosis by the newborn's cells and increased susceptibility to infection.

Immune Complex Clearance

Another important role of C3 fragments and their receptors is solubilization and clearance of immune complexes. Early work by Miller and Nussenzweig (1975) demonstrated that insoluble antigen-antibody complexes can be solubilized by incubation in excess complement. Solubilization is caused by disruption of the ordered antigen-antibody lattice by C3b molecules that become bound during complement activation, resulting in smaller soluble complexes. This process may mobilize immune aggregates that form or localize in critical sites such as glomeruli or joints. In addition, bound C3 fragments are necessary for recognition, binding, and ingestion of immune complexes consisting of IgM or other non-IgG antibodies because the RES macrophages lack Fc receptors for antibodies other than IgG. The importance of this is emphasized by the observations of immune complex deposits and glomerulonephritis in patients with C3 deficiency (Pussell et al., 1980; Berger et al., 1983).

Cytolysis and the Membrane Attack Complex

In contrast to the effects already discussed that require the interaction of complement components with phagocytic cells, the complement system can generate direct cytolytic activity by the formation of the membrane attack complex.

Steps Involved in Membrane Attack Complex Formation

The first step in formation of this complex is the activation of C5 by the classical or alternative pathway C5 convertases, which cleave the α chain of the native molecule at a single site, releasing the small NH_2-terminal peptide C5a. The large fragment, C5b, undergoes conformational changes that increase its lipophilicity and allow it to complex with the next component in the sequence, C6. The C5b is stabilized by binding to C6, and the C5b6 complex can insert into lipid membranes at a distance from the C5 convertase. Because of the affinity of C5b for C3b, however, insertion is most likely to occur at or near the site of activation (Hammer et al., 1976).

In some cases, the C5b generated by a convertase on one cell or in the fluid phase complexes with C6 and deposits on another cell. Because the subsequent steps in the pathway do not involve enzymatic cleavage by earlier components, any cell on which C5b6 deposits can be lysed by the activity of the later components C7 to C9. This phenomenon of *bystander* or *reactive lysis* may be an important mechanism of tissue injury in infectious and immunologic diseases, particularly those in which soluble antigen-antibody complexes are thought to be pathogenic.

C5b6 then acts as an acceptor for C7, which can bind either on the cell surface or in the fluid phase, forming a C5b67 trimolecular complex. This complex is highly hydrophobic and readily inserts into lipid membranes. It can also react with serum lipoproteins or with protein S, also known as *vitronectin,* presumably through hydrophobic interactions, in which case it no longer interacts with cell membranes.

The C5b67 complex is the binding site for C8. If this interaction occurs in the fluid phase, the attachment of C8 reduces the ability of the complex to bind to lipid membranes and thus inhibits its activity (Nemerow et al., 1979). Addition of C8 to membrane-bound C5b67, however, forms an active complex that can cause erythrocyte lysis even in the absence of C9. This complex can bind phospholipids and apparently disrupts the integrity of the phospholipid bilayer and increases the permeability of the cell. At this step in the lytic sequence, there is no morphologically recognizable membrane lesion or pore (Podack et al., 1979).

The assembled membrane attack complex as extracted from membranes is composed of one molecule each of C5b, C6, C7, and C8 and three to six C9 molecules. Thus the C5b-8 complex serves as a nidus for polymerization of C9 (Mayer et al., 1981; Podack et al., 1982; Müller-Eberhard, 1984; Podack and Tschopp, 1984).

Isolated C9 can also polymerize when incubated at elevated temperatures or for a prolonged time. These polymers appear under electron microscopy as hollow rings or donuts that resemble the membrane attack complex; both structures appear to contain disulfide-linked C9 dimers (Ware and Kolb, 1981; Podack and Tschopp, 1984). Binding to C5b-8 causes the C9 molecules to elongate and unfold, exposing previously hidden hydrophobic domains and allowing disulfide exchange to occur. Evidence in favor of conformational changes in C9 is provided by the report of a monoclonal antibody that reacts with polymerized C9 and the membrane attack complex but not with native C9 or other complement components (Falk et al., 1983).

The detergent-extracted complex appears as an annulus, 15 to 20 nm in diameter, that sits above the membrane connected to a somewhat smaller diameter cylindrical stalk 15 to 16 nm long that spans the hydrophobic bilayer of the membrane (Bhakdi and Tranum-Jensen, 1979). When this complex is formed in a cell membrane, it functions as an open channel allowing an influx of water into the cell and leading to osmotic lysis with release of the cellular contents into the medium. In some nucleated cells, the initial membrane damage can be repaired, but with erythrocytes and most bacteria, a single complement hole is sufficient for lysis. Hence the process may be described as a "one-hit" phenomenon.

Although C9 deficiency has not been associated with any clinical problems, recurrent *Neisseria* infections in patients deficient in C5, C6, C7, or C8 suggest that the membrane attack complex may be necessary for defense against gram-negative bacteria even in the presence of normal opsonization and phagocytosis (Ross and Densen, 1984).

Control of Membrane Attack Complex Formation

Although studies with monoclonal antibodies to neoantigens on the membrane attack complex suggest that it is formed during complement activation in a variety of inflammatory processes, there are also proteins that protect autologous cells against damage by this lytic activity. First, lipoproteins, protein S, and other plasma proteins can bind or scavenge C5b-7 in the fluid phase and prevent its attachment to adjacent cell membranes (Podack and Müller-Eberhard, 1978).

In addition, there are two membrane proteins that inhibit formation of the complete membrane attack complex. These are the 20,000-dalton proteins known as CD59, the *membrane inhibitor of reactive lysis* (MIRL), or *protectin;* and a 65,000-dalton protein known as the *homologous restriction factor* (HRF) or *C8-binding protein* (C8bp) (Lachmann, 1991; Morgan and Meri, 1994). These last two proteins act after C8 has become bound to the C5b67 complex and prevent the polymerization and binding of C9, thus interfering with the formation of full lytic complexes. Both CD59 and HRF are linked to the cell membrane by glycolipid phosphatidylinositol anchors, as is DAF.

All three proteins can thus be released from cell membranes by exogenous phosphatidylinositol phospholipase C (PIPLC), which increases the sensitivity of the cell to attack by human complement. The three proteins are deficient on affected red blood cells in the condition known as paroxysmal nocturnal hemoglobinuria, which is now known to be a disorder in which clones of cells cannot make glycolipid anchors efficiently (see Chapter 17).

Virus Neutralization

Another activity of the complement system not requiring the participation of host cells is direct virus neutralization. Complement coats the viral surface, interfering with the ability of the virus to bind to the host cell (Oldstone, 1975; Cooper and Nemerow, 1983). Some viruses, including oncornaviruses, may bind and activate C1 directly and can thus be inactivated by early classical pathway components even in the absence of antibody. Lysis of the lipid coat requiring the later components may also be an important inactivation mechanism of enveloped viruses. The membranes of cultured cells, when infected with certain viruses, may activate the alternative pathway (Cooper and Nemerow, 1983). Complement might then distinguish between normal and infected cells and could lyse the latter directly or facilitate antibody-mediated or lymphocyte-mediated cytotoxicity. The contribution of these activities to host defense is uncertain, inasmuch as severe or disseminated viral infection does not seem to occur in complement-deficient patients.

Immunoregulatory Effects

The complement system may provide important immunoregulatory signals, including a role in the afferent limb of the antibody response. Although earlier investigations suggested normal antibody levels in complement-deficient individuals, some studies indicate that C4 deficiency in humans and guinea pigs diminishes the response to phage antigen φX174 and interferes with the normal switch from IgM to IgG production (Jackson et al., 1979). This defect can be corrected by administration of C4 (to the guinea pigs), indicating that it is not a separate linked defect (Ochs et al., 1983). Möller and Coutinho (1975) found that polyclonal B-cell activators, such as lipopolysaccharide and pneumococcal polysaccharide, caused the proliferation of mouse spleen cells and the generation of immunoglobulin-producing cells in an in vitro plaque-forming assay

at lower doses when they had bound C3 after exposure to fresh serum than when they were exposed to inactivated serum or buffer alone. Presumably, the C3 fragments bound to the activators can also interact with CR1 and CR2 on the lymphocytes, thus anchoring the complex and promoting the interaction of the activator with the cell.

Complement depletion by administration of cobra venom factor to experimental animals also decreases antibody responses, particularly to T-dependent antigens (Pepys, 1976). In this situation, the anamnestic response and the switch to IgG production are affected more than the primary response. Studies with labeled antigen suggest that complement fragments and receptors localize antigens to the dendritic cells in the spleen and lymphoid follicles. After complement depletion, there is decreased persistence of antigen at these sites (Klaus et al., 1980). Because dendritic cells play an important role in antigen presentation and in the generation of immunologic memory, interference with complement-mediated localization of antigen-antibody complexes might impair secondary IgG production more than primary IgM responses.

The anaphylatoxins C3a and C5a may affect T-cell function, with C3a suppressing and C5a enhancing proliferative responses. These effects are highly dependent on the exact mitogen system used and are observed only in serum-free media or in the presence of enzyme inhibitors that block the ability of carboxypeptidase to inactivate the anaphylatoxins (Morgan et al., 1982; Weigle et al., 1983; Fleisher and Berger, 1984). The relevance of these reports as well as observations that C3 degradation products may impair B-cell responses to physiologic immune responses in vitro require further clarification.

MEASUREMENT OF COMPLEMENT AND ITS COMPONENTS

The primary clinical use of complement assays is in the diagnosis and assessment of complement activation in disease (e.g., in systemic lupus erythematosus). Complement levels are also measured in some patients with increased susceptibility to infection (see Chapters 9 and 17). The serum level of a complement component reflects the balance between its synthetic and catabolic rates. Most complement proteins have rapid catabolic rates, with half-lives of about 1 day in most individuals (Ruddy et al., 1975). Although a relatively small increase in catabolic rate of a given component might be expected to lead to a rapid decrease in its serum concentration, this is often not the case because the synthetic rate often increases concomitantly.

Several of the complement components are *acute phase reactants* (Alper, 1974); hence, the presence of normal levels does not exclude involvement of complement in a given disorder. The best method to assess complement metabolism is by using turnover studies with purified radioactively labeled components; such methods are available at only a few research centers. Serum assays for complement fragments that are released during activation such as C3a des-Arg, or for degradation products, such as C3d, may be used to assess complement activation independent of the actual concentration of the native components.

Functional Hemolytic Assays

Complement components can be measured by functional methods, usually in hemolytic assays, or by immunochemical methods (Gaither and Frank, 1979). Hemolytic assays are more sensitive but require special reagents and expertise. In addition, specimens for functional assays must be handled carefully because the components lose activity rapidly at room temperature, and if immune complexes or other activators are present, continued consumption of the components occurs after the sample is obtained. Accordingly, chelators such as ethylenediaminetetra-acetic acid (EDTA) are used, but they can interfere with other functional assays.

The total hemolytic complement activity is measured as the serum dilution that will lyse 50% of a standard preparation of sheep erythrocytes sensitized with specific rabbit antibody. The result is termed the CH_{50} and is usually expressed as the reciprocal of the serum dilution that gives 50% hemolysis. This test is normally used to determine the functional integrity of the classical pathway; however, it is relatively insensitive, and severe depletion of individual components may occur without altering the CH_{50}. A similar assay for the alternative pathway can be performed using unsensitized rabbit erythrocytes, which directly activate the alternative pathway. This is termed the *alternative pathway* H_{50} and gives comparable information on those components. However, falsely elevated readings are obtained in the presence of rabbit erythrocyte antibodies. A rapid semiquantitative assay of classical or alternative complement activity uses glass slides coated with a thin layer of agarose gel in which sensitized sheep erythrocytes or rabbit erythrocytes have been incorporated. A circular zone of hemolysis occurs around a well in which a serum has been added; the size of the circle is proportional to the hemolytic activity of the serum.

Functional titration of individual components is performed by a variation of the basic hemolytic assay. All components other than the one being assayed are present in excess; the serum to be tested supplies the component in question. Often, preformed intermediates, such as $EAC\overline{14}$ or EAC1–7, are used to increase the efficiency and sensitivity of these assays. Sera from humans or animals with isolated single component deficiencies or reagents prepared by mixing appropriate amounts of isolated purified components can also be used to ensure that only a single component is being measured. The results are expressed as the serum dilution that gives a standard degree of hemolysis under defined conditions.

Immunochemical Assays

Immunochemical methods (e.g., radial immunodiffusion and automated nephelometry) are used by most laboratories to determine serum levels of individual components. Specific antisera are used to measure the total level of the component present, and the results are usually expressed as micrograms per unit volume of serum. These immunoassays may be misleading, however, because many of the antisera react with degradation products in addition to intact native components, so the results obtained do not correlate with functional determinations. In the case of C3, crossed immunoelectrophoresis allows direct estimation of the amount of native C3 relative to the amounts of C3c and C3d that might have been formed during activation.

Activation Assays

Commercially available radioimmunoassays have been developed to quantitate anaphylatoxins in serum. They usually employ an acid precipitation step so that the native components are not detected. The inhibition of binding of ^{125}I-C3a, C4a, or C5a to a fixed amount of antibody by unlabeled anaphylatoxin of the test serum is measured (Chenowith and Hugli, 1980). These assays avoid the problems of cross-reactivity of native components and degradation fragments and assess the degree of activation occurring, independent of the total concentration of the component.

Fluorescent-conjugated antibodies to individual components (e.g., C1q, C3, C4, properdin, or factor B) are used to identify sites of complement activation or deposition in tissue sections, and assessment of the pathway by which the activation occurred can sometimes be made. In addition, antibodies to neoantigens exposed during formation of the membrane attack complex have been frequently used to localize deposition of these proteins in a number of diseases (Falk et al., 1983).

Clinical Applications

CH_{50} activity is the best test to indicate whether an individual component of the classical pathway component is lacking and is thus particularly valuable in screening for suspected complement deficiency. In inflammatory or autoimmune diseases, the usual assessment of a patient's complement status, or profile, involves measurement of both CH_{50} and C3 levels. In addition, measurement of factor B or properdin and C4 may allow the determination of which activation pathway is primarily involved. Depression of C4 with a normal factor B indicates that the classical pathway is activated, whereas a normal C4 with depressed factor B or properdin levels indicates alternative pathway activation. In either case, the C3 level and probably the CH_{50} level are usually depressed.

Complement Fixation

Complement fixation tests are widely used to detect and quantitate specific antigens and antibodies in biologic fluids. To determine the presence of antibody, for example, a known amount of antigen is incubated with a sample of fresh serum. If antibody is present, complexes form and the complement in the serum is activated or "fixed." After suitable incubation, sensitized erythrocytes are added. Because the complement activated by the antigen-antibody complexes is no longer available to react with the erythrocytes, a diminished amount of lysis is observed. Complement fixation tests are widely used in the diagnosis of infectious diseases because a common set of reagents can be used to measure many antigen-antibody combinations and the amplification provided by the complement system makes the assays quite sensitive. Obviously, IgA, IgE, and IgG4 antibodies will not be detected by these assays because they do not activate the classical pathway measured in the detection phase.

Immune Complex Assays

Several assays for measuring circulating antigen-antibody or immune complexes use complement components as reagents or assess the binding of complement fragments to the complexes (Lawley and Frank, 1980; Theofilopoulos and Dixon, 1979). The C1q binding assay takes advantage of the ability of the multiple Fc binding sites on the C1q molecule to interact with antigen-antibody complexes. After C1q binding, the complexes are precipitated, leaving free antibodies and nonbound C1q in solution. The use of ^{125}I-C1q permits measurement of the amount of C1q precipitated, which is proportional to the amount of complexed antibody in serum. Only IgG and IgM complexes are detected by this method.

Other assays take advantage of the fact that the C3 fragments become bound to the antigen-antibody complexes during complement activation. Thus, antibodies to C3 and its fragments are coupled to solid phase surfaces, and then conjugated anti–human immunoglobulin reagents are used to detect the antibodies in the complex with radioactive or enzyme-linked assay systems. Similar assays can also be performed using conglutinin, a bovine protein that binds to iC3b, or Raji cells, a human lymphoblastoid cell culture line that bears CR2 receptors, to trap the C3-containing complexes. These methods allow the detection of complexes that activate either the classical or alternative pathway. Another method to measure alternative pathway activation uses enzyme-linked immunosorbent assay (ELISA) techniques and antiproperdin antibodies to detect complexes containing properdin and C3b (Cooper et al., 1983).

COMPLEMENT GENETICS

Several of the complement components have multiple alleles; these allotypes can be distinguished by variations in their electrophoretic mobility (Alper and Rosen, 1976). Although there may be subtle differences, the allotypes are similar in functional activity.

The genes for C2, C4, and factor B are on chromosome 6 as part of the major histocompatibility complex (MHC) (Alper, 1981; Colten et al., 1981). Determina-

tion of an individual's *complotype* (the allotype of each polymorphic protein) correlates with the incidence of certain diseases, such as juvenile diabetes mellitus. The reasons for this association are not known; although it may reflect a functional abnormality in the complement system, it is more likely that the particular complement allotype genes are linked to one or more immune response genes of the MHC that regulate, in turn, the occurrence of abnormal or selectively deficient immune responses.

There are two separate C4 loci in the genome of humans and animals; alleles at both positions have been described. Interestingly, the protein coded for by one of these genes has more hemolytic activity than the other. These two gene products are related to the Chido and Rogers blood group antigens, which represent fragments of two different C4 products.

The human C3 gene is on chromosome 19, and this protein also has multiple alleles. C3, C4, and C5 are apparently encoded by single genes and synthesized as single-chain polypeptide precursors, which are subsequently cleaved before secretion (Hall and Colten, 1977; Colten et al., 1981). As much as 5% of serum C4 may be in the single-chain pro-C4 form; other incompletely cleaved intermediates have also been described. The mechanism by which the unique thioester bond is formed during C3 and C4 synthesis has not yet been elucidated.

Unlike the other multichain components synthesized as single-chain precursors, the three chains of C8 are products of two different, apparently unlinked genes.

The C3b receptor CR1 also has a number of allotypic structural variants; it is not known whether these correlate with the C3 allotypes of the same individual or have different binding affinities or functions (Dykman et al., 1984; Wong et al., 1983). The quantitative expression of this receptor on erythrocytes is apparently also under genetic control; high- and low-expression genotypes give rise to three patterns of receptor expression, high and low homozygotes, and intermediate heterozygotes (Wilson et al., 1982). Although low levels of erythrocyte CR1 expression occur in patients with systemic lupus erythematosus and their families, the role of additional nongenetic factors that govern quantitative CR1 expression have not been elucidated (Iida et al., 1982; Wilson et al., 1982).

As noted earlier, many of the proteins that interact with C3b and C4b and regulate their function share structural homology, and their genes are all grouped within a region of chromosome 1 that has become known as the regulator of complement activation (RCA) cluster. It is not known whether common control elements coordinate the expression of multiple members of this family.

COMPLEMENT SYNTHESIS

Cellular Sources

In vitro organ culture and in vivo tissue localization methods indicate that many types of cells synthesize complement components (Colten, 1976). The intestinal epithelial cells are the most important source of C1 in the body, and parenchymal cells of the liver are the major synthetic site of C3 and most other components. This was nicely demonstrated by observing shifts in the allotypes of these proteins after liver transplantation (Alper et al., 1969). C4 and C2 and the regulatory proteins H and I can be synthesized by monocytes and macrophages (Whaley, 1980). Increased production of these components by activated phagocytic cells during inflammatory reactions may partly explain why these are acute phase reactants. Teleologically, it may be advantageous to synthesize complement components locally so they are available at sites of inflammation. An example is the C3 synthesis by synovial tissue in patients with active rheumatoid arthritis (Ruddy and Colten, 1974).

Complement in the Fetus and Newborn

Complement synthesis by fetal tissues has been observed as early as 5½ weeks of gestational age (Gitlin and Biasucci, 1969; Gitlin and Gitlin, 1975). Studies in complement-deficient mothers and in situations in which the fetus synthesizes a different complement allotype from that of the mother indicate that complement proteins do not cross the placenta. C3, C4, and most other components are detectable in fetal serum by 10 weeks; levels increase progressively with gestational age, reaching about 50 to 75% of the maternal levels at term. As complement levels in the maternal circulation generally rise during pregnancy, this corresponds to 60 to 80% of normal adult levels. This is true for the CH_{50}, most of the early classical components, and factor B, but the levels of C8 and C9 are lower and may reach only 10% of the maternal concentration at term (Ballow et al., 1978). By contrast, C1 esterase inhibitor is present in full adult concentrations as early as the 28th week of gestation.

Preterm and low-birth-weight infants have lower complement levels than do full-term babies, but by 3 months of age, most infants' complement levels are within the normal adult range; (Fireman et al., 1969; Sawyer et al., 1971). The relatively low levels of C3, factor B, and other components of neonates, particularly of low-birth-weight babies, may be responsible for the decreased opsonic activity of their serum and may contribute to their increased susceptibility to infection. Lack of the usual febrile response and leukocytosis accompanying infection in some babies may also be related in part to the low complement component levels (see Chapter 10).

Besides the low complement levels, phagocytic host defenses in newborns may be further compromised by the neonatal neutrophils' partial deficiency of CR3, which results in decreased adherence and complement-dependent phagocytosis when the cells are activated (Abughali et al., 1994, Bruce et al., 1987).

COMPLEMENT IN DISEASE

The role of complement in host defense has been discussed previously; there are also several diseases usually thought of as autoimmune in nature in which complement activation plays a major pathogenic role (see Chapter 17). In these illnesses, the complement cascade functions appropriately but activation is induced by antibody directed against a normal body constituent or as part of an immune complex deposited in otherwise normal tissue, such as DNA–anti-DNA complexes in the kidney in lupus.

Illnesses in which the complement system itself is defective are rare. Examples include patients with deficiencies of the regulatory proteins—C1-esterase inhibitor in hereditary angioedema and factor I (C3 inactivator) in C3 deficiency—and those with the C3 nephritic factor, which causes the alternative pathway to escape from control. In most acute infections, complement levels are normal or elevated, reflecting their role as acute phase reactants. In several of the conditions discussed in this section, the rate of synthesis is lower than the rate of consumption, resulting in decreased complement levels. Serum complement determinations may then be used as a laboratory measure of disease activity. Although many of these illnesses are discussed later (see Chapter 17, Disorders of the Complement System), a brief discussion of complement activation in these diseases may be useful here.

Hemolytic Anemias

Complement fixation on erythrocytes is dependent on the type and affinity of antibodies sensitizing the cell and the number and distribution of antigenic sites on the cell surface (Frank et al., 1977; Rubin, 1977). Many cases of autoimmune hemolytic anemia in childhood are of an acute transient nature caused by IgG antibodies, which bind to erythrocyte Rh antigens at body temperature and are thus called *warm antibodies.* These antibodies fix complement poorly because there are insufficient IgG molecules to form the doublets needed for C1 activation. Thus, fewer than half of these patients have a positive non-gamma Coombs' test for C3 fragments on the erythrocytes. Erythrocyte destruction occurs primarily in the spleen, where the cells are sequestered by binding to the Fc receptors of the macrophages and phagocytosed. If the IgG antibody activates complement, C3 fragments may accelerate destruction of these cells because the complement-coated erythrocytes will bind to C3b receptors in addition to the Fc receptors on the macrophages. Rarely, a patient with a fulminant case presents with acute intravascular hemolysis and hemoglobinuria. The explanation for this appears to relate to the titer, affinity, and specificity of the antibody. Antibodies such as anti-Fya, which generate many complement-fixing sites per cell, lead to marked activation of the complement system and substantial direct lysis.

The rapid therapeutic response to corticosteroids in autoimmune hemolytic anemia patients is due to interference with phagocytic function of the splenic macrophages rather than to interference with antibody production, antibody binding, or complement activation. The effect of chronic corticosteroid therapy may be caused by decreased antibody synthesis over a long period.

Cold Agglutinin Disease

Cold agglutinin disease is uncommon in children but may occur following *Mycoplasma* infections. In this situation, the antibody is usually a polyclonal IgM with anti-I specificity. It is generally self-limited and differs from cold agglutinin disease in adults, which is associated with a monoclonal IgM occurring either in malignancies or arising spontaneously. In cold agglutinin disease, the IgM antibodies bind to the erythrocytes at temperatures below 37°C with complement fixation. Antibody binding and complement fixation may occur in the peripheral circulation of the extremities. The erythrocytes, now coated with complement, return to the central vasculature and are then removed from the circulation by binding to the C3b receptors of the reticuloendothelial system (RES), particularly the hepatic Kupffer cells. The IgM itself does not cause clearance because it elutes from the cell at core body temperature and because macrophages lack Fc receptors for IgM.

Some of the C3b initially bound to the red blood cell undergoes cleavage by factor I with the assistance of factor H or CR1, which also has cofactor activity. Cleavage of C3b may occur on either the erythrocyte or the macrophage before phagocytosis occurs. The erythrocyte is returned to the circulation, where it subsequently has a normal survival even though it will react with Coombs' reagents that recognize C3d.

The fragment of C3 on these erythrocytes is identical to a serum degradation product of C3 termed α2d, a fragment slightly larger than the C3d fragment produced by trypsin cleavage in vitro (Harrison and Lachmann, 1980). The additional segment found on the physiologic fragment is recognizable by a monoclonal antibody that does not react with trypsin-cleaved C3d; hence, α2d has also been designated C3dg (see Fig. 7–2).

Hemolytic Disease of the Newborn

The isoimmune red blood cell destruction in hemolytic disease of the newborn probably does not involve complement; indeed, serum complement levels in babies with this condition are normal for their gestational age (Ewald et al., 1961). The transplacental maternal IgG anti-Rh(D) antibodies fix complement poorly; the cells are destroyed in the RES following Fc-mediated clearance, as previously discussed.

Hemolytic disease of the newborn due to ABO incompatibility probably does not involve complement fixation either, but this has not been examined in detail. Hemolysis in ABO-incompatible blood transfusion stands in marked contrast, however. The sera of most individuals over 9 months of age contains IgM isohemagglutinins against major blood group antigens not found on their own cells. These antibodies fix complement well, and massive intravascular hemolysis may follow mismatched transfusion. Fortunately, IgM antibodies do not cross the placenta, and their presence in the maternal circulation diminishes the risk of maternal sensitization to incompatible fetal erythrocytes.

Paroxysmal Nocturnal Hemoglobinuria

Paroxysmal nocturnal hemoglobinuria (PNH) is a rare disorder in which the red blood cells as well as other blood elements acquire membrane defects rendering them unusually sensitive to complement-induced lysis. Multiple populations of normal and abnormal cells may be present in a single patient at any given time (Rosse, 1973). Antibody is probably not involved in this process, and the abnormal cells are lysed intravascularly. It seems likely that a constant low-level activation of the alternative pathway takes place as a normal result of C3 tickover. Some of the C3b molecules deposit on the surface of normal erythrocytes, but further alternative pathway activation is usually prevented by the action of factor I for which the erythrocyte CR1 can serve as a cofactor (Iida and Nussenzweig, 1981). Erythrocytes also contain a membrane protein (DAF), which promotes dissociation of Bb from C3b and thus also limits the activation of the alternative pathway. Absence of DAF has been reported in PNH (Pangburn et al., 1983; Nicholson-Weller et al., 1983), but there are other defects as well because in addition to bearing increased numbers of C3b molecules, PNH cells also have increased susceptibility to lysis by C5b-9 (Packman et al., 1979). The increased susceptibility to lysis by the membrane attack complex is probably due to deficiencies of the membrane proteins that normally protect against assembly of full lytic complexes containing C9 (see Cytolysis and the Membrane Attack Complex earlier in this chapter).

These proteins, CD59 (protectin or MIRL) and C8 binding protein (homologous restriction factor), are, like DAF, linked to the membrane by glycolipid phosphatidylinositol anchors. It is now recognized that PNH is caused by abnormalities in the synthesis of these anchors (Morgan and Meri, 1994). Because of defects in limiting complement activation at the cell surface, the continuous low-grade alternative pathway activation is sufficient to cause lysis of the PNH erythrocytes (see Chapter 17).

The Ham test involves acidification of serum, facilitating spontaneous activation of the alternative pathway. Lysis of PNH erythrocytes, but not normal erythrocytes, occurs, so the test is diagnostic for PNH. The *sugar water test* induces lysis by the classical pathway by allowing low-avidity autoantibodies (present in all normal sera) to bind to the red blood cells at low ionic strength. Normal erythrocytes are not lysed under either of these conditions because they are relatively resistant to lysis by the membrane attack complex of human complement and, as noted previously, contain a number of protective mechanisms that limit complement activation on their surfaces.

Drug-Induced Hemolytic Anemias

Drug-induced hemolytic anemias occur by three mechanisms (Worlledge, 1973). The most common type of drug-induced sensitization is found in patients taking methyldopa (Aldomet). This drug somehow stimulates production of IgG warm antibodies with anti-Rh specificity. Although a positive Coombs' test is common, significant hemolysis is rare. The hemolytic process, when it occurs, is identical to that associated with other warm antibody hemolytic anemias previously discussed. These patients have a positive IgG Coombs' test during the course of therapy, but the drug itself is not bound to the red blood cell nor does it react with the antibody. The drug's primary mode of action in this disorder seems to be an alteration of immunoregulation, allowing B lymphocytes that produce Rh antibodies to escape from suppression. Most patients have a gradual reversal of their Coombs' positivity over several months after withdrawal of the drug.

A second type of drug-induced hemolytic anemia accompanies high-dose therapy with penicillin or other drugs and is caused by the binding of active drug metabolites to erythrocytes and/or proteins in the circulation. These drug metabolites then act as haptens and induce the production of antibodies that bind to the drug molecule and fix complement on the cell surface. Both the direct antiglobulin Coombs' test and the non-gamma Coombs' test are positive. These antibodies do not bind to erythrocytes in the absence of the drug but do bind to another individual's erythrocytes if the latter have first been reacted with the drug in vitro. In the presence of antibody and complement, these sensitized cells are rapidly cleared from the circulation or lysed intravascularly. Because the drug is responsible for the antibody binding, this condition abates quickly when the drug is discontinued.

The third type occurs with quinine, quinidine, or a similar drug. These compounds attach to serum proteins and act as haptens. When antibodies are produced, soluble immune complexes form that may transiently adhere to the red blood cells and fix complement but then readily dissociate. For the erythrocytes, the results of the non-gamma Coombs' test are positive but no antibody can be detected; they are thus damaged as innocent bystanders (the antibody is not directed to the erythrocytes). Similar mechanisms may occur during infectious diseases that are accompanied by immune complex formation. Because the drug or a microbial product is part of the antigen, this form of hemolytic anemia resolves promptly after therapy is discontinued or the infection is eradicated.

Many autoimmune or drug-related hemolytic anemias are accompanied by thrombocytopenia and/or neutropenia as a result of similar pathophysiologic processes. Postinfectious idiopathic thrombocytopenic purpura may also result from a similar mechanism. The role of complement in antibody-mediated destruction of platelets and neutrophils seems to be exactly analogous to its role in erythrocyte destruction. Thus, at low levels of antibody, complement accelerates clearance by the reticuloendothelial system; at high levels of antibody, however, complement may cause direct intravascular lysis.

Immune Complex Diseases

Circulating or deposited antigen-antibody complexes are implicated in the pathogenesis of a number of clinical problems (Theofilopoulos and Dixon, 1979; Lawley and Frank, 1980). Acute serum sickness is the prototype of immune complex disease, such as that occurring after the administration of heterologous antilymphocyte serum for the treatment of aplastic anemia (Cochrane, 1984; Lawley et al., 1984). The manifestations of serum sickness (fever, rash, arthralgias, adenopathy, proteinuria and, in some cases, glomerulonephritis) result from local deposition of immune complexes. These are formed in moderate antigen excess during the early antibody response to an injected foreign serum protein or to antigens released during an infection. Complement is activated with a fall of CH_{50}, C3, and C4 and an elevation of activation products, such as the C3a anaphylatoxin. The complexes can be detected by any of the assays previously discussed. Circulating leukocytes are attracted by local complement activation and by chemoattractants released from tissue macrophages or other cells; severe local inflammatory damage ensues.

When acute serum sickness follows a single administration of foreign protein, the complexes are cleared from the circulation rapidly and symptoms are transient and self-limited. The process is similar when the host defenses eradicate the organisms responsible for an acute infection. However, if the antigenic stimulus continues, progressive and severe multiple organ damage can occur. Prolonged depression of serum complement results from chronic activation by immune complexes. RES function may become compromised leading to further deposition in sensitive sites such as the kidney. Similarly, primary complement component or receptor deficiency may predispose the individual to suboptimal RES function and tissue deposition of immune complexes (Peters and Lachmann, 1974; Berger et al., 1983). This cascade of events is probably implicated in the development of glomerulonephritis that accompanies bacterial endocarditis, infected ventriculoatrial shunts, and persistent viral infections. The occurrence of immune complex diseases in cases of complement and/or receptor deficiency and in cases in which the antibodies fail to fix complement efficiently emphasizes the important physiologic role of the complement system in normal clearance of antigen-antibody complexes (Schifferli et al., 1986, Fearon; 1988).

Systemic Lupus Erythematosus

Although the underlying cause of systemic lupus erythematosus (SLE) is not known, many clinical manifestations result from the formation of immune complexes containing DNA and other nuclear antigens (Schur, 1975). Such complexes are present in skin, glomeruli, and other involved organs. Immunofluorescent staining reveals the presence of C1q, C4, and C3 associated with these complexes in the tissues and indicates classical pathway activation. Properdin and factor B have been identified at the same sites, suggesting alternative pathway activation also. Immunofluorescent study of unaffected skin in lupus patients shows deposits of antibody and complement at the dermal-epidermal junction, giving a positive lupus band test. The complement membrane attack complex is also present in the skin and glomeruli. Complement consumption is accelerated, outstripping the synthetic rates that are normal or only slightly elevated (Ruddy et al., 1975). Accordingly, serum complement levels are depressed during active systemic lupus erythematosus, particularly if there is renal involvement (see Chapters 24 and 25). Some lupus patients have diminished C3 synthesis during exacerbations, suggesting alterations in the control of component synthesis. Thus, CH_{50}, C3, and C4 levels are of value in the diagnosis and continuing assessment of the disease; normalization of levels indicates remission or a favorable response to therapy. C4 levels may be particularly valuable in this regard.

Juvenile Rheumatoid Arthritis

Immune complexes are not a regular feature of juvenile rheumatoid arthritis (JRA), although many of the clinical manifestations resemble immune complex disorders (see Chapter 24). Serum complement levels are generally normal or elevated, reflecting their role as acute phase reactants. Synovial fluid from inflamed joints contains lower levels of C3 than serum, and the presence of degradation fragments indicates intra-articular complement activation (Rynes et al., 1974). Chemotactic factor generation within the joint leads to leukocyte infiltration; release of lysosomal enzymes leads to a destructive inflammatory process. Similar events may occur in adult rheumatoid arthritis, but there may also be intra-articular deposition of rheumatoid factor (IgM)-IgG complexes (Zvaifler, 1973). By contrast, joint fluids of degenerative arthritides do not reveal evidence of complement activation.

Henoch-Schönlein Purpura

Henoch-Schönlein purpura has many features in common with other immune complex diseases, but besides cutaneous, renal, and joint involvement, gastrointestinal dysfunction with intussusception may occur. In many cases, there is a history of antecedent viral infection, which may be implicated by the elevated serum IgA levels and IgA-containing immune complexes (Levy et al., 1976). CH_{50}, C3, and classical pathway component levels are normal in the disease, but in some cases, properdin and factor B are depressed (Levy et al., 1976; Spitzer et al., 1978). Immunofluorescent studies of renal biopsies show deposition of IgA, C3, and properdin, suggesting that Henoch-Schönlein purpura is an IgA immune complex disorder with unknown antigens. Because IgA does not bind to Fc receptors, bind C1q, or activate the classical complement

pathway, clearance of these complexes may be inefficient. Thus, renal and other tissue injury may result from deposition of these complexes with local activation of the alternative complement pathway (see Chapter 25).

Renal Disease and Transplantation

Many immune complex diseases are associated with nephritis, as evidenced by diminished levels of C3 and other components and immunofluorescent demonstration of complement proteins in renal biopsy sections (Wilson and Dixon, 1979; Cochrane, 1984). The presence of a glomerular receptor for C3b (Gelfand et al., 1975) suggests that complement-containing immune complexes may be specifically bound rather than passively trapped in the kidney. However, the role of this receptor is uncertain because antigen-antibody complexes are also found in the glomeruli of C3-deficient patients and in animals that lack this receptor. Local activation of the classical and/or alternative pathways may result in attraction and activation of leukocytes and release of vasoactive substances and lysosomal enzymes. Direct basement membrane damage caused by the late-acting complement components has been suggested by the presence of neoantigens of the membrane attack complex at this site (Falk et al., 1983). Local activation of the coagulation system may also contribute to the fibrin deposition seen in many nephritides. Mesangial proliferation may also be related to complex deposition or complement activation.

Membranoproliferative Glomerulonephritis and C3 Nephritic Factor

In the 1960s, West and McAdams described children with chronic glomerulonephritis and severely diminished levels of serum complement, which they called hypocomplementemic persistent nephritis (Spitzer et al., 1969; West and McAdams, 1978). Serum from these patients was found to cause rapid consumption of C3 when added to normal serum. The factor responsible for this C3 consumption was termed C3 nephritic factor (C3NeF); it has subsequently been found in the serum of patients with hypocomplementemia and lipodystrophy. C3NeF has been shown to be an IgG antibody to antigens on C3b that become exposed during formation of the alternative pathway C3 convertase $C\overline{3bBb}$ (Davis et al., 1977b). Binding of C3NeF results in abnormal stabilization of the convertase and renders it resistant to inactivation by factors H and I. The C3b formed by this convertase then participates in formation of additional active convertases; hence, there is rapid and unchecked activation of the C3 amplification loop in the fluid phase. Similar autoantibodies that react with and stabilize the classical pathway C3 convertase $C\overline{4b2a}$ have also been described in a few lupus patients (Halbwachs et al., 1980).

Addition of C3NeF to normal serum causes severe depletion of C3 and the later components, but C1, C4, and C2 levels are unaffected. Although it seems clear that this abnormal immunoglobulin is responsible for the hypocomplementemia, its role in the pathogenesis of the renal lesions is uncertain. Indeed, an infant of a mother with circulating C3NeF demonstrated transplacental passage of C3NeF; the infant had severe but self-limited hypocomplementemia but no evidence of nephritis (Davis et al., 1977a). Patients with other types of membranoproliferative glomerulonephritis lack this nephritic factor, although their serum may reveal immune complexes and evidence of classical pathway activation without severe depletion of complement components.

Hypocomplementemic membranoproliferative glomerulonephritis is a major cause of end-stage renal disease in children (see Chapter 25). C3 and C3NeF return to normal levels within 6 weeks after kidney transplantation in those patients who do not experience recurrence or rejection (Curtis et al., 1979). Patients in whom recurrent disease develops in the kidney graft show diminished serum levels of C3 and factor B with a reappearance of high levels of C3NeF. When the serum complement profile before transplantation indicates activation of the classical pathway, recurrence is often heralded by reduced levels of C1, C4, and C2 and depletion of later components.

Poststreptococcal Glomerulonephritis

The acute glomerulonephritis that accompanies streptococcal infections of the skin or pharynx is almost always associated with markedly diminished serum CH$_{50}$ and C3 levels (Nissenson et al., 1979). As the nephritis resolves, the complement levels increase, returning to normal 3 to 4 weeks after the onset of symptoms. The dense glomerular deposits and mesangial cell proliferation seen on electron microscopy resemble those of other immune complex diseases. IgG, properdin, and C3 may be present in these deposits. In this disease, activation of the alternative pathway by complexes containing antibody and an as yet uncharacterized streptococcal antigen probably occurs.

Allograft Rejection

Although kidney transplant rejection is primarily mediated by cellular mechanisms, humoral mechanisms can also play a role (Carpenter, 1974) (see Chapter 32). When a kidney is transplanted into a recipient with preformed antibodies against the donor's tissues, hyperacute rejection occurs, accompanied by severe endothelial damage with local activation of complement and other mediators of inflammation. In chronic or repeated episodes of rejection, antibody and complement may also play a role. Diminished serum levels of both classical and alternative pathway components are noted; turnover studies confirm increased complement catabolism. Immunofluorescent studies confirm that activation of both the classical and alternative pathways can contribute to allograft rejection (Carpenter, 1974; Fearon et al., 1977).

MOLECULAR MIMICRY OF COMPLEMENT PROTEINS BY INFECTIOUS AGENTS

It has been discovered that certain pathogens produce proteins that mimic normal human proteins and

thereby interfere with the inflammatory response (Cooper, 1991; Fishelson, 1994; Moffitt and Frank, 1994). This mimicry goes beyond the sialylation of bacterial capsules that inhibits alternative pathway activation; instead, it involves sequences or structures with homology to complement proteins or receptors. In some cases, the organism mimics a control protein and thus inhibits complement-mediated attack; in other cases, the organism interacts with the complement system in a way that favors its growth.

At least two of the herpesviruses—Epstein-Barr virus (EBV) and herpes simplex (HSV)—use molecular mimicry to facilitate infection of target cells (EBV) and to prevent complement-mediated attack on infected cells (HSV). The Epstein-Barr virus codes for a 350-kD major envelope protein containing a 9–amino acid sequence at its amino terminus that is strikingly similar to the sequence in C3d that interacts with complement receptor type 2 (CR2) (Nemerow et al., 1989). This sequence in gp350 allows the virus to bind to CR2. CR2 serves as the receptor by which the virus binds to B cells and activates the cells to cause internalization of the virus (Tanner et al., 1987). The Epstein-Barr virus also codes for a molecule that can regulate complement activation, similar to those for herpes simplex virus, as described next.

Human cells infected with herpes simplex virus type 1 express receptors for the Fc of IgG as well as a receptor for C3b, which are the products of separate viral genes. One of these is glycoprotein C1 (gC1), which is expressed on the surface of infected cells and can bind C3b and iC3b. Purified gC1 accelerates decay of the alternative pathway C3 convertase C3bBb and decreases the activity of C3bBb complexes (Fries et al., 1986). It can thus protect virus-infected cells from attack by the alternative pathway. It does not accelerate decay of classical pathway convertases or serve as a cofactor for C3b cleavage, but its activity can be blocked by some monoclonal antibodies against human complement receptor type 1 (CR1) (Fries et al., 1986; Kubota et al., 1987).

Herpes simplex virus type 2 codes for a similar protein, gC2, that has somewhat similar activity in that it binds C3b but does not accelerate decay of convertases. Although gC2 apparently is not expressed on the surface of infected cells, it is expressed on the surface of the virus itself; it protects virus-infected cells, but the mechanisms are not clear (McNearney et al., 1987; Harris et al., 1990). Although gC1 and gC2 have only limited sequence homology with members of the RCA group of proteins, some structural motifs are found in these proteins that resemble those of the individual SCRs that make up the RCA proteins. These include (1) conserved cysteine residues and disulfide-linked loops, (2) conserved tryptophan and glycine residues, and (3) a conserved N glycosylation site. It is likely that this structural homology gives rise to the functional homology.

Pox viruses also show molecular mimicry, but in secreted rather than cellular proteins. The 28,600-dalton protein termed *vaccinia control protein* is one of the most abundant products of infected cells and can bind both C3b and C4b. It contains four SCRs and is 38% homologous to the amino terminal half of human C4b-binding protein. Vaccinia control protein can accelerate decay of both classical and alternative pathway convertases and can act as a cofactor for factor I cleavage of both C4b and C3b (McKenzie et al., 1992). Presumably, high concentrations of vaccinia control protein in the milieu of infected cells limits attack on the cells by complement and complement receptor–bearing cells such as monocytes and natural killer cells; animal studies have shown that the presence of vaccinia control protein confers added pathogenicity to the viruses, as evidenced by the size of the skin lesions produced upon injection of the virus.

Candida albicans and other fungi also employ molecular mimicry. The pathogenic mycelial form of *Candida* synthesizes a surface protein that binds iC3b and C3d but not C3b (Edwards et al., 1986). Several monoclonal antibodies to CR2 and CR3 bind to the surface of cultured *Candida* organisms. At least some of the binding of complement fragments and these antibodies involves a protein that shares partial homology with the α chain of CR3 (Edwards, et al., 1986; Eigentler et al., 1989). This fungal receptor not only may interfere with local host defenses but also may help the organism satisfy its iron requirements by binding red blood cells that have been opsonized as bystanders when the alternative pathway of complement is activated by the fungus (Moors et al., 1992).

Histoplasma capsulatum also uses molecular mimicry to facilitate its survival in humans. It produces surface proteins that resemble iC3b, facilitating its entry into host cells via CR3 and other β integrins.

Protozoa have developed similar strategies (Fishelson, 1994). *Trypanosoma cruzi* produces a 60,000-dalton protein that has DAF-like activity and confers resistance to complement-mediated killing. Like DAF, it is linked to the membrane through a glycolipid anchor. *Schistosoma mansoni* can adsorb many proteins from plasma onto its surface in functionally active forms. Binding of complement regulatory proteins thus helps to protect this organism from complement attack. Several intracellular pathogens also use molecules that mimic complement components to facilitate their entry into the cells they parasitize. The surface glycoprotein GP63 of *Leishmania major* binds to CR3 and facilitates its entry into host macrophages. Similarly, legionella and mycobacteria may become opsonized by complement components without being killed and then enter macrophages via CR3 or CR4.

The fact that so many successful pathogens have evolved specific mechanisms to subjugate the complement system or avoid its attack indicates the overall importance of complement in host defense against infection.

SOLUBLE CR1 INHIBITION OF TISSUE INJURY

As noted earlier, nonimmunologic activation of complement can take place in tissues affected by burns (Gelfand et al., 1982) or ischemia (Weisman et al., 1990; Pemberton et al., 1993), presumably because thermal injury alters tissue proteins or exposes structures that are normally intracellular, thus creating surfaces that activate the alternative pathway, C1q, or both. The postischemic complement activation may also occur during reperfusion after temporary vascular occlusion (e.g., in myocardial infarction treated by thrombolytic therapy or during organ transplantation). Complement activation can then cause local injury by attracting neutrophils owing to the release of C5a, by binding and activating neutrophils onto surfaces coated with C3b (i.e., "frustrated" phagocytosis), and by generating membrane attack complexes that damage endothelial and other cells. In addition, the release of large amounts of C5a can cause intravascular aggregation of neutrophils. These aggregates may then lodge in pulmonary capillaries and contribute to the post-burn or post-trauma adult respiratory distress syndrome (ARDS).

In searching among the RCA proteins (Table 7–2) for an inhibitor that might be used therapeutically to ameliorate the effects of complement activation, CR1 seems ideal. CR1 inhibits the alternative and classical pathway C3 and C5 convertases and has cofactor activity for cleavage of C3b and C4b. A soluble form of CR1 (sCR1), which lacks the transmembrane and cytoplasmic domains of the native protein, has been produced by molecular engineering (Weisman et al., 1990). This recombinant protein decreases both local tissue damage and the systemic complications of complement activation in animal models (Weisman et al., 1990; Mulligan et al., 1992; Pemberton et al., 1993).

INHIBITION OF COMPLEMENT-MEDIATED TISSUE DAMAGE BY IVIG

IgG is a high-affinity acceptor for covalent binding of C3b during complement activation. Indeed, a large percentage of the C3b bound to opsonized pneumococci is attached to the IgG rather than to the organism itself (Brown et al., 1983). In vitro studies show that IgG-C3b complexes are resistant to attack by factors H and I and that they are recognized by both Fc receptor and CR1, leading to extremely efficient phagocytosis. In vitro studies show that when complement is activated by antibody-sensitized erythrocytes in the presence of excess nonspecific IgG (intravenous immunoglobulin—IVIG), less C3b is deposited onto the erythrocytes and lysis is inhibited (Berger et al., 1985). This occurs at concentrations of IgG readily achievable during high-dose IVIG therapy and results from the binding of nascent C3b molecules to fluid phase IgG molecules rather than to erythrocyte-bound IgG or to the erythrocyte membrane *per se*. Decreasing the binding of C3b to blood cells, with subsequent inhibition of reticuloendothelial clearance (Basta et al., 1989b), may be a major mechanism for the therapeutic effects of high-dose IVIG in autoimmune cytopenias. Animal models of complement-mediated tissue damage also show that IVIG can decrease the deposition of complement within tissues and can ameliorate antibody-induced complement-mediated reactions, including Forssman shock (Basta et al., 1989a). Thus, the ability to bind C3b may be an important anti-inflammatory mechanism of IVIG.

References

Abughali N, Berger M, Tosi MF. Deficient total cell content of CR3 (CD11b) in neonatal neutrophils. Blood 83:1086–1092, 1994.

Ahearn JM, Fearon DT. Structure and function of the complement receptors, CR1 (CD35) and CR2 (CD21). Adv Immunol 46:183–219, 1989.

Alper CA, Johnson AM, Birtch AG, Moore FD. Human C3: evidence for the liver as the primary site of synthesis, Science 162:286–288, 1969.

Alper CA. Plasma protein measurements as a diagnostic aid. N Engl J Med 291:287–290, 1974.

Alper CA, Rosen FS. Genetics of the complement system. In Advances in Human Genetics, Vol. 7. Harris H, Hirschhorn K, eds. London, Plenum Press, 1976, pp. 141–188.

Alper CA. Complement and the MHC. In Dorff ME, ed. The Role of the Major Histocompatibility Locus in Immunobiology. New York, Garland Press, 1981, pp. 173–220.

Alper CA, Austen KF, Cooper NR, Fearon DT, Gigli I, Hadding U, Lachmann PJ, Lambert PH, Lepow IH, Mayer MM, Müller-Eberhard JH, Nishioka K, Pondman K, Rosen FS, Stroud RM. Nomenclature of the alternative activating pathway of complement. Bull WHO 59:189–191, 1981.

Arnaout MA, Pitt J, Cohen JH, Melamed J, Rosen FS, Colten HR. Deficiency of a granulocyte membrane glycoprotein (gp 150) in a boy with recurrent bacterial infections. N Engl J Med 306:693–699, 1982.

Arnaout MA, Todd RF, Dana N, Melamed J, Schlossman S, Colten HR. Inhibition of phagocytosis of C3 or IgG coated particles and of C3bi binding with monoclonal antibodies to a monocyte/granulocyte membrane glycoprotein (Mo1). J Clin Invest 72:171–179, 1983.

Arnaout MA, Colten HR. Complement C3 receptors: Structure and function. Molec Immunol 21:1191–1199, 1984.

Arroyave CM, Tan EM. Mechanism of complement activation by radiographic contrast media. Clin Exp Immunol 29:89–94, 1977.

Austen KF, Becker EL, Biro CE, Borsos T, Dalmasso AP, Dias DA, Silva W, Isliker H, Klein P, Lachmann PJ, Leon MA, Lepow IH, Mayer MM, Müller-Eberhard HJ, Nelson RA, Nilsson U, Nishioka I, Rapp HP, Brosen FS, Trnka Z, Ward PA, Wardlaw AC. Nomenclature of Complement. Bull WHO 39:935–938, 1968.

Ballow M, Fang F, Good RA, Day NK. Developmental aspects of complement components in the newborn. Clin Exp Immunol 18:257–266, 1978.

Basta M, Kirshbom P, Frank MM, Fries LF. Mechanism of therapeutic effect of high-dose intravenous immunoglobulin. Attenuation of acute, complement-dependent immune damage in a guinea pig model. J Clin Invest 84:1974–1981, 1989a.

Basta M, Langlois PF, Marques M, Frank MM, Fries LF. High-dose intravenous immunoglobulin modifies complement-mediated in vivo clearance. Blood 74:326–333, 1989b.

Beller DI, Springer TA, Schrieber RD. Anti-Mac 1 selectively inhibits the mouse and human type three complement receptor. J Exp Med 156:1000–1009, 1982.

Berger M, Gaither TA, Hammer CH, Frank MM. Lack of binding of human C3 in its native state to C3b receptors. J Immunol 127:1329–1334, 1981.

Berger M, Gaither TA, Frank MM. Complement receptors. Clin Immunol Rev 1:471–545, 1982.

Berger M, Balow JE, Wilson CB, Frank MM. Circulating immune complexes and glomerulonephritis in a patient with congenital absence of the third component of complement. N Engl J Med 308:1009–1012, 1983.

Berger M, O'Shea J, Cross AS, Folks TM, Chused TM, Brown EJ, Frank MM. Human neutrophils increase expression of C3bi as well as C3b receptors upon activation. J Clin Invest 74:1566–1571, 1984.

Berger M, Rosenkranz P, Brown CY. Intravenous and standard im-

mune serum globulin preparations interfere with update of ^{125}I-C3 onto sensitized erythrocytes and inhibit hemolytic complement activity. Clin Immunol Immunopathol 34:227–236, 1985.

Bhakdi S, Tranum-Jensen J. Molecular nature of the complement lesion. Proc Natl Acad Sci U S A 74:5655–5659, 1979.

Blanco C, Griffin FM Jr, Silverstein SC. Studies of the macrophage complement receptor. Alteration of receptor function upon macrophage activation. J Exp Med 141:1278–1290, 1975.

Bora NS, Lublin DM, Kumar BV, Hockett RD, Holers VM, Atkinson JP. Structural gene for human membrane cofactor protein (MCP) of complement maps to within 100 kb of the 3′ end of the C3b/C4b receptor gene. J Exp Med 169:597–602, 1989.

Borsos T, Rapp HJ. Molecular Basis of Complement Action. New York, Appleton-Century-Crofts, 1970, pp. 1–164.

Bowen TJ, Ochs HD, Altman LC, Price TH, van Epps DE, Brautigan DL, Rosin RE, Perkins WD, Babior BM, Klebanoff SJ, Wedgwood RJ. Severe recurrent bacterial infections associated with defective adherence and chemotaxis in two patients with neutrophils deficient in a cell associated glycoprotein. J Pediatr 101:932–940, 1982.

Brown E, Berger M, Joiner K, Frank MM. Classical complement pathway activation by antipneumococcal antibodies leads to covalent binding of C3b to antibody molecules. Infect Immunol 42:594–598, 1983.

Bruce MC, Baley JE, Medvik KA, Berger M. Impaired surface membrane expression of C3bi but not C3b receptors on neonatal neutrophils. Pediatr Res 21:306–311, 1987.

Campbell RD, Dodds AW, Porter RR. The binding of human complement component C4 to antibody-antigen aggregates. Biochem J 189:67–80, 1980.

Carpenter CB. Abnormalities of the complement system in clinical transplantation situations. Transplant Proc 6:83–89, 1974.

Carroll MC, Alicot EM, Katzman PJ, Klickstein LB, Smith JA, Fearon DT. Organization of the genes encoding complement receptors type 1 and 2, decay-accelerating factor, and C4-binding protein in the RCA locus on human chromosome 1. J Exp Med 167:1271–1280, 1988.

Chenowith DE, Hugli TC. Techniques and significance of C3a and C5 measurement. In Nakamura RM, ed. Future Perspectives in Clinical Laboratory Immunoassays. New York, Alan R. Liss, 1980, 443–460.

Chenowith DE, Cooper SW, Hugli TE, Stewart RW, Blackstone EM, Kirklin JW. Complement activation during cardiopulmonary bypass. N Engl J Med 304:497–503, 1981.

Cheung NK, Walter EI, Smith-Mensah WH, Medoff ME. Decay-accelerating factor protects human tumor cells from complement-mediated cytotoxicity in vitro. J Clin Invest 81:1122–1128, 1988.

Cochrane GC. The role of complement in experimental disease models. Springer Semin Immunopathol 7:263–270, 1984.

Colten HR. Biosynthesis of complement. Adv Immunol 22:67–118, 1976.

Colten HR, Alper CA, Rosen FS. Genetics and biosynthesis of complement proteins. N Engl J Med 304:653–656, 1981.

Cooper NR. Activation and regulation of the first complement component. Fed Proc 42:134–138, 1983.

Cooper NR. Complement evasion strategies of microorganisms. Immunol Today 12:327–331, 1991.

Cooper NR, Nemerow GR. Complement, viruses and virus-infected cells. Springer Semin Immunopathol 6:327-348, 1983.

Cooper NR, Nemerow GR, Meyes JT. Methods to detect and quantitate complement activation. Springer Semin Immunopathol 6:195–212, 1983.

Cornacoff JB, Hebert LA, Smead WL, VanAman ME, Birmingham DJ, Waxman FJ. Primate erythrocyte-immune complex-clearing mechanism. J Clin Invest 71:236–247, 1983.

Craddock PR, Fehr J, Brigham KL, Kronenberg RS, Jacob HS. Complement and leukocyte-mediated pulmonary dysfunction in hemodialysis. N Engl J Med 296:769–774, 1977.

Cronstein BN, Weissmann G. The adhesion molecules of inflammation. Arthritis Rheum 36:147–157, 1993.

Crowley CA, Curnutte JT, Rosen RE, Schwartz JA, Gallin JI, Klempner M, Synderman R, Southwick FS, Stossel TP, Babior BM. An inherited abnormality of neutrophil adhesion-genetic transmission and association with a missing protein. N Engl J Med 302:1163–1168, 1980.

Curtis JJ, Wyatt RJ, Bhathena D, Lucas BA, Holland NH, Luke

RG. Renal transplantation for patients with type I and type II membranoproliferative glomerulonephritis. Am J Med 66:216–225, 1979.

Davis AE, Arnaout MA, Alper CA, Rosen FS. Transfer of C3 nephritic factor from mother to fetus. N Engl J Med 297:144–145, 1977a.

Davis AE, Ziegler JB, Gelfand EW, Rosen FS, Alper CA. Heterogeneity of nephritic factor and its identification as an immunoglobulin. Proc Natl Acad Sci U S A 74:3980–3983, 1977b.

Dykman TA, Hatch JA, Atkinson JP. Polymorphism of the human C3b/C4b receptor. J Exp Med 159:691–703, 1984.

Edwards JE Jr, Gaither TA, O'Shea JJ, Rotrosen D, Lawley TJ, Wright SA, Frank MM, Green I. Expression of specific binding sites on candida with functional and antigenic characteristics of human complement receptors. J Immunol 137:3577–3583, 1986.

Edwards MS, Kasper DL, Jennings HJ, Baker CJ, Nicholson-Weller A. Capsular sialic acid prevents activation of the alternative complement pathway by type III, group B streptococci. J Immunol 128:1278–1283, 1982.

Edwards MS, Nicholson-Weller A, Baker CJ, Kasper DL. The role of specific antibody in alternative complement pathway mediated opsonophagocytosis of type III, group B streptococcus. J Exp Med 151:1275–1287, 1980.

Ehlenberger AG, Nussenzweig V. The role of membrane receptors for C3b and C3d in phagocytosis. J Exp Med 145:357–371, 1977.

Eigentler A, Schulz TF, Larcher C, Breitweiser E, Myones BL, Petzer AL, Dierich MP. C3bi-binding protein on *Candida albicans:* Temperature dependent expression and relationship to human complement receptor type 3. Infect Immun 57:616–622, 1989.

Ewald RA, Williams JH, Bowden DH. Serum complement in the newborn: An investigation of complement activity in normal infants and in Rh and AB hemolytic disease. Vox Sang 6:312–319, 1961.

Falk RJ, Dalmasso AP, Kim Y, Tsai CH, Scheinman JI, Gewurz H, Michael AF. Neoantigen of the polymerized ninth component of complement: characterization of a monoclonal antibody and histochemical localization in renal disease. J Clin Invest 72:560–573, 1983.

Fearon DT. Complement, C receptors, and immune complex disease. Hosp Pract 15:63–72, 1988.

Fearon DT. Identification of the membrane glycoprotein that is the C3 receptor of the human erythrocyte, polymorphonuclear leukocyte B lymphocyte and monocyte. J Exp Med 152:20–30, 1980.

Fearon DT. Regulation by membrane sialic acid of B1H-dependent decay dissociation of amplification C3 convertase of the alternative complement pathway. Proc Natl Acad Sci U S A 75:1971–1975, 1978.

Fearon DT. Regulation of the amplification C3 convertase of human complement by an inhibitory protein isolated from human erythrocyte membrane. Proc Natl Acad Sci U S A 76:5867–5871, 1979.

Fearon DT, Austen KF. The alternative pathway of complement: a system for host resistance to microbial infection. N Engl J Med 303:259–263, 1980.

Fearon DT, Collins LA. Increased expression of C3b receptors on polymorphonuclear leukocytes induced by chemotactic factors and by purification procedures. J Immunol 130:370–375, 1983.

Fearon DT, Daha MR, Strom TB, Weiler JM, Carpenter CB, Austen RF. Pathways of complement activation in membranoproliferative glomerulonephritis and allograft rejection. Transplant Proc 9:729–739, 1977.

Fearon DT, Wong W. Complement ligand receptor interactions that mediate biological responses. Ann Rev Immunol 1:243–271, 1983.

Fireman P, Zuckowski DA, Taylor PM. Development of human complement system. J Imunol 103:25–31, 1969.

Fishelson Z. Complement-related proteins in pathogenic organisms. Springer Semin Immunopathol 15:345–368, 1994.

Fleisher TA, Berger M. Immunoregulatory effects of human C3 and its major cleavage fragments. Clin Immunol Immunopathol 33:391–401, 1984.

Frank MM, Schrieber AD, Atkinson JP, Jaffe CJ. Pathophysiology of immune hemolytic anemia. Ann Intern Med 87:210–222, 1977.

Fries LF, Friedman H, Cohen GH, Eisenberg RJ, Hammer CH, Frank MM. Glycoprotein C of herpes simplex virus 1 is an inhibitor of the complement cascade. J Immunol 137:1636–1641, 1986.

Fries LF, Gaither TA, Hammer CH, Frank MM. C3b covalently bound to IgG demonstrates a reduced rate of inactivation by factors H and I. J Exp Med 160:1640–1655, 1984.

Fujita T, Gigli I, Nussenzweig V. Human C4 binding protein: II. Role in proteolysis of C4b by C3b inactivator. J Exp Med 148:1044–1051, 1978.

Gaither TA, Frank MM. Complement. In Henry JB, ed. Clinical Diagnosis and Management by Laboratory Methods. Philadelphia, WB Saunders, 1979, pp. 1245–1261.

Gelfand JA, Donelan M, Hawiger A, and Burke JF: Alternative complement pathway activation increases mortality in a model of burn injury in mice. J Clin Invest 70:1170–1176, 1982.

Gelfand MC, Frank MM, Green I. A receptor for the third component of complement in the human renal glomerulus. J Exp Med 142:1029–1034, 1975.

Gerard C, Hugli TE. Identification of classical anaphylatoxin as the des-Arg form of the C5a molecule: evidence of a modulator role for the oligosaccharide unit in human des-Arg^{71}-C5a. Proc Natl Acad Sci U S A 78:1833–1837, 1981.

Gitlin D, Biasucci A. Development of γG, γA, γM, β_{1C}/β_{1A}, C'1 esterase inhibitor, ceruloplasmin, transferrin, hemopexin, haptoglobin, fibrinogen, plasminogen, antitrypsin, orosomucoid, β-lipoprotein, $\alpha 2$ macroglobulin and prealbumin in the human conceptus. J Clin Invest 48:1433–1446, 1969.

Gitlin D, Gitlin JD. Fetal and neonatal development of human plasma proteins. In Putnam FE, ed. The Plasma Proteins. 2nd ed. New York: Academic Press, 1975, 263–319.

Goers JWF, Porter RR. The assembly of early components of complement on antibody-antigen aggregates and on antibody-coated erythrocytes. Biochem J 175:675–684, 1978.

Goldstein IM, Perez HD. Biologically active peptides derived from the fifth component of complement. Prog Hemost Thromb 5:41–79, 1980.

Goodman EB, Tenner AJ. Signal transduction mechanisms of C1q-mediated superoxide production: evidence for the involvement of temporally distinct staurosporine-insensitive and -sensitive pathways. J Immunol 148:3920–3928, 1992.

Gorski JP, Hugh TE, Müller-Eberhard, HJ. C4a: The third anaphylatoxin of the human complement system. Proc Natl Acad Sci U S A 76:5299–5302, 1979.

Griffin FM Jr, Bianco C, Silverstein SM. Characterization of the macrophage receptor for complement and demonstration of its functional independence from the receptor for immunoglobulin G. J Exp Med 141:1269–1277, 1975.

Griffin JA, Griffin FM Jr. Augmentation of macrophage complement receptor function in vitro: I. Characterization of the cellular interactions required for the generation of a T-lymphocyte product that enhances macrophage complement receptor function. J Exp Med 150:653–675, 1979.

Griffin FM Jr, Mullinax PJ. Augmentation of macrophage complement receptor function in vitro: III. C3b receptors that promote phagocytosis migrate within the plane of the macrophage plasma membrane. J Exp Med 154:291–305, 1981.

Halbwachs L, Leveille M, Lesavre PH, Wattel S, Leibowitch J. Nephritic factor of the classical complement pathway IgG autoantibody directed against the classical pathway C3 convertase enzyme. J Clin Invest 65:1249–1256, 1980.

Hall RE, Colten HR. Cell-free synthesis of the fourth component of guinea pig complement (C4): Identification of a precursor of serum (Pro-C4). Proc Natl Acad Sci U S A 74:1707–1710, 1977.

Hammer CH, Abramovitz AS, Mayer MM. A new activity of complement component C3: Cell-bound C3b potentiates lysis of erythrocytes by C5b6 and terminal components. J Immunol 117:830–834, 1976.

Hammerschmidt DE, Weaver LJ, Hudson LD, Craddock PR, Jacob H. Complement activation and elevated plasma C5a with adult respiratory distress syndrome: pathophysiological relevance and possible prognostic value. Lancet 1:947–949, 1980.

Harris SL, Frank I, Yee A, Cohen GH, Eisenberg RJ, Cohen GH, Friedman HM. Glycoprotein C of herpes simplex virus type 1 prevents complement-mediated cell lysis and virus neutralization. J Infect Dis 162:331–337, 1990.

Harrison RA, Lachmann PJ. The physiological breakdown of the third component of complement. Mol Immunol 17:9–20, 1980.

Harrison RA, Thomas ML, Tack BF. Sequence determination of the thiolester site of the fourth component of human complement. Proc Natl Acad Sci U S A 78:7388–7392, 1981.

Hemler ME. VLA proteins in the integrin family: structures, functions, and their role on leukocytes. Annu Rev Immunol 8:365–400, 1990.

Hogg N. Roll, roll, roll your leucocyte gently down the vein.... Immunol Today 13:113–115, 1992.

Hostetter MK, Thomas ML, Rosen FS, Tack BF. Binding of C3b proceeds by a transesterification reaction at the thiolester site. Nature 298:72–75, 1982.

Hugli TE. Structure and function of the anaphylatoxins. Springer Semin Immunopathol 7:193–220, 1984.

Hugli TE, Müller-Eberhard HJ. Anaphylatoxins: C3a and C5a. Adv Immunol 26:1–53, 1978.

Iida K, Nussenzweig V. Complement receptor is an inhibitor of the complement cascade. J Exp Med 153:1138–1150, 1981.

Iida K, Mornaghi R, Nussenzweig V. Complement receptor (CR1) deficiency in erythrocytes from patients with systemic lupus erythematosus. J Exp Med 153:1427–1438, 1982.

Iida K, Nadler L, Nussenzweig V. Identification of the membrane receptor for complement fragment C3d by means of a monoclonal antibody. J Exp Med 158:1021–1033, 1983.

Inada S, Brown EJ, Gaither TA, Hammer CH, Takahashi T, Frank MM. C3d receptors are expressed on human monocytes after in vitro cultivation. Proc Natl Acad Sci U S A 80:2351–2355, 1983.

Jackson CG, Ochs MD, Wedgwood RJ. Immune response of a patient with deficiency of the fourth component of complement and systemic lupus erythematosus. N Engl J Med 300:1124–1129, 1979.

Jacob HS, Craddock PR, Hammerschmidt DE, Moldow CF. Complement induced granulocyte aggregation. N Engl J Med 302:789–794, 1980.

Kay AB, Glass J, Salter D McG. Leucoattractants enhance complement receptors on human phagocytic cells. Clin Exp Immunol 38:294–299, 1979.

Kazatchkine MD, Fearon DT, Austen KF. Human alternative complement pathway: Membrane-associated sialic acid regulates the competition between B and B1H for cell bound C3b. J Immunol 122:75–81, 1979.

Klaus CGB, Humphrey JH, Kunkl A, Dongworth DW. The follicular dendritic cell—its role in antigen presentation in the generation of immunological memory. Immunol Rev 59:3–28, 1980.

Kolb WP, Lang JH, Lasser EC. Nonimmunologic complement activation in normal human serum induced by radiographic contrast media. J Immunol 121:1232–1238, 1978.

Kubota Y, Gaither TA, Cason J, O'Shea JJ, Lawley TJ. Characterization of the C3 receptor induced by herpes simplex virus type 1 infection of human epidermal, endothelial and A431 cells. J Immunol 138:1137–1142, 1987.

Lachmann PJ. The control of homologous lysis. Immunol Today 12:312–315, 1991.

Lachmann PJ, ed. Biology of Complement. Springer Semin Immunopathol 15:303–431, 1994.

Law SK, Lichtenberg NA, Levine RP. Evidence for an ester linkage between the labile binding site of C3b and receptive surfaces. J Immunol 123:1388–1394, 1979.

Lawley TJ, Frank M. Immune complexes and immune complex diseases. In Parker CT, ed. Clinical Immunology. Philadelphia: WB Saunders, 1980, pp. 143–172.

Lawley TJ, Bielory L, Gascon P, Yancey KB, Young NS, Frank MM. A prospective clinical and immunologic analysis of patients with serum sickness. N Engl J Med 311:1407–1413, 1984.

Levy M, Broyer M, Arsan A, Levy-Bentolila D, Habib R. Anaphylactoid purpura nephritis in childhood: Natural history and immunopathology. Adv Nephrol 6:183–228, 1976.

Lim HW, Poh-Fitzpatrick MB, Gigli I. Activation of the complement system in patients with porphyrias after irradiation in vivo. J Clin Invest 74:1961–1965, 1984.

Marom Z, Shelhamer J, Berger M, Frank M, Kaliner M. The anaphylatoxin C3a enhances mucous glycoprotein release from human airways in vitro. J Exp Med 161:657–668, 1985.

Mayer MM. Complement and complement fixation. In Kabat E, Mayer MF, eds. Experimental Immunochemistry. Springfield, Ill., Charles C Thomas, 1961, pp. 133–240.

Mayer MM, Michaels DW, Ramm LE, Whitlow MB, Willoughby JB, Shin ML. Membrane damage by complement. CRC Crit Rev Immunol 2:133–166, 1981.

McKenzie R, Kotwal GJ, Moss B, Hammer CH, Frank MM. Regulation of complement activity by vaccinia virus complement-control protein. J Infect Dis 166:1245–1250, 1992.

McNearney TA, Odell C, Holers VM, Spear PG, Atkinson JP. Herpes simplex virus glycoproteins gC-1 and gC-2 bind to the third component of complement and provide protection against complement-mediated neutralization of viral infectivity. J Exp Med 166:1525–1535, 1987.

Miller GW, Nussenzweig V. A new complement function: Solubilization of antigen-antibody aggregates. Proc Natl Acad Sci U S A 72:418–422, 1975.

Moffitt MC, Frank MM. Complement resistance in microbes. Springer Seminars Immunopath 15:327–344, 1994.

Möller G, Coutinho AJ. Role of C3 and Fc receptors in B-lymphocyte activation. J Exp Med 141:647–663, 1975.

Moore FD, Fearon DT, Austen KF. IgG on mouse erythrocytes augments activation of the human alternative complement pathway by enhancing deposition of C3b. J Immunol 125:1805–1809, 1981.

Moors MA, Stull TL, Blank KJ, Buckley HR, Mosser DM. A role for complement receptor-like molecules in iron acquisition by *Candida albicans*. J Exp Med 1643–1651, 1992.

Morgan BP, Meri S. Membrane proteins that protect against complement lysis. Springer Semin Immunopathol 15:369–396, 1994.

Morgan EL, Weigle WO, Hugli TE. Anaphylatoxin-mediated regulation of the immune responses. J Exp Med 155:1412–1426, 1982

Müller-Eberhard HJ, ed. Complement: I, II, III. Springer Semin Immunopathol 6:117–258, 259–390; 7:93–270, 1983/1984.

Müller-Eberhard HJ. The membrane attack complex. Springer Semin Immunopathol 7:93–142, 1984.

Müller-Eberhard HJ, Schreiber RD. Molecular biology and chemistry of the alternative pathway of complement. Adv Immunol 29:1–53, 1980.

Mulligan MS, Yeh CG, Rudolph AR, Ward PA. Protective effects of soluble CR1 in complement- and neutrophil-mediated tissue injury. J Immunol 148:1479–1485, 1992.

Myones BL, Dalzell JG, Hogg N, Ross GD. Neutrophil and monocyte cell surface p150,95 has iC3b-receptor (CR4) activity resembling CR3. J Clin Invest 82:640–651, 1988.

Nagasawa S, Stroud RM. Cleavage of C2 and C1s into antigenically distinct fragments C2a and C2b: Demonstration of binding of C2b to C4b. Proc Natl Acad Sci U S A 74:2998–3001, 1977.

Nelson RA. The immune adherence phenomenon: An immunologically specific reaction between micro-organisms and erythrocytes leading to enhanced phagocytosis. Science 118:733–737, 1953.

Nemerow GR, Houghten RA, Moore MD, Cooper NR. Identification of an epitope in the major envelope protein of Epstein-Barr virus that mediates viral binding to the B lymphocyte EBV receptor (CR2). Cell 56:369–377, 1989.

Nemerow GR, Yamamoto K, Lint TF. Restriction of complement-mediated membrane damage by the eighth component of complement. A dual role for C8 in the complement attack sequence. J Immunol 123:1245–1252, 1979.

Nicholson-Weller A, March JP, Rosenfeld SI, Austen KF. Affected erythrocytes of patients with paroxysmal nocturnal hemoglobinuria are deficient in the complement regulatory protein, decay-accelerating factor. Proc Natl Acad Sci U S A 80:5066–5070, 1983.

Nissenson AR, Baraff LJ, Fine RN, Knutson DW. Post-streptococcal acute glomerular nephritis: Fact and controversy. Ann Intern Med 91:76–86, 1979.

Ochs MD, Wedgwood RJ, Frank MM, Heller SP, Hosea SW. The role of complement in induction of antibody responses. Clin Exp Immunol 53:208–216, 1983.

Oldstone MBA. Virus neutralization and virus induced immune complex disease. Prog Med Virol 19:84–119, 1975.

Packman CH, Rosenfeld SI, Jenkins DE, Thiem PA, Leddy JP. Complement lysis of human erythrocytes: Differing susceptibility of two types of paroxysmal nocturnal hemoglobinuria cells to C5b-9. J Clin Invest 64:428–433, 1979.

Pangburn MK, Müller-Eberhard HJ. Relation of a putative thioester bond in C3 to activation of the alternative pathway and the binding of C3b to biological targets of complement. J Exp Med 152:1102–1114, 1980.

Pangburn NK, Schreiber RD, Trombold JS, Müller-Eberhard HJ. Paroxysmal nocturnal hemoglobinuria: Deficiency in factor H-like function of the abnormal erythrocytes. J Exp Med 157:1971–1980, 1983.

Patston PA, Gettins P, Beechem J, Schapira M. Mechanisms of serpin action: evidence that C1 inhibitor function as a suicide substrate. Biochemistry 30:8876–8882, 1991.

Pemberton M, Anderson G, Vetvicka V, Justus DE, Ross GD. Microvascular effects of complement blockade with soluble recombinant CR1 on ischemia/reperfusion injury of skeletal muscle. J Immunol 150:5104–5113, 1993.

Pepys MB. Role of complement in the induction of immunological responses. Transplant Rev 32:93–120, 1976.

Perlmann H, Perlmann P, Schreiber RD, Müller-Eberhard HJ. Interaction of target cell bound C3bi and C3d with human lymphocyte receptors: enhancement of ADCC. J Exp Med 153:1592–1603, 1981.

Peters DK, Lachmann PJ. Immunity deficiency in the pathogenesis of glomerulonephritis. Lancet 1:58–60, 1974.

Pillemer L, Blum L, Lepow IH, Ross OA, Todd EW, Wardlaw AC. The properdin system and immunity I. Demonstration and isolation of a new serum protein, properdin, and its role in immune phenomena. Science 120:279–285, 1954.

Podack ER, Biesecker G, Müller-Eberhard HJ. Membrane attack complex of complement: Generation of high affinity phospholipid binding sites by fusion of five hydrophilic plasma proteins. Proc Natl Acad Sci U S A 76:897–901, 1979.

Podack ER, Müller-Eberhard HJ. Binding of desoxycholate, phosphatidylchol vesicles, lipoprotein and of the S-protein to complexes of terminal complement component. J Immunol 121:1025–1030, 1978.

Podack ER, Tschopp J. Membrane attack by complement. Molec Immunol 21:589–603, 1984.

Podack ER, Tschopp J, Müller-Eberhard HJ. Molecular organization of C9 within the membrane attack complex of complement: Induction of circular C9 polymerization by the C5b-8 assembly. J Exp Med 156:268–282, 1982.

Pommier CG, Inada S, Fries LF, Takahashi T, Frank MM, Brown EJ. Plasma fibronectin enhances phagocytosis of opsonized particles by human peripheral blood monocytes. J Exp Med 157:1844–1854, 1983.

Porter RR, Reid KBM. The biochemistry of complement. Nature 275:699–704, 1978.

Pussell BA, Bourke E, Nayef M, Morris S, Peters DK. Complement deficiency and nephritis: report of a family. Lancet 1:675–677, 1980.

Reid KBM, Porter RR. The proteolytic activation systems of complement. Ann Rev Biochem 50:433–464, 1981.

Ross GD, Newman SL, Lambris JD, Devery-Pocius JE, Cain JA, Lachmann PJ. Generation of three different fragments of bound C3 with purified factor I or serum. II. Location of binding sites in the C3 fragments for factors B and H, complement receptors, and bovine conglutinin. J Exp Med 158:334–352, 1983.

Ross SC, Densen P. Complement deficiency states and infection: Epidemiology, pathogenesis and consequences of neisserial and other infections in an immune deficiency. Medicine 63:243–273, 1984.

Rosse WF. Variations in the red cells in paroxysmal nocturnal hemoglobinuria. Br J Haematol 24:327–334, 1973.

Rother K, Till J, eds. The Complement System. Heidelberg: Springer-Verlag Publishers, 1988.

Rubin H. Autoimmune hemolytic anemia: warm and cold antibody types. Am J Clin Pathol 68(Suppl):638–642, 1977.

Ruddy S, Colten HR. Rheumatoid arthritis: Biosynthesis of complement proteins by synovial tissues. N Engl J Med 290:1284–1288, 1974.

Ruddy S, Carpenter CB, Chin KW, Knostman JN, Soter NA, Gotze O, Müller-Eberhard HJ, Austen KF. Human complement metabolism: an analysis of 144 studies. Medicine 54:165–178, 1975.

Rynes RF, Ruddy S, Schur PH, Spragg J, Austen RF. Levels of complement components, properdin factors and kininogen in patients with inflammatory arthritides. J Rheum 1:413–427, 1974.

Sanchez-Madrid F, Nagy JA, Robbins E, Simon P, Springer TA. A human leukocyte differentiation antigen family with distinct alpha subunits and a common beta subunit: The lymphocyte function-associated antigen (LFA-1), the C3bi complement receptor (OKM1/Mac-1), and the P150, 95 molecule. J Exp Med 158:1785–1803, 1983.

Sawyer MK, Forman ML, Kuplic LS, Stiehm ER. Development aspects of the human complement system. Biol Neonate 19:148–162, 1971.

Schifferli JA, Ng YC, Peters DK. The role of complement and its receptor in the elimination of immune complexes. N Engl J Med 315:488–495, 1986.

Schur PH. Complement in lupus. Clin Rheum Dis 1:519–530, 1975.

Sim RB. The human complement system serine proteases C1r and C1s and their proenzymes. Methods Enzymol 80:26–42, 1981.

Sim RB, Twose TM, Paterson DS, Sim E. The covalent-binding reaction of complement component C3. Biochem J 193:115–127, 1981.

Spitzer RE, Valotta EH, Forristal J, Sudora E, Stitzel A, Davis NC, West CD. Serum C'3 lytic system in patients with glomerulonephritis. Science 164:436–437, 1969.

Spitzer RE, Hirmson JR, Farnett ML, Stitzel AE, Post EM. Alteration of the complement system in children with Henoch-Schonlein purpura. Clin Immunol Immunopathol 11:52–59, 1978.

Stevens P, Huang SNY, Welch WD, Young LS. Restricted complement activation by E. coli with the K-1 capsular serotype: possible role in pathogenicity. J Immunol 121:2174–2180, 1978.

Stossel TP, Field RJ, Gitlin JD, Alper CA, Rosen FS. The opsonic fragment of the third component of human complement. J Exp Med 141:1329–1347, 1975.

Tack BF, Harrison RA, Janatova J, Thomas ML, Prahl JW. Evidence for presence of an internal thiolester bond in third component of human complement. Proc Natl Acad Sci U S A 77:5764–5768, 1980.

Tanner J, Weis J, Fearon D, Whang Y, Kieff E. Epstein-Barr virus gp350/220 binding to the B lymphocyte C3d receptor mediates adsorption, capping and endocytosis. Cell 50:203–213, 1987.

Theofilopoulos AN, Dixon FJ. The biology and detection of immune complexes. Adv Immunol 28:89–220, 1979.

Thomas ML, Janatova J, Gray WR, Tack BF. Third component of human complement: Localization of the internal thiolester bond. Proc Natl Acad Sci U S A 79:1054–1058, 1982.

Ware CF, Kolb WP. Assembly of the functional membrane attack complex of human complement: formation of disulfide linked C9 dimers. Proc Natl Acad Sci U S A 78:6426–6430, 1981.

Weigle WO, Goodman MG, Morgan EL, Hugli TE. Regulation of immune responses by components of the complement cascade and their activated fragments. Springer Semin Immunopathol 6:173–194, 1983.

Weis JJ, Tedder TF, Fearon DT. Identification of a 145,000 MW membrane protein as the C3d receptor of human B lymphocytes. Proc Natl Acad Sci U S A 81:881–885, 1984.

Weis JJ, Toothaker LE, Smith JA, Weis JH, Fearon DT. Structure of the human B lymphocyte receptor for C3d and the Epstein-Barr virus and relatedness to other members of the family of C3/C4 binding proteins. J Exp Med 167:1047–1066, 1988.

Weisman HF, Bartow T, Leppo MK, Marsh HC Jr, Carson GR, Concino MF, Boyle MP, Roux KH, Weisfeldt ML, Fearon DT. Soluble human complement receptor type 1: in vivo inhibitor of complement suppressing post-ischemic myocardial inflammation and necrosis. Science 249:146–151, 1990.

West CS, McAdams AJ. The chronic glomerulonephritides of childhood. J Pediatr 93:1–12, 167–176, 1978.

Whaley K. Biosynthesis of the complement components and the regulatory proteins of the alternative complement pathway by human peripheral blood monocytes. J Exp Med 151:501–516, 1980.

Wilson CB, Dixon FJ. Immunologic mechanisms in nephritogenesis. Hosp Pract 14:57–69, 1979.

Wilson JG, Andriopoulos NA, Fearon DT. CR1 and cell membrane proteins that bind C3 and C4. Immunol Res 6:192–209, 1987.

Wilson JG, Wong W, Schur PH, Fearon DT. Mode of inheritance of decreased C3b receptors on erythrocytes of patients with systemic lupus erythematosus. N Engl J Med 307:981–986, 1982.

Winkelstein JA, Shin HS. The role of immunoglobulin in the interaction of pneumococci and the properdin pathway: evidence for its specificity and lack of requirement for the Fc portion of the molecule. J Immunol 112:1635–1641, 1974.

Wong WW, Wilson JG, Fearon DT. Genetic regulation of a structural polymorphism of human C3b receptor. J Clin Invest 72:685–693, 1983.

Worlledge SM. Immune drug-induced hemolytic anemias. Semin Hematol 10:327–344, 1973.

Wright SD, Silverstein SC. Tumor promoting phorbol esters stimulate C3b and C3b' receptor mediated phagocytosis in cultured human monocytes. J Exp Med 156:1149–1164, 1982.

Wright SD, Rao PE, Van Voorhis WC, Craigmyle LS, Iida K, Talle MA, Westberg EF, Goldstein G, Silverstein SC. Identification of the C3bi receptor of human monocytes and macrophages by using monoclonal antibodies. Proc Natl Acad Sci U S A 80:5699–5703, 1983.

Ziccardi RJ. Activation of the early components of the classical complement pathway under physiologic conditions. J Immunol 126:1769–1773, 1981.

Ziccardi RJ, Cooper NR. Active disassembly of the first component of complement by C1 inactivator. J Immunol 123:788–792, 1979.

Zvaifler NJ. The immunopathology of joint inflammation in rheumatoid arthritis. Adv Immunol 16:265–336, 1973.

Chapter 8

The Mucosal Defense System

Randall M. Goldblum, Lars Å. Hanson,
and Per Brandtzaeg

HISTORICAL BACKGROUND

The mucous membranes are constantly exposed to numerous microorganisms and potentially injurious macromolecules. These sites are the major interface between the antigen-laden external environment and the host defense system. It is no surprise that the mucosal surfaces are also the site of most infections, especially in children. Teleologically, the mucosal epithelium and its secretions should play a major role in local defense. This assumption is supported by pioneering studies on experimental bacterial infections, especially of the gastrointestinal tract.

In 1892, Ehrlich showed that newborn mice that were suckled by immunized mothers were protected against the toxic effects of ricin and abrin in the gastrointestinal tract. In 1919, Besredka demonstrated that

rabbits were protected against dysentery following oral immunization with Shiga's bacilli. In 1922 Davies showed that patients with dysentery had antibodies in the feces (coproantibodies) several days before the antibodies appeared in serum. Later, Burrows and Havens (1948) found that fecal antibodies to *Vibrio cholerae* were not correlated with titers in the serum. Similar studies indicated that antibacterial antibodies are produced locally in the respiratory tract (Bull and McKee, 1929). Subsequent investigations by Fazekas de St. Groth and colleagues (1950, 1951) extended the concept of local immune defense to include viral infections of the respiratory tract; these studies are reviewed by Besredka (1927) and Pierce (1959).

Following the characterization of different types of antibodies, it was shown that the major forms of antibodies of exocrine secretion were different from serum

159

antibodies and that these antibodies were produced locally. Particularly notable was the predominance of immunoglobulin A (IgA) in several external body fluids (Chodirker and Tomasi, 1963) and that this secretory IgA (SIgA) was immunochemically and physicochemically distinct from serum IgA (Hanson, 1961; Hanson and Johansson, 1962; Tomasi et al., 1965). It was soon recognized that SIgA of the external secretions is made of multiple immunoglobulin subunits containing a small joining (J) chain (Halpern and Koshland, 1970; Mestecky et al., 1971) and a larger glycopeptide, unique to secretory IgA, called *secretory component* (Hanson, 1961). These observations accelerated the interest in local immune responses, especially as they related to the control of SIgA formation. Recent studies have elucidated the pathways and mechanisms by which antigen stimulation of a mucosal surface results in the production of specific IgA antibodies at several mucosal sites often with little or no serum antibody response.

Other studies indicate that host defense of the mucosal surfaces also includes T lymphocytes, phagocytes, and innate (nonspecific) immune factors. Since the humoral component of mucosal immunity is understood best, it is emphasized here.

These extensive advances have led to the publication of a complete multiauthor text dedicated to mucosal immunity (Ogra et al., 1994). This chapter provides an overview of the clinically relevant issues in mucosal defenses.

MUCOSAL HUMORAL IMMUNE RESPONSES

Components

The machinery for eliciting antigenically specific immune responses at mucosal surfaces consists of the lymphoid and accessory cells distributed throughout the mucosal tissues. In aggregate, the organized lymphoid nodules at mucosal sites, termed *mucosa-associated lymphoid tissue* (MALT) (Bienenstock et al., 1979), contains many more lymphoid cells than the internal, or systemic, immune system. The majority of the MALT is found in the gastrointestinal tract and is called *gut-associated lymphoid tissue* (GALT). Other concentrations of cells are seen in the bronchi of the respiratory tract and are termed the *bronchus-associated lymphoid tissue* (BALT).

In addition to the lymphocytes of the MALT, other immune cells in mucosae are distributed as solitary nodules, diffusely in the lamina propria, and interspersed between epithelial cells. These cells are termed *interepithelial lymphocytes* (IELs). Some authors consider lymph nodes draining the mucosal sites (e.g., mesenteric and bronchial lymph nodes) part of the MALT. The MALT seems to employ interconnecting migratory pathways that integrate the mucosal immune responses, both locally and distal to the site of antigenic stimulation. Hence, the whole system for mucosal immune responses has been considered a "common" mucosal immune system.

Although many of the processes in mucosal immunity are similar to those of systemic immunity, one characteristic sets it apart. Because of the extensive antigenic exposure at mucosal sites, there is a need to respond to microorganisms and potentially deleterious macromolecules in a way that minimizes inflammatory injury to the host tissue. This is accomplished largely by "pushing" the site of interaction between foreign antigens and specific immune reactants into the lumen of the mucosal organ or, at least, to the epithelial surface, where deleterious inflammatory responses are less likely to injure the underlying and internal tissue. However, the host defense mechanisms of the mucosal sites also function largely without inflammatory mechanisms, particularly complement and phagocytes, which are required to eliminate and destroy pathogens that successfully invade the deeper tissues. Thus, inflammatory injury to mucosal tissue is usually avoided.

Induction of Secretory Immune Responses

Specific mucosal immune responses are usually initiated by antigenic stimulation of specialized lymphoid follicles within certain mucosal tissues (Fig. 8–1). The Peyer's patches of the distal small intestine are the prototype for these organized immunogenic sites. However, anatomically similar lymphoepithelial tissues are present in the bronchi (McDermott et al., 1982), appendix (Bockman et al., 1983), and tonsils (Owen and Nemanic, 1978). The histology of MALT differs from lymph nodes, in that this tissue has no capsule, no medulla, and no afferent lymphatic ducts (Kato and Owen, 1994). This lack of afferent lymphatics suggests that antigens taken up by the epithelium immediately overlying the nodules provide the antigenic stimulation of the follicles.

The epithelium overlying the dome-like structure of the Peyer's patches contains cells that differ from the surrounding enterocytes. These cells, which lack microvilli, are therefore termed *membranous* (M) cells. The basolateral aspects of these cells are also unusual because they have invaginations containing lymphocytes and macrophages that have transversed the fenestrated basal lamina below. This unique anatomic configuration may provide for the efficient transfer of antigenic material from the intestine to the juxtaposed immune cells. Most of the mucosal follicles consist of distinct anatomic regions, including a superficial dome, a corona, and a central germinal center. The germinal centers of Peyer's patches differ from those in peripheral lymph nodes because 75% to 80% of their B cells have surface IgA (sIgA⁺). The surrounding cells are mainly CD4⁺ T cells. These characteristics are in keeping with the role of MALT in the genesis of specific IgA immune responses.

Sampling of Luminal Antigens and Presentation to T Cells

Neutra and Kraehenbuhl (1994) have reviewed the function of the lymphoepithelial structures in sampling and processing luminal antigens for mucosal immune response. The M cells demonstrate some specificity of

Figure 8–1. Hypothetical diagram of the common mucosal immune system in humans. Lymphoid cells, presumably from the bone marrow, enter the Peyer's patches (GALT) through high endothelial venules. Under the local influence of T cells and accessory cells, they express surface IgA. Environmental antigens enter Peyer's patches through pinocytotic and phagocytic M cells and interact with resident accessory, T, and B cells. IgA-committed and antigen-sensitized B cells and lymphoblasts leave Peyer's patches and enter the regional lymph nodes, then the lymph and circulation. Finally, such cells populate various exocrine glands and mucosa-associated tissues, where terminal differentiation into IgA-secreting plasma cells occurs. BALT apparently plays a role analogous to that of GALT. It is thought that tonsils may also contribute to the pool of precursor cells that populate the upper aerodigestive tract. BALT = bronchus-associated lymphoid tissue; GALT = gut-associated lymphoid tissue. (From Mestecky J. The common mucosal immune system and current strategies for induction of immune responses in external secretions. J Clin Immunol 7:265–276, 1987.)

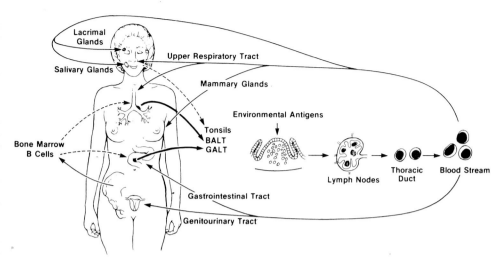

uptake, probably mediated by a number of receptor-ligand pairs. Viable organisms and particulate material are taken up best (Kato and Owen, 1994). Of particular interest is the presence of receptors for immunoglobulins on the apical surface of the M cell (Weltzin et al., 1989), where they may enhance the uptake of antigens combined with luminal antibodies.

The site at which the absorbed luminal antigen is processed for presentation has not yet been defined. The M cells, unlike the subepithelial macrophages and interdigitating dendritic cells, express little or no major histocompatibility complex (MHC) class II molecules (Brandtzaeg and Bjerke, 1990) but have acidic endosomal compartments (Nagura et al., 1991; Allan et al., 1993), which are necessary for antigen processing.

Development of IgA Precursor Cells

Activated CD4[+] T cells are needed to initiate an IgA-predominant mucosal antibody response. However, the detailed way in which the microenvironment in lymphoepithelial structures, like the Peyer's patches, promotes preferential humoral immune responses remains sketchy. The commitment of B cells to production of polymeric IgA and the ability of secretory epithelial cells to transport secretory IgA to the external fluids are the most distinguishing characteristics of the mucosal immune system.

Strober and Ehrhardt (1994) have reviewed the regulation of IgA B-cell development in the GALT. The previous conflict between those who argued that the commitment of Peyer's patch B cells to IgA was due to direct and repeated antigenic stimulation, leading to step-wise B-cell isotype switches, and those who said that soluble factors from local T cells directed the isotype switch to IgA has been largely resolved in favor of the latter view. Differentiation of B cells into IgA precursor cells requires interactions of the antigen-presenting dendritic cells and CD4[+] T cells with the B cells.

Antigenic exposure is required at several steps in this process, but activated T cells and locally secreted cytokines are the most likely mediators of the isotype specificity. Evidence for this concept was provided by Elson and coworkers' (1979) demonstration that antigen-activated T cells from Peyer's patches enhance lipopolysaccharide (LPS)-driven IgA synthesis but suppress IgM and IgG synthesis. Cell lines containing "switch" T cells (Mayer et al., 1985) and clones derived from them (Benson and Strober, 1988) can induce in vitro production of specific Ig isotypes by activated B cells. Although some commitment of Peyer's patch B cells to IgA may be dependent on antigen-stimulated, interdigitating dendritic cells, these cells are ineffective in the absence of T cells (Strober and Ehrhardt, 1994).

The soluble T cell mediators that direct B-cell commitment to IgA have been studied intensively. The sequence and site of the differentiation events are important in understanding this process because some factors enhancing early steps of differentiation may inhibit later steps. All of the steps of differentiation from a virgin (sIgM[+], sIgD[+]) B cell to an IgA-committed cell may not take place in the Peyer's patch follicles. That early steps in the switch process may occur in the bone marrow is in keeping with the relatively high frequency of IgA B cells at that site. Although Peyer's patch is the most important site for the development of B cells that will eventually produce IgA antibodies, there is very little IgA production within the patches. Thus, terminal differentiation to plasma cells must occur near the effector site (e.g., gut lamina propria).

The earliest step of B-cell switch to a "downstream" (e.g., IgA) isotype is increased accessibility of the transcriptional enzymes to the DNA regions 5′ to the C_H genes (Strober and Ehrhardt, 1994). There is no conclusive evidence that this step is either isotype-specific or driven by known soluble stimuli. The next step in the differentiation of an IgA B cell is the production of germline transcripts, encoded by $C\alpha$ genes which have not yet rearranged to a VDJ segment (Stavnezer et al., 1988; Wakatsuki and Strober, 1993). This process suggests that this segment of DNA is also available to the switch recombinase. The same cytokines that induce class switches of other isotype (e.g., interleukin-4 [IL-4] for IgG1) also induce the production of germline transcripts for that isotype. Stravnezer et al. (1988) showed that transforming growth factor-β (TGF-β) induces Cα germline transcripts in a B-cell lymphoma. Thus, TGF-β may be considered a soluble factor that enhances switching to IgA B cells. However, TGF-β is probably not a specific IgA switch factor because it also enhances the switching to other isotypes (McIntyre et al., 1993). IL-4 and IL-10 also enhance B-cell switching to IgA.

Another requirement for isotype switching is activation of the B cells for a proliferative response, an event required for the switch recombinations of DNA that result in productive rearrangements. One effective way to deliver an activation signal for IgA production is through the CD40 membrane structure (Rousset et al., 1991). The natural ligand for CD40 (gp39) is found on activated T cells. Further evidence for the requirement of CD40 ligand for IgA (and IgG) production is the deficiencies of these isotypes in patients with X-linked hyper-IgM syndrome, a congenital deficiency of the CD40 ligand gp39 on T cells (Cutler et al., 1993). The requirement for CD40 ligation for in vitro activation of B cells for IgA production can be replaced by antibodies to CD40. However, for a complete effect, membranes of activated T cells or anti-CD40 on intact B cells (Rousset et al., 1991) are required, which suggests that other accessory membrane signals are also needed.

A unifying, but unproven, concept for commitment of B cells of MALT to IgA is that the process is regulated by the way in which antigen is presented to the T cells in the nodules. This mode of antigen presentation, and/or accessory signals from the antigen-presenting cells (APCs), may activate T cells to perform as switch cells that drive the local B cells to undergo commitment to IgA isotypes. This process may also initiate B-cell migration to mucosal sites. Here the primed B cells, under the influence of memory T cells, differentiate into plasma cells, which produce polymeric IgA. An alternative explanation is that B cells, programmed in the bone marrow to undergo IgA isotype switch, selectively home to mucosal nodules because of unique surface adherence molecules and vascular counter-receptors. Such a vascular determinant, or "mucosal addressin," has been described on the high endothelial venules (HEVs) of Peyer's patches and ordinary venules in the lamina propria (Streeter et al., 1988). The homing receptors for this ligand appear to be L-selection and particularly the integrin α4β7 (Picker, 1994).

Migration, Proliferation, and Differentiation of IgA Cells

The activities of IgA cells have been reviewed by Phillips-Quagliata and Lamm (1994). When antigen-activated IgA-precursor cells leave MALT, they migrate through afferent lymphatics to their regional lymph nodes (see Fig. 8–1). These sites are critical for preparing the B cells for homing to their ultimate effector sites, since the B lymphoblasts from mesenteric lymph nodes migrate preferentially to the gut lamina propria (Phillips-Quagliata et al., 1983). The precise characteristics endowed on B cells during their stay in the regional nodes which promote migration to the lamina propria are not known. However, activation and proliferation are essential. The activated B cells leave the regional nodes via efferent lymphatics and enter the thoracic duct and eventually the venous blood. Some cells extravasate through the vessels near the intestinal crypt or similar sites near other secretory epithelium. The integrin α4β7 may be essential for this process (Picker, 1994). In the gut, the IgA-producing cells then localize in the lamina propria, mainly at the level of the crypt openings. Once migration is complete, further antigenic stimulation is necessary for the B cells to proliferate locally (Husband and Dunkley, 1985).

Within the integrated mucosal immune system, there is regional preference for the sites of final migration of IgA-committed B cells. Mesenteric lymph node cells localize preferentially to the small intestine while bronchial lymph node cells preferentially migrate to the lung (McDermott and Bienenstock, 1979). Even within the gut, there is migratory preference between the small intestine and colon (Pierce and Cray, 1982). Activated B cells from human tonsils may preferentially seed exocrine sites of the upper respiratory tract (Brandtzaeg and Halstensen, 1992). Such preferences may be determined by differences in homing molecules and/or the foreign antigens encountered at the various mucosal sites.

The differentiation and migratory pathway through mucosal nodules and regional nodes may not be the only pathway for mucosal IgA precursors. A less well understood lineage of mucosal B cell, probably arising from the peritoneal cavity, has been described in mice by Herzenberg and associates (1986). These cells, coelomic or B-1 cells, apparently do not migrate through the Peyer's patches (Kroese et al., 1989), and their presence in the lamina propria may be only transient. Reconstitution studies of Kroese and colleagues (1989) suggest that B-1 cells may constitute 30% to 40% of the IgA-producing cells in the murine lamina propria. A similar B-cell population has not been identified in humans.

Terminal Differentiation of B Cells Producing Polymeric IgA

After migration to mucosal effector sites, IgA precursor cells come under the influence of another set of regulatory T cells that, along with direct antigenic exposure, induce B cells to terminally differentiate into IgA-secreting plasma cells. The population of CD4+ T-helper cells responsible for this maturation differ from those of the Peyer's patches or mesenteric lymph nodes because mucosal IgA synthesis is much less prominent than that in the lamina propria.

In vitro stimulation of murine B cells with recombinant cytokines, reviewed by Lebman and Coffman

(1994), suggests that certain cytokines, namely IL-2, IL-4, IL-5, and IL-6, are responsible for IgA B-cell differentiation. Similar studies in humans are limited and mainly performed on tonsillar B cells. In one system, human B cells were stimulated with a CD40 antibody attached through an Fcγ receptor to human fibroblasts (Rousset et al., 1991), thus providing the membrane signals of activated T cells without the associated T-cell cytokines. By the addition of single or mixtures of recombinant cytokines, it was shown in mice that IL-4, in combination with IL-2, IFN-γ, or IL-5, increases IgA production; however, only the IL-2/IL-5 combination selectively enhanced IgA production. The mechanism by which IL-5 induces IgA in this system is not known, but it may selectively stimulate the IgA-committed B cells.

Data in mice provide a clue to the local role of IL-5. Taguchi et al. (1990) examined the pattern of cytokine production from cells derived from mucosal sites; only the gut lamina propria T cells demonstrated cells producing more IL-5 than IFN-γ. Thus, a high frequency of T_H2 T cells at this site is responsible for maturation of IgA-committed B cells. However, since IL-2 and IFN-γ (cytokines typically produced by T_H1 cells) also enhance IgA production, some cooperation with T_H1 cells may also occur.

It is difficult to obtain persistent memory in the secretory immune system. Secretory antibodies from the primary response may exclude the antigens of the booster dose, providing a partial explanation. Both animal (Montgomery et al., 1984) and human (Carlsson et al., 1985) studies show that persistent topical stimulation eventually results in a decreased local IgA response, perhaps because of induction of suppressor T cells. With the exception of cholera toxin (Lycke and Holmgren, 1987), topical induction of a long-lasting secretory immune response requires large and repeated doses of dead antigen (Pierce and Sack, 1977) or the continuous persistence of a replicating antigen (Ogra and Karzon, 1970). Thus, Ogra (1971) found that even 34 months after live oral poliovirus vaccination, there was no decline in nasopharyngeal IgA antibody levels. Similarly, SIgA antibodies against rubella virus persist for several years following live rubella vaccine (Banatvala et al., 1979). On the other hand, SIgA antibodies against poliovirus persist in the saliva without any known antigen re-exposure other than repeated parenteral injections of inactivated poliovirus vaccine (Carlsson et al., 1985). Indeed, functional IgA memory cells have been identified in the Peyer's patches of mice (Lebman et al., 1987).

Studies in dogs and rats demonstrate that parenteral priming and topical boosting is more efficient than topical priming and boosting for the induction of mucosal immune responses (Pierce and Gowans, 1975; Pierce and Sack, 1977; Cebra et al., 1982). Conversely, using *Escherichia coli* antigens in rats and mice, the best SIgA response was obtained by parenteral boosting after mucosal priming (Hanson et al., 1983b). In agreement with this, parenteral vaccination with poliovirus is more efficient in humans in boosting milk SIgA antibodies than peroral vaccination (Svennerholm et

al., 1981; Carlsson et al., 1985). Such parenteral boosting by cholera vaccine occurred only in individuals who had been previously naturally exposed (Svennerholm et al., 1980).

Altogether, these findings indicate considerable interaction between MALT and other lymphoid tissues. In addition to practical problems in eliciting local immunity (Waldman and Ganguly, 1975a), this is an important aspect to consider when immunoprophylaxis is planned, because parenteral immunization will induce IgG antibodies that may decrease antigen penetrability and thus limit vaccine effectiveness (Brandtzaeg and Tolo, 1977).

Characterization of Immunocytes at Secretory Sites

All secretory tissues of adults contain a striking preponderance of IgA-producing immunocytes, including plasma cells and their immediate precursors (Fig. 8–2 and Table 8–1). However, the density of such cells varies greatly, being highest in intestinal mucosa and lacrimal glands (Brandtzaeg, 1983a). Almost 10^{10} IgA-producing cells occur per meter of bowel (Brandtzaeg and Baklien, 1976a), and thus most of the immunocytes of the secretory immune system are located in the gut. The total size of this Ig-producing cell population is considerably greater than 2.5×10^{10} cells, the estimated total number of such cells present in bone marrow, spleen, and lymph nodes combined (Turesson, 1976).

The density of IgA-producing cells correlates with the rate of IgA secretion at various sites. Even though the IgA cell density is not much greater in the lactating human mammary gland than in the parotid, the large size of the former and the local accumulation of IgA between emptying periods explains the large IgA output during milk feedings (Brandtzaeg, 1983a). Although IgM-producing cells contribute significantly to jejunal immunocytes, nasal and bronchial mucosae contain a substantial proportion of IgG-producing cells (see Table 8–1). The reasons for these regional differences are unknown, but differences in antigenic and mitogenic stimulation by the microbial flora in the intestinal and respiratory tracts may influence the development of the local immunocyte populations (Brandtzaeg, 1994).

Ig-producing cells are not normally present in human intestinal mucosa before 10 days of postnatal age (Perkkiö and Savilathi, 1980). However, T and B lymphocytes appear together with dendritic cells in the fetal gut by gestational age of 16 to 19 weeks. IgM and IgD are already expressed at that time (Spencer et al., 1986a, 1986b), suggesting an early capacity for antigenic responses. After birth, a rapid increase in IgM immunocytes occurs; these predominate in the lamina propria for up to one month (Brandtzaeg et al., 1991). Blanco and coworkers (1976) found no increase of IgA-producing cells in children after one year, although the number of IgM immunocytes decreased. A decrease in intestinal IgM immunocytes with age is associated with an increase of IgA cells even beyond 2 years of age (Savilathi, 1972; Maffei et al., 1979).

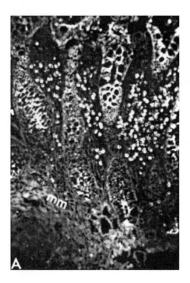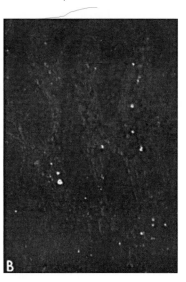

Figure 8–2. Paired immunohistochemical staining of IgA *(A)* and IgG *(B)* in a section of normal human colon mucosa. The two pictures are from the same field after selective filtration of green and red fluorescence, respectively. Most of the extracellular immunoglobulins had been removed from the tissue by washing, but some IgA was retained in the muscularis mucosae (mm) and submucosa. Intracellularly, IgA is present in numerous immunocytes in the lamina propria, in columnar crypt cells, and to a lesser extent in the surface epithelium (at the top). Very few IgG-producing cells are present, and this immunoglobulin is not transported through the columnar epithelial cells. Note that the muscularis mucosae and submucosa are virtually devoid of Ig-producing cells. (× 140.)

Tada and Ishizaka (1970) claim that large numbers of IgE-producing cells are present in mucous membranes and tonsils, but there are many technical problems involved in their identification (Brandtzaeg and Baklien, 1976b; Brandtzaeg, 1984, 1985b). Other studies indicate that their numbers in these tissues are extremely low (Ragnum and Brandtzaeg, 1989).

IgD-producing cells are virtually absent from human intestinal mucosa (Brandtzaeg and Baklien, 1976a; Brandtzaeg 1983a). In the tonsils, however, there are about one third as many IgD-producing cells as those containing cytoplasmic IgM (Brandtzaeg et al., 1978), and in the parotid, lacrimal, and nasal glands (Table 8–1), there are about the same number as the IgM-producing cells (Brandtzaeg et al., 1979; Brandtzaeg, 1983a). This discrepancy is accentuated in IgA deficiency, in which IgA-producing cells are often replaced by IgD immunocytes in the upper aeroalimentary tract, rather than by IgM immunocytes, which predominate in the gut (Brandtzaeg et al., 1979, 1987).

Secretory IgA Production

Extracellular Immunoglobulins in Mucosal Tissues

Immunohistochemical studies of secretory tissues has shown, despite extensive local production of IgA, that

IgG predominates in the extravascular space (Brandtzaeg, 1974; Brandtzaeg and Baklien, 1976a). This finding is compatible with rapid external transport of the locally produced polymeric IgA. Thus, the IgA of the stroma may represent monomeric IgA of local or serum origin. Because local synthesis of IgG is sparse, the intense stromal staining most likely represents serum-derived IgG. Although 50% to 60% of circulating IgA and IgG is extravascular, only 20% of IgM is extravascular (Waldmann and Strober, 1969). Accordingly, the secretory tissue shows little IgM except in basement membrane zones and vessel walls. With antigenic stimulation, the amount of extracellular IgA and IgM may be substantially increased, as in the mucosa of patients with celiac disease (Brandtzaeg and Baklien, 1977b). IgD and IgE cannot usually be demonstrated extracellularly.

Nature of Locally Formed IgA

As reviewed (Brandtzaeg, 1985a), it was initially believed that IgA immunocytes at secretory sites produce monomers, which were then polymerized by complexing with an epithelial glycoprotein called "secretory piece" or "secretory component" (SC) to form dimeric secretory IgA. However, the later finding of J chain in most IgA immunocytes in exocrine tissue strongly

Table 8–1. Distribution of Ig-Producing Immunocytes in Normal Adult Human Glandular Tissue

Tissue Site	IgA (%)	IgM (%)	IgG (%)	IgD (%)	Reference
Lacrimal gland	77	7.2	5.8	9.7	Gjeruldsen and Brandtzaeg, 1978
Parotid gland	91	3.0	3.7	2.5	Korsrud and Brandtzaeg, 1978
Nasal concha	67	7.8	15.8	9.2	Brandtzaeg et al., 1979; Brandtzaeg and Berdal, 1973
Bronchial mucosa	74	N.D.*	29.0	N.D.*	Boye and Brandtzaeg, 1986
Gastric body mucosa	73	13	14	<1.0	Valnes et al., 1986
Gastric antral mucosa	80	8	12	<1.0	Valnes et al., 1986
Jejunum	81	17	2.6	<1.0	Brandtzaeg and Baklien, 1976a
Ileum	83	11	5.0	<1.0	Baklien and Brandtzaeg, 1976
Large bowel	90	6	4.2	<1.0	Baklien and Brandtzaeg, 1975
Lactating mammary gland	68	13	16.0	2.4	Brandtzaeg, 1983a

*N.D. = not determined.

suggested that the IgA dimers were produced within the plasma cells (Brandtzaeg, 1974a, 1983b). SC-affinity tests on tissue sections substantiated that the J-chain–containing IgA as well as IgM is assembled within the plasma cells; this finding, however, does not exclude a concomitant output of some IgA monomers by lamina propria immunocytes (Brandtzaeg, 1994).

Analyses of cultured mononuclear cells from human gut mucosa have not demonstrated conclusively the proportion of IgA monomers and dimers produced (Brandtzaeg, 1985a). However, IgA immunocytes of secretory sites preferentially produce SIgA polymers compared with other lymphoid tissues, such as tonsils or cells from inflammatory foci, where little J-chain production takes place (Brandtzaeg and Korsrud, 1984).

A large fraction of IgA immunocytes (35% to 60%) at secretory sites contain the IgA2 subclass, compared with cells of the tonsils and peripheral lymph nodes (Crago and Mestecky, 1984; Jonard et al., 1984). Production of IgA2 is particularly striking in the ileum and large bowel, where mucosal IgA2 immunocytes often predominate (Kett et al., 1986). Teleologically, this may be advantageous because IgA2 is more resistant to microbial proteases. There is also a relatively high proportion of IgA2 cells in salivary glands (~37%), whereas nasal mucosa contains about 95% IgA1 producers (Kett et al., 1986). Thus, IgA2 predominates where the intensity of bacterial exposure is greatest (Brandtzaeg, 1994).

Active Transfer of Immunoglobulin into External Secretions

Despite the high stromal concentration of IgG, secretory epithelia are virtually devoid of this isotype. IgD and IgE cannot be detected in epithelia, except for IgE that is carried by mast cells (Brandtzaeg, 1984, 1985b).

In contrast, IgA is present at the basal and lateral surfaces of the mucosal epithelial cells and intracellularly in serous-type cells, especially in the apical part of colonic and rectal crypt cells (Brandtzaeg, 1974b; Brandtzaeg and Baklien, 1977b). The epithelial distribution of IgM mimics that of IgA, although it is much less prominent and is readily demonstrable only in the large bowel (Brandtzaeg, 1975b). The predominance of polymeric Ig isotypes (dimeric IgA and pentameric IgM) within epithelial cells suggests that they are selectively transported into or through these cells.

Polymeric Immunoglobulin Receptor

The selective transport of polymeric immunoglobulin into the external secretions is unique to the secretory immune system. The specificity and efficiency of secretory immunoglobulin formation lie in a receptor-ligand interaction. Unlike most receptor-mediated processes, however, the polymeric immunoglobulin receptor (PIgR) remains attached to its ligand (dimeric IgA or pentameric IgM) throughout the transport and secretory process. A fragment of the PIgR, first recognized by Hanson (1961) as a unique structural component of SIgA, was initially termed bound "secretory piece," but is now called simply "bound SC." The PIgR corresponds to transmembrane SC, and fragments of the receptor are released to the lumen as "free SC," structurally identical to bound SC.

With few exceptions, PIgR expression is limited to the serous-type secretory epithelial cells (Figs. 8–3 and 8–4). The PIgR is a member of the Ig supergene family, which consists of seven domains, or functional segments (Mostov et al., 1984; Brandtzaeg, 1994). The five N-terminal domains, which bear strong homology with the immunoglobulin variable domains, form the extracellular segment of the receptor. Following an 8–amino acid hydrophobic transmembrane segment is

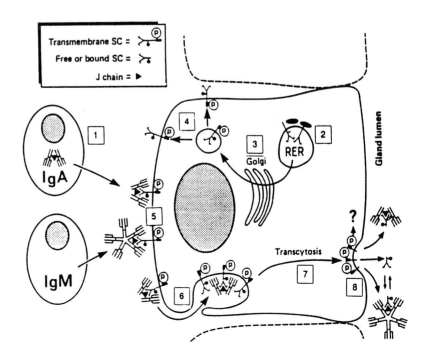

Figure 8–3. Model for local generation of human secretory IgA (SIgA) and secretory IgM (SIgM): 1, Production of J chain–containing poly-IgA and pentameric IgM by gland-associated plasma cells. 2, Synthesis and core glycosylation (——) of transmembrane SC in rough endoplasmic reticulum (RER) of epithelial cell. 3, Terminal glycosylation (—•) in Golgi complex. 4, Phosphorylation (Ⓟ) at some later step. 5, Complexing of SC with J chain–containing poly-Ig on basolateral cell membrane. 6, Endocytosis of complexed and unoccupied SC. 7, Transcytosis of vesicles. 8, Cleavage and release of SIgA, SIgM, and excess free SC. The cleavage mechanism and the fate of the cytoplasmic tail of transmembrane SC are mostly unknown (?). During the external translocation, covalent stabilization of the IgA-SC complexes regularly occurs (two disulfide bridges indicated in SIgA), whereas an excess of free SC in the secretion serves to stabilize the noncovalent SIgM complexes (dynamic equilibrium indicated). (From Brandtzaeg P, Halstensen TS, Huitfeldt HS, et al. Epithelial expression of HLA, secretory component (poly-Ig receptor), and adhesion molecules in the human alimentary tract. Ann N Y Acad Sci 664:61, 1992.)

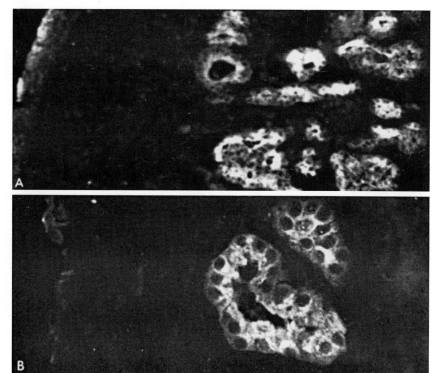

Figure 8–4. Immunohistochemical localization of secretory component (SC) in normal human nasal mucosa from the concha inferior. *A,* Note fluorescence of serous glandular acini, whereas the surface epithelium (to the left) does not contain secretory component except in occasional cells where IgA (not shown) is also present. The mucous coat on the surface has not been retained. *B,* In addition to cytoplasmic localization, secretory component is also present in relation to lateral and basal borders of acinar cells, apparently incorporated into the plasma membrane. Note the absence of secretory component in the connective tissue, where numerous Ig-producing cells (not shown) are present. (*A,* × 60; *B,* × 160.)

a large (~100 amino acids) cytoplasmic tail. After synthesis in the rough endoplasmic reticulum and extensive glycosylation (~20% carbohydrate by weight) in the Golgi complex, the PIgR is selectively targeted to the basal and lateral membranes of the epithelial cells. The molecular information necessary for this targeting resides in a 17–amino acid segment of the cytoplasmic tail (Casanova et al., 1990). Once inserted in the epithelial cell membrane, the extracellular receptor segment becomes available for binding PIg. Bakos et al. (1991) have identified a small segment of the first (N-terminal) domain that is critical for immunoglobulin noncovalent binding. However, studies using synthetic peptides representing this region, and proteolytic fragments of native PIgR, indicate that a more extensive structure is required to achieve specific binding of polymeric IgA and IgM (Bakos et al., 1993).

The portion of the Ig polymer necessary for binding to the PIgR is not known. The striking J-chain expression of immunocytes in secretory tissues suggests that the J chain is involved in binding (Brandtzaeg et al., 1974). J chains enhance IgA and IgM polymer production near the site of external transfer, but the J chain is involved only indirectly in receptor binding, because free J chain has little affinity for SC (Brandtzaeg, 1985b). That J chain is required for PIgR binding is suggested by the finding that monoclonal polymeric IgA and IgM, which are deficient in J chains, do not bind free SC (Brandtzaeg, 1976a) or the transmembrane receptor (Brandtzaeg and Prydz, 1984). Further, antibody to J chain will block the SC-binding site of IgA dimers (Brandtzaeg, 1976b). Thus, the J chain is necessary, but not sufficient, for immunoglobulin to bind avidly and noncovalently to the PIgR.

After ligand binding, the PIgR-ligand complexes are internalized via clatharine-coated pits into intracellular vesicles (see Fig. 8–3). The transport of PIgR through the epithelial cell is called *transcytosis.* The migration of these vesicles across the epithelial cells is regulated by signaling information present in the cytoplasmic tail of the PIgR (Mostov et al., 1984). In some tissues, the PIgR-ligand complexes accumulate in vesicles near the apical surface of the cell. These complexes may serve as a reservoir of secretory immunoglobulin (SIg) that can be rapidly secreted when needed. Indeed, there may be a highly regulated mechanism for rapid release of the SIg (Mostov, 1994).

The final steps of SIg formation entail fusion of the vesicles with the epithelial apical membrane and by an enzyme cleavage of the extracellular segment of the PIgR within the apical membrane (Musil and Baenziger, 1988). This process releases SIg (polymeric immunoglobulin and its bound SC) into the lumen.

Secretory IgA Formation

Several elements of SIg formation deserve further comment. During transcytosis, a disulfide bond is formed between the IgA polymers and the PIgR. Only one of the subunits of IgA is involved in this reaction (Underdown et al., 1977; Garcia-Pardo et al., 1979). The mechanisms and intracellular site of this covalent bond formation have been studied (Lindh and Björk, 1976; Chintalacharuvu, et al., 1993). Although intracellular enzymes may be involved in this process, the same bonds can be formed in vitro in the absence of any enzymes (Brandtzaeg, 1977a). Interchain disulfide bonds do not form between IgM and SC because of the lack of a free sulfhydryl group on IgM. The importance of the disulfide bond on IgA-SC integrity and function has not been studied in detail, but covalently bound SC may enhance the resistance of SIgA against proteolytic degradation.

The process of transcytosis of the PIgR does not require the binding of immunoglobulin polymers. In the absence of a ligand, the proteolytic product of PIgR number is free SC. This fragment can also be found in the secretions in which SIgA is normally found. This suggests that epithelial transport is constitutive and that PIgR is not a rate-limiting factor for SIgA formation. Free SC can be found in secretions of young infants and other patients who are IgA-deficient (South et al., 1966) in amounts similar to the total (free and bound) SC in healthy subjects (Brandtzaeg, 1974a). This suggests that polymers are not necessary for PIgR expression by secretory epithelia. The presence of free SC in body fluids (e.g., amniotic fluid) has been used as a marker for the presence of secretory epithelium capable of SIgA formation (Cleveland et al., 1991).

Secretory immunoglobulin formation by epithelial cells is highly regulated. Mostov (1994) has examined the signals for entry of the PIgR into the transcytotic pathway and the release of SIg from the apical membrane. The expression of PIgR also seems to be regulated, at least in some tissues. Evidence for the enhanced PIgR expression after stimulation by pro-inflammatory cytokines (TNF-α, IFN-γ, and IL-4) is derived from in vitro studies using a single human colon carcinoma cell line (Phillips et al., 1990). Increased epithelial expression of PIgR, however, is present in several diseases in which these cytokines can be expected to be produced (Brandtzaeg et al., 1992). Some studies suggest that the modulation occurs at the messenger ribonucleic acid (mRNA) level (Krajci et al., 1993; Piskurich et al., 1993). A small effect of TGF-β on SC production has also been demonstrated in a rat epithelial cell line (McGee et al., 1991).

In vivo regulation of the PIgR expression to increase SIgA production at sites of intensified mucosal immune responses may focus the output of the secretory immune system. Thus, increased amounts of SIgA, free SC, or both may indicate enhanced local immunity. Examples include high levels of SIgA in the urine of patients with pyelonephritis (Fliedner et al., 1986) and in duodenal secretions in untreated celiac disease (Brandtzaeg et al., 1993).

Passive Transfer of Immunoglobulin into External Secretions

In addition to selective external transport of IgA and IgM polymers, passive intercellular epithelial diffusion contributes to the immunoglobulin content of exocrine fluids, as indicated by the immunohistochemical demonstration of IgG. A similar but brighter staining pattern is shown for albumin. Intercellular epithelial diffusion is more pronounced in respiratory and intestinal surface epithelia than in pure glandular epithelia. Thus, the composition of an exocrine fluid is also dependent on extraglandular extravasation, which may be influenced by inflammation and local immunoglobulin production (Brandtzaeg et al., 1970; Haneberg and Aar-

skog, 1975). The trace amounts of IgE in external secretions may be the result of passive diffusion or IgE release from interepithelial mast cells (Brandtzaeg, 1984, 1985b).

STRUCTURE AND FUNCTION OF IMMUNOGLOBULINS IN EXOCRINE SECRETIONS

Secretory IgA Structure

Most serum IgA molecules are monomers composed of two identical heavy and two light chains arranged as in IgG. Only about 15% to 20% of normal serum IgA molecules are dimers and larger polymers of IgA (Delacroix et al., 1983; Neukirk et al., 1983). The proportion of polymeric IgA is considerably higher in infancy (Delacroix et al., 1983; Splawski et al., 1984). Conversely, polymeric forms predominate in the secretions and monomeric IgA makes up only 5% to 20% (Brandtzaeg et al., 1970; Sørensen, 1982; Jonard et al., 1984). Variation of the monomer:polymer ratio in different secretions may be due to different degrees to which the IgA is transported by the PIgR or leaks through the epithelium. Both processes are influenced by inflammation and local immunoglobulin production (Brandtzaeg et al., 1970; Haneberg and Aarskog, 1975).

Secretory IgA polymers are heterogeneous in size, but most are dimers. The proportion of larger polymers varies; some authors have found 5% to 20% (Tomasi et al., 1965; Rossen et al., 1966; Newcomb et al., 1968; Hurlimann et al., 1969; Delacroix and Vaerman, 1982), others found considerably higher percentages (Brandtzaeg et al., 1970; Mestecky and Kraus, 1970). Variable degrees of aggregation following SIgA purification may explain these discrepancies.

IgA and IgM polymers also contain a polypeptide J chain of about 15 (kD) (Halpern and Koshland, 1970; Mestecky et al., 1971). This J chain is disulfide-linked to the penultimate cysteine of the C-terminal octapeptide of the heavy chains (Mestecky, 1976). Regardless of the size of the polymer, there is one J chain that acts as a "clasp" connecting only two Ig subunits, whereas the remaining subunits of polymers larger than dimers are mutually connected by inter–heavy-chain disulfide bridges (Inman and Mestecky, 1974; Koshland, 1975; Garcia-Pardo et al., 1981; Bastian et al., 1992). However, J chains are prone to degradation, and exact quantification is difficult. Immunochemical studies suggest that there may be two J chains per IgA dimer and three per IgM pentamer (Brandtzaeg, 1975a, 1975b).

Secretory IgA also differs from serum polymeric IgA by its content of bound SC. The majority of SIgA consists of a dimer of IgA, one or two J chains, and one SC. The resulting molecule has a molecular weight of 375 kD estimated by gel filtration and 390 kD by ultracentrifugation (Newcomb et al., 1968; Tomasi and Czerwinski, 1968; Hurlimann et al., 1969).

Secretory component endows SIgA with unique antigenic properties. Thus, antibodies to SC distinguish between the serum IgA and SIgA; these antibodies are used extensively in studies of clinical samples and molecular structure. Degradation of SIgA, followed by antigenic analyses of the split products, provides information about the tertiary and quaternary structure of the intact molecule. Disruption of only the noncovalent bonds results in only minor release of IgA monomers and SC (Tomasi and Bienenstock, 1968; Brandtzaeg, 1971b). In human SIgA, 70% to 80% of SC is bound by disulfide bridges, secondarily stabilized by noncovalent bonds. Thus, when complexed with IgA, part of the SC is inaccessible to antibodies or enzymes. Moreover, formation of SIgA results in extensive configurational changes on SC because most epitopes of free SC are not detectable on SIgA (Brandtzaeg et al., 1970; Brandtzaeg, 1971b; Iscaki et al., 1978; Woodard et al., 1984, Bakos et al., 1993). The enhanced stability and resistance to enzymatic degradation of SIgA may result from masking the labile segments of IgA and free SC (Bakos et al., 1993).

Secretory IgA Stability

The external secretions are potentially more destructive to proteins than are the plasma and interstitial tissue spaces. Thus, enhanced resistance of SIg to degradation favors protection of the host. Most in vitro studies showing increased resistance of SIgA to proteolytic digestion do not identify whether the effect is due to the presence of a dimeric structure or presence of SC (Ghetie and Mota, 1973; Underdown and Dorrington, 1974, Lindh, 1975). In either case, these results suggest that SIgA can function in the protease-containing external secretions. In vivo evidence for this is derived from studies showing that human milk SIgA traverses the infant gut with its antibody activity intact (Kenny et al., 1967; Gindrat et al., 1972; Haneberg, 1974a; Schanler et al., 1986). Most of these studies did not assess the amount of antibody the infants were receiving or other properties of human milk (e.g., its high buffering capacity), but it is believed that SIgA persists and functions well, even in the harsh environment of the gastrointestinal tract.

Some bacteria can counter the attack of SIgA antibodies. As in the mammalian liver (Hanson et al., 1973), some *Escherichia coli* have nucleotide-dependent reductases that can split colostral IgA (Moore et al., 1964), thus degrading SIgA antibodies attached to *E. coli* bacteria in the intestine. Other pathogenic oral, enteric, and upper respiratory tract bacteria have proteases with high specificity and activity for IgA1, cleaving it to Fc and Fab fragments (Plaut, 1983; Kilian and Reinholdt, 1986; Kilian and Russell, 1994). IgA1 normally constitutes about 80% of serum IgA, whereas SIgA consists of 60% to 70% IgA1 (Delacroix and Vaerman, 1982), depending on the production site (Brandtzaeg, 1994). This IgA2 enrichment in secretions may provide enhanced protection, especially in the colon and mouth, where IgA2 isotype is highest and bacteria are plentiful. However, *Clostridium ramosum* protease has specificity for both IgA1 and IgA2 of the A2m(1) but not the A2m(2) allotype (Fujiyama et al.,

1985). Furthermore, yeasts of the species *Torulopsis* and *Candida* as well as *Pseudomonas aeruginosa* make proteases that can degrade IgA1, IgA2, and SIgA (Reinholdt et al., 1987; Kilian and Russell, 1994).

Thus, an absolute resistance of SIgA against in vivo proteolytic degradation does not occur. Humans often make SIgA antibody to certain microbial enzymes, thereby inhibiting their activity (Gilbert et al., 1983). Serum IgA and SIgA are often resistant to IgA proteases as a result of antibodies that neutralize the enzymes (Kobayashi et al., 1987). However, neither fluid contains neutralizing antibodies to the *Clostridium* enzyme that degrades IgA1 and IgA2 (Fujiyama et al., 1985). The fact that some 20% to 80% of milk SIgA can be recovered undegraded in the stool of breast-fed babies (Schanler et al., 1986; Davidson and Lönnerdal, 1987) suggests that the overall balance of this microbe-host defense battle favors the host. The most effective SIgA antibodies are those that bind to the pathogenic microorganisms; these may be particularly susceptible to microbial proteases (Kilian and Russell, 1994).

Function of Secretory IgA

The first issue regarding the function of SIgA is whether these antibodies in secretions are indeed protective. Despite evidence that SIgA antibodies appear in the secretions after oral immunization, that their presence is correlated with protection against toxic substances and pathogenic microorganisms, and that most of the immunoglobulin produced is released into the secretions, direct evidence that SIgA mediates immune protection is limited. Indeed, most patients with severe isolated IgA deficiency have no obvious increase in mucosal infections. The best explanation for this observation is that SIgA is so important that compensatory mechanisms, including SIgM and certain IgG subclasses, compensate for deficiencies in the SIgA system (see Chapter 14).

Several studies provide evidence for a protective role of SIgA. The most convincing have examined the effects of passively transferred IgA, thus excluding a contribution by other components of the immune system. Glass and coworkers (1983) demonstrated that infants ingesting maternal milk containing cholera antibodies have fewer symptoms after exposure to cholera than infants ingesting maternal milk lacking such antibodies. Other studies have confirmed these findings for other enteric organisms (reviewed by Carlsson and Hanson, 1994). In most of these studies, IgA antibodies reduced the frequency and severity of symptoms rather than reducing the incidence of infection. Thus, the immune factors in secretions seem to limit epithelial cell infection and intoxication without initiating an inflammatory reaction rather than completely preventing infection (Goldman et al., 1986).

The efficacy of SIgA antibodies in experimental models also demonstrates that passive transfer of specific polymeric IgA prevents infection following challenge with the live homologous organism. Winner and coauthors (1991) demonstrated serotype-specific protection against oral challenge of mice with *Vibrio cholerae* by subcutaneous implantation of a hybridoma producing polymeric IgA directed against the lipopolysaccharide of that organism. Renegar and Small (1991) showed that intravenous polymeric IgA but not monomeric IgA antibodies against influenza virus protected against challenge of the respiratory tract with influenza virus. The role of SIgA in the resolution of ongoing mucosal infections is less clear. In sum, human and animal studies indicate that mucosal antibody responses are effective at preventing mucosal infections.

The next issue is whether SIgA protection is mediated solely by the specificity of the antibodies or whether it requires the unique biochemical properties of SIgA. Kilian and Russell (1994) divide the functions of SIgA into those mediated solely by (Fab portion) antigen binding and those dependent on Fc and/or secretory specific portions of the SIgA (Kilian et al., 1988). This distinction may be particularly important for SIgA1 in secretions frequently exposed to pathogenic bacteria that produce IgA1 proteases. Despite cleavage into Fc and Fab fragments, some of IgA1 antibody functions may be preserved.

The Fab portion of SIgA by itself can neutralize some toxins and virulence enzymes of microorganisms at the mucosal surfaces. Antibodies against cholera toxin (Lycke et al., 1987) and to glucosyltransferase of streptococci that synthesize adherent glucans (Smith et al., 1985) are examples of virulence factors neutralized by the Fab portion of IgA. Single Fab units of IgA may also prevent viral attachment to their cellular receptors.

Most functions of SIgA require the intact molecule. This includes viral neutralization, inhibition of bacterial adherence, and immune exclusion (Brandtzaeg and Korsrud, 1984; Newby, 1984). SIgA antibodies neutralize viruses efficiently (Hanson and Johansson, 1970; Newcomb and Sutoris, 1974; Taylor and Dimmock, 1985), with a broader antibody specificity than serum antibodies (Waldman et al., 1970; Shvartzman et al., 1977). This broad neutralizing activity may be advantageous in coping with the antigenic drift of microorganisms growing on mucosal surfaces.

Secretory IgA antibodies may also inhibit internalization or even intracellular replication of certain viruses (Armstrong and Dimmock, 1992). Polymeric IgA may even be able to inhibit replication of viruses that have previously entered cells (Mazanac et al., 1992). This activity may be mediated by polymeric IgA antibodies entering infected epithelial cells via the PIgR. Thus, a virus entering an epithelial cell at its apical (luminal) face might be neutralized by antibodies from the transcytotic pathway, thus extending the range of IgA-mediated protection. Finally, a virus that breaches the epithelial cell may combine with IgA antibodies to form immune complexes that are transported to the lumen by other IgR-expressing cells (Kaetzel et al., 1991).

Prevention of bacterial adherence and colonization by SIgA is one of its most crucial functions (Williams and Gibbons, 1972; Tramont, 1977; Svanborg Edén and Svennerholm, 1978; Svanborg Edén, 1994). The mechanisms by which SIgA prevents bacterial adherence are multiple. Binding of the surface adherence factors on the bacteria by the Fab region of SIgA may have some neutralizing effects. The hydrophilic nature of the intact IgA provided by the extensive glycosylation of both α chains of IgA2 and SC may reduce the ability of bacteria to interact with epithelial cell membranes. The multiple combining sites of SIgA polymers promote agglutination of microorganisms (Newcomb and DeVald, 1969) and enhance their removal by peristalsis. SIgA may also interact directly with mucin (Clamp, 1977) or, by their hydrophilicity, may make the bacteria more "mucophilic" and susceptible to mucociliary clearance (Magnusson and Stjernström, 1982).

In vivo coating of bacteria by SIgA can be demonstrated by immunofluorescence (Fig. 8–5), but this may be mediated, in part, by nonspecific binding of type 1 pili of gram-negative bacteria to mannose residues of SIgA. This binding, which is reversed by mannose, may agglutinate bacteria, thus augmenting mucosal defense (Wold et al., 1988). Moreover, several types of bacteria express Fcα receptors that may bind SIgA.

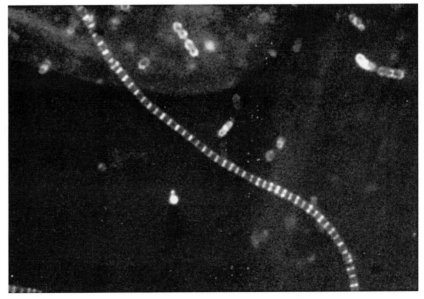

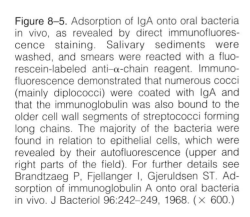

Figure 8–5. Adsorption of IgA onto oral bacteria in vivo, as revealed by direct immunofluorescence staining. Salivary sediments were washed, and smears were reacted with a fluorescein-labeled anti–α-chain reagent. Immunofluorescence demonstrated that numerous cocci (mainly diplococci) were coated with IgA and that the immunoglobulin was also bound to the older cell wall segments of streptococci forming long chains. The majority of the bacteria were found in relation to epithelial cells, which were revealed by their autofluorescence (upper and right parts of the field). For further details see Brandtzaeg P, Fjellanger I, Gjeruldsen ST. Adsorption of immunoglobulin A onto oral bacteria in vivo. J Bacteriol 96:242–249, 1968. (× 600.)

Immune exclusion refers to the ability of SIgA antibodies to hamper microbial colonization and the penetration of macromolecules through the mucous membranes (Walker et al., 1972, 1974, 1975; André et al., 1974; Stokes et al., 1975; Lim and Rowley, 1982). This concept is supported by the observation that IgA-deficient individuals have increased levels of antibodies to dietary antigens and circulating immune complexes containing such antigens (Cunningham-Rundles et al., 1979). The mechanisms involved in immune exclusion are probably similar to those that inhibit viral and bacterial invasion.

In sum, SIgA antibodies act as a "first line of defense" because of their physical attributes and largely their ability to inhibit microbes and antigens from interacting with the mucosa (see Fig. 8–5). This is done without promoting an inflammatory response. Certain cells and soluble components of the secretory system may also interact with SIgA, enhancing its activity.

Structure and Function of Secretory IgM

Only small amounts of IgM are found in the external secretions of normal adults, but their levels are increased in young infants and in individuals with selective IgA deficiency (Brandtzaeg et al., 1968a; Girard and de Kalbermatten, 1970; Brandtzaeg, 1971a; Savilathi, 1973; Mellander et al., 1984, 1986b). It was originally thought that IgM in serum and secretions was identical; later it was shown that 60% to 70% of secretory IgM (SIgM) contains bound SC (Brandtzaeg, 1975b). Pentameric IgM shows better in vitro affinity for SC than does dimeric IgA (Brandtzaeg, 1977, 1985a). This may reflect the fact that IgM probably served the function of protecting mucosal surfaces before the evolution of dimeric IgA (Portis and Coe, 1975). Alternatively, because the SC-IgM complex is not stabilized by disulfide bonds, a higher avidity may be required for survival during transcytosis or in the secretions. However, both rabbit SIgA of the subclass g, which lacks SC-IgA disulfide bonds (Knight et al., 1975), and human SIgM are sensitive to proteolytic digestion (Haneberg, 1974a). Thus, the disulfide bond in human SIgA may have a stabilizing effect that cannot be fully overcome by strong noncovalent binding forces. This property of the disulfide bonds in SIgA may contribute to its evolution as the major secretory antibody in mammals.

Secretory IgM also has antibody activity (Ogra et al., 1974; Haneberg and Aarskog, 1975; Mellander et al., 1984, 1986b) and is extremely efficient at promoting phagocytosis, complement-mediated bacteriolysis, and protection against intestinal infection (Heddle and Rowley, 1975). Some of these effects are markedly enhanced by complement (Girard and de Kalbermatten, 1970). Further, local IgM production in the upper respiratory tract of IgA-deficient patients may confer resistance to infection (Brandtzaeg et al., 1987b). However, SIgM may not be stable enough to provide sufficient antigen exclusion in every IgA-deficient individual. Thus, although SIgM may contribute to a first line of defense of infants and IgA-deficient individuals, it cannot completely replace SIgA (Hanson et al., 1983b).

Other Immunoglobulin Classes in External Secretions

Traces of IgG, IgD, and IgE are found in most normal human secretions. The low concentrations relative to SIgA and even SIgM in mammary and parotid gland secretions and lack of association with SC indicate that the external transfer of the other immunoglobulin classes is passive (Brandtzaeg et al., 1971a). Fluids collected from surfaces of mucous membranes contain relatively more IgG, indicating extraglandular external diffusion. More than 90% of IgG in nasal fluid is of serum origin (Mygind et al., 1975). Such leakage of IgG is enhanced by inflammatory processes (Brandtzaeg et al., 1970). However, there may be preferential local synthesis of certain IgG subclasses (Keller et al., 1983). Even serum-derived IgG may exert some external protective functions, particularly in respiratory secretions. In fact, IgG seems to be the major antibody class of the lower respiratory tract (Newhouse et al., 1976). IgG-mediated immune complex formation at the mucosa may promote inflammation that enhances penetration of foreign substances (Brandtzaeg and Tolo, 1977; Lim and Rowley, 1982).

Early studies suggested that IgE was actively transported into the external secretions, but this conclusion was based on IgE measurement that overestimated its secretory concentration (Johansson and Deuschl, 1976; Underdown et al., 1976, Turner et al., 1977; Magnusson and Masson, 1985). Moreover, SC shows no affinity for IgE in vitro (Brandtzaeg, 1977a) and is not associated with exocrine IgE (Newcomb and Ishizaka, 1970; Bennich and Johansson, 1971). Thus, when there is an enrichment of IgE in some exocrine fluids, this is probably due to passive diffusion through the epithelium (Nakajima et al., 1975) combined with local contribution of IgE—to some extent synthesized by local plasma cells, but mainly from mast cells armed with IgE in regional lymph nodes (Mayrhofer et al., 1976; Brandtzaeg, 1984, 1985b). The biologic significance of IgE in external secretions is unknown; it is rapidly degraded in intestinal fluid (Brown et al., 1975), appearing in the feces as a 40-kd fragment (Kolmannskog et al., 1985). In mucosal membranes, IgE is of major importance for defense against parasites, by arming macrophages, platelets, and eosinophils (Capron et al., 1982, 1987).

Like IgG and IgE, IgD has no affinity for SC (Brandtzaeg, 1977a). Nevertheless, one study indicated preferential appearance of IgD in human colostrum compared with IgG (Keller et al., 1985). The fact that IgD appears in colostrum and saliva but not in intestinal juice (Sewell et al., 1979) indicates that exocrine IgD is of local origin. Indeed, IgD-producing cells are absent in the gastrointestinal tract, in contrast to other secretory sites (Brandtzaeg, 1983a). Exocrine IgD can exhibit antibody activities (Keller et al., 1985), but its biologic significance is unknown. In some patients with IgA deficiency, a striking increase of IgD-producing immunocytes has been noted in nasal mucosa. This IgD was not transported into the lumen, and these patients, unlike patients with an increase of IgM-producing cells, still had frequent infections (Brandtzaeg et al., 1987b).

Quantification of Secretory Immunoglobulins

The biologic activity of an immunoglobulin depends on its total quantity, antigenic specificity, and binding affinity. Measurement of immunoglobulin production is more difficult in secretions than in serum, since the rates of formation, under basal and stimulated states, must also be considered. An additional problem is loss during sample storage, particularly pronounced in unstimulated and dilute exocrine fluids (e.g., parotid fluid and urine) (Brandtzaeg, 1971a; Sohl-Åkerlund et al., 1977).

Quantification of Total Immunoglobulins in Secretions

Depending on the exocrine site and method used to collect the secretion, the IgA may vary from essentially all SIgA to a mixture of SIgA and transudated serum IgA. However, since serum IgA and SIgA are antigenically different and dissimilar in size, immunoassays can allow specific quantification of SIgA. This approach is preferable for assessment of secretory immunity. Such assays utilize antibodies against α chain and SC and a purified SIgA standard in successive steps of a solid-phase immunosorbent assay, for example, the enzyme-linked immunosorbent assay (ELISA) (Sohl-Åkerlund et al., 1977; Goldblum and van Bavel, 1978; Goldblum et al., 1980; Hamaguchi et al., 1982). Particular care must be taken when testing secretions containing free SC, monomeric IgA, and polymeric IgA with and without bound SC and SIgM. Another assay approach uses monoclonal antibodies, which recognize combinatorial epitopes formed from SC-PIg complexes (Woodard et al., 1984; Vincent and Revillard, 1988). By using such antibodies as the capture phase of the immunoassay, one can avoid competition with non–secretory immunoglobulins and free SC (Vincent and Revillard, 1988). Theoretically, SIgA and SIgM can also be quantified independently by using different isotype-specific detecting reagents. However, it is not possible to obtain a reliable estimate of SIgM because of its lack of covalent association with SC (Feltelius et al., 1994).

Few methodologic studies have evaluated the different assay methods and standards in the quantification of IgM, IgG, IgE, and IgD in secretions. Theoretically, it should be acceptable to use a serum-derived immunoglobulin as a reference. However, degradation of these immunoglobulins in secretions is common and immunoglobulin fragments can interfere in most immunoassays. In addition, quantification in secretions of low immunoglobulin levels (such as IgE and IgD) with highly sensitive methods is often subject to nonspecific interference that may lead to overestimation (Johansson and Deuschl, 1976; Underdown et al., 1976; Turner

et al., 1977; Mygind, 1978; Magnusson and Masson, 1985).

Quantification of Specific Secretory IgA Antibodies

Many of the same considerations as described for measurement of total SIgA apply to SIgA antibodies. Isotype-specific antibody assays are often based on a solid-phase immunoassay (e.g., ELISA) in which the specific antigen is attached to the solid phase prior to adding dilutions of the secretion. After unbound material is removed by washing, specific antibodies to SC are added. This approach avoids interference from free SC but does not allow a distinction between SIgA and SIgM (Mellander et al., 1984). These assays are also susceptible to competition for antigen-binding sites by high concentrations of antibodies of other isotypes. The latter concern might be overcome if SIg-specific antibodies were used as the capture phase and the isotope-specific antibody detected by their binding of labeled antigen. Assays of this type, called *antigen capture immunoassays* are cumbersome.

The other major limitation in assessing specific SIgA antibodies is the lack of a good standard. Ideally, affinity-purified human antibodies can be obtained and their quantity determined in an immunoassay for total SIgA. However, this is rarely feasible because of the limited availability of specific antibodies. Often a pool of high-titered biologic fluid is used as the standard, and the antibody concentration in the unknown is expressed as a proportion of the antibody content in that pool. Without providing an absolute measurement, this approach allows comparison of the antibody concentration before and after infection or immunization.

The total SIgA or SIgA antibody concentration may vary, depending on how the sample was obtained. Washings of mucosal membranes are particularly susceptible to differences in the amount of solution applied and the proportion that is recovered. Even with naturally flowing secretions, such as saliva or urine, the concentration of antibody often depends on the flow rate (Brandtzaeg, 1971c). The best way to express the concentration of SIgA antibodies is as a ratio to the total SIgA in the same sample. This provides a measure of the specific activity of the SIgA as an indicator of the intensity of the local immune response.

Variables That Influence Immunoglobulin Concentrations in Secretions

In view of these technical limitations, normal levels of SIgA or SIgA antibodies in various secretions is limited and usually not confirmed by multiple laboratories. Some values for secretions from healthy individuals are presented in Table 8–2. The IgG:IgA ratio in most secretions is much lower than in serum and is probably dependent on the amount of contamination from transudated serum proteins. The IgG:IgM ratio in colostrum and saliva is also reduced compared with serum. This is more evident in IgA-deficient individuals

Table 8–2. Immunoglobulins in Serum and Secretions from Healthy Adults

Tested Material	Reference	No. of Samples	Immunoglobulin Levels (gm/L)			Ratio	
			IgA	IgM	IgG	IgG:IgA	IgG:IgM
Serum	a	pool	3.28	1.32	12.30	3.750	9.32
Colostrum, 1–2 days	a	pool	12.34	0.61	0.10	0.008	0.16
Milk, 2–5 days	c	pool	0.99	0.34	0.08	0.081	0.24
Milk, 5–44 days	c	13	0.468	0.14	0.04	0.085	0.29
Milk, 55–147 days	c	3	0.88	0.14	0.05	0.057	0.36
Stimulated parotid saliva	b	10	0.0149	—	—	—	—
Stimulated parotid saliva	a	9	0.0395	0.00043	0.00036	0.009	0.84
Nasal secretion	d	17	0.846	—	0.304	0.359	—
Urine, adults	b	13	0.00062	—	—	—	—
Duodenal fluid	e	40	0.313	0.207	0.104	0.33	0.50
Jejunal fluid	f	5	0.276	—	0.340	1.230	—
Colonic fluid	f	3	0.827	—	0.860	1.040	—

a. Brandtzaeg et al., 1970 (radial immunodiffusion with correction factor for IgA).
b. Sohl-Åkerlund et al., 1977 (enzyme-linked immunosorbent assay specific for secretory IgA).
c. Wadsworth et al., 1977a (spot immunoprecipitate assay, SIA).
d. Mygind et al., 1975 (radial immunodiffusion).
e. Girard and de Kalbermatten, 1970 (radial immunodiffusion).
f. Bull et al., 1971 (radial immunodiffusion).

whose secretions often have increased amounts of IgM, although they may also have elevated levels of IgG (Hanson, 1968; Brandtzaeg, 1971a; Hanson et al., 1983a).

The wide anatomic and functional differences between glandular structures account for part of the variations in the concentrations and proportions of the secreted immunoglobulin; additional variations occur as a result of fluctuations in the flow rate. Thus, the concentration of IgA in parotid saliva decreases three to fourfold after stimulation, although the actual IgA excretion rate increases twofold to threefold (Brandtzaeg, 1971a). The marked diurnal variation in nasal IgA points to the importance of collecting secretions at a fixed time of the day (Mygind et al., 1975; Mygind, 1978).

The SIgA concentration in human milk also depends on the flow rate and the volume produced. The high concentration of IgA and specific antibodies in the small volume of colostrum produced during the first few days of lactation rapidly diminishes in parallel with an increase in volume during the transition to mature milk. Consequently, the total daily output of SIgA antibodies stays high and relatively constant throughout lactation (Goldman et al., 1986). During nursing, when the flow rate is high, the concentration is relatively constant (Sohl-Åkerlund et al., 1977; Prentice, 1987; Prentice et al., 1984), and the titers of E. coli antibodies remain fairly stable (Hanson et al., 1975). However, Haneberg (1974b) found 30% to 40% higher IgA levels at the end of a feeding than before the infant started to nurse. Per weight of secretory tissue, the IgA output from the lactating breast is similar to that of the parotid gland (Brandtzaeg, 1983a).

Influence of Age

Ontogeny has a striking impact on the immunoglobulin levels in secretions. Age-matched controls must therefore be used when studies are performed in young patients (Burgio et al., 1980). The timing of SIgA appearance in the infant has been reviewed by Hanson et al. (1980) and Brandtzaeg et al. (1991). In one study, SIgA and SIgM antibodies to E. coli and poliovirus were found in the saliva during the first days of life. Although these antibodies may represent maternal IgA and IgM, there was evidence that they may also be of fetal origin; such antibodies were, in fact, found in the saliva and meconium of a newborn of a hypogammaglobulinemic mother whose IgA and IgM levels were undetectable (Mellander et al., 1986a).

In developing countries, infants exposed to poliovirus develop salivary SIgA antibodies against poliovirus antigens by 1 month of age, and the antibody concentration reaches adult levels by the age of 6 months (Carlsson et al., 1985). Infants heavily exposed to E. coli from the time of birth had significantly increased salivary SIgA antibody levels by 2 to 3 weeks of age, rapidly reaching adult levels (Mellander et al., 1985). In less exposed infants, such levels were not attained until about 12 months of age for both SIgA and SIgA antibodies to E. coli O antigens. A slower increase in the levels of such antibodies was found by Gleeson and colleagues (1987).

Other studies show that SIgM antibodies predominate in the secretions of infants (Girard and de Kalbermatten, 1970; Gleeson et al., 1982). SIgM antibodies to E. coli were consistently found in the saliva of young infants (Mellander et al., 1984, 1985, 1986a, 1986b). As the synthesis and transport of SIgA antibodies into the saliva increased during the first 1 to 3 months of age, levels of the SIgM antibodies decreased in parallel, suggesting competition for the same SC-dependent transfer mechanism or replacement of the local IgM-producing cells by IgA producers.

The perinatal ontogeny of SIg formation in the parotid, as studied immunohistologically by Thrane and coworkers (1991), confirmed that the IgM-producing cells that predominated were replaced by IgA-producing cells during the first 6 months of life. Prenatally, most IgA-producing cells were of the IgA1 isotype and contained J chains. However, IgA2-producing cells reached adult proportions (~40% of IgA producers) soon after birth. The early ability to transport the polymeric immunoglobulins into the lumen of the parotid gland was indicated by the prenatal expression of SC. However, anti-SC staining increased rapidly after birth, concomitant with a rapid increase in IgA-producing cells, which suggested that these events are driven by the presence of microbial flora or other antigens.

Influence of Nutrition

The increased susceptibility to infections of undernourished children may be explained by an impaired local immune system. SIgA concentrations are more sensitive to malnutrition than are serum IgA, IgG, or IgM. A reduction in IgA concentrations has been reported in duodenal, nasal, and salivary secretions of children with severe protein-calorie malnutrition (Chandra, 1975; Sirisinha et al., 1975; Reddy et al., 1976; McMurray et al., 1977). Conversely, Beatty and colleagues (1983) have shown that the intestinal immune system of undernourished children responds to bacterial overgrowth with enhanced IgA synthesis and secretion. Furthermore, total salivary SIgA and salivary antibody responses of chronically undernourished children are equal to those of better nourished children (Glass et al., 1986). Renourishment after acute malnutrition rapidly restored the secretory immunoglobulin concentration (Reddy et al., 1976). Severe protein undernutrition in mice resulted in decreased total IgA concentration in intestinal washes, whereas serum IgA levels were increased (McGee and McMurray, 1988). The IgA plaque-forming cell response to an orally administered antigen was unchanged, although this response was decreased in the spleens from the most severely underfed. Refeeding resulted in normalized IgA levels and responses.

In severely undernourished mothers, the SIgA *E. coli* antibody titers in milk were comparable to those of healthy mothers, but because their milk volumes were smaller, their total output of milk SIgA was diminished (Carlsson et al., 1976). The effects of two different levels of protein supplementation on SIgA concentration and daily excretion in milk of undernourished mothers were examined by Herias and coworkers (1993). The higher protein supplementation prevented the fall in SIgA production seen in mothers who received less protein, suggesting that nutritional protein is a rate-limiting factor for SIgA production. Interestingly, there were no differences in the concentrations or avidities of three different specific antibodies between early and late gestation or with the different supplementations (Herias et al., 1993).

There is considerable interest in the effects of vitamin A on the mucosal immune responses. Rats that were made vitamin A–deficient have lower serum and biliary IgA concentrations and markedly reduced IgA responses to oral immunization with cholera toxin (Wiedermann et al., 1993). Most of these effects were reversed by supplementation with vitamin A, which suggested that the immune defects were a direct effect of the vitamin deficiencies rather than a secondary effect of poor food intake. The deficient IgA response was due to a suppression of T_H2 cells, associated with

an increase in IFN-γ and IL-2 production in vitro, suggesting enhanced T_H1 activity (Wiedermann et al., 1993).

Secretory Immunoglobulins in Serum

Trace quantities of secretory IgA can be detected in human serum (Thompson et al., 1969; Brandtzaeg, 1971c). Studies using solid-phase radioimmunoassay (Delacroix and Vaerman, 1981), an immunofluorescence assay (Goldblum et al., 1980), or ELISA (Iscaki et al., 1979; Kvale and Brandtzaeg, 1986) have produced somewhat discrepant results; however, most indicate that about 1% of the serum IgA is normally SIgA. SIgM has also been detected in normal serum (Delacroix and Vaerman, 1982; Kvale and Brandtzaeg, 1986). Elevated serum levels of SIgA and SIgM in patients with various mucosal or liver diseases may have some diagnostic value (Goldblum et al., 1980; Delacroix et al., 1982; Kvale and Brandtzaeg, 1986), but the difficulty of the assays has limited their widespread use.

ORAL TOLERANCE

Most intestinal antigens, particularly food antigens, are not injurious to the host. Teleologically, an immune response to these antigens not only would be wasteful but also might result in adverse reactions with every re-exposure. Indeed, oral administration of soluble antigens that produce an immune response, if given parenterally, results in weak or absent secretory immune responses. Furthermore, after oral exposure to such antigens, both cellular and humoral immune response to subsequent parenteral challenges with the same antigen are markedly diminished.

Mechanisms of Oral Tolerance

Although multiple mechanisms are probably involved in such "oral tolerance" (Chernokhvostova, 1984; Elson, 1985; Mowat, 1987; Kagnoff, 1988), its induction seems to depend primarily on antigen handling by an intact gut epithelium (Nicklin and Miller, 1983). The epithelial presentation of antigen to T cells may induce a general or antigen-specific hyporesponsiveness (Bland and Warren, 1986a, 1986b; Mayer and Shlien, 1987). Coadministrations of factors that activate macrophages and enhance antigen presentation can prevent the development of oral tolerance (Zhang and Michael, 1990). These findings may explain why microbial and other particulate antigens produce a secretory immune response whereas soluble antigens tend to produce tolerance. The differences in physical form may determine whether the antigens are picked up by the M cells of the Peyer's patches or by the absorptive epithelium.

Transfer of Oral Tolerance

Studies in the 1970s and 1980s demonstrated that oral tolerance could be transferred to naive animals by administering CD8$^+$ T cells from orally immunized animals (Kagnoff 1978; Miller and Hanson, 1979). The origin of these T-suppressor cells, the site of their interaction with the orally administered antigens, and their mode of action has not been elucidated, in part due to the inability to develop cell lines or clones with suppressor characteristics. Other explanations for oral tolerance include deletion or anergy of responsive T cells, production of a suppressive cytokine or cytokine mixtures, or suppressive antibodies or other humoral factors.

Clinical Significance of Oral Tolerance

Defects in the development or maintenance of oral tolerance may occur in patients who have hypersensitivity reactions to food proteins (Stokes et al., 1987). Factors that predispose to these reactions, including intestinal infections, early feeding of intact proteins, and early weaning, are known to inhibit the development of oral tolerance.

It is not known whether oral tolerance is operative in humans, but support is derived from the finding that serum IgG antibodies to common dietary antigens decrease with increasing age (Scott et al., 1985). Persistence of microbial antigens likewise may lead to systemic hyporesponsiveness, although it is usually limited to IgM (Chernokhvostova, 1984). Oral immunization of lactating mothers with a food protein or live poliovirus vaccine decreases prevaccination milk SIgA antibody levels (Carlsson et al., 1985; Cruz and Hanson, 1986).

The propensity to induce oral tolerance in humans is relevant to the current efforts to develop oral immunization to prevent mucosal and systemic infections and toxin exposures. If these regimens induce tolerance, rather than immunity, they will fail. Conversely, there are currently clinical trials of feeding antigens involved in antigen-specific autoimmunity in hopes of preventing the onset of or suppressing ongoing pathologic autoimmune responses (e.g., multiple sclerosis) (Marx, 1991).

MUCOSAL LYMPHOCYTES

The three major sites of T cells in the mucosal tissue are the organized MALT, the lamina propria, and the epithelium (e.g., the interepithelial lymphocytes [IELs]). These T cells have not been investigated in the same detail as the mucosal B cells have, but there is some evidence that intestinal T cells follow a migration pathway similar to that of the IgA-committed B cells. The mucosal T cells are phenotypically and functionally different from those in the blood or systemic lymphoid tissues (James and Zietz, 1994). Even lamina propria T cells and IELs differ. These differences are understandable, since mucosal T cells are constantly exposed to foreign antigens and must have their responses muted to prevent chronic, inflammatory tissue injury. This is compatible with the concept that the mucosal immune system must maintain its barrier function without developing deleterious inflammatory reactions.

Lamina Propria Lymphocytes

The primary role of the lamina propria T cells is to support terminal differentiation and immunoglobulin production by lamina propria B cells.

Lamina propria T cells are phenotypically different from circulating T cells (James and Zietz, 1994). While the CD4:CD8 ratio is similar to that of peripheral blood, most lamina propria T cells have the surface markers of primed memory cells, as indicated by the RO isoform of the CD45 molecule. The CD45RO molecule, typical of memory cells, is present on essentially all of the lamina propria T cells (Halstensen et al., 1990). Only half of the adult blood T cells express this isoform; the rest display the CD45RA, the isoform of naive T cells. In addition, about 40% of lamina propria T cells express the integrin $\alpha4\beta7$; this marker is present on freshly isolated lymphocytes from other tissue sites (Cerf-Bensussan et al., 1987). However, $\alpha4\beta7$ can be induced on other lymphocyte populations by in vitro activation, which again suggests that the lamina propria T cells are stimulated, perhaps in a tissue-specific fashion (Schieferdecker et al., 1990).

Other markers of activation, such as IL-2R (CD25), are rarely present on lamina propria T cells (Halstensen and Brandtzaeg, 1993b). Consistent with inherent priming, lamina propria T cells express more mRNAs for the cytokines IFN-γ, IL-2, IL-4, and IL-5 after nonspecific stimulation than do circulating T lymphocytes. Surface antigens involved in cell migration (e.g., L-selectin), present on about half of the blood T cells, are absent on lamina propria lymphocytes (James and Zietz, 1994); this is consistent with the fact that L-selectin is lost with activation or migration to the lamina propria.

An intriguing characteristic of lamina propria lymphocytes is their limited capacity to proliferate (Brandtzaeg and Halstensen, 1992) or become cytotoxic killer cells. Lamina propria T cells show weak proliferative responses to specific antigen, mitogens, or even anti-CD3 antibodies (James and Zeitz, 1994). However, after antigenic or pokeweed mitogen stimulation, these T cells can act as helpers for B-cell antibody production (James and Zeitz, 1994). This suggests that lamina propria T cells predominantly enhance local immunoglobulin production rather than proliferate or injure surrounding structures.

Interepithelial Lymphocytes

The IELs are strategically located to respond to antigenic stimulation by luminal antigens while minimizing tissue injury. Because epithelial cells are rapidly replenished, immunologic identification and destruction of infected or otherwise abnormal villus cells may protect the internal environment without detrimental effects to normal tissues. Although this is an attractive hypothesis, the exact function of the IEL remains obscure (Lefrancois, 1994).

The origin and function of the IELs are suggested by their surface phenotype because it differs extensively from those of circulating T cells. Unlike the murine (mouse) situation, in which the $\gamma\delta$ form of the T cell receptor (TCR) predominates, most human small intestinal IELs express the $\alpha\beta$ form of TCR, typical of T cells in the blood and lymphoid tissues (Brandtzaeg et al., 1989a). However, most IELs express the CD8 marker (Parrott et al., 1983; Brandtzaeg et al., 1989) associated with suppressive and cytotoxic activities. The few IELs that express CD4 co-express CD8. These double-positive cells are extremely rare in other tissues except the thymus. This finding suggests that some of the murine IELs are derived not from the thymus but from a prethymic population that migrates to the gut and differentiates there.

Another characteristic of IELs is the limited repertoire of their TCR (Balk et al., 1991; Van Kerckhove et al., 1992). This is in marked distinction to peripheral T cells, in which essentially each cell has a unique TCR structure. The IEL must recognize a limited number of antigens, perhaps autologous antigens that become expressed when the enterocyte becomes infected or otherwise stressed. The functional activities of IELs, once activated, may be to release cytokines that destroy damaged enterocytes (Lefrancois, 1994).

OTHER MUCOSAL DEFENSE MECHANISMS

In addition to antigen-specific mucosal immune responses, other more primitive soluble and cellular defense mechanisms protect the mucosal surfaces. These factors may function alone to prevent or control microbial colonization or infections or to augment T-cell and B-cell immunity at these sites.

Soluble Factors

Lactoferrin, an iron-binding protein present in secretions, inhibits the growth of many pathologic bacteria and fungi. This activity, which is potentiated by antibodies (Bullen et al., 1972), including human milk IgA antibodies (Rogers and Synge, 1978), is probably due to neutralization of iron-binding compounds from the bacteria (Bullen et al., 1974; Griffiths and Humphreys, 1977), thereby further depriving the microorganisms of growth-promoting iron. However, a bactericidal peptide of lactoferrin (lactoferricin) may also be important in mucosal defense by lactoferrin (Bellamy et al., 1992).

External secretions also contain the enzyme lysozyme (muramidase), which can cleave the cell wall of gram-positive bacteria. The concentration of lysozyme is particularly high (0.5 to 2g/L) in human milk (Chandan et al., 1964; Hanson and Johansson, 1970; Goldman et al., 1982a, 1982b, 1983b). SIgA antibodies may become bacteriolytic by activating complement in combination with lysozyme (Adinolfi et al., 1966; Hill and Porter, 1974), but this has not been verified (Eddie et al., 1971; Heddle et al., 1975). Indeed all forms of human IgA, including both subclasses, lack classical complement-activating properties (Pfaffenbach et al., 1982; Johnson et al., 1984; Russel-Jones et al., 1984; Nikolova et al., 1994). In the rat, IgA immune complexes can activate complement via the alternative pathway (Rits et al., 1988).

The lactoperoxidase of various secretions may also be effective in the defense against infections (Mata and Wyatt, 1971; Goldman and Smith, 1973; Gothefors, 1975; Gothefors and Marklund, 1975). Lactoperoxidase may not be present in human milk (Moldoveanu et al., 1982). SIgA may enhance the effect of the lactoperoxidase system independently of antibody specificity (Tenovuo et al., 1982).

Interferon-α may be another important nonspecific defense factor. Its synthesis is stimulated by infection or topical application of virus vaccines. Interferons appear in nasal secretions within 24 hours of viral infections (Danielescu et al., 1975) and therefore may play a decisive role in the initial phase of infection.

Immune reactions at epithelial surfaces may stimulate release of mucus from goblet cells, thereby enhancing this mechanical barrier of macromolecules and microorganisms (Walker et al., 1982). Furthermore, the development of goblet cells may depend on functional T lymphocytes in humans (Karlsson et al., 1985) and animals (Mayrhofer, 1979; Ahlstedt et al., 1988). Antigens of immune complexes trapped in the mucous layer are more rapidly degraded by proteolytic enzymes (Walker et al., 1975).

Most mucosal infections begin with attachment of the microorganism to epithelial cells, often mediated by specific receptors on the epithelium. For instance, in the urinary tract, Svanborg Edén and coworkers (1983) have shown that E. coli, which causes acute pyelonephritis, often have fimbrial receptors for the P antigen on urinary epithelium. Receptor analogs, present in exocrine secretions such as milk, may prevent bacterial attachment (Holmgren et al., 1981, 1983; Svanborg Edén et al., 1983; Otnaess et al., 1983; Andersson et al., 1985, 1986). This topic has been reviewed by Svanborg Edén (1994).

Phagocytes

Under normal conditions, few polymorphonuclear leukocytes (PMNs) are present in mucosal tissues; however, certain secretions, notably milk, do contain PMNs. PMNs are critical in the control of microbial colonization at highly contaminated mucosal sites, such as the gingiva. Since PMN function is dependent on opsonins for optimal phagocytosis, their interaction with IgA is of interest.

The role of secretory IgA in opsonizing bacteria for phagocytosis is controversial. Fcα receptors are present on human neutrophils (Lawrence et al., 1975) and show much better binding activity for dimeric than for monomeric IgA (Fanger et al., 1980). In vitro phagocytosis-promoting effect of purified SIgA antibodies depends on the presence of lysozyme (Girard and de Kalbermatten, 1970). In vivo experiments, however, have produced discrepant results (Eddie et al., 1971; Heddle and Rowley, 1975), possibly because of differences in the bacteria or the type of phagocyte involved. In human saliva, IgA coats certain bacteria (see Fig. 8–5), but it is unknown whether the coating is directly bacteriostatic. Growing chains of streptococci occur in the mouth, and some of the IgA-coated bacteria are engulfed by neutrophils mainly derived from the gingival crevices (Sharry and Krasse, 1960; Brandtzaeg et al., 1968b).

A prompt immune-mediated emigration of neutrophils takes place in the gut lumen after epithelial exposure to antigen to which there is serum antibody (Bellamy and Nielsen, 1974). These cells may then limit further antigen penetration. However, the reaction of serum antibodies with luminal antigen may enhance penetration of other macromolecules. This is probably caused by adverse effects on the mucosa exerted by lysosomal enzymes released from the phagocytes (Brandtzaeg and Tolo, 1977; Lim and Rowley, 1982). Formation of immune complexes outside the epithelium does not induce chemotaxis of neutrophils (Bellamy and Nielsen, 1974). Cultured epithelial cells of the respiratory and gastrointestinal tracts infected with viruses or bacteria can induce the production and release of IL-8, a potent chemoattractant for PMNs (Garofalo et al., 1995).

Certain lymphocytes, eosinophils, and monocytes also express Fcα receptors and, in conjunction with IgA, mediate antibody-dependent cellular cytotoxicity (ADCC) against bacteria and parasites to assist in mucosal defense (Lowell et al., 1980). Intraepithelial lymphocytes from the murine gut exert antibacterial ADCC with SIgA antibodies from rabbit intestinal juice (Tagliabue et al., 1984). Bacterial killing by SIgA antibodies and T lymphocytes occurs in the human gut after vaccination against *Salmonella typhi* (Tagliabue et al., 1986).

The acidity of the gastric juices, the flow of urine in the urinary tract, the flow of saliva in the oral cavity, intestinal peristalsis, the coughing reflex, and mucociliary transport in the respiratory tract also contribute to local defense by inactivating or removing microorganisms.

CLINICAL SIGNIFICANCE OF THE MUCOSAL DEFENSE SYSTEM

Immunologic Homeostasis of Mucosa

Immunologic homeostasis is normally maintained in the mucosa through a critical balance between the level of local antibodies of the various isotypes (Fig. 8–6). Dimeric IgA (and pentameric IgM) may act as the first line of defense by excluding antigen at the mucosal surface. Antigens that bypass this trapping mechanism, however, may meet non-IgA antibodies in the lamina propria. Because IgG and IgM antibodies can activate complement and because complement permeates the lamina propria (Baklien and Brandtzaeg, 1974), an inflammatory cascade may be initiated. However, this may be moderated by "blocking" activities of dimeric and monomeric IgA of local or systemic origin (Hall et al., 1971; Griffis and Goroff, 1983; Russel-

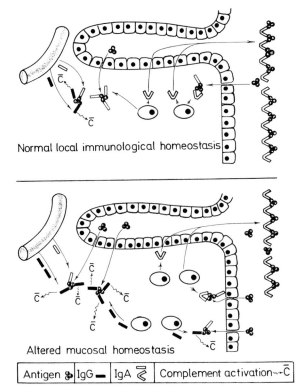

Normal local immunological homeostasis

Altered mucosal homeostasis

Antigen 🦠	IgG ▬	IgA ⟶	Complement activation~C̄

Figure 8–6. It is postulated *(top)* that a normal immunologic homeostasis is maintained in the mucosa through a critical balance between humoral available antibodies. Dimeric IgA acts in a "first line of defense" by antigen exclusion at the mucosal surface (to the right). Antigens that bypass this trapping mechanism may meet corresponding serum-derived IgG antibodies in the lamina propria. The immune complexes formed will activate complement, and inflammatory mediators are thus generated in the mucosa. Such a development is moderated by "blocking" antibody activities in the lamina propria exerted by serum-derived or locally produced monomeric or dimeric IgA. This homeostasis is altered *(bottom)* when there is undue antigen stimulation because of increased mucosal penetrability or excessive antigen exposure. A "second line of defense" is then set up in the mucosa by local production of IgG as part of the "pathotopic potentiation" of mucosal immunity (see Fig. 8–7) to limit dissemination of foreign substances. However, because of the phlogistic properties of IgG antibodies, a vicious circle may develop with further increase of mucosal antigen penetrability, intensified complement activation and cytotoxic reactions, massive attraction of phagocytic cells, and release of their lysosomal enzymes. This results in aggravation and perpetuation of inflammation and thus leads to disease.

Jones et al., 1984; Nikolova et al., 1994). In vitro studies (Kaetzel et al., 1991) suggest that immune complexes containing IgA formed in the vicinity of secretory epithelia can be transported externally by the PIg receptor mechanism and released into the lumen. This transport system may also include mixed immune complexes with IgG and dimeric IgA, acting as a backup for the immune exclusion process (Mazanec et al., 1993).

Conversely, excessive IgG and possibly IgM antibodies may attract phagocytes to mucosal sites (Bellamy and Nielsen, 1974). Release of their lysosomal enzymes may enhance mucosal permeability (Brandtzaeg and Tolo, 1977; Lim and Rowley, 1982). However, leukocyte migration is suppressed by dimeric IgA, which inhibits leukocyte chemotaxis (van Epps and Williams,

1976; Reed et al., 1979; Kemp et al., 1980). IgA may also inhibit the release of proinflammatory cytokines from mucosal phagocytes and inhibit production of toxic oxygen radicals (Wolf et al., 1994a, 1994b).

In addition to antibodies and complement, beneficial (or detrimental) effects may be mediated by activated T cells, macrophages, mast cells, goblet cells, and natural killer (NK) cells at local tissue sites. The effectiveness of these backup systems for mucosal immunity is evidenced in patients with X-linked agammaglobulinemia and common variable immunodeficiency, most of whom have no clinical, functional, or structural abnormalities in the gut (Eidelman, 1976).

Primary and Secondary Mucosal Defense Lines

Deviations from the normal polymeric immunoglobulin-dominant pattern of mucosal defenses may occur transiently or permanently. In most cases, the SIgA response (first line of defense) neutralizes noxious influences and maintains local immunologic homeostasis. Transient shifts to a backup mode may result in proinflammatory mechanisms with deleterious, although reversible, changes of the mucosa, as seen, for example, in celiac disease (Brandtzaeg et al., 1985a). However, when the secretory immune system fails to cope with persistent mucosal antigen, a pronounced local IgG response may occur, possibly combined with an IgE response in atopic individuals. Through the phlogistic properties, these antibodies, "pathotopic potentiation" of local immunity (see Fig. 8–7), may develop. This may be considered the "second line of defense" of the mucosa to neutralize noxious factors. However, the local consequence may be severe alteration of mucosal

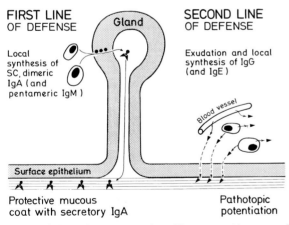

FIRST LINE OF DEFENSE

Gland

SECOND LINE OF DEFENSE

Local synthesis of SC, dimeric IgA (and pentameric IgM)

Exudation and local synthesis of IgG (and IgE)

Blood vessel

Surface epithelium

Protective mucous coat with secretory IgA

Pathotopic potentiation

Figure 8–7. Schematic representation of human nasal mucosa. Two basic principles of antibody protection are visualized. The "first line of defense" primarily consists of secretory IgA, which is produced as J chain–containing dimers by immunocytes adjacent to glandular structures; the dimers are then conjugated with epithelial "secretory component" (SC) during selective transmission through the glandular epithelium and are subsequently included in a protective mucous coat on the surface epithelium. The "second line of defense" is associated with a local inflammatory reaction, giving rise to passive external diffusion of serum-derived and locally produced IgG and perhaps influx of IgE bound to mast cell; the latter events represent "pathotopic potentiation" of local immunity.

immunologic homeostasis (see Fig. 8–6), with aggravation and perpetuation of an inflammatory reaction. This is probably the underlying mechanism leading to chronic inflammatory disease of mucous membranes.

Antimicrobial Activities of the Mucosal Immune System

Viral Infections

Immune responses to viral infections of the mucosal surfaces have been reviewed (Murphy, 1994). Once a viral infection has started, resolution is mediated by cellular mechanisms, including NK cells (Biron et al., 1989), MHC class I restricted CD8[+] cytotoxic T cells, and CD4[+] helper cells (Murphy, 1994). Each cell must recognize the viral or viral-induced structures on the host cell and combat the viral infection by destroying the host cells. For rapidly dividing viruses, specific cellular immunity may not have much effect until after the peak of virus production (Greenberg et al., 1978). Thus, other host responses must limit the early phase of viral replication. These include production of interferon by multiple cell types and possibly the intracellular neutralization in secretory epithelial cells by internalized polymeric antibodies, as described earlier (Mazanec et al., 1992a).

Prevention of mucosal reinfection is largely mediated by antibodies. At some sites, notably the lungs and upper respiratory tract, IgG antibodies may diffuse passively from the systemic circulation to provide some protection (Murphy, 1994). In contrast, protection in the gastrointestinal tract is mostly mediated by SIgA. The effectiveness of antibodies in preventing viral reinfection has been demonstrated experimentally by passive administration of antibodies directly on the mucosal surface (Mazanec et al., 1992b) or intravenously as polymeric IgA antibodies (Renegar and Small, 1991). These experiments indicate that antibodies directed against a virus can prevent or markedly reduce mucosal viral replication. Human breast milk antibodies largely diminish symptoms of natural viral infections (Carlsson and Hanson, 1994; Murphy, 1994). This outcome is similar to the first reinfection with a respiratory virus, when residual levels of endogenous SIgA antibodies are low. Only after multiple infections are titers of mucosal antibodies high enough to prevent subsequent infection (Murphy, 1994).

Bacterial Infections

Secretory antibodies may protect against bacterial infections (Gay, 1924; Pierce, 1959; Artenstein, 1975). The specificity of these secretory antibodies reflects the local nature of the antigenic stimulus. Thus, gonococcal antibodies are found in genital secretions (Kearns et al., 1973); *Streptococcus pneumoniae* and *Haemophilus influenzae* (Gump et al., 1973), *Mycoplasma pneumoniae* (Biberfeld and Sterner, 1971), and *Neisseria meningitidis* (Wenzel et al., 1973) antibodies are found in respiratory secretions; *Streptococcus mutans* and other oral bacterial antibodies are found in saliva (Arnold et al.,

1976); and *E. coli* (Girard and de Kalbermatten, 1970; Michael et al., 1971), *V. cholerae* (Waldman et al., 1972) and *Shigella* (Reed and Williams, 1971) antibodies are found in intestinal contents. The presence of antibodies in the nasal secretion against diphtheria toxoid in individuals with high serum antibody titers indicates some transfer of serum antibodies (Remington et al., 1964) that may be increased during infection (see Fig. 8–3). To demonstrate this, it is necessary to utilize specific methods that will distinguish between SIgA and serum IgG responses.

Parasitic Infections

Certain parasites (e.g., *Trichinella spiralis*) can be trapped in mucus by either the complement-conglutinin system or by secretory or serum antibodies (Lee and Ogilvie, 1982). Although IgA antibodies against several parasites are present in secretions, their protective role is unclear. Milk of immunized mothers protects infant mice against *Giardia muris* infection (Andrews and Hewlett, 1981).

Antibody-dependent cellular cytotoxicity may be of major importance for host defense against parasites (Capron et al., 1982). Eosinophils, neutrophils, and macrophages (but not NK cells) participate in antiparasitic reactions through their IgG and especially IgE Fc receptors. IgE antibodies may also protect against parasites by binding to and activating platelets. Such IgE platelet-mediated hypersensitivity may contribute to the pathogenesis of mucosal atopic reactions (Capron et al., 1987).

Many parasitic infections are immunosuppressive. *T. spiralis* infection, for example, depresses serum antibody responses and Ig-producing cells in the lamina propria following oral immunization with cholera toxin (Ljungström et al., 1980). A similar immunosuppression was observed for cellular immune responses during *Nippostrongylus brasiliensis* infection, especially in MALTs (McElroy et al., 1983).

Intestinal infections with some parasites cause local inflammation. Infection with *N. brasiliensis* or *T. spiralis* causes mice to mount a strong T$_H$2 response in the spleens and mesenteric lymph nodes, resulting in increased levels of IL-4 and IL-5 and decreased levels of IFN-γ and IL-2 (Pond et al., 1989). This results in increased levels of circulating eosinophils and IgE, which may contribute to the expulsion of the parasites. Clearance of some parasites is blocked by the injection of anti–IL-4 antibodies (Urban et al., 1991).

Gastroenterologic Mucosal Immunity

Oral Cavity

Oral mucosal immunity has been reviewed by Challacombe and Shirlaw (1994). Both local and systemic immune factors help stabilize the bacterial flora, thus preventing acute infections and chronic oral inflammation of the mouth. The salivary glands are the source of oral SIgA, including the parotid (40%); submandibular (40%); sublingual (10%); and minor salivary glands (10%) (Challacombe and Shirlaw, 1994). Serum-derived components of saliva enter through the junctions between the teeth and the mucosa.

Secretory oral antibodies can be demonstrated by the presence of bacteria coated with IgA (see Fig. 8–5). These antibodies, demonstrated by Brandtzaeg and co-workers (1968b), may prevent bacterial adherence to oroepithelial cells (Williams and Gibbons, 1972) and teeth, thereby promoting the disposal of oral microorganisms. Oral colonization with *Streptococcus mutans,* the major causative organism of dental caries, may be inhibited by salivary SIgA antibodies (Gregory et al., 1985). These antibodies can be induced in humans by oral immunization (Mestecky et al., 1978; Gregory and Filler, 1987). The SIgA response in experimental animals may be enhanced by administering antigens or bacteria in liposomes or by adding adjuvants such as muramyl dipeptide (Michalek et al., 1985). In rats, control of caries can be achieved by vaccination. In humans, resistance to dental caries is related to natural salivary IgA antibodies against *S. mutans* (Lehtonen et al., 1984). An efficient and safe caries vaccine is not yet available.

The salivary SIgA may function in the oral cavity through its interactions with innate immune factors, including mucin, lactoferrin, lysozyme, and lactoperoxidase. In addition, because the phagocytes that enter the saliva have enhanced expression of Fcα receptors, these cells may effectively phagocytize IgA-coated (opsonized) bacteria (Fanger et al., 1980).

Intestines and Gastroenteritis

The secretory IgA responses against bacterial and viral infections of the gastrointestinal tract have been examined extensively. In experimental cholera, Fubara and Freter (1972) showed that SIgA antibodies were protective by diminishing the adherence of *V. cholerae* to the intestinal wall (Lange and Holmgren, 1978; Svennerholm et al., 1978). Effective immunity following immunization correlated with number of lamina propria plasma cells producing antibodies to cholera toxin (Lange et al., 1980). Antibodies against cholera enterotoxin and lipopolysaccharide have a synergistic protective effect (Svennerholm and Holmgren, 1976). Antibacterial antibodies presumably keep bacteria from adhering to the gut epithelium, and antitoxin antibodies neutralize or prevent the toxin from binding to its specific epithelial receptor.

In humans, long-lasting immunity to cholera occurs despite a short-lived local SIgA response. This may be related to a long-lasting SIgA immunologic memory response to cholera toxin (Lange et al., 1980; Pierce and Cray, 1982; Lycke and Holmgren, 1987). The cholera toxin is a remarkably potent immunogen because of its special binding capability and physiologic activities. Oral toxin induces SIgA as well as serum IgG and IgA responses (Elson and Falding, 1984). The serum IgA and IgG responses have their origin in Peyer's patches (Elson and Falding, 1984; Dahlgren et al., 1986, 1987).

The nontoxic receptor-binding beta-subunit of cholera toxin is a good immunogen that efficiently induces toxin-neutralizing antibodies. An oral beta-subunit/whole cell cholera vaccine stimulates a good mucosal antibody response and has been successful in large-scale field trials (Svennerholm et al., 1984; Clemens et al., 1986). This vaccine also protects against *E. coli* enterotoxin-induced diarrhea (Clemens et al., 1988a). This vaccination results in a decreased diarrheal morbidity and mortality (Clemens et al., 1988b). Oral administration of GM_1 ganglioside, the epithelial cell receptor for cholera toxin, also prevents toxin-induced diarrhea in experimental animals, but this has not been studied in humans (Glass et al., 1984).

Passive transfer of SIgA in animals confirms the efficacy of local SIgA against enteric infection. Winner et al. (1991) implanted mice with hybridoma that produced polymeric IgA antibodies to the LPS of *V. cholerae*. These mice demonstrated a high level of strain-specific resistance to oral challenge with the cholera organisms. Interestingly, there was no protection with antibodies to the cholera toxin itself (Apter et al., 1991). This difference is presumably due to the ability of the LPS antibodies to prevent colonization or the inability of antitoxin to neutralize locally produced toxin (Kraehenbuhl and Neutra, 1994).

Specific antibody is not the only mechanism against intestinal toxins. Desensitization of intestinal adenylate cyclase occurs after immunization with cholera toxin, presumably because of the production of an "antisecretory factor" found in bile, milk, and intestinal mucosa (Lönnroth and Lange, 1981; Lange and Lönnroth, 1986). This factor, a 60-kd protein, is induced by hyperosmotic solutions of monosaccharides and amino acids (Lönnroth and Lange, 1987). The protective effects of antisecretory factor may explain the lack of correlation between the protection against toxin and the titers of antitoxin (Lange et al., 1984).

For some enteric bacteria, immune cells may also be involved in the protection. Tagliabue and colleagues (1984) demonstrated SIgA-mediated ADCC against *Salmonella* strains and *Shigella* X16 (a hybrid between *Shigella flexneri* and *E. coli*). Whereas IgG armed splenic lymphocytes for ADCC better, SIgA functioned better in ADCC with lymphocytes from Peyer's patches, mesenteric lymph nodes, gut epithelium, and lamina propria. Such SIgA antibodies have also been described in humans (Tagliabue et al., 1986).

For intracellular intestinal infections, such as those caused by *Salmonella*, T-cell mediated mechanisms similar to those that mediate the clearing of other viral infections may be involved. MHC class I–restricted cytotoxic lymphocytes may be crucial in these responses (Kaufmann, 1988).

Liver and Gall Bladder

Unlike the liver of some animals, the human liver does not efficiently transport polymeric IgA from the circulation into the bile (Brown et al., 1982). This difference is due to the lack of expression of the PIgR by human hepatocytes (Brandtzaeg, 1982, 1985a;

Vaerman et al., 1982), although some discrepant information has been reported. Some SC-independent binding of IgA to hepatocytes may take place, and this along with transport through SC-expressing duct epithelium may explain why 50% of the small amounts of polymeric IgA of human bile is derived from the circulation (Delacroix and Vaerman, 1983; Brandtzaeg, 1985a). However, only about 2% of injected polymeric IgA appears in bile after 24 hours (Delacroix and Vaerman, 1983). Thus, polymeric IgA (without bound SC) can accumulate in extremely high concentrations (about 6000 mg/dl) in the blood of patients with excessive intestinal IgA production, even when liver function is normal (Brandtzaeg and Baklien, 1977a). Although serum IgA is often increased in various liver disorders, it is not known whether this reflects increased IgA production in the intestinal mucosa, decreased hepatic uptake or catabolism of circulating IgA or IgA-containing immune complexes, or reflux of biliary IgA into the blood.

Respiratory Mucosal Immunity

Mucosal immunity is more important in the upper respiratory tract and perhaps in the bronchi than in the lower respiratory tract, notably the lungs, where systemic immunity predominates. Immunity to respiratory infections has been reviewed by Welliver (1994).

Upper Respiratory Tract

Mucosal immune responses to respiratory viruses, particularly respiratory syncytial virus (RSV) and influenza, has been studied in detail. Secretory IgA antibodies specific for RSV have been demonstrated after primary infection (McIntosh et al., 1979), but their role in clearing the infection is uncertain (McIntosh et al., 1979). While systemic administration of IgG antibodies to RSV does not decrease viral shedding in infected infants (Hemming et al., 1987), the presence of neutralizing serum antibodies correlates with resistance to infection (Hall et al., 1991). Repeated infections also result in accelerated production of local RSV-specific antibodies (Kaul et al., 1980). Thus, the relative contributions of local and systemic antibodies to resolution and prevention of reinfection with RSV remains unclear. However, because some individuals with high levels of serum antibodies can become infected (Hall et al., 1991), rapid production of local antibodies after re-exposure may be a major determinant in resistance to reinfection.

Renegar and Small (1991) demonstrated that intravenous administration of a monoclonal IgA antibody to influenza virus in mice resulted in resistance to infection after intranasal challenge. Much larger amounts of IgG antibodies were required to achieve the same degree of protection, which suggested that specific polymeric IgA antibodies selectively transported into the respiratory tract are more effective than transudated serum IgG.

Resolving ongoing RSV infections is probably dependent on the development of specific cytotoxic T cells.

Such cells have been demonstrated in the blood of infants at about the time when viral shedding begins to wane (Issacs et al., 1987; Chiba et al., 1989). These same T cells may be involved in the lung disease that develops in some of these infants (Welliver et al., 1979).

Middle Ear Immunity and Otitis Media

The mucosal immunity of the middle ear and eustachian tube have been reviewed (Lim and Mogi, 1994). The surfaces of the eustachian tube and middle ear are lined largely with ciliated respiratory epithelium, but secretory glands are also found in the proximal eustachian tube and to a lesser extent in the tympanic cavity and antrum (Lim, 1974). Only a few immunocompetent cells are normally associated with the middle ear mucosa (Lim, 1974) and mast cells predominate. In experimental models of middle ear infection, immune-induced inflammation, cells the monocyte/macrophage lineage and T and B lymphocytes accumulate in the middle ear mucosa over a period of weeks (Ichimiya et al., 1990; Takahashi et al., 1992).

The noninfected human middle ear contains minimal fluid; however, in chronic serous and acute purulent otitis media, the fluid that accumulates may contain antibodies to pneumococci and *H. influenzae* (Howie et al., 1973; Sloyer et al., 1975). Although IgG and IgM antibodies are present, SIgA antibodies dominate. The role of locally produced IgA antibodies in protection against reinfection is unknown, but bacteria were isolated less often from those ear effusions with high levels of SIgA than from those with low titers (Howie et al., 1973). It has been proposed that the tonsils and adenoids are a major source of the antibody-producing cells of the middle ear (Brandtzaeg, 1984). In guinea pigs, however, systemic priming, followed by intraduodenal or intratracheal challenge, also results in IgA-specific antibodies in the inflamed middle ear (Watanabe et al., 1988).

Serum IgG antibodies may also help to protect against middle ear infection. It has been found that patients with recurrent otitis media had much higher serum IgG titers of strain-specific antibodies than those of the IgM or IgA class. Over time, persistent titers of these type-specific antibodies in the serum correlated with decreased infection. However, these studies did not exclude the possibility that a rapid local response to re-exposure in the middle ear mediated the protection. In experimental animal models, serum antibodies and complement can themselves produce otitis media after antigen is introduced into the middle ear (Lim and Mogi, 1994).

The bacteria that cause otitis media enter through the eustachian tube after colonization and/or infection of the nasopharynx. Strains of *H. influenzae* and pneumococci, which are common causes of otitis media, adhere efficiently to retropharyngeal epithelium (Andersson et al., 1981; Porras et al., 1985). Antibodies present in exocrine secretions (such as milk or saliva) may inhibit attachment of the bacteria, decrease colonization, and prevent ear infection (Andersson et al.,

1985, 1986). Indeed, breast-feeding seems to reduce nasopharyngeal carriage of these bacteria (Aniansson et al., 1987, 1988).

Lower Respiratory Tract Infection

Locally formed antibodies against several respiratory bacterial pathogens have been demonstrated in humans (Artenstein, 1975; Brandtzaeg, 1984). It has been claimed that the presence of local IgA antibodies to *M. pneumoniae* may confer resistance (Brunner and Chanock, 1973). Antibodies against the P1 protein, which functions as an adhesin for *M. pneumoniae* to ciliated epithelium, may be protective by blocking its adhesion (Hu et al., 1983). Immunization of the respiratory tract with an M protein vaccine may confer local protection against challenge with streptococci (Waldman et al., 1975. Ingestion of *H. influenzae* can induce IgA and IgG antibodies in exocrine secretions, such as saliva and tears (Clancy and Cripps, 1983).

Acute bacterial infections of the lower respiratory tract frequently follow viral infections. Several different mechanisms have been invoked to explain this relationship, but none are fully proven (Welliver, 1994). The resolution of bacterial lung infections does not seem to depend on the mucosal immune response. Specific serum antibodies and the complement system seem to be the major factors in resolution of pneumonia and prevention of reinfection. The fact that administration of large doses of IgG can prevent upper and lower respiratory tract infections, including pneumonia, in patients with severe antibody deficiencies suggests that serum IgG can compensate for a lack of both serum and local antibody responses.

Urogenital Tract Mucosal Immunity

Urinary Tract Infection

Recurrent and chronic infections are common in the urinary tract and in the female and male reproductive tracts. The host mechanisms involved in resolution and prevention of reinfections at these sites are poorly understood. However, the recognition of human immunodeficiency virus (HIV) as a sexually and vertically transmitted infection has expanded the interest in prevention of genital tract infections.

Urinary IgG and especially SIgA antibodies against *E. coli* O and K antigens appear in patients with acute urinary tract infections (Jodal et al., 1974). In noninfected children, SIgA dominates, but during infection, total IgG and monomeric IgA as well as SIgA levels increase (Uehling and Stiehm, 1971; Svanborg Edén et al., 1985; Fliedner et al., 1986). Such urinary SIgA antibodies may prevent *E. coli* adherence to uroepithelial cells (Svanborg Edén et al., 1976). This activity may be of biologic significance, since bacteria with the capacity to adhere are isolated commonly from the urine of patients with acute pyelonephritis, whereas bacteria from patients with "asymptomatic" bacteriuria adhere poorly or not at all (Svanborg Edén et al., 1983).

The urinary antibodies may therefore protect against symptomatic infection. It is possible that antibodies induce changes in the urinary bacteria in patients with long-standing bacteriuria, resulting in less virulent asymptomatic infections (Hanson et al., 1977a). However, one study has also shown that girls with normal urinary tracts but recurrent symptomatic bacteriuria have abnormally low levels of urinary SIgA between infections (Fliedner et al., 1986), perhaps leading to recurrent infections.

Local immunity to urinary tract infections can be induced in rats (Hanson et al., 1977a; Kaijser et al., 1978). In mice, resistance to ascending urinary tract infection was linked to the LPS response gene, whereas genetic defects in T and B lymphocytes and C5 had little effect on the clearance of bacteria from the kidneys (Svanborg Edén et al., 1984; Hagberg et al., 1984a). These data suggest that the inflammatory mechanisms induced by LPS are important in the host defense against pyelonephritis.

Children with the blood group P_1 were found to be more susceptible to recurrent pyelonephritis in the absence of reflux. This enhanced susceptibility is most likely because the P globoside structure, expressed on the epithelium of the urinary tract, can serve as a receptor for pyelonephritogenic *E. coli* (Lomberg et al., 1983). In the presence of reflux, P-dependent adherence may not be required to induce renal infection. The secretory status of the host may also influence bacterial attachment to the epithelium, since the released A and B glycoconjugates can block binding of bacteria to these receptors (Lomberg et al., 1986a). However, the overrepresentation of nonsecretors among patients with urinary tract infection who have renal scarring (May et al., 1989) and the low frequency of adhering strains in this group of patients, regardless of the presence of reflux (Lomberg et al., 1986b), suggest an altered balance between host and organism unrelated to adherence. Instead, a more generalized host defense defect may be present (Waissbluth and Langman, 1971; Grundbacher, 1972). A wide range of infections have been found to be overrepresented among nonsecretors (Kilian et al., 1983; Blackwell et al., 1988).

Oligosaccharide analogs for the *E. coli*–specific receptor have been shown to prevent ascending urinary infections in mice (Hagberg et al., 1984b). It is not yet known whether such approaches can be applied in humans.

Genital Tract Infections

Infections of the reproductive tract are uncommon in young children but are an increasing problem of adolescence. The topic of mucosal immunity of the reproductive tracts has been reviewed by Parr and Parr (1994). One of the major dilemmas in understanding the immune mechanisms that induce mucosal immune responses in the female genital tract is that local immunity to sperm and seminal fluid can result in infertility (Bronson et al., 1984). Thus, if immune responses are to be stimulated at the vaginal cervical site, they must be limited to organisms that, unlike sperm, penetrate the epithelial barrier. Given the lack of organized lymphoid tissue at these sites, it is likely that vaginal immune responses can be induced more efficiently by antigen stimulation of GALT in the rectum (Forrest et al., 1990) or at more distant mucosal surfaces.

BREAST MILK AND BREAST-FEEDING

Breast milk can be considered a specialized mucosal secretion. Its main function is to transfer nutrients from the mother to the infant during a period when the infant is adapting to other sources of nutrition. Mucosal immune factors of the milk are important in protecting the mammary gland and infant against infection. Both roles may enhance the adaptation of the nursing infant to the extrauterine environment. The immunologic role of human milk in protecting the infant has been reviewed by Goldblum and Goldman (1994) and Carlsson and Hanson (1994).

Many of the immunologic factors in human milk are the same as those in other secretions, although the concentration is usually higher in milk. However, these concentrations decline as lactation proceeds, in a temporal relationship with increases in the infant's own production of the same factors. This finding suggests a dynamic regulation tuned to the infant's needs. The immunologic factors in milk are well adapted to protect the mucosal surfaces, where they function without inciting tissue-injuring inflammatory reactions. Human milk also contains growth factors and cytokines that may modulate the development of the infant's immune system.

Breast Milk Immunoglobulins

Secretory IgA in Human Milk

Secretory IgA is the predominant Ig in human milk throughout lactation. Indeed, the observation that mother's milk contained predominantly IgA that differed structurally from serum IgA led to the first descriptions of SIgA (Hanson, 1961; Hodes et al., 1964; Tomasi et al., 1965). Subsequent studies showed that milk SIgA antibodies develop after maternal intestinal antigenic exposure (Allardyce et al., 1974; Bohl and Saif, 1975; Goldblum et al., 1975; Montgomery et al., 1979) and that natural milk SIgA antibodies are directed against intestinal microorganisms and food antigens. Experimental animal studies later demonstrated that lymphoid cells from the Peyer's patches migrate specifically to the lactating mammary gland (Roux et al., 1977; Dahlgren et al., 1986, 1987). Together this information led to the concept of the enteromammary pathway of secretory immune response (see Fig. 8–1). Additional studies showed that exposure of the mother's respiratory tract to live organisms also resulted in specific SIgA antibodies in the milk (Theodore et al., 1982; Cumella and Ogra, 1986), providing evidence for a similar bronchomammary pathway.

Most milk antibodies are synthesized within the mammary gland. Brandtzaeg (1983a) showed that the lactating human mammary gland has sufficient numbers of IgA-producing cells to account for the daily output of milk SIgA. The concentration of Ig in human milk varies throughout breast-feeding (Hanson et al., 1971; Ogra and Ogra, 1978; Reddy et al., 1977; McClelland et al., 1978; Goldman et al., 1982a). The concentration of SIgA is highest in the colostrum but decreases to a relatively stable level, around 1.0 mg/ml, after the first few weeks. Since the milk volumes increase, the fully breast-fed infant obtains at least 500 mg of SIgA per day, corresponding to about 75 to 125 mg/kg/day for the first 4 months of life (Butte et al., 1984). By comparison, this is many times the IgG given intravenously to patients with hypogammaglobulinemia (~100 mg/kg/week). The high concentrations of SIgA in milk persist, even during a second year of lactation (Goldman et al., 1983a). During weaning, there is a slight increase in SIgA concentration and SIgA titers against *E. coli* O antigens (Goldman et al., 1983b). Lower SIgA levels with increasing parity were observed in Gambian (Prentice et al., 1983) but not British mothers (Lewis-Jones et al., 1985).

Milk from mothers of premature infants has significantly higher concentrations of SIgA than milk from term mothers and shows a further increase toward the 12th week of lactation, as do specific *E. coli* SIgA antibodies (Goldman et al., 1982b; Suzuki et al., 1983). Malnutrition may also decrease breast milk SIgA antibodies (see Influence of Nutrition, earlier).

Breast Milk Antibodies and Response to Immunization

Because of the enteromammary pathway, human milk is rich in SIgA antibodies against microorganisms present in the mother's intestine. As a result, infants ingest antibodies against the microorganisms that they are most likely to encounter. Thus, the Pakistani infant receives SIgA antibodies against *V. cholerae* and *E. coli* enterotoxin from the mother's milk, but the Swedish infant does not (Holmgren et al., 1976).

Typically, human milk contains antibodies to the common colonizing bacteria of the species *E. coli, Klebsiella, Clostridium, Bacteroides,* streptococci, and *Lactobacillus* and against a number of bacterial pathogens, viruses, fungi, and dietary proteins (Vahlquist, 1958; Ogra et al., 1983; Hanson et al., 1983a; Pickering and Ruiz-Palacios, 1986). The presence in human milk of SIgA antibodies to bacterial adhesins, such as somatic pili of *E. coli* (Svanborg Edén et al., 1979) and CFA/I of toxin-producing *E. coli* (Castrignano et al., 1988), *Klebsiella* (Davis et al., 1982), and *Bordetella pertussis* (Oda et al., 1985), may be of particular value to the infant, since they may prevent colonization and infection with potentially pathogenic, piliated enterobacteria.

One approach to disease prevention in newborns would be to immunize their lactating mothers, who could provide passive protective antibodies. The nature of the enteromammary immune response limits this approach, particularly following oral immunization. Although parenteral vaccination with cholera vaccine boosts the milk SIgA response (Svennerholm et al.,

1977), this occurred only in previously exposed Pakistani mothers, not in unexposed Swedish mothers (Svennerholm et al., 1980). This finding agrees with rodent experiments showing that optimal secretory IgA responses follow parenteral boosting after mucosal priming (Hanson et al., 1983a). Indeed, oral immunization with polio vaccine during lactation caused an unexplained decrease in the level of SIgA antibody to poliovirus in the milk (Hanson et al., 1979; Svennerholm et al., 1981). Subcutaneous or intranasal immunization with attenuated rubella virus gave small but consistent milk IgA responses (Losonsky et al., 1982).

Fate of Secretory IgA in Ingested Milk

Because human milk antibodies ingested by the infant are not absorbed into the circulation, the advantages of ingesting SIgA on local immunity were not appreciated until recently. Some milk SIgA passes through the gastrointestinal tract of the infant undigested (see Secretory IgA Stability, earlier). Antibodies have been found in the stool of breast-fed babies (Kenny et al., 1967; Gindrat et al., 1972; Schanler et al., 1986) and as much as 20% to 80% of the milk SIgA can be detected in the stool (Ogra et al., 1977; Davidson and Lönnerdal, 1987; Schanler et al., 1986; Prentice, 1987). Some additional SIgA, not measured in the stool, may be bound to fecal bacteria. Much of the SIgA that escapes proteolysis in the small intestines is degraded by bacterial IgA proteases and reductases in the colon (Hanson et al., 1973; Kilian et al., 1983; Plaut et al., 1983; Kilian and Reinholdt, 1986). Some of the Fab fragments of SIgA produced by these enzymes may still be active, e.g., against poliovirus (Hanson and Johansson, 1970).

IgG and IgM in Milk

Human milk also contains small amounts of IgG and IgM antibodies. The IgG concentration is less than 3% of the serum IgG value and the IgM is about 10% of the serum IgM level (McClelland et al., 1978). Thus, the daily intake of the breast-fed infant is never more than 100 mg of IgG and 70 mg of IgM, and these immunoglobulins become undetectable in milk after the 50th day of lactation. Some milk IgG and IgM is locally produced (Brandtzaeg, 1983a; Cox et al., 1985; Dahlgren et al., 1986). Transfer experiments in rats (Dahlgren et al., 1987) indicate that none of the IgA or IgM antibodies injected into the serum appears in the milk (Nilsson et al., 1988b).

Other Soluble Immunologic Factors

Human milk contains other soluble factors important in host defense of the nursing infant and the mammary gland (Goldblum and Goldman, 1994). This part of the text emphasizes those factors most likely to provide immunologic protection to the infant. Hormones, growth factors, and cytokines are also present in human milk and may play regulatory roles in the development of the infant's own immune system (Goldblum and Goldman, 1994). Soluble milk factors are classified as follows:

- Those that have direct host defense activity
- Those that inhibit inflammatory reactions
- Those that modulate the infant's own protective responses

Direct-Acting Milk Factors

Lactoferrin

Lactoferrin is a major protein of human milk (1 to 6 mg/ml). The bacteriostatic activity of lactoferrin depends on its capacity to bind iron, thereby eliminating this as a growth factor for most aerobic bacteria (except lactobacilli). The described synergy between SIgA antibodies and unsaturated lactoferrin in inhibiting the growth of *E. coli* (Adinolfi et al., 1966) may be related to the presence of specific antibodies against the bacterial iron-binding proteins or to the targeting of bacteria by lactoferrin-IgA complexes (Jorieux et al., 1984; Watanabe et al., 1984). Despite this in vivo activity its in vitro value is not precisely known. A growth-promoting activity of lactoferrin for epithelial cells, described by Nichols et al., (1987), may also enhance resistance of the infant's mucosae to injury.

Lysozyme

The enzyme lysozyme, with activity against the cell wall of gram-positive bacteria, is present in milk throughout lactation (~ 0.1 mg/ml). Unlike other factors, lysozyme concentration increases late in lactation (Goldman et al., 1982a, 1983a, 1983b). The effect of lysozyme in the gastrointestinal tract is not known.

Mucins

Mucin, a highly glycosylated protein that is present in human milk, protects against experimental rotavirus infections in mice (Yolken et al., 1992). This activity may be crucial, since rotavirus is the most common cause of infectious enteritis in infants and children. Mucins associated with the milk fat globules of human milk may interfere with the binding of S-fimbriated *E. coli* to the infant's mucous membranes (Schroten et al., 1992).

Glycocompounds

Human milk contains glycocompounds that may function as analogs to mucosal receptors for bacteria. Bacterial hemagglutination by *V. cholerae* and *E. coli* as well as enterotoxin-binding are inhibited by non-Ig fractions of milk, which contain glycoprotein and/or oligosaccharide (Holmgren et al., 1981, 1983). The inhibitory activity of milk on *E. coli* and *V. cholerae* enterotoxin is related to a glycolipid fraction (Otnaess and Orstavik, 1981; Otnaess and Svennerholm, 1982) that resembles the GM1 ganglioside, the receptor for those toxins (Otnaess et al., 1983). Cleary et al., (1983) detected a human milk component, presumably an oligosaccharide, that prevents fluid loss in mice caused by *E. coli* heat-stable enterotoxin. An antisecretory factor

found in rat milk that inhibits enterotoxin (Lange and Lönnroth, 1986) may be related to this factor.

Prevention of the attachment of pneumococci to retropharyngeal cells by human milk is mediated, at least in part, by low-molecular-weight substances that contain the disaccharide N-acetylglucosamine $(1 \rightarrow 3)$-β-galactose, the minimal component of the *Pneumococcus* receptor (Hanson et al., 1983a; Svanborg Edén et al., 1983; Andersson et al., 1986). Mucosal attachment of *H. influenzae* is inhibited by a high-molecular-weight non-Ig component (Andersson et al., 1985, 1986). A carbohydrate-containing constituent of milk, thought to be a glucosaminoglycan, has been found to inhibit binding of HIV to its lymphocyte CD4 receptor (Newburg et al., 1992). A protective role for receptor analogs is suggested by animal studies (Cleary et al., 1983), but their role in human milk is not established.

Lipolytic Products

Human milk contains both triglycerides and lipolytic enzymes that combine to produce lipolytic products with antimicrobial activity. The infant's own lingual lipase may be important in initiating the lipolysis (Hamosh, 1990). Fatty acids and monoglycerides produced from milk fats by bile salt–stimulated lipases or lipoprotein lipase may prevent intestinal coronavirus infections (Resta et al., 1985). Enveloped viruses may also be disrupted by these products (Stock and Francis, 1940; Welsh et al., 1979; Issacs et al., 1986; Thromar et al., 1987). Killing of *Giardia lamblia* is also dependent on bile salt–stimulated lipase (Gillin et al., 1985), which causes the release of fatty acids (Hernell et al., 1986).

Anti-inflammatory Factors

Human milk, like other secretions, seems to provide protection against infection without inducing an inflammatory reaction, as seen in protection against rotavirus infections (Duffy et al., 1986). Breast-fed infants have fewer symptoms of rotavirus infection than do cow milk–fed infants. This anti-inflammatory activity might be due to decreased levels of inflammatory agents or active anti-inflammatory factors in the milk (Goldman et al., 1986).

Inflammatory factors absent in human milk include coagulation factors, kallikrein-kininogen, many complement components, IgE, basophils, and mast cells. In addition, the macromolecules of human milk rarely provoke an immunologic response by the infant. By avoiding exposure to most foreign food antigens, breast-fed infants do not become sensitized to multiple food antigens (Kramer, 1988; Lucas et al., 1990a), thereby reducing intestinal inflammation.

Other anti-inflammatory substances of human milk contain antioxidants, including ascorbate-like compounds, uric acid (Buescher and McIlheran, 1992), α-tocopherol, and β carotene (Chapell et al., 1985). Epithelial growth factors may make the mucosal surfaces more resistant to injury by oxidations.

Growth Factors

Factors in human milk that enhance the growth and differentiation of epithelial cells include: epithelial growth factor (Carpenter, 1980), lactoferrin (Nichols et al., 1987), polyamines (Sanguansermsri et al., 1974; Romain et al., 1992), and cortisol (Kulski and Hartmann, 1981). These and other factors in human milk may accelerate the development of the infant's gut, making it less permeable to foreign macromolecules and microbes. This effect may account for the lowered incidence of necrotizing enterocolitis in breast-fed infants (Lucas and Cole, 1990).

Factors Modulating Protective Responses

The ability of human milk to modulate the development of the infant's own mucosal and perhaps systemic immune systems are just now being explored. The impetus for this examination are epidemiologic studies suggesting that breast-fed infants have a lower risk for type 1 diabetes mellitus (Mayer et al., 1988), lymphomas (Davis et al., 1988), and Crohn's disease (Koletzko et al., 1989) long after breast-feeding has ceased. The lowered risk may be due to prevention of infections during breast-feeding but, more likely, is related to effects on the infant's immune system. During breast-feeding, infants produce higher blood levels of interferon-α in response to respiratory syncytial virus infections (Chiba et al., 1987) and have higher levels of fibronectin (Friss et al., 1988) in blood than infants fed cow milk formulas. In addition, breast-fed infants have a more vigorous antibody response to systemic immunization to protein antigens (Stephens et al., 1984) and higher levels of secretory immunoglobulins, including urinary SIgA excretion (Goldblum et al., 1989).

Leukocytes of human milk are activated more often than those in peripheral blood (see The Cells of Breast Milk next). They may become activated during migration through the epithelium of the mammary gland or may be responding to immunomodulatory factors in the milk. The first evidence for the leukocyte activation by milk was the finding of enhanced mobility of peripheral blood monocytes incubated with human milk in vitro. That activity was abrogated by adding antibodies to TNF-α to the milk (Mushtaha et al., 1989). The presence of immunoreactive TNF-α in human milk was subsequently verified (Rudloff et al., 1992).

Other cytokines have been discovered in human milk, including IL-1β (Munoz et al., 1990), IL-6 (Saito et al., 1991; Rudloff et al., 1993), IL-8 (Palkowetz et al., 1994), IL-10 (Garofalo et al., 1995), and TGF-β (Palkowetz et al., 1994). This list is expanding rapidly. The effect of these cytokines on the developing infant remains to be elucidated.

The Cells of Breast Milk

Milk differs from most other secretions, in that it contains numerous viable cells, especially during the first few weeks of lactation. This was first reported by Donné in 1844 and later detailed by Smith and Goldman (1968). Enumeration of the cells in milk is complicated by the presence of numerous cell-like particles, mainly milk fat globules. The neutrophils and macrophages are difficult to recognize because they contain cytoplasmic vacuoles consisting of phagocytosed milk fat globules and casein micelles (Paape and Wergin, 1977; Ho and Lawton, 1978). These inclusions also make the milk phagocytes difficult to separate (Paape and Keller, 1985).

Colostrum and early milk contain 1 to 3 × 10^6 leukocytes/ml, falling to about 1 × 10^5 cells/ml 2 to 3 months later (Ogra and Ogra, 1979; Goldman et al., 1982a). Of these cells, 18% to 23% are neutrophils, 59% to 63% are monocytes/macrophages, and 7% to 13% are lymphocytes, as determined by conventional and monoclonal antibody staining techniques (Söderström et al., 1988).

Neutrophils and Macrophages in Milk

The mechanism by which leukocytes enter the mammary secretions is poorly understood. The finding that both milk neutrophils and macrophages have markers of cellular activation suggests that their migration may be similar to those present at sites of inflammation. Thus, relative to blood neutrophils, milk neutrophils demonstrate decreased adherence, decreased response to chemotactic factors, decreased motility (Thorpe et al., 1986; Özkaragöz et al., 1988), and decreased uptake and killing of *Staphylococcus aureus* (Pickering et al., 1980). These functional differences may be associated with prior PMN activation (Keeney et al., 1993). By contrast, milk macrophages, which also demonstrate markers of activation (Keeney et al., 1993) are more motile than blood monocytes (Özkaragöz et al., 1988).

Human milk leukocytes contain considerable amounts of SIgA (Pittard et al., 1977), which suggests that they transport some of the SIgA antibodies to the milk. However, the amount of IgA in leukocytes varies considerably (Moro et al., 1983; Clemente et al., 1986) and release of intact IgA remains controversial.

The role of the milk macrophages in the synthesis of cytokines present in human milk is currently being explored. IL-1 and interferon are produced by milk macrophages (Emödi and Just, 1974; Söder, 1987).

Lymphocytes in Milk

Milk contains small numbers of lymphocytes, 80% of which are T cells (Wirt et al., 1992). Some studies using flow cytometry on unfractionated cells suggest a slight predominance of CD8+ cells (Wirt et al., 1992) in agreement with a finding of a CD4:CD8 ratio of less than 1.0 in 17 of 22 milk samples (Söderström et al., 1988). Earlier studies suggested differential antigen reactivity of milk T cells and circulating T cells (Parmely et al., 1976; Richie et al., 1980), but other reports show similarities in antigen responsiveness (Keller et al., 1980) and production of monocyte chemotactic factor and interferon (Emödi and Just, 1974; Keller et al., 1981, 1984). Cytotoxic lymphocytes have been identified in milk, as have cells mediating weak ADCC (Kohl et al., 1980; Steinmetz et al., 1981) and NK cell activity (Moro et al., 1985). As with milk phagocytes, the T cells display surface activation markers (CD45RO, IL-2 receptor and MHC class II antigens) (Wirt et al., 1992).

The lymphocyte fraction may also contain IgA-producing B cells (Smith and Goldman, 1968; Murillo and Goldman, 1970). IgA synthesis was also shown by Goldblum and van Bavel (1978) and by Hanson (1982) in some but not all milk cell cultures. However, a later series of papers pointed out that the presence of particles and cell fragments that carry IgA make the agar plaque technique unreliable in assessing IgA production. Other workers did not demonstrate in vitro antibody synthesis by milk lymphocytes (Crago et al., 1979; Laven et al., 1981; Moro et al., 1983; Crago and Mestecky, 1984). However, colostral lymphocytes transformed by Epstein-Barr virus produced IgM, IgA, and IgG (Hanson et al., 1985, Söderström et al., 1988). The IgM- and IgA-producing cells contained J chain in high frequency and were of the IgA1 isotype (Söderström et al., 1988). In addition, Shinmoto and coworkers (1986) identified an 80-kd factor from human colostrum that provided selective help for IgA production by peripheral lymphocytes. Whether this factor is responsible for the IgA-enhancing activity of colostrum reported by Pittard and Bill (1979) remains unclear. Thus, human milk may contain IgA-producing cells, cells containing ingested IgA, and factors that stimulate IgA production.

The biologic role of milk phagocytes is not known; they may protect the mammary gland or aid in the host defense of the infants. The T and B lymphocytes of milk may enhance antigen-specific reactivity of the infant. Several groups have reported that human milk feeding can transfer tuberculin sensitivity (Mohr, 1973; Schlesinger and Covelli, 1977), at least temporarily (Ogra et al., 1977). However, because intrauterine transfer of tuberculin sensitivity may also occur (Masters, 1982), transfers of specific cellular sensitivity by humoral factors in the milk (e.g., anti-idiotypic antibodies) cannot be excluded.

Immunologic Protection by Breast-Feeding

Immunologic protection by human milk has been reviewed by Carlsson and Hanson (1994). The diversity and high concentrations of some host defense factors in human milk should protect the breast-fed infant against various infections and perhaps, through modulation of the infant's immune response, should diminish the frequency of immune-mediated disease.

Protection Against Infection

Specific SIgA antibodies in milk can prevent or attenuate bacterial and viral gastrointestinal infections (Carlsson and Hanson, 1994) (see Function of Secretory IgA earlier). The remainder of the evidence for protection against acute infections is derived from epidemiologic studies that compare the frequency of these infections in breast and bottle-fed infants. Thus, most studies indicate some protective effect but do not address which component of breast-feeding is responsible for the differences in the groups. For instance, avoidance of contaminated foods and reduced exposure to other infected infants during early infancy may reduce

the incidence of infections in the breast-fed infants, unrelated to the immune factors in the milk. On the other hand, infants from developing countries often receive foods and fluids that are contaminated with microbes prior to initiation and during breast-feeding (Ashraf, 1993). The inclusion of these infants in the breast-feeding groups of epidemiologic studies may reduce the apparent protective effect of breast-feeding. The methodologic problems in the epidemiologic studies of breast-feeding have been reviewed by Kramer (1987).

The most positive effect of breast-feeding on acute infections relates to the frequency and severity of gastroenteritis. These studies provide evidence that breast-feeding is protective, especially in developing countries and also in disadvantaged subpopulations of developed countries (Mata and Urrutia, 1971; Larsen and Homer, 1978; Cunningham, 1977, 1979; Chandra, 1979; Fergusson et al., 1978, 1981; Rowland et al., 1980; Mittal et al., 1983; Forman et al., 1984; Clemens et al., 1986). However, protection may be difficult to demonstrate, even in the fully breast-fed infants, because of extremely heavy microbial inocula (Hanson et al., 1986; Jalil et al., 1995). Further, the effects of breast-feeding in viral gastroenteritis may not be complete prevention, since only the severity of rotavirus-induced diarrhea is reduced (Jason et al., 1984; Duffy et al., 1986).

Several studies also indicate that breast-feeding protects against respiratory infections (Downham et al., 1976; Fergusson et al., 1978, 1981; Chandra, 1979). Breast-feeding also protects against otitis media (Chandra, 1979; Cunningham, 1979; Timmermans and Gerson, 1980; Saarinen, 1982; Aniansson et al., 1988).

The protective effects of breast-feeding against neonatal sepsis and meningitis (Winberg and Wessner, 1971) seems to be particularly apparent in infants at very high risk (Narayanan et al., 1980, 1981, 1982; Ashraf et al., 1991).

Breast-Feeding and Allergic Disease

Walker and coworkers (1974) showed that locally formed antibodies in animals diminish the absorption of ingested native antigens, presumably by binding to the antigens and enhancing their intraluminal degradation. Infants who are directly transferred from breast-feeding to cow's milk formulas have higher serum IgG antibodies to cow's milk proteins than infants who were weaned to cow's milk formula over 3 or more weeks (Hanson et al., 1977b). Serum IgG antibodies to cow's milk antigen were correlated with early introduction of cow's milk (Fällström et al., 1984). As much as 27% of the serum IgG antibody levels could be attributed to introduction of cow's milk (Hanson et al., 1986). These studies suggest that the breast milk feeding not only reduces the exposure to foreign milk proteins but also modulates the response to these antigens, thus reducing the incidence and/or delaying the onset of food intolerance. However, epidemiologic studies of the effect of breast-feeding on milk allergy are limited (Gerrard et al., 1973; Stintzing et al., 1979). Some studies demonstrate a reduced frequency of eczema in atopic infants after 6 months of this regimen (Matthew et al., 1977). Further, Blair (1977) found that breast-feeding correlated with a better prognosis of asthma in a 20-year follow-up study. Businco and coworkers (1983), Kajosaari and Saarinen (1983), and Chandra and associates (1985) also demonstrated a protective effect of prolonged breast-feeding. However, others have not shown a decrease in atopic disease (Peters et al., 1985). It has been shown that prolonged breast-feeding does delay the onset of the atopic disease. These various studies have been reviewed (Atherton, 1983; Björkstén, 1983; Kovar et al., 1984; Kjellman, 1987). One explanation for these diverse results is that tiny amounts of food proteins are present in human milk from the maternal diet and these may sensitize and elicit symptoms of hypersensitivity in the infant.

MUCOSAL INFLAMMATORY DISEASES

A genetic deficiency of the local immune response is not responsible for mucosal inflammatory disease. However, aberrant immune response, a result of genetic predisposition, may be a factor in some of these disorders (Brandtzaeg et al., 1989).

Celiac Disease

In patients with celiac disease, there is a twofold to threefold increase in the number of IgA- and IgM-producing cells in the proximal small intestinal mucosa. There is also increased local formation of IgG, which may include the gluten antibodies present in this disorder (Brandtzaeg and Baklien, 1976a; Brandtzaeg et al., 1993). Because IgG antibodies are not actively transferred to the secretions, they will be of little value in excluding gluten antigens from the mucosa. Those gluten antibodies may be pathogenetic by formation of complement-activating immune complexes and promotion of cytotoxicity. In addition, activated, gluten-specific CD4[+] T cells (and activated macrophages) in the lamina propria may be involved in the pathogenesis and explain many of the immunopathologic features of the active lesion (Brandtzaeg et al., 1993). Mucosal T-cell activation appears to be directly related to the strong HLA Dq2 association of celiac disease (Halstensen et al., 1993).

Inflammatory Bowel Disease

Severe alterations of the local immunologic homeostasis are seen in Crohn's disease and ulcerative colitis (Brandtzaeg et al., 1989) (see Chapter 23). The stimulatory antigens or mitogens have not been identified. Perhaps an initial break in the mucosal barrier is caused by a viral (transmissible agent) or bacterial infection, possibly combined with nutritional factors and genetic predisposition. However, the pronounced increase in local production of IgG may be of pathogenetic importance.

Although the local IgG-cell responses generally rep-resent an attempt to establish a second line of defense against a battery of foreign substances entering the mucosa, elimination of antigenic material may be unsuccessful in inflammatory bowel diseases. Persistent excessive local production of IgG, combined with massive exudation of IgG from serum, may result in adverse local reactions. First, complement-activating immune complexes may form, and these aggravate and perpetuate the inflammatory reaction. Second, several cell types (for example, monocytes and certain lymphocytes) show affinity for the Fc portion of IgG, which participate in ADCC reactions. Third, a striking shift from local IgA2 to IgA1 and IgG production and a marked decrease in cellular J-chain expression indicate deterioration of the SIgA system in inflammatory bowel disease (Brandtzaeg et al., 1992).

The local overprotection of IgG may represent a specific immune abnormality, particularly the preferential overprotection of IgG1 antibodies in ulcerative colitis. This includes the production of autoantibodies to an epithelial apical 40-kD protein (tropomyosin). Complement-mediated attack on the surface epithelium from the luminal side may also contribute to its pathogenesis (Halstensen and Brandtzaeg, 1993a).

References

Adinolfi M, Glynn AA, Lindsay M, Milne CM. Serological properties of gamma A antibodies to *Escherichia coli* present in human colostrum. Immunology 10:517–526, 1966.

Ahlstedt S, Enander I, Johansen K. Immunoglobulin regulation of the appearance of goblet cells in the mucosa. In Hanson LA, Svanborg-Edén C, eds. Nobel Symposium 68: Mucosal Immunobiology. Monographs in Allergy Basel, Karger, 1988, pp. 71–77.

Allan CH, Mendrick DL, Trier JS. Rat intestinal M cells contain acidic endosomal-lysosomal compartments and express class II major histocompatibility complex determinants. Gastroenterology 104:698–708, 1993.

Allardyce RA, Shearman DJC, McClelland DBL, Marwick K, Simpson AJ, Laidlaw RB. Appearance of specific colostrum antibodies after clinical infection with *Salmonella typhimurium*. Br Med J 3:307–309, 1974.

Andersson B, Eriksson B, Falsen E, Foch A, Hanson LA, Nylén O, Svanborg Edén C. Adhesion of *Streptococcus pneumoniae* to human pharyngeal cells *in vitro*: differences in adhesive capacity among strains isolated from subjects with otitis media, septicemia or meningitis or from healthy carriers. Infect Immun 32:311–317, 1981.

Andersson B, Porras O, Hanson LA, Lagergard T, Svanborg Edén C. Inhibition of attachment of *Streptococcus pneumoniae* and *Haemophilus influenzae* by human milk and receptor oligosaccharides. J Infect Dis 153:232–237, 1986.

Andersson B, Porras O, Hanson LA, Svanborg Edén C, Leffler H. Nonantibody containing fractions of breast milk inhibit epithelial attachment of *Streptococcus pneumoniae* and *Haemophilus influenzae*. Lancet 1:643, 1985.

André C, Lambert R, Bazin H, Heremans JF. Interference of oral immunization with the intestinal absorption of heterologous albumin. Eur J Immunol 4:701–704, 1974.

Andrews JS, Hewlett EL. Protection against infection with *Giardia muris* by milk containing antibody to *Giardia*. J Infect Dis 143:242–246, 1981.

Aniansson G, Andersson B, Alm B, Larsson P, Nylén O, Pettersson H, Rignér P, Svanborg Edén C. Reduced nasopharyngeal carriage of bacteria in breast-fed babies. Abstract. Proceedings of International Symposium on Otitis Media, 1987.

Aniansson G, Alm B, Andersson B, Larsson P, Nylén O, Pettersson H, Rignér P, Svanborg M, Svanborg Edén C. Reduced frequency of acute otitis media in breast-fed infants. Abstract. Proceedings of the American Society of Microbiology, 1988.

Apter FM, Lencer WI, Mekalanos JJ, Neutra MR. Analysis of epithelial protection by monoclonal IgA antibodies directed against cholera toxin B subunit *in vivo* and *in vitro* (abstract). J Cell Biol 115:399, 1991.

Armstrong SJ, Dimmock NJ. Neutralization of influenza virus by low concentrations of hemagglutinin-specific polymeric immunoglobulin A inhibits viral fusion activity, but activation of the ribonucleoprotein is also inhibited. J Virol 66:3823–3832, 1992.

Arnold RJ, Mestecky J, McGhee J. Naturally occurring secretory immunoglobulin A antibodies to *Streptococcus mutans* in human colostrum and saliva. Infect Immun 14:355–362, 1976.

Artenstein MS. Antibacterial aspects of local immunity. In Neter E, Milgrom F, eds. The Immune System and Infectious Diseases. Basel, Karger, 1975, pp. 366–375.

Ashraf RN, Jalil F, Zaman S, Karlberg J, Khan SR, Lindblad BS, Hanson LA. Breastfeeding and protection against neonatal sepsis in a high risk population. Arch Dis Child 66:488–490, 1991.

Ashraf RN, Jalil F, Khan SR, Zaman S, Karlberg J, Lindblad BS, Hanson LA. Early child health in Lahore, Pakistan: V. Feeding patterns. Acta Paediatr 390:47–61, 1993.

Ashraf RN, Jalil F, Hanson LA, Karlberg J. Giving additional water during breastfeeding affects diarrhoeal incidence and early short term growth in poor environment. In press, 1995.

Atherton DJ. Breast-feeding and atopic eczema. Br Med J 287:775–776, 1983.

Baklien K, Brandtzaeg P. Immunohistochemical localization of complement in intestinal mucosa. Lancet 2:1087–1088, 1974.

Baklien K, Brandtzaeg P. Comparative mapping of the local distribution of immunoglobulin-containing cells in ulcerative colitis and Crohn's disease of the colon. Clin Exp Immunol 22:197–209, 1975.

Baklien K, Brandtzaeg P. Immunohistochemical characterization of local immunoglobulin formation in Crohn's disease of the ileum. Scand J Gastroenterol 11:447–457, 1976.

Bakos M, Kurosky A, Czerwinski EW, Goldblum RM. A conserved binding site on the receptor for polymeric Ig is homologous to CDR1 of Ig V_k domains. J Immunol 151:1346–1352, 1993.

Bakos M, Kurosky A, Goldblum RM. Characterization of a critical binding site for human polymeric Ig on secretory component. J Immunol 147:3419–3426, 1991.

Balk SP, Ebert EC, Blumenthal RL, McDermott FV, Wucherpfennig KW, Lanndau SB, Blumberg RS. Oligoclonal expansion and CD1 recognition by human intestinal intraepithelial lymphocytes. Science 253:1411–1415, 1991.

Banatvala JE, Best JM, O'Shea S, Harcourt GC. Rubella immunity gap: is intranasal vaccination the answer? Lancet 1:970, 1979.

Bastian A, Kratzin H, Eckart K, Hilschmann N. Intra- and interchain disulfide bridges of the human J chain secretory immunoglobulin. Biol Chem Hoppe Seyler 373:1255–1263, 1992.

Beatty DW, Napier B, Sinclair-Smith CC, McCabe K, Hughes EJ. Secretory IgA synthesis in kwashiorkor. J Clin Lab Immunol 12:31–36, 1983.

Bellamy JEC, Nielsen NO. Immune-mediated emigration of neutrophils into the lumen of the small intestine. Infect Immun 9:615–619, 1974.

Bellamy W, Takase M, Yamauchi K, Wakabayashi H, Kawase K, Tomita M. Identification of the bactericidal domain of lactoferrin. Biochim Biophys Acta 1121:130–136, 1992.

Bennich H, Johansson SGO. The structure and function of human immunoglobulin E. Adv Immunol 13:1–57, 1971.

Benson EB, Strober W. Regulation of IgA secretion by T cell clones derived from the human gastrointestinal tract. J Immunol 140:1874–1882, 1988.

Besredka A. Du mécanisme de l'infection dysentérique de la vaccination contre la dysentérie par la voie buccale et de la nature de l'immunité antidysentérique. Ann Inst Pasteur 33:301–317, 1919.

Besredka A. Local Immunization. Baltimore: Williams & Wilkins, 1927.

Biberfeld G, Sterner G. Antibodies in bronchial secretions following natural infection with *Mycoplasma pneumoniae*. Acta Pathol Microbiol Scand 79:599–605, 1971.

Bienenstock J, McDermott M, Befus D. A common mucosal immune system. In Ogra PL, Dayton D, eds. Immunology of Breast Milk. New York, Raven Press, 1979, pp. 91–107.

Biron CA, Byron KS, Sullivan JL. Severe herpes virus infections in an adolescent without natural killer cells. N Engl J Med 320:1731–1735, 1989.

Björkstén B. Does breast-feeding prevent the development of allergy? Immunol Today 4:215–217, 1983.

Blackwell CC, Thom SM, Weir DM, Kinane DF, Johnstone FD. Host-parasite interactions underlying non-secretion of blood group antigens and susceptibility to infections by *Candida albicans.* In Lark D, ed. Protein-Carbohydrate Interactions in Biological Systems. London, Academic Press, 1988.

Blair H. Natural history of childhood asthma: 20-year follow up. Arch Dis Child 52:613–619, 1977.

Blanco A, Linares P, Andion R, Alonso M, Villares ES. Development of humoral immunity system of the small bowel. Immunopathology 4:235–240, 1976.

Bland PW, Warren LG. Antigen presentation by epithelial cells of the rat small intestine. I. Kinetics, antigen specificity and blocking by anti-Ia antisera. Immunology 58:1–7, 1986a.

Bland PW, Warren LG. Antigen presentation by epithelial cells of the rat small intestine. II. Selective induction of suppressor cells. Immunology 58:9–14, 1986b.

Bockman DE, Boydston WR, Beezhold DH. The role of epithelial cells in gut-associated immune reactivity. Ann N Y Acad Sci 49:129–143, 1983.

Bohl EH, Saif LJ. Passive immunity in transmissible gastroenteritis in swine: immunoglobulin characteristics of antibodies in milk after inoculating virus by different routes. Infect Immun 11:23–32, 1975.

Brandtzaeg P. Human secretory immunoglobulins: III. Immunochemical and physiochemical studies of secretory IgA and free secretory piece. Acta Pathol Microbiol Scand 79:165–188, 1971a.

Brandtzaeg P. Human secretory immunoglobulins: VII. Concentrations of parotid IgA and other secretory proteins in relation to the rate of flow and duration of secretory stimulus. Arch Oral Biol 16:1295–1310, 1971b.

Brandtzaeg P. Human secretory immunoglobulins: I. Salivary secretions from individuals with selectively excessive or defective synthesis of serum immunoglobulins. Clin Exp Immunol 8:69–85, 1971c.

Brandtzaeg P. Presence of J chain in human immunocytes containing various immunoglobulin classes. Nature 252:418–420, 1974a.

Brandtzaeg P. Mucosal and glandular distribution of immunoglobulin components: immunohistochemistry with a cold ethanol-fixation technique. Immunology 26:1101–1114, 1974b.

Brandtzaeg P. Purification of J chain after mild reduction of human immunoglobulins. Scand J Immunol 4:309–320, 1975a.

Brandtzaeg P. Human secretory immunoglobulin M: an immunochemical and immunohistochemical study. Immunology 29:559–570, 1975b.

Brandtzaeg P. Complex formation between secretory component and human immunoglobulins related to their content of J chain. Scand J Immunol 5:411–419, 1976a.

Brandtzaeg P. Studies of J chain and binding site for secretory component in circulating human B cells: II. Cytoplasm. Clin Exp Immunol 25:59–66, 1976b.

Brandtzaeg P. Human secretory component. VI. Immunoglobulin-binding properties. Immunochemistry 14:179–188, 1977.

Brandtzaeg P. Review and discussion of IgA transport across mucosal membranes. In Strober W, Hanson L, Sell KW, eds. Recent Advances in Mucosal Immunity. New York, Raven Press, 1982, pp. 267–285.

Brandtzaeg P. The secretory immune system of lactating human mammary glands compared with other exocrine organs. Ann N Y Acad Sci 409:353–381, 1983a.

Brandtzaeg P. The oral secretory immune system with special emphasis on its relation to dental caries. Proc Finn Dent Soc 79:71–84, 1983b.

Brandtzaeg P. Immune functions of human nasal mucosa and tonsils in health and disease. In Bienenstock J, ed. Immunology of the Lung and Upper Respiratory Tract. New York, McGraw-Hill, 1984, pp. 28–95.

Brandtzaeg P. Research in gastrointestinal immunology: state of the art. Scand J Gastroenterol 20:137–156, 1985a.

Brandtzaeg P. Role of J-chain and secretory component in receptor-mediated and hepatic transport of immunoglobulins in man. Scand J Immunol 22:111–146, 1985b.

Brandtzaeg P. Distribution and characteristics of mucosal immunoglobulin-producing cells. In Ogra PL, Mestecky J, Lamm ME,

Strober W, McGhee JR, Bienenstock J, eds. Handbook of Mucosal Immunology. San Diego, Academic Press, 1994, pp. 251–262.

Brandtzaeg P. Autoimmunity and ulcerative colitis: can two enigmas make sense together? Gastroenterology (in press) 1995.

Brandtzaeg P, Baklien K. Immunohistochemical studies of the formation and epithelial transport of immunoglobulins in normal and diseased human intestinal mucosa. Scand J Gastroenterol 11:1–45, 1976a.

Brandtzaeg P, Baklien K. Inconclusive immunohistochemistry of human IgE in mucosal pathology. Lancet 1:1297–1298, 1976b.

Brandtzaeg P, Baklien K. Characterization of the IgA immunocyte population and its product in a patient with excessive intestinal formation of IgA. Clin Exp Immunol 30:77–88, 1977a.

Brandtzaeg P, Baklien K. Intestinal secretion of IgA and IgM: a hypothetical model. In Immunology of the Gut, Ciba Foundation, Symposium 46. Amsterdam, Elsevier/Excerpta Medica/North Holland, 1977b, pp. 77–113.

Brandtzaeg P, Baklien K, Bjerke K, Rognum TO, Scott H, Valnes K. Nature and properties of the human gastrointestinal immune system. In Miller K, Nicklin S, eds. Immunology of the Gastrointestinal Tract. Vol. 1. Boca Raton, Fla., CRC Press, 1987a, pp. 1–85.

Brandtzaeg P, Berdal P. Mucosal immunohistochemistry in the characterization of immunodeficiency states. Scand J Immunol 2:215, 1973.

Brandtzaeg P, Bjerke K. Immunomorphological characteristics of human Peyer's patches. Digestion 46:262–273, 1990.

Brandtzaeg P, Fjellanger I, Gjeruldsen ST. Immunoglobulin M: Local synthesis and selective secretion in patients with immunoglobulin A deficiency. Science 160:789–791, 1968a.

Brandtzaeg P, Fjellanger I, Gjeruldsen ST. Adsorption of immunoglobulin A onto oral bacteria in vivo. J Bacteriol 96:242–249, 1968b.

Brandtzaeg P, Fjellanger I, Gjeruldsen ST. Human secretory immunoglobulins: I. Salivary secretions from individuals with normal or low levels of serum immunoglobulins. Scand J Haematol Suppl 12:1–83, 1970.

Brandtzaeg P, Gjeruldsen ST, Korsrud F, Baklien K, Berdal P, Ek J. The human secretory immune system shows striking heterogeneity with regard to involvement of chain-positive IgD immunocytes. J Immunol 122:503–510, 1979.

Brandtzaeg P, Halstensen TS. Immunology and immunopathology of tonsils. Adv Otorhinolaryngol 47:64–75, 1992.

Brandtzaeg P, Halstensen TS, Hvatum M, Kvale D, Scott H. The serologic and mucosal immunologic basis of celiac disease. In Walker WA, Harmatz PR, Wershil BK, eds. Immunophysiology of the Gut. London, Academic Press, 1993, pp. 295–333.

Brandtzaeg P, Halstensen TS, Kett K, Krajci P, Kvale D, Rognum TS, Scott H, Sollid LM. Immunobiology and immunopathology of human gut mucosa: humoral immunity and intraepithelial lymphocytes. Gastroenterology 97:1562–1584, 1989.

Brandtzaeg P, Halstensen TS, Huitfeldt HS, Krajci K, Kvale D, Scott H, Thrane PS. Epithelial expression of HLA, secretory component (poly-Ig receptor), and adhesion molecules in the human alimentary tract. Ann N Y Acad Sci 664:157–179, 1992.

Brandtzaeg P, Halstensen TS, Scott H, Sollid LM, Valnes K, Bosnes V. Epithelial homing of gamma/delta T cells? Nature 341:113–114, 1989.

Brandtzaeg P, Karlsson G, Hansson G, Petrusson B, Bjorkander J, Hanson L. The clinical condition of IgA-deficient patients is related to the proportion of IgD- and IgM-producing cells in their nasal mucosa. Clin Exp Immunol 67:626–636, 1987b.

Brandtzaeg P, Korsrud FR. Significance of different J chain profiles in human tissues: generation of IgA and IgM with binding site for secretory component is related to the J chain expressing capacity of the total local immunocyte population, including IgG and IgD producing cells, and depends on the clinical state of the tissue. Clin Exp Immunol 58:709–718, 1984.

Brandtzaeg P, Nilssen DE, Rognum TO, Thrane PS. Ontogeny of the mucosal immune system and IgA deficiency. In MacDermott RP, Elson CO, eds. Mucosal Immunology I: Basic Principles. Gastroenterol Clin North Am 20:397–439, 1991.

Brandtzaeg P, Prydz H. Direct evidence for an integrated function of J chain and secretory component in epithelial transport of immunoglobulin. Nature 311:71–73, 1984.

Brandtzaeg P, Surjan L, Berdal P. Immunoglobulin systems of human tonsils: I. Control subjects of various ages: quantifications of Ig-producing cells, tonsillar morphometry, and serum Ig concentrations. Clin Exp Immunol 31:367–381, 1978.

Brandtzaeg P, Tolo K. Serum derived antibodies may enhance mucosal penetrability. Nature 266:262–263, 1977.

Bronson RA, Cooper GW, Rosenfeld DL. Sperm antibodies: their role in infertility. Fertil Steril 42:171–183, 1984.

Brown WR, Borthistle BK, Chen ST. Immunoglobulin E (IgE) and IgE-containing cells in human gastrointestinal fluid and tissues. Clin Exp Immunol 20:227–237, 1975.

Brown WR, Smith PD, Lee E, McCalmon RT, Nagura H. A search for an enriched source of polymeric IgA in human thoracic duct lymph, portal vein blood and aortic blood. Clin Exp Immunol 48:85–90, 1982.

Brunner H, Chanock RM. A radioimmunoprecipitation test for the detection of Mycoplasma pneumoniae antibody. Proc Soc Exp Biol Med 143:97–105, 1973.

Buescher SE, McIlheran SM. Colostral antioxidants: separation and characterization of two activities in human colostrum. J Pediatr Gastroenterol Nutr 14:47–56, 1992.

Bull CG, McKee CM. Respiratory immunity in rabbits: resistance to intranasal infection in absence of demonstrable antibodies. Am J Hyg 9:490–499, 1929.

Bull DM, Bienenstock J, Tomasi TB. Studies on human intestinal immunoglobulin A. Gastroenterology 60:370–380, 1971.

Bullen JJ, Rogers HJ, Griffiths E. Bacterial iron metabolism in infection and immunity. In Neilands JB, ed. Microbial Iron Metabolism. New York, Academic Press, 1974, pp. 517–551.

Bullen JJ, Rogers HJ, Leigh L. Iron-binding proteins in milk and resistance to Escherichia coli infection in infants. Br Med J 1:69–75, 1972.

Burgio GR, Lanzavecchia A, Plebani A, Jayakar S, Ugazio A. Ontogeny of secretory immunity: levels of secretory IgA and natural antibodies in saliva. Pediatr Res 14:1111–1114, 1980.

Burrows W, Havens I. Studies on immunity to Asiatic cholera: V. The absorption of immune globulin from the bowel and its excretion in the urine and feces of experimental animals and human volunteers. J Infect Dis 82:231–250, 1948.

Businco L, Ioppi M, Morse NL, Nisini R, Wright S. Breast milk from mothers of children with newly developed atopic eczema has low levels of long chain polyunsaturated fatty acids. J Allergy Clin Immunol 9:1134–1139, 1983.

Butte NF, Goldblum RM, Fehl LM, Loftin K, Smith EO, Garza C, Goldman AS. Daily ingestion of immunologic components in human milk during the first four months of life. Acta Paediatr Scand 73:296–301, 1984.

Capron A, Dessaint JP, Hague A, Capron M. Antibody-dependent cell mediated cytotoxicity against parasites. In Kallos P, ed. Immunity and Concomitant Immunity in Infectious Diseases. Progress Allergy. Basel, Karger, 1982, pp. 234–267.

Capron A, Joseph M, Ameisen JC, Capron M, Pancre V, Auriault C. Platelets as effectors in immune and hypersensitivity reactions. Int Arch Allergy Appl Immunol 82:307–312, 1987.

Carlsson B, Ahlstedt S, Hanson LA, Lidin-Janson G, Lindblad BS, Sultana R. Escherichia coli O antibody content in milk from healthy Swedish mothers and mothers from a very low socioeconomic group of a developing country. Acta Paediatr Scand 65:417–423, 1976.

Carlsson B, Hanson L. Immunologic effects of breast-feeding on the infant. In Ogra PL, Lamm ME, McGhee JR, Mestecky J, Strober W, Bienenstock J, eds. Handbook of Mucosal Immunology. San Diego, Academic Press, 1994, pp. 653–660.

Carlsson B, Zaman S, Mellander L, Jalil F, Hanson L. Secretory and serum immunoglobulin class specific antibodies against poliovirus type 1: vaccination in areas with and without natural exposure. J Infect Dis 152:1238–1244, 1985.

Carpenter G. Epidermal growth factor is a major growth-promoting agent in human milk. Science 210:198–199, 1980.

Casanova JE, Breitfeld PP, Ross AS, Mostov KE. Phosphorylation of the polymeric immunoglobulin receptor required for its efficient transcytosis. Science 248:742–745, 1990.

Castrignano SB, Carlsson B, Jalil F, Hanson L. The ontogeny of serum and secretory antibodies to Escherichia coli CFA/I and other types of pili in Pakistani infants. Unpublished data, 1988.

Cebra JJ, Fuhrman JA, Horsfall DJ, Shatin RD. Natural and deliberate priming of IgA responses to bacterial antigens by the mucosal route. In Weinstein L, Fields B, eds. Seminars in Infectious Diseases. Bacterial Vaccines. Vol. 4. Robbins JB, Hill JC, Sadoff JC, eds. New York, Thieme-Stratton, 1982, pp 6–12.

Cerf-Bensussan N, Jarry A, Brousse NL, Liskowska-Grospierre B, Guy-Grand D, Griscelli C. A monoclonal antibody (HML-1) defining a novel membrane molecule present on human intestinal lymphocytes. Eur J Immunol 17:1279–1285, 1987.

Challacombe SJ, Shirlaw PJ. Immunology of diseases of the oral cavity. In Ogra PL, Lamm ME, McGhee JR, Mestecky J, Strober W, Bienenstock J, eds. Handbook of Mucosal Immunology. San Diego, Academic Press, 1994, pp. 607–624.

Chandan RC, Shahani KM, Holly RG. Lysozyme content of human milk. Nature 204:76–77, 1964.

Chandra RK. Reduced secretory antibody response to live attenuated measles and poliovirus vaccines in malnourished children. Br Med J 2:583–585, 1975.

Chandra RK. Nutritional deficiency and susceptibility to infection. Bull WHO 57:167–177, 1979.

Chandra RK, Puri S, Cheema PS. Predictive value of cord blood IgE in the development of atopic disease and role of breast-feeding in its prevention. Clin Allergy 15:517–522, 1985.

Chapell JE, Francis T, Clandinin MT. Vitamin A and E content of human milk at early stages of lactation. Early Hum Dev 11:157–167, 1985.

Chernokhvostova EV. Orally induced immunologic tolerance. Immunol Clin Sper 3:171–183, 1984.

Chiba Y, Minagawa T, Mito K, Nakane A, Suga K, Honjo T, Nako T. Effect of breast feeding on responses of systemic interferon and virus-specific lymphocyte transformation in infants with respiratory syncytial virus infection. J Med Virol 21:7–14, 1987.

Chiba Y, Higashidate Y, Suga K, Honjo K, Tsutsumi H, Ogra PL. Development of cell-mediated cytotoxic immunity to respiratory syncytial virus in human infants following naturally acquired infection. J Med Virol 28:133–139, 1989.

Chintalacharuvu KR, Tavill AS, Louis LN, Vaerman JP, Lamm ME, Kaetzel CS. Disulfide bond formation between dimeric immunoglobulin A and the polymeric immunoglobulin receptor during hepatic transcytosis. Hepatology 19:162–173, 1994.

Chodirker WB, Tomasi TB, Jr. Gamma-globulins: quantitative relationships in human serum and nonvascular fluids. Science 142:1080–1081, 1963.

Clamp JR. The relationship between secretory immunoglobulin A and mucus. Biochem Soc Trans 5:1579–1581, 1977.

Clancy R, Cripps A. Specific immune response in the respiratory tract after administration of an oral polyvalent bacterial vaccine. Infect Immun 39:491–496, 1983.

Cleary TG, Chambers JP, Pickering LK. Protection of suckling mice from heat-stable enterotoxin of *Escherichia coli* by human milk. J Infect Dis 148:1114–1119, 1983.

Clemens JD, Sack DA, Harris JR, Chakraborty J, Khan MR, Stanton BF, Kay BA, Khan MU, Yunus M, Atkinson W, Svennerholm A-M, Holmgren J. Field trial of oral cholera vaccines in Bangladesh. Lancet 2:124–127, 1986.

Clemens JD, Sack DA, Harris JR, Chakraborty J, Neogy PK, Stanton B, Huda N, Khan MU, Kay BA, Khan MR, Yunus M, Rao MR, Svennerholm AM, Holmgren J. Cross-protection by B subunit–whole cell cholera vaccine against diarrhea associated with heat-labile toxin-producing enterotoxigenic *Escherichia coli*: results of a large-scale field trial. J Infect Dis 158:372–377, 1988a.

Clemens JD, Sack DA, Harris JR, Chakraborty J, Neogy PK, Stanton B, Huda N, Khan MU, Kay BA, Khan MR, Yunus M, Rao MR, Svennerholm A-M, Holmgren J. Impact of B subunit–killed whole cell and killed whole cell only oral vaccines against cholera upon diarrhoeal illnesses and mortality in an area endemic for cholera. Lancet 1:1375–1379, 1988b.

Clemente J, Leyva-Cobián F, Hernandez M, Garcia-Alonso A. Intracellular immunoglobulins in human milk macrophages: ultrastructural localization and factors affecting the kinetics of immunoglobulin release. Int Arch Allergy Appl Immunol 80:291–299, 1986.

Cleveland MG, Bakos M, Pyron DL, Rajaraman S, Goldblum RM. Characterization of secretory component in amniotic fluid: identification of a new form of secretory IgA. J Immunol 147:181–188, 1991.

Cox DS, Furman S, Muench D. Affinity of antibody of a secretory site in the rat. Immunol Invest 14:151–159, 1985.

Crago SS, Mestecky J. Human colostral cells: II. Response to mitogens. Cell Immunol 86:222–229, 1984.

Crago SS, Prince SJ, Pretlow TG, McGhee JR, Mestecky J. Human colostral cells: I. Separation and characterization. Clin Exp Immunol 38:585–597, 1979.

Cruz JR, Hanson LÅ. Specific milk immune response of rural and urban Guatemalan mothers. J Pediatr Nutr Gastroenterol 5:450–454, 1986.

Cumella JC, Ogra PL. Pregnancy associated hormonal milieu and bronchomammary cell traffic. In Hamosh M, Goldman AS, eds. Human Lactation. 2. Maternal and Environmental Factors. New York, Plenum Press, 1986, pp. 507–524.

Cunningham AS. Morbidity in breast-fed and artificially fed infants. J Pediatr 90:726–729, 1977.

Cunningham AS. Morbidity in breast-fed and artificially fed infants: II. J Pediatr 95:685–689, 1979.

Cunningham-Rundles C, Brandeis WE, Good RA, Day NK. Bovine antigens and the formation of circulating immune complexes in selective immunoglobulin A deficiency. J Clin Invest 64:272–279, 1979.

Cutler AR, Armitage RJ, Conley ME, Rosenblatt H, Jenkins NA, Copeland NG, Bedell MA, Edelhoff S, Disteche CM, Simoneaux DK, Fanslow WC, Belmont J, Spriggs MK. CD40 ligand gene defects responsible for X-linked hyper IgM syndrome. Science 259:990–993, 1993.

Dahlgren U, Ahlstedt S, Hanson L. Origin and kinetics of IgA, IgG and IgM milk antibodies in primary and secondary responses of rats. Scand J Immunol 23:273–278, 1986.

Dahlgren U, Ahlstedt S, Hanson L. The localization of the antibody response to milk or bile depends on the nature of the antigen. J Immunol 138:1397–1402, 1987.

Danielescu G, Barbu C, Sorodoc Y, Cajal N, Sarateanu D, Petrescu A, Motas C, Ganea E. The presence of interferon and type A immunoglobulins in the nasopharyngeal secretions of volunteers immunized with an inactivated influenza vaccine. Acta Virol 19:245–249, 1975.

Davidson LA, Lönnerdal B. Persistence of human milk proteins in the breast-fed infant. Acta Paediatr Scand 76:733–740, 1987.

Davies A. An investigation into the serological properties of dysentery stools. Lancet 2:1009–1012, 1922.

Davis CP, Houston CW, Fader RC, Goldblum RM, Weaver EA, Goldman AS. Immunoglobulin A and secretory immunoglobulin A antibodies to purified type 1 *Klebsiella pneumoniae* pili in human colostrum. Infect Immun 38:496–501, 1982.

Davis MK, Savitz DA, Grauford B. Infant feeding in childhood cancer. Lancet 2:365–368, 1988.

Delacroix DL, Jonard P, Dive C, Vaerman JP. Serum IgM-bound secretory component (SIgM) in liver diseases: comparative molecular state of the secretory component in serum and bile. J Immunol 129:133–138, 1982.

Delacroix DL, Lirous E, Vaerman JP. High proportion of polymeric IgA in young infants' sera and independence between IgA-size and IgA-subclass distributions. J Clin Immunol 3:51–56, 1983.

Delacroix DL, Vaerman JP. A solid phase, direct competition, radioimmunoassay for quantitation of secretory IgA in human serum. J Immunol Methods 40:345–358, 1981.

Delacroix DL, Vaerman JP. Secretory component (SC): preferential binding to heavy (>11S) IgA polymers and IgM in serum, in contrast to predominance of 11S and free SC forms in secretions. Clin Exp Immunol 49:717–724, 1982.

Delacroix DL, Vaerman JP. Function of the human liver in IgA homeostasis in plasma. Ann N Y Acad Sci 409:383–400, 1983.

Donné A. *Cours de Microscopie.* Paris, Bailliére, 1844.

Downham MAPS, Scott R, Sims DG, Webb JKG, Garner PS. Breast-feeding protects against respiratory syncytial virus infections. Br Med J 2:274–276, 1976.

Duffy LC, Riepenhoff-Talty M, La Scolea LJ, Zielezny MA, Dryja DM, Ogra PR. Modulation of rotavirus enteritis during breastfeeding. Am J Dis Child 140:1164–1168, 1986.

Eddie DS, Schulkind ML, Robbins JB. The isolation and biologic activities of purified secretory IgA and IgG anti–*Salmonella typhimurium* O antibodies from rabbit intestinal fluid and colostrum. J Immunol 106:181–190, 1971.

Ehrlich P. Über Immunität durch Vererbung und Säugung. Z Hyg Infektionskrankheiten 12:183–203, 1892.

Eidelman S. Intestinal lesions in immune deficiency. Hum Pathol 7:427–434, 1976.

Elson CO, Heck JA, Strober W. T cell regulation of murine IgA synthesis. J Exp Med 149:632–643, 1979.

Elson CO. Induction and control of the gastrointestinal immune system. Scand J Gastroenterol 20:1–15, 1985.

Elson CO, Falding W. Generalized systemic and mucosal immunity in mice after mucosal stimulation with cholera toxin. J Immunol 132:2736–2741, 1984.

Emödi G, Just M. Interferon production by lymphocytes in human milk. J Immunol 3:157–160, 1974.

Fanger MW, Shen L, Pugh J, Bernier GM. Subpopulations of human peripheral granulocytes and monocytes express receptors for IgA. Proc Natl Acad Sci U S A 77:3640–3644, 1980.

Fazekas de St. Groth S, Donnelley M. Studies in experimental immunology of influenza: IV. The protective value of active immunization. Aust J Exp Biol Med Sci 28:61–75, 1950.

Fazekas de St. Groth S, Donnelley M, Graham DM. Studies in experimental immunology of influenza: VIII. Pathotopic adjuvants. Aust J Exp Biol Med Sci 29:323–337, 1951.

Fällström SP, Ahlstedt S, Carlsson B, Wettergren B, Hanson LA. Influence of breast feeding on the development of cow's milk protein antibodies and the IgE level. Int Arch Allergy Appl Immunol 75:87–91, 1984.

Fälth-Magnusson K, Kjellman N-IM. Development of atopic disease in babies whose mothers were on exclusive diet during pregnancy—a randomized study. J Allergy Clin Immunol 80:868–876, 1987.

Feltelius N, Hvatum M, Brandtzaeg P, Knutson L, Hallgren R. Increased jejunal secretory IgA and IgM in ankylosing spondylitis: normalization after treatment with sulphasalazine. J Rheumatol 21:2076–2081, 1994.

Fergusson DM, Horwood LJ, Shannon FT, Taylor B. Infant health and breast-feeding during the first 16 weeks of life. Aust Pediatr J 14:254–258, 1978.

Fergusson DM, Horwood LJ, Shannon FT, Taylor B. Breast-feeding, gastrointestinal and lower respiratory illness in the first two years. Aust Pediatr 17:191–195, 1985.

Fliedner M, Mehls O, Rauterberg EW, Ritz E. Urinary SIgA in children with urinary tract infection. J Pediatr 109:416–421, 1986.

Forman MR, Graubard B, Hoffman HJ, Beren R, Harley EE, Bennett P. The Pima infant feeding study: breastfeeding and gastroenteritis in the first year of life. Am J Epidemiol 119:335–349, 1984.

Forrest BD, Shearman DJC, LaBrooy JT. Specific immune response in humans following rectal delivery of live typhoid vaccine. Vaccine 8:209–212, 1990.

Friss HE, Rubin LG, Carsons S, Baranowski J, Lipsitz PJ. Plasma fibronectin concentrations in breast fed and formula fed neonates. Arch Dis Child 63:528–532, 1988.

Fubara ES, Freter R. Protection against enteric bacterial infection by secretory IgA antibodies. J Immunol 111:395–403, 1972.

Fujiyama Y, Kobayashi K, Senda S, Benno Y, Bamba T, Hosoda S. A novel IgA protease from Clostridium sp. capable of cleaving IgA1 and IgA2 A2m(1) allotype but not IgA2 A2m(2) allotype paraproteins. J Immunol 134:573–576, 1985.

Garcia-Pardo A, Lamm ME, Plaut AG, Frangione B. J chain is covalently bound to both monomer subunits in human secretory IgA. J Biol Chem 256:11734–11738, 1981.

Garcia-Pardo A, Lamm ME, Plaut AG, Franzione B. Secretory component is covalently bound to a single subunit in human secretory IgA. Mol Immunol 16:477–482, 1979.

Garofalo R, Chheda S, Mei F, Palkowetz KH, Rudloff HE, Schmalstieg FC Jr, Rassin DK, Goldman AS. Interleukin-10 in human milk. Pediatr Res 37:444–449, 1995.

Gay FP. Local resistance and local immunity to bacteria. Physiol Rev 4:191–214, 1924.

Gerrard JW, Mackenzie JWA, Goluboff N, et al. Cow's milk allergy: prevalence and manifestations in an unselected series of newborns. Acta Paediatr Scand (Suppl.) 234:1–21, 1973.

Ghetie V, Mota G. The decrease of human colostral immunoglobulin A resistance to papain action after gradual release of the secretory component. Immunochemistry 10:839–844, 1973.

Gilbert JV, Plaut AG, Longmaid B, Lamm ME. Inhibition of microbial IgA proteases by human secretory IgA and serum. Mol Immunol 20:1039–1049, 1983.

Gillin FD, Reiner DS, Gault MJ. Cholate-dependent killing of Giardia lamblia by human milk. Infect Immun 47:619–622, 1985.

Gindrat JJ, Gothefors L, Hanson L, Winberg J. Antibodies in human milk against E. coli of the serogroups most commonly found in neonatal infections. Acta Paediatr Scand 61:587–590, 1972.

Girard JP, de Kalbermatten A. Antibody activity in human duodenal fluid. Eur J Clin Invest 1:188–195, 1970.

Gjeruldsen ST, Brandtzaeg P. Immunoglobulin-producing cells in human lacrimal glands: accumulation of IgD immunocytes in IgA deficiency. Scand J Immunol 8:156–157, 1978.

Glass RI, Svennerholm AM, Stoll BJ, Khan MR, Belayet Hossain KM, Huq MI, Holmgren J. Protection against cholera in breast-fed children by antibodies in breast milk. N Engl J Med 308:1389–1392, 1983.

Glass RI, Holmgren J, Khan MR, Belayet Hossain KM, Imdadul Huq M, Greenough WB. A randomized controlled trial of the toxin-blocking effects of B subunit in family members of patients with cholera. J Infect Dis 149:495–500, 1984.

Glass RI, Stoll BJ, Wyatt RG, Banu H, Kapikian AZ, Huda S: Observations questioning a protective role for breast-feeding in severe rotavirus disease. Acta Paediatr Scand 75:713–718, 1986.

Gleeson M, Cripps AW, Clancy RL, Wlodarczyk JH, Dobson AJ, Hensley MJ. The development of IgA-specific antibodies to Escherichia coli O antigen in children. Scand J Immunol 26:639–643, 1987.

Goldblum RM, Ahlstedt S, Carlsson B, Hanson L, Jodal U, Lidin-Janson G, Sohl-Akerlund A. Antibody-forming cells in human colostrum after oral immunisation. Nature 257:797–799, 1975.

Goldblum RM, Goldman AS. Immunological components of milk: formation and function. In Ogra PL, Lamm ME, McGhee JR, Mestecky J, Strober W, Bienenstock J, eds. Handbook of Mucosal Immunology. San Diego, Academic Press, 1994, pp. 643–652.

Goldblum RM, Powell GK, Van Sickle G. Secretory IgA in the serum of infants with obstructive jaundice. J Pediatr 97:33–36, 1980.

Goldblum RM, Schanler RJ, Garza C, Goldman AS. Human milk feeding enhances the urinary excretion of immunologic factors in low birth weight infants. Pediatr Res 25:184–188, 1989.

Goldblum RM, van Bavel J. Immunoglobulin A production by human colostral cells: quantitative aspects. In Mestecky J, Babb JL, eds. Secretory Immunity and Infection. New York, Plenum, 1978a, pp. 87–94.

Goldblum RM, Van Bavel J. Immunoglobulin A production by human colostral cells: quantitative aspects. Adv Exp Med Biol 107:87–94, 1978b.

Goldman AS, Garza C, Nichols BL, Johnson CA, O'Brian Smith E, Goldblum RM. Effects of prematurity on the immunologic system in human milk. J Pediatr 101:901–905, 1982a.

Goldman AS, Garza C, Nichols BL, Goldblum RM. Immunologic factors in human milk during the first year of lactation. J Pediatr 100:563–567, 1982b.

Goldman AS, Goldblum RM, Garza C. Immunologic components in human milk during the second year of lactation. Acta Paediatr Scand 72:461–462, 1983a.

Goldman AS, Goldblum RM, Garza C, Nichols BL, O'Brian Smith E. Immunologic components in human milk during weaning. Acta Paediatr Scand 72:133–134, 1983b.

Goldman AS, Smith WC. Host resistance factors in human milk. J Pediatr 82:1082–1090, 1973.

Goldman AS, Thorpe LW, Goldblum RM, Hanson L. An hypothesis: anti-inflammatory properties of human milk. Acta Paediatr Scand 75:689–695, 1986.

Gothefors L. Studies of antimicrobial factors in human milk and bacterial colonization of the newborn. Doctoral dissertation, Umea University, 1975.

Gothefors L, Marklund S. Lactoperoxidase activity in human milk and in saliva of the newborn infant. Infect Immun 11:10–15, 1975.

Greenberg SB, Criswell BS, Six HR, Couch RB. Lymphocyte cytotoxicity to influenza virus–infected cells: response to vaccination in virus infection. Infect Immun 20:640–645, 1978.

Gregory RL, Schöller M, Filler SJ, Crago SS, Prince SJ, Allansmith MR, Michalek SM, Mestecky J, McGhee JR. IgA antibodies to oral and ocular bacteria in human external secretions. In Peeters H, ed. Protides of the Biological Fluids. Oxford, Pergamon Press, 1985, pp. 53–56.

Gregory RL, Filler SJ. Protective secretory immunoglobulin A antibodies in humans following oral immunization with *Streptococcus mutans.* Infect Immun 55:2409–2415, 1987.

Griffis JM, Goroff DK. IgA blocks IgM- and IgG-initiated immune lysis by separate molecular mechanisms. J Immunol 130:2882–2885, 1983.

Griffiths E, Humphreys J. Bacteriostatic effect of human milk and bovine colostrum on *Escherichia coli:* the importance of bicarbonate. Infect Immun 15:396–401, 1977.

Grundbacher FJ. Immunoglobulins, secretor status and the incidence of rheumatic heart disease. Hum Hered 25:399–404, 1972.

Gump DW, Christmas WA, Forsyth BR, Phillips CA, Stouch WH. Serum and secretory antibodies in patients with chronic bronchitis. Arch Intern Med 132:847–851, 1973.

Hagberg L, Leffler H, Svanborg Edén C. Non-antibiotic prevention of urinary tract infection. Infection 12:132–137, 1984a.

Hagberg L, Hull R, Hull S, McGhee JR, Michalek SM, Svanborg Edén C. Difference in susceptibility to gram-negative urinary tract infection between C3H/HeJ and C3H/HeN mice. Infect Immun 46:839–844, 1984b.

Hall CB, Walsh EE, Long CE, Schnabel KC. Immunity to and frequency of reinfection with respiratory syncytial virus. J Infect Dis 163:693–698, 1991.

Hall WH, Manion RE, Zinneman HH. Blocking serum lysis of *Brucella abortus* by hyperimmune rabbit immunoglobulin A. J Immunol 107:41–46, 1971.

Halpern MS, Koshland MR. Novel subunit in secretory IgA. Nature 228:1276–1278, 1970.

Halstensen TS, Scott H, Brandtzaeg P. Human CD8$^+$ intraepithelial T lymphocytes are mainly CD45RA-RB$^+$ and show increased co-expression of CD45RO in celiac disease. Eur J Immunol 20:1825–1830, 1990.

Halstensen TS, Brandtzaeg P. Mucosal complement deposition in inflammatory bowel disease. Can J Gastroenterol 7:91–101, 1993a.

Halstensen TS, Brandtzaeg P. Activated T lymphocytes in the celiac lesion; non-proliferative activation (CD25) of CD4$^+$ α/β cells in the lamina propria but proliferation (Ki-67) of α/β and γ/δ cells in the epithelium. Eur J Immunol 23:505–510, 1993b.

Halstensen TS, Scott H, Fausa O, Brandtzaeg P. Gluten stimulation of coeliac mucosa *in vitro* induces activation (CD25) of lamina propria CD4$^+$ T cells and macrophages but no crypt cell hyperplasia. Scand J Immunol 38:590, 1993.

Hamaguchi Y, Ohi M, Sakakura Y, Mukojima T. Quantitation of nasal secretory IgA by enzyme-linked immunosorbent assay. Int Arch Allergy Appl Immunol 69:1–6, 1982.

Hamosh M. Lingual and gastric lipases. Nutrition 6:421–428, 1990.

Haneberg B. Immunoglobulins in feces from infants fed human or bovine milk. Scand J Immunol 3:191–197, 1974a.

Haneberg B. Human milk immunoglobulins and agglutinins to rabbit erythrocytes. Int Arch Allergy Appl Immunol 47:716–729, 1974b.

Haneberg B, Aarskog D. Human faecal immunoglobulins in healthy infants and children, and in some with diseases affecting the intestinal tract or the immune system. Clin Exp Immunol 22:210–222, 1975.

Hanson L. Comparative immunological studies of the immune globulins of human milk and of blood serum. Int Arch Allergy 18:241–267, 1961.

Hanson L. Review and discussion of mammary gland and mucosal immunity. In Strober W, Hanson L, Sell KW, eds. Recent Advances in Mucosal Immunity. New York, Raven Press, 1982, pp. 417–424.

Hanson L, Ahlstedt S, Fasth A, Jodal U, Kaijser B, Larsson P, Lindberg U, Olling S, Sohl-Akerlund A, Svanborg Edén C. Antigens of *Escherichia coli*, human immune response and the pathogenesis of urinary tract infections. J Infect Dis 136:S144–S149, 1977a.

Hanson LÅ, Ahlstedt S, Carlsson B, Fällström SP. Secretory IgA antibodies to cow's milk and their possible effect in mixed feeding. Int Arch Allergy Appl Immunol 54:457–462, 1977b.

Hanson L, Carlsson B, Cruz JR, Garcia B, Holmgren J, Khan SR, Lindblad BS, Svennerholm A-M, Svennerholm B, Urrutia JJ. Immune response in the mammary gland. In Ogra PL, Dayton D, eds. Immunology of Breast Milk. New York, Raven Press, 1979, pp. 145–157.

Hanson L, Borssen R, Holmgren J, Jodal U, Johansson BG, Kaijser B. Secretory IgA. In Kagan B, Stiehm ER, eds. Immunologic Incompetence. Chicago, Year Book Medical Publishers, 1971, pp. 39–59.

Hanson L, Johansson BG. Immunological characterization of chromatographically separated protein fractions from human colostrum. Int Arch Allergy Appl Immunol 20:65–79, 1962.

Hanson L, Johansson BG. Immunological studies of milk. In McKenzie H, ed. Milk Proteins, Chemistry and Molecular Biology. New York, Academic Press, 1970, pp. 45–123.

Hanson L, Motas C, Barrett J, Wadsworth C, Jodal U. Studies of the main immunoglobulin of human milk: secretory IgA. In Immunology of Reproduction. Sofia, Bulgarian Academy Science Press, 1973, pp. 687–692.

Hanson LA. Aspects of the absence of IgA system. In Bergsma D, Good RA, eds. Immunologic Deficiency Diseases in Man. Baltimore, Williams & Wilkins, 1968, pp. 292–297.

Hanson LA, Ahlstedt S, Andersson B, Carlsson B, Fallström SP, Mellander L, Porras O, Söderström T, Svanborg Edén C. Protective factors in milk and development of the immune system. J Pediatr 75:172–175, 1985.

Hanson LA, Jalil F, Hasan R, Khan SR, Karlberg J, Carlsson B, Lindblad BS, Adlerbert I, Mellander L, Söderström T. Breast-feeding in reality. In Hamosh M, Goldman AS, eds. Human Lactation 2: Maternal and Environmental Factors in Human Lactation. New York, Plenum Press, 1986, pp. 1–12.

Hanson L, Ahlstedt S, Andersson B, Carlsson B, Cole MF, Cruz JR, Dahlgren U, Ericsson TH, Jalil F, Raza Khan S, Mellander L, Schneerson R, Svanborg Edén C, Söderström T, Wadsworth C. Mucosal immunity. Ann N Y Acad Sci 409:1–21, 1983a.

Hanson LA, Bjorkander J, Oxelius VA. Selective IgA deficiency. In Chandra RK, ed. Primary and Secondary Immunodeficiency Disorders. New York, Churchill Livingstone, 1983b, pp. 62–84.

Hanson LA, Carlsson B, Ahlstedt S, Svanborg C, Kaijser B. Immune defense factors in human milk. In Milk and Lactation. Basel, Karger, 1975, pp. 63–72.

Hanson LA, Carlsson B, Dahlgren U, Mellander L, Svanborg ED. The secretory IgA system in the neonatal period. In Excerpta Medica. Amsterdam, Ciba Foundation Symposium, 1980, pp. 187–204.

Heddle RJ, Knop J, Steele EJ, Rowley D. The effect of lysozyme on the complement-dependent bactericidal action of different antibody classes. Immunology 28:1061–1066, 1975.

Heddle RJ, Rowley D. Dog immunoglobulins: II. The antibacterial properties of dog IgA, IgM and IgG antibodies to *Vibrio cholerae.* Immunology 29:197–208, 1975.

Hemming VG, Rodriguez W, Kim HW, Brandt CD, Parrott RH, Burch B, Prince GA, Baron PA, Fink RJ, Reaman G. Intravenous immunoglobulin treatment of respiratory syncytial virus infections in infants and young children. Antimicrob Agents Chemother 12:1882–1886, 1987.

Herias MV, Cruz JR, Gonzalez-Cossio T, Nave F, Carlsson B, Hanson LA. The effect of caloric supplementation on selected milk protective factors in undernourished Guatemalan mothers. Pediatr Res 34:217–221, 1993.

Hernell O, Ward H, Blackberg L, Pereira ME. Killing of *Giardia lamblia* by human milk lipases: an effect mediated by lipolysis of milk lipids. J Infect Dis 153:715–720, 1986.

Herzenberg LA, Stall AM, Lalor PA, Sideman C, Moore WA, Parks DR. The Ly-1 B cell lineage. Immunol Rev 93:81–102, 1986.

Hill IR, Porter P. Studies of bactericidal activity to *Escherichia coli* of porcine serum and colostral immunoglobulins and the role of lysozyme with secretory IgA. Immunology 26:1239–1250, 1974.

Ho PC, Lawton JW. Human colostral cells: phagocytosis and killing of *E. coli* and *C. albicans.* J Pediatr 93:910–915, 1978.

Ho PC, Powell DA, Albright F, Gardner DE, Collier AM, Clyde WA. A solid-phase radioimmunoassay for detection of antibodies against *Mycoplasma pneumoniae.* J Clin Lab Immunol 11:209–213, 1983.

Hodes HL, Berger R, Ainbender E, Hevizy MM, Zepp HD, Kochwa S. Proof that colostrum polio antibody is different from serum antibody. J Pediatr 65:1017–1018, 1964.

Holmgren J, Hanson L, Carlsson B, Lindlad BS, Rahimtolla J. Neutralizing antibodies against *E. coli* and *V. cholerae* enterotoxins in human milk from a developing country. Scand J Immunol 5:867–871, 1976.

Holmgren J, Svennerholm AM, Ahren C. Nonimmunoglobulin fraction of human milk inhibits bacterial adhesion (hemagglutination) and enterotoxin binding of *Escherichia coli* and *Vibrio cholerae.* Infect Immun 33:136–141, 1981.

Holmgren J, Svennerholm AM, Lindblad M. Receptor-like glycocompounds in human milk that inhibit classical and El Tor *Vibrio cholerae* cell adherence (hemagglutination). Infect Immun 39:147–154, 1983.

Howie VM, Ploussard JH, Sloyer JL, Johnston RB. Immunoglobulins of the middle ear fluid in acute otitis media: relationship of serum immunoglobulin concentrations and bacterial cultures. Infect Immun 7:589–593, 1973.

Hurlimann J, Waldesbuhl M, Zuber C. Human salivary immunoglobulin A: some immunological and physiochemical characteristics. Biochem Biophys 181:393–409, 1969.

Husband AJ, Dunkley ML. Lack of site of origin effects on distribution of IgA-antibody–containing cells. Immunology 54:215–221, 1985.

Ichimiya I, Kawauchi H, Mogi G. Analysis of immunocompetent cells in the middle ear mucosa. Arch Otolaryngol Head Neck Surg 116:324–330, 1990.

Inman FP, Mestecky J. The J chain of polymeric immunoglobulins. In Ada GL, ed. Contemporary Topics in Molecular Immunology. Vol. 3. New York, Plenum Press, 1974, pp. 111–141.

Iscaki S, Geneste C, d'Azambuja S, Pillot J. Human secretory component: II. Easy detection of abnormal amounts of combined secretory component in human sera. J Immunol Methods 28:331–339, 1979.

Iscaki S, Geneste C, Pillot J. Human secretory component: I. Evidence for a new antigenic specificity. Immunochemistry 15:401–408, 1978.

Issacs CE, Thromar H, Pessolano T. Membrane-disruptive effect of human milk: inactivation of enveloped viruses. J Infect Dis 154:966–971, 1986.

Issacs D, Bangham CRM, McMichael AJ. Cell-mediated cytotoxic response to respiratory syncytial virus in infants with bronchiolitis. Lancet 2:769–771, 1987.

Jalil F, Mahmud A, Ashraf RN, Zaman S, Khan SR, Hanson LA, Karlberg J, Lindblad BS. Breastfeeding and diarrhoeal disease: dependence of protection on age, season of the year and population group. Submitted, 1995.

James SP, Graeff AS, Zeitz M, Kappus E, Quinn TC. Cytotoxic and immunoregulatory function of intestinal lymphocytes in LGV proctitis of non-human primates. Infect Immun 55:1137–1143, 1987.

James SP, Zeitz M. Human gastrointestinal mucosal T cells. In Ogra PL, Lamm ME, McGhee JR, Mestecky J, Strober W, Bienenstock J, eds. Handbook of Mucosal Immunology. San Diego, Academic Press, 1994, pp. 275–285.

Jason JM, Nieburg P, Marks JS. Mortality and infectious disease associated with infant-feeding practices in developing countries. Pediatrics 74:702–727, 1984.

Jodal U, Ahlstedt S, Carlsson B, Hanson L, Lindberg U, Sohl A. Local antibodies in childhood urinary tract infection: a preliminary study. Int Arch Allergy Appl Immunol 47:537–546, 1974.

Johansson SGO, Deuschl H. Immunoglobulins in nasal secretion with special reference to IgE: I. Methodological studies. Int Arch Allergy Appl Immunol 52:364–375, 1976.

Johnson KJ, Wilson BS, Till GO, Ward PA. Acute lung injury in rat caused by immunoglobulin A immune complexes. J Clin Invest 74:358–369, 1984.

Jonard PP, Rambaud JC, Dive C, Vaerman JP, Galian A, Delacroix DL. Secretion of immunoglobulins and plasma proteins from the jejunal mucosa: transport rate and origin of polymeric immunoglobulin. Am J Clin Invest 74:525–535, 1984.

Jorieux S, Mazurier J, Montreuil J, Spik G. Characterization of lactotransferrin complexes in human milk. In Peeters H, ed. Protides of the Biological Fluids. Oxford, Pergamon Press, 1984, pp. 115–118.

Kaetzel CS, Robinson JK, Chintalacharuvu KR, Vaerman JP, Lamm ME. The polymeric immunoglobulin receptor (secretory component) mediates transport of immune complexes across epithelial cells: a local defense function for IgA. Proc Natl Acad Sci USA 88:8796–8800, 1991.

Kagnoff M. Oral tolerance. In Hanson L, Svanborg Edén C, eds. Nobel Symposium 68: Mucosal Immunobiology Monograph. Basel, Karger, 1988, pp. 222–226.

Kagnoff MF. Effects of antigen-feeding on intestinal and systemic immune responses: II. Suppression of delayed type hypersensitivity reactions. J Immunol 120:1509–1513, 1978.

Kaijser B, Larsson P, Olling S. Protection against ascending *Escherichia coli* pyelonephritis and significance of local immunity. Infect Immun 20:78–81, 1978.

Kajosaari M, Saarinen UM. Prophylaxis of atopic disease by six months total solid food elimination. Acta Paediatr 72:411–415, 1983.

Karlsson G, Hansson HA, Petrusson B, Björkander J, Hanson L. Goblet cell number in the nasal mucosa relates to cell-mediated immunity in patients with antibody deficiency syndrome. Int Arch Allergy Appl Immunol 78:86–91, 1985.

Kato T, Owen RL. Structure and function of intestinal mucosal epithelium. In Ogra PL, Lamm ME, McGhee JR, Mestecky J, Strober W, Bienenstock J, eds. Handbook of Mucosal Immunology. San Diego, Academic Press, 1994, pp. 11–26.

Kaul MN, Misra RC, Agarwal SK, Saha K. Decreased gut-associated IgA levels in patients with typhoid fever. Scand J Immunol 11:623–628, 1980.

Kaufmann SHE. CD8$^+$ T lymphocytes in intracellular microbial infections. Immunol Today 9:168–174, 1988.

Kearns DH, O'Reilly RJ, Lee L, Welch BG. Secretory IgA antibodies in the urethral exudate of men with uncomplicated urethritis due to *Neisseria gonorrhoeae*. J Infect Dis 127:99–101, 1973.

Keeney SE, Schmalstieg FC, Palkowetz KH, Rudloff HE, Goldman AS. Activated neutrophils and neutrophil activators in human milk: increased expression of CD11b and decreased expression of L-selectin. J Leukoc Biol 54:97–104, 1993.

Keller MA, Heiner DC, Kidd RM, Myers AS. Local production of IgG4 in human colostrum. J Immunol 130:1654–1657, 1983.

Keller MA, Heiner DC, Myers AS, Reisinger DM. IgD in human colostrum. Pediatr Res 19:122–126, 1985.

Keller MA, Kidd RM, Bryston YJ, Turner JL, Carter J. Lymphokine production by human milk lymphocytes. Infect Immun 32:632–636, 1981.

Keller MA, Kidd RM, Stewart DD. PDD-induced monocyte chemotactic factor production by human milk cells. Acta Paediatr Scand 79:465–470, 1984.

Keller MA, Turner JL, Stratton JA, Miller ME. Breast milk lymphocyte response to K1 antigen of *Escherichia coli*. Infect Immun 27:903–909, 1980.

Kemp AS, Cripps AW, Brown S. Suppression of leucocyte chemokinesis and chemotaxis by human IgA. Clin Exp Immunol 40:388–395, 1980.

Kenny JF, Boesman MI, Michaels RH. Bacterial and viral coproantibodies in breast-fed infants. Pediatrics 39:202–223, 1967.

Kett K, Brandtzaeg P, Radl J, Haaijman JJ. Different subclass distribution of IgA-producing cells in human lymphoid organs and normal secretory tissues. J Immunol 136:3631–3635, 1986.

Kilian M, Mestecky J, Russell MW. Defense mechanisms involving Fc-dependent functions of immunoglobulin A and their subversion by bacterial immunoglobulin A proteases. Microbiol Rev 52:296–303, 1988.

Kilian M, Reinholdt J. Interference with IgA defense mechanisms by extracellular bacterial enzymes. In Easmon GSF, Jeljaszewicz J, eds. Medical Microbiology. London, Academic Press, 1986, pp. 173–208.

Kilian M, Russell MW. Function of mucosal immunoglobulins. In Ogra PL, Lamm ME, McGhee JR, Mestecky J, Strober W, Bienenstock J, eds. Handbook of Mucosal Immunology. San Diego, Academic Press, 1994, pp. 127–137.

Kilian M, Thomsen B, Petersen TE, Bleeq HS. Occurrence and nature of bacterial IgA proteases. Ann N Y Acad Sci 409:612–623, 1983.

Kjellman N-IM. Food allergy: treatment and prevention. Ann Allergy 59:168–174, 1987.

Knight KL, Vetter M, Malek TR. Distribution of covalently bound and non-covalently bound secretory component on subclass of rabbit secretory IgA. J Immunol 115:595–598, 1975.

Kobayashi K, Fujiyama Y, Hagiwara K, Kondoh H. Resistance of normal serum IgA and secretory IgA to bacterial IgA proteases: evidence for the presence of enzyme-neutralizing antibodies in both serum and secretory IgA, and also in serum IgG. Microbiol Immunol 31:1097–1106, 1987.

Kohl S, Pickering LK, Cleary TG, Steinmetz KD, Loo LS. Human colostral cytotoxicity: II. Relative defects in colostral leucocyte cytotoxicity and inhibition of peripheral blood leucocyte cytotoxicity by colostrum. J Infect Dis 142:884–891, 1980.

Koletzko S, Sherman P, Corey M, Griffiths A, Smith C. Role of infant feeding practices in development of Crohn's disease in childhood. BMJ 298:1617–1618, 1989.

Kolmannskog S, Marhaug G, Haneberg B. Fragments of IgE antibodies in human feces. Int Arch Allergy Appl Immunol 78:358–363, 1985.

Korsrud F, Brandtzaeg P. Quantification of immunoglobulin-producing cells in human parotid glands with special reference to IgD immunocytes. Scand J Immunol 8:161–162, 1978.

Koshland ME. Structure and function of the J chain. Adv Immunol 20:41–69, 1975.

Kovar MG, Serdula MK, Marks JS, Fraser DW. Review of the epidemiologic evidence for an association between infant feeding and infant health. Pediatrics 74:615–638, 1984.

Kraehenbuhl JP, Neutra MR. Monoclonal secretory IgA for protection of the intestinal mucosa against viral and bacterial pathogens. In Ogra PL, Lamm ME, McGhee JR, Mestecky J, Strober W, Bienenstock J, eds. Handbook of Mucosal Immunology. San Diego, Academic Press, 1994, pp. 403–410.

Krajci P, Tasken K, Kvale D, Brandtzaeg P. Interferon-gamma stimulation of messenger RNA for human secretory component (poly-Ig receptor) depends on continuous intermediate protein synthesis. Scand J Immunol 37:251–256, 1993.

Kramer MS. Breast feeding and child health: methodologic issues in epidemiologic research. In Goldman AS, Atkinson SA, Hanson LA, eds. Human Lactation 3. New York, Plenum Press, 1987, pp. 339–360.

Kramer MS. Infant feeding, infection, and public health. Pediatrics 81:164–166, 1988.

Kroese HGM, Butcher EC, Stall AM, Lalor PA, Adams S, Herzenberg LA. Many of the IgA producing plasma cells in murine gut are from self-replenishing precursors in the peritoneal cavity. Int Immunol 1:75–84, 1989.

Kulski JK, Hartmann PE. Changes in the concentration of cortisol in milk during different stages of human lactation. Aust J Exp Biol Med Sci 59:769–780, 1981.

Kvale D, Brandtzaeg P. An enzyme-linked immunosorbent assay for immunoglobulins of the isotypes A and M in human sera. J Immunol Methods 86:107–114, 1986.

Lange S, Holmgren J. Protective antitoxic cholera immunity in mice: influence of route and number of immunizations and mode of action of the protective antibodies. Acta Pathol Microbiol Scand [C], 86:145–154, 1978.

Lange S, Lönnroth I. Bile and milk from cholera toxin treated rats contain a hormone-like factor which inhibits diarrhoea induced by the same toxin. Int Arch Allergy Appl Immunol 79:270–275, 1986.

Lange S, Lönnroth I, Nygren H. Intestinal resistance to cholera toxin in mouse: antitoxic antibodies and desensitization of adenylate cyclase. Int Arch Allergy Appl Immunol 74:221–225, 1984.

Lange S, Nygren H, Svennerholm AM, Holmgren J. Antitoxic cholera immunity in mice: influence of antigen deposition on antitoxin-containing cells and protective immunity in different parts of the intestine. Infect Immun 28:17–23, 1980.

Larsen SA, Homer DR. Relation of breast versus bottle feeding to hospitalization for gastroenteritis in a middle class U.S. population. J Pediatr 92:417–418, 1978.

Laven GT, Crago SS, Kutteh WH, Mestecky J. Hemolytic plaque formation by cellular and noncellular elements of human colostrum. J Immunol 127:1967–1972, 1981.

Lawrence DA, Weigle WO, Spiegelberg HL. Immunoglobulins cytophilic for human lymphocytes, monocytes, and neutrophils. J Clin Invest 55:368–376, 1975.

Lebman D, Griffin PM, Cebra JJ. Relationship between expression of IgA by Peyer's patch cells and functional IgA memory cells. J Exp Med 166:1405–1418, 1987.

Lebman DA, Coffman RL. Cytokines in the mucosal immune system. In Ogra PL, Lamm ME, McGhee JR, Mestecky J, Strober W, Bienenstock J, eds. Handbook of Mucosal Immunology. San Diego, Academic Press, 1994, pp. 243–250.

Lee GB, Ogilvie BM. The intestinal mucus layer in *Trichinella spiralis*–infected rats. In Strober W, Hanson LA, Sell KW, eds. Recent Advances in Mucosal Immunity. New York, Raven Press, 1982, pp. 319–329.

Lefrancois L. Basic aspects of intraepithelial lymphocyte immunobiology. In Ogra PL, Lamm ME, McGhee JR, Mestecky J, Strober W, Bienenstock J, eds. Handbook of Mucosal Immunology. San Diego, Academic Press, 1994, pp. 287–297.

Lehtonen PPJ, Grangstromhn EM, Stangstromlberg TH, Laitinen LA. Amount and avidity of salivary and serum antibodies against *Streptococcus mutans* in two groups of human subjects with different dental caries susceptibility. Infect Immun 43:308–313, 1984.

Lewis-Jones DI, Lewis-Jones MS, Connolly RC, Lloyd DC, West CR. The influence of parity, age and maturity of pregnancy on antimicrobial proteins in human milk. Acta Paediatr Scand 74:655–659, 1985.

Lim DJ. Functional morphology of the lining membranes of the middle ear and Eustachian tube. Ann Otol Rhinol Laryngol 83:5–22, 1974.

Lim PL, Mogi G. Mucosal immunology of the middle ear and eustachian tube. In Ogra PL, Lamm ME, McGhee JR, Mestecky J, Strober W, Bienenstock J, eds. Handbook of Mucosal Immunology. San Diego, Academic Press, 1994, pp. 599–606.

Lim PL, Rowley D. The effect of antibody on the intestinal absorption of macromolecules and on intestinal permeability in adult mice. Int Arch Allergy Appl Immunol 68:41–46, 1982.

Lindh E. Increased resistance of immunoglobulin A dimers to proteolytic degradation after binding of secretory component. J Immunol 114:284–286, 1975.

Lindh E, Bjork I. Binding of secretory component to dimers of immunoglobulin A *in vitro*. Mechanism of covalent bond formation. Eur J Biochem 62:263–270, 1976.

Ljungström I, Holmgren J, Huldt G, Lange S, Svennerholm AM. Changes in intestinal fluid transport and immune responses to enterotoxins due to concomitant parasitic infection. Infect Immun 30:734–740, 1980.

Lomberg H, Cedergren B, Leffler H, Nilsson B, Carlström AS, Svanborg Edén C. Influence of blood group on the availability of receptors for attaching *Escherichia coli*. Infect Immun 51:919–926, 1986a.

Lomberg H, Hanson LA, Jacobsson U, Jodal U, Leffler H, Svanborg Edén C. P blood group phenotype, vesicoureteric reflux and the susceptibility to recurrent pyelonephritis. N Engl J Med 308:1189–1192, 1983.

Lomberg H, Hellström M, Jodal U, Svanborg Edén C. Renal scarring and non-attaching *Escherichia coli*. Lancet, ii:1341, 1986b.

Losonsky, GA, Fishaut JM, Strussenberg J, Ogra PL. Effect of immunization against rubella on lactation products: I. Development and characterization of specific immunologic reactivity in breast milk. J Infect Dis 145:654–660, 1982.

Lowell GH, Smith LF, Griffiss JM, Brandt BL. IgA-dependent, monocyte-mediated antibacterial activity. J Exp Med 152:452–457, 1980.

Lönnroth I, Lange S. A new principle for resistance to cholera: desensitization to cyclic AMP-mediated diarrhea induced by cholera toxin in the mouse intestine. J Cycl Nucl Res 7:247–257, 1981.

Lönnroth I, Lange S. Intake of IgA monosaccharides or amino acids induces pituitary gland synthesis of proteins regulating intestinal fluid transport. Biochem Biophys Acta 925:117–123, 1987.

Lucas A, Brooke OG, Morley R, Cole JT, Bamford MF. Early diet of preterm infants and the development of allergic or atopic disease: randomized prospective study. Br Med J 300:837–840, 1990.

Lucas A, Cole TJ. Breast milk and neonatal necrotising enterocolitis. Lancet 336:1519–1523, 1990.

Lycke N, Eriksen L, Holmgren J. Protection against cholera toxin after oral immunization is thymus-dependent and associated with intestinal production of neutralizing IgA antitoxin. Scand J Immunol 25:413–419, 1987.

Lycke N, Holmgren J. Strong adjuvant properties of cholera toxin on gut mucosal immune responses to orally presented antigens. Immunology 59:301–308, 1987.

Maffei HVL, Kingston D, Hill ID, Shimer M. Histopathologic changes and the immune response within the jejunal mucosa in infants and children. Pediatr Res 13:733–736, 1979.

Magnusson CGM, Masson PL. A reappraisal of IgE levels in various human secretions by particle counting immunoassay combined with pepsin digestions. Int Arch Allergy Appl Immunol 77:292–299, 1985.

Magnusson KE, Stjernström I. Mucosal barrier mechanisms: interplay between secretory IgA (SIgA), IgG and mucins on the surface properties and association of *salmonellae* with intestine and granulocytes. Immunology 45:239–248, 1982.

Marx J. Testing of autoimmune therapy begins. Science 252:27–28, 1991.

Masters PL. Maternal transmission of skin sensitivity to tuberculin. Lancet 2:276–277, 1982.

Mata LJ, Urrutia JJ. Intestinal colonization of breast-fed children in a rural area of low socioeconomic level. Ann N Y Acad Sci 176:93–109, 1971.

Mata LJ, Wyatt RG. The uniqueness of human milk. Host resistance to infection. Am J Clin Nutr 24:976–986, 1971.

Matthew DJ, Taylor B, Norman AP, Turner MW, Soothill JF. Prevention of eczema. Lancet 1:321–324, 1977.

May SJ, Blackwell CC, Brettle RP, MacCallum CJ, Weir DM. Nonsecretion of ABO blood group antigens: a host factor predisposing to recurrent urinary tract infections and renal scarring. FEMS Microbiol Immunol 1:383–387, 1989.

Mayer EJ, Hamman RF, Gay EC, Lezotte DC, Savitz DA, Klingensmith GJ. Reduced risk of IDDM among breast fed children: the Colorado IDDM registry. Diabetes 37:1625–1632, 1988.

Mayer L, Posnett DN, Kunkel HG. Human malignant T cells capable of inducing an immunoglobulin class switch. J Exp Med 161:134–144, 1985.

Mayer L, Shlien R. Evidence for function of Ia molecules on gut epithelial cells in man. J Exp Med 166:1471–1483, 1987.

Mayrhofer G. The nature of the thymus dependency of mucosal mast cells: II. The effect of thymectomy and of depleting recirculating lymphocytes on the response to Nippostrongylus brasiliensis. Cell Immunol 47:312–322, 1979.

Mayrhofer G, Bazin H, Gowans JL. Nature of cells binding anti-IgE synthesis in regional nodes and concentration in mucosal mast cells. Eur J Immunol 6:537–545, 1976.

Mazanec MB, Kaetzel CS, Lamm ME, Fletcher D, Nedrud JG. Intracellular neutralization of virus by immunoglobulin A antibodies. Proc Natl Acad Sci USA 89:6901–6905, 1992a.

Mazanec MB, Lamm ME, Lyn D, Portner A, Nedrud JG. Comparison of IgA versus IgG monoclonal antibodies for passive immunization of the murine respiratory tract. Virus Res 23:7–12, 1992b.

Mazanec MB, Nedrud JG, Kaetzel CS, Lamm ME. A three-tiered view of the role of IgA in mucosal defense. Immunol Today 14:430–435, 1993.

McClelland DBL, McGrath J, Samson RR. Antimicrobial factors in human milk: studies of concentration and transfer to the infant during the early stages of lactation. Acta Paediatr Scand 67:1–20, 1978.

McDermott MR, Befus AD, Bienenstock J. The structural basis for immunity in the respiratory tract. Int Rev Exp Pathol 23:47–112, 1982.

McDermott MR, Bienenstock J. Evidence for a common mucosal immunologic system: I. Migration of B immunoblasts into intestinal, respiratory and genital tissues. J Immunol 122:1892–1898, 1979.

McElroy PJ, Szewczuk MR, Befus AD. Regulation of heterologous IgM, IgG and IgA antibody responses in mucosal-associated lymphoid tissues of Nippostrongylus brasiliensis–infected mice. J Immunol 130:435–441, 1983.

McGee DW, Aicher WK, Eldridge JH, Peppard JV, Mestecky J, McGhee JR. Transforming growth factor-beta enhances secretory component and major histocompatibility complex class I antigen expression on rat IEC-6 intestinal epithelial cells. Cytokine 3:543–550, 1991.

McGee DW, McMurray DN. The effect of protein malnutrition on the IgA immune response in mice. Immunology 63:25–29, 1988.

McIntosh K, McQuillin J, Gardner PS. Cell-free and cell-bound antibody in nasal secretions from infants with respiratory syncytial virus infection. Infect Immun 23:276–281, 1979.

McIntyre TM, Klinman DR, Rothman P, Lugo M, Dasch JR, Mond JJ, Snapper CM. Transforming growth factor β1 selectivity stimulates immunoglobulin G2b secretion by lipopolysaccharide-activated murine B cells. J Exp Med 177:1031–1037, 1993.

McMurray DN, Rey H, Casazza LJ, Watson RR. Effect of moderate malnutrition on concentration of immunoglobulins and enzymes in tears and saliva of young Colombian children. Am J Clin Nutr 30:1944–1948, 1977.

Mellander L, Bjorkander J, Carlsson B, Hanson L. Secretory antibodies in IgA-deficient and immunosuppressed individuals. J Clin Immunol 6:284–291, 1986a.

Mellander L, Carlsson B, Hanson L. Appearance of secretory IgM and IgA antibodies to Escherichia coli in saliva during early infancy and childhood. J Pediatr 104:564–568, 1985.

Mellander L, Carlsson B, Hanson LA. Secretory IgA and IgM antibodies to E. coli and poliovirus type I antigens occur in amniotic fluid, meconium and saliva from newborns: a neonatal immune response without antigenic exposure—a result of anti-idiotypic induction? Clin Exp Immunol 107:430–433, 1986b.

Mellander L, Carlsson B, Jalil F, Söderström T, Hanson LA. Secretory IgA antibody response against Escherichia coli antigens in infants in relation to exposure. J Pediatr, 107:430–433, 1985.

Mestecky J. Structural aspects of human polymeric IgA. LaRicerca Clin Lab 6:87–95, 1976.

Mestecky J. The common mucosal immune system and current strategies for induction of immune responses in external secretions. J Clin Immunol 7:265–276, 1987.

Mestecky J, Kraus FW. Heterogeneity of human secretory immunoglobulin (abstract). Int Assoc Dent Res 1970.

Mestecky J, McGhee JR, Arnold RR, Michalek SM, Prince SJ, Babb JL. Selective induction of an immune response in human external secretions by ingestion of bacterial antigen. J Clin Invest 61:731–737, 1978.

Mestecky J, Zikan J, Butler W. Immunoglobulin M and secretory immunoglobulin A: evidence for a common polypeptide chain different from light chains. Science 171:1163–1165, 1971.

Michalek SM, Morisaki I, Gregory RL, Kimuva S, Harmon CC, Hamada S, Kotani S, McGhee JR. Oral adjuvants enhance salivary IgA responses to purified Streptococcus mutans antigens. In Peeters H, ed. Protides of the Biological Fluids. Oxford, Pergamon Press, 1985, pp. 53–56.

Miller SD, Hanson DG. Inhibition of specific immune responses by feeding protein antigens: IV. Evidence for tolerance and specific active suppression of cell-mediated immune responses to ovalbumin. J Immunol 123:2344–2350, 1979.

Mittal SK, Kanwar A, Varghese A, Ramachandran VG. Gut flora in breast and bottlefed infants with and without diarrhea. Indian Pediatr 20:21–26, 1983.

Mohr JA. The possible induction and/or acquisition of cellular hypersensitivity associated with ingestion of colostrum. J Pediatr 82:1062–1064, 1973.

Moldoveanu Z, Tenovuo J, Mestecky J, Pruitt KM. Human milk peroxidase is derived from milk leukocytes. Biochem Biophys Acta 718:103–108, 1982.

Montgomery PC, Cohen C, Skandera CA, Connelly KM. Evidence for an IgA anamnestic response in rabbit mammary secretions. In Ogra PL, Dayton D, eds. Immunology of Breast Milk. New York, Raven Press, 1979, pp. 115–127.

Montgomery PC, Majumdar AS, Shandera CA, Rockey JH. The effect of immunization route and sequence of stimulation on the induction of IgA antibodies in tears. Curr Eye Res 3:861–865, 1984.

Moore EC, Reichard P, Thelander L. Enzymatic synthesis of deoxyribonucleotides: V. Purification and properties of thioredoxin reductase from Escherichia coli. Br J Biol Chem 239:3445–3452, 1964.

Moro I, Abo T, Crago SS, Komiyama K, Mestecky J. Natural killer cells in human colostrum. Cell Immunol 93:467–474, 1985.

Moro I, Crago SS, Mestecky J. Localization of IgA and IgM in human colostral elements using immunoelectron microscopy. J Clin Immunol 3:382–391, 1983.

Mostov KE. Transepithelial transport of immunoglobulins. Annu Rev Immunol 12:63–84, 1994.

Mostov KE, Friedlander M, Blobel G. The receptor for transepithelial transport of IgA and IgM contains multiple immunoglobulin-like domains. Nature 308:34–43, 1984.

Mowat AM. The regulation of immune responses to dietary protein antigens. Immunol Today 8:93–98, 1987.

Munoz C, Endres S, van der Meer J, Schlesinger L, Arevalo M, Dinarello C. Interleukin-1β in human colostrum. Res Immunol 141:501–513, 1990.

Murillo GJ, Goldman AS. The cells of human colostrum: II. Synthesis of IgA and beta 1c. Pediatr Res 4:71–75, 1970.

Murphy BR. Mucosal immunity to viruses. In Ogra PL, Lamm ME, McGhee JR, Mestecky J, Strober W, Bienenstock J, eds. Handbook of Mucosal Immunology. San Diego, Academic Press, 1994, pp. 333–343.

Mushtaha AA, Schmalstieg FC, Hughes TK Jr, Rajaraman S, Rudloff HE, Goldman AS. Chemokinetic agents for monocytes in human milk: possible role of tumor necrosis factor–alpha. Pediatr Res 1989:629–633, 1989.

Musil LS, Baenziger JU. Proteolytic processing of rat liver membrane secretory component: cleavage activity is localized to bile canalicular membranes. J Biol Chem 263:15799–15808, 1988.

Mygind N. Nasal Allergy. Oxford, Blackwell, 1978.

Mygind N, Weeke B, Ullman S. Quantitative determination of immunoglobulins in nasal secretion. Int Arch Allergy Appl Immunol 49:99–107, 1975.

Nagura H, Ohtani H, Masuda T, Kimura M, Nakamura S. HLA-DR expression on M cells overlying Peyer's patches is a common feature of human small intestine. Acta Pathol Jpn 41:818–823, 1991.

Nakajima S, Gillespie DN, Gleich GJD. Differences between IgA and IgE as secretory proteins. Clin Exp Immunol 21:306–317, 1975.

Narayanan I, Bala S, Prakash K, Verma RK, Gujral VV. Partial supplementation with expressed breastmilk for prevention of infection in low-birth-weight infants. Lancet 2:561–563, 1980.

Narayanan I, Prakash K, Gujral VV. The value of human milk in the prevention of infection in the high-risk low-birth-weight infant. J Pediatr 99:496–498, 1981.

Narayanan I, Prakash K, Gujral VV. A planned prospective evaluation of the anti-infective property of varying quantities of expressed human milk. Acta Paediatr Scand 71:441–445, 1982.

Neukirk MM, Klein MH, Katz A, Fischer MM, Underdown BM. Estimation of polymeric IgA in human serum: an assay based on binding of radiolabelled human secretory component with applications in the study of IgA nephropathy, IgA monoclonal gammopathy, and liver disease. J Immunol 130:1176–1181, 1983.

Neutra MR, Kraehenbuhl JP. Cellular and molecular basis for antigen transport in the intestinal epithelium. In Ogra PL, Lamm ME, McGhee JR, Mestecky J, Strober W, Bienenstock J, eds. Handbook of Mucosal Immunology. San Diego, Academic Press, 1994, pp. 27–39.

Newburg DS, Viscidi RP, Ruff A, Yolken RH. A human milk factor inhibits binding of human immunodeficiency virus to the CD4 receptor. Pediatr Res 31:22–28, 1992.

Newby TJ. Protective immune responses in the intestinal tract. In Newby TJ, Stokes CR, eds. Local Immune Responses of the Gut. Boca Raton, Fla.: CRC Press, 1984, pp. 143–198.

Newcomb RW, DeVald BL. Antibody activities of human exocrine gamma A diphtheria antitoxin. Fed Proc 28:765, 1969.

Newcomb RW, Ishizaka K. Physiochemical and antigenic studies on the human gamma E in respiratory fluids. J Immunol 105:85–89, 1970.

Newcomb RW, Normansell D, Stanworth DR. A structural study of human exocrine IgA globulin. J Immunol 101:905–914, 1968.

Newcomb RW, Sutoris CA. Comparative studies on human and rabbit exocrine IgA antibodies to an albumin. Immunochemistry 11:623–632, 1974.

Newhouse M, Sanchis J, Bienenstock J. Lung defense mechanism. N Engl J Med 295:1045–1052, 1976.

Nichols BL, McKee KS, Henry JF, Putnam M. Human lactoferrin stimulates thymidine incorporation into DNA of rat crypt cells. Pediatr Res 21:563–567, 1987.

Nicklin S, Miller K. Local and systemic immune response to intestinally presented antigen. Int Arch Allergy Appl Immunol 72:87–90, 1983.

Nikolova EB, Tomana M, Russell MW. All forms of human IgA antibodies bound to antigen interfere with complement (C3) fixation induced by IgG or by antigen alone. Scand J Immunol 39:275–280, 1994.

Nilsson K, Dahlgren UIH, Hanson L. Origin of IgG and IgM antibodies appearing in bile and milk of rats. Unpublished data, 1988.

Oda M, Cowell JL, Burstyn DG, Thaib S, Manclark CR. Antibodies to *Bordetella pertussis* in human colostrum and their protective activity against aerosol infection in mice. Infect Immun 47:441–445, 1985.

Ogra PL. Effect of tonsillectomy and adenoidectomy on nasopharyngeal antibody response to poliovirus. N Engl J Med 284:59–64, 1971.

Ogra PL, Coppola PR, MacGillivray MH, Dzierba JL. Mechanism of mucosal immunity to viral infections in gamma A immunoglobulin-deficiency syndromes. Proc Soc Exp Biol Med 145:811–816, 1974.

Ogra PL, Losonsky GA, Fishaut M. Colostrum-derived immunity and maternal-neonatal interaction. Ann N Y Acad Sci 409:82–95, 1983.

Ogra SS, Ogra PL. Immunologic aspects of human colostrum and milk: I. Distribution, characteristics and concentrations of immunoglobulins at different times after the onset of lactation. J Pediatr 92:546–549, 1978.

Ogra SS, Weintraub D, Ogra PL. Immunologic aspects of human colostrum and milk: III. Fate and absorption of cellular and soluble components in the gastrointestinal tract of the newborn. J Immunol 119:245–248, 1977.

Ogra PL, Lamm ME, McGhee JR, Mestecky J, Strober W, Bienenstock J, eds. Handbook of Mucosal Immunity. San Diego, Academic Press, 1994.

Otnaess A, Svennerholm A. Non-immunoglobulin fraction of human milk protects against enterotoxin-induced intestinal fluid secretion. Infect Immun 35:738–740, 1982.

Otnaess AB, Laegreid A, Ertresvag K. Inhibition of enterotoxin from *Escherichia coli* and *Vibrio cholerae* by gangliosides from human milk. Infect Immun 40:563–569, 1983.

Otnaess AB, Orstavik I. Effect of fractions of Ethiopian and Norwegian colostrum on rotavirus and *Escherichia coli* heat labile enterotoxin. Infect Immun 33:459–466, 1981.

Owen RL, Nemanic P. Antigen processing structures of the mammalian intestinal tract: a SEM study of lymphoepithelial organs. Scan Electron Microsc 2:367–378, 1978.

Özkaragöz F, Rudloff HE, Rajaraman S, Mushtaha AA, Schmalstieg FC, Goldman AS. The motility of human milk macrophages in collagen gels. Pediatr Res 23:449–452, 1988.

Paape MJ, Keller M. Determination of numbers and function of cells in human milk. In Jensen RG, Neville MC, eds. Human Lactation. Milk Components and Methodologies. New York, Plenum Press, 1985, pp. 53–60.

Paape MJ, Wergin WS. Scanning and transmission electron microscopy of polymorphonuclear leucocytes (PMN) isolated from milk. Fed Proc 36:1201, 1977.

Palkowetz KH, Royer CL, Garofalo R, Rudloff HE, Schmalstieg FC Jr, Goldman AS. Production of interleukin-6 and interleukin-8 by human mammary gland epithelial cells. J Reprod Immunol 26:57–64, 1994.

Parmely MJ, Beer AE, Billingham RE. *In vitro* studies on the T-lymphocyte population of human milk. J Exp Med 144:358–370, 1976.

Parr MB, Parr EL. Mucosal immunity in the female and male reproductive tracts. In Ogra PL, Lamm ME, McGhee JR, Mestecky J, Strober W, Bienenstock J, eds. Handbook of Mucosal Immunology. San Diego, Academic Press, 1994, pp. 677–689.

Parrott DMV, Tait C, MacKenzie S, Mowat AM, Davies MDJ, Micklem HS. Analysis of the effector functions of different populations of mucosal lymphocytes. Ann N Y Acad Sci 409:307–320, 1983.

Perkkiö M, Savilathi E. Time of appearance of immunoglobulin-containing cells in the mucosa of the neonatal intestine. Pediatr Res 14:953–955, 1980.

Peters T, Golding J, Butler NR. Breast-feeding and childhood eczema. Lancet 1:49–50, 1985.

Pfaffenbach G, Lamm ME, Gigli I. Activation of the guinea pig alternative complement pathway by mouse IgA immune complexes. J Exp Med 155:231–247, 1982.

Phillips JO, Everson MP, Moldoveanu Z, Lue C, Mestecky J. Synergistic effect of IL-4 and IFN-γ on the expression of polymeric Ig receptor (secretory component) and IgA binding by human epithelial cells. J Immunol 145:1740–1744, 1990.

Phillips-Quagliata JM, Lamm ME. Lymphocyte homing to mucosal effector sites. In Ogra PL, Lamm ME, McGhee JR, Mestecky J, Strober W, Bienenstock J, eds. Handbook of Mucosal Immunology. San Diego, Academic Press, 1994, pp. 225–239.

Phillips-Quagliata JM, Roux ME, Arney M, Kelly-Hatfield P, McWilliams M, Lamm ME. Migration and regulation of B-cells in the mucosal immune system. Ann N Y Acad Sci 409:194–202, 1983.

Picker LJ. Control of lymphocyte homing. Curr Opin Immunol 6:394–406, 1994.

Pickering LK, Cleary TG, Kohl S. Polymorphonuclear leucocytes of human colostrum: I. Oxidative metabolism and kinetics of killing radiolabelled *Staphylococcus aureus*. J Infect Dis 142:685–698, 1980.

Pickering LK, Ruiz-Palacios G. Antibodies in milk directed against specific enteropathogens. In Hamosh M, Goldman AS, eds. Human

Lactation 2. Maternal Environmental Factors. New York, Plenum Press, 1986, pp. 499–506.

Pierce AE. Specific antibodies at mucous surfaces. Vet Rev Annot 5:17–36, 1959.

Pierce NF, Cray WC. Determinants of the localization, magnitude and duration of a specific mucosal IgA plasma cell response in enterically immunized rats. J Immunol 128:1311–1315, 1982.

Pierce NF, Gowans JL. Cellular kinetics of the intestinal immune response to cholera toxoid in rats. J Exp Med 142:1550–1563, 1975.

Pierce NF, Sack RB: Immune response of the intestinal mucosa to cholera toxoid. J Infect Dis 136:S113–S117, 1977.

Piskurich JF, France JA, Tamer CM, Willmer CA, Kaetzel CS, Kaetzel DM. Interferon-gamma induces polymeric immunoglobulin receptor mRNA in human intestinal epithelial cells by a protein synthesis dependent mechanism. Mol Immunol 30:413–421, 1993.

Pittard WB, Polmar SH, Fanaroff AA. The breast milk macrophage: a potential vehicle for immunoglobulin transport. J Reticuloendothel Soc 22:597–604, 1977.

Pittard WB III, Bill K. Differentiation of cord blood lymphocytes into IgA-producing cells in response to breast milk stimulatory factor. Clin Immunol Immunopathol 13:430–434, 1979.

Plaut AG. The IgA1 proteases of pathogenic bacteria. Ann Rev Microbiol 37:603–622, 1983.

Pond L, Wassom DL, Hayes CE. Evidence for differential induction of helper T cell subsets during *Trichinella spiralis* infection. J Immunol 143:4232–4237, 1989.

Porras O, Svanborg Edén C, Lagergard T, Hanson LA. Method for testing adherence of *Haemophilus influenzae* to human buccal epithelial cells. Eur J Clin Microbiol 4:310–315, 1985.

Porter P, Kenworthy R, Noakes DE, Allen WD. Intestinal antibody secretion in the young pig in response to oral immunization with *Escherichia coli*. Immunology 27:841–853, 1974.

Portis JL, Coe JE. IgM, the secretory immunoglobulin of reptiles and amphibians. Nature 258:547–548, 1975.

Prentice A. Breast feeding increases concentrations of IgA in infant's urine. Arch Dis Child 62:792–795, 1987.

Prentice A, Prentice AM, Cole TJ, Paul AA, Whitehead RG. Breast-milk antimicrobial factors of rural Gambian mothers: I. Influence of stage of lactation and maternal plan of nutrition. Acta Paediatr Scand 73:796–802, 1984.

Prentice A, Prentice AM, Cole TJ, Whitehead RG. Determinants of variations in breast milk protective factor concentrations of rural Gambian mothers. Arch Dis Child 58:518–522, 1983.

Ragnum TO, Brandtzaeg P. IgE-positive cells in human intestinal mucosa are mainly mast cells. Int Arch Allergy Appl Immunol 89:256–260, 1989.

Reddy V, Bhaskaram C. Raghuramulu N, Jagadeesan V. Antimicrobial factors in human milk. Acta Paediatr Scand 66:229–234, 1977.

Reddy V, Raghuramulu N, Bhaskaram C. Secretory IgA in protein-calorie malnutrition. Arch Dis Child 51:871–874, 1976.

Reed KJ, van Epps DE, Williams RC. Inhibition of human eosinophil chemotaxis by IgA paraproteins. Inflammation 3:405–416, 1979.

Reed WP, Williams RC Jr. Intestinal immunoglobulins in shigellosis. Gastroenterology 61:35–45, 1971.

Reinholdt J, Krogh P, Holmstrup P. Degradation of IgA1, IgA2 and S-IgA by *Candida* and *Torulopsis* species. Acta Pathol Microbiol Immunol Scand 95:265–274, 1987.

Remington JS, Vosti KL, Lietze A, Zimmerman AL. Serum proteins and antibody activity in human nasal secretions. J Clin Invest 43:1613–1624, 1964.

Renegar KB, Small PA. Passive transfer of local immunity to influenza virus infection by IgA antibody. J Immunol 146:1972–1978, 1991.

Resta S, Luby JP, Rosenfeld CR, Siegel JD. Isolation and propagation of human enteric coronavirus. Science 229:978–981, 1985.

Richie ER, Steinmetz KD, Meistrich ML, Ramirez I, Hilliard HK. T lymphocytes in colostrum and peripheral blood: difference in their capacity to form thermostable E-rosettes. J Immunol 125:2344–2346, 1980.

Rits M, Hiematra PS, Bazin H, van Es LA, Daha M, Vaerman JP. Activation of rat complement by soluble and insoluble immune complexes of rat IgA. In Hanson LA, Svanborg-Edén C, eds. Nobel

Symposium 68: Mucosal Immunobiology. Monographs in Allergy. Basel, Karger, 1988, pp. 129–133.

Rogers HJ, Synge C. Bacteriostatic effect of human milk on *Escherichia coli*: The role of IgA. Immunology 34:19–28, 1978.

Romain N, Dandrifosse G, Jeusette F, Forget P. Polyamine concentration in rat milk and food, human milk, and infant formula. Pediatr Res 32:58–63, 1992.

Rossen RD, Alford RH, Butler WT, Vannier WE. The separation and characterization of proteins intrinsic to nasal secretion. J Immunol 97:369–378, 1966.

Rousset F, Gracia E, Banchereau J. Cytokine-induced proliferation and immunoglobulin production of human B lymphocytes triggered through their CD40 antigen. J Exp Med 173:705–710, 1991.

Roux ME, McWilliams M, Phillips-Quagliata JM, Weisz-Carrington P, Lamm ME. Origin of IgA-secreting plasma cells in the mammary gland. J Exp Med 146:1311–1322, 1977.

Rowland MGM, Cole TJ, Tully M, Dolby JM, Honow P. Bacteriostasis of *Escherichia coli* by milk: VI. The *in vitro* bacteriostatic property of Gambian mothers' breast milk in relation to the *in vivo* protection of their infants against diarrhoeal disease. J Hyg (Cambridge) 85:405–413, 1980.

Rudloff HE, Schmalstieg FC, Mushtaha AA, Palkowetz KH, Liu SK, Goldman AS. Tumor necrosis factor-α in human milk. Pediatr Res 31:23–33, 1992.

Rudloff HE, Schmalstieg FC, Palkowetz KH, Paszkiewicz EJ, Goldman AS. Interleukin-6 in human milk. J Reprod Immunol 23:13–20, 1993.

Russel-Jones GJ, Ey PL, Reynolds BL. The ability of IgA to inhibit complement consumption by complement-fixing antigens and antigen-antibody complexes. Aust J Exp Biol Med Sci 62:1–10, 1984.

Saarinen UM. Prolonged breast feeding as prophylaxis for recurrent otitis media. Acta Paediatr Scand 71:567–571, 1982.

Saito S, Maruyama M, Kato Y, Moriyama I, Ichijo M. Detection of IL-6 in human milk and its involvement in IgA production. J Reprod Immunol 20:267–276, 1991.

Sanguansermsri J, György P, Zilliken F. Polyamines in human and cow's milk. Am J Clin Nutr 59:859–870, 1974.

Savilathi E. Immunoglobulin-containing cells in the intestinal mucosa and immunoglobulins in the intestinal juice in children. Clin Exp Immunol 11:415–425, 1972.

Savilathi E. IgA deficiency in children: immunoglobulin-containing cells in the intestinal mucosa, immunoglobulins in secretions, and serum IgA levels. Clin Exp Immunol 13:395–406, 1973.

Schanler RL, Goldblum RM, Garza C, Goldman AS. Enhanced fecal excretion of selected immune factors in very low birth-weight infants fed fortified human milk. Pediatr Res 20:711–715, 1986.

Schieferdecker HL, Ullrich R, Weiss-Breckwoldt AN, Schwarting R, Stein H, Riecken EO, Zeitz M. The HML-1 antigen of intestinal lymphocytes is an activation antigen. J Immunol 144:2541–2549, 1990.

Schlesinger JJ, Covelli HD. Evidence for transmission of lymphocyte response to tuberculin by breast-feeding. Lancet 2:529–532, 1977.

Schroten J, Hanisch FF, Plogmann R, Hacker J, Uhlernbruch G, Nobis-Bosch R, Wahn V. Inhibition of adhesion of S-fimbriated *Escherichia coli* to buccal epithelial cells by human milk fat globule membrane components: a novel aspect of the protective function of mucins in the nonimmunoglobulin fraction. Pediatr Res 32:58–63, 1992.

Scott H, Rognum TO, Midtvedt T, Brandtzaeg P. Age-related changes of human serum antibodies to dietary and colonic bacterial antigens measured by an enzyme-linked immunosorbent assay. Acta Pathol Microbiol Immunol Scand 93:65–70, 1985.

Sewell HF, Matthews JB, Flack V, Jefferis R. Human immunoglobulin D in colostrum, saliva and amniotic fluid. Clin Exp Immunol 36:183–188, 1979.

Sharry JJ, Krasse B. Observations on the origins of salivary leukocytes. Acta Odontol Scand 18:347–358, 1960.

Shinmoto H, Kawakami H, Dosako S, Sogo Y. IgA specific helper factor (αHF) in human colostrum. Clin Exp Immunol 66:223–230, 1986.

Shvartzman YS, Agranovskaya EN, Zykov MP. Formation of secretory and circulating antibodies after immunization with live inactivated influenza virus vaccines. J Infect Dis 135:697–705, 1977.

Sirisinha S, Suskind R, Edelman R, Asvapaka C, Olson RE. Secretory and serum IgA in children with protein-calorie malnutrition. Pediatrics 55:166–170, 1975.

Sloyer JL, Cote CC, Howie VM, Ploussard JH, Johnston RB. The immune response to acute otitis media in children: II. Serum and middle ear fluid antibody in otitis media due to *Hemophilus influenzae*. J Infect Dis 132:685–688, 1975.

Smith DJ, Taubman MA, Ebersole JL. Salivary IgA antibody to glucosyltransferase in man. Clin Exp Immunol 61:416–424, 1985.

Smith HW, Goldman AS. The cells of human colostrum: I. *In vitro* studies of morphology and functions. Pediatr Res 2:103–109, 1968.

Söder O. Isolation of interleukin-1 from human milk. Int Arch Allergy Appl Immunol 83:19–23, 1987.

Söderström T, Lundberg A, Söderström R, Hanson LA. Characterization of fresh and Epstein-Barr virus transformed human colostral cells. Unpublished, 1988.

Sohl-Åkerlund A, Hanson LA, Ahlstedt S, Carlsson B. A sensitive method for specific quantitation of secretory IgA. Scand J Immunol 6:1275–1282, 1977.

South MA, Cooper MD, Wollheim FA, Hong R, Good RA. The IgA system: I. Studies of the transport and immunochemistry of IgA in the saliva. J Exp Med 123:615–627, 1966.

Spencer J, Dillon SB, Isaacson PG, MacDonald TT. T cell subclasses in fetal human ileum. Clin Exp Immunol 65:553–558, 1986a.

Spencer J, MacDonald TT, Finn TT, Isaacson PG. Development of gut associated lymphoid tissue in the terminal ileum of fetal human intestine. Clin Exp Immunol 64:536–543, 1986b.

Splawski JB, Woodard CS, Denney RM, Goldblum RM. Rapid development of polymeric IgA in the serum of infants. Clin Res 31:902A, 1984.

Stavnezer J, Radcliffe G, Lin YC, Nietupski J, Berggren L, Sitia R, Severinson E. Immunoglobulin heavy-chain switching may be directed by prior induction of transcripts from constant-region genes. Proc Natl Acad Sci USA 85:7704–7708, 1988.

Steinmetz KD, Kohl S, Richie ER. Separation of cytotoxic leucocyte populations of human peripheral blood and colostrum on PVP-silica (Percoll) density gradients. J Immunol Methods 42:157–170, 1981.

Stephens S, Kennedy CR, Lakhani PK, Brenner MK. *In-vivo* immune responses of breast- and bottle-fed infants to tetanus toxoid antigen and to normal gut flora. Acta Paediatr Scand 73:426–432, 1984.

Stintzing G, Zetterstrom R. Cow's milk allergy, incidence and pathogenetic role of early exposure to cow's milk formula. Acta Paediatr Scand 68:383–387, 1979.

Stock CC, Francis T Jr. The inactivation of the virus of epidemic influenza by soaps. J Exp Med 71:661–681, 1940.

Stokes CR, Miller BG, Bourne FJ. Animal models of food sensitivity. In Brostoff J, Challacombe SJ, eds. Food Allergy and Intolerance. Eastbourne, England, WB Saunders, 1987, pp. 286–300.

Stokes CR, Soothill JF, Turner MW. Immune exclusion is a function of IgA. Nature 255:745–746, 1975.

Streeter PR, Berg EL, Rouse BTN, Bargatze RF, Butcher EC. A tissue-specific endothelial cell molecule involved in lymphocyte homing. Nature 331:41–46, 1988.

Strober W, Ehrhardt RO. Regulation of IgA B cell development. In Ogra PL, Lamm ME, McGhee JR, Mestecky J, Strober W, Bienenstock J, eds. Handbook of Mucosal Immunology. San Diego, Academic Press, 1994, pp. 159–176.

Suzuki S, Lucas A, Coombs RRA. Immunoglobulin concentrations and bacterial antibody titres in breast milk from mothers of "preterm" and "term" infants. Acta Paediatr Scand 72:671–677, 1983.

Svanborg Edén C, Carlsson B, Hanson LA, Jann B, Jann K, Korhonen T, Wadström T. Anti-pili antibodies in breast milk. Lancet 2:1235, 1979.

Svanborg Edén C, Andersson B, Hagberg L, Leffler H, Magnusson G, Noori G, Dahmén J, Söderström T. Receptor analogues and anti-pili antibodies as inhibitors of bacterial attachment *in vivo* and *in vitro*. Ann N Y Acad Sci 409:580–591, 1983.

Svanborg Edén C, Briles D, Hagberg L, McGhee J, Michalec S. Genetic factors in host resistance to urinary tract infection. Infection 12:118–123, 1984.

Svanborg Edén C, Hanson L, Jodal U, Lindberg U, Sohl-Åkerlund A. Variable adherence to normal human urinary tract epithelial cells of *Escherichia coli* strains associated with various forms of urinary tract infection. Lancet 2:490–492, 1976.

Svanborg Edén C, Kulhavy R, Prince SJ, Mestecky J. Urinary immunoglobulins in healthy individuals and children with acute pyelonephritis. Scand J Immunol 21:305–313, 1985.

Svanborg Edén C. Bacterial adherence and mucosal immunity. In Ogra PL, Lamm ME, McGhee JR, Mestecky J, Strober W, Bienenstock J, eds. Handbook of Mucosal Immunology. San Diego, Academic Press, 1994, pp. 71–75.

Svanborg Edén C, Svennerholm AM. Secretory immunoglobulin A and G antibodies prevent adhesion of *Escherichia coli* to human urinary tract epithelial cells. Infect Immun 22:790–797, 1978.

Svennerholm AM, Hanson LA, Holmgren J, Lindblad BS, Nilsson B, Quereshi F. Different secretory IgA antibody response to cholera vaccination in Swedish and Pakistani women. Infect Immun 30:427–430, 1980.

Svennerholm AM, Holmgren J. Synergistic protective effect in rabbits of immunization with *Vibrio cholerae* lipopolysaccharide and toxin/toxoid. Infect Immun 13:735–740, 1976.

Svennerholm AM, Hanson LÅ, Holmgren L, Lindblad BS, Khan SR, Nilsson A, Svennerholm B. Milk antibodies to live and killed polio vaccines in Pakistani and Swedish mothers. J Infect Dis 143:707–711, 1981.

Svennerholm AM, Holmgren J, Hanson LA, Lindblad BS, Quereshi F, Rahimtoola RJ. Boosting of secretory IgA antibody responses in man by parenteral cholera vaccination. Scand J Immunol 6:1345–1349, 1977.

Svennerholm AM, Jertborn M, Gothefors L, Karim AMMM, Sack DA, Holmgren J. Mucosal antitoxic and antibacterial immunity after cholera disease and after immunization with a combined B subunit–whole cell vaccine. J Infect Dis 149:884–893, 1984.

Svennerholm AM, Lange S, Holmgren J. Correlation between synthesis of specific immunoglobulin A and protection against experimental cholera in mice. Infect Immun 21:1–6, 1978.

Tada T, Ishizaka K. Distribution of gamma E–forming cells in lymphoid tissues of the human and monkey. J Immunol 104:377–387, 1970.

Tagliabue A, Boraschi D, Villa L, Keren DF, Lowell GH, Rappuoli R, Nencioni L. IgA-dependent cell-mediated activity against enteropathogenic bacteria: distribution, specificity, and characterization of the effector cells. J Immunol 133:988–992, 1984.

Tagliabue A, Villa L, de Magistris TM, Romano M, Silvestri S, Boraschi D, Nencioni L. IgA-driven T cell–mediated anti-bacterial immunity in man after live oral Ty-21a vaccine. J Immunol 137:1504–1510, 1986.

Taguchi T, McGhee JR, Coffman RL, Beagley KW, Eldridge JH, Takatsu K, Kiyono H. Analysis of Th1 and Th2 cells in murine gut-associated tissues: frequencies of CD4+ and CD8+ T cells that secrete IFN-gamma and IL-5. J Immunol 145:68–75, 1990.

Takahashi M, Kanai N, Watanabe A, Oshima O, Ryan AF. Lymphocyte subsets in immune-mediated otitis media with effusion. Eur Arch Oto-Rhino-Laryngol 249:24–27, 1992.

Taylor HP, Dimmock NJ. Mechanism of neutralization of influenza virus by secretory IgA is different from that of monomeric IgA or IgG. J Exp Med 161:198–209, 1985.

Tenovuo J, Moldoveanu Z, Mestecky J, Pruitt KM, Rahemtulla BM. Interaction of specific and innate factors of immunity: IgA enhances the antimicrobial effect of the lactoperoxidase system against *Streptococcus mutans*. J Immunol 128:726–731, 1982.

Theodore CM, Losonsky G, Peri B, Fishaut M, Rothberg RM, Ogra PL. Immunologic aspects of colostrum and milk: Development of antibody response to respiratory syncytial virus and bovine serum albumin in the human and rabbit mammary gland. In Strober W, Hanson LA, Sell K, eds. Recent Advances in Mucosal Immunity. New York, Raven Press, 1982, pp. 393–403.

Thompson RAP, Asquith P, Cooke WT. Secretory IgA in serum. Lancet 2:517–519, 1969.

Thorpe LW, Rudloff HE, Powell LC, Goldman AS. Decreased response of human milk leucocytes to chemoattractant peptides. Pediatr Res 20:373–377, 1986.

Thrane PS, Rognum TO, Brandtzaeg P. Ontogenesis of the secretory immune system and innate defense factors in human parotid glands. Clin Exp Immunol 86:342–348, 1991.

Thromar H, Issacs CE, Brown HR, Barshatzky MR, Pessolano T. Inactivation of enveloped viruses and killing of cells by fatty acids and monoglycerides. J Am Soc Microbiol 32:27–31, 1987.

Timmermans FJW, Gerson S. Chronic granulomatous otitis media in bottle-fed Inuit children. Can Med Assoc J 122:545–547, 1980.

Tomasi TB Jr, Bienenstock J. Secretory immunoglobulins. Adv Immunol 9:1–96, 1968.

Tomasi TB Jr, Czerwinski DS. The secretory IgA system. In Bergsma D, Good RA, eds. Immunologic Deficiency Diseases in Man. Baltimore, Williams & Wilkins, 1968, pp. 270–275.

Tomasi TB Jr, Tan EM, Solomon A, Prendergast RA. Characteristics of an immune system common to certain external secretions. J Exp Med 121:101–124, 1965.

Tramont EC. Inhibition of adherence of *Neisseria gonorrhoeae* by human genital secretions. J Clin Invest 59:117–124, 1977.

Turesson I. Distribution of immunoglobulin-containing cells in human bone marrow and lymphoid tissues. Acta Med Scand 199:293–304, 1976.

Turner MW, McClelland DBL, Medlen AR, Stokes CR. IgE in human urine and milk. Scand J Immunol 6:343–348, 1977.

Uehling DT, Stiehm ER. Elevated urinary secretory IgA in children with urinary tract infection. Pediatrics 47:40–46, 1971.

Underdown BJ, DeRose J, Plaut A. Disulfide bonding of secretory component to a single monomer subunit in human secretory IgA. J Immunol 118:1816–1821, 1977.

Underdown BJ, Dorrington KJ. Studies on the structural and conformational basis for the relative resistance of serum and secretory immunoglobulin A to proteolysis. J Immunol 112:949–959, 1974.

Underdown BJ, Knight A, Papsin FR. The relative paucity of IgE in human milk. J Immunol 116:1435–1438, 1976.

Urban JF Jr, Katona IM, Paul WE, Finkelman FD. Interleukin 4 is important in protective immunity to a gastrointestinal nematode infection in mice. Proc Natl Acad Sci USA 88:5513–5517, 1991.

Vaerman JP, Lemaitre-Coelho I, Limet J, Delacroix DL. Hepatic transfer of polymeric IgA from plasma to bile in rats and other mammals: a survey. In Strober W, Hanson LA, Sell KW, eds. Recent Advances in Mucosal Immunity. New York, Raven Press, 1982, pp. 233–250.

Vahlqvist B. The transfer of antibodies from mother to offspring. Adv Pediatr 10:305–338, 1958.

Valnes K, Brandtzaeg P, Elgjo K, Stave R. Quantitative distribution of immunoglobulin-producing cells in gastric mucosa: relation to chronic gastritis and glandular atrophy. Gut 27:505–519, 1986.

van Epps DE, Williams RC. Suppression of leucocyte chemotaxis by human IgA myeloma components. J Exp Med 144:1227–1242, 1976.

Van Kerckhove C, Russell GJ, Deusch K, Reich K, Bhan AK, DerSimonian H, Brenner MB. Oligoclonality of human intestinal intraepithelial T cells. J Exp Med 175:57–63, 1992.

Vincent C, Revillard JP. Sandwich-type ELISA for free and bound secretory component in human biological fluids. J Immunol Methods 106:153–160, 1988.

Wadsworth C. A rapid spot immunoprecipitate assay method applied to quantitating C-reactive protein (CRP) in pediatric sera. Scand J Immunol 6:1263–1273, 1977.

Waissbluth JG, Langman JS. ABO blood group, secretor status, salivary protein, and serum and salivary immunoglobulin concentrations. Gut 12:646–649, 1971.

Wakatsuki Y, Strober W. Effect of down-regulation of germline transcripts on IgA isotype differentiation. J Exp Med 178:7, 1993.

Waldman RH, Bencic Z, Sinha R, Deb BC, Sakazaki R, Tamura K, Mukerjee S, Ganguly R. Cholera immunology: II. Serum and intestinal secretion antibody response after naturally occurring cholera. J Infect Dis 126:401–407, 1972.

Waldman RH, Ganguly R. Techniques for eliciting mucosal immune response. Acta Endocrinol 78(Suppl. 194):262–280, 1975a.

Waldman RH, Ganguly R. Cell-mediated immunity and the local immune system. In Neter E, Milgrom F, eds. The Immune System and Infectious Diseases. Basel, Karger, 1975b, pp. 334–346.

Waldman RH, Lee JD, Polly SM, Dorfman A, Fox EN. Group A streptococcal M protein vaccine: protection following immuniza-

tion via the respiratory tract. Develop Biol Standard 28:429–434, 1975c.

Waldman RH, Wigley FM, Small PA Jr. Specificity of respiratory secretion antibody against influenza virus. J Immunol 105:1477–1483, 1970.

Waldmann TA, Strober W. Metabolism of immunoglobulins. Progr Allergy 13:1–110, 1969.

Walker WA, Isselbacher KJ, Bloch KJ. Intestinal uptake of macromolecules: effect of oral immunization. Science 177:608–610, 1972.

Walker WA, Isselbacher KJ, Bloch KJ. Immunologic control of soluble protein absorption from the small intestine: a gut-surface phenomenon. Am J Clin Nutr 27:1434–1440, 1974.

Walker WA, Lake AM, Bloch KJ. Immunologic mechanisms for goblet cell mucous release: possible role in mucosal host defense. In Strober W, Hanson LA, Sell KW, eds. Recent Advances in Mucosal Immunity. New York, Raven Press, 1982, pp. 331–351.

Walker WA, Wu M, Isselbacher KJ, Bloch KJ. Intestinal uptake of macromolecules: III. Studies on the mechanisms by which immunization interferes with antigen uptake. J Immunol 115:854–861, 1975.

Watanabe N, Yoshimura H, Mogi G. Induction of antigen-specific IgA forming cells in the middle ear mucosa. Arch Otolaryngol Head Neck Surg 114:758–762, 1988.

Watanabe T, Nagura H, Watanabe K, Brown WR. The binding of human milk lactoferrin to immunoglobulin A. FEBS Lett 168:203–207, 1984.

Welliver RC. Respiratory infections. In Ogra PL, Lamm ME, McGhee JR, Mestecky J, Strober W, Bienenstock J, eds. Handbook of Mucosal Immunology. San Diego, Academic Press, 1994, pp. 551–559.

Welliver RC, Kaul A, Ogra PL. Cell mediated immune response to respiratory syncytial virus infection: relationship to the development of reactive airway disease. J Pediatr 94:370–519, 1979.

Welsh JK, Arsenakis M, Coelen RJ, May JT. Effect of antiviral lipids, heat, and freezing on the activity of viruses in human milk. J Infect Dis 140:332–338, 1979.

Weltzin R, Lucia-Jandris P, Michetti P, Fields BN, Kraehenbuhl JP, Neutra MR. Binding and transepithelial transport of immunoglobulins by intestinal M cells: demonstration using monoclonal IgA antibodies against enteric viral proteins. Cell Biol 108:1673–1685, 1989.

Wenzel RP, Mitzel JR, Davies JA, Edwards EA, Berling C, McCormick DP, Beam WE Jr. Antigenicity of a polysaccharide vaccine from *Neisseria meningitidis* administered intranasally. J Infect Dis 128:31–40, 1973.

Wiedermann U, Hanson LA, Holmgren J, Kahu H. Impaired mucosal antibody response to cholera toxin in vitamin A–deficient rats immunized with oral cholera vaccine. Infect Immun 61:3952–3957, 1993.

Williams RC, Gibbons RJ. Inhibition of bacterial adherence by secretory immunoglobulin A: a mechanism of antigen disposal. Science 177:697–699, 1972.

Winberg J, Wessner G. Does breast milk protect against septicemia in the newborn? Lancet 1:1091–1094, 1971.

Winner L, Mack J, Weltzin R, Mekalanos JJ, Kraehenbuhl JP, and Neutra MR. New model for analysis of mucosal immunity: intestinal secretion of specific monoclonal immunoglobulin A from hybridoma tumors protects against *Vibrio cholerae* infection. Infect Immun 59:977–982, 1991.

Wirt DP, Adkins LT, Palkowetz KH, Schmalstieg FC, Goldman AS. Activated-memory T lymphocytes in human milk. Cytometry 13:282–290, 1992.

Wold A, Mestecky J, Svanborg Edén C. Agglutination of *E. coli* by secretory IgA—a result of interaction between bacterial mannose-specific adhesins and immunoglobulin carbohydrate? In Hanson L, Svanborg Edén C, eds. Nobel Symposium 68: Mucosal Immunobiology. Monographs in Allergy. Basel, Karger, 1988, pp. 307–309.

Wolf HM, Fischer MB, Puhringer H, Samstag A, Vogel E, Eibl MM. Human serum IgA downregulates the release of inflammatory cytokines (tumor necrosis factor–alpha, interleukin-6) in human monocytes. Blood 83:1278–1288, 1994a.

Wolf HM, Vogel E, Fischer MB, Rengs H, Schwarz HP, Eibl MM.

Inhibition of receptor-dependent and receptor-independent generation of the respiratory burst in human neutrophils and monocytes by human serum IgA. Pediatr Res 36:235–243, 1994b.

Woodard CS, Splawski JB, Goldblum RM, Denney RM. Characterization of epitopes of human secretory component on free secretory component, secretory IgA, and membrane-associated secretory component. J Immunol 133:2116–2125, 1984.

Yolken RH, Peterson JA, Vonderfecht SL, Fouts ET, Midthun K, Newburg DS. Human milk mucin inhibits rotavirus replication and prevents experimental gastroenteritis. J Clin Invest 90:1984–1991, 1992.

Zeitz M, Green WC, Peffer NJ, James SP. Lymphocytes isolated from the intestinal lamina propria of normal non-human primates have increased expression of genes associated with T cell activation. Gastroenterology 94:647–655, 1988.

Zhang Z, Michael JG. Orally inducible immune unresponsiveness is abrogated by IFN–gamma treatment. J Immunol 144:4163–4165, 1990.

PART II

IMMUNODEFICIENCY DISORDERS

Chapter 9

Immunodeficiency Disorders: General Considerations

Mary Ellen Conley and E. Richard Stiehm

HISTORICAL ASPECTS

Primary immunodeficiency disorders, the naturally occurring defects of the immune system, were not identified until after the introduction of antibiotics, since morbidity and mortality from infection even in normal subjects was so high. Only after the "expectation of cure" of pneumonia, meningitis, cellulitis, and other severe infections with antibiotics could individuals be identified.

Nevertheless, several syndromes of immunodeficiency with characteristic clinical features were described before 1940, including mucocutaneous candidiasis by Thorpe and Handley in 1924, ataxia-telangiectasia by Syllaba and Henner in 1926, and Wiskott-Aldrich syndrome by Wiskott in 1937.

A patient with defective cellular immunity was initially described by Glanzmann and Riniker in 1950. In 1958 the combination of antibody deficiency with defective cellular immunity was identified in a Swiss infant, Swiss-type agammaglobulinemia (Hitzig et al., 1958).

Two years after Bruton's description of congenital agammaglobulinemia in 1952, acquired agammaglobulinemia (common variable immunodeficiency) in an adult was described in 1954 by Sanford and coworkers.

A phagocytic immunodeficiency was first described in 1957 as chronic granulomatous disease by Berendes and associates in 1957. A complement deficiency (C2 deficiency) was initially described in 1965 by Klemperer and associates.

EPIDEMIOLOGY

The immunodeficiency disorders are a diverse group of illnesses that, as a result of one or more abnormalities of the immune system, increase susceptibility to infection. Although the possibility of an immunodeficiency should be considered in any individual with "too many" infections, these are relatively uncommon disorders and it is thus important to consider other conditions that lead to infection (Table 9–1). A consideration of nonimmunologic causes of recurrent infection is beyond the scope of this volume; most of these

conditions can be readily suspected after a careful history and physical examination and can be confirmed by appropriate laboratory tests.

When there is no apparent explanation for the recurrent infections, a primary defect in host defense must be considered. The primary immunodeficiencies generally are congenital and hereditary, so that most of the affected patients are infants or children. The following represents a typical case.

A CASE REPORT

A boy, 8 years old, was well until the age of 4 years, when pneumonia with rubeola developed. The birth, developmental history, and family history were normal; a male sibling was well. At age 4½ years, the patient experienced chills, fever, and pain in the left knee. Physical examination was unremarkable except for a few petechiae on the arms and tenderness of the knee. The white blood cell (WBC) count was 16,400/mm³ with 88% neutrophils; blood culture findings were normal. The pain and fever disappeared with administration of penicillin.

Two weeks later, fever recurred; pneumonia was diagnosed, and sulfadiazine was given. Four days later, mumps and gastroenteritis developed, and the boy was admitted to the hospital. He experienced a prolonged febrile course, complicated by recurrent otitis. The throat, blood, and ear cultures were positive for type XIV pneumococcal infection.

After being treated with penicillin for 10 days, the boy improved. Otitis media developed 2 months later. Two days after antibiotics were discontinued for an ear infection, fever and left shoulder pain developed. The WBC count was 25,000/mm³ with 91% neutrophils. Antibiotics were again administered. Six months later, fever recurred, and type XXXIII pneumococci were recovered from the blood stream.

After recovery, a tonsillectomy and adenoidectomy were performed in the hope of decreasing the number of infections. During the next 4 years, however, the patient experienced 15 episodes of high fever resulting from sepsis; on seven occasions, pneumococci specimens from the blood were obtained for culture. He also had two episodes of pneumonia, three episodes of otitis, and two episodes of mumps. Prophylactic sulfadiazine and pneumococcal vaccine were ineffective in controlling the infections.

This is the first recorded case of agammaglobulinemia (Bruton, 1952); it demonstrates many of the major characteristics of this disorder, including male sex, early onset, recurrent major pyogenic infection, and ineffectiveness of most forms of therapy. The study of antibody immunodeficiencies in pediatric patients and hypergammaglobulinemic states in adults (e.g., multiple myeloma) first served to stimulate the specialty of clinical immunology.

Since Bruton's description of agammaglobulinemia, about 50 primary immunodeficiencies have been delineated. This chapter describes these disorders, a classification, some etiologic mechanisms, the laboratory diagnosis, general approaches to treatment, and prognosis.

Table 9–1. Disorders With Increased Susceptibility to Infection and Examples

Type of Disorder	Examples
Circulatory disorders	Sickle cell disease, diabetes, nephrosis, congenital cardiac defect
Obstructive disorders	Ureteral or urethral stenosis, bronchial asthma, allergic rhinitis, blocked eustachian tube, cystic fibrosis, foreign body
Integumental defects	Eczema, burn, skull fracture, midline sinus tract, ciliary abnormalities
Unusual microbiologic factors	Antibiotic overgrowth, chronic infections with resistant organism, continuous reinfection (contaminated water supply, infectious contact, contaminated inhalation therapy equipment)
Foreign bodies	Ventricular shunt, central venous catheter, artificial heart valve, urinary catheter, aspirated foreign body
Secondary immunodeficiencies	Malnutrition, prematurity, lymphoma, splenectomy, uremia, immunosuppressive therapy, protein-losing enteropathy
Primary immunodeficiencies	X-linked agammaglobulinemia, DiGeorge anomaly, chronic granulomatous disease, C3 deficiency

Other reviews are available (Hong, 1990; Buckley, 1972, 1992; Iseki and Heiner, 1993).

Classification

The immune system is conveniently divisible into distinct classifications:

- B-lymphocyte (antibody) system
- T-lymphocyte (cellular immune) system
- Phagocytic (polymorphonuclear and mononuclear) system
- Complement (opsonic) system

This division provides the easiest and most common way to classify the immunodeficiencies and is used here.

The World Health Organization Expert Committee (Rosen et al., 1995) has used a more complicated scheme to classify the primary immunodeficiencies (Table 9–2). This takes into account the frequent interactions of the B-cell and T-cell systems and the multiple variants of several syndromes. The inheritance patterns of the illnesses are also shown. Several immunodeficiency syndromes omitted from this classification are also considered in this book.

The approximate relative frequency of the immunodeficiencies is shown in Figure 9–1. This figure combines the Japanese experience (Hayakawa et al., 1981), the Swiss experience (Ryser et al., 1988), and our own experience; it excludes asymptomatic selective IgA deficiency, which is more common than all the others combined. The antibody deficiencies constitute about 50% of all cases of primary immunodeficiencies (see Chapter 11). They include disorders in which immunoregulatory T-cell abnormalities are present (e.g., immunodeficiency with hyper-IgM) but in which the major defect is poor antibody function.

Separate chapters are devoted to disorders of IgA (see Chapter 14) and IgE (see Chapter 13). IgA abnormalities, including selective IgA deficiency, are common, heterogeneous, and immunologically unique and justify separate coverage. Similarly, the IgE disorders

are distinct, with many associated immunologic abnormalities and unique therapeutic approaches.

T-cell (cellular) immunodeficiencies compose the next largest group, making up about 30% of total primary immunodeficiencies (see Chapter 12). Two thirds (20% of the total) of these patients have associated B-cell (antibody) deficiencies, termed *combined immunodeficiencies.* Many combined immunodeficiencies exhibit clinical features that constitute a distinct syndrome (e.g., ataxia-telangiectasia, Wiskott-Aldrich syndrome) or are associated with thymic hypoplasia or dysplasia.

Phagocytic immunodeficiencies, about 18% of the total, involve the polymorphonuclear phagocytic system (see Chapter 15), the mononuclear phagocytic (monocyte/macrophage) system (see Chapter 16), or both. Defects of locomotion, phagocytosis, and intracellular killing are recognized. Primary disorders of the complement system are unusual and make up only 2 to 5% of immunodeficiencies (see Chapter 17).

Two other groups of immunodeficiencies are considered in this section. Immunodeficiency as a result of immaturity affects many components of the immune system and leads to a high incidence of infection in early life, particularly in the premature. The immunodeficiencies of immaturity, considered separately in Chapter 10, are of particular importance to pediatricians. The secondary immunodeficiencies (see Chapter 19) result when there is interference with immune function as a result of other illness, injury, or treatment (Table 9–3). These are quite common; indeed, nearly every serious illness interferes with the immune system to some degree. These illnesses can affect one or more components of the immune system. An increasing cause of secondary immunodeficiency relevant to children in the United States is human immunodeficiency virus (HIV) infection. Because of this infection, an entire chapter is devoted to pediatric acquired immunodeficiency syndrome (AIDS) and HIV infection (see Chapter 18).

Terminology

The names of the immunodeficiencies were initially based on place of discovery, name of discoverer, immunoglobulin patterns, or possible pathogenic mechanisms. In addition, several names were applied to the same disorder, leading to considerable confusion and ambiguity. The terminology for the primary immunodeficiencies, continuously being recodified by the World Health Organization (Fudenberg et al., 1971; Rosen et al., 1983, 1984, 1986, 1992, 1995), is used in this book. It minimizes eponyms, designation of country, numbers based on immunoglobulin pattern, and hypothetical pathogenic mechanisms; it stresses the mode of genetic transmission and distinctive features. Thus, Bruton's agammaglobulinemia is renamed *X-linked agammaglobulinemia.* Because certain eponyms are well established (such as Swiss-type agammaglobulinemia for severe "combined immunodeficiency disease" [SCID]), they also are provided.

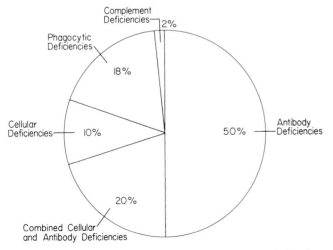

Figure 9–1. Relative distribution of the primary immunodeficiencies.

Table 9–2. 1995 WHO Classification of Primary and Secondary Immunodeficiencies

Groups	Inheritance*	Groups	Inheritance*
A. *Predominantly Antibody Deficiencies*		F. *Complement Deficiencies* Continued	
1. X-linked agammaglobulinemia	XL	38. C6 deficiency	AR
2. Hyper-IgM syndrome		39. C7 deficiency	AR
a. X-linked	XL	40. C8α + C8γ deficiency	AR
b. Other	AR, unknown	41. C8β deficiency	AR
3. Ig heavy-chain gene deletions	AR	42. C9 deficiency	AR
4. κ-chain deficiency	AR	43. C1 inhibitor deficiency	AD
5. Selective deficiency of IgG subclasses (with or without IgA deficiency)	Unknown	44. Factor I deficiency	AR
		45. Factor H deficiency	AR
		46. Factor D deficiency	
6. Antibody deficiency with normal Igs	Unknown	47. Properdin deficiency	XL
7. Common variable immunodeficiency	Various: AR, AD, or unknown	G. *Immunodeficiency Associated With or Secondary to Other Diseases*	
8. IgA deficiency	Various: AR, unknown	CHROMOSOMAL INSTABILITY OR DEFECTIVE REPAIR	
9. Transient hypogammaglobulinemia of infancy	Unknown	48. Bloom syndrome	
		49. Fanconi anemia	
B. *Combined Immunodeficiencies*		50. ICF syndrome	
10. Severe combined immunodeficiency (SCID)		51. Nijmegen breakage syndrome	
		52. Seckel syndrome	
a. X-linked	XL	53. Xeroderma syndrome	
b. Autosomal recessive	AR	CHROMOSOMAL DEFECTS	
11. Adenosine deaminase (ADA) deficiency	AR	54. Down syndrome	
12. Purine nucleoside phosphorylase (PNP) deficiency	AR	55. Turner syndrome	
		56. Chromosome 18 rings and deletions	
13. MHC class II deficiency	AR	SKELETAL ABNORMALITIES	
14. Reticular dysgenesis	AR	57. Short-limbed skeletal dysplasia	
15. CD3γ or CD3ε deficiency	AR	58. Cartilage-hair hypoplasia	
16. CD8 deficiency	AR	IMMUNODEFICIENCY WITH GENERALIZED GROWTH RETARDATION	
C. *Other Well-Defined Immunodeficiency Syndromes*		59. Schimke immuno-osseous dysplasia	
17. Wiskott-Aldrich syndrome	XL	60. Immunodeficiency with absent thumbs	
18. Ataxia-telangiectasia	AR	61. Dubowitz syndrome	
19. DiGeorge anomaly	Unknown	62. Growth retardation, facial anomalies, and immunodeficiency	
D. *Other Primary Immunodeficiency Diseases*		63. Progeria (Hutchinson-Gilford syndrome)	
20. Primary CD4 deficiency		IMMUNODEFICIENCY WITH DERMATOLOGIC DEFECTS	
21. Primary CD7 deficiency		64. Partial albinism	
22. IL-2 deficiency		65. Dyskeratosis congenita	
23. Multiple cytokine deficiency		66. Netherton syndrome	
24. Signal transduction deficiency		67. Acrodermatitis enteropathica	
E. *Defects of Phagocytic Function*		68. Anhidrotic ectodermal dysplasia	
25. Chronic granulomatous disease (CGD)		69. Papillon-Lefèvre syndrome	
a. X-linked CGD (deficiency of 91 kD binding chain of cytochrome b)	XL	HEREDITARY METABOLIC DEFECTS	
b. Autosomal recessive CGD	AR	70. Transcobalamin 2 deficiency	
(1) p22 phox		71. Methylmalonic acidemia	
(2) p47 phox		72. Type 1 hereditary orotic aciduria	
(3) p67 phox		73. Biotin-dependent carboxylase deficiency	
26. Leukocyte adhesion defect (deficiency of β chain (CD18) of LFA-1, Mac-1, p150,95)	AR	74. Mannosidosis	
		75. Glycogen storage disease, type 1b	
27. Leukocyte adhesion defect 2 (failure to convert GDP mannose to fucose)		76. Chédiak-Higashi syndrome	
28. Neutrophil G6PD deficiency	XL	HYPERCATABOLISM OF IMMUNOGLOBULIN	
29. Myeloperoxidase deficiency	AR	77. Familial hypercatabolism	
30. Secondary granule deficiency	AR	78. Intestinal lymphangiectasia	
31. Shwachman syndrome	AR	OTHER	
F. *Complement Deficiencies*		79. Hyper-IgE syndrome	
32. C1q deficiency	AR	80. Chronic mucocutaneous candidiasis	
33. C1r deficiency	AR	81. Hereditary or congenital hyposplenia or asplenia	
34. C4 deficiency	AR		
35. C2 deficiency	AR	82. Ivermark syndrome	
36. C3 deficiency	AR		
37. C5 deficiency	AR		

Abbreviations: AD = autosomal dominant; AR = autosomal recessive; GDP = guanosine diphosphate; G6DP = glucose 6-phosphate dehydrogenase; LFA = leukocyte function associated antigen; Mac = macrophage; phox = phagocyte oxidase; XL = X-linked.

Modified from Rosen FS, Wedgwood RJ, Eibl M, et al. Primary immunodeficiency diseases: report of a WHO Scientific Group. Clin Exp Immunol 1(Suppl. 99):1–24, 1995.

Table 9–3. Factors Associated With Secondary Immunodeficiency

Premature and Newborn
Hereditary and Metabolic Diseases
　Chromosomal abnormalities (Down syndrome, others)
　Uremia
　Diabetes mellitus
　Malnutrition
　Vitamin and mineral deficiencies
　Protein-losing enteropathies
　Nephrotic dystrophy
　Myotonic dystrophy
　Sickle cell disease

Immunosuppressive Agents
　Radiation
　Immunosuppressive drugs
　Corticosteroids
　Antilymphocyte or antithymocyte globulin
　Anti–T cell monoclonal antibodies

Infectious Diseases
　Congenital rubella
　Viral exanthems—measles, varicella
　HIV infection, AIDS
　Cytomegalovirus
　Infectious mononucleosis
　Bacterial infections
　Mycobacterial, fungal, or parasitic disease

Infiltrative and Hematologic Diseases
　Histiocytosis
　Sarcoidosis
　Hodgkin's disease and lymphoma
　Leukemia
　Myeloma
　Agranulocytosis and aplastic anemia
　Lymphoma in immunocompromised transplant recipients

Surgery and Trauma
　Burns
　Splenectomy
　Anesthesia
　Head injury

Miscellaneous
　Lupus erythematosus
　Chronic active hepatitis
　Alcoholic cirrhosis
　Aging

Incidence

Since 1952, more than 2000 cases of primary immunodeficiency have been reported; many more have remained undiagnosed or unreported. Recognition of these disorders is increasing because of the wider availability of immunologic laboratory tests throughout the community, the increasing ability of physicians to recognize the disorders, and the description of new syndromes heretofore unrecognized. Since the last edition of this book (1988), several new primary immunodeficiencies have been delineated (e.g., interleukin-2 [IL-2] deficiency, signal transduction defects), and many others have been subdivided into biochemical or genetic variants (e.g., multiple variants of chronic granulomatous disease).

The incidence of primary immunodeficiency was first estimated to be about one case per 100,000 population, based on a 1969 report of the Medical Research Council Working Party from the United Kingdom. Because this report did not include cases of cellular immunode-

ficiency and used strict criteria for diagnosis (an IgG level less than 200 mg/dl), this is a minimal figure. More recent studies from Japan (Hayakawa et al., 1981) and Australia (Roberton et al., 1983; Hosking and Roberton, 1983) suggest that the incidence is closer to one per 10,000, excluding asymptomatic IgA deficiency (which occurs at a rate of 20 per 10,000). The incidence of some specific disorders in the Australian study includes X-linked agammaglobulinemia—1:103,000; the DiGeorge anomaly—1:66,000; severe combined immunodeficiency—1:66,000; common variable immunodeficiency—1:83,000, chronic mucocutaneous candidiasis—1:103,000, and chronic granulomatous disease—1:181,000. These figures agree with the prevalence of congenital and acquired hypogammaglobulinemia in Northern Ireland reported by McCluskey and Boyd (1991). There were 12 patients with congenital agammaglobulinemia (11 cases were X-linked), and 11 patients with acquired agammaglobulinemia in this extremely stable population of 1.5 million.

The overall 1:10,000 incidence of primary immunodeficiency is one-fourth that of cystic fibrosis (1:2500), one-half that of congenital hypothyroidism (1:5000), and somewhat more common than phenylketonuria (1:14,000). Regional differences based on differing populations and environmental factors affect the relative incidence of each disorder. This can be appreciated by comparison of the immunodeficiency registries of four countries (Table 9–4).

According to these figures, there are about 400 new cases of primary immunodeficiency in children born annually in the United States (4.0 million live births) and somewhere between 5000 and 10,000 total cases (assuming a shortened life span). Such calculations are of particular value when the frequency of undiagnosed immunodeficiency in patients receiving potentially fatal live virus vaccines is determined, when the need for bone marrow transplant facilities is calculated, or when the need for intravenous immunoglobulin administration is estimated.

Among hospitalized patients, the frequency of immunodeficiency is considerably higher. Hobbs (1966) noted that 138 of 6000 patients (2.3%) admitted to a general hospital in the United Kingdom demonstrated total γ-globulin levels lower than 400 mg/dl. Only 20 of 6000 (0.3%) had a primary immunodeficiency. The remaining patients had hypogammaglobulinemia of immaturity (20 patients) or secondary hypogammaglobulinemia (98 patients). Other secondary immunodeficiencies, mostly those affecting cellular immunity, are also common among hospitalized patients.

In the outpatient setting, patients with less severe immunodeficiency syndromes are identified. Palma-Carlos and Palma-Carlos (1991) identified 37 primary immunodeficiencies in 5100 outpatients followed in an allergy and clinical immunology clinic (0.74%), including 27 patients with selective IgA deficiency.

Age and Sex

The age of onset, based on the time of diagnosis, can be estimated from British studies (Medical Research

Table 9–4. Comparison of Frequency of Major Antibody and Cellular Immunodeficiencies in
Four Different Countries*

Diagnosis	Italy		Japan		Switzerland		Sweden	
	Total	%	Total	%	Total	%	Total	%
X-linked agammaglobulinemia	33	4.7	72	13.7	15	6.3	12	8.0
IgA deficiency	354	50.1	80	15.2	79	32.2	75	5.0
Common variable immunodeficiency	117	16.6	111	21.1	49	20.4	19	12.7
Combined immunodeficiency (all types)	113	14.6	60	11.2	31	13.0	17	11.4
Wiskott-Aldrich syndrome	14	2.0	46	8.8	14	5.8	8	5.3
Ataxia-telangiectasia	50	7.1	58	11.0	4	1.7	8	5.3
DiGeorge anomaly	8	1.1	36	6.9	6	2.5	5	5.3
Total specific immunodeficiencies	706		525		123		150	
Population of country	55×10^6		111×10^6		6.6×10^6		8.3×10^6	
Overall frequency	1 in 77,000		1 in 200,000		1 in 54,000		1 in 55,000	

*Excludes phagocytic and complement immunodeficiencies, IgG subclass deficiencies, and mucocutaneous candidiasis.
Data from Ryser O, Morell A, Hitzig WH. Primary immunodeficiencies in Switzerland: first report of the national registry in adults and children. J Clin Immunol 8:479–485, 1988.

Council, 1969), Japanese studies (Hayakawa et al., 1981), and the Swiss Registry (Ryser et al, 1988). This, of course, varies from illness to illness. Overall, however, about 40% of cases are diagnosed in the first year, another 40% by age 5 years, another 15% by age 16, and only 5% in adulthood. About 10% of registered cases are adults, and the diagnosis was established before age 16 in most of these cases. Most of the new late-onset patients exhibit common variable immunodeficiency.

In the Japanese study, 72% of the cases occurred in males, 28% in females. The only immunodeficiency that was more common in females was chronic mucocutaneous candidiasis (7 of 11 were female). In the British study, 62% of cases occurred in males; in children under age 12 months, 82% occurred in males. In all affected children under the age of 15 years, 83% were males. In adults, the sex difference is lost; indeed, 60% of the adults in Britain were female. This is due to the frequent occurrence of late-onset common variable immunodeficiency in females. In the Swiss registry (Ryser et al, 1988), males represented 63% of all cases and 68% of pediatric cases.

There is a family history of a similar deficiency in about 25% of patients with immunodeficiency. This is more common in affected males (33%) than in females (5.5%). These age and sex differences are largely accounted for by the many boys with X-linked immunodeficiencies with early-onset disease.

ETIOLOGY

Immunodeficiencies are a heterogeneous group of disorders that include both systemic defects and defects limited to a single protein produced by a specific cell lineage (Table 9–5). When confronting a spectrum of clinical and laboratory abnormalities of the immune system, one may sometimes find it difficult to distinguish primary and secondary defects. In addition, primary defects are often accompanied by secondary defects. For example, patients with a primary B-cell defect, X-linked agammaglobulinemia, may secondarily have T-cell or monocyte populations that suppress immunoglobulin production by normal B cells (Krantman et al., 1981; Rozynska et al., 1989). Attempts to determine the cause of a specific defect are further complicated by the fact that the same panorama of clinical and laboratory findings may be the result of different gene defects or a different constellation of factors. As an example, IgA deficiency can be attributed to many factors (see Chapter 14). In contrast, different mutations of the same gene—for example, the gene for adenosine deaminase (ADA)—can cause disease of widely varying severity (Hirschhorn, 1990).

In the past, attempts to determine the causes of immunodeficiencies first led to grouping them ac-

Table 9–5. Pathogenesis of Immunodeficiency and
Examples

Genetic Defects
Single-gene defects expressed in multiple tissues (e.g., ataxia-telangiectasia; adenosine deaminase deficiency)
Single-gene defects specific to the immune system (e.g., tyrosine kinase defect in X-linked agammaglobulinemia; ε chain of TCR abnormality)
Multifactorial disorders with genetic susceptibility (e.g., common variable immunodeficiency)

Drugs or Toxins
Immunosuppressives (e.g., corticosteroids, cyclosporine)
Anticonvulsants (e.g., phenytoin [Dilantin])

Nutritional and Metabolic Disorders
Malnutrition (e.g., kwashiorkor)
Protein-losing enteropathy (e.g., intestinal lymphangiectasia)
Vitamin deficiency (e.g., biotin or transcobalamin II deficiency)
Mineral deficiency (e.g., zinc deficiency in acrodermatitis enteropathica)

Infection
Transient immunodeficiency (e.g., varicella, rubeola)
Permanent immunodeficiency (e.g., HIV infection, congenital rubella)

Chromosome Abnormalities
DiGeorge anomaly (e.g., deletion of 22q11)
Selective IgA deficiency (e.g., trisomy 18)

Abbreviation: TCR = T-cell antigen receptor.

cording to whether they affected T cells, B cells, phagocytes, or complement and then to making subgroups dependent on the point in differentiation at which the abnormality could first be demonstrated. This system is useful clinically, but it has its drawbacks. Many immunodeficiencies do not easily fit into this scheme, and the designations can be misleading. For example, X-linked hyper-IgM syndrome results in antibody deficiency, but the defective gene, which encodes the ligand for CD40, is expressed by activated T cells (Allen et al., 1993).

There has been an increasing emphasis on examining disorders from the point of view of defects in cell biology—for example, deoxyribonucleic acid (DNA) replication, signal transduction, or cell adhesion. This shift can be attributed to the rapid progress in understanding the processes involved in normal cell development and in the identification of several of the genes responsible for specific immunodeficiencies. As more genes involved in immunodeficiencies are identified, it will become increasingly important to make accurate genetic diagnoses to permit informative genetic counseling and to design appropriate therapy.

Single Gene Defects of the Immune System

Several primary immunodeficiencies are associated with abnormal genes localized to certain regions of specific chromosomes (Table 9–6). Single gene defects of the immune system can be divided into those that are expressed in multiple tissues and those that are specific to the immune system. Examples of the former include ataxia-telangiectasia, in which there is defective recognition or repair of DNA damage (Kastan et al., 1992), and defects in the enzymes adenosine deam-

Table 9–6. Chromosome Locations of Abnormal Genes of Some Primary Immunodeficiencies

	Gene Location
X-linked (XL) Disorders	
XL chronic granulomatous disease (gp91 phox)*	Xp21 (56%)†
Wiskott-Aldrich syndrome (WASP)	Xp11
Properdin deficiency	Xp21
XL severe combined immunodeficiency (IL-2Rγ)	Xq13
XL agammaglobulinemia (Btk)	Xq22
XL lymphoproliferative syndrome	Xq25
XL hyper-IgM syndrome (CD40 ligand)	Xq27
Autosomal Recessive (AR) Disorders	
AR chronic granulomatous disease	
p22-phox	16q24 (6%)†
p47-phox	7q11.23 (33%)†
p67-phox	1q25 (5%)†
Adenosine deaminase deficiency	20q13.11
Purine nucleoside phosphorylase deficiency	14q13.1
Ataxia-telangiectasia (ATM)	11q22-23 (97%)†
Leukocyte adhesion defect type 1 (CD18)	21q22.3
HLA class II deficiency (CIITA)	16q
Other Disorders	
C1 esterase deficiency	11q11
DiGeorge anomaly	22q11.2 (90%)†
Immunoglobulin heavy-chain deletion	14q32.3
κ-chain deficiency	2p11

*Genetic abnormality.
†Percent of patients with abnormal gene.
Abbreviations: ATM = ataxia-telangiectasia mutated; Btk = Bruton's tyrosine kinase; phox = phagocytic oxidase; WASP = Wiskott-Aldrich syndrome protein.

inase or purine nucleoside phosphorylase. Because lymphocytes must undergo rapid DNA replication, associated with extensive proliferation, and DNA rearrangement to produce functional antigen receptor genes, it is not surprising that they are exquisitely sensitive to derangements in DNA metabolism. Other metabolic defects that may result in immunodeficiency include biotinidase deficiency (Hurvitz et al., 1989), biotin-dependent carboxylase deficiency (Cowan et al., 1979), and transcobalamin II deficiency (Kaikov et al., 1991).

Defects specific to the immune system may affect specialized functions of the immune system. These include defects in production of complement components, abnormalities of superoxide production (as seen in chronic granulomatous disease), and defects in antigen receptor gene rearrangements, as seen in one variant of severe combined immunodeficiency (SCID) (Schwarz et al., 1991). Some defects relate to genes required for growth, development, or regulation of lymphocytes. X-linked agammaglobulinemia results from a defective tyrosine kinase that is required for normal B-cell development (Tsukada et al., 1993). Defects in cytokines and their receptors result in decreased number or function of lymphocytes. Because immune cells must circulate and home to appropriate targets, defects of adhesion or recognition cause immunodeficiency. Leukocyte adhesion defect–1 and the bare lymphocyte syndrome are examples of these defects.

Multigene Defects of the Immune System

Several primary immunodeficiencies do not follow a single specific pattern of inheritance but are clearly influenced by genetic factors. In the families of patients with common variable immunodeficiency, there is an increased incidence of IgA deficiency and autoimmune disorders (Cunningham-Rundles, 1989). Studies from several laboratories have demonstrated that patients with either common variable immunodeficiency or IgA deficiency are more likely to have certain unusual human leukocyte antigen (HLA) haplotypes (Schaffer et al., 1989; Olerup et al., 1990). These haplotypes appear to function as susceptibility genes. Not every member of a family who inherits the haplotype associated with risk will go on to have an immunodeficiency. This suggests that additional genetic or environmental factors must be present to cause immunodeficiency.

Other disorders that may occur in more than one member of a family, but not according to a consistent pattern of inheritance, are chronic mucocutaneous candidiasis (Herrod, 1990) and hyper-IgE syndrome. The lack of a consistent pattern of inheritance suggests that the disorder is the result of either several different genetic defects, each of which has its own pattern of inheritance, or several susceptibility genes acting together.

Drugs, Toxins, and Nutrient Deficiency

Certain immunodeficiencies may result from exposure to a toxin or drug. The ingestion of phenytoin

(Dilantin) or one of several other anticonvulsant drugs can be associated with selective IgA deficiency or hypogammaglobulinemia (Ruff et al., 1987; Ishizaka et al., 1992). Maternal alcohol consumption during pregnancy has been associated with some cases of DiGeorge anomaly (Ammann et al., 1982b); indeed, in most children with fetal alcohol syndrome, T-cell function is depressed (Johnson et al., 1981).

A lack of vitamins, minerals, calories, or protein may adversely affect the immune system and may be responsible for an immune defect. Zinc deficiency has been associated with acrodermatitis enteropathica, which in turn has been associated with combined immunodeficiency. Vitamin B_{12} deficiency, as a result of transcobalamin II deficiency, may lead to hypogammaglobulinemia (Kaikov et al., 1991). Severe protein-calorie malnutrition leads to a profound but reversible T-cell immunodeficiency. Intrauterine malnutrition secondary to placental insufficiency may result in permanent cellular immunodeficiency (Chandra, 1975).

Infection

Infectious agents can cause or exacerbate immunodeficiency. It is now well recognized that the cause of AIDS is infection with a retrovirus, HIV-1. Congenital rubella infection is associated with a variety of immunodeficiency syndromes, including IgA deficiency and hyper-IgM syndrome. Both congenital rubella and HIV infection can result in permanent immunodeficiency. Infection with other microorganisms, including varicella and rubeola, can cause a transient increased susceptibility to infection.

Chromosomal Abnormalities

Chromosomal abnormalities are noted in several immunodeficiencies. Deletions in the long arm of chromosome 22 and other deletions and translocations are seen in a high proportion of patients with the DiGeorge anomaly (Driscoll et al., 1992, Greenberg et al., 1986). Defects in chromosome 18 are sometimes associated with IgA deficiency (see Chapter 14). Chromosomal breakage syndromes, including ataxia-telangiectasia and Nijmegen breakage syndrome, are associated with hypogammaglobulinemia and T-cell abnormalities (Taalman et al., 1989).

CLINICAL GENETICS

Genetic Counseling

Because many primary immunodeficiencies are single or multiple gene defects, complete care for an affected child should include genetic counseling, not only for the child's parents but also for siblings and the extended family. It may be helpful to refer the family to a genetic counselor who has experience in providing complex information in an unbiased and easily understood manner. However, it is also important to confirm the diagnosis using the most specific and accurate technology possible. Genetic counseling based on an incorrect diagnosis is misleading.

Shortly after the patient is diagnosed as having a particular primary immunodeficiency, the pattern of inheritance should be described to the family and the potential for carrier detection and prenatal diagnosis can be discussed. The patient's siblings should be screened to ensure that they do not have the same disorder. In families with X-linked or autosomal dominant disorders, it is wise to discuss genetic risks again when the patient or the siblings reach reproductive age.

Genetic counseling issues vary, depending on the mode of inheritance of the immunodeficiency. In families who carry an autosomal recessive gene defect, such as adenosine deaminase deficiency, ataxia-telangiectasia, or C3 deficiency, the major concern is prenatal diagnosis for the parents' future children. All of the autosomal recessive immunodeficiencies are sufficiently rare that one would not expect the patient or the patient's siblings to be at risk of having affected children. Although it is often possible to determine which family members are heterozygous for the autosomal recessive disorders, it is usually not clinically important. The issues are somewhat different in families with X-linked immunodeficiencies. Because the sisters, cousins, and aunts of boys with X-linked immunodeficiencies are at risk of having affected children, carrier detection as well as prenatal diagnosis is a concern for these families.

In other immunodeficiencies that follow less clearly defined patterns of inheritance, genetic issues should also be addressed. DiGeorge anomaly is associated with a high incidence of chromosomal defects, particularly partial monosomy of chromosome 22 (Driscoll et al., 1992). Most cases are sporadic, but in occasional families one of the parents carries a balanced translocation or another silent defect. Thus, it is important to screen all patients with the DiGeorge anomaly for chromosomal defects. If abnormalities are found, the parents and siblings should be studied. Hyper-IgE syndrome can follow both autosomal recessive and autosomal dominant patterns of inheritance, making it difficult to provide genetic counseling for affected families. Family members of patients with common variable immunodeficiency and IgA deficiency have an increased risk of antibody deficiencies and autoimmune disorders, although data are insufficient to document the exact risk.

Approximately 25% to 35% of patients seen in an immunodeficiency clinic have clearly demonstrated abnormalities of the immune system that do not fall into any well-described syndrome. These patients may have disorders that are secondary to in utero infection or a toxic exposure, or they may have genetic disorders that have not previously been described. It is reasonable to assume that the parents of these children do have a risk of having another similarly affected child, although the risk is probably less than 25%.

Prenatal Diagnosis

A variety of approaches can be used to provide prenatal diagnosis (Table 9–7). The technology of genetic

Table 9–7. Techniques Used in Prenatal Diagnosis

Approaches	Indication (Example)
Immunologic studies on fetal blood	The defective gene is not known, but the disorder has a characteristic phenotype (severe combined immunodeficiency with no T or B cells)
Functional assay to measure the activity of the gene product in fetal blood or tissue	Assays are available to assess directly the function of the defective gene (adenosine deaminase activity on chorionic villus samples)
Mutation detection	The defective gene has been identified, and the mutation in the family at risk is known (a C to T base pair substitution in codon 520 in *Btk*, the defective gene in X-linked agammaglobulinemia)
Linkage analysis	The defective gene has been mapped to a specific site on a single chromosome, and sufficient family members are available to identify haplotypes carrying the mutation (X-linked lymphoproliferative syndrome when DNA is available on the proband)

analysis and prenatal diagnosis is evolving rapidly, so that a review of the current literature may be required to ensure that the patient is receiving the most up-to-date management. When the defective gene is not known but the disorder has a characteristic immunologic or histologic phenotype, as in Chédiak-Higashi syndrome, fetal blood samples can be obtained to make a specific diagnosis. For some disorders (e.g., adenosine deaminase deficiency), the activity of the gene product in amniocytes or chorionic villus samples can be measured. This has several advantages. It can be performed early in pregnancy, it does not require extended family studies, and it is rapid.

DNA analysis, particularly polymerase chain reaction (PCR) (Rose, 1991), is being used with increasing frequency to provide prenatal diagnosis and carrier detection. When the family is known to carry a specific mutation, for example, a base-pair alteration in the gene for gp91-phagocytic oxidase (phox), resulting in X-linked chronic granulomatous disease—it is possible to develop probes that bind selectively to the normal or mutant allele in PCR-amplified samples of DNA (Bolscher et al., 1991). Alternatively, one can track the mutation, using a technique called *single-strand conformation polymorphism* (Sheffield et al., 1993). These studies can also be performed early in pregnancy, but detailed information is needed about the mutation carried by the family being studied. Sometimes the defective gene is known, but the specific mutation in a particular family has not been identified. In other cases, the defective gene has not been identified but has been mapped to a specific locus on a particular chromosome. In both situations, anonymous DNA probes that identify polymorphisms near the gene of interest can be used to identify the disease-carrying haplotype (Puck et al., 1990). This type of assay is called *linkage analysis*,

and it is dependent on the availability of DNA from essential members of the family.

Carrier Detection

Although most of the techniques used for prenatal diagnosis can also be used for carrier detection, the DNA-based assays, including mutation analysis and linkage studies, are likely to be the most reliable. As noted earlier, carrier detection is particularly important for X-linked disorders. There are at least seven X-linked disorders of the immune system. All seven have been mapped to specific sites on the X chromosome (see Table 9–6), and in families with a family history of the disorder, it is possible to use linkage analysis to provide carrier detection. However, as is true with all X-linked disorders that are lethal without medical intervention, only about 50% of the patients who have the phenotypic characteristics of one of the X-linked immunodeficiencies have a family history of that disorder. The remaining patients are either the first manifestation in their family of a new mutation of the gene causing the X-linked disorder, or the patient has an unrelated genetic disorder with similar clinical and laboratory findings. The new mutation may have occurred in the gamete that gave rise to the patient, but it may have occurred in earlier generations. Thus, it is important to determine whether the patient's mother and grandmother are carriers of a particular immunodeficiency in order to know whether the patient's sisters and other family members are at risk of carrying the gene.

In X-linked chronic granulomatous disease and in properdin deficiency, the assays used to detect carriers are the same as those used to diagnose an affected patient. The phagocytes from carriers of chromic granulomatous disease are usually intermediate between those from controls and from affected patients in their ability to produce superoxide radicals (see Chapter 15). Carriers of properdin deficiency have approximately half the normal serum concentration of properdin (Sjöholm et al., 1988). In contrast, carriers of X-linked agammaglobulinemia, X-linked severe combined immunodeficiency, and Wiskott-Aldrich syndrome are normal by all immunologic criteria. However, in cell lineages primarily affected by the gene defect (i.e., B cells in X-linked agammaglobulinemia, T and B cells in X-linked severe combined immunodeficiency, and all hematopoietic cell lineages in Wiskott-Aldrich syndrome), carrier women exhibit selective use of the nonmutant X chromosome as the active X chromosome (Conley, 1992). This can be explained by the fact that the cells that express the defective gene; that is, cells with the mutant X chromosome active are at a disadvantage in cell proliferation or differentiation. As a result, all cells of that lineage are derived from precursors that have the normal X chromosome as the active X.

Several techniques have been used to analyze patterns of X chromosome inactivation. One PCR-based assay takes advantage of the fact that the active and inactive X vary in methylation, particularly in regions near housekeeping genes (Allen et al., 1994).

CLINICAL FEATURES

Major Symptoms

All infants and children referred for "too many" infections must be carefully evaluated. Most turn out to be normal or to have respiratory allergy. Indeed, we estimate that among children referred for evaluation for immunodeficiency, 50% turn out to be normal, 30% have allergy, 10% have a serious but nonimmunologic disorder, and only 10% have an immunodeficiency, either primary or secondary.

The major manifestation of immunodeficiency is increased susceptibility to infection. This may mean (1) increased frequency of infection, (2) increased severity of infection, (3) prolonged duration of infection, (4) repeated infections without a symptom-free interval, (5) increased dependency on antibiotics, (6) unexpected or severe complications of infection, or (7) infection with an unusual organism, usually an opportunistic one. In many immunodeficiencies, there is an increased frequency of infection plus one or more of the other characteristics previously listed. A poster (Fig. 9–2) distributed by the Modell Foundation and the American Red Cross alerts parents to early warning signs of immunodeficiency.

Some common clinical findings of primary immunodeficiencies are summarized in Table 9–8. These include features that are common to several disorders,

Table 9–8. Clinical Features in Immunodeficiency

Usually Present
Recurrent upper respiratory infections
Severe bacterial infections
Persistent infections with incomplete
 or no response to therapy

Often Present
Failure to thrive or growth retardation
Infection with an unusual organism
Skin lesions (e.g., rash, seborrhea, pyoderma, necrotic
 abscesses, alopecia, eczema, telangiectasia,
 severe warts)
Recalcitrant thrush
Diarrhea and malabsorption
Persistent sinusitis, mastoiditis
Recurrent bronchitis, pneumonia
Evidence of autoimmunity
Paucity of lymph nodes and tonsils
Hematologic abnormalities; aplastic anemia, hemolytic
 anemia, neutropenia, thrombocytopenia

Occasionally Present
Weight loss, fevers
Chronic conjunctivitis
Periodontitis
Lymphadenopathy
Hepatosplenomegaly
Severe viral disease
Chronic liver disease
Arthralgia or arthritis
Chronic encephalitis
Recurrent meningitis
Pyoderma gangrenosa
Cholangitis and/or hepatitis
Adverse reaction to vaccines
Bronchiectasis
Urinary tract infection
Delayed umbilical cord detachment
Chronic stomatitis

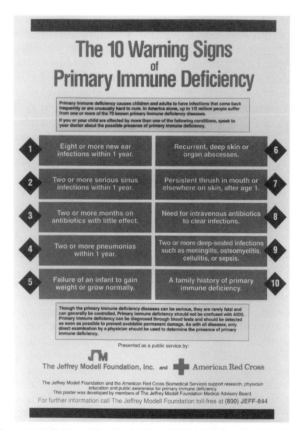

Figure 9–2. Poster of the Modell Foundation detailing the 10 warning signs of primary immunodeficiency. (Courtesy of the Jeffrey Modell Foundation, New York.)

grouped as to their relative frequency. Excluded are specific features associated with specific disorders.

Respiratory Infection

In subjects with immunodeficiency, repeated respiratory infections lead to chronic sinusitis, otitis, mastoiditis, and bronchitis. This often is accompanied by continuous purulent nasal discharge, postnasal drip, sputum production, and a diminished gag reflex. Bronchiectasis at an early age may result. Indeed, many hypogammaglobulinemic adults present in the chest clinic with early-onset bronchiectasis. Cigarette smoke is particularly aggravating to these patients. The persistence of respiratory pathogens, such as *Streptococcus, pneumococcus,* or *Haemophilus influenzae,* in the sputum should suggest immunodeficiency.

A careful history helps to separate the immunologically normal child brought to the physician for too many colds from the immunodeficient child. Many children experience six to eight respiratory infections per year, and this number is increased if there is exposure to older siblings or other children at nursery school. In the immunologically normal child, the respiratory infections are usually mild, without fever, and lasting only a few days. Furthermore, the normal child recovers completely between infections.

When symptoms suggestive of respiratory infections occur repeatedly as the sole infectious manifestation, allergy must also be suspected. Allergic disorders, in contrast to immunodeficiency, are characterized by (1) absence of fever, (2) clear nonpurulent discharge, (3) prior history of colic, food intolerance, eczema, or other allergic symptoms, (4) a positive family history of allergy, (5) a characteristic seasonal or exposure pattern, (6) a poor response to antibiotics, and (7) a good response to antihistamines or bronchodilators.

Pneumonia is common in immunodeficiency. In patients who have pneumonia unresponsive to antibiotic therapy and associated with a low P_{O_2} and rapid respirations, *Pneumocystis carinii* infection must be suspected. Because this infection is interstitial, rales often are minimal or absent. A tracheal brushing, open-lung biopsy, or needle biopsy must usually be performed to confirm the diagnosis.

Other Manifestations

Severe bacterial infections (pneumonia, sepsis, meningitis, osteomyelitis) may accompany respiratory infections in immunodeficiency. Although one such severe infection may occur in a normal child, a second occurrence should alert the physician to possible immunodeficiency. In antibody immunodeficiency, the organisms responsible for infections usually are the major encapsulated pathogens; most viral infections are tolerated well. In cellular deficiencies, the organisms responsible for infection usually are gram-negative bacteria or the fungi, protozoa, viruses, or mycobacteria. Infections caused by staphylococci, *Nocardia,* and gram-negative bacteria are common in phagocytic deficiencies. Recurrent neisserial infection is characteristic of patients with C6, C7, and C8 complement deficiencies. Infections with certain opportunistic organisms (e.g., *P. carinii, Cryptosporidia,* and *Mycoplasma*) may occur in several types of immunodeficiencies.

Diarrhea, malabsorption, and vomiting are common in immunodeficiency. Occasionally, a specific organism can be implicated (e.g., *Escherichia coli* in diarrhea, *Giardia lamblia* in malabsorption). These gastrointestinal symptoms are often aggravated by antibiotics or concomitant respiratory infection. Patients with severe cellular immunodeficiency are particularly likely to have chronic diarrhea. Liver disease and cholangitis are not uncommon. Indeed, eight of 56 patients with sclerosing cholangitis had primary immunodeficiency (Debray et al., 1994).

Prior to diagnosis, failure to thrive is frequent. Immunodeficient children often are underweight and short of stature, and developmental milestones are delayed as a result of chronic infection. The mother may describe the child as shy or quiet. The active, robust child climbing all over the office is a less likely candidate for a serious immunodeficiency.

Past History

The birth history should be explored for maternal illness, gestational length, birth weight, and neonatal illness. A history of delayed umbilical cord attachment (>3 weeks) suggests a leukocyte adhesion defect. The immunization record should be obtained to determine any adverse reactions. The nature and severity of past infectious diseases should be detailed; an unusually severe course of measles or chickenpox is common in cellular immunodeficiency. The rash of a viral exanthem or rhus dermatitis (poison ivy or oak) suggests intact cellular immunity. The occurrence of autoimmune type of features (e.g., thrombocytopenia, hemolytic anemia, arthritis, parotitis, chronic active hepatitis) should be sought.

The current medications that the child is or has been taking should be recorded. Immunodeficiency is associated with certain drugs (phenytoin, immunosuppressives), and allergy is often associated with exposure to medication.

The past history should be explored for earlier surgery, including tonsillectomy, adenoidectomy, or splenectomy. A review of the histology of the removed organs is sometimes valuable in establishing a retrospective diagnosis. Previous radiation therapy for the thymus or nasopharynx; prior blood transfusion; earlier antibiotic or gamma globulin therapy (and their apparent clinical benefit); and adverse reactions to blood, plasma, or gamma globulin injections should be noted. A history of marked clinical benefit from small doses of gamma globulin can be attributed to a placebo effect.

An immunization history should be obtained. Live virus vaccines, particularly oral polio vaccine, may cause progressive disease in a profoundly immunodeficient child, but an uneventful vaccination with a normal antibody response suggests intact immunity. An immunization history is crucial when one is evaluating antibody or T cell responses to vaccine antigens; tetanus antibody or skin testing is of value in children who have received these immunizations.

An environmental history of smoking and of exposure to animals (including farm animals), birds, and unusual chemicals should be obtained. Recent travel to foreign countries, camp, or rural areas may result in exposure to unusual organisms, bites, or a contaminated water supply. A recent change in the patient's schedule or home environment may increase exposure to infectious agents (from a new housekeeper or a new day care center), allergens, or toxins.

Family History

The family history of patients with possible immunodeficiency should be explored for severe infections or early deaths of near and distant relatives. If the history is positive, a genetic tree should be constructed. The racial and national background, a history of consanguinity, and the occurrence of arthritis, collagen disease, allergy, hypersensitivity, or lymphoreticular malignancy in other family members should be sought.

A parental history of blood or plasma infusions or lifestyle suggestive of illicit drug use, promiscuity, or bisexuality may suggest exposure to HIV via an infected mother.

Table 9–9. Characteristic Clinical Patterns in Some Primary Immunodeficiencies

Features	Diagnosis
In Newborns and Young Infants (0 to 6 Months)	
Hypocalcemia, heart disease, unusual facies	DiGeorge anomaly
Delayed umbilical cord detachment, leukocytosis, recurrent infections	Leukocyte adhesion defect
Diarrhea, pneumonia, thrush, failure to thrive	Severe combined immunodeficiency
Maculopapular rash, alopecia, lymphadenopathy	Severe combined immunodeficiency with graft-versus-host disease
Scaly, generalized dermatitis, severe diarrhea	Leiner's syndrome, erythroderma, failure to thrive, diarrhea (EFD syndrome)
Bloody stools, draining ears, eczema	Wiskott-Aldrich syndrome
Mouth ulcers, neutropenia, recurrent infections	Immunodeficiency with hyper-IgM
In Infancy and Young Children (6 Months to 5 Years)	
Severe progressive infectious mononucleosis	X-linked lymphoproliferative syndrome
Paralytic disease following oral poliovirus immunization	X-linked agammaglobulinemia
Recurrent cutaneous and systemic staphylococcal infections, coarse features	Hyper-IgE syndrome
Persistent thrush, nail dystrophy, endocrinopathies	Chronic mucocutaneous candidiasis
Short stature, fine hair, severe varicella	Cartilage hair hypoplasia with short-limbed dwarfism
Oculocutaneous albinism, recurrent infection	Chédiak-Higashi syndrome
Lymphadenopathy, dermatitis, pneumonia, osteomyelitis	Chronic granulomatous disease
In Older Children (Over 5 Years) and Adults	
Progressive dermatomyositis with chronic enterovirus encephalitis	X-linked agammaglobulinemia
Sinopulmonary infections, neurologic deterioration, telangiectasia	Ataxia-telangiectasia
Recurrent neisserial meningitis	C6, C7, or C8 deficiency
Sinopulmonary infections, malabsorption, splenomegaly, autoimmunity	Common variable immunodeficiency
Candidiasis with raw egg ingestion	Biotin-dependent cocarboxylase deficiency

Physical Examination

Patients with immunodeficiencies, particularly those with T-cell immunodeficiencies, characteristically appear chronically ill and exhibit pallor, irritability, reduced subcutaneous fat, and a distended abdomen. Examination of the skin may reveal macular rashes, pyoderma, eczema, petechiae, severe warts, alopecia, or telangiectasia. Conjunctivitis is frequently noted. Cervical lymph nodes are typically absent, despite recurrent throat infections; occasionally, the lymph nodes may be enlarged or suppurative. The tympanic membranes are often scarred or perforated; purulent ear drainage is common. The nostrils are often excoriated and crusted, indicative of a purulent nasal discharge.

Candidiasis of the mucous membranes, roof of the mouth, tongue, or corners of the mouth is common. Periodontitis and dental decay are noted in some disorders, particularly granulocytic disorders. Diffuse ulceration of the mucous membranes and discrete necrotizing lesions of the tongue or mucous membranes (noma) are noted in some forms of immunodeficiency (Rotbart et al., 1986). The tonsils may be atrophic and may appear to have been surgically removed. Often, there is a deep cough or chest rattle; rales are frequently heard.

The liver and spleen may be enlarged. Muscle mass is diminished, and the fat deposits of the buttocks are atrophied. There may be excoriation around the anus as a result of chronic diarrhea. There may be joint swelling, limitation of joint motion, and subcutaneous nodules as a result of arthritis. Neurologic abnormalities may include slow development or ataxia. In very early cases, none or only a few of these are present.

Table 9–10. Initial Screening Tests for Immunodeficiency

Blood Count
Hemoglobin, white blood cell count, lymphocyte morphology, differential count, platelet estimation or count

Quantitative Immunoglobulins
IgG, IgM, IgA, and IgE levels

Antibody Responses to Previous Vaccines
Tetanus, diphtheria, rubella, *Haemophilus influenzae* titers (for IgG function)

Isoagglutinin (Anti-A and Anti-B) Titers
For IgM function

Total Hemolytic Complement
Tests classical complement pathway

Infection Evaluation
Erythrocyte sedimentation rate, appropriate cultures, appropriate roentgenograms

Clinical Patterns

Certain clinical patterns among the primary immunodeficiencies are sufficiently characteristic to suggest the diagnosis to the astute clinician (Table 9–9). These are based on age of onset, type of infection, sex, and other characteristic clinical findings. For example, in a 1-year-old boy with recurrent pneumococcal infections since the age of 6 months whose tonsils are absent and who has no palpable lymph nodes, a diagnosis of X-linked agammaglobulinemia is suggested. For a definitive diagnosis in all instances, laboratory tests are required.

LABORATORY DIAGNOSIS

Because the clinical findings in immunodeficiency are rarely distinctive, the diagnosis must be established by appropriate laboratory procedures. In this portion of the text, the initial screening and advanced tests for the evaluation of each group of immunodeficiencies are outlined. These are summarized in Tables 9–10 and 9–11.

General Laboratory Tests

As with other ill patients, certain nonspecific laboratory tests are often indicated, including a complete blood count (CBC), erythrocyte sedimentation rate, urinalysis, tuberculin test, and chest and sinus x-rays. Specific laboratory tests are sometimes indicated to exclude cystic fibrosis (sweat test), malabsorption (xylose tolerance test), malnutrition (protein, vitamin, and albumin levels), and allergy (immediate skin tests, nasal smear for eosinophils).

Chronic diarrhea may be accompanied by electrolyte imbalance. Autoantibodies (antinuclear antibodies, rheumatoid factor) may be present. Liver enlargement is an indication for obtaining liver function tests and tests for viral hepatitis (e.g., hepatitis B surface antigen [HBsAg]; cytomegalovirus [CMV] culture and antibody; HIV antibody; hepatitis C virus [HCV] antibody).

Table 9–11. Laboratory Tests in Immunodeficiency

Screening Tests	Advanced Tests	Research/Special Tests
B-Cell Deficiency		
IgG, IgM, IgA levels	B-cell enumeration (CD19 or CD20)	Advanced B-cell phenotyping
Isoagglutinin titers	IgG subclass levels	Biopsies: e.g., lymph nodes
Ab response to vaccine antigens:	IgD and IgE levels	Ab responses to special antigens: e.g., ϕX, KLH
e.g., tetanus, diphtheria, rubeola,	Natural Ab titers, e.g., anti-streptolysin O,	In vivo Ig survival
Haemophilus influenzae	*Escherichia coli*	Secretory Ig levels
	Ab responses to new vaccines: e.g.,	In vitro Ig synthesis
	typhoid, pneumococcal vaccines	Cell activation analysis
	Lateral pharyngeal x-ray for adenoidal	Mutation analysis
	tissue	
T-Cell Deficiency		
Lymphocyte count and morphology	T-cell subset enumeration (CD3, CD4,	Advanced T-cell phenotyping
Chest x-ray for thymic size*	CD8)	Cytokine and receptor assays, e.g., IL-2, IFN-γ,
Delayed skin tests: e.g.,	Proliferative responses to mitogens,	TNF-α
Trichophyton, mumps, *Candida,*	antigens, allogeneic cells	Cytotoxic assays: e.g., NK, ADCC, CTL
tetanus toxoid, multitest panel	HLA typing	Enzyme assays: e.g., ADA, PNP
	Chromosome analysis	Biopsies: e.g., skin, liver, thymus
		Thymic hormone assays
		Cell-activation analysis
		Mutation analysis
Phagocytic Deficiency		
WBC count, morphology	Chemiluminescence	Adhesion molecule assays,
NBT dye test	WBC turnover	e.g., CD11b/CD18, selectin ligand
IgE level	Special morphology	Rebuck skin window
	Random mobility and chemotaxis	Deformability, adherence, and aggregation
	Phagocytosis assays	Oxidative metabolism
	Bactericidal assays	Enzyme assays: e.g., MPO, G6PD, NADPH oxidase
		Mutation analysis
Complement Deficiency		
CH_{50} activity	Opsonic assays	Alternative pathway activity
C3 level	Component assays	Functional assays: e.g., chemotactic factor, immune
C4 level	Activation assays: e.g., C3a, C4a, C4d,	adherence
	C5a	In vivo component survival
		C allotype analysis

*In infants only.
Abbreviations: Ab = Antibody; ADA = adenosine deaminase; ADCC = antibody-dependent cellular cytotoxicity; C = complement; CH = hemolytic complement; CTL = cytotoxic T lymphocyte; DR = Class II histocompatibility antigen; G6PD = glucose-6-phosphate dehydrogenase. IFN = interferon; Ig = immunoglobulin; KLH = keyhole limpet hemocyanin antigen; MIF = migration inhibition factor; MPO = myeloperoxidase; NADPH = nicotinamide adenine dinucleotide phosphate; NBT = nitroblue tetrazolium; NK = natural killer, PNP = purine nucleoside phosphorylase; ϕX = phage antigen.

Special cultures or stain for specific organisms may be necessary in certain situations. Of particular importance are *P. carinii* and cytomegalovirus in the lung; *G. lamblia,* rotavirus, cryptosporidia, and poliomyelitis virus (particularly in recently vaccinated patients) in the stool (Lopez et al., 1974); and cytomegalovirus in the urine or blood.

Some rare nonimmunologic disorders should be excluded in certain clinical situations. Absence of the spleen should be suspected if a patient has repeated episodes of sepsis and bizarre red blood cell (RBC) forms or Howell-Jolly bodies on peripheral smear. Asplenia is confirmed by ultrasonography. Immobile cilia may be present in some patients with sinusitis and bronchiectasis, owing to a lack of dynein arms within the cilia (Afzelius, 1976). Sperm motility is also decreased in these patients and can be used to diagnose the defect. This deficiency may be present in patients with Kartagener's syndrome. Complete absence of nasal cilia has also been reported (Welch et al., 1984).

Certain laboratory findings should suggest specific immunodeficiencies. These include an elevated level of alpha$_2$-fetoprotein, present in ataxia-telangiectasia; (Waldmann and McIntire, 1972), presence of megaloblastic anemia in infancy (transcobalamin II deficiency), abnormal chromosome 18 or 22 (associated with IgA deficiency and the DiGeorge anomaly, respectively), increased chromosomal breakage (ataxia-telangiectasia), inability to grow chromosomes for karyotyping (severe combined immunodeficiency [SCID] with lack of proliferation to phytohemagglutinin [PHA]), and situs inversus on chest x-ray (Kartagener's syndrome).

Initial Screening Evaluation

The initial screening evaluation for suspected immunodeficiency includes a CBC; quantitation of serum IgG, IgM, and IgA levels; assessment of antibody function; measurement of total hemolytic complement (CH$_{50}$); and an infection evaluation (see Table 9–10).

Blood Count

The CBC, including hemoglobin level, leukocyte count, differential count, platelet enumeration, and examination of the blood smear, establishes the presence of anemia, thrombocytopenia, leukopenia, or leukocytosis; the latter, with a shift to the left, suggests the presence of acute or chronic infection. The total lymphocyte count should be calculated (WBC × percent lymphocytes); the normal lymphocyte count is 2000 to 6000 cells/μl (see Table 9–15). Lymphopenia is *suggested* if the lymphocyte count is less than 2000 cells/μl and is *present* if the count is less than 1500 cells/μl. When lymphopenia is suggested, several counts over a period of several weeks are indicated. Persistent lymphopenia, generally associated with a paucity of small lymphocytes on the peripheral smear, is present in many cellular immunodeficiencies. By contrast, large lymphocytes with pale cytoplasm, reminiscent of monocytes rather than darkly stained small lymphocytes, are often present.

The peripheral smear should also be examined for the presence of Howell-Jolly bodies and other unusual red blood cell forms; these are characteristic features of asplenia. The granulocytes may also disclose morphologic abnormalities, such as the giant vacuoles of the Chédiak-Higashi syndrome (Blume et al., 1968) or the bilobed or kidney-shaped nuclei of the secondary granule deficiency syndrome (Strauss et al., 1974).

Immunoglobulin Assays

Quantitative determination of serum IgG, IgM, IgA, and IgE levels should be performed; IgD levels are not part of the initial screening. Levels of IgG, IgM, and IgA are often determined by radial immunodiffusion, a procedure available in most hospitals and commercial laboratories (Mancini et al., 1965). Reagent kits with agar plates and standards are available from several companies. Alternatively, nephelometric techniques are used in many large clinical laboratories. IgE assays require radioimmunoassay.

Quantitative immunoglobulin assays are recommended, inasmuch as immunoelectrophoresis or plasma electrophoresis do not provide exact information about the levels of individual immunoglobulins. A gamma globulin level by plasma electrophoresis below 600 mg/dl should be further studied by quantitative immunoglobulin assays.

The immunoglobulin levels must be interpreted with care because of marked alterations with each age (Stiehm and Fudenberg, 1966b). All infants aged 3 to 6 months are hypogammaglobulinemic if adult normal values are used. Therefore, comparison of each immunoglobulin value with its age-matched control is essential (Tables 9–12 and 9–13).

Premature infants have particularly low levels of immunoglobulins in the first year of life. Ballow and colleagues (1986) have published values for premature infants and young children at various birth weights and ages. An immunoglobulin level within two standard deviations of the mean for age is considered normal. In older children and adults, a total immunoglobulin level above 600 mg/dl with normal screening antibody tests excludes antibody deficiency. By contrast, total immunoglobulins (IgG + IgM + IgA) under 400 mg/dl or an IgG globulin level under 200 mg/dl usually indicates antibody immunodeficiency. Total immunoglobulin levels of 400 to 600 mg/dl and IgG levels of 200 to 400 mg/dl are nondiagnostic and must be correlated with functional antibody tests.

Antibody Function Tests

Tetanus, rubella, measles, diphtheria, *H. influenzae B,* and isoagglutinin titers are simple antibody functional tests recommended for the initial screening. The first five tests are valid only if the patient has previously been immunized to these agents. These titrations are available at many hospital laboratories or reference laboratories. Negative titers (particularly if obtained by

Table 9–12. Levels of Immunoglobulins in Sera of Normal Subjects by Age*

Age	IgG		IgM		IgA		Total Immunoglobulin	
	mg/dl	% of Adult Level	mg/dl	% of Adult Level	mg/dl	% of Adult Level	mg/dl	% of Adult Level
Newborn	1031 ± 200†	89 ± 17	11 ± 5	1.1 ± 5	2 ± 3	1 ± 2	1044 ± 201	67 ± 13
1–3 mo	430 ± 119	37 ± 10	30 ± 11	30 ± 11	21 ± 13	11 ± 7	481 ± 127	31 ± 9
4–6 mo	427 ± 186	37 ± 16	43 ± 17	43 ± 17	28 ± 18	14 ± 9	498 ± 204	32 ± 13
7–12 mo	661 ± 219	58 ± 19	54 ± 23	55 ± 23	37 ± 18	19 ± 9	752 ± 242	48 ± 15
13–24 mo	762 ± 209	66 ± 18	58 ± 23	59 ± 23	50 ± 24	25 ± 12	870 ± 258	56 ± 16
25–36 mo	892 ± 183	77 ± 16	61 ± 19	62 ± 19	71 ± 37	36 ± 19	1024 ± 205	65 ± 14
3–5 yr	929 ± 228	80 ± 20	56 ± 18	57 ± 18	93 ± 27	47 ± 14	1078 ± 245	69 ± 17
6–8 yr	923 ± 256	20 ± 22	65 ± 25	66 ± 25	124 ± 45	62 ± 23	1112 ± 293	71 ± 20
9–11 yr	1124 ± 235	97 ± 20	79 ± 33	80 ± 33	131 ± 60	66 ± 30	1334 ± 254	85 ± 17
12–16 yr	946 ± 124	82 ± 11	59 ± 20	60 ± 20	148 ± 63	74 ± 32	1153 ± 169	74 ± 12
Adults	1158 ± 305	100 ± 26	99 ± 27	100 ± 27	200 ± 61	100 ± 31	1457 ± 353	100 ± 24

*The values were divided from measurements made in 296 normal children and 30 adults. Levels were determined by the radial diffusion technique using specific rabbit antisera to human immunoglobulins.
†One standard deviation.
From Stiehm ER, Fudenberg HH. Serum levels of immune globulins in health and disease. A survey. Pediatrics 37:715, 1966.

hemagglutinin inhibition or neutralization methods), despite a positive immunization history, suggest functional antibody deficiency. These are usually IgG antibodies and thus test IgG function. We use tetanus and *H. influenzae* antibody titers as the preferred initial antibody tests.

The saline isoagglutinin (anti-A, anti-B, or both) titers measure IgM globulin function. In most immunologically normal individuals older than 6 months of age (with the exception of those of blood group AB), titers are at least 1:8 to A₁ and B cells, respectively. These titers are available in hospital blood banks, since the method is identical to that used to identify low titer O blood for exchange transfusion. Isoagglutinins are selectively deficient in older children with Wiskott-Aldrich syndrome; these patients often have low IgM globulin levels (Stiehm and McIntosh, 1967). Soothill (1962) showed correlation between serum IgM globulin levels and the isoagglutinin titers in normal subjects. If isoagglutinins and other antibody test results are all abnormal, an antibody immunodeficiency probably exists.

Total Hemolytic Complement Activity

Most complement component defects can be identified by a low CH_{50}; this test assesses the ability of the patient's serum to lyse antibody-coated sheep erythrocytes by the classical complement pathway. Values must be compared with standards used in the laboratory.

Infection Evaluation

Patients with immunodeficiency often have chronic infection. The erythrocyte sedimentation rate is usually elevated in proportion to the severity of the chronic infection. The condition should be investigated by appropriate x-rays and cultures of the suspected site(s).

If these screening tests are all normal, immunodeficiency is usually excluded and the patient can be assured that γ-globulin or other long-term therapy is not indicated. However, if the screening tests are positive, if chronic infection is documented but unexplained, or if the history is unusually suggestive for immunodeficiency, advanced tests are indicated (see Table 9–11).

Table 9–13. Serum IgE Levels in 425 White Subjects by Age Groups

Age (Years)	N	Natural Log Means	Natural Log SD	Antilog Means (IU/ml)	Antilog Means + 1 SD (IU/ml)	Antilog Means + 2 SD (IU/ml)
1–2	29	2.98	1.18	20	64	208
3–5	31	3.55	1.23	35	119	405
6–15	45	3.92	1.09	51	150	446
16–20	59	3.63	1.18	38	123	401
21–30	114	3.29	1.32	27	100	376
31–40	38	3.53	1.19	34	113	372
Over 40	109	3.52	1.21	34	114	382
Total	425	3.47	1.21	32	108	386

Abbreviations: IU = international unit; N = Number; SD = standard deviation.
From Wittig HJ, Belloit J, DeFillippi I, Royal G. Age-related serum immunoglobulin E levels in healthy subjects and in patients with allergic disease. J Allergy Clin Immunol 66:305–313, 1980.

Tests for Antibody Deficiencies

Initial Tests

Immunoglobulin levels and functional antibody tests are part of the screening evaluation for immunodeficiency (see Table 9–10); in the antibody immunodeficiencies, one or more test results is abnormal. If the immunoglobulin levels are very low (total < 100 mg/dl), a diagnosis of antibody immunodeficiency is established and further tests are done only to assess the degree of antibody impairment and the involvement of other components of the immune system.

B-Cell Enumeration

B cells are the precursors of the antibody-producing plasma cells and are characterized by the presence of one or more classes of surface membrane immunoglobulin (SMIG) and certain B cell–related surface antigens,

such as CD19, CD20, and CD21 (Tables 9–14 and 9–15). B-cell enumeration is indicated when immunoglobulins are very low or absent; it is rarely indicated in the presence of normal or elevated immunoglobulins except to look for unusual surface immunoglobulin isotope distribution or density, which is characteristic of some antibody deficiencies.

B cells are usually measured by automated immunofluorescence (flow cytometry—see T-cell enumeration, later) with an antibody to either the CD19 or CD20 B-cell surface antigen. This assay is often performed in conjunction with CD3, CD4, and CD8 T-cell enumeration. B cells make up 10 to 20% of the total lymphocytes but vary with age (see Table 9–15).

Alternatively, B cells can be assessed by measuring surface membrane immunoglobulin using immunofluorescence and a polyvalent antihuman immunoglobulin antisera with specificity for all immunoglobulin subclasses and κ and λ chains (WHO/IARC Tech-

Table 9–14. Principal Cell Surface Antigens (Cluster Designation) Used to Identify Cells of the Human Immune System

Cluster Designation	Predominant Reactivity	Names of Monoclonal Antibody Clones	Other Cellular Reactivity
All Leukocytes			
CD45	Tyrosine phosphatase	Anti-HLe-1	
T Cells			
IMMATURE T CELLS			
CD1a	Corticothymocytes	Leu-6, OKT6	Pre-B, dendritic cells
CD38	Immature cells	Leu-17, OKT10	Pre-B, plasma, NK, B subset
PAN-T CELLS			
CD2	Sheep erythrocyte, LFA-3 receptor	Leu-5, OKT11, CT-2	NK subset
CD3	T-Cell receptor complex	Leu-4, OKT3	
CD5	Mature T cells	Leu-1, OKT1, T101	B subset
SUBSETS OF T CELLS			
CD4	Helper/inducer T cells	Leu-3, OKT4	Mono
CD8	Cytotoxic/suppressor T cells	Leu-2, OKT8	NK subset
ACTIVATED T CELLS			
CD25	IL-2α receptor	Tac	B subset
CD38	Immature cells	Leu 17, OKT10	Pre-B, plasma, NK, B subset
CD71	Transferrin receptor	OKT9	Act B, Mono
—*	HLA-DR (class II MHC)		B, Mono
B Cells			
EXCLUSIVE B-CELL MARKERS			
CD19	Pan-B cell	Leu-12, B4	
CD20	Pan-B cell	Leu-16, B1	
CD21	CR2, EBV receptor	B2	
CD22	Pan-B cell	Leu-14	
NON-EXCLUSIVE B-CELL MARKERS			
CD35	CR1, C3b receptor		Mono, RBC, PMN
—*	HLA-DR (class II MHC)		Mono, Act T
—*	HLA-DP (class II MHC)		Mono, Act T
—*	HLA-DQ (class II MHC)		Mono, Act T
Monocytes			
CD11b	CR3, C3bi receptor	Leu-15, OKM1, Mac-1, Mo-1	NK, PMN, T subset
CD11c	CR4 receptor	Leu-M5	NK, T subset
CD14	Monocytes	Leu-M3, Mo-2	
Natural Killer Cells			
CD16	FcγRIII	Leu-11	Mono, PMN
CD11b	CR3, C3bi receptor	Leu-15, OKM1, Mac-1, Mo-1	Mono, PMN, T subset
CD56	N-CAM	Leu-19, NKH-1	T subset
CD57	Large granular lymphocytes	Leu-7, HNK-1	T subset

*No CD assigned.
Abbreviations: Act = activated; CD = cluster designation; CR = complement receptor; EBV = Epstein-Barr virus; FcR = Fc receptor; LFA = leukocyte function associated antigen; MHC = major histocompatibility complex; mono = monocytes; N-CAM = neural cell adhesion molecule; NK = natural killer; PMN = polymorphonuclear leukocytes.

Table 9–15. Normal Human Blood Lymphocyte Subpopulations at Various Ages

Subpopulations (Cells/µl)	Cord Blood	2–3 Months	4–8 Months	12–23 Months	2–5 Years	7–17 Years	Adult
TOTAL LYMPHOCYTES							
Median (%)	5400 (41%)	5680 (66%)	5990 (64%)	5160 (59%)	4060 (50%)	2400 (40%)	2100 (32%)
Confidence intervals (%)	4200 (35%) to	2920 (55%) to	3610 (45%) to	2180 (44%) to	2400 (38%) to	2000 (36%) to	1600 (28%) to
	6900 (47%)*	8840 (78%)	8840 (79%)	8270 (72%)	5810 (64%)	2700 (43%)*	2400 (39%)*
CD3 T CELLS							
Median (%)	3100 (55%)	4030 (72%)	4270 (71%)	3300 (66%)	3040 (72%)	1800 (70%)	1600 (73%)
Confidence intervals (%)	2400 (49%) to	2070 (55%) to	2280 (45%) to	1460 (53%) to	1610 (62%) to	1400 (66%) to	960 (61%) to
	3700 (62%)*	6540 (78%)	6450 (79%)	5440 (81%)	4230 (80%)	2000 (76%)*	2600 (84%)*
CD4 T CELLS							
Median (%)	1900 (35%)	2830 (52%)	2950 (49%)	2070 (43%)	1800 (42%)	800 (37%)	940 (46%)
Confidence intervals (%)	1500 (28%) to	1460 (41%) to	1690 (36%) to	1020 (31%) to	900 (35%) to	700 (33%) to	540 (32%) to
	2400 (42%)*	5116 (64%)	4600 (61%)	3600 (54%)	2860 (51%)	1100 (41%)*	1660 (60%)*
CD8 T CELLS							
Median (%)	1500 (29%)	1410 (25%)	1450 (24%)	1320 (25%)	1180	800 (30%)	520 (27%)
Confidence intervals (%)	1200 (26%) to	650 (16%) to	720 (16%) to	570 (16%) to	630 (22%) to	600 (27%) to	270 (13%) to
	2000 (33%)*	2450 (35%)	2490 (34%)	2230 (38%)	1910 (38%)	900 (35%)*	930 (40%)*
B CELLS (CD19 or CD20)†							
Median (%)	1000 (20%)†	900 (23%)	900 (23%)	900 (23%)	900 (24%)	400 (16%)†	246 (13%)†
Confidence intervals (%)	200 (14%) to	500 (19%) to	500 (19%) to	500 (19%) to	700 (21%) to	300 (12%) to	122 (10%) to
	1500 (23%)*	1500 (31%)	1500 (31%)	1500 (31%)	1300 (28%)	500 (22%)*	632 (31%)
CD4:CD8 RATIO							
Median	1.2	2.2	2.1	1.6	1.4	1.3	1.7
Confidence intervals	0.8 to 1.8	1.3 to 3.5	1.2 to 3.5	1.0 to 3.0	1.0 to 2.1	1.1 to 1.4	0.9 to 4.5

Confidence intervals given are the 5th to 95th percentiles except where indicated (*); these are the 25th to 75th percentiles. B cells use the CD20 antigen except where indicated (†); these use the CD19 antigen. The lymphocyte % is the percentage of total leukocytes. The CD3, CD4, CD8, and B cell (CD19 or CD20) % is the percentage of total lymphocytes.

Combined data from Erkellor-Yuksel FM, et al. J Pediatr 120:216–222, 1992 (cord blood, 7–17 yrs; B cells); Denny T, et al. JAMA 267:1484–1488, 1992 (2–3 mo to 5 yr); Fahey JL, cited in Giorgi JV et al. In Rose NR, et al. Manual of Clinical Laboratory Immunology, 4th ed. Washington, D.C., American Society for Microbiology, 1992, pp. 174–181 (adults).

Each subgroup contains at least 22 normal subjects.

nical Report, 1974). B cells with specifically µ or δ chain or both are most common. Distribution of surface membrane immunoglobulin is shown in Figure 3–13.

In the past, B cells were enumerated by rosetting techniques using sheep red blood cells coated with antibody or with antibody and complement. These react with the fragment (Fc) and C3 receptors of the B cells to form erythrocyte-antibody (EA) and erythrocyte-antibody-complement (EAC) rosettes, respectively. Since Fc and C3 receptors are also present on monocytes, some null cells, and some T cells, this method is inexact and is no longer recommended.

Pre-B cells are usually enumerated on a bone marrow aspirate with fluorescein-labeled antibodies to heavy chains. Pre-B cells are lymphocytes without surface membrane immunoglobulin but with small quantities of cytoplasmic µ heavy chains. Most pre-B cells are also CD10+.

B cells are low in X-linked agammaglobulinemia and in some forms of SCID and are slightly reduced (2% to 6%) in transient hypogammaglobulinemia of infancy. In most antibody immunodeficiencies, B cells are present in normal quantities, indicating that the defect is one of differentiation rather than a lack of the precursor cells. B-cell enumeration is of particular value in infant boys in whom X-linked agammaglobulinemia is suspected; the absence of B cells favors this diagnosis, and their presence favors a diagnosis of transient hypogammaglobulinemia, common variable hypogammaglobulinemia, or hyper-IgM syndrome.

Abnormal distribution of SMIG, such as the presence of several isotypes or selective increase or decrease of one isotype, may provide some diagnostic information in selective immunoglobulin deficiency (e.g., IgA deficiency, hyper-IgM syndrome) or in B-cell malignancies.

IgG Subclass Levels

Selective deficiency of one of the four subclasses of IgG may occur in antibody deficiency (Schur et al., 1970). The relative contributions of IgG1, IgG2, IgG3, and IgG4 to the total IgG are 70, 20, 7, and 3%, respectively (see Chapter 3). Specific antisera for quantitative measurements are now available; normal levels of IgG subclasses for age are presented in Table 9–16. Several reference laboratories offer these assays, but reproductivity and standardization are less than optimal.

Such measurements are indicated when IgG levels are normal or near-normal but when functional antibody deficiency is present (Yount et al., 1970). IgG subclasses should also be measured in patients with selective IgA deficiency who exhibit increased susceptibility to infection. Many IgA-deficient patients have IgG2 subclass deficiency (Oxelius et al., 1981). Some patients with chronic lung disease have been reported with IgG4 subclass deficiency (Heiner et al., 1983), but isolated IgG4 deficiency also occurs in normal subjects.

A reasonable guideline for diagnosis of subclass deficiency is a value less than 2 standard deviations (SD) below the mean for age or an IgG1 less than 250

Table 9–16. Levels of IgG subclasses in Sera of Normal Subjects by Age*

Age (Years)	No. of Subjects	IgG	IgG1	IgG2	IgG3	IgG4‡
0–1	22	420† (250–690)	340 (190–620)	59 (30–140)	39 (9–62)	19 (6–63)
1–2	42	470 (270–810)	410 (230–710)	68 (30–170)	34 (11–98)	13 (4–43)
2–3	36	540 (300–980)	480 (280–830)	98 (40–240)	28 (6–130)	18 (3–120)
3–4	52	600 (400–910)	530 (350–790)	120 (50–260)	30 (9–98)	32 (5–180)
4–6	31	660 (440–1000)	540 (360–810)	140 (60–310)	39 (9–160)	39 (9–160)
6–8	24	890 (560–1400)	560 (280–1120)	150 (30–630)	48 (40–250)	81 (11–620)
8–10	21	1000 (530–1900)	690 (280–1740)	210 (80–550)	85 (22–320)	42 (10–170)
10–13	33	910 (500–1660)	590 (270–1290)	240 (110–550)	58 (13–250)	60 (7–530)
13–16	19	910 (580–1450)	540 (280–1020)	210 (60–790)	58 (14–240)	60 (11–330)

*Levels were determined by radial diffusion using monospecific antisera.
†Geometric means are presented for each Ig at every age. The normal bounds, given in parentheses, are obtained by taking the mean logarithm.
‡IgG4 levels appear to be absent in 10% of individuals.
± 2 SD of the logarithms and then take the antilogs of the results.
Data from Schur PH, Rosen F, Norman ME. Immunoglobulin subclasses in normal children. Pediatr Res 13:181–183, 1979.

mg/dl, an IgG2 less than 50 mg/dl, and an IgG3 less than 25 mg/dl. An isolated IgG4 deficiency is not usually clinically significant.

IgD and IgE Levels

Determinations of IgD and IgE levels are indicated in the complete evaluation of suspected antibody immunodeficiency. IgD levels are determined by radial immunodiffusion, radioimmunoassay, or enzyme-linked immunosorbent assay (ELISA). IgE levels, because they are so low, are usually performed by radioimmunoassay or ELISA. Commercial kits are available. Table 9–13 (shown earlier) provides normal levels of IgE at different ages.

Abnormalities of IgD and IgE levels, both high and low values, are not uncommon in incomplete antibody deficiency syndromes. IgE levels often parallel IgA levels, and IgD levels often parallel IgM levels.

Isolated deficiencies of IgD and IgE are rare and of minimal significance. When other immunoglobulin levels are extremely low, levels of IgD and IgE are often low (Buckley and Fiscus, 1975). In partial cellular immunodeficiencies (e.g., Nezelof syndrome, Wiskott-Aldrich syndrome, DiGeorge anomaly), moderately elevated levels of IgE are commonly noted. In certain immunodeficiencies (e.g., hyper-IgE syndrome), IgE levels are markedly elevated (see Chapter 13).

A rare syndrome of elevated levels of IgD (IgD > 150 international units (IU)/ml [>20 mg/dl]) characterized by periodic bouts of fever, lymphadenitis, and occasional bouts of arthritis has been described; recurrent infection was not seen. (Haraldson et al., 1992; Van der Meer et al., 1984; Drenth et al., 1994) (see Chapter 11).

In allergic and parasitic disorders, IgE levels are markedly elevated. IgE levels above 50 IU/ml before age 1 year, above 100 IU/ml before age 2 years, or higher than 400 IU/ml after age 3 years are considered elevated (Wittig et al., 1980).

Natural Antibody Levels

The function of the antibody system can be assessed by measuring the antibody response to ubiquitous and injected antigens. Natural antibodies (those present without deliberate antigenic challenge) that are conveniently measured, in addition to anti-A and anti-B isoagglutinins, include the heterophile titer (antibody to sheep erythrocytes) and the streptolysin O titer. Nearly all normal individuals have antibodies at low titers (>1:10) to these antigens because of their widespread presence in food, inhaled particles, and the respiratory flora. Other natural antibodies that can be assayed are those to *E. coli* (Webster et al., 1974) or endotoxin (Gupta and Reed, 1968).

Specific Antibody Responses

If the patient has not been immunized with diphtheria or tetanus toxoids, immunization with these agents (two or three injections), followed by antibody titers within 2 to 3 weeks after the last injection, is the preferred test for antibody function. The antibody response to tetanus toxoid is particularly valuable because delayed cutaneous hypersensitivity and in vitro proliferative responses to tetanus antigen can also be assessed following vaccine, thus providing information on T-cell responsiveness (Borut et al., 1980). ELISAs to tetanus antibodies that measure both IgG and IgM responses are available.

The antibody response to *H. influenzae* type B vaccine is also of value. The newer conjugate vaccines produce a good antibody response even in infants younger than

1 year of age. Titers to tetanus, diphtheria, and *H. influenzae* are often used together in the immunized infants for the initial antibody screening.

The antibody response to typhoid vaccine can also be used to assess antibody function. These antibody titers are performed in most hospital laboratories. The antibody response to the H and O antigens measures IgG and IgM globulin function, respectively. Serum is obtained before and 3 weeks after three subcutaneous injections of 0.5 ml of typhoid vaccine (at 1- to 2-week intervals). Agglutinin titers to both antigens over 1:40 are normal; lower titers indicate poor antibody responses.

The antibody response to pneumococcal or meningococcal polysaccharide vaccines can also be used, particularly in subjects in whom the antibody response to polysaccharides is suspect (e.g., Wiskott-Aldrich syndrome, IgG2 subclass deficiency). The weak responses of normal infants to these antigens limit this procedure to children older than age 2 years.

The antibody response to viral antigens can also be assessed. Rubella or rubeola or varicella-zoster titers following measles-rubella vaccinations or following natural chickenpox infection are used. Antibody to hepatitis B virus following administration of vaccine is also of value. Poliomyelitis titers following vaccination are less valuable in our experience because of low postimmunization titers even in normal subjects. As noted elsewhere, live virus vaccines to test for immunodeficiency are contraindicated because of the risk of disseminated infection.

Other antigens used to assess antibody responses include the special antigens, keyhole-limpet hemocyanin (KLH), and the bacteriophage ϕX174. The antibody response to ϕX antigen clearance is an extremely sensitive test for low levels of antibody; both the primary and secondary responses can be identified (see Chapter 11).

Lateral Pharyngeal X-ray

A lateral radiograph of the pharynx may show a marked decrease in adenoidal tissues, indicative of poor lymphoid development and immunodeficiency (Baker et al., 1962). This finding was first described in Wiskott-Aldrich syndrome; it is also present in other antibody and cellular immunodeficiencies. By contrast, many immunologically normal children with recurrent upper respiratory tract infections have enlarged adenoids.

Biopsies

Biopsies are occasionally of value in patients with antibody immunodeficiencies if the diagnosis is equivocal; they are rarely necessary and entail some risk of infection at the biopsy site. A biopsy specimen should be obtained after local antigenic stimulation. A diphtheria-pertussis-tetanus (DPT) or typhoid immunization is given in the anterior thigh, and an inguinal node is obtained from the same side 5 to 7 days later. Lymph nodes are examined to assess the thymus-de-

pendent paracortical areas, the medullary plasma cells, and the cortical germinal centers. Immunofluorescent studies using antibodies to T- and B-cell surface antigens can identify the exact cells present in the biopsy.

Nodes from patients with antibody immunodeficiencies show a paucity of plasma cells, a diminished number of primary lymphoid follicles, a thin cortex, absence of germinal centers, and cellular disorganization. An increased number of histiocytes and other reticuloendothelial elements may be present. Biopsy results are especially valuable in immunodeficient patients with lymphadenopathy to exclude reticuloendothelial malignancy. In immunodeficiency with hyper-IgM and in Wiskott-Aldrich syndrome, the cervical lymph nodes are characteristically large with abundant plasma cells; however, the overall architecture is abnormal.

The rectal mucosa is the preferred biopsy site of some investigators (Davis et al., 1971). A decreased number of plasma cells in the lamina propria of the submucosa is noted in antibody deficiency. The diagnostic value of this procedure is enhanced if immunofluorescence for B cells and immunoglobulins is performed concomitantly.

Examination of the bone marrow in antibody deficiency also shows a paucity of plasma cells and sometimes of pre-B cells. The few plasma cells in normal marrow ($<0.1\%$) and the lack of precise morphologic criteria for differentiating plasma cells from other mononuclear cells limit the value of this procedure except to exclude other hematologic disorders.

Immunoglobulin Survival Studies

Metabolic studies are of value when it is suspected that immunoglobulin is being lost through the gastrointestinal tract or when there is hypercatabolism of IgG. This is suggested by hypoalbuminemia or the presence of alpha$_1$-antitrypsin in the stools. The easiest way to estimate IgG survival (in the presence of low IgG level) is to give a sufficient quantity of intravenous immunoglobulin (IVIG) to increase the IgG to a near-normal level. This may require up to 800 mg/kg of IVIG. Then daily IgG levels are obtained, and a curve of the disappearance rate can be constructed to estimate the IgG half-life.

For a more sophisticated and exact measurement, purified IgG (or IgM or IgA) isolated from the patient or another subject is radioiodinated and a tiny dose is injected intravenously (Waldmann and Strober, 1969). Serial blood samples are obtained for several weeks for radioactive measurements and immunoglobulin levels so that the catabolic rate can be calculated. The normal IgG half-life is 25 days; IgM and IgA half-lives are 5 and 7 days, respectively. The net synthetic rate of the immunoglobulin under study can be calculated and compared with normal values (see Chapter 3).

Secretory Antibody Studies

Secretory IgA deficiency occurs concomitantly with selective serum IgA deficiency (see Chapter 14). Most patients with selective IgA deficiency are asymptomatic; the absence of IgA in the secretions is usually compensated for by secretion of IgM (Brandtzaeg et al., 1968). Measurement of immunoglobulins in such secretions as saliva, tears, nasal fluid, or gastric juice is hampered by low concentrations, technical difficulty in obtaining the samples (particularly in uncooperative infants), and lack of normal values at each age. An easy way to obtain a saliva sample is to have the patient chew on a cotton ball; after it is saturated, it is compressed in a 5-ml syringe, and the filtrate is assessed for immunoglobulin levels. Salivary IgA levels are near normal by age 6 months.

The mean IgA globulin level in parotid secretions is 0.6 mg/dl (South et al., 1967); the IgG level is about 0.04 mg/dl (Brandtzaeg et al., 1968). Specific antibodies in secretions can be assessed, including natural antibodies (e.g., isoagglutinins) and viral antibodies after antigenic challenge (e.g., influenza or poliovirus antibodies) (see Chapter 8).

Advanced B-Cell Phenotyping

Advanced B-cell phenotyping that uses flow cytometry with two-color and three-color staining is of interest in patients with antibody deficiencies but who have detectable B cells. For example, Saxon et al. (1989) have identified a differentiation defect in B cells from some patients with common variable immunodeficiency. Often this requires activating the cells before analysis. These patients may also have abnormalities of regulatory T cells, identifiable by advanced T-cell phenotyping.

In Vitro Immunoglobulin Synthesis

The regulation of immunoglobulin synthesis and secretions can also be assessed in vitro in antibody deficiencies; the effect of autologous or normal T cells can also be measured (Waldmann et al., 1974; Buckley et al., 1976a). The B cells are incubated with pokeweed mitogen, and free (secreted) and bound immunoglobulins or specific antibody is measured by radioimmunoassay. Waldmann and coworkers (1974) have shown that T cells from some patients with common variable immunodeficiency suppress immunoglobulin synthesis of normal B cells.

Seeger and associates (1976) described a T–helper cell defect in a patient with combined immunodeficiency with B cells; addition of normal T cells to the patient's B cells activate immunoglobulin synthesis. B cells from patients with X-linked hyper-IgM syndrome can be stimulated to secrete IgG, IgA, and IgE when cultured with antibody to CD40 and cytokines (Durandy et al., 1993). These and other similar studies indicate that in certain immunodeficiencies T-cell regulatory subpopulations are abnormal.

Immunization with special antigens, such as φX174 or KLH, followed by in vitro studies of antibody synthesis is indicated under special circumstances. Characteristic abnormal primary or secondary antibody responses can occur in various immunodeficiencies. Administration of special antigens generally necessitates special permission from the institutional review board because they are not licensed vaccines and it is considered a research procedure.

Mutation Analysis

In patients suspected of having X-linked agammaglobulinemia or X-linked hyper-IgM syndrome, it is sometimes possible to evaluate the mutant gene, mutant transcript, or mutant gene product directly. Occasional patients have small deletions that can be detected by Southern blot analysis (Vetrie et al., 1993). Other patients have mutations that result in the absence of the transcript of interest (Tsukada et al., 1993). This is demonstrated by analyzing ribonucleic acid (RNA) from cells that should express the transcript with a probe that contains the gene. In many patients, however, the mutations permit the production of normal amounts of transcript of normal size. To detect the mutation in these patients, it is necessary to sequence the complementary deoxyribonucleic acid (cDNA) or genomic DNA for the gene.

Other Procedures

Immunoelectrophoresis or polysaccharide gel electrophoresis may disclose homogeneous immunoglobulins of limited electrophoretic heterogeneity (paraproteins) in certain antibody deficiencies, such as Wiskott-Aldrich syndrome, and in SCID patients who have undergone bone marrow transplantation. Abnormal κ/λ light chain ratios, low-molecular-weight IgM, autoimmune antibodies, and specific deletions of portions of the immunoglobulin molecule are also encountered in rare instances.

Tests for Cellular Immunodeficiencies

Initial Tests

Estimation of the total lymphocyte count and lymphocyte morphology is the first step in the diagnosis of cellular immunodeficiency. Serial lymphocyte counts must be done to establish the presence of significant (<1600/mm³) and persistent lymphopenia. Lymphocyte counts decrease with age; levels are very high in newborns and young infants (see Table 9–15).

Chest radiographs (posteroanterior and lateral views) to determine the presence of a thymic shadow should be obtained; a narrowing of the anterior mediastinum is suggestive of thymic hypoplasia. A right-sided aortic arch is often seen in congenital thymic hypoplasia (DiGeorge anomaly). Ultrasonograms of the chest may confirm absence of the thymus. If hereditary cellular or combined immunodeficiency disease is suspected in a neonate, it is particularly important to obtain an early chest x-ray prior to the development of infection or other stress that will shrink the thymus. We recommend a chest film immediately after the newborn is stabilized.

Skin Tests

Delayed cutaneous hypersensitivity tests are used to evaluate T-cell function by assessing pre-existing immunity to microbial agents or vaccine antigens. Cellular immunity to mumps, *Trichophyton*, purified protein derivative (PPD), *Candida albicans*, and fluid tetanus toxoid are measured by injecting 0.1 ml of these antigens intradermally and recording the erythema and induration at 24 and 48 hours. The antigens used include 0.1 ml of mumps skin test antigen (1 mg/ml solution),* PPD (intermediate strength), *Trichophyton* (1:30),† *Candida* (1:100),‡ fluid tetanus toxoid (1:100), or combined diphtheria-tetanus toxoid (DT) (1:100).‡ If the skin test results are negative, higher concentrations should be used; the PPD is repeated at second strength dilution, and the tetanus and *Candida* tests are repeated at 1:10 dilutions (Gordon et al., 1983). The use of tetanus toxoid as a skin test reagent is particularly valuable in infants and children (Borut et al., 1980). A multitest system (Merieux)§ with seven recall antigens already diluted is also available for delayed hypersensitivity screening (Corriel et al., 1985) and is particularly useful if only occasional office testing is performed.

Skin tests of children older than 2 years and nearly all adults will be positive for one or more of these antigens (Gordon et al., 1983). In individuals who show no positive skin test results, especially those with histories of mumps, tuberculosis, bacille Calmette-Guérin (BCG) injection, or tetanus immunization, cellular immunodeficiency is suspected. In children younger than 2 years of age, these skin tests are of limited value because of lack of prior sensitization. In the infant with long-standing thrush whose *Candida* skin test is negative, cellular immunodeficiency, of course, is suspected.

Active sensitization with 2,4-dinitrochlorobenzene (DNCB) has been used in the past to assess cellular immunity. Because unpleasant burns and scars may occur during sensitization, this procedure is recommended only in special circumstances. A vesicant dose of DNCB, 0.05 ml of a 10% solution in acetone (30% in adults) is applied to the volar surface of the forearm on a filter paper 1 cm in diameter. A test dose (0.05 ml of 0.1% solution of DNCB in acetone) is applied at the same time as a presensitization control. The filter papers are removed after 24 hours; the control is read at 48 hours after application for the degree of erythema, induration, and vesiculation. Patients are challenged 14 to 21 days later with the test dose. The filter paper (1 cm in diameter) is applied to a different area and kept in place for 24 hours; the reaction is read 48 hours after application. Skin reactions are graded as follows:

- (0), no reaction
- (+), erythema only
- (+ +), erythema and induration
- (+ + +), vesiculation
- (+ + + +), bullae and ulceration

Only (+ +) reactions or greater are accepted as evidence of sensitization. Subsequent testing is indicated if the initial test is negative. A positive result is seen in 95% of normal subjects.

T-Cell Subset Enumeration

The first advanced test for T-cell immunodeficiency is enumeration of the total number of T cells (CD3$^+$ cells) and major T-cell subsets (CD4$^+$ and CD8$^+$ cells) in the peripheral blood. Both the percentage and absolute number of these cells should be recorded and the ratio between CD4 and CD8 cells calculated. The percentage and the CD4:CD8 ratio tends to be more constant over a period of time and is of particular value in determining long-term trends. Absolute numbers of T cells, although dependent on the total white blood cell count, better reflect the degree of T-cell immunodeficiency.

Flow Cytometry

The preferred method for T-cell (and B-cell) enumeration is automated immunofluorescence with fluorochrome-tagged specific monoclonal antibodies and flow cytometry. Manual immunofluorescence techniques can be used, but they are laborious and imprecise. The flow cytometer, also known as the fluorescence-activated cell scanner, analyzes the properties of single cells as they pass through an orifice at high velocity. A laser beam is passed through each cell, and light scatter, absorption, and wave length are measured to determine the proportion of cells of different size, volume, granularity, and specific fluorescence.

To assess fluorescence, the cells are stained ahead of time with monoclonal antibodies with an attached fluorochrome. A fluorochrome is a dye (e.g., fluorescein, Texas red) that emits a certain wave length of light when activated by a beam of white light. The dye can be attached directly to a monoclonal antibody (direct fluorescence) or to an antibody to the mouse monoclonal antibody (indirect immunofluorescence). Using two or three different fluorochromes attached to different monoclonal antibodies, one can analyze cells for the presence of two or three different antigens simultaneously. The instrument can calculate the proportion of cells that are stained with one, two (dual-stained), or three (triple-stained) fluorochromes.

Current methods for CD3, CD4, CD8, and CD19 (B-cell) analysis may use whole blood. The erythrocytes, monocytes, and granulocytes can be "gated out" of the analysis electronically. For advanced flow cytometry simultaneously using multiple monoclonal antibodies, it is usually preferable to use isolated lymphocytes.

CD3, CD4, and CD8 Assays

The preferred cell marker to identify total T cells is CD3, an antigen associated with the T-cell receptor

---

*Mumps skin test antigen, Eli Lilly, Indianapolis, IN 46206.

†Hollister-Stier Laboratories, P.O. Box 3145, Terminal Annex, Spokane, WA 99220.

‡Pediatric diphtheria and tetanus toxoid, Wyeth Laboratories, P.O. Box 8299, Philadelphia, PA 19101.

§Merieux, distributed by Connaught Laboratories, Swiftwater, PA 18370.

complex present on all mature T cells. Other markers used for total T cells are CD2 and CD5 (see Table 9–14); these are less specific because some NK and B cells share these antigens. Normal values of CD3$^+$ T cells are given (see Table 9–15); T-cell numbers are greatly increased in newborns and young infants, so that values must be compared with age-matched normals.

CD3 cells are further divided into CD4 *helper/inducer* and CD8 *suppressor/cytotoxic phenotypes* using monoclonal antibodies to these antigens. Within each of these subdivisions are phenotypic and functionally distinct subtypes based on the presence of other antigens; most CD8$^+$ suppressor cells stain with CD11, whereas CD8$^+$ cytotoxic cells are usually CD11$^-$. Since CD4 and CD8 are also expressed on other (non-T) cells, the recommended way to enumerate CD4 and CD8 T cells is to enumerate CD3$^+$ cells that are CD4$^+$ and CD8$^+$; this requires dual staining techniques. Normal levels of T-cell subsets by age are given in Table 9–15.

The best single laboratory test to assess the T-cell system is the total number of T-helper/inducer (CD3$^+$, CD4$^+$) cells. A CD4 count of less than 500 cells is generally associated with impaired cellular immunity; profound depression is associated with a CD4 count less than 200 cells. A CD4:CD8 ratio is also of some value; ratios less than 1.0 are abnormal, and ratios less than 0.3 are associated with profound T-cell deficiency. The CD4:CD8 ratio is independent of the total leukocyte count and is of particular value in following HIV infection. In children with common variable immunodeficiency, the CD4:CD8 ratio is often increased as a result of decreased CD8 cells (Conley et al., 1986).

Early studies measured total T cells by their ability to form rosettes with fresh sheep erythrocytes. (WHO/IARC, 1974). These are termed *erythrocyte rosette–forming cells*. Rosetting is based on the presence of the sheep-cell receptor (CD2 antigen) on most T cells (and some natural killer cells), but the technique is laborious and less precise than immunofluorescence with monoclonal antibodies. E-rosetting is still used in the laboratory to isolate T cells.

Lymphocyte Proliferation

Cellular immunity is also evaluated by determining the ability of the patient's lymphocytes to proliferate and enlarge (transform) in vitro under the influence of antigens, allogeneic cells, mitogens such as phytohemagglutinin (PHA) or pokeweed (Oppenheim et al., 1975), or monoclonal antibodies to T–cell surface antigens involved in signal transduction (e.g., CD3, CD28, CD43). Mitogens activate lymphocytes nonspecifically by receptors on the cell membrane (Table 9–17).

Lymphocyte reactivity can be assayed morphologically or by measuring the incorporation of radioactive thymidine into dividing cells. In the latter assay, a known number of peripheral blood mononuclear cells are cultured under sterile conditions in the presence of mitogen (and saline control). Such preparations contain monocytes, which are necessary for antigen processing and lymphocyte activation. After 48 to 72 hours (5 to 7 days for allogeneic cells or antigens) at 37°C, the cells are harvested. In the morphologic assay, the cells are exposed to hypotonic media, fixed on slides, stained, and counted; the number of transformed cells should exceed 50%; less than this suggests defective cellular immunity.

Alternatively, tritiated thymidine is added to the 72-hour culture and incubated 6 more hours. The cells or their nucleic acids are separated from the incubation mixture, washed, and counted in a scintillation counter to determine incorporation of labeled precursor into DNA. The absolute count and the ratio of counts to the unstimulated control (the *stimulation index*) are recorded. The stimulation index of PHA-activated lymphocytes should be at least 20 to 100, but comparison with controls for each laboratory must be used.

The lymphocytes from patients with profound cellular immunodeficiencies may show no increase in thymidine incorporation with PHA, whereas others have intermediate values. Using PHA at several dilutions may aid in identifying patients with partial immune defects (Oppenheim et al., 1970).

Techniques for using whole blood to measure mitogen responsiveness have been developed but are considerably less sensitive (Fletcher et al., 1987). Newer techniques that assess lymphocyte proliferation by the appearance of activation antigens using flow cytometry (e.g., IL-2 receptor [CD25]) or by the in vitro production of IL-2 are also available (Prince and John, 1986).

The response to mitogens does not indicate the ability to respond to specific antigens; this can be determined by substituting allogeneic lymphocytes (from an unrelated person) or an antigen to which the patient

Table 9–17. T- and B-Cell Stimulants

T-Cell Stimulants	T-Dependent B-Cell Stimulants	T-Independent B-Cell Stimulants
Phytohemagglutinin	Pokeweed mitogen	Endotoxin
Concanavalin-A	Polysaccharides	Anti-immunoglobulin
Pokeweed mitogen	Antigens (e.g., PPD, bacteria, viruses, fungi)	Epstein-Barr virus
Alloantigens (DR)		Staphylococcal protein A
Anti-CD3 monoclonal antibody		*Nocardia* mitogen
Antithymocyte and antilymphocyte globulin		
Antigens (e.g., PPD, bacteria, virus, fungi)		
Superantigens (e.g., staphylococcal enterotoxin)		

Abbreviations: DR = major histocompatibility complex class II antigen; PPD = purified protein derivative.

has been previously exposed. Allogeneic lymphocytes are treated with mitomycin or x-irradiation so that they cannot react to the cells being tested in the mixed leukocyte culture (MLC). Every normal individual reacts to histocompatibility antigens that he or she lacks, even without prior sensitization (a positive MLC). A positive stimulation index in an MLC and in an antigen-stimulated culture is usually 2 to 20, considerably less than the response to a mitogen.

Because the response to a specific antigen requires prior sensitization, it indicates cellular immunodeficiency only when prior contact with the antigen has been established. For example, a failure of response to *Candida* antigen in a patient with widespread mucocutaneous candidiasis indicates a T-cell defect to this antigen. Superantigens can also be used to assess lymphocyte proliferation. Superantigens are bacterial products (e.g., staphylococcal toxins) that stimulate a large fraction of T cells without prior sensitization (Takei et al., 1993).

Because serum factors may modulate the response to mitogens or antigens, a decreased proliferative response may be further studied by culturing the washed lymphocytes in the presence of normal serum. If this improves the response and if the addition of the patient's serum depresses the response of normally responsive lymphocytes, an inhibitor is present. This inhibition can be specific—that is, to one or a few related antigens—or nonspecific. Specific inhibitors are usually antibodies to the antigens; they have been observed in miliary tuberculosis, atypical measles, and mucocutaneous candidiasis (Oppenheim et al., 1975).

Nonspecific inhibitors include antibodies directed against lymphocytes; they may occur in systemic lupus erythematosus, pregnancy, and multitransfused blood recipients. Nonspecific inhibitors, poorly characterized but nonantibody in nature, are seen in uremia, certain malignancies, leprosy, hepatitis, and ataxia-telangiectasia.

Cytokine and Cytokine Receptor Assays

Cytokines are low-molecular-weight (20,000 to 30,000 MW) proteins or glycoproteins produced primarily by immune cells that affect many cells in an antigen-nonspecific fashion through specific cell surface receptors (see Appendix 2). They can be considered the hormones of the immune system. One cytokine can have multiple biologic functions and multiple cytokines can have overlapping biologic functions. The cytokines include the interleukins (IL-1 to IL-15), the hematopoietic colony-stimulating factors (CSFs), the interferons (IFNs α, β, and γ), tumor necrosis factors (TNFs α and β), and various growth factors, such as transforming growth factor–β (TGF-β), platelet-derived growth factor, epidermal growth factor and fibroblast growth factor. Some cytokines induce differentiation and maturation; others augment inflammatory responses and recruit other cells; and some have direct effects in other cells (e.g., promote viral resistance, lyse tumor cells). Some are made by specific cells (e.g., IL-5 by activated T-helper cells), whereas others are

made by a variety of cells. Because of their low molecular weight, they usually have very brief lives in the circulation and thus are measured in cultures of stimulated cells.

Elevations of some cytokines can be detected transiently in the blood after therapeutic administration, during the acute phase of an illness, or in certain chronic infections. They can also be elevated in body fluids, such as joint fluid or cerebrospinal fluid.

The four most common cytokine assays used clinically are IL-1, IL-2, TNF-α, and IFN-γ (Table 9–18). Biological and commercial radioimmunoassays are available. Assays are generally performed on leukocyte cultures following mitogen or antigen activation. Production of IL-2 is decreased in many T-cell immunodeficiencies, including HIV (Prince et al., 1984). A small number of children with SCID have a specific defect in IL-2 production (Weinberg and Parkman, 1990). A primary defect in the production of IFN-γ has also been reported in a few children (Lipinski et al., 1980). IL-1 and TNF-α levels are increased in HIV and the CSF of several central nervous system disorders (e.g., meningitis) (Saez-Llorens et al., 1990; Arditi et al., 1991).

The cytokine profile has been used to define T_H1 and T_H2 responses in various diseases, particularly AIDS. T_H1 responses are characterized by IL-2, IFN-γ, and IL-12 secretion and are associated with a cellular (T-cell) immune response, whereas T_H2 responses are characterized by IL-4, IL-5, IL-6, and IL-10 secretion with enhanced antibody responses and suppression of T_H1 responses (see Chapter 2).

Because of the increased availability of these assays, cytokine abnormalities in various immunodeficiencies will be further identified.

Receptor Assays

Soluble cytokine and leukocyte antigen receptor assays are available for several factors, including IL-2 receptor, TFN-γ receptor, soluble CD4, soluble CD8, soluble CD23, soluble Fc receptor (FcR), and soluble intracellular adhesion molecule (ICAM-1 [CD54]). Assays of serum, plasma, body fluids (e.g., cerebrospinal fluid, joint fluid), or supernatants of active lymphocytes can be done by radioimmunoassay. Alterations are present in a wide variety of inflammatory diseases, autoimmune diseases, and graft-versus-host disease. Since these factors are regulators of the immune system, alterations in many immunodeficiencies may be expected. For example, Jyonouchi and coworkers (1991) found normal levels of soluble FcεRII in the serum of patients with common variable immunodeficiency but elevated levels in the serum of patients with ectodermal dysplasia.

Cytotoxic Assays

Determining the ability of a mononuclear cell to lyse a target is a valuable assay of lymphocyte function. In these assays, a target cell is isotopically labeled (e.g., with ^{51}Cr), and the amount of radioactivity released after exposure to the effector cell is used as a measure

Table 9–18. Cytokines Used in Clinical Immunology

Cytokine	Principal Cell Source	Principal Action	Comment
IL-1	MΦ, other cells	Stimulates T cells, augments inflammation, fever	↑ in inflammatory diseases, infections
IL-2	T, NK	T and B growth factor; LAK, NK stimulant	↓ in T cell IDD, HIV
IL-4	T	B-cell, IgE stimulant	↑ in hyper IgE
IL-5	T	B-cell, eosinophil, IgA stimulant	↑ in eosinophilia
IL-6	Multiple cells	B-cell stimulant	↑ in HIV, Castleman's disease
TNF-α	T	Augments inflammation, tumoricidal	↑ in inflammatory diseases
IFN-α	Leukocytes	Antiviral	↓ in hepatitis, cancer
IFN-β	Fibroblasts	Antiviral	↓ in hepatitis, cancer
IFN-γ	T, NK	Antiviral, immune enhancer	↓ in IFN-IDD

Abbreviations: IDD = immunodeficiency disease; IFN = interferon; Ig = immunoglobulin; IL = interleukin; LAK = lymphokine-activated killer cells; MΦ = macrophage; NK = natural killer cells; TNF = tumor necrosis factor.

of cell lysis. Several types of cytotoxicity have been identified (Table 9–19) based on the effector cell involved, the type of target cell lysed, and the participation of soluble factors (e.g., antibodies, interferon, interleukins).

Natural killer (NK) cells are non-T, non-B, large granular lymphocytes that lyse tumor or viral-infected target cells without presensitization. These cells are identified by the CD16 and CD56 antigens (and sometimes CD57), using monoclonal antibodies or lysis of the K562 tumor cell line (Table 9–20). Natural killer deficiency is present in some patients with SCID, AIDS, Chédiak-Higashi syndrome, leukocyte adhesion defect type 1, X-linked lymphoproliferative syndrome, lymphohistiocytosis syndrome, Griscelli syndrome, and primary NK deficiency (Stiehm, 1992). In two patients with SCID, levels of NK cells were unusually high (Sindel et al., 1984).

Antibody-dependent cellular cytotoxicity (ADCC) involves lysis of an antibody coated target cell. The nonspecific effector cell is often termed a *killer cell*, although the cell has an NK phenotype. The specificity of the cytotoxic reaction comes from the antibody coat.

Sanel and Buckley (1978), using antibody-coated human lymphocytes as targets, noted profound ADCC defects in X-linked agammaglobulinemia and combined immunodeficiency; using human lymphocytes or chicken or human erythrocytes as targets, they noted less severe ADCC defects in common variable immunodeficiency and immunodeficiency with hyper-IgM. Albrecht and Hong (1976) noted decreased cytotoxicity toward antibody-coated human erythrocytes in primary monocyte defects. Patients with leukocyte adhesion defect–1 also exhibit low ADCC (and NK) because their effector cells do not adhere well to target cells.

Antigen-specific cytotoxic T-cell reactions, in which CD8+ T cells have been presensitized to a virus or an alloantigen (cell-mediated lympholysis) are deficient in primary cellular immunodeficiencies, such as SCID and ataxia-telangiectasia, and in severe viral infection. Antigen-nonspecific cytotoxic reactions of T cells include lectin-dependent cytotoxicity (Lubens et al., 1982) and lymphokine-activated cytotoxicity (Grimm and Rosenberg, 1984). These cytotoxic reactions tend to be decreased in newborns, in patients with cellular immunodeficiency, and in patients following bone marrow ablative procedures.

Enzyme Assays

When combined immunodeficiency is suspected, assays should be performed for adenosine deaminase (ADA) and purine nucleoside phosphorylase (PNP), inasmuch as absence of these enzymes identifies variants of autosomal recessive combined immunodeficiency (Meuwissen et al., 1975; Giblett et al., 1975). ADA catalyzes the conversion of adenosine to inosine, and PNP catalyzes the conversion of inosine to hypoxanthine. Their absence may lead to intracellular accumulation of adenosine, inosine, deoxyadenosine, and deoxyinosine, which exert an immunosuppressive action (see Chapter 12). Radiologic abnormalities of the ribs and long bones may be seen in patients with this type of enzymatic deficiency. ADA and PNP are best

Table 9–19. Types of Cytotoxic Reactions

Types	Cell	Activating or Enhancing Agent	Specificity
Natural killer (NK)	NK (CD16, CD56)	Interferon	Nonspecific
Antibody-dependent cellular cytotoxicity	NK, (M/MΦ), granulocyte	IgG antibody on target surface	Specificity dependent on antibody
Cytotoxic T cell	T	Viral or tumor antigens, haptens	Specific, HLA-restricted
Cell-mediated lympholysis	T	Alloantigens	Specific, HLA-restricted
Lymphokine-activated	K, NK, T, M/MΦ	IL-2	Nonspecific
Lectin-dependent	K, T, M/MΦ	Mitogens	Nonspecific

Abbreviations: HLA = human leukocyte antigen; Ig = immunoglobulin; IL = interleukin; K = killer cell; M/MΦ = monocyte/macrophage.

Table 9–20. Age-related Changes in Natural Killer Cells and Natural Killer Lytic Activity

| Age | n | Phenotypic Markers | | | | | | K562 Lysis* | |
| | | CD16 | | CD56 | | CD57 | | | |
		%	CELLS/ul	%	CELLS/ul	%	CELLS/ul	n	%
Birth	11	13.8 ± 4.3	709 ± 316	9.1 ± 4.3	481 ± 198	1.2 ± 0.7	60 ± 40	26	15 ± 6
1–5 mo	6	12.7 ± 4.6	790 ± 352	10.6 ± 5.4	627 ± 308	1.4 ± 0.8	80 ± 40	7	36 ± 12
6–12 mo	7	12.5 ± 4.9	714 ± 300	12.2 ± 6.0	676 ± 295	1.7 ± 1.5	120 ± 110	12	42 ± 9
1–4 yr	8	12.9 ± 4.6	573 ± 264	13.1 ± 5.6	586 ± 310	2.6 ± 1.9	120 ± 90	23	41 ± 8
5–8 yr	6	14.4 ± 5.2	418 ± 134	15.0 ± 6.7	431 ± 181	12.5 ± 6.7	360 ± 170	13	40 ± 8
9–13 yr	7	15.2 ± 4.2	408 ± 196	16.5 ± 5.9	438 ± 181	15.8 ± 6.9	410 ± 190	19	38 ± 8
Adult	12	15.5 ± 5.4	318 ± 191	16.4 ± 6.5	343 ± 214	20.5 ± 5.5	400 ± 150	42	38 ± 8

Values are means ± 1 SD.
*Percent specific lysis of K562 tumor cells using a 20:1 target/effector ratio and a 4-hr chromium release assay.
Data derived from Yabuhara A, Kawai H, Komiyama A. Development of natural killer cytotoxicity during childhood: Marked increases in number of natural killer cells with adequate cytotoxic abilities during infancy to early childhood. Pediatr Res 28:316–322, 1990.

measured on hemolyzed erythrocytes (Scott et al., 1974). Heterozygotes have half-normal levels. Intra-uterine diagnosis of ADA deficiency has been accomplished by showing decreased levels in cultured amniotic fluid cells (Hirschhorn et al., 1975). A complete discussion is presented in Chapter 12.

Several infants with deficiency of biotin-dependent carboxylase have been noted to have T-cell immunodeficiency, primarily manifested by mild mucocutaneous candidiasis (Cowan et al., 1979). Biotin is necessary for the catabolism of isoleucine and leucine; its absence causes organic aciduria with alopecia and central nervous system abnormalities.

HLA Typing

HLA typing is of value to identify potential bone marrow transplant donors; siblings and parents are HLA typed along with the patient. A mixed leukocyte culture (MLC) between individuals of the same HLA type can confirm the existence of HLA identity between the patient and the donor.

HLA typing can also be used to detect *chimerism.* Certain infants with profound T-cell deficiencies may have lymphoid chimerism as a result of engraftment of maternal cells in utero or engraftment from a blood or plasma transfusion (Kadowaki et al., 1965; Parkman et al., 1974). In some infants, there is evidence of graft-versus-host disease with alopecia, rash, diarrhea, hepatitis, and gastrointestinal disturbances but in most the engraftment is silent.

The presence of more than two HLA antigens at any one locus or HLA antigens not present in either parent usually indicates engraftment with a second population of cells, either from the mother or from a blood donor. A few instances of multiple weak HLA antigens not caused by chimerism have been reported in SCID (Terasaki et al., 1972). Some patients with SCID have no class I or class II antigens, which is the bare lymphocyte syndrome (Touraine et al., 1978; Touraine and Betuel, 1983; Klein et al., 1993; de la Salle et al., 1994).

Karyotype analysis or DNA studies can also be used to identify chimerism or engraftment (Conley et al., 1984).

Chromosome Analysis

Chromosome analysis is of value in the diagnosis of certain immunodeficiencies, notably the DiGeorge anomaly and ataxia-telangiectasia (see Chapter 12). Chimerism may also be diagnosed by the simultaneous presence of XX and XY cell lines in routine chromosome counts of peripheral blood. If there is no response to PHA, there may be an insufficient number of mitoses for karyotyping, and severe combined immunodeficiency should be suspected. HLA typing can also be used to detect chimerism.

Biopsies

Biopsies may also be helpful in the exact diagnosis of cellular immunodeficiency. Bone marrow and lymph node biopsies were discussed earlier. A lymph node biopsy is of value in cellular immunodeficiency if the laboratory evaluation is equivocal. However, there is some risk of infection, particularly if a specimen is obtained in the groin area. The lymph node architecture of patients with cellular immunodeficiency shows considerable disorganization without a clear demarcation between cortical and medullary areas. Germinal centers are absent, and the lymphoid follicles are rudimentary. Lymphoid and plasma cells may be entirely absent if there is a combined B-cell and T-cell defect. Stromal cells, monocytes, and histiocytes predominate. Criteria for morphologic assessment of lymph nodes have been published (Cottier et al., 1972). Immunohistologic study to identify T and B subsets within the lymph nodes may help to identify the immunopathogenesis of the disorder.

A thymic biopsy can also provide useful diagnostic and therapeutic information in special cases. This type of biopsy should be performed by someone with special skills in the procedure. There is not complete correlation between thymic morphology and functional capacity (Borzy et al., 1979b). Autopsies of children with suspected immunodeficiency should always include a histologic examination of the thymus gland, lymph nodes, and lymphatic tissue of the gastrointestinal system.

Intestinal biopsy can provide valuable information in the presence of a protein-losing enteropathy and may aid in establishing an exact diagnosis, such as intestinal lymphangiectasia or infiltrative disorder. Organisms such as *Cryptosporidia* and *Giardia* can also be identified.

A skin biopsy is sometimes of value in immunodeficiency when graft-versus-host disease is suspected or when histiocytosis X or another dermatosis must be excluded.

Thymic Hormone Assays

Several factors from thymic epithelial cells with biologic activity have been isolated, including thymulin, thymosin, thymopoietin, and *facteur thymique sérique* (FTS) (Hadden, 1993). Radioimmunoassays for thymosin and bioassays for FTS and thymopoietin have been reported but are not generally available (Dardenne and Bach, 1975; Incefy et al., 1977; Goldstein et al., 1966).

Thymic hormone levels are typically high at birth and early childhood, decreasing slowly with age. Thymic hormones are absent or greatly depressed in combined immunodeficiency and the DiGeorge anomaly (Lewis et al., 1977). For atypical patients in which these diagnoses are being considered, assay of thymic activity may be of some diagnostic value. Serial assays may also be of use in following response to reconstitution or other therapies.

Cell Activation Analysis

A complete analysis of certain T-cell immunodeficiencies requires assessment of T-cell activation, including the integrity of the T-cell receptor (TCR) and the signal transduction pathway (Gelfand, 1993). Defects in T-cell activation or the TCR have been reported in a few patients with T-cell immunodeficiencies (Alarcon et al., 1988; Rijkers et al., 1991; Arpaia et al., 1994; Le Deist et al., 1995). Such patients may have normal numbers of T cells and variable susceptibility to infection but poor proliferative responses to mitogens, antigens, or anti–CD3 monoclonal antibody (Stiehm, 1993).

T-cell activation includes antigen processing and presentation, an intact TCR, participation by CD45 phosphatase, inositol phospholipid turnover, translocation of protein kinase C (PKC) from cytosol to the plasma membrane, and activation of several protein tyrosine kinases (PTKs) (see Chapter 2). The PKC and PTK pathways are linked insofar as phospholipase C, which initiates phospholipid turnover, requires tyrosine phosphorylation for its activation. Phospholipase C converts phosphatidylinositol 4,5-diphosphate (PIP_2) to inositol 1,4,5-triphosphate (IP_3), and diacylglycerol (DG). IP_3 leads to intracellular Ca^{2+} mobilization, and DG activates phosphokinase C.

These alterations open the Ca^{2+} channels and this in turn activates IL-2 gene expression in conjunction with a nuclear factor (NF-AT). Finally, IL-2 receptor expression occurs. IL-2 gene transcription also requires the participation of several proto-oncogenes (e.g., *C-Fos, C-Jun*), a tyrosine protein kinase, and TCR ζ-chain phosphorylation.

Assessment of activation utilizes various stimulants or inhibitors, such as phorbol myristate acetate (PMA), ionophores, and CD3 antisera, which stimulate or bypass certain pathways. Following these steps, IL-2 production, IL-2 receptor expression, intracellular calcium, biochemical events (enzyme levels, cyclic adenosine monophosphate [cAMP] levels), and specific DNA and RNA assays for various components (e.g., ζ-chains of CD3, IL-2, PTK) are performed. Such assays are available in only a few research laboratories.

Alternate activation pathways may also exist. For example, activation of CD43 (sialophorin) by anti-CD43 antibody occurs and can be abnormal in Wiskott-Aldrich syndrome. CD28 activation by anti-CD28 antibody can also be assessed; this is an important coreceptor for cellular growth versus tolerance or apoptosis.

Tests for Phagocytic Deficiencies

Initial Tests

An investigation for phagocytic and complement disorders is indicated when a patient with a convincing history of recurrent bacterial infections is shown to have normal antibody (B-cell) and cellular (T-cell) function. The screening tests for a phagocytic disorder (involving either granulocytes or monocytes) include the total WBC count, the differential, the morphologic appearance of the granulocytes and monocytes, the nitroblue tetrazolium (NBT) dye reduction test, and an IgE level (see Table 9–10).

A white blood cell count consistently below 3000/mm^3 or above 12,000/mm^3 is abnormal. Patients with leukocyte adhesion defect–1 have persistent leukocytosis. Leukopenia, unusual vacuolization, or the presence of myelocytes in the peripheral blood should be investigated further by bone marrow aspiration. Toxic Döhle bodies are present in the granulocytes of patients with severe infections; the presence of these cells may be correlated with poor chemotaxis.

Nitroblue Tetrazolium Test

The NBT dye test for chronic granulomatous diseases (CGDs) is based on the increased metabolic activity of normal granulocytes during phagocytosis and on the absence of such an increase in CGD. Although nonphagocytizing leukocytes slowly reduce colorless NBT to purple formazan, addition of latex particles to normal leukocytes markedly increases the rate of dye reduction. This color change can be estimated visually, microscopically, or spectrophotometrically. The leukocytes of patients with CGD or leukocyte glucose-6-phosphate dehydrogenase (G6PD) deficiency cannot reduce NBT in the normal fashion; this defect is correlated with their inability to generate superoxide and hydrogen peroxide and to kill certain microorganisms.

The simplest NBT screening test is a histochemical slide test in which resting (unstimulated) leukocytes are incubated with NBT, and the percentage of granulocytes containing formazan granules is estimated microscopically (Park et al., 1969). This test can be made more sensitive by using an endotoxin-coated slide (Ochs and Igo, 1973). In normal subjects, the percentage of NBT-positive granulocytes is above 90%; patients with CGD have less than 1% NBT-positive granulocytes.

In another screening test, peripheral leukocytes in autologous plasma are incubated with NBT and latex particles; a normal result is indicated by the appearance of bluish-purple granules in the leukocytes and a change in the color of the supernatant from yellow to gray or purple. An abnormal finding consists of the complete absence of blue or purple color in the granules or supernatant after 25 minutes (Johnston, 1969).

IgE Levels

Elevated levels of IgE are seen in several phagocytic deficiency syndromes, particularly those with chemotactic defects (see Chapter 13). The finding of a high IgE (see Table 9–13 for normal standards) in the presence of recurrent infection should signal the need for an evaluation of leukocyte mobility.

Chemiluminescence

Allen and associates (1972) showed that human neutrophils during phagocytosis produce chemiluminescence (chemically produced light). A direct correlation between chemiluminescence and intracellular bacterial killing was suggested when Stjernholm and colleagues (1973) demonstrated that granulocytes from patients with chronic granulomatous disease produced no chemiluminescence during phagocytosis of opsonized bacteria.

During phagocytosis, normal neutrophils and monocytes produce free oxygen radicals, including singlet oxygen, hydroxyl radical, superoxide, and hydrogen peroxide (see Chapter 5). These react with oxidizable substrates on microbes, such as unsaturated lipids, nucleic acids, and peptides, to form unstable intermediates. When these intermediates return to their ground state, light energy measurable as chemiluminescence is released (Allen et al., 1972).

Because chemiluminescence is readily measured with a beta-scintillation spectrophotometer or a chemiluminometer, it has become a valuable assay of oxidative metabolism during phagocytosis and an aid in the diagnosis of CGD (Johnston et al., 1975a). It is a sensitive and reliable way to diagnose the CGD carrier state (Mills et al., 1978). An increased chemiluminescent response to soluble stimuli (e.g., phorbol myristate acetate) but a reduced one to particulate stimuli (e.g., zymosan) is characteristic of leukocyte adhesion defect–1 (see Chapter 15) (Anderson et al., 1984).

White Blood Cell Turnover

In neutropenic states, particularly when the bone marrow shows myeloid precursors, serial WBC counts should be done to determine the presence of cyclic neutropenia. Then the peripheral WBC response to the administration of corticosteroids, epinephrine, or endotoxin can be tested (Cline et al., 1976). The response to corticosteroid measures bone marrow reserve, whereas the response to epinephrine and endotoxin assesses the marginating pool (Metcalf et al., 1986). If increased leukocyte destruction is suggested by an active marrow, the presence of leukocyte antibodies should be sought (Lalezari and Bernard, 1966). A trial of intravenous immunoglobulin to evaluate whether such treatment can correct the neutropenia should be considered (Pollack et al., 1982).

Special Morphology

Staining of granulocytes by histochemical techniques is used to demonstrate alkaline phosphatase, myeloperoxidase, and esterase activities. Absence of these enzymes should be followed by quantitative assays for each enzyme. Whereas ordinary light microscopy has the capability of detecting certain intrinsic disorders of granulocytes (such as bilobed nuclei and the giant vacuoles of Chédiak-Higashi syndrome), phase and electron microscopy are able to detect defects in granule formation, spreading, pseudopod formation, and mobility as seen in specific granule deficiency or leukocyte adhesion defect type 1 (Anderson et al., 1984).

Bone marrow aspiration can be done to assess the morphology of the granulocyte precursors, to exclude other hematopoietic disorders, and to obtain a culture for unusual organisms.

Random Mobility and Chemotaxis

Random mobility and chemotaxis assays are usually performed on granulocytes, but purified monocytes and eosinophils can also be studied. The three assays used are the Boyden chamber technique; the double microfilter radioimmunoassay, using ^{51}Cr-labeled cells; and the under agarose/gel plate technique. In the Boyden procedure (Boyden, 1962), isolated granulocytes are placed in the upper chamber, separated by a Millipore filter from a chemotactic stimulus placed in the lower chamber. The number of cells migrating toward a chemotactic stimulus (or spontaneously, in random migration) is assessed by microscopy of the lower side of the filter. The counting procedure can be automated by use of an image analyzer. Alternatively, the radioactivity in the lower filter can be assessed as an indicator of the number of migrating cells (Gallin et al., 1973).

Random mobility and chemotaxis can also be assessed under agarose gel from a well toward a second well filled with a chemotactic factor (Nelson et al., 1975). The usual chemotactic stimulus is human serum to which endotoxin, zymosan, or antigen-antibody complexes have been added; these stimuli cause C3 and C5 to release the low-molecular-weight peptides C3a and C5a, which are strong chemotactic substances. Other chemotactic substances are particle-activated plasma (through release of kallikrein and plasminogen activator), bacteria, or lymphocyte-derived chemotactic factor from antigen-activated lymphocytes. Chemotactic values must be compared with age-matched controls.

Monocyte chemotactic abnormalities are less common but have been observed in one form of candidiasis (Snyderman et al., 1973), in Wiskott-Aldrich syndrome (Altman et al., 1974), and in newborns (Klein et al., 1977).

Chemotactic defects are usually secondary to an intrinsic defect of the cell, but occasionally a serum inhibitor of chemotaxis can be implicated in some patients with primary immunodeficiency, Hodgkin's disease, and cirrhosis (Ward and Schlegel, 1969; Miller, 1975).

Phagocytosis Assays

Phagocytosis measures the ability of granulocytes or other cells to recognize and ingest particles or microbial agents. Phagocytes show considerable selectivity as to which particles they will ingest; this depends on the surface of the particle, its age (particularly erythrocytes), and the presence of substances that resist ingestion, such as the capsules of certain microorganisms. Particles that are coated with antibody or complement are engulfed with much greater avidity, primarily because phagocytes have Fc and complement receptors. Indeed, most phagocytic disorders are the result of opsonic defects rather than intrinsic abnormalities of the leukocytes.

Opsonic defects are tested by using the patient's serum with normal granulocytes in a phagocytic assay. In the phagocytic assay, the patient's isolated leukocytes, in the presence of normal serum, are exposed to particles (baker's yeast, polystyrene beads, paraffin-oil particles), microorganisms, or radiolabeled immune complexes, and ingestion is assessed by microscopy (for baker's yeast, polystyrene, or bacteria) (Miller and Nilsson, 1970), spectrophotometry (paraffin-oil particles) (Stossel, 1973), or scintillation counting (labeled bacteria, immune complexes) (Keusch et al., 1972).

Because ingestion must precede killing, a phagocytic defect is indirectly excluded if leukocyte microbial killing is present.

Bactericidal Assays

The most definitive test for a functional defect of the granulocytes is the quantitative bacterial killing assay of Quie and associates (1967). This test is used to measure serum opsonic activity, phagocytosis, and bactericidal activity. Peripheral blood leukocytes are isolated, washed, counted, and suspended in a medium containing normal serum (as an opsonic source) and an equal number of freshly grown bacteria (usually *Staphylococcus aureus*, *E. coli*, or *Serratia marcescens*). During incubation and agitation at 37°C for 2 hours, aliquots are removed at 0, 30, 60, and 120 minutes from the leukocyte-bacteria suspension, and the number of viable bacteria is assayed by pour-plate technique. After 120 minutes, the mixture is centrifuged so that the leukocytes (and any phagocytized bacteria) are in the cell button and free bacteria are in the supernatant.

Both the cell button and the supernatant are then assayed for viable bacteria.

Leukocytes from a normal subject phagocytize and kill 95% of the bacteria within 120 minutes. Leukocytes from a patient with chronic granulomatous disease kill less than 10% of the bacteria in this period; further, the viable bacteria are within the leukocyte, indicating that phagocytosis has occurred but that intracellular killing is deficient. In a phagocytic defect, killing is deficient, but the viable bacteria remain in the supernatant fluid. An opsonic defect can also be identified with this assay by using normal cells and the test serum as an opsonic source.

Alternatively, histochemical and autoradiographic methods are available to obtain semiquantitative estimates of killing by individual cells of fungi (Lehrer and Cline, 1969a) or bacteria (Cline, 1973).

Adhesion Molecule Assays

Adhesion molecule assays should be done when two syndromes associated with defective leukocyte adhesion (leukocyte adhesion defect types 1 and 2 [LAD-1,-2]) are suspected (see Chapter 15). Both are characterized by leukocytosis, recurrent soft tissue infections, and defective chemotaxis. LAD-1, the most common form, is associated with a deficiency of leukocyte function–associated antigen–1 (LFA-1) integrin. Integrins are a group of structurally related heterodimer molecules (an α and a β chain) on various leukocytes responsible for cell-cell and cell-tissue interactions. In LAD-2 there is a deficiency of a leukocyte ligand for selectin; a selectin is an adhesive molecule related to epidermal growth factor present on endothelial cells that adheres to leukocytes (Etzioni et al., 1992).

Defects of these glycoproteins on the granulocyte surface are best assessed by flow cytometry using specific monoclonal antibodies. In LAD-1 there is a deficiency of both CD11b (CR3–Mac-1) and CD18, the α and β chains, respectively, of LFA-1. In LAD-2 an anti–sialyl-Lewis X monoclonal antibody can be used to identify a defect in the selectin ligand (see Chapter 15).

The degree of deficiency of the LFA-1 molecule can be used to identify mild and severe phenotypes and heterozygotes of LAD-1. Leukocyte activation by ionophore prior to flow cytometry can greatly enhance the expression of these glycoproteins in order to magnify the differences between healthy subjects and patients (Todd et al., 1988).

Rebuck Skin Window

The Rebuck skin window is an in vivo procedure to assess the mobility of leukocytes. Defects of mobility may be associated with lack of pus formation at the site of infection; conversely, the presence of pus provides clinical evidence that leukocyte mobility and chemotactic factor production are intact.

The Rebuck procedure is used to assess the morphology and in vivo motility of cells in the inflammatory response (Rebuck and Crowley, 1955). The skin is abraded superficially with a scalpel blade over an area of 4 mm², and cover slips are placed over the site; the cover slips are changed at 30-minute intervals for 24 hours. The leukocytes migrate to the abrasion and adhere to the slides, which are stained and analyzed. An initial influx of polymorphonuclear granulocytes should occur within 2 hours; these cells should be replaced by mononuclear cells within 12 hours.

Deformability, Adherence, and Aggregation

When random mobility or chemotaxis is abnormal, advanced tests to identify the exact nature of the defect are available. These include assays of deformability (Miller, 1975), adherence (MacGregor et al., 1974), or aggregation (Hammerschmidt et al., 1980). If findings are abnormal, tests for spreading, chemotactic orientation, and membrane fluidity can be undertaken (Anderson et al., 1984).

Etzioni and colleagues (1992) utilized a qualitative assay of leukocyte adherence by measuring the binding of IL-1–activated granulocytes to umbilical vein endothelium to identify LAD-2.

White Blood Cell Oxidative Metabolism

Ingestion of organisms by phagocytes and intracellular killing is accompanied by a number of metabolic changes, including increased oxygen consumption, activation of the hexose-monophosphate shunt, increased nicotinamide adenine dinucleotide phosphate, reduced form (NADPH) oxidase activity, increased glucose metabolism, and generation of activated oxygen species. The latter have important bactericidal functions and are closely linked to the activity of NADPH oxidase (Stossel, 1974). Several assays are available that measure the oxidative response of leukocytes during phagocytosis and killing that can be used as correlative assays of bactericidal activity. These include:

1. Chemiluminescence.
2. Quantitative NBT dye reduction.
3. Quantitative iodination.
4. Direct assays of oxygen consumption, hexose–monophosphate shunt activation, and superoxide or hydrogen peroxide production.

A quantitative NBT dye reduction test can be used to assess the oxidase activity of granulocytes (Baehner and Nathan, 1968). In this procedure, washed isolated leukocytes are incubated at 37°C with and without latex particles in the presence of NBT dye. After 15 minutes, the reaction is stopped and the reduced NBT is extracted with pyridine and measured spectrophotometrically. The difference (Δ) in optical density at 515 mμ/2.5 $\times$ 10^6 phagocytes between the resting (no latex particles) and phagocytizing cells is calculated; the normal value is 0.233 $\pm$ 0.103. Values in affected patients with CGD range from 0.034 to 0.045. Heterozygote carriers have intermediate values.

A combination of the NBT test with the phagocytosis of paraffin oil particles containing oil red O and coated with *E. coli* polysaccharide has been described (Stossel, 1973). After incubation, uningested particles are separated from the phagocytes by differential centrifugation; ingested oil red O and reduced NBT (formazan) are extracted from the washed cell pellets with dioxane. The optical densities of oil red O and formazan differ, allowing spectrophotometric quantitation of the two compounds in the dioxane extracts. The ratio of NBT reduction to ingestion is calculated; abnormal oxidative metabolism can be differentiated from abnormal ingestion.

Quantitative Iodination. Pincus and Klebanoff (1971) have used leukocyte iodination to assess microbicidal activity. In this reaction, inorganic iodide is fixed to bacteria (or a yeast particle) by myeloperoxidase in the presence of hydrogen peroxide generated by the hexose monophosphate shunt. Because of the failure of peroxide production, this reaction is defective in CGD. The assay employs radioactive inorganic iodide, isolated leukocytes, zymosan or bacteria, and serum; it can be used to detect CGD, CGD heterozygotes, or myeloperoxidase deficiency.

Oxygen Metabolism. Metabolic assays have been used to assess phagocytic function associated with killing. These include assessment of glucose metabolism, increased oxygen consumption, hexose monophosphate shunt activation, and hydrogen peroxide production in phagocytizing leukocytes (Holmes et al., 1967). Several studies have shown that defects in NADPH oxidase, superoxide production, and singlet oxygen formation are present in CGD (Hohn and Lehrer, 1975; Johnston et al., 1975a).

Enzyme Assays

Enzyme defects associated with defective granulocyte function include NADPH oxidase deficiency, myeloperoxidase deficiency, alkaline phosphatase deficiency, and G6PD. When CGD is suspected, certain laboratories can identify the exact enzymatic defect leading to the NADPH oxidase deficiency (Curnutte, 1993). When CGD has been excluded, the other enzyme defects should be sought. In myeloperoxidase deficiency, killing is abnormal, leukocyte iodination is abnormal, and hydrogen peroxide is normal (Klebanoff and Pincus, 1971). Specific diagnosis depends on demonstrating lack of myeloperoxidase activity (Lehrer and Cline, 1969b).

A complete lack of leukocyte G6PD was described in a patient in whom the neutrophils failed to kill staphylococci (Cooper et al., 1972). There was also deficient generation of hydrogen peroxide, and the case clinically resembled CGD. Most patients with erythrocyte G6PD deficiency have sufficient G6PD levels in the leukocytes for normal microbicidal activity.

A deficiency of glutathione peroxidase has been noted in some (Holmes et al., 1970), but not all, girls with CGD (DeChatelet et al., 1976). This enzyme is normal in males with CGD, indicating a different molecular defect despite phenotypic similarity. Lysosomal enzymes can also be assessed, including lysozyme, glucuronidase, and B$_{12}$ binding protein (Roberts and Gallin, 1983).

Tuftsin Assay

Tuftsin is a phagocytosis-stimulating tetrapeptide of IgG immunoglobulin; deficiency has been noted in a few patients with recurrent infections and following splenectomy (Constantopoulos et al., 1972). Tuftsin is assayed by its ability to stimulate phagocytosis of opsonized *S. aureus* bacteria of isolated granulocytes (Najjar and Constantopoulos, 1972).

Tests for Complement Immunodeficiencies

Initial Tests

The initial tests for complement abnormalities are measurement of serum total hemolytic complement expressed in 50% hemolytic units (CH_{50}) and serum C3 and C4 levels in mg/dl (see Chapter 7).

CH_{50} is assessed by the hemolysis of sheep erythrocytes by antibody (hemolysin) when test serum is used as a complement source (Gewurz and Suyehira, 1976). There is a wide range of normal values (from 20 to 100 CH_{50} units), depending on the cells and hemolysin used, so that normal levels must be established by each laboratory. Hemolytic complement assays are laborious, and all reagents, including the test serum, must be fresh. Hemolytic complement can also be estimated by radial diffusion in agar impregnated with sensitized sheep erythrocytes; this serves as a valuable screening test (Gewurz and Suyehira, 1976).

A normal CH_{50} generally indicates integrity of the complete system. However, decreases in the concentrations of individual components of up to 50% may not be reflected in this test. A low or absent CH_{50} indicates a profound defect at one or more locations of the classical complement cascade and is an indication for further studies. High levels of CH_{50} are often seen in inflammatory states.

Levels of C3 and C4 are measured immunochemically by radial immunodiffusion or nephelometry, using known standards. C3 has the highest serum level of any of the complement components, with a mean of 150 mg/dl and a range of 110 to 190 mg/dl. Levels of C3 generally parallel the total hemolytic complement activity. The mean C4 level is 25 mg/dl, with a range of 10 to 40 mg/dl. Very low or absent levels of C3 and C4 result from primary complement immunodeficiencies affecting these components; the CH_{50} will then also be low.

Levels of C3 are also depressed in acute glomerulonephritis, chronic membranous glomerulonephritis, lupus erythematosus, immune complex disease, serum sickness, Coombs' positive hemolytic anemia, and cryoglobulinemia (see Chapters 7 and 17).

Levels of C4 are decreased in hereditary angioneurotic edema. Low levels of CH_{50} or individual components are not necessarily associated with increased susceptibility to infection.

Opsonic Assays

The complement system is the chief source of nonspecific opsonic activity of the serum. Antibodies are also specific opsonins. Complement activity, unlike IgG opsonins, is heat-labile. "Pure" phagocytic defects (defective ingestion, normal killing) are usually due to opsonic defects rather than to primary granulocytic disorders. The C3b and C3d fragments and the C567 trimolecular complex are particularly active in bacterial opsonization, and C5 is active in fungal opsonization (Johnston and Stroud, 1977). Assays for phagocytic function are readily modified for opsonic assays. Defects in opsonization should be correlated with defects of individual complement components and activity of the classic and alternate pathway.

The microbicidal assay using isolated granulocytes, washed bacteria, and dilutions of test serum (instead of normal serum) assesses opsonization by the decrease in number of bacteria (as measured by colony counts) with time (Forman and Stiehm, 1969). Certain strains of *E. coli* or *S. marcescens* that cannot be phagocytized in the absence of complement are used for the test organism. Baker's yeast particles have been used to assess C5 function (Miller and Nilsson, 1970); particle uptake is assessed microscopically. Zymosan particle uptake can also be used to assess opsonic function; opsonic-dependent phagocytosis by normal granulocytes can be assessed by quantitative iodination (Pincus and Klebanoff, 1971) or chemiluminescence. Opsonization of oil red O coated with *E. coli* polysaccharide by test serum can be assessed in normal granulocytes by spectrophotometry (Stossel et al., 1973).

Complement Component Assays

Individual assays of the classical and alternative pathway components and of the inhibitor proteins should be done if there is abnormality of the complement screening tests or if there is evidence that a complement-mediated function is abnormal. Complement components can be assayed either by hemolytic titration or by immunoassay. Titration assays of individual complement components require reagents containing individual complement components purified to the extent that they are free of other component activity. When these reagents are used, antibody-coated erythrocytes are maximally sensitized up to the step that is to be measured and are exposed to the test serum; a mixture of all later-acting components is used to produce hemolysis (Alper and Rosen, 1975). The hemolysis achieved is then dependent on the functional activity of the test serum.

Alternatively, complement component levels can be measured by immunoassay, using antisera to C1q, C1r, C1s, C2, C3, C4, C5, C6, C7, C8, B, P, and D. Many of these antisera are commercially available. Patients with deficiencies of each of these components have now been described (see Chapter 17). Functional and immunoassays for C1 inactivator are of value in the diagnosis of hereditary angioneurotic edema.

A complement component profile indicates which complement pathway is activated. Classical pathway activation is generally associated with extremely low levels of C1, C4, C2, C3, and C5 and to a lesser extent, C6, C7, C8, and C9. By contrast, alternative pathway activation is associated with normal levels of C1, C4, and C2 but with low levels of C3. In addition, factors B, D, and P are reduced in alternative pathway activation. For screening purposes, low C4 with normal factor B indicates classical pathway activation and low factor B with normal C4 indicates alternative pathway activation.

Complement Activation Assays

Certain complement deficiencies result from increased catabolism; in some other illnesses, complement activation may be occurring with only slight or transient decreases in complement levels. Complement activation is suggested by the presence of complement breakdown products, particularly of C3. These are distinguishable from the native molecule by alterations of the immunoelectrophoretic pattern or by the appearance of low-molecular-weight breakdown products on crossed electrophoresis. For such analyses, serum must be collected in such a way as to prevent in vitro breakdown. Alper and Rosen (1975) recommend:

1. Using plasma from an atraumatic venipuncture.
2. Discarding the first 3 ml.
3. Preserving the sample in edetic acid (EDTA)
4. Immediate centrifugation.
5. Storage in aliquots at $-65°C$.
6. Minimal thawing and refreezing.

Immunoassays are available for C3a, C4a, and C5a anaphylotoxins and other complement split products, such as C4d. Because these are of low molecular weight and disappear rapidly from the circulation, they are present only during an ongoing or very recent event.

C3 activation can be observed in immunoelectrophoresis by total or partial replacement of the C3 (β_{1c}) arc by a faster arc (β_{1A}) and the appearance of low molecular weight (β_{1d}) in proportion to the degree of activation. In crossed electrophoresis, electrophoresis in gel is performed in one direction, followed by electrophoresis perpendicular to the first path in gel containing antiserum to a specific protein (e.g., C3). C3 activation is indicated by two or more C3 peaks (converted and native). Excess breakdown of C3 is associated with the presence of C3 nephritic factor in membranoproliferative glomerulonephritis (see Chapter 25). This disorder should be suspected when C3 is low, C4 is normal, and activation products are present in the circulation. Functional assays for C3 nephritic factor are also available.

Alternative Pathway Assays

Functional activity of the alternative pathway can be assessed by pneumococcal opsonic activity assay (Johnston et al., 1973), hemolysis of sheep cells in the presence of EGTA* (Fine et al., 1972), or antibody-independent hemolysis of rabbit erythrocytes (Platts-Mills and Ishizaka, 1974; Polhill et al., 1975). Radial

---

*Ethyleneglycol tetraacetic acid chelates calcium and blocks the classical pathway.

diffusion agar kits using rabbit erythrocytes are available for screening alternative pathway activity.

Alternative pathway abnormalities are noted in sickle cell disease, including pneumococcal opsonic defects (Johnston et al., 1973; Winkelstein and Drachman, 1968), and low levels of factor B (Wilson et al., 1976) in splenectomized patients (Polhill and Johnston, 1975) and in newborns (Stossel et al., 1973).

Other Complement Functional Assays

Serum chemotactic activity is assessed by activating the patient's serum complement with endotoxin, antigen-antibody complexes, or zymosan, using normal granulocytes or monocytes as the chemotaxing cells (Miller, 1975). A comparison with a normal serum and a known deficient serum must be performed. Chemotactic factor generation from serum is dependent on the formation of C3a, C5a, and the C567 trimolecular complex, and thus is abnormal in C3 and C5 deficiency (Johnston and Stroud, 1977). C6-deficient subjects generate adequate chemotactic activity.

Other functional assays of complement that can be used to evaluate a complement immunodeficiency are the measurements of immune adherence (Nishioka, 1963), serum bactericidal activity (Skarnes and Watson, 1956), virus neutralization (Daniels et al., 1970), and enhancement of antibody-dependent cellular cytotoxicity (Perlmann et al., 1975).

Complement Component Survival

The metabolic rate of a number of the complement components (e.g., C3, C4, C1q, C5, B, P) are known; thus, the turnover of purified labeled components can provide an exact determination of their metabolism. Component metabolism is increased in any disorder associated with complement activation; in one illness (factor I deficiency), C3 metabolism is selectively increased. It is characterized by low levels of C3, rapid turnover of C3, and pyogenic infections (Alper et al., 1970a, 1970b); this results from a deficiency of C3 inactivator, an essential regulator of the alternative pathway (Ziegler et al., 1975a). In patients with partial lipodystrophy, C3 levels are low, pyogenic infections are common, and hypercatabolism of C3 occurs because of the presence of a C3-cleaving nephritic factor (see Chapter 17) (Sissons et al., 1976).

Complement Allotypes

Complement allotyping for various components with allotypy (C2, C4, factor B) is sometimes of value in identifying the familial nature of a complement deficiency.

TREATMENT

Prevention

Prevention of immunodeficiency is limited to averting certain viral infections that cause immunodeficiency, genetic counseling, and in utero prenatal diagnosis with interruption of pregnancy. However, a maximum effort in all these areas would have minimal effect on the prevalence of congenital immunodeficiencies. Nevertheless, rubella vaccination programs have resulted in the disappearance of immunodeficiency secondary to congenital rubella. Prevention of HIV infections would decrease the incidence of AIDS. Genetic counseling is of value only when the genetic pattern is established.

Patients with a personal or family history of hereditary immunodeficiency should be counseled as to the risks of occurrence in their offspring as described earlier. Prenatal diagnosis is available for many illnesses if early treatment or therapeutic abortion are possibilities.

Immunoglobulin and complement levels should be obtained in the immediate family of patients with antibody or complement deficiencies to determine a familial pattern. In disorders in which procedures are available for heterozygosity testing (e.g., LAD-1, CGD), the parents, siblings, and children of the affected subject can be tested. If other family members have suggestive histories, they should also be studied. Newborn siblings of an affected patient are followed carefully from birth for manifestations of a similar disorder.

Neonatal Management

If a previous sibling has had combined immunodeficiency and the mother is again pregnant and about to deliver, prior planning is imperative. Cesarean section may be considered if a difficult labor is anticipated; however, it is not routinely indicated. At birth, cord blood should be obtained for blood count, immunoglobulin assays, B-cell and T-cell enumeration, phytohemagglutinin stimulation, and HLA typing to detect chimerism. The newborn infant with suspected immunodeficiency should be placed in a sterile isolator and maintained on reverse isolation until his or her immunologic status is clarified. A chest x-ray for thymic size should be done as soon as possible (see Chapter 10).

Newborns with combined immunodeficiency should remain in a protective environment with reverse isolation or in an isolator with food and liquid sterilized until definitive therapy is completed.

Gastrointestinal sterilization (with nonabsorbable antibiotics) and *P. carinii* prophylaxis (with trimethoprim-sulfamethoxazole) should be considered for patients suspected of combined immunodeficiency.

General Treatment

Patients with immunodeficiency require extraordinary amounts of pediatric care to maintain general health and nutrition, to prevent emotional problems related to their illness, and to manage their numerous infectious episodes. No special dietary limitations are necessary; the aim is to provide a well-rounded, nutritious diet.

Patients with immunodeficiencies should be protected from unnecessary exposure to infection. They should sleep in their own beds, preferably with rooms of their own, and should be kept away from individuals with respiratory or other infections.

Since many patients with immunodeficiency have a normal life span on immunoglobulin or other therapy, the parents must avoid making the patient an emotional cripple by overprotection. The child is encouraged to be outdoors, to play with other children in small groups, and to attend nursery and regular school. The aim is to teach such children to live in a near-normal fashion with their disease, in much the same way as the diabetic child. Killed vaccines (DPT, inactivated poliomyelitis) should be given if there is evidence of some antibody synthesis. Unless the child is anergic, tuberculin testing should be done every 2 years. The teeth should be kept in good repair.

The accompanying chronic infections, such as mastoiditis, sinusitis, bronchitis, and bronchiectasis, should be managed as in other patients. Long-term chronic antibiotic therapy may be of value (Sweinberg et al., 1991). Patients with B-cell, T-cell, or phagocyte defects should have pulmonary function tests performed at regular intervals and should have a home treatment plan of physiotherapy and inhalation therapy similar to that used in cystic fibrosis. Vigorous exercise, including team sports, should be strongly encouraged. Special attention must be directed toward such problems as hearing loss, the need for tutors to make up for school absences, and financial help for the family. The National Immune Deficiency Foundation is a valuable resource for patients and their families.

Precautions

Patients with suspected or proven T-cell immunodeficiencies should not be given routine blood transfusions because of the possibility of a graft-versus-host reaction from heterologous lymphocytes. If transfusion is necessary, the blood should be irradiated prior to administration. The authors use 2500 rad, but higher and lower doses have been used (Strauss et al., 1993). Because of the risks of cytomegalovirus (CMV) from blood products, it is advisable to use CMV-negative donors. Tonsillectomy and adenoidectomy should be performed rarely and then only with strict indications. Splenectomy is contraindicated, except in unusual circumstances, because the addition of a phagocytic defect (absence of the spleen) to the already existing immunodeficiency may result in sudden overwhelming sepsis. Continuous antibiotics are indicated in the splenectomized immunodeficient subject (see Chapter 19). Corticosteroids should be used in these patients only with extreme caution.

Vaccines

Live attenuated vaccines (smallpox, poliomyelitis, measles, mumps, rubella, BCG) should be avoided in all severe antibody or cellular immunodeficiencies because of the risk of vaccine-induced infection. The authors have given live virus vaccines to patients with selective IgA deficiency, mucocutaneous candidiasis with intact cellular immunity to other antigens, and phagocytic and complement immunodeficiencies and to children fully reconstituted following bone marrow transplantation. The risk from smallpox vaccination is especially great, and many infants with cellular immunodeficiencies were initially diagnosed as a result of a complication of smallpox vaccine. Paralytic poliomyelitis and prolonged poliovirus shedding from the gastrointestinal tract is a recognized complication of oral poliomyelitis vaccination in immunodeficiency. Parents, siblings, and other household members should not be given live poliomyelitis vaccine because of the increased risk of spread to the patient. Yearly influenza vaccination is also recommended for immunodeficient children who can make an antibody response and for family members of the immune-deficient child.

Following chicken pox exposure in T-cell and antibody-deficient children, varicella-zoster immunoglobulin (VZIG) or acyclovir prophylaxis is indicated. For the antibody-deficient child with normal T-cell immunity receiving regular intravenous immunoglobulin, VZIG is generally unnecessary, inasmuch as IVIG contains antibody to varicella-zoster virus, and chickenpox, even if not prevented, is attenuated by the IVIG infusions.

Antibiotics and Antivirals

Antibiotics are lifesaving in the treatment of the infectious episodes of patients with immunodeficiency. Before their availability, most patients with immunodeficiencies probably succumbed from early infection. The choice and dosage of antibiotics for specific infections are identical to those used in normal subjects. However, because these patients may succumb rapidly to infection, fevers or other manifestations of infection are assumed to be secondary to bacterial infection, and antibiotic treatment is begun immediately. Throat, blood, and other culture specimens deemed appropriate are obtained prior to therapy; these are especially important if the infection does not respond promptly to the initial antibiotic chosen.

Patients should be "overtreated" for infectious episodes, even if this necessitates frequent or chronic antibiotics and occasional unnecessary hospitalizations. If the infection does not respond to antibiotics, the physician should consider the possibility of fungal, mycobacterial, viral, or protozoal (*P. carinii*) infection. Because certain of these infections can be treated only with special drugs (e.g., pentamidine or trimethoprim-sulfamethoxazole for *P. carinii* infection, ribavirin for parainfluenza infection), an exact microbiologic diagnosis is imperative.

P. carinii *Pneumonia Prophylaxis*

P. carinii pneumonia (PCP) prophylaxis is recommended for children with significant primary and secondary cellular (T-cell) immunodeficiencies. The guidelines for children with HIV infection can be followed (Centers for Disease Control, 1991). Prophylaxis is recommended for infants less than 12 months of age with a CD4 count less than 1500 cells/μl, for young children aged 12 to 23 months with a CD4 count less than 750 cells/μl, for children 2 to 5 years with a CD4 count less than 500 cells/μl, and for children over 5 years of age and adults with a CD4 count less than 200 cells/μl. In addition, any patient with a CD4 count less than 25% of the total lymphocytes or a past history of PCP is a candidate for prophylaxis. Prophylaxis consists of trimethoprim-sulfamethoxazole (TMP/SMX) 160 mg/M^2/day of the TMP and 750 mg/M^2/day of SMX given orally in divided doses twice per day 3 times per week, with frequent checks of the WBC count. Alternative drugs for PCP prophylaxis include pentamidine and dapsone.

Continuous prophylactic antibiotics often are of benefit in immunodeficiencies. They are especially useful in disorders characterized by rapid overwhelming infections (e.g., in Wiskott-Aldrich syndrome), in antibody immunodeficiencies when recurrent infections occur despite optimal immunoglobulin therapy, and in phagocytic disorders in which no other form of therapy is available. In these instances, penicillin, ampicillin, or dicloxacillin given orally, 0.5 to 1.0 g/day in divided doses, is recommended. If diarrhea or vomiting results, lower doses or other drugs are used. The continuous use of antibiotics in the antibody immunodeficiencies is not an adequate substitute for immunoglobulin therapy but can be used if patients refuse immunoglobulin on religious grounds. In chronic granulomatous disease, the continuous use of sulfisoxazole or trimethoprim-sulfamethoxazole is indicated not only because of its antimicrobial activity but because it may increase the bactericidal activity of the phagocytes (Johnston et al., 1975b).

Antiviral therapy can be used effectively in some immunodeficiencies. Exposure to influenza or early symptomatic influenza infection can be managed with amantidine. Severe herpes simplex, chickenpox, or herpes zoster can be treated with acyclovir. Ribavirin aerosols have been used in the treatment of respiratory syncytial virus and parainfluenza viral infections in SCID (McIntosh et al., 1984). Acyclovir can also be used in the incubation period to modify or prevent chickenpox (Asano et al., 1993).

Human Immune Serum Globulin

Indications

Many antibody immunodeficiencies are treated successfully with repeated injections or infusions of human immune serum globulin (HISG, gamma globulin). This treatment allows many patients to be symptom-free, similar to the well-controlled diabetic on insulin therapy. Others given immunoglobulin remain chronically ill or undergo a progressive downhill course; often these patients have other immunologic or hematologic deficits. Immunoglobulin is not of value in the treatment of cellular, phagocytic, or complement immunodeficiencies, and it is of only limited value in combined antibody and cellular immunodeficiencies. Two forms of HISG are available: intramuscular immunoglobulin (ISG) and intravenous immunoglobulin (IVIG) (Table 9–21).

Table 9–21. Comparison of Intramuscular (ISG) and Intravenous (IVIG) Human Immune Serum Globulins for Therapeutic Use

	ISG	IVIG
Strength	16.5% (165 mg/ml)	3%, 5%, 10%, or 12%
Buffer	0.1 M glycine	Various sugars*
Preservative	Thimerosal	None
How supplied	2- and 10-ml vials	Powder for reconstitution or 5%–12% solution of various sizes*
Indications	Prophylaxis of specific infections; antibody immunodeficiency	Antibody immunodeficiency: immune thrombocytopenic purpura, Kawasaki disease, other immunoregulatory disorders
Major advantages	Convenience of administration; infrequent side effects	Predictable blood levels; high dosage feasible
Major disadvantages	Unreliable blood levels; discomfort at injection sites; large doses not feasible	Long duration of administration: more frequent side effects; higher cost
Frequency of side effects	10/1000 injections	50/1000 infusions
Most frequent side effects	Pain at injection site	Flushing, nausea, back pain
Minimal dose in immunodeficiency/mo	100 mg/kg (0.7 ml/kg)	200 mg/kg (4 ml/kg) of 5% solution
Approximate cost per dose for 25-kg child	$100 (20 ml of 16%)	$340 (100 ml of 5%)
Unit cost	$30/g	$68/g

*See Table 9–22.

Immunoglobulin for Intramuscular or Subcutaneous Use

Pharmacology

Immune serum globulin (ISG) is prepared by alcohol fractionation of pooled human serum by the Cohn alcohol fractionation procedure (thus deriving its alternative name of Cohn fraction II). In this procedure, most other serum proteins and live viruses (e.g., hepatitis B virus, HIV) are removed, thus providing a sterile product for intramuscular or subcutaneous injection. ISG is reconstituted as a sterile 16.5% solution (165 mg/ml) with thimerosal as a preservative.* It contains a wide spectrum of antibodies to viral and bacterial antigens.

ISG is 95% IgG globulin, but trace quantities of IgM and IgA globulins and other serum proteins are present. The IgM and IgA globulins are therapeutically insignificant because of their rapid half-lives (about 7 days) and their low concentrations in ISG. ISG contains multiple IgG allotypes (Gm and Km types).

ISG is approved only for intramuscular or subcutaneous use, and intravenous injection of ISG is contraindicated. It aggregates in vitro to large-molecular-weight complexes (9.5 to 40 Svedberg units) that are strongly anticomplementary. These aggregates are probably responsible for the occasional systemic reactions to ISG. The incidence of these reactions is increased if the recipient has received gamma globulin previously or if ISG is given intravenously. Agammaglobulinemic boys with affected male relatives (suggesting X-linked inheritance) may experience a lower incidence of reactions (Medical Research Council Working Party, 1969). Small intradermal injections of ISG are not of value (except as a placebo), and they are also contraindicated.

Dosage

The usual dose of ISG for antibody immunodeficiency is 100 mg/kg per month, about equivalent to 0.7 ml/kg/month of the commercially available 16.5% (165 mg/ml) product. A double or triple dose is given at the onset of therapy, often over a 3- to 5-day period. The maximum dose should not exceed 20 or 30 ml/week. Few studies of the optimal dose are available; however, the Medical Research Council Working Party (1969) found that 25 mg/kg/week (100 mg/kg/month) was equivalent therapeutically to 50 mg/kg/week but that 10 mg/kg/week was inadequate.

The ISG should be given at multiple sites in order to avoid giving more than 5 ml at any one site (10 ml in a large adult). The buttocks are the preferred sites, but the anterior thighs can also be used. Tenderness, sterile abscesses, fibrosis, and sciatic nerve injury may result from these injections. The danger of sciatic nerve injury is especially great in a small malnourished infant with inadequate muscle and fat in the gluteal regions. ISG injections should not be given to patients with thrombocytopenia because of the risk of hematoma and infection.

The injections are initially given at monthly intervals. If the patient continues to have infection or if a characteristic symptom recurs at the end of the injection period (such as cough, conjunctivitis, diarrhea, arthralgia, or purulent nasal discharge), the interval between doses is decreased to 3 or 2 weeks. Older patients often report that they can tell when the IgG level is low and when they need another injection. During acute infections, gamma globulin catabolism increases, so extra injections of ISG are given. Many adults needing large doses (e.g., 40 ml/month) prefer to get weekly injections of 10 ml.

Because no specific serum level of IgG must be maintained, serial immunoglobulin assays are unnecessary in assessing the effectiveness of treatment. The maximum increase of the serum IgG level after a standard

---

*In the United States; in many other countries, ISG is preservative-free.

ISG injection varies from patient to patient and from dose to dose because of different rates of absorption, local proteolysis at the injection site, and distribution within the tissues. An intramuscular injection of 100 mg/kg of ISG usually raises the IgG serum level by 100 to 125 mg/dl after 2 to 4 days (Stiehm et al., 1966; Liese et al., 1992). Thus, a recent ISG injection usually does not obscure the diagnosis of hypogammaglobulinemia.

Adverse Effects of ISG

Although ISG is one of the safest biologic products available, rare anaphylactic reactions to intramuscular injections have been reported, particularly in patients requiring repeat injections (Ellis and Henney, 1969). The Medical Research Council Working Party (1969) noted such reactions in 33 of 175 patients (19%) treated over a 10-year period. In all, there were 85 reactions to about 40,000 injections; in eight patients, the injections were stopped because of these adverse effects, and one death was recorded. Such reactions occurred at all stages of treatment and were unrelated to any particular lot number of gamma globulin or to its anticomplementary activity. The symptoms include anxiety, nausea, vomiting, malaise, flushing, facial swelling, cyanosis, and loss of consciousness. Immediate treatment with epinephrine and antihistamines is indicated.

Individuals who experience such reactions should be evaluated before a repeat injection. Skin testing, using several lots of ISG, should be done (Ellis and Henney, 1969). A skin test that is positive for an old but not a new lot of ISG may indicate a particular idiosyncratic reaction to a particular unit. Under these circumstances, incremental doses of ISG from a new lot are recommended. In other patients, IgE antibodies to IgG develop, resulting in positive immediate skin tests. In others, no cause of the reactions can be found. Some of these patients tolerate repeated small doses of ISG, particularly if they are premedicated with aspirin, diphenhydramine, or corticosteroids. Finally, a few patients have developed IgG or IgE antibodies to the IgA present in minute quantities in the ISG; these IgA antibodies can be detected by serologic means in several laboratories. IVIG with low IgA content or IgA-deficient plasma can be used under these circumstances (Burks et al., 1986).

Immunologically normal patients given gamma globulin (or plasma) may develop antibodies to a genetic gamma globulin type different from their own (usually anti-Gm antibodies). These are clinically insignificant. Allen and Kunkel (1966) found anti-Gm antibodies in 17 of 24 thalassemic children given repeated blood transfusions. Stiehm and Fudenberg (1965) noted anti-Gm antibodies in normal children given single gamma globulin injections and in hypogammaglobulinemic children given repeated gamma globulin injections. In patients with severe antibody immunodeficiency, such antibodies do not develop. One plasma transfusion reaction was attributed to a Gm/anti-Gm interaction (Fudenberg and Fudenberg, 1964). Patients with antibodies to IgA may have a reaction to gamma globulin

as a result of the trace quantities of IgA in ISG or IVIG (Vyas et al., 1968). However, some patients with combined IgA and IgG2 deficiency with anti-IgA antibodies tolerate treatment with IVIG, particularly IVIG with low levels of IgA (Björkander et al., 1987).

Administration of exogenous immunoglobulin may theoretically inhibit the endogenous synthesis of immunoglobulin. Premature infants given ISG monthly in the first year of life had lower IgG levels at 1 year of age than albumin-treated controls (Amer et al., 1963). In immunodeficiency with hyper-IgM, intramuscular IgG results in diminution of IgM levels, suggesting inhibition of endogenous IgM synthesis (Stiehm and Fudenberg, 1966a). The authors have noted depressed IgG levels that return to normal when the injections are stopped in a few patients with transient hypogammaglobulinemia given immunoglobulin from early infancy.

Late side effects with ISG injections are uncommon; in a few patients, fibrosis of the buttocks or localized subcutaneous atrophy develops at the site of repeated injections. Repeat injections of ISG may result in high levels of mercury because of the thimerosal preservative. Although acrodynia developed in one patient as a result of such therapy (Matheson et al., 1980), most patients remain asymptomatic.

Slow Subcutaneous ISG Injections

As an alternative to intramuscular injections, ISG can be given to immunodeficient patients by slow (0.05 to 0.20 ml/kg/hr) subcutaneous injections (Berger et al., 1980). The usual maintenance dose is 100 mg/kg/wk, preceded by several consecutive days of therapy as a loading dose. These injections are self-administered into the abdominal wall with the use of a battery-operated pump (Autosyringe). These injections are well tolerated and enable the patient to obtain increased quantities of ISG and maintain higher serum levels of IgG. In some patients, when the cost of IVIG is prohibitive, ISG infusions are used regularly (Gardulf et al., 1991, Waniewski et al., 1993). The authors have used this method successfully in patients with anaphylactic reactions to intramuscular ISG or IVIG (Welch and Stiehm, 1983).

Intravenous Immunoglobulin

IVIG is indicated in the management of several primary and secondary immunodeficiency syndromes (Table 9–22). There are several advantages to the administration of immunoglobulin by the intravenous route (see Table 9–21), including:

1. Ease of administering large doses.
2. More rapid action.
3. No loss in the tissues from proteolysis.
4. Avoidance of painful intramuscular injections.

Although regular ISG has been used intravenously (Barandun et al., 1962), severe reactions are common, and thus intravenous use of ISG is contraindicated.

Intravenous immunoglobulin is prepared from Cohn fraction II by eliminating high-molecular-weight com-

Table 9–22. Some Immunodeficiencies in Which Intravenous Immunoglobulin May Be of Benefit

Antibody Deficiencies
  X-linked agammaglobulinemia
  Common variable immunodeficiency
  Immunodeficiency with hyper-IgM
  Transient hypogammaglobulinemia of infancy (sometimes)
  IgG subclass deficiency ± IgA deficiency (sometimes)
  Antibody deficiency with normal immunoglobulins

Combined Deficiencies
  Severe combined immunodeficiencies (all types)
  Wiskott-Aldrich syndrome
  Ataxia-telangiectasia
  Short-limbed dwarfism
  X-linked lymphoproliferative syndrome

Secondary Immunodeficiencies
  Malignancies with antibody deficiencies; multiple myeloma,
    chronic lymphocytic leukemia, other cancers
  Protein-losing enteropathy with hypogammaglobulinemia
  Nephrotic syndrome with hypogammaglobulinemia
  Pediatric acquired immunodeficiency syndrome
  Intensive care patients: trauma/surgery/shock
  Post-transplantation period
  Post–bone marrow transplantation
  Burns
  Prematurity

plexes and their resultant anticomplementary activity. Methods to accomplish this have utilized:

1. Physical removal of aggregates by ultracentrifugation or gel filtration.
2. Treatment with proteolytic enzymes.
3. Treatment with chemicals that reduce sulfhydryl bonds, followed by alkylation of the free SH bonds.
4. Incubation at low pH.

Although physical removal of aggregates is impractical, the other methods have been used with considerable success. Indeed, nine IVIGs have been licensed in the United States (Table 9–23), and others are in use elsewhere in the world.

The first IVIG licensed in the United States was a reduced (dithiothreitol) and alkylated (iodoacetamide) product formulated as a 5% solution in 10% maltose (Gamimune, Cutter Laboratories). This is no longer available because it was low in IgG3 and IgG4 subclasses. The second licensed IVIG (1984) was an acidified, pepsin-treated powder reconstituted to a 3% or 6% solution in 5% or 10% sucrose (Sandoglobulin, Sandoz Laboratories). Several other IVIGs are now available. For patients with anti-IgA antibodies, Gammagard is the preparation of choice because it has the lowest level of IgA (Apfelzweig et al., 1987).

All of these preparations offer acceptable serum half-lives (18 to 25 days), contain all IgG subclasses, have minimal anticomplementary activity, have a good and diverse antibody content, and are negative for hepatitis B surface antigen (HBsAg), hepatitis C virus (HCV), and HIV. A few cases of hepatitis C following experimental IVIG have been recorded (Lever et al., 1984). Gammagard was recently associated with several cases of HCV infection and was removed from the market temporarily (Centers for Disease Control, 1994). Do-

nors are now screened for HCV antibodies and HIV antibodies.

Dosage

Studies with IVIG preparations indicate that they are equally effective in preventing serious infections in antibody-deficient subjects and are as effective as equivalent quantities of intramuscular ISG injections (Ammann et al., 1982a). For adults requiring large volumes of intramuscular ISG injections, IVIG therapy is much better tolerated, and in patients with thrombocytopenia (e.g., with Wiskott-Aldrich syndrome or during bone marrow transplantation), IVIG avoids intramuscular injections. Another advantage of IVIG is the large quantities of IgG that can be administered; indeed, IgG levels can be normalized with repeated infusions.

High-dose IVIG may be of benefit in some immunodeficient patients who continue to have repeated infections while receiving the usual doses of IVIG (100 to 200 mg/kg/month) (Ochs et al., 1984; Bernatowski et al., 1987; Liese et al., 1992). IVIG is given at doses of 400 to 600 mg/kg to bring the trough IgG level to the normal range (i.e., >600 mg/dl). This may require weekly or biweekly infusions and frequent monitoring of IgG levels. The level of IgG usually increases 250 mg/dl immediately and 125 mg/kg after 3 to 4 weeks for each 100 mg/kg IVIG infused (Ochs et al., 1984). These large doses are not recommended for all antibody-deficient subjects because of the increased expense, lack of proven efficacy, and variation of metabolism among different patients (Schiff et al., 1984; Schiff and Rudd, 1986).

Adverse Reactions

Adverse reactions to IVIG are unusual, usually preventable, and easily treated. The pain of needle insertion can be minimalized by applying Emla cream, a local anesthetic, to the infusion site an hour before the infusion. The most common adverse reactions to IVIG are nonanaphylactic reactions, occurring in about 5% of infusions, usually in the first 30 minutes of administration and consisting of backache, abdominal pain, headache, chills, fever, and mild nausea. Most reactions can be minimized by pretreatment with aspirin or diphenhydramine (or occasionally steroids) and treated by slowing the infusion. True anaphylactic reactions are extremely rare. Some of these reactions may be due to the presence of anti-IgA antibodies in the patient reacting with trace amounts of IgA present in the preparations.

Long-term side effects of IVIG are unusual. A few cases of aseptic meningitis have been noted shortly after the administration of IVIG; most are in patients with immune thrombocytopenic purpura (ITP) (Rao et al., 1992). A few cases of transient or permanent renal insufficiency (Miller et al., 1992; Schifferli et al., 1991; Barton et al., 1987); pulmonary insufficiency (Rault et al., 1991); hemolytic anemia, Coombs' positivity, or both (Copeland et al., 1986; Moscow et al., 1987); and thrombotic events (Comenzo et al., 1992; Woodruff et al., 1986) have been reported. Non-A, non-B hepatitis

Table 9–23. Intravenous Immunoglobulin (IVIG) Preparations Available in the United States

Trade Name, Year Released, Manufacturer	Isolation Method	Product Form (Stabilizers)	pH	IgA Content	Comments
Sandoglobulin (1984) Sandoz Pharmaceuticals E. Hanover, N.J.	Acid and pepsin	Lyophilized; reconstituted as 3, 6, and 12% solution; Available in 1-, 3-, and 6-g bottles (5% sucrose).	6.6	VH	Reaction rates may be somewhat higher than other IVIG products; store room temperature
Gammagard (1986) Baxter HealthCare Co. Hyland Division, Glendale, Calif.	PEG and ultrafiltration	Lyophilized; reconstituted as a 5% solution; 0.5-, 2.5-, 5-, and 10-g bottles (glycine, albumin, and 2% glucose)	6.8	L	A number of hepatitis C cases reported;* temporarily withdrawn from the market in 1994; recommended for patients with absent IgA; a detergent-treated form has been available since 1995; store room temperature
Gamimune-N (1986—5%) (1992—10%) Cutter Laboratories Berkeley, Calif.	Acid and diafiltration	Liquid; reconstituted as a 5% or 10% solution; available in 0.5-, 2.5-, 5- and 12.5-g bottles (10% maltose)	4.25	H	Low rate of side effects; store refrigerated
Iveegam (1988) Immuno-US Rochester, Mich.	Trypsin and PEG	Lyophilized; reconstituted as 5% solution; available in 0.5-, 1, 2.5-, and 5-g bottles (5% glucose)	6.8	VL	First used in Kawasaki syndrome trials; no longer available in the United States; refrigerate
Venoglobulin-I (1988) Alpha Therap. Corp. Los Angeles, Calif.	PEG-DEAE-sephadex fractionation	Lyophilized; reconstituted as 5% solution; available in 0.5-, 2.5-, 5-, and 10-g bottles (albumin 2% mannitol)	6.8	L	Store room temperature
Polygam (1988) American Red Cross Washington, D.C.	PEG, ultrafiltration	Lyophilized; reconstituted as 5% solution; available in 2.5-, 5-, and 10-g bottles (glycine, albumin, and 2% glucose)	6.8	L	Manufactured for the American Red Cross by Baxter Pharmaceuticals from volunteer donors; no cases of hepatitis C reported; however, temporarily removed from the market in 1994 along with Gammagard;* store room temperature
Gammar-IV (1989) Armour Pharmaceuticals Chicago, Ill.	Low-ionic-strength ethanol fractionation	Lyophilized; reconstituted as 5% solution; available in 1-, 2.5-, and 5-g bottles (albumin and 5% sucrose)	7.0	L	Store room temperature
CytoGam (1991) Med Immune, Inc. Gaithersburg, Md.	PEG and ultrafiltration	Lyophilized; reconstituted as 5% solution; available in 2.5-g bottles (5% sucrose and albumin)	NA	NA	Enriched for CMV antibodies; manufactured by the Massachusetts Public Health Biologic Laboratories for Med Immune, Inc.; store room temperature
Venoglobulin-S (1992) Alpha Therapeutics Los Angeles, Calif.	PEG and DEAE-sephadex fractionation followed by solvent detergent treatment	Liquid; reconstituted as 5% solution; available in 2.5-, 5-, and 10-g bottles (5% D-sorbitol)	5.2	L	Store room temperature

*Centers for Disease Control. Outbreak of hepatitis C associated with intravenous immunoglobulin administration—United States, Oct 1993–June 1994. MMWR 43:505–509, 1994.
   Abbreviations: CMV = cytomegalovirus; DEAE = diethylaminoethyl; H = high; L = low; PEG = polyethylene glycol; VH = very high; VL = very low.

(hepatitis C) has been noted following infusions of experimental lots of IVIG (Ochs et al., 1985; Lever et al., 1984; Trepo et al., 1986) and following infusions of Gammagard in 1993 and 1994. Gammagard and Polygam—the latter made by the same manufacturer (Baxter) for the American Red Cross—were temporarily removed from the market (Centers for Disease Control, 1994).

Home Administration

IVIG can be given at home by a home-care service, by the parents, or by another adult patient. Home infusion is much more convenient, with considerable cost and time savings (Kobayashi et al., 1990; Daly et al., 1991). This also gives the patients (or parents) a feeling that they are in charge of their own (or their child's) health. The initial infusions should be given in the hospital or clinic; if the outcome is uneventful, the infusions can be administered at home subsequently. Home infusions are not recommended for patients with

difficult venous access or those with significant side effects from the infusions. Home infusions should never be administered without a responsible adult present. The patient should be under continued supervision, including periodic examinations by a physician.

Special Uses of IVIG in Immunodeficiency

Infections. During infections or prolonged fever, IgG catabolism increases, and consumption of antibody to the offending microorganism is consumed. Thus, it is prudent to give extra IVIG infusions during severe infections so as to maintain IgG levels. In severe diarrhea, IgG may be lost in the stool and extra doses of immunoglobulin should be considered. In refractory severe infections in immunodeficient subjects, particularly if neutropenia is present, high-dose IVIG therapy in addition to antimicrobial agents may be effective.

Enterovirus Encephalitis and Polymyositis. Chronic meningocephalitis and polymyositis resulting from echovirus or coxsackievirus characteristically occur in patients with X-linked agammaglobulinemia. Treatment with high doses of intravenous immunoglobulin at frequent intervals may modify the severity of infection and improve survival (Mease et al., 1981). A review of published reports shows that 8 of 11 patients treated with IVIG survived compared with only 2 of 10 patients given intramuscular immunoglobulin or immune plasma and 0 of 4 patients who received no treatment (Stiehm, 1992). Two patients who received intraventricular immunoglobulin as well as IVIG showed resolution of cerebrospinal fluid (CSF) pleocytosis with eradication of the echovirus from the CSF. However, most other patients, including two others given intraventricular immunoglobulin, have had a chronic fluctuating course with persistent CSF pleocytosis and positive CSF cultures.

Respiratory Viral Infections. In patients with immunodeficiency, severe respiratory viral infections may develop. IVIG preparations contain antibodies to several common respiratory tract viral pathogens, including adenovirus, influenza, and parainfluenza, and may be of value in management of these diseases (Stiehm et al., 1986). Adenovirus pneumonia has occurred in immunodeficient children lacking neutralizing antibody to adenovirus, and one child recovered after receiving intramuscular immunoglobulin.

In contrast, IVIG failed to eradicate parainfluenza in a child with SCID and in one child with advanced HIV disease. A respiratory syncytial virus (RSV) hyperimmune IVIG is under clinical trial (Groothuis et al., 1993) and may be of value in the treatment of RSV infection in immunocompromised individuals.

Parvovirus Infection. Parvovirus B19 infection causes aplastic anemia in immunodeficient and immunocompromised subjects. Kurtzman and colleagues (1989) reported cure of pure red blood cell aplasia caused by parvovirus in a 24-year-old man. After intensive IVIG therapy, the virus disappeared permanently from the marrow and peripheral blood. The IVIG treatments were then discontinued without relapse. Others have reported similar experiences.

Oral Immunoglobulin. Human immunoglobulin has been used orally in immunodeficiency to diminish or abolish the shedding of rotavirus, poliovirus, or coxsackievirus (Losonsky et al., 1985). It has also been used in *Cryptosporidium* infection. The recommended dose is 150 mg/kg given at 4- to 6-hour intervals of an IVIG preparation.

Hypercatabolism. IVIG can be used to study the metabolism of IgG in hypogammaglobulinemic patients suspected of gastrointestinal or urinary tract loss or hypercatabolism. A large dose of IVIG (2 g/kg) is given rapidly to raise the IgG levels acutely, and then serial IgG levels are studied to determine the rate of disappearance from the circulation. Patients with primary hypogammaglobulinemia have a normal or increased IgG half-life (>20 days), whereas patients with loss or hypercatabolism have a shortened IgG half-life (<15 days).

Autoimmune Diseases. Patients with immunodeficiency may develop immunoregulatory disorders such as autoimmune hemolytic anemia, immune thrombo-

cytopenic purpura, or vasculitis that will benefit from large-dose IVIG. They can be treated with the larger doses of IVIG recommended for these disorders.

Pregnancy. IVIG has been used in pregnancy with safety and efficacy for immunodeficiency, thrombocytopenic purpura, and threatened abortion. The profound transient hypogammaglobulinemia of the newborn of a mother with agammaglobulinemia can be prevented by large doses of IVIG during late pregnancy; however, IVIG can also be given to the infant at birth. A few of these children have done well without immunoglobulin therapy (Kobayashi et al., 1980).

Other Uses of Intravenous Immunoglobulin

Secondary Immunodeficiencies. IVIG is of value in a number of secondary immunodeficiencies that have a significant antibody deficiency (see Table 9–22). Patients are good candidates for IVIG if they are having frequent infections and one or more of the following:

- Significant hypogammaglobulinemia (a serum IgG level < 200 mg/dl or total immunoglobulin (IgG + IgM + IgA) < 400 mg/dl
- Low levels of natural antibodies to ubiquitous antigens
- Poor antibody responses to vaccine antigen challenges

Refractory Infection. Patients with refractory or severe overwhelming infection may be benefited by concomitant administration of IVIG along with antibiotics. Likely situations include sepsis in newborn (particularly premature infants), refractory staphylococcal infection, severe gram-negative infections in surgical or trauma patients, and severe viral infections, notably CMV infections.

Immunoregulatory Disorders. High-dose IVIG has immunosuppressive and anti-inflammatory effects that make it a valuable agent in the treatment of several autoimmune or inflammatory disorders (Table 9–24). High-dose IVIG (1 to 2 g/kg/week) may work by the following mechanisms (Ballow, 1994):

1. Inhibits antibody synthesis (possibly by a direct effect on proliferating B cells).
2. Combines directly with autoimmune antibodies (because it contains anti-idiotypic antibodies).
3. Blocks the uptake of antibody-coated cells in the spleen and liver (Fc receptor blockade of antibody-dependent cellular cytotoxicity).
4. Down-regulates immune activation by decreasing inflammatory cytokine release or action.
5. Combines with bacterial superantigens that may be present in certain inflammatory disorders (e.g., toxic shock syndrome)
6. Inhibits complement mediated tissue injury.

The best-documented uses of high-dose IVIG as an immunoregulator are in the treatment of Kawasaki disease (see Chapter 24) and immune thrombocytopenic purpura (see Chapter 27). In most other disorders, the reports of efficacy are based on small, uncontrolled studies or case studies.

Table 9–24. Other (Noninfectious) Uses of
Intravenous Immunoglobulin

Proven Benefit*
  Kawasaki syndrome
  Immune thrombocytopenic purpura
  Guillain-Barré syndrome
  Dermatomyositis

Probable Benefit†
  Neonatal isoimmune or autoimmune thrombocytopenic purpura
  Postinfectious thrombocytopenic purpura
  Immune neutropenia (including neonatal)
  Autoimmune hemolytic anemia
  Chronic inflammatory demyelinating polyneuropathy
  Myasthenia gravis

Possible Benefit‡
  Anticardiolipin antibody syndrome
  Toxic shock syndrome
  Coagulopathy with factor VIII inhibitor
  Bullous pemphigoid
  Churg-Strauss vasculitis

Unproven Benefit§
  Intractable seizures
  Movement disorders
  Steroid-dependent asthma
  Eczema
  Juvenile rheumatoid arthritis
  Lupus erythematosus
  Recurrent abortion
  Hemolytic-uremic syndrome

*Controlled studies demonstrate efficacy.
†Several case reports or uncontrolled series are convincing.
‡Preliminary studies are encouraging but incomplete.
§Preliminary studies are limited or equivocal.

Special Immune Serum Globulins

Special preparations of ISG for intramuscular use are available for the prevention and treatment of certain infectious diseases. These include varicella-zoster immunoglobulin (VZIG), rabies immunoglobulin (RIG), tetanus immunoglobulin (TIG), and hepatitis B immunoglobulin (HBIG). These have been prepared from immunized or convalescing donors, and their antibody content has been standardized. Pharmacologically, these preparations are identical to standard ISG preparations (see Chapter 29 for indications and dosage).

Other special immunoglobulins are under clinical trial but not yet licensed. These include group B streptococcus antibody–enriched immunoglobulin (GBS-IVIG), *Pseudomonas* antibody–enriched immunoglobulin, bacterial polysaccharide immunoglobulin (BPIG), respiratory syncytial virus–intravenous immunoglobulin (RSV-IVIG), botulism immunoglobulin, and HIV-intravenous immunoglobulin (HIVIG). Most are used in the treatment of severe infections. HIVIG is under trial to prevent transmission of HIV from HIV-infected pregnant women to their newborns.

The intravenous administration of monoclonal antibodies from other species (e.g., mice) is limited by their short half-life and the risk of serum sickness. Nevertheless, they have been used in certain situations, such as in the treatment of acute graft-versus-host disease or graft rejection with OKT3 (anti–CD3 antibody) and tumor localization (anti–tumor cell antibody). The production and clinical use of human monoclonal antibodies are also under development (Bron et al., 1984).

Plasma

Periodic plasma infusions can be used to administer IgG, IgM, and IgA by the intravenous route to patients with antibody immunodeficiencies (Stiehm et al., 1966; Buckley, 1972). In addition to supplying large quantities of undenatured γ globulin, plasma supplies complement components and other proteins of possible importance in combating infection. Plasma infusions have been reported to be of particular benefit in the Wiskott-Aldrich syndrome (Stiehm and McIntosh, 1967), hypogammaglobulinemia with diarrhea (Binder and Reynolds, 1967), and ataxia-telangiectasia (Ammann et al., 1969). Plasma may also be used in complement component immunodeficiencies. Cannon and coworkers (1982) described two infants with diarrhea, malabsorption, and hypoproteinemia who were initially diagnosed as having SCID and who recovered with intensive plasma therapy. Hyperimmune plasma for HIV-positive donors has been used in the therapy of advanced HIV infection.

Because plasma therapy may transmit hepatitis, CMV, or HIV, the plasma from a single hepatitis-free, CMV, and HIV antibody–negative donor, usually a relative, is recommended. This is collected by plasmapheresis, aliquoted in plasma bags, and frozen before use; freezing destroys lymphocytes that may cause graft-versus-host disease. A minor cross-match of the donor plasma with the patient's red blood cells must be negative. The usual dose of plasma is 20 ml/kg, which contains about 200 ml/kg of IgG, 40 ml/kg of IgA, and 20 ml/kg of IgM. Larger doses may be given if this dose is ineffective; in these instances, large quantities of plasma can be obtained from the recipient by plasmapheresis. Patients may experience tingling and paresthesias of the lips and a slight tightening of the chest during plasma infusions; these have not been severe enough to terminate the infusion. Such reactions are often minimized by pretreating the patient with aspirin or Benadryl.

Leukocyte Transfusions

In patients with phagocytic immunodeficiencies, notably chronic granulomatous disease (CGD) granulocytes from a normal donor may permit resolution of an infection not responsive to antibiotic therapy (Raubitschek et al., 1973; Fanconi et al., 1985). Although compatible leukocytes of the same HLA type are not imperative, they result in fewer reactions and have a longer half-life within the recipient. The separated granulocytes must be given within 3 to 4 hours of procurement, and repeated courses of therapy are generally necessary (Boggs, 1974).

In patients with cellular immunodeficiencies, donor granulocytes should be irradiated to remove the risk of graft-versus-host disease from contaminating lymphocytes. Granulocyte infusions can cause febrile reactions, hepatitis, CMV and HIV infections, and the development of antigranulocyte antibodies. CMV antibody–negative donors are recommended.

Pharmacologic Agents

Certain drugs have been used in an attempt to alter the basic immunologic defect in a few immunodeficiency syndromes.

Levamisole, an antihelminthic agent that enhances cutaneous reactivity by nonspecifically stimulating T lymphocytes and macrophages, has been used in immunodeficient subjects. Despite some restoration of immune function (Lieberman and Hsu, 1976), no clinical benefit has been observed in patients with Wiskott-Aldrich syndrome or mucocutaneous candidiasis. Some reports suggest therapeutic benefit of levamisole in the hyper-IgE syndrome by enhancing chemotaxis (DeCree et al., 1974; Wright et al., 1970); its efficacy is unproven.

Vitamin C enhances the chemotaxis of normal granulocytes, probably by increasing the intracellular levels of cyclic 3′,5′-guanosine monophosphate (cGMP), and improves the in vitro bactericidal capacity of the granulocytes from patients with the Chédiak-Higashi syndrome. Accordingly, high-dose vitamin C may benefit certain patients with this syndrome (Boxer et al., 1976; Gallin et al., 1979; Weening et al., 1981). Vitamin B_{12} is beneficial in the treatment of transcobalamin II deficiency.

Antihistamines may also enhance phagocytic chemotaxis under some circumstances. Hill and Quie (1974) found that patients with elevated IgE levels exhibit defective chemotaxis secondary to high levels of intracellular histamine, which in turn affects immune function. Histamine may modify levels of cyclic adenosine monophosphate (cAMP) and cGMP. Other drugs that influence cAMP and cGMP (e.g., theophylline) may have a therapeutic role in disorders associated with abnormal nucleotide regulation.

Cimetidine, an antihistamine with primarily H_2-blocking activity that is widely used in peptic ulcer disease, diminishes suppressor-cell activity and enhances delayed cutaneous hypersensitivity in immunologically normal subjects (Avella et al., 1978). One patient with common variable immunodeficiency had increased immunoglobulin synthesis following its use (White and Ballow, 1985).

Immunostimulants

Several agents that stimulate the immune system nonspecifically are available, but their value in primary immunodeficiency is limited at best. These include microbial products (BCG and other bacterial or fungal extracts), thymus-derived T cell stimulants, thymomimetic drugs, muramyl peptides, lipid A analogs, levamisole, isoprinosine, tuftsin, and interferon inducers (e.g., ampligen) (Hadden, 1993). Several are licensed in other countries, and clinical trials in cancer, HIV, and recurrent infections are under way. None shows proven clinical benefit in primary immunodeficiency. Indeed, in most patients with primary immunodefi-

ciency, excessive antigenic stimulation is present as a result of chronic infection, so that their compromised immune system is already maximally activated.

Cytokine Therapy

Cytokine therapy has been used successfully in selected primary immunodeficiencies. The best example is the use of IFN-γ in patients with chronic granulomatous disease (Gallin, 1991) (see Chapter 15). IFN-γ given weekly subcutaneously enhanced respiratory burst activity in some of these patients and nonoxidative bactericidal activity with a 72% reduction in infections in a double-blind placebo-controlled study. IFN-γ may also be of value in hyper-IgE syndrome, glycogen storage disease type 1b (McCawley, et al., 1993), and primary interferon immunodeficiency (Lipinski et al., 1980).

A second cytokine of proven value is granulocyte–colony stimulating factor (G-CSF), used in the treatment of congenital neutropenia (Kostmann's syndrome), cyclic neutropenia, or other primary immunodeficiencies with neutropenia (e.g., X-linked hyper-IgM immunodeficiency) (Bonilla et al., 1989).

IL-2 therapy may benefit children with SCID who have had selective IL-2 deficiency (Weinberg and Parkman, 1990; Paganelli et al., 1983). IL-2 conjugated to polyethylene glycol (PEG–IL-2) is also under study in common variable immunodeficiency (Cunningham-Rundles et al., 1994).

Soluble cytokine receptors and monoclonal antibodies to cytokines or their receptors are being tested for their immunosuppressive, inflammatory, or antitumor effects.

Transfer Factor

Transfer factor (TF) is a dialyzable extract of immune leukocytes that is used to transfer cellular immunity from a skin test–positive donor to a skin test–negative recipient (Lawrence, 1969). It is often referred to as *dialyzable leukocyte extract* (DLE). Concomitantly, there may be the acquisition of proliferative responses and mediator production to a specific antigen. Transfer factor is a low-molecular-weight (1110- to 1600-MW) nucleopeptide that is heterogeneous in column chromatography. Its exact mechanism of action is uncertain. It is nonantigenic and can be lyophylized and stored for many years.

Transfer factor has been used in a variety of immunodeficiencies with limited success. In some cases of Wiskott-Aldrich syndrome treated with TF, there has been some clinical benefit, as evidenced by decreased infection and eczema and lessening of the thrombocytopenia for up to 6 months (Spitler et al., 1972). Repeated injections were necessary when skin tests became negative.

Some patients with mucocutaneous candidiasis have benefited, particularly when concomitant antifungal therapy is given to reduce the antigenic load (Schulkind et al., 1972). An occasional patient with combined immunodeficiency may show clinical improvement

(Strauss and Hake, 1974). Several patients with combined deficiency have been given TF in conjunction with fetal thymus transplantation with engraftment of T cells from the fetal thymus (Ammann et al., 1973; Rachelefsky et al., 1975b). In general, TF therapy is of doubtful value in cellular immunodeficiency (see Chapter 12).

Thymic Hormone Therapy

The thymic epithelium synthesizes a number of soluble factors that regulate and differentiate T lymphocytes. These include thymosin, *facteur thymique sérique* (FTS), and thymopoietin. These can be assayed by biologic or immunoassays.

Thymosin, a 28–amino acid peptide extracted from bovine thymus, has been the most widely used therapeutically. Wara and Ammann (1976) treated 17 patients with cellular immunodeficiency with thymosin injections. No responses were noted in combined immunodeficiency and ataxia-telangiectasia, but some clinical benefit and restoration of immunologic function in vitro was noted in some patients with the Wiskott-Aldrich, Nezelof, and DiGeorge syndromes.

Another thymic polypeptide in clinical use is thymic pentapeptide (TP5), a polypeptide that includes the active site (amino acids 32 to 36) of the intact thymopoietin molecule. Aiuti and colleagues (1983) have reported some clinical benefit in the DiGeorge and Nezelof syndromes. Therapeutic benefits in immunodeficiency for synthetic FTS (Bordigoni et al., 1982), and thymostimulin (Aiuti et al., 1984) have been reported.

Fetal Tissue Transplantation

Fetal Thymus Transplantation

Thymus transplantation (into either the subcutaneous tissue or the peritoneum) from a fetus of less than 16 weeks' gestation has restored cellular immunity to several patients with DiGeorge anomaly (Cleveland et al., 1968; August et al., 1970), combined immunodeficiency (Rachelefsky et al., 1975b), and Nezelof syndrome (Ammann et al., 1973; Shearer et al., 1978). In the DiGeorge anomaly, fetal thymus brings about rapid reconstitution (within days), which appears to be permanent, and lymphoid chimerism is absent; the mechanism in this syndrome appears to result from the presence of an inducer that activates the patient's own thymic precursor cells (Wara and Ammann, 1976).

In combined immunodeficiency, including the Nezelof syndrome, fetal thymus transplantation resulted in slow reconstitution of T-cell immunity, mild graft-versus-host manifestations, and lymphoid chimerism derived from the implanted thymocytes. Transfer factor has been given concurrently with fetal thymus; its contribution is not clear. The timing and temporary reconstitution distinguishes this effect from the reconstitution in DiGeorge anomaly. Fetal thymic tissue is often difficult to obtain; intact fetuses are available only after hysterectomies, prostaglandin-induced abortions, or at laparotomy for the removal of an unruptured tubal pregnancy. Thus, the popularity of this procedure has waned.

Transplantation of Cultured Thymic Epithelium

Thymic epithelial transplantation has been used in combined immunodeficiency by Hong and coworkers (1976). Thymic fragments removed from normal infants undergoing heart surgery are held for several weeks in tissue culture, during which time most of the lymphoid cells die while the epithelial elements persist. The cultured thymic tissue is implanted intraperitoneally or intramuscularly. After this procedure, increased immunoglobulin levels, antibody production, and restoration of T-cell numbers and proliferative responses associated with mild to moderate clinical improvement have been noted. The incomplete nature of the immunologic reconstitution and the occurrence of lymphomas in three (of 30) patients given thymic epithelial transplants have reduced the enthusiasm for this procedure (Borzy et al., 1979a).

Fetal Liver Transplantation

The fetal liver is a source of stem cells and can reconstitute lethally irradiated mice. Keightley and coworkers (1975) and Buckley and associates (1976b) have reported successful reconstitution in combined immunodeficiency using large numbers (8.4×10^7 to 3.0×10^8) of fresh liver cells from fetuses of less than 10 weeks' gestation. Another successful reconstitution utilized both fetal liver and thymus (Ackeret et al., 1976). Graft-versus-host reactions and chimerism have been observed in some of these cases. The good results with haploidentical T-cell depleted marrow and the incomplete nature of the immune reconstitution have diminished the applicability of this procedure.

Enzyme Replacement

In some children with combined immunodeficiency with adenosine deaminase (ADA) deficiency, partial restoration of immune function and clinical improvement with erythrocyte transfusions containing adequate amounts of ADA have occurred (Polmar et al., 1976). Other ADA-deficient children have not shown clinical benefit from transfusions (Schmalsteig et al., 1978).

Hershfield and associates (1987) first reported that the weekly intramuscular injection of bovine ADA conjugated with polyethylene glycol resulted in correction of the metabolic abnormalities, clinical improvement, and increased T cells in two children with ADA-deficient combined immunodeficiency. Since then, 17 additional children have been successfully treated with this approach (Chaffee et al., 1992).

Bone Marrow Transplantation

HLA-Matched Transplants

Bone marrow transplantation from an HLA-A, HLA-B identical, mixed leukocyte culture (MLC), nonreactive (i.e., HLA-D identical) sibling is the treatment of choice for patients with combined immunodeficiency and the Wiskott-Aldrich syndrome (Goldsobel et al.,

1985). It has also been used in a limited number of patients with reticular dysgenesis (Levinsky and Tiedeman, 1983), chronic granulomatous (disease) (Rappeport et al., 1982), leukocyte adhesion defect type 1 (Kamani et al., 1984), Chédiak-Higashi syndrome (Virelizier et al., 1982), Omenn's syndrome (Fischer et al., 1994) and DiGeorge anomaly (Goldsobel et al., 1985), X-linked lymphoproliferative disorder (Williams et al., 1993; Vowels et al., 1993), and several other immunodeficiencies (see Chapter 32).

More than 200 infants with SCID and more than 20 infants and children with Wiskott-Aldrich syndrome have been restored to health since the initial bone marrow transplants in 1969 (Gatti et al., 1968; Bach et al., 1969). Dramatic and permanent (up to 23 years) restoration of both cellular and antibody functions ensues with evidence of engraftment. Graft-versus-host reactions vary in severity, and some patients have succumbed from infection during this period. The graft-versus-host reaction is usually self-limited, and following its disappearance, the child is usually restored to a state of good health. Some patients have chronic graft-versus-host reactions with persistent dermatitis, hepatitis, or diarrhea.

Because each sibling of the patient has only a 1-in-4 chance of being HLA-identical, most patients will not have an HLA matched donor (see Chapter 32). When a sibling donor is not available, parents and relatives should be examined for HLA identity.

Bone marrow transplantation for immunodeficiency is available in many major medical centers. If transplantation is contemplated, the parents and all siblings should be HLA-A and HLA-B typed, and if any are identical to the patient, a mixed leukocyte culture (MLC) is warranted. All MLC identical matches should be confirmed by repeat testing. The MLC identical donor is hospitalized at the time of transplantation, and the marrow is obtained under anesthesia. It is enumerated, filtered, and injected intravenously (Thomas and Storb, 1970). No immunosuppression is necessary if there is a complete lack of cellular immunity. *P. carinii* prophylaxis is used before and throughout the procedure, and the CMV antibody status of the donor and recipient are identified to determine whether CMV prophylaxis is indicated.

In patients with intact or slightly decreased T-cell immunodeficiency, Wiskott-Aldrich syndrome, or SCID with some degree of cellular immunity present, as indicated by a positive MLC reaction to an unrelated donor, immunosuppression before transplantation is necessary to ensure T-cell engraftment, and in the Wiskott-Aldrich syndrome, to ensure hematopoietic engraftment. One regimen is oral busulfan (3 to 4 mg/kg/day) for 4 days, and intravenous cyclophosphamide (50 mg/kg/day) for 4 days, followed by transplantation on day 10. After the transplant, cyclosporine is usually given to suppress a graft-versus-host reaction. Antithymocyte globulin and corticosteroids are also sometimes used.

Haploidentical Transplants

When an HLA-identical donor is unavailable for a patient with SCID, a haploidentical, T cell–depleted marrow transplantation (half-matched) can be undertaken. In this procedure, mature T cells are removed from the donor marrow before infusion; the less mature T cells then reconstitute the patient without the occurrence of life-threatening graft-versus-host disease. Two techniques are used for T-cell depletion: (1) removal by agglutination with soybean lectin and (2) lysis of T cells with monoclonal anti–T cell antibody plus complement. The former has been used in more than 100 cases (O'Reilly, et al., 1983; Cowan et al., 1985; Friedrich et al., 1985; Buckley et al., 1986), the latter method in more than 30 cases (Reinherz et al., 1982; Parkman, 1986; Fischer et al., 1994) with little or no graft-versus-host disease and a 60% to 80% survival.

Immunosuppression is sometimes necessary to ensure T-cell engraftment. B-cell engraftment with antibody function is not always achieved, and graft-versus-host responses may still occur. Despite these limitations, this technique has been associated with many impressive successes and has replaced fetal liver or cultured thymic epithelial transplants for the SCID patient without a matched donor.

Matched Unrelated Transplants

An alternative to a T-depleted haploidentical bone marrow transplant is an unrelated HLA, phenotypically identical, and (usually) MLC-identical nonrelated donor, usually identified through the National Marrow Donor Program. This has been used with success in eight children with SCID, two children with Chédiak-Higashi syndrome, and six children with the Wiskott-Aldrich syndrome (Filipovich et al., 1992; Lenarsky et al., 1993). Powerful immunosuppressives before and after the procedure are necessary, since the marrow is not T-depleted.

Gene Therapy

Gene therapy has been used with encouraging results in the treatment of a few children with adenosine deaminase–SCID. Successful gene therapy necessitates identification and cloning of the gene lacking or abnormal in the disorder under question, such as ADA deficiency, purine nucleoside phosphorylase deficiency, CGD, and leukocyte adhesion defect type 1 (LAD). The gene is inserted into peripheral leukocytes or bone marrow stem cells, using a Maloney-murine leukemia-based retrovirus vector. The cells are then infused back into the patient at regular intervals (Blaese, 1993) with improved ADA activity and T-cell function and numbers. The patients remain on polyethylene glycol–ADA, however.

As genes are identified in other immunodeficiencies, gene therapy may be used for other diseases, such as X-linked agammaglobulinemia and immunodeficiency with hyper-IgM.

PROGNOSIS

The short-term prognosis depends on the severity of the infectious complications. The long-term prognosis is determined by the nature of the defect. Patients with cellular and combined immunodeficiencies usually have the poorest prognosis unless successful transplantation is achieved. Although acute infectious episodes can be controlled with antibiotics, chronic tissue damage, such as necrotizing colitis or bronchiectasis, may not be prevented.

The long-term prognosis for patients with immunodeficiency is continually changing. Gabrielson and associates (1969) estimate that one third of their patients died prematurely from infectious complications. Among patients with antibody immunodeficiency studied by the Medical Research Council Working Party (1969), the overall mortality was 29% (51 of 176 patients) and 14% died within 6 months of diagnosis. All 11 patients with combined immunodeficiency succumbed rapidly. The mortality for infants under 1 year of age was 45%, compared with 11% for older patients. Among eight patients older than age 2 years who stopped receiving gamma globulin therapy, five died shortly thereafter. Cunningham-Rundles (1989) reported an overall mortality rate of 22% in 103 patients with common variable immunodeficiency followed over a 13-year period. Males died at an earlier age (28.9 years) than females (55.4 years).

COMPLICATIONS

Complications other than bacterial infections include arthritis, amyloidosis, chronic hepatitis, sclerosing cholangitis, chronic lung disease, malignancy, and psychosocial problems. If live vaccines are given, systemic bacille Calmette-Guérin infection, vaccinia gangrenosa, paralytic poliomyelitis, or giant cell (measles) pneumonia may develop in these patients.

There is a high incidence of lymphoreticular malignancy in certain primary immunodeficiencies, notably ataxia-telangiectasia, Wiskott-Aldrich syndrome, and common variable immunodeficiency. Indeed, malignancy is the second leading cause of death after infections in immunodeficiency (see Chapter 27). Occasionally, the onset of immunodeficiency and malignancy is simultaneous; usually, however, the immunodeficiency precedes the malignancy by several years.

RECOVERY

An occasional adult may spontaneously recover the ability to synthesize antibody. In three (of 176) adult females in the Medical Research Council Working Party (1969) study, antibody function returned. One 36-year-old man with common variable hypogammaglobulinemia, diagnosed at age 24, showed normalization of antibody responsiveness and immunoglobulin levels following acquisition of HIV infection at age 30 (Wright et al., 1987). Several patients with selective IgA deficiency may undergo spontaneous cure; most of these have low but measurable IgA and are children under the age of 5 years (Blum et al., 1982). In general, the primary immunodeficiencies are lifelong, incurable, and associated with a guarded prognosis for extended life.

SUPPORT ORGANIZATIONS

Two organizations are active for patients with primary immunodeficiency in the United States. These are the parent-based Immune Deficiency Foundation, Courthouse Square, 3565 Ellicott Drive, Unit B2, Ellicott City, MD 21043 (1-800-296-4433) and the Jeffrey Modell Foundation, 43 W. 47th Street, New York, 10036 (1-800-JEFF-844).

The Immune Deficiency Foundation (IDF) has regional chapters in many areas and offers free publications for physicians, nurses, and patients (including children) on immunodeficiency. Both groups sponsor parent support groups, research meetings, and physician fellowships. The IDF also provides scholarships for patients and helps with insurance and access to care issues.

References

Ackeret C, Pluss HJ, Hitzig WH. Hereditary severe combined immunodeficiency and adenosine deaminase deficiency. Pediatr Res 10:67–70, 1976.

Afzelius BA. A human syndrome caused by immobile cilia. Science 193:317–319, 1976.

Aiuti F, Businco L, Fiorilli M, Galli E, Quinti I, Rossi P, Seminara R, Goldstein G. Thymopoietin pentapeptide treatment of primary immunodeficiencies. Lancet 1:551–554, 1983.

Aiuti F, Sirianni MC, Fiorilli M, Paganelli R, Stella A, Turbessi G. A placebo-controlled trial of thymic hormone treatment of recurrent herpes simplex labialis infection in immunodeficient host: Results after a 1-year follow-up. Clin Immunol Immunopathol 30:11–18, 1984.

Alarcon B, Regueiro JR, Arnaiz-Villena A, Terhorst C. Familial defect in the surface expression of the T-cell receptor-CD3 complex. N Engl J Med 319:1203–1208, 1988.

Albrecht RM, Hong R. Basic and clinical consideration of the monocyte-macrophage system in man. J Pediatr 88:751–765, 1976.

Aliabadi H, Gonzalez R, Quie PG. Urinary tract disorders in patients with chronic granulomatous disease. New Engl J Med 321:706–708, 1989.

Allen JC, Kunkel HG. Antibodies against gamma-globulin after repeated blood transfusions in man. J Clin Invest 45:29–39, 1966.

Allen RC, Armitage RJ, Conley ME, Rosenblatt H, Jenkins NA, Copeland NG, Bedell MA, Edelhoff S, Disteche CM, Simoneaux DK, Fanslow WC, Belmont JW, Spriggs MK. CD40 Ligand gene defects responsible for X-linked hyper-IgM syndrome. Science 259:990–993, 1993.

Allen RC, Nachman RC, Rosenblatt HM, Belmont JW. Application of carrier testing to genetic counseling for X-linked agammaglobulinemia. Am J Hum Genet 54:25–35, 1994.

Allen RC, Stjernholm RL, Steele RH. Evidence for the generation of an electronic excitation state in human polymorphonuclear leukocytes and its participation in bactericidal activity. Biochem Biophys Res Comm 47:679–684, 1972.

Allison AC, Watts RWE, Hovi T, Webster ADB. Immunological observation on patients with Lesch-Nyhan syndrome, and on the role of de novo purine synthesis in lymphocyte transformation. Lancet 2:1179–1182, 1975.

Alper CA, Rosen FS. Complement in laboratory medicine. In Laboratory Diagnosis of Immunologic Disorders. Vyas GN, Stites DP, Brecher G, eds. New York, Grune & Stratton, 1975, pp. 47–68.

Alper CA, Abramson N, Johnston RB Jr, Jandl JH, Rosen FS. Increased susceptibility to infection associated with abnormalities of complement-mediated function and of the third component of complement C3. N Engl J Med 282:350–354, 1970a.

Alper CA, Abramson N, Johnston RB Jr, Jandl JH, Rosen FS. Studies in vivo and in vitro on an abnormality in the metabolism of C3 in a patient with increased susceptibility to infection. J Clin Invest 49:1975–1985, 1970b.

Altman LC, Snyderman R, Blaese RM. Abnormalities of chemotactic lymphokine synthesis and mononuclear leukocyte chemotaxis in Wiskott-Aldrich syndrome. J Clin Invest 54:486–493, 1974.

Amer J, Ott E, Ibbott FA, O'Brien D, Kempe H. The effect of monthly gamma-globulin administration on morbidity and mortality from infection in premature infants during the first year of life. Pediatrics 32:4–9, 1963.

Ammann AJ, Ashman RF, Buckley RH, Hardie WR, Krantman HJ, Nelson J, Ochs H, Stiehm ER, Tiller T, Wara DW, Wedgwood R. Use of intravenous gamma globulin in antibody immunodeficiency. Results of a multicenter controlled trial. Clin Immunol Immunopath 22:60–67, 1982a.

Ammann AJ, Good RA, Bier D, Fudenberg HH. Long-term plasma infusions in a patient with ataxia-telangiectasia and deficient IgA and IgE. Pediatrics 44:672–676, 1969.

Ammann AJ, Wara DW, Cowan MJ, Barrett DJ, Stiehm ER. The DiGeorge syndrome and the fetal alcohol syndrome. Am J Dis Child 136:906–908, 1982b.

Ammann AJ, Wara DW, Salmon S, Perkins HL. Thymus transplantation: permanent reconstitution of cellular immunity in a patient with sex-linked combined immunodeficiency. N Engl J Med 289:5–9, 1973.

Anderson DC, Schmalstieg FC, Arnaout MA, Kohl S, Tosi MF, Dapa N, Buffone GJ, Hughes BJ, Brinkley BR, Dickey WD, Abramson JS, Springer T, Boxer LA, Hollers JM, Smith CW. Abnormalities of polymorphonuclear leukocyte function associated with a heritable deficiency of high molecular weight surface glycoproteins (GP138): common relationship to diminished cell adherence. J Clin Invest 74:536–551, 1984.

Anderson WF. Prospects of human gene therapy. Science 226:401–409, 1984.

Apfelzweig R, Piszkiewicz D, Hooper JA. Immunoglobulin A concentrations in commercial immune globulins. J Clin Immunol 7:46–50, 1987.

Arditi M, Kabat W, Togev BS, Yogev R. Serum tumor necrosis factor alpha, interleukin 1-beta, p24 antigen concentrations and CD4+ cells at various stages of human immunodeficiency virus 1 infection in children. Pediatr Infect Dis J 10:450–455, 1991.

Arnaiz-Villena A, Timon M, Corell A, Perez-Aciego P, Martin-Villa JM, Regueiro JR. Primary immunodeficiency caused by mutations in the gene encoding the CD3-γ subunit of the T-lymphocyte receptor. N Engl J Med 327:529–533, 1992.

Arpaia E, Sharar M, Dadi H, Cohen A, Roifman CM. Defective T-cell receptor signaling and CD8+ thymic selection in humans lacking Zap-70 kinase. Cell 76:947–958, 1994.

Asano Y, Yoshikawa T, Suga S, Kobayashi I, Nakashima T, Yazaki T, Ozaki T, Yamada A, Imanishi J. Postexposure prophylaxis of varicella in family contact by oral acyclovir. Pediatrics 92:219–222, 1993.

August CS, Levey RH, Berkel AI, Rosen FS. Establishment of immunological competence in a child with congenital thymic aplasia by a graft of fetal thymus. Lancet 1:1080–1083, 1970.

Avella J, Madsen JE, Binder HJ, and Askenase PW. Effect of histamine H2-receptor antagonists on delayed hypersensitivity. Lancet 1:624–626, 1978.

Bach FH, Albertini RJ, Anderson JL, Joo P, Bortin MM. Bone-marrow transplantation in a patient with the Wiskott-Aldrich syndrome. Lancet 2:1364–1366, 1968.

Baehner RL, Nathan DG. Quantitative nitroblue tetrazolium test in chronic granulomatous disease. N Engl J Med 278:971–980, 1968.

Baker DH, Parmer EA, Wolff JA. Roentgen manifestation of the Aldrich syndrome. Am J Roentgenol 88:458–465, 1962.

Ballow M. Mechanisms of action of intravenous immune globulin therapy. Pediatr Inf Dis J 13:806–811, 1994.

Ballow M, Cater KL, Rowe JC, Goetz C, Desbonnet C. Development of the immune system in very low birth weight (less than 1500 g) premature infants: concentrations of plasma immunoglobulins and patterns of infections. Pediatr Res 20:899–904, 1986.

Barandun S, Kistler P, Jeunet F, Isliker H. Intravenous administration of human γ-globulin. Vox Sang 7:157–174, 1962.

Barton JC, Herrera GA, Galla JH, Bertoli LF, Work J, Koopman WJ.

Acute cryoglobulinemic renal failure after intravenous infusion of gamma globulin. Am J Med 82:624–629, 1987.

Berendes H, Bridges RA, Good RA. A fatal granulomatous disease of childhood: the clinical study of a new syndrome. Minn Med 40:309–312, 1957.

Berger M, Cupps TR, Fauci A. Immunoglobulin replacement therapy by slow subcutaneous infusion. Ann Intern Med 93:55–56, 1980.

Bernard A, Boumsell L. The clusters of differentiation (CD) defined by the first international workshop on human leucocyte differentiation antigens. Hum Immunol 11:1–10, 1984.

Bernatowska E, Madalinski K, Janowicz W, Weremowicz R, Gutkowski P, Wolf HM, Eibl MM. Results of a prospective controlled two-dose crossover study with intravenous immunoglobulin and comparison (retrospective) with plasma treatment. Clin Immunol Immunopath 43:153–162, 1987.

Biggar WD, Park BH, Good RA. Compatible bone marrow transplantation and immunologic reconstitution of combined immunodeficiency disease. In Bergsma D, Good RA, Finstad J, eds. Immunodeficiency in Man and Animals. New York, Sinauer, 1975, pp. 385–390.

Binder HJ, Reynolds RD. Control of diarrhea in secondary hypogammaglobulinemia by fresh plasma infusions. N Engl J Med 277:802–803, 1967.

Björkander J, Hammarström L, Smith CIE, Buckley RH, Cunningham-Rundles C, Hanson LA. Immunoglobulin prophylaxis in patients with antibody deficiency syndromes and anti-IgA antibodies. J Clin Immunol 7:8–15, 1987.

Blaese RM. Development of gene therapy for immunodeficiency: adenosine deaminase deficiency. Pediatr Res (Suppl 33):S49–S55, 1993.

Blaese RM, Lawrence EC. Development of macrophage function and the expression of immunocompetence. In Cooper MD, Dayton DH, eds. Development of Host Defenses. New York, Raven Press, 1977, pp. 201–211.

Blum PM, Hong R, Stiehm ER. Spontaneous recovery of selective IgA deficiency: additional case report and a review. Clin Pediatr 21:77–80, 1982.

Blume RS, Beanett JM, Yankee RA, Wolff SM. Defective granulocyte regulation in the Chédiak-Higashi syndrome. N Engl J Med 279:1009–1015, 1968.

Boggs DP. Transfusions of neutrophils as prevention or treatment of infection in patients with neutropenia. N Engl J Med 290:1055–1062, 1974.

Bolscher BGJM, de Boer M, de Klein A, Weening RS, Roos D. Point mutations in the β-subunit of cytochrome b_{558} leading to X-linked chronic granulomatous disease. Blood 77:2482–2487, 1991.

Bonforte RJ, Topilsky M, Siltzbach LE, Glade PR. Phytohemagglutinin skin test: a possible in vivo measure of cell-mediated immunity. J Pediatr 81:775–780, 1972.

Bonilla MA, Gillio AP, Ruggeiro M, Kernan NA, Brochstein JA, Abboud M, Fumagalli L, Vincent M, Gabrilove JL, Welte K, Souza LM, O'Reilly RJ. Effects of recombinant human granulocyte colony-stimulating factor on neutropenia in patients with congenital agranulocytosis. N Engl J Med 320:1574–1580, 1989.

Bordigoni P, Faure G, Bene MC, Dardenne M, Bach JF, Duheille J. Improvement of cellular immunity and IgA production in immunodeficient children after treatment with synthetic serum thymic factor (FTS). Lancet 2:293–297, 1982.

Borowitz SM, Saulsbury FT. Treatment of chronic cryptosporidial infection with orally administered human serum immune globulin. J Pediatr 119:593–595, 1991.

Borut TC, Ank BJ, Gard SE, Stiehm ER. Tetanus toxoid skin test in children: Correlation with in vitro lymphocyte stimulation and monocyte chemotaxis. J Pediatr 97:567–573, 1980.

Borzy MS, Hong R, Horowitz SD, Gilbert E, Kaufman D, DeMendonca W, Oxelius VA, Dictor M, Pachman L. Fatal lymphoma after transplantation of cultured thymus in children with combined immunodeficiency disease. N Engl J Med 301:565–568, 1979a.

Borzy MS, Ridgway D, Noya FJ, Shearer WT. Successful bone marrow transplantation with split lymphoid chimerism in DiGeorge syndrome. J Clin Immunol 9:386–392, 1989.

Borzy MS, Schulte-Wissermann H, Gilbert E, Horowitz SD, Pellett J, Hong R. Thymic morphology in immunodeficiency diseases: results of thymic biopsies. Clin Immunol Immunopathol 12:31–51, 1979b.

Boulos GN, Rosenau W, Goldberg ML. Comparison and yield of

antigen- or mitogen-induced human lymphotoxins. J Immunol 112:1347–1353, 1974.

Bowen TJ, Ochs HD, Altman LC, Price TH, Van Epps DE, Brautigan DL, Rosin RE, Perkins WD, Babior BM, Klebanoff SJ, Wedgwood RJ. Severe recurrent bacterial infections associated with defective adherence and chemotaxis in two patients with neutrophils deficient in a cell-associated glycoprotein. J Pediatr 101:932–940, 1982.

Boxer LA, Hedley-Whyte ET, Stossel TP. Neutrophil actin dysfunction and abnormal neutrophil behavior. N Engl J Med 291:1093–1099, 1974.

Boxer LA, Watanabe AM, Rister M, Besch HR Jr, Allen J, Baehner RL. Correction of leukocyte function in Chédiak-Higashi syndrome by ascorbate. N Engl J Med 293:1041–1045, 1976.

Boyden S. The chemotactic effect of mixtures of antibody and antigen on polymorphonuclear leukocytes. J Exp Med 115:453–466, 1962.

Brandtzaeg P, Fjellanger I, Gjeruldsen ST. Immunoglobulin M: local synthesis and selective secretion in patients with immunoglobulin A deficiency. Science 160:789–791, 1968.

Broder S, Humphrey R, Durm M, Blackman M, Meade B, Goldman C, Strober W, Waldmann T. Impaired synthesis of polyclonal (non-paraprotein) immunoglobulins by circulating lymphocytes from patients with multiple myeloma. N Engl J Med 293:887–892, 1975.

Bron D, Feinberg MB, Teng NN, Kaplan HS. Production of human monoclonal IgG antibodies against Rhesus (D) antigen. Proc Natl Acad Sci U S A 81:3214–3217, 1984.

Bruton OC. Agammaglobulinemia. Pediatrics 9:722–728, 1952.

Buckley RH. Plasma therapy in immunodeficiency diseases. Am J Dis Child 124:376–381, 1972.

Buckley RH. Immunodeficiency diseases. JAMA 268:2797–2806, 1992.

Buckley RH, Gilbertsen RB, Schiff RI, Ferreira E, Sanal SO, Waldmann TA. Heterogeneity of lymphocyte subpopulations in severe combined immunodeficiency. J Clin Invest 58:130–136, 1976a.

Buckley RH, Schiff SE, Sampson HA, Schiff RI, Markert ML, Knutsen AP, Hershfield MS, Huang AT, Mickey GH, Ward FE. Development of immunity in human severe primary T cell deficiency following haploidentical bone marrow stem cell transplantation. J Immunol 136:2398–2407, 1986.

Buckley RH, Whisnant JK, Schiff RI, Gilbertsen RB, Huang AT, Platt MS. Correction of severe combined immunodeficiency by fetal liver cells. N Engl J Med 294:1076–1082, 1976b.

Burks AW, Sampson HA, Buckley RH. Anaphylactic reactions after gamma globulin administration in patients with hypogammaglobulinemia. N Engl J Med 314:560–564, 1986.

Cannon RA, Blum PM, Ament ME, Byrne WJ, Soderberg-Warner M, Seeger RC, Saxon AE, Stiehm ER. Reversal of enterocolitis-associated combined immunodeficiency by plasma therapy. J Pediatr 101:711–717, 1982.

Carroll RR, Noyes WD, Rosse WF, Kitchens CS. Intravenous immunoglobulin administration in the treatment of severe chronic immune thrombocytopenic purpura. Am J Med 76(3A):181–186, 1984.

Carson DA, Seegmiller JE. Effect of adenosine deaminase inhibition upon human lymphocyte blastogenesis. J Clin Invest 57:274–282, 1976.

Centers for Disease Control. Guidelines for prophylaxis against *Pneumocystis carinii* pneumonia for children infected with human immunodeficiency virus. MMWR 40:1–11, 1991.

Centers for Disease Control. Outbreak of hepatitis C associated with intravenous immunoglobulin administration—United States Oct 1993—June 1994. MMWR 43:505–509, 1994.

Chaffee S, Mary A, Stiehm ER, Girault D, Fischer A, Hershfield MS. IgG antibody response to polyethylene glycol-modified adenosine deaminase in patients with adenosine deaminase deficiency. J Clin Invest 89:1643–1651, 1992.

Chandra RK. Fetal malnutrition and postnatal immunocompetence. Am J Dis Child 129:450–454, 1975.

Chang TW, McKinney S, Liu V, Kung PC, Vileek J, Lee J. Use of monoclonal antibodies as sensitive and specific probes for biologically active human gamma-interferon. Proc Natl Acad Sci U S A 81:5219–5222, 1984.

Charache P, Rosen FS, Janeway CA, Craig JM, Rosenberg HA. Acquired agammaglobulinemia in siblings. Lancet 1:234–237, 1965.

Chatila T, Wong R, Young M, Miller R, Terhorst C, Geha RS. An immunodeficiency characterized by defective signal transduction in T lymphocytes. N Engl J Med 320:696–702, 1989.

Chenoweth DE, Cooper SW, Hugli TE, Stewart RW, Blackstone EH, Kirklin JW. Complement activation during cardiopulmonary bypass: evidence for generation of C3a and C5a anaphylatoxins. N Engl J Med 304:497–503, 1981.

Cleveland WW, Fogel BJ, Brown WT, Kay HEM. Foetal thymic transplant in a case of DiGeorge's syndrome. Lancet 2:1211–1214, 1968.

Cline MJ. A new white cell test which measures individual phagocyte function in a mixed leukocyte population. I. A neutrophil defect in acute myelocytic leukemia. J Lab Clin Med 81:311–316, 1973.

Cline MJ, Opelz G, Saxon A, Fahey JL, Golde DW. Autoimmune panleukopenia. N Engl J Med 295:1489–1493, 1976.

Collet J-P, Cucruet T, Kramer MS, Haggerty J, Floret D, Chomel J-J, Durr F, and the Epicrèche Research Group. Stimulation of nonspecific immunity to reduce the risk of recurrent infections in children attending day-care centers. Pediatr Inf Dis J 12:648–652, 1993.

Comenzo RL, Malachowski ME, Meissner HC, Fulton DR, Berkman EM. Immune hemolysis, disseminated intravascular coagulation, and serum sickness after large doses of immune globulin given intravenously for Kawasaki disease. J Pediatr 120:926–928, 1992.

Conley ME. Molecular approaches to analysis of X-linked immunodeficiencies. Annu Rev Immunol 10:215–238, 1992.

Conley ME. Nowell PC, Henle G, Douglas SD. XX T cells and XY B cells in two patients with severe combined immune deficiency. Clin Immunol Immunopathol 31:87–95, 1984.

Conley ME, Park CL, Douglas SD. Childhood variable immunodeficiency with autoimmune disease. J Pediatr 108:915–922, 1986.

Constantopoulos A, Najjar V, Smith JW. Tuftsin deficiency: a new syndrome with defective phagocytosis. J Pediatr 80:564–572, 1972.

Cooper MD, Chase HP, Lowman JT, Krivit W, Good RA. Wiskott-Aldrich syndrome: immunologic deficiency disease involving the afferent limb of immunity. Am J Med 44:499–513, 1968.

Cooper MR, DeChatelet LD, LaVia MF, McCall CE, Spurr CL, Baehner RL. Complete deficiency of leukocyte glucose-6-phosphate dehydrogenase with defective bactericidal activity. J Clin Invest 51:769–778, 1972.

Cooper NR. The complement system. In Stites DP, Stobot JD, Fudenberg HH, Wells JV, eds. Basic and Clinical Immunology, 5th ed. Los Altos, Calif, Lange, 1984, pp. 119–131.

Copeland EA, Strohm PL, Kennedy MS, Tutschka PJ. Hemolysis following intravenous immune globulin therapy. Transfusion 26:410–412, 1986.

Corriel RN, Kniker WT, McBryde JL, Lesourd BM. Cell-mediated immunity in school children assessed by multitest skin testing. Am J Dis Child 139:146, 1985.

Cottier H, Turk J, Sobin L. Propositions en vue de standardiser la description histologique du ganglion lymphatique humain dans ses rapports avec la fonction immunologique. Bull WHO 47:409–417, 1972.

Cowan MJ, Wara DW, Packman S, Ammann AJ. Multiple biotin-dependent carboxylase deficiencies associated with defects in T cell and B cell immunity. Lancet 2:117–119, 1979.

Cowan MJ, Wara DW, Weintrub PS, Pabst H, Ammann AJ. Haploidentical bone marrow transplantation for severe combined immunodeficiency disease using soybean agglutinin-negative, T-depleted marrow cells. J Clin Immunol 5:370–376, 1985.

Cunningham-Rundles C. Clinical and immunologic analyses of 103 patients with common variable immunodeficiency. J Clin Immunol 9:22–33, 1989.

Cunningham-Rundles C, Kazbay K, Hassett J, Zhou Z, Mayer L. Enhanced humoral immunity in common variable immunodeficiency after long-term treatment with polyethylene glycol–conjugated interleukin-2. N Engl J Med 331:918–921, 1994.

Curnutte JT. Chronic granulomatous disease: the solving of a clinical riddle at the molecular level. Clin Immunol Immunopathol 67:S2–S15, 1993.

Dagan R, Schwartz RH, Insel RA, Meregus HA. Severe diffuse adenovirus or pneumonia in a child with combined immunodeficiency: possible therapeutic effect of human immune serum globulin containing specific neutralizing antibody. Pediatr Infect Dis 3:246–251, 1984.

Daly PB, Evans JH, Kobayashi RH, Kobayashi AL, Ochs HD, Fischer

SH, Pirofsky B, Sprouse C. Home-based immunoglobulin infusion therapy: quality of life and patient health perceptions. Ann Allergy 67:504–510, 1991.

Daniels CA, Borsos T, Rapp HJ, Snyderman R, Notkins AL. Neutralization of sensitized virus by purified components of complement. Proc Nat Acad Sci U S A, 65:528–535, 1970.

Dardenne M, Bach JF. The sheep cell rosette assay for the evaluation of thymic hormones. In Biologic Activity of Thymic Hormones. Rotterdam, Kooyker Scientific Publications, 1975, pp. 235–243.

David JR, Al-Askarr S, Lawrence HS, Thomas L. Delayed hypersensitivity in vitro. I. The specificity of inhibition of cell migration by antigen. J Immunol 93:264–273, 1964.

Davis SD, Schaller J, Wedgwood RJ. Antibody deficiency syndromes. In Kagan BM, and Stiehm ER, eds. Immunologic Incompetence: Chicago, Year Book Medical Publishers, 1971, pp. 179–189.

Debray D, Pariente D, Urvoas E, Hadchouel M, Bernard O. Sclerosing cholangitis in children. J Pediatr 124:49–56, 1994.

DeChatelet LP, Shirley PS, McPhail LC. Normal leukocyte glutathione peroxidase activity in patients with chronic granulomatous disease. J Pediatr 89:598–600, 1976.

DeCree J, Verhaegen H, DeCock W, Vanheule R, Brugmans J, Schuermans V. Impaired neutrophil phagocytosis. Lancet 2:294–295, 1974.

de la Salle H, Hanau D, Fricker D, Urlacher A, Kelly A, Salamero J, Powis SH, Donato L, Bausinger H, Laforet M, Jeras M, Spehner D, Bieber T, Falkenrodt A, Cazenave JP, Trowsdale J, Tongio MM. Homozygous human TAP peptide transporter mutation in HLA class 1 deficiency. Science 265:237–241, 1994.

Drenth JPH, Haagsma CJ, van der Meer JWM, the International Hyper-IgD Study Group. Hyperimmunoglobulinemia D and periodic fever syndrome: the clinical spectrum in a series of 50 patients. Medicine 73:133–144, 1994.

Driscoll DA, Budarf ML, Emanuel BS. A genetic etiology for DiGeorge syndrome: consistent deletions and microdeletions of 22q11. Am J Hum Genet 50:924–933, 1992.

Dumonde DC. Lymphocyte-produced substances in immunopharmacology and immunotherapy. EOS J Immunol Immunopharmacol 4:77–84, 1984.

Dunn KD, Lubens R, Stiehm ER. Reversal of neutropenia in X-linked immunodeficiency by large doses of plasma. Clin Res 30:125A, 1982.

Durandy A, Dumez Y, Guy-Grand D, Oury C, Henrion R, Griscelli C. Prenatal diagnosis of severe combined immunodeficiency. J Pediatr 101:995–997, 1982.

Durandy A, Schiff C, Bonnefoy JY, Forveille M, Rousset F, Mazzei G, Milili M, Fischer A. Induction by anti-CD40 antibody or soluble CD40 ligand and cytokines of IgG, IgA, and IgE production by B cells from patients with X-linked hyper-IgM syndrome. Eur J Immunol 23:2294–2299, 1993.

Edwards NL, Magilavy DB, Cassidy JT, Fox IH. Lymphocyte ecto-5'-nucleotidase deficiency in agammaglobulinemia. Science 201:628–630, 1978.

Eibl MM, Cairns L, Rosen FS. Safety and efficacy of a monomeric, functionally intact intravenous IgG preparation in patients with primary immunodeficiency syndromes. Clin Immunol Immunopathol 31:151–169, 1984.

Eibl MM, Mannhalter JW, Zlabinger G, Mayr WR, Tilz GP, Ahmad R, Zielinski CC. Defective macrophage function in a patient with common variable immunodeficiency. N Engl J Med 307:803–806, 1982.

Ellis EF, Henney CS. Adverse reactions following administration of human gammaglobulin. J Allergy 43:45–54, 1969.

Etzioni A, Frydman M, Pollack S, Avidor I, Phillips ML, Paulson JC, Gershoni-Baruch R. Recurrent severe infections caused by a novel leukocyte adhesion deficiency. N Engl J Med 237:1789–1792, 1992.

Fanconi S, Seger R, Gmür J, Willi U, Schaer G, Spiess H, Otto R, Hitzig WH. Surgery and granulocyte transfusions for life-threatening infections in chronic granulomatous disease. Helv Paediat Acta 40:277–284, 1985.

Fearon ER, Winkelstein JA, Civin CI, Pardoll DM, Vogelstein B. Carrier detection in X-linked agammaglobulinemia by analysis of X-chromosome inactivation. N Engl J Med 316:427–431, 1987.

Felsburg PJ, Edelman R. The active E-rosette test: a sensitive in vitro correlate for human delayed-type hypersensitivity. J Immunol 118:62–66, 1977.

Ferreira A, García Rodriguez MC, Fontán G. Follow-up of anti-IgA antibodies in primary immunodeficient patients treated with γ-globulin. Vox Sang 56:218–222, 1989.

Fletcher MA, Baron GC, Ashman MR, Fischl MA, Kimas NG. Use of whole blood methods in assessment of immune parameters in immunodeficiency states. Diagn Clin Immunol 5:69–81, 1987.

Filipovich AH, Shapiro RS, Ramsay NKC, Kim T, Blazar B, Kersey J, McGlave P. Unrelated donor bone marrow transplantation for correction of lethal congenital immunodeficiencies. Blood 80:270–276, 1992.

Filipovich AH, Zerbe D, Spector BD, Kersey JH. In Magrath IT, O'Conor GT, Ramot B, eds. Lymphomas in Persons with Naturally Occurring Immunodeficiency Disorders. Pathogenesis of Leukemia and Lymphomas: Environmental Influences. New York, Raven Press, 1984, pp. 225–234.

Fine DP, Marynwy SR Jr, Calley DG, Sergent JS, Des Pres RM. C3 shunt activation in human serum chelated with EGTA. J Immunol 109:807–809, 1972.

Fischer A, Landais P, Friedrich W, Gerritsen B, Fasth A, Porta F, Vellodi A, Benkerrou M, Jais JP, Cavazzana-Calvo M, Souillet G, Bordigoni P, Morgan G, VanDijken P, Vossen J, Locateli F, di Bartolomeo P. Bone marrow transplantation (BMT) in Europe for primary immunodeficiencies other than severe combined immunodeficiency: a report from the European group for BMT and the European group for immunodeficiency. Blood 83:1149–1154, 1994.

Fischer GW, Weisman LB, Hemming VG, London WT, Hunter KW, Bosworth JM, Sever JL, Wilson SR, Curfman BL. Intravenous immunoglobulin in neonatal group B streptococcal disease. Pharmacokinetic and safety studies in monkeys and humans. Am J Med 76(3A):117–123, 1984.

Forman ML, Stiehm ER. Impaired opsonic activity but normal phagocytosis in low-birth-weight infants. N Engl J Med 281:926–931, 1969.

Friedrich W, Goldman SF, Ebell W, Blutters-Sawatzki R, Gaedicke G, Raghavachar A, Peter HH, Belohradsky B, Kreth W, Kubanek B, Kleihauer E. Severe combined immunodeficiency: treatment by bone marrow transplantation in 15 infants using HLA-haploidentical donors. Eur J Pediatr 144:125–130, 1985.

Fudenberg H, German JL III, Kunkel HG. The occurrence of rheumatoid factor and other abnormalities in families of patients with agammaglobulinemia. Arthritis Rheum 5:565–588, 1962.

Fudenberg HH, Fudenberg BR. Antibody to hereditary human gamma-globulin (Gm) factor resulting from maternal-fetal incompatibility. Science 145:170, 1964.

Fudenberg HH, Good RA, Goodman HC, Hitzig W, Kunkel HG, Roitt IM, Rosen FS, Rowe DS, Seligmann M, Soothill JR. Primary immunodeficiencies. Report of a World Health Organization Committee. Pediatrics 47:927–946, 1971.

Fudenberg HH, Wybran J. Experimental immunotherapy. In Stites DP, Stobo JD, Fudenberg HH, Wells JV, eds. Basic Clinical Immunology, 5th ed. Los Altos, Calif., Lange, 1984, pp. 744–761.

Furucho K, Kamiya T, Nakano H, Kiyosawa N, Shinomiya K, Hayashidera T, Tamura T, Hirose O, Manabe Y, Yokoyama T. High-dose intravenous gammaglobulin for Kawasaki disease. Lancet 2:1055–1058, 1984.

Gabrielson AE, Cooper MD, Peterson RDA, Good RA. The primary immunologic deficiency diseases. In Meischer PA, Müller-Eberhard HJ, eds. Textbook of Immunopathology, Vol. 2. New York, Grune & Stratton, 1969, pp 385–405.

Gallin JI. Interferon-γ in the treatment of the chronic granulomatous diseases of childhood. Clin Immunol Immunopath 61:S100–S105, 1991.

Gallin JI, Clark RA, Kimball HR. Granulocyte chemotaxis: an improved in vitro assay employing ^{51}Cr-labeled granulocytes. J Immunol 110:233–240, 1973.

Gallin JI, Elin RJ, Hubert RT, Fauci AS, Kaliner MA, Wolff SM. Efficacy of ascorbic acid in Chédiak-Higashi syndrome (CHS). Studies in humans and mice. Blood 53:226–234, 1979.

Gardulf A, Hammarström L, Smith CIE. Home treatment of hypogammaglobulinemia with subcutaneous gammaglobulin by rapid infusion. Lancet 338:162–166, 1991.

Gatti R. Ataxia-telangiectasia: immune dysfunction is one of many defects. Immunol Today, 5:121–123, 1984.

Gatti RA, Meuwissen HJ, Allen HD, Hong R, and Good RA. Immunological reconstitution of sex-linked lymphopenic immunological deficiency. Lancet 2:1366–1369, 1968.

Geha RS, Malakian A, Lefranc G, Chayban D, Serre JL. Immunologic reconstitution in severe combined immunodeficiency following transplantation with parental bone marrow. Pediatrics 58:451–455, 1976.

Geisler C, Pallesen G, Platz P, Odum N, Dickmeiss E, Ryder LP, Svejgaard A, Plesner T, Larsen JK, Koch C. Novel primary thymic defect in T lymphocytes expressing T-cell receptor. J Clin Pathol 42:705–711, 1989.

Gelfand EW. Transmembrane signalling and T-cell immunodeficiency. Pediatr Res (33 Suppl):S16–S23, 1993.

Gewurz H, Suyehira LA. Complement. In Rose NR, Friedman H, eds. Manual of Clinical Immunology. Washington, DC, American Society of Microbiology, 1976, pp. 36–47.

Giblett ER, Ammann AJ, Wara DW, Sandman R, Diamond LK. Nucleoside-phosphorylase deficiency in a child with severely defective T-cell immunity and normal B-cell immunity. Lancet 1:1010–1014, 1975.

Girot R, Hamet JL, Perignon JL, Guesnu M, Fox RM, Cartier P, Durandy A, Griscelli C. Cellular immunodeficiency in two siblings with hereditary orotic aciduria. N Engl J Med 308:700–704, 1983.

Glanzmann E, Riniker P. Essentielle lymphocytophthise. Ein neues Krankheitsbild aus der Säuglings-pathologie. Ann Paediatr (Basel) 175:1–32, 1950.

Goldsobel AB, Ehrlich RM, Mendoza GR, Stiehm ER. Bone marrow transplantation for Wiskott-Aldrich syndrome: report of 2 cases with use of 2-mercaptoethane sulfonate and review of the literature. Transplantation 59:568–570, 1985.

Goldstein AL, Slater FD, White A. Preparation, assay, and partial purification of a thymic lymphocytopoietic factor (thymosin). Proc Natl Acad Sci U S A 56:1010–1017, 1966.

Goodwin JS, Messner RP, Bankhurst AD, Peake GT, Saiki J, Williams RC. Prostaglandin producing suppressor cells in Hodgkin's disease. N Engl J Med 297:963–968, 1977.

Gordon EH, Krause A, Kinney JL, Stiehm ER, Klaustermeyer WB. Delayed cutaneous hypersensitivity in normals: choice of antigens and comparison to in vitro assays of cell-mediated immunity. J Allergy Clin Immunol 72:487–494, 1983.

Greenberg F, Valdes C, Rosenblatt HM, Kirkland JL, Ledbetter DH. Hypoparathyroidism and T cell immune defect in a patient with 10p deletion syndrome. J Pediatr 109:489–492, 1986.

Grimm EA, Rosenberg SA. The human lymphokine-activated killer cell phenomenon. In Pick E, Landy M, eds. Lymphokines, Vol. 19. New York, Academic Press, 1984, pp. 279–311.

Groothuis JR, Simoes EAF, Levin MJ, Hall CB, Long CE, Rodriguez WJ, Arrobio J, Meissner HC, Fulton DR, Welliver RC, Tristram DA, Siber GR, Prince GA, VanRaden M, Hemming VG, and the Respiratory Syncytial Virus Immune Globulin Study Group. Prophylactic administration of respiratory syncytial virus immune globulin to high-risk infants and young children. N Engl J Med 329:1524–1530, 1993.

Groshong T, Horowitz S, Lovchik J, Davis A, Hong R. Chronic cytomegalovirus infection, immunodeficiency, and monoclonal gammopathy—antigen-driven malignancy? J Pediatr 88:217–223, 1976.

Gupta JD, Reed CE. Natural antibodies to Salmonella enteritidis endotoxin in maternal and cord sera and in patients with immunologic deficiency diseases. Int Arch Allergy 34:324–330, 1968.

Hadden JW. Immunostimulants. Immunol Today 14:275–280, 1993.

Hammerschmidt PE, Bowers TK, Kammi-Kepfe CJ, Jacob HS, Craddock PR. Granulocyte aggregometry: a sensitive technique for the detection of C5a and complement activation. Blood 55:898–902, 1980.

Haraldson A, Weemaes CMR, De Boer AW, Bakkeren JAJM, Stoelinga GBA. Immunological studies in the hyper-immunoglobulin D syndrome. J Clin Immunol 12:424–428, 1992.

Hayakawa H, Iwata T, Yata J, Kobayashi N. Primary immunodeficiency syndrome in Japan. I. Overview of a nationwide survey on primary immunodeficiency syndrome. J Clin Immunol 1:31–39, 1981.

Heiner DC, Myers AS, Beck CS. Deficiency of IgG4: Disorder associated with frequent infections and bronchiectasis which may be familial. Clin Rev Allergy 1:259–266, 1983.

Herrod HG. Chronic mucocutaneous candidiasis in childhood and complications of non-Candida infection: a report of the Pediatric Immunodeficiency Collaborative Study Group. J Pediatr 116:377–382, 1990.

Hersh EM, Reuben JM, Rios A, Mansell PWA, Newell GR, McClure JE, Goldstein AL. Elevated serum alpha-1-thymosin levels associated with evidence of immune dysregulation in male homosexuals with a history of infectious diseases or Kaposi's sarcoma. N Engl J Med 308:45–46, 1983.

Hershfield MS, Buckley RH, Greenberg ML, Melton AL, Schiff R, Hatem C, Kurtzberg J, Markert ML, Kobayashi RH, Kobayashi AL, Abuchowski A. Treatment of adenosine deaminase deficiency with polyethylene glycol–modified adenosine deaminase. N Engl J Med 316:589–596, 1987.

Hershfield MS, Chaffee S, Sorenson RU. Enzyme replacement therapy with polyethylene glycol–adenosine deaminase in adenosine deaminase deficiency: overview and case reports of three patients, including two now receiving gene therapy. Pediatr Res (33 Suppl):S42–S48, 1993.

Hill HR, Quie PG. Raised serum-IgE levels and defective neutrophil chemotaxis in three children with eczema and recurrent bacterial infections. Lancet 1:183–187, 1974.

Hirschhorn R. Adenosine deaminase deficiency. Immunodefic Rev 2:175–198, 1990.

Hirschhorn R, Beratis N, Rosen FS, Parkman R, Stern R, Polmar S. Adenosine-deaminase deficiency in a child diagnosed prenatally. Lancet 1:73–75, 1975.

Hitzig WH, Biro A, Bosch H, Huser HJ. Agammaglobulinamie und Almphozytose mit Schwund des lymphatischen Gewebes. Helv Paediat Acta 13:551–585, 1958.

Hitzig WH, Grob PJ. Therapeutic uses of transfer factor. Prog Clin Immunol 2:69–100, 1976.

Hobbs JR. Disturbances of the immunoglobulins. Sci Basis Med, pp 106–127, 1966.

Hohn DC, Lehrer RI. NADPH oxidase deficiency in X-linked chronic granulomatous disease. J Clin Invest 55:707–713, 1975.

Holder IA, Naglich JG. Experimental studies of the pathogenesis of infections due to Pseudomonas aeruginosa. Treatment with intravenous immunoglobulin. Am J Med 76(3A):168–174, 1984.

Holland PV, Alter HJ, Purcel RH, Lander JT, Sgouris JT, Schmidt JP. Hepatitis B antigen (HBAg) and antibody (anti-ABAg) in cold ethanol fractions of human plasma. Transfusion 12:363–370, 1972.

Holmes B, Page AR, Good RA. Studies of the metabolic activity of leukocytes from patients with a genetic abnormality of phagocytic function. J Clin Invest 46:1422–1432, 1967.

Holmes B, Park BH, Malawista SE, Quie PG, Nelson DL, Good RA. Chronic granulomatous disease in females. A deficiency of leukocyte glutathione peroxidase. N Engl J Med 283:217–221, 1970.

Hong R. Update on the immunodeficiency diseases. Am J Dis Child 144:983–992, 1990.

Hong R, Santosham M, Schulte-Wisserman H, Horowitz S, Hsu SH, Winkelstein JA. Reconstitution of B and T lymphocyte function in severe combined immunodeficiency disease following transplantation with thymic epithelium. Lancet 2:1270–1272, 1976.

Hoofnagle JH, Waggoner JG. Hepatitis A and B virus markers in immune serum globulin. Gastroenterology 78:259–263, 1980.

Hornbrook MC, Dodd RY, Jacobs P, Friedman LI, Sherman KE. Reducing the incidence of non-A, non-B post-transfusion hepatitis by testing donor blood for alanine aminotransferase. N Engl J Med 307:1315–1321, 1982.

Horowitz S, Groshong T, Albrecht R, Hong R. The "active" rosette test in immunodeficiency diseases. Clin Immunol Immunopath 4:405–414, 1975a.

Horowitz SD, Groshong T, Bach FH, Hong R, Yunis EJ. Treatment of severe combined immunodeficiency with bone marrow from an unrelated mixed-leukocyte culture nonreactive donor. Lancet 2:431–433, 1975b.

Hosking CS, Roberton DM. Epidemiology and treatment of hypogammaglobulinemia. Birth Defects, Original Articles Series 19:223–227, 1983.

Hurvitz H, Ginat-Israeli T, Elpeleg ON, Klar A, Amir N. Biotinidase deficiency associated with severe combined immunodeficiency. Lancet 2:228–229, 1989.

Incefy G, Dardenne M, Pahwa S, Grimes E, Pahwa PN, Smithwick E, O'Reilly R, Good RA. Thymic activity in severe combined immunodeficiency diseases. Proc Natl Acad Sci U S A 74:1250–1253, 1977.

Iseki M, Heiner DC. Immunodeficiency disorders. Pediatr Rev 14:226-236, 1993.

Ishizaka A, Nakanishi M, Kasahara E, Mizutani K, Sakiyama Y, Matsumoto S. Phenytoin-induced IgG2 and IgG4 deficiencies in a patient with epilepsy. Acta Paediatr 81:646–648, 1992.

Johnson S, Knight R, Marmer DJ, Steele RW. Immune deficiency in fetal alcohol syndrome. Pediatr Res 15:908–911, 1981.

Johnston RB Jr. Screening test for the diagnosis of chronic granulomatous disease. Pediatrics 43:122–124, 1969.

Johnston RB Jr, Stroud RM. Complement and host defense against infection. J Pediatr 90:169–179, 1977.

Johnston RB Jr, Keele BB Jr., Misra HP, Lehmeyer JE, Webb LE, Baehner RL, Rajagopalan, KV. The role of superoxide anion generation in phagocyte bactericidal activity. Studies with normal and chronic granulomatous disease leukocytes. J Clin Invest 55:1357–1372, 1975a.

Johnston RB Jr, Newman SL, Struth AG. An abnormality of the alternate pathway of complement activation in sickle cell disease. N Engl J Med 288:803–808, 1973.

Johnston RB Jr, Wilfert CM, Buckley RH, Webb LS, DeChatelet LR, McCall CE. Enhanced bactericidal activity of phagocytes from patients with chronic granulomatous disease in the presence of sulphisoxazole. Lancet 1:824–827, 1975b.

Jyonouchi H, Voss RM, Krishna S, Urval K, Sjahli H, Welty PB, Good RA. Soluble FcεR II levels in normal children and patients with immunodeficiency diseases. J Clin Immunol Allergy 87:965–970, 1991.

Kadowaki J, Zuelzer WW, Brough AJ, Thompson RI, Wooley PV Jr., Gruber D. XX/XY lymphoid chimaerism in congenital immunological deficiency syndrome with thymic alymphoplasia. Lancet 2:1152–1155, 1965.

Kaikov Y, Wadsworth LD, Hall CA, Rogers PCJ. Transcobalamin II deficiency: case report and review of the literature. Eur J Pediatr 150:841–843, 1991.

Kamani N, August CS, Douglas SD, Burkey E, Etzioni A, Lischner HW. Bone marrow transplantation in chronic granulomatous disease. J Pediatr 105:42–46, 1984.

Kastan MB, Zhan Q, el-Deiry WS, Carrier F, Jacks T, Walsh WV, Plunkett BS, Vogelstein B, Fornace AJ. A mammalian cell cycle checkpoint pathway utilizing p53 and GADD45 is defective in ataxia-telangiectasia. Cell 71:587–597, 1992.

Keightley RG, Lawton AR, Cooper MD. Successful fetal liver transplantation in a child with severe combined immunodeficiency. Lancet 2:850–853, 1975.

Kelley RI, Zackai EH, Emanuel BS, Kistenmacher M, Greenberg F, Punnett HH. The association of the DiGeorge anomalad with partial monosomy of chromosome 22. J Pediatr 101:197–200, 1982.

Kersey JH, Fish LA, Cox ST, August CS: Severe combined immunodeficiency with response to calcium ionophore: a possible membrane defect. Clin Immunol Immunopathol 7:62–68, 1977.

Keusch GT, Douglas SD, Mildvan D, Hirschman SZ. ^{14}C-glucose oxidation in whole blood: a clinical assay for phagocyte dysfunction. Infect Immun 5:414–415, 1972.

Kevy SV, Tefft M, Vawter GF, Rosen FS. Hereditary splenic hypoplasia. Pediatrics 42:752–757, 1968.

Klebanoff SJ, Pincus SH. Hydrogen peroxide utilization in myeloperoxidase-deficient leukocytes: a possible microbicidal control mechanism. J Clin Invest 50:2226–2129, 1971.

Klein RB, Fischer TJ, Gard SE, Biberstein M, Rich KC, Stiehm ER. Decreased mononuclear and polymorphonuclear chemotaxis in human newborns, infants, and young children. Pediatrics 60:467–472, 1977.

Klein C, Lisowska-Grospierre B, Le Deist F, Fischer A, Griscelli C. Major histocompatibility complex class II deficiency. Clinical manifestations, immunologic features and outcome. J Pediatr 123:921–928, 1993.

Klemperer MR, Woodworth HC, Rosen FS, Austen KF. Hereditary deficiency of the second component of human complement: transmission as an autosomal codominant trait (abstract). J Lab Clin Med 66:886, 1965.

Kniker WT, Anderson CT, Roumiantzeff M. The multi-test system: a standardized approach to evaluation of delayed hypersensitivity and cell-mediated immunity. Ann Allergy 43:73–79, 1979.

Kobayashi N, Gohya N, Matsumoto S. Clinical trial of sulfonated immunoglobulin preparation for intravenous administration. Eur J Pediatr 136:159–165, 1981.

Kobayashi RH, Hyman CJ, Stiehm ER. Immunologic maturation in an infant born to a mother with agammaglobulinemia. Am J Dis Child 134:942–944, 1980.

Kobayashi RH, Kobayashi AD, Lee N, Fischer S, Ochs HD. Home self-administration of intravenous immunoglobulin therapy in children. Pediatrics 85:705–709, 1990.

Krantman HJ, Saxon A, Stevens RH, Stiehm ER. Phenotypic heterogeneity in X-linked infantile agammaglobulinemia with in vitro monocyte supression of immunoglobulin synthesis. Clin Immunol Immunopathol 20:170–178, 1981.

Kretschmer R, Janeway CA, Rosen FS. Immunologic amnesia. Pediatr Res 2:7–16, 1968.

Kurtzman G, Frickhofen N, Kimball J, Jenkins DW, Nienhuis AW, Young NS. Pure red-cell aplasia of 10 years duration due to persistent parvovirus B19 infection and its cure with immunoglobulin therapy. N Engl J Med 321:519–521, 1989.

Lalezari P, Bernard GE. An isologous antigen-antibody reaction with human neutrophils related to neonatal neutropenia. J Clin Invest 45:1741–1750, 1966.

Lawlor GJ Jr, Stiehm ER, Kaplan MS, Sengar DPS, Terasaki PI. Phytohemagglutinin (PHA) skin test in the diagnosis of cellular immunodeficiency. J Allergy Clin Immunol 52:31–37, 1973.

Lawrence HW. Transfer factor. Adv Immunol 11:195–266, 1969.

Le Deist F, Hivroz C, Partiseti M, Thomas C, Buc HA, Oleastro M, Belohradsky B, Choquet D, Fischer A. A primary T-cell immunodeficiency associated with defective transmembrane calcium flux. Blood 85:1053–1062, 1995.

Lehrer RI, Cline MJ. Interaction of *Candida albicans* with human leukocytes and serum. J Bacteriol 98:996–1004, 1969a.

Lehrer RI, Cline MJ. Leukocyte myeloperoxidase deficiency and disseminated candidiasis. The role of myeloperoxidase in resistance to *Candida* infection. J Clin Invest 48:1478–1488, 1969b.

Lenarsky C, Weinberg K, Kohn DB, Parkman R. Unrelated donor BMT for Wiskott-Aldrich syndrome. Bone Marrow Transplant 12:145–147, 1993.

Leung DYM, Brozek C, Frankel R, Geha RS. IgE-specific suppressor factors in normal human serum. Clin Immunol Immunopathol 32:339–350, 1984.

Leung DYM, Frankel R, Wood N, Geha RS. Potentiation of human immunoglobulin E synthesis by plasma immunoglobulin E binding factors from patients with the hyperimmunoglobulin E syndrome. J Clin Invest 77:952–957, 1986.

Lever AM, Webster ADB, Brown D, Thomas HC. Non-A, non-B hepatitis occurring in agammaglobulinaemic patients after intravenous immunoglobulin. Lancet 2:1062–1064, 1984.

Levinsky RJ, Tiedeman K. Successful bone marrow transplantation for reticular dysgenesis. Lancet 1:671–673, 1983.

Lewis V, Twomey JJ, Goldstein G, O'Reilly R, Smithwick E, Pahwa R, Pahwa S, Good RA, Schulte-Wisserman H, Horowitz S, Hong R, Jones J, Sieber O, Kirkpatrick C, Polmar S, Bealmear P. Circulating thymic hormone activity in congenital immunodeficiency. Lancet 2:471–475, 1977.

Lieberman R, Hsu M. Levamisole-mediated restoration of cellular immunity in peripheral blood lymphocytes of patients with immunodeficiency diseases. Clin Immunol Immunopathol 5:142–146, 1976.

Liese JG, Wintergerst U, Tympner KD, Belohradsky B. High- vs. low-dose immunoglobulin therapy in the long-term treatment of X-linked agammaglobulinemia. Am J Dis Child 146:335–339, 1992.

Lillie MA, Yang LC, Honig PJ, August CS. Erythroderma, hypogammaglobulinemia, and T-cell lymphocytosis. Arch Dermatol 119:415–418, 1983.

Lipinski M, Virelizier JL, Tursz T, Griscelli C. Natural killer and killer cell activities in patients with primary immunodeficiencies or defects in immune interferon production. Eur J Immunol 10:246–249, 1980.

Lisowska-Grospierre B, Fondaneche MC, Rols MP, Griscelli C, Fischer A. Two complementation groups account for most cases of inherited MHC class II deficiency. Hum Mol Genet 3:953–958, 1994.

Lopez C, Biggar WD, Park BH, Good RA. Nonparalytic poliovirus infections in patients with severe combined immunodeficiency disease. J Pediatr 84:497–502, 1974.

Losonsky GA, Johnson JP, Winkelstein JA, Yolken RH. Oral administration of human serum immunoglobulin in immunodeficient patients with viral gastroenteritis. J Clin Invest 76:2362–2367, 1985.

Lubens RG, Gard SE, Soderberg-Warner M, Stiehm ER. Lectin-dependent T lymphocyte and natural killer cytotoxic deficiencies in human newborns. Cell Immunol 74:40–53, 1982.

MacGregor RR, Spagnuolo PJ, Lentnek AL. Inhibition of granulocyte adherence by ethanol, prednisone, and aspirin, measured with an assay system. N Engl J Med 291:642–646, 1974.

Maderazo EG, Ward PA, Quintiliani R. Defective regulation of chemotaxis in cirrhosis. J Lab Clin Med 85:621–630, 1975.

Mancini G, Carbonara AO, Heremans JF. Immunochemical quantitation of antigens by single radial diffusion. Int J Immunochem 2:235–254, 1965.

Matheson DS, Clarkson TW, Gelfand EW. Mercury toxicity (acrodynia) induced by long-term injection of gamma globulin. J Pediatr 97:153–155, 1980.

McCawley LJ, Korchak HM, Cutilli JR, Stanley CA, Baker L, Douglas SD, Kilpatrick L. Interferon-γ corrects the respiratory burst defect in vitro in monocyte-derived macrophages from glycogen storage disease type 1b patients. Pediatr Res 34:265–269, 1993.

McCluskey DR, Boyd NAM. Prevalence of primary hypogammaglobulinemia in a well-defined population in the UK. In Chapel HM, Levinsky RJ, Webster ADB. Progress in Immune Deficiency, 3rd ed. Royal Society of Medicine Services, International Congress and Symposium Series No. 173, London, 1991, pp. 100–101.

McIntosh K, Kurachek SC, Cairns LM, Burns JC, Goodspeed B. Treatment of respiratory viral infection in an immunodeficient infant with ribavirin aerosol. Am J Dis Child 138:305–308, 1984.

Mease PJ, Ochs HD, Wedgwood RJ. Successful treatment of Echovirus meningoencephalitis and myositis-fasciitis with intravenous immune globulin therapy in a patient with X-linked agammaglobulinemia. N Engl J Med 304:1278–1281, 1981.

Medical Research Council Working Party. Hypogammaglobulinemia in the United Kingdom. Lancet 1:163–169, 1969.

Metcalf JA, Gallin JI, Nauseef WM, Root RK. Laboratory Manual of Neutrophil Function. New York, Raven Press, 1986.

Meuwissen HJ, Pollara B, Pickering RJ. Combined immunodeficiency disease associated with adenosine deaminase deficiency. J Pediatr 86:169–181, 1975.

Meyers PA, Carmel R. Hereditary transcobalamin II deficiency with subnormal serum cobalamin levels. Pediatrics 74:866–871, 1984.

Miller FW, Leitman SF, Plotz PH. High-dose intravenous immune globulin and acute renal failure. N Engl J Med 327:1032–1033, 1992.

Miller ME. Pathology of chemotaxis and random mobility. Semin Hematol 12:59–82, 1975.

Miller ME, Nilsson UR. A familial deficiency of the phagocytosis-enhancing activity of serum related to a dysfunction of the fifth component of complement. N Engl J Med 282:354–358, 1970.

Mills EL, Rholl K, Quie PG. Chemiluminescence, a rapid sensitive method for detection of patients with chronic granulomatous disease (abstract). Pediatr Res 12:454, 1978.

Moscow JA, Casper AJ, Kodis C, Fricke WA. Positive direct antiglobulin test results after intravenous immune globulin administration. Transfusion 27:248–249, 1987.

Najjar VA, Constantopoulos A. A new phagocytosis-stimulating tetrapeptide hormone, tuftsin, and its role in disease. J Reticuloendothel Soc 12:197–215, 1972.

Nathenson G, Schorr JB, Litwin B. Gm factor fetomaternal gamma-globulin incompatibility. Pediatr Res 5:2–9, 1971.

Nelson RD, Quie PG, Simmons RL. Chemotaxis under agarose: a new and simple method for measuring chemotaxis and spontaneous migration of human polymorphonuclear leukocytes and monocytes. J Immunol 115:1650–1656, 1975.

Newburger JW, Takahashi M, Burns JC, Beiser AS, Chung KJ, Duffy E, Glode MP, Mason WH, Reddy V, Sanders SP, Shulman ST, Wiggins JW, Hicks RV, Fulton DR, Lewis AB, Leung DYM, Colton T, Rosen FS, Melish ME. The treatment of Kawasaki syndrome with intravenous gamma globulin. N Engl J Med 315:341–347, 1986.

Nishioka A. Measurements of complement by agglutination of human erythrocytes reacting in immune-adherence. J Immunol 90:86–97, 1963.

Ochs H, Fischer SH, Virant FS, Lee ML, Kingdon HS, Wedgwood RJ. Non-A, non-B hepatitis and intravenous immunoglobulin. Lancet 1:404–405, 1985.

Ochs HD, Fischer SH, Wedgwood RJ, Wara DW, Cowan MJ, Ammann AJ, Saxon A, Budinger MD, Alfred RU, Rousell RH. Comparison of high-dose and low-dose intravenous immunoglobulin therapy in patients with primary immunodeficiency diseases. Am J Med 76(3A):78–82, 1984.

Ochs HD, Igo RP. The NBT slide test: a simple screening method for detecting chronic granulomatous disease and female carriers. J Pediatr 83:77–82, 1973.

Olerup O, Smith CIE, Hammarström L. Different amino acids at position 57 of the HLA-DQβ chain associated with susceptibility and resistance to IgA deficiency. Nature 347:289–290, 1990.

Oppenheim JJ, Blaese RM, Waldmann TA. Defective-lymphocyte transformation and delayed hypersensitivity in Wiskott-Aldrich syndrome. J Immunol 104:835–844, 1970.

Oppenheim JJ, Dougherty S, Chan SP, Baker J. Use of lymphocyte transformation to assess clinical disorders. In Vyas GN, Stites DP, Brecher G, eds. Laboratory Diagnosis of Immunologic Disorder. New York, Grune & Stratton, 1975, pp. 87–109.

O'Reilly RJ, Kapoor N, Kirkpatrick D, Cunningham-Rundles S, Pollack MS, Dupont B, Hodes MZ, Good RA, Reisner Y. Transplantation for severe combined immunodeficiency using histoincompatible parental marrow fractionated by soybean agglutinin and sheep red blood cells: experience in six consecutive cases. Transplant Proc 15:1431–1435, 1983.

Oster G, Kilburn KH, Siegal FP. Chemically induced congenital thymic dysgenesis in the rat: a model of the DiGeorge syndrome. Clin Immunol Immunopathol 28:128–134, 1983.

Oxelius V, Laurell A, Lindquist B, Golebiowska H, Axelsson U, Björkander J, Hanson LA. IgG subclasses in selective IgA deficiency: importance of IgG2-IgA deficiency. N Engl J Med 304: 1476–1478, 1981.

Paganelli R, Aiuti F, Beverley PC, Levinsky RJ. Impaired production of interleukins in patients with cell-mediated immunodeficiencies. Clin Exp Immunol 51:338–344, 1983.

Palma-Carlos AG, Palma-Carlos ML. Incidence of primary and acquired immunodeficiencies in an outpatient population. In Chapel HM, Levinsky RJ, Webster ADB, eds. Progress in Immune Deficiency, 3rd ed. London Royal Society of Medicine Services, International Congress and Symposium Series No. 173, 1991, pp. 100–101.

Park BH, Holmes B, Rodey GE, Good RA. Nitro-blue tetrazolium test in children with fatal granulomatous disease and newborn infants. Lancet 1:157, 1969.

Parkman R. Antibody-treated bone marrow transplantation for patients with severe combined immune deficiency. Clin Immunol Immunopathol 40:142–146, 1986.

Parkman R, Mosier D, Umansky I, Cochran W, Carpenter CB, Rosen FS. Graft-versus-host disease after intrauterine and exchange transfusions for hemolytic disease of the newborn. N Engl J Med 290:359–363, 1974.

Parkman R, Remold-O'Donnell E, Kenney DM, Perrine S, Rosen FS. Surface protein abnormalities in lymphocytes and platelets from patients with Wiskott-Aldrich syndrome. Lancet 2:1387–1389, 1981.

Paryani SG, Arvin AM, Koropchak CM, Wittek AE, Amylon MD, Dodkin MB, Budinger MD. Varicella zoster antibody titers after the administration of intravenous immune serum globulin or varicella zoster immune globulin. Am J Med 76(3A):124–127, 1984.

Perlmann P, Perlmann H, Müller-Eberhard HJ. Cytolytic lymphocytic cells with complement receptor in human blood: induction of cytolysis by IgG antibody but not by target cell-bound C3. J Exp Med 141:287–296, 1975.

Perlmutter RM. Molecular dissection of lymphocyte signal transduction pathways. Pediatr Res (33 Suppl):S9–S15, 1993.

Peterson RDA, Cooper MD, Good RA. The pathogenesis of the immunologic deficiency diseases. Am J Med 38:579–604, 1965.

Pidot ALR, O'Keefe G III, McManus N, McIntyre OR. Human leukocyte interferons: the variation in normal and correlation with PHA transformation. Proc Soc Exp Biol Med 140:1263–1269, 1972.

Pincus SH, Klebanoff SJ. Quantitative leukocyte iodination. N Engl J Med 284:744–750, 1971.

Platts-Mills TAE, Ishizaka K. Activation of the alternate pathway of human complement by rabbit cells. J Immunol 113:348–358, 1974.

Polhill RB Jr., Johnston RB Jr. Diminished alternative complement pathway (ACP) activity after splenectomy (abstract). Pediatr Res 9:333, 1975.

Polhill RB Jr., Pruitt KM, Johnston RB Jr. Assessment of alternate complement pathway activity in a continuously monitored hemolytic system (abstract). Fed Proc 34:982, 1975.

Pollack S, Cunningham-Rundles C, Smithwick EM, Barundun S, Good RA. High-dose intravenous gamma globulin for autoimmune neutropenia (letter). N Engl J Med 307:253, 1982.

Polmar SH, Stern RC, Schwartz AL, Wetzler EM, Chase PA, Hirschhorn R. Enzyme replacement therapy for adenosine deaminase deficiency and severe combined immunodeficiency. N Engl J Med 295:1337–1343, 1976.

Prince HE, John JK. Early activation marker expression to detect impaired proliferative responses to pokeweed mitogen and tetanus toxoid: studies in patients with AIDS and related disorders. Diagn Immunol 4:306–311, 1986.

Prince HE, Kermani-Arab V, Fahey JL. Depressed interleukin-2–receptor expression in acquired immune deficiency and lymphadenopathy syndromes. J Immunol 133:1313–1317, 1984.

Puck JM, Krauss CM, Puck SM, Buckley RH, Conley ME. Prenatal test for X-linked severe combined immunodeficiency by analysis of maternal X-chromosome inactivation and linkage analysis. N Engl J Med 322:1063–1066, 1990.

Quie PG, White JG, Holmes B, Good RA. In vitro bactericidal capacity of human polymorphonuclear leukocytes: diminished activity in chronic granulomatous disease of childhood. J Clin Invest 46:668–679, 1967.

Rachelefsky GS, McConnachie PR, Ammann AJ, Terasaki PI, Stiehm ER. Antibody-dependent lymphocyte killer function in human immunodeficiency diseases. Clin Exp Immunol 19:1–9 1975a.

Rachelefsky GS, Stiehm ER, Ammann AJ, Cederbaum SD, Opelz G, Terasaki PI. T-cell reconstitution by thymus transplantation and transfer factor in severe combined immunodeficiency. Pediatrics 54:114–118, 1975b.

Rao SP, Teitlebaum J, Miller ST. Intravenous immune globulin and aseptic meningitis. Am J Dis Child 146:147, 1992.

Rappeport JM, Newburger PE, Goldblum RM, Goldman AS, Nathan DG, Parkman R. Allogeneic bone marrow transplantation for chronic granulomatous disease. J Pediatr 101:952–955, 1982.

Raubitschek AA, Levin AS, Stites DP, Shaw EB, Fudenberg HH. Normal granulocyte infusion therapy for aspergillosis in chronic granulomatous disease. Pediatrics 51:230–233, 1973.

Rault R, Piraino B, Johnston JR, Oral A. Pulmonary and renal toxicity of intravenous immunoglobulin. Clin Nephrol 26:83–86, 1991.

Rebuck JW, Crowley JH, A method of studying leukocytic functions in vivo. Ann NY Acad Sci 59:757–805, 1955.

Reinhart WH, Berchtold PE. Effect of high-dose intravenous immunoglobulin therapy on blood rheology. Lancet 339:662–664, 1992.

Reinherz EL, Geha R, Rappeport JM, Wilson M, Penta AC, Hussey RE, Fitzgerald KA, Daley JR, Levine J, Rosen FS, Schlossman SF. Reconstitution after transplantation with T lymphocyte–depleted HLA haplotype–mismatched bone marrow for severe combined immunodeficiency. Proc Natl Acad Sci U S A 79:6047–6051, 1982.

Reinherz EL, Geha R, Wohl ME, Morimoto C, Rosen RS, Schlossman SF. Immunodeficiency associated with loss of T4+ inducer T-cell function. N Engl J Med 304:822–816, 1981.

Rijkers GT, Scharenberg JGM, Van Dongen JJM, Neijens HJ, Zegers BJ. Abnormal signal transduction in a patient with severe combined immunodeficiency disease. Pediatr Res 29:306–309, 1991.

Roberton DM, Shelton MJ, Hosking CS. Incidence of primary immunodeficiency disorders in childhood (abstract). Fifth International Congress of Immunology, 1983.

Roberts RL, Gallin JI. The phagocytic cell and its disorders. Ann Allergy 50:330–345, 1983.

Rocklin RE. Inhibition of cell migration as a correlate of cell mediated immunity. In Vyas GN, Stites DP, Brecher G, eds. Laboratory Diagnosis of Immunologic Disorders. New York, Grune & Stratton, 1975, pp. 111–126.

Roord JJ, Van der Meer JWM, Kuis W, de Windt GE, Zegers BJM, Van Furth R, Stoop JW. Home treatment in patients with antibody deficiency by slow subcutaneous infusion of gamma globulin. Lancet 2:689–690, 1982.

Rose EA. Applications of the polymerase chain reaction to genome analysis. FASEB J 5:46–54, 1991.

Rosen FS, Aiuti F, Cooper MD, Good RA, Hanson LA, Hitzig WH, Matsumoto S, Seligmann M, Soothill JF, Waldmann TA, Wedg-

wood RJ. Primary immunodeficiency diseases. Report prepared for the WHO by a scientific group on immunodeficiency. Clin Immunol Immunopathol 28:450–475, 1983.

Rosen FS, Charache P, Pensky J, Donaldson V. Hereditary angioneurotic edema: two genetic variants. Science 148:957–958, 1965.

Rosen FS, Cooper MD, Wedgwood RJP. The primary immunodeficiencies. N Engl J Med 311:235–310, 1984.

Rosen FS, Wedgwood RJ, Eibl M. Primary immunodeficiency diseases: report of a World Health Organization Scientific Group. Clin Immunol Immunopathol 40:166–196, 1986.

Rosen FS, Wedgwood RJ, Eibl M, Griscelli C, Seligmann M, Aiuti F, Kishimoto T, Matsumoto S, Khakhalin LN, Hanson LA, Hitzig WH, Thompson RA, Cooper MD, Good RA, Waldmann TA. Primary immunodeficiency diseases: report of a WHO scientific group. Immunodefic Rev 3:195–236, 1992.

Rosen FS, Wedgwood RJP, Eibl M, Griscelli C, Seligmann M, Aiuti F, Kishimoto T, Matsumoto S, Reznik IB, Hanson LA, Thompson RA, Cooper MD, Geha RS, Good RA, Waldmann TA. Primary immunodeficiency diseases: report of a WHO Scientific Group. Clin Exp Immunol 1(Suppl 99):1–24, 1995.

Ross SC, Densen P. Complement deficiency states and infection: epidemiology, pathogenesis and consequences of Neisserial and other infections in an immune deficiency. Medicine 63:243–273, 1984.

Rotbart HA, Levin MJ, Jones JF, Hayward AR, Allan J, McLane MF, Essex M. Noma in children with severe combined immunodeficiency. J Pediatr 109:596–600, 1986.

Rozynska KE, Spickett GP, Millrain M, Edwards A, Bryant A, Webster ADB, Farrant J. Accessory and T cell defects in acquired and inherited hypogammaglobulinemia. Clin Exp Immunol 78:1–6, 1989.

Ruff ME, Pincus LG, Sampson HA. Phenytoin-induced IgA depression. Am J Dis Child 141:858–861, 1987.

Ryser O, Morell A, Hitzig WH. Primary immunodeficiencies in Switzerland: first report of the national registry in adults and children. J Clin Immunol 8:479–485, 1988.

Saez-Llorens X, Ramilo O, Mustafa MM, Mertsola J, McCracken GH. Molecular pathophysiology of bacterial meningitis: current concepts and therapeutic implications. J Pediatr 116:671–684, 1990.

Sanel SO, Buckley RH. Antibody-dependent cellular cytotoxicity in primary immunodeficiency diseases and with normal leukocyte subpopulations. J Clin Invest 61:1–10, 1978.

Sanford JP, Favour CB, Tribeman MS. Absence of serum gamma globulins in an adult. N Engl J Med 250:1027–1029, 1954.

Sato M, Hayashi Y, Yoshida H, Yanagawa T, Yura Y. A family with hereditary lack of T4+ inducer/helper T cell subsets in peripheral blood lymphocytes. J Immunol 132:1071–1073, 1984.

Saxon A, Giorgi JV, Sherr EH, Kagan JM. Failure of B cells in common variable immunodeficiency to transit from proliferation to differentiation is associated with altered B cell surface–molecule display. J Allergy Clin Immunol 84:44–53, 1989.

Schaffer FM, Palermos J, Zhu ZB, Barger BO, Cooper MD, Volanakis JE. Individuals with IgA deficiency and common variable immunodeficiency share polymorphisms of major histocompatibility complex class III genes. Proc Natl Acad Sci U S A 86:8015–8019, 1989.

Schiff RI, Rudd C. Alterations in the half-life and clearance of IgG during therapy with intravenous gamma globulin in 16 patients with severe primary humoral immunodeficiency. J Clin Immunol 6:256–264, 1986.

Schiff RI, Rudd C, Johnson R, Buckley RH. Use of a new chemically modified intravenous IgG preparation in severe primary humoral immunodeficiency: clinical efficacy and attempts to individualize dosage. Clin Immunol Immunopathol 31:13–23, 1984.

Schifferli J, Favre H, Nydegger U, Leski M, Imbach P, Davies K. High-dose intravenous IgG treatment and renal function. Lancet 337:457–458, 1991.

Schimke RN, Bolano C, Kirkpatrick CH. Immunologic deficiency in the congenital rubella syndrome. Am J Dis Child 118:626–633, 1969.

Schlievert PM. Role of superantigens in human disease. J Infect Dis 167:997–1002, 1993.

Schmalsteig FC, Mills GC, Nelson JA, May LT, Goldman AS, Goldblum RM. Limited effect of erythrocyte and plasma infusions in adenosine deaminase deficiency. J Pediatr 93:597–603, 1978.

Schmidt AD, Taswell HF, Gleich GT. Anaphylactic transfusion reactions associated with anti-IgA antibody. N Engl J Med 280:188–193, 1969.

Schulkind ML, Adler WM, Altemeier WA, Ayoub EM. Transfer factor in the treatment of a case of chronic mucocutaneous moniliasis. Cell Immunol 3:606–615, 1972.

Schur PH, Borel H, Gelfand EW, Alper CA, Rosen FS. Gamma-G globulin deficiencies in patients with recurrent pyogenic infections. N Engl J Med 283:631–634, 1970.

Schur PH, Rosen F, Norman ME. Immunoglobulin subclasses in normal children. Pediatr Res 13:181–183, 1979.

Schwarz K, Hansen-Hagge TE, Knobloch C, Friedrich W, Kleihauer E, Bartram CR. Severe combined immunodeficiency (SCID) in man: B cell-negative (B−) SCID patients exhibit an irregular recombination pattern at the J_H locus. J Exp Med 174:1039–1048, 1991.

Scott CR, Chen SH, Giblett ER. Detection of the carrier state in combined immunodeficiency associated with adenosine deaminase deficiency. J Clin Invest 53:1194–1196, 1974.

Seeger RC, Robins RA, Stevens RH, Klein RB, Waldman DJ, Zeltzer PM, Kessler SW. Severe combined immunodeficiency with B lymphocytes: in vitro correction of defective immunoglobulin production by addition of normal T lymphocytes. Clin Exp Immunol 26:1–10, 1976.

Segal AW, Cross AR, Garcia RC, Borregaard N, Valerius NH, Soothill JF, Jones OTG. Absence of cytochrome b_{245} in chronic granulomatous disease. N Engl J Med 308:245–251, 1983.

Seto B, Coleman WJR, Iwarson S, Gerety RJ. Detection of reverse transcriptase activity in association with the NANB hepatitis agents. Lancet 2:941–943, 1984.

Shearer WT, Wedner HJ, Strominger DB, Kissane J, Hong R. Successful transplantation of the thymus in Nezelof's syndrome. Pediatrics 61:619–624, 1978.

Sheffield VC, Beck JS, Kwitek AE, Sandstrom DW, Stone EM. The sensitivity of single-strand conformation polymorphism analysis for the detection of single-base substitutions. Genomics 16:325–332, 1993.

Siegel RL, Issekutz T, Schwaber J, Rosen FS, Geha RS. Deficiency of T helper cells in transient hypogammaglobulinemia of infancy. N Engl J Med 305:1307–1313, 1981.

Sindel LJ, Buckley RH, Schiff SE, Ward FE, Mickey GH, Huang AT, Naspitz C, Koren H. Severe combined immunodeficiency with natural killer-cell predominance: abrogation of graft-versus-host disease and immunologic reconstitution with HLA-identical bone marrow cells. J Allergy Clin Immunol 73:829–836, 1984.

Sissons JGP, West RJ, Fallows J, Williams DG, Boucher BJ, Amos N, Peters DK. The complement abnormalities of lipodystrophy. N Engl J Med 294:461–465, 1976.

Sjöholm AG, Kuijper EJ, Tijssen CC, Jansz A, Bo P, Spanjaard L, Zanen HC. Dysfunctional properdin in a Dutch family with meningococcal disease. N Engl J Med 319:33–37, 1988.

Skarnes RC, Watson DW. Characterization of leukin: an antibacterial factor from leukocytes active against gram-positive pathogens. J Exp Med 104:829–845, 1956.

Snyderman R, Altman LC, Frankel A, Blaese RM. Defective mononuclear chemotaxis: a previously unrecognized immune dysfunction: studies in a patient with chronic mucocutaneous candidiasis. Ann Intern Med 78:509–513, 1973.

Soberg M. In vitro detection of cellular hypersensitivity in man. Specific inhibition of white blood cells from brucella-positive persons. Acta Med Scand 182:167–174, 1967.

Soothill JF. The concentration of gamma-macroglobulin in the serum of patients with hypogammaglobulinemia. Clin Sci 23:27–35, 1962.

Sorrell TC, Forbes IJ, Burness FR, Rischbieth RHC. Depression of immunological function in patients treated with phenytoin sodium (sodium diphenylhydantoin). Lancet 2:1233–1235, 1971.

South MA, Warwick WJ, Wollheim FA, Good RA. The IgA system. III. IgA levels in the serum and saliva of pediatric patients—evidence for a local immunological system. J Pediatr 71:645–653, 1967.

Spitler LE, Levin AS, Stites DP, Fudenberg HH, Pirofsky B, August CS, Stiehm ER, Hitzig WH, Gatti RA. The Wiskott-Aldrich syndrome: results of transfer factor therapy. J Clin Invest 51:3216–3224, 1972.

Stiehm ER. Passive immunization. In Feigen RW, Cherry JD, eds. Textbook of Pediatric Infectious Diseases, 3rd ed. Philadelphia, WB Saunders, 1992, pp. 2261–2288.

Stiehm ER. New and old immunodeficiencies. Pediatr Res (33 Suppl) S2–S8, 1993.

Stiehm ER, Fudenberg HH. Antibodies to gamma-globulin in infants and children exposed to isologous gamma-globulin. Pediatrics 35:229–235, 1965.

Stiehm ER, Fudenberg HH. Clinical and immunologic features of dysgammaglobulinemia type I: report of a case diagnosed in the first year of life. Am J Med 40:805–815, 1966a.

Stiehm ER, Fudenberg HH. Serum levels of immune globulins in health and disease: a survey. Pediatrics 37:715–727, 1966b.

Stiehm ER, Chin TW, Haas A, Peerless AG. Infectious complications of the primary immunodeficiencies. Clin Immunol Immunopathol 40:69–86, 1986.

Stiehm ER, McIntosh RM, Wiskott-Aldrich syndrome: review and report of a large family. Clin Exp Immunol 2:179–189, 1967.

Stiehm ER, Vaerman JP, Fudenberg HH. Plasma infusions in immunologic deficiency states: metabolic and therapeutic studies. Blood 28:918–938, 1966.

Stjernholm RL, Allan RC, Steele RH, Waring WW, Harris JA. Impaired chemiluminescence during phagocytosis or opsonized bacteria. Infect Immun 7:313–314, 1973.

Stossel TP. Evaluation of opsonic and leukocyte function with a spectrophotometric test in patients with infection and with phagocytic disorders. Blood 42:121–130, 1973.

Stossel TP. Phagocytosis. N Engl J Med 290:717–723, 774–780, 833–839, 1974.

Stossel TP, Alper CA, Rosen FS. Opsonic activity in the newborn: role of properdin. Pediatrics 53:134–137, 1973.

Strauss RG, Bove KE, Jones JF, Mauer AM, Fulginiti VA. An anomaly of neutrophil morphology with impaired function. N Engl J Med 290:478–484, 1974.

Strauss RG, Hake DA. Combined immunodeficiency disease with response to transfer factor. J Pediatr 85:680–682, 1974.

Strauss RG, Levy GJ, Sotelo-Avila C, Albanese MA, Hume H, Schloz L, Blazina JB, Werner A, Barrasso C, Blanchette V, Warkentin PI, Pepkowitz S, Mauer AM, Hines D. National survey of neonatal transfusion practices: II. Blood component therapy. Pediatrics 91:530–536, 1993.

Strober S, Bobrove AM. Assays for T and B cells. In Vyas GN, Stites DP, Brecher G, eds. Laboratory Diagnosis of Immunologic Disorders. New York, Grune & Stratton, 1975, pp. 71–86.

Strober W, Krakauer R, Klaeveman HL, Reynolds HY, Nelson DL. Secretory component deficiency: a disorder of the IgA immune system. N Engl J Med 294:351–356, 1976.

Sweinberg SK, Wodell RA, Grodofsky MP, Greene JM, Conley ME. Retrospective analysis of the incidence of pulmonary disease in hypogammaglobulinemia. J Allergy Clin Immunol 88:96–104, 1991.

Syllaba L, Henner K. Contribution à l'indépendance de l'athetose double idiopathique et congénitale: atteinte familiale, syndrome dystrophique, signe du réseau vasculaire conjonctival, intégrité psychique. Rev Neurol (Paris) 1:541–562, 1926.

Taalman RDFM, Hustinx TWJ, Weemaes CMR, Seemanová E, Schmidt A, Eberhard P, Scheres JMJC. Further delineation of the Nijmegen breakage syndrome. Am J Med Genet 32:425–431, 1989.

Tabor E, Gerety RJ. Transmission of hepatitis B by immune serum globulin. Lancet 2:1293, 1979.

Takahara S. Progressive oral gangrene probably due to lack of catalase in the blood (acatalasemia). Lancet 2:1101–1104, 1952.

Takei S, Arora YK, Walker SM. Intravenous immunoglobulin contains specific antibodies inhibitory to activation of T cells by staphylococcal superantigens. J Clin Invest 91:602–607, 1993.

Terasaki PI, Miyajima R, Sengar DPS, Stiehm ER. Extraneous lymphocytic HLA antigens in severe combined immunodeficiency disease. Transplantation 13:250–255, 1972.

Thomas ED, Storb R. Technique for human marrow grafting. Blood 36:507–515, 1970.

Thorpe ES, Handley HE. Chronic tetany and chronic mycelial stomatitis in a child aged four and one-half years. Am J Dis Child 38:328–338, 1929.

Todd RF III, Fegen DR. The CD11/CD18 leukocyte glycoprotein deficiency. Hematol Oncol Clin North Am 4:13–31, 1988.

Touraine JL, Betuel H. The bare lymphocyte syndrome: immunodeficiency resulting from the lack of expression of HLA antigens. Birth Defects, Original Article series, 19:83–85, 1983.

Touraine J-L, Betuel H, Souillet G, Jeune M. Combined immunodeficiency disease associated with absence of cell-surface HLA-A and -B antigens. J Pediatr 93:47–51, 1978.

Touraine J-L, Touraine F, Kiszkiss DF, Choi YS, Good RA. Heterologous specific antiserum for identification of human T lymphocytes. Clin Exp Immunol 16:503–510, 1974.

Trepo C, Degos F, Vivitski L, Carlson R, Chossegros P, Pichoud C, Hantz O, Chevallier P, Chevre JC, Simon N, Peyrol S, Grimaud A, Felman G, Sepetjan M, Wands J. Evidence for a transmissible non-A non-B agent inextricably linked with hepatitis B virus. In Vyas GJ, Dienstag JL, Hoofnagle JH, eds. Viral Hepatitis and Liver Disease, Grune & Stratton, New York, 1984, pp. 355–365.

Trepo C, Hantz O, Jacquier MF, Nemoz G, Cappel R, Trepo D. Different fates of hepatitis B virus markers during plasma fractionation. Vox Sang 35:143–148, 1978.

Trepo C, Hantz O, Vitvitski L. Non-A, non-B hepatitis after intravenous gammaglobulin. Lancet 1:322, 1986.

Tsukada S, Saffran DC, Rawlings DJ, Parolini O, Allen RC, Klisak I, Sparkes RS, Kubagawa H, Mohandas T, Quan S, Belmont JW, Cooper MD, Conley ME, Witte ON. Deficient expression of a B-cell cytoplasmic tyrosine kinase in human X-linked agammaglobulinemia. Cell 72:279–290, 1993.

Valdimarsson H, Higgs JM, Wells RS, Yamamura M, Hobbs JR, Holt PJL. Immune abnormalities associated with chronic mucocutaneous candidiasis. Cell Immunol 6:348–361, 1973.

Van der Meer JWM, Vossen JM, Radl J, Van Nieuwkoop JA, Meijer CJLM, Lobatto S, Van Furth R. Hyperimmunoglobulinemia D and periodic fever: a new syndrome. Lancet 1:1087–1090, 1984.

Vetrie D, Vorechovsky I, Sideras P, Holland J, Davies A, Flinter F, Hammarström L, Kinnon C, Levinsky R, Bobrow M, Smith CIE, Bentley DR. The gene involved in X-linked agammaglobulinemia is a member of the *src* family of protein-tyrosine kinases. Nature 361:226–233, 1993.

Virelizier JL, Lagrue A, Durandy A, Arenzana F, Oury C, Griscelli C. Reversal of natural killer defect in a patient with Chédiak-Higashi syndrome after bone-marrow transplantation. N Engl J Med 306:1055–1056, 1982.

Vowels MR, Lam-Poo-Tang R, Berdoukas V, Ford D, Thierry D, Purtilo D, Gluckman E. Correction of X-linked lymphoproliferative disease by transplantation of cord-blood stem cells. N Engl J Med 22:1623–1625, 1993.

Vyas GH, Perkins HA, Fudenberg HH. Anaphylactoid transfusion reaction associated with anti-IgA. Lancet 2:312–315, 1968.

Vyas GN, Perkins HA, Yaug YM, Basantanix GK. Healthy blood donors with selective absence of immunoglobulin A: Prevention of anaphylactic transfusion reactions caused by antibodies to IgA. J Lab Clin Med 85:838–842, 1975.

Waldmann TA, McIntire KR. Serum alpha-fetoprotein levels in patients with ataxia-telangiectasia. Lancet 2:1112–1115, 1972.

Waldmann TA, Strober W. Metabolism of immunoglobulins. Prog Allergy 13:1–110, 1969.

Waldmann TA, Broder S, Blaese RM, Durin M, Blackman M, Strober W. Role of suppressor T cells in pathogenesis of common variable hypogammaglobulinaemia. Lancet 2:609–613, 1974.

Waldmann, TA, Strober W, Blaese RM. T and B cell immunodeficiency diseases. In Parker CW, ed. Clinical Immunology. Philadelphia, WB Saunders, 1980, pp. 314–375.

Waniewski J, Gardulf A, Hammarström L. Bioavailability of γ-globulin after subcutaneous infusions in patients with common variable immunodeficiency. J Clin Immunol 14:90–97, 1993.

Wara DW, Ammann AJ. Thymic cells and humoral factors as therapeutic agents. Pediatrics 57:643–646, 1976.

Ward KN, Morgan G, Ashworth K, Bremner J, O'Callaghan A, Teo CG. Spurious outbreak of HCV in bone marrow recipients treated with cytomegalovirus immunoglobulin. Lancet 340:1290–1291, 1992.

Ward PA, Schlegel RJ. Impaired leucotactic responsiveness in a child with recurrent infections. Lancet 2:344–347, 1969.

Warrier AI, Lusher JM. Intravenous gamma globulin treatment of chronic idiopathic thrombocytopenic purpura in children. Am J Med 76(3A):193–198, 1984.

Webster ADB, Lever AML. Non-A, non-B hepatitis after intravenous gammaglobulin. Lancet 1:322, 1986.

Webster ADB, Efter T, Asherson GL. *Escherichia coli* antibody: a screening test for immunodeficiency. Br Med J 3:16–18, 1974.

Weening RS, Schoorel EP, Roos D, van Schaik MLJ, Voetman AA, Bot AAM, Batenburg-Plenter AM, Willems CH, Zeijlemaker WP, Astaldi A. Effect of ascorbate on abnormal neutrophil, platelet, and lymphocyte function in a patient with the Chédiak-Higashi syndrome. Blood 57:856–865, 1981.

Weinberg K, Parkman R. Severe combined immunodeficiency due to a specific defect in the production of IL-2. N Engl J Med 322:1718–1720, 1990.

Weiss Arthur. T Lymphocyte activation. In Paul WE, ed. Fundamental Immunology. Raven Press, New York, 1989, pp. 259–284.

Welch MJ, Stiehm ER. Slow subcutaneous immunoglobulin: therapy in a patient with reactions to intramuscular immunoglobulin. J Clin Immunol 3:285–286, 1983.

Welch MJ, Stiehm ER, Dudley JP. Isolated absence of nasal cilia: a case report. Ann Allergy 52:32–34, 1984.

Westminster Hospital Bone Marrow Transplant Team. Bone-marrow transplant from an unrelated donor for chronic granulomatous disease. Lancet 1:210–213, 1977.

White WB, Ballow M. Modulation of suppressor-cell activity in cimetidine in patients with common variable hypogammaglobulinemia. N Engl J Med 312:198–202, 1985.

WHO/IARC Technical Report. Identification enumeration and isolation of B and T lymphocytes from human peripheral blood. Scand J Immunol 3:521–532, 1974.

Williams LL, Rooney CM, Conley ME, Brenner MK, Krance RA, Heslop HE. Correction of Duncan's syndrome by allogeneic bone marrow transplantation. Lancet 342:587–588, 1993.

Wilson WA, Hughes GRV, Lachmann PJ. Deficiency of factor B of the complement system in sickle cell anemia. Br Med J 1:367–369, 1976.

Winkelstein JA, Drachman RH. Deficiency of pneumococcal serum opsonizing activity in sickle-cell disease. N Engl J Med 279:459–466, 1968.

Winston DJ, Ho WG, Lin CH, Budinger MD, Champlin RM, Gale RP. Intravenous immune globulin for modification of cytomegalovirus infections associated with bone marrow transplantation. Preliminary results of a controlled trial. Am J Med 76(3A):128–133, 1984.

Wiskott A. Familiarer, angeborener Morbus Werihofii? Aschr Kinderheilk 68:212–216, 1937.

Wittig HJ, Belloit J, De Filippi I, Royal G. Age-related serum immunoglobulin E levels in healthy subjects and in patients with allergic disease. J Allergy Clin Immunol 66:305–313, 1980.

Wollheim F. Inherited "acquired" hypogammaglobulinemia. Lancet 1:316–317, 1961.

Woodruff RK, Grigg AP, Firkin FC, Smith IL. Fatal thrombotic events during treatment of autoimmune thrombocytopenia with intravenous immunoglobulin in elderly patients. Lancet 2:217–218, 1986.

Wright DG, Kirkpatrick CH, Gallin JI. Effects of levamisole on normal and abnormal leukocyte locomotion. J Clin Invest 59:941–950, 1970.

Yabuhara A, Kawai H, Komiyama A. Development of natural killer cytotoxicity during childhood: marked increases in number of natural killer cells with adequate cytotoxic abilities during infancy to early childhood. Pediatr Res 28:316–322, 1990.

Yount WJ, Hong R, Seligmann M, Good RA, Kunkel HG. Imbalances of gammaglobulin subgroups and gene defects in patients with primary hypogammaglobulinemia. J Clin Invest 49:1957–1966, 1970.

Ziegler JB, Alper CA, Rosen FS, Lachmann PJ, Sherington L. Restoration by purified C3b inactivator of complement-mediated function in vivo in a patient with C3b inactivator deficiency. J Clin Invest 55:668–672, 1975a.

Ziegler JB, Rosen FS, Alper CA, Grupe W, Lepow IH. Metabolism of properdin in normal subjects and patients with renal disease. J Clin Invest 56:761–765, 1975b.

Chapter 10

The Physiologic Immunodeficiency of Immaturity

Christopher B. Wilson, David B. Lewis,
and Laurie A. Penix

Ontogenetic studies of the immune system provide insight into normal development of the immune system, the cellular and molecular basis for the physiologic immunodeficiency of the human neonate, and the resultant increase in susceptibility of the fetus and neonate to severe infection. This chapter focuses on the ontogeny of the cellular and humoral components of the immune system and their function in the human fetus and neonate. Antigen presentation and antigen-specific immunity are discussed first, followed by innate mechanisms of host defense. The relationship between deficiencies in immune function in the neonate and fetus and their increased susceptibility to bacterial, viral, and protozoan infections along with the current and potential application of this knowledge for immunotherapy in the fetus and neonate is examined next. Finally, clues to the recognition of primary immunodeficiency in the neonate are presented.

ESTABLISHMENT OF HEMATOPOIESIS AND IMMUNOPOIESIS IN THE FETUS

The immune system is composed of hematopoietic cells, including lymphocytes, mononuclear phagocytes, and granulocytes; products secreted by these cells; and certain humoral factors produced by non-hematopoietic cells. The hematopoietic cells are derived from stem cells that originate in the yolk sac. As a principal source of hematopoietic cells, the yolk sac is replaced by the liver at 6 to 8 weeks of gestation and subsequently by the bone marrow at 5 months of gestation.

Macrophages are detectable as early as 4 weeks of gestation in the human fetal yolk sac (Kelemen and Janossa, 1980), and these phagocytes are the first detectable element of the immune system. The early appearance of cells of this lineage may be critical for normal embryogenesis, since tissue-specific ablation of macrophages in transgenic mice results in abnormalities in the development of those tissues (Lang and Bishop, 1993). Precursors of neutrophilic phagocytes are detectable in the yolk sac and then in the liver but appear somewhat later than macrophages. Moreover, mature neutrophils are not detected until 14 to 16 weeks of gestation (Playfair et al., 1963; Christensen, 1989). The first cells of the lymphoid lineage to develop are the natural killer (NK) cells, which are detectable in the liver at 6 weeks of gestation (Phillips et al., 1992). Precursors of T and B lymphocytes are detectable in the liver by 7 to 8 weeks of gestation (Gathings et al., 1977; Haynes et al., 1988). The thymic rudiment is colonized by T-cell precursors at 8.5 weeks of gestation (Lobach et al., 1985; Haynes et al., 1988), and the bone marrow contains pre-B cells by 13 weeks of gestation (Gathings et al., 1977). Thus, all the major lineages of cells that will develop into a functional immune system are present in the human by the onset of the second trimester.

ANTIGEN PROCESSING AND PRESENTATION

T lymphocytes recognize antigen in the form of short peptides bound in a cleft in host major histocompatibility complex (MHC) molecules. CD8 T cells preferentially recognize antigen in association with class I MHC (human leukocyte antigens [HLA]-A, -B, and -C in humans), which consists of a polymorphic α chain and an invariant chain, β_2-microglobulin. CD4 T cells preferentially recognize antigen in association with class II MHC (HLA-DR, -DQ, and -DP in humans), which consists of a variable α and β chain.

Peptides bound to class I MHC molecules are derived from proteins synthesized *de novo* within the antigen-presenting cell (APC) (Townsend and Bodmer, 1989). A specific peptide transporter/pump apparently shuttles peptides formed in the cytoplasm to the endoplasmic reticulum, where peptide binding to recently synthesized class I MHC can take place (Van Kaer et al., 1992). In contrast to class I MHC, peptides that bind to class II MHC proteins are mostly derived from phagocytosis or endocytosis of soluble or membrane-bound proteins (Morrison et al., 1986; Nuchtern et al., 1990; Harding et al., 1991; Hunt et al., 1992). Newly synthesized class II MHC molecules associate in the endoplasmic reticulum with a protein called the invariant chain that impedes their binding of endogenous peptides in this compartment.

This effectively separates peptides binding to class I and to class II MHC into two separate pools (Roche and Creswell, 1990; Teyton et al., 1990). Where endocytosed protein is processed into antigenic peptide and where peptide associates with class II MHC remains uncertain, but endosomal or lysosome-like compartments or both are likely to be involved (Guagliardi et al., 1990; Harding et al., 1991; Long, 1992). An additional pathway for antigen presentation by class I MHC may operate when mononuclear phagocytes phagocytose bacteria, such as *Escherichia coli* or *Salmonella* (Pfeifer et al., 1993).

Class I MHC and the cell components required for peptide generation, transport, and class I binding are virtually ubiquitous in the cells of vertebrates (Daar et al., 1984; Yewdell and Bennink, 1990; Bahram et al., 1991). This is advantageous for the host, allowing cytotoxic CD8 T cells to recognize and lyse cells infected with intracellular pathogens in most tissues. Interestingly, class I MHC HLA-A, -B, and -C molecules are absent from the trophoblast of the placenta. This may serve to limit the recognition of these fetal-derived cells as foreign by maternal T cells. Human trophoblast does express HLA-G, a monomorphic molecule that is otherwise quite similar to class I MHC in its structure and association with β_2-microglobulin (Lata et al., 1992). As discussed later in the section Development and Function of Natural Killer Cells, cells lacking expression of class I MHC are highly susceptible to lysis by NK cells. It has been hypothesized that the expression of HLA-G may serve to prevent lysis of the trophoblast cells by maternal NK cells. Large numbers of maternal NK cells are found nearby in the decidua. Their immunologic function is uncertain.

In contrast to trophoblast, the expression of class I and class II MHC molecules by a variety of fetal tissues is evident by 12 weeks of gestation (Hofman et al., 1984; Oliver et al., 1989). At this time, all of the major "professional" antigen-presenting cells (macrophages, B cells, Langerhans cells, dendritic cells) are present and their expression of class II MHC molecules appears comparable with that in the adult (Edwards et al., 1985; Foster and Hollbrook, 1989; Harvey et al., 1990b). Likewise, at term the fraction of blood monocytes from neonates that express HLA-DR, -DP and -DQ antigens is similar to that in adults (Edwards et al., 1985; Glover et al., 1987), although a subset that expresses less HLA-DR than adult monocytes do is observed (Stiehm et al., 1984; Glover et al., 1987). These results in humans are in marked contrast to results in studies of neonatal rodents, in which expression of MHC at birth is clearly diminished.

Although the efficiency of antigen presentation by fetal and neonatal APCs has not been analyzed in depth (e.g., no data exist regarding expression of the peptide transporter proteins that serve to facilitate protein loading on class I molecules), it appears to be grossly intact. Monocytes from newborns are able to present soluble and particulate antigens to maternal T cells as effectively as can maternal monocytes, a response that is presumably class II MHC–restricted (Hoffman et al., 1981; Zlabinger et al., 1983; Chilmonczyk et al., 1985). Fetal tissues are frequently vigorously rejected after transplantation into non–MHC-matched hosts. This indicates that the level of surface MHC expression on fetal tissue is sufficient to initiate a vigorous allogeneic response by the host in which the foreign cells are killed by cytotoxic T cells, predominantly of the CD8 subset. There is growing evidence that most allogeneic responses of T cells are directed against peptide/allogeneic MHC molecule complexes rather than against the MHC molecules alone (Benoist and Mathis, 1991; Heath et al., 1991). Thus, the vigor of rejection of fetal allografts suggests that antigen presentation (at least of endogenous antigens) by class I MHC for the generation of cytolytic T cells is largely intact.

DEVELOPMENT AND FUNCTION OF THE T-CELL LINEAGE

Thymic Ontogeny

Phenotype of Thymocytes

Lymphoid cells with a prothymocyte phenotype (i.e., CD7+) but lacking other surface markers characteristic of thymocytes or T cells are found in the yolk sac and liver of the human fetus at 7 weeks of gestation, before first colonization of the thymic rudiment by lymphocytes (Haynes et al., 1988). These cells are probably the sources of prothymocytes at this age. The extent to which prothymocytes are committed to differentiate along the T lineage prior to thymic entry remains con-

troversial. For example, a small number of fetal liver cells express CD3-ε within the cytoplasm, suggesting commitment to the T lineage, prior to 15 weeks of gestation (Campana et al., 1989). Lymphocytes expanded in vitro from fetal liver of this gestational age have also been shown to contain CD3-δ and CD3-γ within the cytoplasm (Lanier et al., 1992a). However, it is unclear whether these cytoplasmic CD3+ cells can reconstitute human thymocyte development—for example, in the severe combined immunodeficiency (SCID) mouse–human thymus chimera system (Peault et al., 1991).

Because thymocyte development proceeds rapidly after lymphoid colonization at about 8 weeks, lymphoid cells in the fetal liver and bone marrow after 10 weeks of gestation with markers suggestive of T lineage, such as CD3 or CD2 (Campana et al., 1989; Terstappen et al., 1992), may be post-thymic emigrants rather than prothymocytes or cells undergoing extrathymic T-lineage differentiation. Putative prothymocyte cells from the yolk sac, fetal liver, or bone marrow, as well as CD7+CD34+ thymocytes, can be induced to express T-cell receptor (TCR) and other T-lineage proteins or, alternatively, to differentiate into natural killer cells or cells of the myeloid lineage (Kurtzberg et al., 1989; Peault et al., 1991; Chabannon et al., 1992; Lanier et al., 1992b; Poggi et al., 1993) depending on the conditions of culture. This suggests that these cells may be capable of T, NK, or myeloid differentiation even after their entry into the thymic microenvironment.

Shortly after colonization of the human fetal thymus with CD7+ cells at approximately 8½ weeks of gestation (Lobach et al., 1985; Haynes et al., 1988), thymocytes begin to express a group of proteins characteristic for T-lineage cells, including CD2, CD4, CD8, and components of the T-cell receptor. By 12 weeks of gestation, a clear architectural separation between the thymic cortex and medulla is apparent (Horst et al., 1990), and Hassall's corpuscles are evident shortly thereafter (Gilhus et al., 1985). By 14 weeks, the three major human thymocyte subsets are found in their usual location for the postnatal thymus (Harvey and Jones, 1990) (Fig. 10–1): The subcapsular region contains type I thymocytes, large blasts cells that do not express CD3, CD4, or CD8. The cortex contains smaller thymocytes that express CD3, CD4, and CD8, whereas the medulla predominantly contains cells that express CD3 and CD4 or CD8. By this age, the pattern of expression of a number of other proteins expressed by thymocytes, such as CD2, CD5, CD38, and the CD45 isoforms, matches that in the postnatal thymus. CD4 and CD8 T cells are found in the fetal liver and spleen by 14 weeks of gestation, indicating that the emigration of mature T-lineage cells from the thymus is established by this age (Asma et al., 1983).

Thymic cellularity increases dramatically during the last trimester. The thymus continues to increase in cellularity during postnatal life, reaching a peak size at about 10 years of age. It subsequently involutes, the cortex and medulla being gradually replaced with fat. The single CD4 or CD8 mature thymocytes within the

Cell Type	Major Developmental Events
Prothymocyte	Migration into thymus from bone marrow
Type I Thymocyte	Proliferation, TCR gene rearrangement
Type II Thymocyte	Selection of the αβ-TCR repertoire
Type III Thymocyte	Emigration to periphery
Peripheral CD4+ and CD8+ T cells	

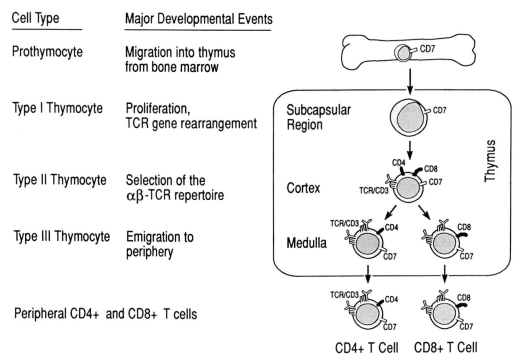

Figure 10–1. Putative stages of human thymocyte development. Prothymocytes from the bone marrow enter the thymus and give rise to three major stages of progressively mature αβ T cell receptor (TCR)–lineage thymocytes, defined by their pattern of expression of the αβ-TCR/CD3 complex, CD4, and CD8. TCR-α and TCR β-chain genes are rearranged during stage I, thymic selection occurs mainly during stage II, and emigration from the thymus occurs at stage III. (From Lewis DB, Wilson CB. In Remington JS, Klein JO, eds. Infectious Diseases of the Fetus and Newborn Infant, 4th ed. Philadelphia, WB Saunders, 1994, p. 25.)

medulla are relatively spared during the involutionary process compared with the immature, double-positive cortical thymocytes (Baroni et al., 1983).

Diversity of the Fetal Thymic T-Cell Receptor Repertoire

The fetal thymus expresses at least 22 different variable (V_β) segments at midgestation (Vanderkerckhove et al., 1992), indicating that the TCR repertoire is probably not significantly limited by restricted use of V segments at this age. However, the fetal thymus at 8 weeks of gestation demonstrates reduced diversity of sequences at the junctions between the V, D, and J segments of the TCR-β chain. Most striking is the shorter length of the hypervariable region formed at the junction of V with D and J, the equivalent of the CDR3 hypervariable region of immunoglobulin molecules (Jores et al., 1990; George and Schroeder, 1992). This is apparently due to decreased activity of terminal deoxynucleotidyl transferase (TdT), an enzyme that is responsible for the addition of extra nucleotides of random sequence at these joins (Gilfillan et al., 1993; Komori et al., 1933). The addition of extra nucleotides increases thereafter, reaching close to adult levels at 16 weeks of gestation (George and Schroeder, 1992). This enhancement is paralleled by gradual increases in the amount of TdT found in the thymus during gestation (Bodger et al., 1983; Asma et al., 1986; Campana et al., 1989; George and Schroeder, 1992). Since the CDR3-equivalent region of the TCR chains appears to be critical in determining antigen specificity (Danska et

al., 1990), decreased diversity in this region could compromise the ability of the first-trimester fetal TCR repertoire to recognize antigens.

Ontogeny of Peripheral T Cells

Cell Number, Peripheral T-Cell Phenotype, and Generation of Primed, or Memory, T Cells

From the second trimester onward, the number of T cells in the fetal circulation gradually increases during pregnancy (Hohlfeld et al., 1990). This increase continues for about 6 months after birth and is followed by a gradual decline to adult levels during childhood (European Collaborative Study, 1992; Erkeller-Yuksel et al., 1992). The ratio of CD4 to CD8 T cells in the circulation is high during fetal life (about 3.5:1) and gradually declines with age; most studies (Hohlfeld et al., 1990; European Collaborative Study, 1992), but not all (Erkeller-Yuksel et al., 1992), have found that the adult value of approximately 2:1 is reached at 4 years of age.

Unlike resting adult T cells, virtually all peripheral fetal and neonatal T cells express the CD38 (OKT10) molecule (Wilson, 1985). CD38 is also found on most thymocytes, suggesting that peripheral T cells in the fetus and neonate may represent an immature transitional population. In contrast to circulating fetal and neonatal T cells, a significant fraction of T cells in the fetal spleen between 14 and 20 weeks of gestation are CD38⁻ (Asma et al., 1983). The precursor-product relationship between CD38$^+$ and CD38$^-$ peripheral T cells in humans is unknown. In premature or term neonates who are stressed, a portion of circulating T-lineage cells are CD3^{low}, express CD1, and coexpress both CD4 and CD8, a phenotype characteristic of double-positive thymocytes (see Fig. 10–1) (Wilson et al., 1985; Lanier et al., 1986). It is likely that stress results in the premature release of cortical thymocytes into the circulation.

In adults, T cells capable of rapid proliferation in response to previously administered antigens are contained predominantly within a subset of putative memory cells constituting approximately 40% of the circulating $\alpha\beta$ CD4 T cells (Sanders et al., 1988a, 1988b; Akbar et al., 1988). A reciprocal population, which makes up about 60% of adult peripheral blood T cells, appears to contain naive or virgin CD4 T cells that have not previously encountered their cognate antigen (Sanders et al., 1988b; Akbar et al., 1988; Tedder et al., 1985). After mature T cells have participated in a primary response to an antigen and have ceased to proliferate, their phenotype and function remain significantly altered. Previously activated, or "primed," cells are larger with increased ribonucleic acid (RNA) content compared with antigenically naive cells and express increased levels of molecules involved in adhesion to the APC and to endothelium (Sanders et al., 1988a, 1988b). These previously primed memory cells exhibit enhanced adhesion and ability to migrate across endothelium in nonlymphoid tissues. Naive T cells appear preferentially to migrate from the blood to peripheral lymphoid tissue, whereas memory cells in the circulation preferentially adhere to and migrate across the endothelium of inflamed tissues (Arai et al., 1990; Pitzalis et al., 1991).

Primed T cells are less dependent on costimulatory signals from APC, which are necessary for activation of antigenically naive T cells. These and other alterations may account for the ability of the host upon rechallenge with antigen to mount a more rapid and expanded secondary response in terms of T-cell proliferation, cytokine production, and cytotoxicity. Enhanced secondary responses by T cells can be observed months to decades after an initial single exposure to antigen, indicating that the initial response has generated a population of memory T cells. The duration over which such primed or memory T cells are maintained in vivo in the absence of continual or intermittent exposure to the original or to a cross-reactive antigen remains controversial (Gray, 1993).

Putative memory CD4$^+$ T cells mostly express on their surface the low-molecular-weight isoform of the CD45 protein, CD45RO, and relatively high levels of CD29 (Sanders et al., 1988b; Akbar et al., 1988). Naive CD4$^+$ T cells express the high-molecular-weight isoform of CD45 (CD45RA) but not the low-molecular-weight isoform (CD45RO) and have lower amounts of CD29 (Tedder et al., 1985; Sanders et al., 1988a, 1988b; Akbar et al., 1988). The phenotype of neonatal T cells is almost completely that of the antigenically naive T cells in the adult (CD45RA$^+$CD45RO$^-$CD29^{low}), consistent with the limited exposure of the neonate to foreign antigens (Tedder et al., 1985; Sanders et al.,

1988b; George and Schroeder, 1992). Circulating fetal T cells also bear this antigenically naive surface phenotype (Peakman et al., 1992). It is hypothesized that CD45RA$^+$CD29^{low} naive T cells are the precursors of CD45RO$^+$CD29^{hi} memory cells (Tedder et al., 1985; Sanders et al., 1988a, 1988b; Akbar et al., 1988). A precursor-product relationship between CD45RA and CD45RO T cells during postnatal ontogeny is suggested by the fact that the proportion of $\alpha\beta$ T cells with a putative memory surface phenotype increases with age, presumably as a result of cumulative antigenic exposure and T-cell activation (de Paoli et al., 1988; Hayward et al., 1989). However, this pathway of differentiation, if correct, may not be unidirectional, since some CD45RO$^+$ T cells appear to become CD45RA$^+$ in vivo (Michie et al., 1992).

For CD8 T cells, it is controversial whether selective expression of CD45RA and CD45RO clearly demarcates the naive and memory populations (De Jong et al., 1991; Okumura et al., 1993). A number of other proteins are differentially expressed by memory versus naive CD4 and CD8 T cells (Sanders et al., 1988b). Neonatal CD8 T cells also lack a CD28$^-$CD11b$^+$ that may contribute to memory cytotoxic T cell (CTL) activity (Azuma et al., 1993). The proportion of circulating CD8 T cells with this CD28$^-$CD11b$^+$ phenotype gradually increases with age, consistent with this population's mediating memory cell responses (Hoshino et al., 1993). The levels of expression of the CD3, CD4, CD5, and CD8 proteins of fetal and neonatal T cells are similar to those of adult T cells.

Activation and Lymphokine Production by Neonatal T Cells

Neonatal T cells synthesize interleukin-2 (IL-2), express high-affinity IL-2 receptors, and proliferate in response to mitogens or allogeneic cells as effectively as adult T cells (Olding et al., 1977; Hayward and Kurnick, 1981; Wilson et al., 1986). Together, these findings indicate that IL-2–mediated autocrine or paracrine proliferation is intact in neonatal T cells. However, neonatal T cells do not proliferate as well as unfractionated adult T cells after activation by anti-CD2 or anti-CD3 monoclonal antibodies (Gerli et al., 1989; Pirenne et al., 1992). Decreased proliferation with these stimuli is also observed with adult naive T cells (Byrne et al., 1988, 1989; Sanders et al., 1989), indicating that it is a property of antigenically naive cells at all ages rather than an intrinsic immaturity peculiar to neonatal T cells. This idea is supported by the fact that with age, the proportion of peripheral blood T cells that are memory cells increases in parallel with the ability of peripheral blood T cells to respond to anti-CD2 or anti-CD3 monoclonal antibodies (Pirenne et al., 1992).

In contrast to IL-2, the production of other cytokines or expression of their cognate mRNAs by neonatal T cells is either slightly (tumor necrosis factor [TNF]-α) (English et al., 1988), moderately (granulocyte-macrophage colony–stimulating factor [GM-CSF]), or markedly reduced (interleukin-3, -4, -5; interferon γ [IL-3,

IL-4, IL-5; IFN-γ]) compared with adult T cells (Ehlers and Smith, 1991; Lewis et al., 1991; English et al., 1992) (Table 10–1). Since naive T cells from adults also have a reduced capacity to produce these cytokines, the apparent cytokine deficiency of neonatal T cells may reflect their antigenically naive status rather than an intrinsic immaturity in function. This idea is supported by the ability of neonatal T cells activated and cultured in vitro to acquire a memory T-cell surface phenotype and the capacity to produce cytokines such as IL-4 and IFN-γ (Sanders et al., 1989; Ehlers and Smith, 1991; Wilson, 1991), to provide help for antibody production (Clement et al., 1988), and to proliferate vigorously in response to anti-CD3 monoclonal antibody (Koulova et al., 1990). In addition, they become predominantly CD45RO+CD29hi (Sanders et al., 1988b; Akbar et al., 1988). However, an analysis of antigen-specific proliferation and IFN-γ production by T cells ex vivo suggests that the generation of T cells with antigen-specific memory function is markedly delayed in neonates compared with adults after primary infection with herpes simplex virus (HSV) (Burchett et al., 1992). The basis for this delay remains to be determined but could result from problems with any or all of these—initial activation, proliferation, or activation-induced differentiation—or perhaps with limitations in the TCR repertoire of neonatal T cells in vivo (Chilmonczyk et al., 1985).

T-Cell Help for Antibody Production

T cells are important in the regulation of B-cell proliferation and enhanced immunoglobulin secretion. This help is provided both by contact-dependent mechanisms and through secretion of soluble lymphokines. The contact-dependent interactions between T and B cells include both cognate recognition through the TCR of antigenic peptides associated with major histocompatibility complex molecules on B cells and those mediated by pairs of receptor-ligand molecules (Ochs et al., 1993). The importance of contact-dependent T-cell help is clearly illustrated by the phenotype of patients with X-linked hyper-IgM who have genetic defects in the expression of the CD40 ligand (gp39) (Aruffo et al., 1993). The marked paucity of immunoglobulin isotypes other than IgM and the inability to generate memory B-cell responses in these patients indicate that these responses critically depend on the CD40 molecule of the B cell binding to CD40 ligand (gp39) on the T cell (Noelle et al., 1992; Aruffo et al., 1993). The identi-

Table 10–1. Properties of Lymphokines, Cytokines, and Colony-Stimulating Factors

Name	Biochemical Characteristics (Human)	Principal Cell Source	Major Biologic Effects	Production by Neonatal* versus Adult Cells
Interleukin-1 (lymphocyte-activating factor, endogenous pyrogen)	Two proteins: α and β both Mr ~ 17.5 kD; α more acidic than β	Many cell types; mononuclear phagocytes are a major cause	Fever, inflammatory response, cofactor in T-cell and B-cell growth and bone marrow stem cell growth and differentiation	Normal—term and premature
Interleukin-2 (T-cell growth factor)	Glycoprotein Mr ~ 15 kD	T cells, NK cells	T-cell > B-cell growth, increased T-cell lymphokine production and cytotoxicity T and NK cells	Normal to most stimuli; ↓ to anti-CD3
Interleukin-3 (multi-CSF)	Glycoprotein 14–28 kD	T cells	Growth of early hematopoietic precursors	10%–25% of adult
Interleukin-4 (B-cell stimulating factor, B-cell growth factor I)	Glycoprotein ~ 20 kD	T cells, mast cells, basophils	Cofactor in B- and T-cell growth, required for IgE synthesis, enhances T-cell cytotoxicity, enhances class II MHC expression, mast cell growth factor; inhibits most macrophage inflammatory functions	< 10% of adult
Interleukin-5 (B-cell growth factor II, T cell–replacing factor)	Glycoprotein ~ 18 kD (circulates as a homodimer)	T cells, mast cells, basophils, eosinophils	Growth and immunoglobulin secretion by activated B cells; eosinophil growth and differentiation	↓ ↓ by mRNA analysis
Interleukin-6 (B-cell stimulating factor I, B-cell differentiation factor)	Glycoprotein 21–29 kD	Mononuclear phagocytes, fibroblasts, T cells	Hepatic acute phase protein synthesis, fever, induction of immunoglobulin production in activated B cells, support marrow precursors growth, T-cell growth	Term—normal to slightly ↓; premature ~ 25% of adult
Interleukin-7	Glycoprotein ~ 25 kD	Stromal cells—bone marrow and other sites	Supports growth of B-cell precursors, mature T cells, CTL differentiation	Not known
Interleukin-8	8 kD protein	Macrophages, endothelial cells, fibroblasts, T lymphocytes, epithelial cells	Chemotaxis and activation of neutrophils, chemotaxis of subset memory T cells	See text, Mononuclear Phagocytes, Production of Cytokines
Interleukin-9	Glycoprotein 30–40 kD	CD4+ T cells	Growth of CD4+ T-cell clones, mast cell growth	Not known
Interleukin-10	Glycoprotein 17–21 kD	TH2 CD4 T cells, B cells, macrophages	Inhibits production of IFN-γ > IL-2, IL-3, TNF by T cells; inhibits macrophage inflammation functions	Not known
Interleukin-11	20 kD	Marrow stromal cells	B cell/plasma cell growth; hematopoietic cell growth	Not known
Interleukin-12 (NKSF)	30, 40 kD	Macrophages, B cells	Induces IFN-γ secretion from NK+ T cells, enhances T-cell and NK cytotoxicity; T-cell growth	Not known
Interleukin-13	10 kD	T cells	Similar to IL-4	Not known
Interferon-α	Family of 18–20-kD peptides	Mononuclear phagocytes, lymphocytes	Interfere with viral replication, decrease cell replication, increase class I MHC expression, increase NK cell function	Term—normal; premature—? ↓

Table 10–1. Properties of Lymphokines, Cytokines, and Colony-Stimulating Factors *Continued*

Name	Biochemical Characteristics (Human)	Principal Cell Source	Major Biologic Effects	Production by Neonatal* vs Adult Cells
Interferon-β	Glycoprotein 23 kD	Fibroblasts, epithelial cells	Interfere with viral replication, decrease cell replication, increase class I MHC expression, increase NK cell function	Normal
Interferon-γ	Glycoprotein 20–25 kD	T cells, NK cells	Same as IFN-α and IFN-β; also increase class II MHC expression, enhance macrophage functions, inhibit IgE production	< 10% of adult
Tumor necrosis factors				
TNF-α (cachectin)	17-kD peptide	Mononuclear phagocytes T cells, NK cells	Fever and inflammatory response effects similar to IL-1, shock, hemorrhagic necrosis of tumors, altered endothelial cell function, induce catabolic state	Term—T cells, monocytes: ~ 50% of adult Macrophages, preterm monocytes: ~ 25% adult
TNF-β (lymphotoxin)	Glycoprotein 25 kD	T cells, NK cells	Same as TNF-α	Normal
Colony-Stimulating Factors				
GM-CSF	Glycoprotein 14–35 kD	T cells, endothelial cells, mononuclear phagocytes, fibroblasts	Growth of GM precursors, enhance GM function	T cells ~ 50% adult Monocytes—normal
M-CSF (CSF1)	Glycoprotein two forms: 35–45-kD, 20–25-kD (one gene) (both circulate as homodimers)	Monocytes, fibroblasts, endothelial cells	Growth of monocytes, enhance macrophage function	Normal
G-CSF	Glycoprotein 19 kD	Mononuclear phagocytes; epithelial cells; fibroblasts	Promotes proliferation of granulocytes; enhances granulocyte function	Normal or slight ↓
Steel factor	Glycoprotein 31–36 kD	Bone marrow stromal cells	Early hematopoietic precursor growth (? stem cells); mast cell growth	Not known
Chemokines α FAMILY (C-X-C) IL-8 human GRO	~ 8-kD protein	Mononuclear phagocytes, endothelium fibroblasts	Neutrophil chemoattractant	Not known (see above for IL-8)
Others β FAMILY (C-C) MIP-1α, β (human LD78, ACT-2)	~ 8-kD protein	Mononuclear phagocytes, T-cells	Monocyte and T-cell subset chemoattractant, fever	Not known
Monocyte chemoattractant protein (MCP or MCAF, murine = JE)		Blood mononuclear cells, endothelial cells, fibroblasts, epithelial cells	Monocyte and T-cell subset chemoattractant	Not known
RANTES		T cells	Monocyte and CD4+ memory, T-cell chemoattractant	Not known

*Unless otherwise indicated, results are with cells from the blood of term neonates.
Abbreviations: CSF = colony-stimulating factor; G = granulocyte; GM = granulocyte-macrophage; M = macrophage; MCAF = monocyte chemotactic activating factor; MCP = monocyte chemoattractant protein; MHC = major histocompatibility complex; MIP = macrophage inflammatory peptides; NK = natural killer cells.
Adapted from Lewis DB, Wilson CB. Developmental immunology and role of host defenses in neonatal susceptibility to infection. In Remington JS, Klein JO, eds. Infectious Diseases of the Fetus and Newborn, 4th ed. Philadelphia, WB Saunders, 1994.

fied CD40 ligand, gp39, which is expressed only on activated T cells, is a membrane-bound cytokine with homology to TNF (Hollenbaugh et al., 1992). Engagement of CD40 on the B cell in conjunction with other signals provided by cytokines, such as IL-4, can markedly enhance immunoglobulin production in vitro and promote class switching (Rousset et al., 1991). Other ligand pairs, such as B7/CD28 and leukocyte function–associated antigen-1 (LFA-1)/CD54, may promote interaction between B and T cells during the immune response and may enhance activation of these cells (Clark and Lane, 1991; Ochs et al., 1993).

Soluble cytokines produced by activated T cells influence B-cell immunoglobulin production. Experiments in mice in which the IL-2, IL-4, or IFN-γ receptor genes have been disrupted by gene targeting suggest that these cytokines, which are derived largely from T cells, are not essential for B-cell development but are important for the proper regulation of B-cell immuno-

globulin isotype expression. Inactivation of the IL-4 gene prevents all IgE production (Kühn et al., 1991); inactivation of the IL-2 gene results in a marked elevation of IgE and IgG1 from normal levels (Schimpl et al., 1992); inactivation of the IFN-γ receptor gene leads to diminished production of IgG2a in response to specific antigen (Huang et al., 1993). In activated B cells, IL-2 promotes IgM secretion by inducing secretion of the J chain necessary for the assembly of IgM into functional pentamers (Blackman et al., 1986). IL-6, a product of multiple cell types, including T cells, may serve as an autocrine factor for the differentiation factor of mature B cells and the proliferation of plasma cells (Xia et al., 1989). IL-6 has also been shown to enhance the production of antibodies against thymus-independent type II antigens in vitro (Ambrosino et al., 1990).

In the neonate, studies indicate that T-cell help for B cells is diminished, under many but not all conditions.

When T and B cells are activated with stimuli that are not suppressive in vitro (e.g., *Staphylococcus* protein A or Epstein-Barr virus), total immunoglobulin production by B cells is similar or moderately reduced compared with adult T cells (Tosato et al., 1980; Andersson et al., 1981; Hayward, 1981; Miyawaki et al., 1981b). This response correlates with the normal to modestly reduced antibody response of neonates to immunization with protein antigens that require T-cell help. Supernatants from neonatal T cells are also able to support the production of antibodies against pneumococcal polysaccharide, a thymus-independent type II antigen, by adult but not by neonatal B cells (Banchereau et al., 1991). As discussed later, this is consistent with the hypothesis that the neonate is deficient in the population of B cells that responds to polysaccharide antigens in the absence of cognate T-cell help.

Despite these observations, there is now increasing evidence to suggest that neonatal T cells are immature in their ability to provide contact-dependent and lymphokine factors required to help B cells undergo efficient class switching and differentiation into memory B cells. Recent studies suggest that neonatal B cells in the presence of adult T cells (Splawski and Lipsky, 1991) or recombinant CD40 ligand and cytokines (e.g., IL-4, IL-10, or both) (Nonoyama et al., 1995) have the capacity to switch isotypes and secrete each of the immunoglobulin classes, including IgG, IgA, and IgE. In the presence of IL-4 and recombinant CD40 ligand, IgE secretion by neonatal B cells was comparable with that by adult B cells. Activated neonatal T cells alone fail to support these responses. This appears to reflect in part the inability of neonatal T cells to express the CD40 ligand following activation (Nonoyama, et al., 1995) and in part the decreased production of the critical cytokines, such as IL-4, by neonatal T cells (Lewis et al., 1991).

It is important to note that the diminished expression of CD40 ligand and critical lymphokines by neonatal T cells appears to be due to their antigenically naive status rather than an intrinsic developmental immaturity. Thus, when primed by exogenous stimulation in vitro, these cells have an ability to efficiently express CD40 ligand (Nonoyama, 1994) similar to their enhanced capacity to secrete lymphokines that modulate B cell responses (as noted earlier in Activation and Lymphokine Production by Neonatal T Cells). These differences may account, at least in part, for the delayed response or the need for additional doses of antigens in young infants that are required to achieve antibody levels comparable with those elicited in older individuals (see Antibody Response to Specific T Cell–Dependent and T Cell–Independent Antigens).

In addition to the immaturity in neonatal T-cell help for B-cell responses, under certain conditions neonatal T cells may inhibit or suppress B-cell responses, whereas adult T cells do not. Neonatal T cells that are stimulated with pokeweed mitogen, a T- and B-cell mitogen, suppress immunoglobulin production by neonatal or adult B cells compared with production observed in adult T cells (Hayward and Merrill, 1981; Hayward and Kurnick, 1981; Andersson et al., 1983).

Suppression in this system may require both CD8 and CD4 T cells. The subpopulation of adult CD4 T cells with a naive phenotype (CD45RA$^+$CD45RO$^-$CD29^{low}) also suppresses antibody production in this assay and has been termed the suppressor-inducer subset (Morimoto et al., 1985, 1986; Kingsley et al., 1988). Virtually all neonatal CD4 T cells express this phenotype (de Paoli et al., 1988), showing that suppressor activity induced by pokeweed mitogen correlates with the surface phenotype of CD4 T cells in both neonates and adults. Although these results have been interpreted as showing that neonatal T cells have increased suppressor function compared with adult T cells, this suppressor-like activity depends on the stimulus—for example, it is not observed with other mitogens, such as concanavalin A, or with activation by Epstein-Barr virus (Morito et al., 1979; Miyawaki et al., 1981a, 1981b). It is also unclear whether pokeweed mitogen is an accurate mimic of the physiologic activation of T and B cells and of the T- and B-cell interaction induced by antigen.

As discussed earlier, there is growing evidence that the CD45RA$^+$CD45RO$^-$ subset of T cells in the neonate and adult may represent antigenically naive cells that are precursors of memory T cells rather than a separate suppressor-inducer lineage (Sanders et al., 1988a; Clement et al., 1988; Ehlers and Smith, 1991; Lewis et al., 1991; Pirenne et al., 1992). The suppressive effect in the pokeweed mitogen system could therefore represent a developmental feature of all CD4 T cells rather than the function of a separate suppressor T-cell lineage. Consistent with this idea, when CD45RA$^+$CD45RO$^-$ cells from adults or neonates are activated in vitro and propagated, they acquire the ability to provide help rather than suppression in the pokeweed mitogen system for antibody production (Clement et al., 1990). To determine the relevance of this in vitro system to immune responses by the neonate will require a greater understanding of the cellular and molecular nature of suppression by T cells in vivo.

T Cell–Mediated Cytotoxicity

Studies of T cell–mediated cytotoxicity (CTL) activity in the neonate are limited. After sensitization in vitro, CTL activity by neonatal T cells against allogeneic targets has been found in different studies to range from approximately 50% to 100% of adult activity (Granberg et al., 1979; Rayfield et al., 1980). Allogeneic CTL activity by fetal blood T cells obtained at 15 to 22 weeks' gestation varies from no detectable activity to values similar to those for adult blood T cells (Rayfield et al., 1980). Reduced CTL activity against human or murine cell targets has also been found with lectin-activated cord lymphocytes, particularly if purified T cells are used (Campbell et al., 1974; Andersson et al., 1981; Lubens et al., 1982). Part of this apparent deficiency could reflect the absence of memory T cells in the neonatal samples, because memory CD8 T cells kill more efficiently than naive T cells after stimulation with lectin or anti-CD3 mAb (Phillips and Lanier, 1986; De Jong et al., 1991; McFarland et al., 1992).

In studies of CTL activity against human immunodeficiency virus (HIV-1), decreased MHC-restricted activity was found in infants who had acquired infection through vertical transmission compared with older children who had acquired infection by transfusion (Luzuriaga et al., 1991). Although this finding suggests that CTL activity may be decreased during the immediate postnatal period, the interpretation is complicated by the likely suppression of multiple aspects of antigen-specific immunity by HIV-1 in these patients, particularly when infected at a younger age. Using mononuclear cells from infants with acute respiratory syncytial virus (RSV) infection, cytolytic activity was found against RSV-infected targets in two studies (Isaacs et al., 1987; Chiba et al., 1989). In one of these studies, the percentage of children with cellular cytotoxicity to RSV was lower in infants under 5 months of age than in those 6 to 24 months of age (Chiba et al., 1989). However, neither of these studies definitively showed what proportion of the killing was mediated by T cells and was appropriately MHC-restricted. Further studies will be necessary to determine more precisely the postnatal ontogeny of CTL activity following viral infection.

Gamma Delta T Cells and Their Ontogeny

T cells expressing $\gamma\delta$ T-cell receptor are rarer than $\alpha\beta$ T cells in most human tissues, with a few exceptions, such as the intestinal epithelium (Bucy et al., 1989). In the thymus and peripheral blood of most individuals only about 2% to 5% of T-lineage cells express $\gamma\delta$ TCR (Kabelitz, 1992). The human γ and δ TCR genes undergo a programmed rearrangement of dispersed segments analogous to that of the α and β TCR genes shortly after colonization of the thymus with lymphoid cells during fetal gestation (McVay et al., 1991; Kabelitz, 1992). Differentiation of $\gamma\delta$ thymocytes occurs by a pathway largely or completely independent of that for $\alpha\beta$ thymocytes (Philpott et al., 1992; Itohara et al., 1993). Unlike $\alpha\beta$ T cells, whose development absolutely requires an intact thymus, at least a portion of $\gamma\delta$ T cells can develop by a thymic-independent pathway (Borst et al., 1991). For example, normal numbers of $\gamma\delta$ cells are found in cases of complete thymic aplasia (Borst et al., 1991). Also, $\gamma\delta$ T cells may not undergo the same selection process that is obligatory for $\alpha\beta$ T cells (Bigby et al., 1993). Most $\gamma\delta$ cells lack both CD4 and CD8, suggesting that they do not undergo positive selection analogous to that required for $\alpha\beta$ thymocytes.

The percentage of circulating $\gamma\delta$ T cells is lower in the neonate than in the adult (Yachie et al., 1989). The percentage of $\gamma\delta$ T cells in the circulation appears to gradually increased after birth, with adult values achieved by approximately 1 year of age (Yachie et al., 1989; Smith et al., 1990b). Circulating neonatal $\gamma\delta$ T cells mostly lack expression of a cytotoxicity-associated marker, serine esterase, whereas adult peripheral blood $\gamma\delta$ T cells are uniformly serine esterase–positive (Smith et al., 1990b). Although these observations raise the possibility that $\gamma\delta$ T cell–mediated immune responses in the neonate may be decreased compared with those in the adult, this has not been directly shown.

Although there is potential for the formation of a highly diverse $\gamma\delta$ TCR repertoire (Davis and Bjorkman, 1988), the actual diversity of γ and δ V segments found on $\gamma\delta$ T cells in humans is strikingly less than that observed for $\alpha\beta$ T cells. From midgestation onward, $\gamma\delta$ thymocytes that express $V_\delta 1$ predominate. Interestingly, at birth, $\gamma\delta$ T cells that express $V_\delta 1$ also predominate in the circulation. However, during childhood there is an increase in $\gamma\delta$ cells expressing $V_\gamma 9/V_\delta 2$ TCR, so that by adulthood, this becomes the predominant circulating $\gamma\delta$ T cell population (Parker et al., 1990). It has been proposed that these changes during postnatal ontogeny in the peripheral $\gamma\delta$ population reflect the preferential expansion of $V_\gamma 9/V_\delta 2$ as a result of encountering a ubiquitous antigen or antigens (Kabelitz, 1992). In mice, $\gamma\delta$ T cells that express different V region gene segments develop and are released in distinct ontogenetically determined waves to particular tissues. In the human thymus, there appears to be a preferential expression of a particular repertoire of V_γ gene segments during fetal development (Krangel et al., 1990; McVay et al., 1991), but it is unclear if cells bearing these receptors are released in distinct waves and preferentially home to particular tissues.

Although some $\gamma\delta$ T cells can recognize antigens presented by conventional class I MHC and occasionally by class II MHC (Kozbor et al., 1989), this is probably not true for the majority (Kabelitz et al., 1990). $\gamma\delta$ T cells also appear to be enriched in cells that can recognize antigens presented by "nonclassical" MHC molecules, such as CD1 and CD48 (Porcelli et al., 1989; Mami-Chouaib et al., 1990). Lipid- or carbohydrate-enriched extracts from a variety of bacteria, including mycobacteria and the important neonatal pathogen, *Listeria monocytogenes,* can activate $\gamma\delta$ T cells (De Libero et al., 1991; Goerlich et al., 1991; Kabelitz et al., 1991; Tsuyuguchi et al., 1991). Neonatal $\gamma\delta$ T cells proliferate in response to lipid-enriched extracts from *Mycobacteria* as effectively as adult $\gamma\delta$ T cells (Tsuyuguchi et al., 1991). $\gamma\delta$ T cells appear to contribute to the initial clearance of *Listeria* in mice (Skeen and Ziegler, 1993), although they are not absolutely necessary, since mice deficient in $\gamma\delta$ cells as a result of a selective gene targeting clear *Listeria* effectively (Mombaerts et al., 1993); however, the nature of the inflammatory response is altered. The role of $\gamma\delta$ T cells in other neonatal infections remains to be determined.

Practical Aspects of T-Cell Function in the Neonate

Delayed Cutaneous Hypersensitivity and Graft Rejection

Skin test reactivity to cell-free antigens assesses a form of delayed type hypersensitivity (DTH), which requires the function of antigen-specific CD4 T cells. Skin test reactivity to common antigens, such as *Candida,* streptokinase-streptodornase, and tetanus toxoid, is usually not detectable in neonates (Steele et al., 1976; Franz et al., 1976; Munoz and Limbert, 1977). This primarily reflects a lack of antigen-specific sensitization because in vitro reactivity to these antigens is also absent. However, when leukocytes and presumably antigen-specific CD4 T cells from sensitized adults are adoptively transferred to neonates, children, or adults, only neonates fail to respond to antigen-specific skin tests (Warwick et al., 1960). As discussed later, this indicates that the neonate may be deficient in other components of the immune system required for DTH, such as monocyte chemotaxis. Such deficiencies may account, in least in part, for diminished skin reactivity by the neonate compared with that in the adult after specific sensitization or after intradermal injection with T-cell mitogens (Uhr et al., 1960; Bonforte et al., 1972). Diminished skin reactivity after sensitization appears to persist postnatally until approximately 1 year of age (Kniker et al., 1985).

Nevertheless, neonates, including those that are premature, are capable of rejecting foreign grafts (Fowler et al., 1960). Blood transfusions rarely induce graft-versus-host disease in the term neonate. However, exceptional cases of persistence of donor lymphocytes and of graft-versus-host disease have developed subsequent to intrauterine transfusion in the last trimester and in transfused premature neonates (Naiman et al., 1969; Parkman et al., 1974; Berger and Dixon, 1989; Flidel et al., 1992). The precise age-related risk for this complication is not known. The infusion of fresh leukocytes in the neonate has been shown to induce a state of partial tolerance to skin grafts (Fowler et al., 1960). The induction of tolerance for transfused lymphocytes may occur by a similar mechanism, predisposing the fetus or neonate to graft-versus-host disease. Together, these observations suggest a partial immaturity in T-cell and inflammatory mechanisms required for DTH and graft rejection.

T-Cell Reactivity to Specific Antigens

Lymphocyte reactivity, measured in vitro by proliferation or by production of lymphokines, has been detected at birth or during the first week of life in response to tuberculin purified protein derivative (PPD) (Schlesinger and Covelli, 1977; Shiratsuchi and Tsuyuguchi, 1981), *Mycobacterium leprae* (Barnetson et al., 1976), and measles and rubella virus antigens (Thong et al., 1974; Gallagher et al., 1981). Infants with detectable lymphocyte reactivity were uncommon (usually <20%) among those born to mothers without evidence of active infection with these agents; the data were interpreted to suggest possible transfer of maternal cellular immunity to the fetus (Leikin and Oppenheim, 1971). The mechanism by which this might have occurred is not known, although transfer of maternal lymphocytes has been proposed. Rarely, apparent reactivity to tetanus and diphtheria toxoids has been observed in cells from neonates with (Leikin and Oppenheim, 1971) or without (Leikin, 1975) maternal reactivity. In vitro reactivity of neonatal T cells to various whole preparations of gram-negative bacteria or *Staphylococcus aureus* has been reported with variable frequency (Brody and Oski, 1968; Ivanyi and Lehner, 1977; Rubin et al., 1981). In some cases, these findings

have not been reproduced in other laboratories—for example, reactivity to tetanus or influenza virus antigens was not demonstrated with cells from neonates of reactive mothers (Englund et al., 1993). The magnitude of the responses observed in each of these cases is low and, at least in some cases, may represent artifacts. It is difficult to exclude in utero exposure of the fetus to the antigens in question.

The interpretation is further confounded by the potential of some of the stimuli tested to act as mitogens or superantigens rather than as MHC-restricted peptide antigens. For example, T cells, including those from the neonate, are activated by superantigen toxins produced by *S. aureus* and other bacteria (Choi et al., 1989). Bacterial superantigens polyclonally activate T cells based on the expression of particular TCR V_β gene segments rather than through variable region antigen-MHC binding sites. Mycobacterial products, such as PPD tuberculin or *M. leprae* extracts, can activate many $\gamma\delta$ T cells in the absence of specific prior sensitization and without MHC restriction; the $\gamma\delta$ TCR appears to recognize heat-shock proteins, carbohydrate-like compounds expressed by these bacteria, or both (Haregewoin et al., 1989; Holoshitz et al., 1989). Thus, reports of neonatal T-cell responses resulting from transfer of maternal immunity remain suspect, unless the T-cell population that mediated the response is identified and its antigen specificity and MHC restriction have been demonstrated. Overall, antigen-specific cell-mediated immunity is probably rare in the neonate in the absence of fetal infection.

Specific cellular immunity, as demonstrated by antigen-specific lymphocyte proliferation or IFN production, is usually not detectable at birth and in the first months of life in infants with congenital syphilis (Friedmann, 1977), rubella virus (Buimovici-Klein, et al., 1979), or cytomegalovirus (CMV) infections (Gehrz et al., 1977; Reynolds et al., 1979; Starr et al., 1979). The lack of response in infants with congenital rubella persists longer in those infected early in gestation. Cellular immunity develops later in infants with persistent active or severe congenital CMV infection. In the first months of life, proliferative responses of T cells from neonates to *Toxoplasma* antigen are often not detectable above background, although most develop a detectable response thereafter (Wilson et al., 1980; McLeod et al., 1990). In a study by McLeod et al. (1990), none of eight congenitally infected infants studied in the first 15 months of life had blood mononuclear cells that produced detectable IFN-γ or IL-2, even though antigen-specific proliferative responses were detectable in some. More detailed analysis is needed to determine the basis for the protracted impairment in the development of effective T cell–mediated responses in these infants.

The ability to mount a cellular immune response to infection acquired perinatally is also delayed in neonates compared with adults. Thirty percent of neonates with primary HSV infection have detectable lymphocyte proliferation in response to viral antigen within 4 weeks of onset, compared with 100% of adults (Sullender et al., 1987). The lag in the acquisition of a proliferative response is paralleled by a similar delay in acquisition of antigen-specific IFN-γ production (Burchett et al., 1992). Delayed acquisition of antigen-specific cellular immunity in the neonate may account in part for the more severe clinical disease in neonates infected with HSV and the other perinatal pathogens noted earlier compared with older individuals who have these infections.

Summary

Overall, T-cell function in the fetus and neonate is impaired compared with that in adults. Diminished functions include T cell–mediated lymphokine production, cytotoxicity, delayed type hypersensitivity (DTH), and help for B-cell differentiation. The lack of memory T cells in the antigenically naive fetus and neonate compared with T cells from more mature individuals may account in part for many of these differences. Limitations in the numbers of T cells and in the available repertoire of αβ TCR do not appear to play a major role in the diminished immune responses by the neonate, although they are likely to do so in the fetus before mid-gestation. Following infection, the acquisition of detectable T cell–dependent antigen-specific responses is delayed. The basis for this delay remains to be defined. There is no compelling evidence that the mother transfers T cell–specific immunity to the fetus.

DEVELOPMENT OF B CELLS AND IMMUNOGLOBULINS

Phenotype of Fetal and Neonatal B Cells

Pre-B cells are detected in the human fetal liver and omentum by 8 weeks of gestation and in fetal bone marrow by 13 weeks of gestation (Gathings et al., 1977; Solvason and Kearney, 1992). After 30 weeks of gestation, pre-B cells are found only in bone marrow. B cells expressing surface IgM are detectable as early as 10 weeks of gestation (Gathings et al., 1977), and at midgestation, marrow pre-B cells expressing surface IgM with surrogate light chains have been detected (Nishimoto et al., 1991). The expression of surrogate light chains during early B-cell development is postulated to allow the M heavy chain to transit through the endoplasmic reticulum without degradation and is essential for B-cell development in mice (Kitamura et al., 1992). The surface IgM and surrogate light-chain complex may generate intracellular signals required for subsequent B-cell development (Brouns et al., 1993). Unlike surface IgM–positive adult B cells found in the peripheral lymphoid organs, which also express surface IgD, fetal B cells at this stage express IgM without IgD (Gupta et al., 1976; Gathings et al., 1977). Experiments in mice have shown that exposure of IgM⁺IgD⁻ B cells to antigens functionally inactivates them (induces clonal anergy) (Lawton et al., 1972; Raff et al., 1975; Metcalf and Klinman, 1976). Engagement of the surface IgM molecule at this stage of B-cell development appears to deliver a tolerogenic intracellular signal distinct from that which leads to B-cell activation (Yellen et al., 1991). Thus, antigen exposure in utero may

induce specific tolerance in the fetus rather than an antibody response. This may account for the observation that early congenital infection, such as with rubella, can result in pathogen-specific defects in antibody production (Fitzgerald et al., 1988). For antibody production that requires T-cell help, such antigen-specific defects could also reflect the induction of T-cell tolerance. It is hypothesized that the susceptibility of IgM⁺IgD⁻ cells to clonal anergy throughout life helps to maintain B-cell tolerance to soluble self-antigens present at high concentrations.

Between 10 and 12 weeks of gestation in the human, B cells bearing surface immunoglobulin of the IgA, IgG, and IgD isotypes appear. The frequency of B cells in tissues then rapidly increases, so that by 22 weeks' gestation, the proportion of B cells in the spleen, blood, and bone marrow is similar to that in the adult (Hayward and Ezer, 1974; Gupta et al., 1976; Gathings et al., 1977; DeBiagi et al., 1985). In contrast to adult B cells, which bear IgM plus IgD or IgG or IgA alone, many neonatal B cells, and probably fetal B cells, express three surface immunoglobulins, IgG or IgA with IgM and IgD (Gathings et al., 1977) (Fig. 10–2). Coexpression of three isotypes on a single cell is probably accomplished by alternative RNA processing, since isotype switching to IgG or IgA would preclude the expression of IgM or IgD. It is not known whether these striking differences between neonate and adult in B-cell isotype expression are accounted for by lineage differences, developmental differences, or recent activation (presumably by self-antigens). Germinal centers in the spleen are absent during fetal life but appear in the first months after birth, presumably as a result of postnatal antigenic stimulation (Timens et al., 1989).

Another major difference in the fetal B-cell repertoire is the relative preponderance of B cells expressing CD5 (also known as Ly-1⁺ or B1 cells) (Bofill et al., 1985; Herzenberg et al., 1986; Punnonen et al., 1992). More than 40% of B cells in the fetal spleen, omentum, and circulation at midgestation are CD5⁺ (Antin et al., 1986; Solvason and Kearney, 1992; Bhat et al., 1992), but lesser numbers are found in the fetal liver and bone marrow (Antin et al., 1986). The preponderance of CD5⁺ B cells noted in the fetus is also observed in the neonatal circulation (Erkeller-Yuksel et al., 1992). The percentage of B cells that are CD5⁺ in the peripheral lymphoid organs gradually declines with postnatal age (Griffiths-Chu et al., 1984; Hoover et al., 1985; Small et al., 1989; Bhat et al., 1992). Since activation of CD5⁻ B cells in vitro induces CD5 surface expression (Werner-Favre et al., 1989), it has been suggested that CD5⁺ and CD5⁻ B cells may represent different stages of activation of a common B-cell population. However, a variety of evidence in the mouse indicates that CD5⁺ or B1 cells represent a separate lineage, precursors for which are found only early during development (Herzenberg et al., 1986; Hardy, 1991). Moreover, human CD5⁺ B cells that predominate in the fetus and neonate lack most surface markers characteristic of previously activated B cells (Antin et al., 1986). Unlike conventional (B2) B cells that depend on continued replenishment from immature bone marrow–derived

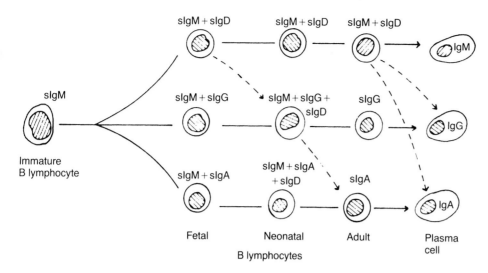

Figure 10–2. Pattern of isotype switching during B-cell maturation in the fetus, neonate, and adult. (From Lawton AR. In Twomey J, ed. The Pathophysiology of Human Immunologic Disorders. Baltimore, Urban & Schwarzenberg, 1982, pp. 11–27.)

cells, B1 cells are capable of self-renewal. B1 cells, including those in the newborn, typically produce antibodies that are often directed against self-antigens (autoantibodies), such as anti-DNA (Barbouche et al., 1992). It has been suggested that they play a role in regulation and development of the immune system in early ontogeny, perhaps in the induction of tolerance to self-antigens.

The Immunoglobulin Repertoire

The primary, or preimmune, immunoglobulin repertoire is more limited during the initial stages of B-cell development in the fetus than in the adult. In early to midgestation in the human fetus, the set of variable region (V) segments used to generate the heavy-chain gene is markedly restricted compared with that in the adult (Schroeder et al., 1987; Cuisinier et al., 1989). The V segments that are expressed are scattered throughout the heavy-chain gene locus (Schutte et al., 1992; Willems van Dijk et al., 1992). The length of the heavy chain's third complementarity-determining region (CDR3), which is formed at the junction of the V segment with the D and J segments, is shorter than at birth (Raaphorst et al., 1992). This could be due to decreased activity of TdT, the enzyme involved in random nucleotide addition at V-D and D-J junctions. The CDR3 region is the most hypervariable portion of immunoglobulins, and a short CDR3 region significantly reduces the diversity of the fetal immunoglobulin repertoire (Sanz, 1991).

The B-cell repertoire increases during gestation (Cuisinier et al., 1990), and by birth it is substantially more diverse in the use of heavy-chain V segments and in length of the CDR3 region for IgM and IgA but not for IgG transcripts (Mortari et al., 1993). Some limitations in V-segment repertoire may persist through the neonatal period, since some heavy-chain V segments expressed by the adult repertoire are not found in the neonate (Sanz, 1991; Mortari et al., 1992). The V regions used by heavy chains in B cells of the germinal centers of the tonsil may be more limited in the first three years of life than in later childhood (Valles-Ayoub et al., 1990). Although neonatal and fetal immunoglobulin heavy-chain gene variable regions appear not to have undergone somatic mutation (Raaphorst et al., 1992; Mortari et al., 1992; van Es et al., 1992), these conclusions are true only of IgM, an isotype in which somatic mutation is uncommon in the adult. In contrast, somatic mutations in IgG and IgA transcripts are common in neonatal B cells, indicating that somatic mutation is operative at birth (Mortari et al., 1993). Differences in repertoire, along with functional differences, may play a role in limiting the capacity of the fetus and neonate to produce antibodies to certain antigens.

B-Cell Differentiation into Immunoglobulin-Secreting Plasma Cells and Immunoglobulin Class Switching

Immunoglobulin-secreting plasma cells appear later in gestation than do B cells. Plasma cells secreting IgM are detectable by the fifteenth week of gestation, and those secreting IgG and IgA are first observed at the twentieth and thirtieth weeks, respectively (Gathings et al., 1981). First synthesis of IgM and IgG has been detected as early as 12 weeks in fetal organ cultures (Gitlin and Biasucci, 1969). In general, neonatal B cells can differentiate into IgM-secreting plasma cells as efficiently as adult cells. Unlike adult B cells, neonatal B cells do not differentiate into plasma cells that secrete IgG or IgA in most assay systems (Durandy et al., 1990); these functions are not mature until the ages of approximately 2 years (IgG) and 5 years (IgA), respectively and are reflected in the postnatal increase in the levels of these isotypes in serum (Table 10–2). As described earlier in the section T-Cell Help for Antibody Production, several recent studies suggest that the paucity of isotypes other than IgM in the neonate results at least in part from the inability of the neonate's naive T cells to provide contact-dependent help, including the CD40 ligand, and cytokines (e.g., IL-4), rather than an inherent inability of neonatal B cells to switch to other classes of immunoglobulin. Fetal B cells from as early as 12 weeks' gestation were able to undergo class switching when provided with the necessary

T cell–derived cofactors, although IgA production was not observed (Punnonen et al., 1992). Nevertheless, the net result of the differences in capacity for T-cell help and intrinsic differences in B-cell phenotype is a clearly diminished ability to efficiently switch to the production of isotypes other than IgM in vitro and in vivo.

Antibody Response to Specific T Cell–Dependent and T Cell–Independent Antigens

The ability to respond with antibody production to specific antigens develops chronologically; the capacity to respond to antigens requiring contact-dependent T-cell help (generally protein antigens) precedes the development of the capacity to respond to those not requiring such cognate help (e.g., capsular polysaccharides). Whether this reflects B- or T-cell immaturity remains unclear. Some data support the former possibility. The acquisition of competence to respond to bacterial polysaccharides at approximately 2 to 3 years of age closely correlates with the appearance of B cells in a particular area of the spleen, the marginal zone (Timens et al., 1987). The origin of these B cells and their functional characteristics remain to be defined. Although macrophages within the marginal zone were proposed as playing a key role in the induction of B-cell responses to polysaccharides, recent studies suggest this may not be true (Kraal et al., 1989). Nevertheless, the amount and isotype of antibodies produced in response to those antigens not requiring cognate help are significantly influenced by T cells, in part by secretion of cytokines—for example, the switch to IgE production induced by IL-4 (Kühn et al., 1991) and the apparent enhancement of responses to bacterial capsular polysaccharides by IFN-γ (Peeters et al., 1992). The limited capacity of naive neonatal T cells to produce these lymphokines may contribute to the poor antibody response of neonates to polysaccharide vaccines and to capsulated bacteria such as group B streptococci (Fink et al., 1962; Smith et al., 1964; Baker et al., 1981).

Antibody responses by the fetus have been documented in response to maternal immunization with tetanus toxoid in the latter half of gestation; although the response was primarily IgM, it did appear to prime for a secondary antibody response later rather than to induce tolerance (Gill et al., 1983, 1991). In addition, specific antibody production has been documented in response to a variety of intrauterine infections. However, not all fetuses mount a detectable antibody response to intrauterine infection. Specific IgM antibody was absent in 34% of infants with congenital rubella (Enders, 1985), 19% of infants with congenital *Toxoplasma* infection (Naot et al., 1981), and 11% of infants with congenital CMV infection (Griffiths et al., 1982). Similar results have been obtained by measuring IgA antibodies. Interestingly, IgA antibodies are detectable in a somewhat greater fraction of infants with congenital *Toxoplasma* infection (89%) than are IgM antibodies, indicating that fetal infection can lead to antibody production and to class switching from IgM to IgA antibodies in the fetus (DeCoster et al., 1992).

It is important to note that these results were obtained at term or in early infancy and that fetal antibody production as detected by IgM or IgA antibodies to the infecting pathogens is detected in fewer than 25% to 50% of infants with established congenital *Toxoplasma* infection at 20 to 30 weeks' gestation (Desmonts et al., 1985; Stepick-Biek et al., 1990; DeCoster et al., 1992). Together, these results suggest that production of antibodies by the fetus may be absent or delayed in development relative to adults. Once responses develop, the capacity to undergo class switching is present by the latter part of gestation, at least in those cases in which the antigens are proteins and are presumably dependent on cognate T-cell help. This is consistent with the notion that the limitation in ability of neonatal T cells to provide help is not due to intrinsic immaturity but rather due to the lack of priming by exposure to foreign antigen.

Immunization or infection of neonates elicits a protective response to most protein antigens, including tetanus and diphtheria toxoids (Dengrove et al., 1986), inactivated or live poliovirus vaccine (Smolen et al.,

Table 10–2. Levels of Immunoglobulins in Sera of Normal Subjects, by Age*

Age	IgG mg/dl	IgG Percentage of Adult Level	IgM mg/d	IgM Percentage of Adult Level	IgA mg/dl	IgA Percentage of Adult Level	Total Immunoglobulins mg/dl	Total Immunoglobulins Percentage of Adult Level
Newborn	1031 ± 200†	89 ± 17	11 ± 5	11 ± 5	2 ± 3	1 ± 2	1044 ± 201	67 ± 13
1–3 mo	430 ± 119	37 ± 10	30 ± 11	30 ± 11	21 ± 13	11 ± 7	481 ± 127	31 ± 9
4–6 mo	427 ± 186	37 ± 16	43 ± 17	43 ± 17	28 ± 18	14 ± 9	498 ± 204	32 ± 13
7–12 mo	661 ± 219	58 ± 19	54 ± 23	55 ± 23	37 ± 18	19 ± 9	752 ± 242	48 ± 15
13–24 mo	762 ± 209	66 ± 18	58 ± 23	59 ± 23	50 ± 24	25 ± 12	870 ± 258	56 ± 16
25–36 mo	892 ± 183	77 ± 16	61 ± 19	62 ± 19	71 ± 37	36 ± 19	1024 ± 205	65 ± 14
3–5 yr	929 ± 228	80 ± 20	56 ± 18	57 ± 18	93 ± 27	47 ± 14	1078 ± 245	69 ± 17
6–8 yr	923 ± 256	80 ± 22	65 ± 25	66 ± 25	124 ± 45	62 ± 23	1112 ± 293	71 ± 20
9–11 yr	1124 ± 235	97 ± 20	79 ± 33	80 ± 33	131 ± 60	66 ± 30	1334 ± 254	85 ± 17
12–16 yr	946 ± 124	82 ± 11	59 ± 20	60 ± 20	148 ± 63	74 ± 32	1153 ± 169	74 ± 12
Adult	1158 ± 305	100 ± 26	99 ± 27	100 ± 27	200 ± 61	100 ± 31	1457 ± 353	100 ± 24

*The values were derived from measurements made for 296 normal children and 30 adults. Levels were determined by the radial diffusion technique using specific rabbit antisera to human immunoglobulins.

†One standard deviation.

From Stiehm ER, Fudenberg HH. Serum levels of immune globulins in health and disease: a survey. Pediatrics 37:715, 1966.

1983), enteroviruses (Alford et al., 1975), *Salmonella* flagellar antigen (Fink et al., 1962; Smith et al., 1964), and bacteriophage φX174 (Uhr et al., 1962). However, the response to some vaccines may be less than that of older children or adults. The response of neonates to influenza vaccine, a T-dependent antigen, appears to be limited because of the lower frequency of B cells that recognize antigen (Yarchoan and Nelson, 1983). The lower frequency of B-cell precursors for influenza may reflect a lack of expansion of the precursor pool because of lack of exposure to cross-reactive antigens, an inherently smaller precursor pool in neonates, or both. As discussed earlier, this does not appear to reflect a limitation in the expression of immunoglobulin variable regions, at least for the heavy-chain gene. However, the heavy- and light-chain V segments involved in the response to influenza remain to be defined. A study of young infants immunized with a single dose of diphtheria or tetanus toxoid found lower and delayed production of specific antibody in 2-week-olds compared with older infants; by 2 months of age, the response was similar to that of 6-month-old infants (Dancis et al., 1953), suggesting that postnatally there was rapid maturation of thymus-dependent responses. The switch from IgM to IgG production may also be delayed as, for example, with *Salmonella* H vaccine (Smith et al., 1964).

Interestingly, neonates given pertussis vaccine may have a poor initial response to that vaccine, and their response to subsequent immunization may be less than that of children immunized at 1 month of age or older, which suggests the induction of tolerance by early immunization (Peterson and Christie, 1951; Provenzano et al., 1965; Baraff et al., 1984). In contrast, as discussed later, pertussis immunization of premature infants (28 to 36 weeks' gestation) at 2 months of age elicited responses similar to that of 2-month-olds born at term (Smolen et al., 1983). This suggests that the tolerogenic period for vaccination with proteins rapidly wanes during the postnatal period. The tolerogenic effect may also be antigen-dependent. No inhibitory effect on antibody titer at 6 months of age was found when diphtheria or tetanus toxin was administered at 4 days of age rather than at 2 months (Dengrove et al., 1986), and oral polio vaccine given to neonates enhanced rather than inhibited the response to subsequent oral immunization during infancy (Schoub et al., 1988). These findings notwithstanding, most studies of the immunization response to thymus-dependent antigens have not evaluated antibody affinity, a reflection of somatic mutation, or isotype expression, which may be important determinants of the protective effects of antibodies.

In contrast to the responses to protein antigens, the response to many polysaccharide antigens is absent or severely blunted, as demonstrated by the inability of neonates to mount a response to *Haemophilus influenzae* type b PRP vaccine or to group B streptococcal type-specific capsular antigens after infection. In humans the response to some polysaccharide antigens can be demonstrated by 6 months of age (e.g., type 3 pneumococcus capsular polysaccharide), but the response to

vaccination with *H. influenzae* polysaccharides remains poor until approximately 18 to 24 months (Smith et al., 1973). The basis for the inability of infants to respond to polysaccharides may be multifactorial but does not appear to involve a lack of the appropriate antibody repertoire, at least for *H. influenzae* (Adderson et al., 1991). Coupling of the *H. influenzae* capsular polysaccharide to protein carriers converts it from a thymic-independent antigen to one that elicits cognate T-cell help. This renders it immunogenic in infants as young as 2 to 6 months of age, although multiple doses are required to achieve the concentrations observed in older children and adults following a single dose (see *Haemophilus*, MMWR, 1991). This requirement is not caused by a change in the repertoire of the antibodies produced in response to the conjugate as compared with the free polysaccharide (Adderson et al., 1991). It is as yet unknown whether this is also true for other polysaccharide antigens that are poorly immunogenic in infants.

Preterm neonates of 24 weeks' or more gestation produce antibody in response to protein antigens, such as diphtheria toxoid, as do term neonates or infants, and they respond appropriately to the diphtheria-pertussis-tetanus and oral and inactivated poliovirus vaccines when these are administered at the usual intervals of 2, 4, and 6 months (Smolen et al., 1983; Bernbaum et al., 1985; Koblin et al., 1988; Adenyi-Jones et al., 1992). However, the response of premature infants to multiple doses of hepatitis vaccine initially administered at birth may be more reduced than in term infants (Lau et al., 1992; del Canho et al., 1993). Small-for-gestational age infants also appear to respond adequately to immunization, although antibody responses to a single dose of oral poliovirus vaccine were slightly less in one study (Chandra, 1975). Thus, infants born prematurely or those small for gestational age respond to most immunizations as well as term infants of similar postnatal age. B cells from preterm infants also synthesize antibody in vitro as well as B cells from term infants (Pittard et al., 1985). As in term infants, the ability to respond to polysaccharide antigens remains diminished during the first two years of life.

Concentrations of Immunoglobulin Isotypes in the Fetus and Infant

IgG. IgG is the predominant immunoglobulin isotype at all ages (Stiehm and Fudenberg, 1966). IgG transport across the placenta can be detected as early as 8 weeks of gestation, but circulating fetal concentrations of IgG remain below 100 mg/dl until about 17 to 20 weeks (Fig. 10–3). After this time the levels rise steadily, reaching half of the term serum concentration by about 30 weeks; the term neonate's IgG level usually exceeds the maternal level by 5% to 10% (Kohler and Farr, 1966). The fetus synthesizes little IgG, so that the concentration in utero reflects maternally derived antibody (Martensson and Fudenberg, 1965). Accordingly, prematurity is reflected in proportionately lower neonatal IgG concentrations. Small-for-gestational-age neonates

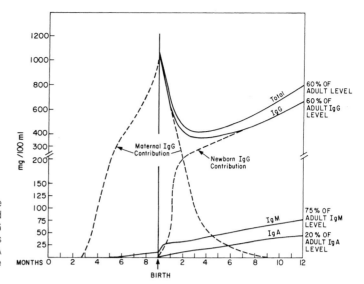

Figure 10–3. Immunoglobulin (IgG, IgM, and IgA) levels in the fetus and infant in the first year of life. The IgG of the fetus and newborn infant is solely of maternal origin. The maternal IgG disappears by the age of 9 months, by which time endogenous synthesis of IgG by the infant is well established. The IgM and IgA of the neonate are entirely endogenously synthesized because maternal IgM and IgA do not cross the placenta.

may have somewhat lower IgG concentrations (Yeung and Hobbs, 1968; Shapiro et al., 1981), perhaps related to impaired placental transport, although this was not observed in one study (Einhorn et al., 1987).

All IgG subclasses cross the placenta, and in most studies, the relative amounts of IgG1, IgG2, IgG3, and IgG4 in cord serum are comparable with those in maternal serum. However, in other studies, preferential transport of IgG1 and IgG3 was observed, possibly reflecting the higher affinity of the trophoblast Fc receptor for these IgG subclasses than for the others (Table 10–3) (McNobb et al., 1976; Einhorn et al., 1987; van de Winkel and Anderson, 1991). IgG1 levels tend to be higher in fetal than in maternal sera at the end of gestation (Lee et al., 1986). Because the half-life of IgG3 (7 days) is less than that of the other three subclasses (25 days), the relative subclass concentrations in infants soon differ from those in adults. IgM, IgA, IgD, and IgE do not cross the placenta.

Passively derived maternal IgG is the source of virtually all of the IgG subclasses detected in the normal fetus and neonate, and levels of these fall rapidly after birth (see Fig. 10–3). By 2 months of life, the amount of circulating IgG synthesized by the infant equals the amount derived from transplacental transfer; by 10 to 12 months of age, the IgG is nearly all derived from

synthesis by the infant. As a consequence of the fall in passively derived IgG and increased synthesis of IgG, values reach a nadir of approximately 400 mg/dl in term infants at 3 to 4 months of age and rise thereafter (see Table 10–2). The premature infant has proportionally lower IgG concentrations at birth, and values reach an even lower point; at 3 months of age, values of 60 and 104 mg/dl, are observed in infants born at 25 to 28 and 29 to 32 weeks of gestation, respectively (Ballow et al., 1986). Values for premature infants remain below those for term infants throughout the first year of life.

The slow onset of IgG synthesis in the neonate appears to reflect intrinsic B-cell development rather than maternal factors—for example, by idiotypic networking—because a similar pattern was observed in a neonate born to a mother with agammaglobulinemia (Kobayashi et al., 1980). By the age of 1 year, the total IgG concentration in term neonates is approximately 60% of that of adults. IgG3 and IgG1 subclasses reach adult concentrations by 8 years, whereas IgG2 and IgG4 do so by 10 and 12 years of age, respectively (Ochs and Wedgwood, 1987). The slow rise in IgG2 concentrations parallels the poor antibody response to bacterial polysaccharide antigens (e.g., *H. influenzae*), antibodies to which following natural infection are predominantly IgG2 (Granoff et al., 1986). Interestingly,

Table 10–3. Properties of IgG Subclasses

Subtype	Biologic Half-Life (Days)	Classical Pathway Complement Activation	Fc Receptor* Binding			Placental Transfer†
			Type I	*Type II*	*Type III*	
IgG1	25	+ +	+ +	±	+ +	+ +
IgG2	23	+	±	+	±	+
IgG3	9	+ +	+ +	+ +	+ +	+ +
IgG4	25	—‡	+	±	±	+

*Cells expressing FcR: FcRI—monocytes, macrophages, IFN-γ–treated neutrophils; FcRII—monocytes, macrophages, all granulocytes, B cells; FcRIII—some monocytes, macrophages, neutrophils, eosinophils, NK cells (rare T cells), trophoblast.
†See text.
‡Activates alternative pathway.
From Lewis DB, Wilson CB. Developmental immunology and role of host defenses in neonatal susceptibility to infection. In Remington JS, Klein JO, eds. Infectious Diseases of the Fetus and Newborn, 4th ed. Philadelphia, WB Saunders, 1994.

the order in which the adult levels of isotype expression are achieved after birth closely parallels the order of the heavy-chain gene segments that encode these isotypes. This raises the possibility that there may be postnatal developmental regulation of isotype switching, mediated in part at the level of the heavy-chain gene locus.

IgM. IgM increases from a mean of 6 mg/dl in premature neonates less than 28 weeks of gestation to 11 mg/dl at term (Cederqvist et al., 1978). As opposed to its usual pentameric functional form, some of this IgM may be monomeric and therefore nonfunctional (Allansmith et al., 1968; Perchalski et al., 1968). However, IgM is relatively more abundant in secretions of neonates than in those of adults. Serum concentrations in umbilical cord blood are usually 0.1 to 5.0 mg/dl, levels undetectable by conventional methods and are similar in term and preterm neonates. Postnatally, presumably in response to antigenic stimulation, IgM concentrations rise rapidly for the first month and then more gradually thereafter (see Fig. 10–3). By the age of 1 year, values are approximately 60% of those in adults. IgM concentrations in premature infants are lower than in infants for the first six months of life (Ballow et al., 1986). Elevated (>20 mg/dl) IgM concentrations in cord blood suggest possible intrauterine infections (Alford et al., 1975), but many infants with congenital infections have normal IgM concentrations in cord blood (Griffiths et al., 1982).

IgA. IgA does not cross the placenta, and serum concentrations in cord blood are usually 0.1 to 5.0 mg/dl. Concentrations are similar in term and premature neonates (Cederqvist et al., 1978), and both IgA1 and IgA2 are present. At birth, the frequencies of IgA1-bearing and IgA2-bearing B cells are equivalent. Subsequently, there is a preferential expansion of IgA1-bearing cells, presumably as a result of postnatal exposure to environmental antigens (Conley et al., 1980). Concentrations in serum increase to 20% of those in adults by 1 year of age and rise progressively through adolescence. Concentrations in preterm infants are less than in term infants for the first six months of life (Ballow et al., 1986). Increased cord blood IgA concentrations are observed in some infants with congenital infection (Alford et al., 1975). Elevated IgA is common in young infants infected by vertical transmission with HIV.

Secretory IgA. Secretory IgA is undetectable at birth but can be detected by 1 week to 2 months of age in tears, nasopharyngeal secretions, and saliva (Haworth and Dilling, 1966; McKay and Thom, 1969; Burgio et al., 1980; Mellander et al., 1984) and reaches adult values by 6 to 8 years of age. The more rapid relative increase in secretory compared with circulating IgA presumably reflects local production. Synthesis of IgA rather than secretory component appears to be the limiting factor in the development of IgA concentrations in secretions (Remington and Sheafer, 1968; Burgio et al., 1980). Secretory IgA increases more rapidly in infants with more intensive antigenic exposure or mucosal infections (Smith et al., 1964; Mellander et al., 1984). The greater abundance of IgM in secretions of neonates than those of more mature individuals may

provide some compensatory protection (Mellander et al., 1984), as may breast milk (Yap et al., 1979).

IgD and IgE. IgD is detected by sensitive techniques in cord blood in most term and preterm neonates (0.4 mg/dl) and concentration increases during the first year of life (Cederqvist et al., 1978; Josephs and Buckley, 1980). IgE synthesis is detectable in the fetus, but concentrations in the blood are generally below the limit of detectability at birth (Young and Geha, 1985). The rate of postnatal increase in IgE varies, depending on the predisposition of the individual to allergy and on exposure to allergens (Bazaral et al., 1971; Young and Geha, 1985).

Summary

The neonate receives passive protection by placental transfer of maternal IgG in the latter part of pregnancy. Immunoglobulin concentrations similar to or higher than maternal concentrations are achieved after 34 weeks of gestation. However, neonatal resistance to bacterial pathogens to which the mother has little or no IgG antibody is particularly compromised by an inability to produce antibodies to bacterial polysaccharides. This most likely depends on the lack of B cells able to respond to polysaccharides, responses that are independent of cognate T-cell help. In contrast, the neonatal response to protein antigens appears relatively intact for IgM production. Limitations in isotype expression by B cells after immunization with T cell–dependent antigens appear primarily to reflect limitations in T-cell help rather than an intrinsic limitation of the B cell.

DEVELOPMENT AND FUNCTION OF NATURAL KILLER CELLS

Natural killer (NK) cells are a lymphocyte subset, originally identified by their morphologic appearance as large granular lymphocytes, having the capacity to kill certain tumor and virus-infected cells in a manner not restricted by MHC antigens and not requiring presensitization. Recent evidence suggests that this involves a novel and more phylogenetically and ontogenetically primitive system for self and non-self discrimination. NK cells appear to recognize the absence of self-MHC expression (Versteeg, 1992; Raulet, 1992), in contrast to T cells, which recognize foreign antigen in the context of self-MHC or the presence of foreign MHC. In humans, NK cells can be identified by the expression of the CD16, CD56 surface antigens, or both and the absence of surface expression of the CD3 complex (Phillips et al., 1992; Lanier et al., 1992b). Most NK cells in the adult express CD57 and many express CD2. The latter is a marker also expressed on all T lymphocytes.

Cells with an NK phenotype appear to make up a considerable percentage of mononuclear cells in the fetal liver, where they can be detected as early as 6 weeks of gestation (Phillips et al., 1992). The percentage of CD16-expressing NK cells in the blood of neonates at term is similar (~15% of total lymphocytes) to that in the blood of adults, and the total number of NK cells exceeds that of adults by approximately two-fold (Phillips et al., 1992; Moretta et al., 1992). However, the fraction of NK cells that express another NK cell marker, CD57, is markedly diminished, and the fraction that expresses CD56 is reduced by about 50% (Yabuhara et al., 1990; Sancho et al., 1991; Phillips et al., 1992). The cytolytic function of NK cells increases progressively during fetal life to reach values approximately 50% (a range of 15% to 60% in various studies) of those in adult cells at term, as determined in assays using either unpurified (Toivanen et al., 1981; Lubens et al., 1982; Tarkkanen and Saksela, 1982; Ueno et al., 1985; Seki et al., 1985; Baley and Schacter, 1985; Nair et al., 1985) or NK cell–enriched preparations (Tarkkanen and Saksela, 1982; Kaplan et al., 1982; Seki et al., 1985; Sancho et al., 1991; McDonald et al., 1992; Phillips et al., 1992). Full function is not achieved until at least 9 to 12 months of age (see Chapter 9). The reduced cytolytic activity appears to reflect primarily diminished postbinding cytotoxic activity and diminished recycling to kill multiple targets. This parallels the reduced numbers of CD56$^+$ NK cells in the neonate and is consistent with the poor cytolytic activity of CD56$^-$ NK cells. When only CD56$^+$ neonatal NK cells are studied, their cytolytic activity is similar to that of adult NK cells (Sancho et al., 1991; Phillips et al., 1992).

As with adult NK cells, the cytolytic activity of neonatal NK cells is augmented by IL-2 and IFN-α, -β, and -γ. However, the enhancement of cytotoxicity by IL-2 is relatively greater and by IFN is relatively less with neonatal NK cells than with adult NK cells. The net result is that IL-2–treated NK cells from adults and neonates have similar levels of activity, whereas IFN-treated cells from neonates have much less activity than similarly treated cells from adults (Seki et al., 1985; Baley and Schacter, 1985; Sancho et al., 1991; McDonald et al., 1992; Phillips et al., 1992). It has been suggested that immature CD56$^-$ NK cells are preferentially affected by IL-2, whereas CD56$^+$ cells are the ones that respond to IFN. Consistent with this, neonates with higher percentages of CD56$^+$ NK cells have greater enhancement of activity with IFN treatment.

Paralleling the reduction in natural cytotoxic activity of neonatal cells, the activity of these cells in assays measuring antibody-dependent cell-mediated cytotoxicity (ADCC) is also reduced, averaging approximately 50% of that of cells of adults. Deficits in neonatal NK cell cytotoxicity against virus-infected targets have also been observed. The cytotoxic activity of human cord blood mononuclear cells against HSV-infected cells in vitro is consistently diminished, even with the addition of IL-2. ADCC activity against HSV-infected cells is also reduced, as is NK activity against CMV-infected target cells (Harrison and Waner, 1985).

In summary, although NK cells appear early during gestation and are present in normal numbers by mid to late gestation, the phenotype of about 50% of these cells is immature (CD56$^-$). These immature cells have decreased cytotoxic activity compared with cells from

adults, which are uniformly CD56$^+$. This immaturity is associated with diminished functional activity, including diminished activity against cells infected with herpes group viruses.

NEUTROPHILS IN THE FETUS AND NEONATE

Neutrophil Production and Release

The most critical deficiency in the phagocytic defense mechanisms of the fetus and neonate is the limited capacity to accelerate neutrophil production in response to infection. This appears to result from a limited neutrophil storage pool and a near-maximal level of neutrophil production in the normal fetus and neonate.

Neutrophil precursors are first detected in the yolk sac and then in the liver, spleen, and bone marrow, appearing somewhat later than macrophage precursors (Playfair et al., 1963; Christensen, 1989). Mature neutrophils are first detected by 14 to 16 weeks of gestation. The numbers of circulating neutrophil precursors, or colony-forming units–granulocyte/macrophage (CFU-GM), are 10- to 20-fold higher in the fetus and neonate than in adults, and neonatal bone marrow also contains increased numbers of neutrophil precursors (Shapiro and Bassen, 1941; Christensen, 1989). However, particularly in premature neonates, the fraction of granulocyte precursors is less than the number of monocyte precursors (Playfair et al., 1963), and although it has not been possible to directly measure the total body pool of CFU-GMs in human term or preterm neonates, the total body pool of CFU-GM is likely to be less than in adults. Further, the rate of proliferation of these circulating neutrophil precursors appears to be near maximal in normal neonates (Christensen and Rothstein, 1984; Laver et al., 1990). This suggests that these CFU-GMs may be incapable of increasing in number in response to infection. The increased numbers of circulating precursor cells and the high rate of spontaneous proliferation of these cells may result from the increased concentration of circulating colony-stimulating factors (CSFs) in neonatal blood (Christensen, 1989; Laver, et al., 1990).

In the fetus through 22 to 24 weeks of gestation, neutrophils constitute less than 10% of circulating leukocytes, rising to values of 50% to 60% at term. Within hours of birth, the numbers of circulating neutrophils increase sharply in term and preterm neonates (Manroe et al., 1979). The fraction of neutrophils that are immature (bands) remains constant at about 15% (Fig. 10–4). These values are influenced by a number of factors. Most important is the response to sepsis. Sepsis in premature neonates is commonly accompanied by neutropenia (Manroe et al., 1979). However, other perinatal complications, including maternal hypertension, periventricular hemorrhage, and severe asphyxia, can cause neutropenia, and septic infants may also have normal or increased neutrophil counts. Severe or fatal sepsis is more often associated with persistent neutropenia (Squire et al., 1979; Christensen and

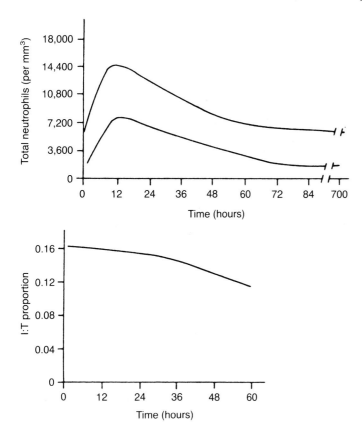

Figure 10–4. Change in total number of neutrophils and in ratio of immature to total neutrophils (I:T proportion) in the neonate. (Adapted from Manroe BL, Weinberg AG, Rosenfeld CR, Browne R. The neonatal blood count in health and disease. I. Reference values for neutrophilic cells. J Pediatr 95:89–98, 1979.)

Rothstein, 1980). Neutropenia may be associated with increased margination of circulating neutrophils, which occurs early in response to infection (Walker and Willemze, 1980). However, neutropenia that is sustained often reflects depletion of the postmitotic neutrophil storage pool. Christensen and Rothstein (1980) have found that those neutropenic infants in whom bone marrow examination revealed depletion of the neutrophil storage pool often died rapidly of fatal infection; neutropenic infants with normal storage pools survived. More rapid depletion of neutrophils may also reflect diminished survival of neonatal neutrophils, which has been observed in vitro.

Although the human neutrophil pool is not amenable to study, investigations with neonatal rats indicate that the storage pool in neonates, especially premature neonates, is approximately 20% to 30% of that in adults (Christensen, 1989). Inflammatory stimulation or infection caused a greater release and depletion of neutrophil stores in neonatal rats compared with adult rats (Christensen et al., 1980; Erdmann et al., 1982; Zeligs et al., 1982). Preliminary studies of neonatal rats suggest that both recombinant human granulocyte (G)-CSF and recombinant human granulocyte-macrophage (GM)-CSF induce a brisk increase in blood neutrophil counts within 6 hours of administration (Cairo, 1989); whether this is also associated with an expansion in the neutrophil storage pool or merely reflects an accelerated release of mature cells is not known. More information is needed regarding the effects of such cytokines on neutrophil kinetics to determine their

potential for ameliorating the neonate's deficit in neutrophil supply.

The available data suggest that the ability of the human neonate to increase neutrophil production in response to infection may be limited. Whether this limited response reflects near maximal output in even healthy neonates, inefficient granulopoiesis (which might be amenable to manipulation with exogenous CSF), or both remains to be determined. This may be an important factor in neonatal susceptibility to overwhelming pyogenic infection. Answers to these questions are needed because their implications for potential immunologic treatment differ.

Adhesion and Chemotaxis

Although adhesion of neonatal neutrophils has been evaluated in a variety of assays, the relevance of these in vitro assays to the in vivo ability of these cells to adhere and migrate through endothelium is not always clear. These studies generally suggest that adhesion of unstimulated cells is normal or at most modestly impaired, whereas adhesion of activated cells is deficient (Anderson et al., 1981, 1984; Rao et al., 1981; Krause et al., 1982). Re-evaluation since recognition of the combined roles of selectins, β_2 integrins, and their ligands suggests that there are dual deficits in adhesion of neonatal leukocytes. Adhesion to activated endothelium under conditions of flow similar to those found in capillaries or postcapillary venules is variable, but on average is only 40% to 45% of that observed with adult neutrophils (Anderson et al., 1991; Smith et al., 1992).

This appears to reflect at least in part a deficiency in the abundance of L-selectin on the surface of neonatal neutrophils. In addition, multiple groups (Bruce et al., 1987; Anderson et al., 1990, 1991; Jones et al., 1990; Smith et al., 1992) with one exception (Adinolfi et al., 1988) find that despite comparable resting levels of the β_2 integrins Mac-1 and LFA-1, neonatal cells do not up-regulate expression of these integrins with activation as is seen with adult neutrophils. This failure is associated with a parallel decrease in adhesion to activated endothelium or purified intracellular adhesion molecule (ICAM)-1 (Anderson et al., 1990). The net effect is that neonatal neutrophils are impaired in their ability to bind initially to activated endothelial cells and subsequently to bind with high avidity in the presence of local chemotactic factors. The deficit in adhesion appears to be a major factor underlying the diminished ability of neonatal neutrophils to migrate through endothelium into tissues (Anderson et al., 1990, 1991).

Although there is variability in the results from study to study, deficient chemotaxis is the most consistent abnormality observed in neutrophils from neonates compared with those from adults (Table 10–4) (Pahwa et al., 1977; Klein et al., 1977; Tono-Oka et al., 1979; Anderson et al., 1981; Fontan et al., 1981; Raghunathan et al., 1982; Boner et al., 1982; Hill, 1987). In premature neonates, chemotaxis is further impaired but within a few weeks after birth is similar to that of cells from term neonates (Usmani et al., 1991; Kamran et al., 1993). When compared directly, chemotaxis of peripheral blood neutrophils is more impaired than is that of cord blood neutrophils from human neonates (Pahwa et al., 1977). Chemotaxis appears to reach adult competence only after 2 years of age (Pahwa et al., 1977; Klein et al., 1977). Assay conditions affect the magnitude of the differences between adult and neonatal neutrophils, this difference being greater in Boyden chamber assays (particularly with filters with smaller pore diameter) than when assayed under agarose.

Receptors for the bacterial chemotactic agent formyl-methionylleucyl-phenylalanine (FMLP) are similar in adult and neonatal neutrophils (Anderson et al., 1981; Strauss and Snyder, 1984; Sacchi and Hill, 1984), although one study found them to be decreased (Nunoi et al., 1983). Receptors for other chemotactic factors have not been studied directly. In contrast to the binding of chemotactic factors, postreceptor binding events are impaired, including

1. The induced increase in intracellular calcium and change in cell membrane potential (Sacchi and Hill, 1984).

2. Adherence and redistribution of sites of adhesion allowing effective diapedesis through the endothelium (Anderson et al., 1981).

3. Orientation in the chemotactic gradient (Anderson et al., 1981, 1984).

Not all changes in response to chemotactic factors are abnormal: up-regulation of the type I complement receptor (CR1) is normal or at most slightly impaired (Bruce et al., 1987; Smith et al., 1990b). However, when taken as a whole, the data suggest that the abnormal chemotaxis of neonatal neutrophils is due in large part to abnormalities in events following binding of chemotactic factors to membrane receptors. A relative deficiency of specific or gelatinase-containing granules in neonates offers one possible mechanism (Anderson et al., 1985; Jones et al., 1990). The pool of β_2 integrins in these types of granules is a major source of the increase in plasma membrane expression of these adhesins induced by chemotactic agents in adult neutrophils. The smaller size of this pool in neonatal neutrophils may limit the increased expression induced by chemotactic agents and thereby impair adherence and chemotaxis. This is consistent with the greater impairment of stimulated than of unstimulated adherence and migration of neonatal neutrophils (Anderson et al., 1981; Krause et al., 1982). Differences in cytoskeletal components of neonatal neutrophils may be an additional factor. Although the total content of tubulin (Anderson et al., 1984) and of G-actin is normal, che-

Table 10–4. Chemotaxis of Neonatal Granulocytes

Cell Source	Assay	Stimulus	% of Adult Response	Comment
Cord blood	3-μm Nuclepore filter	EAS	79	Normal random motility
Peripheral blood	Agarose	ZAS	27	Low until age 2 y
Cord blood	3-μm Nuclepore filter	EAS	125	
Peripheral blood			53	Still low at age 6 mo; normal chemokinesis
Cord blood	Agarose	ZAS	≤30	More severe with lower concentrations of ZAS
Peripheral blood	5-μm cellulose filter, whole blood	ZAS	79	Ill neonates = 62%
Cord blood	Cellulose filter, 3, 5, or 8 μm	Casein	37–60	Normal random motility, normal chemokinesis
Cord blood	Agarose	Bacterial factor or EAS	60–80	Normal random motility
	3-μm cellulose		<15	
Peripheral blood	5-μm cellulose filter	ZAS	88	

Abbreviations: EAS = endotoxin-activated serum; ZAS = zymosan-activated serum; FMLP = formylated bacterial peptide.
From Lewis DB, Wilson CB. Developmental immunology and role of host defenses in neonatal susceptibility to infection. In Remington JS, Klein JO, eds. Infectious Diseases of the Fetus and Newborn, 4th ed. Philadelphia, WB Saunders, 1994.

motactic factor–induced polymerization of actin is reduced compared with that in adult cells (Raghunathan et al., 1982; Hill, 1987). These data suggest that there is not a primary cytoskeletal abnormality but rather impaired reorganization of the cytoskeleton in response to stimulation.

Because neonatal neutrophil chemotaxis is relatively more impaired at low than at high concentrations of chemotactic factors (Boner et al., 1982), decreased generation of chemotactic factors in neonatal serum (Pahwa et al., 1977; Boner et al., 1982) may compound the intrinsic deficits of neonatal neutrophils (see Complement section, later). However, the generation of other chemotactic agents (e.g., leukotriene B_4) by neonatal neutrophils appears to be normal (Kikawa et al., 1986).

A recent report described three neonates in whom the expression of the CD11b/CD18 β_2 integrin on neutrophils was markedly but transiently decreased to levels of 11% to 25% of controls (Shigeoka and Wittwer, 1993). The expression of the other β_2 integrins (CD11a and CD11c) was less severely reduced. The reduced β_2 integrin expression was associated with persistence of the umbilical cord beyond 2 months of age in two of the neonates and a perirectal abscess in the other. In two of the mothers, variable decreases in expression of CD11b/CD18 were observed, suggesting that the abnormality may have been transmitted from mother to fetus by an autoantibody to this adhesin.

Phagocytic and Microbicidal Activity

Under conventional in vitro conditions, neutrophils from neonates bind and ingest bacteria as well as or only slightly less well than do cells from adults (Gluck and Silverman, 1957; McCracken and Eichenwald, 1971; Harris et al., 1983). The numbers of Fc receptors for IgG and of receptors for C3b (CR1) also are similar (Bruce et al., 1987; Smith et al., 1990a). In contrast, under suboptimal conditions, such as limiting concentrations of opsonins, neonatal neutrophils phagocytose bacteria less well (Miller, 1979). This may be clinically relevant since neonatal serum is frequently deficient in opsonins. The mechanism for the diminished ingestion with limiting opsonin concentrations is not known, although the diminished up-regulation of the CR3 receptor for C3bi (the β_2 integrin Mac-1) may be a factor (Bruce et al., 1987; Jones et al., 1990; Smith et al., 1990a).

Killing of phagocytosed bacteria and yeast (Candida) by neonatal neutrophils is generally normal (Dosset et al., 1969; Park et al., 1970; McCracken and Eichenwald, 1971; Wright et al., 1975; Oseas and Lehrer, 1979; Shigeoka et al., 1979), although in some studies modest differences in killing of some bacteria have been observed (Cocchi and Marianelli, 1967; Coen et al., 1969; Becker et al., 1981; Stroobant et al., 1984). If the ratio of bacteria to phagocytes is increased or if the neutrophils are obtained from sick or stressed neonates, killing of microbes is diminished compared with neutrophils from healthy adults (Wright et al., 1975; Shigeoka et al., 1979; Mills et al., 1979b). This

appears to reflect impaired killing rather than impaired phagocytosis. It should be noted that neutrophils from ill adults may also have diminished microbicidal activity. It is not known whether neutrophils from ill neonates have more impaired function than those from adults.

The basis for the difference in microbicidal activity is not fully clear. In most studies, the rates of generation of superoxide anion by adult, neonatal (Ambruso et al., 1979; Shigeoka et al., 1981), or fetal (Newburger, 1982) neutrophils were similar. Generation of the more toxic hydroxyl radical may be diminished (Ambruso et al., 1979), as is chemiluminescence (Strauss et al., 1980; Sacchi and Hill, 1984). Variable results have been obtained in other assays that assess generation of reactive oxygen metabolites (e.g., nitroblue tetrazolium reduction, oxygen consumption) (Coen et al., 1969; McCracken and Eichenwald, 1971; Anderson et al., 1974; Tovo and Ponzone, 1977).

Oxygen-independent microbicidal mechanisms of neonatal neutrophils remain poorly characterized. Their ability to release the lysosomal enzymes lysozyme and β-glucuronidase appears to be intact (Yasui et al., 1988). However, neonatal neutrophil content of specific granules (Ambruso et al., 1984; Jones et al., 1990) and the release of specific granule content on activation appear to be reduced. Because a diminished content of microbicidal defensins has been observed in individuals with inherited specific granule deficiency, it is possible that neonatal neutrophils may have reduced amounts of defensins.

Modulation of Function by Cytokines

Studies performed in vitro indicate that IFN-γ and GM-CSF enhance the chemotactic response of neonatal neutrophils (Frenck et al., 1989; Cairo, 1989; Cairo et al., 1989; Hill et al., 1991). However, GM-CSF inhibits chemotaxis at higher concentrations than are associated with enhancement of oxygen radical production (Frenck et al., 1989; Cairo et al., 1989). Similarly, the methylxanthine pentoxifylline exhibits a biphasic enhancement of chemotaxis by neonatal neutrophils (Hill, 1987). None of these agents results in a full normalization of chemotaxis compared with that by cells of adults. Of potential concern, indomethacin, which is used clinically to facilitate ductal closure in premature neonates, impairs chemotaxis of cells from term and preterm neonates (Kamran et al., 1993).

Summary

The most clearly defined deficits in neonatal phagocytic defenses are the diminished neutrophil storage pool and diminished ability of neonatal neutrophils to adhere and to migrate in response to chemotactic stimuli. Deficiencies in phagocytosis and killing appear to be less significant but may be exacerbated by a limitation in opsonins or a high local bacterial density.

EOSINOPHILIC GRANULOCYTES IN THE FETUS AND NEONATE

In adults and older children, eosinophils represent a small percentage of the circulating granulocytes. Their numbers are increased in allergic states, in patients with parasitic (particularly metazoan) infections, and in certain autoimmune or malignant disease states. In the fetus and neonate, eosinophils commonly represent a sizable fraction of the total number of circulating granulocytes. At 18 to 30 weeks of gestation, total granulocytes represent only about 10% of total circulating leukocytes, but eosinophils constitute 10% to 20% of total granulocytes (Forestier et al., 1986).

Similarly, in premature neonates the numbers of eosinophils are increased relative to those in term neonates, often reaching values of 1500 to 3000 cells/mm³ and representing up to one third of total granulocytes in the first month of life (Bhat and Scanlon, 1981; Rothberg et al., 1983). The postnatal increase of eosinophils lags behind that of neutrophils, peaking at the third to fourth weeks of postnatal life. There is a relative increase in the abundance of eosinophils in inflammatory exudates in neonates, paralleling their greater numbers in the circulation (reviewed in Smith et al., 1992). In addition to prematurity, certain conditions have been associated with a relatively greater degree of eosinophilia; these include total parenteral nutrition and transfusions (Bhat and Scanlon, 1981). In contrast to conditions such as allergic and parasitic diseases, neonatal eosinophilia is not associated with increased amounts of circulating IgE (Rothberg et al., 1983). The basis or the significance of the eosinophilic tendency of the neonate is not known. Certain of the functional deficits observed in neonatal neutrophils, such as the diminished expression of adhesion molecules important in leukocyte migration into tissues, have been observed in neonatal eosinophils (Smith et al., 1992).

MONONUCLEAR PHAGOCYTES IN THE FETUS AND NEONATE

Production and Differentiation

Macrophages are detected by 4 weeks of fetal life in the yolk sac, soon thereafter in the fetal liver, and then in the bone marrow (Kelemen and Janossa, 1980). Production of macrophage colonies from fetal liver, bone marrow, or cord blood is equal to or greater than that achieved in adult bone marrow (Ueno et al., 1981). The number of monocytes per volume of blood is also at least as great in the neonate as in the adult.

The numbers of tissue macrophages are uncertain. The lung in lower mammals and in monkeys contains few macrophages until shortly before term (Jacobs et al., 1983; Wilson, 1984), and this is probably also true in humans (Alenghat and Esterly, 1984). Postnatally, the number of alveolar macrophages increases rapidly to adult levels by 24 to 48 hours in term monkeys but not in those with hyaline membrane disease (Jacobs et al., 1983). An indirect measure of splenic (and perhaps of liver) macrophage number and function is provided by the assessment of the numbers of pitted erythrocytes in the blood. These damaged erythrocytes are increased in the blood of neonates born before 36 weeks of gestation but are similar in term neonates and adults (Freedman et al., 1980).

Adhesion and Chemotaxis

The influx of monocytes into sites of inflammation and cellular immune reactions is diminished in neonates. After dermal abrasion, the influx of monocytes is delayed and remains below that of adults even after 24 hours (Sheldon and Caldwell, 1963; Bullock et al., 1969). Similarly, delayed hypersensitivity responses are diminished in neonates, even when in vitro tests indicate that the neonate responds to the test antigen (Warwick et al., 1960; Fowler et al., 1960). The poor response in vivo may be due in part to poor immigration of monocytes and lymphocytes into dermal tissue. This may reflect in part diminished monocyte chemotaxis (Table 10–5). However, chemotaxis of monocytes from neonates in vitro is less clearly impaired than is that of neonatal neutrophils. In general, studies that have used peripheral blood as a source of neonatal monocytes more consistently show impaired chemotaxis than do those that used cord blood (Weston et al., 1977; Klein et al., 1977; Raghunathan et al., 1982). Monocyte chemotaxis did not reach adult competence until 6 to 10 years of age in the one study available (Klein et al., 1977). The basis for these differences has not been studied in as much detail as it has been for neutrophils.

Data regarding adhesion molecules on monocytes from neonates are limited to two conflicting reports on the expression of the β_2 integrins. One study reported increased amounts of the β_2 integrin Mac-1 (CD11b/CD18) on resting and activated neonatal monocytes (Adinolfi et al., 1988). In response to activation with chemotactic agents, adult cells increased expression of this integrin more in response to one agent, but their response remained less than neonatal cells in response to another. These results conflict with those of another group that examined expression of each of the β_2 integrins and found them to be modestly less on monocytes from neonates than on monocytes from adults before and after activation of the cells (Marwitz et al.,

Table 10–5. Delayed Monocyte Response in Rebuck Skin Windows in Human Neonates and Adults

Population	% Monocytes			
	2 hr	*4 hr*	*6 hr*	*24 hr*
Premature*	4	13	18	30
Term <24 h	4	9	13	20
Term 24–108 hr	2	7	11	19
Adult	5	21	38	76

From Lewis DB, Wilson CB. Developmental immunology and role of host defenses in neonatal susceptibility to infection. In Remington JS, Klein JO eds. Infectious Diseases of the Fetus and Newborn, 4th ed. Philadelphia, WB Saunders, 1994.

1988). The affinity and function of these receptors were not evaluated directly. Resolution of this discrepancy and a more detailed analysis of adhesion molecule expression and function (e.g., the L-selectin and β_1 integrins) of neonatal monocytes are needed.

Monocyte chemotaxis, like that of polymorphonuclear leukocytes, is induced by activated complement components, bacterial factors, leukotriene B$_4$, and the chemokine monocyte chemotactic factor (MCP) (see Table 10–1). Production of this factor by neonatal cells appears to be normal, although studies done to assess this used bioassays that do not detect MCP specifically (Kretschmer et al., 1976; Hawes et al., 1980).

Phagocytic and Microbicidal Activity

Monocytes from human neonates ingest and kill *S. aureus, E. coli,* and group B streptococci as well as do monocytes from adults (Kretschmer et al., 1976; Orlowski et al., 1976; Weston et al., 1977; Hawes et al., 1980; Becker et al., 1981), although the rate at which they ingest unopsonized latex particles is lower (Schuit and Powell, 1980). The production of microbicidal oxygen metabolites by neonatal and adult monocytes is similar (Hawes et al., 1980; Speer et al., 1985). The ability of neonatal monocyte–derived macrophages (monocytes culture in vitro) to phagocytose bacteria or other particles through receptors for microbial mannose-fucose, IgG, complement, and opsonin-independent pathways appears not to differ from that of similarly prepared cells from adults (Conley and Speert, 1991). Neonatal monocytes have comparable oxygen radical generation and microbicidal activity against staphylococci (Speer et al., 1988; Conley and Speert, 1991).

There are few studies of the microbicidal activity of tissue macrophages from neonates because such cells are difficult to obtain. Because tissue macrophages are derived from monocytes, it could be assumed that these functions of neonatal tissue macrophages would also be mature. However, local tissue conditions in neonates may differ from those in adults and may be reflected by differences in macrophage function. Studies with alveolar macrophages are illustrative.

One study compared macrophages obtained from aspirated bronchial fluid of neonates with alveolar macrophages obtained by bronchoalveolar lavage from adults. A qualitative difference in killing of *Candida* was observed. Cells from neonates killed the yeast form less well, but total killing was normal since surviving yeast cells then formed intracellular pseudohyphae, which cells from neonates killed normally (D'Ambola et al., 1988); concern must be raised that the cell preparations were not truly equivalent. However, parallel studies with macrophages from neonatal and adult rabbits obtained by bronchoalveolar lavage showed similar qualitative differences and are consistent with a deficit in phagocytosis and killing of *Candida* yeast observed with alveolar macrophages from neonatal Rhesus monkeys (Kurland et al., 1988).

Overall, studies from monkeys, rabbits, and rats present a relatively consistent picture. There is a marked paucity in numbers of alveolar macrophages at birth, particularly in preterm neonates; when the animals are challenged with a wide variety of bacteria in vivo, the rate at which alveolar macrophages ingest the bacteria is diminished, particularly in the premature neonates (Coonrod et al., 1987; Martin et al., 1988, 1992; Sherman et al., 1992); phagocytosis in vitro is diminished in most but not all studies (Martin et al., 1992; Sherman et al., 1992); and the microbicidal activity of macrophages is impaired to a modest degree (Becker et al., 1981; Jacobs et al., 1983; Wilson, 1984; D'Ambola et al., 1988; Kurland et al., 1988). This correlates with diminished generation of microbicidal oxygen metabolites (Bellanti et al., 1979; Sherman and Lehrer, 1985) and a lower content of microbicidal defensins in alveolar macrophages of neonatal rabbits (Ganz et al., 1985). In one study of rabbits, decreased killing of *Candida albicans* could be induced by exposure of adult alveolar macrophages to crude surfactant containing material from the alveoli of neonates, suggesting that deficits in killing of *Candida* by alveolar macrophages from neonates may be secondary to their ingestion of surfactant (reviewed in Bellanti et al., 1979); more recent data suggest that the deleterious effects of surfactant may be due in part to impaired assembly of the phagocyte oxidase (Geertsma et al., 1993).

In contrast to the extracellular pathogens described previously, viruses and certain nonviral intracellular pathogens survive and replicate within cells. Control of infection with these organisms may be effected either by limiting the entry of these microbes into the cells in which they replicate or by the capacity of the host cells to kill or inhibit their intracellular replication. Of the nonviral intracellular pathogens, *Toxoplasma gondii* and *L. monocytogenes* are pathogens in neonates. Neonatal monocytes ingest and kill these organisms as well as do cells from adults (Berman and Johnson, 1978; Wilson and Haas, 1984; CB Wilson, unpublished data).

To a much greater degree than with neutrophils, the microbicidal activity of macrophages can be primed by exposure to products derived from stimulated T or NK cells; IFN-γ appears to be the most important cytokine, although in some cases TNF-α or GM-CSF may play a contributing or even dominant role. Human neonatal macrophages can be activated by IFN-γ to kill or inhibit the growth of these microbes with efficiency similar to that of adult cells. Further, macrophages from neonates or fetal macrophages from the placenta are similar to adult cells in their permissiveness for the replication of another neonatal pathogen, HSV (Mintz et al., 1980; Plaeger-Marshall et al., 1989). Exogenous IFN-γ induces resistance to *Listeria* infection in neonatal rats and to HSV infection in neonatal mice. This suggests that in these species the antimicrobial activity of host macrophages (and other host cells mediating resistance to these microbes) can be enhanced sufficiently to protect, given the provision of this cytokine (Bortolussi et al., 1989, 1992; Kohl, 1990). This also implies that the deficit in production of IFN-γ and perhaps certain other cytokines (e.g., TNF-α) that facilitate resistance to these microbes may be the major factor in increased susceptibility of the neonate to these pathogens (see the following and the discussion of viral host defenses in the fetus and neonate).

Production of Cytokines

Production of IL-1, IL-6, and TNF-α has been investigated in some detail with cells from humans (summarized in Table 10–1). IL-1 production by monocytes and macrophages from term and premature neonates appears to be equivalent to that of adult cells in response to various agonists. In contrast, for both IL-6 and TNF-α, production by cells from term neonates appears to be equal to or at most modestly less (under 50%) than that by monocytes from adults. However, cells from preterm neonates produce about 75% less IL-6 and TNF-α. Furthermore, production of TNF-α by monocyte-derived and tissue (placental) macrophages from term neonates is reduced to a greater extent than that by blood monocytes and appears to be upregulated less by IFN-γ than by cells from adults. This is similar to results in neonatal rats challenged with lipopolysaccharide or *L. monocytogenes* (Bortolussi et al., 1989, 1992); in rats less than 8 days of age, TNF-α production is not detectable in vivo, and it reaches adult levels in response to these agonists only after 16 days of age; IFN-γ does not enhance TNF-α production in the less mature animals. Deficient production of IFN-γ by neonatal T cells may further compound the deficit in TNF-α production in humans, and decreased production of IFN-γ by NK and T cells in neonatal rats may be a contributing factor in the decreased production of TNF-α and diminished resistance to *Listeria* (Bortolussi et al., 1992).

Production of IFN-α by neonatal mononuclear cells and monocytes appears to be relatively normal in response to a variety of inducers, including HSV and other viruses (Ray, 1970; Handzel et al., 1983; Kohl and Harmon, 1983), although one study suggested that production in response to HSV may be diminished (Cederblad et al., 1990). Production of GM-, M- and G-CSFs has been examined in monocytes to a limited extent and appears to be normal (English et al., 1992). There has been no direct assessment of chemokine production by neonatal monocytes or macrophages. However, in preterm and term human neonates born to mothers with amnionitis, considerable amounts of IL-8 are detectable in the circulation (Shimoya et al., 1992). Although the source of the IL-8 was not determined, these amounts are in the range of concentrations observed in baboons following injection of *E. coli* or lipopolysaccharide (van Zee et al., 1991), suggesting that the overall capacity of the neonate to produce this chemokine is mature.

Summary

Monocytes from term neonates are normal in number and as competent as those from adults in phagocytosis and microbicidal activity. Chemotactic activity may be impaired and may be a factor in the clearly diminished influx of monocytes in sites of inflamma-

tion and in the delayed hypersensitivity responses in neonates. The data regarding function of tissue macrophages from human neonates are consistent with those from other species and suggest that phagocytosis, microbicidal activity, and antigen presentation by macrophages from tissues may not be fully competent. The capacity to produce certain cytokines (i.e., TNF-α and IL-6) may be modestly reduced, particularly in cells from preterm neonates. This modestly reduced cytokine production may be further compromised by the diminished production of IFN-γ by neonatal T cells, since IFN-γ acts to enhance not only the killing of intracellular organisms but also the production of proinflammatory cytokines by macrophages.

HUMORAL MEDIATORS OF INFLAMMATION

Complement

Fetal complement component synthesis commences by 6 to 14 weeks of gestation, depending on the component and tissue examined (Gitlin and Biasucci, 1969; Kohler, 1973). There is little or no transfer of complement across the placenta.

The activity of the classical and alternative complement pathways and the abundance of individual components in neonates are summarized in Table 10–6. There is substantial variability in some of the reports and within patients, such that many term neonates have amounts of individual components and both classical pathway hemolysis (CH_{50}) and alternative pathway activity (AP_{50}) within the adult range. Overall, the abundance of components and activity of the alternative pathway are consistently diminished relative to those in the classical pathway. A marked deficiency in the terminal complement component C9 is associated

Table 10–6. Summary of Published Complement Levels in Neonates

Complement Component	Mean % of Adult Levels	
	Term Neonate	Preterm Neonate
CH_{50}	56–90 (4)*	45–71 (3)
AP_{50}	49–65 (3)	40–51 (2)
C1q	65–90 (3)	
C4	60–100 (4)	27–58 (2)
C2	76–100 (2)	42–91 (3)
C3	60–100 (5)	96 (1)
C5	75 (1)	—
C6	47 (1)	—
C7	67 (1)	—
C8	~20 (1)	
C9	<20 (2)	—
B	35–59 (8)	36–50 (3)
P	33–71 (5)	13–65 (2)
H	61 (1)	—
C3bi	55 (1)	—

*Number of studies.

From Lewis DB, Wilson CB. Developmental immunology and role of host defenses in neonatal susceptibility to infection. In Remington JS, Klein JO, eds. Infectious Diseases of the Fetus and Newborn, 4th ed. Philadelphia, WB Saunders, 1994.

with poor killing of gram-negative bacteria with serum from neonates (Lassiter et al., 1992). In addition to the quantitative deficiency of C9, poor cross-linking of C3 despite efficient deposition on the surface of the microbe may contribute to the decreased lytic and opsonic activity of neonatal serum (Zach and Hostetter, 1989). Generation of the chemotactic fragment of C5, C5a, is diminished in serum from term neonates (Miller, 1971; Pahwa et al., 1977).

Preterm neonates have more clearly and consistently diminished activity of both pathways (Johnston et al., 1979). In contrast, mature but small-for-gestational-age infants have activity in both pathways, similarly to term neonates (Notarangelo et al., 1984). Postnatally, the concentration of most complement components increases, approaching values of adults by 6 to 18 months of age (Davis et al., 1979).

Fibronectin

Fibronectin contributes to leukocyte adherence and migration and may play an ancillary role in opsonization. Plasma concentrations of fibronectin are diminished in neonates, particularly premature neonates (Gerdes et al., 1983; Barnard and Arthur, 1983; Yoder et al., 1983). Sepsis and other serious conditions (e.g., asphyxia or respiratory distress syndrome) are associated with a further reduction in fibronectin concentrations, although these illness-induced changes are not unique to neonates (Gerdes et al., 1983; Yoder et al., 1983; McCafferty et al., 1983). The lower concentrations of plasma fibronectin may reflect in part diminished synthesis by neonatal monocytes.

C-reactive Protein

C-reactive protein has opsonic activity for pneumococci. This protein does not cross the placenta, but concentrations in the serum are similar to those in adults (Ainbender et al., 1982), and they increase in response to infection or inflammation as do those in adults (Squire et al., 1979).

Mannose- and Lipopolysaccharide-Binding Proteins

With rare exceptions, glycoproteins containing high amounts of mannose are not found on extracellular proteins in mammals, since they are modified in the endoplasmic reticulum before transport through the Golgi complex. In contrast, high-mannose sugars are integral components of the membranes of gram-negative bacteria, mycobacteria, and yeast. Tissue macrophages contain mannose-fucose receptors, which bind high-mannose carbohydrates, mediate phagocytosis, and trigger the microbicidal processes of these cells. In contrast, neutrophils and blood monocytes lack these mannose-fucose receptors. However, the liver produces a homologous secreted protein that binds to and opsonizes these microbes for subsequent ingestion by neutrophils and monocytes and also enhances activation of complement on the surface of such organisms

(Kuhlman et al., 1989). This protein is an acute-phase protein, so that its concentration in blood increases in inflammation. This mechanism is impeded by capsular polysaccharides of most virulent gram-negative pathogens. Approximately 5% to 7% of the general population is deficient in mannose-binding protein (Ainbender et al., 1982); although some individuals with this deficiency may experience increased numbers of infections, most do not, suggesting that mannose-binding protein plays an auxiliary rather than a critical role in host defense. The concentration of mannose-binding protein in the blood of infants appears to be similar to that in adults, although reports of analysis restricted to neonates or premature neonates have not been published (Super et al., 1989). The lipopolysaccharide-binding protein is also produced by the liver constitutively and as an acute-phase protein. It facilitates binding of lipopolysaccharide to the high-affinity CD14 receptor expressed by mononuclear phagocytes and to a lesser extent by neutrophils (Wright, 1991). This plays an important role in activation of macrophages by lipopolysaccharide and promotes binding of gram-negative bacteria by these cells. There are no published data regarding content of lipopolysaccharide-binding protein in the blood of neonates.

Opsonization

Variable production of specific antibody to pathogenic microbes and decreased amounts of nonspecific opsonins may combine to markedly diminish microbial opsonization and the generation of complement-derived chemotactic factors in the neonate. Although opsonic activity against *Staphylococcus aureus* is generally normal in the neonate, opsonization of group B streptococci, *Streptococcus pneumoniae*, and gram-negative bacteria (e.g., *E. coli*) is more commonly found to be diminished (Dossett et al., 1969; Park et al., 1970; Winkelstein et al., 1979; Edwards et al., 1983; Geelen et al., 1990). Greater deficits are commonly observed with microbes for which alternative pathway complement opsonization appears to be most important (Mills et al., 1979a; Marodi et al., 1985). The deficits in opsonization are predictably greater when sera from preterm neonates are tested.

Summary

Compared with adults, neonates have moderately diminished alternative complement pathway activity, slightly diminished classical pathway activity, and decreased activity of the terminal complement components C8 and C9. Fibronectin concentrations are also slightly lower. These deficiencies along with variable amounts of antibody to specific microbes are associated with diminished ability of neonatal sera to opsonize certain organisms efficiently. Generation of complement-derived chemotactic activity is also modestly diminished. In concert with deficiencies in phagocyte production and migration to sites of infection, these factors may contribute to the delayed inflammatory response and impaired clearance of pyogenic microbes in the neonate.

CONDITIONS AFFECTING NEONATAL IMMUNITY

Intrauterine Growth Retardation

As has been observed in older individuals with malnutrition, intrauterine growth retardation (IUGR) appears primarily to affect T cells. These infants have a smaller thymus (Naeye et al., 1971) and lower circulating concentrations of thymic hormones (Chandra, 1981). The number of T cells assessed by sheep erythrocyte rosetting is also diminished (Ferguson et al., 1974; Chandra, 1975; Bhaskaram et al., 1977), as are delayed hypersensitivity responses after sensitization with dinitrochlorobenzene (Chandra, 1975) or injection of phytohemagglutinin (Bhaskaram et al., 1977). Lymphocyte proliferation in response to mitogens may be diminished. In studies from India, infants with IUGR had diminished responses to mitogens (Chandra, 1975; Bhaskaram et al., 1977), whereas in studies in Italy and Canada, this was not found (Ferguson, 1978), perhaps reflecting greater severity of IUGR in the Indian infants. These abnormalities in cell-mediated immunity appear to persist for at least the first year of life. In general, numbers of other lymphocyte subsets and of serum immunoglobulins have differed little from those of non–growth-retarded neonates (Evans and Smith, 1963; Yeung and Hobbs, 1968; Catty et al., 1977; Bhaskaram et al., 1977; Ferguson, 1978; Anderson et al., 1983).

Hyperbilirubinemia

Severe hyperbilirubinemia appears to be associated with several alterations in immune function, including impaired neutrophil microbicidal activity; diminished lymphocyte proliferation; and decreased antibody response to subsequent immunization with diphtheria, pertussis, and tetanus antigens but not in response to naturally encountered *E. coli* antigens (Nejedla, 1970; Rubaltelli et al, 1977; Oseas and Lehrer, 1979; Mills et al., 1979b). Whether these findings are a result of hyperbilirubinemia or of the underlying conditions that lead to increased bilirubin is not known, although bilirubin may directly impair lymphocyte proliferation in vitro (Rola-Pleszcynski et al., 1975; Sevjcar et al., 1984). However, there is no clear evidence that these findings are associated with increased predisposition to infection.

Maternal Medications and Drug Abuse

Antenatal administration of glucocorticoids in a brief pulse in an effort to prevent the respiratory distress syndrome does not affect the lymphocyte count or immunoglobulin production by the neonate (Ryhanen et al., 1980; Gleicher et al., 1981), although slight impairment of phagocytosis was noted in one study (Lazzarin et al., 1977). Administration of hydrocortisone in two doses on the first day of life did not affect subsequent lymphocyte counts, immunoglobulin or complement concentrations, or antibody response to immunization when the child was assessed at 5 years of age. These infants did have a lower fraction of T cells (53% versus 69%), but the biological significance of this is not clear (Gunn et al., 1981). In general, there is little to suggest that such brief courses of glucocorticoids have a biologically significant effect on the immune system of neonates. A child born to a mother who received azathioprine and prednisone during pregnancy to prevent renal allograft rejection was born with a defect in T-cell signal transduction. However, the biochemical basis for this has not been elucidated, and the relationship to the treatment is not clear (Chatila et al., 1989).

Intravenous drug abuse by the mother—of heroin, cocaine, amphetamines, or any combination of these—has been associated with a diminished absolute lymphocyte count, decreased percentage of CD4 cells, and decreased proliferation in response to phytohemagglutin (PHA) by blood mononuclear cells at birth in one study of 17 infants (Culver et al., 1987). However, no association was found between maternal intravenous drug abuse and lymphocyte or CD4 numbers in two large European studies of infants at risk for HIV infection (de Maurizio et al., 1991; European Collaborative Study, 1992). Maternal alcoholism has been associated with a diminished percentage of T cells and T-cell proliferation in response to mitogens (Chatila et al., 1989), and the abnormalities were reported to persist until 10 years of age. Maternal smoking has not been associated with detectable abnormalities in neonatal immune responses (Paganelli et al., 1979).

HOST DEFENSES IN THE FETUS AND NEONATE

Pyogenic Bacterial Infections

The first line of defense preventing the establishment of infection is the mucocutaneous barrier. Compared with adult epithelium, there may be unique characteristics of neonatal epithelium that allow virulent strains of pathogens to gain an advantage. It has been suggested that the greater capacity of pathogenic type III group B streptococci to adhere to mucosal epithelial cells of neonates, particularly ill neonates, may facilitate colonization (Fischer et al., 1982). The mechanism for this difference is not known at present and awaits identification of the critical ligands. The lack of secretory IgA in the first week of life may also contribute to an increased risk of colonization. Nevertheless, the most clearly defined factor in the risk of the neonate for colonization and infection by capsulated pyogenic bacteria, such as group B streptococci, is the absence of passively acquired maternal antibody. This may be compounded by the failure of most colonized or infected neonates to synthesize antibodies in response to group B streptococci. Those that do produce antibody synthesize only IgM and do so transiently (Edwards et al., 1990).

After colonization has been established, the paucity of alveolar macrophages in the lungs of term, and particularly preterm, neonates at birth and the diminished rates of phagocytosis and killing of bacteria by these cells may allow greater multiplication of bacteria invading through the respiratory tract. Furthermore, limited generation of chemotactic factors may delay recruitment of neonatal neutrophils that are themselves deficient in adhesion and chemotaxis. Once the neutrophils reach the site of infection, limitations in opsonins may further impede the ability of neutrophils to clear the bacteria. Rapid dissemination of infection may then deplete the limited neutrophil reserve in the marrow of the neonate. Thus, several defined deficiencies in host defense are likely to be contributing factors predisposing the neonate to severe infection with these pyogenic microbes.

Viral Infections

The neonate experiences more severe or rapidly progressive infection with certain viruses, most notably HSV, CMV, HIV, and enteroviruses. Viruses replicate intracellularly; thus, it is not surprising that mechanisms that act to control or block infection within cells and/or spread of virus from cell to cell are critical for effective host defense. With the exception of the enteroviruses, the most important components of the immune response are cellular. Because it is a prototype of a viral infection that is unduly severe in the neonate, much of the discussion focuses on defenses operative against HSV, mentioning relevant information specific to other viral infections. Neonatal defense against HIV has been recently reviewed (Koup and Wilson, 1994) and is not discussed in detail.

The antiviral immune response can generally be divided into an early, nonspecific phase (the first 5 to 7 days in HSV infection) and a later, antigen-specific phase (Kohl, 1989). In the early phase, infection may be contained by innate host defenses or proceed to disseminate throughout the host. Antigen-specific immunity during the later phase acts to eliminate active infection by either eradication of the virus or the establishment of latency. Characteristically, HSV infection in neonates is rapidly fulminant and disseminated, so that the early containment phase of the response may be the most critical; indeed, deficits in the early nonspecific phase of viral resistance have been reported in neonatal humans and animals.

The basis for these findings is suggested by the differences in function of neonatal macrophages and NK cells. Initial data suggesting that a greater permissiveness for replication of HSV in mononuclear phagocytes from human neonates have not been corroborated in more recent studies. Yet considerable data indicate that the cytotoxic activity of neonatal blood mononuclear cells, monocytes, and purified NK cells against a variety of targets, including those infected with HSV, is impaired. Such deficits have been apparent in assays measuring natural cytotoxicity and antibody-dependent cell-mediated cytotoxicity (ADCC). The deficit in NK cell function is likely to be related in large part to their poor cytolytic function.

The ability of neonatal NK cells to produce IFN-γ in response to the combination of live HSV and IL-2, although modest, appeared not to differ from that of cells of adults in one study (Hayward et al., 1986). However, indirect evidence for a deficit in the production of IFN-γ by human neonatal NK cells comes from the failure of IL-2 and human neonatal blood mononuclear cells to mediate adoptive protection in neonatal mice. In contrast, adult mononuclear cells mediate adoptive protection in combination with IL-2; this protection is dependent on IL-2–facilitated IFN-γ production by the transferred mononuclear cells (Kohl et al., 1989a). Although human adult mononuclear cells in combination with antibody, IFN-α, IFN-γ, or IL-2 will protect neonatal mice from HSV, human neonatal mononuclear cells protect only in combination with IFN-γ (Kohl, 1990). In contrast to the deficit in production of IFN-γ by neonatal T cells, the capacity of neonatal mononuclear cells to produce IFN-α has been normal in all but one study, and individual case reports have demonstrated the presence of IFN-α in the body fluids of human neonates with HSV infection.

Compounding the poor ability of the neonate to contain HSV infection in the early nonspecific phase, antigen-specific T cell–mediated immune responses are commonly diminished or delayed or both in their development in human neonates compared with adults with primary HSV infection. Multiple studies have shown a delay in development of antigen-specific responses as detected by lymphocyte proliferation (Yeager et al., 1980; Sullender et al., 1987; Kohl, 1989). In a longitudinal analysis, a 3-week delay was found in the development of HSV antigen–specific lymphocyte proliferation in neonates as compared with adults having primary HSV infection, and this was paralleled by a delay in antigen-specific production of IFN-γ (Burchett et al., 1992).

The basis for this delay is not completely clear. Hayward and his colleagues have shown that this may reflect in part the lower precursor cell frequency for antigen-responsive cells in HSV-infected neonates (Hayward et al., 1984; Chilmonczyk et al., 1985); similar findings were made in infants with congenital CMV infection. Once human infants who were infected as neonates developed HSV antigen–specific T cells, as indicated by a detectable proliferative response, antigen-specific IFN-γ production was usually detectable as well (Burchett et al., 1992). This is consistent with the notion that the lack of antigen-specific memory T cells is the major cause of the deficit in production of IFN-γ (and certain other cytokines) by neonatal T cells (see discussion under Activation and Lymphokine Production by Neonatal T Cells earlier).

This delay in the acquisition of antigen-specific T cells and cytokine production may be an important factor in the neonate's greater susceptibility to infections with HSV and pathogens against which such defenses play an important role. It is unknown if this is accompanied by a similar delay or deficit in T cell–

mediated antigen-specific cytotoxicity. However, it seems likely that antiviral cytotoxicity would be impaired as is cytotoxicity to other targets (see T Cell–Mediated Cytotoxicity discussion, earlier).

The data on antiviral cytotoxicity of neonatal cells to virus-infected targets are limited and lack clear evidence for antigen-specific, MHC-restricted T cell–mediated cytotoxicity (Isaacs et al., 1987; Chiba et al., 1989), with the exception of two studies in infants and young children with perinatal HIV infection. In the latter study (Luzuriaga et al., 1991), only 3 of 12 infants, compared with 4 of 5 individuals who acquired HIV infection later in life, exhibited CD8-mediated cytotoxicity to viral antigen–expressing target cells. In the other study (Buseyne et al., 1993), most of the perinatally infected children were studied at an older age. These infants commonly had cytotoxic T cells directed to HIV envelope proteins but rarely had such activity against targets expressing the *gag* or *pol* proteins. In the two who were initially studied in infancy, similar spontaneous cytolytic activity was not detected to any viral antigen at less than 11 months of age.

These results suggest that there may be a delay in the development of cytotoxic activity compared with adults and, additionally, that the nature of the target antigens recognized by neonatal cytotoxic T cells may be more limited. It remains to be determined whether neonates have similar deficits in development of cytotoxic T cells directed to other viruses. Together, the diminished and delayed T cell–mediated responses to viral antigens along with deficits in NK function are likely to be important factors in the predisposition of the neonate.

In addition to the neonate's own immune response, antibody-mediated protection can be provided passively from the mother. The risks of transmission of HSV from mother to infant in cases of primary or initial maternal infection are much higher (~35%) than in cases of recurrent maternal infection. This may reflect in part lesser amounts of virus in the maternal genital tract in recurrent infection but also appears to correlate with HSV type-specific antibody, particularly to glycoprotein G (gpG) (Ashley et al., 1992). Kohl and colleagues (1989b) have also shown that of HSV-infected infants, those with greater concentrations of ADCC antibody had less severe disease. It is important to note that healthy adults and older children with primary HSV infection, who by definition lack antibody to HSV, do not develop severe disease, as do neonates with primary infection. This indicates that the deficits intrinsic to the neonate are the important factors predisposing the neonate to severe infection. Nevertheless, passively acquired antibody may play a role in decreasing transmission or ameliorating disease severity.

It is noteworthy that HSV and enterovirus infections are severe in term infants infected at the time of parturition, as well as in the uncommon cases acquired in utero. In contrast, congenital infection with CMV produces considerably greater damage when primary maternal infection and thereby fetal infection occur in the first half of gestation (Stagno et al., 1986). When infection is acquired after midgestation, severe sequelae are uncommon, although some sequelae, particularly sensorineural hearing loss, may result. Similarly, congenital rubella virus infection produces sequelae essentially only when maternal infection occurs in the first 16 weeks of gestation. Infections that occur in the first 10 weeks of gestation do so at a time when the fetus has few detectable T or B cells, and if infection begins before the sixth week of gestation NK cells also will be absent. Furthermore, the numbers and repertoire for antigen recognition of T cells, B cells, and antibody-secreting plasma cells are low in the first half of gestation.

Thus, it is reasonable to suggest that the extraordinary susceptibility to infection with these agents in the first half of gestation reflects quantitative deficits in these cells of the immune system. The less severe sequelae of congenital CMV infection, when infection occurs after midgestation, may result from qualitative, rather than quantitative, deficiencies in the fetal and neonatal immune systems, as described above for HSV infection. For enterovirus infections, the absence of protective neutralizing antibody appears to be the major predisposing factor (Modlin et al., 1981; Hammond et al., 1985), although it is likely that T cell–mediated immune responses also play a role in defense with these agents.

Nonviral Intracellular Pathogens

In addition to viruses, several other intracellular pathogens are capable of causing severe infection in neonates, including *L. monocytogenes, Salmonella,* and *Mycobacterium tuberculosis,* which are facultative intracellular pathogens, and *T. gondii* and *Chlamydia trachomatis,* which are obligate intracellular pathogens. Based to a large extent on experiments performed in rodent models, the principal mechanisms of host defense against these pathogens appear to be a concerted and sequential interaction between two components of the innate immune system, NK cells and macrophages, and later in infection, antigen-specific T lymphocytes and the cytokines produced by these cells. These are in many ways analogous to the components acting in defense against viruses. The common feature of infections with both agents appears to be the necessity to recognize organisms residing within host cells and to eliminate the organisms and the infected cells.

The factors resulting in the poor ability of the neonate to contain infections caused by intracellular pathogens are likely to include immaturity in NK cell function and perhaps the somewhat slower migration of neonatal monocytes into sites of infection. However, it seems more likely that the critical factors in the neonate are the deficits in production of IFN-γ and to some extent of TNF-α. Such a conclusion is supported by studies in neonatal rodents, which are highly susceptible to infection with *Listeria.* In neonatal mice and rats, administration of recombinant IFN-γ prior to or at the time of infection protects from acute infection and allows the development of protective immunity (Chen et al., 1989; Bortolussi et al., 1989, 1992). In adult animals, TNF-α or agents that induce TNF-α enhance resistance, whereas this is not observed in the neonates. Coadministration of suboptimal doses of IFN-γ and TNF-α protects neonatal rats. Acquisition of resistance to infection correlates with the acquisition of adult competence for TNF-α production (Bortolussi et al., 1992); acquiring resistance is also likely to correlate with competence for IFN-γ production, but this was not tested.

Although the maturity of the neonatal rodent immune system is different from that of human neonates, these results appear to parallel those in human neonates. As noted earlier, there is a clear deficit in the production of IFN-γ in the human neonate, but once antigen-specific memory T cells develop, antigen-induced IFN-γ production appears to approximate that of cells from older individuals. This fact suggests that the poor IFN-γ production reflects at least in large part the paucity and delay in development of memory T cells in neonates.

Gestational age influences the severity of neonatal infection in a pathogen-specific way. Infection with *Toxoplasma,* like that with CMV, is much more likely to produce severe untoward infection when the mother acquires primary infection early in pregnancy. The most severely damaged infants are likely to have acquired infection when the numbers of T cells and their repertoire for recognition of antigens are limited compared with the fetus in the latter half of gestation. However, severe sequelae in infants with congenital *Toxoplasma* infection may occur in infants born to mothers who acquired infection in mid-to-late gestation, and the majority of infants infected at any time during gestation will ultimately develop sequelae. Similarly, *Listeria* infection occurring in infants in the latter part of gestation is usually severe. This suggests that mechanisms acting to contain *Toxoplasma* and *Listeria* infections are still immature in late gestation and at term relative to older individuals.

As discussed earlier under T-Cell Reactivity to Specific Antigens, studies of congenital *Toxoplasma* infection suggest that infection of the fetus in utero may in some cases further impede the development of memory T cells and that in such cases, cells capable of producing protective cytokines may not always develop in parallel with antigen-specific T-cell proliferation (McLeod et al., 1990). Impairment in the development of antigen-specific T-cell responses has also been observed in infants with congenital syphilis (Friedmann, 1977), CMV (Gehrz et al., 1977; Reynolds et al., 1979; Starr et al., 1979) or rubella (Buimovici-Klein et al., 1979). These findings contrast with the less persistent delay in development of antigen-specific T-cell responses in children infected with HSV at term and raise the possibility that infection occurring at a time of greater immunologic immaturity may lead to a state of relative anergy, as observed in rodents.

IMMUNOTHERAPY IN THE NEONATE

Adjunctive Therapy in Pyogenic Infections

The principal deficits in the neonate relevant to defenses against pyogenic pathogens appear to be a deficiency of opsonins, particularly protective antibodies,

and a limited capacity to increase neutrophil production and mobilize neutrophils to sites of infection. Both deficits have been addressed by targeted immunologic interventions. However, evidence supporting the routine use of any form of immunologic augmentation either for prevention or as an adjunct to antimicrobial therapy of infections in the neonate is currently lacking.

Intravenous Immunoglobulin

In an early retrospective, uncontrolled study, fresh whole blood containing type-specific antibody, but not blood lacking type-specific antibody, improved survival in human neonates with group B streptococcal sepsis (Shigeoka et al., 1978). In addition to the obvious limitations of study design, the relative role of antibody, complement, or leukocytes was unclear; nevertheless, this study provided an impetus for a number of subsequent trials designed to test the role of antibody preparations in neonatal sepsis. Such studies were also predicated on the development of preparations of immunoglobulin for intravenous use (IVIG) and a series of animal studies. It is important to note that these antibody studies suggested that the quantity and quality of antibodies to specific pathogens varied considerably among preparations of IVIG and that both efficacy and deleterious effects could be observed in animal models of infection, depending on this and other variables. The results of clinical studies are mixed, perhaps reflecting differences in the study designs and populations, the preparation of IVIG, and dosage.

A number of prospective studies have evaluated the use of IVIG to prevent nosocomial or late-onset infections in premature neonates, a group at increased risk of infection (reviewed in Schreiber and Berger, 1992; and in Hill, 1993). Of these studies, only that by Baker and colleagues (1992) has shown clear benefit. This study enrolled prospectively 588 neonates of 500 to 1750 g birth weight and postnatal age of 3 to 7 days. Neonates received IVIG or an albumin placebo at a predetermined schedule based on earlier pharmacologic studies. The IVIG recipients had fewer first infections, coagulase-negative and -positive staphylococci being the most common cause of infection in both groups. However, there was no significant difference in overall survival or duration of hospitalization between the groups.

Four other multicenter, randomized studies failed to show an effect of prophylactic IVIG in similar patient populations:

- A study in Paris of 235 premature neonates who received a different preparation (not available in the United States) and dosage schedule of IVIG found no benefit; when both proved and probable infections were included, a significantly increased risk of infection was observed in the IVIG group (Magny et al., 1991).
- A study of 170 infants of varying birth weight (108 weighed <1500 g) received 750 mg/kg within 72 hours of birth and every 154 days thereafter. There

were no differences in infections, duration of hospital stay, or mortality between those receiving IVIG and those receiving placebo (Kinney et al., 1991).

• A study in multiple military institutions in the United States that used IVIG lots selected for high titers of antibody to group B streptococci, which included all infants younger than 34 weeks of age and less than 2 kg birth weight, and initiated therapy before 12 hours postnatal age, was terminated after enrollment of 753 infants because no prophylactic efficacy was evident (Weisman et al., 1992).

• The NIH supported a multicentered, two-phase, controlled study of 2416 newborns weighing 500 to 1500 g. These were given 700 or 900 mg/kg of IVIG or placebo every 14 days until they weighed 1800 g or were transferred to another institution; they showed no reduction in incidence of hospital-acquired infection (Fanaroff et al., 1994).

Although the results are mixed, the preponderance of the evidence at the present time suggests that IVIG administered to low-birth-weight infants in an attempt to prevent subsequent nosocomial infection is not usually efficacious. Whether modifications in patient selection or in the nature of the IVIG preparation would result in greater general efficacy is not known.

In contrast to the large placebo-controlled studies seeking to identify a prophylactic role for IVIG, those studies investigating this material as adjunctive therapy for neonatal sepsis are limited. This reflects concerns raised by some animal studies, in which a deleterious effect with high concentrations of IVIG was found; this may have reflected blockade of macrophage Fc receptors, although this is unproven (reviewed in Schreiber and Berger, 1992). Nevertheless, the efficacy observed in other models against group B streptococci and *E. coli* K1 have prompted a number of pilot studies in humans. Three such pilot studies, each of which evaluated a different population of patients and each of which used different preparations of IVIG or, in one study, a preparation of mixed immune globulins, concluded that mortality was reduced. However, because of the small numbers of neonates studied, lack of controls, or absence of a prospective design, these studies do not provide sufficient information to form a meaningful conclusion regarding efficacy (Hill, 1993).

There was no evidence of toxicity of the IVIG in these or in two more recent prospective, controlled studies (Christensen et al., 1991; Weisman et al., 1992). In the controlled studies, improvement in neutrophil counts (perhaps reflecting improved mobilization of storage pools) and opsonic capacity was observed in IVIG-treated but not in albumin placebo–treated neonates with clinical or proven sepsis in one study (Christensen et al., 1991); there was no mortality in either group. In the study by Weisman and associates (1992), which also assessed prophylactic efficacy (described previously), all premature neonates were randomly assigned to receive IVIG selected for high titers of antibody to group B streptococci or albumin placebo within 12 hours of birth. Although no efficacy in prevention of late-onset infection was found, IVIG

may have been beneficial among the 31 patients with early-onset sepsis; sepsis was most commonly caused by group B streptococci. Among these 31, 5 of 16 placebo recipients died within the first 7 days of life, in contrast to none of 14 IVIG-treated neonates ($P < .05$). However, two late deaths occurred in the IVIG group, so that survival rates at 8 weeks of age did not differ between the two groups, although the trend still favored the IVIG group. The treatment arm of the study was terminated early, because the monitoring group concluded that the prophylactic arm of the trial did not show efficacy of IVIG.

Thus, at the present time data are insufficient to recommend the use of IVIG for adjuvant therapy. Further studies are needed to determine if these preliminary results can be replicated in other centers and with other lots of IVIG. The long-term effects of neonatal IVIG therapy on subsequent production of antibody in infants must also be assessed.

Monoclonal Antibodies

An alternative to IVIG, a biologic agent with varying concentrations and quality of antibodies to specific neonatal pathogens, is the use of monoclonal antibody preparations. Murine monoclonal antibodies to group B streptococci (Harris et al., 1982; Christensen et al., 1983; Shigeoka et al., 1984) and *E. coli* K1 (raised against cross-reacting group B meningococci) (Raff et al., 1991) provide protection in animal models. Because of concern regarding efficacy or development of antibody to the murine preparations, human or humanized monoclonal antibodies have been or are being developed. Differences in efficacy of the antibodies with identical antigen-binding domains have also been observed when the Fc domain, which determines valency, complement fixation, and binding to Fc receptors, has been switched (Raff et al., 1991). Clinical trials with such preparations have yet to be undertaken.

Oral Immunoglobulin

A novel formulation of oral immunoglobulin, enriched in IgA, reduced the risk of necrotizing enterocolitis in premature infants for whom breast milk was not available (Eibl et al., 1988). Although this study was published in 1988, it does not appear to have been replicated to date, and such a preparation is not available clinically.

Leukocyte Transfusions

In animal models of neonatal sepsis, neutrophil transfusions can enhance survival (Santos et al., 1980). An initial uncontrolled trial of neutrophil transfusions in neonates with nonfulminant sepsis suggested striking efficacy; mortality was 2 of 20 in the group receiving neutrophils and 13 of 18 in those not receiving neutrophils (Cairo et al., 1984). However, more recent studies have yielded more mixed results (reviewed in Krause et al., 1989). The study by Christensen and coworkers (1982) examined a group of neonates that was restricted to those with severe early-onset sepsis, neutropenia, and neutrophil storage pool depletion, more representative of those with high morbidity and mortality in most centers. The numbers studied were small (Table 10–7) but included seven neonates with group B streptococcal sepsis. Statistical significance in favor of neutrophil transfusions was achieved but only by pooling both randomized and nonrandomized patients with sepsis caused by a variety of bacterial species. The other studies noted in Table 10–7 have yielded mixed results.

It is clear that many of the infants with early-onset sepsis who survive do not have neutrophil storage pool depletion despite being neutropenic; in most studies such infants have a high probability of survival with antimicrobial therapy alone and do not benefit from neutrophil transfusions. The difficulty in ascertainment of neutrophil storage pool size in clinical practice and the failure of this to predict outcome in some studies make this measure an imperfect one in clinical practice.

A later study from Cairo and colleagues (1992), which compared the efficacy of IVIG to that of neutrophil transfusions in infants with either early- or late-onset infection, concluded that neutrophil transfusions (five transfusions given over 3 days) were more efficacious in that population. However, no untreated control group was included in this study. Overall, the results of neutrophil transfusion studies fail to establish this as a generally useful approach in neonates with suspected or proven sepsis. The utility of neutrophil transfusions is further compromised by logistical difficulties in obtaining neutrophils in a timely fashion and the potential complications of transfusions, including the risk of infection. They cannot be recommended for routine use in the management of neonatal sepsis at the present time.

Colony-Stimulating Factors

An alternative approach to neutrophil transfusions is the use of recombinant cytokines or hematopoietic growth factors to augment the numbers or function of neonatal neutrophils. Several related in vitro studies that were described earlier (see the section on Neutrophil Production and Release) suggest that such an approach might be efficacious. Limited studies in animal models also support this approach. When administered concomitantly or prior to infection and given in conjunction with specific antimicrobial therapy, recombinant human granulocyte colony–stimulating factor (G-CSF), which has activity in rodents as well, or recombinant murine granulocyte-macrophage (GM)–CSF enhanced survival compared with antimicrobial therapy alone in neonatal rats infected with group B streptococci or *Staphylococcus aureus* (Frenck et al., 1989; Cairo, 1989). In one study, administration of recombinant human GM-CSF up to 19 hours after infection of neonatal rats with group B streptococci improved survival; however, the bacteria and the GM-CSF were given into the same site, raising concern that the effects may have been related to a local effect (Frenck et al., 1989). Others have not found that recombinant human G-CSF enhances survival in neonatal rats infected with group B streptococci (Iguchi et al., 1991). These CSFs are marketed for the treatment of neutropenia in older individuals with chemotherapy-induced or primary forms of neutropenia, conditions for which they appear to be efficacious.

One published report exists that demonstrates increased blood neutrophils in response to recombinant human G-CSF in a premature neonate with neutropenia and recurrent sepsis. However, it is not clear that the G-CSF contributed to the cessation of the septic episodes in this child (Roberts et al., 1991). There are at this time no other published data regarding the use of hematopoietic growth factors in human neonates.

Immunotherapy for Viral and Nonviral Intracellular Pathogens

The studies cited previously raise the possibility that neonates can be passively protected by administration of antibody to HSV, particularly antibody that would facilitate antibody-dependent cell-mediated cytotoxic-

Table 10–7. Clinical Trials of Polymorphonuclear Neutrophil Leukocyte Transfusion in Newborn Infants with Sepsis

Study	Experimental Group	Number of Infants	Number of PMNs Transfused	Number of Transfusions	Mortality Rate (%)
Laurenti et al. (1981)	Treatment	20	$0.5–1 \times 10^9$	2–15	10
	Control	18	0	0	72
Christensen et al. (1982)	Treatment	7	$0.1–1 \times 10^9$	1	0
	Control	9	0	0	89
Cairo et al. (1984)	Treatment	13	$0.5–1 \times 10^9$	5	0
	Control	10	0	0	40
Laing et al. (1983)	Treatment	6	$0.05 \times 1.8 \times 10^8$	1	50
Cairo et al. (1987)	Treatment	21	$0.5 \times 1 \times 10^9$	5	5
	Control	14	0	0	36
Wheeler et al. (1987)	Treatment	4	$0.3–0.7 \times 10^9$	1	50
	Control	5	0	0	60
Baley et al. (1987)	Treatment	12	$0.1–0.9 \times 10^9$	1–3	33
	Control	13	0	0	23

Abbreviation: PMN = polymorphonuclear neutrophil leukocyte.
From Krause PJ, Herson VC, Eisenfeld L, Johnson GM. Enhancement of neutrophil function for treatment of neonatal infections. Pediatr Infect Dis J 8:382–389, 1989.

ity. The unique capacity of IFN-γ to endow human neonatal blood mononuclear cells with the ability to protect neonatal mice from infection suggests that exogenous IFN-γ may also be a potentially useful means to enhance the human neonate's resistance to HSV. However, in the experimental models described by Kohl (1989), it is necessary that passive immunotherapy be given before or at the time of infection. This raises the concern that such therapy, if administered once infection is established, may be less effective, at least in controlling the damage from the acute infection. Nevertheless, such approaches are under active discussion by the National Institute for Allergy and Infectious Disease Collaborative Antiviral Studies Group. Ultimately, facilitating the development of antigen-specific T cells with appropriate effector function would be a more physiologic approach, thus allowing localization of such cells and their cytokines to the sites of infection. Further elucidation of the cellular and molecular events governing these processes may provide the means to address these problems.

The efficacy of immunoglobulin in the prevention of neonatal echovirus infection was suggested by its use in control of a nursery outbreak (Report of the Committee on Infectious Diseases, 1991). Hyperimmune immunoglobulin also has a proven role, along with active immunization in the prevention of hepatitis B virus infection in the neonate (Report of the Committee on Infectious Diseases, 1991).

Regarding infections caused by nonviral intracellular neonatal pathogens, such as *T. gondii*, the findings in human neonates in concert with the results of studies in rodents suggest that correction of the deficits in NK function, cytokine production, and T-cell response could facilitate treatment of these infections. However, several limitations are apparent. For example, treatment of neonatal rats with IFN-γ or TNF-α after establishment of infection with *Listeria* is not effective, whereas concomitant or pretreatment is effective (Bortolussi et al., 1991). This perhaps is not surprising given the evidence that IFN-γ is important only in the early phase of this infection. In the case of congenital infection with *Toxoplasma*, therapy would need to be initiated in utero when maternal infection is often asymptomatic, and there is no obvious way by which this could be safely targeted to the fetus. After birth it may be possible to provide exogenous IFN-γ (or perhaps TNF-α), but the same caveats noted for treatment in cases of viral infection would apply. If studies in other populations (e.g., of acquired immunodeficiency syndrome [AIDS]) provide evidence that IFN-γ (or TNF-α) can contribute to resolution of established disease in conjunction with antimicrobial therapy, its use in neonates might be considered. Alternatively, approaches that seek to modify the deficit in development of antigen-specific effector T cells may be a more useful approach.

Immunoprophylaxis in the Neonate Born to a Mother with Hypogammaglobulinemia

Although the results of studies on whether to provide broad immunoprophylaxis in high-risk neonates do not support this approach at present, infants born to mothers who have hypogammaglobulinemia may benefit from prophylactic administration of IVIG, depending on whether maternal IgG concentrations are maintained at concentrations near term that result in adequate levels in the neonate.

PRIMARY IMMUNODEFICIENCIES IN THE NEONATE

Clinical and Laboratory Features

Recognition of primary immunodeficiency, particularly forms other than those limited to defects of humoral immunity, may be possible in the neonate and young infant (see Chapter 9). Several syndromes have characteristic features that permit early recognition: thrombocytopenia in Wiskott-Aldrich syndrome; hypocalcemia, characteristic facies, and congenital heart disease in the DiGeorge syndrome; and short-limb dwarfism and paucity of hair in cartilage-hair hypoplasia. Leukocyte adhesion defect may come to attention because of delay in separation of the umbilical cord. It is important to recognize that with contemporary umbilical cord care, separation may not occur by 3 weeks of age in as many as 10% of infants (Wilson et al., 1985). However, separation delayed beyond 2 months or associated infection of the umbilical cord suggests the possibility of leukocyte adhesion defect.

Patients with severe combined immunodeficiency may present with severe or recalcitrant mucocutaneous candidiasis, protracted diarrhea, *Pneumocystis carinii* pneumonia, severe eczema, or both. Severe erythroderma, eosinophilia, and progressive lymphadenopathy and splenomegaly may suggest the Omenn syndrome form of severe combined immunodeficiency and must be differentiated from early-onset HIV-related disease. Unusually severe, recalcitrant, or recurrent infections or those related to opportunistic organisms of low virulence suggest immunodeficiency, particularly when they occur without other known predisposing factors—for example, prematurity, protracted use of assisted ventilation, indwelling catheters, or antibiotic therapy. A family history of immunodeficiency may suggest the diagnosis.

Normal term neonates lack detectable delayed cutaneous hypersensitivity responses and in vitro proliferative responses to antigens, have IgG and IgG subclass values similar to those in their mothers, but have little or no detectable circulating IgM and IgA. These laboratory tests have little utility in evaluation of the immune response in the neonatal period and in early infancy. Useful screening tests to evaluate lymphocyte function at this age include

1. Chest radiograph to assess thymic size.
2. Enumeration of total lymphocyte, T- and B-cell numbers, and T-cell subsets by flow cytometry.
3. Lymphocyte proliferative responses to mitogens, allogeneic cells, and certain bacterial superantigens.
4. Assessment of NK cell numbers by flow cytometry and cytolytic function (see Chapter 9).

It is important that results in these tests be considered in the context of the numeric and functional differences that vary with age, as described earlier in the discussions of T cells, B cells, and NK cells. The principal genetic disorders of neutrophil function—chronic granulomatous disease and leukocyte adhesion defect type I—may be detected by testing for defects in the neutrophil respiratory burst, using nitroblue tetrazolium reduction or flow cytometric detection of hydrogen peroxide production, and by testing for expression of the β_2 integrin, CD18, by flow cytometry, respectively.

Transient Hypogammaglobulinemia of Infancy

Following birth there is a diminution in the concentration of IgG, reflecting the loss of maternally derived IgG and the gradual accumulation of IgG synthesized by the infant. The physiologic low point is normally reached at 3 to 4 months. In infants who were born prematurely, the nadir will be proportionately lower because of the diminished amount of IgG received from the mother, and values may remain less than those of term infants throughout the first year of life. Concentrations of IgM and IgA also are characteristically low at this age, rising gradually thereafter; the values in premature infants are lower than those of term infants until 10 months of age. See earlier, Concentrations of Immunoglobulin Isotypes in the Fetus and Infant, for details.

Transient hypogammaglobulinemia of infancy is characterized by diminished concentrations of one or more classes of immunoglobulin, which subsequently rise with age to approach or reach normal values. B cells are present in normal or near normal numbers.

The underlying basis for this disorder is unknown and may be heterogeneous. It is most commonly thought to be a variant of the normal age-related acquisition of the capacity to produce immunoglobulins. This notion is consistent with the congruence between the frequency of the disorder and the predicted frequency for low values of a given immunoglobulin isotype. Statistical considerations dictate that 2.5% of all immunoglobulin isotype determinations will be below 2 standard deviations (S.D.). Since there are three isotypes, there is a probability of 7.5% that one of the three major immunoglobulin isotypes will be considered abnormal on any assessment. Since two abnormal determinations are required, the probability of a consistently decreased value for one isotype is 0.6%, and for a given isotype, such as IgG, the probability would be 0.06%. The latter figure is similar to the observed incidence of less than 1/1000 observed at two different centers and represents less than 5% of the primary immunodeficiencies diagnosed at these centers (Tiller and Buckley, 1978; Dressler et al., 1989). Along with the notion that most of these patients represent the extremes of normal variability rather than a true abnormality of the immune system, there are no consistent immunologic defects in these patients other than the low values for immunoglobulins.

The criteria for the diagnosis are not standardized. A rigorous definition requires that concentrations of one or more isotypes be more than 3 standard deviations below those of age-matched controls on two or more determinations (Siegel et al., 1981), although most use 2 standard deviations as the criterion (Tiller and Buckley, 1978; McGeady, 1987; Dressler et al., 1989). The frequency with which different isotypes have been diminished varies from one report to another. The WHO classification includes diminished IgG and IgA in the defining criteria (World Health Organization, 1992). Diminished values of IgG are generally considered to be invariant and when evaluated these have not been restricted to specific IgG subclasses (Dressler et al., 1989). In contrast, the incidence of diminished IgA and IgM concentrations has ranged from 0% to 100% (Siegel et al., 1981; McGeady, 1987) and 14% (McGeady, 1987) to 63% (Siegel et al., 1981) in different reports. In those patients who are evaluated because of clinical symptoms or signs suggesting humoral immune deficiency, diminished concentrations of IgA may persist beyond 5 years of age in as many as one half of the patients (Tiller and Buckley, 1978; McGeady, 1987; Dressler et al., 1989), and some may have persistent IgA deficiency (Tiller and Buckley, 1978; McGeady, 1987).

Immunization with tetanus and diphtheria toxoids induces a readily detectable antibody response in these patients, although absolute amounts of antibody may be somewhat less than those observed in controls (Tiller and Buckley, 1978; McGeady, 1987; Dressler et al., 1989). Isohemagglutinin values are also detectable and generally are in the normal range for age in these patients. The numbers of B and T cells and T-cell responses to mitogens are normal. One study found that the numbers and percentage of CD4 T cells were diminished (Siegel et al., 1981), but this has not been observed by others (Dressler et al., 1989). There does not appear to be an intrinsic defect in their B cells (Siegel et al., 1981), and abnormal CD4 T-cell numbers and function suggested in one study (Siegel et al., 1981) have not been confirmed (Dressler et al., 1989).

Among the patients in whom evaluation was undertaken because of an apparently increased incidence of infections, the types of infections observed are usually not life-threatening. Rather, an increased frequency of otitis media, sinusitis and bronchitis, and occasionally mucocutaneous candidiasis, is observed. Infections with opportunistic organisms and severe infections with capsulated bacterial pathogens suggest another diagnosis. It is also uncommon for patients to exhibit any increased susceptibility to infection beyond the ages of 2 to 3 years, even if the immunoglobulin concentrations have not fully normalized. This may reflect the fact that antigen-specific responses are intact in this condition.

In general, supportive therapy and appropriate antimicrobial therapy for specific infections are sufficient. Immunoglobulin replacement therapy is generally not warranted and has not been shown to be beneficial. In cases in which infections are severe or refractory to conventional management, immunoglobulin therapy may be considered. However, it is important under these circumstances that a thorough evaluation be performed to exclude other, more serious forms of immunodeficiency.

Transient Deficiency of CD11b/CD18

Three infants with transient deficiency of neutrophil CD11b/CD18, which is one of the β_2 integrins and is also known as Mac-1, or complement receptor 3, have been described (Shigeoka and Wittwer, 1993). Two of these infants presented with a delay in separation of the umbilical cord beyond 2 months of age, and the third had a perirectal abscess. These abnormalities were transient. This appears to be an acquired rather than a genetic defect in β_2 integrin expression, possibly related to a maternal autoantibody.

Leiner's Disease and Erythroderma/Failure to Thrive/Diarrhea Syndrome

In 1908 Leiner described a series of infants in whom severe generalized erythroderma, diarrhea, and failure to thrive were noted as early as 1 month of age, persisting for weeks to months. There was substantial mortality in these patients. More recently Miller and Nilsson (1970, 1974) described C5 dysfunction in infants with a similar presentation in whom recurrent infections commonly developed but in whom the disorder resolved by 2 months of age. Infusions of fresh plasma were thought to be of clinical benefit. The rationale for the plasma infusions was the finding by these workers of an apparent functional deficiency in the complement component C5 in these infants, whereas C5 concentrations were normal by immunochemical analysis.

For several reasons there is now doubt as to whether this represents a distinct nosological entity and whether C5 dysfunction is a tenable illness. The dermatologic manifestations of Leiner's disease place it within in the spectrum of seborrheic dermatitis of infancy (Bonifazi and Meneghini, 1989) rather than as a distinct disease. Furthermore, patients with genetic deficiency in C5 have not exhibited these clinical manifestations but rather have suffered later in life from recurrent infections caused by *Neisseria meningitidis* or *Neisseria gonorrhoeae* (Ross and Densen, 1984).

Glover and colleagues (1988) described a syndrome of erythema, failure to thrive, and diarrhea in a group of infants with similar clinical features but were unable to detect a functional deficit in C5. In the five infants they described, a variety of immunologic defects were observed, including severe combined immunodeficiency, hypogammaglobulinemia, and increased IgE with chemotactic defects; these last patients may have had unusually severe atopic dermatitis or the hyper-IgE syndrome. This study illustrates the frequencies with which eczematoid or seborrhea-like dermatitis are observed in patients with immunodeficiency of various causes and casts doubt on the role of C5 dysfunction in the pathogenesis of this clinical syndrome.

References

Adderson EE, Shackelford PG, Quinn A, Carroll WL. Restricted Ig H chain V gene usage in the human antibody response to *Haemophilus influenzae* type b capsular polysaccharide. J Immunol 147:1667–1674, 1991.

Adenyi-Jones SCA, Faden H, Ferdon MB, Kwong MS, Ogra PL. Systemic and local immune responses to enhanced-potency inactivated poliovirus vaccine in premature and term infants. J Pediatr 120:686–689, 1992.

Adinolfi M, Cheetham M, Lee T, Rodin A. Ontogeny of human complement receptors CR1 and CR3: expression of these molecules on monocytes and neutrophils from maternal, newborn, and fetal samples. Eur J Immunol 18:565–569, 1988.

Ainbender E, Cabatu EE, Guzmann DM, Sweet AY. Serum C–reactive protein and problems of newborn infants. J Pediatr 101:438–440, 1982.

Akbar AN, Terry L, Timms A, Beverly PC, Janossy G. Loss of CD45R and gain of UCHL1 reactivity is a feature of primed T cells. J Immunol 140:2171–2178, 1988.

Alenghat E, Esterly JR. Alveolar macrophages in perinatal infants. Pediatrics 74:221–224, 1984.

Alford CA, Stagno S, Reynolds DW. Diagnosis of chronic perinatal infections. Am J Dis Child 129:455–463, 1975.

Allansmith M, McClennan BH, Butterworth M, Maloney JR. The development of immunoglobulin levels in man. J Pediatr 72:276–290, 1968.

Ambrosino DM, Delaney NR, Shamberger RC. Human polysaccharide-specific B cells are responsive to pokeweed mitogen and IL-6. J Immunol 144:1221–1226, 1990.

Ambruso DR, Altenburger KM, Johnston RB. Defective oxidative metabolism in newborn neutrophils: discrepancy between superoxide anion and hydroxyl radical generation. Pediatrics 64:722–725, 1979.

Ambruso DR, Bentwood B, Henson PM, Johnston RB Jr. Oxidative metabolism of cord blood neutrophils: relationship to content and degranulation of cytoplasmic granules. Pediatr Res 18:1148–1153, 1984.

Anderson DC, Abbassi O, Kishimoto TK, Koenig JM, McIntire LV, Smith CW. Diminished lectin-, epidermal growth factor-, complement binding domain-cell adhesion molecule-1 on neonatal neutrophils underlies their impaired CD18-independent adhesion to endothelial cells in vitro. J Immunol 146:3372–3379, 1991.

Anderson DC, Freeman KB, Hughes BJ, Buffone GJ. Secretory determinants of impaired adherence and motility of neonatal PMNs. Pediatr Res 19:257A, 1985.

Anderson DC, Hughes BJ, Smith CW. Abnormal mobility of neonatal polymorphonuclear leukocytes. J Clin Invest 68:863–874, 1981.

Anderson DC, Hughes BJ, Wible GJ, Perry GJ, Smith CW, Brinkley BR. Impaired motility of neonatal PMN leukocytes: relationship to abnormalities of cell orientation and assembly of microtubules in chemotactic gradients. J Leukocyte Biol 36:1–15, 1984.

Anderson DC, Krishna GS, Hughes BJ, Mace ML, Mintz AA, Smith CW, Nichols BL. Impaired polymorphonuclear leukocyte motility in malnourished infants: relationship to functional abnormalities of cell adherence. J Lab Clin Med 101:881–895, 1983.

Anderson DC, Pickering LK, Feigin RD. Leukocyte function in normal and infected neonates. J Pediatr 85:420–425, 1974.

Anderson DC, Rothlein R, Marlin SD, Krater SS, Smith CW. Impaired transendothelial migration by neonatal neutrophils: abnormalities of Mac-1 (CD11b/CD18)-dependent adherence reactions. Blood 76:2613–2621, 1990.

Andersson U, Bird AG, Britton S, Palacios R. Humoral and cellular immunity in humans studied at the cell level from birth to two years of age. Immunol Rev 57:6–38, 1981.

Andersson U, Britton S, de Ley M, Bird G. Evidence for the ontogenic precedence of suppressor T cell functions in the human neonate. Eur J Immunol 13:6–13, 1983.

Antin JH, Emerson SG, Martin P, Gadol N, Ault KA. LEU-1$^+$ (CD5$^+$) B cells. A major lymphoid subpopulation in human fetal spleen: phenotypic and functional studies. J Immunol 136:505–510, 1986.

Arai K-I, Lee F, Miyajima A, Miyatake S, Arai N, Yokota T. Cytokines: coordinators of immune and inflammatory responses. Annu Rev Biochem 59:783–836, 1990.

Aruffo A, Farrington M, Hollenbaugh D, Li X, Milatovich A, Nonoyama S, Bajorath J, Grosmaire LS, Stenkamp R, Neubauer M, Roberts RL, Noelle RJ, Ledbetter JA, Francke U, Ochs HD. The CD40 ligand, gp39, is defective in activated T cells from patients with X-linked hyper-IgM syndrome. Cell 72:291–300, 1993.

Ashley RL, Dalessio J, Burchett S, Brown Z, Berry S, Mohan K, Corey L. Herpes simplex virus-2 (HSV-2) type-specific antibody correlates of protection in infants exposed to HSV-2 at birth. J Clin Invest 90:511–514, 1992.

Asma GEM, van den Bergh RL, Vossen JM. Characterization of early lymphoid precursor cells in the human fetus using monoclonal antibodies and anti-terminal deoxynucleotidyl transferase. Clin Exp Immunol 64:356–363, 1986.

Asma GEM, van den Bergh RL, Vossen JM. Use of monoclonal antibodies in a study of the development of T lymphocytes in the human fetus. Clin Exp Immunol 53:429–436, 1983.

Azuma M, Phillips JH, Lanier LL. CD28$^-$ T lymphocytes. Antigenic and functional properties. J Immunol 150:1147–1159, 1993.

Bahram S, Arnold D, Bresnahan M, Strominger JL, Spies T. Two putative subunits of a peptide pump encoded in the human major histocompatibility complex class II region. Proc Natl Acad Sci U S A 88:10094–10098, 1991.

Baker CJ, Edwards MS, Kasper DL. Role of antibody to native type III polysaccharide of group B streptococcus in infant infection. Pediatrics 68:544–549, 1981.

Baker CJ, Melish ME, Hall RT, Casto DT, Vasan U, Givner LB. Intravenous immune globulin for the prevention of nosocomial infection in low-birth-weight neonates. N Engl J Med 327:213–219, 1992.

Baley JE, Schacter BZ. Mechanisms of diminished natural killer cell activity in pregnant women and neonates. J Immunol 134:3042–308, 1985.

Baley JE, Stork EK, Warentin PI, Shurin SB. Buffy coat transfusions in neutropenic neonates with presumed sepsis: a prospective randomized trial. Pediatrics 80:712–720, 1987.

Ballow M, Cates KL, Rowe JC, Goetz C, Desbonnet C. Development of the immune system in very low birth weight (less than 1500 g) premature infants: concentrations of plasma immunoglobulins and patterns of infection. Pediatr Res 20:899–904, 1986.

Banchereau J, de Paoli P, Vallé Garcia E, Rousset F. Long-term human B cell lines dependent on interleukin-4 and antibody to CD40. Science 251:70–72, 1991.

Baraff LJ, Leake RD, Burstyn DG, Payne T, Cody CL, Manclark CR, St. Geme JW Jr. Immunologic response to early and routine DTP immunization in infants. Pediatrics 73:37–42, 1984.

Barbouche R, Forveille M, Fischer A, Avrameas S, Durandy A. Spontaneous IgM autoantibody production in vitro by B lymphocytes of normal human neonates. Scand J Immunol 35:659–667, 1992.

Barnard DR, Arthur MM. Fibronectin (cold insoluble globulin) in the neonate. J Pediatr 102:453–455, 1983.

Barnetson RSC, Bjune G, Duncan ME. Evidence for a soluble lymphocyte factor in the transplacental transmission of T-lymphocyte responses to *Mycobacterium leprae.* Nature 260:150–151, 1976.

Baroni CD, Valtieri M, Stoppacciaro A, Ruco LP, Uccini S, Ricci C. The human thymus in aging: histologic involution paralleled by increased mitogen response and by enrichment of OKT3$^+$ lymphocytes. Immunology 50:519–528, 1983.

Bazaral M, Orgel HA, Hamburger RN. IgE levels in normal infants and mothers and an inheritance hypothesis. J Immunol 107:794–801, 1971.

Becker ID, Robinson OM, Bazan TS, Lopez-Osuna M, Kretschmer RR. Bactericidal capacity of newborn phagocytes against group B beta-hemolytic streptococci. Infect Immun 34:535–539, 1981.

Bellanti JA, Nerurkar LS, Zeligs BJ. Host defenses in the fetus and neonate: studies of the alveolar macrophage during maturation. Pediatrics 64:726–739, 1979.

Benoist C, Mathis D. Demystification of the alloresponse. Curr Biol 1:143–144, 1991.

Berger RS, Dixon SL. Fulminant transfusion-associated graft-versus-host disease in a premature infant. J Am Acad Dermatol 20:945–950, 1989.

Berman JD, Johnson WD Jr. Monocyte function in human neonates. Infect Immun 19:898–902, 1978.

Bernbaum JC, Daft A, Anolik R, Samuelson J, Barkin R, Douglas S, Polin R. Response of preterm infants to diphtheria-tetanus-pertussis immunizations. J Pediatr 107:P184–188, 1985.

Bhaskaram C, Raghuramulu N, Reddy V. Cell-mediated immunity and immunoglobulin levels in light-for-date infants. Acta Paediatr Scand 66:617–619, 1977.

Bhat AM, Scanlon JW. The pattern of eosinophilia in premature infants: a prospective study in premature infants using the absolute eosinophil count. J Pediatr 98:612–616, 1981.

Bhat NM, Kantor AB, Bieber MM, Stall AM, Herzenberg LA, Teng NM. The ontogeny and functional characteristics of human B-1 (CD5$^+$ B) cells. Int Immunol 4:243–252, 1992.

Bigby M, Markowitz JS, Bleicher PA, Grusby MJ, Simha S, Siebrecht M, Wagner M, Nagler-Anderson C, Glimcher LH. Most $\gamma\delta$ T cells develop normally in the absence of MHC class II molecules. J Immunol 141:4465–4475, 1993.

Blackman MA, Tiggest MA, Minie ME, Koshland ME. A model system for peptide hormone action in differentiation: interleukin 2 induces a B lymphoma to transcribe the J chain gene. Cell 47:609–617, 1986.

Bodger MP, Janossy G, Bollum FJ, Burford GD, Hoffbrand AV. The ontogeny of terminal deoxynucleotidyl transferase positive cells in the human fetus. Blood 61:1125–1131, 1983.

Bofill M, Janossy G, Janossa M, Burford GD, Seymour GJ, Wernet P, Kelemen E. Human B cell development. II. Subpopulations in the human fetus. J Immunol 134:1531–1538, 1985.

Boner A, Zeligs BJ, Bellanti JA. Chemotactic responses of various differential stages of neutrophils from human cord and adult blood. Infect Immun 35:921–928, 1982.

Bonforte RJ, Topilsky M, Siltzbach LE, Glade PR. Phytohemagglutinin (PHA) skin test: a possible in vivo measure of cell-mediated immunity. J Pediatr 81:775–780, 1972.

Bonifazi E, Meneghini CL. Atopic dermatitis in the first six months of life. Acta Derm Venereol 144(Suppl.):20–22, 1989.

Borst J, Broom TM, Bos JD, van Dongen JJM. Tissue distribution and repertoire selection of human $\gamma\delta$ T cells: comparison with the murine system. Curr Top Microbiol Immunol 173:41–46, 1991.

Bortolussi R, Burbridge S, Durnford P, Schellekens H. Neonatal *Listeria monocytogenes* infection is refractory to interferon. Pediatr Res 29:400–402, 1991.

Bortolussi R, Issekutz T, Burbridge S, Schellekens H. Neonatal host defense mechanisms against *Listeria monocytogenes* infection: the role of lipopolysaccharides and interferons. Pediatr Res 25:311–315, 1989.

Bortolussi R, Rajaraman K, Serushago B. Role of tumor necrosis factor-α and interferon-γ in newborn host defense against *Listeria monocytogenes* infection. Pediatr Res 32:460–464, 1992.

Brody JI, Oski FA. Neonatal lymphocyte reactivity as an indicator of intrauterine bacterial contact. Lancet 1:1396–1398, 1968.

Brouns GS, de Vries E, van Noesel CJM, Mason DY, van Lier RAW, Borst J. The structure of the μ/pseudo light chain complex on human pre-B cells is consistent with a function in signal transduction. Eur J Immunol 23:1088–1097, 1993.

Bruce MC, Baley JE, Medvik KA, Berger M. Impaired surface membrane expression of C3bi but not C3b receptors on neonatal neutrophils. Pediatr Res 21:306–311, 1987.

Bucy RP, Chan C-LH, Cooper MD. Tissue localization and CD8 accessory molecule expression of T$\gamma\delta$ cells in humans. J Immunol 142:3045–3049, 1989.

Buimovici-Klein E, Lang PB, Ziring PR, Cooper LZ. Impaired cell-mediated immune response in patients with congenital rubella: correlation with gestational age at time of infection. Pediatrics 64:620–626, 1979.

Bullock JD, Robertson AF, Bodenbender JG, Kontras SB, Miller CE. Inflammatory responses in the neonate reexamined. Pediatrics 44:58–61, 1969.

Burchett SK, Corey L, Mohan KM, Westall J, Ashley R, Wilson CB. Diminished interferon-γ and lymphocyte proliferation in neonatal and postpartum primary herpes simplex virus infection. J Infect Dis 165:813–818, 1992.

Burgio GR, Lanzavecchia A, Plebani A, Jayakar S, Ugazio AG. Ontogeny of secretory immunity: levels of secretory IgA and natural antibodies in saliva. Pediatr Res 14:1111–1114, 1980.

Buseyne F, Blanche S, Schmitt D, Griscelli C, Riviere Y. Detection of HIV-specific cell-mediated cytotoxicity in the peripheral blood from infected children. J Immunol 150:3569–3581, 1993.

Byrne JA, Butler JL, Cooper MD. Differential activation requirements for virgin and memory T cells. J Immunol 141:3249–3257, 1988.

Byrne JA, Butler JL, Reinherz EL, Cooper MD. Virgin and memory T cells have different requirements for activation via the CD2 molecule. Int Immunol 1:29–35, 1989.

Cairo MS. Review of G-CSF and GM-CSF effects on neonatal neutrophil kinetics. Am J Pediatr Hematol Oncol 11:238–244, 1989.

Cairo MS, Rucker R, Bennetts GA, Hicks D, Worcester C, Amlie R, Johnson S, Katz J. Improved survival of newborns receiving leukocyte transfusions for sepsis. Pediatrics 74:887–892, 1984.

Cairo MS, van de Ven C, Toy C, Mauss D, Sender L. Recombinant human granulocyte-macrophage colony-stimulating factor primes neonatal granulocytes for enhanced oxidative metabolism and chemotaxis. Pediatr Res 26:395–399, 1989.

Cairo MS, Worcester C, Rucker R, Bennetts GA, Amlie R, Perkin R, Anas N, Hicks D. Role of circulating complement and polymorphonuclear leukocyte transfusion in treatment and outcome in critically ill neonates with sepsis. J Pediatr 100:935–941, 1987.

Cairo MS, Worcester CC, Rucker RW, Hanten S, Amlie RN, Sender L, Hicks DA. Randomized trial of granulocyte transfusions versus intravenous immune globulin therapy for neonatal neutropenia and sepsis. J Pediatr 120:281–285, 1992.

Campana D, Janossy G, Coustan-Smith E, Amlot PL, Tian WT, Ip S, Wong L. The expression of T cell receptor–associated proteins during T cell ontogeny in man. J Immunol 142:57–66, 1989.

Campbell AC, Waller C, Wood J, Aynsley-Green A, Yu V. Lymphocyte subpopulations in the blood of newborn infants. Clin Exp Immunol 18:469–482, 1974.

Catty D, Seger R, Drew R, Stroder J, Metze H. IgG subclass concentrations in cord sera from premature, full-term, and small-for-dates babies. Eur J Pediatr 125:89–96, 1977.

Cederblad B, Risenfeld T, Alm GV. Deficient herpes simplex virus–induced interferon-α production by blood leukocytes of preterm and term newborn infants. Pediatr Res 27:7–10, 1990.

Cederqvist LL, Ewool LC, Litwin SD. The effect of fetal age, birth weight, and sex on cord blood immunoglobulin values. Am J Obstet Gynecol 131:520–525, 1978.

Chabannon C, Wood P, Torok-Storb B. Expression of CD7 on normal human myeloid progenitors. J Immunol 149:2110–2113, 1992.

Chandra RK. Fetal malnutrition and postnatal immuno-competence. Am J Dis Child 129:450–454, 1975.

Chandra RK. Serum thymic hormone activity and cell-mediated immunity in healthy neonates, preterm infants, and small for gestational age infants. Pediatrics 67:407–411, 1981.

Chatila T, Wong R, Young M, Miller R, Terhorst C, Geha RS. An immunodeficiency characterized by defective signal transduction in T lymphocytes. N Engl J Med 320:696–702, 1989.

Chen Y, Nakane A, Minagawa T. Recombinant murine gamma interferon induces enhanced resistance to *Listeria monocytogenes* infection in neonatal mice. Infect Immun 57:2345–2349, 1989.

Chiba Y, Higashidate Y, Suga K, Honjo K, Tsutsumi H, Ogra PL. Development of cell-mediated cytotoxic immunity to respiratory syncytial virus in human infants following naturally acquired infection. J Med Virol 28:133–129, 1989.

Chilmonczyk BA, Levin MJ, McDuffy R, Hayward AR. Characterization of the human newborn response to herpesvirus antigen. J Immunol 134:4184–4188, 1985.

Choi Y, Kotzin B, Herron L, Callahan J, Marrack P, Kappler J. Interaction of *Staphylococcus aureus* toxin "superantigens" with human T cells. Proc Natl Acad Sci U S A 86:8941–8945, 1989.

Christensen RD. Hematopoiesis in the fetus and neonate. Pediatr Res 26:531–535, 1989.

Christensen RD, Rothstein G. Exhaustion of mature marrow neutrophils in neonates with sepsis. J Pediatr 96:316–318, 1980.

Christensen RD, Rothstein G. Pre- and postnatal development of granulocytic stem cells in the rat. Pediatr Res 18:599–602, 1984.

Christensen RD, Brown MS, Hall DC, Lassiter HA, Hill HR. Effect on neutrophil kinetics and serum opsonic capacity of intravenous administration of immune globulin to neonates with clinical signs of early-onset sepsis. J Pediatr 118:606–614, 1991.

Christensen RD, Rothstein G, Anstall HB, Bybee B. Granulocyte transfusions in neonates with bacterial infection, neutropenia, and depletion of mature marrow neutrophils. Pediatrics 70:1–6, 1982.

Christensen RD, Rothstein G, Hill HR, Pincus SH. The effect of hybridoma antibody administration upon neutrophil kinetics during experimental type III group B streptococcal sepsis. Pediatr Res 17:795–799, 1983.

Christensen RD, Shigeoka AO, Hill HR, Rothstein G. Circulating and storage neutrophil changes in experimental type II group B streptocococcal sepsis. Pediatr Res 14:806–808, 1980.

Clark EA, Lane PJL. Regulation of human B-cell activation and adhesion. Annu Rev Immunol 9:97–127, 1991.

Clement LT, Vink PE, Bradley GE. Novel immunoregulatory functions of phenotypically distinct subpopulations of CD4+ cells in the human neonate. J Immunol 145:102–108, 1990.

Clement LT, Yamashita N, Martin AM. The functionally distinct subpopulations of human CD4+ helper/inducer T lymphocytes defined by anti-CD45R antibodies derive sequentially from a differentiation pathway that is regulated by activation-dependent postthymic differentiation. J Immunol 141:1464–1470, 1988.

Cocchi P, Marianelli L. Phagocytosis and intracellular killing of *Pseudomonas aeruginosa* in premature infants. Helv Paediatr Acta 22:110–118, 1967.

Coen R, Grusch O, Kauder E. Studies of bactericidal activity and metabolism of the leukocyte in full-term neonates. J Pediatr 75:400–406, 1969.

Conley ME, Speert DP. Human neonatal monocyte-derived macrophages and neutrophils exhibit normal nonopsonic and opsonic receptor-mediated phagocytosis and superoxide anion production. Biol Neonate 60:361–366, 1991.

Conley ME, Kearney JF, Lawton AR III, Cooper MD. Differentiation of human B cells expressing the IgA subclasses as demonstrated by monoclonal hybridoma antibodies. J Immunol 125:2311–2316, 1980.

Coonrod JD, Jarrells MC, Bridges RB. Impaired pulmonary clearance of pneumococci in neonatal rats. Pediatr Res 22:736–742, 1987.

Cuisinier A-M, Fumoux F, Moinier D, Boubli L, Guigou V, Milili M, Schiff C, Fougereau M, Tonelle C. Rapid expansion of human immunoglobulin repertoire (V_H, V_κ, V_λ) expressed in early fetal bone marrow. New Biol 2:689–699, 1990.

Cuisinier A-M, Guigou V, Boubli L, Fougereau M, Tonelle C. Preferential expression of V_H5 and V_H6 immunoglobulin genes in early human B-cell ontogeny. Scand J Immunol 30:493–497, 1989.

Culver KW, Ammann AJ, Partridge JC, Wong DF, Wara DW, Cowan MJ. Lymphocyte abnormalities in infants born to drug-abusing mothers. J Pediatr 111:230–235, 1987.

Daar AS, Fuggle SV, Fabre JW, Ting A, Morris PJ. The detailed distribution of HLA-A, B, C antigens in normal human organs. Transplantation 38:287–292, 1984.

D'Ambola JB, Sherman MP, Tashkin DP, Gong H Jr. Human and rabbit newborn lung macrophages have reduced anti-candida activity. Pediatr Res 24:285–290, 1988.

Dancis J, Osborn JJ, Kunz HW. Studies of the immunology of the newborn infant. Pediatrics 12:151–156, 1953.

Danska JS, Livingstone AM, Paragas V, Ishihara T, Fathman CG. The presumptive CDR3 regions of both T cell receptor α and β chains determine T cell specificity for myoglobin peptides. J Exp Med 172:27–33, 1990.

Davis CA, Vallota EH, Forristal J. Serum complement levels in infancy: age-related changes. Pediatr Res 13:1043–1046, 1979.

Davis MM, Bjorkman PJ. T-cell antigen receptor genes and T-cell recognition. Nature 334:395–402, 1988.

DeBiagi M, Andreani M, Centis F. Immune characterization of human fetal tissues with monoclonal antibodies. Prog Clin Biol Res 193:89–94, 1985.

DeCoster A, Darcy F, Caron A, Vinatier D, Houze de l'Aulnoit G, Vittu G, Niel G, Heyer F, Lecolier B, Delcroix M, Monnier JC, Duhamel M, Capron A. Anti-P30 IgA antibodies as prenatal markers of congenital toxoplasma infection. Clin Exp Immunol 87:310–315, 1992.

De Jong R, Brouwer M, Miedema F, van Lier RAW. Human CD8+ T lymphocytes can be divided into CD45RA+ and CD45RO+ cells with different requirements for activation and differentiation. J Immunol 146:2088–2094, 1991.

De Libero G, Cassorati G, Giachino C, Carbmara C, Migone N, Matzinger P, Lanzavecchia A. Selection by two powerful antigens may account for the presence of the major population of human peripheral γδ+ T-cells. J Exp Med 173:1311–1322, 1991.

de Maurizio D, Tovo P-A, Galli L, Gabiano C, Cozzani S, Gotta C, Scarlatti G, Fiocchi A, Cocchi P, Marchisio P, Canino R, Mautone A, Chiappe F, Campelli A, Consolini R, Izzi G, Laverda A, Alberti S, Tozzi AE, Duse M. Prognostic significance of immunologic changes in 675 infants perinatally exposed to human immunodeficiency virus. J Pediatr 119:702–709, 1991.

de Paoli P, Battistin S, Santini GF. Age-related changes in human lymphocyte subsets: progressive reduction of the CD4 CD45R (suppressor-inducer) population. Clin Immunol Immunopathol 48:290–296, 1988.

del Canho R, Grosheide PM, Gerards LJ, Heijtink RA, Schalm SW. Hepatitis B vaccination and preterm infants. Pediatr Infect Dis J 12:407–408, 1993.

Dengrove J, Lee EJ, Heiner DC, St. Geme JW Jr, Leake R, Baraff LJ, Ward JI. IgG and IgG subclass–specific antibody responses to diphtheria and tetanus toxoids in newborns and infants given DTP immunization. Pediatr Res 20:735–739, 1986.

Desmonts G, Daffos F, Forestier F, Capella–Pavlosky M, Thulliez PH, Chartier M. Prenatal diagnosis of congenital toxoplasmosis. Lancet 1:500–504, 1985.

Dossett JH, William RC Jr, Quie PG. Studies on interaction of bacteria, serum factors, and polymorphonuclear leukocytes in mothers and newborns. Pediatrics 44:49–57, 1969.

Dressler F, Peter HH, Muller W, Rieger ChHL. Transient hypogammaglobulinemia of infancy. Five new cases: review of the literature and redefinition. Acta Paediatr Scand 78:767–774, 1989.

Durandy A, Thuillier L, Forveille M, Fischer A. Phenotypic and functional characteristics of human newborns' B lymphocytes. J Immunol 144:60–65, 1990.

Edwards JA, Durant BM, Jones DB, Evans PR, Smith JL. Differential expression of HLA class II antigens in fetal human spleen: relationship of HLA-DP, DQ, and DR to immunoglobulin expression. J Immunol 137:490–497, 1985.

Edwards MS, Buffone GJ, Fuselier PA, Weeks JL, Baker CJ. Deficient classical complement pathway activity in newborn sera. Pediatr Res 17:685–688, 1983.

Edwards MS, Hall MA, Rench MA, Baker CJ. Patterns of immune response among survivors of group B streptococcal meningitis. J Infect Dis 151:65–70, 1990.

Ehlers S, Smith KA. Differentiation of T cell lymphokine gene expression. The in vitro acquisition of T cell memory. J Exp Med 173:25–36, 1991.

Eibl MM, Wolf HM, Fürnkranz H, Rosenkranz A. Prevention of necrotizing enterocolitis in low-birth-weight infants by IgA-IgG feeding. N Engl J Med 319:1–7, 1988.

Einhorn MS, Granoff DM, Nahm MH, Quinn A, Shackelford PG. Concentrations of antibodies in paired maternal and infant sera: relationship to IgG subclass. J Pediatr 111:783–788, 1987.

Enders G. Serologic test combination for safe detection of rubella infections. Rev Infect Dis 7:S113–S122, 1985.

English BK, Burchett SK, English JD, Ammann AJ, Wara DW, Wilson CB. Production of lymphotoxin and tumor necrosis factor by human neonatal mononuclear cells. Pediatr Res 24:717–722, 1988.

English BK, Hammond WP, Lewis DB, Borwn CB, Wilson CB. Decreased granulocyte-macrophage colony-stimulating factor production by human neonatal blood mononuclear cells and T cells. Pediatr Res 31:211–216, 1992.

Englund JA, Mbawuike IN, Hammill H, Holleman MC, Baxter BD, Glezen WP. Maternal immunization with influenza or tetanus toxoid vaccine for passive antibody protection in young infants. J Infect Dis 168:647–656, 1993.

Erdmann SH, Christensen RD, Bradley PP, Rothstein, G. Supply and release of storage neutrophils. Biol Neonate 41:132–137, 1982.

Erkeller-Yuksel FM, Deneys V, Yuksel B, Hannet I, Hulstaert F, Hamilton C, Mackinnon H, Stokes LT, Munhyeshol V, Vanlangendonck F, deBruyere M, Bach BA, Lydyard, PM. Age-related changes in human blood lymphocyte subpopulations. J Pediatr 1120:216–222, 1992.

European Collaborative Study. Age-related standards for T lymphocyte subsets based on uninfected children born to human immunodeficiency virus 1–infected women. Pediatr. Infect Dis J 11:1018–1026, 1992.

Evans DG, Smith JWG. Response of the young infant to active immunization. Br Med Bull 19:225–229, 1963.

Fanaroff AA, Korones SB, Wright LL, Wright EC, Poland RL, Bauer CB, Tyson JE, Philips JB, Edwards W, Lucey JF, Catz CS, Shankaran S, Oh W (for the National Institute of Child Health and Human Development Neonatal Research Network). A controlled trial of intravenous immune globulin to reduce nosocomial infec-

tions in very-low-birth-weight infants. N Engl J Med 330:1107–1113, 1994.

Ferguson AC. Prolonged impairment of cellular immunity in children with intrauterine growth retardation. J Pediatr 93:52–56, 1978.

Ferguson AC, Lawlor GJ Jr, Neumann CG, Oh W, Stiehm ER. Decreased rosette-forming lymphocytes in malnutrition and intrauterine growth retardation. J Pediatr 85:717–723, 1974.

Fink CW, Miller WE, Dorward B, LoSpalluto J. The formation of macroglobulin antibodies. II. Studies on neonatal infants and older children. J Clin Invest 41:1422–1428, 1962.

Fischer GW, Wilson SR, Hunter KW. Functional characteristics of a modified immunoglobulin preparation for intravenous administration: summary of studies of opsonic and protective activity against group B streptococci. J Clin Immunol 2:31S–35S, 1982.

Fitzgerald MG, Pullen GR, Hosking CS. Low-affinity antibody to rubella antigen in patients after rubella infection in utero. Pediatrics 81:812–814, 1988.

Flidel O, Barak Y, Lipschitz–Mercer B, Frumkin A, Mogilner BM. Graft-versus-host disease in extremely low birth weight neonate. Pediatrics 89:689–690, 1992.

Fontan G, Lorente F, Rodriguez MCG, Ojeda JA. In vitro human neutrophil movement in umbilical cord blood. Clin Immunol Immunopathol 20:224–230, 1981.

Forestier F, Daffos F, Galactéros F, Bardakjian J, Rainaut M, Beuzard Y. Hematological values of 163 normal fetuses between 18 and 30 weeks of gestation. Pediatr Res 20:342–346, 1986.

Foster CA, Hollbrook KA. Ontogeny of Langerhans cells in human embryonic and fetal skin: cell densities and phenotypic expression relative to epidermal growth. Am J Anat 184:157–164, 1989.

Fowler R, Schubert WK, West CD. Acquired partial tolerance to homologous skin grafts in the human infant at birth. Ann NY Acad Sci 87:403–428, 1960.

Franz ML, Carella JA, Galant SP. Cutaneous delayed hypersensitivity in a healthy pediatric population: diagnostic value of diphtheria-tetanus toxoids. J Pediatr 88:975–978, 1976.

Freedman RM, Johnston D, Mahoney M, Pearson HA. Development of splenic reticuloendothelial function in neonates. J Pediatr 96:466–468, 1980.

Frenck RW Jr, Buescher ES, Vadhan-Raj S. The effects of recombinant human granulocyte-macrophage colony stimulating factor in in vitro cord blood granulocyte function. Pediatr Res 26:43–48, 1989.

Friedmann PS. Cell-mediated immunological reactivity in neonates and infants with congenital syphilis. Clin Exp Immunol 30:271–276, 1977.

Gallagher MR, Welliver R, Yamanaka T, Eisenberg B, Sun M, Ogra PL. Cell-mediated immune responsiveness to measles. Am J Dis Child 135:48–51, 1981.

Ganz T, Sherman MP, Selsted ME, Lehrer RI. Newborn rabbit alveolar macrophages are deficient in two microbicidal cationic peptides, MCP-1 and MCP-2. Am Rev Respir Dis 132:901–904, 1985.

Gathings WE, Kubugawa H, Cooper MD. A distinctive pattern of B cell immaturity in perinatal humans. Immunol Rev 57:107–126, 1981.

Gathings WE, Lawton AR, Cooper MD. Immunofluorescent studies of the development of pre-B cells, B lymphocytes, and immunoglobulin isotype diversity in humans. Eur J Immunol 7:804–810, 1977.

Geelen SPM, Fleer A, Bezemer AC, Gerards LJ, Rijkers GT, Verhoef J. Deficiencies in opsonic defense to pneumococci in the human newborn despite adequate levels of complement and specific IgG antibodies. Pediatr Res 27:514–518, 1990.

Geertsma MF, Broos HR, van den Barselaar MT, Nibbering PH, van Furth R. Lung surfactant suppresses oxygen-dependent bactericidal functions of human blood monocytes by inhibiting the assembly of the NADPH oxidase. J Immunol 150:2391–2400, 1993.

Gehrz RC, Knorr SO, Marker SC, Kalis JM, Balfour HH Jr. Specific cell-mediated immune defect in active cytomegalovirus infection of young children and their mothers. Lancet 2:844–847, 1977.

George JF Jr, Schroeder HW Jr. Developmental regulation of D_β reading frame and junctional diversity in T cell receptor–β transcripts from human thymus. J Immunol 148:1230–1239, 1992.

Gerdes JS, Yoder MC, Douglas SD, Polin RA. Decreased plasma fibronectin in neonatal sepsis. Pediatrics 72:877–881, 1983.

Gerli R, Bertotto A, Crupi S, Arcangeli C, Marinelli I, Spinozzi F,

Cernetti C, Angelella P, Rambotti P. Activation of cord T lymphocytes. I. Evidence for a defective T cell mitogenesis induced through the CD2 molecule. J Immunol 142:2583–2589, 1989.

Gilfillan S, Dierich A, Lemeur M, Benoist C, Mathis D. Mice lacking TdT: mature animals with an immature lymphocyte repertoire. Science 261:1175–1178, 1993.

Gilhus NE, Matre R, Tonder O. Hassall's corpuscles in the thymus of fetuses, infants, and children: Immunological and histochemical aspects. Thymus 7:123–135, 1985.

Gill TJ, Repetti CF, Metlay LA, Rabin BS, Taylor FH, Thompson DS, Cortese AL. Transplacental immunization of the human fetus to tetanus by immunization of the mother. J Clin Invest 72:987–996, 1983.

Gill TJ III, Karasic RB, Antoncic J, Rabin BS. Long-term follow-up of children born to women immunized with tetanus toxoid during pregnancy. Am J Reprod Immunol 25:69–71, 1991.

Gitlin D, Biasucci A. Development of γG, γA, γM, β1C–β1A, C1 esterase inhibitor, ceruloplasmin, transferrin, hemopexin, haptoglobin, fibrinogen, plasminogen, α_1-antitrypsin, orosomucoid, β-lipoprotein, α_2-macroglobulin, and prealbumin in the human conceptus. J Clin Invest 48:1433–1446, 1969.

Gleicher N, Siegel I, Cederqvist LL. Do glucocorticosteroids affect the fetal immune system? Am J Reprod Immunol 1:185–186, 1981.

Glover DM, Growstein D, Burchett S, Larsen A, Wilson CB. Expression of HLA class II antigens and secretion of interleukin-one by monocytes and macrophages from adults and neonates. Immunology 61:195–201, 1987.

Glover MT, Atherton DV, Levinsky RJ. Syndrome of erythroderma, failure to thrive, and diarrhea in infancy: a manifestation of immunodeficiency. Pediatrics 81:66–72, 1988.

Gluck L, Silverman WA. Phagocytosis in premature infants. Pediatrics 20:951–957, 1957.

Goerlich R, Hacker G, Pfeffer K, Heeg K, Wagner H. *Plasmodium falciparum* merozoites primarily stimulate the Vγ9 subset of human $\gamma\delta$ T cells. Eur J Immunol 21:2613–2616, 1991.

Granberg C, Hirvonen T, Toivanen P. Cell-mediated lympholysis by human maternal and neonatal lymphocytes: mother's reactivity against neonatal cells and vice versa. J Immunol 123:2563–2567, 1979.

Granoff DM, Shackelford PG, Pandey JP, Boies EG. Antibody responses to *Haemophilus influenzae* type b polysaccharide vaccine in relation to Km(1) and G2m(23) immunoglobulin allotypes. J Infect Dis 154:257–264, 1986.

Gray D. Immunologic memory. Annu Rev Immunol 11:49–78, 1993.

Griffiths PD, Stagno S, Pass RF, Smith RJ, Alford CA Jr. Congenital cytomegalovirus infection: diagnostic and prognostic significance of the detection of specific immunoglobulin M antibodies in cord serum. Pediatrics 69:544–550, 1982.

Griffiths-Chu S, Patterson JAK, Berger CL, Edelson RL, Chu AC. Characterization of immature T cell subpopulations in neonatal blood. Blood 64:396–300, 1984.

Guagliardi L, Koppelman B, Blum JS, Marks MS, Creswell P, Brodsky FM. Co-localization of molecules involved in antigen processing and presentation in an early endocytic compartment. Nature 343:133–139, 1990.

Gunn T, Reece ER, Metrakos K, Colle E. Depressed T cells following neonatal steroid treatment. Pediatrics 67:61–67, 1981.

Gupta S, Pahwa R, O'Reilly R, Good RA, Siegal FP. Ontogeny of lymphocyte subpopulations in human fetal liver. Proc Natl Acad Sci. U S A 73:919–922, 1976.

Haemophilus b conjugate vaccines for prevention of *Haemophilus influenzae* type b disease among infants and children two months of age and older. MMWR Morb Mortal Wkly Rep 40:1–7, 1991.

Hammond GW, Lukes H, Wells B, Thompson L, Low DE, Cheang M. Maternal and neonatal neutralizing antibody titers to selected enteroviruses. Pediatr Infect Dis J 4:32–35, 1985.

Handzel ZT, Levin S, Dolphin A, Schlesinger M, Hahn T, Altman Y, Schechter B, Shneyour A, Trainin N. Immune competence of newborn lymphocytes. Pediatrics 65:461–463, 1983.

Harding CV, Collins DS, Slot JW, Geuze HJ, Unanue ER. Liposome-encapsulated antigens are processed in lysosomes, recycled, and presented to T cells. Cell 64:393–401, 1991.

Hardy RR. CD5 B cells: a separate lineage at last? Curr Biol 1:290–292, 1991.

Haregewoin A, Soman G, Hom RC, Finberg RW. Human $\gamma\delta^+$ T cells respond to mycobacterial heat-shock protein. Nature 340:309–312, 1989.

Harris MC, Douglas SD, Kolski GB, Polin RA. Functional properties of anti–group B streptococcal monoclonal antibodies. Immunol Immunopathol 24:342–350, 1982.

Harris MC, Stroobant J, Cody CS, Douglas SD, Polin RA. Phagocytosis of group B streptococcus by neutrophils from newborn infants. Pediatr Res 17:358–361, 1983.

Harrison CJ, Waner JL. Natural killer cell activity in infants and children excreting cytomegalovirus. J Infect Dis 151:301–307, 1985.

Harvey JE, Jones DB. Distribution of LCA protein subspecies and the cellular adhesion molecules LFA-1, 1CAM-1 and p150,95 within human foetal thymus. Immunology 70:203–209, 1990.

Harvey J, Jones DB, Wright DH. Differential expression of MHC- and macrophage-associated antigens in human fetal and postnatal small intestine. Immunology 69:409–415, 1990.

Hawes CS, Kemp AS, Jones WR. In vitro parameters of cell-mediated immunity in the human neonate. Clin Immunol Immunopathol 17:530–536, 1980.

Haworth JC, Dilling L. Concentration of gamma A–globulin in serum, saliva, and nasopharyngeal secretions of infants and children. J Lab Clin Med 67:922–933, 1966.

Haynes BF, Martin ME, Kay HH, Kurtzberg J. Early events in human T cell ontogeny. Phenotypic characterization and immunohistologic localization of T cell precursors in early human fetal tissues. J Exp Med 168:1061–1080, 1988.

Hayward AR. Development of lymphocyte responses and interactions in the human fetus and newborn. Immunol Rev 57:61–87, 1981.

Hayward AR, Ezer G. Development of lymphocyte populations in the human foetal thymus and spleen. Clin Exp Immunol 17:169–178, 1974.

Hayward AR, Kurnick J. Newborn T cell suppression: early appearance, maintenance in culture, and lack of growth factor suppression. J Immunol 126:50–53, 1981.

Hayward AR, Merrill D. Requirement for OKT8$^+$ suppressor cell proliferation for suppression by human newborn T cells. Clin Exp Immunol 45:468–474, 1981.

Hayward AR, Herberger MJ, Groothuis J, Levin MR. Specific immunity after congenital or neonatal infection with cytomegalovirus or herpes simplex virus. J Immunol 133:2469–2473, 1984.

Hayward AR, Herberger M, Saunders D. Herpes simplex virus–stimulated γ-interferon production by newborn mononuclear cells. Pediatr Res 20:398–401, 1986.

Hayward AR, Lee J, Beverley PCL. Ontogeny of expression of UCHL1 antigen on TcR-1$^+$ (CD4/8) and TcRδ^+ T cells. Eur J Immunol 19:771–773, 1989.

Heath WR, Kane KP, Mescher MF, Sherman LA. Alloreactive T cells discriminate among a diverse set of endogenous peptides. Proc Natl Acad Sci U S A 88:5101–5105, 1991.

Herzenberg LA, Stall AM, Lalor PA, Sidman C, Moore WA, Parks DR, Herzenberg LA. The LY-1 B cell lineage. Immunol Rev 93:81–102, 1986.

Hill HR. Biochemical, structural, and functional abnormalities of polymorphonuclear leukocytes in the neonate. Pediatr Res 22:375–382, 1987.

Hill HR. Intravenous immunoglobulin use in the neonate: role in prophylaxis and therapy of infection. Pediatr Infect Dis J 12:549–559, 1993.

Hill HR, Augustine NH, Jaffee HS. Human recombinant interferon γ enhances neonatal polymorphonuclear leukocyte activation and movement and increases free intracellular calcium. J Exp Med 173:767–770, 1991.

Hoffman AR, Hayward AR, Kurnick JT, Defreitas EC, McGregor J, Harbeck RJ. Presentation of antigen by human newborn monocytes to maternal tetanus toxoid–specific T-cell blasts. J Clin Immunol 1:217–221, 1981.

Hofman FM, Danilovs JA, Taylor CR. HLA-DR (1a)-positive dendritic-like cells in human fetal nonlymphoid tissues. Transplantation 27:590–594, 1984.

Hohfeld P, Forestier F, Marion S, Thulliez P, Marcon P, Daffos F. *Toxoplasma gondii* infection during pregnancy: T lymphocyte subpopulations in mothers and fetuses. Pediatr Infect Dis J 9:878–881, 1990.

Hollenbaugh D, Grosmaire LS, Kullas CD, Chalupny NJ, Braesch-

Andersen S, Noelle RJ, Stamenkovic I, Ledbetter JA, Aruffo A. The human T cell antigen gp39, a member of the TNF gene family, is a ligand for the CD40 receptor: expression of a soluble form of gp39 with B cell co-stimulatory activity. EMBO J 11:4313–4321, 1992.

Holoshitz J, Koning F, Coligan JE, DeBruyn J, Strober S. Isolation of CD4⁻ CD8⁻ mycobacteria-reactive T lymphocyte clones from rheumatoid arthritis synovial fluid. Nature 339:226–229, 1989.

Hoover ML, Chapman SW, Cuchens MA. A procedure for the isolation of highly purified populations of B cells, T cells, and monocytes from human peripheral and umbilical cord blood. J Immunol Methods 78:71–85, 1985.

Horst E, Meijer CJLM, Duijvestijn AM, Hartwig N, Van der Harten HJ, Pals ST. The ontogeny of human lymphocyte recirculation: high endothelial cell antigen (HECA-452) and CD44 homing receptor expression in the development of the immune system. Eur J Immunol 20:1483–1489, 1990.

Hoshino T, Yamada A, Hionda J, Imai YL, Nakao M, Inoue M, Sagawa K, Yokoyama MM, Oizumi K, Itoh K. Tissue-specific distribution and age-dependent increase of human CD11b⁺ T cells. J Immunol 151:2237–2246, 1993.

Huang S, Hendriks W, Althage A, Hemmi S, Bluethmann H, Kamijo R, Vilcek J, Zinkernagel RM, Aguet M. Immune response in mice that lack the interferon-γ receptor. Science 259:1742–1745, 1993.

Hunt DF, Michel H, Dickinson TA, Shabanowitz J, Cox AL, Sakaguchi K, Appella E, Grey HM, Sette A. Peptides presented to the immune system by the murine class II major histocompatibility complex molecule I-Aᵈ. Science 256:1817–1820, 1992.

Iguchi K, Inous S, Kamar A. Effect of recombinant human granulocyte colony–stimulating factor administration in normal and experimentally infected newborn rats. Exp Hematol 19:352–358, 1991.

Isaacs D, Bangham CRM, McMichael AJ. Cell-mediated cytotoxic response to respiratory syncytial virus in infants with bronchiolitis. Lancet 2:769–771, 1987.

Itohara S, Mombaerts P, Lafaille J, Iacomini J, Nelson A, Clarke AR, Hooper ML, Farr A, Tonegawa S. T cell receptor δ gene mutant mice: independent generation of αβ T cells and programmed rearrangements of γδ TCR genes. Cell 72:337–348, 1993.

Ivanyi L, Lehner T. Interdependence of in vitro responsiveness of cord and maternal blood lymphocytes to antigens from oral bacteria. Clin Exp Immunol 30:252–258, 1977.

Jacobs RF, Wilson CB, Smith AL, Haas JE. Age-dependent effects of aminobutyryl muramyl dipeptide on alveolar macrophage function in infant and adult macaca monkeys. Am Rev Respir Dis 128:862–867, 1983.

Johnston RB, Altenburger KM, Atkinson AW, Curry RH. Complement in the newborn infant. Pediatrics 64:781–786, 1979.

Jones DH, Schmalstieg FC, Dempsey K, Krater SS, Nannen DD, Smith CW, Anderson DC. Subcellular distribution and mobilization of MAC-1 (CD11b/CD18) in neonatal neutrophils. Blood 75:488–498, 1990.

Jores R, Alzari PM, Meo T. Resolution of hypervariable regions in T-cell receptor β chains by a modified Wu-Kabat index of amino acid diversity. Proc Natl Acad Sci U S A 87:9138–9142, 1990.

Josephs SH, Buckley RH. Serum IgD concentrations in normal infants, children, and adults and in patients with elevated IgE. J Pediatr 96:417–420, 1980.

Kabelitz D. Function and specificity of human γ/δ-positive T cells. Crit Rev Immunol 11:281–303, 1992.

Kabelitz D, Bender A, Prospero T, Wesselborg S, Janssen O, Pechhold K. The primary response of human γδ⁺ T-cells to mycobacterium tuberculosis is restricted to Vγ9-bearing cells. J Exp Med 173:1331–1338, 1991.

Kabelitz D, Bender A, Schondelmaier S, da Silva Lobo ML, Janssen O. Human cytotoxic lymphocytes. V. Frequency and specificity of γδ⁺ cytotoxic lymphocyte precursors activated by allogeneic autologous stimulator cells. J Immunol 145:2827–2832, 1990.

Kamran S, Usmani SS, Wapnir RA, Mehta R, Harper RG. In vitro effect of indomethacin on polymorphonuclear leukocyte function in preterm infants. Pediatr Res 33:32–35, 1993.

Kaplan J, Shope TC, Bollinger RO, Smith J. Human newborns are deficient in natural killer activity. J Clin Immunol 2:350–355, 1982.

Kelemen E, Janossa M. Macrophages are the first differentiated blood cells formed in human embryonic liver. Exp Hematol 8:996–1000, 1980.

Kikawa Y, Shigematsu Y, Sudo M. Leukotriene B₄ biosynthesis in polymorphonuclear leukocytes from blood of umbilical cord, infants, children, and adults. Pediatr Res 20:402–406, 1986.

Kingsley G, Pitzalis C, Waugh AP, Panayi GS. Correlation of immunoregulatory function with cell phenotype in cord blood lymphocytes. Clin Exp Immunol 73:40–45, 1988.

Kinney R, Mundorf L, Gleason C, Lee C, Townsend T, Thibault R, Nussbaum A, Abby H, Yolken R. Efficacy and pharmacokinetics of intravenous immune globulin administration to high-risk neonates. Am J Dis Child 145:1233–1238, 1991.

Kitamura D, Kudo A, Schaal S, Muller W, Melchers F, Rajewsky K. A critical role of λ5 protein in B cell development. Cell 69:823–831, 1992.

Klein RB, Fischer TJ, Gard SE, Biberstein M, Rich KC, Stiehm ER. Decreased mononuclear and polymorphonuclear chemotaxis in human newborns, infants, and young children. Pediatrics 60:467–472, 1977.

Kniker WT, Lesourd BM, McBryde JL, Corriel RN. Cell-mediated immunity assessed by multitest CMI skin testing in infants and preschool children. Am J Dis Child 139:840–845, 1985.

Kobayashi R, Hyman CJ, Stiehm ER. Immunologic maturation in an infant born to a mother with agammaglobulinemia. Am J Dis Child 134:922–924, 1980.

Koblin BA, Townsend TR, Munoz A, Onorato I, Wilson M, Polk BF. Response of preterm infants to diphtheria-tetanus-pertussis vaccine. Pediatr Infect Dis J 7:704–711, 1988.

Kohl S. The neonatal human's immune response to herpes simplex virus infection: a critical review. Pediatr Infect Dis J 8:67–74, 1989.

Kohl S. Protection against murine neonatal herpes simplex virus infection by lymphokine-treated human leukocytes. J Immunol 144:307–312, 1990.

Kohl S, Harmon MW. Human neonatal leukocyte interferon production and natural killer cytotoxicity in response to herpes simplex virus. J Interferon Res 3:461–463, 1983.

Kohl S, Loo LS, Drath DB, Cox P. Interleukin-2 protects neonatal mice from lethal herpes simplex virus infection: a macrophage-mediated, γ interferon–induced mechanism. J Infect Dis 159:239–247, 1989a.

Kohl S, West MS, Prober CG, Sullender WM, Loo LS, Arvin AM. Neonatal antibody-dependent cellular cytotoxicity antibody levels are associated with the clinical presentation of neonatal herpes simplex virus infection. J Infect Dis 160:770–776, 1989b.

Kohler PF. Maturation of the human complement system. I. Onset time and sites of fetal C1q, C4, C3, and C5 synthesis. J Clin Invest 52:671–678, 1973.

Kohler PF, Farr RS. Elevation of cord over maternal IgG immunoglobulin: evidence for an active placental IgG transport. Nature 210:1070–1071, 1966.

Komori T, Okada A, Stewart V, Alt FW. Lack of N regions in antigen receptor variable region genes of TdT-deficient lymphocytes. Science 261:1171–1175, 1993.

Koulova L, Yang SY, Dupont B. Identification of the anti–CD3-unresponsive subpopulation of CD4⁺, CD45RA⁺ peripheral T lymphocytes. J Immunol 145:2035–2043, 1990.

Koup RA, Wilson CB. Clinical immunology of HIV-infected children. In Pizzo P, Wilfert C.M., eds. Pediatric AIDS: The Challenge of HIV Infection in Infants, Children, and Adolescents, 2nd ed. Baltimore, Williams & Wilkins, 1994, pp. 129–157.

Kozbor D, Trinchieri G, Monos DS, Isobe M, Russo G, Haney JA, Zmijewski C, Croce CM. Human TCR-γ⁻/δ⁻, CD8⁻ T lymphocytes recognize tetanus toxoid in a MHC-restricted fashion. J Exp Med 169:1847–1851, 1989.

Kraal G, Ter Hart H, Meelhuizen C, Venneker G, Claassen E. Marginal zone macrophages and their role in the immune response against T-independent type 2 antigens: modulation of the cells with specific antibody. Eur J Immunol 19:675–680, 1989.

Krangel MS, Yssel H, Brocklehurst D, Spits H. A distinct wave of human T-cell receptor lymphocytes in the early fetal thymus: evidence for controlled gene rearrangement and cytokine production. J Exp Med 172:847–859, 1990.

Krause PJ, Herson VC, Eisenfeld L, Johnson GM. Enhancement of neutrophil function for treatment of neonatal infections. Pediatr Infect Dis J 8:382–389, 1989.

Krause PJ, Maderazo EG, Scroggs M. Abnormalities of neutrophil adherence in newborns. Pediatrics 69:184–188, 1982.

Kretschmer RR, Stewardson PR, Papierniak CK, Gotoff SP. Chemotactic and bactericidal capacities of human newborn monocytes. J Immunol 117:1303–1307, 1976.

Kuhlman M, Joiner K, Ezekowitz RAB. The human mannose-binding protein functions as an opsonin. J Exp Med 169:1733–1745, 1989.

Kühn R, Rajewsky K, Müller W. Generation and analysis of interleukin-4–deficiency mice. Science 254:707–710, 1991.

Kurland G, Cheung ATW, Miller ME, Ayin SA, Cho MM, Ford EW. The ontogeny of pulmonary defenses: alveolar macrophage function in neonatal and juvenile rhesus monkeys. Pediatr Res 23:292–297, 1988.

Kurtzberg J, Denning SM, Nycum LM, Singer KH, Haynes BF. Immature human thymocytes can be driven to differentiate into nonlymphoid lineages by cytokines from thymic epithelial cells. Proc Natl Acad Sci U S A 86:7575–7579, 1989.

Laing IA, Boulton FE, Hume R. Polymorphonuclear leukocyte transfusion in neonatal septicaemia. Arch Dis Child 58:1003–1005, 1983.

Lang RA, Bishop JM. Macrophages are required for cell death and tissue remodeling in the developing mouse eye. Cell 74:453–462, 1993.

Lanier LL, Allison JP, Phillips JH. Correlation of cell surface antigen expression on human thymocytes by multi-color flow cytometric analysis: implications for differentiation. J Immunol 137:3501–2507, 1986.

Lanier LL, Change C, Spits H, Phillips JH. Expression of cytoplasmic CD3ε proteins in activated human adult natural killer (NK) cells and CD3γ,δ,ε complexes in fetal NK cells. Implications for the relationship of NK and T lymphocytes. J Immunol 149:1876–1880, 1992a.

Lanier LL, Spits H, Phillips JH. The relationship between NK and T cells. Immunol. Today 13:392–395, 1992b.

Lassiter HA, Watson SW, Seifring ML, Tanner JE. Complement factor 9 deficiency in serum of human neonates. J Infect Dis 166:53–57, 1992.

Lata JA, Tuan RS, Shepley KJ, Mulligan MM, Jackson LG, Smith JB. Localization of major histocompatibility complex class I and II mRNA in human first-trimester chorionic villi by in situ hybridization. J Exp Med 175:1027–1032, 1992.

Lau Y-L, Tam AYC, Ng KW. Clinical laboratory observations. Response of preterm infants to hepatitis B vaccine. J Pediatr 121:962–965, 1992.

Laurenti F, Ferro R, Giancarlo I, Isacchi G, Panero A, Savignoni PG, Malagnino F, Palermo D, Mandelli F, Bucci G. Polymorphonuclear leukocyte transfusion for the treatment of sepsis in the newborn infant. J Pediatr 98:118–123, 1981.

Laver J, Duncan E, Abboud M, Gasparetto C, Sahdev I, Warren D, Bussel J, Auld P, O'Reilly RJ, Moore MA. High levels of granulocyte and granulocyte-macrophage colony–stimulating factors in cord blood of normal full-term neonates. J Pediatr 116:627–632, 1990.

Lawton AR III, Asofsky R, Hylton MB, Cooper MD. Suppression of immunoglobulin class synthesis in mice. I. Effects of treatment with antibody to μ-chain. J Exp Med 135:277–297, 1972.

Lazzarin A, Capsoni F, Moroni M, Pardi G, Marini A. Leucocyte function after antenatal betamethasone given to prevent respiratory distress (letter to the editor). Lancet 2:1354–1355, 1977.

Lee SI, Heiner DC, Wara D. Development of serum IgG subclass levels in children. Mongr Allergy 19:108–121, 1986.

Leikin S. Differences in transformation of adult and newborn lymphocytes stimulated by antigens in mother and child. Clin Exp Immunol 22:457-460, 1975.

Leikin S, Oppenheim JJ. Differences in transformation of adult and newborn lymphocytes stimulated by antigen, antibody, and antigen-antibody complexes. Cell Immunol 1:468–475, 1971.

Lewis DB, Yu CC, Meyer J, English BK, Kahn SJ, Wilson CB. Cellular and molecular mechanisms for reduced interleukin-4 and interferon-γ production by neonatal T cells. J Clin Invest 87:194–202, 1991.

Lobach DF, Hensley LL, Ho W, Haynes BF. Human T cell antigen expression during the early stages of fetal thymic maturation. J Immunol 135:1752–1759, 1985.

Long EO. Antigen processing for presentation to CD4+ T cells. New Biol 4:274–282, 1992.

Lubens RG, Gard SE, Soderberg-Warner M, Stiehm ER. Lectin-dependent T-lymphocyte and natural killer cytotoxic deficiencies in human newborns. Cell Immunol 74:40–53, 1982.

Luzuriaga K, Koup RA, Pikora CA, Brettler DB, Sullivan JL. Deficient human immunodeficiency virus type 1–specific cytotoxic T cell responses in vertically infected children. J Pediatr 119:230–236, 1991.

Magny J-F, Bremard-Oury C, Brault D, Menguy C, Voyer M, Landais P, Dehan M, Gabilan JC. Intravenous immunoglobulin therapy for prevention of infection in high-risk premature infants: report of a multicenter, double-blind study. Pediatrics 88:437–443, 1991.

Mami-Chouaib F, Miossec C, Del Porto P, Flament C, Triebel F, Hercend T. T-cell target 1 (TCT 1): A novel target molecule for human non–major histocompatibility complex-restricted T lymphocytes. J Exp Med 172:1071–1082, 1990.

Manroe BL, Weinberg AG, Rosenfeld CR, Browne R. The neonatal blood count in health and disease. I. Reference values for neutrophilic cells. J Pediatr 95:89–98, 1979.

Marodi L, Leijh PCJ, Braat A, Daha MR, Van Furth R. Opsonic activity of cord blood sera against various species of microorganism. Pediatr Res 19:433–436, 1985.

Martensson L, Fudenberg HH. Gm genes and gamma G-globulin synthesis in the human fetus. J Immunol 94:514–520, 1965.

Martin TR, Rubens CE, Wilson CB. Lung antibacterial defense mechanisms in infant and adult rats: implications for the pathogenesis of group B streptococcal infections in the neonatal lung. J Infect Dis 147:91–100, 1988.

Martin TR, Ruzinski JT, Rubens CE, Chi EV, Wilson CB. The effect of type-specific polysaccharide capsule on the clearance of group B streptococci from the lungs of infant and adult rats. J Infect Dis 165:306–314, 1992.

Marwitz PA, Van Arkel VE, Rijkers GT, Zegers BJ. Expression and modulation of cell surface determinants on human adult and neonatal monocytes. Clin Exp Immunol 72:260–266, 1988.

McCafferty MH, Lepow M, Saba TM, Cho E, Meuwissen H, White J, Zuckerbrod SF. Normal fibronectin levels as a function of age in the pediatric population. Pediatr Res 17:482–485, 1983.

McCracken GH, Eichenwald HF. Leukocyte function and the development of opsonic and complement activity in the neonate. Am J Dis Child 121:120–126, 1971.

McDonald T, Sneed J, Valenski WR, Dockter M, Cooke R, Herrod HG. Natural killer cell activity in very low birth weight infants. Pediatr Res 31:376–380, 1992.

McFarland HI, Nahill SR, Maciaszek JW, Welsh RM. CD11b (Mac-1): a marker for CD8+ cytotoxic T cell activation and memory in virus infection. J Immunol 149:1326–1333, 1992.

McGeady SJ. Transient hypogammaglobulinemia of infancy: need to reconsider name and definition. J Pediatr 110:47–50, 1987.

McKay E, Thom H. Observations on neonatal tears. J Pediatr 75:1245–1256, 1969.

McLeod R, Mack DG, Boyer K, Mets M, Roizen N, Swisher C, Patel D, Beckmann E, Vitullo D, Johnson D, Meier P. Phenotypes and functions of lymphocytes in congenital toxoplasmosis. J Lab Clin Med 116:623–635, 1990.

McNabb T, Koh TY, Dorrington KJ, Painter RH. Structure and function of immunoglobulin domains. V. Binding of immunoglobulin G and fragments to placental membrane preparations. J Immunol 117:882–888, 1976.

McVay LD, Carding SR, Bottomly K, Hayday AC. Regulated expression and structure of T cell receptor γ/δ transcripts in human thymic ontogeny. EMBO J 10:83–91, 1991.

Mellander L, Carlsson B, Hanson LA. Appearance of secretory IgM and IgA antibodies to *Escherichia coli* in saliva during early infancy and childhood. J Pediatr 104:564–568, 1984.

Metcalf ES, Klinman NR. In vitro tolerance induction of neonatal murine B cells. J Exp Med 143:13270–1340, 1976.

Michie CA, McLean A, Alcock C, Beverley PCL. Lifespan of human lymphocyte subsets defined by CD45 isoforms. Nature 360:264–265, 1992.

Miller ME. Chemotactic function in the human neonate: humoral and cellular aspects. Pediatr Res 5:487–492, 1971.

Miller ME. Phagocyte function in the neonate: selected aspects. Pediatrics 64:709–712, 1979.

Miller ME, Nilsson UR. A familial deficiency of the phagocytosis enhancing activity of serum related to a dysfunction of the fifth component of complement (C5). N Engl J Med 282:354–358, 1970.

Miller ME, Nilsson UR. A major role for the fifth component of complement (C5) in the opsonization of yeast particles. Partial dichotomy of functional and immunochemical measurement. Clin Immunol Immunopathol 2:246–255, 1974.

Mills EL, Bjorksten B, Quie PG. Deficient alternative complement pathway activity in newborn sera. Pediatr Res 13:1341–1344, 1979a.

Mills EL, Thompson T, Bjorksten B, Filipovich D, Quie PG. The chemiluminescence response and bactericidal activity of polymorphonuclear neutrophils from newborns and their mothers. Pediatrics 63:429–434, 1979b.

Mintz L, Drew WL, Hoo R, Finley TN. Age-dependent resistance of human alveolar macrophages to herpes simplex virus. Infect Immun 28:417–420, 1980.

Miyawaki T, Kubo M, Nagaoki T, Moriya N, Yukoi T, Mukai M, Taniguchi N. Developmental changes in humoral suppressor activity released from concanavalin A–stimulated human lymphocytes on B cell differentiation. J Immunol 126:1720–1723, 1981a.

Miyawaki T, Moriya N, Takeshi N, Taniguchi N. Maturation of B-cell differentiation ability and T-cell regulatory function in infancy and childhood. Immunol Rev 57:61–87, 1981b.

Modlin JF, Polk BF, Horton P, Etkind P, Crane E, Spiliotes A. Perinatal echovirus infection: risk of transmission during a community outbreak. N Engl J Med 305:368–371, 1981.

Mombaerts P, Arnoldi J, Russ F, Tonegawa S, Kaufmann SHE. Different roles of α/β and γ/δ T cells in immunity against an intracellular bacterial pathogen. Nature 365:53–56, 1993.

Moretta L, Ciccone E, Moretta A, Hoglund P, Ohlen C, Karre K. Allorecognition by NK cells: non-self or no self? Immunol Today 13:300–306, 1992.

Morimoto C, Letvin NL, Distaso JA, Aldrich WR, Schlossmann SF. The isolation and characterization of the human suppressor inducer T cell subset. J Immunol 134:1508–1515, 1985.

Morimoto C, Letvin NL, Distaso JA, Brown HM, Schlossman SF. The cellular basis for the induction of antigen-specific T8 suppressor cells. Eur J Immunol 16:198–204, 1986.

Morito T, Bankhurst AD, Williams RC. Studies of human cord blood and adult lymphocyte interactions with in vitro immunoglobulin production. J Clin Invest 64:990–995, 1979.

Morrison LA, Lukacher AE, Braciale VL, Fan DP, Braciale TJ. Differences in antigen presentation to MHC class I- and class II-restricted influenza virus-specific cytolytic T lymphocyte clones. J Exp Med 163:903–921, 1986.

Mortari F, Newton JA, Wange JY, Schroeder HW Jr. The human cord blood antibody repertoire. Frequent usage of the V$_H$7 gene family. Eur J Immunol 22:241–245, 1992.

Mortari F, Wang J-Y, Schroeder HW Jr. Human cord blood antibody repertoire: mixed population of V$_H$ gene segments and CDR3 distribution in the expressed Cα and Cγ repertoires. J Immunol 150:1348–1357, 1993.

Munoz AI, Limbert D. Skin reactivity to *Candida* and streptokinase-streptodornase antigens in normal pediatric subjects: influence of age and acute illness. J Pediatr 88:975–978, 1977.

Naeye RL, Diener MM, Harcke HT Jr, Blanc WA. Relation of poverty and race to birth weight and organ and cell structure in the newborn. Pediatr Res 5:17–22, 1971.

Naiman JL, Punnett HH, Lischner HW, Destine ML, Arey JB. Possible graft-versus-host reaction after intrauterine transfusion for Rh erythroblastosis fetalis. N Engl J Med 281:697–701, 1969.

Nair MPN, Schwartz SA, Menon M. Association of decreased natural and antibody-dependent cellular cytotoxicity and production of natural killer cytotoxic factor and interferon in neonates. Cell Immunol 94:159–171, 1985.

Naot YD, Desmonts G, Remington JS. IgM enzyme-linked immunosorbent assay test for the diagnosis of congenital toxoplasma infection. J Pediatr 98:32–36, 1981.

Nejedla Z. The development of immunological factors in infants with hyperbilirubinemia. Pediatrics 45:102–104, 1970.

Newburger PE. Superoxide generation by human fetal granulocytes. Pediatr Res 16:373–376, 1982.

Nishimoto N, Kubugawa H, Ohno T, Gartland GL, Stankovic AK, Cooper MD. Normal pre-B cells express a receptor complex of μ heavy chains and surrogate light-chain proteins. Proc Natl Acad Sci U S A 88:6284–6288, 1991.

Noelle RJ, Ledbetter JA, Aruffo A. CD40 and its ligand, an essential ligand-receptor pair for thymus-dependent B-cell activation. Immunol Today 13:431–433, 1992.

Nonoyama S, Penix LA, Edwards CP, Aruffo A, Wilson CB, Ochs HD. Diminished expression of CD40 ligand (gp39) by activated neonatal T cells. J Clin Invest 95:66–75, 1995.

Notarangelo LD, Chirico G, Chiara A, Colombo A, Rondini G, Plebani A, Martini A, Ugazio AG. Activity of classical and alternative pathways of complement in preterm and small for gestational age infants. Pediatr Res 18:281–285, 1984.

Nuchtern JG, Biddison WE, Klausner RD. Class II MHC molecules can use the endogenous pathway of antigen presentation. Nature 343:74–76, 1990.

Nunoi H, Endo F, Chikazawa S, Namikawa T, Matsuda I. Chemotactic receptor of cord blood granulocytes to the synthesized chemotactic peptide N-formyl-methionyl-leucyl-phenylalanine. Pediatr Res 17:57–60, 1983.

Ochs HD, Wedgwood RJ. IgG subclass deficiencies. Annu Rev Med 38:325–340, 1987.

Ochs HD, Nonoyama S, Zhu Q, Farrington M, Wedgwood RJ. Regulation of antibody responses: the role of complement and adhesion molecules. Clin Immunol Immunopathol 67:S33–S40, 1993.

Okumura M, Fujii Y, Inada K, Nakahara K, Matsuda H. Both CD45RA$^+$ and CD45RA$^-$ subpopulations of CD8$^+$ T cells contain cells with high levels of lymphocyte function–associated antigen-1 expression, a phenotype of primed T cells. J Immunol 150:429–437, 1993.

Olding LB, Murgita RA, Wigzell H. Mitogen-stimulated lymphoid cells from human newborns suppress the proliferation of maternal lymphocytes across a cell-impermeable membrane. J Immunol 119:1109–1114, 1977.

Oliver AM, Sewell HF, Abramovich DR, Thomson AW. The distribution and differential expression of MHC class II antigens (HLA-DR, DP, and DQ) in human fetal adrenal, pancreas, thyroid, and gut. Transplant Proc 21:651–652, 1989.

Orlowski JP, Sieger L, Anthony BF. Bactericidal capacity of monocytes of newborn infants. J Pediatr 89:797–801, 1976.

Oseas R, Lehrer RI. A micromethod for measuring neutrophil candidicidal activity in neonates. Pediatr Res 12:828–829, 1979.

Paganelli R, Ramadas D, Layward L, Harvey BA, Soothhill JF. Maternal smoking and cord blood immunity function. Clin Exp Immunol 36:256–259, 1979.

Pahwa SG, Pahwa R, Grimes E, Smithwick E. Cellular and humoral components of monocyte and neutrophil chemotaxis in cord blood. Pediatr Res 11:677–680, 1977.

Park BH, Holmes B, Good RA. Metabolic activities in leukocytes of newborn infants. J Pediatr 76:237–241, 1970.

Parker CM, Groh V, Band H, Porcelli SA, Morita C, Fabbi M, Glass D, Strominger JL, Brenner MB. Evidence for extra-thymic changes in the T-cell receptor γδ repertoire. J Exp Med 171:1597–1612, 1990.

Parkman R, Mosler D, Unmansky I, Cochran W, Carpenter CB, Rosen FS. Graft-versus-host disease after intrauterine and exchange transfusions for hemolytic disease of the newborn. N Engl J Med 290:359–363, 1974.

Peakman M, Buggins AGS, Nicolaides KH, Layton DM, Vergani D. Analysis of lymphocyte phenotypes in cord blood from early gestation fetuses. Clin Exp Immunol 90:345–350, 1992.

Peault B, Weissman IL, Baum C, McCune JM, Tsukamoto A. Lymphoid reconstitution of the human fetal thymus in SCID mice with CD34$^+$ precursor cells. J Exp Med 174:1283–1286, 1991.

Peeters CCAM, Tenbergen-Meekes A-M, Heijnen CJ, Poolman JT, Zegers BJM, Rijkers GT. Interferon-γ and interleukin-6 augment the human in vitro antibody response to the *Haemophilus influenzae* type b polysaccharide. J Infect Dis 165(Suppl 1):S161–S162, 1992.

Perchalski JE, Clem LW, Small PA. 7S gamma-M immunoglobulin in normal human cord serum. Am J Med Sci 256:107–111, 1968.

Peterson JC, Christie A. Immunization in the young infant: Response to combined vaccines: I–IV. Am J Dis Child 81:484–491, 1951.

Pfeifer JD, Wick MJ, Roberts RL, Findlay K, Normark SJ, Harding CV. Phagocytic processing of bacterial antigens for class I MHC presentation to T cells. Nature 361:359–362, 1993.

Phillips JH, Lanier LL. Lectin-dependent and anti-CD3 induced cytotoxicity are preferentially mediated by peripheral blood cytotoxic T lymphocytes expressing Leu-7 antigen. J Immunol 136:1579–1585, 1986.

Phillips JH, Hori T, Nagler A, Bhat N, Spits H, Lanier LL. Ontogeny of human natural killer (NK) cells: fetal NK cells mediate cytolytic function and express cytoplasmic CD3ε,δ proteins. J Exp Med 175:1055–1066, 1992.

Philpott KL, Viney JL, Kay G, Rastan S, Gardiner EM, Chae S, Hayday AC, Owen MJ. Lymphoid development in mice congenitally lacking T cell receptor αβ-expressing cells. Science 256:1448–1452, 1992.

Pirenne H, Aujard Y, Eljaafari A, Bourillon A, Qury JF, Le Gac S, Blot P, Sterkers G. Comparison of T cell functional changes during childhood with the ontogeny of CDw29 and CD45RA expression on CD4+ T cells. Pediatr Res 32:81–86, 1992.

Pittard WB, Miller KM, Sorensen RU. Perinatal influences on in vitro B lymphocyte differentiation in human neonates. Pediatr Res 19:655–658, 1985.

Pitzalis C, Kingsley GH, Covelli M, Meliconi R, Markey A, Panayi GS. Selective migration of the human helper-inducer memory T cell subset: confirmation by in vivo cellular kinetic studies. Eur J Immunol 21:369–376, 1991.

Plaeger-Marshall S, Ank BJ, Altenburger KM, Pizer LM, Johnston RB Jr., Stiehm ER. Replication of herpes simplex virus in blood monocytes and placental macrophages from human neonates. Pediatr Res 26:135–139, 1989.

Playfair JHL, Wolfendale MR, Kay HEM. The leucocytes of peripheral blood in the human foetus. Br J Haematol 9:336–344, 1963.

Poggi A, Sargiacomo M, Biassoni R, Pella N, Sivori S, Revello V, Costa P, Valtieri M, Russo G, Mingari MC, Peschle C, Moretta L. Extrathymic differentiation of T lymphocytes and natural killer cells from human embryonic liver precursors. Proc Natl Acad Sci U S A 90:4465–4469, 1993.

Porcelli S, Brenner MB, Greenstein JL, Balk SP, Terhorst C, Bleicher PA. Recognition of cluster of differentiation 1 antigens by human CD4− CD8− T lymphocytes. Nature 341:447–450, 1989.

Provenzano RW, Wetterlow LH, Sullivan CL. Immunization and antibody response in the newborn infant. N Engl J Med 273:959–965, 1965.

Punnonen J, Aversa GG, Vandekerckhove B, Roncarolo MG, de Vries JE. Induction of isotype switching and Ig production by CD5+ and CD10+ human fetal B cells. J Immunol 148:3398–3404, 1992.

Raaphorst FM, Timmers E, Kenter MJH, Van Tol MJD, Vossen JM, Schuurman RKB. Restricted utilization of germ-line V$_H$3 genes and short diverse third complementarity-determining regions (CDR3) in human fetal B lymphocyte immunoglobulin heavy chain rearrangements. Eur J Immunol 22:247–251, 1992.

Raff HV, Bradley C, Brady W, Donaldson K, Lipsich L, Maloney G, Shuford W, Walls M, Ward P, Wolff E, Harris LJ. Comparison of functional activities between IgG1 and IgM class–switched human monoclonal antibodies reactive with group B streptococci or *Escherichia coli* K1. J Infect Dis 163:346–354, 1991.

Raff MC, Owen JJT, Cooper MD, Lawton AR, Megson M, Gathings WE. Difference in susceptibility of mature and immature B lymphocytes to anti–immunoglobulin-induced immunoglobulin suppression in vitro. Possible implications for B-cell tolerance to self. J Exp Med 142:1052–1064, 1975.

Raghunathan R, Miller ME, Everett S, Leake RD. Phagocyte chemotaxis in the perinatal period. J Clin Immunol 2:242–246, 1982.

Rao S, Olesinski R, Doshi U, Vidyasagar D. Granulocyte adherence in newborn infants. J Pediatr 98:622–624, 1981.

Raulet DH. A sense of something missing. Nature 358:21–22, 1992.

Ray CG. The ontogeny of interferon production by human leukocytes. J Pediatr 76:94–98, 1970.

Rayfield LS, Brent O, Rodeck CH. Development of cell-mediated lympholysis in human foetal blood lymphocytes. Clin Exp Immunol 42:561–570, 1980.

Remington JS, Sheafer IA. Transport piece in the urines of premature infants. Nature 217:364–365, 1968.

Report of the Committee on Infectious Diseases, 22nd ed. Elk Grove Village, Ill., American Academy of Pediatrics, 1991.

Reynolds DW, Dean PH, Pass RF, Alford CA. Specific cell-mediated immunity in children with congenital and neonatal cytomegalovirus infection and their mothers. J Infect Dis 140:493–499, 1979.

Roberts RL, Szelc CM, Scates SM, Boyd MT, Soderstrom KM, Davis MW, Glaspy JA. Neutropenia in an extremely premature infant treated with recombinant human granulocyte colony–stimulating factor. Am J Dis Child 145:808–812, 1991.

Roche PA, Cresswell P. Invariant chain association with HLA-DR molecules inhibits immunogenic peptide binding. Nature 345:615–618, 1990.

Rola-Pleszczynski M, Hensen SA, Vincent MM, Bellanti JA. Inhibitory effects of bilirubin on cellular immune responses in man. J Pediatr 86:690–696, 1975.

Ross SC, Densen P. Complement deficiency states and infection: epidemiology, pathogenesis and consequences of neisserial and other infections in an immune deficiency. Medicine 63:243–273, 1984.

Rothberg AD, Cohn RJ, Argent AC, Sher R, Joffe M. Eosinophilia in premature neonates. S A Med J 64:539–541, 1983.

Rousset F, Garcia E, Banchereau J. Cytokine-induced proliferation and immunoglobulin production of human B lymphocytes triggered through their CD40 antigen. J Exp Med 173:705–710, 1991.

Rubaltelli FF, Piovesan AL, Semenzato G, Barbato A, Ongaro G. Immune competence assessment in hyperbilirubinemic newborn before and after phototherapy. Helv Paediatr Acta 32:129–133, 1977.

Rubin HR, Sorensen RU, Polmar SH. Lymphocyte responses of human neonates to bacterial antigens. Cell Immunol 57:307–315, 1981.

Ryhanen P, Kauppila A, Koivisto M. Unaltered neonatal cell-mediated immunity after prenatal dexamethasone treatment. Obstet Gynecol 56:182–185, 1980.

Sacchi F, Hill HR. Defective membrane potential changes in neutrophils from human neonates. J Exp Med 160:1247–1252, 1984.

Sancho L, de la Hera A, Casas J, Vanquer S, Martinez C, Alvarez-Mon M. Two different maturational stages of natural killer lymphocytes in human newborn infants. J Pediatr 119:446–454, 1991.

Sanders ME, Makgoba MW, June CH, Young HA, Shaw S. Enhanced responsiveness of human memory T cells to CD2 and CD3 receptor-mediated activation. Eur J Immunol 19:803–808, 1989.

Sanders ME, Makgoba MW, Shaw S. Human naive and memory T cells: reinterpretation of helper-inducer and suppressor-inducer subsets. Immunol Today 9:195–199, 1988a.

Sanders ME, Makgoba MW, Sharrow SO, Stephany D, Springer TA, Young HA, Shaw S. Human memory T lymphocytes express increased levels of three cell adhesion molecules (LFA-3, CD2, and LFA-1) and three other molecules (UCHL1, CD29, and Pgp-1) and have enhanced IFN-γ production. J Immunol 141:1401–1407, 1988b.

Santos JI, Shigeoka AO, Hill HR. Functional leukocyte administration in protection against experimental neonatal infection. Pediatr Res 14:1408–1410, 1980.

Sanz I. Multiple mechanisms participate in the generation of diversity of human H chain CDR3 regions. J Immunol 147:1720–1729, 1991.

Schimpl A, Schorle H, Holschke T, Horak I. Development and function of T cells in mice rendered IL-2 deficient by targeted disruption of the IL-2 locus (abstract). Cytokine 3:515, 1992.

Schlesinger JJ, Covelli HD. Evidence for transmission of lymphocyte responses to tuberculin by breast-feeding. Lancet 2:529–532, 1977.

Schoub BD, Johnson S, McAnerney J, Gilbertson L, Klaassen KI, Reinach SG. Monovalent neonatal polio immunization: a strategy for the developing world. J Infect Dis 147:836–839, 1988.

Schreiber JR, Berger M. Intravenous immune globulin therapy for sepsis in premature neonates. J Pediatr 121:401–404, 1992.

Schroeder HW Jr., Hillson JL, Perlmutter RM. Early restriction of the human antibody repertoire. Science 238:791–793, 1987.

Schuit KE, Powell DA. Phagocyte dysfunction in monocytes of normal newborn infants. Pediatrics 65:501–504, 1980.

Schutte MEM, Ebeling SB, Akkermans-Koolhaas KE, Logtenberg T. Deletion mapping of Ig V$_H$ gene segments expressed in human CD5 B cell lines. J Immunol 149:3953–3960, 1992.

Seki H, Ueno Y, Taga K, Matsuda A, Miyawaki T, Taniguchi N. Mode of in vitro augmentation of natural killer cell activity by recombinant human interleukin 2: a comparative study of Leu-11+ and Leu-11− cell populations in cord blood and adult peripheral blood. J Immunol 135:2351–2356, 1985.

Sevjcar J, Miler I, Pekarek J. Effects of bilirubin on an in vitro correlate of cell-mediated immunity: the migration inhibition test. J Clin Lab Immunol 3:145–149, 1984.

Shapiro LM, Bassen FA. Sternal marrow changes during the first week of life: correlation with peripheral blood findings. Am J Med Sci 292:341–354, 1941.

Shapiro R, Beatty DW, Woods DL, Malan AF. Serum complement and immunoglobulin values in small-for-gestational-age infants. J Pediatr 99:139–142, 1981.

Sheldon WH, Caldwell JB. The mononuclear cell phase of inflammation in the newborn. Bull Johns Hopkins Hosp 112:258–269, 1963.

Sherman MP, Lehrer RI. Oxidative metabolism of neonatal and adult rabbit lung macrophages stimulated with opsonized group B streptococci. Infect Immun 47:26–30, 1985.

Sherman MP, Johnson JT, Rothlein R, Hughes BJ, Smith CW, Anderson DC. Role of pulmonary phagocytes in host defense against group B streptococci in preterm versus term rabbit lung. J Infect Dis 166:818–826, 1992.

Shigeoka AO, Wittwer CT. Transient deficiency of neutrophil receptor CR3 in early infancy associated with delayed umbilical cord separation or infection: role of maternal anti-neutrophil antibody (abstract). Clin Res 41:24A, 1993.

Shigeoka AO, Charette RP, Wyman ML, Hill HR. Defective oxidative metabolic responses of neutrophils from stressed neonates. J Pediatr 98:392–398, 1981.

Shigeoka AO, Hall RT, Hill HR. Blood-transfusion in group B streptococcal sepsis. Lancet 1:626–638, 1978.

Shigeoka AO, Pincus SH, Rote NS, Hill HR. Protective efficacy of hybridoma type-specific antibody against experimental infection with group B streptococcus. J Infect Dis 149:363–372, 1984.

Shigeoka AO, Santos JI, Hill HR. Functional analysis of neutrophil granulocytes from healthy, infected, and stressed neonates. J Pediatr 95:454–460, 1979.

Shimoya K, Matsuzaki N, Taniguichi T, Jo T, Saji F, Kitajima H, Fujimura M, Nakayama M, Tanizawa O. Interleukin-8 in cord sera: a sensitive and specific marker for the detection of preterm chorioamnionitis. J Infect Dis 165:957–950, 1992.

Shiratsuchi H, Tsuyuguchi I. Tuberculin purified protein derivative-reactive T cells in cord blood lymphocytes. Infect Immun 33:651–657, 1981.

Siegel RL, Issekutz T, Schwaber J, Rosen FS, Geha RS. Deficiency of T helper cells in transient hypogammaglobulinemia of infancy. N Engl J Med 305:1307–1313, 1981.

Skeen MJ, Ziegler HK. Induction of murine peritoneal γ/δ T cells and their role in resistance to bacterial infection. J Exp Med 178:971–984, 1993.

Small TN, Keever C, Collins N, Dupont B, O'Reilly RJ, Flomenberg N. Characterization of B cells in severe combined immunodeficiency disease. Human Immunol 25:181–193, 1989.

Smith DH, Peter G, Ingram DL, Harding AL, Anderson P. Responses of children immunized with the capsular polysaccharide of *Haemophilus influenzae.* Pediatrics 52:637–644, 1973.

Smith JB, Campbell DE, Ludomirsky A, Polin RA, Douglas SD, Garty BZ, Harris MC. Expression of the complement receptors CR1 and CR3 and the type III Fcγ receptor on neutrophils from newborn infants and from fetuses with Rh disease. Pediatr Res 28:120–126, 1990a.

Smith JB, Kunjummen RD, Kishimoto TK, Anderson DC. Expression and regulation of L-selectin on eosinophils from human adults and neonates. Pediatr Res 32:465–471, 1992.

Smith MD, Worman C, Yuksel F, Yuksel B, Moretta L, Ciccone E, Grossi CE, MacKenzie L, Lydyard PM. Tγδ-cell subsets in cord and adult blood. Scand J Immunol 32:491–495, 1990b.

Smith RT, Eitzman DV, Catlin ME, Wirtz EO, Miller BE. The development of the immune response. Pediatrics 33:163–183, 1964.

Smolen P, Bland R, Heiligenstein E, Lawless MR, Dillard R, Abramson J. Antibody response to oral polio vaccine in premature infants. J Pediatr 103:917–920, 1983.

Solvason N, Kearney JF. The human fetal omentum: a site of B cell generation. J Exp Med 175:397–404, 1992.

Speer CP, Ambruso DR, Grimsley J, Johnston RB Jr. Oxidative metabolism in cord blood monocytes and monocyte-derived macrophages. Infect Immun 50:919–921, 1985.

Speer CP, Gahr M, Wieland M, Eber S. Phagocytosis-associated functions in neonatal monocyte-derived macrophages. Pediatr Res 24:213–216, 1988.

Splawski JB, Lipsky PE. Cytokine regulation of immunoglobulin secretion by neonatal lymphocytes. J Clin Invest 88:967–977, 1991.

Squire E, Favara B, Todd J. Diagnosis of neonatal bacterial infection: hematologic and pathologic findings in fatal and nonfatal cases. Pediatrics 64:60–64, 1979.

Stagno S, Pass RF, Cloud G, Britt WJ, Henderson RE, Walton PD, Veren DA, Page F, Alford CA. Primary cytomegalovirus infection in pregnancy. JAMA 256:1904–1908, 1986.

Starr SE, Tolpin MD, Friedman HM, Paucker K, Plotkin SA. Impaired cellular immunity to cytomegalovirus in congenitally infected children and their mothers. J Infect Dis 140:500–505, 1979.

Steele RW, Suttle DE, LeMaster PC, Patterson FD, Canales L. Screening for cell-mediated immunity in children. Am J Dis Child 130:1218–1221, 1976.

Stepick-Biek P, Thulliez P, Araujo FG, Remington JS. IgA antibodies for diagnosis of acute congenital and acquired toxoplasmosis. J Infect Dis 162:270–273, 1990.

Stiehm ER, Fudenberg HH. Serum levels of immune globulins in health and disease: a survey. Pediatrics 37:715–726, 1966.

Stiehm ER, Sztein MB, Steeg PS, Mann D, Newland C, Blaese M, Oppenheim JJ. Deficient DR antigen expression human cord blood monocytes: reversal with lymphokines. Clin Immunol Immunopathol 30:430–436, 1984.

Strauss R, Snyder E. Chemotactic peptide binding by intact neutrophils from human neonates. Pediatr Res 18:63–66, 1984.

Strauss RG, Rossenberger TG, Wallace PD. Neutrophil chemiluminescence during the first month of life. Acta Haematol 63:326–329, 1980.

Stroobant J, Harris MC, Cody CS, Polin RA, Douglas SD. Diminished bactericidal capacity for group B streptococcus in neutrophils from "stressed" and healthy neonates. Pediatr Res 18:634–637, 1984.

Sullender WM, Miller JL, Yasukawa LL, Bradley JS, Black SB, Yeager AS, Arvin AM. Humoral and cell-mediated immunity in neonates with herpes simplex virus infection. J Infect Dis 155:28–37, 1987.

Super M, Thiel S, Lu J, Levinsky RJ, Turner MW. Association of low levels of mannan-binding protein with a common defect of opsonisation. Lancet 2:1236–1239, 1989.

Tarkkanen J, Saksela E. Umbilical cord blood–derived suppressor cells of the human natural killer cell activity are inhibited by interferon. Scand J Immunol 15:149–157, 1982.

Tedder TF, Clement LT, Cooper MD. Human lymphocyte differentiation antigens HB-10 and HB-11. I. Ontogeny of antigen expression. J Immunol 134:2983–2988, 1985.

Terstappen LWMM, Huang S, Picker LJ. Flow cytometric assessment of human T-cell differentiation in thymus and bone marrow. Blood 79:666–677, 1992.

Teyton L, O'Sullivan D, Dickson PW, Lotteau V, Sette A, Fink P, Peterson PA. Invariant chain distinguishes between the exogenous and endogenous antigen presentation pathways. Nature 348:39–44, 1990.

Thong YH, Hurtado RC, Rola-Pleszczynski M, Hensen SA, Vincent MM, Micheletti SA, Bellanti JA. Transplacental transmission of cell-mediated immunity. Lancet 1:1286–1287, 1974.

Tiller TL Jr., Buckley RH. Transient hypogammaglobulinemia of infancy: review of the literature, clinical and immunologic features of 11 new cases, and long-term follow-up. J Pediatr 92:347–553, 1978.

Timens W, Boes A, Rozeboom-Uiterwijk T, Poppema S. Immaturity of the human splenic marginal zone in infancy. Possible contribution to the deficient infant immune response. J Immunol 143:3200–3206, 1989.

Timens W, Rozeboom T, Poppema S. Fetal and neonatal development of human spleen: an immunohistological study. Immunology 60:603–609, 1987.

Toivanen P, Uksila J, Leino A, Lassila O, Hirvonen T, Ruuskanen O. Development of mitogen-responding T cells and natural killer cells in the human fetus. Immunol Rev 57:89–105, 1981.

Tono-Oka T, Nakayama M, Uehara H, Matsumoto S. Characteristics of impaired chemotactic function in cord blood leukocytes. Pediatr Res 13:148–151, 1979.

Tosato G, Magrath IT, Koski IR, Dooley NJ, Blaese RM. B cell differentiation and immunoregulatory T cell function in human cord blood lymphocytes. J Clin Invest 66:383–388, 1980.

Tovo PA, Ponzone A. Cellular and humoral factors involvement in the enhanced NBT reduction by neutrophil leucocytes of newborn infants. Acta Paediatr Scand 66:549–552, 1977.

Townsend A, Bodmer H. Antigen recognition by class I–restricted T lymphocytes. Annu Rev Immunol 7:601–624, 1989.

Tsuyuguchi I, Kawasumi H, Ueta C, Yano I, Kishimoto S. Increase of T-cell receptor γ/δ-bearing T cells in cord blood of newborn babies obtained by in vitro stimulation with mycobacterial cord factor. Infect Immun 59:3053–3059, 1991.

Ueno Y, Koizumi S, Yamagami M, Miura M, Taniguchi N. Characterization of hemopoietic stem cells (CFU$_c$) in cord blood. Exp Hematol 9:716–711, 1981.

Ueno Y, Miyawaki T, Seki H, Matsuda A, Taga K, Sato H, Taniguchi N. Differential effects of recombinant human interferon-γ and interleukin 2 on natural killer cell activity of peripheral blood in early human development. J Immunol 135:180–184, 1985.

Uhr JW, Dancis J, Franklin EC, Finkelstein MS, Lewis EW. The antibody response to bacteriophage in newborn premature infants. J Clin Invest 41:1509–1513, 1962.

Uhr JW, Dancis J, Neumann CG. Delayed-typed hypersensitivity in premature neonatal humans. Nature 187:1130–1131, 1960.

Usmani SS, Schlessel JS, Sia CG, Kamran S, Orner SD. Polymorphonuclear leukocyte function in the preterm neonate. Pediatrics 87:675–679, 1991.

Valles-Ayoub Y, Govan HL III, Braun J. Evolving abundance and clonal pattern of human germinal center B cells during childhood. Blood 76:17–23, 1990.

Vanderkerkhove BAE, Baccala R, Jones D, Kono DH, Theofilopoulos AN, Roncarolo MG. Thymic selection of the human T cell receptor Vβ repertoire in SCID-hu mice. J Exp Med 176:1619–1624, 1992.

van de Winkel JGJ, Anderson CL. Biology of human immunoglobulin G Fc receptors. J Leukoc Biol 49:511–524, 1991.

van Es JH, Gmelig FHJ, Logtenberg T. High frequency of somatically mutated IgM molecules in the human adult blood B cell repertoire. Eur J Immunol 22:2761–2764, 1992.

Van Kaer L, Ashton-Rickardt PG, Ploegh HL, Tonegawa S. TAP1 mutant mice are deficient in antigen presentation, surface class I molecules, and CD4$^-$ 8$^+$ T cells. Cell 71:1205–1214, 1992.

van Zee KJ, DeForge LE, Fischer E, Marano MA, Kenney JS, Remick DG, Lowry SF, Moldawer LL. IL-8 in septic shock, endotoxemia, and after IL-1 administration. J Immunol 146:3478–3482, 1991.

Versteeg R. NK cells and T cells: mirror images? Immunol Today 13:244–247, 1992.

Walker RI, Willemze R. Neutrophil kinetics and the regulation of granulopoiesis. Rev Infect Dis 2:282–292, 1980.

Warwick WJ, Good RA, Smith RT. Failure of passive transfer of delayed hypersensitivity in the newborn human infant. J Lab Clin Med 56:139–147, 1960.

Weisman LE, Stoll BJ, Kueser TJ, Rubio TT, Frank CG, Heiman HS, Subramanian KN, Hankins CT, Anthony BF, Cruess DF, Hemming VG, Fischer GW. Intravenous immune globulin therapy for early-onset sepsis in premature neonates. J Pediatr 121:434–443, 1992.

Werner-Favre C, Vischer TL, Wohlwend D, Zubler RH. Cell surface antigen CD5 is a marker for activated human B cells. Eur J Immunol 19:1209–1213, 1989.

Weston WL, Carson BS, Barkin RM, Slater GD, Dustin RD, Hecht SK. Monocyte-macrophage function in the newborn. Am J Dis Child 131:1241–1242, 1977.

Wheeler JG, Chauvenet AR, Johnson CA, Block SM, Dillard R, Abramson JS. Buffy coat transfusion in neonates with sepsis and neutrophil storage depletion. Pediatrics 79:422–425, 1987.

Willems van Dijk K, Milner LA, Sasso EH, Milner ECB. Chromosomal organization of the heavy chain variable region gene segments comprising the human fetal antibody repertoire. Proc Natl Acad Sci U S A 89:10430–10434, 1992.

Wilson CB. Lung antimicrobial defenses in the newborn. Semin Respir Med 6:149–155, 1984.

Wilson CB. The role of T-cell immaturity in the physiologic immunodeficiency of the fetus and neonate. In Report of the 101st Ross Conference on Pediatric Research December 1991, pp. 64–74, Columbus, Ohio.

Wilson CB, Haas JE. Cellular defenses against *Toxoplasma gondii* in newborns. J Clin Invest 73:1606–1616, 1984.

Wilson CB, Desmonts G, Couvreur J, Remington JS. Lymphocyte transformation in the diagnosis of congenital toxoplasma infection. N Engl J Med 302:785–788, 1980.

Wilson CB, Ochs HD, Almquist J, Dassel S, Mauseth R, Ochs UH.

When is umbilical cord separation delayed? J Pediatr 107:292–294, 1985a.

Wilson CB, Westall J, Johnston L, Lewis DB, Alpert AR. Decreased production of interferon-gamma by human neonatal cells. J Clin Invest 77:860–867, 1986.

Wilson M. Immunology of the fetus and newborn: lymphocyte phenotype and function. Clin Immunol Allergy 5:271–286, 1985.

Wilson M, Rosen FS, Schlossman SF, Reinherz EL. Ontogeny of human T and B lymphocytes during stressed and normal gestation: phenotypic analysis of umbilical cord lymphocytes from term and preterm infants. Clin Immunol Immunopathol 37:1–12, 1985b.

Winkelstein JA, Kurlandsky LE, Swift AJ. Defective activation of the third component of complement in the sera of newborn infants. Pediatr Res 13:1093–1096, 1979.

World Health Organization. Primary immunodeficiency diseases: report of a WHO scientific group. Immunodefic Rev 3:195–236, 1992.

Wright SD. Multiple receptors for endotoxin. Curr Opin Immunol 3:83–90, 1991.

Wright WC, Ank BJ, Herbert J, Stiehm ER. Decreased bactericidal activity of leukocytes of stressed newborn infants. Pediatrics 56:579–584, 1975.

Xia X, Lee H-K, Clark SC, Choi YS. Recombinant interleukin (IL)-2–induced human B cell differentiation is mediated by autocrine IL-6. Eur J Immunol 19:2275–2281, 1989.

Yabuhara A, Kawai T, Komiyama A. Development of natural killer cytotoxicity during childhood: marked increases in number of natural killer cells with adequate cytotoxic abilities during infancy to early childhood. Pediatr Res 28:316–322, 1990.

Yachie A, Ueno Y, Takano N, Miyawaki T, Taniguchi N. Developmental changes of double-negative (CD3$^-$ 4$^-$ 8$^-$) T cells in human peripheral blood. Clin Exp Immunol 76:258–261, 1989.

Yap PL, Pryde A, Latham PJ, McLelland DB. Serum IgA in the neonate. Acta Paediatr Scand 68:695–700, 1979.

Yarchoan R, Nelson DL. A study of the functional capabilities of human neonatal lymphocytes for in vitro specific antibody production. J Immunol 131:1222–1228, 1983.

Yasui K, Masuda M, Matsuoka T, Yamazaki M, Komiyama A, Akabane T, Hasui M, Kobayashi Y, Murata K. Abnormal membrane fluidity as a cause of impaired functional dynamics of chemoattractant receptors on neonatal polymorphonuclear leukocytes: lack of modulation of the receptors by a membrane fluidizer. Pediatr Res 24:442–446, 1988.

Yeager AS, Arvin AM, Urbani LJ, Kemp JA. Relationship of antibody to outcome in neonatal herpes simplex virus infections. Infect Immun 29:532–538, 1980.

Yellen AJ, Gleen W, Sukhatme VP, Cao X, Monroe JG. Signaling through surface IgM in tolerance-susceptible immature murine B lymphocytes: Developmentally regulated differences in transmembrane signaling in splenic B cells from adult and neonatal mice. J Immunol 146:1446–1454, 1991.

Yeung CY, Hobbs JR. Serum γ-globulin levels in normal, premature, post-mature, and "small-for-dates" newborn babies. Lancet 1:1167–1170, 1968.

Yewdell JW, Bennink JR. The binary logic of antigen processing and presentation to T cells. Cell 62:203–206, 1990.

Yoder MC, Douglas SD, Gerdes J, Kline J, Polin RA. Plasma fibronectin in healthy newborn infants: respiratory distress syndrome and perinatal asphyxia. J Pediatr 102:777–780, 1983.

Young MC, Geha RS. Ontogeny and control of human IgE synthesis. In Rosen, F.S, ed. Clinics in Immunology and Allergy. Developmental Immunology. Philadelphia, W.B. Saunders, 1985, pp. 339–349.

Zach TL, Hostetter MK. Biochemical abnormalities of the third component of complement in neonates. Pediatr Res 26:116–120, 1989.

Zeligs BJ, Armstrong DC, Walser JB, Bellanti JA. Age-dependent susceptibility of neonatal rats to group B streptococcal type II infection: correlation of severity of infection and response to myeloid pools. Infect Immun 37:255–263, 1982.

Zlabinger GJ, Mannhalter JW, Eibl MM. Cord blood macrophages present bacterial antigen (*Escherichia coli*) to paternal T cells. Clin Immunol Immunopathol 28:405–412, 1983.

Chapter 11

Disorders of the B-Cell System

Hans D. Ochs and Jerry Winkelstein

INTRODUCTION

The largest number of patients with a primary immunodeficiency have an illness associated with a significant and predominant defect in B-lymphocyte function. In some of these disorders, the defect is intrinsic to the B lymphocyte (e.g., X-linked agammaglobulinemia). In others, the B-lymphocyte defect is secondary to abnormalities of other cells and/or proteins of the immune system (e.g., X-linked immunodeficiency with hyper-IgM). This chapter describes those primary immunodeficiency diseases in which, regardless of the cause, the major clinical manifestations are defective B-lymphocyte function and deficient humoral immunity.

Development of the B-Lymphocyte System

Antibody-producing lymphocytes (B lymphocytes) originate and proliferate within the bursa of Fabricius in birds (Cooper et al., 1965) and in the ''bursa equivalent'' (fetal liver, Peyer's patches, bone marrow) in mammals (Owen et al., 1974). During the subsequent phase of B-lymphocyte development, a peripheral B-lymphocyte pool is established in the spleen and lymph nodes and autoreactive B lymphocytes are deleted by negative selection (Nemazee and Bürki, 1989). Finally, during the last phase of B-lymphocyte development, an antigen-dependent process, surface immunoglobulin positive (Ig^+) cells undergo positive selection in germinal centers and develop into memory B lymphocytes (see Chapter 2).

B lymphocytes are derived from pluripotent hematopoietic stem cells. Commitment to the B lineage of lymphocytes is achieved before the formation of progenitor B lymphocytes. Proliferation and differentiation of progenitor B lymphocytes occur in close contact with a microenvironment containing a diversity of cells referred to as *stromal cells*. At this stage, progenitor B-lymphocyte development is dependent on cell-cell contact and on cytokines secreted by stromal cells. Progenitor B lymphocytes do not express B lineage-specific markers and have not begun to rearrange the Ig genes (Rolink and Melchers, 1991).

During B-lymphocyte differentiation at the pre-B and B-lymphocyte stage, the genes encoding heavy (H) and light (L) chains are assembled by sequential rearrangements, respectively (Tonegawa, 1983). The H chain locus consists of multiple copies of variable (V_H), diversity (D_H), and joining (J_H) genes. The V-D-J region is linked to a cluster of C_H (constant) genes that encode the different H chain classes (μ, δ, $\gamma3$, $\gamma1$, $\alpha1$, $\gamma2$, $\gamma4$, ϵ, $\alpha2$). Each H chain class defines an Ig isotype/class with distinct biologic function, such as half-life, passage across the placenta, and complement fixation. During the pre-B lymphocyte stage, cytoplasmic μ chains are expressed (Levitt and Cooper, 1980); but the gene segments encoding L chains are not yet rearranged (Maki et al., 1980). To be transported to the cell surface, H chains have to be associated with L chains. In the absence of (κ) and (λ) L chains, the μH chains expressed by pre-B lymphocytes associate with surrogate L chains, encoded by genes located on the same chromosome that carries the λ L chain loci. The resulting complexes are transported to the cell surface and the surrogate L chains are subsequently replaced by κ and λ L chains (Rolink and Melchers, 1991).

Membrane-bound immunoglobulins act as B-lymphocyte antigen receptors, providing specific antigen recognition and initiating a cascade of events that lead to B-lymphocyte activation. Membrane-associated immunoglobulin (mIg) has a very short intracytoplasmic process that is unsuitable for signal transduction. Co-purification experiments demonstrate that mIgM forms a complex with a heterodimer consisting of two glycoproteins ($\sim$34 kD and 39 kD) designated IgM-α and Ig-β. These constitutively expressed components of the mIgM antigen receptor complex are encoded by the B-cell lineage-specific genes, mb-1 (IgM-α) and B29 (Ig-β) (Reth et al., 1991). Structures homologous to the murine glycoproteins have been identified in association with human mIgM, although the molecular mass of the subunits differs slightly (Van Noesel, et al., 1990). Both mIgM-associated glycoproteins have long cytoplasmic tails that provide binding sites to one or more nonreceptor kinases involved in transmitting signals to the nucleus of B lymphocytes.

Lymphocytes with markers characteristic of B cells are abundant in lymph nodes, spleen, tonsil, appendix and Peyer's patches and circulate in the peripheral blood. Following exposure to antigen, positive selection of antigen-specific B lymphocytes is initiated and further diversity generated by somatic hypermutation. The germinal center formation in lymph nodes and spleen plays a central role in T-dependent and T-independent antigenic challenge (MacLennan et al., 1992). Within germinal centers, B lymphocytes interact closely with T lymphocytes and follicular dendritic cells (FDCs) and undergo oligoclonal proliferation. The FDCs trap and store antigen in the form of antigen-antibody-complement complexes and, together with T lymphocytes, provide the milieu for the continuous development of memory B lymphocytes and isotype switching. A major role in T-cell/B-cell interaction within germinal centers is played by the ligand-receptor pair, CD40 ligand (CD40L, gp39), expressed by activated T cells, and CD 40, expressed by B cells (Foy et al., 1994; Hollenbaugh et al., 1994a; Kawabe et al., 1994).

Regulation of B-Lymphocyte Function

The antigen-specific antibody response is dependent on a series of complex events associated with the cognate interaction of T and B lymphocytes (Fig. 11-1). (Noelle and Snow, 1990; Ochs and Aruffo, 1993; Aruffo et al., 1993, 1994; Hollenbaugh et al., 1994a). As a consequence, B lymphocytes differentiate into immunoglobulin-secreting plasma cells designed to produce large quantities of specific antibody of different isotypes. Following binding to membrane-associated IgM, protein antigen is internalized and peptides generated. Antigen-derived peptides form a complex with MHC class II molecules and, after transport to the B-lymphocyte membrane, are presented to antigen-specific $CD4^+$

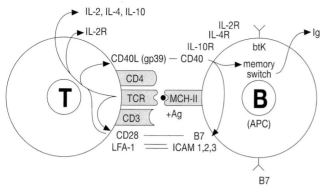

Figure 11–1. Schematic of events involved in T-B cell interaction. Bruton's agammaglobulinemia tyrosine kinase (btK) is required for the maturation of pre-B cells to naive B cells expressing surface IgM and IgD. After cognate binding to surface antibody (antigen binding complex), the antigen is internalized, and digested, and the resulting peptides presented by the major histocompatibility complex II (MHC-II) to T lymphocytes via the T-cell receptor (TCR/CD4/CD3) complex. This interaction requires direct cell-cell contact, which is strengthened by the adhesion molecules, leukocyte function–associated antigen (LFA-1) and intracellular adhesion molecules (ICAM-1, -2, -3). As a result of this interaction, CD4+ T cells express the activation molecule CD40 ligand (gp39) and produce and secrete lymphokines, which bind to the appropriate lymphokine receptors expressed by T and B lymphocytes. This results in lymphocyte proliferation and B-cell maturation. In addition, B-cell activation via CD40 directly affects the expression of B7, which improves antigen presentation by B cells via TCR and initiates additional activation of T lymphocytes via its ligand, CD28. APC = antigen-presenting cell; Ig = immunoglobulin; IL = interleukin.

T lymphocytes. Recognition of the MHC II–associated peptides by antigen-specific T cell receptors (TCRs) leads to the physical binding of the two cell types.

This relatively weak binding is strengthened by the interaction of other ligand-receptor pairs, including CD4-MHC class II and LFA-1/ICAM-1. Antigen presentation to the TCR complex initiates T-lymphocyte activation and the rapid expression of CD40L (a T-cell membrane glycoprotein that interacts with B lymphocytes via CD40), the secretion of several lymphokines and the expression of the high-affinity IL-2 receptor complex (IL-2R α, β, γ). The CD40-dependent and lymphokine-modified pathway is crucial for B-lymphocyte proliferation, differentiation, and secretion of antigen-specific antibody of various isotypes and subclasses (Marshall et al., 1993; Hollenbaugh et al., 1994a; Kawabe et al., 1994).

Committed B lymphocytes can be stimulated in vitro via CD40 and antigen in the presence of IL-10 to produce antigen-specific antibody (Nonoyama et al., 1993b). Anti-CD40 activated B lymphocytes exposed to IL-10 synthesize large quantities of immunoglobulins (Rousset et al., 1992); exposure to IL-4 induces anti-CD40 activated B lymphocytes to switch to the production of IgE (Gascan et al., 1991). Other lymphokines may down-regulate immunoglobulin synthesis, as exemplified by the suppressive effect of interferon-gamma on in vitro IgE synthesis (Pène et al., 1988).

Histology of Lymphoid Organs

The lymphoid organs provide the milieu for the development and the interaction of lymphocytes and ac-

cessory cells. They can be divided into three main functional units:

1. Pluripotential stem cells, primarily located in the bone marrow.
2. Primary lymphoid organs (thymus, bone marrow, liver).
3. Secondary lymphoid organs (lymph nodes; tonsils; adenoids; spleen; lymphoid tissue of the gastrointestinal tract and exocrine glands; and peripheral blood).

Progenitor B lymphocytes, pre-B lymphocytes, and immature B cells expressing only surface IgM, are primarily located in the sinusoidal spaces near the central sinuses of the bone marrow, where they are in close contact with stromal cells and may undergo apoptosis if self antigens are recognized.

B-lymphocyte proliferation and differentiation preferentially occurs in germinal centers of lymph nodes and spleen (MacLennan et al., 1992). Histologically, three distinct regions can be differentiated in the lymph nodes (Fig. 11–2):

1. Follicles and germinal centers of the cortex, consisting predominantly of B lymphocytes.
2. The paracortical area, which is rich in thymus-dependent (T) lymphocytes.
3. The medulla, showing an abundance of plasma cells.

Antigens enter the lymph node from the periphery through the afferent lymph channels, forming antigen/antibody-complement complexes that are trapped within the germinal centers by follicular dendritic cells. This allows germinal center B lymphocytes to take up and present antigen-to-antigen–specific T cells, which after activation express CD40L (gp39) and interact with CD40, constitutively expressed by B lymphocytes. B lymphocytes forming germinal centers are oligoclonal. *Plasma cells,* the end stage of B-cell differentiation, are abundant in the medulla.

The white pulp of the spleen is formed by periarterial lymphatic sheets (predominantly T lymphocytes) and lymphoid nodules and follicles (malpighian bodies), which consist predominantly of B lymphocytes. Mature plasma cells are found in abundance throughout the marginal zone and the red pulp, which corresponds to the medulla of the lymph nodes. B lymphocytes are also found in abundance in the tonsils, adenoids, Peyer's patches, appendices, and the solitary nodules located in the mucosa of the digestive and respiratory tracts.

Laboratory Evaluation of B-Lymphocyte Disorders

A discussion of laboratory methods useful for the diagnosis of immunodeficiency syndromes is provided in Chapter 9. If the clinical findings suggest the possibility of a defect in B-lymphocyte function, the most cost-effective screening test is the quantitative determination of serum immunoglobulin (IgG, IgA, IgM) levels. A more sophisticated approach to the pathophysiologic basis for defective B-lymphocyte function and to

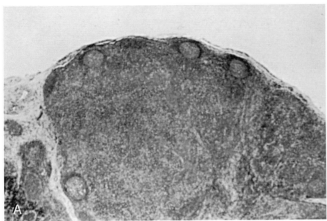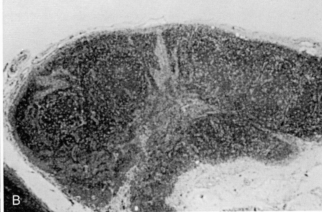

Figure 11–2. *A,* Normal lymph node obtained at herniorrhaphy from a healthy 4-month-old boy. Note the differentiation into cortex and medulla and the well-formed germinal centers with cuffs of lymphocytes. (×27.5.) *B,* Lymph node from a 10-year-old boy with X-linked agammaglobulinemia. Note the absence of differentiation into cortex and medulla; there are no germinal centers or lymphoid follicles. Plasma cells are absent. (×27.5.) (*A* and *B* courtesy of Dr. David Lagunoff.)

the assessment of B-lymphocyte function is discussed next.

Assessment of B-Lymphocyte Subpopulations

Pre-B cells can be clearly identified in the bone marrow and in the peripheral blood as cells containing cytoplasmic μ chains. Mature B lymphocytes express the immunoglobulin antigen receptor complex and the B-lymphocyte specific markers, CD19, CD20, and B7.

The enumeration of B- and T-lymphocyte subsets is useful in differentiating and classifying primary immunodeficiency syndromes. Patients with disorders affecting the B-cell system and antibody synthesis may have normal or low numbers or nearly absent B lymphocytes. Disorders in which B lymphocytes are markedly diminished include patients with XLA, a small proportion of patients with CVI, and most patients with autosomal recessive severe combined immunodeficiency disease (SCID) (Seeger and Stiehm, 1975).

The preferred technique for enumerating B lymphocytes in human peripheral blood is by flow cytometry using monoclonal antibodies recognizing the B-lymphocyte markers CD19 or CD20. Normal values at different ages are given in Chapter 9. Surface immunoglobulin positive B lymphocytes can be identified with similar techniques using antibody against Ig isotypes. Mature B lymphocytes also express CD40 and the receptor for Epstein-Barr virus (EBV), CD21 (CR2).

In Vitro Assessment of B-Lymphocyte Function

If cultured in vitro in the presence of T lymphocytes and pokeweed mitogen, B lymphocytes proliferate and secrete immunoglobulin of all isotypes. If B lymphocytes are cultured in vitro in the presence of anti-CD40 or soluble CD40 ligand (sgp39), they produce IgG, IgM and IgA if exposed to IL-10 and IgE if exposed to IL-4 (Nonoyama et al., 1993a). In the presence of anti-

CD40 and IL-4, normal B lymphocytes proliferate in vitro (Banchereau et al., 1991). These characteristic in vitro functions may be absent in patients with intrinsic B-cell abnormalities. In contrast, patients with abnormal antibody responses secondary to T-cell deficiencies may have normal B-lymphocyte function in assay systems not requiring T lymphocytes (Nonoyama et al., 1993a). T- and B-lymphocyte interaction can also be assessed by measuring in vitro antibody synthesis by peripheral blood lymphocyte (PBLs) from individuals previously exposed in vivo to a given antigen (e.g., tetanus toxoid, bacteriophage φX174) (Stevens et al., 1983; Bohnsack et al., 1985; Nonoyama et al., 1993b).

In Vivo Assessment of B-Lymphocyte Function

Determination of in vivo antibody responses to selected antigens can provide useful information to classify and to optimally treat patients with immunodeficiency syndromes. If previously fully immunized, patients may be challenged with a recall antigen booster (e.g., diphtheria or tetanus toxoid, conjugated *Haemophilus influenzae* vaccine or hepatitis B vaccine). To test for responses to polysaccharide antigens that are less T-cell–dependent, pneumococcal polysaccharide or meningococcal polysaccharide vaccines are available. However, polysaccharide antigens are poor immunogens in normal children younger than 2 years of age. A preimmunization sample and a sample collected 3 to 4 weeks after immunization are assayed simultaneously for antibody titers. If these screening tests suggest a primary or secondary antibody deficiency or if the patient has received plasma or immunoglobulin infusions, other antigens, e.g., bacteriophage φX174, a T-cell–dependent neoantigen (Wedgwood et al., 1975; Pyun et al., 1989), may be selected.

Bacteriophage is a potent antigen; the antibody assays, phage neutralization or enzyme-linked immunosorbent assay (ELISA), are sensitive, quantitative, and reproducible. Bacteriophage φX174 has a molecu-

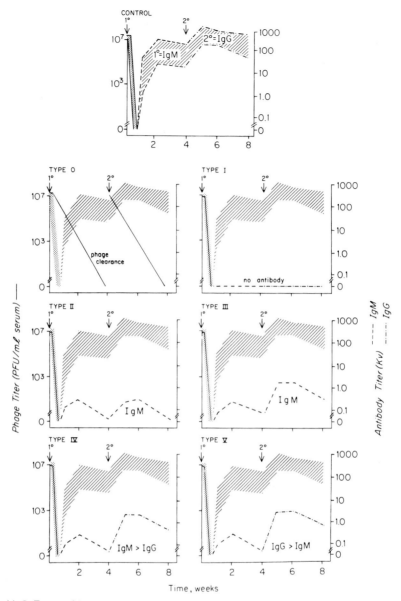

Figure 11–3. Types of immune responses to bacteriophage φX174 in patients with X-linked agammaglobulinemia. The phage injections, given at time 0 (1°) and at 4 weeks (2°), are indicated by a downward *arrow* (↓). Normal phage clearance is accomplished within 3 to 4 days after primary immunization *(stippled area)*. Patients with prolonged phage clearance *(solid line)* are assigned to the type 0 category. All other types have normal clearance of phage. Range of antibody titers observed in a control population is shown by the *hatched area* (1° = primary antibody response, 2° = secondary antibody response). Patients classified as types 0 and I do not produce antibody to phage; those classified as type II make small amounts of IgM antibody without expressing immunologic memory. Patients classified as types III to V demonstrate immunologic memory but have either a qualitative (types III and IV with no or reduced amounts of IgG antibody) or a quantitative (type V) deficiency of antibody response. Of 50 X-linked agammaglobulinemic patients immunized with φX174, 25 had a type 0 response, 4 had a type I response, 9 had a type II response, 6 had a type III response, and 6 had a type IV response.

lar mass of 6×10^6 and is retained in the intravascular space until it is cleared from the circulation immunologically within 3 to 4 days after administration. After phage clearance, antibody activity can be demonstrated in the serum of normal individuals. The primary response peaks at 2 weeks and consists predominantly of IgM antibody. The secondary response, consisting of equal proportions of IgG and IgM antibody, is brisk, peaks at 1 week, then declines slowly. A third immuni-

zation results in a further increase of the antibody titer and consists exclusively of IgG. Thus, there are quantitative and qualitative differences between primary, secondary and tertiary responses to this antigen.

In the immunologically normal individual, the following components of the immune response to bacteriophage φX174 can be distinguished:

1. Antigen clearance.

Table 11–1. Immune Responses of 317 Patients with Primary Immunodeficiency Syndromes to Bacteriophage φX174

Immunodeficiency Syndrome	No. of Patients	Type of Response						
		0	I	II	III	IV	V	Normal
X-linked agammaglobulinemia	50	25	4	9	6	6		
X-linked hyper-IgM syndrome	5		5					
Antibody deficiency with normal or hypergammaglobulinemia	18			4	3	11		
Common variable immunodeficiency	132		4	24	34	48	22	
Selective IgM deficiency	8			2		1	2	3
Selective IgA deficiency	3						1	2
Antibody deficiency and transcobalamin II deficiency	6			2	4			
Antibody deficiency and complement (C4, C2, C3) deficiency	5			2	3			
Immunodeficiency with thymoma	1		1					
DiGeorge anomalad	8			1	3	3	1	
T-cell defects (unclassified)	10			3	3	3	1	
Severe combined immunodeficiency (n = 44)								
"Sporadic" (unclassified)	23	2	2	15	1	3		
X-linked	2			2				
Autosomal recessive (n = 19)								
Unclassified	5	3		2				
ADA deficiency	4			4				
PNP deficiency	1				1			
Omenn syndrome	3				3			
Cartilage-hair hypoplasia	4			2	1	1		
Short-limbed skeletal dysplasia	1			1				
MHC-II deficiency (bare lymphocyte syndrome)	1			1				
Ataxia-telangiectasia	16			1	4	7	1	3
Wiskott-Aldrich syndrome	11			7	2		2	
Pediatric AIDS	12			10		2		
Totals	317	30	11	87	68	83	30	8

Abbreviations: AIDS = acquired immunodeficiency syndrome; ADA = adenosine deaminase; MHC = major histocompatibility complex; PNP = purine nucleoside phosphorylase.

2. The primary IgM response.

3. The secondary response demonstrating amplification, immunologic memory and limited isotype switch.

4. The tertiary response characterized by amplification, a complete switch from IgM to IgG and persistent memory

The generation of memory cells and the process of isotype switching is T-cell–dependent. The early antiphage IgG antibody produced by normal subjects is of the IgG3 and IgG1 subclasses; later, antiphage antibodies of the other IgG subclasses appear in the serum. The persisting antibody after multiple immunizations is of the IgG1 class (Pyun et al., 1989).

Theoretically, six types of quantitatively and qualitatively abnormal immune responses to immunization with bacteriophage φX174 are possible (Fig. 11–3). Examples of all such aberrant responses have been observed (Table 11–1) (Wedgwood et al., 1975).

1. Patients in whom the antigen is not cleared in a normal fashion and who produce no antibody (type 0).

2. Patients with normal (accelerated) antigen clearance but absent antibody activity (type I).

3. Patients with normal antigen clearance, followed by production of small amounts of IgM antibody without immunologic memory (type II).

4. Patients with normal antigen clearance, antibody formation limited to IgM, some immunologic memory and limited amplification (type III).

5. Patients with normal antigen clearance, low antibody titers, immunologic memory, and production of some, but limited, IgG antibody (type IV).

6. Patients with normal antigen clearance and low antibody production consisting predominantly of IgG, intact memory, and amplification, suggesting a qualitatively normal but quantitatively depressed response (type V).

Most patients (60%) with X-linked agammaglobulinemia have a markedly prolonged phage clearance or an inability to make antibody to bacteriophage. A considerable proportion of X-linked agammaglobulinemia patients, however, can clear phage normally and produce small amounts of IgM and, occasionally, IgG antibody. Five of 44 patients (two boys and three girls) with SCID were unable to clear phage and failed to produce detectable antibody to phage. Most patients with common variable immunodeficiency produce antibody but are unable to switch from IgM to IgG after secondary immunization (see Table 11–1).

Treatment of B-Cell Deficiencies

General aspects of treatment of patients with immunodeficiency disorders are discussed in Chapter 9. Patients with a significant B-cell abnormality respond favorably to lifelong treatment with immunoglobulin injections or infusions. The intramuscular injection of 100 mg/kg (0.7 ml/kg of a 16% immunoglobulin solution, Cohn fraction II) per month of human immune serum globulin, as recommended in the past, is often not sufficient to keep these patients symptom-free. Absorption of intramuscular IgG from the injection site may be delayed and incomplete, and proteolytic degradation at the injection site occurs. The preparations for intramuscular use available in the United States contain a mercury compound as a preservative, and long-term exposure is cumulative; occasionally, symptoms of mercury poisoning have been observed (Matheson et al., 1980).

Immunoglobulin (Ig) administration by slow subcutaneous infusion at a rate of 1 to 2 ml/hour is well tolerated; if immunoglobulin is given several times per week, high serum IgG levels may be achieved (Berger et al., 1980; Roord et al., 1982; Ugazio et al., 1982; Leahy, 1986). Human immune serum globulin for intramuscular use (ISG), if properly processed, is free of hepatitis A, B, and C, and human immunodeficiency virus (HIV) (Centers for Disease Control, 1986; Zuck et al., 1986). The fractionation process generally used to isolate immunoglobulin (predominantly IgG) inactivates and partitions up to 13 cumulative logs of HIV-1 as determined by in vitro studies (Wells et al., 1986).

Preparations of Cohn fraction II contain IgG aggregates and are strongly anticomplementary, often causing severe anaphylactic reactions if they are given intravenously. The need for a safe intravenous immunoglobulin preparation was recognized in the 1970s (Eibl and Wedgwood, 1989), resulting in the development of new preparations. Several methods to modify immune serum globulin for use as intravenous immunoglobulin (IVIG) by preventing IgG aggregate formation have been developed, including:

- Formulation at pH 4.25 in maltose (Gamimune N, Cutter Biological, Miles Pharmaceutical Division).
- Exposure to acid pH in the presence of trace amounts of pepsin (Sandoglobulin, Sandoz).
- Ultracentrifugation and ion exchange adsorption (Gammagard S/D, Hyland Division, Baxter Healthcare Division)
- Treatment with polyethylene glycol and ion exchange adsorption (Venoglobulin-1, Venoglobulin-S, Alpha Therapeutics Corporation)
- Stabilization with glucose (Iveegam, Immuno-U.S.)
- Sucrose and human albumin (Gammar IV, Armour Pharmaceutical Company)

To further increase the safety margin against viral contamination, solvent-detergent treated IVIG preparations have become available (Venoglobulin-S, Gammagard S/D, Polygam S/D). Exposure of virus-spiked IgG to low pH markedly reduces the amount of infectious virus (see Table 9–23). All of these preparations are derived from large pools of prescreened (HIV and hepatitis C antibody, hepatitis B antigen negative) plasma units. To be suitable for prophylactic treatment of patients with antibody-deficiency, IVIG must be free of viral contaminants, must have a low incidence of adverse effects, must retain a half-life of IgG not significantly different from that of conventional immune serum globulin (Cohn fraction II), must represent all IgG subclasses in physiologic concentration, must have

protective levels of antibody to a variety of infective agents, and must maintain its biologic activity during the modification process.

Intravenous infusion allows substantial increases in the quantity of immunoglobulin that can be given. In clinical trials with IVIG, the postinfusion serum IgG concentration increases initially by approximately 250 mg/dl for each 100 mg/kg of IgG infused. In patients receiving 300 to 400 mg/kg every 4 weeks, but not in those receiving only 100 mg/kg, there is a stepwise increase in their trough and peak IgG levels until a new plateau is reached (Ochs et al., 1984).

To provide consistent protection for patients with antibody deficiency syndromes throughout the intervals between their IVIG infusions, the trough serum IgG concentration should be maintained at a level at least 300 mg/dl above the "base line" IgG level found in the patient's serum prior to immunoglobulin therapy. Sorensen and Polmar (1984) have noted that serum IgG levels <400 mg/dl are associated with an increased number of infections. At the National Institutes of Health Consensus Development Conference on Intravenous Immunoglobulin in May 1990, data were presented suggesting a markedly diminished incidence of echovirus-induced dermatomyositis-meningoencephalitis in patients with X-linked agammaglobulinemia since the wide use of IVIG.

There is considerable variation among patients between the dose of IVIG given and the serum IgG levels achieved. Thus, the frequency of infusion and dose of IVIG must be individualized and adjusted by following serum IgG levels. Generally, patients initially require a dose of 300 to 400 mg/kg/month (Ochs et al., 1984). More frequent infusions, for example, 150 to 200 mg/kg every other week, reduce the fluctuation between peak and trough levels, resulting in more stable physiologic serum IgG levels. In selected cases, the cost and inconvenience of hospital and office infusions can be reduced by teaching patients to self-administer IVIG in the home (Ashida and Saxon, 1986; Ochs et al., 1987).

In immunodeficient patients with chronic lung disease as a sequela of frequent respiratory infections, pulmonary function may improve after IVIG infusions of 600 to 800 mg/kg/month are given (Roifman et al., 1985, 1987). Similarly, large doses of IVIG may be required for the treatment of disseminated viral infections (e.g., echovirus infection in X-linked agammaglobulinemia) (Mease et al., 1981, 1985). To prevent development of chronic lung disease and bronchiectasis, early diagnosis of antibody deficiency and initiation of prophylactic treatment before age 1 year with IVIG are of great importance. In some instances, bacterial infections develop in spite of optimal IVIG prophylaxis, necessitating the addition of broad-spectrum antibiotics at effective doses to eradicate the infection. Sometimes, these measures must be continued indefinitely.

X-LINKED AGAMMAGLOBULINEMIA

X-linked agammaglobulinemia is a primary immunodeficiency disease in which the underlying defect is limited to cells of the B-lymphocyte lineage. The disorder is characterized by a profound deficiency of B cells and arrest in B-lymphocyte development, resulting in severe hypogammaglobulinemia (Rosen et al., 1984; Lederman and Winkelstein, 1985).

The disorder was one of the first of the primary immunodeficiency diseases to be identified (Bruton, 1952) and remains the prototypic example of a primary immunodeficiency disease in which the defect is limited to B lymphocytes and their function. As a consequence, observations in patients with this disorder have provided valuable insights into the physiologic processes necessary for normal B-lymphocyte development and the role of antibody in host defense and inflammation.

Etiology

X-linked agammaglobulinemia (XLA) is caused by mutations of the B cell specific tyrosine kinase, *Btk* (Tsukada et al., 1993; Vetrie et al., 1993) and is inherited as an X-linked recessive disorder (Rosen et al., 1984). The *Btk* gene maps to the long arm of the X chromosome at Xq22 and is closely linked to a number of polymorphic markers (Kwan et al., 1986, 1990; Mensink et al., 1986b; Malcolm et al., 1987; Guioli et al., 1989; Parolini et al., 1993; Lovering et al., 1993). One of these polymorphic markers, DXS 178, maps very close to the XLA locus, since there have been no recombinations between the XLA locus and the DXS 178 locus in more than 70 affected families (Kwan et al., 1986, 1990; Guioli et al., 1989; Parolini et al., 1993).

B-Lymphocyte Development

The molecular defect in X-linked agammaglobulinemia interferes with the development and function of B lymphocytes and their progeny (Conley, 1992). The major consequence of the defect appears to be at the stage of development of pre-B lymphocytes to B lymphocytes. Patients have pre-B lymphocytes in their bone marrow (Pearl et al., 1978) but have few if any B lymphocytes in their blood and lymphoid tissues (Siegal et al., 1971; Aiuti et al., 1972; Cooper and Lawton, 1972; Bentwich and Kunkel, 1973; Preud'Homme et al., 1973; Geha et al., 1973; Schiff et al., 1974). As one would expect, the progeny of B lymphocytes—plasma cells—are also absent in tissues where they are normally present (i.e., bone marrow, lymph nodes and the lamina propria of intestinal mucosa) (Figs. 11–2 and 11–4) (Good, 1955; Gitlin et al., 1959; Ament et al., 1973).

However, the defect may also affect B-lymphocyte development at more than one level and may not be limited to the stage of pre-B lymphocyte to B-lymphocyte development. For example, bone marrow samples from patients with XLA have a predominance of cytoplasmic (c) μ⁻, terminal deoxynucleotidyl transferase (TdT)⁺ pro-B lymphocytes and fewer cytoplasmic μ⁺ pre-B lymphocytes than expected. In addition, those cytoplasmic μ⁺ pre-B lymphocytes that are present

have reduced proliferative responses (Campana et al., 1990).

In other studies, patients with XLA have small numbers of B lymphocytes (0.01% to 0.03% of all lymphocytes) in their circulation (Conley, 1985), but the B lymphocytes that are present have an immature phenotype; this finding suggests that they too have been arrested at a relatively early stage of development (Conley, 1985; Golay and Webster, 1986; Leickley and Buckley, 1986). When variable-diversity-joining (V-D-J) rearrangements do occur in B lymphocytes from patients with XLA, they are normal and representative of clonal diversity (Mensink et al., 1986a; Anker et al., 1989; Timmers et al., 1991; Milili et al., 1993).

There is evidence that the defect in XLA is not only operative at many levels of B-lymphocyte development but that the block is also incomplete. As noted, small numbers of B lymphocytes can be detected in peripheral blood and immunoglobulin can be demonstrated in culture supernatants of lymphocytes (Cooperband et al., 1968; Stites et al., 1971; Levitt et al., 1984). Further, nearly all patients with XLA have some immunoglobulin of one or another isotype in their serum (Wedgwood and Ochs, 1980; Rosen et al., 1984; Lederman and Winkelstein, 1985).

X-Chromosome Inactivation Analysis

Studies of X-chromosome inactivation analysis in female carriers of X-linked agammaglobulinemia have provided important evidence that the defect in XLA is intrinsic to the B-lymphocyte lineage (Conley et al., 1986a; Fearon et al., 1987; Conley and Puck; 1988). The B-lymphocyte population in normal women is composed of one population in which the maternal X-chromosome is active and another population in which the paternal X-chromosome is active. In contrast, the B lymphocytes of female carriers of XLA contain only one population of B lymphocytes with respect to the active X-chromosome. The active X-chromosome in the B lymphocytes of female carriers of XLA is always the X-chromosome that carries the normal allele. Presumably, B lymphocytes in which the active X-chromosome carries the normal allele are at a selective advantage, proliferate, and make up most of the mature B lymphocytes, whereas B lymphocytes in which the active X-chromosome carries the mutant allele are at a selective disadvantage and do not develop. Other hematopoietic cell lineages in female carriers of XLA, such as T lymphocytes and monocytes, are normal with respect to X-chromosome inactivation analysis; that is, they show two populations of cells with respect to X-chromosome inactivation. Thus, the defect in XLA seems to be restricted to, or be intrinsic to, cells of the B-lymphocyte lineage.

The Btk Gene

Studies from two independent groups have identified the gene responsible for X-linked agammaglobulinemia (Tsukada et al., 1993; Vetrie et al., 1993). The gene, a member of the src-related tyrosine kinase family, has

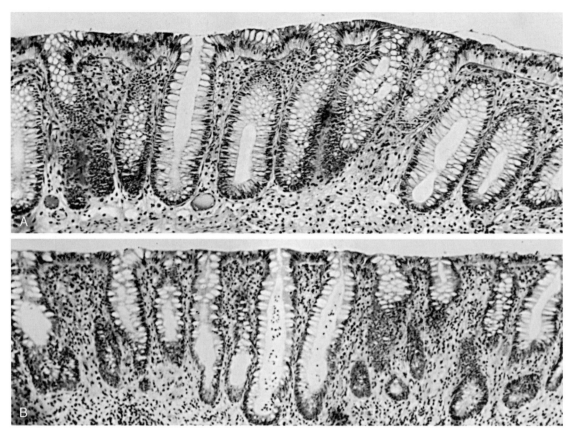

Figure 11–4. Rectal biopsy specimen from a healthy adult *(top panel)*. The architecture is normal, and plasma cells are plentiful. (×115.) *B*, Rectal biopsy specimen from a patient with X-linked agammaglobulinemia. The architecture is normal except for glands filled with polymorphonuclear leukocytes. Plasma cells are absent. (×115.) *(A and B courtesy of Dr. Marvin Ament.)*

been named *Btk* in honor of Dr. Bruton (Bruton agammaglobulinemia tyrosine kinase) (Kinnon et al., 1993). One group identified the gene using *positional cloning*, in which DNA from the relevant position of the X-chromosome was cloned in yeast artificial chromosomes and B-cell specific complementary deoxyribonucleic acids (cDNAs) isolated (Vetrie et al., 1993). The other group identified the gene using the *candidate gene approach*, in which the human analog of a mouse gene known to be important in B-lymphocyte development was identified (Tsukada et al., 1993). More recently, the genomic organization of *Btk* has been characterized; the gene, approximately 37 kb in length, consists of 19 exons (Ohta et al., 1994; Hagemann et al., 1994).

The evidence that the *Btk* gene is responsible for XLA rests on four observations. First, *Btk* is expressed in all stages of the B-lymphocyte lineage (except plasma cells) but not in T lymphocytes (Smith et al., 1994). Second, it maps to the same chromosomal location as the XLA locus. Third, most patients with XLA have reduced levels of *Btk* messenger ribonucleic acid (mRNA), reduced *Btk* protein and *Btk* kinase activity in their pre-B lymphocyte and B-lymphocyte lines. Finally, as of 1994, mutations in the *Btk* gene were identified in 30 families with XLA (Vetrie et al., 1993; Bradley et al., 1994; de Weers et al., 1994; Saffran et al., 1994; Zhu et al., 1994a, 1994b) and the mutations segregate with the X-chromosome carrying the XLA allele within each of the families. The fact that Btk is

expressed throughout B-lymphocyte development is compatible with the observations that the defect in XLA may involve more than a single step in B-lymphocyte development (Conley, 1985; Kinnon et al., 1993).

Mutation Analysis

Mutation analysis of the *Btk* gene has revealed considerable heterogeneity from family to family, affecting every domain of the gene. Point mutations have been the most frequent defects identified, resulting in amino acid substitutions, premature stop codons, exon skipping resulting from splice junction mutations, and "non-start" from initiation codon mutations (Vetrie et al., 1993; Bradley et al., 1994; Conley et al., 1994a; de Weers et al., 1994; Hagemann et al., 1994; Saffran et al., 1994; Zhu et al., 1994a, 1994b). Of 14 consecutively sequenced *Btk* mutations, all but two were caused by point mutations within genomic DNA (Zhu et al., 1994b). Of the 30 mutations published during 1993 and 1994, two involve the initiation codon, 4 are in the pleckstrin homology (PH) and Tec homology (TH) domain, 3 are in the SH3 domain, 5 are in the SH2 domain, and 16 are in the SH1 domain, which contains the enzyme activity and adenosine triphosphate (ATP) binding site (Fig. 11–5).

The location and type of mutation do not seem to correlate with the clinical phenotype of XLA, although several families with a "leaky" XLA phenotype have been observed (Saffran et al., 1994; Zhu et al., 1994b). Patients presenting with classic XLA symptoms and clinical findings had mutations located within every Btk domain. For instance, a B-lymphoblastoid cell line derived from a patient with a classic XLA phenotype and a deletion within SH3 resulting in a truncated protein had normal *Btk* mRNA and normal kinase activity; this suggests that Btk domains not directly involved in kinase activity are important for Btk function, possibly by initiating protein-protein interaction (Zhu et al., 1994a). Furthermore, because there can be considerable phenotypic variation within XLA families (Wedgwood and Ochs, 1980), it is difficult to correlate a clinical phenotype with the location of the mutation.

Clinical Manifestations

Because IgG is actively transported across the placenta, newborns with XLA have normal levels of serum IgG at birth and few, if any, symptoms. However, as the maternally derived IgG is catabolized, panhypogammaglobulinemia and an increased susceptibility to infection develop. Thus, most patients with XLA are asymptomatic for the first few months of life and begin to have recurrent infections between 4 and 12 months of age (Lederman and Winkelstein, 1985). However, not all patients are symptomatic in the first year of life. In one series of 96 patients with XLA reported from the United States and Canada, nearly 20% experienced their initial clinical symptoms after their first birthday and about 10% after 18 months of age (Lederman and Winkelstein, 1985). In another series of 44 XLA patients reported from United Kingdom, as many as 21% first presented clinically as late as 3 to 5 years of age (Hermaszewski and Webster, 1993).

Bacterial Infections

Infections are the most common clinical manifestation of X-linked agammaglobulinemia, both before the diagnosis is made and after therapy with immunoglobulin has been instituted (Lederman and Winkelstein, 1985; Liese et al., 1992; Hermaszewski and Webster, 1993). The infections are usually caused by pyogenic encapsulated bacteria, such as *Streptococcus pneumoniae, Haemophilus influenzae, Staphylococcus aureus,* and *Pseudomonas* species, organisms for which antibody is an important opsonin. For example, these four organisms alone account for most of the cases of sepsis, pyogenic meningitis, and septic arthritis in patients with XLA (Lederman and Winkelstein, 1985). Other bacterial species, such as *Salmonella* and *Campylobacter,* have also been seen (Wyatt et al., 1977; Lederman and Winkelstein, 1985; Van der Meer et al., 1986; Chusid et al., 1987; Hermaszewski and Webster, 1993).

The infections may be localized to the respiratory tract (e.g., otitis, sinusitis, pneumonia), skin (e.g., pyoderma), or gastrointestinal tract (e.g., diarrhea), or they may be systemic and blood-borne (e.g., sepsis, meningitis, septic arthritis). Although any single infection may be limited to one anatomic location, it usually occurs in multiple locations over time. For example, in a large multi-institutional series of patients with XLA, 74% of patients had infections of the upper respiratory tract (e.g., otitis, sinusitis) before diagnosis, but of these, more than two thirds had also had infections of the lower respiratory tract (e.g., pneumonia, bronchiolitis) and/or gastrointestinal tract (Lederman and Winkelstein, 1985).

Although respiratory and gastrointestinal tract infections are the most common infections seen in patients with XLA, other infections occur with regularity as well (Lederman and Winkelstein, 1985; Hermaszewski and Webster, 1993). Blood-borne systemic infections, such as sepsis, meningitis, osteomyelitis and septic arthritis, are relatively uncommon and are seen more frequently in patients before diagnosis than after immunoglobulin therapy has been instituted (Lederman and Winkelstein, 1985). When such infections do occur, they

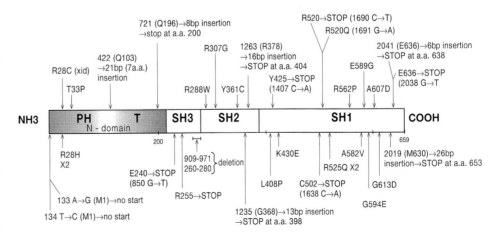

Figure 11–5. Schematic representation of the domains of Bruton's agammaglobulinemia tyrosine kinase (Btk). The pleckstrin homology (PH) and Tec homology (TH) domains are at the N-terminal site followed by src homology domains SH3, SH2, and SH1. The adenosine triphosphate (ATP) binding site and kinase activity are located within SH1. Mutations of Btk from 32 families with X-linked agammaglobulinemia (XLA) are indicated (see Vetrie et al., 1993; Bradley et al., 1994; de Weers et al., 1994; Saffran et al., 1994; and Zhu et al., 1994a, 1994b). Numbers without a designating letter represent base pairs (bp). Letters (by convention) represent amino acids (a.a.), and the subsequent number indicates the location of the amino acids within the normal Btk protein; the letter after the amino acid number stands for the mutated amino acid (i.e., R28C indicates that amino acid number 28, an arginine, is substituted by a cysteine in this mutation). (R28C) (xid) is a mutation causing X-linked immunodeficiency in mice. The same amino acid (arginine) has been substituted (by histidine) in two nonrelated families with XLA. Only one other Btk mutation (R525Q) has been observed in more than one family. At least one member of each of the families represented has a classic form of XLA, except a family with two affected brothers with G613D substitution who both have a common variable immunodeficiency (CVI)–like phenotype.

most often are secondary complications of infections in other sites. Gastroenteritis is also seen and in some instances is secondary to chronic infections with *Giardia lamblia* (Fig. 11–6) (Ochs et al., 1972; LoGalbo et al., 1982), rotavirus (Saulsbury et al., 1980), or *Campylobacter* (Melamed, et al., 1983).

Enteroviral Infections

Although resistance to viral infections is generally intact in patients with XLA (Janeway et al., 1953; Good and Zak, 1956), there are some important exceptions. The patients are unusually susceptible to infections with enteroviruses, such as echovirus, coxsackievirus and poliovirus (McKinney et al., 1987). These viruses usually cause primary infections in the gastrointestinal tract, with spread to the blood stream and secondary infection of the central nervous system in some individuals. Because antibody is important in neutraliza-

tion of these viruses during their passage through the blood stream (Hammon et al., 1952), patients with XLA lack an important mechanism of resistance to this family of viruses.

Poliovirus

A number of patients with XLA have vaccine-related poliomyelitis after immunization with the live polio virus vaccine (Wright et al., 1977; Lederman and Winkelstein, 1985). Vaccine-related disease in these patients is usually characterized by a prolonged incubation period (often greater than 30 days), an unusually high mortality rate and failure of the vaccine strain to revert to wild type virus (Wyatt, 1973).

Echovirus and Coxsackievirus

Before the wide use of intravenous immunoglobulin, a significant proportion of patients with XLA used to have chronic and disseminated infections with echovi-

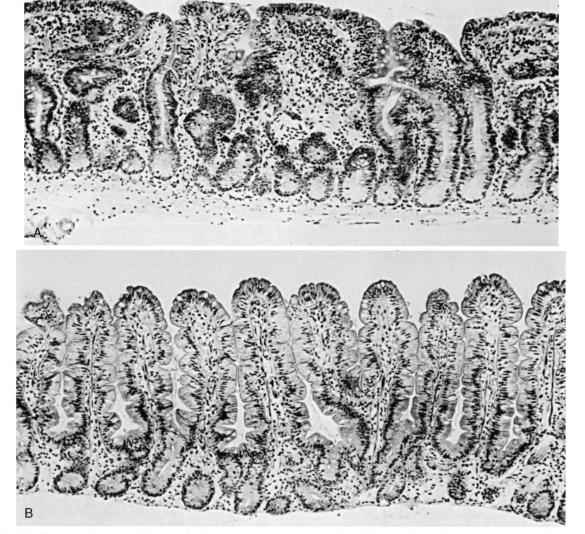

Figure 11–6. *A*, Representative peroral biopsy specimen taken near the duodenojejunal junction of a patient with common variable immunodeficiency, gastrointestinal symptoms, and malabsorption caused by *Giardia lamblia* infestation. The villus architecture is markedly abnormal. (H and E, ×150.) *B*, Biopsy specimen taken 4 weeks after completion of treatment to eradicate giardiasis; the villus architecture is normal. (H and E, ×150.) (*A* and *B* courtesy of Dr. Marvin Ament.)

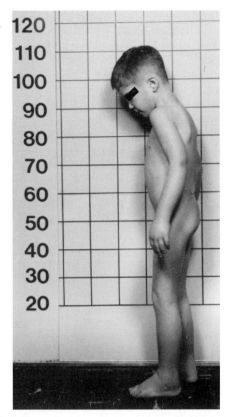

Figure 11–7. The patient is a 6-year-old boy with X-linked agammaglobulinemia and the dermatomyositis-like syndrome caused by disseminated echovirus 24 infection. Note the edema of the patient's extremities, especially the hands and feet, the gluteal wasting, and the flexion contractures of his arms and legs.

rus and coxsackievirus (Bardelas et al., 1977; Wilfert et al., 1977; McKinney et al., 1987). The infections may involve a number of different organs (e.g., the central nervous system, skin, subcutaneous tissue, muscle, heart and liver), leading to a syndrome of chronic meningoencephalitis (Wilfert et al., 1977), dermatomyositis (Gotoff et al., 1972; Bardelas et al., 1977) and/or hepatitis (Ziegler and Penny, 1975; Bardelas et al., 1977) (Fig. 11–7).

The chronic meningoencephalitis is often insidious in its onset with slowly progressive neurologic symptoms, including emotional lability and personality changes, episodic confusional states, loss of some cognitive functions, lethargy, weakness, ataxia, and paresis. In some patients, the onset is more acute and manifested initially by fever, headache, and seizures. The course is usually protracted, with some patients showing evidence of infection for nearly 10 years (Mease et al., 1985; McKinney et al., 1987) even when they have been treated with high doses of IVIG (see Treatment). In some patients, isolation of the virus from the cerebrospinal fluid (CSF) may be difficult or delayed until after symptoms and signs of central nervous system (CNS) infection have progressed. Isolation of coxsackie A virus is especially difficult and may require inoculation of suckling mice (O'Neil et al., 1988b). Newer detection systems, which depend on identification of viral genomic material by polymerase chain reaction

(PCR), have proved especially useful in documenting infection in some patients (Rotbart et al., 1990; Webster et al., 1993). In any case, CSF findings are generally typical of a viral meningoencephalitis with a mononuclear pleocytosis, elevated protein levels, and, occasionally, hypoglycorrhachia. However, some patients may have normal or near-normal CSF findings and may still have clinical evidence of encephalitis (Webster et al., 1993).

Patients with the *dermatomyositis-like syndrome* usually present with brawny edema of their extremities, an erythematous rash, and biopsy evidence of fasciitis and myositis. Affected areas show perivascular mononuclear infiltrates. In cases in which the technique has been attempted, virus can be isolated from the skin, muscle, or liver (Ziegler and Penny, 1975; Bardelas et al., 1977; Mease et al., 1981; Junker and Dimmick, 1982).

Other Infections

Resistance to other infections, presumed to be dependent on intact T-lymphocyte function (tuberculosis, histoplasmosis, varicella zoster), appears to be intact. When these infections occur, they are no more serious than in normal patients and they are self-limited. Although infection with *Pneumocystis carinii* has been observed in a few patients with XLA, it has usually occurred in patients who are also debilitated or otherwise compromised (Saulsbury et al., 1979; Lederman and Winkelstein, 1985).

Arthritis

Patients with XLA also may have arthritis. In some cases, the arthritis is caused by pyogenic bacteria and is typical of septic arthritis (Lederman and Winkelstein, 1985; Hermaszewski and Webster, 1993). However, there is also a form of arthritis that is not clearly septic in nature (Janeway et al., 1956; Good et al., 1957; Gitlin et al., 1959; Good and Rotstein, 1960; McLaughlin et al., 1972). It characteristically affects the large joints, and although hydrarthrosis and limited range of motion are common, pain is infrequent. There usually is no evidence of joint destruction, erythrocyte sedimentation rates are normal, and, as expected, serologic tests for rheumatoid factor and antinuclear antibodies are negative. The arthritis may improve when treatment with immunoglobulin is initiated or when the dose is increased, suggesting an infectious cause. In fact, in some patients the arthritis has been shown to be due to infection with enteroviruses or *Mycoplasma* (Hermaszewski and Webster, 1993; Ackerson et al., 1987), although in many the cause remains obscure. As newer techniques become available for the diagnosis of viruses and fastidious microorganisms, more cases of apparent noninfectious arthritis may in fact be identified as infectious.

Other Manifestations

A number of other less common clinical manifestations have also been described in patients with XLA. These include:

- Neutropenia (Buckley and Rolands, 1973; Lederman and Winkelstein, 1985; Hermaszewski and Webster, 1993)
- Alopecia totalis (Ipp and Gelfand, 1976), Glomerulonephritis (Avasthi et al., 1975)
- Protein-losing enteropathy (Norman et al., 1975)
- Malabsorption with disaccharidase deficiency (Dubois et al., 1970)
- Amyloidosis (Ziegler and Penny, 1975; Hermaszewski and Webster, 1993)

Physical Examination

Abnormalities on physical examination that are directly related to XLA include markedly hypoplastic or absent tonsils, adenoids, and lymph nodes, tissues that are normally rich in B lymphocytes (Fig. 11–8). Other abnormal physical findings are usually secondary to specific infections. In patients who have been diagnosed and treated after recurrent or severe infections have already occurred, evidence of chronic otitis, sinusitis and mastoiditis, or bronchiectasis may be present. However, in patients who are diagnosed and treated before permanent structural damage has occurred, the physical examination is normal and growth and development are age-appropriate.

Laboratory Findings

Immunoglobulins and Antibodies

Patients with XLA have markedly reduced levels of all three major classes of immunoglobulins in their serum (Rosen et al., 1984; Lederman and Winkelstein, 1985). Serum IgG levels are generally below 100 mg/dl and in some cases may be so low as to be nearly undetectable. However, in no patient is there a complete absence of IgG when highly sensitive assays are employed. In contrast, in some patients with XLA, levels of IgG may be as high as 200 to 300 mg/dl, although levels of IgG this high are relatively uncommon. Serum levels of IgA, IgM, and IgE are also markedly reduced or not detectable.

Along with their profound panhypogammaglobulinemia, patients with XLA fail to make antibody following antigenic stimulation. Antibody responses to ubiquitous antigens (e.g., anti-A and anti-B isohemagglutinins) are absent, and responses to known antigenic challenges are markedly decreased. Thus, antibody responses to the usual childhood vaccines (such as tetanus, diphtheria, pertussis, and *H. influenzae* type b) are all markedly reduced or undetectable (Rosen et al., 1984). In addition, their response to other immunogens (such as pneumococcal polysaccharide and typhoid vaccines) are also markedly abnormal. When immunized with a potent antigen to which the patient has never been exposed, such as bacteriophage ϕX-174, 60% of patients with XLA demonstrate an absolute inability to respond (see Fig. 11–3; Table 11–1) (Ching et al., 1966; Wedgwood et al., 1975). They do not clear phage from the blood stream in an accelerated manner and produce no detectable antibody. However, as many as 40% of patients with XLA clear phage from their blood stream in less than 1 week and produce small amounts of antigen-specific IgM antibody.

B and T Lymphocytes

Assessment of lymphocyte populations in peripheral blood and tissues generally reflects the underlying defect in the maturation of B lymphocytes. B-lymphocyte precursors (pre-B lymphocytes) are found in the bone marrow of patients with XLA (Pearl et al., 1978). How-

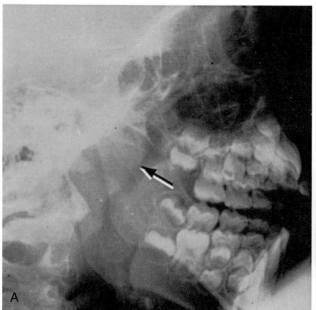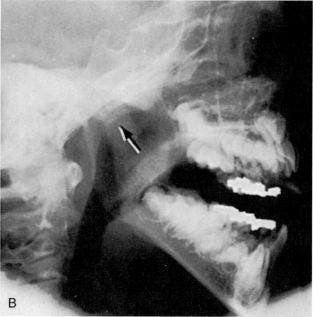

Figure 11–8. *A*, Lateral roentgenogram of the nasopharynx of a normal 10-year-old boy. Adenoidal tissue is present *(arrow)*. *B*, Lateral roentgenogram of the nasopharynx of a 10-year-old boy with X-linked agammaglobulinemia. Adenoidal tissue is absent *(arrow)*.

ever, such patients have few, if any, B lymphocytes in their peripheral blood or tissues, whether assessed by staining for the presence of surface immunoglobulin or by staining with B lymphocyte–specific monoclonal antibodies (anti-CD19, anti-CD20) (Siegal et al., 1971; Aiuti et al., 1972; Cooper and Lawton, 1972; Bentwich and Kunkel, 1973; Geha et al., 1973; Preud'Homme et al., 1973; Schiff et al., 1974). Because patients with XLA lack B lymphocytes, they also lack plasma cells in the bone marrow, the lamina propria of rectal mucosa (see Fig. 11–4) and lymph nodes (Good, 1955; Gitlin et al., 1959; Ament et al., 1973). Similarly, areas of lymph nodes that are usually rich in B lymphocytes and plasma cells, such as lymphoid follicles and germinal centers of lymph nodes, are markedly hypoplastic or absent altogether (see Fig. 11–2).

As expected, T-lymphocyte numbers and functions are normal. In vivo delayed-type hypersensitivity skin tests to ubiquitous antigens (e.g., *Candida*) or to known antigenic sensitization (e.g., mumps) are also normal.

The diagnosis of XLA in the newborn period and in the first few months of life is obscured by the presence of passively acquired maternal IgG. In addition, serum levels of IgA and IgM are low in normal infants during the first few months of life (Stiehm and Fudenberg, 1966a) and thus are not very helpful in making the diagnosis either. However, because normal infants have normal numbers of B lymphocytes in their peripheral blood at birth and patients with XLA have markedly reduced numbers (<1%), the diagnosis may be suggested by enumeration of B lymphocytes in peripheral blood at any age, even in the newborn.

Carrier Detection

Until recently, carrier detection was not possible in patients with XLA. In the last few years however, three new tools have made carrier detection a reality.

The first method relies on the fact that female carriers of XLA have altered patterns of X-chromosome inactivation in their B lymphocytes. Circulating B lymphocytes of noncarrier females contain two populations, one in which the maternal X-chromosome is active and one in which the paternal X-chromosome is active. In contrast, the B lymphocytes of female carriers of XLA contain only one population of B lymphocytes with respect to the active X-chromosome; the active X-chromosome is always the one that carries the normal allele at the XLA locus (see X-chromosome Inactivation Analysis). In one approach, methylation patterns are used to discriminate between the active and inactive X-chromosome (Fearon et al., 1987). In another approach, X-chromosome inactivation patterns are determined by examination of somatic cell hybrids that have selectively retained the active X-chromosome (Conley and Puck, 1988). The advantages of X-chromosome inactivation analysis for carrier detection are that the precise mutation responsible for the XLA does not need to be known and a previously affected family member need not be available for testing, as is the case in linkage analysis (Winkelstein and Fearon, 1990; Conley, 1992).

The second method relies on the ability to predict the presence of the mutant gene for XLA based on the presence of specific alleles of closely linked genes on the same chromosome (i.e., linkage analysis). Unfortunately, in order for linkage analysis to be useful, there must be a previously affected family member in whom a specific allele of the closely linked gene and the gene for XLA are present on the same chromosome. A number of polymorphic loci (e.g., DXS178) are closely linked to the XLA locus and have been useful in carrier detection (Kwan et al., 1986, 1990; Mensink et al., 1986a; Malcolm et al., 1987; Guioli et al., 1989; Parolini et al., 1993).

Finally, the discovery that XLA is due to mutations in the *Btk* gene (Tsukada et al., 1993; Vetrie et al., 1993) (see The *Btk* Gene) has allowed mutational analysis to be used as a direct method of carrier detection in families with known mutations (Vorechkovsky et al., 1993; Zhu et al., 1994a).

Prenatal Diagnosis

Prenatal diagnosis is possible by linkage analysis of amniotic fluid cells and/or enumeration of B lymphocytes in fetal cord blood. Prenatal diagnosis of an affected fetus has been performed using both techniques (Ochs, unpublished observation); these techniques have also been used to exclude the diagnosis in fetuses at risk (Journet et al., 1992; Kwan et al., 1994). In addition, just as mutational analysis has proved useful in carrier detection, it should also prove useful in prenatal diagnosis.

Treatment

The primary goal of treating patients with X-linked agammaglobulinemia is to replace immunoglobulin. Although intramuscular injection of immunoglobulin G (ISG) was initially the only form of replacement therapy, a number of different preparations of immunoglobulin suitable for intravenous infusion (IVIG) are available. Not only has IVIG allowed patients to achieve normal or near-normal serum levels of IgG; IVIG has also significantly improved the clinical course of patients with XLA (Sweinberg et al., 1991; Liese et al., 1992; Hermaszewski and Webster, 1993). In one study comparing different doses of IVIG to immune serum globulin (ISG) (Liese et al., 1992), patients who received relatively high doses of IVIG (>400 mg/kg every 3 weeks) and maintained trough levels of IgG at or near the lower limit of normal (>500 mg/dl) had significantly fewer hospitalizations and infections than patients who received lower doses of IVIG (<200 mg/kg every 3 weeks) or ISG. The effect of the higher dose of IVIG on the incidence of pneumonia, bacterial meningitis, and gastrointestinal infections, was particularly evident when treatment was initiated early in life.

Of particular concern in the treatment of patients with XLA is the prevention of or therapy for disseminated enterovirus infections (McKinney et al., 1987). Since the introduction of IVIG, the incidence of disseminated enteroviral infections has dropped dramatically;

however, it still may occur in some patients receiving IVIG (Rotbart et al., 1990; Misbah et al., 1992) or in children in whom the diagnosis of XLA is not recognized until after the enteroviral infection has occurred. Most patients with XLA and disseminated enteroviral infection have been treated with relatively high doses of IVIG aimed at maintaining the serum level of IgG above 1000 mg/dl. In many instances, specific lots of IVIG, with relatively high titers of antibody against the specific serotype of virus, have been employed. In some instances, IVIG has also been given by the intraventricular route in an attempt to deliver IgG to the site of CNS infection (Erlendsson et al., 1985).

Unfortunately, none of these therapies has proved completely successful in every patient. In some patients, relapses occurred (Mease et al., 1985; McKinney et al., 1987), indicating that despite clinical improvement, the infection did not resolve. In other patients, neurologic signs persisted (Ciliberti et al., 1994) or progressed despite high-dose IVIG given by both the intravenous and intraventricular routes (Johnson et al., 1985; O'Neil et al., 1988a; McKinney et al., 1987; Webster et al., 1993), albeit more slowly than in untreated patients, indicating that immunoglobulin therapy is not completely adequate in all cases once the infection has been established.

Although immunoglobulin therapy has been a major advance in the treatment of patients with XLA, it has some limitations. IVIG only replaces IgG and is unable to correct the defect in secretory immunity. In addition, the use of nonselected lots of IVIG does not provide high levels of specific antibody and, by definition, does not establish active immunity. Therefore, although IVIG significantly lowers the frequency and severity of infections in patients with XLA, it cannot prevent all infections in every patient. Treatment of acute bacterial infections with specific antibiotics may be necessary in some patients. In other patients, especially those in whom structural damage to the sinuses and/or lungs developed before treatment was instituted, chronic infections may necessitate long-term, broad-spectrum antibiotics and postural drainage.

Live viral vaccines are contraindicated in patients with XLA because vaccine-related infections, such as poliomyelitis (Wyatt, 1973; Wright et al., 1977; Lederman and Winkelstein, 1985; Hermaszewski and Webster, 1993), may develop. Killed vaccines are ineffective and are used only to test for antibody or T-cell responses.

Prognosis and Complications

Before antibiotics and immunoglobulin replacement therapy were available, few, if any, patients with XLA survived past infancy or early childhood. However, early diagnosis, regular immunoglobulin therapy, and prompt use of antibiotics have improved prognosis dramatically. In a series of 44 patients with XLA, age-related survival was significantly improved in those patients who had been diagnosed and treated more recently (Hermaszewski and Webster, 1993). Many patients with XLA have reached adulthood, have re-

mained free of long-term complications, and are productive members of society.

Nevertheless, complications may develop in some patients, especially in patients in whom the diagnosis has been delayed or in older patients who initially did not have the benefit of high-dose IVIG therapy. For example, in a series largely made up of patients who were diagnosed and treated before the introduction of IVIG, approximately 75% of the patients over 20 years of age had chronic lung disease, either obstructive disease alone or combined obstructive and restrictive disease, and 5% to 10% had cor pulmonale (Lederman and Winkelstein, 1985). Long-term disability may also result from chronic otitis media and hearing loss, which in turn may lead to delayed acquisition of speech and learning disorders.

Other less common complications of XLA include chronic disseminated enteroviral infections, vaccine-related poliomyelitis, and amyloidosis (Hermaszewski and Webster, 1993).

Finally, there has been some suggestion that patients with XLA have an increased prevalence of lymphoreticular malignancies (Page et al., 1963) (see Chapter 27). In one series, lymphoreticular malignancies developed in 2 of 96 patients (2%) with XLA (Lederman and Winkelstein, 1985), a figure very close to the estimate reported from the Immunodeficiency-Cancer Registry (0.7%) (Spector et al., 1978). In one study, 3 of 52 patients with XLA from the Netherlands developed colorectal cancer as young adults (25 to 36 years of age), an incidence 30-fold greater than expected (van der Meer et al., 1993). It is unknown whether this increased prevalence of colorectal cancer in patients with XLA is related to the absence of plasma cells in the gut mucosa or to persistent asymptomatic inflammation, as suggested by the presence of multiple crypt abscesses and polymorphonuclear leukocyte infiltrates in the lamina propria (see Fig. 11–4) (Ament et al., 1973). In another large series of patients with XLA, however, none of the 44 patients with XLA had a malignancy (Hermaszewski and Webster, 1993).

X-LINKED HYPOGAMMAGLOBULINEMIA WITH GROWTH HORMONE DEFICIENCY

In 1980, Fleisher and associates reported a family in which the combination of hypogammaglobulinemia and growth hormone deficiency were inherited as an X-linked recessive disorder (Fleisher et al., 1980). Since that original report, three additional unrelated families have been identified (Sitz et al., 1990; Conley et al., 1991; Monafo et al., 1991), suggesting that X-linked hypogammaglobulinemia with growth hormone deficiency is a distinct clinical entity rather than the coincidental occurrence in the same patients of two unrelated inherited disorders. However, the more recent report of growth hormone deficiency in a boy with immunodeficiency and increased IgM (Ohzeki et al., 1993) and the finding of isolated growth hormone deficiency and antibody deficiency in a girl with Mulibrey nanism (Haraldsson et al., 1993) support the alternative explanation of a nonspecific growth hormone deficiency that may develop in patients suffering from recurrent infections and an abnormal immune system.

Etiology

The cause of X-linked hypogammaglobulinemia with growth hormone deficiency is unknown. Studies in two of the families using X-chromosome inactivation analysis of female carriers have shown that the immunologic defect is intrinsic to the B-lymphocyte lineage (Conley et al., 1991). Other studies in these same two families using linkage analysis have also shown that the defect maps to a region of the X-chromosome that encompasses the gene for the more typical X-linked agammaglobulinemia (XLA) (Conley et al., 1991).

These findings suggest that X-linked hypogammaglobulinemia with growth hormone deficiency is either an allelic variant of the more typical XLA, which in some fashion affects both B-lymphocyte development and growth hormone production, or is a small, contiguous gene deletion syndrome that includes both the gene for XLA and another closely linked gene involved in growth hormone production. In this regard, it is interesting to note that although the structural gene for growth hormone is located on the long arm of chromosome 17 (George et al., 1981), there is also an X-linked gene that controls growth hormone production (Najiar et al., 1990; Phillips and Vnencak-Jones, 1989). Mutation analysis of *Btk* will be required to determine whether this entity is a variant of XLA or whether the two entities are unrelated disorders.

Clinical Manifestations

Patients with X-linked hypogammaglobulinemia with growth hormone deficiency have generally presented with many of the same problems seen in patients with more typical XLA. Individual patients have presented with recurrent upper respiratory infections, pneumonia, sepsis, recurrent otitis media, conjunctivitis, dacryocystitis, and monarticular arthritis. Their growth hormone deficiency has been manifested by short stature and, in those patients of an appropriate age, delayed onset of puberty.

Laboratory Findings

Most patients have presented with marked panhypogammaglobulinemia and absent B lymphocytes in the peripheral blood. However, one patient from the original kindred had normal levels of IgA and IgM and reduced but detectable (3%) numbers of B lymphocytes (Fleisher et al., 1980). Affected males do not respond to immunization with either protein or polysaccharide antigens. T-lymphocyte function is intact. Growth hormone deficiency is manifested by retarded bone age and deficient growth hormone responses to insulin, arginine, and L-dopa (Sitz et al., 1990; Conley et al., 1991; Monafo et al., 1991). As expected, levels of circulating somatomedin are also reduced (Fleisher et al., 1980). Other tests of endocrine function, includ-

ing cortisol responses to insulin-induced hypoglycemia and gonadal function, are normal (Fleisher et al., 1980).

Treatment

As with other patients with significant defects in B-lymphocyte function and humoral immunity, intravenous immunoglobulin (IVIG) remains the mainstay of therapy. Growth retardation appears to respond appropriately to exogenous growth hormone therapy.

Prognosis and Complications

Patients with X-linked hypogammaglobulinemia with growth hormone deficiency appear to have an excellent prognosis. In fact, many of the patients had not been identified as hypogammaglobulinemic until they were of school age or older (Fleisher et al., 1980; Sitz et al., 1990; Conley et al., 1991; Monafo et al., 1991), suggesting that the clinical expression of their immunodeficiency may be milder than in the more typical XLA. However, in one member of the original kindred, chronic disseminated echovirus infection developed and was manifested clinically as chronic meningoencephalitis and dermatomyositis (Wagner et al., 1989).

IMMUNOGLOBULIN DEFICIENCY WITH INCREASED IgM (HYPER-IgM SYNDROME)

Immunoglobulin deficiency with increased IgM is characterized by recurrent infections associated with low serum levels of IgG, IgA, and IgE and normal or increased IgM (Notarangelo et al., 1992). First described in 1961 (Burtin, 1961; Rosen et al., 1961), the syndrome is most commonly observed in males, and the most common mode of inheritance is X-linked (Krantman et al., 1980; Benkerrou et al., 1990; Notarangelo et al., 1991). However, the observation of women with immunoglobulin deficiency and increased IgM (Stiehm and Fudenberg, 1966b; Pascual-Salcedo et al., 1983; Benkerrou et al., 1990) suggests that there may be genetic heterogeneity with some cases of autosomal recessive or autosomal dominant inheritance (Beall, 1980; Brahmi et al., 1983). Secondary hyper-IgM syndromes (e.g., secondary to congenital rubella [Benkerrou et al., 1990] or the use of anti-epileptic drugs [Mitsuya et al., 1979]), are not discussed here.

Etiology

Although the dominant feature of the hyper-IgM syndrome is antibody deficiency, a number of clinical and laboratory observations have suggested that the abnormality is secondary to an intrinsic T-lymphocyte defect rather than due to an intrinsic defect of B lymphocytes. For example, the susceptibility of hyper-IgM patients to *Pneumocystis carinii* infections and autoimmune diseases is more commonly associated with T- than with B-lymphocyte defects. Other observations have suggested that the defect directly affects the T-lymphocyte–driven switch from IgM to other isotype synthesis. For example, when immunized with T-dependent antigens, such as bacteriophage φX174, hyper-IgM patients have depressed antibody responses and do not switch from IgM to IgG synthesis (Nonoyama et al., 1993b).

Several hypotheses have been considered to explain the inability of hyper-IgM B lymphocytes to switch from IgM to other immunoglobulin isotypes. An intrinsic B-lymphocyte defect was initially suggested by the finding that allogeneic T cells from healthy controls were unable to induce in vitro IgG or IgA synthesis by B lymphocytes from hyper-IgM patients, whereas hyper-IgM syndrome T cells readily induced IgG and IgA synthesis by normal B lymphocytes (Geha et al., 1979; Levitt et al., 1983). However, the subsequent finding that cultured T lymphoblasts obtained from a patient with a Sézary-like syndrome provided a signal for IgG and IgA secretion if cocultured with B lymphocytes from hyper-IgM patients suggested that a specific T cell–mediated switch signal may be lacking (Mayer et al., 1986).

CD40 Ligand Defect

These speculations were resolved by the discovery of the molecular defect for the X-linked form of the hyper-IgM syndrome. Five groups using different strategies independently assigned the defect to the gene encoding the T-cell activation protein CD40 ligand CD40L (gp39). CD40, the receptor for CD40L, is expressed constitutively by antigen-presenting cells, including B lymphocytes (Allen et al., 1993; Aruffo et al., 1993; DiSanto et al., 1993; Fuleihan et al., 1993; Korthäuer et al., 1993).

CD40 plays a major role in B-lymphocyte proliferation and differentiation (Clark and Lane, 1991); the interaction of CD40 with its ligand, gp39, induces the formation of memory B lymphocytes and the switch from IgM to other immunoglobulin isotypes (Lane et al., 1992; Noelle et al., 1992). With the use of fluores-

cence chromosomal in situ hybridization, the gene for CD40 ligand (gp39) was placed at band q26 of the X chromosome (Allen et al., 1993; Aruffo et al., 1993) precisely at the location where the gene for the hyper-IgM syndrome (HIGM1) had been mapped by restriction fragment length polymorphism (Mensink et al., 1987; Hendriks et al., 1991). When a soluble recombinant of CD40 (CD40-Ig), the physiologic receptor for CD40 ligand (gp39), was used, most activated peripheral blood T lymphocytes from normal individuals expressed CD40 ligand (Noelle et al., 1992). In contrast, activated T lymphocytes from 17 male patients with the clinical presentation of hyper-IgM syndrome did not bind the soluble CD40-Ig construct.

These findings suggest that all patients have in common a functional defect of CD40 ligand (gp39) (Allen et al., 1993; Aruffo et al., 1993; DiSanto et al., 1993; Fuleihan et al., 1993; Korthäuer et al., 1993). Three patients were also studied with a polyclonal antiserum to CD40 ligand (gp39) and, in two, a cross-reactive protein on the membrane of activated T cells was demonstrated; a third patient's T cells lacked CD40 ligand (gp39) protein (Korthäuer et al., 1993); this patient was the only one with a point mutation resulting in a positive charge located within the transmembrane domain, presumably preventing the protein from associating with the cell membrane.

All patients with hyper-IgM who were evaluated had detectable CD40 ligand (gp39) messenger RNA, either at normal or at moderately decreased levels. DNA sequencing revealed a wide spectrum of defects in the CD40 ligand gene (Fig. 11–9), including point mutations affecting the extracellular domain and resulting in amino acid substitutions that presumably interfere with the receptor binding site. In addition, there were point mutations resulting in stop codons or in deletions secondary to splice site mutations (Villa et al., 1994). The finding that patient-derived soluble CD40 ligand (gp39) failed to activate normal B lymphocytes to proliferate in the presence of interleukin-4 (IL-4) (Allen et al., 1993; Aruffo et al., 1993) demonstrates that these mutations were functionally of importance.

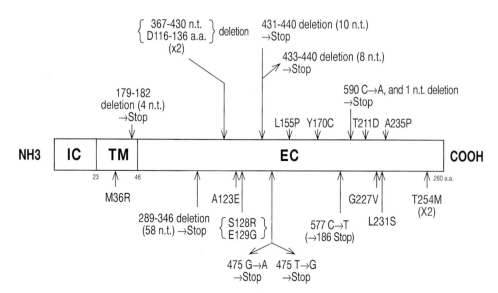

Figure 11–9. Schematic representation of the domains of CD40 ligand (gp39) expressed by activated T lymphocytes. The mutations published to date (Dec 1994) are localized throughout the coding region of gp39 and include point mutations affecting the extracellular domain and resulting in amino acid substitutions that may interfere directly with the receptor binding site. In addition, there are point mutations resulting in stop codons or in deletions secondary to splice site mutations. The nomenclature is explained in Figure 11–5. IC = intracellular domain; TM = transmembrane domain; EC = extracellular domain.

As a direct consequence of defective CD40 ligand (gp39) expression, activation signals cannot be efficiently delivered from T to B lymphocytes via the CD40 ligand (gp39)/CD40 system. This explains the fact that the circulating B lymphocytes of X-linked hyper-IgM patients express only IgM and IgD and make antibodies restricted to the IgM isotype. In accordance with this concept, B lymphocytes obtained from X-linked hyper-IgM patients proliferate and produce normal amounts of immunoglobulin, including IgM, IgG, IgA, and IgE, if appropriately stimulated in vitro with anti-CD40 and lymphokines (Allen et al., 1993; Aruffo et al., 1993; Korthäuer et al., 1993).

Further evidence of the importance of the CD40 ligand (gp39)/CD40 engagement on B-cell differentiation and isotype switch was provided by CD40 ligand deficient mice generated by gene targeting (CD40L knockout mice) (Xu et al., 1994). The mutant mice were able to mount IgM responses to T-dependent antigens, but not IgG, IgA, or IgE responses. Germinal center formation was defective in the mutant mice (in analogy to patients with X-linked hyper-IgM syndrome), demonstrating that CD40 ligand (gp39) expression is essential for T cell–dependent immunoglobulin class switching and germinal center formation. The observation of a similar phenotype in CD40-deficient mice (Kawabe et al., 1994) raises the possibility that a primary defect of CD40 may be the cause of hyper-IgM syndrome in some patients. Such a mechanism was suggested by the finding that 4 of 17 boys with the clinical phenotype of the hyper-IgM syndrome expressed normal amounts of CD40 ligand on their activated T lymphocytes (Conley et al., 1994b). In these patients, however, there were abnormal responses of B lymphocytes to stimulation with anti-CD40, which suggests that their immune defect was due to abnormal CD40-mediated signal transduction in their B lymphocytes.

In addition to its effect on regulating B-lymphocyte proliferation and differentiation, CD40 may also play an important role in the functional responses of other cell types. For example, CD40 is expressed on the surface of monocytes, follicular dendritic cells, basal epithelial cells, and thymic epithelial cells; the contribution of the CD40 ligand (gp39)/CD40 interaction between these cell types and activated T cells may be important for other host defense mechanisms. The frequently observed neutropenia, the common infection with *P. carinii*, and the increased incidence of malignancies characteristic for the hyper-IgM syndrome may be causally related to impaired cell-cell interaction.

Clinical Manifestations

Most patients with the hyper-IgM syndrome are males, have X-linked inheritance, and a defect in the gene encoding CD40 ligand (gp39). As a group, hyper-IgM patients present with characteristic clinical symptomatology and laboratory findings (Notarangelo et al., 1992). As with most primary immunodeficiency syndromes, hyper-IgM patients have in common an in-

creased susceptibility to infections, which is first observed at 6 months to 2 years of age, coinciding with the decline of maternally derived antibodies. Recurrent upper respiratory infections, otitis media, and pneumonia are observed in the majority of patients.

The predominant infective agents are bacterial. However, *P. carinii* pneumonia can be the presenting feature early in life of affected infants (Levitt et al., 1983; Benkerrou et al., 1990). Gastrointestinal complaints and malabsorption are frequently reported and in a subgroup of patients may become a major problem requiring parenteral nutrition (Kyong et al., 1978; Stiehm et al., 1986; Benkerrou et al., 1990). *G. lamblia* infection has been reported in a few cases (Barth et al., 1965; Benkerrou et al., 1990) and *Cryptosporidium* infection has been identified as causing protracted watery diarrhea (Stiehm et al., 1986). Cutaneous and soft tissue infections are occasionally present, and peritonsillar and peritracheal soft tissue infections may become life-threatening (Kyong et al., 1978; Barkin et al., 1975).

Lymphoid hyperplasia, including enlargement of tonsils, lymph nodes, spleen, and liver, is a common feature of X-linked hyper-IgM syndrome and may be a result of constant antigenic stimulation of a B-lymphocyte system limited to IgM production. The appearance of autoantibodies has been associated with the development of thrombocytopenia, hemolytic anemia, and hypothyroidism (Pascual-Salcedo et al., 1983; Benkerrou et al., 1990). Arthritis and arthralgias observed in the hyper-IgM syndrome and in other primary immunodeficiency disorders may be a result of chronic infection or the production of autoantibody.

The mechanisms for the intermittent or persistent neutropenia, which may develop in more than 50% of the patients with X-linked hyper-IgM and cause persistent stomatitis and recurrent oral ulcers, are unknown. There have been families observed with several affected males, some with and some without neutropenia. Most hyper-IgM patients with neutropenia present with either a block at the myelocyte-promyelocyte stages or a reduced number of cells within the myeloid series, including early myeloid progenitors (Notarangelo et al., 1992).

The susceptibility to *P. carinii* pneumonia (Levitt et al., 1983; Benkerrou et al., 1990), cryptosporidium infection (Stiehm et al., 1986), the observation of extensive verruca vulgaris lesions (Rosen and Janeway, 1966), and the increased risk of malignancies (Filipovitch et al., 1987), rarely observed in other antibody deficiency syndromes, have been used as an argument for a T-cell defect, a suggestion that has been confirmed in the X-linked form of the hyper-IgM syndrome.

Laboratory Findings

One can establish the diagnosis of X-linked hyper-IgM syndrome unequivocally by demonstrating the inability of activated CD4$^+$ T cells to express CD40 ligand (gp39), using either a soluble form of the physiologic receptor for the CD40 ligand (a recombinant of CD40, CD40-Ig) or a monoclonal antibody recognizing the extracellular domain of CD40 ligand and flow cytometry. Both techniques can also be used in the attempt to identify carrier females (Hollenbaugh et al., 1994b). The diagnosis of X-linked hyper-IgM syndrome is confirmed by demonstration of a mutation within the CD40 ligand gene.

Several characteristic immunologic abnormalities differentiate the X-linked form of the hyper-IgM syndrome from other immunodeficiencies, such as XLA. The number of peripheral blood B lymphocytes is normal, and they express surface IgM, IgD, or both, but rarely other isotypes (Levitt et al., 1983). As a correlate, serum IgG, IgA, and IgE are absent or very low. Serum IgM levels may be normal or as high as 1000 mg/dl. In contrast to Waldenström's macroglobulinemia, multiple myeloma and benign monoclonal gammopathy with IgM paraproteinemia (Rosen and Janeway, 1966), the elevated IgM concentration in the hyper-IgM syndrome is not due to a monoclonal component; rather, it reflects a polyclonal increase of serum IgM and consists of both κ and λ chains. Serum IgM may in part be low molecular weight (7S) IgM and may lead to inappropriate high estimates of IgM if radioimmunodiffusion techniques are used (Notarangelo et al., 1992).

Specific antibodies that usually are of the IgM isotype (isohemagglutinins, antityphoid O, Forssman antibodies) are frequently present in patients with primary or secondary hyper-IgM syndrome (Pascual-Salcedo et al., 1983; Benkerrou et al., 1990). If immunized with a T cell–dependent antigen, for example, bacteriophage φX174 (see Table 11–1), patients with hyper-IgM syndrome demonstrate a low normal primary and depressed secondary antibody response consisting of IgM only and either absent or markedly reduced amplification (Aruffo et al., 1993; Nonoyama et al., 1993a). In the X-linked form of the hyper-IgM syndrome, the quantitative (lack of amplification and memory) and qualitative (failure to switch) defect characteristically observed is a direct consequence of the genetic defect, the inability to express functional CD40 ligand on activated T lymphocytes. If stimulated in vitro with anti-CD40 or with soluble CD40 ligand (gp39) and in the presence of IL-10, hyper-IgM B lymphocytes produce predominantly IgM. However, if stimulated with anti-CD40 and IL-4, B lymphocytes from hyper-IgM patients switch normally to IgE production and can produce some IgG and IgA (Allen et al., 1993; Aruffo et al., 1993; Korthäuer et al., 1993).

Although lymphoid hyperplasia is a constant finding, germinal centers are absent and follicles are rarely observed (Stiehm and Fudenberg, 1966b; Benkerrou et al., 1990). The number of T lymphocytes, T-lymphocyte subsets, and in vitro proliferation of lymphocytes are normal in most patients (Geha et al., 1979; Benkerrou et al., 1990).

In addition to the immunologic abnormalities, patients with the hyper-IgM syndrome frequently have abnormalities of other hematopoietic lineages. Of the patients with X-linked hyper-IgM, 50% present with persistent or cyclic neutropenia (Benkerrou et al., 1990; Notarangelo et al., 1992). Anemia is present in approximately 25% and may be a direct result of

autoantibodies (Notarangelo et al., 1992; Pascual-Salcedo et al., 1983). Production of autoantibodies has been observed in hyper-IgM patients and may lead to nephritis, hemolytic anemia, and thrombocytopenia.

Treatment and Prognosis

The complex clinical presentation of the hyper-IgM syndrome is reflected in an equally complex therapeutic approach that consists of several goals. Regular infusions of IVIG at a dose of 300 to 500 (or more) mg/kg per month is the most important single therapeutic step in reducing the frequency and severity of infections. If the patient is not well controlled on monthly IVIG infusions, the interval between infusions may be shortened. Regular IVIG infusions often result in a reduction or normalization of serum IgM levels (Benkerrou et al., 1990). In many instances, patients resume normal growth and become asymptomatic after the institution of IVIG therapy. In some patients, neutropenia has improved during treatment with high doses of IMIG/plasma or IVIG (Rieger et al., 1974; Banatvala et al., 1994). Infants with the X-linked form of hyper-IgM syndrome are especially susceptible to *P. carinii* pneumonia and should receive prophylaxis with trimethoprim-sulfamethoxazole (Banatvala et al., 1994).

Patients with persistent neutropenia have responded to granulocyte–colony-stimulating factor (G-CSF) therapy (Banatvala et al., 1994). Patients with lymphoid hyperplasia and arthritis or other autoimmune disorders who are not responding to IVIG may benefit from steroid therapy. In some cases, malabsorption is a major complication, necessitating total parenteral nutrition (Stiehm et al., 1986; Benkerrou et al., 1990). Progressive sclerosing cholangitis developed in five patients (Banatvala et al., 1994; Stiehm, personal communication, 1995).

Although patients with the hyper-IgM syndrome, unlike those with XLA, are not susceptible to severe enteroviral infections and can make specific IgM antibody, their overall prognosis is not better, and may even be worse, than the outcome for patients with XLA. The high incidence of autoimmune disorders, bowel disease, and neutropenia, and the increased incidence of malignancies are responsible for additional morbidity and mortality. However, because of more benign therapeutic options, bone marrow transplantation is generally not indicated. In patients with the CD40 ligand defect, gene therapy may be an option in the future.

ANTIBODY DEFICIENCY WITH NORMAL OR ELEVATED IMMUNOGLOBULINS

There have been patients identified in whom there is clear evidence of deficient antibody formation and an increased susceptibility to infection in spite of normal serum levels of immunoglobulin isotypes and subclasses. Cellular immunity is intact.

Etiology

The cause and pathogenesis of antibody deficiency with normal levels of immunoglobulins are unclear. It is known, however, that the antibody response to immunization with specific antigens varies from individual to individual within a population, and it is possible that some of the causes for that variation are responsible, at least in part, for this immunodeficiency. For example, the magnitude of an antibody response and the ability to form any antibody at all to some antigens are related to immune response genes located within the major histocompatibility locus (Klein et al., 1983) or to the presence of certain immunoglobulin allotypes (Granoff et al., 1984; Ambrosino et al., 1985).

Developmental defects may also be a contributing factor, since, even in normal individuals, the ability to form antibody against polysaccharides is markedly diminished in the first year or two of life (Peltola et al., 1977; Douglas et al., 1983).

Finally, environmental factors may also contribute because exposure to high doses of antigen at an early stage of development can induce specific tolerance and lack of antibody formation on later exposure to that antigen (Nossal, 1983).

Thus, it is likely that this disorder does not represent a single entity. All reported cases have been sporadic with no familial clustering.

Clinical Manifestations

Patients with antibody deficiency and normal immunoglobulin levels present with the same infections as patients with common variable immunodeficiency. Recurrent otitis, sinusitis, and pneumonia are relatively common (Blecher et al., 1968; Rothbach et al., 1979; Saxon et al., 1980; Ambrosino et al., 1987), and recurrent pneumococcal sepsis has also been described (Gigliotti et al., 1988; Germain-Lee et al., 1990). In some instances, persistent lymphadenopathy has also been noted (Rothbach et al., 1979; Saxon et al., 1980).

This immunodeficiency may be more common than is generally appreciated. A number of investigators have examined patients with recurrent respiratory tract infections who had normal levels of serum immunoglobulin classes and subclasses for the presence of antibody deficiency (Ambrosino et al., 1988; Herrod et al., 1989; Shapiro et al., 1991; Sanders et al., 1993). In each series, a significant number of patients were identified who did not respond to immunization with pneumococcal and/or *H. influenzae* type b, capsular polysaccharide vaccines, although the frequency of individuals who failed to respond (between 10 and 20%) varied from series to series.

Laboratory Findings

The hallmark of this type of antibody deficiency is the inability to form antibody against specific antigens. Most patients reported have shown significant responses to some antigens, even though they did not respond to others (Blecher et al., 1968; Rothbach et

al., 1979; Saxon et al., 1980; Ambrosino et al., 1987). Thus, it is critical that a patient suspected of having this disorder be immunized with a battery of antigens, including both proteins (e.g., tetanus) and purified polysaccharides (e.g., pneumococcal capsular polysaccharide). Patients have had abnormal responses to some protein antigens and to some polysaccharide antigens (Blecher et al., 1968; Rothbach et al., 1979; Saxon et al., 1980), but other patients had normal responses to all protein antigens tested but did not respond to polysaccharides (Ambrosino et al., 1987; Gigliotti et al., 1988; Germain-Lee et al., 1990). It is of interest that in some of the latter patients, immunization with polysaccharide antigen coupled to protein carriers overcame the defect (Gigliotti et al., 1988; Herrod et al., 1989); in others, it did not (Germain-Lee et al., 1990).

Because the serum levels of immunoglobulin classes and subclasses are normal or elevated and the numbers of B lymphocytes and T lymphocytes in the peripheral blood are normal, the diagnosis can be confirmed only by assessing in vivo antibody responses to a battery of T-dependent and less T-dependent antigens.

Treatment

Treatment of this type of antibody deficiency is similar to that of patients with other B-lymphocyte deficiencies. Regular infusions with IVIG have been of benefit and have decreased the frequency and severity of infections. In contrast to the situation in patients with hypogammaglobulinemia, however, using IgG levels after infusions as a guide to establishing the proper dose of IVIG is of little benefit because these patients, by definition, have normal levels of IgG before therapy.

COMMON VARIABLE IMMUNODEFICIENCY

Common variable immunodeficiency (CVI) refers to a heterogeneous group of patients who may present at any age; often, however, onset is after puberty, usually in the second or third decade of life, with recurrent bacterial infections, hypogammaglobulinemia, and impaired antibody responses (Rosen and Janeway, 1966; Cunningham-Rundles, 1989; Hermaszewski and Webster, 1993; Sneller et al., 1993; Strober et al., 1993). Most patients have normal or moderately decreased numbers of circulating B lymphocytes and normal cell-mediated immunity. However, careful analysis of T-lymphocyte function has revealed abnormalities in a large proportion of patients with CVI (Reinherz et al., 1979; Cunningham-Rundles et al., 1981).

Etiology

The diagnosis of common variable immunodeficiency is dependent on excluding other well-defined immunodeficiency syndromes. Patients with the hyper-IgM syndrome (Aruffo et al., 1993) or with a milder form of X-linked agammaglobulinemia (Vorechkovsky et al., 1993; Zhu et al., 1994b) can be clearly identified by demonstrating the characteristic molecular defect involving CD40 ligand (gp39) and *Btk*, respectively. Because there is great variability in the age of onset, a broad spectrum of clinical findings and laboratory abnormalities, and an unpredictable genetic component (Ashman et al., 1992; Volanakis et al., 1992), it is to be expected that CVI is not caused by a single defect. Indeed, in spite of intensive investigation, a precise molecular defect resulting in the clinical entity of CVI has not yet been discovered.

Studies of T and B lymphocytes from patients with CVI, both in vitro and in vivo, have revealed a wide variety of abnormalities. Although most patients with CVI have normal numbers of mature B lymphocytes in the peripheral blood and lymphoid tissue, B lymphocytes from patients with CVI are unable to differentiate into immunoglobulin-secreting plasma cells. Because normal B-lymphocyte differentiation is influenced greatly by T lymphocytes, either through direct interaction or through the secretion of lymphokines, the immunodeficiency observed in CVI may be due to an intrinsic B-lymphocyte defect (Farrant et al., 1989), a T-lymphocyte defect (Jaffe et al., 1993), or an accessory cell defect (Eibl et al., 1982a, 1982b; Farrant et al., 1985).

B-Cell Defect

A B-lymphocyte defect as a cause of CVI is suggested by the observation that in a small proportion of CVI patients, peripheral B lymphocytes are low in number or undetectable (Preud'Homme et al., 1973; Farrant et al., 1989). Male patients with the clinical diagnosis of CVI and low numbers of B lymphocytes may in fact have atypical X-linked agammaglobulinemia and should be studied for mutations of the *Btk* gene (Vorechkovsky et al., 1993; Zhu et al., 1994b). In contrast to the mature memory B cells observed in normal people, circulating CVI B cells have the phenotypic characteristics of immature B lymphocytes—increased size, use of specific V_H gene families, and lack of somatic mutation of variable heavy-chain genes (Braun et al., 1992).

During earlier studies of B-lymphocyte function in CVI, in vitro immunoglobulin synthesis in response to polyclonal activators was measured. From these studies, it appeared that most patients had an intrinsic B-lymphocyte defect, as suggested by the observation that if cocultured with normal allogeneic T lymphocytes, CVI B lymphocytes did not produce or secrete immunoglobulin. Conversely, T lymphocytes from most of these patients supported immunoglobulin production by normal B lymphocytes (De la Concha et al., 1977; Ashman et al., 1980). When partially purified B lymphocytes were activated with mitogens in the presence of soluble T-cell factors, three subgroups of patients with CVI could be identified. One group of patients failed to produce any immunoglobulin; a second group produced only IgM, with little or no IgG; and a third group produced IgM and IgG in normal quantities (Bryant et al., 1990). Similar findings were reported by Saiki et al. (1982), DeGast et al. (1980), Mitsuya et al. (1981), Mayer et al. (1984), and Saxon et al. (1989).

These studies suggest that most patients with CVI have B lymphocytes that can secrete immunoglobulin, although often limited to IgM, if given the appropriate in vitro stimulation. To date, no evidence has been provided for any specific intrinsic B-lymphocyte abnormality in CVI affecting immunoglobulin genes, immunoglobulin gene rearrangement, or isotype switching. These results support the hypothesis that B lymphocytes from most patients with CVI are not intrinsically abnormal and that their dysfunction may be a result of the lack of appropriate external stimuli, causing a differentiation arrest at an immature B-lymphocyte level (Braun et al., 1991, 1992).

T-Cell Defect

The concept of a primary T-lymphocyte defect in CVI has been favored in recent years and is based on in vitro analysis of T- and B-lymphocyte subsets and their function. Although most CVI patients have normal T-cell subsets (Jaffe et al., 1993) a subgroup of CVI patients (25% to 30%) have increased numbers of CD8⁺ lymphocytes, normal or decreased numbers of CD4⁺ lymphocytes and, as a result, reduced CD4/CD8 ratios (Jaffe et al., 1993; Aukrust et al., 1994). A decrease in the CD4⁺ CD45RA⁺ population observed in a subgroup of CVI patients by several investigators (Lebranchu et al., 1990, 1991; Baumert et al., 1992; Richards et al., 1992) suggests the possibility of persistent activation of circulating naive T cells to the more mature CD45RO population, or, alternatively, preferential homing of the CD45RA⁺ lymphocytes into chronically infected tissues. A functional T-lymphocyte defect was suggested by the observation of decreased proliferation of CVI-derived peripheral blood lymphocytes when stimulated in vitro with mitogens or specific antigens (Cunningham-Rundles et al., 1981; North et al., 1991). Furthermore, lymphocytes from a subgroup of CVI patients, when activated in vitro by various agents, produced markedly decreased amounts of interleukin-specific messenger RNA and of functional interleukins, including IL-2 (Kruger et al., 1984; Eisenstein et al., 1993; Farrington et al., 1994); IL-2 and IL-4 (Pastorelli et al., 1989a); IFN-γ (Paganelli et al., 1988); and IL-2, IL-4, IL-5, and IFN-γ (Sneller and Strober, 1990).

The existence of a subgroup of CVI patients whose symptoms of splenomegaly and lymphadenopathy suggest chronic immune activation was supported by the detection of serum immunoreactive IL-4 and IL-6 in more than one third of all CVI patients tested (Aukrust et al., 1994). These lymphokines could not be demonstrated in normal control serum or in serum from patients with classic XLA with similar infections. Elevated IL-4 and IL-6 serum levels in the patients were accompanied by elevated serum levels of neopterin and of soluble CD8 and by low numbers of CD4⁺ T lymphocytes and CD19⁺ B lymphocytes. It is interesting to speculate that this clinical phenotype is caused by an as yet unknown chronic viral infection and that the overproduction of cytokines plays a role in the pathogenesis of CVI. The persistence of measurable IL-4 in serum of some CVI patients may be of significance, since IL-4 can suppress in vitro immunoglobulin production by activated CVI lymphocytes (Pastorelli et al., 1989b).

Suppressor T-Cell Defect

The concept of suppressor T cells playing a role in the pathogenesis of common variable immunodeficiency was first proposed in 1974 by Waldmann et al. In some series, the proportion of CVI patients with CD8[+] T lymphocytes that had a suppressive effect on B-cell differentiation and immunoglobulin secretion was considerable (Siegal et al., 1976; Rodriguez et al., 1983). Other reports suggest that suppressor T cells play a minor role, if any, in the pathogenesis of CVI (Siegal et al., 1978). It is, however, possible that the overabundance of T cell subsets predominantly secreting lymphokines that suppress immunoglobulin synthesis (e.g., gamma-interferon), contribute to the immunodeficiency observed in CVI.

Activation Defect

CD40 ligand (gp39), expressed by activated CD4[+] lymphocytes, is of pivotal importance in inducing B-cell proliferation and differentiation. The observation that gp39 mRNA as well as functional gp39 protein expression by activated lymphocytes from 40% of all CVI patients (who have a normal gp39 gene) studied was significantly depressed compared with normal controls suggests that inefficient signaling via CD40 may be responsible, in part, for the lack of B-cell differentiation in this subgroup of CVI patients (Farrington et al., 1994).

The observation that B cells from CVI patients, when cultured in vitro in the presence of anti-CD40 and IL-4, undergo normal proliferation and synthesize normal quantities of IgE further supports the hypothesis that most patients with CVI have B lymphocytes capable of normal function (Nonoyama et al., 1993a). Furthermore, if cultured with anti-CD40 and IL-10, B cells from every CVI patient studied produced immunoglobulin. Four patterns of in vitro Ig isotype synthesis by CVI B cells were observed. One third of CVI patients produced normal amounts of IgM, IgG and IgA; 25% produced normal quantities of IgM and IgG, but no IgA. Of the remaining 12 patients who did not synthesize IgG and IgA, eight produced normal amounts of IgM and four synthesized decreased amounts (Nonoyama et al., 1993a).

Genetic Abnormality

Although common variable immunodeficiency is not usually inherited as a single gene defect, there is evidence for a genetic component in some patients. For example, there is a small group of CVI patients with a positive family history, suggesting a genetic predisposition. In fact, in the same families, some patients may have CVI whereas others have IgA deficiency. The existence of a genetic predisposition for CVI is further supported by the association of CVI and familial IgA deficiency with specific major histocompatibility complex (MHC) haplotypes (Ashman et al., 1992; Volanakis et al., 1992).

In summary, CVI is probably a heterogeneous group of disorders that may have an intrinsic B-cell defect; more likely, it is a B-cell dysfunction that is caused by abnormal T-B cell interaction caused by a primary T-cell defect. The precise molecular defect is unknown and may include abnormal lymphokine production or, perhaps, defective activation of one or more genes involved in lymphokine function.

Clinical Manifestations

As is characteristic of all primary immunodeficiency diseases affecting antibody production, patients with CVI present foremost with recurrent sinopulmonary infections. Symptoms may first appear during childhood or, more often, after puberty. Bronchiectasis may develop if optimal therapy is delayed. In fact, unrecognized CVI cases often are identified in "chest" or pulmonary clinics; this finding indicates that individuals with unexplained bronchiectasis must be evaluated for immunodeficiency.

The organisms most often involved are *H. influenzae*, *S. pneumoniae*, and staphylococci. In rare situations, infections may develop and involve such unusual organisms as *P. carinii*, *Mycobacterium*, or fungi (Esolen et al., 1992; Sneller et al., 1993). Prolonged and persistent infection with *Mycoplasma pneumoniae* is not infrequent (Foy et al., 1973; Taylor-Robinson et al., 1980; Lee et al., 1993). Recurrent attacks of herpes simplex are frequently observed, and herpes zoster eventually develops in up to 20% of CVI patients (Asherson et al., 1980).

Gastrointestinal involvement is common in patients with CVI. A chronic malabsorption syndrome characterized by steatorrhea, folate and vitamin B_{12} deficiency, lactose intolerance, generalized disaccharidase deficiency, protein-losing enteropathy, and abnormalities of villus architecture, is seen frequently in CVI patients (Ament et al., 1973). *G. lamblia* was present in seven of eight symptomatic individuals. Eradication of the parasites with metronidazole resulted in disappearance of the gastrointestinal symptoms, including malabsorption, and in normalization of villus architecture (see Fig. 11–6).

Nodular lymphoid hyperplasia is frequently observed. Endoscopic examination of the small bowel reveals large lymphoid follicles with germinal centers within the lamina propria, causing protrusion of the overlying mucosa and nodular or polypoid appearance on radiographs (Hermans et al., 1966). Plasma cells of the lamina propria are usually absent or markedly reduced. Most patients with nodular lymphoid hyperplasia are asymptomatic unless they are infected with *G. lamblia*; eradication of the parasites improves symptomatology but does not change the extent of nodular lymphoid hyperplasia. In addition to *G. lamblia* infection, patients with CVI are at risk for gastrointestinal infections with enteropathogens, including *Salmonella, Shigella, Campylobacter,* and such rare organisms as dysgonic fermenter-3 (DF-3), a gram-negative bacterium (Sneller et al., 1993).

Autoimmune disorders are more frequent in patients with CVI and in their relatives than in a normal control population (Fudenberg et al., 1962; Friedman et al., 1977; Conley et al., 1986b; Lee et al., 1993). Disorders resembling rheumatoid arthritis, dermatomyositis, scleroderma, and systemic lupus erythematosus have been described in adult CVI patients. Autoimmune hemolytic anemia, idiopathic thrombocytopenic purpura, autoimmune neutropenia, pernicious anemia, chronic active hepatitis, parotitis, and Guillain-Barré syndrome have also been observed (Good and Yunis, 1974; Conley et al., 1986b; Lee et al., 1993). In adult patients, especially those living in the southeastern part of the United States, noncaseating granulomas of the lung, spleen, and liver, a condition resembling sarcoidosis, may develop (Bronsky and Dunn, 1965; Davis et al., 1970; Sharma and James, 1971). Inflammatory bowel disease (both Crohn's and ulcerative colitis) occurs in CVI with increased frequency (Ament et al., 1973).

There is an unusually high incidence of lymphoreticular and gastrointestinal malignancies in older patients with CVI. Gastric carcinoma is increased 50-fold and lymphoma is increased 300-fold compared with the general population (Kinlen et al., 1985; Cunningham-Rundles et al., 1987).

Laboratory Findings

Serum immunoglobulin levels are consistently depressed but are generally higher in patients with CVI than in patients with XLA. IgG concentrations rarely exceed 300 mg/dl but occasionally may reach 500 mg/dl. IgM and IgA levels are low or undetectable in most patients. Isohemagglutinin titers and specific antibody levels are depressed or absent. Following immunization with bacteriophage φX174, all CVI patients studied have cleared antigen and the majority of patients produced neutralizing antibody. However, a large proportion of CVI patients exhibit low titers, abnormal amplification, and a depressed switch from IgM to IgG (see Table 11–1).

Lymphocyte subsets in the peripheral blood, as determined by surface markers, are normal in the majority of patients, including the presence of normal or only moderately decreased numbers of B lymphocytes. However, up to one third of patients with CVI have an abnormally low CD4/CD8 ratio (<1.0), primarily as a result of a significant increase in $CD8^+$ T lymphocytes. This subset of $CD8^+$ T cells, preferentially expressed by patients with splenomegaly and bronchiectasis, co-express HLA-DR and IL-2 receptor, suggesting in vivo activation (Wright et al., 1990; Jaffe et al., 1993).

The standard tests to assess T-cell function, including in vitro proliferation in response to mitogens, antigens, and allogeneic cells, are subnormal in up to 50% of CVI patients, with a small subgroup of patients having very low responses (Kopp et al., 1968; Douglas et al.,

1970; Lieber et al., 1971). In addition, as pointed out earlier, a number of investigators have demonstrated a decreased production of lymphokines and abnormally low expression of T-lymphocyte activation markers (e.g., CD40 ligand) in a subgroup of CVI patients (Kruger et al., 1984; Paganelli et al., 1988; Pastorelli et al., 1989a; Sneller and Strober, 1990; Farrington et al., 1994).

In vitro assessment of B cells with techniques that eliminate the need of direct T-cell contact suggests that B cells from most CVI patients are either normal or less mature, similar to cord blood B lymphocytes (Nonoyama et al., 1993a).

Treatment

In the absence of a clinically relevant T-lymphocyte defect, treatment of CVI patients with immunoglobulin infusions improves the clinical course and often ensures a normal life style. Dose and infusion schedule are similar to those described for XLA. Those patients with an increase in $CD8^+$ T cells, often associated with splenomegaly, may not respond as well to IVIG as do CVI patients without signs of in vivo activation of the immune system. The standard dose is 400 mg/kg per month; more frequent infusions with an appropriately reduced dose may be more effective. Some patients with chronic lung disease require up to 600 to 800 mg/kg per month (Roifman et al., 1987). Most patients with immunodeficiency and arthritis, including CVI, respond favorably to adequate treatment with intravenous immunoglobulin (McLaughlin et al., 1972).

Because treatment with immunoglobulin does not always reverse chronic infections, long-term treatment with broad-spectrum antibiotics may be needed in some patients. To avoid the development of resistant organisms, antibiotics should be rotated, with preparations changed every 2 weeks.

The presence of chronic bronchiectasis may require physical therapy and postural drainage. Patients with gastrointestinal symptoms and malabsorption should be evaluated for the presence of *G. lamblia;* since stool evaluation is often unreliable, a negative result should be followed up by a *Giardia*-specific ELISA test or by small-bowel biopsy to be examined for *Giardia* trophozoites. In most instances, treatment with metronidazole results in marked improvement of the gastrointestinal complaints.

Steroids or other immunosuppressive drugs should be used with caution and given only in autoimmune disorders that result in significant disease. In general, a short course of steroid therapy is well tolerated. Occasionally, if splenomegaly is excessive and there are signs of hypersplenism, splenectomy may be indicated. This results in an increased risk for septicemia, and therefore prophylactic antibiotic therapy is indicated.

Because of the observation that lymphocytes from a subgroup of patients with CVI, when activated in vitro, produce markedly decreased amounts of IL-2 (Pastorelli et al., 1983a; Kruger et al., 1984; Sneller and Strober, 1990; Eisenstein et al., 1993; Farrington et al., 1994), an experimental preparation of IL-2 conjugated with polyethylene glycol (PEG) was given to a select group of CVI patients (Cunningham-Rundles et al., 1992, 1994). After several months of therapy, in vitro immunoglobulin secretion by the patients' B cells increased significantly and an increase in the in vitro production of IL-2 and the production of serum antibody was observed. One of the CVI patients who seemed to improve clinically was kept on weekly subcutaneous injection of PEG-conjugated IL-2 at a dose of 250,000 IU per square meter of body surface area. This prolonged treatment resulted in improved cellular immune functions, including an increase in T-cell proliferation in response to mitogens and antigens, restoration of lymphokine secretion of IL-2, IL-6 and a B-cell differentiation factor, an increase in serum immunoglobulin levels, and the production of antibody to pneumococcal polysaccharide, tetanus, and diphtheria toxoid. Carefully controlled clinical studies need to be performed to determine whether regular injections of lymphokines are useful for the long-term treatment of patients with CVI.

Treatment with 13-cis retinoic acid given longitudinally in an attempt to induce B-cell differentiation has not improved the clinical course of patients with CVI, although in vivo maturation of B cells has been promoted in individual CVI patients (Saxon et al., 1993).

Prognosis

The prophylactic use of immunoglobulin infusions and antibiotic therapy for acute infections have greatly improved the prognosis of patients with CVI. In many individuals with CVI, however, chronic sinopulmonary diseases develop, progressing to chronic lung disease and bronchiectasis. The causes of premature death include chronic lung disease with or without cor pulmonale, liver failure due to viral hepatitis, sequelae of chronic gastroenteritis, and malignancies, including carcinoma and lymphoma (Kersey et al., 1973; Filipovich et al., 1987; Cunningham-Rundles et al., 1987; Cunningham-Rundles, 1989).

Female patients over age 45 seem to be especially susceptible to malignancy. Nevertheless, males with CVI have higher mortality than females do. In one large series, the average age of women with CVI at the time of death was 55 years and the average age of males was 29 years (Cunningham-Rundles, 1989). Many years of follow-up are required to determine whether the long-term outcome of CVI can be improved by optimal therapy with IVIG.

HYPER-IMMUNOGLOBULIN D SYNDROME (HYPER-IgD SYNDROME)

IgD is the least understood serum immunoglobulin, but it may play a role in immunological memory (Lafrenz et al., 1982; Blattner and Tucker, 1984) and in immune regulation (Coico et al., 1985). The hyper-IgD syndrome is a rare disorder originally observed in several unrelated Dutch families (Van der Meer et al., 1984; Hiemstra et al., 1989; Haraldsson et al., 1992).

In a subsequently published review, 50 patients with hyper-IgD syndrome, mainly from Western Europe, and a single case from Japan were described in detail (Drenth et al., 1994).

The observations that many children with the hyper-IgD syndrome have a history of adverse reactions to childhood immunizations, that some have had characteristic attacks following treatment with trimethoprim-sulfamethoxazole, and that skin lesions resembling vasculitis are not uncommon in affected patients (Haraldsson et al., 1992), suggest the possibility of a hyper-reactive immune response perhaps associated with the production of certain lymphokines (e.g., IL-1, tumor necrosis factor). However, no experimental evidence for this hypothesis has been provided.

Clinical Features

The clinical features of the hyper-IgD syndrome include recurrent febrile attacks associated with abdominal pain, diarrhea, vomiting, lymphadenopathy, splenomegaly, arthralgia or arthritis, and erythematous macules or papules. The arthritis is benign, asymmetric, and painful and affects predominantly larger joints, in particular the knees, ankles, wrists, and elbows. The synovial fluid is mucoid and loaded with neutrophils; culture specimens are always negative.

The first attacks are usually observed during the first year of life. Typical attacks occur every 4 to 8 weeks and last 3 to 7 days; however, individual variations are common. The episodes resemble familial Mediterranean fever, but the two syndromes can be clearly distinguished on clinical and laboratory grounds (van der Meer, 1984). In one third to one half of the affected individuals, the hyper-IgD syndrome is familial, affecting males and females equally. Several patients, observed longitudinally, had clinical symptoms prior to elevated IgD levels, suggesting that both the clinical symptoms and the raised IgD concentration are the results of the same underlying pathologic event. No specific microorganisms have been identified as a potential cause.

Diagnosis and Treatment

In all patients studied, serum IgD was significantly increased, with levels ranging from 145 to 5300 U/ml (normal $\leq$100 U/ml). In most patients with hyper-IgD syndrome, IgA levels were also elevated and IgG and IgM concentrations were increased in one third of the patients. In one report, the serum IgD kappa-lambda ratio was elevated up to ten times that of normal controls; in contrast, the serum total light-chain ratio and IgG, IgA and IgM kappa/lambda ratios were normal (Haraldsson et al., 1992). The absolute number of B lymphocytes in the peripheral blood of hyper-IgD patients is normal; when the patients were immunized with specific antigens, normal or elevated titers of specific antibody were observed (Haraldsson et al., 1992). Cellular immunity did not differ from that in normal controls (Drenth et al., 1994). Bone marrow evaluation revealed an abnormally high percentage of cytoplasmic

IgD-containing lymphocytes, the number of which correlated with serum IgD levels (Hiemstra et al., 1989).

Early diagnosis of the hyper-IgD syndrome is difficult and should be considered in children with characteristic clinical features, elevated sedimentation rate, neutrophilia, and persistently elevated serum IgD levels (>100 U/ml). The occurrence of febrile attacks following childhood immunizations provides an additional clue to early diagnosis. The attacks tend to diminish with age, but symptoms may occur throughout life. The attacks are self-limiting, and patients are symptom-free between episodes. Colchicine, corticosteroids, cyclosporine, and IVIG ameliorated the severity or affected the frequency of the attacks. However, none of the medical therapies were convincingly effective (Drenth et al., 1994).

IMMUNODEFICIENCY WITH THYMOMA

Immunodeficiency with thymoma, first described by Good in 1954 (*Good's syndrome*), is a disorder of adults, commonly seen between ages 40 and 70. To date, only one child with this syndrome has been reported, an 8-year-old boy who died of complications of chickenpox 4 months after removal of a benign thymoma (Watts and Kelly, 1990). The immunodeficiency is characterized by recurrent sinopulmonary infections of gradual onset and, occasionally, by chronic mucocutaneous candidiasis or cytomegalovirus infection. The thymic tumors are predominantly of the spindle cell type and are usually benign, rarely malignant. The immunodeficiency associated with thymoma affects both B and T lymphocytes.

Pathogenesis

The pathogenesis of the association between immunodeficiency and thymoma is unknown. Two mechanisms of pathogenesis have been proposed: (1) the thymoma is primary and the immune deficiency is secondary, and (2) the immunodeficiency is the primary defect that allows the development of the thymoma. A viral cause, autoantibodies (Jeunet and Good, 1968), secretion of a substance by the thymoma that suppresses immunoglobulin synthesis (Peterson et al., 1965; Goldstein and Mackay, 1969), and chronic stimulation of the thymus by an activated immune system (Peterson et al., 1965) have been proposed as possible mechanisms.

Several studies have identified patients with this syndrome who had excessive CD8$^+$ suppressor cells that seemed to interfere with in vitro immunoglobulin synthesis by normal B cells (Moretta et al., 1977; Hayward et al., 1982); this suppressor effect can be removed by eliminating CD8$^+$ cells from the culture system. Most patients with immunodeficiency and thymoma completely lack both pre-B cells in the bone marrow and B cells in the peripheral blood (Pearl et al., 1978; Hayward et al., 1982). This has led to the hypothesis that the suppressor T cells generated in the thymoma interfere with B-cell maturation to immunoglobulin-secreting plasma cells. However, the description of a thymoma patient with hypogammaglobulinemia and normal numbers of B cells and no evidence of suppressor T-cell activity (Brenner et al., 1984) suggests that more than one mechanism for the pathogenesis of this syndrome exists. Finally, a striking prevalence of autoimmune disorders in thymoma patients demonstrates that autoimmune mechanisms play a major role in the clinical presentation of this syndrome (Souadjian et al., 1974).

Clinical Manifestations

The incidence of hypogammaglobulinemia and immunodeficiency in patients with thymoma is estimated to be between 4% and 12% (Waldmann et al., 1967; Souadjian et al., 1974; Otto, 1978; Gray and Gutowski, 1979). Thymoma and hypogammaglobulinemia are usually detected simultaneously, either during the initial investigation of hypogammaglobulinemia or when a mediastinal mass is detected on a chest film. Occasionally, the thymoma may be present for many years before symptoms of immune deficiency are noticed and hypogammaglobulinemia is diagnosed (Chapin, 1965; TeVelde et al., 1966). Removal of the thymoma does not affect hypogammaglobulinemia; the onset of immunodeficiency may even occur several years after thymomectomy (Lambie et al., 1957).

Symptoms of recurrent sinopulmonary infections, weight loss, and malaise appear gradually (Jeunet and Good, 1968; Goldstein and Mackay, 1969). Chronic diarrhea, often associated with candidiasis and persistent viral infection (Gupta et al., 1985), is present in 20% to 30% of patients with thymoma and hypogammaglobulinemia. Malabsorption is generally mild, villus architecture is intact, but plasma cells are absent. Anemia is frequently associated with the syndrome and may be due to pure red blood cell aplasia (Al-Mondhiry et al., 1971) or malabsorption of vitamin B$_{12}$ (Jeandel et al., 1994). Muscle weakness due to myasthenia gravis is a frequent complication (Gehrmann and Engstfeld, 1965). Other clinical findings associated with thymoma and immunodeficiency include thrombocytopenia (Peterson et al., 1965), neutropenia (Degos et al., 1982), arthritis (Webster, 1976), alopecia areata (Tan, 1974), and pemphigus vulgaris (Safai et al., 1978).

Infections commonly associated with cellular immunodeficiency have frequently been reported in patients with this syndrome, including invasive candidiasis (Kirkpatrick and Windhorst, 1979; Gupta et al., 1985), generalized cytomegalovirus infection (Jacox et al., 1964; Mongan et al., 1966; Bernadou et al., 1972; Kauffman et al., 1979; Gupta et al., 1985), cutaneous and systemic herpes simplex infection (Beck et al., 1981; Gupta et al., 1985), and *P. carinii* pneumonia (TeVelde et al., 1966).

Laboratory findings

Every patient with a mediastinal mass should be studied for possible immunodeficiency. Typically, immunoglobulin levels of all isotypes are low, antibody responses to immunization with specific antigens are depressed, and in vitro immunoglobulin synthesis by peripheral blood lymphocytes is decreased because of the absence of functional B lymphocytes (Pearl et al., 1978; Litwin et al., 1979; Hayward et al., 1982), or the presence of CD8$^+$ suppressor lymphocytes (Moretta et al., 1977; Hayward et al., 1982).

When tested at the time of diagnosis, most patients with thymoma and immunodeficiency have abnormal T-cell function. Skin tests for delayed-type hypersensitivity are negative, in vitro lymphocyte responses to mitogens and specific antigens are often impaired and the number of T cells is low, with a reverse CD4/CD8 ratio. Anemia, thrombocytopenia, neutropenia, and autoantibodies may be present.

Pathology

The mediastinal mass associated with this syndrome is characteristically a neoplasm of the thymic epithelium; lymphoma and other malignancies of the mediastinum should be excluded. The histology of a typical thymoma has been reviewed in detail (Goldstein and Mackay, 1969; Gray and Gutowski, 1979).

Thymomas associated with hypogammaglobulinemia cannot be distinguished histologically from other thymomas. Most thymomas arise from the anterior mediastinum and weigh up to 250 g; the maximum diameter is 4 to 20 cm. Two thirds of the tumors are encapsulated and benign, and one third are invasive (Gray and Gutowski, 1979). In a large series, 50% of the tumors consisted of round epithelial cells, 25% were of the spindle cell type, and 25% were of mixed type.

Lymphocytes are present in most thymomas and are usually T cells. Functionally, they are similar to lymphocytes from a normal thymus (Lauriola et al., 1981; Musiani et al., 1982). Bone marrow lacks both pre-B lymphocytes and plasma cells, and lymph nodes and spleen are hypocellular with absence of germinal centers and decreased numbers of plasma cells.

Treatment

To identify the nature of the tumor, the thymoma must be removed surgically. Removal of the thymoma does not correct the hypogammaglobulinemia, but it may improve the cellular immune defect. Symptoms of myasthenia gravis and other autoimmune diseases frequently improve after excision of the thymoma. Immunoglobulin therapy is effective in controlling recurrent bacterial infections and may alleviate chronic diarrhea (Conn and Quintiliani, 1966), but its effect on neutropenia or thrombocytopenia is unknown.

Prognosis

The prognosis of a benign thymoma by itself is excellent, with a 5-year survival of between 80% and 90% (Bernatz et al., 1973; Batata et al., 1974). However, the clinical course of patients with thymoma and immunodeficiency is less favorable. Immunologic deterioration is observed frequently, resulting in recurrent pulmonary infections that may progress to chronic lung disease and pulmonary insufficiency. Neutropenia, thrombocytopenia, and severe anemia are serious complications. The nature of the tumor is of prognostic importance. If it is malignant, the clinical course is usually rapidly fatal.

SELECTIVE DEFICIENCY OF IMMUNOGLOBULIN ISOTYPES

Selective IgA Deficiency

Selective IgA deficiency is the most common primary immunodeficiency disease affecting B-lymphocyte function; 1 in 400 to 1 in 800 individuals are affected. As originally defined by the World Health Organization, selective IgA deficiency is characterized by a serum IgA level lower than 5 mg/dl, normal levels of IgG and IgM, normal antibody responses to T-dependent antigens, and intact T-lymphocyte function (Fudenberg et al., 1971). In recent years, however, there has been a growing appreciation that the immunologic defect in some patients with "selective" IgA deficiency is broader than originally appreciated. Some patients with IgA deficiency have a concurrent IgG2 deficiency and may respond poorly to polysaccharide antigens (see IgG Subclass Deficiencies later). An association with certain MHC complotypes has been reported (Ashman et al., 1992; Volanakis et al., 1992). For a more detailed discussion of selective IgA deficiency, see Chapter 14.

Selective IgM Deficiency

Isolated IgM deficiency has been reported in 0.03% to 1.0% of populations screened (Hobbs et al., 1967; Cassidy and Nordby, 1975). Afflicted individuals may have recurrent bacterial infections or may be clinically healthy (Ross and Thompson, 1976). By definition, serum IgM levels in patients with this diagnosis are lower than 20 mg/dl and other Ig isotypes are normal. Cellular immunity is normal in most, but not all, patients with selective IgM deficiency.

Hobbs and colleagues (1967) reported two unrelated boys with selective IgM deficiency who died of meningococcal sepsis. The father of both of these children had low serum IgM levels but no clinical symptoms. Subsequent reports associated selective IgM deficiency with a variety of clinical findings, including severe recurrent sinopulmonary infections, urinary tract infections, disseminated molluscum contagiosum, chronic eczema, atopic dermatitis, steatorrhea, autoimmune hemolytic anemia, and systemic lupus erythematosus (Stoelinga et al., 1969; Faulk et al., 1971; De la Concha et al., 1982; Mayumi et al., 1986; Ohno et al., 1987; Guill et al., 1989).

Considering the ontogeny of B-cell maturation, the selective absence of IgM is difficult to explain, especially because most patients studied have normal numbers of circulating surface μ^+ B lymphocytes. When in vitro systems were used, B-cell defects (Ohno et al., 1987) or T-cell defects (De la Concha et al., 1982) that selectively interfere with in vitro IgM synthesis were reported. After in vivo immunization, depressed antibody responses to diphtheria-tetanus antigen and to pneumococcal polysaccharide antigens were observed in a group of selective IgM-deficient patients, despite normal serum IgG levels (Guill et al., 1989). After immunization with bacteriophage φX174, some patients with selective IgM deficiency had normal responses, some had a primary antibody response of predominantly IgG (in contrast to predominantly IgM in normal controls), and some patients had suppressed primary and secondary responses, lack of amplification, and failure to switch from IgM to IgG (Guill et al., 1989). A possible explanation of these findings is the observation by Inoue et al. (1986), who used an in vitro coculture technique, that a subgroup of patients with selective IgM deficiency have isotype-specific suppressor T cells in their peripheral blood.

In view of the heterogeneity of this syndrome, treatment should be adjusted to the need of individual patients, their immune defects, and their clinical problems. Immunoglobulin therapy and the use of prophylactic antibiotics may be helpful in patients who have a broader antibody deficiency.

Selective IgE Deficiency

Individuals with selective IgE deficiency have been identified, but the clinical significance of the deficiency has been difficult to determine. Two patients with isolated IgE deficiency (as assessed by reverse passive cutaneous anaphylaxis), normal levels of other serum immunoglobulins, normal T-lymphocyte function, and severe chronic pulmonary disease have been described (Cain et al., 1969; Hong, 1971). Both patients, however, had significant lymphopenia, which suggested that they may have had a broader immune defect that may have contributed to their pulmonary disease.

Isolated IgE deficiency has also been described in healthy individuals (Levy and Chen, 1970; Gleich et al., 1971; Polmar et al., 1972). In one series, selective IgE deficiency (IgE < 15 ng/ml) was reported as frequently as 7 of 73 healthy adult individuals (Polmar et al., 1972). Selective IgE deficiency and other disorders of the IgE system are presented in more detail in Chapter 13.

IgG SUBCLASS DEFICIENCIES

Selective IgG subclass deficiency is defined as a situation in which a single IgG subclass is deficient in a patient with a normal total serum IgG concentration (Herrod, 1993a). This definition is problematic because IgG4 may be below the level of detection in normal infants and because a deficiency of IgG1 (60% of total IgG) will present as hypogammaglobulinemia G. Indeed, the first reports describing selective IgG subclass deficiencies in patients with recurrent pyogenic infections would be considered common variable immunodeficiencies (CVIs), since most patients had hypogammaglobulinemia involving IgG and other immunoglobulin isotypes (Schur et al., 1970; Yount et al., 1970). A more practical definition of IgG subclass deficiency, therefore, includes patients with low levels (below 2 standard deviations of the age-adjusted geometric mean (see Table 9–6) of one or more IgG subclasses, including patients with low IgG who have normal IgM and IgA levels and who have depressed antibody responses. For children older than age 2, this means that the IgG1 level should be less than 250 mg/dl, the IgG2 level less than 50 mg/dl, and the IgG3 level less than 25 mg/dl; the IgG4 level may be nondetectable in normal children if less sensitive detection methods are used (see Chapter 9).

Pathogenesis

Each of the four IgG subclasses, defined by unique primary structures of the constant region of the heavy-chain molecule (Grey et al., 1964; Terry and Fahey, 1964), have clear biologic and functional differences (Ochs and Wedgwood, 1987; Shackelford, 1993). For instance, purified IgG1 and IgG3 myeloma proteins bind C1 efficiently and can activate the classic pathway of complement. In contrast, IgG2 fixes C1 poorly and IgG4 does not fix C1 at all. There are differences in the degree to which IgG subclasses cross the placenta. All IgG subclasses except IgG3 combine with staphylococcal protein A, a characteristic of the Fc portion of the molecule. Differences in the regulation of IgG subclass expression are evident by the strikingly different subclass levels in serum and characteristic differences in ontogeny. In infants, IgG1 and IgG3 levels increase quickly with age; IgG2 and IgG4 display a slower increase and reach adult levels at puberty (Fig. 11–10). The order of appearance of the IgG subclasses in chil-

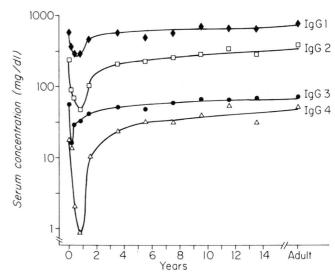

Figure 11–10. Serum IgG subclass levels in healthy infants and children. The means for each age group were obtained from data published by Oxelius. Time 0 represents cord blood values. (Modified from Oxelius V-A. IgG subclass levels in infancy and childhood. Acta Paediatr Scand 68:23–27, 1979.)

dren follows precisely the downstream order of the Ig heavy chain constant region gene segments on chromosome 14 (. . . γ3, γ1, . . . γ2, γ4) (Flanagan and Rabbitts, 1982).

Ig subclass restriction has been reported for antibodies against many bacterial and viral antigens. Antibody titers to pneumococcal polysaccharides correlate best with serum IgG2 concentrations (Siber et al., 1980). In adults, antibody activity to polysaccharides is found predominantly in the IgG2 fraction (Freijd et al., 1984); in children and in IgG2-deficient individuals, antibody to polysaccharides is predominantly IgG1 (Freijd et al., 1984; Hammarström et al., 1984). Antitetanus toxoid antibody is found predominantly in the IgG1 subclass (Stevens et al., 1983) and the high titers of antibody noted in patients with chronic schistosomiasis (Iskander et al., 1981) and filariasis (Ottesen et al., 1985) are limited to the IgG4 subclass. Following antigen exposure, a characteristic pattern of IgG subclass appearance has been observed. After the initial IgM response, IgG1 and IgG3 appear first, followed by IgG2 and IgG4 during the secondary immune response, an order of appearance that recapitulates ontogeny (Pyun et al., 1989).

A major problem in studying IgG subclass deficiencies has been the difficulty of developing sensitive, specific, and reliable assays. Because of a high degree of homology within the IgG subclass constant regions, it is difficult to produce specific antisera in animals and to develop discriminating monoclonal antibodies. Furthermore, there is a need for international standards and establishment of normal ranges for each laboratory, which are wide and dependent on age, sex, and Gm types. IgG4 may be very low in normal infants and children, with values that may be less than 1 μg/ml (Heiner et al., 1983). Thus, establishing a diagnosis of IgG4 deficiency in young children may be very difficult. (Preud'Homme and Hanson, 1990).

Isolated or combined deficiencies of IgG1, IgG2, and IgG3 have been associated with increased risk of infection. Selective low or unmeasurable serum levels of IgG4 are not uncommon in children and in most cases are not associated with increased risk of infection; in contrast, the combination deficiency of IgG2 and IgG4 has been found in patients with frequent infections (Oxelius et al., 1981). However, skepticism as to a direct correlation between IgG subclass deficiencies and infections has remained in view of reports of (1) healthy individuals who have deletions of one or more genes encoding IgG2, IgG4, and IgA, (2) healthy children who have low serum IgG2 concentrations, and (3) symptomatic children who have "selective" IgG2 deficiency associated with broader immune defects (Shackelford, 1993). There is a general consensus that the absence of one or more IgG subclasses is relevant only if this deficiency is associated with abnormal antibody responses that may be important for normal host defense (Shackelford, 1993; Herrod, 1993a, 1993b).

Clinical Manifestations

The most frequently reported symptoms associated with IgG subclass deficiency are recurrent upper respi-

ratory tract infections, including sinusitis, otitis, and rhinitis. Patients usually do not present with life-threatening infectious episodes. Studies carried out in Scandinavia suggest that children more frequently have IgG2 deficiency than do adults, who more commonly have IgG3 deficiency (Hanson et al., 1988). The results of these studies also suggest that in children with IgG subclass deficiency, there is a prevalence of boys, and that in adults, there is a prevalence of women.

Although the clinical findings associated with IgG subclass deficiencies have been heterogeneous, some characteristic findings have been observed by a number of investigators.

IgG1 Deficiency

IgG1 deficiency is invariably associated with other Ig subclass deficiencies and usually presents with low serum IgG levels (Schur et al., 1970; Smith et al., 1984; Stanley et al., 1984). Patients classified with IgG1 deficiency may in fact represent common variable immunodeficiency, especially if combined with other IgG subclass deficiencies. Often there is a lifelong history of susceptibility to pyogenic infections, and persistent, progressive lung disease may develop.

IgG2 Deficiency

Frequently, but not always, IgG2 deficiency is associated with IgG4 and IgA deficiencies (Oxelius et al., 1981; Braconier et al., 1984; Morell et al., 1986). In children with frequent respiratory infections, an association between IgG2 deficiency and impaired responses to polysaccharide antigens has been clearly established (Umetsu et al., 1985; Insel and Anderson, 1986; Geha, 1988). Antibody responses to diphtheria and tetanus toxoid antigens are usually normal (Geha, 1988). It is of interest that from a group of children with a similar clinical presentation, a subgroup was identified who had normal IgG subclasses but abnormal responses to polysaccharide antigens (Geha, 1988). This suggests that low IgG2 levels may be a marker and that these children have in common a defective response to certain antigens, but not to others. In addition to the clinical symptoms of upper respiratory infection, patients may also present with recurrent meningitis caused by *Neisseria meningitidis* (Bass et al., 1983) or disseminated pneumococcal disease. Most patients with selective IgG2 deficiency have normal serum immunoglobulin levels.

IgG3 Deficiency

Antibodies to proteins, including viral proteins, are mainly of the IgG1 or IgG3 subclass. IgG3 antibodies may be the most efficient virus neutralizing antibodies (Hanson et al., 1988). Deficiency of this subclass has been associated with the history of recurrent infections leading to chronic lung disease (Björkander et al., 1985; Oxelius et al., 1986). In a Swedish study, a low serum IgG level was present in 313 samples of sera collected from 6580 patients (1864 children and 4716 adults) with a history of recurrent infections (Oxelius et al., 1986). Of these 313 individuals, 186 had an isolated IgG3 deficiency, 113 presented in addition with IgG1 deficiency, 14 presented in addition with IgG2 deficiency, and 11 presented with IgG3 and IgG4 deficiency.

IgG4 Deficiency

The diagnosis of IgG4 deficiency is difficult to establish because a large proportion of infants and children have IgG4 serum levels that cannot be detected with standard methods. Only studies in which more sensitive techniques were used (e.g., radioimmunoassay, ELISA) have unequivocally identified patients with selective IgG4 deficiency (IgG4 concentration <0.05 µg/ml) who presented with severe recurrent respiratory tract infections, including bronchiectasis (Heiner et al., 1983; Heiner, 1984). In one patient with selective IgG4 deficiency and a history of pulmonary infections recurrent chalazia developed (Insler and Gordon, 1984).

Most IgG4-deficient patients have normal or elevated concentrations of total IgG, of other IgG subclasses, IgA, IgM, and IgE. In a small group of patients, IgG4 deficiency was associated with both IgG2 and IgA deficiency (Schur et al., 1970; Oxelius, 1974; Oxelius et al., 1981; Heiner et al., 1983). However, the significance of IgG4 deficiency is not clear, since very low concentrations of IgG4 have been reported in a substantial proportion of normal children (Herrod, 1993a, 1993b).

Treatment

The most important aspect in the management of children who have acute or chronic infections due to antibody deficiency from any cause is the appropriate use of antibiotics (Geha, 1988; Shackelford, 1993). A child identified as having IgG subclass deficiency should receive protein-conjugated polysaccharide vaccines. Most investigators recommend that administration of intravenous immunoglobulin be reserved for children with significant clinical symptoms and insufficient response to treatment with antibiotics (Geha, 1988; Herrod, 1993a). The recommended dose is 200 to 400 mg/kg per month, similar to that for patients with other primary antibody deficiencies. Those patients who also lack IgA should be carefully monitored for the production of anti-IgA antibody.

IgG Subclass Imbalances in Primary Immunodeficiencies

Deficiencies of one or more IgG subclasses have been observed in patients with common variable immunodeficiency (CVI) (Yount et al., 1970; Wedgwood et al., 1986). The most frequently and severely deficient IgG subclass in patients with CVI is IgG4, followed by IgG2, IgG1, and IgG3 (Wedgwood et al., 1986). These findings support the hypothesis that the immunologic defects in CVI represent an impediment of heavy-chain constant (C) region gene rearrangements and follow

the order of the heavy-chain gene located on chromosome 14 (Flanagan and Rabbitts, 1982). In sera from patients with ataxia-telangiectasia, IgG2 and IgG4 levels are frequently deficient (Oxelius et al., 1982; Wedgwood et al., 1986). In contrast, all IgG subclass levels are proportionally low in patients with XLA and the Wiskott-Aldrich syndrome (Wedgwood et al., 1986). A transient imbalance of immunoglobulin classes and subclasses has also been observed in patients with severe combined immunodeficiency disorder (SCID) treated with bone marrow transplantation (Rádl et al., 1972; Morell et al., 1975).

DELETIONS OF IMMUNOGLOBULIN HEAVY-CHAIN CONSTANT REGION GENES

The observation that homozygous deletions of one or multiple immunoglobulin heavy-chain constant (C) region genes could be demonstrated in healthy individuals, but not in antibody-deficient patients, was unexpected—and informative. A series of different multigene deletion haplotypes have been identified involving the deletion of a single or multiple immunoglobulin isotype or subclass genes (Lefranc et al., 1991). Some individuals were found to lack the entire set of genes for IgG1, IgA1, IgG2, and IgG4; others lacked IgG2, IgG4, IgE, and IgA2 entirely. The selective absence of the gene for IgG1, IgG2, or IgA1 was demonstrated in other individuals. However, 15 of 16 individuals with deletions were totally asymptomatic (Lefranc et al., 1991; Olsson et al., 1993; Smith et al., 1989); only one patient with a selective IgG1 deletion and asthma had become symptomatic.

A large survey conducted in Italy suggests that the gene frequency of haplotypes with deletions of one or more immunoglobulin heavy-chain genes is 2.7%, suggesting an expected frequency of homozygous deletion of these genes to be 1 in 1400 normal individuals (Plebani et al., 1993). Yet none of 33 patients with common variable immunodeficiency had a homozygous deletion of one or more immunoglobulin heavy-chain genes (Olsson et al., 1991), and symptomatic patients with immunoglobulin subclass deficiencies do not have gene deletions (Lefranc et al., 1991).

The identification of individuals with multiple gene deletions has made it possible to study the importance of the missing genes for the overall immune response. In addition to the lack of clinical symptoms, individuals with Ig heavy-chain C region gene deletions produced antibody to protein and to polysaccharides, utilizing immunoglobulin isotypes and subclasses not affected by the deletion.

KAPPA AND LAMBDA CHAIN DEFICIENCIES

During normal B-cell development, an attempt is made to match a kappa light chain (of which there are two allotypes) coded by genes on chromosome 2 to the heavy chain derived from the gene rearrangement on chromosome 14. If the attempt is unsuccessful, a lambda light-chain transcript, coded by genes on chromosome 22, is tried and kappa chain synthesis stops (Korsmeyer et al. 1981).

Deficiencies of kappa- or lambda-type immunoglobulins have been reported in immune-deficient individuals. Bernier and colleagues (1972) described a selective decrease of serum levels of kappa-type immunoglobulin in a patient with recurrent respiratory infections and diarrhea. Subsequently, Barandun and co-workers (1976) described two patients, one with a severe deficiency of kappa-type immunoglobulin and the other with severe deficiency of lambda-type immunoglobulin. Pernicious anemia had developed in both patients, and both had hypogammaglobulinemia.

In 1976, Zegers and coworkers described a patient with complete absence of kappa-type immunoglobulin without excessive susceptibility to infection, even though cystic fibrosis and selective IgA deficiency were present. Kappa-type immunoglobulin could not be detected in the patient's serum, and the peripheral blood B lymphocytes and bone marrow–derived B lymphocytes expressed only lambda-type light chains. Antibody responses to several antigens were adequate, and the half-life of injected kappa-type immunoglobulin was normal. Sequence analysis of the patient's constant κ chain region genes revealed two different point mutations, one in each allele, resulting in substitution of a single amino acid in each kappa light-chain molecule (Stavnezer-Nordgren et al., 1985).

OTHER B-CELL DEFECTS

Antibody Deficiency with Transcobalamin II Deficiency

Hereditary transcobalamin II (TCII) deficiency is a rare autosomal recessive disorder (Hakami et al., 1971) caused by a mutation of the TCII gene located on chromosome 22 (Arwert et al., 1986). TCII is required for absorption of cobalamin from the bowel and transport to vitamin B_{12}–requiring tissues. Cobalamin is taken up by cells only when bound to TCII (Hall, 1981). Typically, patients with TCII deficiency present in the first few months of life with failure to thrive, diarrhea, ulcers of oral mucous membranes, lethargy, irritability, delayed neurologic development, severe macrocytic anemia, and neutropenia. In addition, most patients present with decreased serum IgG levels and cannot produce specific antibodies following childhood immunization (Hitzig and Kenny, 1975). Absolute numbers of T- and B-lymphocyte subsets in the peripheral blood are no different from those in controls, and in vivo and in vitro T-cell functions are normal (Hitzig et al., 1974; Kaikov et al., 1991). Following parenteral treatment with high-dose (1 mg given subcutaneously once or twice a week) of vitamin B_{12}, patients recover completely clinically, hematologically, and immunologically. Some patients have remained symptom-free on oral maintenance therapy with hydroxocobalamin at 1 to 2 mg daily (Zeitlin et al., 1985).

The observation by Hitzig and associates (1974) that immunization attempts initially failed to induce specific antibody production, but that patients began to produce specific antibody without further immunization as soon as vitamin B_{12} was provided parenterally suggests that antigen exposure initated the differentiation of antigen-specific memory cells in the absence of vitamin B_{12} utilization. These findings indicate that rapidly replicating cell systems, such as intestinal mucosa and the hematopoietic and lymphoid systems, are dependent on a continuous supply of vitamin B_{12}.

Antibody Deficiency in Down Syndrome

Patients with Down syndrome have frequent bacterial infections, an increase in autoimmune disorders (Burgio et al., 1983), a high risk of lymphoproliferative malignancies (Robinson et al., 1984), and persistence of hepatitis B antigenemia (Sutnik et al., 1972; Ugazio et al., 1977). Immunologic evaluation of such patients has suggested deficiencies in humoral and cell-mediated immunity as well as in phagocytic function (see Chapter 19).

Serum IgG levels in newborns with Down syndrome are significantly lower than maternal levels at delivery and lower than in normal infants (Miller et al., 1969). Older children, adolescents, and adults with Down syndrome generally have high IgG levels, whereas IgM and IgA levels are variable (Stiehm and Fudenberg, 1966a; Adinolfi et al., 1967; Sutnik et al., 1972).

A study of institutionalized patients with Down syndrome reported high serum IgG, decreased IgM, and normal IgA levels (Lopez et al., 1975). In 11 of 17 patients studied, the primary antibody response to bacteriophage ϕX174 was impaired, whereas the secondary immune response was normal in one, moderately impaired in seven, and very low in nine patients. Those with a moderately impaired secondary immune response had a normal, predominantly IgG antibody response to a third immunization, and those with a very low secondary response had a poor tertiary response, predominantly of the IgM isotype; this suggests abnormal T- and B-lymphocyte interaction.

Antibody responses to common antigens, including tetanus toxoid, typhoid, and influenza, were depressed in some studies (Siegal, 1948; Gordon et al., 1971) and normal in others (Leibovitz and Yannet, 1942; Griffith and Sylvester, 1967). Isohemagglutinin titers and natural antibodies to *Escherichia coli* were normal (Adinolfi et al., 1967).

The antibody deficiency observed in Down syndrome may in part be the result of defective T-cell function. Published data, although conflicting, include decreased numbers of circulating T lymphocytes, normal or increased numbers of CD8+ cells (Burgio et al., 1983), and decreased numbers of CD4+ cells (Karttunen et al., 1984; Phillip et al., 1986). In vitro lymphocyte proliferation in response to mitogens were both normal and depressed, but responses to specific antigens were consistently abnormal (Phillip et al., 1986). Furthermore, histologic evidence of an abnormal thymus has been reported in Down syndrome of all ages, including a reduced size with poor corticomedullary differentiation, anomalous Hassall's corpuscles, and lymphocyte depletion (Levin et al., 1979).

The controversies in the literature related to the extent of the immunodeficiency in Down syndrome may be caused by differences in age of the patients and institutionalization. Premature aging observed in patients with Down syndrome (Haberland, 1969; Schneider and Epstein, 1972) may result in diminution of cellular and humoral immune responses (immunosenescence), and defects in antibody responses were consistently observed in institutionalized patients (Lopez et al., 1975).

An intriguing hypothesis has been proposed by Epstein and Epstein (1980). The gene coding for the interferon receptor has been assigned to chromosome 21 (Revel et al., 1976). As a result of gene dosage, trisomic T lymphocytes are several times more sensitive to interferon than normal cells and may respond abnormally to interferon, perhaps by down-regulating the immune response.

Transient Hypogammaglobulinemia of Infancy

Transient hypogammaglobulinemia of infancy is a self-limited defect in immunoglobulin synthesis that occurs during the first few years of life. The condition needs to be clearly differentiated from *physiologic* hypogammaglobulinemia, a term that describes the normal physiologic nadir in serum IgG levels experienced by every infant between 3 and 6 months of life.

Physiologic hypogammaglobulinemia occurs as maternal IgG in the infant's serum decreases and the infant's serum IgG level increasingly reflects its own synthesis of IgG. During this period, the infant's serum IgG level reaches a nadir but begins to increase after 6 months of age, climbing progressively to near adult levels by age 5 years.

In contrast, infants with transient hypogammaglobulinemia cannot synthesize normal amounts of IgG. As a consequence, after the serum IgG level reaches its nadir between 3 and 6 months of age, it does not increase at the expected rate and remains relatively low for age until between 18 and 36 months of age. In spite of this relative hypogammaglobulinemia, antibody function is generally intact and B- and T-lymphocyte values are normal (Rieger et al., 1977; Tiller and Buckley, 1978). In some patients, defective T-helper function has been observed (Siegal et al., 1981). Unfortunately, by definition, the diagnosis of transient hypogammaglobulinemia cannot be established with complete confidence until after the child's immunoglobulin levels have reached age-appropriate levels. Until that time, every effort should be made to differentiate "transient" hypogammaglobulinemia from other primary immunodeficiency diseases characterized by hypogammaglobulinemia such as X-linked agammaglobulinemia and common variable immunodeficiency. Thus, long-term follow-up and frequent re-evaluation of the child's clinical status and immune system are usually required. A more complete discussion of transient hypogammaglobulinemia can be found in Chapter 10.

Antibody Deficiency in Complement Component or Receptor Deficiencies

There is evidence that certain components of the complement system and their receptors are critical in the development of a normal antibody response. Cells of the monocyte/macrophage series, B lymphocytes, and a subset of T lymphocytes all have receptors for C3 and/or C5 cleavage products on their cell membranes (Fearon and Wong, 1983). In fact, a variety of in vitro studies have shown that cleavage products of C3 (C3a and C3b) and of C5 (C5a) can either enhance or inhibit cellular functions affecting the normal antibody response (Weiler et al., 1982; Egwang and Befus, 1984). The in vivo significance of these studies has been difficult to predict because the inhibitory and enhancing effects of these cleavage products operate at different steps in a complex series of cell-to-cell interactions.

However, studies using experimental animals pharmacologically depleted of C3 (Pepys, 1972), or animals with genetically determined deficiencies of C4 (Ochs et al., 1983a), C2 (Böttger et al., 1985; Ochs et al., 1986) or C3 (Böttger et al., 1986; O'Neil et al., 1988a), have all shown that the complement system is important in generating a normal antibody response in vivo. It appears that the antibody response to T-dependent antigens is relatively more dependent on an intact complement system than is the response to T-independent antigens. In addition, an intact complement system facilitates the isotype switch from IgM to IgG.

The ability to generate a normal antibody response after immunization with the neoantigens bacteriophage ϕX174 and keyhole limpet hemocyanin has been studied in a few patients with genetic deficiencies of individual components of complement and the iC3b receptor, CR3. Patients with deficiencies of C3, C4, or C2 (components necessary for the activation of C3) and patients with deficiencies of CR3 (leukocyte adhesion defect type 1) have reduced titers of antibody after primary immunization, poor immunologic memory, and incomplete switching from IgM to IgG production after repeated immunizations (Ochs et al., 1986, 1993). Interestingly, as one might expect, patients with deficiencies of C7, a component not needed for the activation of C3 or C5, appear to have normal antibody responses. It is not known to what degree the defect in antibody production contributes to these patients' increased susceptibility to infection.

Antibody Deficiency in Asplenic Patients

An asplenic state may be the consequence of surgical removal of the spleen, functional asplenia (e.g., in sickle cell disease), or *congenital asplenia* (see Chapter 19). Overwhelming bacterial infections with a high rate of mortality have been noted in children and adults with *anatomical* or *functional asplenia* (Eraklis et al., 1967; Singer, 1973; Balfanz et al., 1976). Although all asplenic infants, children, and adults are at increased risk for fulminant bacteremia, susceptibility is influenced considerably by the underlying disease and the patient's age. In comparison with healthy children, the incidence of mortality from septicemia is increased 50-fold in children who have had splenectomy after trauma, approximately 350-fold in children with sickle cell disease, and even higher in children who have had a splenectomy for thalassemia or Hodgkin's disease. The risk of bacteremia is higher in younger than in older children and may be greater in the years right after splenectomy (American Academy of Pediatrics, 1994). *Streptococcus pneumoniae, Haemophilus influenzae,* type b, and *N. meningitidis* are the most frequent pathogens observed in asplenic children.

As part of the reticuloendothelial system, the spleen plays a major role in the clearance of bacteria from the blood stream both in experimental animals and in humans (Brown et al., 1981). In congenitally asplenic patients or in those whose spleen has been removed surgically, the liver is unable to compensate completely for the loss of phagocytic activity. The result is delayed clearance of particulate matter from the blood stream, including Fc-mediated clearance of sensitized autologous erythrocytes (Wang and Hsieh, 1991). Furthermore, the spleen is a major lymphoid organ that is important in antibody synthesis, especially in response to circulating antigens.

Decreased serum IgM levels (Schumacher, 1970; Drew et al., 1984) and impaired capacity to produce antibody against heterologous erythrocytes (Rowley, 1950) and pneumococci (Hosea et al., 1981) have been reported in splenectomized patients. Antibody responses to subcutaneously injected pneumococcal polysaccharides have been normal or depressed (Ammann et al., 1977; Sullivan et al., 1978; Giebink et al., 1980; Hosea et al., 1981). A significant decline in antibody titers to pneumococcal polysaccharide antigens has been reported in children who had undergone splenectomy because of trauma compared with non-splenectomized controls (Giebink et al., 1984). When immunized with the T-cell–dependent antigen, bacteriophage φX174, asplenic patients mounted a quantitatively and qualitatively abnormal antibody response; those who had a splenectomy for staging of Hodgkin's disease responded with more depressed titers than those who underwent splenectomy following trauma (Sullivan et al., 1978).

The observation that peripheral blood lymphocytes from splenectomized patients are unable to differentiate into immunoglobulin-secreting cells in mitogen-driven culture systems suggests the possibility of decreased T-helper function or the presence of T suppression (Müller et al., 1984; Drew et al., 1984). However, the abnormalities in T-lymphocyte subsets and in in vitro lymphocyte proliferation in response to mitogens observed in children with congenital asplenia (Wang and Hsieh, 1991) and in patients with post-traumatic splenectomy (Kreuzfelder et al., 1991) may reflect the loss of the spleen as a reservoir of lymphocytes rather than a direct T-cell abnormality.

The clinical observations and laboratory findings of suppressed immune functions in congenitally asplenic,

functionally asplenic, or splenectomized patients have led to the recommendation to immunize all asplenic patients 2 years and older with polyvalent pneumococcal vaccine. Immunization against *H. influenzae* type b infections should be initiated in infancy, as recommended for otherwise healthy young children, using a conjugate vaccine. Quadrivalent meningococcal polysaccharide vaccine is indicated in asplenic children 2 years and older. Daily prophylaxis with antimicrobial agents is strongly recommended for all asplenic children younger than 5 years of age, and should be considered for older children and adults, especially if they have conditions that are associated with a high risk of fulminant infections. For antimicrobial prophylaxis, oral penicillin V (120 mg twice daily for children younger than 5 years and 250 mg twice daily for children 5 years and older) is usually recommended. Amoxicillin (20 mg/kg/day) or trimethoprim-sulfamethoxazole for children younger than 5 years may be more effective.

Antibody Deficiency with Viral Infections

Epstein-Barr virus (EBV), cytomegalovirus (CMV), human T-cell leukemia virus (HTLV-I), and human immunodeficiency virus (HIV) are known to infect lymphoid cells and thus have the potential to interfere with normal immune functions. Evidence for abnormal antibody responses has been observed in patients affected with any of these lymphotropic viruses.

Epstein-Barr Virus

A group of healthy college students presenting with signs and symptoms of acute infectious mononucleosis were studied for in vivo and in vitro antibody responses to bacteriophage φX174. Antibody titers were depressed, and in vitro experiments revealed the presence of suppressor T cells and impairment of antibody responses; the results suggest that uncomplicated infectious mononucleosis is associated with a broad-based transient immune deficiency that resolves within 6 to 8 weeks after onset of the disease (Junker et al., 1986).

A disastrous response to EBV infection has been observed in boys with X-linked lymphoproliferative syndrome (XLP), also known as *Duncan disease,* or *Purtilo syndrome* (see Chapter 12). These apparently healthy individuals, if infected with EBV, may develop fatal infectious mononucleosis and overwhelming hepatitis, marrow aplasia, B-cell lymphoma, or agammaglobulinemia (Purtilo et al., 1977, 1982; Provisor et al., 1975; Grierson and Purtilo, 1987). The outcome of the EBV infection appears related to the age when exposure to EBV occurs; the median age of onset for fatal infectious mononucleosis is 1.7 years; for lymphoma, 4.9 years; and for hypogammaglobulinemia, 6.9 years (Grierson and Purtilo, 1987).

Before exposure to EBV, affected individuals are clinically normal, B-cell and T-cell functions appear adequate, and natural killer cell numbers are normal. During acute EBV infection, serum Ig levels increase, lymphocyte proliferation in response to mitogen and antigen stimulation decreases, and natural killer cell activity increases. After infection with EBV, a decrease of B lymphocytes in the peripheral blood of affected males is observed, serum immunoglobulin values decrease to low levels, antibody responses to immunization with bacteriophage φX174 are severely depressed (Ochs et al., 1983b), and natural killer cell activity is descreased (Sullivan et al., 1983). X-linked lymphoproliferative (XLP) syndrome patients with agammaglobulinemia and reduced numbers of B lymphocytes may be difficult to distinguish from patients with X-linked agammaglobulinemia. Although the XLP gene has been mapped to Xq24-26, with tight linkage to DXS42 (Skare et al., 1987), the molecular defect responsible for XLP is not yet known. Because the gene involved in XLA *(Btk)* has recently been cloned and sequenced (see section on X-linked agammaglobulinemia), assessment of Btk should clarify the diagnosis. If agammaglobulinemia and abnormal antibody responses are predominant findings, treatment with immunoglobulin is indicated (see X-linked agammaglobulinemia).

Human Immunodeficiency Virus

Acquired immunodeficiency syndrome (AIDS) is associated with a profound defect in cell-mediated immunity owing to destruction of CD4 T-helper cells; however, B-cell immunity is also affected. Depressed antibody responses to KLH and pneumococcal polysaccharide vaccine are observed in homosexual men with AIDS (Ammann et al., 1984). Antibody responses to bacteriophage φX174 were significantly depressed in pediatric patients with AIDS (Bernstein et al., 1985) and in homosexual men with the lymphadenopathy complex (Ochs et al., 1988). As one would predict from these studies, infusions of IVIG at a dose of 400 mg/kg every 4 weeks significantly reduced serious and minor bacterial and viral infections in children with CD4 counts $\geq$ 200/mm³ (Mofenson et al., 1992). An additional benefit from IVIG therapy is a slowing of CD4⁺ count decline in the treated cohort of children (Mofenson et al., 1993). See Chapter 18 for a further discussion of pediatric HIV infection.

Rubella

Congenital rubella may be associated with hypogammaglobulinemia affecting all three major immunoglobulin isotypes (Plotkin et al., 1966; Soothill et al., 1966; Hancock et al., 1968). Immunodeficiency with elevated IgM, low IgG, and absent IgA levels has been noted during early infancy as the result of congenital rubella (Soothill et al., 1966). The immunoglobulin abnormalities may return to normal at the same time as virus excretion diminishes or ceases (Michaels, 1969). During virus excretion, patients with congenital rubella and congenital cytomegalovirus infection have an abnormal antibody response to bacteriophage φX174, including low antibody titers and failure to switch from IgM to IgG.

Measles

During acute infection with measles virus, viral antigens are expressed on peripheral blood lymphocytes and infectious virus can be recovered from monocytes, B lymphocytes, and CD4⁺ and CD8⁺ T lymphocytes. Infection of human peripheral blood mononuclear cells with measles virus does not alter lymphocyte survival and is not associated with cytolysis. However, if infected in vitro with measles virus, peripheral blood mononuclear cells do not proliferate and fail to synthesize immunoglobulins in response to mitogen stimulation (Casali et al., 1984).

Drug-Induced Immunodeficiency

Immunosuppressive agents, including corticosteroids, alkylating agents, purine antagonists, and other drugs that interfere with cell proliferation and DNA synthesis, may have a profound effect on cellular immunity and may interfere with antibody production. The abnormalities associated with these agents are usually reversible if treatment is discontinued.

A lupus-like syndrome, lymphotoxic autoantibodies, lymphopenia, defective cell-mediated immunity, IgA deficiency, and lymphoma-like lesions have been reported in patients treated with phenytoin (Dilantin) for epilepsy (Sorrell et al., 1971; Grob and Herold, 1972; Ooi et al., 1974; Slavin et al., 1974; Li et al., 1975; Seager et al., 1975; Sorrell and Forbes, 1975).

Reversible hypogammaglobulinemia associated with recurrent infections developed in a child treated with phenytoin and the tranquilizer hydroxyzine. Hypogammaglobulinemia and recurrent infections disappeared when treatment was stopped (De Gast et al., 1974). Abnormal suppressor T cells and hypogammaglobulinemia were observed in an 11-year-old boy who was treated with phenytoin for post-traumatic seizures. After 12 months of therapy, generalized edema, a desquamating erythematous rash, generalized lymphadenopathy, and fever developed. He had draining ears, a diffusely erythematous pharynx, and productive cough. Lymphocyte studies performed while he was receiving phenytoin showed normal values and adequate function of T lymphocytes but severely reduced levels of B lymphocytes. In vitro experiments revealed suppressed synthesis of specific antibody attributed to the presence of spontaneous suppressor T cells. These abnormalities resolved within 10 weeks after discontinuation of phenytoin. The presence of both suppressor cell activity and antibody deficiency may indicate that the two phenomena are causally related (Dosch et al., 1982).

Laxative abuse by a 64-year-old patient has been associated with extreme wasting, hypogammaglobulinemia, and absence of circulating B lymphocytes. The immunologic abnormalities were corrected after laxative intake was stopped and after lean body mass was restored (Levine et al., 1981).

References

Ackerson BK, Raghunathan R, Keller MA, Bui RHD, Phinney PR, Imagawa DT. Echovirus 11 arthritis in a patient with X-linked agammaglobulinemia. Pediatr Infect Dis 6:485–488, 1987.

Adinolfi M, Gardner B, Martin W. Observations on the levels of γG, γA, and γM globulins, anti-A and anti-B agglutinins and antibodies to *Escherichia coli* in Down's anomaly. J Clin Pathol 20:860–864, 1967.

Aiuti F, Lacava V, Fiorilli M. B lymphocytes in agammaglobulinemia. Lancet 2:761, 1972.

Al-Mondhiry H, Zanjani ED, Spivack M, Zalusky R, Gordon AS. Pure red cell aplasia and thymoma: loss of serum inhibitor of erythropoiesis following thymectomy. Blood 38:576–582, 1971.

Allen RC, Armitage RJ, Conley ME, Rosenblatt H, Jenkins NA, Copeland NG, Bedell MA, Edelhoff S, Disteche CM, Simoneaux DK, Fanslow WC, Belmont J, Spriggs MK. CD40 ligand gene defects responsible for X-linked hyper-IgM syndrome. Science 259:990–993, 1993.

Ambrosino DM, Schiffman G, Gotschlich EC, Schur PH, Rosenberg GA, DeLange GG, Van Logheme E, Siber GR. Correlation between G2m(n) immunoglobulin allotype and human antibody response and susceptibility to polysaccharide encapsulated bacteria. J Clin Invest 75:1935–1942, 1985.

Ambrosino DM, Siber GR, Chilmonczyk BA, Jernberg JB, Finberg RW. An immunodeficiency characterized by impaired antibody responses to polysaccharides. N Engl J Med 316:790–793, 1987.

Ambrosino DM, Umetsu DT, Siber GR, Howie G, Goularte TA, Michaels R, Martin P, Schur PH, Noyes J, Schiffman G, Geha RS. Selective defect in the antibody response to *Haemophilus influenzae* type b in children with recurrent infections and normal serum IgG subclass levels. J Allergy Clin Immunol 81:1175–1179, 1988.

Ament ME, Ochs HD, Davis SD. Structure and function of the gastrointestinal tract in primary immunodeficiency syndromes: a study of 39 patients. Medicine 52:227–248, 1973.

American Academy of Pediatrics. In Peter G., ed. 1994 Red Book: Report of the Committee on Infectious Diseases, 23rd ed., Elk Grove Village, Ill., 1994, pp. 57–59.

Ammann AJ, Addiego J, Wara DW, Lubin B, Smith WB, Mentzer WC. Polyvalent pneumococcal-polysaccharide immunization of patients with sickle-cell anemia and patients with splenectomy. N Engl J Med 297:897–900, 1977.

Ammann AJ, Schiffman G, Abrams D, Volberding P, Ziegler J, Conant M. B-cell immunodeficiency in acquired immune deficiency syndrome. JAMA 251:1447–1449, 1984.

Anker R, Conley ME, Pollor BA. Clonal diversity in the B cell repertoire of patients with X-linked agammaglobulinemia. J Exp Med 169:2109–2119, 1989.

Aruffo A, Farrington M, Hollenbaugh D, Li X, Milatovich A, Nonoyama S, Bajorath J, Grosmaire L, Stenkamp R, Neubauer M, Roberts RL, Noelle RJ, Ledbetter JA, Francke U, Ochs HD. The CD40 ligand, gp39, is defective in activated T cells from patients with X-linked hyper-IgM syndrome. Cell 72:291–300, 1993.

Aruffo A, Hollenbaugh D, Wu LH, Ochs HD. The molecular basis of X-linked agammaglobulinemia, hyper-IgM syndrome, and severe combined immunodeficiency in humans. Curr Opin Hematol 1:12–18, 1994.

Arwert F, Porck HJ, Frater-Schroder M, Brahe C, Geurts van Kessel A, Westerveld A, Meera Khan P, Zang K, Frants RR, Korbeek HT, Eriksson AW. Assignment of human transcobalamin II (TCII) to chromosome 22 using somatic cell hybrids and monosomic meningioma cells. Hum Genet 73:378–381, 1986.

Asherson GL, Webster ADB. Late onset hypo-gammaglobulinemia. In Asherson GL, Webster ADB, eds. Diagnosis and Treatment of Immunodeficiency Diseases. Oxford, England, Blackwell Scientific Publishers, 1980, pp. 37–60.

Ashida ER, Saxon A. Home intravenous immunoglobulin therapy by self-administration. J Clin Immunol 6:306–309, 1986.

Ashman RF, Saxon A, Stevens RH. Profile of multiple lymphocyte functional defects in acquired hypogammaglobulinemia, derived from in vitro cell recombination analysis. J Allergy Clin Immunol 65:242–256, 1980.

Ashman RF, Schaffer FM, Kemp JD, Yokoyama WM, Zhu Z-B, Cooper MD, Volanakis JE. Genetic and immunologic analysis of a family containing five patients with common-variable immune deficiency or selective IgA deficiency. J Clin Immunol 12:406–414, 1992.

Aukrust P, Müller F, Froland SS. Elevated serum levels of interleukin-4 and interleukin-6 in patients with common variable immunodeficiency (CVI) are associated with chronic immune activation

and low numbers of CD4+ lymphocytes. Clin Immunol Immunopathol 70:217–224, 1994.

Avasthi PS, Avasthi P, Tung KSK. Glomerulonephritis in agammaglobulinemia. Br Med J 2:478, 1975.

Balfanz JR, Nesbit ME Jr, Jarvis C, Krivit W. Overwhelming sepsis following splenectomy for trauma. J Pediatr 88:458–460, 1976.

Banatvala N, Davies J, Kanariou M, Strobel S, Levinsky R, Morgan G. Hypogammaglobulinaemia associated with normal or increased IgM (the hyper IgM syndrome): a case series review. Arch Dis Child 71:150–152, 1994.

Bancherau J, de Paoli P, Vallé A, Garcia E, Rousset F. Long-term human B cell lines dependent on interleukin-4 and antibody to CD40. Science 251:70–72, 1991.

Barandun S, Morell A, Skvaril F, Oberdorfer A. Deficiency of kappa- or gamma-type immunoglobulins. Blood 47:79–89, 1976.

Bardelas JA, Winkelstein JA, Seto DS, Tsai T, Roger AD. Fatal ECHO 24 infection in a patient with hypogammaglobulinemia: relationship to dermatomyositis-like syndrome. J Pediatr 90:396–398, 1977.

Barkin RM, Bonis SL, Elghammer RM, Todd JK. Ludwig angina in children. J Pediatr 87:563–565, 1975.

Barth WF, Asofsky R, Liddy TJ, Tanaka Y, Rowe DS, Fahey JL. An antibody deficiency syndrome: selective immunoglobulin deficiency with reduced synthesis of gamma and alpha immunoglobulin polypeptide chains. Am J Med 39:319–334, 1965.

Bass JL, Nuss R, Mehta KA, Morganelli P, Bennet L. Recurrent meningococcemia associated with IgG2-subclass deficiency (letter). N Engl J Med 309:430, 1983.

Batata MA, Martini N, Huvos AG, Aguilar RI, Beattie EJ: Thymomas: clinicopathologic features, therapy, and prognosis. Cancer 34:389–396, 1974.

Baumert E, Wolff-Vorbeck G, Schlesier M, Peter HH. Immunophenotypical alterations in a subset of patients with common variable immunodeficiency (CVID). Clin Exp Immunol 90:25–30, 1992.

Beall GN, Ashman RF, Miller ME, Easwaran C, Raghunathan R, Louie J, Yoshikawa T. Hypogammaglobulinemia in mother and son. J Allergy Clin Immunol 65:471–481, 1980.

Beck S, Slater D, Harrington CI. Fatal chronic cutaneous herpes simplex associated with thymoma and hypogammaglobulinaemia. Br J Dermatol 105:471–474, 1981.

Benkerrou M, Gougeon ML, Griscelli C, Fischer A. Hypogammaglobulinémie G et A avec hypergammaglobulinémie M: a propos de 12 observations. Arch Fr Pediatr 47:345–349, 1990.

Bentwich Z, Kunkel HG. Specific properties of human B and T lymphocytes and alterations in disease. Transplant Rev 16:29–50, 1973.

Berger M, Cupps TR, Fauci AS. Immunoglobulin replacement therapy by slow subcutaneous infusion. Ann Intern Med 93:55–56, 1980.

Bernadou A, Devred C, Diebold J, Bilski-Pasquier G, Bousser J. Thymome fuso-cellulaire associé à une érythroblastopénie, une mégacaryocytopénie et une maladie des inclusions cytomégaliques. Semin Hôp Paris 48:3443–3449, 1972.

Bernatz PE, Khonsari S, Harrison EG Jr, Taylor WF. Thymoma: factors influencing prognosis. Surg Clin North Am 53:885–892, 1973.

Bernier GM, Gunderman JR, Ruymann FB. Kappa-chain deficiency. Blood 40:795–805, 1972.

Bernstein LJ, Ochs HD, Wedgwood RJ, Rubinstein A. Defective humoral immunity in pediatric acquired immune deficiency syndrome. J Pediatr 107:352–357, 1985.

Björkander J, Bake B, Oxelius V-A, Hanson LA. Impaired lung function in patients with IgA deficiency and low levels of IgG2 or IgG3. N Engl J Med 313:720–724, 1985.

Blattner FR, Tucker PW. The molecular biology of immunoglobulin D. Nature 307:417–422, 1984.

Blecher TE, Soothill JF, Voyce MA, Walker WHC. Antibody deficiency syndrome: a case with normal immunoglobulin levels. Clin Exp Immunol 3:47–56, 1968.

Bohnsack J, Ochs HD, Wedgwood RJ, Heller SR. Antibody to bacteriophage φX 174 synthesized by cultured human peripheral blood lymphocytes. Clin Exp Immunol 59:673–678, 1985.

Böttger EC, Hoffman T, Hadding U, Bitter-Suermann D. Influence of genetically inherited complement deficiencies on humoral immune response in guinea pigs. J Immunol 135:4100–4107, 1985.

Böttger EC, Metzger S, Bitter-Suermann D, Stevenson G, Kleindienst S, Burger R. Impaired humoral immune response in complement C3-deficient guinea pigs: absence of secondary antibody response. Eur J Immunol 16:1231–1235, 1986.

Braconier JH, Nilsson B, Oxelius V-A, Karup-Pederson F. Recurrent pneumococcal infections in a patient with lack of specific IgG and IgM pneumococcal antibodies and deficiency of serum IgA, IgG2 and IgG4. Scand J Infect Dis 16:407–410, 1984.

Bradley LAD, Sweatman AK, Lovering RC, Jones AM, Morgan G, Levinsky RJ, Kinnon C. Mutation detection in the X-linked agammaglobulinemia gene, *BTK*, using single strand conformation polymorphism analysis. Hum Mol Genet 3:79–83, 1994.

Brahmi Z, Lazarus KH, Hodes ME, Baehner RL. Immunologic studies of three family members with the immunodeficiency with hyper-IgM syndrome. J Clin Immunol 3:127–134, 1983.

Braun J, Berberian L, King L, Sanz I, Govan HL. Restricted use of fetal VH3 immunoglobulin genes by unselected B cells in the adult: predominance of 56p1-like VH genes in common variable immunodeficiency. J Clin Invest 89:1395–1402, 1992.

Braun J, Galbraith L, Valles-Ayoub Y, Saxon A. Human immunodeficiency resulting in a maturational arrest of germinal center B cells. Immunol Lett 27:205–208, 1991.

Brenner MK, Reittie JGE, Chadda HR, Pollock A, Asherson GL. Thymoma and hypogammaglobulinaemia with and without T suppressor cells. Clin Exp Immunol 58:619–624, 1984.

Bronsky D, Dunn YOL. Sarcoidosis with hypogammaglobulinemia. Am J Med Sci 250:11–18, 1965.

Brown EJ, Hosea SW, Frank MM. The role of the spleen in experimental pneumococcal bacteremia. J Clin Invest 67:975–982, 1981.

Bruton OC.: Agammaglobulinemia. Pediatrics 9:722–728, 1952.

Bryant A, Calver NC, Toubi E, Webster ADB, Farrant J. Classification of patients with common variable immunodeficiency by B cell secretion of IgM and IgG in response to anti-IgM and interleukin-2. Clin Immunol Immunopathol 56:239–248, 1990.

Buckley RH, Rowlands DT Jr. Agammaglobulinemia, neutropenia, fever, and abdominal pain. J Allergy Clin Immunol 51:308–318, 1973.

Burgio GR, Ugazio A, Nespoli L, Maccario R. Down syndrome: a model of immunodeficiency. In Wedgwood RJ, Rosen FS, Paul NW, eds. Primary Immunodeficiency Diseases. New York, Alan R. Liss, 1983, pp. 325–327.

Burtin P. Un exemple d'agammaglobulinémie atypique (un cas de grande hypogammaglobulinémie avec augmentation de la β2-macroglobuline). Rev Franc Étud Clin et Biol 6:286–289, 1961.

Cain WA, Ammann AJ, Hong R, Ishizaka K, Good RA. IgE deficiency associated with chronic sinopulmonary infection (abstract). J Clin Invest 48:12a, 1969.

Campana D, Farrant J, Inamdar N, Webster ADB, Janossy G. Phenotypic features and proliferative activity of B cell progenitors in X-linked agammaglobulinemia. J Immunol 145:1675–1680 1990.

Casali P, Rice GPA, Oldstone MBA. Viruses disrupt functions of human lymphocytes. J Exp Med 159:1322–1337, 1984.

Cassidy JT, Nordby GL. Human serum immunoglobulin concentrations: prevalence of immunoglobulin deficiencies. J Allergy Clin Immunol 55:35–48, 1975.

Centers for Disease Control. Safety of therapeutic immune globulin preparations with respect to transmission of human T-lymphotropic virus type III/lymphadenopathy-associated virus infection. MMWR Morb Mortal Wkly Rep 35:231–233, 1986.

Chapin MA. Benign thymoma, refractory anemia and hypogammaglobulinemia—case report. J Maine Med Assoc 56:83–87, 1965.

Ching YC, Davis SD, Wedgwood RJ. Antibody studies in hypogammaglobulinemia. J Clin Invest 45:1593–1600, 1966.

Chusid MJ, Coleman CM, Dunne WM. Chronic asymptomatic campylobacter bacteremia in a boy with X-linked hypogammaglobulinemia. Pediatr Infect Dis J 6:943–944, 1987.

Ciliberti MD, Zweiman B, Atkins PC, Levinson AI, Mittl RL, Phillips DM. Chronic enteroviral meningoencephalitis in X-linked agammaglobulinemia: prolonged survival with the use of intrathecal therapy. Immunol Allergy Prac 16:7–10, 1994.

Clark EA, Lane PJ. Regulation of human B-cell activation and adhesion. Annu Rev Immunol 9:97–127, 1991.

Coico RF, Xue B, Wallace D, Pernis B, Siskind GW, Thorbecke GJ. T cells with receptors for IgD. Nature 316:744–746, 1985.

Conley ME. B cells in patients with X-linked agammaglobulinemia. J Immunol 134:3070–3074, 1985.

Conley ME. Molecular approaches to analysis of X-linked immunodeficiencies. Ann Rev Immunol 10:215–238, 1992.

Conley ME, Brown P, Pickard AR, Buckley RH, Miller DS, Raskind WH, Singer JW, Fialkow PJ. Expression of the gene defect in X-linked agammaglobulinemia. N Engl J Med 315:564–567, 1986a.

Conley ME, Burks AW, Herrod HG, Puck JM. Molecular analysis of X-linked agammaglobulinemia with growth hormone deficiency. J Pediatr 119:392–397, 1991.

Conley ME, Fitch-Hilgenberg ME, Cleveland JL, Parolini O, Rohrer J. Screening of genomic DNA to identify mutations in the gene for Bruton's tyrosine kinase. Hum Mol Genet 3:1751–1756, 1994a.

Conley ME, Larche M, Bonagura VR, Lawton AR, Buckley RH, Fu SM, Coustan-Smith E, Herrod HG, Campana D. Hyper-IgM associated with defective CD40-mediated B cell activation. J Clin Invest 94:1404–1409, 1994b.

Conley ME, Park CL, Douglas SD. Childhood common variable immunodeficiency with autoimmune disease. J Pediatr 108:915–922, 1986b.

Conley ME, Puck JM. Carrier detection in typical and atypical X-linked agammaglobulinemia. J Pediatr 112:688–694, 1988.

Conn HO, Quintiliani R. Severe diarrhea controlled by gamma globulin in a patient with agammaglobulinemia, amyloidosis, and thymoma. Ann Intern Med 65:528–541, 1966.

Cooper MD, Lawton AR. Circulating B-cells in patients with immunodeficiency. Am J Pathol 69:513–528, 1972.

Cooper MD, Peterson RDA, Good RA. Delineation of the thymic and bursal lymphoid systems in the chicken. Nature 205:143–146, 1965.

Cooperband SR, Rosen FS, Kibrick S. Studies on the in vitro behavior of agammaglobulinemic lymphocytes. J Clin Invest 47:836–847, 1968.

Cunningham-Rundles C. Clinical and immunologic analyses of 103 patients with common variable immunodeficiency. J Clin Immunol 9:22–33, 1989.

Cunningham-Rundles C, Kazbay K, Hassett J, Zhou A, Mayer L. Brief report: enhanced humoral immunity in common variable immunodeficiency after long-term treatment with polyethylene glycol-conjugated interleukin-2. N Engl J Med 331:918–921, 1994.

Cunningham-Rundles C, Mayer L, Sapira E, Mendelsohn L. Restoration of immunoglobulin secretion in vitro in common variable immunodeficiency by in vivo treatment with polyethylene glycol-conjugated human recombinant interleukin-2. Clin Immunol Immunopathol 64:46–56, 1992.

Cunningham-Rundles C, Siegal FP, Cunningham-Rundles S, Lieberman P. Incidence of cancer in 98 patients with common varied immunodeficiency. J Clin Immunol 7:294–299, 1987.

Cunningham-Rundles S, Cunningham-Rundles C, Ma DI, Siegal SP, Kosloff C, Good RA. Impaired proliferative response to B lymphocyte activators in common variable immunodeficiency. J Clin Immunol 1:65–72, 1981.

Davis SD, Eidelman S, Loop JW. Nodular lymphoid hyperplasia of the small intestine and sarcoidosis. Arch Intern Med 126:668–672, 1970.

DeGast GC, The TH, Viersma JW, Marrink J, Arisz LA. Reversible hypogammaglobulinaemia after diphenylhydantoin and hydroxyzine therapy. Neth J Med 17:261–269, 1974.

DeGast GC, Wilkins SR, Webster ADB, Rickinson A, Platts-Mills TAE. Functional "immaturity" of isolated B cells from patients with hypogammaglobulinemia. Clin Exp Immunol 42:535–544, 1980.

De la Concha EG, Garcia-Rodriguez MC, Zabay JM, Laso MT, Alonso F, Bootello A, Fontan G. Functional assessment of T and B lymphocytes in patients with selective IgM deficiency. Clin Exp Immunol 49:670–676, 1982.

De la Concha EG, Oldham G, Webster ADB, Asherson GL, Platts-Mills TAE. Quantitative measurements of T- and B-cell function in "variable" primary hypogammaglobulinemia: evidence for a consistent B-cell defect. Clin Exp Immunol 27:208–215, 1977.

de Weers M, Mensink RGJ, Kraakman MEM, Schuurman RKB, Hendriks RW. Mutation analysis of the Bruton's tyrosine kinase gene in X-linked agammaglobulinemia: identification of a mutation which affects the same codon as is altered in immunodeficient *xid* mice. Hum Mol Genet 3:161–166, 1994.

Degos L, Faille A, Housset M, Boumsell L, Rabian C, Parames T.

Syndrome of neutrophil agranulocytosis, hypogammaglobulinemia, and thymoma. Blood 60:968–972, 1982.

DiSanto JP, Bonnefoy JY, Gauchat JF, Fischer A, De Saint Basile G. CD40 ligand mutations in X-linked immunodeficiency with hyper IgM. Nature 361:541–543, 1993.

Dosch H-M, Jason J, Gelfand EW. Transient antibody deficiency and abnormal T suppressor cells induced by phenytoin. N Engl J Med 306:406–409, 1982.

Douglas RM, Paton JC, Duncan SJ, Hansman DJ. Antibody response to pneumococcal vaccination in children younger than five years of age. J Infect Dis 148:131–137, 1983.

Douglas SD, Goldberg LS, Fudenberg HH. Clinical, serologic and leukocyte function studies on patients with idiopathic "acquired" agammaglobulinemia and their families. Am J Med 48:48–53, 1970.

Drenth JP, Haagsma CJ, van der Meer JW. Hyperimmunoglobulinemia D and periodic fever syndrome: the clinical spectrum in a series of 50 patients. International Hyper IgD Study Group. Medicine 73:133–144, 1994.

Drew PA, Kiroff GK, Ferrante A, Cohen RC. Alterations in immunoglobulin synthesis by peripheral blood mononuclear cells from splenectomized patients with and without splenic regrowth. J Immunol 132:191–196, 1984.

Dubois RS, Roy CC, Fulginiti VA, Merrill DA, Murray RL. Disaccharidase deficiency in children with immunologic deficits. J Pediatr 76:377–385, 1970.

Egwang TG, Befus AD. The role of complement in the induction and regulation of immune responses. Immunology 51:207–224, 1984.

Eibl MM, Mannhalter JW, Zielinksi CC, Ahmad R. Defective macrophage–T-cell interaction in common varied immunodeficiency. Clin Immunol Immunopathol 22:316–322, 1982a.

Eibl MM, Mannhalter JW, Zlabinger G, Mayr WR, Tilz GP, Ahmad R, Zielinski CC. Defective macrophage function in a patient with common variable immunodeficiency. N Engl J Med 307:803–806, 1982b.

Eibl MM, Wedgwood RJ. Intravenous immunoglobulin: a review. Immunodeficiency Rev 1(Suppl):1–42, 1989.

Eisenstein EM, Jaffe JS, Strober W. Reduced interleukin-2 (IL-2) production in common variable immunodeficiency is due to a primary abnormality of CD4+ T cell differentiation. J Clin Invest 13:247–258, 1993.

Epstein LB, Epstein CJ. T lymphocyte function and sensitivity to interferon in trisomy 21. Cell Immunol 51:303–318, 1980.

Eraklis AJ, Kevy SV, Diamond LK, Gross RE. Hazard of overwhelming infection after splenectomy in childhood. N Engl J Med 276:1225–1229, 1967.

Erlendsson K, Swartz T, Dwyer JM. Successful reversal of echovirus encephalitis in X-linked hypogammaglobulinemia by intraventricular administration of immunoglobulin. N Engl J Med 312:351–353, 1985.

Esolen LM, Fasano MB, Flynn J, Burton A, Lederman HM. *Pneumocystis carinii* osteomyelitis in a patient with common variable immunodeficiency. N Engl J Med 326:999–1001, 1992.

Farrant J, Bryant A, Almandoz F, Spickett G, Evans SW, Webster ADB. B cell function in acquired "common-variable" hypogammaglobulinemia: proliferative responses to lymphokines. Clin Immunol Immunopathol 51:196–204, 1989.

Farrant J, Bryant A, Lever AML, Edwards AJ, Knight SC, Webster ADB. Defective low-density cells of dendritic morphology from the blood of patients with common variable hypogammaglobulinemia: low immunoglobulin production on stimulation of normal B cells. Clin Exp Immunol 61:189–194, 1985.

Farrington M, Grosmaire LS, Nonoyama S, Fischer SH, Hollenbaugh D, Ledbetter JA, Noelle RJ, Aruffo A, Ochs HD. CD40 ligand expression is defective in a subset of patients with common variable immunodeficiency. Proc Natl Acad Sci U S A 91:1099–1103, 1994.

Faulk WP, Kiyasu WS, Cooper MD, Fudenberg HH. Deficiency of IgM. Pediatrics 47:399–404, 1971.

Fearon ER, Winkelstein JA, Civin CI, Pardoll DM, Vogelstein B. Carrier detection in X-linked agammaglobulinemia by analysis of X-chromosome inactivation. N Engl J Med 316:427–431, 1987.

Fearon DT, Wong WW. Complement ligand-receptor interactions that mediate biological responses. Annu Rev Immunol 1:243–271, 1983.

Filipovich AH, Heinitz KJ, Robison LL, Frizzera G. The immunodeficiency cancer registry: a research resource. Am J Pediatr Hematol Oncol 9:183–184, 1987.

Flanagan JG, Rabbitts TH. Arrangement of human immunoglobulin heavy chain constant region genes implies evolutionary duplication of a segment containing gamma, epsilon, and alpha genes. Nature 300:709–713, 1982.

Fleisher TA, White RM, Broder S, Nissley SP, Blaese RM, Mulvihill JJ, Olive G, Waldmann TA. X-linked hypogammaglobulinemia and isolated growth hormone deficiency. N Engl J Med 302:1429–1434, 1980.

Foy HM, Ochs H, Davis SD, Kenny GE, Luce RR. *Mycoplasma pneumoniae* infections in patients with immunodeficiency syndromes: report of four cases. J Infect Dis 127:388–393, 1973.

Foy TM, Laman JD, Ledbetter JA, Aruffo A, Claassen E, Noelle RJ. gp39-CD40 interactions are essential for germinal center formation and the development of B cell memory. J Exp Med 180:157–163, 1994.

Freijd A, Hammarström L, Persson MAA, Smith CIE. Plasma anti-pneumococcal antibody activity of the IgG class and subclasses in otitis prone children. Clin Exp Immunol 56:233–238, 1984.

Friedman JM, Fialkow PJ, Davis SD, Ochs HD, Wedgwood RJ. Autoimmunity in the relatives of patients with immunodeficiency diseases. Clin Exp Immunol 28:375–388, 1977.

Fudenberg H, German JL, Kunkel HG. The occurrence of rheumatoid factor and other abnormalities in families of patients with agammaglobulinemia. Arthritis Rheum 5:565–588, 1962.

Fudenberg H, Good RA, Goodman HC, Hitzig W, Kunkel HG, Roitt IM, Rosen FS, Rose DS, Seligmann M, Soothill JR. Primary immunodeficiencies: report of a World Health Organization Committee. Pediatrics 47:927–946, 1971.

Fuleihan R, Ramesh N, Loh R, Jabara H, Rosen FS, Chatila T, Fu SM, Stamenkovic I, Geha RS. Defective expression of the CD40 ligand in X chromosome-linked immunoglobulin deficiency with normal or elevated IgM. Proc Natl Acad Sci U S A 90:2170–2173, 1993.

Gascan H, Gauchat JF, Aversa G, Van Vlasselaer P, De Vries JE. Anti-CD40 monoclonal antibodies or CD4+ T cell clones and IL-4 induce IgG4 and IgE switching in purified human B lymphocytes via different signaling pathways. J Immunol 147:8–13, 1991.

Geha RS. IgG antibody response to polysaccharides in children with recurrent infections. Monogr Allergy 23:97–102, 1988.

Geha RS, Hyslop N, Alami S, Farah F, Schneeberger EE, Rosen FS. Hyper immunoglobulin M immunodeficiency (dysgammaglobulinemia). J Clin Invest 64:385–391, 1979.

Geha RS, Rosen FS, Merler E. Identification and characterization of subpopulations of lymphocytes in human peripheral blood after fractionation on discontinuous gradients of albumin: the cellular defect in X-linked agammaglobulinemia. J Clin Invest 52:1726–1734, 1973.

Gehrmann G, Engstfeld G. Thymoma and agammaglobulinemia. German Med Monthly 10:281–283, 1965.

George DL, Phillips JA, Francke U, Seeburg PH. The genes for growth hormone and chorionic somatomammotropin are on the long arm of human chromosome 17 in region q21→(q21→qter). Hum Genet 57:138–141, 1981.

Germain-Lee EL, Schiffman G, Mules EH, Lederman HM. Selective deficiency of antibody responses to polysaccharide antigens in a child mosaic for partial trisomy 1 {46,XX,dir dup (1)(q12→q23)/46,XX}. J Pediatr 117:96–99, 1990.

Giebink GS, Foker JE, Kim Y, Schiffman G. Serum antibody and opsonic response to vaccination with pneumococcal capsular polysaccharide in normal and splenectomized children. J Infect Dis 141:404–412, 1980.

Giebink GS, Le CT, Schiffman G. Decline of serum antibody in splenectomized children after vaccination with pneumococcal capsular polysaccharides. J Pediatr 105:576–582, 1984.

Gigliotti F, Herrod HG, Kalwinsky DK, Insel RA. Immunodeficiency associated with recurrent infections and an isolated in vivo inability to respond to bacterial polysaccharides. Pediatr Infect Dis 7:417–420, 1988.

Gitlin D, Janeway CA, Apt L, Craig JM. Agammaglobulinemia. In Lawrence HS, ed. Cellular and Humoral Aspects of the Hypersensitivity States: A Symposium. New York, Hoeber–Harper, 1959, pp. 375–441.

Gleich GJ, Averbeck AK, Swedlung HA. Measurement of IgE in normal and allergic serum by radioimmunoassay. J Lab Clin Med 77:690–698, 1971.

Golay JT, Webster ADB. B cells in patients with X-linked and "common variable" hypogammaglobulinaemia. Clin Exp Immunol 65:100–104, 1986.

Goldstein G, Mackay IR, eds. The Human Thymus. St. Louis, Warren H. Green, 1969, pp. 194–227.

Good RA. Agammaglobulinemia—a provocative experiment of nature. Bull Univ Minn Med Found 26:1–19, 1954.

Good RA. Studies on agammaglobulinemia: II. Failure of plasma cell formation in the bone marrow and lymph nodes of patients with agammaglobulinemia. J Lab Clin Med 46:167–181, 1955.

Good RA, Rotstein J. Rheumatoid arthritis and agammaglobulinemia. Bull Rheum Dis 10:203–206, 1960.

Good RA, Rotstein J, Mazzitello WF. The simultaneous occurrence of rheumatoid arthritis and agammaglobulinemia. J Lab Clin Med 49:343–357, 1957.

Good RA, Yunis E. Association of autoimmunity, immunodeficiency and aging in man, rabbits and mice. Fed Proc 33:2040–2050, 1974.

Good RA, Zak SJ. Disturbances in gamma globulin synthesis as "experiments of nature." Pediatrics 18:109–149, 1956.

Gordon MC, Sinha SK, Carolson SD. Antibody responses to influenza vaccine in patients with Down's syndrome. Am J Ment Deficiency 75:391–399, 1971.

Gotoff SP, Smith RD, Sugar O. Dermatomyositis with cerebral vasculitis in a patient with agammaglobulinemia. Am J Dis Child 123:53–56, 1972.

Granoff DM, Pandy JP, Boies E, Squires J, Munson RS, Suarez B. Response to immunization with *Haemophilus influenzae* type b polysaccharide-pertussis vaccine and risk of *Haemophilus* meningitis in children with the Km(1) immunoglobulin allotype. J Clin Invest 74:1708–1714, 1984.

Gray GF, Gutowski WT. Thymoma: a clinicopathologic study of 54 cases. Am J Surg Pathol 3:235–249, 1979.

Grey HM, Kunkel HG. H chain subgroups of myeloma proteins and normal 7S gamma-globulin. J Exp Med 120:253–266, 1964.

Grierson H, Purtilo DT. Epstein-Barr virus infections in males with the X-linked lymphoproliferative syndrome. Ann Intern Med 106:538–545, 1987.

Griffiths AW, Sylvester PE. Mongols and nonmongols compared in their response to active tetanus immunization. J Ment Deficiency 11:263–266, 1967.

Grob PJ, Herold GE. Immunological abnormalities and hydantoins. Br Med J 2:561–563, 1972.

Guill MF, Brown DA, Ochs HD, Pyun KH, Moffitt JE. IgM deficiency: clinical spectrum and immunologic assessment. Ann Allergy 62:547–552, 1989.

Guioli S, Arveiler B, Bardoni B, Notarangelo LD, Panina P, Duse M, Ugazio A, Oberle I, de Saint Basile G, Mandel JL, Camerino G. Close linkage of probe p212 (DXS178) to X-linked agammaglobulinemia. Hum Genet 84:19–21, 1989.

Gupta S, Saverymuttu SH, Gibbs JSR, Evans DJ, Hodgson HJF. Watery diarrhea in a patient with myasthenia gravis, thymoma, and immunodeficiency. Am J Gastroenterol 80:877–881, 1985.

Haberland C. Alzheimer's disease in Down syndrome: clinical-neuropathological observations. Acta Neurol Belg 69:369–380, 1969.

Hagemann TL, Chen Y, Rosen FS, Kwan S-P. Genomic organization of the Btk gene and exon scanning for mutations in patients with X-linked agammaglobulinemia. Hum Mol Genet 3:1743–1749, 1994.

Hakami N, Neiman PE, Canellos GP, Lazerson J. Neonatal megaloblastic anemia due to inherited transcobalamin II deficiency in two siblings. N Engl J Med 285:1163–1170, 1971.

Hall CA. Congenital disorders of vitamin B_{12} transport and their contribution to concept. II. Yale Biol Med 54:485–495, 1981.

Hammarström L, Granström M, Oxelius V, Persson MAA, Smith CIE. IgG subclass distribution of antibodies against *S. aureus* teichoic acid and alpha-toxin in normal and immunodeficient donors. Clin Exp Immunol 55:593–601, 1984.

Hammon WMcD, Coriell LL, Stokes J. Evaluation of red cross immunoglobulin as a prophylaxis agent for poliomyelitis. JAMA 150:739–760, 1952.

Hancock MP, Huntley CC, Sever JL. Congenital rubella syndrome with immunoglobulin disorder. J Pediatr 72:636–645, 1968.

Hanson LA, Söderström R, Avanzini A, Bengtsson U, Björkander J, Söderström T. Immunoglobulin subclass deficiency. Pediatr Infect Dis J 7:S17–S21, 1988.

Haraldsson A, van der Burgt CJAM, Weemaes CMR, Otten B, Bakkeren JAJM, Stoelinga GBA. Antibody deficiency and isolated growth hormone deficiency in a girl with Mulibrey nanism. Eur J Pediatr 152:509–519, 1993.

Haraldsson A, Weemaes CMR, De Boer AW, Bakkeren JAJM, Stoelinga GBA. Immunological studies in the hyper-immunoglobulin D syndrome. J Clin Immunol 12:424–428, 1992.

Hayward AR, Paolucci P, Webster ADB, Kohler P. Pre-B cell suppression by thymoma patient lymphocytes. Clin Exp Immunol 48:437–442, 1982.

Heiner DC. Significance of immunoglobulin G subclasses. Am J Med 76:1–6, 1984.

Heiner DC, Myers AS, Beck CS. Deficiency of IgG4: disorder associated with frequent infections and bronchiectasis that may be familial. Clin Rev Allergy 1:259–266, 1983.

Hendriks RW, Sandkuyl LA, Kraakman MEM, Espanol T, Schuurman RKB. RFLP linkage and X chromosome inactivation analysis in X-linked immunodeficiency with hyperimmunoglobulinemia M. In Chapel HM, Levinsky RJ, Webster ADB, eds. Progress in Immune Deficiency. III. London, Royal Society of Medicine, 1991, pp. 266–271.

Hermans PE, Huizenga KA, Hoffman HN, Brown AL, Markowitz H. Dysgammaglobulinemia associated with nodular lymphoid hyperplasia of the small intestine. Am J Med 40:78–89, 1966.

Hermaszewski RA, Webster ADB. Primary hypogammaglobulinaemia: a survey of clinical manifestations and complications. Q J Med 86:31–42, 1993.

Herrod HG. Clinical significance of IgG subclasses. Curr Opin Pediatr 5:696–699, 1993a.

Herrod HG. Management of the patient with IgG subclass deficiency and/or selective antibody deficiency. Ann Allergy 70:3–11, 1993b.

Herrod HG, Gross S, Insel R. Selective antibody deficiency to *Haemophilus influenzae* type B capsular polysaccharide vaccination in children with recurrent respiratory tract infection. J Clin Immunol 9:429–434, 1989.

Hiemstra I, Vossen JM, van der Meer JWM, Weemaes CMR, Out TA, Zegers BJM. Clinical and immunological studies in patients with an increased serum IgD level. J Clin Immunol 9:393–400, 1989.

Hitzig WH, Dohmann U, Pluss HJ, Vischer D. Hereditary transcobalamin II deficiency: clinical findings in a new family. J Pediatr 85:622–628, 1974.

Hitzig WH, Kenny AB. The role of vitamin B_{12} and its transport globulins in the production of antibodies. Clin Exp Immunol 20:105–111, 1975.

Hobbs JR, Milner RDG, Watt PJ. Gamma-M deficiency predisposing to meningococcal septicaemia. Br Med J 4:583–586, 1967.

Hollenbaugh D, Ochs HD, Noelle RJ, Ledbetter JA, Aruffo A. The role of CD40 and its ligand in the regulation of the immune response. Immunol Rev 138:23–37, 1994a.

Hollenbaugh D, Wu LH, Ochs HD, Nonoyama S, Grosmaire LS, Ledbetter JA, Noelle RJ, Hill H, Aruffo A. The random inactivation of the X chromosome carrying the defective gene responsible for X-linked hyper IgM syndrome (X-HIM) in female carriers of HIGM1. J Clin Invest 94:616–622, 1994b.

Hong R. The biological significance of IgE in chronic respiratory infections. In Dayton DH Jr, Small PA Jr, Chanock RM, et al., eds. The Secretory Immunologic System. Washington, DC, U.S. Government Printing Office, 1971, pp. 433–445.

Hosea SW, Burch CG, Brown EJ, Berg RA, Frank MM. Impaired immune response of splenectomised patients to polyvalent pneumococcal vaccine. Lancet 1:804–807, 1981.

Inoue T, Okumura Y, Shirahama M, Ishibashi H, Kashiwagi S, Okubo H. Selective partial IgM deficiency: functional assessment of T and B lymphocytes in vitro. J Clin Immunol 6:130–135, 1986.

Insel RA, Anderson PW. Response to oligosaccharide-protein conjugate vaccine against *Hemophilus influenzae b* in two patients with IgG2 deficiency unresponsive to capsular polysaccharide vaccine. N Engl J Med 315:499–503, 1986.

Insler MS, Gordon RA. Absolute IgG4 deficiency and recurrent bacterial blepharo-kerato-conjunctivitis. Am J Ophthalmol 98:243–244, 1984.

Ipp MM, Gelfand EW. Antibody deficiency and alopecia. J Pediatr 89:728–731, 1976.

Iskander R, Das PK, Aalberse RC. IgG4 antibodies in Egyptian patients with schistosomiasis. Int Arch Allergy Appl Immunol 66:200–207, 1981.

Jacox RF, Mongan ES, Hanshaw JB, Leddy JP. Hypogammaglobulinemia with thymoma and probable pulmonary infection with cytomegalovirus. N Engl J Med 271:1091–1096, 1964.

Jaffe JS, Eisenstein E, Sneller MC, Strober W. T-cell abnormalities in common variable immunodeficiency. Pediatr Res 33(Suppl):S24–S28, 1993.

Janeway CA, Apt L, Gitlin D. "Agammaglobulinemia." Trans Assoc Am Physicians 66:200–202, 1953.

Janeway CA, Gitlin D, Craig JM, Grice DS. "Collagen disease" in patients with congenital agammaglobulinemia. Trans Assoc Am Physicians 69:93–97, 1956.

Jeandel C, Gastin I, Blain H, Jouanny P, Laurain MC, Penin F, Saunier M, Nicolas JP, Guéant JL. Thymoma with immunodeficiency (Good's syndrome) associated with selective cobalamin malabsorption and benign IgM-κ gammopathy. J Intern Med 235:179–182, 1994.

Jeunet FS, Good RA. Thymoma, immunologic deficiencies and hematological abnormalities. In Bergsma D, Good RA, eds. Immunologic Deficiency Diseases in Man. Baltimore, Williams & Wilkins, 1968, pp. 192–206.

Johnson PR Jr, Edwards KM, Wright PF. Failure of intraventricular gamma globulin to eradicate echovirus encephalitis in a patient with X-linked agammaglobulinemia. N Engl J Med 313:1546–1547, 1985.

Journet O, Durandy A, Doussau M, Le Deist F, Couvreur J, Griscelli C, Fischer A, de Saint-Basile G. Carrier detection and prenatal diagnosis of X-linked agammaglobulinemia. Am J Med Genet 43:885–887, 1992.

Junker AK, Dimmick JE. Progressive generalized edema in an 8-year-old boy with agammaglobulinemia. J Pediatr 101:147–153, 1982.

Junker AK, Ochs HD, Clark EA, Puterman ML, Wedgwood RJ. Transient immune deficiency in patients with acute Epstein-Barr virus infection. Clin Immunol Immunopathol 40:436–446, 1986.

Kaikov Y, Wadsworth LD, Hall CA, Rogers PCJ. Transcobalamin II deficiency: case report and review of the literature. Eur J Pediatr 150:841–843, 1991.

Karttunen R, Nurmi T, Ilonen J, Surcel H-M. Cell-mediated immunodeficiency in Down's syndrome: normal IL-2 production but inverted ratio of T cell subsets. Clin Exp Immunol 55:257–263, 1984.

Kauffman CA, Linnemann CC Jr, Alvira MM. Cytomegalovirus encephalitis associated with thymoma and immunoglobulin deficiency. Am J Med 67:724–727, 1979.

Kawabe T, Naka T, Yoshida K, Tanaka T, Fujiwara H, Suematsu S, Yoshida N, Kishimoto T, Kikutani H. The immune responses in CD40-deficient mice: impaired immunoglobulin class switching and germinal center formation. Immunity 1:167–178, 1994.

Kersey JH, Spector BD, Good RA. Primary immunodeficiency-cancer registry. Int J Cancer 12:333–347, 1973.

Kinlen IJ, Webster ADB, Bird AG, Haile R, Peto J, Soothill JF, Thompson RA. Prospective study of cancer in patients with common variable hypogammaglobulinemia. Lancet 1:263–266, 1985.

Kinnon C, Hinshelwood S, Levinsky RJ, Lovering RC. X-linked agammaglobulinemia—gene cloning and future prospects. Immunol Today 14:554–558, 1993.

Kinnon C, Levinsky R. The molecular basis of X-linked immunodeficiency disease. J Inherit Metab Dis 15:674–682, 1992.

Kirkpatrick CH, Windhorst DB. Mucocutaneous candidiasis and thymoma. Am J Med 66:939–945, 1979.

Klein J, Figueroa F, Nogy ZA. Genetics of the major histocompatibility complex. Ann Rev Immunol 1:119–142, 1983.

Kopp WL, Trier JS, Stiehm ER, Foroozan P. "Acquired" agammaglobulinemia with defective delayed hypersensitivity. Ann Intern Med 69:309–317, 1968.

Korsmeyer SJ, Hieter PA, Ravetch J, Poplack DG, Waldmann TA, Leder P. Developmental hierarchy of immunoglobulin gene rearrangements in human leukemic pre-B cells. Proc Natl Acad Sci U S A 78:7096–7100, 1981.

Korthäuer U, Graf D, Mages HW, Brière F, Padayachee M, Malcolm S, Ugazio AG, Notarangelo LD, Levinsky RJ, Kroczek RA. Defective expression of T-cell CD40 ligand causes X-linked immunodeficiency with hyper IgM. Nature 361:539–543, 1993.

Krantman HJ, Stiehm ER, Stevens RH, Saxon A, Seeger RC. Abnormal B cell differentiation and variable increased T cell suppression in immunodeficiency with hyper-IgM. Clin Exp Immunol 40:147–156, 1980.

Kreuzfelder E, Obertacke U, Erhard J, Funk R, Steinen R, Scheiermann N, Thraenhart O, Eigler FW, Schmit-Neuerburg KP. Alterations of the immune system following splenectomy in childhood. J Trauma 31:358–364, 1991.

Kruger G, Welte K, Ciobanu N, Cunningham-Rundles C, Ralph P, Venuta S, Feldman S, Koziner B, Wang CY, Moore MAS, Mertelsmann R. Interleukin-2 correction of defective in vitro T-cell mitogenesis in patients with common varied immunodeficiency. J Clin Immunol 4:295–303, 1984.

Kwan S-P, Kunkel L, Bruns G, Wedgwood RJ, Latt S, Rosen FS. Mapping of the X-linked agammaglobulinemia locus by use of restriction fragment-length polymorphism. J Clin Invest 77:649–652, 1986.

Kwan S-P, Terwilliger J, Parmley R, Raghu G, Sandkuyl LA, Ott J, Ochs H, Wedgwood R, Rosen F. Identification of a closely linked DNA marker, DXS178, to further refine the X-linked agammaglobulinemia locus. Genomics 6:238–242, 1990.

Kwan S-P, Walker AP, Hagemann T, Gupta S, Vayuvegula B, Ochs HD. A new RFLP marker, SP282, at the *btk* locus for genetic analysis in X-linked agammaglobulinaemia families. Prenat Diagn 14:493–496, 1994.

Kyong CU, Virella G, Fudenberg HH, Darby CP. X-linked immunodeficiency with increased IgM: clinical, ethnic, and immunologic heterogeneity. Pediatr Res 12:1024–1026, 1978.

Lafrenz D, Teale JM, Strober S. Role of IgD in immunological memory. Ann NY Acad Sci, 399:375–388, 1982.

Lambie AT, Burrows BA, Sommers SC. Clinicopathologic conference: refractory anemia, agammaglobulinemia and mediastinal tumor. Am J Clin Pathol 27:444–452, 1957.

Lane P, Traunecker A, Hubele S, Inui S, Lanzavecchia A, Gray D. Activated human T cells express a ligand for the human B cell-associated antigen CD40 which participates in T cell-dependent activation of B lymphocytes. Eur J Immunol 22:2573–2578, 1992.

Lauriola L, Maggiano N, Marino M, Carbone A, Piantelli M, Musiani P. Human thymoma: immunologic characteristics of the lymphocytic component. Cancer 48:1992–1995, 1981.

Leahy MF. Subcutaneous immunoglobulin home treatment in hypogammaglobulinemia. Lancet 2:48, 1986.

Lebranchu Y, Thibault G, Degenne D, Bardos P. Deficiency of CD4+ CD45R+ T lymphocytes in common variable immunodeficiency. N Engl J Med 323:276–277, 1990.

Lebranchu Y, Thibault G, Degenne D, Bardos P. Abnormalities in CD4+ T lymphocyte subsets in patients with common variable immunodeficiency. Clin Immunol Immunopathol 61:83–92, 1991.

Lederman HM, Winkelstein JA. X-linked agammaglobulinemia: an analysis of 96 patients. Medicine 64:145–156, 1985.

Lee AH, Levinson AI, Schumacher HR Jr. Hypogammaglobulinemia and rheumatic disease. Semin Arthritis Rheum 22:252–264, 1993

Lefranc M-P, Hammarström L, Smith CIE, Lefranc G. Gene deletions in the human immunoglobulin heavy chain constant region locus: molecular and immunological analysis. Immunodefic Rev 2:265–281, 1991.

Leibovitz A, Yannet H. The production of humoral antibodies by the mongolian. Am J Ment Defic 46:304–309, 1942.

Leickley FE, Buckley R. Variability in B cell maturation and differentiation in X-linked agammaglobulinemia. Clin Exp Immunol 65:90–99, 1986.

Levin S, Schlesinger M, Handzel Z, Hahn T, Altman Y, Czernobilsky B, Boss J. Thymic deficiency in Down's syndrome. Pediatrics 63:80–87, 1979.

Levine D, Goode AW, Wingate DL. Purgative abuse associated with reversible cachexia, hypogammaglobulinaemia, and finger clubbing. Lancet 1:919–920, 1981.

Levitt D, Cooper MD. Mouse pre-B lymphocytes synthesize and secrete μ heavy chains but not light chains. Cell 19:617–625, 1980.

Levitt D, Haber P, Rich K, Cooper MD. Hyper IgM immunodeficiency: a primary dysfunction of B lymphocyte isotype switching. J Clin Invest 72:1650–1657, 1983.

Levitt D, Ochs HD, Wedgwood RJ. Epstein-Barr virus-induced lymphoblastoid cell lines derived from the peripheral blood of patients with X-linked agammaglobulinemia can secrete IgM. J Clin Immunol 4:143–150, 1984.

Levy DA, Chen J. Healthy IgE-deficient person. N Engl J Med 283:541–542, 1970.

Li FP, Willard DR, Goodman R, Vawter G. Malignant lymphoma after diphenylhydantoin (Dilantin) therapy. Cancer 36:1359–1362, 1975.

Lieber E, Douglas SD, Fudenberg HH. In vitro cytotoxicity of lymphocytes from patients with "acquired" and sex-linked agammaglobulinaemia. Clin Exp Immunol 9:603–609, 1971.

Liese JG, Wintergerst U, Tympner KD, Belohradsky BH. High- vs low-dose immunoglobulin therapy in the long-term treatment of X-linked agammaglobulinemia. Am J Dis Child 146:335–339, 1992.

Litwin SD. Immunodeficiency with thymoma: failure to induce Ig production in immunodeficient lymphocytes cocultured with normal T cells. J Immunol 122:728–732, 1979.

LoGalbo PR, Sampson HA, Buckley RH. Symptomatic giardiasis in three patients with X-linked agammaglobulinemia. J Pediatr 101:78–80, 1982.

Lopez V, Ochs HD, Thuline HC, Davis SD, Wedgwood RJ. Defective antibody response to bacteriophage ϕX174 in Down syndrome. J Pediatr 86:207–211, 1975.

Lovering R, Middleton-Price HR, O'Reilly MA, Genet SA, Parkar M, Sweatman AK, Bradley LD, Alterman LA, Malcolm S, Morgan G. Genetic linkage analysis identifies new proximal and distal flanking markers for the X-linked agammaglobulinemia gene locus, refining its localization in Xq22. Hum Mol Genet 2:139–141, 1993.

MacLennan IC, Liu YJ, Johnson GD. Maturation and dispersal of B-cell clones during T cell-dependent antibody responses. Immunol Rev 126:143–161, 1992.

Maki R, Kearney J, Paige C, Tonegawa S. Immunoglobulin gene rearrangement in immature B lymphocytes. Science 209:1366–1369, 1980.

Malcolm S, de Saint Basile G, Arveiler B, Lau YL, Szabo P, Fischer A, Griscelli C, Debre M, Mandel JL, Callard RE, Robertson ME, Goodship JA, Pembrey ME, Levinsky RJ. Close linkage of random DNA fragments from Xq 21.3–22 to X-linked agammaglobulinaemia (XLA). Hum Genet 77:172–174, 1987.

Marshall LS, Aruffo A, Ledbetter JA, Noelle RJ. The molecular basis for T cell help in humoral immunity: CD40 and its ligand, gp39. J Clin Immunol 13:165–174, 1993.

Marshall WC, Weston HJ, Bodian M. *Pneumocystis carinii* pneumonia and congenital hypogammaglobulinaemia. Arch Dis Child 39:18–25, 1964.

Matheson DS, Clarkson TW, Gelfand EW. Mercury toxicity (acrodynia) induced by long-term injection of gammaglobulin. J Pediatr 97:153–155, 1980.

Mayer L, Fu SM, Cunningham-Rundles C, Kunkel HG. Polyclonal immunoglobulin secretion in patients with common variable immunodeficiency using monoclonal B cell differentiation factors. J Clin Invest 74:2115–2120, 1984.

Mayer L, Kwan SP, Thompson C, Ko HS, Chiorazzi N, Waldmann T, Rosen F. Evidence for a defect in "switch" T cells in patients with immunodeficiency and hyperimmunoglobulinemia M. N Engl J Med 314:409–418, 1986.

Mayumi M, Yamaoka K, Tsutsui T, Mizue H, Doi A, Matsuyama M, Ito S, Shinomiya K, Mikawa H. Selective immunoglobulin M deficiency associated with disseminated molluscum contagiosum. Eur J Pediatr 145:99–103, 1986.

McKinney RE, Katz SL, Wilfert CM. Chronic enteroviral meningoencephalitis in agammaglobulinemic patients. Rev Infect Dis 9:334–356, 1987.

McLaughlin JF, Schaller J, Wedgwood RJ. Arthritis and immunodeficiency. J Pediatr 81:801–803, 1972.

Mease PJ, Ochs HD, Wedgwood RJ. Successful treatment of echovirus meningoencephalitis and myositis-fasciitis with intravenous immune globulin therapy in a patient with X-linked agammaglobulinemia. N Engl J Med 304:1278–1281, 1981.

Mease PJ, Ochs HD, Corey L, Dragavon J, Wedgwood RJ. Echovirus encephalitis/myositis in X-linked agammaglobulinemia (letter). N Engl J Med 312:758, 1985.

Melamed I, Bujanover Y, Igra YS, Schwartz D, Zakuth V, Spirer Z. *Campylobacter* enteritis in normal and immunodeficiency children. Am J Dis Child 137:752–753, 1983.

Mensink EJB, Schuurman RKB, Schot JDL, Thompson A, Alt FW. Immunoglobulin heavy chain gene rearrangements in X-linked agammaglobulinemia. Eur J Immunol 16:963–967, 1986a.

Mensink EJB, Thompson A, Sandkuyl LA, Kraakman ME, Schot JD, Espanol T, Schuurman RKB. X-linked immunodeficiency with hyperimmunoglobulinemia M appears to be linked to the DXS42 restriction fragment length polymorphism locus. Hum Genet 76:96–99, 1987.

Mensink EJBM, Thompson A, Schot JDL, van de Greef WMM, Sandkuyl LA, Schuurman, RKB. Mapping of a gene for X-linked agammaglobulinemia and evidence for genetic heterogeneity. Hum Genet 73:327–332, 1986b.

Michaels RH. Immunologic aspects of congenital rubella. Pediatrics 43:339–350, 1969.

Milili M, Le Deist F, de Saint-Basile G, Fischer A, Fougereau M, Schiff C. Bone marrow cells in X-linked agammaglobulinemia express pre-B-specific genes (lambda-like and V pre-B) and present immunoglobulin V-D-J gene usage strongly biased to a fetal-like repertoire. J Clin Invest 91:1616–1629, 1993.

Miller ME, Mellman WJ, Cohen MM, Kohn G, Dietz WH Jr. Depressed immunoglobulin G in newborn infants with Down's syndrome. J Pediatr 75:996–1000, 1969.

Misbah SA, Spickett GP, Ryba PCJ, Hockaday JM, Kroll JS, Sherwood C, Kurtz JB, Moxon ER, Chapel HM. Chronic enteroviral meningoencephalitis in agammaglobulinemia: case report and literature review. J Clin Immunol 12:266–270, 1992.

Mitsuya H, Osaki K, Tomino S, Katsuki T, Kishimoto S. Pathophysiologic analysis of peripheral blood lymphocytes from patients with primary immunodeficiency: I. Ig synthesis by peripheral blood lymphocytes stimulated with either pokeweed mitogen or Epstein-Barr virus in vitro. J Immunol 127:311–315, 1981.

Mitsuya H, Tomino S, Hisamitsu S, Kishimoto S. Evidence for the failure of IgA specific T helper activity in a patient with immunodeficiency with hyper IgM. J Clin Lab 2:337–342, 1979.

Mofenson LM, Bethel J, Moye J Jr, Flyer P, Nugent R. Effect of intravenous immunoglobulin (IVIG) on CD4$^+$ lymphocyte decline in HIV-infected children in a clinical trial of IVIG infection prophylaxis. J AIDS 6:1103–1113, 1993.

Mofenson LM, Moye J Jr, Bethel J, Hirschhorn R, Jordan C, Nugent R. Prophylactic intravenous immunoglobulin in HIV-infected children with CD4$^+$ counts of 0.20 × 10^9/L or more: effect on viral, opportunistic, and bacterial infections: The National Institute of Child Health and Human Development Intravenous Immunoglobulin Clinical Trial Study Group. JAMA 268:483–488, 1992.

Monafo V, Maghnie M, Terracciano L, Valtorta A, Massa M, Severi F. X-linked agammaglobulinemia and isolated growth hormone deficiency. Acta Paediatr Scand 80:563–566, 1991.

Mongan ES, Kern WA Jr, Terry R. Hypogammaglobulinemia with thymoma, hemolytic anemia, and disseminated infection with cytomegalovirus. Ann Intern Med 65:548–554, 1966.

Morell A, Muehlheim E, Schaad U, Skvaril F, Rossi E. Susceptibility to infections in children with selective IgA- and IgA-IgG subclass deficiency. Eur J Pediatr 145:199–203, 1986.

Morell A, Skvaril F, Rádl J, Dooren LJ, Barandun S. IgG subclass abnormalities in primary immunodeficiency diseases. In Bergsma D, ed. Immunodeficiency in Man and Animals. Sunderland, Mass., Sinauer Associates, 1975, pp. 108–120.

Moretta L, Mingari MC, Webb SR, Pearl ER, Lydyard PM, Grossi CE, Lawton AR, Cooper MD. Imbalances in T cell subpopulations associated with immunodeficiency and autoimmune syndromes. Eur J Immunol 7:696–700, 1977.

Müller C, Mannhalter JW, Ahmad R, Zlabinger G, Wurnig P, Eibl MM. Peripheral blood mononuclear cells of splenectomized patients are unable to differentiate into immunoglobulin-secreting cells after pokeweed mitogen stimulation. Clin Immunol Immunopathol 31:118–123, 1984.

Musiani P, Lauriola L, Maggiano N, Tonali P, Piantelli M. Functional properties of human thymoma lymphocytes: role of subcellular factors in blastic activation. J Natl Cancer Inst 69:827–831, 1982.

Najiar JL, Phillips JA, Manness KJ, Teague D, Summar ML, Lorenz RA. Some cases of non-classical growth hormone deficiency may be due to an X-linked disorder (abstract). Presented at the Seventy-second Annual Meeting of the Endocrine Society, Atlanta, June 20–23, 1990.

Nemazee DA, Bürki K. Clonal deletion of B lymphocytes in a transgenic mouse bearing anti-MHC class I antibody genes. Nature 337:562–566, 1989.

Noelle RJ, Snow EC. Cognate interactions between helper T cells and B lymphocytes. Immunol Today 11:361–368, 1990.

Noelle RJ, Meenakshi R, Shepherd DM, Stamenkovic I, Ledbetter JA, Aruffo A. A 39-kDa protein on activated helper T cells binds CD40 and transduces the signal for cognate activation of B cells. Proc Natl Acad Sci U S A 89:6550–6554, 1992.

Nonoyama S, Farrington M, Ishida H, Howard M, Ochs HD. Activated B cells from patients with common variable immunodeficiency proliferate and synthesize immunoglobulin. J Clin Invest 92:1282–1287, 1993a.

Nonoyama S, Hollenbaugh D, Aruffo A, Ledbetter JA, Ochs HD. B cell activation via CD40 is required for specific antibody production by antigen-stimulated human B cells. J Exp Med 178:1097–1102, 1993b.

Norman ME, Hansell JR, Holtzapple PG, Parks JS, Waldmann TA. Malabsorption and protein-losing enteropathy in a child with X-linked agammaglobulinemia. Clin Immunol Immunopathol 4:157–164, 1975.

North ME, Webster ADB, Farrant J. Defects in proliferative responses of T cells from patients with common variable immunodeficiency on direct activation of protein kinase C. Clin Exp Immunol 85:198–201, 1991.

Nossal GJV. Cellular mechanisms of immunologic tolerance. Ann Rev Immunol 1:33–62, 1983.

Notarangelo LD, Duse M, Ugazio AG. Immunodeficiency with hyper-IgM (HIM). Immunodefic Rev 3:101–122, 1992.

Notarangelo LD, Mantuano E, Bione S, Gimbo E, Giliani S, Caraffini A, Purtilo D, Farr C, Ugazio AG, Toniolo D. Molecular analysis of X-linked immunodeficiency with hyper-IgM and X-linked lympho-proliferative syndrome. Immunodeficiency 4:225–229, 1993.

Notarangelo LD, Parolini O, Albertini A, Duse M, Mazzolari E, Plebani A, Camerino G, Ugazio AG. Analysis of X-chromosome inactivation in X-linked immunodeficiency with hyper-IgM (HIGM1): evidence for involvement of different hematopoietic cell lineages. Hum Genet 88:103–134, 1991.

Ochs HD, Ament ME, Davis SD. Giardiasis with malabsorption in X-linked agammaglobulinemia. N Engl J Med 287:341–342, 1972.

Ochs HD, Aruffo A. Advances in X-linked immunodeficiency diseases. Curr Opin Pediatr 5:684–691, 1993.

Ochs HD, Fischer SH, Wedgwood RJ, Wara DW, Cowan MJ, Ammann AJ, Saxon A, Budinger MD, Allred RU, Rousell RH. Comparison of high-dose and low-dose intravenous immunoglobulin therapy in patients with primary immunodeficiency diseases. Proceedings of a Symposium: Intravenous Immune Globulin and the Compromised Host. Am J Med 76:78–82, 1984.

Ochs HD, Junker AK, Collier AC, Virant FS, Handsfield HH, Wedgwood RJ. Abnormal antibody responses in patients with persistent generalized lymphadenopathy. J Clin Immunol 8:57–63, 1988.

Ochs HD, Lee ML, Fischer SH, Delson ES, Chang BS, Wedgwood RJ. Self-infusion of intravenous immunoglobulin by immunodeficient patients at home. J Infect Dis 156:652–654, 1987.

Ochs HD, Nonoyama S, Zhu Q, Farrington M, Wedgwood RJ. Regulation of antibody responses: the role of complement and adhesion molecules. Clin Immunol Immunopathol 67:S33–S40, 1993.

Ochs HD, Sullivan JL, Wedgwood RJ, Seeley JK, Sakamoto K, Purtilo DT. X-linked lymphoproliferative syndrome: abnormal antibody responses to bacteriophage φX174. In Wedgwood RJ, Rosen FS, Paul NW, eds. Primary Immunodeficiency Diseases, Vol. 19. Birth Defects: Original Article Series, 1983b, pp. 321–323.

Ochs HD, Wedgwood RJ. IgG subclass deficiencies. Ann Rev Med 38:325–340, 1987.

Ochs HD, Wedgwood RJ, Frank MM, Heller SR, Hosea SW. The role of complement in the induction of antibody responses. Clin Exp Immunol 53:208–216, 1983a.

Ochs HD, Wedgwood RJ, Heller SR, Beatty PG. Complement, membrane glycoproteins and complement receptors: their role in regulation of the immune response. Clin Immunol Immunopathol 40:94–104, 1986.

Ohno T, Inaba M, Kuribayashi K, Masuda T, Kanoh T, Uchino H. Selective IgM deficiency in adults: phenotypically and functionally altered profiles of peripheral blood lymphocytes. Clin Exp Immunol 68:630–637, 1987.

Ohta Y, Haire RN, Litman RT, Fu SM, Nelson RP, Kratz J, Kornfeld SJ, De La Morena M, Good RA, Litman GW. Genomic organization and structure of Bruton agammaglobulinemia tyrosine kinase: localization of mutations associated with varied clinical presentations and course in X chromosome-linked agammaglobulinemia. Proc Natl Acad Sci U S A, 91:9062–9066, 1994.

Ohzeki T, Hanaki K, Motozumi H, Ohtahara H, Hayashibara H, Harada Y, Okamoto M, Shiraki K, Tsuji Y, Emura H. Immunodeficiency with increased immunoglobulin M associated with growth hormone insufficiency. Acta Paediatr 82:620–623, 1993.

Olsson PG, Hofker MH, Walter MA, Smith S, Hammarström L, Smith CIE, Cox DW. IgH chain variable and C region genes in common variable immunodeficiency: characterization of two new deletion haplotypes. J Immunol 147:2540–2546, 1991.

Olsson PG, Rabbani H, Hammarström L, Smith CIE. Novel human immunoglobulin heavy chain constant region gene deletion haplotypes characterized by pulsed-field electrophoresis. Clin Exp Immunol 94:84–90, 1993.

O'Neil KM, Ochs HD, Heller SR, Cork LC, Morris JM, Winkelstein JA. Role of C3 in humoral immunity: defective antibody production in C3-deficient dogs. J Immunol 140:1939–1945, 1988a.

O'Neil KM, Pallansch MA, Winkelstein JA, Lock TM, Modlin JF. Chronic group A coxsackie virus infection in agammaglobulinemia: demonstration of genomic variation of serotypically identical isolates persistently excreted from the same patient. J Infect Dis 157:183–186, 1988b.

Ooi BS, Kant KS, Hanenson IB, Pesce AJ, Pollak VE. Lymphocytotoxins in epileptic patients receiving phenytoin. Clin Exp Immunol 30:56–61, 1977.

Ottesen EA, Skvaril F, Tripathy SP, Poindexter RW, Hussain R. Prominence of IgG4 in the IgG antibody response to human filariasis. J Immunol 134:2707–2711, 1985.

Otto HF. Klinisch-pathologische Studie zur Klassifikation und Prognose von 57 Thymustumoren: II. Prognostische Kriterien. Z Krebsforsch 91:103–115, 1978.

Owen JJT, Cooper MD, Raff MC. In vitro generation of B lymphocytes in mouse foetal liver, a mammalian ''bursa equivalent.'' Nature 249:361–363, 1974.

Oxelius V-A. Chronic infections in a family with hereditary deficiency of IgG2 and IgG4. Clin Exp Immunol 17:19–27, 1974.

Oxelius V-A. IgG subclass levels in infancy and childhood. Acta Paediatr Scand, 68:23–27, 1979.

Oxelius V-A, Laurell A-B, Lindquist B, Golebiowska H, Axelsson U, Björkander J, Hanson LA. IgG subclasses in selective IgA deficiency: importance of IgG2-IgA deficiency. N Engl J Med 304:1476–1477, 1981.

Oxelius V-A, Berkel AI, Hanson LA. IgG2 deficiency in ataxia-telangiectasia. N Engl J Med 306:515–517, 1982.

Oxelius V-A, Hanson LA, Björkander J, Hammarström L, Sjoholm A. IgG3 deficiency: common in obstructive lung disease. Hereditary in families with immunodeficiency and autoimmune disease. In Hanson LA, Söderström T, Oxelius VA, eds. Immunoglobulin Subclass Deficiencies. Mongr Allergy 20:106–115, 1986.

Paganelli R, Capobianchi MR, Ensoli B, D'Offizi GP, Facchini J, Dianzani F, Aiuti F. Evidence that defective gamma interferon production in patients with primary immunodeficiencies is due to intrinsic incompetence of lymphocytes. Clin Exp Immunol 72:124–129, 1988.

Page AR, Hansen AE, Good RA. Occurrence of leukemia and lymphoma in patients with agammaglobulinemia. Blood 21:197–206, 1963.

Parolini O, Hejtmancik JF, Allen RC, Belmont JW, Lassiter GL, Henry MJ, Barker DF, Conley ME. Linkage analysis and physical mapping near the gene for X-linked agammaglobulinemia at Xq22. Genomics 15:342–349, 1993.

Pascual-Salcedo D, de la Concha EG, Garcia-Rodriguez MC, Zabay JM, Sainz T, Fontan G. Cellular basis of hyper IgM immunodeficiency. J Clin Lab Immunol 10:29–34, 1983.

Pastorelli G, Roncarolo MG, Touraine JL, Peronne G, Tovo PA, De Vries JE. Peripheral blood lymphocytes of patients with common variable immunodeficiency (CVI) produce reduced levels of interleukin-4, interleukin-2 and interferon-gamma, but proliferate normally upon activation by mitogens. Clin Exp Immunol 78:334–340, 1989a.

Pastorelli G, Roncarolo MG, Touraine JL, Rousset F, Pene J, De Vries JE. Interleukin-4 suppresses immunoglobulin production by peripheral blood lymphocytes of patients with common variable immunodeficiency (CVI) induced by supernatants of T cell clones. Clin Exp Immunol 78:341–347, 1989b.

Pearl ER, Vogler LB, Okos AJ, Crist WM, Lawton AR III, Cooper MD. B lymphocyte precursors in human bone marrow: an analysis of normal individuals and patients with antibody deficiency states. J Immunol 120:1169–1175, 1978.

Peltola H, Kayhty H, Sivonen A, Makela H. *Haemophilus influenzae* type b capsular polysaccharide vaccine in children: a double-blind field study of 100,000 vaccinees 3 months to 5 years of age in Finland. Pediatrics 60:730–737, 1977.

Pène J, Rousset F, Brière F, Chrétien I, Bonnefoy J-Y, Spits H, Yokota T, Arai N, Arai K-I, Bancherau J. IgE production by normal human lymphocytes is induced by interleukin 4 and suppressed by interferons γ and α and prostaglandin E₂. Proc Natl Acad Sci U S A, 85:6880–6884, 1988.

Pepys MB. Role of complement in the induction of the allergic response. Nature (New Biol) 237:157–159, 1972.

Peterson RDA, Cooper MD, Good RA. The pathogenesis of immunologic deficiency diseases. Am J Med 38:579–604, 1965.

Phillip R, Berger AC, McManus N, Warner NH, Epstein LB. Abnormalities of the in vitro cellular and humoral responses to tetanus and influenza antigens with concomitant numerical alternation in lymphocyte subsets in Down's syndrome (trisomy 21). J Immunol 136:1661–1667, 1986.

Phillips JA, Vnencak-Jones CL. Genetics of growth hormone and its disorders. Adv Hum Genet 18:305–363, 1989.

Plebani A, Ugazio AG, Meini A, Ruggeri L, Negrini A, Albertini A, Leibovitz M, Duse M, Bottaro A, Brusco R, Cariota U, Boccazzi C, Carbonara AO. Extensive deletion of immunoglobulin heavy chain constant region genes in the absence of recurrent infections: when is IgG subclass deficiency clinically relevant? Clin Immunol Immunopathol 68:46–50, 1993.

Plotkin SA, Klaus RM, Whitely JP. Hypogammaglobulinemia in an infant with congenital rubella syndrome: failure of 1-adamantanamine to stop virus excretion. J Pediatr 69:1085–1091, 1966.

Polmar SH, Waldmann TA, Balestra ST, Jost MC, Terry WD. Immunoglobulin E in immunologic deficiency diseases: I. Relation of IgE and IgA to respiratory tract disease in isolated IgE deficiency, IgA deficiency and ataxia-telangiectasia. J Clin Invest 51:326–330, 1972.

Preud'Homme JL, Griscelli C, Seligmann M. Immunoglobulins on the surface of lymphocytes in fifty patients with primary immunodeficiency diseases. Clin Immunol Immunopathol 1:241–256, 1973.

Preud'Homme J-L, Hanson LA. IgG subclass deficiency. Immunodefic Rev 2:129–150, 1990.

Provisor AJ, Iacuone JJ, Chilcote RR, Neiburger RG, Crussi FG, Baehner RL. Acquired agammaglobulinemia after a life-threatening illness with clinical and laboratory features of infectious mononucleosis in three related male children. N Engl J Med 293:62–65, 1975.

Purtilo DT, DeFlorio D Jr, Hutt LM, Bhawan J, Yang JPS, Otto R, Edwards W. Variable phenotypic expression of an X-linked recessive lymphoproliferative syndrome. N Engl J Med 297:1077–1081, 1977.

Purtilo DT, Sakamoto K, Barnabei V, Seeley J, Bechtold T, Rogers G, Yetz J, Harada S, collaborators. Epstein-Barr virus-induced diseases in boys with the X-linked lymphoproliferative syndrome (XLP). Am J Med 73:49–56, 1982.

Pyun KH, Ochs HD, Wedgwood RJ, Yang X, Heller SR, Reimer CB. Human antibody responses to bacteriophage φX174: sequential induction of IgM and IgG subclass antibody. Clin Immunol Immunopathol 51:252–263, 1989.

Rádl J, Dooren LJ, Eijsvoogel VP, Van Went JJ, Hijmans W. An immunological study during post-transplantation follow-up of a case of severe combined immunodeficiency. Clin Exp Immunol 10:367–382, 1972.

Reinherz EL, Rubinstein A, Geha RS, Strelkauskas AJ, Rosen FS, Schlossman SF. Abnormalities of immunoregulatory T cells in disorders of immune function. N Engl J Med 301:1018–1021, 1979.

Reth M, Hombach J, Wienands J, Campbell KS, Chien N, Justement LB, Cambier JC. The B-cell antigen receptor complex. Immunol Today 12:196–205, 1991.

Revel M, Bash D, Ruddle FH. Antibodies to a cell surface component coded by human chromosome 21 inhibit action of interferon. Nature 260:139–141, 1976.

Richards SJ, Scott CS, Cole JC, Gooi HC. Abnormal CD45R expression in patients with common variable immunodeficiency and X-linked agammaglobulinemia. Br J Haematol 81:160–166, 1992.

Rieger CHL, Moohr JW, Rothberg RM, Todd JK. Correction of neutropenia associated with dysgammaglobulinemia. Pediatrics 54:508–511, 1974.

Rieger CHL, Nelson LA, Peri BA, Lustig JV, Level C, Shahidi N, Kennedy A, Hammond D, Newcomb RW. Transient hypogammaglobulinemia of infancy. J Pediatr 91:601–603, 1977.

Robinson LL, Nesbit ME, Sather HN, Level C, Shahidi N, Kennedy A, Hammond D. Down syndrome and acute leukemia in children: a 10-year retrospective study from Children's Cancer Study Group. J Pediatr 105:235–242, 1984.

Rodriguez MA, Bankhurst AD, Williams RC Jr. Characterization of the suppressor activity in lymphocytes from patients with common variable hypogammaglobulinemia: evidence for an associated primary B-cell defect. Clin Immunol Immunopathol 29:35–50, 1983.

Roifman CM, Lederman HM, Lavi S, Stein LD, Levison H, Gelfand EW. Benefit of intravenous IgG replacement in hypogammaglobulinemic patients with chronic sinopulmonary disease. Am J Med 79:171–174, 1985.

Roifman CM, Levison H, Gelfand EW. High-dose versus low-dose intravenous immunoglobulin in hypogammaglobulinaemia and chronic lung disease. Lancet 1:1075–1077, 1987.

Rolink A, Melchers F. Molecular and cellular origins of B lymphocyte diversity. Cell 66:1081–1094, 1991.

Roord JM, van der Meer JWM, Kuis W, de Windt GE, Zegers BJM, van Furth R, Stoop JW. Home treatment in patients with antibody deficiency by slow subcutaneous infusion of gammaglobulin. Lancet i:689–690, 1982.

Rosen FS, Cooper MD, Wedgwood RJP. The primary immunodeficiencies. N Engl J Med 311:235–242, 300–310, 1984.

Rosen FS, Janeway CA. The gamma globulins: III. The antibody deficiency syndromes. N Engl J Med 275:769–775, 1966.

Rosen FS, Kevy SV, Merler E, Janeway CA, Gitlin D. Recurrent bacterial infections and dysgammaglobulinemia: deficiency of 7S gammaglobulins in the presence of elevated 19S gammaglobulins. Pediatrics 28:182–195, 1961.

Ross IN, Thompson RA. Severe selective IgM deficiency. J Clin Pathol 29:773–777, 1976.

Rotbart HA, Kinsella JP, Wasserman RL. Persistent enterovirus infection in culture-negative meningoencephalitis: demonstration by enzymatic RNA amplification. J Infect Dis 161:787–791, 1990.

Rothbach C, Nagel J, Rabin B, Fireman P. Antibody deficiency with normal immunoglobulins. J Pediatr 94:250–253, 1979.

Rousset F, Garcia E, Defrance T, Péronne C, Vezzio N, Hsu D-H, Kastelein R, Moore KW, Bancherau J. Interleukin-10 is a potent growth and differentiation factor for activated human B lymphocytes. Proc Natl Acad Sci U S A 89:1890, 1992.

Rowley DA. The effect of splenectomy on the formation of circulating antibody in the adult male albino rat. J Immunol 64:289–295, 1950.

Ryser O, Morell A, Hitzig WH. Primary immunodeficiencies in Switzerland: first report of the national registry in adults and children. J Clin Immunol 8:479–485, 1988.

Safai B, Gupta S, Good RA. Pemphigus vulgaris associated with a syndrome of immunodeficiency and thymoma: a case report. Clin Exp Dermatol 3:129–134, 1978.

Saffran DC, Parolini O, Fitch-Hilgenberg ME, Rawlings DJ, Afar DEH, Witte ON, Conley ME. A point mutation in the SH2 domain of Bruton's tyrosine kinase in atypical X-linked agammaglobulinemia. N Engl J Med 330:1488–1491, 1994.

Saiki O, Ralph P, Cunningham-Rundles C, Good RA. Three distinct stages of B cell defects in common varied immunodeficiency. Proc Natl Acad Sci U S A 79:6008–6012, 1982.

Sanders LAM, Rijkers GT, Kuis W, Tenbergen-Meekes AJ, de Graeff-Meeder BR, Hiemstra I, Zegers BJM. Defective antipneumococcal polysaccharide antibody response in children with recurrent respiratory tract infections. J Allergy Clin Immunol 91:110–119, 1993.

Saulsbury FT, Bernstein MTW, Winkelstein JA. *Pneumocystis carinii* pneumonia as the presenting infection in congenital hypogammaglobulinemia. J Pediatr 95:559–561, 1979.

Saulsbury FT, Winkelstein JA, Yolken RH. Chronic rotavirus infection in immunodeficiency. J Pediatr 97:61–65, 1980.

Saxon A, Giorgi JV, Sherr EH, Kagan JM. Failure of B cells in common variable immunodeficiency to transit from proliferation to differentiation is associated with altered B cell surface-molecule display. J Allergy Clin Immunol 84:44–55, 1989.

Saxon A, Keld B, Braun J, Dotson A, Sidell N. Long-term administration of 13-cis retinoic acid in common variable immunodeficiency: circulating interleukin-6 levels, B-cell surface molecule display, and in vitro and in vivo B-cell antibody production. Immunology 80:477–487, 1993.

Saxon A, Kobayashi RH, Stevens RH, Singer AD, Stiehm ER, Siegel SC. In vitro analysis of humoral immunity in antibody deficiency with normal immunoglobulins. Clin Immunol Immunopathol 17:235–244, 1980.

Schiff RI, Buckley RH, Gilbertsen RB, Metzgar RS. Membrane receptors and in vitro responsiveness of lymphocytes in human immunodeficiency. J Immunol 112:376–386, 1974.

Schneider EL, Epstein CJ. Replication rate and lifespan of cultured fibroblasts in Down's syndrome. Proc Soc Exp Biol Med 141:1092–1094, 1972.

Schumacher MJ. Serum immunoglobulin and transferrin levels after childhood splenectomy. Arch Dis Child 45:114–117, 1970.

Schur PH, Borel H, Gelfand EW, Alper CA, Rosen FS. Selective gamma-G globulin deficiencies in patients with recurrent pyogenic infections. N Engl J Med 283:631–634, 1970.

Seager J, Jamison DL, Wilson J, Hayward AK, Soothill JF. IgA deficiency, epilepsy, and phenytoin treatment. Lancet 2:632–635, 1975.

Seeger RC, Stiehm ER. T and B lymphocyte subpopulations. Pediatrics 55:157–160, 1975.

Shackelford PG. IgG subclasses: importance in pediatric practice. Pediatr Rev 14:291–296, 1993.

Shapiro GG, Virant FS, Furukawa CT, Pierson WE, Bierman CW. Immunologic defects in patients with refractory sinusitis. Pediatrics 87:311–316, 1991.

Sharma OP, James DG. Hypogammaglobulinemia, depression of delayed type hypersensitivity and granuloma formation. Am Rev Respir Dis 104:228–231, 1971.

Siber GR, Schur PH, Aisenberg AC, Weitzman SA, Schiffman G. Correlation between serum IgG2 concentrations and the antibody response to bacterial polysaccharide antigens. N Engl J Med 303:178–182, 1980.

Siegal FP, Pernis B, Kunkel HG. Lymphocytes in human immunodeficiency states: a study of membrane-associated immunoglobulins. Eur J Immunol 1:482–486, 1971.

Siegal FP, Siegal M, Good RA. Role of helper, suppressor and B-cell defects in the pathogenesis of the hypogammaglobulinemias. N Engl J Med 299:172–178, 1978.

Siegal FP, Siegal M, Good RA. Suppression of B-cell differentiation by leukocytes from hypogammaglobulinemic patients. J Clin Invest 58:109–122, 1976.

Siegal M. Susceptibility of mongoloids to infection: II. Antibody response to tetanus toxoid and typhoid vaccine. Am J Hyg 48:63–73, 1948.

Siegal RL, Issekutz T, Schwaber J, Rosen FS, Geha RS. Deficiency of T helper cells in transient hypogammaglobulinemia of infancy. N Engl J Med 305:1307–1313, 1981.

Singer DB. Postsplenectomy sepsis. In Rosenberg HS, and Bolande RP, eds. Perspectives in Pediatric Pathology, Vol. 1. Chicago, Year Book Medical Publishers, 1973, pp. 285–311.

Sitz KV, Burks AW, Williams LW, Kemp SF, Steele RW. Confirmation of X-linked hypogammaglobulinemia with isolated growth hormone deficiency as a disease entity. J Pediatr 116:292–294, 1990.

Skare JC, Milunsky A, Byron KS, Sullivan JL. Mapping the X-linked lymphoproliferative syndrome. Proc Natl Acad Sci U S A 84:2015–2018, 1987.

Slavin BN, Fenton GM, Laundy M, Reynolds EH. Serum immunoglobulins in epilepsy. J Neurol Sci 23:353–357, 1974.

Smith CIE, Baskin B, Humire-Greiff P, Zhou J-N, Olsson PG, Maniar HS, Kjellen P, Lambris JD, Christensson B, Hammarström L, Bentley D, Vetrie D, Islam KB, Vorechovsky I, Sideras P. Expression of Bruton's agammaglobulinemia tyrosine kinase gene, *BTK*, is selectively down-regulated in T lymphocytes and plasma cells. J Immunol 152:557–565, 1994.

Smith CIE, Hammarström L, Henter J-I, De Lange GG. Molecular and serologic analysis of IgG1 deficiency caused by new forms of the constant region of the Ig H chain gene deletions. J Immunol 142:4514–4519, 1989.

Smith TF, Morris EC, Bain RP. IgG subclasses in nonallergic children with chronic chest symptoms. J Pediatr 105:896–900, 1984.

Sneller MC, Strober W. Abnormalities of lymphokine gene expression in patients with common variable immunodeficiency. J Immunol 144:3762–3769, 1990.

Sneller MC, Strober W, Eisenstein E, Jaffe JS, Cunningham-Rundles C. New insights into common variable immunodeficiency. Ann Intern Med 118:720–730, 1993.

Soothill JF, Hayes K, Dudgeon JA. The immunoglobulins in congenital rubella. Lancet 1:1385–1388, 1966.

Sorensen RU, Polmar SH. Efficacy and safety of high-dose intravenous immune globulin therapy for antibody deficiency syndromes. Am J Med 76(3A):83–90, 1984.

Sorrell TC, Forbes IJ. Depression of immune competence by phenytoin and carbamazepine: studies in vivo and in vitro. Clin Exp Immunol 20:273–285, 1975.

Sorrell TC, Forbes IJ, Burness FR, Rischbieth RHC. Depression of immunological function in the patients treated with phenytoin sodium (sodium diphenylhydantoin). Lancet 2:1233–1235, 1971.

Souadjian JV, Enriquez P, Silverstein MN, Pépin J-M. The spectrum of diseases associated with thymoma: coincidence or syndrome? Arch Int Med 134:374–379, 1974.

Spector BD, Perry GS III, Kersey JH. Genetically determined immunodeficiency diseases (GDID) and malignancy: report from the Immunodeficiency-Cancer Registry. Clin Immunol Immunopathol 11:12–29, 1978.

Stanley PJ, Corbo G, Cole PJ. Serum IgG subclasses in chronic and recurrent respiratory infections. Clin Exp Immunol 58:703–708, 1984.

Stavnezer-Nordgren J, Kekish O, Zegers BJM. Molecular defects in a human immunoglobulin κ chain deficiency. Science 230:458–461, 1985.

Stevens R, Dichek D, Keld B, Heiner D. IgG1 is the predominant subclass of in vivo and in vitro produced anti-tetanus toxoid antibodies and also serves as the membrane IgG molecule for delivering inhibitory signals to antitetanus toxoid antibody-producing B cells. J Clin Immunol 3:65–69, 1983.

Stiehm ER, Chin TW, Haas A, Peerless AG. Infectious complications of the primary immunodeficiencies. Clin Immunol Immunopathol 40:69–86, 1986.

Stiehm ER, Fudenberg HH. Serum levels of immune globulins in health and disease: a survey. Pediatrics 37:715–727, 1966a.

Stiehm ER, Fudenberg HH. Clinical and immunologic features of dysgammaglobulinemia Type I: report of a case diagnosed in the first year of life. Am J Med 40:805–815, 1966b.

Stites DP, Levin AS, Austin KE, Fudenberg HH. Immunobiology of human lymphoid cell lines. J Immunol 107:1376–1381, 1971.

Stoelinga GBA, Van Munster PJJ, Slooff JP. Antibody deficiency syndrome and autoimmune haemolytic anemia in a boy with isolated IgM deficiency dysimmunoglobulinaemia type 5. Acta Paediatr Scand 58:352–362, 1969.

Strober W, Eisenstein E, Jaffe JS, Cunningham-Rundles C. New insights into common variable immunodeficiency. Ann Intern Med 118:720–730, 1993.

Sullivan JL, Byron KS, Brewster FE, Baker SM, Ochs HD. X-linked lymphoproliferative syndrome: natural history of the immunodeficiency. J Clin Invest 71:1765–1778, 1983.

Sullivan JL, Ochs HD, Schiffman G, Hammerschlag MR, Miser J, Vichinsky E, Wedgwood RJ. Immune response after splenectomy. Lancet 1:178–181, 1978.

Sutnick AI, London WT, Blumberg BS, Gerstley BJ. Persistent anicteric hepatitis with Australia antigen in patients with Down's syndrome. Am J Clin Pathol 57:2–12, 1972.

Sweinberg SK, Wodell RA, Grodofsky MP, Greene JM, Conley ME. Retrospective analysis of the incidence of pulmonary disease in hypogammaglobulinemia. J Allergy Clin Immunol 88:96–104, 1991.

Tan RS-H. Thymoma, acquired hypogammaglobulinaemia, lichen planus, alopecia areata. Proc R Soc Med 67:196–198, 1974.

Taylor-Robinson D, Webster ADB, Furr PM. Prolonged persistence of *Mycoplasma pneumoniae* in a patient with hypogammaglobulinaemia. J Infect 2:171–175, 1980.

Te Velde K, Huber J, Van der Slikke LB. Primary acquired hypogammaglobulinemia, myasthenia, and thymoma. Ann Intern Med 65:554–559, 1966.

Terry WD, Fahey JL. Subclasses of human gamma-2-globulin based on differences in the heavy polypeptide chains. Science 146:400–401, 1964.

Tiller TL Jr, Buckley RH. Transient hypogammaglobulinemia of infancy: review of the literature, clinical and immunological features of 11 new cases and long-term follow-up. J Pediatr 92:347–353, 1978.

Timmers E, Kenter M, Thompson A, Kraakman MEM, Berman JE, Alt FW, Schuurman RKB. Diversity of immunoglobulin heavy chain gene segment rearrangement in B lymphoblastoid cell lines from X-linked agammaglobulinemia patients. Eur J Immunol 21:2355–2363, 1991.

Tonegawa S. Somatic generation of antibody diversity. Nature 302:575–581, 1983.

Tsukada S, Saffran DC, Rawlings DJ, Parolini O, Allen RC, Klisak I, Sparkes RS, Kubagawa H, Mohandas T, Quan S, Belmont JW, Cooper MD, Conley ME, Witte ON. Deficient expression of a B cell cytoplasmic tyrosine kinase in human X-linked agammaglobulinemia. Cell 72:279–290, 1993.

Ugazio AG, Duse M, Re R, Mangili G, Burgio GR. Subcutaneous infusion of gammaglobulins in management of agammaglobulinemia (letter). Lancet 1:226, 1982.

Ugazio AG, Jayakar S, Marcioni AF, Duse M, Monafo V, Pasquali F, Burgio GR. Immunodeficiency in Down's syndrome: relationship between presence of human thyroglobulin antibodies and HBs Ag carrier status. Eur J Pediatr 126:139–146, 1977.

Umetsu DT, Ambrosino DM, Quinti I, Siber GR, Geha RS. Recurrent sinopulmonary infection and impaired antibody response to bacterial capsular polysaccharide antigen in children with selective IgG-subclass deficiency. N Engl J Med 313:1247–1251, 1985.

van der Meer JWM, Mouton RP, Daha MR, Schuurman KB. *Campylobacter jejuni* bacteremia as a cause of recurrent fever in a patient with hypogammaglobulinaemia. J Infect 12:235–239, 1986.

van der Meer JWM, Vossen JM, Radl J, van Nieuwkoop JA, Meyer CJLM, Lobatto S, van Furth R. Hyperimmunoglobulinaemia D and periodic fever: a new syndrome. Lancet 1:1087–1090, 1984.

van der Meer JWM, Weening RS, Schellekens PTA, Van Munster IP, Nagengast FM. Colorectal cancer in patients with X-linked agammaglobulinemia. Lancet 341:1439–1440, 1993.

van Noesel CJM, Borst J, De Vries EF, Van Lier RA. Identification of two distinct phosphoproteins as components of the human B cell antigen receptor complex. Eur J Immunol 20:2789–2793, 1990.

Vetrie D, Vorechovsky I, Sideras P, Holland J, Davies A, Flinter F, Hammarström L, Kinnon C, Levinsky R, Bobrow M, Smith CIE, Bentley DR. The gene involved in X-linked agammaglobulinaemia is a member of the src family of protein-tyrosine kinases. Nature 361:226–233, 1993.

Villa A, Notarangelo LD, Di Santo JP, Macchi PP, Strina D, Frattini A, Lucchini F, Patrosso CM, Giliani S, Mantuano E, Agosti S, Nocera G, Kroczek RA, Fischer A, Ugazio AG, De Saint Basile G, Vezzoni P. Organization of the human CD40L gene: implications for molecular defects in X chromosome-linked hyper-IgM syndrome and prenatal diagnosis. Proc Natl Acad Sci U S A 91:2110–2114, 1994.

Volanakis JE, Zhu Z-B, Schaffer FM, Macon KJ, Palermos J, Barger BO, Go R, Campbell RD, Schroeder HW Jr, Cooper MD. Major histocompatibility complex class III genes and susceptibility to immunoglobulin A deficiency and common variable immunodeficiency. J Clin Invest 89:1914–1922, 1992.

Vorechkovsky I, Zhou JN, Vetrie D, Bentley D, Björkander J, Hammarström L, Smith CIE. Molecular diagnosis of X-linked agammaglobulinemia (letter). Lancet 341:1153, 1993.

Wagner DK, Marti GE, Jaffe ES, Straus SE, Nelson DL, Fleisher TA. Lymphocyte analysis in a patient with X-linked agammaglobulinemia and isolated growth hormone deficiency after development of echovirus dermatomyositis and meningoencephalitis. Int Arch Allergy Appl Immunol 89:143–148, 1989.

Waldmann TA, Durm M, Broder S, Blackman M, Blaese RM, Strober W. Role of suppressor T cells in pathogenesis of common variable hypogammaglobulinaemia. Lancet 2:609–613, 1974.

Waldmann T A, Strober WS, Blaese MR, Strauss AJL. Thymoma, hypogammaglobulinemia and absence of eosinophils. J Clin Invest 46:1127–1128, 1967.

Wang J-K, Hsieh K-H. Immunologic study of the asplenic syndrome. Pediatr Infect Dis J 10:819–822, 1991.

Watts RG, Kelly DR. Fatal varicella infection in a child associated with thymoma and immunodeficiency (Good's syndrome). Med Pediatr Oncol 18:246–251, 1990.

Webster ADB. Thymoma, polyarthropathy and hypogammaglobulinaemia. Proc R Soc Med 69:58–59, 1976.

Webster ADB, Rotbart HA, Warner T, Rudge P, Hyman N. Diagnosis of enterovirus brain disease in hypogammaglobulinemic patients by polymerase chain reaction. Clin Infect Dis 17:657–661, 1993.

Wedgwood RJ, Ochs HD. Variability in the expression of X-linked agammaglobulinemia: the co-existence of classic X-LA (Bruton type) and "common variable immunodeficiency" in the same families. In Seligmann, M, and Hitzig, W H, eds.: Primary Immunodeficiencies INSERM Symposium No 16, New York, Elsevier/North-Holland Biomedical Press, 1980, pp. 69–78.

Wedgwood RJ, Ochs HD, Davis SD. The recognition and classification of immunodeficiency diseases with bacteriophage φX174. In Bergsma, D, ed. Immunodeficiency in Man and Animals. Birth Defects: Original Article Series, Vol. XI, No. 1. Sunderland, Mass, Sinauer Associates, 1975, pp. 331–338.

Wedgwood RJ, Ochs HD, Oxelius V-A. IgG subclass levels in the serum of patients with primary immunodeficiency. In Hanson, LA, Soderstrom T, Oxelius VA, eds. Immunoglobulin Subclass Deficiencies. Monogr Allergy 20:80–89, 1986.

Weiler JM, Ballas ZK, Needleman BW, Hobbs MV, Feldbush TL. Complement fragments suppress lymphocyte immune responses. Immunol Today 3:238–243, 1982.

Wells MA, Wittek AE, Epstein JS, Marcus-Sekura C, Daniel S, Tankersley DL, Preston MS, Quinnan GVJ. Inactivation and partition of human T-cell lymphotropic virus, type III, during ethanol fractionation of plasma. Transfusion 26:210–213, 1986.

Wilfert CM, Buckley RH, Mohanakumar T, Griffith JF, Katz SL, Whisnant JK, Eggleston PA, Moore M, Treadwell E, Oxman MN, Rosen FS. Persistent and fatal central-nervous-system ECHOvirus infections in patients with agammaglobulinemia. N Engl J Med 296:1485–1489, 1977.

Winkelstein JA, Fearon ER. Carrier detection of the X-linked immunodeficiency diseases using X-chromosome inactivation analysis. J Allergy Clin Immunol 85:1090–1096, 1990.

Wright JJ, Wagner DK, Blaese RM, Hagengruber C, Waldmann TA, Fleisher TA. Characterization of common variable immunodeficiency: identification of a subset of patients with distinctive immunophenotypic and clinical features. Blood 76:2046–2051, 1990.

Wright PF, Hatch MH, Kasselberg AG, Lowry SP, Wadlington WB, Karzon DT. Vaccine-associated poliomyelitis in a child with sex-linked agammaglobulinemia. J Pediatr 91:408–412, 1977.

Wyatt HV. Poliomyelitis in hypogammaglobulinemics. J Infect Dis 128:802–806, 1973.

Wyatt RA, Younoszai K, Anuras S, Myers MG. *Campylobacter fetus* septicemia and hepatitis in a child with agammaglobulinemia. J Pediatr 91:441–442, 1977.

Xu J, Foy TM, Laman JD, Elliott EA, Dunn JJ, Waldschmidt TJ, Elsemore J, Noelle RJ, Flavell RA. Mice deficient for the CD40 ligand. Immunity 1:423–431, 1994.

Yount WJ, Hong R, Seligmann M, Good R, Kunkel HG. Imbalances of gamma globulin subgroups and gene defects in patients with primary hypogammaglobulinemia. J Clin Invest 49:1957–1966, 1970.

Zegers BJM, Maertzdorf WJ, van Loghem E, Mul NAJ, Stoop JW, van der Laag J, Vossen JJ, Ballieux RE. Kappa-chain deficiency: an immunoglobulin disorder. N Engl J Med 294:1026–1030, 1976.

Zeitlin HC, Sheppard K, Baum JD, Bolton FG, Hall CA. Homozygous transcobalamin II deficiency maintained on oral hydroxocobalamin. Blood 66:1022–1027, 1985.

Zhu Q, Zhang M, Rawlings DR, Vihinen M, Hagemann T, Saffran DC, Kwan S-P, Nilsson L, Smith CIE, Witte ON, Chen S-H, Ochs HD. Deletion within the Src homology domain 3 of Bruton's tyrosine kinase resulting in X-linked agammaglobulinemia (XLA). J Exp Med 180:461–470, 1994a.

Zhu Q, Zhang M, Winkelstein J, Chen S-H, Ochs HD. Unique mutations of Bruton's tyrosine kinase in fourteen unrelated X-linked agammaglobulinemia families. Hum Mol Genet 3:1899–1900, 1994b.

Ziegler JB, Penny R. Fatal ECHO 30 virus infection and amyloidosis in X-linked hypogammaglobulinemia. Clin Immunol Immunopathol 3:347–352, 1975.

Zuck TF, Preston MS, Tankersley DL, Wells MA, Wittek AE, Epstein JE, Daniel S, Phelan M, Quinnan GV Jr. More on partitioning and inactivation of AIDS virus in immune globuln preparations (letter). N Engl J Med 314:1454–1455, 1986.

Chapter 12

Disorders of the T-Cell System

Richard Hong
with contributions by Loran T. Clement,
Richard A. Gatti, and Charles H. Kirkpatrick

T cells (or T lymphocytes) are produced by maturation, differentiation and selection processes in the thymus gland (see Chapter 2). Along with the B cells, they constitute the lymphocyte component of the immune system. B-cell function is to a large part dependent on helper function of T cells, so that any major loss or dysfunction of T cells causes secondary B-cell deficiency. Thus, a number of disorders show the clinical manifestations of combined B- and T-cell deficiency even though the only pathology is in the T cell or its site of origin, the thymus. Stated another way, in terms of infectious susceptibility, isolated T-cell diseases usually show the same clinical picture as if the lesion involved both T- and B-cell lineages. However, the converse situation, that of isolated B-cell disorders, shows patients who can handle organisms primarily controlled by the T cells (e.g., varicella, cytomegalovirus) in a completely normal fashion.

This chapter discusses one disease of the thymus and a series of lymphocyte defects. The thymic disorder is a part of the DiGeorge anomaly and is considered to result from total absence of the gland. The lymphocyte defects involve the myriad of cellular processes now known to be necessary to generate an immune response (reviewed in Rosen et al., 1992; Abbas et al, 1994a, 1994b; Janeway and Travers, 1994).

DiGEORGE ANOMALY (Thymic Hypoplasia, Third and Fourth Pouch/Arch Syndrome, Cellular Immunodeficiency with Hypoparathyroidism)

DiGeorge anomaly (DGA) is a congenital immunodeficiency characterized clinically by hypocalcemic tetany, congenital heart disease, unusual facies, and increased susceptibility to infection. Pathologically, the disorder is marked by the absence or hypoplasia of the thymus and parathyroid glands and cardiac or aortic arch abnormalities. An immune system defect is present in only 25% of patients (Bastian et al., 1989).

The terms *partial DiGeorge syndrome* and *complete DiGeorge syndrome* have been used in the past but in a confusing manner. In some cases, the modifier "partial" was used to denote that an immune system defect was present but mild, the inference being that ultimate spontaneous improvement was likely. Alternatively, "partial" was used to mean that the immune system was intact, and "complete" DiGeorge syndrome meant that immunologic deficiency was present in addition to other features of the anomaly. I prefer the latter convention for the use of the terms "complete" and "partial" because it focuses attention on the required clinical responses. Reserving the designations "complete DGA" for those patients with immune system deficiency and "partial DGA" for those with intact immunity sets the tone for therapeutic approaches. Patients with complete DGA require correction of the immune defect; irradiated blood products must be given to avoid graft-versus-host disease (GVHD) and intravenous immunoglobulin therapy is usually necessary.

Historical Aspects

The association of congenital absence of the thymus with seizures and abnormal third and fourth pharyngeal pouch development was recorded as early as 1829 (Harrington, 1829). In 1965, DiGeorge described the association of infection, absent thymus, and congenital hypoparathyroidism in three infants (DiGeorge, 1965). One of these patients, while still alive, underwent immunologic studies that revealed absent T-cell immunity, normal immunoglobulin levels, and deficient antibody production (Lischner and DiGeorge, 1969). The characteristic features of the syndrome, including the abnormal facies, were delineated as additional cases were described (Taitz et al., 1966; Kretschmer et al., 1968).

With the recognition that the immunologic defect might be due to deficient thymic function, restoration of T-cell function was achieved by fetal thymus transplantation. Two successful transplants, utilizing intact fetal thymus glands, were reported (Cleveland et al., 1968; August et al., 1968). Steele and colleagues (1972) accomplished successful T-cell reconstitution with a fetal thymus contained within a Millipore diffusion chamber.

Pathogenesis

Lammer and Opitz (1986) classified DGA as a field defect, a type of malformation in which the clinical manifestations consistently involve a group of tissues (the field) that develop normally together as a unit during embryogenesis. Coordinate development of the field dependends on appropriate integration of a determining influence at the correct time. In a field defect, there is a group of similar clinical manifestations but the specific causes are many and varied. By con-

trast, in a syndrome, the multiple commonly associated clinical features result from a single cause. The field in DGA, which includes many structures of the face as well as the derivatives of the branchial arches, depends on contribution from cephalic neural crest cells (Bockman and Kirby, 1984; LeDouarin, 1986).

Although emphasis in original descriptions was placed on the third and fourth pharyngeal pouches, defects involving the first to sixth pouches occur. Any intrauterine insult to the facial neural crest can result in features of the DiGeorge anomaly. The association of DGA with multiple causes can be thus explained (Table 12–1).

Abnormalities of chromosome 22 largely explain the heart abnormalities. Most patients with DiGeorge anomaly who have heart defects and a related disorder, the velocardiofacial (Shprintzen) syndrome, show chromosome 22q11 deletions (Carey et al., 1990, 1992; Scambler et al., 1992, Driscoll et al., 1992). Indeed, such deletions were transmitted from parent to child in five families who manifested familial heart outflow tract defects (Wilson et al., 1992). A deletion 17p13 defect was found in a stillborn child with a double-outlet right ventricle and thymic hypoplasia; the heart anomaly was attributed to a possible effect of 17p13 deletion on neural crest development.

Originally, the T-cell defect was considered to be the result of small thymic mass. Small, morphologically normal, undescended glands were found at autopsy in patients dying of causes unrelated to immune deficiency. This finding, associated with the observation that the T-cell deficiency was only partial or transient,

---

Table 12–1. Associations of DiGeorge Anomaly

Teratogens
  Maternal diabetes
  Alcohol
  Bisdiamine
  Retinoids

Mendelian disorders
  Autosomal dominant inheritance
    Autosomal dominant DiGeorge anomaly
    Velo-cardio-facial syndrome and conotruncal anomaly face
      syndrome
  Autosomal recessive inheritance
    Cerebro-hepato-renal syndrome of Zellweger
    Autosomal recessive disorder of fetal death, growth
      retardation, and DiGeorge anomaly
  X-linked inheritance

Cytogenetic abnormalities
  Monosomy 22
  Deletion (22q)
  Duplication (8q22→qter)
  Monosomy 10p
  Anomalies of chromosome 1
  Deletion (5) (p13)

Other
  Kallmann syndrome
  CHARGE association*
  Arrhinencephaly and holoprosencephaly

---

*C, coloboma; H, heart anomalies; A, atresia of choanae; R, retardation, mental and somatic; G, genital hypoplasia; E, ear anomalies.
From Lammer EJ, Opitz JM. The DiGeorge anomaly as a developmental field defect. Am J Med Genet 2(Suppl.):113–127, 1986. ©1986, Reprinted by permission of Wiley-Liss, a subsidiary of John Wiley & Sons, Inc.

supported the concept of a small gland requiring time to grow to generate normal T-cell function. Much of the confusion about the degree and permanence of T-cell deficiency in DGA is due to inadequate characterization of the immune system in the days before availability of the more discriminating and sensitive techniques now available.

Bastian and coworkers (1989) reviewed 18 patients with DGA in a multi-institution study. Since all patients had cardiac surgery or were examined at autopsy, direct visualization of the thymus was possible. In only three patients was the thymus present in the mediastinum.

Furthermore, in my own series of thymus biopsies involving more than 50 patients with primary immune deficiency (Borzy et al., 1979 and unpublished data), I have never failed to find thymus tissue for examination, except in the DiGeorge anomaly. I therefore conclude that failure of descent is nearly always present in DGA. Because undescended thymuses reside in sites such as the tongue, thyroid, and middle ear, they cannot attain a very large size, or else they would show symptoms or be clinically notable. Since only 25% of DGA patients have T-cell deficiency, these small thymuses can provide competent T-cell functions. I believe that the immune defect in DGA is the result of a completely absent thymus and is not accounted for by a tiny (~1 to 3 g), but otherwise normal, gland.

The disease is usually a sporadic event but may be inherited. Most familial cases are associated with a deletion of chromosome 22. Unfortunately, high-resolution chromosome analysis is not sufficient to detect these deletions and more sensitive DNA probing is required. Careful examination of the parents and search for suggestive symptomatology (history of hypocalcemic syndromes) is necessary to detect more subtle familial varieties (Greenberg et al., 1984; Rohn et al., 1984; Keppen et al., 1988; Carey et al., 1992).

Clinical Manifestations

Most patients with DiGeorge anomaly are recognized by characteristic external features. These include hypertelorism, antimongoloid slant of the eyes, low-set prominent ears with notched pinnae and reduced helix formation, and micrognathia (Fig. 12–1). A short philtrum of the upper lip, a bifid uvula, a high arched palate, and nasal speech have also been described. Rarely, esophageal atresia and an imperforate anus may be found. Urinary tract abnormalities, particularly hydronephrosis, are common (Conley et al., 1979). In the presence of cleft palate and learning difficulties, the patient probably has velocardiofacial syndrome, a closely related disorder, also associated with chromosome 22 abnormality.

Tetany secondary to hypocalcemia usually occurs within the first 24 to 48 hours of life. Serum calcium levels are low, the phosphorus level is elevated, and parathyroid hormone (parathormone) is absent.

The combination of parathyroid and thymic deficiencies has also been described in the *Zellweger syndrome* (Conley et al., 1979; Hong et al., 1981). The

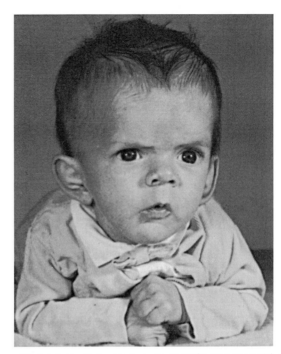

Figure 12–1. Infant with thymic hypoplasia (DiGeorge anomaly). Note the hypertelorism, antimongoloid slant of the eyes, ear malformation, and peculiar mouth. (Courtesy of Dr. Russell W. Steele, Washington, D.C.)

relationship between the two disorders is unclear. However, clinical differentiation is important because the fundamental fault in the Zellweger syndrome is in peroxisomes; thus, thymic or lymphoid replacement therapy would be useless. If the infants survive the neonatal period, increased susceptibility to infection occurs, manifested by chronic rhinitis, recurrent pneumonia (including *Pneumocystis carinii* pneumonia), oral candidiasis, and diarrhea. The patients are weak, fail to thrive, and are susceptible to sudden death.

The appreciation of DGA as a field defect explains the unique type of pathology seen in the heart and great vessels. Conley and colleagues (1979) and Lodewyk and associates (1986) reported a high frequency of interrupted aortic arch (IAA) type B. In a survey of 161 patients with DGA, more than 50% of the heart lesions resulted from two rare disorders—IAA type B and truncus arteriosus. Of all patients with IAA type B, 68% had DGA; of patients with truncus arteriosus, 33% had DGA. These heart lesions are due to failure of neural crest and branchial arch integration. In contrast, only 2% of the other congenital heart lesions seen in this clinic had concomitant DGA (Lodewyk et al., 1986). Right-sided aortic arch is also a common defect.

As in many cases of T-cell deficiency, dysregulation of the immune system results in autoimmune disorders. Graves' disease occurred in a long-term survivor (Ham Pong et al., 1985). Severe intractable eczema is encountered in some DGA patients (Archer et al., 1990); aplastic anemia followed an adenovirus infection in another instance (Tuvia et al., 1988). Durandy and coworkers (1968) found that DGA patients' lymphocytes spontaneously produced immunoglobulin in vitro; this was associated with low numbers of CD8[+] cells. With time, the CD8[+] number increased and in vitro immunoglobulin synthesis disappeared. The interpretation was that deficient control of the immune system was present for a short time but spontaneously returned to normal. Muller and associates (1989) found increased levels of antibodies to bovine serum albumin in DGA patients. Increased levels of milk antibody proteins are characteristic of another disease in which thymic dysregulation and autoimmunity occur—Wiskott-Aldrich syndrome (see that section, later in this chapter.).

A single case of glioma was reported by Asamoto and Furata (1977). Two cases of B-cell lymphoproliferative disorder have been encountered in my experience: one during a period of observation to see whether the immune deficit would spontaneously improve, and the other after thymus transplantation (Hong, unpublished).

Most cases of the DiGeorge syndrome are sporadic, but several instances of familial occurrence are known (Rohn et al., 1984). Analysis of these cases does not reveal a single mode of inheritance. The report of Rohn and colleagues (1984) emphasizes the importance of studying the extended family. In this study, the father and two siblings had hypocalcemia; both infants had truncus arteriosus, but only one had associated severe immunodeficiency. The marked heterogeneity of clinical symptoms is well illustrated by this kindred.

Laboratory Findings

A low serum calcium level, an elevated phosphorus level, and an absent-to-low parathormone level confirm a parathyroid deficiency. These findings also occur in familial neonatal hypoparathyroidism; however, this disorder is rare and the condition is usually transient. Hypoparathyroidism may be latent or subclinical, in which case a challenge with disodium edetate is informative. This test is of particular value in older relatives of patients with DGA who have either facial or cardiac stigmata of DGA without immune system manifestations (Gidding et al., 1988; Masswinkel-Mooij et al., 1989).

Chest radiographs may show an absent thymus shadow, but this is not a reliable indicator of T-cell competence. X-ray features of conotruncal abnormalities, such as right-sided aortic arch, pulmonary overvascularity, and cardiomegaly, may be present.

Much of the confusion about the permanence and the degree of immunodeficiency present in DGA patients has been due to the less sensitive and less precise methods of immune assessment available in earlier studies. Bastian and colleagues (1989) studied 18 patients with DGA to determine predictors of a persistent immune defect. The most reliable were a mitogen response to phytohemagglutinin of less than 10 times background and a total of less than 400 CD4[+] T lymphocytes/mm³. Data were insufficient to assess other tests of the immune system for predictive value. Although the total number of patients studied by modern methods remains small, the available data suggest that in vitro proliferative responses to other mitogens (con-

canavalin A and pokeweed mitogen) are also diminished. Serum immunoglobulin levels are usually normal, but specific antibody responses are diminished. B-cell numbers are elevated. Natural killer activity is normal. Most patients are not lymphopenic (Muller et al., 1989; Hong, 1991). An inability to respond to pneumococcal polysaccharide has been reported in one family (Schubert and Moss, 1992).

There is a deficiency of thyroid C cells as a result of fifth pharyngeal pouch maldevelopment (Burke et al., 1987). Wells and coworkers (1986) found a lack of ossification of the hyoid bone during the first month of life to be a common feature of DGA; the thyroid cartilage is a derivative of the fourth branchial arch.

Approximately 90% of DGA patients show chromosome abnormalities; most involve chromosome 22 (monosomy 22q11). Defects of other chromosomes (1, 5, 10, 12, 17, and 18) have been described (reviewed in Greenberg et al., 1988a, 1988b). Chromosomal analysis is indicated in all patients with DGA; if an unbalanced translocation of chromosome 22 is found, the likelihood is greater for familial transmission. A sensitive fluorescent assay is now available (Desmaze et al., 1993).

Treatment

The cardiac malformation is usually the most serious and life-threatening feature of DiGeorge anomaly. It should be treated as aggressively as necessary. The patients are not more difficult to manage because of any possible immune defect. The important caveat is that irradiated blood and blood products should be used at all times. Correction should not be deferred or delayed pending immune system evaluation or immune system reconstitution.

Hypocalcemia should be treated with calcium, vitamin D, and low-phosphorus diets. Parathyroid hormone injections may be necessary.

If an immune system defect is found, trimethoprim-sulfamethoxazole prophylaxis is indicated. The CD4 guidelines for *Pneumocystis carinii* prophylaxis in pediatric human immunodeficiency (HIV) infection can be utilized (see Chapter 31, Table 31–9). Also, gamma globulin replacement is nearly always indicated, and live virus vaccines should not be given to the patient nor to any family members.

Thymus transplantation can be corrective if an immune defect is confirmed. Fetal thymus or postnatal thymus can be employed. Any fetal thymus from a donor older than 14 weeks of age can contain sufficient mature T lymphocytes to cause graft-versus-host disease. Culture of thymus tissue for at least 1 week in the presence of deoxyguanosine destroys the mature lymphocytes, and the tissue can be transplanted. My preference is for postnatal thymus, but there are insufficient data to favor one type of tissue over another.

In a review of thymus transplantation results, Goldsobel and associates (1987) found that only one third of patients receiving a thymus transplant (17 fetal, 3 postnatal) were alive and clinically well over a span of 15 years. Accordingly, the authors performed a bone marrow transplantation from an HLA-matched sibling. T-cell and B-cell reconstitution was accomplished, and the patient has remained well since. A similar experience was reported by Borzy and coworkers (1989). From a therapeutic standpoint, this is a highly promising approach; however, from a theoretical standpoint, the results are puzzling. If the thymic defect in DGA is complete absence, transplantations such as those performed could still produce the observed results with the T cells being transplanted along with the marrow. However, a T cell–depleted transplantation, such as has been employed for haploidentical donors, would not work in DGA, and only matched donors could be employed. One T cell–depleted transplantation was unsuccessful, with no evidence of engraftment even after three attempts (Rosenblatt, 1993, personal communication). The use of non–T cell–depleted marrows from matched unrelated donors might be an option in this case (Filipovitch et al., 1992). Further experience with bone marrow transplantation should resolve these issues.

Prognosis

The oldest known survivor is the patient originally reported by Cleveland (1968), who has remained free of infections following fetal thymus transplantation. Although immunologic studies are normal, the patient continues to have hypoparathyroidism. Mental retardation is present in this patient and in several other patients, possibly as a result of the neonatal seizures.

A major determinant in the prognosis of DiGeorge anomaly is the severity of the congenital heart disease. It is usually easier to cure the immunodeficiency than to control the hypoparathyroidism or to correct the congenital heart disease surgically.

RETICULAR DYSGENESIS

Reticular dysgenesis is a severe congenital cellular and antibody deficiency associated with agenesis of the granulocytic precursors of the bone marrow; it leads to death shortly after birth. It is considered to be a variant of severe combined immunodeficiency.

Historical Aspects

De Vaal and Seynhaeve described the disorder in newborn male twins in 1959. Gitlin and colleagues reported another patient in 1964. A fourth patient was described by Alonso and coworkers in 1972. Brothers were reported by Español and associates (1979). Other early cases were reported by Ownby and colleagues (1976) and Haas and coworkers (1977).

Clinical Manifestations

The disorder manifests within the first few days of life with failure to thrive, vomiting, diarrhea, or localized infection. The course is rapidly progressive, and the six reported patients died on the third, fifth, eighth, 16th, 50th, and 90th days of life.

The outstanding laboratory finding in all cases is the marked leukopenia (no cells in two patients, 200 to 600 cells/mm,^{3} in the third, 1200 to 1800 cells/mm^3 in the fourth, 3800 to 4000 cell/mm^3 in the fifth, and 500 to 3200 cells/mm^3 in the sixth). Hemoglobin and platelets are normal or slightly reduced. Total gamma globulin levels reflect transplacental maternal IgG. IgM and IgA levels were not reported in four cases. In the fifth immunoglobulin levels were IgG, 170 mg/dl; IgM, 7 mg/dl; and IgA, 20 mg/dl after a 75-ml blood transfusion (Alonso et al., 1972). In the sixth patient, cord immunoglobulins were IgG, 530 mg/dl; IgA and IgM, absent. E-rosette assay was found to be 66%, but the lymphocytes did not stimulate with phytohemagglutinin. Lymphocyte and erythrocyte adenosine deaminase levels were elevated in this patient.

The autopsy findings were similar to those of severe combined immunodeficiency; a small dysplastic thymus without Hassall's corpuscles; depletion of lymphoid tissue of the spleen, lymph nodes, and gastrointestinal tract; and abnormal lymphoid architecture. In addition, an absence or marked deficiency of granulocytic precursors was noted in the bone marrow. The marrow does contain megakaryocytes or reticular and erythroid precursors. Erythrophagocytosis was noted in two cases (De Vaal and Seynhaeve, 1959; Ownby et al., 1976). One infant had congenital cytomegalovirus disease (Ownby et al., 1976).

The family history of the affected infants was generally negative for immunologic disease except for a maternal uncle with selective IgA deficiency in one case (Ownby et al., 1976) and occurrence in brothers (Español et al., 1979). The occurrence in both males (four) and females (two) suggests autosomal inheritance.

Reticular dysgenesis is thought to be caused in most instances by an interruption of bone marrow differentiation about or before the 10th week of gestation. The presence of normal numbers of T cells in one case (Ownby et al., 1976) suggests that the T-cell defect may not always be caused by a primordial stem cell defect but instead may result from a metabolic defect that prevents mature lymphocytes from proliferating.

Treatment

Bone marrow transplantation from an HLA-identical sibling was curative (Levinsky and Tiedeman, 1983). Two successful haploidentical marrow transplants have also been recorded (Haas et al., 1986; Stephan et al., 1993). During acute overwhelming infections, granulocyte transfusions may also be helpful; these should be irradiated to prevent GVH disease.

COMBINED IMMUNODEFICIENCY (Severe Combined Immunodeficiency [SCID], Swiss-Type Agammaglobulinemia, Lymphopenic Agammaglobulinemia, Thymic Alymphoplasia, Hereditary Thymic Dysplasia, and Cellular Immunodeficiency with Abnormal Immunoglobulin Synthesis [Nezelof Syndrome])

This part of the text groups together a number of disorders that have significant impairment of both T-cell and B-cell immunity; for the most part, they require the same treatment. Rather than focus on differences in laboratory tests as the basis for a classification, I prefer to characterize the different disorders as manifestations of a defect in one or more of the steps required to generate a competent immune response. Table 12-2 places the various diseases within this context. With this framework in mind, the reader can have a more global view of the immune response and can see disease as a breakdown in normal developmental or physiologic pathways. Also, one can predict where new diseases can occur.

Some of the combined deficiencies—adenosine deaminase deficiency, Wiskott-Aldrich syndrome, ataxia-telangiectasia, and bare lymphocyte syndrome—are considered in greater detail in other parts of the chapter because they illustrate informative variations of pathogenesis. Severe combined immunodeficiency (SCID) is not considered as a separate entity, since this clinical phenotype may be associated with many different causes. SCID is not differentiated from combined immunodeficiency (CID) because the arbitrary criterion of death before 2 years of age does not precisely denote a specific cause. Furthermore, as the diseases become defined genetically, it is apparent that children within the same family show quite differing phenotypic expressions of the same genetic defect. With more precise definition of the specific cause, differentiation based on clinical symptomatology becomes less useful.

Historical Aspects

At first the T and B lymphocytes were considered to be completely independent of each other in terms of development and function. By implication, therefore, genetically determined combined T-cell and B-cell immunodeficiency disorders were either stem cell defects or a result of a defect common to both cell lineages. Because the likelihood of occurrence of the latter event on the basis of a single gene defect was rare, most combined deficiency disease was thought to result from a stem cell defect (Good, 1971).

As more insight was gained into the details of the immune response, the original view gave way to an appreciation of the extreme heterogeneity of the combined T-cell and B-cell disorders. The concept of T-cell regulation (Waldmann et al., 1974; Waldmann and Broder, 1977) and the development of monoclonal antibodies to define lymphocyte subsets (Reinherz et al., 1980) greatly increased the number of potential mechanisms for combined immunodeficiency diseases. Giblett and colleagues (1972) described the first immunodeficiency disorder secondary to an enzyme defect (adenosine deaminase). The roles of cytokines in the immune process began with the elucidation of interleukin-1 (IL-1) (Dinarello, 1984). Since then, well over a dozen cytokines have been discovered (see Chapters 2 and 4). In 1988, a defect in interleukin-2 (IL-2) responses was reported as a cause of SCID, and replace-

Table 12–2. Classification of T-Cell Immunodeficiencies

Function/Process at Fault	Defect	Disease/Comment
Stem cell generation	Cell lineage defect	Reticular dysgenesis; complete lymphocyte and hematopoietic deficiency ? Most lymphopenic forms of SCID
Thymic differentiation	Absence of gland Cell lineage defect	DiGeorge anomaly CD8+ absence; lineage defects due to Zap-70 defect
Surface receptor expression and transduction	Defect in CD3/T-cell receptor Defect in transduction Defect in Ca++ movement Defect in gp39 Defect in CD43 (gp115) Zap-70 defect MHC defects Failure to respond to a single agent	 Hyper-IgM; accounts for T-helper defect (gp 39 = CD40 ligand) Wiskott-Aldrich syndrome CD8 deficiency Bare lymphocyte syndrome Chronic mucocutaneous candidiasis; some cases caused by multiple cocarboxylase deficiency
Cytokine response or secretion	Interleukin-1 defect Interleukin-2 defect* Interleukin-2 receptor defect	 γ chain defect in X-linked SCID
Homing		None described yet
Maintenance of normal cell number	Loss due to infection Loss due to toxins	AIDS Adenosine deaminase, purine nucleoside phosphorylase deficiencies
Unknown		Cartilage-hair hypoplasia Omenn syndrome Cartilage-hair hypoplasia; short-limbed dwarfism Ataxia-telangiectasia X-linked lymphoproliferative syndrome

*May be a multicytokine defect.
Abbreviations: AIDS = acquired immunodeficiency syndrome; SCID = severe combined immunodeficiency.

ment therapy with IL-2 was successfully instituted the following year (Doi et al., 1988; Pahwa et al., 1989).

Bone marrow transplantation was first accomplished successfully in severe combined immunodeficiency (Gatti et al., 1968) and simultaneously in Wiskott-Aldrich syndrome (Bach et al., 1968). This experience was followed soon by the establishment of bone marrow transplantation as first-line therapy in many hematopoietic malignancies, culminating in the award of the Nobel Prize to E. Donnall Thomas, the pioneer of bone marrow transplantation.

The addition of molecular biology approaches brought new technology to diagnosis and treatment of immunodeficiency (reviewed by Conley, 1992; Blaese, 1993). Genetic analyses now permit detection of carriers of X-linked disorders, and the loci for Wiskott-Aldrich syndrome and X-linked severe combined immunodeficiency have been mapped (de Saint-Basile et al., 1989; Puck et al., 1989; Peacocke and Siminovitch, 1987; Kwan et al., 1988). Anderson and his colleagues (Anderson, 1992; Blaese, 1993) transferred the gene for adenosine deaminase into peripheral blood lymphocytes, producing a sustained clinical benefit for the first time by using gene transfer. Repeated infusions were required. Subsequently, bone marrow cells, into which the genes were transferred, were used to treat two newborns and to attempt a permanent cure. The identification of a gene causing X-linked SCID was described in early 1993 (Noguchi et al, 1993b; Puck et al., 1993). The next decade should see genetic replacement supplanting many bone marrow transplants.

Pathogenesis

The causes and potential causes of combined immunodeficiency diseases are legion, and the number grows rapidly. Rather than simply contribute to an ever growing list, I have organized the diseases into a conceptual framework based on steps required for a complement–T cell response. I have divided these steps into six broad categories and have grouped the different diseases according to the step at fault (Table 12–2). The six functions are:

1. Stem cell generation.
2. Thymic differentiation.
3. Surface receptor expression and transduction.
4. Cytokine response or secretion.
5. Homing.
6. Maintenance of cell number.

The first five steps encompass the series of events that must be synchronized and integrated appropriately to generate competent T cells of sufficient diversity to recognize the universe of antigens we encounter throughout our lifetimes. The details of these functions are considered in Chapter 2 (see also Abbas et al., 1994a, 1994b, 1994c; Janeway and Travers, 1994). Failure of the T-cell system at any one of these points results in a disease state.

Stem Cell Generation

Stem cells arise early in the yolk sac, migrate to the fetal liver and then to the bone marrow; after the first

few months of intrauterine life, the bone marrow is the major repository for stem cells. Precise mechanisms for failure of lymphocyte stem cells to develop have not yet been defined. The lymphocyte stem cells and hematopoietic stem cells arise from a common stem cell precursor in the bone marrow. The commonality of origin provides one explanation for the frequent association of hematopoietic disorders with primary immunodeficiency. In the most extreme example, there is a severe deficiency of both hematopoietic and lymphoid cells in the periphery—reticular dysgenesis (De Vaal and Seynhaeve, 1959).

A defect analogous to, but not identical to, stem cell failure would result in a failure of differentiation of the stem cells. A murine model, SCID mouse, lacks T and B cells because of impaired coding joint formation as V-D-J rearrangement of the T-cell and immunoglobulin receptor genes occurs (Carroll and Bosma, 1991; Phillips and Spaner, 1991). This defect has also been observed in the recombination pattern of D_H to J_H elements of pre–B cells of human SCID patients who lack T and B cells (Schwarz et al., 1991). Thus, combined immunodeficiency without T or B cells may be a human analog of the SCID mouse.

Thymic Differentiation

In stem cell defects, the thymus is alymphoid but becomes repopulated after bone marrow transplant. Therefore, in a stem cell deficiency, thymic differentiation capacity is apparently normal. Absence of thymic differentiation occurs in the DiGeorge anomaly, in which I have inferred that the thymus is completely absent (see earlier). The details of thymic differentiation are given in Chapters 1 and 2 and have been reviewed (Boyd et al., 1993; Ritter and Boyd, 1993). Negative and positive selection of bone marrow–derived T-cell precursors yields the ultimate mature repertoire of T cells. These processes involve cellular interactions and secreted hormones and cytokines; most, if not all, selection is mediated through the T-cell receptor.

In humans, only two examples of aberrant thymic differentiation have been described. Acrodermatitis enteropathica is caused by zinc deficiency, and the thymic hormone, thymulin, is known to be a zinc-dependent metallohormone. Except for that, however, no disease has been shown to result from a hormone deficiency, and therapy with thymic hormone fractions has resulted only in equivocal benefit.

CD8 Deficiency (ZAP 70 Defect). Another example of thymic differentiation fault was described by Roifman and coworkers (1989). This patient manifested a selective absence of CD8$^+$ cells. Study of the thymus showed the presence of CD4$^+$/CD8$^+$ double-positive early thymocytes in the cortex. However, the medulla contained only CD4$^+$ singly marked cells. Apparently, there was a block in the development of mature single-positive CD8$^+$ cells from the double-marked positives. As anticipated, antibody function (dependent on CD4$^+$ T cells) was normal and infectious susceptibility was characteristic of defective T-cell cytotoxicity. The failure to generate CD8$^+$ T cells is due to a mutation in the Zap-70 kinase gene. Zap-70 kinase, one of three protein-tyrosine kinases that are activated when the T-cell receptor is stimulated, is associated with the ζ-chain of CD3, forming a part of the CD3–T-cell receptor (TCR) complex. In the absence or mutation of Zap-70, $CD4^+CD8^+$ (double-positive) T-cell precursors cannot be further differentiated to single-positive mature $CD8^+$ T cells, and only $CD4^+$ mature cells develop (Arpaia et al., 1994).

Surface Receptor/Transduction Defects. The TCR imparts antigen specificity to the immune response. The initial intercellular contacts of T lymphocytes involve weak interactions including the adhesion molecules CD11a-CD18, CD43, and CD45RO. Mutations of CD18 cause the bulk of adhesion molecule defects. Although this defect, leukocyte adhesion defect type I, results in profound granulocyte impairment and life-threatening infections, the effect on T-lymphocyte function is surprisingly minimal and these patients do not suffer from the infectious susceptibility to opportunistic agents seen in lymphopenic forms of CID (Anderson and Springer, 1987; Springer et al., 1987).

The T-cell receptor is expressed as a complex with CD3, a molecule consisting of four polypeptide chains (gamma, delta, epsilon, and zeta) (Oettgen and Terhorst, 1987). Mutations in these chains lead to abnormal or absent expression of the T-cell receptor (Thornes et al., 1990; Arnaiz-Villena et al., 1992a). Surprisingly, the defects so far described do not lead to complete absence of TCR-bearing cells. The 10% to 20% of TCR^+ cells found in these patients may show a decreased TCR expression, however (Arnaiz-Villena et al., 1992a, 1992b).

The external signals must be internally transduced in order for the next stages of the T-cell response to occur—namely, activation, proliferation, or both. Details of signal transduction are given in Chapter 2. Two patients have been described who demonstrated poor signal transduction. In one, the T-cell receptor was unable to transduce external signals, which is similar to the defect found in the mutant Jurkat cell line derived from a human T-cell leukemia (Goldsmith and Weiss, 1987; Chatila et al., 1989). In the other, the mechanism of the defect was unclear (Rijkers et al., 1991).

As mentioned above, a defect in ZAP-70 resulted in isolated $CD8^+$ T-cell deficiency, implicating its role in thymic differentiation of precursor cells. As ZAP-70 is a T-cell receptor–associated protein tyrosine kinase, transduction of antigen signals would be affected in mature T cells as well. In studies of other children with symptoms of combined immunodeficiency demonstrating the unusual profile of normal total numbers of T cells with virtually all of the cells expressing only CD4, ZAP-70 deficiency was found (Chan et al., 1994; Elder et al., 1994). Characteristically, the T cells responded to phorbol ester and calcium ionophore in vitro as this pathway bypasses the T-cell receptor, whereas stimulation using antibody to CD3, which reacts with the CD3/TcR complex, was nonstimulatory. Some T-cell activity was present, with attainment of normal immunoglobulin levels. The residual T-cell function can be attributed to other transduction pathways, such as *Lck* and *Fyn* tyrosine kinases. Natural killer activity was normal. The disease is inherited as an autosomal recessive disorder.

gp39 Deficiency (X-Linked Hyper-IgM). The ligand of the CD40 B-cell antigen is gp39, expressed by activated T cells. T-cell gp39 can induce B-cell proliferation and differentiation. With IL-4 or IL-10, gp39 drives human B cells to IgE and IgA or IgG and IgM synthesis, respectively (Spriggs et al., 1992; Aruffo et al., 1993). Thus, the gp39/CD40 complex plays a major role in the T-cell helper activities of isotype switching and immunoglobulin secretion. Synthesis of gp39 is defective in patients with X-linked hyper-IgM syndrome, usually considered a B-cell disease. This finding clearly defines X-linked hyper-IgM syndrome as a T-cell disorder (Aruffo et al., 1993). Two clinical observations had suggested a T-cell defect, the high incidence of *Pneumocystis carinii* pneumonia, and a description of severe histoplasmosis in this syndrome (Tu et al., 1991). This disorder is further discussed in Chapter 11.

Cytokine Defects. Cytokines enhance the proliferation events necessary for expansion of the responding population in an immune response. In addition, further maturation, secretion, and numerous inflammatory events are mediated by cytokines (reviewed in Rosen et al., 1992; Abbas et al., 1994c; Janeway and Travers, 1994; see Chapter 3).

Defective IL-1 synthesis was described by Chu and associates (1984). Several cases of inability to synthesize IL-2 have been described (Doi et al., 1988; Weinberg and Parkman, 1990; Disanto et al., 1990; Arnaiz-Villena et al., 1992b; Sorensen et al., 1992). In one case, the nuclear factor of activated T cells (NF-AT), an IL-2 gene regulator protein was structurally abnormal (Arnaiz-Villena et al., 1992b). This patient had a multiple cytokine defect with impaired ability to synthesize IL-2, IL-4, and interferon-γ (Castigli et al., 1993). The molecular defect in the other patients was not defined.

IL-2 Receptor Defect (X-Linked Severe Combined Immunodeficiency). Mutations of the gamma-chain (γ_c) of the IL-2 receptor have been found in 7 of 7 patients with X-linked SCID tested so far (Noguchi et al., 1993b; Puck et al., 1993). The marked lymphopenia seen in patients with X-linked SCID stands in marked contrast to the relatively normal numbers seen in IL-2–deficient patients. This observation suggests that the IL-2 receptor may play a more global role in lymphocyte development than IL-2. The IL-2 receptor is a member of the cytokine receptor superfamily, which includes myeloid cell growth factor receptors (Minami et al., 1993). Some studies show the IL-2 receptor gamma-chain to be a functional component of IL-4 and IL-7 receptors. Thus, the IL-2 gamma-chain receptor is common to multiple cytokine receptors (hence *c* for *common* in γ_c), and its absence or abnormality results in defective responses to multiple cytokines. Other T-cell growth factors (e.g., IL-9) may also use γ_c (Kondo et al., 1993; Noguchi et al., 1993a; Russell et al., 1993). A defect in the IL-2 receptor could thus affect cells of myeloid lineages as well, explaining the high incidence of associated hematopoietic cell defects in some forms of combined immunodeficiency (Voss et al., 1994).

Other Combined Immunodeficiency Disorders

A number of diseases have been described, mostly in single case reports. The pathogenesis is unclear, and they cannot fit easily into the schema above. Various clinical clues that help to identify them are shown in Table 12–3, which lists a number of phenotypic characteristics of various combined immunodeficiency disorders.

OKT4 Epitope Deficiency. CD4 is a surface molecule expressed by T cells that binds to class II major histocompatibility complex (MHC) molecules (see Chapter 2). In so doing, it augments antigen recognition by T cells responding to peptides carried in the class II MHC molecule cleft. Two different epitopes of CD4 are distinguished by the monoclonal antibodies OKT4 and Leu-3a. In 1981, Bach and colleagues described patients whose CD4$^+$ cells did not react with OKT4 but did bind to Leu-3a.

Since then, numerous examples have been described (Fukuda et al., 1984; Sato et al., 1984; Aozasa et al., 1985; Gill et al., 1985; Levinson et al., 1985; Stohl et al., 1985), and the disorder is known as OKT4 epitope deficiency (OED). Analysis of these patients' immunity has increased the knowledge of CD4 structure and function relationships. Patients lacking the OKT4 epi-

Table 12–3. Characeristics of Newly Described Forms of Combined Immunodeficiency Disorders

Reference/Comment	T Cells*	B Cells*	Clinical Features*
A new X-linked immunodeficiency Brooks et al., 1990	CD3$^+$CD4$^+$ low CD3$^+$CD8$^+$ low CD45RA$^+$CD45RO$^+$ very low CD45RA$^+$CD45RO$^-$ very low Mitogen response low IL-2 production low	CD19/20 nl Total Ig levels nl IgG ab responses low IgM, IgA ab responses nl	X-linked Severe varicella Warts Ages from 2½ to 34 yrs
A new X-linked immunodeficiency de Saint-Basile et al., 1992	CD3$^+$CD4$^+$ nl† CD3$^+$CD8$^+$ nl† CD45$^+$ nl Mitogen response sl low Alloantigen response low	SIg$^+$ cells nl Total Ig levels high Specific ab formation poor	X-linked Intractable diarrhea Overwhelming sepsis
CID associated with cyclic hematopoietic defect Junker et al., 1991	T-cell counts vary from low to nl Mitogen response low to nl	Total B-cells nl number Total Ig levels very low	Cyclic hematopoiesis *Pneumocystis* pneumonia
CD4 decrease without AIDS; idiopathic CD4-lymphocytopenia Smith et al., 1993 Ho et al., 1993 Spira et al., 1993 Duncan et al., 1993 Fauci, 1993	CD4$^+$ less than 300/mm³ or less than 20% of total	Ig levels normal or low	HIV negative; risk factors + in <50% Immunologic studies tend to remain stable Age 16 yr or over Wasting syndrome Extrapulmonary cryptococcosis, atypical *Mycobacterium* infection Kaposi's sarcoma Some asymptomatic
IL-I defect Chu et al., 1984	Lymphocytosis (8470/mm³) CD3$^+$CD4$^+$ high CD3$^+$CD8$^+$ high	Total Ig levels normal	Failure to thrive Severe herpes zoster
Multiple cytokine defects; IL-2 defect Doi et al., 1989 Pahwa et al., 1989 Castigli et al., 1993 Weinberg and Parkman, 1990 Disanto et al., 1990	Lymphocytes nl to high CD2$^+$ nl CD3$^+$CD4$^+$ low to nl CD3$^+$CD8$^+$ low to nl Mitogen and antigen response low; correctable by exogenous IL-2	CD20$^+$ nl All Ig levels very low	Oral thrush
Calcium flux defect Le Deist et al., 1995 Gehrz et al., 1980	Lymphocytes nl Normal phenotype CD4 RO/RA distribution nl	IgA elevated IgM elevated IgG restricted heterogeneity	Protracted diarrhea CMV pneumonia
An X-linked disease with genetic proximity to Wiskott-Aldrich, mapped to Xp11.2, and T-cell activation Shigeoka et al., 1993 Powell et al., 1983	Activated (DR$^+$) T cells common		X-linked Insulin-dependent diabetes constant Other autoimmune disorders common Diarrhea and fatal infection may occur

*Underlined characteristic most distinguishing feature of disorder.

†T lymphocyte counts low until the age of 4 months but thereafter became normal.

Abbreviations: ab = antibody; CID = combined immunodeficiency; nl = normal; + = positive; sl = slightly.

tope generally have normal ability to resist infectious agents that are susceptible to T-cell control. Their T cells respond to mitogens, and delayed hypersensitivity skin tests are normal. A slight defect in T-helper function support of immunoglobulin production may be present (Fukuda et al., 1984; Sato et al., 1984; Aozasa et al., 1985; Levinson et al., 1985; Stohl et al., 1985). Thus, most of the physiologic functions of CD4 are subserved by the Leu-3a epitope. Of interest, Leu-3a is an HIV receptor, serving as one of the portals of entry into the T lymphocytes; OKT4 is unnecessary (Hoxie et al., 1986).

Many patients with OED are asymptomatic, but autoimmune problems such as Graves' disease and systemic lupus erythematosus have been described (Fukuda et al., 1984; Stohl et al., 1985). Another patient with thymoma, hypogammaglobulinemia, and red blood cell aplasia was reported by Levison and coworkers (1985).

The disorder is inherited as an autosomal codominant trait. Homozygotes lack completely OKT4$^+$ cells. Heterozygotes show normal numbers of OKT4$^+$ cells, but they express the markers at approximately 50% of the density of normal persons (Takenaka et al., 1993; Aozasa et al., 1985). The trait is common in blacks (8.3%), but rare in whites and Japanese (<1%) (Takenaka et al., 1993; Aozasa et al., 1985).

Idiopathic CD4 Lymphocytopenia. In this group of diseases, CD4$^+$ lymphocytes are profoundly depressed but HIV infection cannot be proven. Approximately 40% of the patients exhibit some risk factor for acquired immunodeficiency syndrome (AIDS). Levels below the ninety-fifth percentile for age, or less than 20% of the total T-lymphocyte count, define the disease. Infection with opportunistic agents is common; only a few patients are otherwise symptomatic, however. The disorder is extremely rare, 0.0002% in one study (Smith et al., 1993). Most of the patients are adults, but the lymphocytopenia has been found in 10 children and a few adolescents.

Exhaustive investigation has not uncovered evidence for infection by HIV (neither HIV-1 or HIV-2), nor for T-cell lymphotropic viruses (HTLV-I or HTLV-II). The syndrome differs somewhat clinically from HIV infections, in that hypergammaglobulinemia is not seen and the CD4$^+$ counts tend to stabilize rather than continue in a downward progression. In fact, the CD4$^+$ T-cell lymphocytopenia has reversed in some patients. The patient group involved differs from that ordinarily associated with HIV infections; one third are women, and the geographic and age distributions are much wider than those seen with AIDS.

The causes of CD4$^+$ T–lymphocytopenia are many and varied; no definite etiology has been determined as yet (Duncan et al., 1993; Fauci, 1993; Ho et al., 1993; Smith et al., 1993; Spira et al., 1993).

Griscelli Syndrome. A number of immunodeficiency patients with characteristic silvery hair fall into the category of Griscelli syndrome. These patients were originally described by Griscelli and colleagues (1978) and Siccardi and associates (1978). The hair color is due to defective melanosome transfer. In addition, the patients suffer widespread histiocytic infiltrations, resulting in a multisystem disorder. Hepatosplenomegaly, lymphadenopathy, and pulmonary infiltrations are common. Erythrophagocytosis and progressive neurologic deterioration are other features in this usually fatal disease.

Microscopic examination of the hair reveals pigment clumps; engorged melanocytes are found in the basal layer of the epidermis. Lymph node architecture is obliterated. Lymphocyte counts are normal, but the CD3$^+$ cells may be decreased in number. Mitogen responses are normal to minimally depressed. Some studies show deficient T-cell help for immunoglobulin production in vitro. However, serum immunoglobulin levels may be either normal or depressed.

The physical appearance of the patients is similar to that seen in Chédiak-Higashi syndrome. However, Griscelli syndrome patient leukocytes lack the characteristic large azurophilic granules seen in granulocytes of Chédiak-Higashi syndrome patients. Natural killer activity, which is diminished in patients with Chédiak-Higashi syndrome, has not been evaluated in those with Griscelli syndrome.

Bone marrow transplant has been accomplished in Griscelli syndrome and is curative (Schneider et al., 1990).

CD7 Deficiency. A patient with both CID and CD7 deficiency has been reported. CD7 is an early marker of lymphocytes associated with commitment to the T-cell lineage (Rosen et al., 1992).

Nezelof Syndrome. Also known as cellular immunodeficiency with immunoglobulins, this syndrome was first described by Nezelof in 1964. In addition to profound T-cell immunodeficiency, immunoglobulin levels are either normal or elevated; antibody function, however, is decreased or absent (Nezelof et al., 1968). IgE levels are also elevated. Often these patients have a less severe clinical course than other patients with CID (Lawlor et al., 1974). However, most regard this disorder as a variant of CID with the associated thymic dysplasia. Nezelof syndrome is probably not a single entity. It must be differentiated from childhood HIV infection, since both disorders have elevated immunoglobulins, poor antibody function, and decreased T-cell immunity.

Clinical Manifestations

Generally, the clinical presentation of the CID patient does not correlate with the more precise delineation of the defect provided by in vitro T-cell assessment. For example, oral candidiasis, highly resistant to therapy, is observed in some, but not all, patients with profound T-cell defects. There is no laboratory test that will distinguish between these patients that do or do not present with such symptomatology, however. Similarly, freedom from infections during the first few months or even the first year of life does not necessarily indicate a milder defect. The frequency of infections is often controlled by such a trivial event as exposure. Ultimately, many such patients experience undue frequency of serious infections, both the bacterial infections that characterize B-cell deficiency and the viral complications (varicella or cytomegalovirus pneumonia) or the opportunistic infections seen in T-cell deficiency.

Normal infants frequently experience oral thrush, particularly when the diaper area is infected or after a course of antibiotics. Oral candidiasis caused by T-cell deficiency occurs in the absence of the previously described predisposing factors and characteristically does not respond to simple therapy (oral antifungal agents). Either the infection recurs immediately on cessation of therapy or does not respond at all. When attenuated infectious agents are used for vaccinations, life-threatening or fatal infections can occur. This was commonly seen with vaccinia virus when smallpox vaccination was routine and is a complication of immunization with bacille Calmette-Guérin. Interestingly, vaccine strains of polio are usually nonsymptomatic in CIDs; paradoxically, in agammaglobulinemia, they cause paralysis.

Pneumocystis carinii pneumonia is a common mode of initial presentation, and the underlying immunodeficiency disease is completely unsuspected until that episode. With the increasing incidence of tuberculosis, it is anticipated that overwhelming pneumonia caused by this organism will be seen more often. Atypical *Mycobacterium* can cause chronic infections that can ultimately result in fatality. Parainfluenza and adenovirus, in addition to measles, may cause severe giant cell pneumonia in these compromised hosts.

Skin disorders are common. In the short-limbed dwarfism type of CID, the skin is redundant, hanging in loose folds; large umbilical hernias and lax joints are associated. The hair may be sparse; in some cases there is total alopecia. Seborrheic dermatitis may be severe, sometimes causing confusion with Letterer-Siwe or graft-versus-host disease. Ectodermal dysplasia has been described (Feigen et al., 1971). Persistent deep ulcers of the buccal mucosa, tongue, and perineum occur.

The clinical symptoms may be quite variable, even among those sharing the same defect. One of two siblings with CD3–gamma-chain deficiency had a series of severe autoimmune problems and ultimately died of giant cell pneumonia, probably caused by parainfluenza 3 virus. The other sibling was healthy. A child with CD3–epsilon-chain deficiency had only mild respiratory infections. Antibody production to protein antigens was normal, but there were no polysaccharide responses (Alarcon et al., 1988; Arnaiz-Villena et al., 1992a, 1992b).

These laboratory-clinical correlations emphasize the redundancy of signaling mechanisms in the immune system, which permits amazingly good health in face of what would appear to be a lethal defect. Few clear-cut inferences concerning the pathogenesis can be drawn from the clinical presentation. Nevertheless, I have listed some characteristics of recently described and rarer varieties of combined deficiencies (see Table 12–3). These may help the clinician to categorize the continually increasing numbers and varieties of CID being described.

Gastrointestinal manifestations can be severe. Chronic hepatitis secondary to cytomegalovirus or unknown agents is common. A characteristic form of liver involvement involves the bile ducts, causing focal disappearance. This may be a variant of sclerosing cholangitis (Fig. 12–2) described in familial B-cell deficiency (Record et al., 1973) and in combined immunodeficiency (Thomas et al., 1974). The most life-threatening gastrointestinal complication is chronic diarrhea, refractory to disaccharide-free diets or predigested formulas. A search for chronic rotavirus or *Campylobacter* infection or parasitic infestation, such as *Giardia* or *Cryptosporidia,* should be made. The malabsorption can be so severe that the resultant wasting is lethal. Hyperalimentation is often necessary and can be life-saving.

Hematologic abnormalities, including neutropenia, red blood cell aplasia, and megaloblastic anemia resistant to vitamin B_{12} or folic acid, are common. Eosinophilia and monocytosis may signal an unusual infection, such as with *Pneumocystis*. Thrombocytosis or thrombocytopenia may occur; the latter is often associated with intercurrent infection.

Chronic encephalopathy was observed in 11 of 24 autopsy cases reviewed by Dayan (1971). In one child with a mild form of combined immunodeficiency, chronic progressive multifocal leukoencephalopathy developed at age 4. Postmortem examination revealed Jamestown Canyon virus in the brain (ZuRhein et al., 1978). Previously, this disorder had been recorded only in adults, usually in association with some underlying immune dysfunction (Richardson, 1970; Mathews et al., 1976).

Patients with Nezelof syndrome may have somewhat milder clinical courses, despite chronic diarrhea and recurrent pneumonia. A series of six patients was well characterized by Lawlor and coworkers (1974).

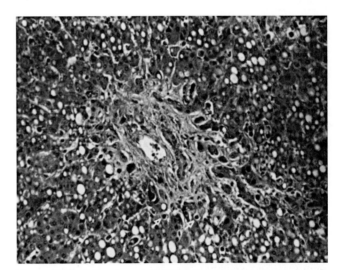

Figure 12–2. Sclerosing cholangitis characteristic of immunodeficiency. The patient had had combined immunodeficiency and secreted cytomegalovirus from early infancy. Transient hyperbilirubinemia and increase of liver enzymes were observed at 3 months of age. A liver biopsy at the time showed no bile ducts. At autopsy (2 months later), some bile ducts were seen, but the portal area was extensively fibrosed and biliary stasis was present. Inclusion bodies of cytomegalovirus infection are seen *(white arrows)*.

Variable patterns of serum immunoglobulins were observed; only one patient had normal levels of all immunoglobulins. She had normal levels of isohemagglutinins, abnormal response to keyhole limpet hemocyanin, and no antibody response to pneumococcal polysaccharide. The lymphocyte response was reduced to phytohemagglutinin but normal to allogeneic cells. The other five patients had a profound T-cell deficiency. This heterogeneity makes generalizations difficult, except that all were unable to form functional antibody to all antigens.

Laboratory Findings

Quantitative assessment of the T-cell system involves enumeration and characterization on the basis of cell surface characteristics (see Chapter 9). Competent lymphocytes accomplish their roles in immune responses by reacting to external signals and interacting with other cells, including tissue components, such as endothelial cells, and mobile members of the immune system, such as B-cells and macrophages. These multiple interactions require cell surface molecules to control adhesion, homing, and transduction events. Accordingly, the mature T lymphocyte displays on its surface the molecules that control its destiny. Demonstration of these surface markers (see Chapters 2 and 9) indicates the competence of the cell and often provides some indication of its state of activation (i.e., whether it is responding to an antigen or resting in a quiescent state). Particularly with X-linked SCID, there is marked lymphopenia, and virtually no cells with the mature T-cell phenotype (i.e., $CD3^+/CD4^+$ or $CD3^+/CD8^+$) exist. In other disorders, the patterns are highly variable. When lymphocytes are abundant, they often show the phenotype of immature thymocytes (e.g., $CD3^+/CD4^-/CD8^-$ or $CD3^-/CD1^+$ profiles), indicating a developmental arrest.

Qualitative measurements provide a closer correlate to the actual protective capability of the T lymphocytes. The most informative assessment in this regard is the in vitro proliferative response to specific antigen (Lane et al., 1985). Because this test requires prior sensitization, it is not a useful assay in early life. In the latter portion of the first year, in vitro responses to tetanus toxoid should be present if the child has been immunized. Delayed hypersensitivity skin tests are the in vivo analogs of the antigen proliferation assays; they tend to be less sensitive than the in vitro responses. Furthermore, positive skin tests may not be seen until 2 to 3 years of age in normal children.

Mitogens (phytohemagglutinin, concanavalin A, and pokeweed mitogen) and allogeneic lymphocytes (mixed leukocyte culture) stimulate the T cells in a global manner; thus, proliferation induced by these agents is less sensitive for detection of more subtle, yet clinically significant deficiency states. When absent, mitogen responses indicate a profound T-cell defect; if present, these responses do not absolutely exclude susceptibility to infection. Failure to respond to a specific antigen, even in the face of adequate mitogen responses, usually means clinical disease.

Immunoglobulin levels usually are extremely low; IgA and IgM are usually nondetectable by routine immunologic assays, and IgG is usually less than 200 mg/dl. Antibody responses to vaccines are usually absent. Some patients show unusual elevation of IgM levels as present in dysgammaglobulinemia (Fireman et al., 1966). Some patients show monoclonal paraproteins (M components) of restricted heterogeneity; they do not have an antibody response to administered antigens. Some patients with Nezelof syndrome have this type of immunoglobulin. Because these patients have no functional antibody, they have CID and their clinical course is similar to those with low or absent immunoglobulins. They are more likely to have palpable or enlarged lymph nodes. Patients with monoclonal paraproteins may show marked immunoglobulin elevations, with values up to 8 g/dl recorded (Groshong et al., 1976).

Additional evaluation of the T cells is provided by measurement of cytokines elaborated during the immune response and assessment of cytolytic activity against various cellular targets. Cytotoxic function is usually deficient in the lymphocytes of patients with CID. This involves specific T-cell cytotoxicity, antibody-dependent cellular cytotoxicity, and natural killer (NK) cytotoxicity. In some patients with CID, however, one or more of these are intact and, indeed, Sindel and colleagues (1984) describe a patient with SCID who showed increased NK cytotoxicity, both functionally and by the use of NK-reactive monoclonal antibodies.

Thymic biopsy has been advocated by Hong and Horowitz (1975). Borzy and coworkers (1979) described several histologic patterns in biopsy specimens from infants with CID (Figs. 12–3 to 12–6). The subject has been extensively reviewed (Nezelof, 1992). Monoclonal antibodies have defined three types of thymic epithelium: type 1, cortical, and medullary (Haynes et al., 1984, 1988; reviewed in Boyd et al., 1993).

Unfortunately, these antibodies have not been used extensively to assess thymic tissue in primary immunodeficiency. In one study, differences in expression of

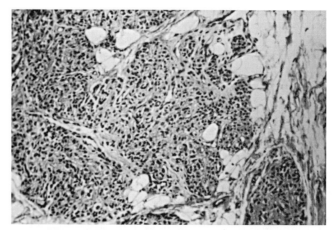

Figure 12–3. A typical dysplastic thymus of combined immunodeficiency. The lobules are small and consist of only small, spindle-shaped epithelial cells. No lymphocytes or Hassall's corpuscles are present; corticomedullary differentiation is lacking. ($\times$ 100.)

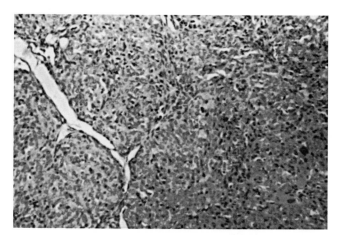

Figure 12–4. Partial dysplasia of the thymus. The lobules are bigger and the predominant cell type is plumper with abundant eosinophilic cytoplasm. Again, Hassall's corpuscles and corticomedullary differentiation are absent. (× 100.)

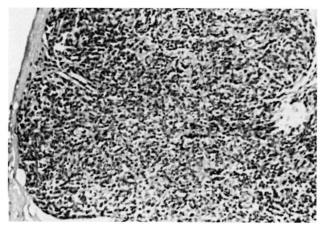

Figure 12–6. Late fetal pattern of the thymus gland. The lobules are of moderate size. There is a suggestion of corticomedullary differentiation with a few monocyte lymphocyte clusters at the lobule edge. Hassall's corpuscles are still absent. (× 100.)

thymic epithelial antigens were found between patients with SCID and the Nezelof syndrome (Haynes et al., 1983). More studies are required to see whether an informative pattern emerges.

An unexplained but consistent serum defect found in CID is a decreased level of a subunit of the first component of complement, C1q. C1q levels are about one third of normal and increase after successful bone marrow transplantation (Ballow et al., 1973). This defect may be an associated genetic defect or a metabolic abnormality of the C1q component.

In Utero Diagnosis and Carrier Detection

It is now possible to use chorionic villus biopsies with gene probing or DNA fingerprinting techniques to make in utero diagnoses of immunodeficiency within the first trimester (Lau and Levinsky, 1988). Chorionic villus biopsies carry a slight risk of miscarriage (0.5%), and occasional injury to the fetus has been reported (Jackson et al., 1992; Platt and Carlson, 1992). After 18

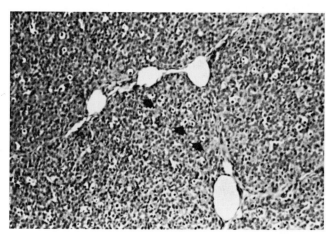

Figure 12–5. Partial dysplasia of the thymus with phagocytosis. The plump epithelial cell is again the major cell type, but phagocytosis (arrows) is a prominent feature. (× 100.)

weeks' gestation, fetal blood samples can be obtained reliably and analyzed by flow cytometry, lymphocyte function tests, and biochemistry (Durandy et al., 1982).

Carriers of X-linked immunodeficiency diseases can be defined on the basis of nonlyonization of target cell populations. This is accomplished most commonly by restriction fragment length polymorphism (RFLP) analysis of the X chromosome. By RFLP analysis, one can detect which X chromosome (paternal or maternal) is being used. In the normal population, approximately one half of the cells use the paternal X and one half use the maternal (Lyon effect). If affected cell populations (for example, T cells) in the obligate heterozygote are examined for X chromosome usage, they show restriction to the normal paternally derived X (nonlyonization). The inference is that because the affected chromosome cannot maintain cell survival, such cells are lost with time. Use of both maternal and paternal X chromosomes in a random manner can be demonstrated in unaffected (e.g., granulocyte) cell populations (Fearon et al., 1987; Conley et al., 1988; Goodship et al., 1988; Puck et al., 1990a; Conley, 1992).

One can also work backward from examination of maternal cells and infer that the disorder in an affected male is X-linked, if nonlyonization is found in the mother. This is a useful analysis when the disease occurs for the first time in a male with the inheritance pattern unclear (de Saint-Basile et al., 1992).

Treatment

Bone Marrow Transplantation

Optimal treatment for combined immunodeficiency is a bone marrow transplant (BMT) from a histocompatible sibling, matched at the HLA-A, -B, and -D loci. Survival with complete restoration of B-cell and T-cell systems can be expected in 70% of cases (O'Reilly et al., 1978, 1989; Fischer et al., 1986; Lenarsky and Parkman, 1990). Lifetime cure is expected, since the first BMT patient, transplanted in 1968, is alive today with normal immunity (Gatti et al., 1968). Occasionally, subsequent repeated transplants are necessary.

In the absence of an HLA-matched sibling donor, various therapies have been tried, including transplants of fetal liver, fetal liver and thymus, fetal thymus, and cultured thymus fragments. In general, most of these strategies have failed and are not in general use today. Bacchetta and colleagues (1993) reported on two notable exceptions—two children, ages 5 and 18, who received several fetal liver and fetal thymus injections in early life. The persisting T cells were of donor origin, whereas the B cells were the patient's. One patient receives intravenous immunoglobulin, but the other does not. These same workers (Touraine et al., 1989, 1991; Touraine, 1990) have reported on in utero infusions of cells derived from fetal thymus and fetal liver. One child had bare lymphocyte syndrome and the other had SCID. Some evidence of engraftment of the fetal cells was seen, but there was an insufficient number to achieve significant correction of the defects. Both children received further infusions of fetal cells after birth. The child with the bare lymphocyte syndrome has acquired proliferative responses to antigens, but the other patient has shown no signs of improvement (Touraine et al., 1989, 1991; Touraine, 1990).

An exciting advance in the treatment of patients with primary immunodeficiency has been the successful engraftment of haplotype-mismatched marrow, usually from one of the patient's parents. Two major strategies have been employed, both with the object of removing sufficient mature T cells from the inoculum to prevent fatal graft-versus-host disease (GVHD).

The lectin separation method, pioneered by Reisner and associates (1983), depends on the agglutination of mature T cells by soybean lectin and sheep erythrocytes. The agglutinated cells are then removed by centrifugation, and the stem cell–rich remainder of the inoculum is infused. Some children have shown full reconstitution following this procedure, but one experienced severe GVHD. Many of the children show persistent B-cell deficiency and require gamma globulin replacement therapy (Friedrich et al., 1984, 1985). Others have achieved full engraftment (Cowan et al., 1985).

The second approach uses a monoclonal antibody directed against mature T cells (Reinherz et al., 1982; Trigg et al., 1984). Incubation of the marrow with the antibody in the presence of complement lyses the mature T cells; the marrow is then infused. This technique has also permitted transplantation across a haplotype-mismatch barrier. Most children receiving transplantation by this approach have shown full T- and B-cell reconstitution (Moen et al., 1987).

An alternative approach is based on finding an HLA match outside the family by searching a large donor pool. The likelihood of two unrelated individuals matching at the major HLA loci is of the order of 1 in 20,000; thus, a large pool must be searched. In a registry of 200,000 white donors, 50% to 75% of them will find an HLA-A, -B, -DR match. However, if the patient possesses rare HLA antigens, matching becomes much more difficult. When minorities are involved, a match becomes even more unlikely. At present, finding a matched-unrelated donor is a difficult and time-consuming task.

Even so, Filipovitch and coworkers (1992) successfully employed transplantations in 10 children and used matched unrelated donors. Of the recipients, eight had severe combined immunodeficiency, two had Wiskott-Aldrich syndrome, and two had Chédiak-Higashi syndrome. Two of the SCID patients died of pretransplant opportunistic infections. Graft-versus-host disease occurred in only four children and was successfully treated in all.

A surprising finding in the treatment of combined immunodeficiency by haplotype-mismatched marrow is that ablation of host cells is often necessary. Before the use of this form of therapy, bone marrow transplantation (except in adenosine deaminase deficiency) from matched sibling donors always resulted in engraftment if the patient survived long enough. Failure to engraft occurs frequently when haplotype-mismatched donors are used. The cell population responsible for this rejection has not been identified. It may represent NK-type cells. The determination of which children require ablation before transplantation is an important area presently being investigated. When required, the regimen used for children with normal immunity (e.g., leukemic patients) has been employed. This means that in addition to the risks of BMT *per se*, the additional side effects of strong chemotherapeutic ablation and, in some cases, total body irradiation must be considered in the risk-benefit ratios of the therapy proposed.

In this regard, the most toxic regimens employ irradiation. Total-body irradiation is associated with diminished growth velocity, dental abnormalities, delayed pubescence, gonadal failure, and hypothyroidism; cataracts usually occur. Fortunately, BMT for immunodeficiency does not require complete host cell elimination as does BMT for malignancy; hence, cyclophosphamide can be used as an alternative for immunosuppression. Long-term systemic effects are minimal when cyclophosphamide alone is used, but the addition of busulfan causes gonadal damage.

Cyclophosphamide conditioning regimens may not *a priori* result in sterility. In a Seattle study, 15 men and 14 women had 33 children after receiving cyclophosphamide for BMT preparation. Of those who received cyclophosphamide alone, 14 men fathered 16 children and 14 women delivered 14 live births. One man fathered 3 children after receiving both cyclophosphamide and total-body irradiation (Sanders et al., 1989).

It is still too early to compare the ultimate results of either method to see whether significant differences will develop. However, the initial responses are so gratifying that BMT, even from nonmatched donors, is the next best form of treatment for combined immunodeficiency when a matched sibling (or close relative) is not available as a bone marrow donor. Replacement therapy by fetal or cultured tissues can no longer be recommended as primary treatment.

Lymphoproliferative Disease. B-cell lymphoproliferative disease (BCLD) is a complication of transplantation. Its frequency after organ transplantation is reported from 0.6% to 5% (Hanto et al., 1985), but BCLD is a rare complication of matched allogeneic BMT—0.23% to 0.45% (Shapiro et al., 1988b; Zutter et al., 1988).

Three major factors predispose to the development of BCLD:

- Nonidentity at HLA
- Depletion of T cells from the marrow
- Treatment of the recipient with antiserum directed against T cells.

Antibodies directed against T cells are used to enhance engraftment or treat GVDH. Mismatching alone increases BCLD frequency to 10%, but T-cell depletion of the graft or the administration of T-cell antibody to the host will double the incidence to more than 20% (Shapiro et al., 1988a).

As a complication of BMT, B-cell lymphoproliferative disease carries a poor prognosis; it is nearly always fatal (Shapiro et al., 1988b; Zutter et al., 1988; Fischer et al., 1991a). By contrast, BCLD that develops after organ transplantation may resolve in as many as 40% of patients, particularly when immunosuppression is stopped (Hanto et al., 1985). The difference is that the immunodeficiency in organ transplant recipients is not as profound as in primary immunodeficiency and can easily revert toward normality when the immunosuppressive drugs are stopped. In primary immunodeficiency disorders treated by BMT, there is minimal, if any, immune capability. What exists is further compromised by ablative regimens and graft-versus-host disease.

Most, if not all, of the tumors are caused by Epstein-Barr virus (EBV), and they are of both host and donor origin (List et al., 1987). Only one description of a non–EBV-associated B-cell lymphoproliferation has been described (Garcia et al., 1987). When human B cells are infected by EBV, some cells carry the virus permanently as a latent infection. These cells are immortalized, and in vitro, would grow spontaneously as long cell lines. They do not develop continuous growth in vivo in normal persons because they are held in check by a functional T-cell system. With ablative preparation for the transplant, any host T cells are destroyed. When the mature T cells in the bone marrow inoculum are also removed, the passive transfer of T-cell immunity is abrogated. Any latently EBV-infected B cells, either in the host or transplanted along with the marrow, are now freed from constraining T cells. They may also be activated by the antigenic differences between the host and the donor and by the secretion of cytokines such as IL-6 (Tosato et al., 1993). They expand rapidly, and the clinical course can be as short as a few weeks from the first clinical sign (usually high fever) to death. Virtually every organ is invaded by the tumor; massive hepatosplenomegaly and lymphadenopathy occur. Infiltration of the gastrointestinal tract may lead to uncontrollable hemorrhage.

Treatment is, by and large, unsuccessful. Occasional success has been reported with alpha-interferon and intravenous immunoglobulin (Shapiro et al., 1988a)

and anti–B-cell monoclonal antibodies (Fischer et al., 1991a); in general, however, fatality is the rule.

Gene Therapy

Gene therapy is discussed later (see Adenosine Deaminase Deficiency).

Other Therapeutic Considerations

Varicella pneumonia or encephalitis is a potentially lethal complication in CID. Varicella-zoster immunoglobulin is effective if injected within 72 hours of the exposure (Gershon et al., 1974; Hattori et al., 1976). With established infection, acyclovir should be given. Varicella is readily controlled. If the patient has had a previous bone marrow transplant, usually adequate immunity develops after the infection and protective titers of varicella antibody are attained.

The administration of whole blood or blood products may cause GVHD in children with CID. Thus, all blood products should be irradiated with 25 Gy before administration; this will not interfere with the functional capability of the erythrocytes or granulocytes. Blood products should come from cytomegalovirus antibody–negative donors, if possible.

P. carinii pneumonia can be treated effectively by pentamidine isethionate or trimethoprim-sulfamethoxazole. Prophylaxis with trimethoprim-sulfamethoxazole should be used until reconstitution has been accomplished (Hughes et al., 1977).

Live virus vaccinations are contraindicated for the patient and all family members.

Prognosis

The prognosis is poor unless a suitable bone marrow donor is identified. Better supportive care and the recognition of milder variants negate the popular notion that all children with CID will expire before age 2. An extensive review of a single center's experience reveals a generally favorable outcome (Stephan et al., 1993).

BARE LYMPHOCYTE SYNDROME (MHC Class I and Class II Deficiencies)

The bare lymphocyte syndrome (BLS) refers to a heterogeneous collection of combined immunodeficiency diseases that are associated with deficient expression of major histocompatibility complex (MHC) class I (HLA-A, -B, and -C) antigens, class II (HLA-DR, -DQ, and -DP) MHC antigens, or both. Although this syndrome is heterogeneous in many respects, three main phenotypic subtypes have been proposed (Touraine et al., 1985).

Historical Aspects

Patients with immunodeficiency and abnormalities of MHC class I antigen expression were first recognized by Touraine and colleagues (1978) and Schuurman and coworkers (1979). The absence of MHC class I antigen expression was discovered using serologic histocompatibility typing methods with leukocytes from patients being evaluated for bone marrow transplantation. Touraine initially proposed the use of the term *bare lymphocyte syndrome* for this form of combined immune deficiency. Subsequent studies of these and other patients with bare lymphocyte syndrome have demonstrated that this syndrome more frequently involves defective expression of the class II (HLA-DR, -DQ, and -DP) MHC antigens, with or without an associated defect in class I antigen expression (Hadam et al., 1984; Touraine et al., 1985). The immunodeficiency disease associated with absent class II antigens is often referred to as the MHC class II deficiency syndrome. More than 100 affected individuals have now been reported.

Pathogenesis

Considerable progress has been made in defining the normal biologic role of class I and class II MHC antigens, particularly in regard to the efficient functioning of the immune system. Class I MHC antigens are normally expressed by all nucleated cells. In contrast, class II MHC membrane antigens are constitutively expressed only by B cells and monocyte lineage cells, although these antigens can also be expressed under certain circumstances by a variety of other cell types. Class I and class II MHC antigens both serve as recognition structures for the interactions among immunocompetent cells that are vital for initiating an effective immune response. In addition, class II antigen–bearing cells mediate the intrathymic maturation and "education" of T cells (Kruisbeek et al., 1985).

The molecular lesions responsible for the defective expression of membrane MHC antigens in this syndrome appear to be heterogeneous. There is considerable evidence that BLS results from autosomal recessive genetic defects affecting regulatory genes involved in the coordinate expression of MHC antigens. Cells from individuals with defective class II MHC antigen expression have most extensively been studied. DNA hybridization studies have shown that the structural genes encoding for the molecules that form MHC antigens are present in cells from BLS patients (Payne et al., 1983; Marcadet et al., 1985). However, the transcription of these structural genes is defective in cells from class II–deficient BLS patients (Lisowska-Grospierre et al., 1985; de Preval et al., 1988). The defects in gene transcription can be corrected by somatic cell hybridization of BLS B-cell lines with various normal or mutant cell types (Yang et al., 1988).

Although complementation studies suggest that at least four different types of defects can produce this syndrome (Benichou and Strominger, 1991), most BLS patients studied to date fall within two complementation groups (Lisowska-Grospierre et al., 1994). The transcription of class II MHC structural genes is coordinately regulated by two or more *trans*-acting genes that are not linked to the MHC (Salter et al., 1985; de Preval et al., 1985). A splicing mutation of one such gene, the class II transactivator (CIITA) gene, has been shown to be present in some patients with BLS

(Steimle et al., 1993). Other regulatory genes produce DNA-binding proteins that bind to conserved *cis*-active upstream promoter elements (X and Y boxes) and thus initiate gene transcription. A deficiency of one such binding protein, RF-X, has been reported in a subset of patients with BLS (Reith et al., 1988).

In other BLS patients, defective production of accessory proteins that organize class II promoters into a configuration that is accessible to binding proteins or otherwise enhance the stable association of DNA-binding proteins with the X box promoter sequence has been demonstrated (Stimac et al., 1991; Kara and Glimcher, 1993). Although the nature of the one or more defects leading to defective expression of class I MHC molecules is less well understood, defective production of transporter associated with antigen-processing (TAP) proteins can produce this syndrome (de la Salle et al., 1994).

In most patients with BLS, the defect in MHC antigen expression is complete and affects all relevant cell types. In some affected individuals, however, the defect may be incomplete and low levels of class I or class II antigens may be expressed, either constitutively (Payne et al., 1983; Rijkers et al., 1987) or after exposure to agents that up-regulate MHC antigen expression (i.e., Epstein-Barr virus or interferon) (Lisowska-Grospierre et al., 1985; Plaeger-Marshall et al., 1988; de Preval et al., 1988). Furthermore, the defect may differentially affect tissue-specific regulatory elements that control class II antigen expression (Maffei et al., 1987; Plaeger-Marshall et al., 1988). These disparate findings again highlight the heterogeneous nature of the defects that may produce this syndrome.

Because MHC antigens serve as recognition structures for interactions among immunocompetent cells, the primary basis for the immunodeficiency in this syndrome resides in the inability of cells to recognize foreign antigens in the context of self-MHC molecules. However, MHC antigens also mediate certain aspects of the differentiation or function or both of T and B lymphocytes, thereby compounding the defects in cellular and humoral immunity. For example, the deficiency of peripheral CD4+ T cells seen in many class II–deficient patients appears to be a consequence of the absence of intrathymic accessory cells expressing class II, which are necessary for the generation of mature CD4+ CD8− cells (Blue et al., 1985; Kruisbeek et al., 1985; Grusby et al., 1991). The post-thymic differentiation of phenotypically and functionally distinct subsets of CD4+ cells may also be abnormal (Clement et al., 1988a).

Clinical Manifestations

Although the first reported cases of the bare lymphocyte syndrome involved children from North African or Turkish families, this syndrome has now been identified in a wide variety of ethnic populations. Many of the first reported cases were born following consanguineous unions, and an autosomal recessive inheritance pattern has been seen in several kindreds analyzed. However, the recognition of sporadic cases without a positive family history has increased as awareness of this disorder has widened.

In its most severe form, this syndrome is a combined immunodeficiency typically manifesting within the first 8 months of life. Affected individuals are susceptible to severe or recurrent systemic infections by a wide variety of bacterial, viral, protozoan, and fungal pathogens, including *P. carinii, Candida,* and herpes-type viruses. The spectrum of infectious agents seen in the most severely affected patients does not differ significantly from that characteristic of other severe combined immunodeficiencies. Failure to thrive and oral candidiasis are frequent presenting symptoms. In addition, chronic, severe diarrhea and malabsorption (resulting from *Giardia lamblia* infestations or unknown agents) is a characteristic feature of this disorder (Hadam et al., 1984). In contrast to patients with some combined immune deficiency syndromes, patients with BLS often have normal or enlarged peripheral lymph nodes, and a thymus shadow is usually seen on radiographs of the chest.

Although most patients present with a severe combined immune deficiency, a minority of patients appear to be less susceptible to severe, life-threatening infections. Although the basis for this is not firmly established, at least some of these individuals appear to have defects that lead to partial, rather than complete, deficiencies of MHC antigen expression (Payne et al., 1983; Rijkers et al., 1987). The degree to which quantitative variations in MHC antigen expression may correlate with the magnitude of the defect in immune function remains to be established.

Laboratory Findings

Because MHC antigens serve as recognition structures for interactions among immunocompetent cells, the primary basis for the immune deficiency in this syndrome resides in the inability of cells to recognize antigens in the context of self-MHC molecules. In addition, defects in lymphocyte differentiation and function compound the defects in cellular and humoral immunity.

Assessment of Lymphocyte Subpopulations

The lymphocyte count in patients with bare lymphocyte syndrome is typically normal or only moderately reduced. Although the number of circulating surface immunoglobulin–bearing B cells is typically normal, decreased numbers have been found in some patients. Phenotypic evidence of arrested B-cell differentiation at an immature stage has been described in many patients with BLS (Hadam et al., 1984; Rijkers et al., 1987; Clement et al., 1988b). In lymph nodes, follicle development is poor, and germinal centers are absent. Virtually no plasma cells are found in tissues or bone marrow.

Although the total number of circulating T cells is normal in most patients, the number of CD4+ T cells is often significantly reduced particularly in patients who lack class II MHC antigen expression (Griscelli et al., 1981; Hadam et al., 1984; Clement et al., 1988a).

This may be associated with a relative or absolute increase in the CD8+ cytotoxic/suppressor subset of T cells, thereby resulting in a reversed CD4:CD8 cell ratio.

Abnormalities in the differentiation of functionally and phenotypically distinct subsets of CD4+ and CD8+ T cells may also occur. In the one patient in whom CD4+ cell maturation has been examined, virtually all of the CD4+ cells present expressed the immature CD4+ CD45RA+ phenotype (Clement et al., 1988a). This patient also lacked the subset of CD8+ CD28−CD11b+ T cells that mediate suppressor functions.

The thymus morphology in BLS patients is relatively normal with reasonable corticomedullary demarcation. However, the cortical area is sparse, and Hassall's corpuscles are diminished (Schuurman et al., 1985).

Assessment of Lymphocyte Functions

Virtually all individuals with the class II MHC antigen deficiency syndrome have panhypogammaglobulinemia, and specific antibody production following immunization is severely diminished in most patients. As noted earlier, however, the defects in class II antigen expression may be incomplete in some patients. This may be associated with a mitigation of the humoral deficits, and patients with less severe forms of BLS may produce some antibody in vivo and in vitro (Rijkers et al., 1987). Thus, heterogeneity of the molecular lesions may produce variability in the magnitude of both the class II deficiency and the B-cell functional impairment.

Delayed type hypersensitivity skin test reactions to recall antigens are weak or absent, and primary sensitization to dinitrochlorobenzene (DNCB) cannot be accomplished. In vitro T-cell proliferative responses induced by polyclonal mitogens, such as phytohemagglutinin and anti-CD3 antibodies, are normal or only modestly reduced for most patients. In like fashion, T cells from most affected individuals proliferate in mixed leukocyte reaction (MLR) cultures when stimulated with allogeneic cells. Cells from patients with BLS, including cells from class II–deficient individuals, may be potent stimulator cells in MLR cultures (Jin and Yang, 1990). In contrast, responses of CD4+ T cells to specific soluble antigens, such as tetanus toxoid or *Candida,* are markedly reduced or absent, even in previously immunized patients. Thus, T cells from affected individuals are able to respond to stimuli that do not require class II antigen–bearing accessory cells, but they do not respond to specific antigens that must be recognized in the context of class II MHC antigens on the surface of antigen-presenting cells.

Studies of the ability of CD4+ T cells in BLS patients to provide help for in vitro antibody secretion by normal B cells have yielded mixed results; T-helper cell function has been found in some, but not all, affected individuals. The basis for this heterogeneity is unknown. In contrast, attempts to induce the differentiation of class II–deficient B cells in T helper cell–dependent assays has been uniformly negative.

In summary, the defects in T cell–mediated immune functions found in the MHC class II deficiency syndrome appear to result from several diverse but interdependent pathogenetic mechanisms, involving the production, differentiation, and/or cellular interactions of T cells. First, the absence of intrathymic class II antigens may result in deficient production of the CD4+ cells that emigrate from the thymus. Furthermore, as a result of the defects in class II antigen expression by antigen-presenting cells, the CD4+ cells that do emerge from the thymus are not induced to undergo post-thymic maturation into CD4+ CD45RA cells with helper capabilities (Clement et al., 1988a).

Diagnosis

The diagnosis of the bare lymphocyte syndrome requires definitive demonstration of severely diminished or absent constitutive expression of class I or class II MHC antigen expression or both by mononuclear cells from an individual with clinical and laboratory evidence of immune dysfunction. This is most readily achieved by immunofluorescent membrane antigen analyses of blood lymphocytes using monoclonal antibodies reactive with nonpolymorphic regions of human class I and class II MHC antigens and flow cytometry. Confirmation by serologic cytotoxicity techniques using a panel of different antibody reagents can also be performed. Successful antenatal detection of affected fetuses has been achieved (Durandy et al., 1982, 1985).

Treatment and Prognosis

Supportive treatment with intravenous immunoglobulin, antibiotics for documented infections, and prophylaxis against *P. carinii* should be provided to all patients with bare lymphocyte syndrome. At present, the best definitive therapeutic option is stem cell replacement by bone marrow transplantation. Ideally, cells should be obtained from an HLA-identical sibling, and methods using DNA probes for the genotypic typing of BLS patients and potential donors are available (Marcadet et al., 1985). Because T cells capable of responding against alloantigens are present in these patients, the potential risk of graft rejection exceeds that for patients with other severe combined immunodeficiency disorders, and pre-transplant immune ablation is indicated (Touraine et al., 1992a). In the absence of this potential life-saving procedure, death is common within the first few years of life.

In utero transplantation of fetal liver cells has been reported to be beneficial (Touraine et al., 1992b). Because the antenatal diagnosis of BLS is possible, in utero stem cell transplantation offers an exciting and potentially beneficial therapeutic option deserving future consideration.

Contributed by Loran T. Clement

IMMUNODEFICIENCY WITH ENZYME DEFICIENCY (Adenosine Deaminase and Nucleoside Phosphorylase Deficiencies)

Immunodeficiency is associated with two enzyme deficiencies of the purine metabolic pathway: (1) adenosine deaminase (ADA) deficiency and (2) purine nucleoside phosphorylase (PNP) deficiency. The immunodeficiency of ADA deficiency is a combined one, consisting of complete or partial deficiency of both T- and B-cell immunity. The immunodeficiency of PNP deficiency is associated with normal B-cell immunity but absent or severely depressed T-cell immunity.

ADA deficiency accounts for approximately 40% of autosomal recessive combined immunodeficiency, or 20% of all cases of CID; PNP accounts for 4% of patients with CID (Hirschhorn, 1990; Markert, 1991).

Historical Aspects

Giblett and colleagues (1972) first described a deficiency of the enzyme ADA in the red blood cells of two patients with CID. One patient had experienced from birth recurrent infections associated with severe lymphopenia. She had a depressed lymphocyte response to PHA and allogeneic cells, low levels of IgG and IgM, but some specific antibody responses. The second patient had a history of recurrent infection associated with severely depressed responses to PHA and allogeneic cells. Immunoglobulin levels were normal, and some antibody to bacterial and viral antigens was present. The red blood cell ADA levels in the parents of patients varied from one half to two thirds of normal values.

In 1975, Giblett and coworkers described a patient with normal B-cell but absent T-cell immunity with complete absence of PNP in the red blood cells, white blood cells, and fibroblasts. PNP levels approximately one half of normal were found in both parents, indicating an autosomal recessive inheritance (Sandman et al., 1977). The second patient described with PNP deficiency had normal immune function at birth (Stoop et al., 1976), but there was gradual immunologic deterioration; by the age of 2 years, severe depression in T-cell immunity with intact B-cell immunity was observed. Additional patients with PNP deficiency with immunodeficiency have been described (Hamet et al., 1977; Biggar et al., 1978; Carpella-DeLuca et al., 1978; Rich et al., 1978).

Pathogenesis

The purine salvage pathway is illustrated in Figure 12–7. ADA enzyme is an amino hydrolase that deaminates adenosine to yield inosine. Inosine is converted to hypoxanthine by PNP enzyme. Hypoxanthine then follows either of two pathways: salvage by hypoxanthine guanine phosphoribosyltransferase (HGPRT) to inosine monophosphate or conversion to uric acid for excretion.

Although ADA and PNP are present in all cells, the primary effects of the deficiency are seen in the lymphocytes. Furthermore, in PNP deficiency, the B cells are relatively spared. This paradox has not been fully explained, but the selective toxicity in different tissues is thought to be due to variability of intracellular accumulation of toxic metabolites and differential effects of deoxyadenosine and deoxyguanosine. Deoxyadenosine

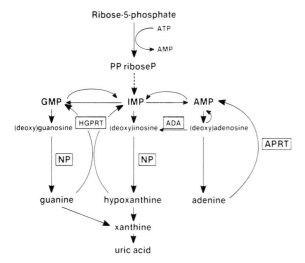

Figure 12–7. Biochemical pathways in purine metabolism, illustrating the role of adenosine deaminase and nucleoside phosphorylase. ADA = adenosine deaminase; AMP = adenosine monophosphate; APRT = adenine phosphoribosyl transferase; ATP = adenosine triphosphate; HGPRT = hypoxanthine-guanine phosphoribosyl transferase; NP = nucleoside phosphorylase; PPriboseP = phosphoribosyl pyrophosphate; IMP = inosine monophosphate; GMP = guanosine monophosphate.

is derived primarily from cells with rapid turnover. Thus, the major contributors to the deoxyadenosine pool are epithelial cells and lymphocytes such as those undergoing thymic maturation, of which 99% die in situ. ATP breakdown and cell death provide the major sources for adenosine.

A number of metabolites are elevated because of ADA deficiency. Adenosine and adenine accumulate in the plasma; adenosine triphosphate (ATP) collects in erythrocytes; and adenosine diphosphate (ADP), guanosine triphosphate (GTP), and ATP in lymphocytes. The elevated levels of deoxyadenosine, in the presence of a high lymphocyte deoxycytidine kinase activity, lead to formation of excessive amounts of deoxyadenosine triphosphate. DeoxyATP cannot equilibrate with the external milieu and attains toxic levels that inhibit ribonucleotide reductase, an enzyme essential for the synthesis of DNA precursors (Moore and Herlbert, 1966; Cohen et al., 1978). Parallel changes in deoxyGTP levels occur, with similar consequences, in PNP deficiency. Subsequently, S-adenosyl homocysteine hydrolase is inactivated, leading to further toxicity by inhibition of methylation (Kredich and Martin, 1977; Hirschhorn et al., 1982; Hirschhorn, 1993).

One can surmise that thymocytes, because of their high death rate, generate markedly increased levels of deoxyATP and deoxyGTP in the thymic milieu, accounting for selective, increased destruction of T-cells. The preservation of B-cell function in PNP deficiency can be explained by differing effects of deoxyadenosine and deoxyguanosine on resting lymphocytes; deoxyadenosine can lyse resting T and B lymphocytes in 4 days (Carson et al., 1982; Carson and Carerra, 1990). Deoxyguanosine, which accumulates in PNP deficiency, has little effect.

A T-cell activation molecule, CD26, binds to ADA. Thus, in contrast to the usual view of its simple housekeeping role, ADA may play a direct role in T-cell activation. Further insight into the biologic significance of CD26-ADA interactions should clarify the full impact of ADA deficiency on immune functions (Kameoka et al., 1993).

The elevated levels of adenosine have less effect on cell proliferation but may play a role in neurologic symptoms, such as lethargy and visual-following defects (Hirschhorn, 1993).

Only small amounts of ADA are necessary for competent immunity. Somewhere between 1% and 5% of normal levels is adequate (Hirschhorn and Ellenbogen, 1986; Hirschhorn, 1993).

A number of mutations of the ADA locus have been described. Most of the defects described earlier were missense mutations resulting in unstable or inactive enzymes. Some mutations are associated with milder forms of ADA deficiency, with enzyme levels varying from 8% to 42% of normal—not profound immunodeficiency—termed *partial ADA deficiency* (Hirschhorn, 1993). Santisteban and colleagues (1993) have defined other mutations in varieties of ADA deficiency associated with late or delayed onset of symptoms. These patients show novel splicing, missense, and deletion mutations, resulting in higher enzyme levels and lower tissue levels of toxic metabolites.

In PNP deficiency, two mutations associated with disease have been described, one missense and one frameshift (Williams et al., 1987; Andrews and Markert, 1992). The gene is located on the long arm of chromosome 14.

Clinical Manifestations

Adenosine Deaminase Deficiency

Four phenotypes of ADA deficiency have been described. Most (80% to 90%) of the patients present with the clinical course of SCID—early onset of life-threatening infections and marked lymphopenia. In a few, onset of serious infections does not occur until the latter part of the first year of life. B-cell immunity may still be detected, and usually diagnosis is delayed. Some present even later in life, and diagnosis is made after the age of 4 years. This group is probably underdiagnosed. Some of the patients with HIV-negative CD4[+] lymphopenia may fall in this category. Autoimmunity is more commonly seen in the second and third varieties (Notarangelo et al., 1992).

Finally, there are approximately a dozen children who were found to have ADA deficiency incidentally, as a result of population screening. This last group has normal immunity. The groups are denoted (1) ADA-SCID, (2) delayed-onset ADA deficiency, (3) late-onset ADA deficiency, and (4) partial ADA deficiency (Hirschhorn and Ellenbogen, 1986; Hirschhorn, 1990, 1993; Santisteban et al., 1993).

Purine Nucleoside Phosphorylase Deficiency

Thus far, all patients homozygous for PNP deficiency have been symptomatic. The history consists primarily

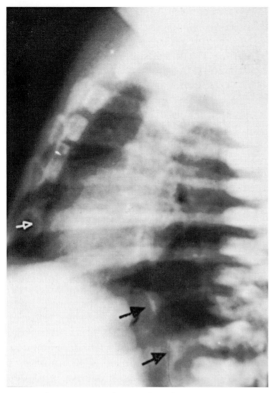

Figure 12–8. Lateral view of chest in adenosine deaminase (ADA) deficiency with combined immunodeficiency indicating lack of a thymus. Flaring and cupping of the ends of the ribs are apparent *(arrows)*.

ity in red blood cells. Two male siblings who had approximately 5% of normal PNP activity have been reported; both had severe T-cell deficiency.

Characteristic x-ray findings are seen in about half the cases of ADA deficiency (Figs. 12–8 to 12–11). These include cupping and flaring of the ribs and abnormalities of the transverse processes of the vertebrae and the scapula. Unique histologic abnormalities accompany these alterations (Fig. 12–12), permitting distinction from short-limbed dwarfism (Cederbaum et al., 1976).

Ratech and associates (1985a) examined the autopsy findings in eight ADA patients and reported lesions of the kidney and adrenals. Seven of the eight showed mesangial sclerosis, and six showed adrenal gland sclerosis. In addition, one of three pituitary glands examined showed sclerosis. The findings were similar to those found in mice given the ADA inhibitor deoxycoformycin (Ratech et al., 1985b). Also, pathologic changes were diminished or absent in patients receiving enzyme therapy by blood transfusions. Ratech and coworkers (1985a) therefore concluded that toxic metabolite accumulation was responsible for these changes as well. Examination of the thymus, spleen, and lymph nodes revealed marked lymphocyte depletion, as would be expected. A pattern unique to enzyme deficiency was not observed (Ratech et al., 1989).

of recurrent viral, bacterial, and fungal infections. Few physical findings are present except for those related to acute or chronic infection. The development of symptoms attributable to immunodeficiency may be delayed for several years. The patients are prone to disseminated varicella and progressive vaccinia.

Two thirds of patients have evidence of neurologic disorders. Some patients have mental retardation; others show mild developmental delay or muscle spasticity. There also is an increased incidence of hemolytic anemia. Autoimmune thyroiditis, thrombocytopenic purpura, lupus, and cerebral vasculitis have been documented (reviewed by Markert, 1991).

Laboratory Findings

Adenosine deaminase (ADA) deficiency is established by finding low levels or absence of ADA in the patient's erythrocytes, lymphocytes, or fibroblasts. Carriers can be detected by finding half-normal levels of the enzyme in the erythrocytes (Hirschhorn, 1977). In utero diagnosis can be established by measuring enzyme levels in cultured amniotic fluid fibroblasts or tissue obtained by chorionic villus biopsy.

Purine nucleoside phosphorylase (PNP) deficiency is also established by finding low levels or absence of PNP activity in erythrocytes, leukocytes, or fibroblasts (Sandman et al., 1977). Low levels of serum uric acid are characteristic. The carrier state can be detected by finding approximately half-normal levels of PNP activ-

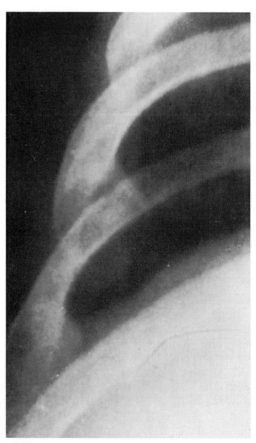

Figure 12–9. Frontal view of the ribs in adenosine deaminase (ADA) deficiency shows cupping deformity of ribs.

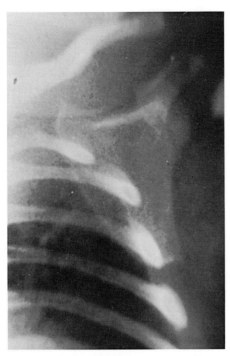

Figure 12–10. "Squaring off" of the tip of the scapula in adenosine deaminase (ADA) deficiency.

Treatment

Bone Marrow Transplantation

Patients with ADA deficiency can successfully receive transplantation with bone marrow from histocompatible siblings with normal ADA activity (Parkman et al., 1975). We successfully transplanted in a 10-month-old ADA-deficient child bone marrow from a 62-year-old HLA-A, B, and D–identical uncle. The child had not previously responded to repeated red blood cell infusions. Successful bone marrow transplantation from haploidentical parents has also been accomplished. Stable immune reconstitution and reversal of skeletal defects have been seen (Moen et al., 1987; Silber et al., 1987; Bluetters-Sawatzki et al., 1989). Several patients with ADA or PNP deficiencies have been treated with fetal liver, fetal thymus transplantation, or both with partial reconstitution.

Enzyme Replacement

Polmar and colleagues (1976) attempted to replace the enzyme in patients with ADA deficiency by blood transfusions. The benefit was only partial in some instances and minimal in the remainder. With time, this approach was replaced by use of an injectable purified enzyme preparation. Bovine adenosine deaminase, modified by polyethylene glycol conjugation (PEG-ADA) to render it less immunogenic and increase its circulation time, has been employed since 1986 (Hershfield et al., 1993). Intramuscular injections are given once or twice a week.

The immune system reconstitution is variable. About 20% of the patients do not respond; the remainder show variable lymphocyte responses. Impressive signs

of reconstitution, such as in vitro responsiveness to antigens, x-ray evidence of thymic enlargement, and increased antibody titers, have been observed. ADA-deficient T-cell progenitors appear to mature in a normal ontogenic pattern after institution of adequate therapy. Clinically, the children show marked improvement in quality of life, and some can attend regular school. Recovery from varicella with the development of antibodies was seen in two patients; rate of growth improved as did pulmonary insufficiency in others. It is likely that PEG-ADA has its greatest benefit in the milder forms of ADA deficiency (Hershfield and Chaffee, 1991; Hershfield et al., 1993; Weinberg et al., 1993).

Gene Therapy

An ADA-deficient patient is an ideal candidate for gene therapy. The enzyme is a single-chain structure, and its expression does not require close regulation to be physiologically effective and safe (Anderson, 1984). Consequently, major efforts to accomplish gene therapy have been focused on this disorder. In 1990 and 1991, peripheral blood T cells, transfected with the ADA gene in vitro, were given to two ADA-deficient patients who were receiving PEG-ADA. Increases in T-cell responsiveness and number, acquisition of a positive skin test, and enlargement of lymphoid tissue were noted. Infusions of cells were given at 4- to 12-week intervals. In one patient, enzyme levels remained elevated at least 6 months after the infusions had stopped and immune benefit continued (Blaese, 1993).

Three neonates have received autologous bone marrow transplants of ADA-transfected stem cells. Advantage was taken of the high numbers of stem cells present in cord blood. The patients were diagnosed in utero, and the cord blood stem cells were harvested at birth, the gene was inserted, and the cells were returned to the patients. Initial evaluation suggests that the procedures have been successful in achieving gene expression in circulating lymphocytes, but the infants keep receiving PEG-ADA injections (Kohn et al., 1995).

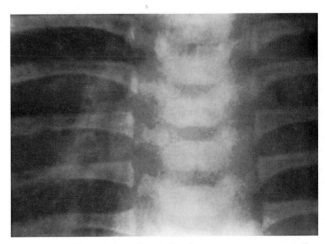

Figure 12–11. Frontal view of posterior rib–transverse process articulation in adenosine deaminase (ADA) deficiency. Some of the transverse processes are concave. The transverse processes do not overlap the ribs so that the articulations form vertical radiolucent bands on either side of the spinal column.

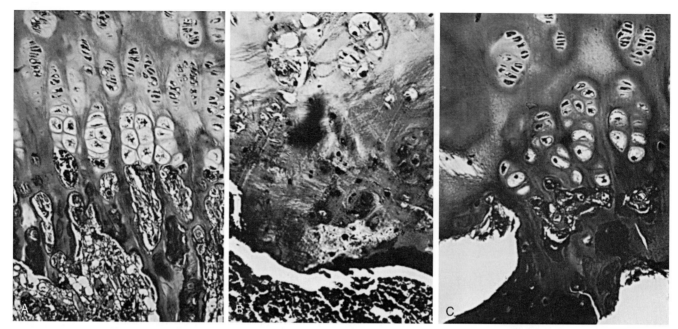

Figure 12–12. Photomicrographs of the costochondral junctions of three children (Masson trichrome stain; × 160). *A,* Normal child. *B,* Adenosine deaminase (ADA) deficiency. *C,* Cartilage-hair hypoplasia (8-year-old girl). *A,* Note the normal linear columns of proliferating cells and hypertrophic cells in the growth plate. *B,* In the patient with ADA deficiency, there is no transition of proliferating to hypertrophic cells, and there are only scattered hypertrophic cells with uninterrupted calcified cartilage formation. *C,* In the patient with cartilage-hair hypoplasia, there are clusters of cells containing both hypertrophic and proliferating cell types. (From Cederbaum SD, Kaitila I, Rimoin DL, Stiehm ER. The chondro-osseus dysplasia of adenosine deaminase deficiency with severe combined immunodeficiency. J Pediatr 89:737–742, 1976).

Two children with PNP deficiency have received haploidentical BMT; one has a partial and the other a complete correction of the immune defect. Three other children, two of whom had matched donors, have died after BMT. The histocompatibility match of the third is unknown. On the basis of so few patients, one cannot generalize about the likelihood of success or the impact of using a nonmatched donor. It is likely that more successful results will be recorded as the total number of transplants increases, with resultant improvement in techniques of support and control of GVHD.

Many attempts to treat ADA and PNP deficiency, using various chemicals to block formation of toxins or otherwise circumvent the biochemical abnormalities, have met with failure.

Prognosis

Patients with ADA or PNP deficiency and combined immunodeficiency disorder have a poor prognosis unless they receive a bone marrow transplant. These patients inevitably die from overwhelming infection. In tarda forms of the disorder, infection may be delayed but patients usually succumb to infection. Patients with more than 5% of ADA activity in tissues are immunologically normal (Hirshhorn, 1977).

In patients with PNP deficiency, recurrent infections develop, which may be delayed or less severe or both. PNP-deficient patients have died from disseminated varicella, progressive vaccinia, lymphosarcoma, and

graft-versus-host disease (Stoop et al., 1976; Ammann et al., 1978; Carpella-DeLuca et al., 1978).

In both ADA and PNP deficiencies, neurologic abnormalities such as progressive spasticity have been described (Hirschhorn, 1977; Stoop et al., 1976). These abnormalities may be related to aberrations in the purine metabolic pathway or may be a consequence of infection.

SHORT-LIMBED DWARFISM WITH IMMUNODEFICIENCY AND CARTILAGE-HAIR HYPOPLASIA

Short-limbed dwarfism with immunodeficiency is an autosomal recessive, predominantly T-cell immunodeficiency associated with metaphyseal or spondyloepiphyseal dysplasia. Cartilage-hair hypoplasia (CHH) is a variant of short-limbed dwarfism in which fine sparse hair is present. Although there is some resemblance to achondroplasia, x-rays of the bones and the presence of immunologic defects readily distinguish the two disorders. The short stature is a result of disproportionate shortening of the extremities.

The immunodeficiency of short-limbed dwarfism may be either a T-cell, B-cell, or combined defect. In short-limbed dwarfism with CHH, T-cell deficiency and combined deficiency—but not isolated B-cell deficiency—have been reported.

Historical Aspects

McKusick and coworkers (1964) first noted unusual susceptibility to varicella virus in Amish children with CHH. Davis (1966) and Alexander and Dunbar (1967) first reported immunodeficiency associated with short-limbed dwarfism.

In a large series of patients reported with progressive vaccinia, one patient had "achondroplasia" (Fulginiti et al., 1968). This patient had antibody to vaccinia virus, emphasizing the predominant T-cell deficiency of short-limbed dwarfism. However, Ammann and colleagues (1974) described two siblings with short-limbed dwarfism who had a predominant antibody deficiency.

T-cell immunodeficiency was described by Hong and colleagues (1972) in a child with CHH. Lux and others (1970) studied two non-Amish children with the condition who had a predominant T-cell defect and neutropenia.

Pathogenesis

The precise defect in the short-limbed dwarfism syndromes is unknown. The bone defects and megaloblastic anemia nonresponsive to folic acid and vitamin B_{12} suggest a biochemical defect. The purine pathway is suspicious because of the occurrence of bone lesions in adenosine deaminase (ADA) deficiency; further, non-responsive megaloblastic anemia occurs in hereditary orotic aciduria. ADA levels, however, are normal in patients with CHH (Kaitila et al., 1975).

Clinical Manifestations

Short-limbed dwarfism is usually evident at birth. The head size is normal; the hands are short and pudgy,

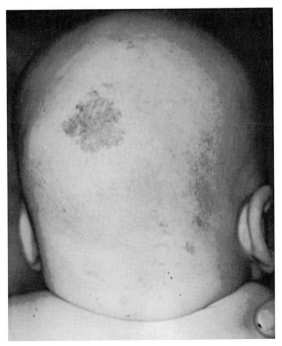

Figure 12–13. Redundant skin folds in the neck of an infant with short-limbed dwarfism.

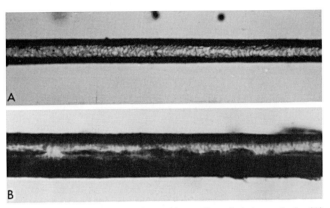

Figure 12–14. Hair of a patient with cartilage-hair hypoplasia *(A)* compared with sample from the normal parent *(B)*. The affected hair lacks the central pigment core, and the diameter is smaller.

the fingernails are short but normal in width, and the joints are loose; however, there is limitation of elbow extension and a peculiar sternal defect (McKusick et al., 1964). At birth and infancy, the skin forms redundant folds (Gatti et al., 1969) around the neck and extremities (Fig. 12–13). In CHH, the hair of the scalp, eyebrows, and eyelashes is light in color, fine (usually less than 55 μ in diameter) and sparse, and lacks a central pigmented core (Fig. 12–14). Malabsorption, celiac disease, and congenital megacolon have also been reported (McKusick et al., 1964). Adult height varies between 42 and 58 inches.

Most patients with short-limbed dwarfism and CHH have a limited susceptibility to infection and live normal lives. Varicella is the most common severe infection; two children died of varicella at 6 and 9 years of age, and five others almost succumbed (McKusick et al., 1964; Lux et al., 1970). Vaccinia and poliovirus vaccine are also potentially lethal (Fulginiti et al., 1968; Hong et al., 1972; Saulsbury et al., 1975). *P. carinii*, cytomegalovirus, and *Candida*, common pathogens in other T-cell deficiencies, have not been reported in CHH or short-limbed dwarfism.

Some patients with short-limbed dwarfism who have combined immunodeficiency have a broad susceptibility to infections and succumb to overwhelming infection during infancy (Davis, 1966; Alexander and Dunbar, 1967; Gatti et al., 1969). Because of the severe T-cell deficiency, these patients are also susceptible to graft-versus-host reactions.

Laboratory Findings

X-ray films of the bones reveal scalloping, irregular sclerosis, and cystic changes of the widened metaphyses (McKusick et al., 1964) (Fig. 12–15). In some patients with short-limbed dwarfism, flaring of the iliac crests is noted (Gatti et al., 1969). The ribs show splayed ends resembling the bone changes of ADA deficiency. Microscopic changes of bone in CHH and ADA deficiency have been compared by Cedarbaum and colleagues (1976) (see Fig. 12–12). In CHH, clusters of hypertrophic and proliferating chondrocytes are found; in ADA deficiency, there is no transition from

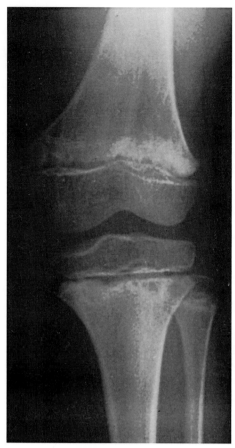

Figure 12–15. X-ray film of the tibia and femur in a child with short-limbed dwarfism. The irregular sclerosis, cystic changes, and scalloped appearance are apparent.

proliferating to hypertrophic cells. Both forms of bone disease show loss of normal column and trabecular formations of the chondrocytes and osteoblasts. Osteoblasts are rare.

The major T-cell abnormalities include decreased T-cell numbers, decreased lymphocyte proliferative responses, lymphopenia, and inability to reject skin grafts (Lux et al., 1970; Hong et al., 1972). T-cell function may decrease with time.

Immunoglobulin levels and antibody responses to injected antigens are usually normal (Lux et al., 1970). In a few cases of non-CHH short-limbed dwarfism, B-cell immunity has been deficient (Gatti et al., 1969; Ammann et al., 1974).

The neutropenia is associated with maturation arrest and decreased mobilization of the marginating pool and bone marrow reserve (Lux et al., 1970). The authors have observed megaloblastic anemia refractory to vitamin B$_{12}$ and folic acid, leading to red blood cell aplasia in one child with CHH.

Treatment

Three thymus transplants did not improve T-cell function in a CHH child with normal B-cell but absent T-cell function (Hong et al., 1972). Bone marrow transplantation in this child later reversed the aregenerative

anemia, malabsorption, chronic diarrhea, and growth failure. The dwarfism has persisted, but general health has been markedly improved (Horowitz and Hong, unpublished data). Bone marrow transplantation in another case of short-limbed dwarfism without CHH to date has resulted in transient improved proliferative responses. After 12 years, the patient's cells are totally his own. He has chronic lung disease but is otherwise well (Horowitz and Hong, unpublished data).

Prognosis

The prognosis for patients with CHH is considerably better than in most T-cell immunodeficiencies because the susceptibility to infection is less. In short-limbed dwarfism associated with combined immunodeficiency disorder (CID), early death may occur (Gatti et al., 1969). In patients with severe immune defects, the ultimate prognosis depends on the ability to treat or prevent potentially lethal infections and to achieve reconstitution by bone marrow transplantation.

OMENN SYNDROME (Combined Immunodeficiency Presenting As Letterer-Siwe Syndrome, Combined Immunodeficiency with Eosinophilia)

Some infants with CID present with a prominent generalized seborrheic skin eruption or scaling erythroderma, enlarged lymph nodes, hepatosplenomegaly, rash, eosinophilia, and histiocytic infiltration of the lymph nodes. This has led to an erroneous diagnosis as the *Letterer-Siwe syndrome*. However, Letterer-Siwe disease is not associated with immunodeficiency (unless immunosuppressive therapy is given).

The Omenn syndrome most likely encompasses a spectrum of T-cell defects somehow resulting in cytotoxic T cells that attack the skin (Fig. 12–16).

Historical Aspects

Omenn (1965) reported on a large family with many instances of this disorder. Lack of Hassall's corpuscles and paucity of lymphoid tissue were observed at autopsy. Immunologic studies performed by Cederbaum and colleagues (1974) established the presence of a combined immunologic defect in these patients.

Pathogenesis

The pathogenesis of Omenn syndrome is unknown. The variability in the assays of lymphocytes suggests that a number of causes are probably involved. Although the skin lesions resemble graft-versus-host disease, direct examination of the skin lesions and search of the peripheral blood for foreign HLA do not support such a diagnosis.

Lymphopenia does not occur, so that the fault does not involve failure of lineage development. However, the cells that are present do not function normally. In one case, a large proportion of the cells lacked CD4

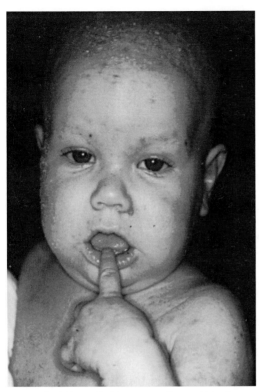

Figure 12–16. An infant with Omenn syndrome. Note the scaly dermatitis and alopecia.

and CD8, molecules important in augmenting T-cell antigen responses. However, these cells constituted the major population infiltrating and attacking the skin, indicating a cytotoxic capacity. Although responsive to mitogenic stimuli, these cells did not react to *Candida* antigen (Wirt et al., 1989). Schandene and coworkers (1993) found a low number of CD4$^+$ cells in their patient, but most also expressed the CD45RO antigen. When the cytokine profile of these cells were examined, they appeared to be T_H2 in type, producing large amounts of IL-4 and IL-5. These observations could explain the hyper-IgE often seen in these patients. Treatment with interferon-γ decreased the IgE levels and the eosinophilia and improved the T-cell in vitro responses.

One patient with Omenn syndrome (and other autosomal recessive CID patients) also demonstrated increased radiosensitivity of granulocyte macrophage colony–forming units and skin fibroblasts, thought to be the result of defective double-strand DNA repair mechanisms (Cavazzana-Calvo et al., 1993). This is a characteristic of SCID mice, whose defect is due to faulty T-cell or immunoglobulin receptor gene rearrangement. However, in that event, there is an absence of T cells and B cells, whereas the Omenn syndrome characteristically does not include lymphopenia. On the other hand, a sibling of a patient with Omenn syndrome showed profound lymphopenia. It has been proposed that Omenn syndrome may represent a "leaky" form of the SCID mouse defect. In SCID mice, with time, mature T cells and B cells appear, but the final repertoire is markedly oligoclonal and lacks the broad het-

erogeneity characteristic of a normal immune system. Thus, it is possible that lymphopenic CID and the Omenn syndrome are the same disease with a different clinical expression, which is a manifestation of time.

This example emphasizes the futility of attempting rigid classifications or definitions of the different forms of immunodeficiency on the basis of laboratory tests or clinical features.

Treatment

Management of Omenn syndrome is identical to that for combined immunodeficiency. Bone marrow transplantation using an HLA-matched sibling, haploidentical parent or HLA-matched unrelated donor marrow has been successful in many cases (Junker et al., 1989; Fischer et al., 1994) (see Chapter 32).

WISKOTT-ALDRICH SYNDROME

Wiskott-Aldrich syndrome (WAS) is an X-linked recessive immunodeficiency characterized by thrombocytopenia, eczema, and recurrent infection. There is defective T-cell function, poor antibody responses to polysaccharide antigens, and a characteristic serum immunoglobulin pattern of markedly elevated levels of IgA and IgE and low levels of IgM.

Historical Aspects

Wiskott first described the syndrome in 1937. Aldrich and coworkers (1954) described a second patient whose family was shown to have an X-linked inheritance. Three years later, Wolff and Bertucio (1957) described the syndrome in a black family, and Huntley and Dees (1957) reported five additional cases; both reports emphasized thrombocytopenia with a probable X-linked inheritance. Huntley and Dees (1957) described eosinophilia, milk sensitivity, and a greatly increased susceptibility to infection if splenectomy was performed.

An immunologic defect in the syndrome was first noted by Krivit and Good (1959), who demonstrated poor antibody responses to selected antigens. The absence of isohemagglutinins was reported 6 years later (Krivit et al., 1966). West and colleagues (1962) first described the characteristic immunoglobulin pattern of decreased serum IgM and increased serum IgA. Cooper and coworkers (1964) first described deficient T-cell immunity. Several other investigators have noted the relationship between the development of malignancies and WAS (Kildeberg, 1961; Amiet, 1963; Bensel et al., 1966; Chaptal et al., 1966; Radl et al., 1967; Brand and Marinkovich, 1969).

Cooper and coworkers (1968) demonstrated poor antibody responses to polysaccharide antigens and postulated a fundamental defect in antigen processing. They also suggested that immunologic attrition occurs with increasing age. Blaese and colleagues (1968) first reported immunologic defects of both the B-cell and T-cell systems. One of the first successful bone marrow transplants for immunodeficiency was successfully accomplished in WAS (Bach et al., 1968). The gene for WAS has now been cloned (Derry et al., 1994). The gene has been named *WASP* (for Wiskott-Aldrich syndrome protein) and is expressed in lymphocytes, megakaryocyte lines, spleen, and thymus.

Pathogenesis

Parkman and associates (1984) reported that Wiskott-Aldrich syndrome and other X-linked immunodeficiencies were associated with a platelet-leukocyte surface molecule defect involving sialophorin (gpL-115, leukosialin, or LSGP), now referred to as CD43. CD43 is a highly O-glycosylated molecule found on all circulating nonerythroid hematopoietic cells, and selective reduction of glycosyltransferases in WAS lymphocytes results in the defective expression (Greer et al., 1989; Higgins et al., 1991). Surface CD43 is stable in normal lymphocytes maintained in culture in vitro, but in cells from patients with the syndrome, after overnight incubation the protein is degraded, yielding a variety of products (Reisinger and Parkman, 1987). The abnormalities of lymphocyte surface architecture, lack of antigen responsivity, and poor differentiation that characterize WAS have been attributed to the CD43 defect.

Molecular characterization of CD43 showed conservation of the amino acid sequence across rat and human species, implying an important biologic role for this protein (Shelley et al., 1989), and the biologic role of CD43 has been elucidated in recent years. The early expression of CD43 in thymocyte ontogeny suggested that it might be important in differentiation, an interpretation supported experimentally. Transfection of a T-cell line with CD43 genes enhanced its antigen responsivity, and antigen-presenting cells were shown to bind specifically to CD43 (Park et al., 1991). Also, monoclonal antibodies to CD43 could activate T cells without involvement of the CD3 T cell–receptor complex, implying a role for CD43 in T-cell activation (Mentzer et al., 1987). More recently, CD43 has been shown to be involved in cytoskeletal structures that form the cleavage furrow during proliferation (Yonemura et al., 1993).

In sum, then, CD43 is involved in lymphocyte maturation, differentiation, and proliferation. However, because the CD43 gene is located on chromosome 16, a primary sialophorin gene defect cannot cause WAS. The primary X chromosome gene at fault was thought to produce the clinical syndrome through an effect on the surface expression of CD43.

In an attempt to obtain cellular representatives of the defect that were not secondarily affected by exposure to the environment of the patient, Molina and colleagues (1992) established long-term T-cell lines from WAS patients. These cell lines did not show the abnormalities of surface CD43 expression found in peripheral blood T cells of WAS patients; therefore, it was concluded that the changes involving CD43 were generated in the circulation of the patient (Remold-O'Donnell et al., 1991; Molina et al., 1992). However,

the cytoarchitectural abnormalities (paucity of microvillus projections) originally described in the peripheral cells of WAS patients were still present in the T-cell lines and were therefore considered an expression of the primary X-linked gene defect (Molina et al., 1992).

Stimulation of the WAS T-cell lines by a variety of stimuli showed selective defects in responsivity. The WAS cell lines proliferated normally to alloantigen, phytohemagglutinin, and phorbol ester plus ionomycin. However, immobilized antibody to CD3 could not stimulate these lines. These observations led Molina and coworkers (1992, 1993) to postulate that the paucity of microvilli was the central defect of WAS. In their absence, CD43, which normally concentrates on the microvilli, could not be properly integrated into the cytoskeletal structures necessary for proliferative responses to certain stimuli. The antigens that are most dependent on this pathway are large, inflexible molecules (such as polysaccharides) and immobilized CD3 antibody, two stimuli that consistently do not induce responses in WAS lymphocytes at times when other antigens are effective (Molina et al., 1993). To date, this hypothesis offers the best explanation for the selective defects in immune responses observed in WAS.

The recent discovery of the gene for WAS (WASP) will soon provide further insight into the pathogenesis. WASP encodes a 501 amino acid proline–rich protein expressed in lymphocytes, megakaryocyte lines, spleen, and the thymus (Derry et al., 1994).

It is possible that a similar disorder involves an autosomal gene. Evans and Holzel (1970) reported the case of a girl with eczema, decreased T-cell immunity, decreased serum IgM, increased IgA, recurrent herpes infections, and pneumococcal meningitis; however, she was not thrombocytopenic.

The ineffective T-cell system probably accounts for other clinical features of WAS, eczema, autoimmunity, and malignancy. The relationships of these phenomena to altered T-cell immunity are not completely defined, but they can probably be explained by T-cell dysregulation or imbalance of T_H1, T_H2, and T-suppressor cells. It is likely that chronic infections with opportunistic organisms or oncogenic viruses are also involved.

One of the early bone marrow transplants for WAS resulted in attainment of normal immunity, even though only T cells were engrafted; this implies that the recipient B cells were competent (Parkman et al., 1978). However, X-inactivation analysis, which demonstrates nonrandom inactivation in all cell lines harboring a gene that may be detrimental to survival or proliferation, reveals nonrandom inactivation of B cells and T cells in WAS carriers. Also, the patients show reduced numbers of $CD23^+$ and increased $CD20^+CD21^-$ B-cell numbers (Morio et al., 1989). Additionally, B-cell lines from these patients do not respond to stimulation by anti-immunoglobulin. Although normal B-cell lines show transmembrane signaling following cross-linking of surface immunoglobulin molecules, WAS B-cell lines showed defective tyrosine phosphorylation and, as a result, no proliferation (Simon et al., 1992). Thus, the WAS defect appears to be multilineage.

Clinical Manifestations

The initial manifestation of the Wiskott-Aldrich syndrome usually is presence of petechiae or a bleeding episode occurring in the first 6 months of life (Fig. 12–17). A typical atopic eczematoid rash of increasing severity appears during this period. Bacterial and viral infections, including otitis with draining ears and pneumonia, also begin to occur. During infections, thrombocytopenia is aggravated, and frank bleeding (e.g., hematemesis, petechiae, melena, or hematuria) may occur.

Infections with cytomegalovirus, *P. carinii*, and varicella may occur, but immunization with bacille Calmette-Guérin (BCG) is tolerated. Herpes simplex infections may be recurrent and, when disseminated, fatal. Severe reactions to immunizations, particularly polysaccharide vaccines, may lead to worsening of the petechiae, eczema, and purpura. Blood loss may be severe enough to require transfusions.

The eczema resembles classic atopic eczema with predilection for the antecubital and popliteal fossae. Splenomegaly, hepatomegaly, and cervical lymphadenopathy are present. The lungs are chronically infected, and rhonchi or rales are usually present. Chronic otitis media with purulent drainage, thickened tympanic membranes, middle ear hemorrhage, perforation, hearing loss, and mastoiditis occurs. Herpetic skin lesions may be present. Chronic herpes conjunctivitis may lead to chronic keratitis. Conjunctival, vitreous, and subconjunctival hemorrhages may result from the thrombocytopenia. Intracranial hemorrhage is not uncommon. Arthritis may occur with upper respiratory infection (Cooper et al., 1968). The nephrotic syndrome has been observed in WAS, once following the use of transfer factor (Fudenberg et al., 1974).

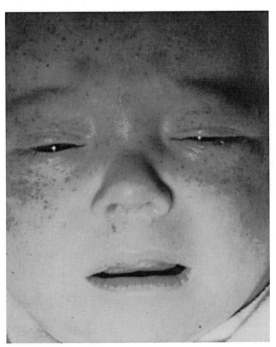

Figure 12–17. An infant with the Wiskott-Aldrich syndrome during an upper respiratory infection that resulted in an exaggeration of the thrombocytopenia and the subsequent appearance of petechiae.

Malignancies occur frequently in children with WAS who are older than 8 years, particularly systemic reticuloendotheliosis and lymphomas (Chaptal et al., 1966; Bensel et al., 1966; Brand and Marinkovich, 1969). These malignancies have a predilection for the brain. Sullivan and colleagues (1994) found in a multi-institutional survey that patients with associated autoimmunity were at greater risk for malignancies.

Variant forms of WAS are described. Canales and Mauer (1967) reported several boys with thrombocytopenia, low isohemagglutins, and increased serum IgA but without recurrent infection or eczema. Stoelinga and colleagues (1969) described a patient with decreased serum IgM, eczema, and inability to form antibody to polysaccharide but without thrombocytopenia; a brother died of pneumococcal meningitis. Mandl and coworkers (1968) reported a 24-year-old man with defective T-cell immunity, recurrent skin infections, and thrombocytopenia but normal immunoglobulin levels and antibody responses, including normal isohemagglutinin levels. A disorder including elevated IgA, IgA nephropathy, and thrombocytopenia has been described as a variant of WAS; a successful renal transplant has been accomplished (Webb et al., 1993).

Another X-linked disorder appears to be related to the syndrome, either by proximity of the affected gene or perhaps as a *forme fruste* version. Powell and associates (1982) described an X-linked syndrome of diarrhea, polyendocrinopathy, and fatal infection. None of the immune abnormalities of WAS were found, and thrombocytopenia was not a feature. Antibody responses to polysaccharides were not measured. Thus, many of the characteristic phenotypic features of WAS were either not present or not sought for. However, the disease was mapped to Xp11.2, close to the locus for WAS and X-linked thrombocytopenia (Shigeoka et al., 1993). Thus, contiguous areas of the X chromosome are involved with features of WAS, thrombocytopenia, and autoimmunity.

Sullivan and colleagues (1994) conducted a multi-institutional survey involving 154 unselected patients with persistent thrombocytopenia. Criteria for inclusion as a WAS patient included persistent thrombocytopenia with one or more of the following:

- Small platelets
- Positive family history
- Associated T-cell or B-cell defect

Viewed in this broader perspective, the classic triad of eczema, draining ears, and thrombocytopenia was seen in only 27% of patients; 20% had only thrombocytopenia before diagnosis.

It seems likely that WAS is part of a spectrum of diseases caused by involvement of a contiguous region in the area of Xp11.22–23. The use of CD43 as a surface marker and genetic analyses will help in defining the relationship of these variants to each other.

Laboratory Findings

Although both T-cell and B-cell defects occur in Wiskott-Aldrich syndrome, the most consistent and characteristic abnormality is the inability to form antibody to polysaccharide antigens. Krivit and Good (1959) first identified this defect as an inability to form isohemagglutinins. Cooper and colleagues (1968) and Blaese and others (1968) showed that WAS patients could not form antibody to such antigens as pneumococcal polysaccharide, lipopolysaccharide VI from *Escherichia coli,* and Forssman antigen. Cooper and coworkers (1968) noted abnormal antibody responses to *Salmonella* antigens, with an inability to make both 19S and 7S antibodies, confirming similar studies by Eitzman and Smith (1960). Ayoub and others (1968) demonstrated that WAS patients had normal antibody responses to streptococcal protein antigens but poor antibody responses to streptococcal polysaccharide antigens.

Other investigators have shown normal antibody responses to viral, bacterial, parasitic, and simple protein antigens (Kildeberg, 1961; Root and Speicher, 1963; Palmgren and Lindberg, 1963; St. Geme et al., 1966; Wolff, 1967; Cooper et al., 1968). Milk precipitins were first demonstrated by Huntley and Dees (1957) and subsequently by Root and Speicher (1963). Blaese and colleagues (1968) showed that, despite documented infection or immunization, many WAS patients have poor antibody responses to viral agents (e.g., herpes simplex or poliomyelitis) and bacterial antigens.

A distinctive immunoglobulin pattern of normal to elevated IgG, extremely high IgA and IgE, and low IgM is present in WAS (Eitzman and Smith, 1960; Kildeberg, 1961; West et al., 1962; Palmgren and Lindberg, 1963; Amiet, 1963; Chaptal et al., 1966). This pattern may not be present until the patient is several years of age. Blaese and colleagues (1971) demonstrated hypercatabolism of immunoglobulins and albumin in WAS; they suggest that this is one of the earliest immunologic abnormalities present. IgG subclass levels are normal, including IgG2 levels, despite their poor response to polysaccharide antigens (Nahm et al., 1986).

Abnormal T-cell function in WAS was reported by Root and Speicher (1963), Wolff (1967), Cooper and coworkers (1968), and Blaese and others (1968). These include a decreased responsiveness to 2,4-dinitro-1-fluorobenzene and other delayed hypersensitivity skin test antigens, diminished but not absent lymphocyte response to phytohemagglutinin, and diminished lymphocyte response to antigens to which the patients have been immunized (Blaese et al., 1968). Blaese and colleagues (1972) showed that the impaired in vitro lymphocyte responses persisted even when macrophages from normal subjects were supplied, thus excluding deficient macrophage function. Oppenheim and coworkers (1973) reported decreased migration inhibition factor and lymphotoxin production and correlated these with the decreased lymphocyte response to mitogens.

Other immunologic findings in WAS include normal interferon production (Blaese et al., 1968), normal clearance of gold by the reticuloendothelial system (Cooper et al., 1968), normal polymorphonuclear leukocyte function (Krivit and Good, 1959; Cooper et

al., 1968), and normal complement levels (Cooper et al., 1968).

Hematologic abnormalities include anemia, lymphopenia, eosinophilia, and thrombocytopenia. Coombs' positive hemolytic anemia may occur spontaneously or in association with transfer factor therapy. When homologous platelets are transfused into WAS patients, there is normal platelet survival (Krivit et al., 1966; Pearson et al., 1966); however, autologous platelets have a shortened survival (Gröttum et al., 1969; Kuramoto et al., 1970). Megakaryocytes in the marrow are usually normal (Huntley and Dees, 1957; Krivit et al., 1966; Pearson et al., 1966; Cooper et al., 1968) but are occasionally decreased (Wolff, 1967). The platelets in WAS are small when compared with those of normal individuals or other patients with thrombocytopenia (Murphy et al., 1972). This finding may be used to make an early diagnosis of WAS when other findings are lacking.

Paraproteins are found in WAS patients, with or without associated malignancy (Radl et al., 1967; Bruce and Blaese, 1974). In most instances, the paraprotein is an IgG.

X-ray studies may reveal chronic lung disease. Subperiosteal hemorrhage is seen occasionally. Decreased lymphoid tissue of the posterior pharynx on lateral films of the skull occurs in this and other primary immunodeficiencies.

The primary pathology is found in the thymus and lymphoid tissue, although the degree of involvement varies considerably. A gradual loss of cellular elements occurs in the thymus and lymphoid organs (Cooper et al., 1968). Lymph nodes from young patients with WAS show only slight depletion of thymic-dependent and thymic-independent areas, and follicular formation is poor or nonexistent. Figures 12–18 and 12–19 compare lymph node biopsy specimens from siblings 4 and 8 years old. The lymphoid tissues and follicles of the gastrointestinal tract are usually normal (Cooper et al., 1968), although gastrointestinal lymphoid depletion may occur (Wolff and Bertucio, 1957).

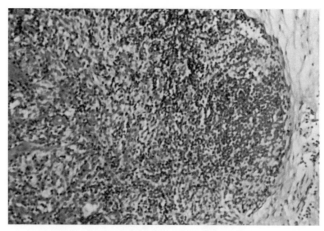

Figure 12–18. A lymph node biopsy specimen taken from a 4-year-old patient with the Wiskott-Aldrich syndrome. There is moderate depletion of lymphoid cells in the thymic-dependent and thymic-independent areas and lack of follicular formation.

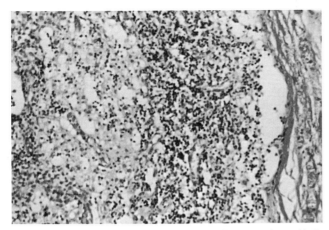

Figure 12–19. Lymph node biopsy specimen from a patient with the Wiskott-Aldrich syndrome. The patient is the older brother (age 8 years) of the patient illustrated in Figure 12–18. There is a greater degree of lymphoid depletion and no evidence of follicular formation.

A variable degree of thymic hypoplasia is present in WAS. Cooper and coworkers (1968) described normal thymic architecture, normal corticomedullary differentiation, and Hassall's corpuscles, despite a small thymus. Wolff (1967) described one patient with a hypoplastic thymus and another with an atrophic thymus. These differences are probably related to the degree of lymphoid involution present, which is usually a function of time.

As mentioned previously, lymphocytes in patients with WAS show absent or deficient expression of CD43. WAS lymphocytes uniformly fail to proliferate in response to periodate, a mitogenic agent reactive with sialic acid residues.

Diagnosis

The diagnosis of WAS is made in male infants with recurrent infections, eczema, thrombocytopenia, and bleeding episodes associated with increased levels of serum IgA and IgE, decreased levels of serum IgM, absent isohemagglutinins, and poor antibody responses to polysaccharide antigens. Because normal infants may not respond to polysaccharide antigens, this assay cannot be used for diagnosis until a child is 18 months of age. Platelet sizing may be useful in the diagnosis of WAS in infancy, inasmuch as small platelets are found almost exclusively in WAS (Murphy et al., 1972). Decreased expression of CD43 on T cells is the outstanding lymphocyte characteristic.

Carrier detection is possible by X-chromosome inactivation analysis (Puck et al., 1990b). In utero diagnosis and carrier detection are facilitated by direct testing, now that the WASP gene has been defined (Derry et al., 1994).

Treatment

The acute bleeding episodes of patients with WAS usually respond to transfusions of fresh platelets, which should be irradiated with 30 Gy to prevent graft-ver-

sus-host reactions. Splenectomy may decrease the bleeding tendency but may result in increased risk of fulminant septicemia (Huntley and Dees, 1957). Lum and coworkers (1980) report that continuous prophylactic antibodies prevented sepsis in splenectomized WAS patients. The risk-benefit ratio of splenectomy should be considered carefully, since bleeding in patients decreases with advancing age. Platelet counts were nearly or completely normal in 17 of 18 splenectomized patients (Lum et al., 1980). Of the 17, 7 were alive with a mean survival of 8 years. None of the patients who died was receiving prophylactic antibiotics, except one whose therapy was stopped 10 days before his death.

In 1968, reconstitution was achieved in a patient by bone marrow transplantation using immunosuppression (Bach et al., 1968). Only T-cell reconstitution was achieved, and thrombocytopenia persisted. However, 20 years later, the patient received a retransplant with complete reconstitution of his immune defect and correction of the thrombocytopenia (Rimm and Rappeport, 1990). Parkman and colleagues (1978) successfully performed a transplantion for two additional patients with WAS. With the use of cytosine arabinoside and cyclophosphamide, only temporary T-lymphocyte engraftment was achieved. Finally, with administration of antithymocyte serum, total-body irradiation, and procarbazine, engraftment and complete immunologic and hematologic reconstitution were achieved. The successful establishment of lymphocyte and hematopoietic cell lines indicates that there is no intrinsic fault of the bone marrow microenvironment.

Although transplants from haploidentical donors yield nearly the same results as HLA-identical donors in most forms of combined immunodeficiency, the results in Wiskott-Aldrich syndrome are clearly inferior. The survival in matched bone marrow transplants in WAS approaches 80%, whereas only 20% to 25% of haploidentical BMT recipients survive (Fischer et al., 1986; Buckley, 1987; O'Reilly et al., 1989; Brochstein et al., 1991). Two reports show results equal to those of matched donors, however (Rumelhart et al., 1990; Fischer et al., 1991b). For unknown reasons, WAS recipients of T-depleted marrow have an extraordinary incidence of B-cell lymphoma which in part accounts for the poor success (Fischer et al., 1991a). Other factors include a high rate of nonengraftment and severe graft-versus-host disease (Brochstein et al., 1991). The recent definition of the WAS gene—WASP—should enhance the possibility for gene replacement in the future (Derry et al., 1994).

Herpes simplex and varicella infections respond to acyclovir therapy. Intravenous gamma globulin therapy may be successful in preventing both viral and bacterial infections. Doses of 100 to 400 mg/kg, given on a monthly basis, are employed.

Antibiotics should be given promptly with each infection to prevent complications and overwhelming sepsis with *Streptococcus pneumoniae, Haemophilus influenzae,* and certain gram-negative organisms. Some patients may need continuous antibiotics.

Systemic steroids should be avoided unless they are

needed to control autoimmune hemolytic anemia or severe bleeding. Local steroids, particularly the fluorinated preparations, are often necessary to control severe eczema.

Prognosis

The average age at death in nontransplanted patients was previously reported as 3½ years (Huntley and Dees, 1957; Cooper et al., 1968). In a review of Sullivan and coworkers (1994), the median age of living patients was reported as 11 years; 16 patients were older than 18 years. The average longevity for untreated patients has been extended to 8 years. The causes of death have remained the same over the years: bleeding (23%), infection (44%), and malignancy (26%). Deaths as a consequence of BMT are excluded from these statistics.

If immunologic reconstitution is successful, the outlook for prolonged life is excellent. Whether the marrow transplant diminishes the risk of hematopoietic malignancies is not known; no such cases have been reported in the patients whose immune systems have been successfully reconstituted. Gene replacement may become an option in the future.

ATAXIA-TELANGIECTASIA

Ataxia-telangiectasia (AT) is an autosomal recessive disorder characterized by telangiectasia, progressive ataxia, sinopulmonary infections, hypersensitivity to ionizing radiation, and a combined immunodeficiency, usually consisting of selective IgA and IgG2 deficiencies, cutaneous anergy, and often depressed but not absent in vitro lymphocyte responsiveness.

Historical Aspects

In 1926, Syllaba and Henner described three siblings, two males and one female, 16 to 20 years of age, who had ataxia and telangiectasia as well as strabismus, athetosis, muscle weakness, goiter, pigmentation of the skin, and hypoplastic genitalia. Recurrent infections were not recorded despite the advanced age of the patients. These authors mentioned a similar case studied by Oppenheim and Vogt and termed the syndrome *Vogt's disease*. Another single nonfamilial case was reported by Louis-Bar in 1941 with typical ataxia, choreoathetosis, and oculocutaneous telangiectasia. The same patient, subsequently followed up by Van Bogaert, expired at age 27 (Martin et al., 1956). In 1957, Wells and Shy described a progressive familial choreoathetosis with oculocutaneous telangiectasia.

The disease was established as a distinct clinicopathologic entity by Boder and Sedgwick (1957), who assigned the term "ataxia-telangiectasia" to the syndrome. They called attention to the recurrent sinopulmonary infections and outlined the distinctive aspects of the disease compared with other forms of ataxia. They also suggested that an immunologic defect might be responsible for recurrent infections. In one

case at autopsy, they noted absence of the thymus and ovaries.

Absence of serum IgA was first described by Thieffry and colleagues (1961). Defective cell-mediated immunity was described by several investigators (Fireman et al., 1964; Young et al., 1964; Peterson et al., 1966). Deficiency of IgE was demonstrated by Ammann and coworkers (1969a) and by Polmar and others (1972). More recently, IgG2 deficiency has been noted in the majority of patients (Rivat-Piran et al., 1981; Oxelius et al., 1982; Gatti et al., 1982).

The widespread pathologic changes in ataxia-telangiectasia became apparent with reports of ovarian dysgenesis (Boder and Sedgwick, 1957, 1963; Aguilar et al., 1968) and testicular atrophy in some patients (Strich, 1966; Aguilar et al., 1968). Other endocrine findings, including abnormalities of the anterior pituitary (Bowden et al., 1963; Strich, 1966; Aguilar et al., 1968), deficient growth hormone response (Ammann et al., 1969b), and an unusual form of insulin-resistant diabetes (Schalch et al., 1970), have also been reported.

In addition to the loss of Purkinje cells in the cerebellum, degenerative lesions have been found in other areas of the central nervous system, along with demyelination of the posterior white columns (Strich, 1966; Centerwall and Centerwall, 1966; Solitare and Lopez, 1967; Aguilar et al., 1968; Terplan and Krauss, 1969). Muscle involvement was reported by Strich (1966), Hassler (1967), and Goodman and colleagues (1969).

Pathogenesis

Although a spectrum of defects in cell-mediated immunity, antibody-mediated immunity, or both, are detected in more than 70% of patients with AT (Peterson et al., 1966; Epstein et al., 1966; Ammann et al., 1969a), it is impossible to define a basic or consistent immunologic defect in this disorder. Any theory concerning the etiology of AT must explain the multisystem involvement, the variable onset of symptoms, and the apparent progression of the disease with time. Peterson and coworkers (1966) suggested that the thymic defect, the telangiectasia, and the gonadal abnormalities might be related to defective embryogenesis of the mesenchyme. This does not explain the consistent involvement of the central nervous system (CNS), where the lesions are degenerative (Gatti et al., 1985) and unassociated with vascular abnormalities. Analysis of collagen from two patients with AT revealed a deficiency of hydroxylysine, suggesting a basic structural component defect (McReynolds et al., 1976).

The endocrine and thymic abnormalities may result from deficiencies of trophic hormones. Lesions in the anterior pituitary and hypothalamus have been described by Bowden and colleagues (1963), Strich (1966), and Aguilar and coworkers (1968). Snell-Bagg dwarf mice are deficient in growth hormone and have immunologic abnormalities (Baroni et al., 1967). However, growth hormone–deficient patients have no immunologic abnormalities, and patients with AT have no consistent growth hormone abnormalities (Ammann et al., 1969b).

The defect in AT may also be a basic thymic abnormality leading to autoimmunity, recurrent infection, or both. Ammann and Hong (1971) found an increased incidence of autoantibodies against endocrine organs and other affected organs, including liver, stomach (parietal cells), and muscle. The degenerative CNS lesions also suggest an autoimmune process (Strich, 1966; Centerwall and Centerwall, 1966; Solitare and Lopez, 1967; Hassler, 1967; Aguilar et al., 1968; Terplan and Kraus, 1969). The presence of an autoimmune process in AT directed against thymus and brain receives support from Kaufman and Miller's (1977) demonstration of a cross-reacting, complement-dependent, cytotoxic IgM serum antibody to both T cells and brain cells.

The elevated alpha-fetoprotein (AFP) in most patients with AT, without evidence of malignancy or chronic liver disease, suggested to Waldmann and McIntire (1972) that the basic defect was one of organ differentiation and maturation. Elevated levels of alpha-fetoprotein are not present in other immunodeficiency disorders, except in an occasional patient with adenosine deaminase (ADA) deficiency and in the elderly. Lectin column chromatography studies indicate that the type of AFP present in the sera of patients with AT is associated with development of liver, not that of yolk sac, tumors (Ishiguro et al., 1986).

Because many cell lineages express the AT defect, it is appropriate to consider that the AT gene may be a housekeeping gene, probably well conserved in phylogeny. Although the gene's impact may be great at the cell surface, its basic site of action is most likely on nuclear DNA. A DNA-binding protein such as a transcription factor may affect many systems at once, including even the expression of a gene such as the AFP gene located on another chromosome (see later). Other DNA-interacting candidate gene products include helicases, polymerases, ligases, topoisomerases, and recombinases. The AT gene product may be a signal transducer; Paterson and Mirzayans (1993) have reported that the radiosensitivity of certain AT cells can be complemented by transfer of soluble cytoplasmic factors.

Patients with ataxia-telangiectasia are extremely sensitive to ionizing radiation (Gotoff et al., 1967; Morgan et al., 1968; Harris and Seeler, 1973). Taylor and associates (1975) demonstrated impaired sensitivity of AT fibroblasts to radiation. Paterson and Mirzayans (1993) postulated a deficiency of functional endonuclease, with inability to initiate excision and repair of DNA; however, this has not been substantiated by others. Defective DNA metabolism after mitomycin-C treatment of cells in patients with AT has also been demonstrated (Hoar and Sargent, 1976). Painter and Young (1980) observed that the normal mitotic delay seen during the cell cycle was shortened in AT cells and suggested that the chromosomal breakage might result from failure of the cells to repair DNA damage before replication.

Kastan and colleagues (1992) showed that the increase in p53 normally observed after irradiating cells with x-rays is not observed in the fibroblasts. p53 is part of a cell cycle checkpoint pathway that allows time for DNA repair and limits the transmission of genetic damage. This might explain the shortened mitotic delay. This faulty pathway may also play a role in the increased incidence of malignancy in patients with AT.

Another consequence of defective cell cycle checkpoint control might be abnormal T-cell receptor (TCR) gene rearrangement or isotype switching as a consequence of damaged DNA replication. This would account for the immunoglobulin deficiencies, low frequencies of $\alpha\beta$ TCR T cells, and high frequency of T cells with interlocus TCRs and chromosome translocations (Lipkowitz et al., 1990; Meyn, 1993). Other cell cycle abnormalities in AT cells have been described (Lavin, 1993; Painter, 1993); however, these changes may simply be another manifestation of the radiation hypersensitivity.

Joncas and coworkers (1977) reported an increased incidence of Epstein-Barr virus (EBV) antibodies in patients with AT. Berkel and colleagues (1984) extended these observations, reporting elevated titers to viral capsid antigen and early antigen but low titers to nuclear antigen. EBV antibodies are also associated with infectious mononucleosis, nasopharyngeal tumors, and Burkitt's lymphoma (Henle et al., 1974).

The variability of the immunologic defects described in AT may result from immunologic attrition (i.e., progressive deterioration with time). This is documented in 10 patients with AT followed for more than 4 years by Ammann and colleagues (1969a). Although two patients showed an increase in serum IgA, eight showed a decrease. Several patients had progressive lymphopenia. Further evidence for immunologic attrition was provided by Cawley and Schenken (1970) in a 5-year study of a patient. Initially, immunoglobulins and lymphocyte counts were normal; subsequently, IgM levels increased and IgA levels decreased. After 5 years, at age 9, IgA disappeared, IgG levels were markedly decreased, IgM became monoclonal, and lymphopenia developed. The cause of immunologic attrition in AT is not known but may be related to "exhaustion" of the immunologic system as a result of chronic infection or to a more basic defect. AFP levels also tend to rise with age.

Family studies suggest a simple autosomal inheritance. In consanguineous matings, autosomal recessive inheritance has been apparent (Tadjoedin and Fraser, 1965; Gimeno et al., 1969). The syndrome has been described in whites, blacks (Haerer et al., 1969), and Asians (Hayakawa et al., 1968; Hatsu and Uno, 1969); it has been reported from Spain (Gimeno et al., 1969), Japan (Hayakawa et al., 1968; Hatsu and Uno, 1969), China (Liang, 1988), India (Dogra and Manchanda, 1967), South Africa (Wagstaff and Joffe, 1969), Argentina (Ammann et al., 1969c), Costa Rica (Porras et al., 1993), Turkey (Ersoy and Berkel, 1974), Europe (Smeby, 1966; Hassler, 1967; Gropp and Flatz, 1967; Hanicki et al., 1967), and the United States (Swift et al., 1986).

At least five complementation groups have been defined (Jaspers et al., 1984, 1988; Bridges et al., 1985). The presence of multiple complementation groups has been taken as evidence for multiple AT genes. However, two lines of evidence caution against this interpretation.

First, several laboratories have now been able to identify AT-complementing genes on different chromosomes (Kapp et al., 1992; Meyn et al., 1993), indicating that complementation, as measured by at least five different end points, can be accomplished by more than just the gene (or genes) that causes AT.

Second, genetic analyses of AT families demonstrate linkage of only a single 2- to 4-centimorgan (cM) region (chromosome 11q22.3–23.1) in 148 of 150 families from nine different countries (Lange et al., 1993). Savitsky and colleagues (1995) have identified a 12 kilobase gene on chromosome 11q 22-23 termed *ATM* (ataxia-telangiectasia mutated) by positional cloning that was found mutated in AT patients from all complementation groups, indicating that it is the sole gene responsible for AT. This discovery may permit identification of AT heterozygotes (carriers), who are at increased risk for cancer.

Clinical Manifestations

There is variability in the time of onset of symptoms (Boder and Sedgwick, 1963; Peterson et al., 1966; Fiorrili et al., 1983). In most patients, ataxia develops during infancy; in others, ataxia may be delayed until 4 or 5 years of age. In all patients, ataxia progresses slowly but relentlessly to severe disability. The ataxia is initially cerebellar in form, involving posture and gait and subsequently including movements of intention (Boder and Sedgwick, 1963). Speech becomes increasingly slurred. Variable choreoathetoid or tic-like movements are present (Syllaba and Henner, 1926; Louis-Bar, 1941; Boder and Sedgwick, 1957).

Eye movements provide a reliable diagnostic finding; apraxia is almost always present. The patient is asked to follow a pencil moving rapidly across the visual field. Typically, the patient moves the entire head faster than the eyes. Other eye movements cause dysconjugate gaze, simulating ophthalmoplegia (Syllaba and Henner, 1926; Louis-Bar, 1941; Boder and Sedgwick, 1957).

Drooling, strabismus, and a mask-like facies are seen. Muscle weakness appears late in AT and is associated with muscle atrophy (Strich, 1966; Hassler, 1967; Goodman et al., 1969).

Mental retardation is present in some patients (Boder and Sedgwick, 1963; Karpati et al., 1965; Solitare and Lopez, 1967; Hatsu and Uno, 1969), whereas most others are of normal intelligence and live functional lives well into their 20s or 30s despite severe physical handicaps. On neurologic examination, cerebellar signs are prominent, as are extrapyramidal and posterior column signs (Syllaba and Henner, 1926; Aguilar et al., 1968; Goodman et al, 1969). Reflexes are diminished, and muscle weakness may be prominent (Goodman et al., 1969). Sensory involvement is uncommon.

Telangiectasia occurs initially on the bulbar conjunctivae and may manifest as early as 1 year or as late as 6 years of age (Fig. 12–20). With time, telangiectasia becomes more prominent and appears in other areas, including the lateral aspect of the nose, the ears, the antecubital and popliteal areas, and the dorsa of the hands and feet. However, some patients have very few telangiectasias. Other skin lesions include progressive cutaneous atrophy, simulating scleroderma (Reed et al., 1966), areas of hypopigmentation and hyperpigmentation, hypertrichosis, atopic dermatitis, nummular eczema, and cutaneous malignancies (Reed et al., 1966). Premature graying of hair and excessive sweating have also been noted (Reed et al., 1966; Aguilar et al., 1968).

Recurrent sinopulmonary infection leading to bronchiectasis is present in many patients (Boder and Sedgwick, 1957; Peterson et al., 1966; Ammann et al., 1969a); it may be the presenting complaint prior to ataxia or telangiectasia. The susceptibility to infection encompasses both viral and bacterial agents, but unlike other immunodeficiency diseases, infections with opportunistic microorganisms are rarely encountered in AT patients (Roifman and Gelfand, 1984). In addition, the severity of sinopulmonary infections varies from country to country, suggesting that pulmonary hygiene and the availability of medical care and antibiotics may play a role in the overall clinical picture.

Patients who survive beyond puberty may not develop secondary sex characteristics (Strich, 1966; Solitare and Lopez, 1967; Ammann et al., 1969b). Menstruation in some female patients may begin, but it usually becomes irregular and often ceases prematurely. Some males have testicular atrophy (Syllaba and Henner, 1926; Strich, 1966; Aguilar et al., 1968). Growth failure may occur with progression of the disease (Dunn et al., 1964; Ammann et al., 1969b). However, most patients grow to normal size and secondary sex characteristics develop. It is not known whether these patients are capable of reproducing; no offspring of bona fide AT homozygotes are known.

Bastianon and associates (1993) performed echocardiography in 11 patients and found cardiac anomalies in 5. Mitral valve prolapse was found in four patients and aortic root dilatation in one. In three of the four patients with mitral valve prolapse, mitral valve regurgitation was present; in one of the three there was also mild pulmonary hypertension.

Numerous malignancies have been reported. The

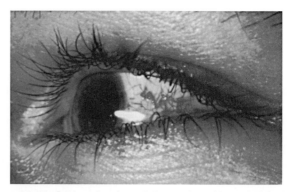

Figure 12–20. Ocular telangiectasis in a patient with ataxia-telangiectasia.

most common is lymphosarcoma (Peterson et al., 1966; Smeby, 1966; Solitare and Lopez, 1967; Harley et al., 1967), but Hodgkin's disease (Boder and Sedgwick, 1963; Harris and Seeler, 1973), leukemia (Harley et al., 1967), adenocarcinoma (Haerer et al., 1969), gonadoblastoma (Goldsmith and Hart, 1975), reticulum cell carcinoma (Feigin et al., 1970), medulloblastoma (Solitare and Lopez, 1967), and dysgerminoma (Solitare and Lopez, 1967) have also been reported. Both B cell and T-cell lymphomas have been observed. As patients with AT live longer, the spectrum of cancers may be changing, with more nonlymphoid types observed. Of the patients who have died, 38% have experienced cancer (Swift, 1984).

Family members of patients may also be at increased risk for development of malignancy. Swift and colleagues (1976) studied 27 family members of patients with AT and found 59 deaths from malignant neoplasms compared with an expected incidence of 43 (P < .02). The incidence of ovarian, gastric, and biliary carcinoma, as well as leukemia, was increased in the families. These data have been subsequently expanded to include 150 additional families in the United States. The risk is approximately eightfold for all cancers; female AT carriers are at a fivefold risk for breast cancer (Swift et al., 1991). Breast cancer has also been observed in several AT homozygotes. In Costa Rica, many families with AT include members with gastric carcinoma (Porras et al., 1993); however, Costa Rica has one of the highest instances of gastric carcinoma in the world. An increased incidence of gastric carcinomas in AT family members has also been reported by Chessa and coworkers (1994).

It is convenient to classify the patients in groupings that reflect the clinical heterogeneity (Lange et al., 1993).

- Type I is the classic syndrome with all manifestations described above.
- Type II patients lack some of the typical findings but show radiosensitivity.
- Type III patients have the classic clinical findings but are not radiosensitive.
- Type IV patients show only some clinical features and are not radiosensitive.

Several methods are available to test radiosensitivity (Huo et al., 1994).

Nijmegen breakage syndrome (NBS) is a related disorder that does not include either ataxia or telangiectasia; however, these patients are radiosensitive and show translocations involving the same sites as AT. (See section titled Nijmegen Breakage Sydrome.) NBS patients are cancer-prone, immunodeficient, microcephalic, and often mentally retarded (Weemaes et al., 1981).

In 1989, Curry and colleagues described twins of Mexican descent who had ataxia, telangiectasia, elevated alpha-fetoprotein, and phenotypic AT (AT$_{Fresno}$). Their fibroblasts corrected all complementation groups of AT but not those of NBS, implying that AT$_{Fresno}$ is caused by the same gene as NBS. Limited data suggest that both AT$_{Fresno}$ and NBS localize to chromosome 11q22–23 (Gatti et al., 1988).

Laboratory Findings

The peripheral blood count usually reveals lymphopenia and eosinophilia. Granulocytopenia has also been described (Feigin et al., 1970). The chest x-ray may reveal chronic lung disease and thymic shadow is usually absent. Sinus x-rays show opacified sinuses.

IgA deficiency is found in about 70% of the patients (Young et al., 1964; Peterson et al., 1966; Epstein et al., 1966; Ammann et al., 1969a). A variety of other abnormalities have been described, including elevated IgA levels (Young et al., 1964; Peterson et al., 1966), decreased IgG levels (Peterson et al., 1966; Gimeno et al., 1969), decreased IgG, IgM, and IgA levels (Peterson et al., 1966; Ammann et al., 1969a), decreased IgE levels (Ammann et al., 1969a; Polmar et al., 1972), decreased IgG and IgA levels (Peterson et al., 1966; Cawley and Schenken, 1970), and IgG2 or combined IgG2 or combined IgG2/IgG4 subclass deficiency (Gatti et al., 1982, Rivat-Peran et al., 1981; Oxelius et al., 1982; Aucouturier et al., 1987).

Antibody responses to viral and bacterial antigens may be deficient (Eisen et al., 1965; Peterson et al., 1966). There is an increased frequency of autoantibodies, including antibodies to IgA and IgG (Strober et al., 1968; Ammann and Hong, 1971).

T-cell immunity is abnormal in about 60% of AT patients. This was first demonstrated by negative delayed hypersensitivity skin tests (Eisen et al., 1965; Peterson et al., 1966; Epstein et al., 1966; Ammann et al., 1969a). The response of peripheral lymphocytes to phytohemagglutinin (PHA) and to specific antigens often is abnormal (Leiken et al., 1966; McFarlin and Oppenheim, 1969). In addition, McFarlin and Oppenheim (1969) have shown a serum inhibitor of transformation of normal lymphocytes.

In addition to reduced proportions of CD4$^+$ cells (Fiorilli et al., 1983), other disturbances of T-cell distribution have been observed. T cells bearing the $\alpha\beta$ T-cell receptor are diminished in favor of $\gamma\delta$ T-cells (Carbonari et al., 1990). CD4$^+$/CD45RA$^+$ lymphocytes (naive) are diminished (Paganelli et al., 1992). Also, an excessive number (70 times normal) of hybrid T-cell receptors composed of TCR-γ variable and TCR-β joining sequences is found in AT patients (Lipkowitz et al, 1990).

Excessive chromosomal breakage has been reported (Gropp and Flatz, 1967), but such studies are limited by the difficulty in inducing AT lymphocytes to proliferate in tissue culture. Reciprocal translocations involving four common breakpoint sites—14q32, 14q12, 7q35, and 7p12—have been noted in lymphocytes (McCaw et al., 1975; Aurias et al., 1980; Kojis et al., 1992). These breakpoints are somatic, not inherited, and correspond with the sites of gene complexes for the immunoglobulin heavy chains and the T-cell receptor chains, alpha, beta, and gamma, respectively. Translocations involving the sites of the two remaining gene complexes that undergo somatic recombinant DNA rearrangements before expression—Ig-κ on chromosome 2p12 and Ig-λ on chromosome 22q11—have also been observed in AT patients (Gatti et al., 1985). Approximately 10% of peripheral lymphocytes show such translocations; fibroblasts show only random chromosomal aberrations (Kojis et al., 1992). Translocations or deletions involving the site of the AT gene at chromosome 11q22.3–23.1 have not been observed.

In one patient, a 14q translocation was identified in leukemic cells. Hecht and coworkers (1973) noted that 1% to 2% of the lymphocytes of an AT patient had a translocation of both 14 chromosomes; after 52 months, this increased to 56% to 78%. Transient clonality of lymphocyte subpopulations has also been observed in other AT patients (Al Saadi et al., 1980; Beatty et al., 1986; Taylor et al., 1993).

There can be decreased urinary excretion of 17-ketosteroids and increased excretion of urinary follicle-stimulating hormone (Dunn et al., 1964; Karpati et al., 1965; Ammann et al., 1969b). Several patients have shown abnormal responses to insulin-induced hypoglycemia (Schalch et al., 1970). This type of insulin-resistant diabetes is also seen in pregnancy and acromegaly. Hyperglycemia and absence of ketosis have also been described (Schalch et al., 1970). Only a few patients need laboratory investigation of their endocrine systems for routine management, however.

Abnormal liver function has been described (Schalch et al., 1970), and antibodies associated with autoimmune liver disease (anti–smooth muscle and antimitochondrial) were found in two patients (Ammann and Hong, 1971). We have not found hepatitis B surface antigen (HBsAg) in our own series of patients. The elevation of AFP is not correlated with the presence or absence of liver disease or malignancy (Waldmann and McIntire, 1972, Ishiguro et al., 1986).

Dilation of the ventricular system and diffuse cerebral atrophy have been demonstrated by pneumoencephalography (Boder and Sedgwick, 1957; Karpati et al., 1965), as well as nuclear magnetic resonance. Electromyograms show fibrillation potentials indicative of anterior horn cell disease (Goodman et al., 1969). Electroencephalograms are diffusely and nonspecifically abnormal (Karpati et al., 1965). Magnetic resonance imaging reveals cerebellar atrophy (Fig. 12–21) (Sedgwick and Boder, 1991).

Pathology

Pathologic studies of the central nervous system in AT reveal a loss of the Purkinje and granular cell layers in the cerebellum (Boder and Sedgwick, 1957; Strich, 1966; Aguilar et al., 1968). The presence of near-normal numbers of basket cells, which only form around pre-existing Purkinje cells, provides evidence that normal numbers of Purkinje cells are probably present at birth in AT patients and undergo progressive degeneration (Gatti and Vinters, 1984). This correlates with the increasing severity of the cerebellar ataxia and dysarthria. The spinal column shows evidence of anterior horn cell degeneration and posterior column demyelination (Strich, 1966; Centerwall and Centerwall, 1966;

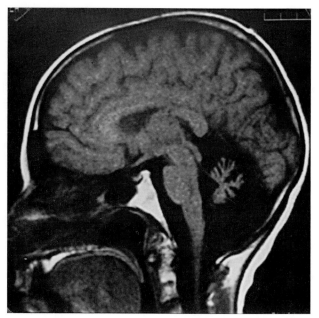

Figure 12–21. Marked cerebellar atrophy of a child with ataxia-telangiectasia on magnetic resonance imaging (MRI) of the brain.

Solitare and Lopez, 1967; Aguilar et al., 1968). Lesions of the thalamus are rare. Degenerative changes in the acidophilic cells of the pituitary are common (Strich, 1966), and lesions of the hypothalamus are occasionally found (Boder and Sedgwick, 1963, Gatti et al., 1991). Skeletal muscle degeneration has been described; in one instance, it was of the central core type (Goodman et al., 1969).

Atrophy of the ovaries or testes has frequently been observed at postmortem examination (Boder and Sedgwick, 1957, 1963; Strich, 1966; Aguilar et al., 1968). The liver may be necrotic with fatty infiltration; the portal areas may be infiltrated with lymphocytes and plasma cells (Schalch et al., 1970; Cawley and Schenken, 1970). There is little or no evidence of fibrosis or chronic hepatitis that would explain the elevated levels of AFP. Diffuse bronchiectasis is common and is usually associated with pneumonia and pulmonary fibrosis (Boder and Sedgwick, 1957; Strich, 1966; Aguilar et al., 1968). Perhaps the most consistent histologic finding is the generalized nucleomegaly or variability in nuclear size (Aguilar et al., 1968). This observation may reflect a defect in cell cycle control, such as the propensity for some AT cells to enter a new cycle without undergoing cell division (Naeim et al., 1994).

The thymus shows various abnormalities (Fireman et al., 1964; Peterson et al., 1966). In some cases, it is atrophic, in others, it is hypoplastic with absence of Hassall's corpuscles and corticomedullary differentiation (Fig. 12–22). Lymphoid tissue is variably hypoplastic. In some patients, abortive follicular formation follows antigenic stimulation (Figs. 12–23 and 12–24).

Genetic Studies

In 1988, linkage analyses localized the AT gene for complementation group A (ATA) to chromosome

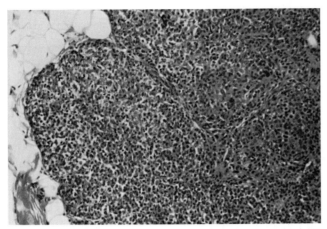

Figure 12–22. Biopsy specimen of a thymus from a patient with ataxia-telangiectasia. Although some degree of cellularity is seen, there is no corticomedullary differentiation and Hassall corpuscles are absent.

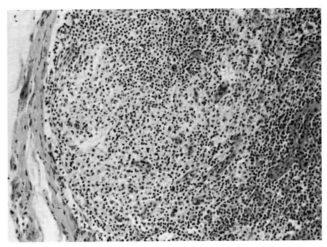

Figure 12–24. A lymph node biopsy specimen taken from an 8-year-old patient with ataxia-telangiectasia. No follicular formation is observed, and there is extensive depletion of lymphocytes in both thymus-dependent and thymus-independent areas. Compare the degree of depletion seen in this specimen with that in Figure 12–22 from a younger patient with ataxia-telangiectasia.

11q22–23 (Gatti et al., 1988). Subsequent analyses have confirmed and refined that localization to a 2- to 4-cM segment defined proximally by the markers STMY, D11S385, and D11S611 and distally by the markers D11S424, D11S132, NCAM, and DRD2x (Sanal et al., 1990; McConville et al., 1990; Foroud et al., 1991). These analyses combined data from all AT families regardless of complementation group assignment. More recently, the highly polymorphic dinucleotide (CA) repeat markers A4(S1819) and A2(S1818) have been used to flank an 850 region K6 (Gatti et al., 1994). The CA markers allow genetic haplotypes to be created, using the polymerase chain reaction; in this way, families with affected children can be analyzed to determine which haplotypes carry the defective AT genes, and genetic counseling can be offered. The recent identification of the *ATM* gene (Savitsky et al., 1995) should simplify heterozygote detection.

Treatment

Although good supportive treatment may prolong survival, there is no cure for this disorder (Perlman, 1993). Propranolol has been used successfully to minimize tremors (Gatti, unpublished data). Infection can be controlled but not eliminated with antibiotics. Gamma globulin is not of proven benefit. In an attempt to provide antibodies of the IgA and IgE classes, infusions of frozen plasma from a single family member were given at 3-week intervals to an AT patient; there was good control of recurrent infection (Ammann et al., 1969c). Such experience with plasma therapy is too limited to draw reliable conclusions; we believe immunoglobulin infusions are unnecessary in most patients. No treatment is effective in halting the CNS degeneration, although some patients have shown temporary improvement with diazepam.

Immune system reconstitution is indicated only when marked susceptibility to infections exists. Fetal thymus transplantation resulted in only transient and incomplete benefit (Lopukhin et al., 1973; Ammann et al., 1975). Because the incidence of severe infections is so variable in AT, bone marrow transplantation is difficult to justify. Also marrow transplantation in AT would require marrow ablation with radiation or radiomimetic drugs for engraftment, a dangerous undertaking in the face of the known radiation sensitivity of these patients. The recent successful accomplishment of a bone marrow transplant in Fanconi anemia, another disease of radiosensitive chromosomes, offers promise for this therapy. Gluckman and colleagues (1983) devised a modified conditioning regimen that is based on low doses of cyclophosphamide and limited thoracoabdominal irradiation. With this preparation regimen, successful transplantation in a patient with Fanconi anemia was accomplished (Gluckman et al., 1989).

Thymosin has been used in a limited fashion in AT. Incubation of AT lymphocytes with thymosin enhances

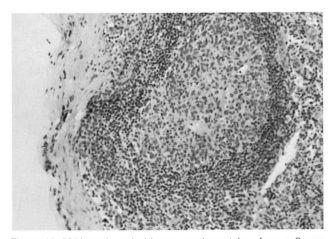

Figure 12–23. Lymph node biopsy specimen taken from a 2-year-old patient with ataxia-telangiectasia. A prominent follicle is observed. There is some depletion of cells in the B-cell-dependent area within the follicles.

T-cell rosettes (Wara et al., 1975). Extended trials of thymosin have not yet been conducted, however.

Because of their undue susceptibility to radiation, treatment of malignancies in patients with AT presents a major challenge. Accordingly, reduced doses of radiation or radiomimetic drugs must be used. Unforeseen complications can occur when the malignancy is the presenting complaint in a family with no previous history of AT.

Prognosis

The clinical variability of AT makes it difficult to state an overall prognosis. There may be early death with malignancy or sinopulmonary infection, or there may be prolonged survival. Some patients have survived into their forties (Goodman et al., 1969; Boder, 1985).

Contributed by Richard A Gatti

NIJMEGEN BREAKAGE SYNDROME

Nijmegen breakage syndrome (NBS) is an autosomal recessive chromosomal instability syndrome characterized by microcephaly with near-normal intelligence, bird-like facies, growth retardation, increased susceptibility to infection, humoral and cellular immunodeficiency, and marked susceptibility to malignancy. It shares many characteristics with ataxia-telangiectasia except that NBS lacks the defining neurocutaneous manifestations indicated in the designation of AT, and the elevated alpha-fetoprotein (AFP) characteristic of AT. The disorder was first described by Weemaes and associates in 1981 in the city of Nijmegen, The Netherlands, in two male siblings whose parents were consanguineous.

Clinical Manifestations

At least 30 patients with NBS have been identified (Weemaes et al., 1994), most of whom are from Eastern Europe, although a case in the United States has been described (Conley et al., 1986). An even sex ratio, consanguinity in one family, and the occurrence of two affected siblings in three families support the hypothesis of an autosomal recessive mode of inheritance.

Patients often have low birth weight for gestational age and persistent, life-long growth retardation. The microcephaly is mild to moderate, but intelligence is normal (in 50%) or slightly to moderately impaired. The face is narrow and bird-like, with a prominent, beaked nose, low-set ears, and a receding chin, but cutaneous depigmentation and café-au-lait spots have been described in some patients.

Most patients with NBS have recurrent respiratory infection, including draining ears, pneumonia, and bronchiectasis (Taalman et al., 1989). Recurrent urinary tract infections are not uncommon. The oldest patient described was a 31-year-old woman with microcephaly, immunodeficiency, and primary amenorrhea (Maraschio et al., 1986).

There is a profound susceptibility to malignancy. In the first 19 patients reported, 7 have developed lymphoma and 1, meningioma (Weemaes et al., 1994). The propensity to malignancy is greater than that in AT.

Laboratory Findings

Immunoglobulin levels are low but not absent, and antibody responses are decreased. IgG subclass and IgD deficiencies have been described (Taalman et al., 1989). T-cell numbers are moderately decreased, and lymphoproliferative responses to antigens and mitogens are reduced but not absent.

On postmortem examination of five patients, the thymus gland was absent or fibrous (Seemanova et al., 1985). AFP levels were consistently normal.

The distinctive laboratory features of NBS are the high percentage of chromosomal breakage and other abnormalities, such as rearrangements and translocations. These often involve chromosomes 7 and 14 at the same bands as found in AT. Their lymphocytes are hypersensitive to ionizing radiation with lessened inhibition of DNA replication, leading to enhanced numbers of chromosomal aberrations.

Complementation studies of fibroblast cell lines from NBS and AT patients indicate that these are distinct disorders (Wegner et al., 1988). Based on such studies, NBS can be divided into two groups, V1 and V2 (Jaspers et al., 1988). Twin girls with phenotypic AT_{Fresno} had complementation studies that indicated a gene defect identical to that of a patient with NBS (Curry et al., 1989) (see section on ataxia-telangiectasia). The location of the NBS gene may map to the AT region of chromosome 11q22 (Gatti et al., 1988).

Treatment and Prognosis

Antibiotics, immunoglobulin, and supportive care may decrease the morbidity of the recurrent infections. Careful observation for malignancy is indicated. Long-term prognosis is guarded. The carrier state has not been defined.

CHRONIC MUCOCUTANEOUS CANDIDIASIS

Chronic mucocutaneous candidiasis is a complex disorder in which patients have persistent or recurrent infections of the skin, nails, and mucous membranes with *Candida* species. In nearly every case, the infections are due to *C. albicans*. The six clinical subgroups of mucocutaneous candidiasis are defined by the extent and location of the infections, genetic factors, and associated disorders, such as polyendocrinopathy, thymomas, autoimmune disorders, and interstitial keratitis (Table 12–4).

Historical Aspects

The first case report is attributed to Thorpe and Handley (1929), who described a child with hypopara-

Table 12–4. Clinical Syndromes of Chronic Mucocutaneous Candidiasis

1. Chronic oral candidiasis
   a. Denture stomatitis
   b. HIV-associated candidiasis
   c. Inhaled corticosteroid therapy
2. Chronic mucocutaneous candidiasis and polyendocrinopathy
3. Chronic localized candidiasis
4. Chronic diffuse candidiasis
5. Chronic candidiasis with thymoma
6. Chronic candidiasis with interstitial keratitis

Abbreviation: HIV = human immunodeficiency virus.

thyroidism and chronic oral candidiasis. In the late 1950s and 1960s, several reports called attention to the presence of chronic candidiasis in patients with hypoparathyroidism, hypoadrenalism, and hypothyroidism (Craig et al., 1955; Whitaker et al., 1956; Hung et al., 1963; Louria et al., 1967; Blizzard and Gibbs, 1968).

Pathogenesis

About this time, reports of immunologic abnormalities in these patients began to appear. Chilgren and coworkers (1967) reported seven patients, aged 6 months to 14 years, who had chronic candidiasis; four patients had endocrinopathies. Three of these patients could not develop delayed type hypersensitivity responses to antigenic extracts from *C. albicans,* and two of these patients did not have anti-*Candida* antibodies in the IgA of their parotid fluids. In 1970, our group described three additional patients (Kirkpatrick et al., 1970). None of the patients could express delayed hypersensitivity to *Candida,* but their responses to other antigens were intact. Lymphocytes from the patients did not have increased thymidine incorporation when they were cultured with *Candida* antigens.

During the 1970s, in vitro tests of cell-mediated immunity were used to further define the immunologic abnormalities in patients with chronic mucocutaneous candidiasis. We described a number of patients whose lymphocytes failed to secrete the lymphokine macrophage migration inhibitory factor (MIF) when they were stimulated with *Candida* extracts (Kirkpatrick et al., 1971a); this finding was quickly confirmed by Lehner and associates (1972) and Valdimarsson and coworkers (1973). Lehner and associates (1972) also noted that peripheral blood lymphocytes from their patients could not be activated to express cytolytic activity against chicken erythrocytes by stimulation with *Candida* extracts.

These findings have led to chronic mucocutaneous candidiasis being classified as an immunodeficiency disease that results from defective function of T lymphocytes. However, as studies from various laboratories are reviewed, it is clear that not all patients have the same immunologic defect and that defects at one of several sites in T cell–mediated immunity may predispose a patient to chronic mucocutaneous candidiasis. The most profound defects are found in patients who develop mucocutaneous candidiasis during infancy and early childhood (Kirkpatrick and Sohnle, 1981) and in patients with extensive candidiasis (Lehner et al., 1972).

Clinical Features

Specific syndromes of chronic mucocutaneous candidiasis are listed in Table 12–5. Patients with chronic oral candidiasis have persistent and recurrent infections of the mucous membranes of the tongue and buccal cavity and usually have perleche. Esophageal candidiasis is uncommon, and the skin and nails are not affected; it is most common in elderly and middle-aged females and has been associated with iron deficiency (Higgs and Wells, 1972). The mucous membranes are covered with a patchy or confluent pseudomembrane that is composed of mycelial-phase *Candida,* inflammatory cells, and debris. The differential diagnosis on these patients should include denture stomatitis, use of inhaled corticosteroids, and HIV infection with immunodeficiency.

The syndrome of chronic mucocutaneous candidiasis with polyendocrinopathy usually begins during infancy with mucous membrane candidiasis and a persistent "diaper rash." The cutaneous infections may become more extensive (Fig. 12–25), and the nails may become involved. It is important to appreciate that the endocrinopathies may develop any time from childhood through adulthood and that patients may have sequential loss of functions of various endocrine organs. A patient with candidiasis who has lost the function of one endocrine organ or who has associated disorders such as alopecia or vitiligo should have regular evaluations of the functions of endocrine organs.

The parathyroids, adrenals, and thyroid are most commonly involved. Females may have impaired ovarian function and infertility. Insulin-dependent diabetes mellitus occurs in approximately 10% of patients. An extensive review of the disorders that occur in patients with the candidiasis-polyendocrinopathy syndrome has been published by Ahonen and associates (1990). They attempted to identify all patients in Finland who had received this diagnosis between 1910 and 1988. The

Table 12–5. Disorders Associated with the Candidiasis-Polyendocrinopathy Syndrome

Disorder	No. Affected Patients/No. Studied
Candidiasis	68/68
Hypoparathyroidism	54/68
Hypoadrenalism	49/68
Hypothyroidism	2/68
Gonadal failure, females	15/25
Gonadal failure, males	4/28
Insulin-dependent diabetes mellitus	8/68
≥1 endocrinopathy	65
≥2 endocrinopathy	41
≥3 endocrinopathy	20

Data from Ahonen P, Myllarniemi S, Sipela I, Perheentupa J. Clinical variation of autoimmune polyendocrinopathy-candidiasis-ectodermal dystrophy (ADECED) in a series of 68 patients. Reprinted with permission from the New England Journal of Medicine 322:1829–1836, 1990.

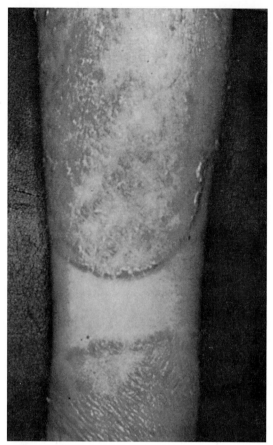

Figure 12–25. Chronic *Candida* infection of the arm in a patient with the granulomatous variety of chronic *Candida* infection. Note the extensive involvement and clearly demarcated borders of uninfected skin.

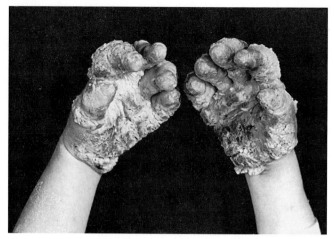

Figure 12–26. An example of the extraordinary hyperkeratosis that characterizes chronic localized mucocutaneous candidiasis.

entry criteria were any two of the following: hypoparathyroidism, hypoadrenalism, and chronic mucocutaneous candidiasis; 68 patients fulfilled the criteria. Their findings illustrate the multiplicity of disorders that are associated with this form of chronic mucocutaneous candidiasis. Fifty-three (78%) of their patients had at least three of the associated components that included candidiasis, hypoparathyroidism, hypoadrenalism, hypogonadism, gastric parietal cell failure, insulin-dependent diabetes mellitus, hypothyroidism, vitiligo, alopecia, hepatitis, intestinal malabsorption, and keratitis. Forty-one patients had at least two endocrinopathies, and three or more endocrine disorders occurred in 20 of the subjects (see Table 12–5). In most of the cases, recurrent candidiasis was the initial event and was present in approximately 50% of the patients by the age of 5 years.

Most studies of pedigrees with the candidiasis-polyendocrinopathy syndrome are suggestive of an autosomal-recessive mode of inheritance. Siblings may have antibodies against endocrine organs even though they do not develop endocrine failure. Thus far, no studies of immunologic or endocrinologic functions in family members have consistently identified carriers. Recently, Aaltonen and associates (1993) reported DNA analyses on members of 15 families with the candidia-

sis-polyendocrinopathy syndrome. They concluded that there was no linkage to the genes coding for the T–cell antigen receptors on chromosomes 7 and 14, the genes coding for immunoglobulin heavy chains (chromosome 14), the gene for the delta chain of CD3 (chromosome 11), or the gene for the alpha chain of CD8 (chromosome 2). These investigators had previously reported that they could not show linkage of the disorder to a single HLA region (Ahonen et al., 1988). However, in the recent report they concluded that there was a fairly high probability (lod score = 3.1) that the gene for the disorder was on chromosome 22 (Aaltonen et al., 1993).

The syndrome of chronic localized candidiasis is unique because the lesions develop marked hyperkeratosis (Fig. 12–26) and may produce cutaneous horn formation (Fig. 12–27). Both sexes are affected equally, and there is no known genetic component.

Patients with chronic diffuse candidiasis have extensive infections of the skin, nails, and mucous membranes. In most reports, only single cases are reported

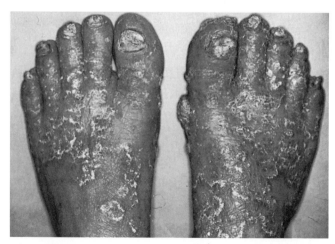

Figure 12–27. Candidiasis of the skin and toenails. Note the cutaneous horn at the base of the right great toe and destruction of the toenails.

in a pedigree, but Wells and associates (1972) have reported eight families in which multiple members were affected. An autosomal dominant mode of inheritance was suggested. A similar family with multiple cases has been reported by Sams and coworkers (1979). Patients with this form of candidiasis do not develop endocrinopathies and may not develop candidiasis until late childhood or adolescence.

The occurrence of chronic mucocutaneous candidiasis in patients with thymomas has been noted in several reports that were summarized in a review (Kirkpatrick and Windhorst, 1979). Both males and females are affected, and no familial predisposition has been described. A unique feature of the disorder is that patients do not develop candidiasis until adulthood or middle age. In addition to candidiasis, many patients with this syndrome also have other thymoma-associated disorders such as myasthenia gravis, aplastic anemia, and hypogammaglobulinemia.

An additional syndrome is the association of chronic mucocutaneous candidiasis with chronic keratitis (Okamoto et al., 1977; Ahonen et al., 1990). It may affect successive members of a pedigree and may be an autosomal dominant trait. Keratopathy was found in 24 of the patients reported by Ahonen and colleagues (1990) and was associated with adrenal insufficiency ($p = 0.048$). The mechanism of the keratitis is unknown, but it may be due to hypersensitivity to *Candida* antigens.

Associated Disorders

In addition to the disorders described previously, patients with chronic mucocutaneous candidiasis are also susceptible to other infectious diseases and to disorders of other organ systems (Table 12–6).

Chipps and associates (1979) noted that patients with chronic candidiasis were susceptible to bacterial and viral infections of the skin and respiratory system. In some cases, the patients developed chronic bronchitis or bronchiectasis, sinusitis, and otitis media. In our review of 58 patients, 26 had significant noncandidal infections (Kirkpatrick and Sohnle, 1981). Recently, Herrod (1990) has described the experience with noncandidal infections in 43 patients at eight medical cen-

ters. Thirty-five patients (81%) had significant infections with a variety of agents that included bacteria, viruses, other fungi, and parasites. Sepsis was common. Seven patients in this series had died, and in each case an infectious disease was the direct cause of death.

Infections with dermatophytes coexist in approximately 20% of patients with chronic mucocutaneous candidiasis (Shama and Kirkpatrick, 1980). These infections may not be appreciated unless cultures are done or potassium hydroxide preparations are studied. There are instances in which failure to recognize a dermatophyte infection has led the physician to incorrectly conclude that his patient has "candidiasis" that is resistant to antifungal drugs.

In addition to their obvious cosmetic significance, vitiligo and alopecia may be important for identification of patients who may develop endocrinopathies. Dysplasia of the dental enamel is a common finding in patients with chronic candidiasis. It was present in 77% of the evaluable patients reported by Ahonen and colleagues (1990) and in 60% of our patients (Kirkpatrick and Sohnle, 1981). The mechanism is unknown, but it does not seem to be related to periodontal disease or to metabolic disorders, such as hypoparathyroidism.

While uncommon, intestinal malabsorption may be a cause of annoying symptoms and the basis for chronic iron deficiency. Patients with parietal cell atrophy may become deficient in Vitamin B_{12}. Little is known about the etiology of hepatitis in candidiasis patients except that it seems to be associated with circulating immune complexes. Hepatitis can lead to liver failure and death.

In addition to the autoimmune endocrinopathies that regularly accompany some syndromes of chronic mucocutaneous candidiasis, other autoimmune disorders are also often associated. The most common is autoimmune hemolytic anemia, present in 4 of 43 patients described by Herrod (1990) and in 3 additional patients reported by Oyefare and associates (1994). Other autoimmune disorders that have been reported include immune thrombocytopenic purpura, autoimmune neutropenia, pernicious anemia, chronic active hepatitis, and juvenile rheumatoid arthritis.

Disorders of other organ systems have been described, but they are infrequent and it is not certain if these events are incidental or components of the syndrome of chronic mucocutaneous candidiasis.

Neoplastic diseases have been described in seven patients with chronic mucocutaneous candidiasis. In six the tumors involved the buccal cavity and in one, the esophagus. Thymomas have been mentioned previously. In the 27 patients with candidiasis and thymoma, 11 of the tumors were malignant and 9 were benign; the others were not described (Kirkpatrick and Windhorst, 1979).

Immunologic Features

T-Cell Function

The predisposition to chronic or recurrent infections of the skin, nails, and mucous membranes with *C.*

Table 12–6. Disorders That May Accompany Chronic Mucocutaneous Candidiasis

Infectious diseases	Hematologic Disorders
Dermatophytosis	Aplastic anemia
Viral infections	Hemolytic anemia
Bacterial infections	Thrombocytopenia
	Neutropenia
Ectodermal Disorders	
Vitiligo	**Musculoskeletal Disorders**
Alopecia	Myopathy
Enamel dysplasia	
	Cancer
Gastrointestinal Disorders	
Malabsorption	
Iron deficiency	
Hepatitis	
Parietal cell failure	

albicans is usually associated with impaired T-lympho-cyte function. However, when patients are subjected to comprehensive evaluations of immunologic functions, a great deal of functional heterogeneity is revealed (Table 12–7).

The early evidence for an association between candidiasis and deficient T-cell function came from clinical observations in patients with syndromes of severe combined immunodeficiency (SCID) or patients with the DiGeorge anomaly (Ammann and Hong, 1989). Patients with these disorders usually have chronic oral candidiasis and may develop candidiasis of the skin and nails. They often are lymphopenic with decreased numbers of T lymphocytes in the peripheral blood (group 1, Table 12–7). Their blood lymphocytes have poor or absent responses to antigens, including *Candida*, and to mitogens such as phytohemagglutinin both for proliferation and for lymphokine secretion. The patients are unable to express delayed type cutaneous hypersensitivity (anergy). This immunologic profile is seen in patients with disorders such as the DiGeorge syndrome, deficiency of purine nucleoside phosphorylase, SCID, infections with the human immunodeficiency virus (HIV), and defects in the T-lymphocyte receptors or signal transduction mechanisms (Arniaz-Villena, et al., 1992b).

Patients in immunologic group 2 have normal numbers of T lymphocytes and normal T-cell subset distribution. Activation of their lymphocytes with mitogens results in normal proliferation and normal cytokine secretion, but when their lymphocytes are activated with an antigen, including *Candida,* only feeble or absent responses are observed. These patients are also unable to express delayed cutaneous hypersensitivity (i.e., are anergic).

The immunologic profile in group 3 is found in approximately 20% of patients with chronic mucocutaneous candidiasis. Their T lymphocytes have normal proliferative responses to mitogens and antigens but do not secrete lymphokines in response to antigens, and do not develop delayed type hypersensitivity.

Patients in groups 4 and 5 are not anergic; they can express delayed hypersensitivity to antigens such as tetanus toxoid, streptococcal proteins, and the mumps skin test antigen but are anergic to *Candida.* Their T lymphocytes do not secrete lymphokines in response

to stimulation with *Candida.* Patients in group 5 differ in that they have normal lymphocyte proliferation responses to *Candida.*

Patients with the immunologic profile of group 6 were first reported by Valdimarsson and associates (1973). Their T lymphocytes respond to activation with *Candida* by secreting MIF, but they do not have proliferation responses. In spite of apparently normal lymphokine production, the patients do not develop delayed hypersensitivity to *Candida.*

Some patients in this group have serum factors that inhibit proliferation responses by T lymphocytes from normal *Candida*-sensitive subjects (Paterson et al., 1971; Lehner et al., 1972; Valdimarsson et al., 1973; Kirkpatrick and Smith, 1974; Twomey et al., 1975; Witkin et al., 1983; Lee et al., 1986). There is impressive evidence that the suppressive factor is a product of *Candida* (Fischer et al., 1978; Lee et al., 1986) or a product of the host that is induced by *Candida.* For example, treatment with antifungal drugs leads to disappearance of the inhibitory substance from the patient's serum (Paterson et al., 1971; Kirkpatrick and Smith, 1974), and the inhibitory factor has been removed from serum with a polyvalent anti-*Candida* antiserum (Lee et al., 1986).

The patients in group 7 have chronic candidiasis of the skin, nails, and mucous membranes that is clinically identical to patients in the other groups. However, the immunologic studies that are informative in patients in the other groups are normal in these subjects.

Phagocytic and Monocytic Function

Other defects in host defense mechanisms have been described in some patients with chronic mucocutaneous candidiasis. For example, several groups have described abnormalities of neutrophil functions. Five patients in our series had deficient chemotactic responses of neutrophils and monocytes to endotoxin-activated serum (Kirkpatrick and Sohnle, 1981). Each of these patients also had pyogenic infections of the skin, the respiratory system, or both, and three of the patients had the hyper-IgE syndrome. Djawari and colleagues (1978) reported five patients, including three members of the same family, who had abnormal neutrophil chemotactic responses. The mother and daughter reported by Van Scoy and coworkers. (1975) also had the hyper-

Table 12–7. Patterns of Abnormalities of Cellular Immunity in Patients with Chronic Mucocutaneous Candidiasis

Group	DTH *(Candida)*	T-Cell Number	Lymphocyte Transformation		MIF Production	
			Candida	*Mitogen*	*Candida*	*Mitogen*
1	Anergy*	Few	SN	SN	SN	SN
2	Anergy	N	SN	N	SN	N
3	Anergy	N	N	N	SN	N
4	Negative	N	SN	N	SN	N
5	Negative	N	N	N	SN	N
6	Negative	N	SN	N	N	?
7	Negative	N	N	N	N	N

*No response to any antigen.
Abbreviations: DTH = delayed type hypersensitivity; MIF = migration inhibitory factor; N = normal response; SN = subnormal or absent; ? = unknown value.

IgE syndrome with impaired chemotaxis and chronic mucocutaneous candidiasis. These patients, too, had repeated infections with pyogenic organisms.

Snyderman and associates (1973) reported a patient with chronic candidiasis and abnormal monocyte chemotaxis. Another example of defective monocyte chemotaxis in both in vivo and in vitro assays was reported in two siblings with chronic candidiasis (Yamazaki et al., 1984). Although it is clear that neutrophils may constitute one mechanism of defense against *Candida* and other filamentous fungi, the fact that most candidiasis patients have normal neutrophil functions argues against a major role for defects in neutrophils as the underlying defect. Abnormalities in neutrophil function may be significant in susceptibility of certain patients to infections with pyogenic organisms.

Abnormal antigen presentation was apparently caused by a defect in macrophage function in a patient reported by Twomey and associates (1975). This patient had multiple abnormalities, including a thymoma and aplastic anemia. Impaired antibody-dependent cellular cytotoxicity by monocytes has been found in a few patients (Rosenblatt et al., 1979).

Drew (1973) reported two siblings with abnormal complement function and chronic candidiasis. However, defects in the complement system are not regularly found in patients with the disorder.

B-Lymphocyte Functions

Some patients with chronic mucocutaneous candidiasis also have repeated pyodermas and viral and bacterial infections of the respiratory tract. As discussed previously, in some patients this may be due to abnormalities in neutrophil functions. Recent work has described immunologic abnormalities involving immunoglobulins and antibody responses. Bentur and associates (1991) reported four candidiasis patients who had repeated bacterial infections and severe pulmonary disease. All four patients lacked cell-mediated immunity against *Candida*. For each patient the absolute values of serum IgG, IgA, and IgM were normal, but all four had subnormal values of the subclasses IgG2 and IgG4. Three patients were immunized with pneumococcal vaccine and one also received *H. influenzae b* vaccine. None of the patients made normal antibody responses. In addition, at least three patients with chronic candidiasis have developed hypogammaglobulinemia with subnormal numbers of B lymphocytes during the years of observation (Hong and Kirkpatrick, unpublished).

The multicenter study of Herrod (1990) points out that B-cell defects are not a common feature of chronic candidiasis. Only 3 of his group of 38 patients had abnormally low values of serum IgG and IgA and only 1 patient had isolated IgA deficiency. Nonetheless, patients with candidiasis who also have repeated bacterial or viral infections or both should be evaluated for other defects in their defense systems.

Asplenia

Another abnormality in patients with chronic candidiasis is asplenia. Parker and colleagues (1990) reported three sisters with the candidiasis-polyendocrinopathy syndrome; two had progressive loss of splenic function. All three patients died in adrenal crisis. The discussion mentions three additional patients with the same syndrome who have hyposplenism. Subsequently, Friedman and coworkers (1991) reported that four of nine patients with chronic mucocutaneous candidiasis and polyendocrinopathy had asplenia. The role of this abnormality in susceptibility to sepsis and other infections needs to be defined.

Immunoregulatory Abnormalities

A number of chronic infectious diseases have immunologic abnormalities that are attributed to abnormal regulatory processes. One of the first lines of evidence that certain chronic fungal infections have underlying immunoregulatory defects was presented by Stobo and coworkers (1976). Only one of their 14 patients had chronic mucocutaneous candidiasis. Nonetheless, their finding that freshly collected T lymphocytes from the patients could suppress proliferation responses by autologous precultured T cells was compatible with a role of suppressor T cells in the patients' immune defects. Another study (Arulanantham et al., 1979) used a different assay for suppressor cell activity to study three children with the candidiasis-polyendocrinopathy syndrome, their parents, and three siblings. Two of the patients and one normal sibling had subnormal suppressor cell activity. In spite of these conflicting results, there is evidence that suppressive factors may contribute to the immunologic abnormalities in some patients with recurrent candidiasis. Jorizzo and coworkers (1980) were able to reverse the immunologic abnormalities and achieve clinical benefits in members of a family with chronic mucocutaneous candidiasis. Witkin et al. (1986) concluded that prostaglandin E_2 was an endogenous immunosuppressant in patients with chronic vaginal candidiasis. They were able to correct the subnormal lymphocyte proliferation responses by their patients by adding cyclooxygenase inhibitors to the cultures.

Treatment

Treatment strategies can be divided into the use of antifungal drugs and those directed at the correction of the underlying immunologic abnormalities. Neither approach is totally satisfactory.

Antifungal Agents

Antifungal medication is the cornerstone of all therapeutic regimens for all variants. Mycostatin, available in many forms, is the first line of treatment because of its virtual absence of side effects. Cases not responding to mycostatin will require clotrimazole (Leiken et al., 1976). Delivery to the oral cavity has been facilitated by a troche form of the medication, which can be very effective except in young children and infants (Kirkpatrick and Alling, 1978). Suppositories inserted into a pacifier were utilized successfully by Mansour and Gelfand (1981).

Fluconazole, ketoconazole, and itraconazole are effective oral agents that succeed in cases not responding to the previously mentioned milder approaches. They provide systemic treatment via the oral route and have become the treatment of choice in most patients (Jones et al., 1981; Stavaren and Stiehm, 1986; Dismukes, 1988; Como and Dismukes, 1994). Flucytosine is also available for oral use.

When intravenous therapy becomes necessary owing to the failure of the previously mentioned drugs, fluconazole or miconazole should be used first because they are better tolerated than amphotericin B. Mild transaminase elevations are sometimes seen with these infusions (Fischer et al., 1977). If there is extensive nail involvement, removal of the nails before therapy or a course of oral antifungals will provide synergistic benefit. In refractory conditions, amphotericin B must be used for control. Amphotericin B is moderately toxic, primarily to the kidneys. Tubular defects, primarily manifested by hypokalemia, and decreased glomerular filtration commonly occur and require close monitoring. Chills and fever frequently accompany the infusions; premedication with diphenhydramine, hydrocortisone, and meperidine is helpful in controlling these side effects. Serum electrolytes, creatinine levels, and liver enzymes should be followed regularly. Although the lesions are usually brought under control with intravenous amphotericin B, return of the disease may occur within several weeks after cessation of therapy.

The shortfalls of this approach are that:

1. Antifungal drugs do not correct the immunologic defects that predispose the patients to recurrent candidiasis.

2. Most patients relapse within weeks or months after cessation of antifungal therapy.

3. Development of infections with drug-resistant organisms may occur.

4. Hepatotoxicity may occur in long-term users of these agents.

On the positive side, the antifungal drugs enable the physician to induce remissions and to undertake immunologic investigations in a timely manner and allow patients to make choices about when and what mode of immunologic therapy they prefer.

Immunotherapies

The results of immunologic therapies depend on the nature of the underlying defect. After transplantation of thymic tissue, a patient with the DiGeorge anomaly of congenital absence of the thymus and parathyroids had spontaneous clearing of oral and cutaneous candidiasis (Cleveland et al., 1968). A similar dramatic clearing of cutaneous and oral candidiasis occurred after thymus transplantation in one of our patients with SCID (unpublished). Clinical and immunologic benefits were noted after thymus transplantation in a patient with the candidiasis-polyendocrinopathy syndrome treated by Levy and colleagues (1971). Immunologic benefits after thymus transplantation have been reported by Ballow and Hyman (1977), Ammann and Hong (1989), and Kirkpatrick and coworkers (1976).

Clinical benefits were observed in Ballow's patient but not in Kirkpatrick's.

Thymic peptides have had limited investigations in patients with chronic candidiasis. Clinical responses were reported in two of four treated patients who received thymosin fraction V (Wara and Ammann, 1978). However, it is unlikely that replacement therapy with thymic hormones will have wide application in chronic candidiasis because most patients have normal numbers of mature T lymphocytes and normal concentrations of thymic hormone in their plasma (Kirkpatrick et al., 1978).

Immunotherapy with peripheral blood leukocytes has also induced remissions in patients with chronic mucocutaneous candidiasis. Valdimarsson and associates (1972a) infused leukocytes from a patient's brother. The recipient acquired the ability to express cellular immunity to *Candida,* and at the time of the report (17 months later), the recipient was in remission. Two of our patients received four daily infusions of peripheral leukocytes that were enriched with lymphocytes from a father (Kirkpatrick et al., 1971b) or a brother (Kirkpatrick, unpublished). The first patient acquired cell-mediated immunity against *Candida* and had a complete remission that lasted 8 months. At this time, the cell-mediated immune responses reverted to negative, and the patient relapsed. The second patient did not acquire cellular immunity against *Candida* but had gradual clinical improvement over the ensuing months.

Bone marrow transplantation was used successfully in a 10-year-old girl with chronic mucocutaneous candidiasis who developed severe aplastic anemia at age 9. She was free of both illnesses 2 years following allogeneic bone marrow transplantation (Deeg et al., 1986).

Transfer factors are peptides that are extracted from T lymphocytes. When a transfer factor is given to an immunodeficient recipient, the recipient acquires the ability to express the cell-mediated immune responses of the donor. This effect is antigen-specific (Petersen et al., 1981). The transfer factor enables the recipient to express delayed type hypersensitivity and to produce MIF in response to the antigens to which the donor has cellular immunity (Kirkpatrick et al., 1972).

Candida-specific transfer factors have corrected the immunologic defects in patients with chronic mucocutaneous candidiasis, but this effect is seen only when the transfer factors come from *Candida*-immune donors (Littman et al., 1978; Kirkpatrick and Greenberg, 1979). Clinical responses have been variable, and the best results are observed when the patient is first treated with an antifungal drug to induce a remission and the transfer factor is then used to prevent relapse.

Specific transfer factors have provided benefits in other clinical settings. Beneficial effects of specific transfer factor therapy have been described in patients with recurrent infections with herpes simplex or other viral infections (reviewed in Kirkpatrick, 1988). However, the role for transfer factors in treatment of immunodeficiency diseases is still uncertain.

Contributed by Charles S. Kirkpatrick

IMMUNODEFICIENCY WITH MULTIPLE CARBOXYLASE DEFICIENCY

Immunodeficiency with multiple carboxylase deficiencies is an autosomal recessive disease manifesting in early infancy or early childhood with severe acidosis, neurologic abnormalities, chronic dermatitis, alopecia, *Candida* infection, and systemic infection with bacteria and viruses. All manifestations of the disease respond to treatment with biotin.

Historical Aspects

Biotin-dependent multiple carboxylase deficiency was initially described as a biochemical disorder associated with severe acidosis in early infancy (Roth, 1976; Packman et al., 1981). The infantile form was frequently associated with bacterial infections, including bacteremia and pneumonia. The delayed form of the disease usually occurs after the first year of life and is frequently associated with dermatitis, mucocutaneous candidiasis, alopecia, and keratoconjunctivitis (Cowan et al., 1979; Charles et al., 1979; Thoene et al., 1979). Although both acute and chronic infection was described in this disorder, a specific immunodeficiency was not recognized until 1979 (Cowan et al., 1979). In vitro laboratory studies of T-cell immunity were usually normal, most likely as a consequence of supplemental biotin, a component of the culture medium used to perform immunologic studies. When biotin was depleted from the medium, the immunologic defect became apparent.

Pathogenesis

A variety of carboxylation reactions require biotin as an essential coenzyme. These reactions involve nucleic acid, fatty acid, carbohydrate, and branched-chain amino acid metabolism. Patients have been described with deficiencies of propionyl-CoA carboxylase, β-methylcrotonyl–CoA carboxylase, and pyruvate carboxylase, all of which are biotin-dependent, suggesting an abnormality in biotin transport of intracellular metabolism (Saunders et al., 1979). In some patients, a nutritional deficiency of biotin may occur, resulting in identical clinical and laboratory abnormalities. Nutritional biotin deficiency has been reported under two circumstances: (1) omission of biotin from total parenteral nutrition, or (2) the inclusion of large amounts of raw egg whites (avidin) in the diet (Baugh et al., 1968; Sweetman et al., 1979).

Experimental evidence suggests that biotin regulates immunologic function and, when deficient, is responsible for abnormal antibody formation, decreased T-cell cytotoxicity, and increased susceptibility to infection. Because biotin-dependent carboxylases are responsible for the metabolism of carbohydrates, amino acids, fatty acids, and purines, immunologic function is probably adversely affected by a deficiency in one or more of these pathways. Although large amounts of organic acids accumulate in the urine of these patients, a "toxic" metabolite for T cells has not been identified.

Clinical Manifestations

Infants with the early-onset form of multiple carboxylase deficiency present with severe acidosis, bacterial infections, bacteremia, and pneumonia. In the delayed form, chronic dermatitis, which is most important when surrounding the eyes, is usually present. Alopecia is prominent. *Candida* infection of the involved skin and the mucous membranes is a common finding. Progressive ataxia and dementia become prominent. The late-onset variety is characterized by a gradual onset and frequent episodes of remission. Untreated, all forms of biotin-dependent multiple carboxylase deficiency are fatal. Patients may succumb to acute viral infections, develop acute bacterial infections, or have fatal reactions following immunization with live virus vaccine.

Detailed immunologic evaluations have been performed in only a few patients. Usually, delayed hypersensitivity skin test responses to *Candida* antigen are absent (Cowan et al., 1979). A patient has been described with selective IgA deficiency and abnormal antibody responses following pneumococcal polysaccharide immunization. If T-cell studies are performed by standard laboratory techniques using culture medium supplemented with biotin, a specific immunologic defect may not be detected. T-cell functional studies should be performed in a culture medium without supplemental biotin.

Other laboratory abnormalities reflect the metabolic effects of multiple carboxylase deficiency and include organic aciduria, ketonuria, lactic acidosis, hypoglycemia, hyperglycinuria, hyperphosphatemia, and hyperammonemia. At autopsy, neuropathologic examination of the brain reveals atrophy and disappearance of the Purkinje layer of the cerebellum (Sander et al., 1980).

A diagnosis of multiple carboxylase deficiency can be established by demonstrating lactic acidosis and elevation of specific organic acids in the plasma or urine. The diagnosis is confirmed by demonstrating enzyme deficiency in cultured leukocytes or fibroblasts. This method may also be used to establish an intrauterine diagnosis using cultured amniotic fluid cells.

Treatment

Biotin is the therapy of choice. Biotin may be administered orally in a dose ranging from 1 to 40 mg/day. Following treatment, neurologic, dermatologic, and immunologic abnormalities are corrected. Biotin must be administered on a continuous basis for an indefinite period of time. Biotin administered to a pregnant woman carrying an affected infant resulted in metabolic correction of the defect at the time of birth. Treatment was temporarily discontinued to confirm the diagnosis and immediately restarted on a long-term basis.

X-LINKED LYMPHOPROLIFERATIVE SYNDROME (Immunodeficiency Following Hereditary Defective Response to Epstein-Barr Virus)

The X-linked lymphoproliferative syndrome (XLP) is characterized by an unusual host response that develops in the wake of an EBV infection. The clinical infection caused by EBV is unusually severe or fatal, and the immune response to EBV is defective. Hypogammaglobulinemia, aplastic anemia, or malignant lymphoma may also be seen. Only males are affected (Seemayer et al., 1993).

Historical Aspects

The disease was first described in 1975 and was designated Duncan disease (Purtilo et al., 1975). Six of 18 boys in the third generation of this kindred died of a fulminating lymphoproliferative disease that occurred following an attack of infectious mononucleosis. Immunoglobulin alterations ranging from hypogammaglobulinemia to polyclonal hypergammaglobulinemia were seen. The variable phenotype and classification of the clinical manifestations as essentially proliferative or aproliferative in nature was emphasized by Purtilo and colleagues (1977a). Sullivan and co-workers (1983) performed a prospective study of two males before they had acquired a fatal EBV infection. Their studies suggested that unregulated anomalous killer and natural killer cell activity against EBV-infected and uninfected cells was the basic defect. Acyclovir therapy was employed by several workers; failure or, at best, equivocal results were seen (Hanto et al., 1982; Sullivan et al., 1982, 1983).

Pathogenesis

Because the disease is X-linked, genetic interactions of this chromosome are involved in the causation of XLP. Purtilo and colleagues (1977a) refer to the relevant area of the X chromosome as the XLP locus. Mothers of patients show elevated titers of antibodies to EBV, suggesting a slight loss of control in the immune response (Purtilo et al., 1982). Initially, Purtilo and others (1977a) proposed that differences in dose, duration, and age of the patient at exposure could account for the varied clinical expression. A lympholytic process secondary to viral infection or excessive T-cell suppression, resulting from cells generated in attempts to clear the viral infection, could result in agammaglobulinemia (Provisor et al., 1975) and other aproliferative syndromes. By contrast, a deficient immune response would not effectively control the viral infection, and the marked lymphostimulatory potential of EBV would be unchecked, resulting in proliferative syndromes. Analysis of lymphocyte function by Lindsten and colleagues (1982) revealed an abnormal T–cell subset distribution, usually with a decrease in CD4 helper cells and decreased in vitro synthesis of immunoglobulins by affected males.

An extensive study by Sullivan and colleagues (1983), involving characterization of the immune status of two children at risk but before either had acquired EBV infection, was particularly informative. Extensive analysis of the immune responses of these two patients showed normal T- and B-cell capability. Appropriate antibody and cytotoxic T-cell responses to EBV virus occurred at the time of infection. However, the normal evolution of the disease with control of actively infected cells and return to the previous state of health did not occur. The EBV-induced cytotoxic T cells were shown to be capable of destruction by autologous lymphoblasts, hepatocytes, and fibroblasts. Analyses of the immune system of four surviving members of this kindred after EBV infection revealed profound defects in proliferative T-cell responses, natural killer cell activity, and secondary antibody responses to bacteriophage ϕX174.

Sullivan and others (1983) showed that the immune system of patients at risk was essentially normal before the EBV infection but that the abnormalities began during the course of and in response to the viral infection. They proposed that the generation of an uncontrolled natural killer and anomalous killer populations (Seeley and Golub, 1978; Vankey et al., 1982; Grimm et al., 1982) is the fundamental fault in XLP. In normal individuals, these populations are generated in response to EBV infections and aid in viral elimination with minimal effects upon the host. In the affected kindreds, an excessively vigorous response at the time of the primary infection leads to death from hepatocytolysis, hematopoietic cell destruction (aplastic anemia), or both. Survivors are left with a weakened immune system as a result of lymphocyte destruction. These patients have variable degrees of hypogammaglobulinemia. The immune deficiency predisposes to subsequent malignancy.

Clinical Manifestations

The clinical manifestations of XLP can be divided into four major phenotypes: infectious mononucleosis, malignant B-cell lymphoma, aplastic anemia, and hypogammaglobulinemia (Purtilo et al., 1982). Patients may have one or more of these. The most common manifestation is infectious mononucleosis, seen in approximately 75% of all cases. Of these, slightly less than half have one or more of the other phenotypic manifestations as well. All patients with aplastic anemia (approximately 20%) also have the infectious mononucleosis picture; early death is the usual outcome. Two thirds of the patients with infectious mononucleosis die of fulminant hepatic failure. Twenty percent of the kindred at risk show hypogammaglobulinemia; of these, infectious mononucleosis occurs concomitantly in half.

Hypogammaglobulinemia in this syndrome is similar in its clinical expression to the primary immunodeficiency states with increased susceptibility to bacterial infections; an appropriate response to replacement therapy is seen. Occasionally, hypogammaglobulinemia precedes the EBV infection. Malignant lymphomas occur in slightly more than one third of cases. Most are found in the ileum (about two thirds), and the remainder are distributed in the liver, kidneys, CNS, thymus, colon, and tonsils. One tumor involved the psoas muscle.

Laboratory Findings

After exposure to infectious mononucleosis, patients show the serologic antibody responses of active EBV infection, namely, elevated titers of antibodies to viral capsid and nuclear antigens (Henle et al., 1974). XLP patients do not maintain antibodies to EBV nuclear antigens, however. Assessment of natural killer function shows progressive fall as the infection progresses. After EBV infections, variable degrees of aberrant immune function and immunodeficiency can be shown. These include abnormal helper T cell to suppressor T cell ratios (usually reversed, e.g., <1:0), diminished antibody responses, and, often, panhypogammaglobulinemia or selective IgA deficiency (Purtilo et al., 1982; Sullivan et al., 1983). Polymorphic lymphoid infiltrates, consisting of lymphocytes, plasmacytoid cells, mature plasma cells, and histiocytes are prominent in the liver, CNS, spleen, and lymph nodes of patients at autopsy. The thymus is usually atrophic, but the changes are more consistent with stress than primary dysplasia (Purtilo et al., 1977b).

Hyperimmunoglobulinemia A, M, G1, and G3, failure of isotype switching following ϕX174 challenge, and inability to maintain antibodies to EBV nuclear antigen provide strong presumptive evidence for the diagnosis of XLP in the appropriate clinical context (Purtilo et al., 1989).

Aplastic anemia may be present. The pathology of the lymphomas varies from American Burkitt's lymphoma to immunoblastic sarcoma (Purtilo et al., 1982).

The gene for XLP is located on the long arm of the X chromosome at Xq24/25 (Wyandt et al., 1989). Using RFLP, carrier and disease status can be determined (Schuster et al., 1993).

Treatment

There is no satisfactory treatment for this disorder. Acyclovir has been given for the EBV infection, but the results are equivocal (Sullivan et al., 1982, 1983). Hypogammaglobulinemia should be treated in the usual manner, with prophylactic antibiotics, IgG replacement therapy, and attention to pulmonary function as necessary. Patients identified before EBV infection may be given gamma globulin in an attempt to prevent this infection (Sullivan, personal communication, 1990). Bone marrow transplant (BMT) has been successfully accomplished (Vowels et al., 1993). In the case of fulminant clinical responses to EBV, it may be necessary to bring the patient into clinical remission before BMT. This has been accomplished with etoposide (Seemayer et al., 1993). Vowels and colleagues (1993) report correction of XLP by transplantation of cord blood stem cells.

Prognosis

The prognosis is guarded. About 75% to 80% of those susceptible die of the primary EBV infection. Of those that survive, hypogammaglobulinemia and malignant lymphoma remain major threats. The malignant lymphoma may respond well to chemotherapy, but it eventually proves fatal, with a mean survival of 19 months. The best prognosis is seen in patients with hypogammaglobulinemia who are given replacement therapy, and of course, those successfully transplanted.

PROTEIN-LOSING ENTEROPATHY WITH IMMUNODEFICIENCY

Protein-losing enteropathy with immunodeficiency results from a loss of lymphocytes, serum proteins, or both from the gastrointestinal tract. There are numerous causes, both congenital and acquired. In some cases, there is no apparent immunodeficiency; in others, there is an antibody immunodeficiency; and in still others, there is both an antibody and a cellular immunodeficiency, the latter associated with lymphopenia. This disorder is also discussed in Chapters 19 and 23.

Historical Aspects

Protein loss through the gastrointestinal (GI) tract was first described by Welch and colleagues (1937) in patients with ulcerative colitis. In 1957, Citrin and coworkers used radiolabeled ^{131}I albumin to demonstrate albumin loss into the GI tract of patients with giant hypertrophy of the gastric mucosa. Holman and others (1959) suggested that certain patients with idiopathic hypoproteinemia might be losing protein into the GI tract. Subsequently, GI protein loss was identified in regional enteritis (Steinfeld et al., 1960), sprue (Parkins, 1960), Whipple's intestinal lipodystrophy (Laster et al., 1966), gastric carcinoma (Jarnum and Schwartz, 1960), allergic gastroenteropathy (Waldmann et al., 1967), intestinal lymphangiectasia (Waldmann et al., 1967), constrictive pericarditis (Waldmann et al., 1961), congenital hypogammaglobulinemia (Waldmann and Schwab, 1965), and iron-deficiency anemia associated with intolerance to cow's milk (Heiner et al., 1964).

Waldmann and colleagues (1961) first clearly demonstrated GI protein loss in 20 patients with idiopathic hypoproteinemia. Twelve of their patients had abnormalities of the lymphatic vessels of the small intestine and mesentery, and they suggested the term *intestinal lymphangiectasia* for this syndrome. In subsequent studies, Strober and coworkers (1967) demonstrated that some of these patients had defects in cell-mediated immunity as well as hypogammaglobulinemia.

Pathogenesis

Lymphopenia that occurs with protein-losing enteropathy in intestinal lymphangiectasia results from lymphocyte loss through the dilated lymphatic vessels. Loss of lymphatic fluid into the GI tract was demonstrated by Stoelinga and others (1963) and Mistilis and colleagues (1965). Jeffries and coworkers (1964) suggested that this loss was due to increased pressure within the lymphatic vessels as a result of increased absorption of long-chain fatty acids. The reduction of protein loss into the intestine with a low-fat diet supports this concept (Jeffries et al., 1964).

Although most of these disorders are probably due to congenital defects of the lymphatic vessels, protein-losing states with lymphopenia also occur in acquired disorders, such as constrictive pericarditis, ulcerative colitis, and Whipple's disease.

In both congenital and acquired forms, dilated lymphatic vessels are observed (Strober et al., 1967). The protein and lymphocyte loss are probably the result of identical mechanisms because both are reversed by surgical treatment of constrictive pericarditis (Barth et al., 1964).

The mechanism of GI protein loss in chronic inflammatory states is obscure. Leakage of protein may occur in areas of inflammation, inasmuch as removal of the involved portions may reverse the protein loss. In allergic gastroenteropathy, the same mechanism may occur; there may be some improvement with corticosteroids, but hypogammaglobulinemia often persists (Waldmann et al., 1967).

Clinical Manifestations

The clinical features of protein-losing enteropathy with immunodeficiency are variable. The hypoproteinemia leads to edema, which may be mild, massive, symmetrical, asymmetrical, chronic, or intermittent. Ascites may be present, often associated with chylothorax, chylous ascites, or both. Diarrhea, vomiting, abdominal pain, and frequent infections may be present. Two infants presented with a clinical picture resembling SCID (Cannon et al., 1982).

Generally, the patients are remarkably free from infections, considering their low immunoglobulin levels; this is because antibody synthesis is maintained and often accelerated. Food hypersensitivities that occur in patients with allergic gastroenteropathy are often associated with asthma and eczema. Other findings are dependent on the underlying disorder—for example, heart failure in constrictive pericarditis, growth failure in ulcerative colitis, GI obstruction in malignancy, and so on.

Laboratory Findings

Immunoglobulin and albumin levels are markedly diminished in protein-losing enteropathy with immunodeficiency. The loss is nonspecific, since both high-molecular-weight (IgM) and low-molecular-weight (IgG, IgA) immunoglobulins are decreased. The immunoglobulin synthetic rate is normal or increased (Strober et al., 1967).

GI protein loss can be documented by demonstrating a shortened survival of various radiolabeled proteins, such as ^{51}Cr-albumin or ^{131}I-polyvinylpyrrolidone (Strober et al., 1967). Lymphangiography can be used to demonstrate the dilated lymphatic vessels of intestinal lymphangiectasia.

These procedures are of particular value in differentiating primary hypogammaglobulinemia from protein-losing enteropathy. In primary hypogammaglobulinemia, there is prolonged IgG survival and decreased IgG synthesis (Waldmann and Schwab, 1965). Further, the antibody response in protein-losing enteropathy is usually normal (Strober et al., 1967).

Lymphopenia is a consistent feature of intestinal lymphangiectasia, but it may also occur in other disorders with dilated intestinal lymphatics, such as constrictive pericarditis, Whipple's disease, and regional enteritis. Strober and colleagues (1967) found that the mean lymphocyte count in intestinal lymphangiectasia was 710 ± 340 lymphocytes/mm^3. The lymphopenia may help to differentiate this disorder from other forms of protein-losing enteropathy, such as allergic gastroenteropathy, ulcerative colitis, and gluten-induced enteropathy, and from congenital hypogammaglobulinemia.

The degree of lymphopenia is directly correlated with the defect of cell-mediated immunity, as measured by the number of T cells, the degree of cutaneous anergy, the ability to become sensitized to 2,4-dinitrofluorobenzene, and the prolongation of homograft survival (Strober et al., 1967).

Radiographic studies may reveal giant hypertrophy of the gastric mucosa, ulcerative colitis, regional enteritis, or intestinal tract malignancy. The x-ray findings of allergic gastroenteropathy or intestinal protein loss with milk intolerance are usually nonspecific.

Intestinal biopsy is invaluable and should be performed in all cases needing a definite diagnosis. Dilated subepithelial lymphatic channels are characteristic of intestinal lymphangiectasis (Strober et al., 1967). Marked eosinophilia in the lamina propria is present in allergic gastroenteropathy. Intestinal biopsy also excludes intestinal tract malignancy.

Diminished serum iron and copper are present in several protein-losing states, especially in infants with edema, hypoproteinemia, and iron deficiency (Wilson et al., 1962) and in cow's milk hypersensitivity (Heiner et al., 1964). Eosinophilia is prominent in allergic gastroenteropathy (Waldman et al., 1967; Greenberger et al., 1967).

Treatment

The immunodeficiency of intestinal lymphangiectasia responds favorably to a diet containing low-fat or medium-chain triglycerides (Stoelinga et al., 1963; Jeffries et al., 1964; Holt, 1964). Successful treatment results in an increase in the serum immunoglobulins and the lymphocyte count.

Allergic gastroenteropathy is treated by identification and elimination of the offending food. In some patients, this is cow's milk (Heiner et al., 1964; Waldmann et al., 1967), although other foods have been implicated (Greenberger et al., 1967). When dietary therapy is unsuccessful, corticosteroids may result in improvement (Waldmann et al., 1967; Greenberger et al., 1967; Lebenthal et al., 1970).

Surgical treatment is indicated for specific abnormalities, such as constrictive pericarditis, localized lymphangiectasia (Ivey et al., 1969), and ulcerative colitis. Success is measured by reversal of the hypoproteinemia and the lymphopenia.

Prognosis

In general, the prognosis in protein-losing enteropathy is dependent on the underlying disorder. These patients rarely succumb from infections despite their marked laboratory abnormalities (Strober et al., 1967). An increased incidence of malignancy or autoimmune disease may result from the impairment of cell-mediated immunity.

NATURAL KILLER CELL DEFICIENCY

Natural killer (NK) cells are non-B, non-T lymphocytes (e.g., null cells) that show cytotoxicity against various targets without prior sensitization. They are not limited to MHC restriction and can be differentiated from classic cytotoxic T cells, granulocytes, and macrophages. NK cells are associated with the large granular lymphocyte population and bear CD56 as a distinguishing surface marker. Their role in body defense is not fully defined; they represent part of the natural defense systems (see review by Herberman and Ortaldo, 1981).

Pathogenesis

Natural killer cells arise from the same pluripotent stems cells as the other cellular components of the immune system. There is no known designated site of differentiation, and details of these processes remain undefined. However, like all cytotoxic cells, they adhere to the target and release cytolytic factors to effect target death. In a general way, NK deficiency results from processes similar to T-cell deficiency.

Only a few cases of NK deficiency have been described. In Chédiak-Higashi syndrome, the NK cells initiate lysis poorly (Targan and Oseas, 1983). In leukocyte adhesion defect type I (LAD-I), lack of adhesion results in poor target binding (Kohl et al., 1984). A complete absence of NK cells was reported by Biron and coworkers (1989). Two siblings showed defective NK cytotoxicity associated with failure of release of natural killer cytotoxic factor (Komiyama et al., 1990).

Clinical Manifestations

The infectious susceptibility of these patients is often minimal. The patient studied by Biron and associates (1989) is illustrative and defines the role of NK cells in defense from infection. Her major susceptibility involved herpesviruses. She was completely asymptomatic until a bout of varicella at age 13; she had been immunized with live attenuated viruses without incident. The varicella infection was complicated by pneumonia, leukopenia, and thrombocytopenia. She improved on acyclovir therapy but was left with severe scarring of the face and trunk. She also experienced a severe episode of cytomegalovirus infection with pneumonia 4 years later. Two siblings studied by Komiyama and colleagues (1990) were essentially asymptomatic.

In other diseases in which NK dysfunction has been reported, Chédiak-Higashi syndrome, LAD-I, chronic neutropenia, and familial hemophagocytic lymphohistiocytosis, the symptoms of the primary disorder overshadow the clinical picture and account for the major symptomatology (Targan and Oseas, 1983; Kohl et al., 1984; Komiyama et al., 1985; Janka, 1983).

Thus, the clinical manifestations of NK deficiency appear to be restricted to a few viruses whose control is particularly dependent on NK cells, but there does not seem to be any global susceptibility. As yet, increased incidence of tumors has not been seen except in Chédiak-Higashi syndrome.

Treatment and Prognosis

The treatment is the treatment of the primary disease and appropriate antiviral therapy. The prognosis seems to be dictated more by the nature of the primary disease than by the defect in NK cells.

GRAFT-VERSUS-HOST DISEASE

Graft-versus-host disease (GVHD) is a T cell–mediated process in which infused (or maternal) histoincompatible T cells react against the recipient of the infusion. Variable destruction, primarily of the skin, liver, and GI tract, is seen. The disease may be fatal. GVHD occurs in acute and chronic forms.

Pathogenesis

The requirements for GVHD were delineated by Billingham in 1966:

1. The graft must contain immunologically competent cells.
2. The recipient must express tissue antigens that are not present in the transplant donor.
3. The recipient must be incapable of mounting an effective response to destroy the transplanted cells.

These requirements are met in many clinical situations. Most commonly, GVHD is seen as a complication of allogeneic bone marrow transplantation. The marrow contains many competent T cells, and the recipient cannot reject the transplant because of ablation or because he or she is genetically immunodeficient. Even when the donor and recipient are "HLA-identical," they most likely differ at minor histocompatibility loci. Because most blood products contain mature immunocompetent T cells, radiation 1500 R (15 Gy) is required for blood, platelet, and granulocyte transfusions. A small-bowel or liver transplant contains many competent lymphocytes and may cause severe GVHD. Because of transplacental passage, infants are exposed to the maternal leukocytes. When the infant has a primary immunodeficiency state, intrauterine GVHD can occur (Kadowaki et al., 1965). Theoretically, a maternal-infant GVH disease can result from the ingestion of maternal lymphocytes during breast-feeding, inasmuch as breast milk contains T cells (Beer and Billingham,

1975). Such a reaction from breast milk has not been reported, however. Other cases of GVHD have been recorded as a complication of intrauterine transfusions and exchange transfusions for erythroblastosis (Hathaway et al., 1965; Naiman et al., 1969; Ammann et al., 1972; Parkman et al., 1974).

In the rare instance in which a blood product donor is homozygous instead of heterozygous for HLA-alleles and his or her haplotypes match one of the recipient's, the recipient finds nothing foreign in the infusion and does not reject the donor leukocytes. The donor T cells, however, will react to the nonmatched recipient haplotype and mount a GVH reaction against the host. In this case, an immunologically normal host can experience GVHD, which may be fatal. This sequence of events has been observed when a parent requests a directed blood transfusion from one of his children (reviewed in Anderson and Weinstein, 1990).

The intensity of the histocompatibility stimulus is most dependent on the HLA-D locus disparity (Dupont et al., 1973; Geha et al., 1976; O'Reilly et al., 1989; Gaschet et al., 1993). In addition to histocompatibility differences, age, the underlying disease for which BMT is performed, and the presence of infection markedly affect the intensity of GVHD. As a general rule, children have milder GVHD than adults. Also, children with primary immunodeficiency have mild to minimal GVHD after HLA-identical BMT; often GVHD prophylaxis is unnecessary. In contrast, children receiving transplants for malignancy will have moderate to severe disease. When haplotype-mismatched BMT is performed, GVHD is more severe, even though the marrow is T-cell depleted; the severity is correlated with the number of mature T cells present in the inoculum (Kernan et al., 1986). For unknown reasons, Wiskott-Aldrich syndrome is associated with a greater likelihood of severe acute and chronic GVHD than the other primary immunodeficiency states. Similarly, among malignancies, chronic myelogenous leukemia is associated with increased risk (Weisdorf et al., 1991).

The addition of microbial antigens (infection) to the MHC stimulation of the donor T cells intensifies their reactivity. This was demonstrated by van Bekkum and coworkers (1974) by showing that mice, even though they differed across major histocompatibility loci, could receive transplants without development of GVHD when the transplantations were carried out under gnotobiotic conditions. Microbial antigens may activate macrophages, γ/δ TCR$^+$ cells, and NK cells, all of which increase the inflammatory response through cytokine release (Ferrara et al., 1989). Infectious agents may also increase T-cell activation through a superantigen effect.

The actual tissue damage may be mediated by direct T-cell cytotoxic attack on the target tissues, but it is likely that major effects also result from cytokine release from T cells, macrophages, and natural killer cells (reviewed by Ferrara and Deeg, 1991). Tumor necrosis factor-α may be the central mediator. In addition, it has also been demonstrated in a mouse model that noncytotoxic T cells account for intestinal GVHD (Thiele et al., 1989). Thus, multiple mechanisms are involved in the tissue destruction of GVHD. The pri-

mary target organs of GVHD are the skin, liver, and GI tract. The lungs, lymphoid, and hematopoietic systems are next most commonly involved. The reason for the localization is not known. One theory is that the target cells are undifferentiated epithelial cells with primitive surface antigens (Sale et al., 1985). However, no tissue is spared.

Clinical Manifestations

GVHD occurs within a few days after the infusion of T cells. The exact time is affected by the circumstances of the infusion and whether or not prophylaxis has been employed. The initial symptom is a papular, erythematous, blotchy eruption that soon spreads to become generalized and involves the palms and soles. In the mildest forms of GVHD, as commonly seen in HLA-matched BMT for primary immunodeficiency, this may be the only involvement, and the skin clears within a week. More often, the skin lesions become more inflamed and are frequently purpuric. Bullous lesions may be seen; in the most extreme form, a "scalded skin" syndrome with total denudation occurs (Peck et al., 1972; Krueger, 1973) (Fig. 12–28).

Liver and gastrointestinal involvement follow within a few days. Mild hepatomegaly and elevation of liver enzymes occur. Hyperbilirubinemia may or may not be seen. GI involvement is manifested by cramping abdominal pain and watery diarrhea. Liver and GI disease may escalate to hepatic failure, profound GI bleeding, and paralytic ileus (Slavin and Santos, 1973; Deeg and Cottler-Fox, 1990). Eye involvement, frequently overlooked, is manifested by conjunctivitis, excess lacrimation, and photophobia.

An arbitrary grading system to denote varying degrees of severity has been used, ranging from Grade 1 with only mild skin involvement to Grade 4, with severe multiorgan disease. Grade 4 is usually fatal (Glucksberg et al., 1974).

Most intrauterine GVHD presents as a chronic scaling erythroderma; alopecia is prominent. Liver and GI involvement are minimal (Kadowaki et al., 1965).

Chronic GVHD may evolve from ongoing acute disease, arise de novo, or ensue after apparent resolution of the acute phase. GVHD occurring 100 days or more after the transplant has been called "chronic," but this is an arbitrary definition; chronic GVHD should be defined on the basis of the clinical picture rather than the time of onset. The most important characteristic of chronic GVHD is its clinical expression as a mixture of autoimmune diseases. The skin texture changes resemble those of scleroderma; joint contractures and atrophic ulcers are prominent. Skin and buccal mucosa lesions resemble lichen planus. A sicca syndrome may affect the mucosae of the eyes, mouth, airways, and esophagus. Eating becomes a chore, and malnutrition frequently results (Deeg and Cottler-Fox, 1990).

A particularly disturbing complication is bronchiolitis obliterans, which may ultimately prove fatal.

The immune system is targeted by the chronic process. In the presence of chronic GVHD, restoration of competent immunity is retarded and the patient re-

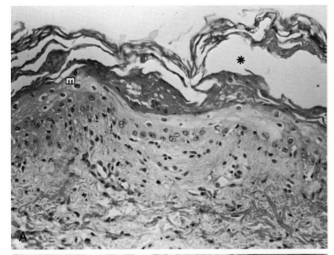

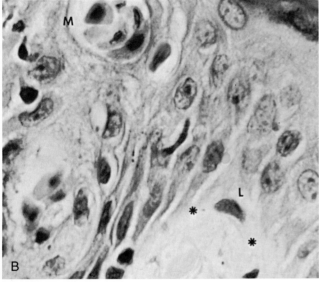

Figure 12–28. Skin in graft-versus-host (GVH) disease. *A*, Distinction of dermis from epidermis is not possible owing to destruction of basal layer. Mummified cells (m) are characteristic of cutaneous GVH disease. In especially severe GVH disease, a "scalded-skin syndrome" is present and intracutaneous separation (*) is seen. (× 100.) *B*, Higher power view. L = liquefaction necrosis, which obscures the normal demarcation of dermis from epidermis (marked by *). M = mummified cell. (× 400.) (*A* and *B* from Horowitz SD, Hong R. The Pathogenesis and Treatment of Immunodeficiency. Basel, S. Karger, 1977.)

mains highly susceptible to infection (Noel et al., 1978). Death from infection is often the terminal event in chronic GVHD.

Laboratory Findings

In acute disease, liver enzymes, particularly γ-glutamyltransferase (GGT), are markedly elevated. Although aspartate and alanine aminotransferase levels are also increased, GGT characteristically is disproportionately high. The degree of hyperbilirubinemia is variable; when it is markedly elevated (more than 20 mg/dl), the prognosis becomes guarded.

The histology shows lesions in intestinal crypts, bile

ducts, and skin. Skin involvement is characterized by lymphocyte invasion of the epidermis with keratinocyte destruction (satellite necrosis). CD8$^+$ cells predominate in the cellular infiltrates (Figs. 12–29 and 12–30) (Slavin and Santos, 1973; Janossy et al., 1982).

In chronic GVHD, the skin lesions show atrophy, characteristic lichenoid lesions, and fibrosis of the hypodermis. The liver shows more advanced lesions with obliteration of bile ducts and marked cholestasis. The lymphoid apparatus is more profoundly disturbed than in acute GVHD. The thymus shows involution, atrophy, and lymphocyte depletion. The lymph nodes are effaced and lack germinal centers. As the process continues, depression of the hematopoietic system with neutropenia and thrombocytopenia is seen. X-rays of the intestine usually show small–bowel wall edema, effacement of ileal folds, stenosis, and poststenotic dilation. Thumbprinting, haustral loss, and ulcerations are seen in the colon (Schuttevaer et al., 1986).

In the usual post-transplantion setting, the demonstration of donor lymphocytes is unnecessary to confirm the diagnosis. After transfusions or in the case of a suspected intrauterine origin, presence of the foreign HLA should be demonstrated. This can be accomplished by usual HLA serotyping, with demonstration of donor HLA in addition to that of the patient. Often, in infants suspected of intrauterine GVHD, there are insufficient numbers of donor cells in the circulation to demonstrate chimerism. In this case, expansion of the lymphocytes with IL-2 and mitogen or search for foreign antigens using DNA probes and sensitive techniques, such as polymerase chain reaction, may be necessary (Ugozzoli et al., 1989; Katz et al., 1990). Infants may also be silently engrafted (i.e., without GVHD) with maternal lymphocytes. Their presence may interfere with subsequent transplantation attempts (Pollack et al., 1982).

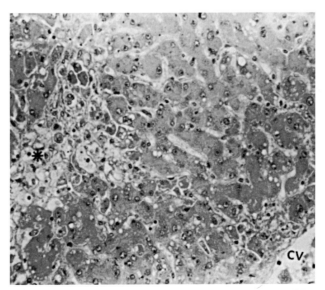

Figure 12–29. Periportal necrosis in graft-versus-host disease. CV = Central vein. (× 400.) (From Horowitz SD, Hong R. The Pathogenesis and Treatment of Immunodeficiency. Basel, S. Karger, 1977.)

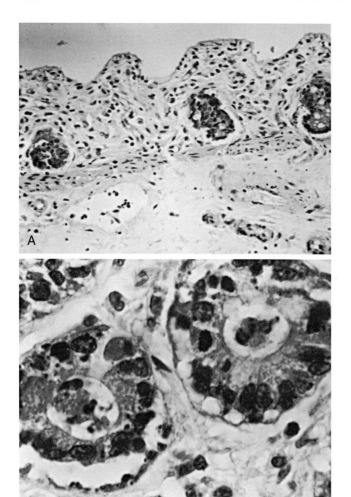

Figure 12–30. Intestinal lesion of graft-versus-host disease. *A,* Flattening of villi and destruction of crypts. (× 100.) *B,* Higher power view of crypt lesion. Epithelial necrosis and debris are present in the lumen. (× 400.) (From Horowitz SD, Hong R. The Pathogenesis and Treatment of Immunodeficiency. Basel, S. Karger, 1977.)

Prevention and Treatment

Prevention is accomplished by interfering with T-cell function. In all transfused blood products, prior irradiation with 2500 R (25 Gy) will destroy the competence of any mature T cells without affecting erythrocyte, neutrophil, or platelet function. T-cell depletion in marrow infusions can essentially eliminate GVHD. Unfortunately, T-cell depletion of matched marrows is associated with a high relapse rate of leukemias (Marmont et al., 1991). When used with mismatched marrows, in addition to the high relapse rate, there is poor engraftment and a high rate of B-cell lymphoma (Shapiro et al., 1988b; Fischer et al., 1991a).

Administration of methotrexate and cyclosporine has evolved as the most optimal regimen for GVHD prophylaxis (Storb et al., 1986). Although GVHD is still seen, the intensity is markedly reduced. Maintenance of the patient in a gnotobiotic environment produces impressive results in animals, but its benefit in human bone marrow transplantation is not clear. It is probably of some benefit in aplastic anemia (Storb et al., 1983).

When overt disease is present, cyclosporine is continued and prednisone may be given. If GVHD is not controlled by these measures, antibodies against T cells are often of benefit. Polyclonal antithymocyte globulin is effective. More recently, toxin-conjugated monoclonal antibodies directed against T cells have shown efficacy. OKT3 directed against the CD3 T–cell receptor complex, which is extremely effective in solid organ transplant rejection crises, is singularly ineffective in GVHD therapy (Ferrara and Deeg, 1991).

Chronic GVHD requires more supportive care. Cyclosporine and prednisone may be continued along with immunosuppressives such as azathioprine. Thalidomide has shown promise in a preliminary trial (Vogelsang et al., 1992). Topical cyclosporine rinses may be of benefit in oral lichen planus (Eisen et al., 1990). The sicca syndrome requires artificial tears; tears made with autologous serum may be more effective (Fox et al., 1984).

Therapy directed against cytokines, particularly tumor necrosis factor, will probably assume greater importance in the future.

Prognosis

Acute GVHD caused by completely unmatched infusions in the absence of prophylaxis (e.g., transfusion-induced GVHD resulting from a homozygous HLA donor or transfusion given to a patient with unsuspected primary immunodeficiency) is usually extremely severe and often fatal.

Acute GVHD, grades 1 and 2, usually responds well to therapy. A fatal outcome becomes more likely with the more severe grades of GVHD. Chronic GVHD may be associated with as high as 50% mortality (Storb et al., 1983; Wingard et al., 1989). Lichenoid skin changes, hyperbilirubinemia, persistent thrombocytopenia, and failure to respond to nine months of therapy predict a dire outcome for chronic GVHD (Wingard et al., 1989; Sullivan et al., 1990).

TREATMENT OF CELLULAR IMMUNODEFICIENCY

Supportive Care

Once a T-cell immunodeficiency disorder has been diagnosed, it is essential that specific treatment, preventive measures, or both be instituted to avoid additional complications before establishing effective immunotherapy. Immunization with live attenuated vaccines is contraindicated. Although routine immunization for smallpox is no longer used in the United States, progressive polio encephalitis, measles encephalitis, and mumps encephalitis have been recorded in immunodeficient patients following routine childhood immunization. Additionally, siblings should not be immunized with live polio vaccines because the virus may be transmitted to the patient. Under these circumstances, if polio immunization is necessary for the normal siblings, killed polio virus may be used.

Special care must be taken in administering blood products to immunodeficient children. All blood given to patients with primary or secondary immunodeficiency should be radiated with 25 Gy to prevent graft-versus-host reaction. Radiation of blood products is a simple procedure and can be accomplished rapidly. Blood administered to immunodeficient patients should also be negative for cytomegalovirus, HIV, and hepatitis virus. Transmission of any of these viral agents to an immunodeficient patient may result in a severe, chronic, or fatal disease.

Broad-spectrum prophylactic antibiotics may be useful in patients with recurrent or chronic bacterial disease. Patients with severe T-cell deficiency should be placed on prophylaxis with trimethoprim-sulfamethoxazole to prevent infection with *P. carinii*. A useful guide is the CD4 recommendation for infants and children with HIV at different ages.

Because most patients with significant T-cell immunodeficiency also have impaired antibody function, they should be evaluated for antibody function; if deficient, they should receive immune globulin therapy. The dose of immune globulin and specific treatment regimens are discussed in Chapter 9.

Participation in a support group such as the Immune Deficiency Foundation provides essential information and help for patients and their families. Medical teams can provide only limited resources to help families cope with the social, economic, emotional, and psychologic issues that these devastating diseases impose on families. Those who experience immunodeficiency disease as patients and their families can offer a perspective not available to most medical personnel. It is from this perspective, however, that patients and their families must develop the wherewithal to accept the impact of immunodeficiency disease on their lives. The address of the Immune Deficiency Foundation is Courthouse Square, 3565 Ellicott Mills Drive, Unit B2, Ellicott City, MD 21043.

Transfer Factor

Transfer of cellular immunity was first achieved with intact cells by Landsteiner and Chase (1940, 1942). Subsequently, Lawrence (1954) demonstrated the transfer of tuberculin hypersensitivity with a nonviable extract of leukocytes obtained from sensitive donors. Transfer of cellular immunity resides in a substance termed transfer factor (TF), which can be extracted from sensitized leukocytes. TF is dialyzable, has a molecular weight of less than 10kD, is not antigenic, and is not an immunoglobulin (Lawrence, 1954, 1963). Transfer factors, peptides extracted from T cells, confer antigen reactivity to nonresponsive recipients (Kirkpatrick, 1972). (See also Chronic Mucocutaneous Candidiasis.)

Transfer factor is prepared as a dialysate of leukocytes obtained from sensitized individuals. It is therefore a crude extract and contains many biologically active moieties. In addition to TF, the dialysate contains thymic hormone activity (Wilson et al., 1983). Thus, the material that is used clinically is more appropriately termed dialyzable leukocyte extract (DLE). DLE contains material that specifically transfers antigen reactivity (i.e., TF), and material that nonspecifically augments the immune response.

Transfer factor was first used clinically in the treatment of T-cell deficiency by Levin and colleagues (1970). Spitler and coworkers (1972) subsequently gave TF to 12 patients with Wiskott-Aldrich syndrome. A large number and variety of patients with such diverse diseases as primary T-cell deficiency, ataxia-telangiectasia, Chédiak-Higashi syndrome, and hypogammaglobulinemia have received TF. Improved results can be expected with better-defined indications for its use (Kirkpatrick, 1988).

The most consistent results with TF are seen in augmentation of host defenses to help eliminate infections. Treatment of chronic mucocutaneous candidiasis has been the most successful. Reduction of the infectious agent burden by prior or concomitant treatment with amphotericin B is generally required (Buckley et al., 1968; Rocklin et al., 1970; Kirkpatrick et al., 1971b; Schulkind et al., 1972; Valdimarsson et al., 1972b, 1973; Fudenberg et al., 1974). Other infections treated with benefit include progressive tuberculosis (Whitcomb and Rocklin, 1973), lepromatous leprosy (Bullock et al., 1972; Silva et al., 1973), cytomegalovirus infection (Rytel et al., 1975), and coccidioidomycosis (Graybill et al., 1973).

Fetal Thymus Transplantation

A dramatic and relatively permanent reconstitution of T-cell immunity has been observed in patients with DiGeorge anomaly (August et al., 1968; Cleveland et al., 1968). The immunologic reconstitution achieved was rapid and unassociated with any GVH. The speed of the recovery implied that humoral factors were involved. A major problem of evaluating therapy in DiGeorge anomaly is the tendency for spontaneous improvement in the immune system (Hong, 1991).

In contrast to these results, the use of fetal thymus in other immunodeficiency states has been less salutary. Hitzig and coworkers (1965) postulated a thymic defect in patients with CID and transplanted a fetal thymus in two patients; one patient was also given bone marrow cells and the other fetal liver cells. Except for a transient increase in the total lymphocyte count, no evidence of immunologic reconstitution was observed in either patient; further, both developed GVHD.

Fetal thymus transplantation reconstituted T-cell immunity in three patients with CID (Ammann et al., 1973; Rachelefsky et al., 1975; Shearer et al., 1978). Reconstitution of T-cell immunity was observed in two patients, as indicated by normal numbers of circulating T cells and normal responsiveness of peripheral blood lymphocytes to mitogens and allogeneic cells. In addition, a transient GVH reaction was observed, showing that fetal thymus alone contains mature immunocompetent T cells. Ammann's patient showed no change in B-cell function and required gamma globulin replacement therapy. Shearer's patient was able to synthesize immunoglobulins but no specific antibody. Both of these patients have subsequently died. Rachelefsky's patient developed a neurologic degenerative disease known as Rett's syndrome (Al-Mateen et al., 1986). Thus, although some benefit is seen, the patients remain at great risk for opportunistic infection.

Thymic Humoral Factors

The observations that cellular immunity could be restored in thymectomized mice by thymic extracts (Goldstein et al., 1972) or by thymus implants in Millipore chambers suggested that immunologic reconstitution might be achieved with thymic hormones. These factors (thymic humoral factor, thymic factor, thymosin, and thymopoietin) have a number of biologic activities, including a maturational effect on T cells, restoration of T-cell immunity following thymectomy, and enhanced resistance to malignancy (Zisblatt et al., 1970; Komuro and Boyse, 1973).

Thymosin, which contains at least 12 polypeptides (Wara and Ammann, 1978), is the thymic extract most intensively studied. Thymosin can increase the number of T cells in vitro in various primary immunodeficiencies (Wara and Ammann, 1978) in various malignancies (Goldstein et al., 1976), and in systemic lupus erythematosus (Scheinberg et al., 1975). In addition, thymosin in vitro can accelerate maturation of T cells in human bone marrow and can reverse depressed mixed leukocyte culture responses (Wara and Ammann, 1978).

Overall, only modest and transient benefit has been seen. One drawback is that thymic hormones act on post-thymic cells; therefore, their benefit in stem cell disease is uncertain.

Cultured Thymus Fragments

In 1976, Hong and co-workers devised a novel approach in the treatment of CID, using cultured thymic epithelial tissue. They found that fragments of thymic tissue grown in organ culture lose lymphocytes and some macrophages, but leave a loose network of thymic epithelium. These epithelial cells retain the capacity to differentiate stem cells into mature thymocytes. Other workers have subsequently shown that thymic epithelium cultures can produce thymic humoral factors (Kruisbeek et al., 1973).

The most startling result of cultured thymic fragment transplantation was the restoration of normal B-cell function, including specific antibody synthesis. This observation convincingly demonstrated the dependency of the B-cell effector function on the thymus and established that combined immunodeficiency could result solely from a thymic defect.

Over an 8-year period, the Wisconsin group performed transplants on 24 patients who were healthy enough at the time of transplant to expect benefit. Four patients survived over 3 years, but their immunity waned, and three died, one of Hodgkin's disease and two during bone marrow transplant. The last patient is alive and completely reconstituted after receiving a haploidentical bone marrow transplant from his father.

Transplantation of cultured fragments has also been used with limited success in milder forms of immunodeficiency, chronic lymphatic leukemia, and chronic mucocutaneous candidiasis (Hong, 1986). In partial T-cell deficiency, immunosuppression appears to be necessary; otherwise, the graft is rejected.

Interferons

Interferons are antiviral substances produced by virtually all animal species. Three major varieties are known; alpha, produced by mononuclear leukocytes; beta, derived from fibroblasts; and gamma, the product of T lymphocytes. Clearly defined states of interferon deficiency have not been observed in primary immunodeficiency with the possible exception of Griscelli syndrome (see Other Combined Immunodeficiency Disorders). However, T cells from patients with AIDS are deficient in interferon production (Murray et al., 1984).

In addition to inhibition of viral reproduction, interferon augments the immune response, enhancing natural killer activity and increasing cytolytic T-cell function. Widespread use of interferon is limited by significant side effects. Fever, nausea, vomiting, diarrhea, and arrhythmias are among the most troublesome. Interferon may be of benefit in life-threatening infections in which alternative therapy has failed (Meyers et al., 1980; Smith et al., 1983). As mentioned previously, interferon-γ was useful in controlling the helper T-cell profile in a patient with Omenn syndrome (Schandene et al., 1993); similar benefit in the hyper-IgE syndrome, ostensibly through its effect on T cells, has been reported (King et al., 1989).

Levamisole

Levamisole is reported to have a number of immunomodulating effects, including suppressor T-cell augmentation and potentiating cytokine activity. Its major clinical benefit is reported to be improving neutrophil chemotaxis. In the hyper-IgE syndrome, however, infections were increased despite the improved neutrophil function (reviewed by Hassner and Adelman, 1991).

Interleukins

The interleukins are a group of factors originally found in tissue culture supernatants and shown to have effects on lymphocyte growth, differentiation, and function. Many of the interleukins have been cloned, and extensive research is being conducted for potential clinical use.

Interleukin-1 (IL-1) has multiple biologic activities and is responsible for a number of important clinical symptoms of acute inflammation. It can produce fever (Beeson, 1948), cartilage resorption (Jasin and Dingle, 1981), and muscle wasting (Clowes et al., 1983). In vitro, it stimulates both T and B lymphocytes and enhances natural killer cytotoxicity. A deficiency of IL-1 was thought to be the cause of common variable immunodeficiency in one case (Eibl et al., 1982). IL-1 has not been used therapeutically (Durum et al., 1985).

IL-3 and IL-6 have potent hematopoietic colony-stimulating activity. IL-3 is a multicolony-stimulating factor acting on early pluripotent progenitors of all hematopoietic lineages (Yang and Clark, 1989). IL-6 induces B-cell differentiation and secretion, cytotoxic T-cell differentiation, and proliferation of committed stem cell progenitors (Kishimoto, 1989). Although IL-3 and IL-6 would be of potential use in support of patients with bone marrow transplant, factors acting on later stages of differentiation, granulocyte-macrophage colony-stimulating factor (GM-GSF) or granulocyte colony–stimulating factor (G-CSF) have been used most widely in the clinic (Nemunaitis et al., 1991).

IL-2 exerts profound effects upon T-cell proliferation and activation of cytotoxic activity (Morgan et al., 1976; Gillis and Smith, 1977; Smith, 1984). Experimentally, it was shown to mature thymocytes, provide T-cell function in athymic nude mice (Wagner et al., 1980; Stotter et al., 1980), and restore T-cell deficits of aging (Thoman and Weigle, 1982). In vitro experiments, using cells from humans with various deficiencies, showed restoration of T-cell helper and cytotoxic functions (Rook et al., 1983; Flomenberg et al., 1983). Recently, after the demonstration of IL-2 deficiency in two children with SCID, cytokine treatments were started, leading to restoration of immunity (Doi et al., 1989; Pahwa et al., 1989).

IL-2 has been used most widely in tumor immunotherapy. Incubation of IL-2 with peripheral blood lymphocytes generates a population of lymphokine-activated killer (LAK) cells. These cells have significant cytotoxic activity against some malignancies. In a large series of patients with far advanced metastatic melanoma or renal carcinoma, 10% showed complete regression of the lesions. These remissions have lasted from 13 to 75 months (Rosenberg, 1992). In an effort to activate more specific lymphocyte populations, Spiess and associates (1987) used IL-2 to expand tumor-infiltrating lymphocytes (TILs). Cells with specific tumor cytotoxicity could be developed in approximately one third of melanoma patients. Cellular therapy for tumors has progressed further by the addition of other cytokines to the incubation (e.g., IL-4), with increased activity. Presently, gene insertion is being used to further increase the therapeutic potential of the cells. For example, insertion of a tumor necrosis-α gene into IL-2–expanded cells provides another dimension for control of the malignancy, by giving the cell the ability to interfere with the vascular supply (reviewed by Rosenberg, 1992). The principles of cellular manipulation employed in these trials can be applied to produce other types of cytotoxic T cells to augment the immune status of patients with primary immunodeficiency states.

Multiple cytokine incubation has been used by others to produce LAK cells with increased cytotoxic potential from the bone marrow. Morecki and colleagues (1993) used a mixture of IL-7, IL-6, and interferon-γ in this manner. Such an approach might help BMT patients during the early period of immunodeficiency that follows the transplant.

T-Cell Clones

The LAK cells previously described represent one version of the cellular analog to intravenous gamma globulin therapy. LAK cells are not MHC-restricted, the distinguishing hallmark of T–lymphocyte antigen recognition. For antibody molecules to protect from infectious agents, specificity for the relevant antigens is necessary. In a similar vein, T cells can provide protection against infectious agents only if they are antigen-specific. When the added requirement of MHC restriction is imposed, the technical problems preclude the development of off-the-shelf preparations for various infections. However, T-cell clones can be developed in anticipation of infectious complications in high-risk situations such as bone marrow transplantation.

Riddell and coworkers (1992) generated in vitro $CD3^+CD8^+$ cytomegalovirus-specific cytotoxic T-cell clones from prospective BMT donors. These were administered weekly to the bone marrow recipient in doses from 3.3×10^7 to 1×10^9 cells/m² of body surface area. Persistence in the recipient for several weeks was confirmed, and cytolytic activity was maintained. The expansion and refinement of this technology offer great promise for adoptive cellular immunotherapy.

Bone Marrow Transplantation

Bone marrow transplantation provides the best treatment for virtually all of the T-cell deficiencies at the present time. With the use of haploidentical or matched unrelated donors, virtually every patient has a donor. This subject is considered in greater detail in Chapter 32. Here I present an overview of general principles and techniques, particularly as they apply to immune deficiency states.

It is important to stress that bone marrow is a heterogeneous mixture of cells, providing cells other than the lymphoid stem cells that form the basis for the ultimate cure of genetic immunodeficiency. Bone marrow provides hematopoietic and lymphoid stem cells, macrophages, and mature T cells to the recipient. The T cells provide immediate protective benefit, and in all probability, they may also provide long-lasting benefit through self-replication. Theoretically, they should also be able to respond to neoantigens, but the size of the transplanted repertoire is unknown. Since the prethymic stem cells repopulate the patient's thymus (Hong, unpublished), normal T-cell diversity and number should be seen with time, except for those children with intrinsic thymic stromal cell defects. On the basis of what is known today, the only case in which the correction may depend entirely on post-thymic T cells contained in the bone marrow inoculum is the DiGeorge anomaly. The inability of T cell–depleted transplants to benefit a patient with DGA supports this view (see the section DiGeorge Anomaly, this chapter). Macrophages may be of import to provide sources of enzyme replacement, thus providing benefit for patients with storage disease. In ADA and PNP deficiency, the enzyme needs to be produced in the lymphocytes, and macrophage production alone would not be expected to provide adequate replacement therapy. Macrophage replacement may be adequate for complement deficiency, however.

In granulocyte disorders, the lymphocytes are unaffected and need not be replaced to obtain correction of the host defense disorder. However, if the T-cell system is not converted to that of the donor, the transplanted hematopoietic precursors will be rejected, and permanent correction will not be achieved. Also, the host precursor cells usually have a selective growth advantage and will ultimately crowd out transplanted stem cells. Thus, ablative therapy to completely empty the recipient marrow and destroy all host ability to reject is necessary.

Ultimate engraftment is, in large part, the outcome of a competition between the transplanted donor cell lines and those present in the recipient. Where there is a complete absence of a patient's cell line, the donated cells will provide replacement and restoration of function. When a normal complement of patient cells is present—for example, the hematopoietic cells—engraftment of that series usually does not occur, and the patient becomes a chimera, retaining his own hematopoietic cells in the presence of the new donor immune system. In patients in whom there is absence of only one lymphoid line (e.g., CID with normal B cells), the donor T cells engraft, the donor B cells usually do not, but competent immunity is provided by cooperation between donor T cells and recipient B cells. It is usually necessary to perform ablation for both the hematopoietic and lymphoid systems to become that of the donor, except that transplantation across the ABO blood group barriers can lead to a conversion of blood types, even in the absence of pre-BMT ablation.

Ablation is probably not required in lymphopenic forms of CID but is usually necessary in virtually all the other forms. There is no general agreement on indications for ablation among the various transplant centers. It is required much more often when T-depleted marrows are used for BMT.

Since only 20% to 30% of patients will have a HLA -A, -B, -D matched donor, alternative donor sources are needed. T-depleted haploidentical donors (usually a parent) provide excellent and equivalent (to matched sibling donor) reconstitution except for Wiskott-Aldrich syndrome, in which failure rates are slightly higher. Matched unrelated donors provide another donor source, and initial reports show excellent results.

Recently, stem cells obtained from peripheral blood have been used instead of bone marrow. Peripheral blood stem cells engraft rapidly and, combined with myeloid growth factors, restore granulocytes and platelets to transfusion-independent numbers within 2 weeks. This type of transplant has been employed primarily in marrow rescue required after high-dose, intensive chemotherapy for tumors (Kessinger et al., 1988; Nemunaitis et al., 1991). To generate sufficient numbers of stem cells in the periphery, the donor usually receives some chemoablative agent (Myers et al., 1992). As the donor usually is also the recipient (i.e., the transplant is autologous), this presents no problem. However, to give such an agent to a normal donor is not a matter to be taken lightly, and one could question its justification. Because autologous stem cell transplantation cannot be performed for treatment of genetic immunodeficiency, peripheral blood stem cell therapy may not be a useful option for these diseases. Also, the total equivalency of peripheral blood stem cells and bone marrow stem cells is as yet incompletely defined (Janssen, 1993). On the other hand, umbilical cord blood contains large numbers of stem cells and has been used successfully in place of bone marrow in the treatment of Fanconi anemia and X-linked lymphoproliferative disease (Broxmeyer et al., 1989; Gluckman et al., 1989; Vowels et al., 1993). With the ability to perform histocompatibility typing and immunologic assessment in utero, the suitability of the fetus as a donor can be determined in time to utilize the cord blood for the transplant.

Gene Therapy

Genes are being defined and cloned on a regular basis, thus making gene insertion a feasible approach to achieving total correction of genetic disease. A number of factors must be considered in selecting the appropriate patient for gene therapy (Anderson, 1984, 1992; Kohn et al., 1989; Levine and Friedmann, 1993). Since long-term benefit derives from long-lived or self-renewing populations, bone marrow stem cells are chosen as the target. A large number of stem cells must be transfected, but only small numbers can be removed by bone marrow aspiration. If genetically corrected cells can be given a growth advantage, however, they will ultimately become the dominant marrow population. Alternatively, the recipient can be given cytoablation and the treated cells can be returned. However, this latter approach does not provide much advantage (if any) over a standard bone marrow transplant performed after marrow ablation. Standard BMT carries a slight risk of graft-versus-host disease, but in a matched sibling transplant for immunodeficiency, GVHD is usually minimal and is often absent. T-cell depletion or GVHD prophylaxis markedly reduces the morbidity of GVHD in haploidentical and matched unrelated transplants. Thus, the choice of gene therapy versus bone marrow transplantation is not an easy one and is most appropriately made on a case by case basis.

Two factors can add greatly to the technical difficulties of gene transfer. One is the degree of control of gene expression required. It is preferable to treat diseases involving genes when only a minimal amount of the gene product is necessary for normal function and when marked overexpression is not detrimental. In other words, the expression of the transferred gene can be highly variable without detriment. Also, the control of synthesis of single-chain gene products is much easier than multichain proteins. For example, to correct sickle cell anemia, the inserted normal beta globin gene needs coordinate expression with the alpha globin gene.

All of the preceding make adenosine deaminase deficiency the ideal candidate for gene therapy. Adenosine deaminase is a single-chain enzyme, and individuals with levels as little as 5% of normal levels show normal immune responses. Individuals with 50-fold excess levels of ADA show only mild hemolytic anemia (Valentine et al., 1977). As mentioned earlier, three children with adenosine deaminase deficiency have been treated with gene therapy.

Gene transfer into bone marrow cells is most readily accomplished by retroviral infection of the stem cells. Other viruses may be more widely utilized with time (Levine and Friedmann, 1993). An alternative approach involves the direct injection of plasmid DNA. Using this technique, stable gene expression in skeletal and cardiac muscle has been achieved (Wolff et al., 1990; Lin et al., 1990; Ascadi et al., 1991). However, this method is inefficient, and unless the drawback is solved, the technique will not help in diseases in which large numbers of cells must be transfected to yield high levels of the product. Also, this method cannot be employed in many immune deficiency diseases in which the gene must be expressed in the lymphocyte. Should the efficiency problem be solved, genetic deficiencies of complement could be appropriate candidate diseases.

The genetic definition of immune deficiency provides an option for parents with a known history of inherited disease. Oocytes fertilized in vitro were analyzed for cystic fibrosis (CF), caused by the ΔF508 deletion. Preimplantation diagnosis, using a single cell from the blastocyst, was used to determine which oocytes were normal or heterozygous for cystic fibrosis. Based on these findings, two oocytes were implanted, one normal and one heterozygous for CF. Subsequently, a normal girl was delivered and her chromosomes were confirmed to be normal (Handyside et al., 1992). This approach should be feasible for other single-gene defects.

References

Aaltonen J, Komulainen J, Vikman A, Palotie A, Wadelius C, Perheentupa J, Peltonen L. Autoimmune polyglandular disease type I: Exclusion map using amplifiable multiallelic markers in a microtiter well format. Eur J Hum Genet 1:164–171, 1993.

Abbas AK, Lichtman AH, Pober JS. Cellular and Molecular Immunology, Philadelphia, WB Saunders, 1994a, pp. 160–166.

Abbas AK, Lichtman AH, Pober JS. Cellular and Molecular Immunology, Philadelphia, WB Saunders, 1994b, pp. 186–204.

Abbas AK, Lichtman AH, Pober JS. Cellular and Molecular Immunology, Philadelphia, WB Saunders, 1994c, pp. 226–242.

Aguilar MJ, Kamoshita S, Landing BH, Boder E, Sedgwick RP. Pathological observations in ataxia-telangiectasia. J Neuropathol Exp Neurol 27:659–676, 1968.

Ahonen P, Koskimies S, Lokki ML, Tiilikainen A, Perheentupa J. The expression of autoimmune polyglandular disease type I appears associated with several HLA-A antigens, but not with HLA-DR. J Clin Endocrinol Metab 66:1152–1157, 1988.

Ahonen P, Myllarniemi S, Sipila I, Perheentupa J. Clinical variation of autoimmune polyendocrinopathy-candidiasis-ectodermal dystrophy (ADECED) in a series of 68 patients. N Engl J Med 322:1829–1836, 1990.

Al-Mateen M, Philippart M, Shields WD. Rett's syndrome: a commonly overlooked progressive encephalopathy in girls. Am J Dis Child 140:761–765, 1986.

Al Saadi A, Palutke M, Kumar GK. Evolution of chromosomal abnormalities in sequential cytogenetic studies of ataxia-telangiectasia. Hum Genet 55:23–29, 1980.

Alarcon B, Regueiro JR, Arnaiz-Villena A, Terhorst C. Familial defect in the surface expression of the T-cell receptor–CD3 complex. N Engl J Med 319:1203–1208, 1988.

Aldrich RA, Steinberg AG, Campbell DC. Pedigree demonstrating a sex-linked recessive condition characterized by draining ears, eczematoid dermatitis and bloody diarrhea. Pediatrics 13:133–139, 1954.

Alexander WJ, Dunbar JS. Unusual bone changes in thymic alymphoplasia. Ann Radiol (Paris) 11:389–394, 1967.

Alonso K, Dew JM, Starke WR. Thymic alymphoplasia and congenital aleukocytosis (reticular dysgenesis). Arch Pathol 94:179–183, 1972.

Amiet A. Aldrich-Syndrome: Beobachtung Zweier Fälle. Ann Paediatr (Basel), 201:315–335, 1963.

Ammann AJ, Cain WA, Ishizaka K, Hong R, Good RA. Immunoglobulin E deficiency in ataxia-telangiectasia. N Engl J Med 281:469–472, 1969a.

Ammann AJ, DuQuesnoy RJ, Good RA. Endocrinological studies in ataxia-telangiectasia and other immunological deficiency diseases. Clin Exp Immunol 6:587–595, 1969b.

Ammann AJ, Good RA, Bier D, Fudenberg HH. Long-term plasma infusions in a patient with ataxia-telangiectasia and deficient IgA and IgE. Pediatrics 44:672–676, 1969c.

Ammann AJ, Hong R. Autoimmune phenomena in ataxia-telangiectasia. J Pediatr 78:821–826, 1971.

Ammann AJ, Hong R. Disorders of the T-cell system. In Stiehm ER, ed. Immunological Disorders in Infants and Children, 3rd ed. Philadelphia, WB Saunders, 1989, pp. 257–315.

Ammann AJ, Sutliff W, Millinchick E. Antibody-mediated immunodeficiency in short-limbed dwarfism. J Pediatr 84:200–203, 1974.

Ammann AJ, Tooley WH, Hong R. Toxic epidermal necrolysis. Lancet 2:484–485, 1972.

Ammann AJ, Wara D, Allen T. Immunotherapy and immunopathologic studies in a patient with nucleoside phosphorylase deficiency. Clin Immunol Immunopathol 10:262–269, 1978.

Ammann AJ, Wara D, Salmon S, Perkins H. Thymus transplantation: permanent reconstitution of cellular immunity in a patient with sex-linked combined immunodeficiency. N Engl J Med 289:5–9, 1973.

Anderson WF. Prospects for human gene therapy. Science 226:401–409, 1984.

Anderson WF. Human gene therapy. Science 256:808–813, 1992.

Anderson DC, Springer TA. Leukocyte adhesion deficiency: an inherited defect in the Mac-1, LFA-1, and p150,95 glycoproteins. Annu Rev Med 38:175–194, 1987.

Anderson KC, Weinstein HJ. Transfusion-associated graft-versus-host disease. N Engl J Med 323:315–321, 1990.

Andrews LG, Markert ML. Exon skipping in purine nucleoside phosphorylase mRNA processing leading to severe immunodeficiency. J Biol Chem 267:7834–7838, 1992.

Aozasa M, Amino N, Iwatani Y, Tamaki H, Watanabe Y, Sato H, Hochito K, Umeda K, Gunji T, Yoshizawa T, Iyama S, Miyai K. Familial OKT4 epitope deficiency: studies on antigen density and lymphocyte function. Clin Immunol Immunopathol 37:48–55, 1985.

Archer E, Chuang T-Y, Hong R. Severe eczema in a patient with DiGeorge's syndrome. Cutis 45:455–459, 1990.

Arnaiz-Villena A, Timon M, Corell A, Perez-Aciego P, Martin-Villa JM, Regueiro JR. Brief report: primary immunodeficiency caused by mutations in the gene encoding the CD3-gamma subunit of the T-lymphocyte receptor. N Engl J Med 326:529–533, 1992a.

Arnaiz-Villena A, Timon M, Rodriguez-Gallego C, Perez-Blas M, Corell A, Martin-Villa JM, Regueiro JR. Human T-cell activation deficiencies. Immunol Today 13:259–265, 1992b.

Arpaia E, Shahar M, Dadi H, Cohen A, Roifman CM. Defective T cell receptor signaling and CD8+ thymic selection in humans lacking zap-70 kinase. Cell 76:947–958, 1994.

Aruffo A, Farrington M, Hollenbaugh D, Li X, Milatovich A, Nonoyama S, Bajorath J, Grosmaire LS, Stenamp R, Neubauer M, Roberts RL, Noelle RJ, Ledbetter JA, Francke U, Ochs HD. The CD40 ligand, gp39, is defective in activated T cells from patients with X-linked hyper-IgM syndrome. Cell 72:291–300, 1993.

Arulanantham K, Dwyer JM, Genel M. Evidence for defective immunoregulation in the syndrome of familial candidiasis endocrinopathy. N Engl J Med 300:164–168, 1979.

Asamoto H, Furuta M. DiGeorge syndrome associated with glioma and two kinds of infection. N Engl J Med 296:1235, 1977.

Ascadi G, Dickson G, Love DR, Jani A, Walsh FS, Gurusinghe A, Wolff JA, Davies KE. Human dystrophin expression in mdx mice after intramuscular injection of DNA constructs. Nature 352:815–818, 1991.

Aucouturier P, Bremard-Oury C, Griscelli C, Berthier M, Preud'Homme JL. Serum IgG subclass deficiency in ataxia-telangiectasia. Clin Exp Immunol 68:392–396, 1987.

August CS, Rosen FS, Filler RM, Janeway CA, Markowski B, Kay HEM. Implantation of a foetal thymus, restoring immunological competence in a patient with thymic aplasia (DiGeorge's syndrome). Lancet 2:1210–1211, 1968.

Aurias A, Dutrillaux B, Buriot D, Lejeune J. High frequencies of inversions and translocations of chromosomes 7 and 14 in ataxia-telangiectasia. Mutat Res 69:369–374, 1980.

Ayoub EB, Dudding BA, Cooper MD. Dichotomy of antibody response to group A streptococcal antigens in Wiskott-Aldrich syndrome. J Lab Clin Med 72:971–979, 1968.

Bacchetta R, Vanderkerckhove BAE, Touraine J-L, Bigler M, Martino S, Gebuhrer L, de Vries JE, Spits H, Roncarolo M-G. Chimerism and tolerance to host and donor in severe combined immunodeficiencies transplanted with fetal liver stem cells. J Clin Invest 91:1067–1078, 1993.

Bach FH, Albertini RJ, Anderson JL, Joo P, Bortin MM. Bone-marrow transplantation in a patient with the Wiskott-Aldrich syndrome. Lancet 2:1364–1366, 1968.

Bach MA, Phan-Dinh-Tuy F, Bach JF, Wallach D, Biddison WE, Sharrow SO, Goldstein G, Kung PC. Unusual phenotypes of human inducer T cells as measured by OKT4 and related mononuclear antibodies. J Immunol 127:980–982, 1981.

Ballow M, Day NK, Biggar WD, Park BH, Yount WJ, Good RA. Reconstitution of C1q after bone marrow transplantation in patients with severe combined immunodeficiency. Clin Immunol Immunopathol 2:28–35, 1973.

Ballow M, Hyman LR. Combination immunotherapy in chronic mucocutaneous candidiasis. Synergism between transfer factor and fetal thymus tissue. Clin Immunol Immunopath 8:504–512, 1977.

Baroni C, Fabris N, Bertoli G. Age-dependency of the primary immune response in the hereditary pituitary dwarf and normal Snell-Bagg mouse. Experientia 23:1059–1060, 1967.

Barth RF, Woehner RD, Waldmann TA, Fahey JL. Metabolism of human gamma macroglobulins. J Clin Invest 43:1036–1048, 1964.

Bastian J, Law S, Vogler L, Lawton A, Herrod H, Anderson S, Horowitz S, Hong R. Prediction of persistent immunodeficiency in the DiGeorge anomaly. J Pediatr 115:391–396, 1989.

Bastianon V, Giglioni E, Buscinco L, Fiorilli M, Chessa L. Cardiac anomalies in ataxia-telangiectasia. Am J Dis Child 147:20–21, 1993.

Baugh CM, Malone JH, Butterworth CE. Human biotin deficiency: a case history of biotin deficiency induced by raw egg white consumption in a cirrhotic patient. Am J Clin Nutr 21:173–182, 1968.

Beatty DW, Arens LJ, Nelson MM. Ataxia-telangiectasia: X,14 translocation, progressive deterioration of lymphocyte numbers and functions, and abnormal in vitro immunoglobulin production. S Afr Med J 69:115–118, 1986.

Beer AE, Billingham, RE. Immunologic benefits and hazards of milk in maternal-perinatal relationship. Ann Intern Med 83:865–871, 1975.

Beeson PB. Temperature-elevating effect of a substance obtained from polymorphonuclear leukocytes (abstract). J Clin Invest 27:324, 1948.

Benichou B, Strominger JL. Class II antigen-negative patients and mutant B cell lines represent at least three, and probably four, distinct genetic defects defined by complementation analysis. Proc Natl Acad Sci U S A 88:4285–4288, 1991.

Bensel TRW, Stadlan EM, Krivit W. The development of malignancy in the course of the Aldrich syndrome. J Pediatr 68:761–767, 1966.

Bentur L, Nisbet-Brown E, Levinson H, Roifman CM. Lung disease associated with IgG subclass deficiency in chronic mucocutaneous candidiasis. J Pediatr 118:82–86, 1991.

Berkel AI, Henle W, Henle G, Ersoy F, Sanal O, Klein G, Yegin O. Immune response to Epstein-Barr virus (EBV) in ataxia-telangiectasia: EBV-specific antibody patterns and their relation to cell-mediated immunity. In Gatti RA, Swift M, eds. Ataxia-Telangiectasia: Genetics, Neuropathology, and Immunology of a Degenerative Disease of Childhood, Vol. 19. New York, Alan R. Liss, 1984, pp. 287–300.

Biggar WD, Giblett ER, Ozere RL, Grover BD. A new form of nucleoside phosphorylase deficiency in two brothers with defective T-cell function. J Pediatr 92:354–357, 1978.

Billingham RE. The biology of graft-versus-host disease. Harvey Lect 62:21–78, 1966.

Biron CA, Byron KS, Sullivan J. Severe herpesvirus infections in an adolescent without natural killer cells. N Engl J Med 320:1731–1735, 1989.

Blaese RM. Development of gene therapy for immunodeficiency: adenosine deaminase deficiency. Pediatr Res 33(Suppl.):S49–S55, 1993.

Blaese RM, Oppenheim JJ, Seeger RC, Waldmann TA. Lymphocyte-macrophage interaction in antigen-induced in vitro lymphocyte transformation in patients with the Wiskott-Aldrich syndrome and other diseases with anergy. Cell Immunol 4:228–242, 1972.

Blaese RM, Strober W, Brown RS, Waldmann TA. The Wiskott-Aldrich syndrome: a disorder with a possible defect in antigen processing or recognition. Lancet 1:1056–1061, 1968.

Blaese RM, Strober W, Levy AL, Waldmann TA. Hypercatabolism of IgG, IgA, IgM and albumin in the Wiskott-Aldrich syndrome. J Clin Invest 50:2331–2338, 1971.

Blizzard RM, Gibbs JH. Candidiasis: studies pertaining to its association with endocrinopathies and pernicious anemia. Pediatrics 42:231–237, 1968.

Blue ML, Daley JF, Levine H, Schlossman SF. Class II major histocompatibility complex molecules regulate the development of T4$^+$T8$^-$ inducer phenotype of cultured human thymocytes. Proc Natl Acad Sci U S A 82:8178–8183, 1985.

Bluetters-Sawatzki R, Friedrich W, Ebell W, Vetter U, Stoess H, Goldmann SF, Kleihauer E. HLA-haploidentical bone marrow transplantation in three infants with adenosine deaminase deficiency: stable immunological reconstitution and reversal of skeletal abnormalities. Eur J Pediatr 149:104–109, 1989.

Bockman DE, Kirby ML. Dependence of thymus development on derivatives of the neural crest. Science 223:498–500, 1984.

Boder E. Ataxia-telangiectasia: an overview. In Gatti RA, Swift M, eds. Ataxia-telangiectasia: Genetics, Neuropathy, and Immunology of a Degenerative Disease of Childhood. New York, Alan R. Liss, 1985, pp. 1–63.

Boder E, Sedgwick RP. Ataxia-telangiectasia: a familial syndrome of progressive cerebellar ataxia, oculocutaneous telangiectasia, and frequent pulmonary infection. Univ S Calif Med Bull 9:15–27, 1957.

Boder E, Sedgwick RP: Ataxia-telangiectasia: a review of 101 cases. In Walsh G, ed. Cerebellum, Posture and Cerebral Palsy. Clinics in Developmental Medicine Series No. 8. London, The National Spastics Society and Heinemann Medical Books, 1963, pp. 110–118.

Borzy MS, Ridgway D, Noya FJ, Shearer WT. Successful bone marrow transplantation with split lymphoid chimerism in DiGeorge syndrome. J Clin Immunol 9:386–392, 1989.

Borzy MS, Schulte-Wissermann H, Gilbert E, Horowitz SD, Pellett J, Hong R. Thymic morphology in immunodeficiency diseases: results of thymic biopsies. Clin Immunol Immunopathol 12:31–51, 1979.

Bowden DH, Danis PG, Sommers SC. Ataxia-telangiectasia: a case with lesions of ovaries and adenohypophysis. J Neuropathol Exp Neurol 22:549–554, 1963.

Boyd RL, Tucek CL, Godfrey DL, Izon DJ, Wilson TJ, Davidson NJ, Bean AGD, Ladyman HM, Ritter MA, Hugo P. The thymic microenvironment. Immunol Today 14:445–459, 1993.

Brand MM, Marinkovich VA. Primary malignant reticulosis of the brain in Wiskott-Aldrich syndrome. Arch Dis Child 44:536–542, 1969.

Bridges BA, Lenoir G, Tomatis L. Workshop on ataxia-telangiectasia: heterozygotes and cancer. Cancer Res 45:3979–3980, 1985.

Brochstein JA, Gillio AP, Ruggiero M, Kernan NA, Emanuel D, Laver J, Small T, O'Reilly RJ. Marrow transplantation from human leukocyte antigen–identical or haploidentical donors for correction of Wiskott-Aldrich syndrome. J Pediatr 119:907–912, 1991.

Brooks EG, Schmalsteig FC, Wirt DP, Rosenblatt HM, Adkins LT, Lookingbill DP, Rudloff HE, Rakusan TA, Goldman AS. A novel X-linked combined immunodeficiency disease. J Clin Invest 86:1623–1631, 1990.

Broxmeyer HE, Douglas GW, Hangoc G, Cooper S, Bard J, English D, Arny M, Thomas L, Boyse EA. Human umbilical cord blood as a potential source of transplantable hematopoietic stem/progenitor cells. Proc Natl Acad Sci U S A 86:3828–3832, 1989.

Bruce RM, Blaese RM. Monoclonal gammopathy in the Wiskott-Alrich syndrome. J Pediatr 85:204–207, 1974.

Buckley RH. Advances in the correction of immunodeficiency by bone marrow transplantation. Pediatr Ann 16:412–421, 1987.

Buckley RH, Lucas ZJ, Hattler BG, Zmijewski CM, Amos DB. Defective cellular immunity associated with chronic mucocutaneous moniliasis and recurrent staphylococcal botryomycosis: immunological reconstitution by allogeneic bone marrow. Clin Exp Immunol 3:153–169, 1968.

Bullock WE, Fields JP, Brandriss MW. An evaluation of transfer factor as immunotherapy for patients with lepromatous leprosy. N Engl J Med 287:1053–1059, 1972.

Burke BA, Johnson D, Gilbert EF, Drut RM, Ludwig J, Wick MR. Thyrocalcitonin-containing cells in the DiGeorge anomaly. Hum Pathol 18:355–360, 1987.

Canales LM, Mauer AM. Sex-linked hereditary thrombocytopenia as a variant of Wiskott-Aldrich syndrome. N Engl J Med 277:899–901, 1967.

Cannon RA, Blum PM, Ament ME, Byrne WJ, Soderberg-Warner M, Seeger RC, Saxon AE, Stiehm ER. Reversal of enterocolitis-associated combined immunodeficiency by plasma therapy. J Pediatr 101:711–717, 1982.

Carbonari M, Cherchi M, Paganelli R, Giannini G, Galli E, Gaetano C, Papetti C, Fiorilli M. Relative increase of T cells expressing the γ/δ rather than the α/β receptor in ataxia-telangiectasia. N Engl J Med 322:73–76, 1990.

Carey AH, Kelly D, Halford S, Wadey R, Wilson D, Goodship J, Burn J, Paul T, Sharkey A, Dumanski J, Nordenskjold M, Williamson R, Scambler PJ. Molecular genetic study of the frequency of monosomy 22q11 in DiGeorge syndrome. Am J Hum Genet 51:964–970, 1992.

Carey AH, Roach S, Williamson R, Dumanski JP, Nordenskjold M, Collins VP, Rouleau G, Blin N, Jalbert P, Scambler PJ. Localization of 27 DNA markers to the region of human chromosome 22q11-pter deleted in patients with the DiGeorge syndrome and duplicated in the der22 syndrome. Genomics 7:1000, 1990.

Carpella-Deluca E, Aiuti F, Lucarelli P, Tozzi MC, Vignetti P, Bruni L, Roos D, Cobo RM, Imperato C. Nucleoside phosphorylase deficiency, autoimmune hemolytic anaemia, and selective T-cell deficiency. Pediatr Res 12:64A, 1978.

Carroll AM, Bosma HJ. T-lymphocyte development in SCID mice is arrested shortly after the initiation of T-cell receptor gene recombination. Genes Dev 5:1357–1366, 1991.

Carson DA, Carrera CJ. Immunodeficiency secondary to adenosine deaminase deficiency and purine nucleoside phosphorylation deficiency. Semin Hematol 27:260–269, 1990.

Carson DA, Wasson DB, Lakow E, Kamatani N. Possible metabolic basis for the different immunodeficient states associated with genetic deficiencies of adenosine deaminase and purine nucleoside phosphorylase. Proc Natl Acad Sci U S A 79:3848–3852, 1982.

Castigli E, Geha RS, Chatila T. Severe combined immunodeficiency with selective T-cell cytokine genes. Pediatr Res 33(Suppl.):S20–S23, 1993.

Cavazzana-Calva M, Le Deist F, de Saint Basile G, Papadopoulo D, De Villartay JP, Fischer A. Increased radiosensitivity of granulocyte-macrophage colony–forming units and skin fibroblasts in human autosomal recessive severe combined immunodeficiency. J Clin Invest 91:1214–1218, 1993.

Cawley LP, Schenken JR. Monoclonal hypergammaglobulinemia of the γM type in a nine-year-old girl with ataxia-telangiectasia. Am J Clin Pathol 54:790–801, 1970.

Cederbaum SD, Kaitila I, Rimoin DL, Stiehm ER. The chondro-osseous dysplasia of adenosine deaminase deficiency with severe combined immunodeficiency. J Pediatr 89:737–742, 1976.

Cederbaum SD, Niwayama G, Stiehm ER, Neerhout RC, Ammann AJ, Berman W Jr. Combined immunodeficiency presenting as the Letterer-Siwe syndrome. J Pediatr 85:466–471, 1974.

Centerwall SA, Centerwall WR. Ataxia-telangiectasia: a familial degenerative disease leading to mental retardation. Am J Ment Defic 71:185–190, 1966.

Chan AC, Kadlecek TA, Elder ME, Filipovich AH, Kuo W-L, Iwashima M, Parslow TG, Weiss A. ZAP-70 deficiency in an autosomal recessive form of severe combined immunodeficiency. Science 264:1599–1601, 1994.

Chaptal J, Royer P, Jean R, Alagille D, Bonnett H, Lagarde E, Robinet M, Rieu D. Syndrome de Wiskott-Aldrich avec survie prolongé (9 ans.). Evolution mortelle par thymosarcoma. Arch Fr Pediatr 23:907–920, 1966.

Charles BM, Hosking G, Green A, Pollitt R, Bartlett K, Taitz LS. Biotin-responsive alopecia and developmental regression. Lancet 2:118–120, 1979.

Chatila T, Wong R, Young M, Miller R, Terhorst C, Geha RF. An immunodeficiency characterized by defective signal transduction in T lymphocytes. N Engl J Med 320:696–702, 1989.

Chessa L, Lisa A, Fiorani O, Zei G. Ataxia-telangiectasia in Italy: genetic analysis. Int J Radiat Biol 6(Suppl):531–533, 1994.

Chilgren RA, Quie PG, Meuwissen HJ, Hong R. Chronic mucocutaneous candidiasis, deficiency of delayed hypersensitivity, and selective local antibody defect. Lancet ii:688–693, 1967.

Chipps BE, Saulsbury FT, Hsu SH, Hughes WT, Winkelstein JA. Non-candidal infections in children with chronic mucocutaneous candidiasis. Johns Hopkins Med J 44:175–179, 1979.

Chu ET, Rosenwasser LJ, Dinarello CA, Rosen FS, Geha RS. Immunodeficiency with defective T-cell response to interleukin 1. Proc Natl Acad Sci U S A 81:4945–4949, 1984.

Citrin Y, Sterling K, Halsted JA. The mechanism of hypoproteinemia associated with giant hypertrophy of the gastric mucosa. N Engl J Med 257:906–912, 1957.

Clement LT, Giorgi JV, Plaeger-Marshall S, Haas A, Stiehm ER, Martin AM. Abnormal differentiation of immunoregulatory T lymphocyte subpopulations in the major histocompatibility complex (MHC) class II antigen deficiency syndrome. J Clin Immunol 8:503–512, 1988a.

Clement LT, Plaeger-Marshall S, Haas A, Saxon A, Martin AM. Bare lymphocyte syndrome: consequences of absent class II major histocompatibility antigen expression for B lymphocyte differentiation and function. J Clin Invest 81:669–675, 1988b.

Cleveland WW, Fogel BJ, Brown WT, Kay HEM. Foetal thymic transplant in a case of DiGeorge's syndrome. Lancet 2:1211–1214, 1968.

Clowes GHA Jr, George BC, Villee CA Jr, Saravis CA. Muscle proteolysis induced by a circulating peptide in patients with sepsis or trauma. N Engl J Med 308:545–552, 1983.

Cohen A, Hirschhorn R, Horowitz SD, Rubenstein A, Polmar SH, Hong R, Martin DW Jr. Deoxyadenosine triphosphate as a toxic metabolite in adenosine deaminase deficiency. Proc Natl Acad Sci U S A 75:472–476, 1978.

Como JA, Dismukes WE. Oral azole drugs as systemic antifungal therapy. N Engl J Med 330:263–272, 1994.

Conley ME. Molecular approaches to analysis of X-linked immunodeficiencies. Ann Rev Immunol 322:1063–1066, 1992.

Conley ME, Beckwith JB, Mancer JFK, Tenckhoff L. The spectrum of the DiGeorge syndrome. J Pediatr 94:883–890, 1979.

Conley ME, Buckley RH, Hong R, Guerra-Hanson C, Roifman CM, Brochstein JA, Pahwa S, Puck JM. X-linked severe combined immunodeficiency: diagnosis in males with sporadic severe combined immunodeficiency and clarification of clinical findings. J Clin Invest 85:1548–1554, 1990.

Conley ME, Lavoie A, Briggs C, Brown P, Guerra C, Puck JM: Nonrandom X chromosome inactivation in B cells from carriers of X chromosome–linked severe combined immunodeficiency. Proc Acad Natl Sci U S A 85:3090–3094, 1988.

Conley ME, Spinner NB, Emanuel BS, Nowell PC, Nichols WW. A chromosomal breakage syndrome with profound immunodeficiency. Blood 67:1251–1256, 1986.

Cooper MD, Chase HP, Lowman JT, Krivit W, Good RA. Wiskott-Aldrich syndrome: immunologic deficiency disease involving the afferent limb of immunity. Am J Med 44:499–513, 1968.

Cooper MD, Krivit W, Peterson RDA, Good RA. An immunological defect in Wiskott-Aldrich patients (abstract). In Transactions American Pediatric Society, 74th Annual Meeting, Seattle, June 16–18, 1964.

Cowan MJ, Wara D, Packman S, Ammann A, Yoshino M, Sweetnam L, Nyhan W. Multiple biotin-dependent carboxylase deficiencies associated with defects in T-cell and B-cell immunity. Lancet 2:115–118, 1979.

Cowan MJ, Wara DW, Weintrub PS, Pabst H, Ammann AJ. Haploidentical bone marrow transplantation for severe combined immunodeficiency disease using soybean agglutinin–negative, T-depleted marrow cells. J Clin Immunol 5:370–376, 1985.

Craig JM, Schiff LH, Boone JE. Chronic moniliasis associated with Addison's disease. Am J Dis Child 89:669–684, 1955.

Curry CJR, O'Lague P, Tsai J, Hutchinson HT, Jaspers NGJ, Wara D, Gatti RA. AT_FRESNO: a phenotype linking ataxia-telangiectasia with the Nijmegen breakage syndrome. Am J Hum Genet 45:270–275, 1989.

Davis JA. A case of Swiss-type agammaglobulinemia and achondroplasia: Clinicopathological Conference. Br Med J 2:1371–1374, 1966.

Dayan AD. Chronic encephalitis in children with severe immunodeficiency. Acta Neuropathol (Berl) 19:234–241, 1971.

de la Salle H, Hanau D, Fricker D, Urlacher A, Kelly A, Salamero J, Powis SH, Donato L, Bausinger H, Laforet M, Jeras M, Spehner D, Bieber T, Falkenrodt A, Cazenave J-P, Trowsdale J, Tongio M-M. Homozygous human TAP peptide transporter mutation in HLA class I deficiency. Science 265:237–240, 1994.

de Preval C, Hadam MR, Mach B. Regulation of genes for HLA class II antigens in cell lines from patients with severe combined immunodeficiency. N Engl J Med 318:1295–1300, 1988.

de Preval C, Lisowska-Grospierre B, Loche M, Griscelli C, Mach B. A trans-acting class II regulatory gene unlinked to the MCH controls expression of HLA class II genes. Nature 318:291–293, 1985.

de Saint-Basile G, Arveiler B, Fraser NJ, Boyd Y, Craig IW, Griscelli C, Fischer A. Close linkage of hypervariable marker DSX255 to disease locus of Wiskott-Aldrich syndrome. Lancet 2:1319–1321, 1989.

de Saint-Basile G, Le Diest F, Caniglia M, Lebranchu Y, Griscelli C, Fischer A. Genetic study of a new X-linked recessive immunodeficiency syndrome. J Clin Invest 89:861–866, 1992.

de Saint-Basile G, Le Diest F, de Villartay J-P, Cerf-Bensussan N, Journet O, Brousse N, Griscelli C, Fischer A. Restricted heterogeneity of T lymphocytes in combined immunodeficiency with hypereosinophilia (Omenn's syndrome). J Clin Invest 87:1352–1359, 1991.

De Vaal OM, Seynhaeve V. Reticular dysgenesia. Lancet 2:1123–1125, 1959.

Deeg HJ, Cottler-Fox M. Clinical spectrum and pathophysiology of acute graft-vs.-host disease. In Burakoff SJ, Deeg HJ, Ferrara J, Atkinson K, eds. Graft-vs.-Host Disease: Immunology, Pathophysiology, and Treatment. New York, Marcel Dekker, pp. 311–336, 1990.

Deeg HJ, Lum LG, Sanders J, Levy GJ, Sullivan KM, Beatty P, Thomas ED, Storb, R. Severe aplastic anemia associated with chronic mucocutaneous candidiasis: immunologic and hematologic reconstitution after allogeneic bone marrow transplantation. Transplantation 41:583–586, 1986.

Derry JMJ, Ochs HD, Francke U. Isolation of a novel gene mutated in Wiskott-Aldrich syndrome. Cell 78:635–644, 1994.

Desmaze C, Scambler P, Priem M, Halford S, Sidi D, LeDiest F, Annias A. Routine diagnosis of DiGeorge syndrome by fluorescent in situ hybridization. Hum Genet 90:663–665, 1993.

Diaz-Buxo JA, Hermans PE, Ritts RE. Wiskott-Aldrich syndrome in an adult. Mayo Clin Proc 49:455–458, 1974.

DiGeorge AM. A new concept of the cellular basis of immunity (discussion). J Pediatr 67:907–908, 1965.

Dinarello CA. Interleukin-1. Rev Infect Dis 6:51, 1984.

Disanto JP, Keever CA, Small TN, Nichols GL, O'Reilly RJ, Flomenberg N. Absence of interleukin 2 production in a severe combined immunodeficiency disease syndrome with T cells. J Exp Med 171:1697–1704, 1990.

Dismukes WE. Azole antifungal drugs. Ann Intern Med 109:177–179, 1988.

Djawari D, Bischoff T, Hornstein OP. Impairment of chemotactic activity of macrophages in chronic mucocutaneous candidosis. Arch Derm Res 262:247–253, 1978.

Dogra KN, Manchanda SS. Ataxia-telangiectasia. Indian Pediatr 4:354–357, 1967.

Doi S, Saiki OH, Sugita T, Ha-Kawa K, Tanaka T, Hara H, Negoro S, Yabuuchi H, Kishimoto S. Administration of recombinant IL-2 augments the level of serum IgM in an IL-2–deficient patient. Eur J Pediatr 148:630–633, 1989.

Doi S, Saiki O, Tanaka T, Ha-Kawa K, Igarashi T, Fujita T, Taniguchi T, Kishimoto S. Cellular and genetic analyses of IL-2 production and IL-2 receptor expression in a patient with familial T-cell–dominant immunodeficiency. Clin Immunol Immunopathol 46:24–36, 1988.

Drew JH. Chronic mucocutaneous candidiasis with abnormal function of serum complement. Med J Austral 2:77–80, 1973.

Driscoll AD, Budarf ML, Emanuel BS. A genetic etiology for DiGeorge syndrome: consistent deletions and microdeletions of 22q11. Am J Hum Genet 50:924–933, 1992.

Duncan RA, von Reyn C, Alliegro GM, Toossi ZS, Levitz SM. Idiopathic CD4+ T-lymphocytopenia—four patients with opportunistic infections and no evidence of HIV infection. N Engl J Med 328:393–398, 1993.

Dunn HG, Meuwissen H, Livingstone CS, Pump KK. Ataxia-telangiectasia. Can Med Assoc J 91:1106–1118, 1964.

Dupont B, Anderson V, Ernst P, Faber V, Good RA, Hansen GS, Henricksen K, Jensen G, Juhl F, Killman SA, Koch C, Muller-Bérat N, Park BH, Svejgaard AS, Thomsen M, Wiik A. Immunological reconstitution in severe combined immunodeficiency with HLA-incompatible bone marrow graft: donor selection by mixed lymphocyte culture. Transplant Proc 5:905–908, 1973.

Durandy A, Dumez Y, Griscelli C. Antenatal diagnosis of severe hereditary immunologic deficiency syndromes. Arch Fr Pediatr 42:163–167, 1985.

Durandy A, LeDiest F, Fischer A, Griscelli C. Impaired T8 mediated suppressive activity in patients with partial DiGeorge syndrome. J Clin Immunol 6:265–270, 1968.

Durandy A, Oury C, Griscelli C, Dumez Y, Oury JF, Henrion R. Prenatal testing for inherited immune deficiencies by fetal blood sampling. Prenat Diagn 2:109–113, 1982.

Durum SK, Schmidt JA, Oppenheim JJ. Interleukin 1: an immunological perspective. Ann Rev Immunol 3:263–287, 1985.

Eibl MM, Mannhalter JW, Zlabinger G, Mayr WR, Tilz GP, Ahmad R, Zielinski CC. Defective macrophage function in a patient with common variable immunodeficiency. N Engl J Med 307:803–806, 1982.

Eisen AH, Karpati G, Laszlo T, Andermann F, Robb JP, Bacal HL. Immunologic deficiency in ataxia-telangiectasia. N Engl J Med 272:18–22, 1965.

Eisen D, Ellis CN, Duell EA, Grifiths CEM, Voorhees JJ. Effect of topical cyclosporine rinse on oral lichen planus. N Engl J Med 323:290–294, 1990.

Eitzman DV, Smith RT. Immunological studies on a patient with Aldrich's syndrome. South Med J 53:1593, 1960.

Elder ME, Lin D, Clever J, Chan AC, Hope TJ, Weiss A, Parslow TG. Human severe combined immunodeficiency due to a defect in ZAP-70, a T cell tyrosine kinase. Science 264:1596–1599, 1994.

Epstein WL, Fudenberg HH, Reed WB, Boder E, Sedgwick RP. Immunologic studies in ataxia-telangiectasia. Int Arch Allergy 30:15–29, 1966.

Ersoy F, Berkel AI. Clinical and immunological studies in twenty families with ataxia-telangiectasia. Turk J Pediatr 16:145–160, 1974.

Español T, Compte J, Alvarez C, Tallada N, Laverde R, Peguero G. Reticular dysgenesis: report of two brothers. Clin Exp Immunol 38:615–620, 1979.

Evans DI, Holzel A. Immune deficiency state in a girl with eczema and low serum IgM: possible female variant of Wiskott-Aldrich syndrome. Arch Dis Child 45:527–533, 1970.

Fauci AS. CD4+ T-lymphocytopenia without HIV infection—no lights, no camera, just facts. N Engl J Med 328:429–430, 1993.

Fearon EF, Winkelstein JA, Civin CI, Pardoll DM, Vogelstein B. Carrier detection in X-linked agammaglobulinemia by chromosome inactivation. N Engl J Med 316:427–431, 1987.

Feigin RD, Middelkamp JN, Kissane JM, Warren RJ. Agammaglobulinemia and thymic dysplasia associated with ectodermal dysplasia. Pediatrics 47:143–147, 1971.

Feigin RD, Vietti TJ, Wyatt RG, Kaufman DG, Smith CH. Ataxia-telangiectasia with granulocytopenia. J Pediatr 77:431–438, 1970.

Ferrara JLM, Deeg HJ: Graft-versus-host disease. N Engl J Med 324:667–674, 1991.

Ferrara JLM, Guillen FJ, van Dijken PJ, Marion A, Murphy GF, Burakoff SJ. Evidence that large granular lymphocytes of donor origin mediate acute graft-versus-host disease. Transplantation 47:50–54, 1989.

Filipovitch AH, Shapiro RS, Ramsay NKC, Kim T, Blazar B, Kersey J, McGlave P. Unrelated donor bone marrow transplantation for correction of lethal congenital immunodeficiencies. Blood 80:270–276, 1992.

Fiorilli M, Businco L, Pandolfi F, Paganelli R, Russo G, Aiuti F. Heterogeneity of immunological abnormalities in ataxia-telangiectasia. J Clin Immunol 3:135–141, 1983.

Fireman P, Boesman M, Gitlin D. Ataxia-telangiectasia: a dysgammaglobulinemia with deficiency of $\gamma_{1A} \beta_{2A}$ globulin. Lancet 1:1193–1195, 1964.

Fireman P, Johnson HA, Gitlin D. Presence of plasma cells and gamma-M-globulin synthesis in a patient with thymic alymphoplasia. Pediatrics 37:485–492, 1966.

Fischer A. Bone marrow transplantation for immunodeficiencies and osteopetrosis. Bone Marrow Transplant 7(Suppl. 3):101–102, 1991.

Fischer A, Ballet J-J, Griscelli C. Specific inhibition of in vitro Candida–induced lymphocyte proliferation by polysaccharide antigens present in the serum of patients with chronic mucocutaneous candidiasis. J Clin Invest 62:1005–1013, 1978.

Fischer A, Blanche S, Le Bidois J, Bordigoni P, Garnier JL, Niaudet P, Morinet F, Le Deist F, Fischer AM, Griscelli C, and Hirn M: Anti-B cell monoclonal antibodies in the treatment of severe B-cell lymphoproliferative syndrome following bone marrow and organ transplantation. N Engl J Med 324:1451–1456, 1991a.

Fischer A, Friedrich W, Fasth A, Blanche S, Le Deist F, Girault D, Veber F, Vossen J, Lopez M, Griscelli C. Reduction of graft failure by a monoclonal antibody (anti-LFA-1 CD11a) after HLA nonidentical bone marrow transplantation in children with immunodeficiencies, osteopetrosis, and Fanconi's anemia: a European Group for Immunodeficiency/European Group for Bone Marrow Transplantation report. Blood 77:249–256, 1991b.

Fischer A, Griscelli C, Friedrich W, Kubanek B, Levinsky R, Morgan G, Vossen J, Wagemaker G, Landais P. Bone marrow transplantation for immunodeficiencies and osteopetrosis: European survey 1968–1985. Lancet 2:1079–1083, 1986.

Fischer A, Landais P, Friedrich W, Gerritsen B, Fasth A, Porta A, Vellodi A, Benkerrou M, Jais JP, Cavazzana-Calvo M, Souillet P, Bordigoni P, Morgan G, Van Dijken P, Vossen J, Locatelli F, di Bartolomeo P. Bone marrow transplantation (BMT) in Europe for primary immunodeficiencies other than severe combined immunodeficiency: A report from the European Group for BMT and the European Group for Immunodeficiency. Blood 83:1149–1154, 1994.

Fischer TJ, Klein RB, Kershnar HE, Borut TC, and Stiehm ER: Miconazole in the treatment of chronic mucocutaneous candidiasis. A preliminary report. J Pediatr 91:815–819, 1977.

Flomenberg N, Welte K, Mertelsmann R, Kernan N, Ciobanu N, Venuta S, Feldman S, Kruger G, Kirkpatrick D, Dupont B, O'Reilly R. Immunologic effects of interleukin-2 in primary immunodeficiency diseases. J Immunol 130:2644–2650, 1983.

Foroud T, Wei S, Ziv Y, Sobel E, Lange E, Chao A, Goradia T, Huo Y, Tolun A, Chessa L, Charmley P, Sanal O, Saiman N, Julier C, Lathrop GM, Concannon P, McConville C, Taylor M, Shiloh Y, Lange K, Gatti RA. Localization of an ataxia-telangiectasia locus to a 4-cm interval on chromosome 11q23 by linkage analyses of an international consortium of 111 families. Am J Hum Genet 49:1263–1279, 1991.

Fox RI, Chan R, Michelson JB, Belmont JB, Michelson PE. Beneficial effect of artificial tears made with autologous serum in patients with keratoconjunctivitis sicca. Arthritis Rheum 27:459–461, 1984.

Friedman TC, Thomas PM, Fleisher TH, Feuillan P, Parker RI, Cassorla F, Chrousos GP. Frequent occurrence of asplenism and cholelithiasis in patients with autoimmune polyglandular disease type I. Am J Med 91:625–630, 1991.

Friedrich W, Goldmann S, Ebell W, Bluters-Sawatzki R, Gaedicke G, Raghavachar A, Peter HH, Belohradsky B, Kreth W, Kubanek B, Kleihauerr E. Severe combined immunodeficiency; treatment by bone marrow transplantation in 15 infants using HLA-haploidentical donors. Eur J Pediatr 144:125–130, 1985.

Friedrich W, Goldmann SF, Vetter U, Fliedner TM, Heymer B, Peter HH, Reisner Y, Kleihauer E. Immunoreconstitution in severe combined immunodeficiency after transplantation of HLA-haploidentical, T-cell–depleted bone marrow. Lancet 1:761–764, 1984.

Fudenberg HH, Levin AS, Spitler LE, Wybran J, Byers V. The therapeutic uses of transfer factor. Hosp Pract 9:95–104, 1974.

Fukuda T, Matsunaga M, Kurata A, Mine M, Ikari N, Katamine S, Kanazawa H, Eguchi K, Nagataki S. Hereditary deficiency of OKT4-positive cells: studies for mode of inheritance and lymphocyte functions. Immunology 53:643–649, 1984.

Fulginiti VA, Kemkpe GH, Hathaway WE, Pearlman DS, Sieber OF, Heller JJ, Joyner JJ, Robinson A. Progressive vaccinia in immunologically deficient individuals. In Bergsma D, Good RA, eds. Immunologic Deficiency Diseases in Man. National Foundation: Birth Defects, Vol. 4, No. 1. Baltimore, Williams & Wilkins, 1968, pp. 129–151.

Garcia CR, Brown NA, Schreck R, Stiehm ER, Hudnall SD. B-cell lymphoma in severe combined immunodeficiency not associated with the Epstein-Barr virus. Cancer 60:2941–2947, 1987.

Gaschet J, Mahe B, Milpied N, Devilder M-C, Dreno B, Bignon J-D, Davodeau F, Hallet M-M, Bonneville M, Vie H. Specificity of T cells invading the skin during acute graft-vs.-host disease after semiallogeneic bone marrow transplantation. J Clin Invest 91:12–20, 1993.

Gatti RA, Aurias A, Griscelli C, Sparkes RS. Translocations involving chromosome 2p and 22q in ataxia-telangiectasia. Dis Markers 3:169–175, 1985.

Gatti RA, Berkel I, Boder E, Braedt G, Charmley P, Concannon P, Ersoy F, Foroud T, Jaspers NGJ, Lange K, Lathrop GM, Leppert M, Nakamura Y, O'Connell P, Paterson M, Salser W, Sanal O, Silver J, Sparkes RS, Susi E, Weeks DE, Wei S, White P, Yoder F. Localization of an ataxia-telangiectasia gene to chromosome 11q22–23. Nature 336:577–580, 1988.

Gatti RA, Bick M, Tam CF, Medici MA, Oxelius VA, Holland M, Goldstein AL, Boder E: Ataxia-telangiectasia: a multiparameter analysis of eight families. Clin Immunol Immunopathol 23:501–516, 1982.

Gatti RA, Boder E, Vinters HV, Sparkes RS, Norman A, Lange K. Ataxia-telangiectasia: an interdisciplinary approach to pathogenesis. Medicine 70:99–117, 1991.

Gatti RA, Lange E, Rotman G. Chen X, Uhrhammer N, Liang T, Chiplunkar S, Yang L, Udar N, Dandekar S, Sheikhavandi S, Wang Z, Yang HM, Polikow J, Elashoff M, Teletar M, Sanal O, Chessa L, McConville C, Taylor M, Shiloh Y, Porras O, Borresen AL, Wegner RD, Curry C, Gerken S, Lange K, Concannon P. Genetic haplotyping of ataxia-telangiectasia families localizes the major gene to an 850 kb region on chromosome 11q23.1. Int J Radiat Biol 6(suppl):S57–S62, 1994.

Gatti RA, Meuwissen HJ, Allen HD, Hong R, Good RA. Immunological reconstitution of sex-linked lymphopenic immunological deficiency. Lancet 2:1366–1369, 1968.

Gatti RA, Platt N, Pomerance HH, Hong R, Langer LO, Kay HEM, Good RA. Hereditary lymphopenic agammaglobulinemia associated with a distinctive form of short-limbed dwarfism and ectodermal dysplasia. J Pediatr 75:675–684, 1969.

Gatti RA, Vinters HV. Cerebellar pathology in ataxia-telangiectasia: the significance of basket cells. In Gatti RA, Swift M, eds. Ataxia-Telangiectasia: Genetics, Neuropathology, and Immunology of a Degenerative Disease of Childhood, Vol. 19. New York, Alan R. Liss, 1984, pp. 225–232.

Geha RA, Malakian A, LeFranc G, Chayban D, Serre JL. Immunologic reconstitution in severe combined immunodeficiency following transplantation with parental bone marrow. Pediatrics 58:451–455, 1976.

Gehrz RC, McAuliffe JJ, Linner KM, Kersey JH. Defective membrane function in a patient with severe combined immunodeficiency disease. Clin Exp Immunol 39:344–348, 1980.

Gershon AA, Steinberg S, Brunnell PA. Zoster immune globulin. N Engl J Med 290:243–245, 1974.

Giblett ER, Ammann AJ, Wara DW, Sandman R, Diamond LK. Nucleoside-phosphorylase deficiency in a child with severely defective T-cell immunity and normal B-cell immunity. Lancet 1:1010–1013, 1975.

Giblett ER, Anderson JE, Cohen F, Pollara B, Meuwissen HJ. Adenosine deaminase deficiency in two patients with severely impaired cellular immunity. Lancet 2:1067–1069, 1972.

Gidding SS, Minciotti AL, Langman CB. Unmasking of hypoparathyroidism in familial partial DiGeorge syndrome by challenge with disodium edetate. N Engl J Med 319:1589–1591, 1988.

Gill JC, Maples J, Nikaein A, Kirchner P, Lockhart D, Snyder AJ, Montgomery RR, Casper JT. Inherited absence of OKT4 lymphocyte antigen in a chronically transfused patient with homozygous sickle cell disease. J Pediatr 107:251–253, 1985.

Gillis S, Smith KA. Long-term culture of cytotoxic T-lymphocytes. Nature 268:154–156, 1977.

Gimeno A, Liano H, Kreisler M. Ataxia-telangiectasia with absence of IgG. J Neurol Sci 8:545–554, 1969.

Gitlin D, Vawter G, Craig JM. Thymic alymphoplasia and congenital aleukocytosis. Pediatrics 33:184–192, 1964.

Glanzmann E, Riniker P. Essentielle Lymphocytophthise. Ein neues Krankheitsbildaus der Sauglings-pathologie. Ann Paediatr (Basel) 175:1–32, 1950.

Gluckman E, Devergie A, Dutreix J: Radiosensitivity in Fanconi anemia: application to the conditioning regimen for bone marrow transplantation. Br J Haematol 54:431–440, 1983.

Gluckman E, Broxmeyer HE, Auerbach AD, Friedman HS, Douglas GW, Devergie A, Esperon H, Thierry D, Socie G, Lehn P, Cooper S, English D, Kurtzberg J, Bard J, Boyse EA. Hematopoietic reconstitution in a patient with Fanconi's anemia by means of umbilical-cord blood from an HLA-identical sibling. N Engl J Med 321:1174–1178, 1989.

Glucksberg H, Storb R, Fefer A, Buckner CD, Neiman PE, Clift RA, Lerner KG, Thomas ED. Clinical manifestations of graft-versus-host disease in human recipients of marrow from HLA-matched sibling donors. Transplantation 18:295–302, 1974.

Goldsmith CI, Hart WR. Ataxia-telangiectasia with ovarian gonadoblastoma and contralateral dysgerminoma. Cancer 36:1838–1842, 1975.

Goldsmith MA, Weiss A. Isolation and characterization of a T-lymphocyte somatic mutant with altered signal transduction by the antigen receptor. Proc Natl Acad Sci U S A 84:6879–6883, 1987.

Goldsobel AB, Haas A, Stiehm ER. Bone marrow transplantation in DiGeorge syndrome. J Pediatr 111:40–44, 1987.

Goldstein AL, Cohen CH, Rossio JL, Thurman GB, Ulrich HT. Use of thymosin in the treatment of primary immunodeficiency diseases and cancer. Med Clin North Am 60:591–606, 1976.

Goldstein AL, Guha A, Zatz MM, Hardy MA, White A. Purification and biological activity of thymosin, a hormone of the thymus gland. Proc Natl Acad Sci U S A 69:1800–1803, 1972.

Good RA. Historical aspects of immunologic deficiency diseases. In Kagan BM, Stiehm ER, eds. Immunologic Incompetence. Chicago, Year Book, 1971, pp. 149–177.

Goodman WN, Cooper WC, Kessler GB, Fischer MS, Gardner MB. Ataxia-telangiectsia: report of two cases in siblings presenting a picture of progressive spinal muscular atrophy. Bull Los Angeles Neurol Sci 34:1–22, 1969.

Goodship J, Malcolm S, Lau YL, Pembrey ME, Levinsky RJ. Use of X-chromosome inactivation analysis to establish carrier status for X-linked severe combined immunodeficiency. Lancet 1:729–732, 1988.

Gotoff SP, Amirmokri E, Liebner EJ. Ataxia-telangiectasia: neoplasia, untoward response to x-irradiation and tuberous sclerosis. Am J Dis Child 114:617–625, 1967.

Graybill JR, Silva J, Alford RH, Thor DE. Immunologic and clinical improvement of progressive coccidioidomycosis following administration of transfer factor. Cell Immunol 8:120–135, 1973.

Greenberg F, Courtney KB, Wessels RA, Huhta J, Carpenter RJ, Rich DC, Ledbetter DH. Prenatal diagnosis of deletion 17p13 associated with DiGeorge anomaly. Am J Med Genet 31:1–4, 1988a.

Greenberg F, Elder FFB, Haffner P, Northrup H, Ledbetter DH. Cytogenetic findings in a prospective series of patients with DiGeorge anomaly. Am J Hum Genet 43:605–611, 1988b.

Greenberg F, Crowder WE, Paschall V, Colon-Linares J, Lubianski B, Ledbetter DH. Familial DiGeorge syndrome and associated partial monosomy of chromosome 22. Hum Genet 65:317–319, 1984.

Greenberger NJ, Tennenbaum JI, Ruppert RD. Protein-losing enteropathy associated with gastrointestinal allergy. Am J Med 43:777–784, 1967.

Greer WL, Higgins E, Sutherland DR, Novogrodsky A, Brockhausen I, Peacocke M, Rubin LA, Baker M, Denis JW, Siminovitch KA. Altered expression of leucocyte sialoglycoprotein in Wiskott-Aldrich syndrome is associated with a specific defect in O-glycosylation. Biochem Cell Biol 67:503–509, 1989.

Grimm EA, Mazumder A, Zhang H, Rosenberg S. Lymphokine-activated killer cell phenomenon. Lysis of natural killer–resistant fresh solid tumor cells by interleukin 2–activated autologous human peripheral blood lymphocytes. J Exp Med 155:1823–1841, 1982.

Griscelli C, Durandy A, Guy-Grand D, Daguillard F, Herzog C, Prunieras M. A syndrome associating partial albinism and immunodeficiency. Am J Med 65:691–702, 1978.

Griscelli C, Durandy A, Virelizier JL, Grospierre B, Oury C, de Saint-Basile G, Couillin P, Niaudet P, Betuel H, Hors J, Lepage V, Colombani J. Impaired cell-to-cell interaction in partial combined immunodeficiency with defective synthesis and membrane expression of HLA antigens. In Touraine JL, Gluckman E, Griscelli C, eds. Bone Marrow Transplantation in Europe II. Amsterdam, Excerpta Medica Elsevier, 1981, pp. 194–200.

Gropp A, Flatz G. Chromosome breakage and blastic transformation of lymphocytes in ataxia-telangiectasia. Humangenetik 5:77–79, 1967.

Groshong T, Horowitz S, Lovchik J, Davis A, Hong R. Chronic cytomegalovirus infection, immunodeficiency and monoclonal immunopathy—antigen-driven malignancy? J Pediatr 88:217–233, 1976.

Gröttum KA, Hovig T, Holmsen H, Abrahamsen F, Jeremic M, Seip M. Wiskott-Aldrich syndrome: qualitative platelet defects and shortened platelet survival. Br J Haematol 17:373–388, 1969.

Grusby MJ, Johnson RS, Papaioannou VE, Glimcher LH. Depletion of CD4$^+$ T cells in major histocompatibility complex class II–deficient mice. Science 253:1417–1420, 1991.

Haas A, Wells J, Chin T, Stiehm ER. Successful treatment of reticular dysgenesis with haploidentical bone marrow transplantation (BMT). Clin Res 34:127A, 1986.

Haas RJ, Neithammer D, Goldman SF, Heit W, Bienzie U, Kleihauer E. Congenital immunodeficiency and agranulocytosis (reticular dysgenesis). Acta Paediatr Scand 66:279–283, 1977.

Hadam MR, Dopfer R, Peter H-H, Niethammer D. Congenital agammaglobulinemia associated with lack of expression of HLA-D region antigens. In Griscelli C, Vossen JM, eds. Progress in Immunodeficiency Research and Therapy I. Amsterdam, Excerpta Medica Elsevier, 1984, pp. 43–50.

Haerer AF, Jackson JF, Evers CG. Ataxia-telangiectasia with gastric adenocarcinoma. JAMA 210:1884–1887, 1969.

Ham Pong AJ, Cavallo A, Holman GH, Goldman AS. DiGeorge syndrome: long-term survival complicated by Graves' disease. J Pediatr 106:619–620, 1985.

Hamet M, Griscelli C, Cartier P, Ballay J, deBruyn C, Hösli P. A second case of inosine phosphorylase deficiency with severe T-cell abnormalities. Adv Exp Med Biol 76A:477–480, 1977.

Handyside AH, Lesko JG, Tarin JJ, Winston RML, Hughes MR. Birth of a normal girl after in vitro fertilization and preimplantation diagnostic testing for cystic fibrosis. N Engl J Med 327:905–909, 1992.

Hanicki Z, Hanicka M, Rembiesowa H. Immunologic aspects of ataxia-telangiectasia. Int Arch Allergy Appl Immunol 32:436–452, 1967.

Hanto DW, Frizzera G, Gajl-Peczalska KJ, Sakamoto K, Purtilo DT, Balfour HH Jr, Simmons RL, Najarian JS. Epstein-Barr virus–induced B-cell lymphoma after renal transplantation: acyclovir therapy and transition from polyclonal to monoclonal B-cell proliferation. N Engl J Med 306:913–918, 1982.

Hanto DW, Frizzera G, Gajl-Peczalska KJ, Simmons RL. Epstein-Barr virus, immunodeficiency, and B cell lymphoproliferation. Transplantation 39:461–472, 1985.

Harley RD, Baird HW, Craven EM. Ataxia-telangiectasia. Arch Ophthalmol 77:582–592, 1967.

Harrington H. Absence of the thymus gland. London Med Gaz 3:314, 1829.

Harris VJ, Seeler RA. Ataxia-telangiectasia and Hodgkin's disease. Cancer 32:1415–1420, 1973.

Hassler O. Ataxia-telangiectasia (Louis-Barr's syndrome). Acta Neurol Scand 43:464–471, 1967.

Hassner A, Adelman DC. Biologic response modifiers in primary immunodeficiency disorders. Ann Intern Med 115:294–307, 1991.

Hathaway WE, Githens JH, Blackburn WR, Fulginiti V, Kempe CH. Aplastic anemia, histiocytosis and erythrodermia in immunologically deficient children. N Engl J Med 273:953–958, 1965.

Hatsu Y, Uno Y. An autopsy case of ataxia-telangiectasia. Acta Pathol Jap 19:229–239, 1969.

Hattori A, Ihara T, Iwasa T, Kamiya H, Sakurai M, Izawa T. Use of live varicella vaccine in children with acute leukemia or other malignancies. Lancet 2:210, 1976.

Hayakawa H, Matsui I, Yoshino K, Hayakawa S, Kobayashi N. Immunopathological aspects of ataxia-telangiectasia. Paediatr Univ Tokyo 16:1–10, 1968.

Haynes BF, Martin ME, Kay HH, Kurtzberg J. Early events in human T cell ontogeny. J Exp Med 168:1061–1080, 1988.

Haynes BF, Scearce RM, Lobach DF, Hensley LL. Phenotypic characterization and ontogeny of mesodermal-derived and endocrine epithelial components of the human thymic microenvironment. J Exp Med 159:1149–1168, 1984.

Haynes BF, Warren RW, Buckley RH, McClure JE, Goldstein AL, Henderson FW, Hensley LL, Eisenbarth GS. Demonstration of abnormalities in expression of thymic epithelial surface antigens in severe cellular immunodeficiency diseases. J Immunol 130:1182–1190, 1983.

Hecht F, McCaw BK, Koler RD. Ataxia-telangiectasia–clonal growth of translocation lymphocytes. N Engl J Med 289:286–291, 1973.

Heiner DC, Wilson JF, Lahey ME. Sensitivity to cow's milk. JAMA 189:563–567, 1964.

Henle W, Henle GE, Horowitz CA. Epstein-Barr virus–specific diagnostic tests in infectious mononucleosis. Hum Pathol 5:551–565, 1974.

Herberman RB, Ortaldo JR. Natural killer cells: their role in defenses against disease. Science 214:24–30, 1981.

Herrod HG. Chronic mucocutaneous candidiasis in childhood and complications of non-Candida infection: a report of the Pediatric Immunodeficiency Collaborative Study Group. J Pediatr 116:377–382, 1990.

Hershfield MS, Chaffee S. PEG enzyme replacement therapy for adenosine deaminase deficiency. In Desnick RJ, ed. Treatment of Genetic Diseases. New York, Churchill Livingstone, 1991, pp. 169–182.

Hershfield MS, Chaffee S, Sorensen RU. Enzyme replacement therapy with polyethylene glycol–adenosine deaminase in adenosine deaminase deficiency: overview and case reports of three patients, including two now receiving gene therapy. Pediatr Res 3(Suppl.):S42–S48, 1993.

Higgins EA, Siminovitch KA, Zhuang D, Brockhausen I, Dennis JW. Aberrant O-linked oligosaccharide biosynthesis in lymphocytes and platelets from patients with the Wiskott-Aldrich syndrome. J Biol Chem 266:6280–6290, 1991.

Higgs JM, Wells RS. Chronic mucocutaneous candidiasis: associated abnormalities of iron metabolism. Br J Dermatol 86(Suppl. 8):88–102, 1972.

Hirschhorn R. Defects of purine metabolism in immunodeficiency disease. Progr Clin Immunol 3:67–83, 1977.

Hirschhorn R. Adenosine deaminase deficiency. Immunodefic Rev 2:175–198, 1990.

Hirschhorn R. Overview of biochemical abnormalities and molecular genetics of adenosine deaminase deficiency. Pediatr Res 3(Suppl.):S35–S41, 1993.

Hirschhorn R, Ellenbogen A. Genetic heterogeneity in ADA deficiency: five different mutations in five new patients with partial ADA deficiency. Am J Hum Genet 38:362–369, 1986.

Hirschhorn R, Ratech H, Rubinstein A, Papageorgiou P, Kesarwala H, Gelfand E, Roegner-Maniscalco V. Increased excretion of modified adenine nucleosides by children with adenosine deaminase deficiency. Pediatr Res 16:362–369, 1982.

Hitzig WH, Kay HEM, Cottier H. Familial lymphopenia with agammaglobulinemia: an attempt at treatment by implantation of foetal thymus. Lancet 2:151–154, 1965.

Ho DD, Cao Y, Zhu T, Farthing C, Wang N, Gu G, Schooley RT, Daar ES. Idiopathic CD4+ lymphocytopenia—immunodeficiency without evidence of HIV infection. N Engl J Med 328:380–385, 1993.

Hoar DI, Sargent P. Chemical mutagen hypersensitivity in ataxia-telangiectasia. Nature 261:590–592, 1976.

Holman H, Nickel WF, Sleisenger MH. Hypoproteinemia antedating intestinal lesions and possibly due to excessive serum protein loss into the intestine. Am J Med 27:963–975, 1959.

Holt P. Dietary treatment of protein loss in intestinal lymphangiec-tasia. The effect of eliminating dietary long-chain triglycerides of albumin metabolism in this condition. Pediatrics 34:629–635, 1964.

Hong R. Reconstitution of T-cell deficiency by thymic hormone or thymus transplant therapy. Clin Immunol Immunopathol 40:136–141, 1986.

Hong R. The DiGeorge anomaly. Immunodefic Rev 3:1–14, 1991.

Hong R, Ammann AJ, Huang SW, Levy RL, Davenport G, Bach ML, Bach FH, Bortin MM, Kay HEM. Cartilage-hair hypoplasia: effect of thymus transplants. Clin Immunol Immunopathol 1:15–26, 1972.

Hong R, Horowitz SD. Thymosin therapy creates a "Hassall." N Engl J Med 292:104–105, 1975.

Hong R, Horowitz SD, Borzy MF, Gilbert EF, Arya S, McLeod N, Peterson RDA. The cerebro-hepato-renal syndrome of Zellweger: similarity to and differentiation from the DiGeorge syndrome. Thymus 3:97–104, 1981.

Hong R, Santosham M, Schulte-Wissermann H, Horowitz S, Hsu SH, Winkelstein JA. Reconstitution of B and T lymphocyte function in severe combined immunodeficiency disease following transplantation with thymic epithelium. Lancet 2:1270–1272, 1976.

Hoxie JA, Flaherty LE, Haggarty BS, Rackowski JL. Infection of T4 lymphocytes by HTLV-III does not require expression of the OKT4 epitope. J Immunol 135:361–363, 1986.

Hughes WT, Kuhn S, Chaudhary S, Feldman S, Verzosa M, Aur RJA, Pratt C, George SL. Successful chemoprophylaxis for Pneumocystis carinii pneumonitis. N Engl J Med 297:1419–1426, 1977.

Hung W, Migeon CJ, Parrott RH. A possible auto-immune basis for Addison's disease in three siblings, one with idiopathic hypoparathyroidism, pernicious anemia and superficial moniliasis. N Engl J Med 269:658–663, 1963.

Huntley CC, Dees SC. Eczema associated with thrombocytopenic purpura and purulent otitis media: report of five fatal cases. Pediatrics 19:351–361, 1957.

Huo YK, Wang Z, Hong J-H, Chessa L, McBride WH, Perlman SL, Gatti RA. Radiosensitivity of ataxia-telangiectasia, X-linked agammaglobulinemia and related syndromes using a modified colony survival assay. Cancer Res 54:2544–2547, 1994.

Ishiguro T, Taketa K, Gatti RA. Tissue of origin of elevated alpha-fetoprotein in ataxia-telangiectasia. Dis Markers 4:293–297, 1986.

Ivey K, Den Besten L, Kent TH, Clifton JH. Lymphangiectasia of the colon with protein loss and malabsorption. Gastroenterology 57:709–714, 1969.

Jackson LG, Zachary JM, Fowler SE, Desnick RJ, Gollbus MS, Ledbetter DH, Mahoney MJ, Pergament E, Simpson JL, Black S, Wapner RJ. A randomized comparison of transcervical and transabdominal chorionic villus sampling. N Engl J Med 327:594–598, 1992.

Janeway CA, Travers P. Immunobiology: The Immune System in Health and Disease. Part IV. The Adaptive Immune Response. New York, Garland Publishing, 1994.

Janka GE. Familial hemophagocytic lymphohistiocytosis. Eur J Pediatr 140:221–230, 1983.

Janossy G, Montano L, Selby WS, Duke O, Panayi G, Lampert I, Thomas JA, Granger S, Bofill M, Tidman N, Thomas HC, Goldstein G. T cell subset abnormalities in tissue lesions developing during autoimmune disorders, viral infection and graft-versus-host disease. J Clin Immunol 2:42S–56S, 1982.

Janssen WE. Peripheral blood and bone marrow hematopoietic stem cells. Are they the same? Semin Oncol 20 (Suppl. 6): 19–27, 1993.

Jarnum S, Schwartz M. Hypoalbuminemia in gastric carcinoma. Gastroenterology 38:769–776, 1960.

Jasin HE, Dingle JT. Human mononuclear cell factors mediate cartilage matrix degradation through chondrocyte activation. J Clin Invest 68:571–581, 1981.

Jaspers NGJ, Gatti RA, Baan C, Linasen PCML, Bootsma D. Genetic complementation analysis of ataxia-telangiectasia and Nijmegen breakage syndrome: a survey of 50 patients. Cytogenet Cell Genet 49:259–263, 1988.

Jaspers NGJ, Painter RB, Paterson MC, Kidson C, Inoue T. Complementation analysis of ataxia-telangiectasia. In Gatti RA, Swift M, eds. Ataxia-Telangiectasia: Genetics, Neuropathology, and Immunology of a Degenerative Disease of Childhood, Vol. 19. New York, Alan R. Liss, pp. 1984, 147–154.

Jeffries GH, Chapman A, Sleisenger MH. Low-fat diet in intestinal lymphangiectasia: its effect on albumin metabolism. N Engl J Med 270:761–766, 1964.

Jin Z, Yang SY. Activation of CD8$^+$ T cells by allogeneic class II–deficient B cell lines derived from patients with bare lymphocyte syndrome. Tissue Antigens 35:136–143, 1990.

Joncas J, LaPointe N, Gervais F, Layritz M. Unusual prevalence of Epstein-Barr virus early antigen (EBV-EA) antibodies in ataxia-telangiectasia. J Immunol 119:1857–1859, 1977.

Jones HE, Simpson JG, Artis WM. Oral ketoconazole: an effective and safe treatment for dermatophytosis. Arch Dermatol 117:129–134, 1981.

Jorizzo JJ, Sams WM, Jegasothy BV, Olansky AJ. Cimetidine as an immunomodulator: chronic mucocutaneous candidiasis as a model. Ann Intern Med 92:192–195, 1980.

Junker AK, Chan KW, Massing BG. Clinical and immune recovery from Omenn syndrome after bone marrow transplantation. J Pediatr 114:596–600, 1989.

Junker AK, Poon M-C, Hoar DI, Rogers PCJ. Severe combined immune deficiency presenting with cyclic hematopoiesis. J Clin Immunol 11:369–377, 1991.

Kadowaki J, Thompson RI, Zuelzer WW, Wooley PV Jr, Brough AJ, Gruber D. XX/XY lymphoid chimaerism in congenital immunological deficiency syndrome with thymic alymphoplasia. Lancet 2:1152–1156, 1965.

Kaitila L, Tanaka KR, Rimoin DL. Normal red cell adenosine deaminase activity in cartilage hair hypoplasia. J Pediatr 87:153–154, 1975.

Kamel OW, van de Rijn M, Weiss LM, Del Zoppo GJ, Hench PK, Robbins BA, Montgomery PG, Warnke RA, Dorfman RF. Brief report: reversible lymphomas associated with Epstein-Barr virus occurring during methotrexate therapy for rheumatoid arthritis and dermatomyositis. N Engl J Med 328:1317–1321, 1993.

Kameoka J, Tanaka T, Nojima Y, Schlossman SF, Morimoto C. Direct association of adenosine deaminase with a T cell activation antigen, CD26. Science 261:466–469, 1993.

Kapp LN, Painter RB, Yu L-C, van Loon N, Richard CW, James MR, Cox DR, Murnane JP. Cloning of a candidate gene for ataxia-telangiectasia group D. Am J Hum Genet 51:45–54, 1992.

Kara CJ, Glimcher LH. Promoter accessibility within the environment of the MHC is affected in class II–deficient combined immunodeficiency. EMBO J 12:187–193, 1993.

Karpati G, Eisen AH, Andermann F, Bacal HL, Robb P. Ataxia-telangiectasia: further observations and report of eight cases. Am J Dis Child 110:51–62, 1965.

Kastan MB, Zhan Q, Wafik SE-D, Carrier F, Jacks T, Walsh WV, Plunkett BS, Vogelstein B, Fornace AJ Jr. A mammalian cell cycle checkpoint pathway utilizing p53 and *GADD45* is defective in ataxia-telangiectasia. Cell 71:587–597, 1992.

Katz F, Malcolm S, Strobel S, Fin A, Morgan G, Levinsky R. The use of locus-specific minisatellite probes to check engraftment following allogeneic bone marrow transplantation for severe combined immunodeficiency disease. Bone Marrow Transplant 5:199–204, 1990.

Kaufman DB, Miller AC. Ataxia-telangiectasia: an autoimmune disease associated with a cytotoxic antibody to brain and thymus. Clin Immunol Immunopathol 7:288–299, 1977.

Keppen LD, Fasules JW, Burks AW, Gollin SM, Sawyer JR, Miller CH. Confirmation of autosomal dominant transmission of the Di-George malformation complex. J Pediatr 113:506–508, 1988.

Kernan NA, Collins N, Juliano L, Cartagena T, Dupont B, O'Reilly RJ. Clonable T lymphocytes in T cell–depleted bone marrow transplants correlate with development of graft-vs-host disease. Blood 68:770–773, 1986.

Kessinger A, Armitage JO, Landmark JD, Smith DM, Weisenburger DD. Autologous peripheral hematopoietic stem cell transplantation restores hematopoietic function following marrow ablative therapy. Blood 71:723–727, 1988.

Kildeberg P. The Aldrich syndrome. Report of a case and discussion of pathogenesis. Pediatrics 27:362–369, 1961.

King CL, Gallin JI, Malech HL, Abramson SL, Nutman TB. Regulation of immunoglobulin production in hyperimmunoglobulin E recurrent-infection syndrome by interferon gamma. Proc Natl Acad Sci U S A 86:10085–10089, 1989.

Kirkpatrick CH. Transfer factor. J Allergy Clin Immunol 81:803–813, 1988.

Kirkpatrick CH, Alling DW. Treatment of chronic oral candidiasis with clotrimazole troches. N Engl J Med 299:1202–1203, 1978.

Kirkpatrick CH, Chandler JW Jr, Schimke RN. Chronic moniliasis with impaired delayed hypersensitivity. Clin Exp Immunol 6:375–386, 1970.

Kirkpatrick CH, Greenberg LE. Treatment of chronic mucocutaneous candidiasis with transfer factor. In Kahn A, Kirkpatrick CH, Hill NO, eds. Immune Regulators in Transfer Factor. New York, Academic Press, 1979, pp. 547–562.

Kirkpatrick CH, Greenberg LE, Chapman SW, Goldstein G, Lewis VM, Twomey JJ. Plasma thymic hormone activity in patients with chronic mucocutaneous candidiasis. Clin Exp Immunol 23:311–317, 1978.

Kirkpatrick CH, Ottesen EA, Smith TK, Wells SA, Burdick JF. Reconstitution of defective cellular immunity with foetal thymus and dialysable transfer factor. Long-term studies in a patient with chronic mucocutaneous candidiasis. Clin Exp Immunol 23:414–428, 1976.

Kirkpatrick CH, Rich RR, Bennett JE. Chronic mucocutaneous candidiasis: model building in cellular immunity. Ann Intern Med 74:955–978, 1971a.

Kirkpatrick CH, Rich RR, Graw RG, Smith TK, Mickenberg ID, Rogentine CN. Treatment of chronic mucocutaneous moniliasis by immunologic reconstitution. Clin Exp Immunol 9:733–748, 1971b.

Kirkpatrick CH, Rich RR, Smith TK. Effect of transfer factor on lymphocyte function in anergic patients. J Clin Invest 51:2948–2958, 1972.

Kirkpatrick CH, Smith TK. Chronic mucocutaneous candidiasis: immunologic and antibiotic therapy. Ann Intern Med 80:310–320, 1974.

Kirkpatrick CH, Sohnle PG. Chronic mucocutaneous candidiasis. In Safai B, Good RA, eds. Immunodermatology. New York, Plenum Medical Book, pp. 495–514, 1981.

Kirkpatrick CH, Windhorst DB. Mucocutaneous candidiasis and thymoma. Am J Med 66:939–945, 1979.

Kishimoto T. The biology of interleukin-6. Blood 74:1–10, 1989.

Klein C, Lisowska-Grospierre B, LeDeist F, Fischer A, Griscelli C. Major histocompatibility complex class II deficiency: clinical manifestations, immunologic features, and outcome. J Pediatr 123:921–928, 1993.

Kohl S, Springer TA, Schmalstieg FC, Loo LS, Anderson DC. Defective natural killer cytotoxicity and polymorphonuclear leukocyte antibody–dependent cellular cytotoxicity in patients with LFA-1/OKM-1 deficiency. J Immunol 133:2972–2978, 1984.

Kohn DB, Anderson WF, Blaese RM. Gene therapy for genetic diseases. Cancer Invest 7:179–192, 1989.

Kohn DB, Weinberg KI, Lenarsky C, Crooks G, Heiss LN, Nolta JA, Wara D, Elder M, Williams-Herman D, Bowen T, Moen RC, Blaese RM, Parkman R. Gene therapy for neonates with ADA deficiency by transfer of the human ADA cDNA into umbilical cord CD34$^+$ cells: Two year follow-up (abstract). Pediatr Res 37:9A, 1994.

Kojis TL, Gatti RA, Sparkes RS. The cytogenetics of ataxia-telangiectasia. Cancer Genet Cytogenet 56:143–156, 1992.

Komiyama A, Kawai H, Yabuhara A, Yanagisawa M, Miyagawa Y, Ota M, Hasekura H, Akabane T. Natural killer cell immunodeficiency in siblings: defective killing in the absence of natural killer cytotoxic factor activity in natural killer and lymphokine-activated killer cytotoxicities. Pediatrics 85:323–330, 1990.

Komiyama A, Kawai H, Yamada S, Aoyama K, Yamazaki M, Saitoh H, Miyagawa Y, Akabane T, Uehara Y. Impaired natural killer cell recycling in childhood chronic neutropenia with morphological abnormalities and defective chemotaxis of neutrophils. Blood 66:99–105, 1985.

Komuro K, Boyse EA. In vitro demonstration of thymic hormone in the mouse by conversion of precursor cells into lymphocytes. Lancet 1:740–743, 1973.

Kondo M, Takeshita T, Ishii N, Nakamura M, Watanabe S, Arai K-I, Sugamura K. Sharing of the interleukin-2 (IL-2) receptor chain between receptors for IL-2 and IL-4. Science 262:1874–1877, 1993.

Kredich NM, Martin DW Jr. Role of S-adenosylhomocysteine in adenosine-mediated toxicity in cultured mouse T lymphoma cells. Cell 12:931–938, 1977.

Kretschmer R, Say B, Brown D, Rosen FS. Congenital aplasia of the thymus gland (DiGeorge's syndrome). N Engl J Med 279:1295–1301, 1968.

Krivit W, Good RA. Aldrich's syndrome (thrombocytopenia, eczema and infection in infants). Am J Dis Child 97:137–153, 1959.

Krivit W, Yunis E, White J. Platelet survival studies in Aldrich syndrome. Pediatrics 37:339–341, 1966.

Krueger GR. Graft-versus-host disease and toxic epidermal necrolysis. Lancet 1:268–269, 1973.

Kruisbeek AM, Kröse TCJM, Zilstra JJ. Increase in T cell mitogen responsiveness in rat thymocytes by thymic epithelium. Eur J Immunol 3:745–748, 1973.

Kruisbeek AM, Mond JJ, Fowlkes BJ, Carmen JA, Bridges S, Longo DL. Absence of the Lyt-2, L3T4$^+$ lineage of T cells in mice treated neonatally with anti-I-A correlates with absence of intrathymic I-A–bearing antigen-presenting cell function. J Exp Med 161:1029–1047, 1985.

Kuramoto A, Steiner MD, Baldini MG. Lack of platelet response to stimulation in Wiskott-Aldrich syndrome. N Engl J Med 282:474–479, 1970.

Kwan SP, Dandkuyl LA, Blaese M, Kunkel LM, Bruns G. Genetic mapping of the Wiskott-Aldrich syndrome with two highly linked polymorphic DNA markers. Genomics 3:39–43, 1988.

Lammer EJ, Opitz JM. The DiGeorge anomaly as a developmental field defect. Am J Med Genet 2(Suppl.):113–127, 1986.

Landsteiner K, Chase MW. Studies on sensitization of animals with simple compounds: VII. Skin sensitization by intraperitoneal injections. J Exp Med 71:237–245, 1940.

Landsteiner K, Chase MW. Experiments on transfer of cutaneous sensitivity to simple compounds. Proc Soc Exp Biol Med 49:688–690, 1942.

Lane HC, Depper JM, Greene WC, Whalen G, Waldmann TA, Fauci AS. Qualitative analysis of immune function in patients with the acquired immunodeficiency syndrome: evidence for a selective defect in soluble antigen recognition. N Engl J Med 313:79–84, 1985.

Lange E, Gatti RA, Sobel E, Concannon P, Lange K. How many A-T genes? In Gatti RA, Painter RB, eds. Ataxia-Telangiectasia. Heidelberg, Springer-Verlag, 1993, pp. 37–54.

Laster L, Waldmann TA, Fenster LF, Singleton JW. Albumin metabolism in patients with Whipple's disease. J Clin Invest 45:637–644, 1966.

Lau YL, Levinsky RJ. Prenatal diagnosis and carrier detection in primary immunodeficiency disorders. Arch Dis Child 63:758–764, 1988.

Lavin RF. Biochemical defects in ataxia-telangiectasia. In Gatti RA, Painter RB, eds. Ataxia-Telangiectasia. Heidelberg, Springer-Verlag, 1993, pp. 235–256.

Lawlor GR Jr, Ammann AJ, Wright WC, LaFranchi SH, Bilstrom D, Stiehm ER. The syndrome of cellular immunodeficiency with immunoglobulins. J Pediatr 84:183–192, 1974.

Lawrence HS. The transfer of generalized cutaneous hypersensitivity of the delayed tuberculin type in man by means of the constituents of disrupted leukocytes. J Clin Invest 33:951–952, 1954.

Lawrence HS. In Amos B, Koprowski H, eds. Conference on Cell-Bound Antibodies. Philadelphia, Wistar Press, pp. 3–6, 1963.

Lebenthal E, Gaifman M, Nitzan ML. Protein-losing gastroenteropathy responding to corticosteroid treatment. Acta Paediatr Scand 59:217–220, 1970.

Le Deist F, Hivroz C, Partiseti M, Thomas C, Buc HA, Oleastro M, Belohradsky B, Choquet D, Fischer A. A primary T-cell immunodeficiency associated with defective transmembrane calcium influx. Blood 85:1053–1062, 1995.

LeDouarin NM. Investigations on the neural crest: methodological aspects and recent advances. Ann NY Acad Sci 486:66–86, 1986.

Lee WM, Holley HP, Stewart J, Galbraith GMP. Refractory esophageal candidiasis associated with a low molecular weight plasma inhibitor of T-lymphocyte function. Am J Med Sci 292:47–52, 1986.

Lehner T, Wilton JMA, Ivanyi L. Immunodeficiencies in chronic mucocutaneous candidiasis. Immunology 22:775–787, 1972.

Leikin SL, Bazelon M, Park KH. In vitro lymphocyte transformation in ataxia-telangiectasia. J Pediatr 68:477–479, 1966.

Lenarsky C, Parkman R. Bone marrow transplantation for the treatment of immune deficiency states. Bone Marrow Transplant 6:361–369, 1990.

Levin AS, Spitler LE, Stites DP, Fudenberg HH. Wiskott-Aldrich syndrome, a genetically determined cellular immunologic deficiency: clinical and laboratory responses to therapy with transfer factor. Proc Natl Acad Sci U S A 67:821–828, 1970.

Levine F, Friedmann T. Gene therapy. Am J Dis Child 147:1167–1174, 1993.

Levinsky RJ, Tiedeman K. Successful bone-marrow transplantation for reticular dysgenesis. Lancet 1:671–673, 1983.

Levinson AI, Hoxie JA, Kornstein MJ, Zembryki D, Matthews DM, Schreiber AD. Absence of the OKT4 epitope on blood T cells and thymus cells in a patient with thymoma, hypogammaglobulinemia, and red blood cell aplasia. J Allergy Clin Immunol 76:433–439, 1985.

Levy RL, Huang SW, Bach ML, Bach FH, Hong R, Ammann AJ, Bortin M, Kay HEM. Thymic transplantation in a case of chronic mucocutaneous candidiasis. Lancet ii:898–900, 1971.

Liang X. Ataxia-telangiectasia. Hereditas 10:34, 1988.

Lin H, Parmacek MS, Marle G, Bolling S, Leiden JM. Expression of recombinant genes in myocardium in vivo after direct injection of DNA. Circulation 82:2217–2221, 1990.

Lindsten T, Seeley JK, Ballow M, Sakamoto K, St. Onge S, Yetz J, Aman P, Purtilo DT. Immune deficiency in the X-linked lymphoproliferative syndrome. J Immunol 129:2536–2540, 1982.

Lipkowitz S, Stern M-H, Kirsch IR. Hybrid T cell receptor genes formed by interlocus recombination in normal and ataxia-telangiectasia lymphocytes. J Exp Med 172:409–418, 1990.

Lischner HW, DiGeorge AM. Role of the thymus in humoral immunity: observations in complete or partial congenital absence of the thymus. Lancet 2:1044–1049, 1969.

Lisowska-Grospierre B, Charron DJ, de Preval C, Durandy A, Griscelli C, Mach B. A defect in the regulation of major histocompatibility complex class II gene expression in human HLA-DR negative lymphocytes from patients with combined immunodeficiency syndrome. J Clin Invest 76:381–385, 1985.

Lisowska-Grospierre B, Fondaneche M-C, Rols M-P, Griscelli C, Fischer A. Two complementation groups account for most cases of inherited MHC class II deficiency. Hum Mol Genet 6:953–958, 1994.

List AF, Greco A, Vogler LB. Lymphoproliferative diseases in immunocompromised hosts: the role of Epstein-Barr virus. J Clin Oncol 5:1673–1689, 1987.

Littman BH, Rocklin RE, Parkman R, David JR. Transfer factor treatment of chronic mucocutaneous candidiasis: requirement of donor reactivity to *Candida* antigen. Clin Immunol Immunopathol 9:97–110, 1978.

Lodewyk HS, Van Mierop MD, Kutsche LM. Cardiovascular anomalies in DiGeorge syndrome and importance of neural crest as a possible pathogenetic factor. Am J Cardiol 58:133–137, 1986.

Lopukhin Y, Morozov Y, Petrov R. Transplantation of neonatal thymus sternum complex in ataxia-telangiectasia. Transplant Proc 5:823–827, 1973.

Louis-Bar D. Sur un syndrome progressif comprenant des télangiectasies capillaires cutanées et conjonctivales symétriques à disposition navoïde et des troubles cérébelleux. Confin Neurol 4:32–42, 1941.

Louria DB, Shannon D, Johnson G, Caroline L, Okas A, Taschdjian C. The susceptibility to moniliasis in children with endocrine hypofunction. Trans Assoc Am Physicians 80:236–248, 1967.

Lum LG, Tubergen DG, Blaese RM. Splenectomy in the management of the thrombocytopenia of the Wiskott-Aldrich syndrome. N Engl J Med 302:892–896, 1980.

Lux SE, Johnston RB, August CS, Say B, Penchaszedeh VB, Rosen FS, McKusick VA. Chronic neutropenia and abnormal cellular immunity in cartilage-hair hypoplasia. N Engl J Med 282:234–236, 1970.

Maffei A, Scarpellino L, Bernard M, Carra G, Jotterand-Bellamo M, Guardiola J, Accolla RS. Distinct mechanisms regulate MHC class II gene expression in B cell and macrophages. J Immunol 139:942–948, 1987.

Mandl MAJ, Watson JI, Rose B. The Wiskott-Aldrich syndrome—immunopathologic mechanisms and a long-term survival. Ann Intern Med 68:1050–1059, 1968.

Mansour A, Gelfand EW. A new approach to the use of antifungal agents in infants with persistent oral candidiasis. J Pediatr 98:161–162, 1981.

Maraschio P, Peretti P, Lambiase S, Low Curto F, Caufin D, Gargantini L, Minoli L, Zuffardi O. A new chromosome instability disorder. Clin Genet 30:353–365, 1986.

Marcadet A, Cohen D, Dausset J, Fischer A, Durandy A, Griscelli C. Genotyping with DNA probes in combined immunodeficiency syndrome with defective expression of HLA. N Engl J Med 312:1287–1292, 1985.

Markert ML. Purine nucleoside phosphorylase deficiency. Immunodefic Rev 3:45–81, 1991.

Marmont AM, Horowitz MM, Gale RP, Sobocinski K, Ash RC, van Bekkum DW, Champlin RE, Dicke KA, Goldman JM, Good RA, Herzig RH, Hong R, Masaoka T, Rimm AA, Ringden O, Speck B, Weiner RS, Bortin MM. T-cell depletion of HLA-identical transplants in leukemia. Blood 78:2120–2130, 1991.

Martin CM, Gordon RS, McCullough NB. Acquired agammaglobulinemia in an adult: report of a case with clinical and experimental studies. N Engl J Med 254:449–456, 1956.

Masswinkel-Mooij PD, Papapoulos SE, Gerritsen EJA, Muddle AH, Van de Kamp JJP. Facial dysmorphia, parathyroid and thymic dysfunction in the father of a newborn with the DiGeorge complex. Eur J Pediatr 149:179–183, 1989.

Mathews T, Wisotzkey H, Moossy J. Multiple central nervous system infections in progressive multifocal leukoencephalopathy. Neurology 26:9–14, 1976.

McCaw B, Hecht F, Harnden DG, Teplitz RL. Somatic rearrangement of chromosome 14 in human lymphocytes. Proc Natl Acad Sci U S A 72:2071–2075, 1975.

McConville CM, Formstone CJ, Hernandez D, Thick J, Taylor AMR. Fine mapping of the chromosome 11q22–23 region using PFGE, linkage and haplotype analysis; localization of the gene for ataxia-telangiectasia to a 5-cm region flanked by NCAM/DRD2 and STMY/CJ52.75, ph2,22. Nucleic Acids Res 18:4334–4343, 1990.

McFarlin DE, Oppenheim JJ. Impaired lymphocyte transformation in ataxia-telangiectasia in part due to a plasma inhibitory factor. J Immunol 103:1212–1222, 1969.

McKusick VA, Elderidge E, Hostetler JA, Ruangwit U, Egeland JA. Dwarfism in the Amish. II. Cartilage-hair hypoplasia. Bull Johns Hopkins Hosp 116:285–326, 1964.

McReynolds EW, Dabbous MK, Hanissian AS, Deunas D, Kimrell R. Abnormal collagen in ataxia-telangiectasia. Am J Dis Child 130:305–307, 1976.

Mentzer SJ, Remold-O'Donnell E, Crimmins MAV, Bierer BE, Rosen FS, Burakoff SJ. Sialophorin, a surface sialoglycoprotein defective in the Wiskott-Aldrich syndrome, is involved in human T-lymphocyte proliferation. J Exp Med 165:1383–1392, 1987.

Meyers JD, McGuffin RW, Neiman PE, Singer JW, Thomas ED. Toxicity and efficacy of human leukocyte interferon for treatment of cytomegalovirus pneumonia after marrow transplantation. J Infect Dis 141:555–562, 1980.

Meyn MS. High spontaneous intrachromosomal recombination rates in ataxia-telangiectasia. Science 260:1327–1330, 1993.

Meyn MS, Lu-Kuo JM, Herzing LSK. Isolation of human cDNAs that complement the ataxia-telangiectasia phenotype in cultured fibroblasts. In Gatti RA, Painter RB, eds. Ataxia-Telangiectasia. Heidelberg, Springer-Verlag, pp. 55–64, 1993.

Minami Y, Kono T, Tadaaki M, Taniguchi T. The IL-2 receptor complex: its structure, function, and target genes. Ann Rev Immunol 11:245–268, 1993.

Mistilis SP, Skyring AP, Stephen DD. Intestinal lymphangiectasia: mechanism of enteric loss of plasma-protein and fat. Lancet 1:77–79, 1965.

Moen RC, Horowitz SD, Sondel PM, Borcherding WR, Trigg ME, Billing R, Hong R. Immune reconstitution after haploidentical bone marrow transplantation for immune deficiency disease: treatment of bone marrow cells with monoclonal antibody CT-2 and complement. Blood 70:664–669, 1987.

Molina IJ, Kenney DM, Rosen FS, Remold-O'Donnell E. T cell lines characterize events in the pathogenesis of the Wiskott-Aldrich syndrome. J Exp Med 176:867–874, 1992.

Molina IJ, Sancho J, Terhorst C, Rosen FS, Remold-O'Donnell E. T cells of patients with the Wiskott-Aldrich syndrome have a restricted defect in proliferative responses. J Immunol 151:4383–4390, 1993.

Moore E, Herlbert L. Regulation of mammalian deoxyribonucleotide biosynthesis by nucleotides as activators and inhibitors. J Biol Chem 41:4802–4807, 1966.

Morecki S, Nagler R, Puyesky Y, Nabet C, Condiotti R, Pick M, Gan G, Slavin S. Effect of various cytokine combinations on induction of non–MHC-restricted cytotoxicity. Lymphokine Cytokine Res 12:159–165, 1993.

Morgan DA, Ruscetti FW, Gallo RC. Selective *in vitro* growth of T lymphocytes from normal human bone marrows. Science 193:1007–1008, 1976.

Morgan JL, Holcomb TM, Morrissey RW. Radiation reaction in ataxia-telangiectais. Am J Dis Child 116:557–558, 1968.

Morio T, Takase K, Okawa H, Oguchi M, Kanbara M, Hiruma F, Yoshino K, Kaneko T, Asamura S, Inoue T. The increase of non-MHC-restricted cytotoxic cells (gamma/delta-TCR–bearing T cells or NK cells) and the abnormal differentiation of B cells in Wiskott-Aldrich syndrome. Clin Immunol Immmunopathol 52:279–290, 1989.

Muller W, Peter HH, Kallfelz HC, Franz A, Rieger CHL. The DiGeorge sequence: II. Immunologic findings in partial and complete forms of the disorder. Eur J Pediatr 149:96–103, 1989.

Murphy S, Oski FA, Haimar JL, Lusch CJ, Goldberg S, Gardner FH. Platelet size and kinetics in hereditary and acquired thrombocytopenia. N Engl J Med 286:499–504, 1972.

Murray HW, Rubin BY, Masur H, Roberts RB. Impaired production of lymphokines and immune (gamma) interferon in the acquired immunodeficiency syndrome. N Engl J Med 310:883–891, 1984.

Myers SE, Williams SG, Geller RB. Cyclophosphamide mobilization of peripheral blood stem cells for use in autologous transplantation after high-dose chemotherapy: clinical results in patients with contaminated or hypocellular bone marrow. J Hematother 1:27–33, 1992.

Naeim A, Repinski C, Huo Y, Hong J-H, Chessa L, Naeim F, Gatti RA. Ataxia-telangiectasia: flow cytometric cell-cycle analysis of lymphoblastoid cell lines in G2/M before and after gamma-irradiation. Mod Pathol 7:587–592, 1994.

Nahm MH, Blaese RM, Crain MJ, Briles DE. Patients with Wiskott-Aldrich syndrome have normal IgG2 levels. J Immunol 137:3484–3487, 1986.

Naiman JL, Punnett HH, Lischner HW, Destine ML, Arey JB. Possible graft-versus-host reaction after intrauterine transfusion for Rh erythroblastosis fetalis. N Engl J Med 281:697–701, 1969.

Nemunaitis J, Rabinowe SN, Singer JW, Bierman PJ, Vose JM, Freedman AS, Onetto N, Gillis S, Oette D, Gold M, Buckner CD, Hansen JA, Ritz J, Appelbaum FR, Armitage JO, Nadler LM. Recombinant granulocyte-macrophage colony-stimulating factor after autologous bone marrow transplantation for lymphoid cancer. N Engl J Med 324:1773–1778, 1991.

Nezelof C. Thymic dysplasia with normal immunoglobulins and immunologic deficiency: pure alymphocytosis. In Bergsma D, ed. Immunologic Deficiency Diseases in Man. Birth Defects (Original Article Series). New York, The National Foundation, Vol. 4, pp. 104–115, 1968.

Nezelof C. Thymic pathology in primary and secondary immunodeficiencies. Histopathology 21:499–511, 1992.

Nezelof C, Jammet ML, Lortholary P, Larbrune B, Lamy, M. L'hypoplasie hereditaire du thymus. Sa place et sa responsabilité dans une observation d'aplasie lymphocytaire, normoplasmocytaire et normoglobulinémique du nourrisson. Arch Fr Pediatr 21:897–920, 1964.

Noel DR, Witherspoon RP, Storb R, Atkinson K, Doney K, Mickelson EM, Ochs H, Warren RP, Weiden PL, Thomas ED. Does graft-versus-host disease influence the tempo of immunologic recovery after allogeneic human marrow transplantation? An observation on 56 long-term survivors. Blood 51:1087–1105, 1978.

Noguchi M, Nakamura Y, Russell SM, Ziegler SF, Tsang M, Cao X, Leonard WJ. Interleukin-2 receptor γ chain: a functional component of the interleukin-7 receptor. Science 262:1877–1880, 1993a.

Noguchi M, Yi H, Rosenblatt HM, Filipovich AH, Adelstein S, Modi WS, McBride OW, Leonard WJ. Interleukin-2 receptor gamma chain mutation results in X-linked severe combined immunodeficiency in humans. Cell 73:147–157, 1993b.

Notarangelo LD, Stoppoloni G, Toraldo R, Mazzolari E, Coletta A, Airo P, Bordignon C, Ugazio AG. Insulin-dependent diabetes mellitus and severe atopic dermatitis in a child with adenosine deaminase deficiency. Eur J Pediatr 151:811–814, 1992.

Oettgen HC, Terhorst C. The T-cell receptor–T3 complex and T-lymphocyte activation. Hum Immunol 18:187–204, 1987.

Okamato GA, Hall JG, Ochs H, Jackson C, Rodaway K, Chandler J. New syndrome of chronic mucocutaneous candidiasis. Birth Defects (Original Article Series). New York, The National Foundation, Vol. 13, pp. 117–125, 1977.

Omenn GS. Familial reticuloendotheliosis with eosinophilia. N Engl J Med 273:427–432, 1965.

Oppenheim JJ, Blaese RM, Horton JE, Thor DE, Granger GA. Production of macrophage migration inhibition factor and lymphotoxin by leukocytes from normal and Wiskott-Aldrich syndrome patients. Cell Immunol 8:63–70, 1973.

O'Reilly RJ, Keever CA, Small TN, Brochstein J. The use of HLA–non-identical T-cell depleted marrow transplants for correction of severe combined immunodeficiency disease. Immunodefic Rev 1:273–309, 1989.

O'Reilly RJ, Pahwa R, Dupont B, Good RA. Severe combined immunodeficiency: transplantation approaches for patients lacking an HLA genotypically identical sibling. Transplant Proc 10:187–199, 1978.

Ownby DR, Pizzo S, Blackmon L, Gall SA, Buckley RH. Severe combined immunodeficiency with leukopenia (reticular dysgenesis) in siblings: immunologic and histopathologic findings. J Pediatr 89:382–387, 1976.

Oxelius VA, Berkel AI, Hanson LA. IgG2 deficiency in ataxia-telangiectasia. N Engl J Med 306:515–517, 1982.

Oyefara BI, Kim HC, Danziger RN, Carroll M, Greene JM, Douglas SD. Autoimmune hemolytic anemia in chronic mucocutaneous candidiasis. Clin Diagn Lab Immunol 1:38–43, 1994.

Packman S, Sweetman L, Wall S. Biotin responsive multiple carboxylase deficiency of infantile onset. J Pediatr 99:421–423, 1981.

Paganelli R, Scala E, Scarselli E, Ortolani C, Cossarizza A, Carmini D, Aiuti F, Fiorilli M. Selective deficiency of CD4$^+$/CD45RA$^+$ lymphocytes in patients with ataxia-telangiectasia. J Clin Immunol 12:84–91, 1992.

Pahwa R, Chatila T, Pahwa S, Paradise C, Day NK, Geha R, Schwartz SA, Slade H, Oyaizu N, Good RA. Recombinant interleukin 2 therapy in severe combined immunodeficiency disease. Proc Natl Acad Sci U S A 86:5069–5073, 1989.

Painter RB. Radiobiology of ataxia-telangiectasia. In Gatti RA, Painter RB, eds. Ataxia-Telangiectasia. Heidelberg, Springer-Verlag, 1993, pp. 257–268.

Painter RB, Young BR. Radiosensitivity in ataxia-telangiectasia: a new explanation. Proc Natl Acad Sci U S A 77:7315–7317, 1980.

Palmgren B, Lindberg T. Immunological studies in Wiskott-Aldrich syndrome. Acta Paediatr (Scand) Suppl 146:116–121, 1963.

Park JK, Rosenstein YJ, Remold-O'Donnell E, Bierer BE, Rosen FS, Burakoff S. Enhancement of T-cell activation by the CD43 molecule whose expression is defective in Wiskott-Aldrich syndrome. Nature 350:706–709, 1991.

Parker RI, O'Shea P, Forman EN. Acquired splenic atrophy in a sibship with the autoimmune polyendocrinopathy-candidiasis syndrome. J Pediatr 117:591–593, 1990.

Parkins RA. Protein-losing enteropathy in sprue syndrome. Lancet 2:1366–1369, 1960.

Parkman R, Gelfand EW, Rosen FS, Sanderson A, Hirschhorn R. Severe combined immunodeficiency and adenosine deaminase deficiency. N Engl J Med 292:714–719, 1975.

Parkman R, Mosier D, Umansky I, Cochran W, Carpenter CB, Rosen FS. Graft-versus-host disease after intrauterine and exchange transfusions for hemolytic disease of the newborn. N Engl J Med 290:359–398, 1974.

Parkman R, Rappaport J, Geha R, Belli J, Cassady R, Levey R, Nathan DG, Rosen FS. Complete correction of the Wiskott-Aldrich syndrome by allogeneic bone marrow transplantation. N Engl J Med 298:921–927, 1978.

Parkman R, Remold-O'Donnell E, Cairns L, Rappaport JM, Cowan M, Ammann AJ, Kenney D, Potter N, Rosen FS. Immunologic abnormalities in patients lacking a lymphocyte surface glycoprotein. Clin Immunol Immunopathol 33:363–370, 1984.

Paterson MC, Mirzayans R. Correction of post–gamma ray DNA repair deficiency in ataxia-telangiectasia complementation group A fibroblasts by cocultivation with normal fibrobalsts. In Gatti RA, Painter RB, eds. Ataxia-Telangiectasia. Heidelberg, Springer-Verlag, 1993, pp. 117–126.

Paterson P, Semo R, Blumenschein G, Swelstad J. Mucocutaneous candidiasis, anergy and a plasma inhibitor of cellular immunity: reversal with amphotericin B. Clin Exp Immunol 9:595–602, 1971.

Payne R, Brodsky FM, Peterlin BM, Young LM. "Bare lymphocytes" without immunodeficiency. Hum Immunol 6:219–227, 1983.

Peacocke M, Siminovitch KA. Linkage of the Wiskott-Aldrich syndrome with polymorphic DNA sequences from the human X chromosome. Proc Natl Acad Sci U S A 84:3430–3433, 1987.

Pearson HA, Schulman NR, Oski FA, Eitzman DV. Platelet survival in Wiskott-Aldrich syndrome. J Pediatr 68:754–760, 1966.

Peck GL, Herzig GP, Elias PM. Toxic epidermal necrolysis in a patient with graft-versus-host reaction. Arch Dermatol 105:561–569, 1972.

Perlman SL. Treatment of ataxia-telangiectasia. In Gatti RA, Painter RB, eds. Ataxia-Telangiectasia. Heidelberg, Springer-Verlag, 1993, pp. 269–278.

Petersen EA, Greenberg LE, Manzara T, Kirkpatrick CH. Murine transfer factor I. Description of the model and evidence for specificity. J Immunol 126:2480–2484, 1981.

Peterson RDA, Cooper MD, Good RA. Lymphoid tissue abnormalities associated with ataxia-telangiectasia. Am J Med 41:342–359, 1966.

Phillips RA, Spaner DE. The SCID mouse: mutation in a DNA repair gene creates recipients useful for studies on stem cells, lymphocyte development and graft-versus-host disease. Immunol Rev 124:63–74, 1991.

Plaeger-Marshall S, Haas A, Clement LT, Giorgi JV, Chen ISY, Quan S, Gatti RA, Stiehm ER. Interferon-induced expression of class II major histocompatibility antigens in the major histocompatibility complex (MHC) class II deficiency syndrome. J Clin Immunol 8:285–295, 1988.

Platt LD, Carlson DE. Prenatal diagnosis—when and how? N Engl J Med 327:636–638, 1992.

Pollack MS, Kirkpatrick D, Kapoor N, Dupont B, O'Reilly RJ. Identification by HLA typing of intrauterine-derived maternal T cells in four patients with severe combined immunodeficiency. N Engl J Med 307:662–666, 1982.

Polmar SH, Stern RC, Schwartz AL, Wetzler EM, Chase PA, Hirschhorn R. Enzyme replacement therapy for adenosine deaminase deficiency and severe combined immunodeficiency. N Engl J Med 295:1337–1343, 1976.

Polmar SH, Waldmann TA, Balestra ST, Jost MC, Terry WE. Immunoglobulin E in immunologic deficiency disease. J Clin Invest 51:326–330, 1972.

Porras O, Arguendas O, Arata M, Barrantes M, Gonzalez L, Saenz E. Epidemiology of ataxia-telangiectasia in Costa Rica. In Gatti, RA, Painter RB, eds. Ataxia-Telangiectasia. Heidelberg, Springer-Verlag, 1993, pp. 199–208.

Powell BR, Buist NRM, Stenzel P. An X-linked syndrome of diarrhea, polyendocrinopathy, and fatal infection in infancy. J Pediatr 100:731–737, 1982.

Provisor AJ, Iacuone JJ, Chilcote RR, Neiburger RG, Crussi FG. Acquired agammaglobulinemia after a life-threatening illness with clinical and laboratory features of infectious mononucleosis in three related male children. N Engl J Med 293:62–65, 1975.

Puck JM, Deschenes SM, Porter JC, Dutra AS, Brown CJ, Willard HF, Henthorn PS. The interleukin-2 receptor γ chain maps to Xq13.1 and is mutated in X-linked severe combined immunodeficiency. Hum Mol Genet 2:1099–1104, 1993.

Puck JM, Krauss CM, Puck SM, Buckley RH, Conley ME. Prenatal test for X-linked severe combined immunodeficiency by analysis of maternal X-chromosome inactivation and linkage analysis. N Engl J Med 322:1063–1066, 1990a.

Puck JM, Nussbaum RL, Smead DL, Conley ME. X-linked severe combined immunodeficiency: localization within the region Xq13.q21.1 by linkage and deletion analysis. Am J Hum Genet 44:724–730, 1989.

Puck JM, Siminovitch KA, Poncz M, Greenberg CR, Rottem M, Conley ME. Atypical presentation of Wiskott-Aldrich syndrome: diagnosis in two unrelated males based on studies of maternal T cell X-chromosome inactivation. Blood 75:2369–2374, 1990b.

Purtilo DT, Cassel CK, Yang JPS, Harper R. X-linked recessive progressive combined variable immunodeficiency (Duncan's disease). Lancet 1:935–940, 1975.

Purtilo DT, DeFlorio D, Hutt LM, Bhawan J, Yang JPS, Otto R, Edwards W. Variable phenotypic expression of an X-linked recessive lymphoproliferative syndrome. New Engl J Med 297:1077–1081, 1977a.

Purtilo DT, Grierson HL, Ochs H. Detection of X-linked lymphoproliferative disease (XLP) using molecular and immunovirological markers. Am J Med 87:421–424, 1989.

Purtilo DT, Sakamoto K, Barnabei V, Seeley J, Bechtold T, Rogers G,

Yetz J, Harada S. Epstein-Barr virus–induced diseases in boys with the X-linked lymphoproliferative syndrome (XLP). Am J Med 73:49–56, 1982.

Purtilo DT, Yang JPS, Allegra S. Hematopathology and pathogenesis of the X-linked recessive lymphoproliferative syndrome. Am J Med 62:225–233, 1977b.

Rachelefsky GS, Stiehm ER, Ammann AJ, Cederbaum SD, Opelz G, Terasaki P. T-cell reconstitution by thymus transplantation and transfer factor in severe combined immunodeficiency. Pediatrics 55:114–118, 1975.

Radl J, Masopust J, Houstek J, Hrodek O. Paraproteinaemia and unusual dys-γ-globulinemia in a case of Wiskott-Aldrich syndrome. Arch Dis Child 42:608–614, 1967.

Ratech H, Alba Greco M, Gallo G, Rimoin DL, Kamino H, Hirschhorn R. Pathologic findings in adenosine deaminase–deficient severe combined immunodeficiency: I. Kidney, adrenal and chondro-osseous tissue alterations. Am J Pathol 120:157–169, 1985a.

Ratech H, Hirschhorn R, Alba Greco M. Pathologic findings in adenosine deaminase deficient–severe combined immunodeficiency: II. Thymus, spleen, lymph node, and gastrointestinal tract lymphoid tissue alterations. Am J Pathol 135:1145–1156, 1989.

Ratech H, Hirschhorn R, Thorbecke GJ. Effects of deoxycoformycin in mice: III. A murine model reproducing multisystem pathology of human deaminase deficiency. Am J Pathol 119:65–72, 1985b.

Record CO, Eddleston ALWR, Shilkin KB, Williams R. Intrahepatic sclerosing cholangitis associated with a familial immunodeficiency syndrome. Lancet 2:18–20, 1973.

Reed WB, Epstein WL, Boder E, Sedgwick R. Cutaneous manifestations of ataxia-telangiectasia. JAMA 195:746–753, 1966.

Reinherz E, Geha R, Rappaport JM, Wison M, Penta AC, Hessey RF, Fitzgerald KA, Daley J, Levine H, Rosen FS, Schlossman SF. Immune reconstitution in severe combined immunodeficiency with T lymphocyte–depleted HLA haplotype–mismatched bone marrow. Proc Natl Acad Sci U S A 79:6047–6051, 1982.

Reinherz EL, Kung PC, Goldstein G, Levey RH, Schlossman SF. Discrete stages of human intrathymic differentiation: analysis of normal thymocytes and leukemic lymphoblasts of T-cell lineage. Proc Natl Acad Sci U S A 77:1588–1592, 1980.

Reisinger D, Parkman R. Molecular heterogeneity of a lymphocyte glycoprotein in immunodeficient patients. J Clin Invest 79:595–599, 1987.

Reisner Y, Kapoor N, Kirkpatrick D, Pollack MS, Cunningham-Rundles S, Dupont B, Hodes MZ, Good RA, O'Reilly RJ. Transplantation for severe combined immunodeficiency with HLA-A, -B, -D, -DR incompatible parental marrow cells fractionated by soybean agglutinin and sheep red blood cells. Blood 61:341–348, 1983.

Reith W, Satola S, Herrero-Sanchez C, Amaldi I, Lisowska-Grospierre B, Griscelli C, Hadam MR, Mach B. Congenital immunodeficiency with a regulatory defect in MHC class II gene expression lacks a specific HLA-DR promoter binding protein, RFX. Cell 53:897, 1988.

Remold-O'Donnell E, Van Brocklyn J, Kenney DM. Effect of platelet calpain on normal T-lymphocyte CD43: hypothesis of events in the Wiskott-Aldrich syndrome. Blood 79:1754–1762, 1992.

Rich K, Arnold W, Fox I, Palella T. Purine nucleoside phosphorylase (PNP) deficiency with cellular immune deficiency. Pediatr Res 12:485A, 1978.

Richardson EP. Progressive multifocal leukoencephalopathy. In Winken PJ, Bruyn GW, eds. Handbook of Clinical Neurology. Amsterdam, North Holland, 1970, pp. 485–499.

Riddell SR, Watanabe KS, Goodrich JM, Li CR, Agha ME, Greenberg PD. Restoration of virus immunity in immunodeficient humans by the adoptive transfer of T-cell clones. Science 257:238–241, 1992.

Rijkers GT, Roord JJ, Koning F, Kuis W, Zegers BJM. Phenotypical and functional analysis of B lymphocytes of two siblings with combined immunodeficiency and defective expression of major histocompatibility complex (MHC) class II antigens on mononuclear cells. J Clin Immunol 7:98–106, 1987.

Rijkers GT, Scharenberg JGM, van Dongen JJM, Neijens HJ, Zegers BJM. Abnormal signal transduction in a patient with severe combined immunodeficiency disease. Pediatr Res 29:306–309, 1991.

Rimm IJ, Rappeport JM. Bone marrow transplantation for the Wiskott-Aldrich syndrome. Transplantation 50:617–620, 1990.

Ritter ML, Boyd RL. Development in the thymus: it takes two to tango. Immunol Today 14:462–469, 1993.

Rivat-Peran L, Buriot D, Salier JP, Rivat C, Dumitresco SM, Griscelli C. Immunoglobulins in ataxia-telangiectasia: evidence for IgG4 and IgA2 subclass deficiencies. Clin Immunol Immunopathol 20:99–110, 1981.

Rocklin RE, Chilgren RA, Hong R, David JR. Transfer of cellular hypersensitivity in chronic mucocutaneous candidiasis monitored in vivo and in vitro. Cell Immunol 1:290–299, 1970.

Rohn RD, Leffell MS, Leadem P, Johnson D, Rubio T, Emanuel BS. Familial third-fourth pharyngeal pouch syndrome with apparent autosomal dominant transmission. J Pediatr 105:47–51, 1984.

Roifman CM, Gelfand EW. Heterogeneity of the immunological deficiency in ataxia-telangiectasia: absence of a clinical-pathological correlation. In Gatti RA, Swift M, eds. Ataxia-Telangiectasia: Genetics, Neuropathology, and Immunology of a Degenerative Disease of Childhood, Vol. 19. New York, Alan R. Liss, 1984, pp. 273–282.

Roifman CM, Hummel D, Martinez-Valdez H, Thorner P, Doherty PJ, Pan S, Cohen F, Cohen A. Depletion of CD8+ cells in human thymic medulla results in selective immune deficiency. J Exp Med 170:2177–2182, 1989.

Rook AH, Masur H, Lane HC, Frederick W, Kasahara T, Macher AM, Djev JV, Manischevitz JF, Jackson L, Fauci AS. Interleukin-2 enhances the depressed natural killer and cytomegalovirus-specific cytotoxic activities of lymphokines from patients with the acquired immune deficiency syndrome. J Clin Invest 72:398–407, 1983.

Root AW, Speicher CE. The trial of thrombocytopenia, eczema, and recurrent infections (Wiskott-Aldrich syndrome) associated with milk antibodies, giant-cell pneumonia and cytomegalic inclusion disease. Pediatrics 31:444–454, 1963.

Rosen F, Wedgwood RJ, Eibl LM, Gross TG, Weisenburger DD, Davis J, Spiegel K, Brichacek B, Sumegi J. Primary immunodeficiency diseases. Report of a WHO scientific group. Immunodeficiency Rev 3:195–236, 1992.

Rosenberg SA. Karnofsky Memorial Lecture. The immunotherapy and gene therapy of cancer. J Clin Oncol 10:180–199, 1992.

Rosenblatt HR, Ladisch S, Albrecht RM, Lehrer RI, Fischer TJ, Hong R, Stiehm ER. Monocyte effector defects in chronic mucocutaneous candidasis (abstract). Pediatr Res 13:454, 1979.

Roth K, Cohn R, Yandrasitz J, Preti G, Dodd P, Segal S. Beta-methylcrotonic aciduria associated with lactic acidosis. J Pediatr 88:229–235, 1976.

Rumelhart SL, Trigg ME, Horowitz SD, Hong R. Monoclonal antibody T-cell–depleted HLA-haploidentical bone marrow transplantation for Wiskott-Aldrich syndrome. Blood 75:1031–1035, 1990.

Russell SM, Keegan AD, Harada N, Nakamura Y, Noguchi M, Leland P, Friedmann MC, Miyajima A, Puri RK, Paul WE, Leonard WJ. Interleukin-2 receptor γ chain: a functional component of the interleukin-4 receptor. Science 262:1880–1883, 1993.

Rytel MW, Aaberg MA, Dee TH, Heim LH. Therapy of cytomegalovirus retinitis with transfer factor. Cell Immunol 19:8–21, 1975.

St. Geme JW Jr, Prince JT, Burke BA, Good RA, Krivit W. Impaired cellular resistance to herpes simplex virus in Wiskott-Aldrich syndrome. N Engl J Med 273:229–234, 1966.

Sale GE, Shulman HM, Galluci BB, Thomas ED. Young rete ridge keratinocytes are preferred targets in cutaneous graft-versus-host disease. Am J Pathol 118:278–287, 1985.

Salter RD, Alexander J, Levine F, Pious D, Cresswell P. Evidence for two trans-acting genes regulating HLA class II antigen expression. J Immunol 135:4235–4238, 1985.

Sams WM, Jorizzo JL, Snyderman R, Jegasothy BV, Ward FE, Wilson JG, Dillard SB. Chronic mucocutaneous candidiasis: immunologic studies in three generations of a single family. Am J Med 67:948–959, 1979.

Sanal O, Wei S, Foroud T, Malhotra U, Concannon P, Charmley P, Salser W, Lange K, Gatti RA. Further mapping of an ataxia-telangiectasia locus to the chromosome 11q23 region. Am J Hum Genet 47:860–866, 1990.

Sander JE, Malamud N, Cowan MJ, Padkman S, Ammann AJ, Wara DW. Intermittent ataxia and immunodeficiency with multiple carboxylase deficiency: a biotin-responsive disorder. Ann Neurol 8:544–547, 1980.

Sanders J, Sullivan K, Witherspoon R, Doney K, Anasetti C, Beatty P, Petersen FB. Long-term effects and quality of life in children and adults after marrow transplantation. Bone Marrow Transplant 4:27–29, 1989.

Sandman R, Ammann AJ, Grose C, Wara DW. Cellular immunodeficiency associated with nucleoside phosphorylase deficiency. Clin Immunol Immunopathol 8:247–253, 1977.

Santisteban I, Arrendondo-Vega FX, Kelly S, Mary A, Fischer A, Hummell DS, Lawton A, Sorensen RU, Stiehm ER, Uribe L, Weinberg K, Hershfield MS. Novel splicing, missense, and deletion mutations in seven adenosine deaminase–deficient patients with late/delayed onset of combined immunodeficiency disease. J Clin Invest 92:2291–2302, 1993.

Sato M, Hayashi Y, Yoshida H, Yanagawa T, Yura Y. A family with hereditary lack of T4⁺ inducer/helper T cell subsets in peripheral blood lymphocytes. J Immunol 132:1071–1073, 1984.

Saulsbury FT, Winkelstein JA, Davis LE, Hsu SH, D'Souza BJ, Gutcher GR, Butler IJ. Combined immunodeficiency and vaccine-related poliomyelitis in a child with cartilage-hair hypoplasia. J Pediatr 86:868–872, 1975.

Saunders M, Sweetman L, Robinson B, Rolth K, Cohn R, Gravel RA. Multiple carboxylase deficiencies and complementation studies with propionicacidemia in cultured fibroblasts. J Clin Invest 64:1695–1701, 1979.

Savitsky K, Bar-Shira A, Gilad S, Rotman G, Ziv Y, Vanagaite L, Tagle DA, Smith S, Uziel T, Sfez S, Ashkenazi M, Pecker I, Frydman M, Harnik R, Patanjali SR, Simmons A, Clines GA, Sartiel A, Gatti RA, Chessa L, Sanal O, Lavin MF, Jaspers NGJ, Taylor AMR, Arlett CF, Miki T, Weissman SM, Lovett M, Collins FS, Shiloh Y. A single ataxia telangiectasia gene with a product similar to PI-3 kinase. Science 268:1749–1753, 1995

Scambler PJ, Kelly D, Lindsay E, Williamson R, Goldberg R, Shprintzen R, Wilson DI, Goodship JA, Cross IE, Burn J. Velo-cardio-facial syndrome associated with chromosome 22 deletions encompassing the DiGeorge locus. Lancet 339:1138–1139, 1992.

Schalch DS, McFarlin DE, Barlow MH. An unusual form of diabetes mellitus in ataxia-telangiectasia. N Engl J Med 282:1396–1402, 1970.

Schandene L, Ferster A, Mascart-Lemone F, Cruisiaux A, Gerard C, Marchart A, Lybin M, Velu T, Sariban E, Goldman M. T helper type 2–like cells and therapeutic effects of interferon-gamma in combined immunodeficiency with hypereosinophilia (Omenn's syndrome). Eur J Immunol 23:53–60, 1993.

Scheinberg MA, Cathcart S, Goldstein AL. Thymosin-induced reduction of "null cells" in peripheral blood lymphocytes of patients with systemic lupus erythematosus. Lancet 1:424–428, 1975.

Schneider LC, Berman RS, Shea CR, Perez-Atayde AR, Weinstein H, Geha RS. Bone marrow transplantation (BMT) for the syndrome of pigmentary dilution and lymphohistiocytosis (Griscelli's syndrome). J Clin Immunol 10:146–153, 1990.

Schubert MS, Moss R. Selective polysaccharide antibody deficiency in familial DiGeorge syndrome. Ann Allergy 69:231–238, 1992.

Schulkind ML, Adler WH, Altemeier WA, Ayoub EM. Transfer factor in the treatment of a case of chronic mucocutaneous candidiasis. Cell Immunol 3:606–615, 1972.

Schuster V, Kress W, Friedrich W, Grim T, Kreth HW. X-linked lymphoproliferative disease: detection of a paternally inherited mutation in a German family using haplotype analysis. Am J Dis Child 147:1303–1305, 1993.

Schuttevaer HM, Kroon HM, Shaw PC. Graft-versus-host disease of the gastrointestinal tract. Diagn Imaging Clin Med 55:254–261, 1986.

Schuurman HJ, van de Wijngaert FP, Huber J, Schuurman RKB, Zegers BJM, Roord JJ, Kater L. The thymus in "bare lymphocyte" syndrome: significance of expression of major histocompatibility complex antigens on thymic epithelial cells in intrathymic T-cell maturation. Hum Immunol 13:69–82, 1985.

Schuurman RKB, van Rood JJ, Vossen JM, Schellekens PTA, Feltkamp-Vroom TM, Doyer E, Gmelig-Meyling F, Visser HKA. Failure of lymphocyte-membrane HLA-A and -B expression in two siblings with combined immunodeficiency. Clin Immunol Immunopathol 14:418–434, 1979.

Schwarz K, Hausen-Hagge TE, Knobloch C, Friedrich W, Kleihauer E. Severe combined immunodeficiency (SCID) in man: B cell–negative (B−) SCID patients exhibit an irregular recombination pattern at the Jₕ locus. J Exp Med 174:1039–1048, 1991.

Sedgwick RP, and Boder E. Ataxia-telangiectasia. In de Jong JMBV, ed. Handbook of Clinical Neurology, Vol. 16: Hereditary Neuropathies and Spinocerebellar Atrophies. Amsterdam, Elsevier Science Publishers BV, 1991, pp 347–423.

Seeley JK, Golub SH. Studies on cytotoxicity generated in human mixed lymphocyte cultures: I. Time course and target spectrum of several distinct concomitant cytotoxic activities. J Immunol 120:1415–1422, 1978.

Seemanova E, Passarge E, Beneskova D, Houstek J, Kasal P, Sevcikova M. Familial microcephaly with normal intelligence, immunodeficiency, and risk for lymphoreticular malignancies: a new autosomal recessive disorder. Am J Med Genet 20:639–648, 1985.

Seemayer TA, Grierson H, Pirruccello SJ, Gross TG, Weisenburger DD, Davis J, Spiegel K, Brichacek B, Sumegi J. X-linked lymphoproliferative disease. Am J Dis Child 147:1242–1245, 1993.

Shama SK, Kirkpatrick CH. Dermatophytosis in patients with chronic mucocutaneous candidiasis. J Am Acad Dermatol 2:285–294, 1980.

Shapiro RS, Chauvenet A, McGuire W, Pearson A, Craft WW, McGlave P, Filipovich A. Treatment of B-cell lymphoproliferative disorders with interferon alpha and intravenous gamma globulin. N Engl J Med 318:1334, 1988a.

Shapiro RS, McClain K, Frizzera G, Gajl-Peczalska KJ, Kersey JH, Blazar BR, Arthur DC, Patton DF, Greenberg JS, Burke B, Ramsay NKC, McGlave P, Filipovich AH. Epstein-Barr virus–associated B cell lymphoproliferative disorders following bone marrow transplantation. Blood 71:1234–1243, 1988b.

Shearer WT, Wedner J, Strominger DB, Kissane J, Hong R. Successful transplantation of the thymus in Nezelof's syndrome. Pediatrics 61:619–624, 1978.

Shelley CS, Remold-O'Donnell E, Davis AE III, Bruns GAP, Rosen FS, Carroll MC, Whitehead AS. Molecular characterization of sialophorin (CD43), the lymphocyte surface sialoglycoprotein defective in Wiskott-Aldrich syndrome. Proc Natl Acad Sci U S A 86:2819–2823, 1989.

Sheppard H. CD4⁺ T-lymphocytopenia without HIV infection. N Engl J Med 328:1847–1848, 1993.

Shigeoka AO, Chance PF, Fain P, Barker DA, Book LS, Rallison ML. An X-linked T cell activation syndrome maps near the Wiskott-Aldrich locus Xp11.1: diarrhea, respiratory infections, autoimmune disease and endocrinopathies in the absence of platelet defects. Clin Res 41:41A, 1993.

Siccardi A, Bianchi E, Calligari A, Clivio A, Fortunato A, Magrini U, Sacchi F. A new familial defect in neutrophil bactericidal activity. Helv Paediatr Acta 33:401–422, 1978.

Silber GM, Winkelstein J, Moen RC, Horowitz SD, Trigg M, Hong R. Reconstitution of T and B cell function after T-lymphocyte–depleted haploidentical bone marrow transplant in severe combined immunodeficiency due to adenosine deaminase deficiency. Clin Immunol Immunopathol 44:317–320, 1987.

Silva C, Lima AO, Andrade LMC, Mattos O. Attempts to convert lepromatous into tuberculoid-type leprosy with blood lymphocyte extracts from sensitized donors. Clin Exp Immunol 15:87–92, 1973.

Simon HU, Mills GB, Hashimoto S, Siminovitch KA. Evidence for defective transmembrane signaling in B cells from patients with Wiskott-Aldrich syndrome. J Clin Invest 90:1396–1405, 1992.

Sindel LJ, Buckley RH, Schiff SE, Ward FE, Mickey GH, Huang AT, Naspitz C, Koren H. Severe combined immunodeficiency with natural killer-cell predominance: abrogation of graft-versus-host disease and immunologic reconstitution with HLA-identical bone marrow cells. J Allergy Clin Immunol 73:829–836, 1984.

Slavin RE, Santos GW. The graft-versus-host reaction in man after bone marrow transplantation: pathology, pathogenesis, clinical features, and implications. Clin Immunol Immunopathol 1:472–498, 1973.

Smeby B. Ataxia-telangiectasia. Acta Paediatr Scand 55:239–243, 1966.

Smith CI, Weissberg J, Bernhardt PB, Gregory PB, Robinson WS, Merigan TC. Acute Dane particle suppression with recombinant leukocyte A interferon in chronic hepatitis B infection. J Infect Dis 148:907–913, 1983.

Smith DK, Neal JJ, Holmberg SD, and Centers for Disease Control, Idiopathic CD4⁺ T-lymphocytopenia Task Force. Unexplained opportunistic infections and CD4⁺ T-lymphopenia with HIV infection—an investigation of cases in the United States. N Engl J Med 328:373–379, 1993.

Smith KA. Interleukin 2. Ann Rev Immunol 2:319–333, 1984.

Snyderman R, Altman LC, Frankel A, Blaese RM. Defective mononuclear leukocyte chemotaxis: a previously unrecognized immune dysfunction. Ann Intern Med 78:509–513, 1973.

Solitare GB, Lopez VF. Louis-Bar's syndrome (ataxia-telangiectasia). Neurology 17:23–31, 1967.

Sorensen RU, Boehm KD, Kaplan D, Berger M. Cryptococcal osteomyelitis and cellular immunodeficiency associated with interleukin-2 deficiency. J Pediatr 121:873–879, 1992.

Spiess PJ, Yang JC, Rosenberg SA. In vivo anti-tumor activity of tumor-infiltrating lymphocytes expanded in recombinant IL-2. J Natl Cancer Inst 79:1067–1075, 1987.

Spira TJ, Jones BM, Nicholson JKA, Lal RB, Rowe T, Mawle AC, Lauter CB, Shulman JA, Monson RA. Idiopathic CD4+ T-lymphocytopenia—an analysis of five patients with unexplained opportunistic infections. N Engl J Med 328:386–392, 1993.

Spitler LE, Levin AS, Stites DP, Fudenberg HH, Pirofsky B, August CS, Stiehm ER, Hitzig WH, Gatti RA. The Wiskott-Aldrich syndrome: results of transfer factor therapy. J Clin Invest 51:3216–3224, 1972.

Spriggs MK, Armitage RJ, Stockbine L, Clifford KN, Macduff BM, Sato TA, Maliszewski CR, Fanslow WC. Recombinant human CD40 ligand stimulates B cell proliferation and immunoglobulin E secretion. J Exp Med 176:1543–1550, 1992.

Springer TA, Dustin ML, Kishimoto TK, Marlin SD. The lymphocyte function–associated LFA-1, CD2, and LFA-3 molecules: cell adhesion receptors of the immune system. Annu Rev Immunol 5:223–252, 1987.

Stavaren AM, Stiehm ER. Chronic mucocutaneous candidiasis: clinical, immunologic and therapeutic considerations. In Moss AJ, ed. Pediatrics Update. New York, Elsevier, 1986, pp. 93–110.

Steele RW, Limas C, Thurman GB, Schuelein M, Bauer H, Bellanti JA. Familial thymic aplasia: attempted reconstitution with fetal thymus in a millipore diffusion chamber. N Engl J Med 287:787–791, 1972.

Steimle V, Otten LA, Zufferey M, Mach B. Complementation cloning of an MHC class II transactivator mutated in hereditary MHC class II deficiency (or bare lymphocyte syndrome). Cell 75:135–146, 1993.

Steinfeld JL, Davidson JD, Gordon RS Jr, Greene FE. Mechanism of hypoproteinemia in patients with regional enteritis and ulcerative colitis (abstract). Am J Med 29:405–415, 1960.

Stephan JL, Vlekova V, Le Deist F, Blanche S, Donadieu J, De Saint-Basile G, Durandy A, Griscelli C, Fischer A. Severe combined immunodeficiency: a retrospective single-center study of clinical presentation outcome in 117 patients. J Pediatr 123:564–572, 1993.

Stimac E, Urieli-Shoval S, Kempkin S, Pious D. Defective HLA DRA X box binding in the class II transactive transcription factor mutant 6.1.6 and in cell lines from class II immunodeficient patients. J Immunol 146:4398–4405, 1991.

Stobo JD, Paul S, Van Scoy RE, Hermans PE. Suppression of thymus-derived lymphocytes in fungal infection. J Clin Invest 57:319–328, 1976.

Stoelinga GB, van Munster PJ. Antibody deficiency syndrome and autoimmune haemolytic anaemia in a boy with isolated IgM deficiency dysimmunoglobulinaemia type 5. Acta Paediatr Scand 58:352–362, 1969.

Stoelinga GBA, van Munster PJ, Sloff JP. Chylous effusions into the intestine in a patient with protein-losing gastroenteropathy. Pediatrics 31:1011–1018, 1963.

Stohl W, Crow MK, Kunkel HG. Systemic lupus erythematosus with deficiency of the T4 epitope on T helper/inducer cells. N Engl J Med 312:4671–4678, 1985.

Stoop JW, Zeger BJM, Hendricky GFM, Siegenbeck van Henkelom LH, Staal GE, DeBree PK, Wadman SK, Ballieux RE. Purine nucleoside phosphorylase deficiency associated with selective cellular immunodeficiency. N Engl J Med 296:651–655, 1976.

Storb R, Deeg HJ, Whitehead J, Appelbaum F, Beatty P, Bensinger W, Buckner CD, Clift R, Doney K, Farewich V, Hansen J. Methotrexate and cyclosporine compared with cyclosporine alone for prophylaxis of acute graft-versus-host disease following marrow transplant for leukemia. N Engl J Med 314:729–735, 1986.

Storb R, Prentice RL, Buckner CD. Graft-versus-host disease and survival in patients with aplastic anemia treated by marrow grafts from HLA-identical siblings: beneficial effect of a protective environment. N Engl J Med 308:302–307, 1983.

Stotter H, Rude E, Wagner H. T cell factor (interleukin-2) allows in vivo induction of T helper cells against heterologous erythrocytes in athymic (nu/nu) mice. Eur J Immunol 10:719–722, 1980.

Strich SJ. Pathologic findings in the three cases of ataxia-telangiectasia. J Neurol Neurosurg Psychiatry 29:489–499, 1966.

Strober W, Wochner RD, Carbone PP, Waldmann TA. Intestinal lymphangiectasia: a protein-losing enteropathy with hypogammaglobulinemia, lymphocytopenia and impaired homograft rejection. J Clin Invest 46:1643–1656, 1967.

Strober W, Wochner RD, Barlow MH, McFarlin DE, Waldmann TA. Immunoglobulin metabolism in ataxia-telangiectasia. J Clin Invest 47:1905–1915, 1968.

Sullivan JL, Byron KS, Brewster FE, Baker SM, Ochs HD. X-linked lymphoproliferative syndrome: natural history of the immunodeficiency. J Clin Invest 71:1765–1778, 1983.

Sullivan JL, Byron KS, Brewster FE, Sakamoto K, Shaw JE, Pagano JS. Treatment of life-threatening Epstein-Barr virus infections with acyclovir. Am J Med 73:262–266, 1982.

Sullivan KE, Mullen CA, Blaese RM, Winkelstein JA. A multi-institutional survey of the Wiskott-Aldrich syndrome. J Pediatr 125:876–885, 1994.

Sullivan KM, Siadak MF, Witherspoon RP. Cyclosporine treatment of chronic graft-versus-host disease following allogeneic bone marrow transplantation. Transplant Proc 22:1336–1338, 1990.

Sweetman L, Shur L, Nyhan WL. Deficiencies of proprionyl-CoA and 3-methylcrotonyl-CoA carboxylases in a patient with a dietary deficiency of biotin. Clin Res 27:118A, 1979.

Swift A, Morrell D, Massey RB, Chase CL. Incidence of cancer in 161 families affected by ataxia-telangiectasia. N Engl J Med 325:1831–1836, 1991.

Swift M. Genetics and epidemiology of ataxia-telangiectasia. In Gatti RA, Swift M, eds. Ataxia-telangiectasia: Genetics, Neuropathology, and Immunology of a Degenerative Disease of Childhood, Vol. 19. New York, Alan R. Liss, 1984, pp. 133–144.

Swift M, Morrell D, Cromartie E, Chamberlain AR, Skolnick MH, Bishop DT. The incidence and gene frequency of ataxia-telangiectasia in the United States. Am J Hum Genet 39:573–583, 1986.

Swift M, Sholman L, Perry M, Chase C. Malignant neoplasms in the families of patients with ataxia-telangiectasia. Cancer Res 36:209–215, 1976.

Syllaba L, Henner K. Contribution a l'indépendance de l'athetose double idiopathique et congenitale: atteinte familiale, syndrome dystrophique, signe du réseau vasculaire conjonctival, intégrité psychique. Rev Neurol (Paris) 1:541–562, 1926.

Taalman RDFM, Hustinx TWJ, Weemaes CMR, Seemanova E, Schmidt A, Passarge E, Scheres JMJC. Further delineation of the Nijmegen breakage syndrome. Am J Med Genet 32:425–431, 1989.

Tadjoedin MK, Fraser FC. Heredity of ataxia-telangiectasia (Louis-Bar syndrome). Am J Dis Child 110:64–68, 1965.

Taitz LS, Zarate-Salvador C, Schwartz E. Congenital absence of the parathyroid and thymus glands in an infant (III and IV pharyngeal pouch syndrome). Pediatrics 38:412–418, 1966.

Takenaka T, Kuribayashi K, Nakamine H, Yoshikawa F, Maeda J, Kishi S, Nakauchi H, Minatogawa Y, Kido R. Autosomal codominant inheritance and Japanese incidence of deficiency of OKT4 epitope and lack of reactivity resulting from a conformational change. J Immunol 151:2864–2870, 1993.

Targan SR, Oseas R. The "lazy" NK cells of Chédiak-Higashi syndrome. J Immunol 130:1671–1674, 1973.

Taylor AMR, Harnden DG, Arlett CF, Harcourt SA, Lehmann AR, Stevens S, Bridges BA. Ataxia-telangiectasia: a human mutation with abnormal radiation sensitivity. Nature 258:427–429, 1975.

Taylor AMR, McConville GM, Woods GW, Byrd PJ, Hernandez D. Clinical and cellular heterogeneity in ataxia-telangiectasia. In Gatti RA, Painter RB, eds. Ataxia-Telangiectasia. Heidelberg, Springer-Verlag, 1993, pp. 209–233.

Terplan KL, Krauss RF. Histopathologic brain changes in association with ataxia-telangiectasia. Neurology 19:446–454, 1969.

Thieffry S, Arthuis M, Aicardi J, Lyon G. L'ataxie-telangiectasie (7 observations personnelles). Rev Neurol (Paris) 105:390–405, 1961.

Thiele DL, Eigenbrodt ML, Bryde SE, Eigenbrodt EH, Lipsky PE. Intestinal graft-versus-host disease is initiated by donor T cells distinct from classic cytotoxic T lymphocytes. J Clin Invest 84:1947–1956, 1989.

Thoene J, Sweetman L, Yoshino M. Biotin-responsive multiple carboxylase deficiency. Am J Hum Gen 31:64A, 1979.

Thoman ML, Weigle WO. Cell-mediated immunity in aged mice: an underlying lesion in IL-2 synthesis. J Immunol 128:2358–2361, 1982.

Thomas IT, Ochs HD, Wedgwood RJ. Liver disease and immunodeficiency syndromes. Lancet 1:311, 1974.

Thornes G, Le Deist F, Fischer A, Griscelli C, Lisowska-Grospierre B. Immunodeficiency associated with defective expression of the T-cell receptor–CD3 complex. N Engl J Med 322:1399, 1990.

Thorpe ES, Handley HE. Chronic tetany and chronic mycelial stomatitis in a child aged four and one-half years. Am J Dis Child 38:228–338, 1929.

Tosato G, Jones K, Breinig MKI, McWilliams HP, McKnight JLC. Interleukin-6 production in posttransplant lymphoproliferative disease. J Clin Invest 91:2806–2814, 1993.

Touraine J-L. Stem cell transplantation in primary immunodeficiency, with special reference to the first prenatal, in utero, transplants. Immunol Clin Sperimentale 9:6509–6510, 1990.

Touraine J-L, Betuel H, Gouillet G, Jeune M. Combined immunodeficiency disease associated with absence of cell-surface HLA-A and -B antigens. J Pediatr 93:47–51, 1978.

Touraine J-L, Marseglia GL-L, Betuel H. Thirty international cases of bare lymphocyte syndrome: biological significance of HLA antigens. Exp Hematol 13(Suppl.):86–87, 1985.

Touraine J-L, Marseglia GL, Betuel LH, Souillet G, Gebuhrer L. The bare lymphocyte syndrome. Bone Marrow Transplant 9(Suppl.):54–56, 1992a.

Touraine J-L, Raudrant D, Rebaud A, Roncarolo MG, Laplace S, Gebuhrer L, Betuel H, Frappaz D, Freycon F, Zabot MT, Touraine F, Souillet G, Philippe N, Vullo C. In utero transplantation of stem cells in humans: immunological aspects and clinical follow-up of patients. Bone Marrow Transplant 9(Suppl. 1):121–126, 1992b.

Touraine J-L, Raudrant D, Royo C, Rebaud A, Barbier F, Roncarolo MG, Touraine F, Laplace S, Gebuhrer L, Betuel H. In utero transplantation of hemopoietic stem cells in humans. Transplant Proc 23:1706–1708, 1991.

Touraine J-L, Raudrant D, Royo C, Rebaud A, Roncarolo MG, Souillet G, Phillippe N, Touraine F, Betuel H. In-utero transplantation of stem cells in bare lymphocyte syndrome. Lancet 1:1382, 1989.

Trigg ME, Billing R, Sondel PM, Dickerman JD, Erickson C, Finlay JL, Bozdech M, Hong R, Padilla-Nash H, Terasaki P. Depletion of T cells from human bone marrow with monoclonal antibody CT-2 and complement. J Biol Resp Mod 3:406–412, 1984.

Tu RK, Peters ME, Gourley GR, Hong R. Esophageal histoplasmosis in a child with immunodeficiency with hyper-IgM. Am J Roentgenol 157:381–382, 1991.

Tuvia JA, Weisselberg B, Shif I, Keren G. Aplastic anaemia complicating adenovirus infection in DiGeorge syndrome. Eur J Pediatr 147:643–644, 1988.

Twomey JJ, Waddell CC, Krantz S, O'Reilly R, L'Esperance P, Good RA. Chronic mucocutaneous candidiasis with macrophage dysfunction, a plasma inhibitor, and co-existent aplastic anemia. J Lab Clin Med 85:968–977, 1975.

Ugozolli L, Baldi L, Delfini C, Lucarelli G, Wallace RB, Ferrara GB. Genotypic analysis of engraftment in thalassemia following bone marrow transplantation using synthetic oligonucleotides. Bone Marrow Transplant 4:173–180, 1989.

Valdimarsson H, Hambleton G, Henry K, McConnell I. Restoration of T-lymphocyte deficiency with dialyzable leucocyte extract. Clin Exp Immunol 16:141–152, 1974.

Valdimarsson H, Higgs JM, Wells RS, Yamamura M, Hobbs JR, Holt PJL. Immune abnormalities associated with chronic mucocutaneous candidiasis. Cell Immunol 6:348–361, 1973.

Valdimarsson H, Moss PD, Holt PJL, Hobbs JR. Treatment of chronic mucocutaneous candidiasis with leukocytes from HLA compatible sibling. Lancet i:469–472, 1972a.

Valdimarsson H, Wood CBS, Hobbs JR, Holt PJL. Immunological features in a case of chronic granulomatous candidiasis and its treatment with transfer factor. Clin Exp Immunol 2:151–163, 1972b.

Valentine WN, Paglia DE, Tartaglia AP, Gilsanz F. Hereditary hemolytic anemia with increased red cell adenosine deaminase (45- to 70-fold) and decreased adenosine triphosphate. Science 195:783–785, 1977.

van Bekkum DW, Roodenburg J, Heidt PJ, van der Waaij D. Mitigation of secondary disease of allogeneic mouse radiation chimeras by modification of the intestinal microflora. J Natl Cancer Inst 52:401–404, 1974.

Van Scoy RE, Hill HR, Ritts RE, Quie PG. Familial neutrophil chemotaxis defect, recurrent bacterial infections, mucocutaneous candidiasis and hyperimmunoglobulin E. Ann Intern Med 82:766–771, 1975.

Vankey J, Gorsky T, Gorsky Y, Masucci MG, Klein E. Lysis of tumor biopsy cells by autologous T lymphocytes activated in mixed cultures and propagated with T-cell growth factor. J Exp Med 155:83–95, 1982.

Vogelsang GB, Farmer ER, Hess AD, Altamonte V, Beschorner WE, Jabs DA, Corio RL, Levin LS, Colvin OM, Wingard JR, Santos GW. Thalidomide for the treatment of chronic graft-versus-host disease. N Engl J Med 326:1055–1058, 1992.

Voss SD, Hong R, Sondel PM. Severe combined immunodeficiency, interleukin-2 (IL-2), and the IL-2 receptor: experiments of nature continue to point the way. Blood 83:626–635, 1994.

Vowels MR, Po-Tang RL, Berdoukas V, Ford D, Thierry D, Purtilo D, Gluckman E. Brief report: correction of X-linked lymphoproliferative disease by transplantation of cord-blood stem cells. N Engl J Med 329:1623–1625, 1993.

Wagner H, Hardt C, Heeg K, Rollinghoff M, Pfizenmaier K. T-cell–derived helper factor allows in vivo induction of cytotoxic T cells in nu/nu mice. Nature 284:278–280, 1980.

Wagstaff LA, Joffe R. Ataxia-telangiectasia in a South African Bantu child. S Afr Med J 43:662–664, 1969.

Waldmann TA, Broder S, Blaese RM, Durm M, Blackman M, Strober W. Role of suppressor T cells in pathogenesis of common variable hypogammaglobulinaemia. Lancet 2:609–614, 1974.

Waldmann TA, Broder S. Suppressor cells in the regulation of the immune response. In Schwartz R, ed. Progress in Clinical Immunology. New York, Grune & Stratton, 1977, pp. 155–199.

Waldmann TA, McIntire KR. Serum alpha-fetoprotein levels in patients with ataxia-telangiectasia. Lancet 2:1112–1115, 1972.

Waldmann TA, Schwab PJ. IgG (7S gamma globulin) metabolism in hypogammaglobulinemia: studies in patients with defective gammaglobulin synthesis, gastrointestinal protein loss or both. J Clin Invest 44:1523–1533, 1965.

Waldmann TA, Steinfield JL, Dutcher TF, Davidson JD, Gordon RS Jr. The role of the gastrointestinal system in "idiopathic hypoproteinemia." Gastroenterology 41:197–207, 1961.

Waldmann TA, Wochner RD, Laster L, Gordon RS Jr. Allergic gastroenteropathy: a cause of excessive gastrointestinal protein loss. N Engl J Med 276:761–769, 1967.

Wara DW, Ammann AJ. Thymosin treatment of children with primary immunodeficiency disease. Transplant Proc 10:203–212, 1978.

Wara DW, Goldstein AL, Doyle E, Ammann AJ. Thymosin activity in patients with cellular immunodeficiency. N Engl J Med 292:70–74, 1975.

Webb MC, Andrews PA, Koffman CG, Cameron JS. Renal transplantation in Wiskott-Aldrich syndrome. Transplantation 56:747–748, 1993.

Weemaes CMR, Hustinx TWJ, Scheres JMJC, Van Munster PJJ, Bakkeren JAJM, Taalman RDFM. A new chromosomal instability disorder: the Nijmegen breakage syndrome. Acta Paediatr Scand 70:557–564, 1981.

Weemaes CMR, Smeets DFCM, Van der Burgt CJAM. Nijmegen breakage syndrome: a progress report. University Hospital, Nijmegen, The Netherlands. Int J Radiat Biol 6(suppl):S185–S188, 1994.

Wegner R-D, Metzger M, Hanefeld F, Jaspers NGJ, Baan C, Magdorf K, Kunze J, Sperling K. A new chromosomal instability disorder confirmed by complementation studies. Clin Genet 33:200–232, 1988.

Weinberg KB, Parkman R. Severe combined immunodeficiency due to a specific defect in the production of interleukin-2. N Engl J Med 322:1718–1723, 1990.

Weinberg K, Hershfield MS, Bastian J, Kohn D, Sender L, Parkman R, Lenarsky C. T lymphocyte ontogeny in adenosine deaminase–deficient severe combined immune deficiency after treatment with polyethylene glycol-modified adenosine deaminase. J Clin Invest 92:596–602, 1993.

Weisdorf D, Hakke R, Blazar B, Miller W, McGlave P, Ramsay N, Kersey J, Filipovich A. Risk factors for acute graft-versus-host disease in histocompatible donor bone marrow transplantation. Transplantation 51:1197–1203, 1991.

Welch CS, Adams M, Wakefield EG. Metabolic studies on chronic ulcerative colitis. J Clin Invest 16:161–168, 1937.

Wells CE, Shy GM. Progressive familial choreoathetosis with oculocutaneous telangiectasia. J Neurol Neurosurg Psychiatry 20:89–104, 1957.

Wells RS, Higgs JM, MacDonald A, Valdimarsson H, Holt PJL. Familial chronic mucocutaneous candidiasis. J Med Genet 9:302–310, 1972.

Wells TR, Gilsanz V, Senac MO, Landing BH, Vachon L, Takahashi M. Ossification centre of the hyoid bone in DiGeorge syndrome and tetralogy of Fallot. Br J Radiol 59:1065–1068, 1986.

West CD, Hong R, Holland NH. Immunoglobulin levels from the newborn period to adulthood and in immunoglobulin deficiency states. J Clin Invest 41:2054–2064, 1962.

Whitaker J, Landing BH, Esselborn VM, Williams RR. The syndrome of familial juvenile hypoadrenocorticism, hypoparathyroidism, and superficial moniliasis. J Clin Endocrinol 16:1374–1387, 1956.

Whitcomb ME, Rocklin RE. Transfer factor therapy in a patient with progressive primary tuberculosis. Ann Intern Med 79:161–166, 1973.

Williams SR, Gekeler V, McIvor RS, Martin RW Jr. A human purine nucleoside phosphorylase deficiency caused by a single base change. J Biol Chem 262:2332–2338, 1987.

Wilson DI, Goodship JA, Burn J, Cross IE, Scambler PJ. Deletions within chromosome 22q11 in familial congenital heart disease. Lancet 340:573–575, 1992.

Wilson GB, Paddock GV, Floyd E, Newell RT, Dopson MH. Immunochemical and physical-chemical evidence for the presence of thymosin alpha$_1$-peptide in dialyzable leukocyte extracts. In Kirkpatrick CH, Lawrence HS, Burger DR, eds. Immunobiology of Transfer Factor. New York, Academic Press, 1983, p. 359.

Wilson JF, Heiner DC, Lahey ME. Studies on iron metabolism. I. Evidence of gastrointestinal dysfunction in infants with iron deficiency anemia: preliminary report. J Pediatr 60:787–800, 1962.

Wingard JR, Piantadosi S, Vogelsang GB, Farmer ER, Jabs DA, Levin LS, Beschorner WE, Cahill RA, Miller DF, Harrison DT. Predictors of death from chronic graft-versus-host disease following allogeneic bone marrow transplantation. Blood 74:1428–1435, 1989.

Wirt DP, Brooks EG, Vaidya S, Klimpel GR, Waldmann TA, Goldblum RM. Novel T-lymphocyte population in combined immunodeficiency with features of graft-versus-host disease. N Engl J Med 321:370–374, 1989.

Wiskott A. Familiarer, angeborener Morbus Werihoff? Wochenschr Kinderheilk 68:212–216, 1937.

Witkin SS, Yu IR, Ledger WJ. Inhibition of Candida albicans–induced lymphocyte proliferation by lymphocytes and sera from women with recurrent vaginitis. Am J Obstet Gynecol 147:809–811, 1983.

Witkin SS, Yu IR, Ledger WJ. A macrophage defect in women with recurrent Candida vaginitis and its reversal in vitro by prostaglandin inhibitors. Am J Obstet Gynecol 155:790–795, 1986.

Wolff JA. Wiskott-Aldrich syndrome: clinical, immunologic and pathologic observations. J Pediatr 70:221–232, 1967.

Wolff JA, Bertucio M. A sex-linked genetic syndrome in a Negro family manifested by thrombocytopenia, eczema, blood diarrhea, recurrent infection, anemia and epistaxis. Am J Dis Child 93:74, 1957.

Wolff JA, Malone RW, Williams P, Chong W, Acsadi G, Jani A, Felgner PL. Direct gene transfer into mouse muscle in vivo. Science 247:1465–1468, 1990.

Wyandt HE, Grierson HL, Sanger WG, Skare JC, Milunsky H, Purtilo DT. Chromosomal deletion of Xq25 in an individual with the X-linked lymphoproliferative disease. Am J Med Genet 33:426–430, 1989.

Yamazaki M, Yasui K, Kawai H, Miyagawa Y, Komiyama A, Akabane T. A monocyte disorder in siblings with chronic candidiasis: a combined abnormality of monocyte mobility and phagocytosis killing ability. Am J Dis Chil 138:192–196, 1984.

Yang YC, Clark SC. Interleukin-3: molecular biology and biologic activities. Hematol Oncol Clin North Am 3:441–452, 1989.

Yang Z, Accolla RS, Pious D, Zegers BJM, Strominger JL. Two distinct genetic loci regulating class II gene expression are defective in human mutant and patient cell lines. EMBO J 7:1965–1972, 1988.

Yonemura S, Nagafuchi A, Sato N, Tsukita S. Concentration of an integral membrane protein, CD43 (leukosialin, sialophorin), in the cleavage furrow through the interaction of its cytoplasmic domain with actin-based cytoskeletons. J Cell Biol 120:437–449, 1993.

Young RR, Austen KR, Moser HW. Abnormalities of serum gamma 1A globulin and ataxia-telangiectasia. Medicine 43:423–433, 1964.

Zisblatt M, Goldstein AL, Lilly F, White A. Acceleration by thymosin of the development of resistance to murine sarcoma–induced tumor in mice. Proc Natl Acad Sci U S A 66:1170–1174, 1970.

ZuRhein GM, Padgett BL, Walker DL, Chun RWM, Horowitz SD, Hong R. Progressive multifocal leukoencephalopathy in a child with severe combined immunodeficiency (letter). N Engl J Med 299:256, 1978.

Zutter MM, Martin PJ, Sale GE, Shulman HM, Fisher L, Thomas ED, Durnam DM. Epstein-Barr virus lymphoproliferation after bone marrow transplantation. Blood 72:520–529, 1988.

Chapter 13

Disorders of the IgE System

Rebecca H. Buckley

Soon after Ishizaka and colleagues discovered the IgE class of immunoglobulins in 1966, elevated serum IgE concentrations were found in several atopic diseases. Sometime later, aberrations of IgE synthesis were noted in many other conditions. Disorders with which alterations in IgE production have been associated include allergic diseases (see Chapter 20); certain bacterial, fungal, and parasitic diseases; graft-versus-host disease; and certain primary and acquired immunodeficiency disorders. Only conditions of the latter three types are considered in this chapter. The diseases discussed include those in which either deficiencies or excesses of IgE production are associated with increased susceptibility to infection, with particular emphasis on the hyper-IgE syndrome.

DISORDERS CHARACTERIZED BY IgE DEFICIENCY

It is difficult to define IgE deficiency because of variability in reported normal ranges from different laboratories. A number of factors contribute to this, including the different methods, standards, nomenclature, sample sizes, and statistical analyses employed. Most laboratories now report IgE levels as international units (IU) per milliliter; 1 IU is equivalent to 2.4 ng (Bazaral and Hamburger, 1972). Serum IgE concentrations in normal individuals vary greatly and do not follow an arithmetic gaussian curve, often having a multimodal distribution (Buckley and Fiscus, 1975). Thus, nonparametric statistics or logarithmic analyses must be used for proper statistical evaluation (Mann and Whitney, 1947). Normal values for IgE have also been found to vary with age (Berg and Johansson, 1969) (see Chapter 9, Table 9–13). In our laboratory, IgE deficiency is defined in children as any value lower than 2 IU/ml

(4.8 ng/ml) and in adults as any value lower than 4 IU/ml (9.6 ng/ml).

Historical Aspects

Interest in the possible role of IgE in host defense was stimulated by the report of Ammann and associates (1969), in which susceptibility to infection in patients with ataxia-telangiectasia was correlated with a combined deficiency of IgA and IgE but not with IgA deficiency alone. This correlation was not confirmed in a larger group of patients with ataxia-telangiectasia studied by Polmar and colleagues (1972a). Indeed, the converse was found—that is, there was a high frequency of respiratory disease in those who were IgA-deficient but not IgE-deficient. Polmar and associates (1972a) as well as others (Buckley and Fiscus, 1975; van der Giessen et al., 1976), however, did find lower than normal mean serum IgE concentrations in patients with ataxia-telangiectasia, as well as in those with other immunodeficiencies (see IgE Deficiency in Primary Immunodeficiency Disorders). Whether IgE deficiency plays any role in these patients' susceptibility to infection is still unknown. Of possible relevance to this question is the report by Levy and Chen (1970) of a healthy IgE-deficient person. We also have identified several healthy IgE-deficient individuals (unpublished). By contrast, several clinical entities are described in which undue susceptibility to infection is associated with abnormally high serum IgE concentrations.

Pathogenic Mechanisms

Since the discovery and delineation of the biologic properties of IgE antibodies (Ishizaka and Ishizaka, 1967), many investigators have searched for their useful function. From a teleologic standpoint, it seems unlikely that IgE would have survived in evolution on the basis of its harmful properties. The predominant production of both IgA and IgE immunoglobulins by plasma cells in lymphoid tissues adjacent to mucosal surfaces suggests that the protective role of IgE antibodies may be that of a "gatekeeper" (Tada and Ishizaka, 1970). Vasoactive substances released following the interaction of antigen with mast cell or basophil-fixed IgE antibodies alter vascular permeability, thus facilitating the passage of other elements of the immune system into sites where they are needed.

Studies in rats experimentally infested with *Schistosoma mansoni* or *Trichinella spiralis* have demonstrated a direct relationship between IgE antibody response and resistance to infection (Capron et al., 1978; Dessein et al., 1981). This resistance appears to be mediated by chemotactic factors for eosinophils elaborated by IgE-sensitized mast cells. These factors include histamine, eosinophil chemotactic factor of anaphylaxis (ECF-A) peptides, platelet activating factor (PAF), and leukotriene B_2 (LTB_2). The eosinophils so attracted are capable of killing schistosomula of *S. mansoni* by both IgE and IgG antibody and complement-dependent mechanisms (Anwar et al., 1979; Capron et al., 1981). The precise mechanism of killing has not been established, although it is known that eosinophil major basic protein can damage schistosomula directly (Butterworth et al., 1979). It is also known that supernatants from cultured mononuclear cell preparations can enhance antibody-dependent eosinophil killing (Veith and Butterworth, 1983).

It has been suggested that genetically determined "high IgE responders" (e.g., members of families with a high incidence of atopic disease) may have had ancestors with a survival advantage in areas of endemic parasitic disease. Once these people moved to an environment relatively free of parasites, the IgE response was then directed against other environmental antigens. Other than the potential disadvantage in handling parasitic infestations, however, there is no evidence that a selective deficiency of IgE leads to a significant host deficit in humans.

IgE Deficiency in Primary Immunodeficiency Disorders

Concentrations of IgE were measured in sera from 165 patients with a variety of well-defined primary immunodeficiency disorders (Buckley and Fiscus, 1975). The mean serum IgE level was significantly below normal in patients who had marked deficiencies in all three major immunoglobulin isotypes, such as those with transient hypogammaglobulinemia of infancy, severe combined immunodeficiency disease, X-linked agammaglobulinemia, and common variable immunodeficiency (Table 13–1). In addition, IgE concentrations were depressed in patients with X-linked immunodeficiency with hyper-IgM and ataxia-telangiectasia. Because there are multiple host deficits in these immunodeficiencies (see Chapters 9, 10, 11, 12, and 14), it is impossible to assign a role for IgE deficiency in these patients' increased susceptibility to infection.

IgE Deficiency, Repeated Infections, and Absence of Eosinophils and Basophils

Juhlin and Michaelson (1977) reported a man in whom eosinophils and basophils were absent in the bone marrow, blood, expectorates, and skin exudates. Mast cells were present in both the bone marrow and skin biopsy specimens. He had a lifelong history of repeated otitis, sinusitis, and pneumonia. As an adult, he had numerous warts, a chronic scabies infestation, and an episode of *Salmonella* gastroenteritis. The serum IgE level was lower than 1 IU/ml and the serum IgA level was low (30 to 50 mg/dl). Because chemotactic

Table 13–1. Serum IgE Concentrations in Patients with Immunodeficiency

Group	Number	Ages	Range (U/ml)	Geometric Mean	P Value (t Test)	Median	P Value (Mann-Whitney)
1. Transient hypogammaglobulinemia	8	(3–20 months)	(2–31)	6	0.05	5	0.0269
2. Severe combined immunodeficiency	9	(3–17 months)	(<1–82)	2	<0.0001	2	0.0018
3. X-linked agammaglobulinemia	10	(3–16 years)	(<1–5)	2	<0.0001	1	<0.0001
4. Non–X-linked agammaglobulinemia	15	(6–35 years)	(1–10)	3	<0.0001	3	<0.0001
5. X-linked immunodeficiency with hyper-IgM	3	(7 months–2 years)	(<1–2)	1	<0.0001	1	0.0016
6. Selective IgA deficiency	74	(5 months–50 years)	(3–3,800)	124	<0.0001	174	0.0001
7. Ataxia-telangiectasia	7	(5–14 years)	(<1–54)	7	<0.0001	10	0.0005
8. Nezelof syndrome	3	(8 months–3 years)	(5–7,000)	55	NS	5	NS
9. Wiskott-Aldrich syndrome	4	(8 months–12 years)	(135–720)	381	<0.0001	487	0.0020
10. Extreme hyperimmunoglobulinemia E	11	(3–31 years)	(2,150–40,000)	11,305	<0.0001	12,362	<0.0001
11. Other variable immunodeficiency	6	(1–14 years)	(11–2,880)	142	NS	70	NS
12. Chronic granulomatous disease	10	(6 months–17 years)	(<1–3,160)	88	NS	100	NS
13. Normal infants	12	(2–19 months)	(3–81)	18 (1–222)*	—	25	—
14. Normal children and adults	106	(2–55 years)	(2–549)	55 (5–621)*	—	55	—

*Confidence interval, 95%.

From Buckley RH, Fiscus SA. Serum IgD and IgE concentrations in immunodeficiency disease. Reproduced from J Clin Invest 55:157–165, 1975. Copyright permission of The American Society for Clinical Investigation.

factors for eosinophils are elaborated as a result of IgE antibody-antigen reactions on the surfaces of either mast cells or basophils, the patient's apparent lack of eosinophils may have been related to his IgE deficiency or his basophil deficiency. The combined deficits present, however, preclude knowing the contribution of the IgE deficiency to his susceptibility to infection.

Diagnosis, Treatment, and Prognosis

Because there are no known characteristic features of selective IgE deficiency, the diagnosis is rarely suspected clinically. It is confirmed by finding low serum IgE levels in the presence of normal levels of other immunoglobulin classes. There is no treatment for IgE deficiency because the rapid catabolic rate of IgE (half-life, 2.7 days) (Iio et al., 1977) and the likelihood of bestowing allergic disease on the recipient make attempts at replacement both futile and risky. The prognosis of IgE deficiency is unknown.

DISORDERS CHARACTERIZED BY EXCESSIVE IgE PRODUCTION

As with IgE deficiency, the definition of excessive IgE production varies from laboratory to laboratory (for reasons outlined earlier). In the author's laboratory, abnormally high IgE concentrations are those greater than 74 IU/ml for infants up to age 2 years and greater than 269 IU/ml for children and adults.

Historical Aspects

The regular association of increased serum IgE concentrations with a particular immunodeficiency disorder was first noted in patients with Wiskott-Aldrich syndrome (Berglund et al., 1968; Waldmann et al., 1972). Later, Buckley and associates (1972) described two adolescent boys with a lifelong history of severe recurrent staphylococcal abscesses involving the skin, lungs, and joints who had exceptionally high serum IgE concentrations but normal concentrations of the other immunoglobulins. Since then, an elevated serum IgE level has been found to be associated with several other genetically determined immunodeficiency diseases.

Pathogenic Mechanisms

The manner in which excessive IgE antibody production can adversely affect host defense is not known. Hill and Quie (1974) postulated that histamine released from basophils or mast cells following IgE antibody-antigen reactions interacts with H_2 receptors on leukocytes to increase intracellular cyclic $3'5'$-adenosine monophosphate (cAMP), resulting in an overall anti-inflammatory effect. In support of their postulate, they reported that histamine in concentrations of 10^{-3} and 10^{-5} M caused significant inhibition of polymorphonuclear chemotactic responsiveness. This finding could not be confirmed by Snyderman and colleagues (1977),

nor could they find inhibition of monocyte chemotaxis by histamine at concentrations ranging from 10^{-3} to 10^{-8} M. Soderberg-Warner and coworkers (1983) noted enhancement of polymorphonuclear chemotaxis by histamine and cimetidine in one patient and depression in the other.

A more attractive hypothesis is that both the infection susceptibility and the augmented IgE production are due to an underlying immunodeficiency involving T cells. Important observations bearing on this point were made by Okumura and Tada (1971), when they demonstrated enhancement of ongoing IgE antibody production in the rat by adult thymectomy and splenectomy. These studies suggested that although T-helper cells are required for the initiation of IgE synthesis, the process is also regulated by T cells or their products.

Studies in mice and humans have demonstrated that two such T-cell products can cause virgin B cells to isotype-switch for IgE production. The first discovered was interleukin-4 (IL-4) (Paul and O'Hara, 1987). This T-cell–derived lymphokine, initially named *B-cell stimulatory factor 1* (BSF-1), was reported by Coffman and Carty in 1986 to induce murine lipopolysaccharide (LPS)-activated B cells to secrete not only large amounts of IgG1 but also 100-fold more IgE. This effect of IL-4 was later shown to occur through the induction of heavy-chain isotype-switching in virgin B lymphocytes (Bergstedt-Lindqvist et al., 1988). In addition to stimulating IgE production, IL-4 has a wide variety of other in vitro activities, including up-regulation of expression of cell surface major histocompatibility complex (MHC) class II molecules and CD23, the low affinity IgE receptor, and promotion of the growth of T, B, and mast cells (Paul and O'Hara, 1987).

In early studies of Coffman and Carty (1986), the effects of IL-4 on murine IgE synthesis in vitro were found to be inhibited by the addition of another T-cell lymphokine, interferon-γ (IFN-γ). Subsequently, IFN-γ, IFN-α, and prostaglandin E_2 (PGE$_2$) were all shown by Pene et al. (1988) to inhibit IL-4–induced human IgE synthesis in vitro. In an effort to identify the cellular sources of these various cytokines, Mosmann and Coffman (1989) examined the types of cytokines produced by cloned murine T-helper (T$_H$) cells. They were able to identify two patterns of cytokine production that distinguished some clones from others and named the two types T$_H$1 and T$_H$2 cells. T$_H$1 clones produced IL-2 and IFN-γ, whereas T$_H$2 clones produced IL-4 and IL-5; both types produced some cytokines, such as IL-3. They postulated that the production of IgE is controlled by these two types of T-helper cells (Fig. 13–1). This led to speculation that excessive IgE production might be due to a predominance of T$_H$2-type cells.

Another cytokine, IL-13, also causes virgin B cells to isotype-switch for IgE production, independent of IL-4 (De Vries et al., 1993; Punonnen et al., 1993; McKenzie et al., 1993). IL-13 has many of the functional properties of IL-4, and their receptors share a common component (Aversa et al., 1993). Unlike IL-4, however, IL-13 does not cause T cells to proliferate. IL-4 is pro-

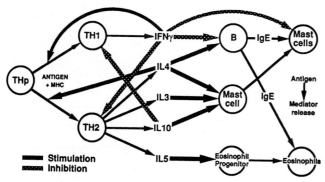

Figure 13–1. Two types of helper T cells. These are distinguished by their cytokine profiles and by their postulated roles in the regulation of IgE synthesis. (From Mosmann TR, Coffman RL. T$_H$1 and T$_H$2 cells: different patterns of lymphokine secretion lead to different functional properties. Annu Rev Immunol 7:145, 1989. Reproduced with permission of Annual Reviews, Inc.)

duced only by T$_H$2 cells; IL-13 is produced by T$_H$0, T$_H$1, and T$_H$2 cells. Prior to isotype-switching, both IL-4 and IL-13 induce germline epsilon (ϵ) chain transcripts in human blood B cells; however, both cytokines require second signals to effect productive immunoglobulin gene rearrangements. These can be provided by the CD40 ligand on activated T cells (Pene et al., 1988; Claassen et al., 1990b; Spriggs et al., 1993), by the Epstein-Barr virus (EBV) interacting with CD21 (Thyphronitis et al., 1989), by hydrocortisone or other corticosteroids (Wu et al., 1991), or by a monoclonal antibody to CD40 (Zhang et al. 1991; Gascan et al., 1991).

The relative importance of these two cytokines in regulating IgE production in humans is as yet unknown, although in vitro studies suggest that IL-13 does not stimulate as much IgE production as does IL-4. Patients with partial T-cell deficiencies may have an increase in T$_H$2-type cells or cytokines for the initiation of IgE antibody formation and a deficiency of T$_H$1-type cells or cytokines, resulting in augmented IgE biosynthesis.

IgE Excess in Primary Immunodeficiency Disorders

In the studies cited earlier (Buckley and Fiscus, 1975), IgE levels were significantly elevated in patients with the Wiskott-Aldrich and Nezelof syndromes, selective IgA deficiency, and the hyper-IgE syndrome (see Table 13–1). In one patient with common variable immunodeficiency, the IgE concentration was also elevated; in all other agammaglobulinemic patients studied, concentrations of IgE were low. In a study of the metabolism of IgE in patients with primary immunodeficiencies, Iio and coworkers (1977) found that IgE levels generally correlated with the IgE synthetic rate and that abnormalities in the catabolic rate did not exert an important effect.

Except for patients with selective IgA deficiency and the single patient with common variable immunodeficiency, all immunodeficiency patients with excessive IgE production have had impaired but not absent cell-mediated immunity (Waldmann et al., 1972; Polmar et

al., 1972a, b; Kikkawa et al., 1973; Buckley and Fiscus, 1975; de Saint-Basile et al., 1991; Schandene et al., 1993). The other characteristic shared by many patients with immunodeficiency who have elevated IgE levels is their tendency to be infected by staphylococcal organisms, raising the question of whether staphylococcal infections stimulate excessive IgE production. Against this possibility is the fact that most patients with chronic granulomatous disease or with cystic fibrosis have normal serum IgE concentrations, despite chronic staphylococcal infections (see Table 13–1); (Buckley and Fiscus, 1975).

Wiskott-Aldrich Syndrome

Characterized by undue susceptibility to infection, dermatitis, and megakaryocytic thrombocytopenic purpura, Wiskott-Aldrich syndrome has been discussed in detail (see Chapter 12). Patients with the Wiskott-Aldrich syndrome consistently have a pruritic eczematoid dermatitis indistinguishable from that of classic atopic eczema except for purpuric lesions often present at sites of excoriation (Fig. 13–2). In keeping with this, serum IgE concentrations are usually elevated (Table 13–1), (Berglund et al., 1968; Waldmann et al., 1972; Buckley and Fiscus, 1975), and immediate skin tests with inhalant and food allergens frequently yield positive results (Huntley and Dees, 1957). Paradoxically, circulating B cells and EBV-transformed B-cell lines from Wiskott-Aldrich syndrome patients were reported by Simon and associates (1993) to have low expression of CD23, the low affinity IgE receptor. This was shown, however, to be the result of post-transcriptional events because messenger RNA (mRNA) for CD23 was increased or normal in these cells. These patients consistently have impaired humoral immune responses to polysaccharide antigens and depressed but not absent T-cell function. In addition to these and other abnormalities already recognized (see Chapter 12), Molina

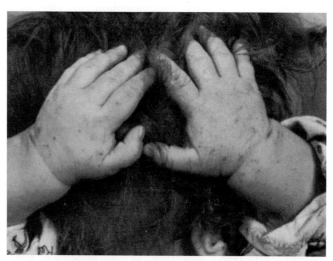

Figure 13–2. Pruritic eczematoid dermatitis over the dorsum of hands of a patient with Wiskott-Aldrich syndrome. Scattered petechiae are seen at sites of excoriation. (From Buckley RH. Allergic eczema. In Kelley's Practice of Pediatrics, Vol. 2. Hagerstown, Md., Harper & Row, 1987, pp 1–29.)

and associates (1993) reported a restricted defect of Wiskott-Aldrich T-cell lines to proliferate in response to immobilized anti-CD3.

Thymic Hypoplasia (DiGeorge Anomaly)

Thymic hypoplasia (third and fourth pharyngeal pouch syndrome) (see Chapter 12), has also been associated with augmented IgE production. Polmar and colleagues (1972b) reported a consistently elevated serum IgE concentration in an infant with DiGeorge anomaly, and the author has observed this in another such patient, who also had eosinophilia and an erythematous, scaly, and pruritic skin rash. Allergic signs or symptoms, however, are not common in these infants. The fact that some (Polmar et al., 1972b) but not all of these infants have had elevated serum IgE concentrations may be related to the degree of thymic hypoplasia. Those with "complete" DiGeorge anomaly may not have sufficient T-helper cell function to initiate IgE antibody formation. On the other hand, those with the more common "partial" form (Lischner and Huff, 1975) who have some (but depressed) T-cell function would be more likely to have increased IgE production because they may have sufficient T_H2-type cells or cytokines but a deficiency of T_H1-type cells or cytokines.

Cellular Immunodeficiency with Immunoglobulins (Nezelof Syndrome)

This thymic dysplasia syndrome, first described by Nezelof (1968), is characterized by a cellular immunodeficiency similar to that seen in severe combined immunodeficiency (SCID) syndromes but clinically less severe. Unlike patients with SCID, those with Nezelof's syndrome usually have normal or elevated serum immunoglobulin levels (see Chapter 12). Greatly elevated concentrations of serum IgE have been described in some but not all of these patients (Kikkawa et al., 1973; Buckley and Fiscus, 1975; Buckley et al., 1986), but allergy has not been a consistent finding. Again, the tendency to augmented IgE production may be related to the degree of thymic dysfunction, with the most severe being incapable of producing IgE.

Omenn Syndrome (Combined Immunodeficiency with Hypereosinophilia)

There has been great interest in the possible role of IgE dysregulation in the profound infection-susceptibility of infants with Omenn's syndrome of combined immunodeficiency with hypereosinophilia (de Saint-Basile et al., 1991; Schandene et al., 1993; Melamed et al., 1994) (see Chapters 12, 15, and 19). This is an autosomal recessive inherited fatal condition characterized by T-cell infiltration of the skin, gut, liver, and spleen, leading to an exfoliative erythroderma, lymphadenopathy, hepatosplenomegaly, and intractable diarrhea (de Saint-Basile et al., 1991). Infants so affected have a persistent leukocytosis with marked eosinophilia; elevated serum IgE level; low IgG, IgA, and IgM

concentrations; and impaired T-cell function because of restricted heterogeneity of the host T-cell repertoire (de Saint-Basile et al., 1991).

A T_H2-like cell dominance has been documented in a patient with Omenn syndrome studied by Schandene and associates (1993); that infant was reportedly treated successfully with IFN-γ. In another such patient, Melamed and colleagues (1994) found a clonally expanded V-β14$^+$ CD3$^+$CD4$^-$CD8$^-$ (double-negative) T-cell population that spontaneously secreted high levels of IL-5 but had low expression of both IL-4 and IFN-γ mRNA.

Selective IgA Deficiency

Selective IgA deficiency (see Chapter 14) is the fifth well-defined primary immunodeficiency disorder in which elevated serum IgE concentrations have been noted (Schwartz and Buckley, 1971; Buckley and Fiscus, 1975). In keeping with this, a high frequency of atopy (55%) was noted in a group of 75 IgA-deficient patients (Buckley, 1975). One should exercise caution in concluding that either allergy or augmented IgE production is a feature of all patients with selective IgA deficiency, however, because these patients were discovered in an allergy clinic. This same reservation should be held about the reported increased incidence of autoimmune and collagen-vascular diseases noted in other series because in the former cases most were discovered in rheumatology clinics (Huntley et al., 1967; Ammann and Hong, 1971).

Possibly related to their propensity to elevated IgE and allergic disorders is the tendency of IgA-deficient patients to have severe or fatal anaphylactic reactions when given blood products containing IgA (Vyas et al., 1968; Vyas and Fudenberg, 1974; Burks et al., 1986). These reactions most likely result from the presence of class-specific IgE antibodies to IgA in these patients (Burks et al., 1986).

The predominant distribution of both IgA-containing and IgE-containing plasma cells is in the paragut and pararespiratory lymphoid tissues (Tada and Ishizaka, 1970). Because IgA antibodies limit mucosal permeability to dietary or inhaled antigens, it is possible that their absence permits greater stimulation of IgE antibody formation, just as it permits the stimulation of IgG antibody to such antigens (Buckley and Dees, 1969). Alternatively, as with the other immunodeficiency states, the augmented IgE production in IgA-deficient patients may result from either a deficiency of T_H1-type cells or cytokines, such as IFN-γ, important in downregulating IL-4–induced IgE production, or from an excess of T_H2-type cells or cytokines, leading to excessive IgE production. In support of the first possibility, Epstein and Ammann (1974) reported impaired IFN-γ production by phytohemagglutinin (PHA)-stimulated lymphocytes from patients with selective IgA deficiency.

THE HYPER-IgE SYNDROME

The hyper-IgE syndrome is a primary immunodeficiency characterized by recurrent staphylococcal abscesses and markedly elevated serum IgE concentrations. These patients have a lifelong history of severe recurrent staphylococcal abscesses involving the skin, lungs, joints, and other sites. In addition, there is a unique tendency to form persistent pneumatoceles following staphylococcal pneumonias. Although there usually is a history of pruritic dermatitis, it is not typical atopic dermatitis, and respiratory allergic symptoms are usually absent.

Laboratory features include the following:

- Exceptionally high serum IgE concentrations (2,150 to 40,000 IU/ml)
- Near-normal serum IgG, IgA, and IgM concentrations
- Elevated IgD concentrations (Josephs and Buckley, 1979)
- Pronounced blood and sputum eosinophilia
- Poor anamnestic antibody responses to booster immunizations (Buckley et al., 1972; Leung et al., 1988; Sheerin and Buckley, 1991)
- Poor antibody and cell-mediated responses to neoantigens (Buckley and Sampson, 1981; Sheerin and Buckley, 1991)
- Decreased mixed leukocyte culture (MLC) responsiveness to genetically disparate family members (Buckley and Sampson, 1981)
- The occasional presence of temporally variable granulocyte chemotactic defects

Historical Aspects

Since the first two patients with the hyper-IgE syndrome were reported by Buckley and associates in 1972, the author has evaluated more than 30 additional patients (Buckley and Sampson, 1981; Sheerin and Buckley, 1991; Claassen et al., 1991). Patients with this syndrome have also been reported from other centers (Clark et al., 1973; Hill et al., 1974; Van Scoy et al., 1975; Church et al., 1976; Blum et al., 1977; Weston et al., 1977; Donabedian and Gallin, 1983; Soderberg-Warner et al., 1983; Geha and Leung, 1989).

Clinical Manifestations

Some general features of 22 of our patients with the hyper-IgE syndrome are listed in Table 13–2. They ranged in age from 2 to 31 years; 15 were male, 7 were female, 8 were black, and 14 were white. They came from a wide geographic area. The hyper-IgE syndrome is a rare disorder, and these are not merely individuals with atopic eczema who have repeated superficial infections of their skin lesions. These patients invariably have recurrent, severe bouts of furunculosis and pneumonia secondary to *Staphylococcus aureus* from early infancy, some from day 1 of life, and in all but one, persistent pneumatoceles developed as a result of recurrent pneumonias (Merten et al., 1979) (Fig. 13–3). Nine patients required thoracic surgery because of giant persistent pneumatoceles that became chronically infected; two underwent complete pneumonectomies, five had lobectomies because of lung abscesses, one had an empyema, and one had an anterior mediastinal *Candida* granuloma.

As shown in Table 13–3, all patients were plagued by infections with *S. aureus*, but some also had recurrent *Haemophilus influenzae*, pneumococcal, group A streptococcal, gram-negative, and fungal infections. The sites of infection are listed in Table 13–4. Infections of the skin and lungs predominated, but the ears, eyes, oral mucosa, sinuses, joints, blood, and even viscera were also involved. A peculiar tendency of the abscesses to localize about the scalp, face, and neck was observed

Table 13–2. General Features of 22 Patients with Hyper-IgE Syndrome

Patient	Age	Sex	Race	Age at First Infection	Dermatitis	Asthma	IgE (IU/ml)
1	14	M	W	6 weeks	+	−	22,300
2	14	M	W	Newborn	+	−	6,600
3	16	M	B	Newborn	+	−	40,000
4	13	M	W	18 months	+	−	6,400
5	11	M	W	Newborn	+	−	9,000
6	6	M	W	Infancy	+	−	5,000
7	12	M	B	10 months	+	−	22,000
8	2	M	W	1 day	+	−	11,600
9	17	M	W	Infancy	+	−	46,000
10	12	M	W	Infancy	+	+	26,500
11	31	F	B	Infancy	+	+	15,600
12	11	F	W	1 months	+	−	38,400
13	7	F	B	Newborn	+	−	25,600
14	13	F	B	Infancy	+	−	2,150
15	3	M	B	4 months	+	−	2,788
16	22	M	W	Infancy	+	−	12,362
17	2	F	W	Infancy	+	−	5,000
18	10	F	B	Infancy	+	−	51,200
19	7	M	W	1 day	+	−	33,000
20	5	F	B	3 weeks	+	−	24,000
21	7	M	W	6 months	+	+	39,500
22	5	M	W	2 weeks	+	−	5,800

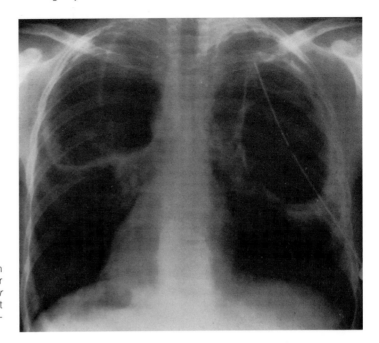

Figure 13–3. Chest roentgenogram of 12-year-old boy with hyper-IgE syndrome. Giant pneumatoceles were present for more than 1 year. A putrid abscess caused by *Enterobacter cloacae* led to chest tube insertion on the right. The left cyst necessitated emergency excision because of massive hemoptysis and was found to contain an aspergilloma.

in infants and younger children. Sites that were not foci of infections included the urinary and gastrointestinal tracts and the bones (except for mastoids). Cryptococcal meningitis was observed in three patients, but bacterial meningitis was not seen.

All 22 patients had either dermatitis at the time of evaluation or, more often, a history of pruritic dermatitis earlier in life. Although the lesions resembled those of an eczematoid dermatitis with lichenified skin, the distribution and characteristics of the lesions were not typical of atopic eczema. No patients had histories of allergic rhinitis, and only three were noted to wheeze; even in these, the wheezing was not a prominent symptom. Two patients without a history of wheezing were given methacholine inhalation challenges without a significant drop in pulmonary function. Thus, there was minimal evidence of respiratory allergy in these patients. None had evidence of parasitic infestation.

Several patients were growth-retarded, mainly those with chronic lower respiratory tract disease, and all but one had coarse facial features (Figs. 13–4 and 13–5). There were no red-haired, fair-skinned females among these 22 patients; red hair and fair skin were physical

features mentioned by Davis and colleagues (1966) in describing two girls with *Job's syndrome* (see Chapter 15). These two patients were also described as having "cold," nontender abscesses. Most abscesses in our patients were tender and warm although many of the patients, despite having large deep-seated abscesses, had minimal systemic toxicity. Job's syndrome was described prior to the discovery of IgE. Although serum IgE concentrations were later found by Hill and co-workers (1974) to be elevated in the two original patients and in two more, it is unclear, from the limited clinical and immunologic data given in these four cases, how Job's syndrome relates to the hyper-IgE syndrome.

Although some features of hyper-IgE patients resemble those present in chronic granulomatous disease (CGD), there are several distinguishing clinical features (see Chapter 15). Unlike CGD patients, hyper-IgE pa-

Table 13–3. Organisms Associated with Infection in 22 Patients With Hyper-IgE Syndrome

Organism	No. of Patients Affected
Staphylococcus aureus, coagulase-positive	22/22
Candida albicans	12/22
Haemophilus influenzae	7/22
Pneumococci	6/22
Streptococci, group A	4/22
Miscellaneous gram-negative organisms	5/22
Aspergillus species	3/22
Trichophyton species	1/22

Table 13–4. Sites of Infections in 22 Patients With Hyper-IgE Syndrome

Site	No. of Patients Affected
Skin	22/22
Abscesses	22/22
Deep cellulitis	3/22
Lung	22/22
Pneumatoceles	21/22
Resection of lobes	5/22
Total pneumonectomy	2/22
Ears	15/22
Mastoidectomy	2/22
Oral mucosa	8/22
Sinuses	9/22
Eyes	10/22
Joints	4/22
Viscera	3/22
Blood	3/22

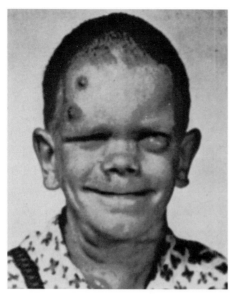

Figure 13–4. Patient with hyper-IgE syndrome showing multiple abscesses of the face and neck and coarse facial features. (From Buckley RH, Wray BB, Belmaker EZ. Extreme hyperimmunoglobulinemia E and undue susceptibility to infection. Pediatrics 49:59–70, 1972. Reproduced with permission from Bristol Laboratories.)

tients may have infections with catalase-negative organisms, such as streptococci and pneumococci. Further, although patients with CGD may also have staphylococcal pneumonias, they rarely have persistent

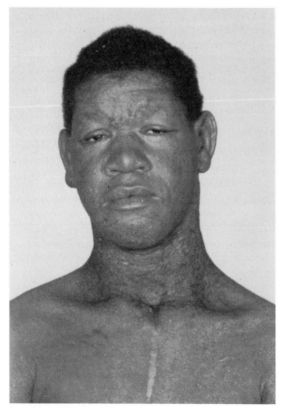

Figure 13–5. Patient with hyper-IgE syndrome, again illustrating coarse facial features. Scar over upper chest is from excision of a *Candida* granuloma of the mediastinum.

pneumatoceles such as those that occur in hyper-IgE patients (Merten et al., 1979). Finally, unlike CGD patients, hyper-IgE syndrome patients rarely have osteomyelitis, urinary tract infections, diarrhea, or intestinal obstruction.

Unexplained osteopenia is present in most patients with the hyper-IgE syndrome, many of whom have problems with recurrent fractures (Kirchner et al., 1985). This problem, which is not correlated with the patient's state of activity or accompanied by any detectable abnormalities in calcium or phosphorus metabolism, was so severe in one of the author's patients that collapses of most vertebral bodies occurred (Buckley et al., 1972). Leung and coworkers (1988) noted that monocytes from hyper-IgE patients were activated to resorb bone in response to the spontaneous release of prostaglandin E_2 (PGE$_2$).

Eight instances of familial occurrence of the hyper-IgE syndrome were noted among the above 22 patients, and there were several additional familial reports (Van Scoy et al., 1975; Blum et al., 1977). The fact that both males and females were affected, as were members of succeeding generations, suggests an autosomal dominant with incomplete penetrance form of inheritance. A summary of the clinical features is presented in Table 13–5.

Laboratory Findings

Hematologic Studies

Eosinophilia of blood and sputum has been a consistent finding in all of our patients. Peripheral eosinophilia as high as 55% to 60% may occur in some infants. In most patients, both the percentage and the absolute number of eosinophils exceeded those seen in the average atopic patient. Total white blood cell counts ranged from normal to markedly elevated (50,000 to 60,000/mm³), but no patients were neutropenic or lymphopenic. Anemia was not uncommon in those with chronic lower respiratory infections but was not present when infection was controlled.

Table 13–5. Major Clinical Features of 22 Patients with Hyper-IgE Syndrome

1. Severe infections of the skin and lower respiratory tract from infancy. All have had *furunculosis*, staphylococcal *pneumonia*, *pneumatoceles*, and over half have required lung surgery. Most have also had infections of ears, sinuses, eyes, and oral mucosa. Fewer have had infections of joints, viscera, or blood.
2. *Staphylococcus aureus*, coagulase-positive, has caused infections in all. *Candida albicans*, *Haemophilus influenzae*, pneumococci and streptococci, group A isolated in from 50 to 25%; miscellaneous gram-negative rods and other fungi in some.
3. Pruritic dermatitis chronically or (more often) in past; little or no respiratory allergy. Rash is *not* typical atopic eczema.
4. Both sexes affected (males, 15; females, 7); 14 were white, 8 were black.
5. Familial occurrence is 8 of 22 families studied; IgE normal in nonaffected relatives. Pattern in families suggests autosomal dominant trait with incomplete penetrance. No increased frequency of any HLA-A or HLA-B locus antigens.

Humoral Immunity

Investigations of humoral immunity consistently showed serum IgE concentrations to be exceedingly high, ranging from 3 to 82 times above the upper limit of normal for our laboratory (see Table 13–2). In addition, serum IgD levels were elevated in a majority, with 14 of 22 patients having values higher than 10 mg/dl and some having levels of 50 to 159 mg/dl (Josephs and Buckley, 1979). Serum concentrations of one or more of the other three immunoglobulin isotypes were also elevated in some patients, but more often they were normal. Serum IgE concentrations were measured in first-degree relatives of nine patients, and all the values were normal.

Poor anamnestic antibody responses to diphtheria and tetanus were noted in the first two patients (Buckley et al., 1972), and they failed to respond to the neoantigen KLH. To investigate further whether an underlying antibody deficiency could account for the infection susceptibility of these patients, Sheerin and Buckley (1991) evaluated 11 additional patients with the hyper-IgE syndrome for their responses to bacteriophage ϕX174, diphtheria and tetanus toxoids, and pneumococcal (Pneumovax) and *H. influenzae* vaccines. Three of nine patients immunized with ϕX174 had normal primary and secondary antibody responses, five had accelerated declines in their titers (after initially normal primary antibody responses) and lower than normal secondary antibody responses, and two of the latter patients did not show normal switching from IgM to IgG antibody production (Table 13–6). Only one of ten tested had normal responses to diphtheria toxoid, and postimmunization antitetanus titers were abnormally low in five of the ten patients tested. Serum antibodies to *H. influenzae* polyribose phosphate were protective in seven of the eight immunized patients. Five of the nine who were given Pneumovax immunizations had poor antibody responses to at least one of the serotypes 7, 9, or 14; all patients responded with protective antibody titers to type 3. Abnormal polysac-

charide antibody responses did not correlate with IgG2 levels.

This heterogeneity in their antibody-forming capacities suggests that antibody deficiency may contribute to the infection susceptibility of some hyper-IgE syndrome patients. Serum antibodies to staphylococcal and *Candida* organisms were detected in the serum of one of the first two patients evaluated (Buckley et al., 1972). Dreskin and colleagues (1985) found normal quantities of IgG and elevated IgM antibodies but a deficiency of IgA antibodies to *S. aureus* in 10 patients with the hyper-IgE syndrome. The titer of IgA anti–*S. aureus* present correlated inversely with the incidence of infection at mucosal surfaces and in adjacent lymph nodes, suggesting a role for a deficient IgA response in their infection susceptibility.

In keeping with their markedly elevated total serum IgE concentrations, our patients all had strongly positive immediate wheal-and-flare responses to a number of inhalant, food, and pollen allergens as well as to *Candida*, staphylococcal, and other bacterial and fungal antigens (Buckley and Sampson, 1981). Schopfer and associates (1979) and Dreskin and coworkers (1985) reported high titers of IgE antibodies to *S. aureus* antigens in hyper-IgE syndrome patients and proposed that such antibodies may have a pathogenic role in their special susceptibility to staphylococci. However, similar antibodies were found in patients with eczema and other atopic diseases who were not susceptible to abscess formation (Walsh et al., 1981; Motala et al., 1986). Moreover, Schmitt and Ballet (1983) and Berger and colleagues (1980) found high titers of IgE antibodies to tetanus and *Candida* antigens in patients with the hyper-IgE syndrome, suggesting that such antibodies are a consequence of their abnormal IgE regulation. IgE isolated from the serum of one of our first two patients contained both kappa (κ) and lambda (λ) chains, excluding the possibility that the IgE was monoclonal.

Cellular Immunity

Although delayed cutaneous anergy to ubiquitous antigens, such as *Candida* and streptokinase-streptodornase, was found in the first two patients described (Buckley et al., 1972), this was a feature in only 50% of the patients. Blood lymphocytes from hyper-IgE patients were reported by Geha and associates (1981) to be deficient in CD8$^+$ T cells. However, our studies and other reports have revealed normal percentages of CD3$^+$, CD4$^+$, and CD8$^+$ lymphocytes and IgE-bearing B lymphocytes (Fig. 13–6). Buckley and coworkers (1991) have found a deficiency of CD3$^+$ T cells bearing the CD45RO isoform (memory T-cell phenotype) in all eight patients with the hyper-IgE syndrome studied. In mice, Luqman and colleagues (1991) have shown this isoform to be present on T$_H$1 but not on T$_H$2 cells. Whether these observations are relevant to these patients' abnormal anamnestic humoral and cellular responses or excessive IgE production is unknown.

In vitro studies of lymphoproliferative responses to the mitogens PHA, concanavalin A (Con A), and pokeweed mitogen (PWM) have been normal in most pa-

Table 13–6. Primary and Secondary Antibody Responses to ϕX174 in the Hyper-IgE Syndrome

Patient No.	Peak Response (kV)		% IgG
	Primary	*Secondary*	
1	9.87*	**79.3**†	**17**
2	6.86*	**6.5**	**1**
3	197	651.0	30†
4	8.70*	**159.0**	39
6	—§	1533.0	68
7	19.80	153.0	93
8	10.00*	**9.9**	68
9	57.00*	**50.5**	53
11	480.00	—	—

*kV normal at 1 week and then decreased.
†Abnormal values are in **boldface**.
‡Borderline.
§Data not available.
From Sheerin KA, Buckley RH. Antibody responses to protein, polysaccharide, and ϕX174 antigens in the hyperimmunoglobulinemia E (hyper-IgE) syndrome. J Allergy Clin Immunol 87:803–811, 1991.

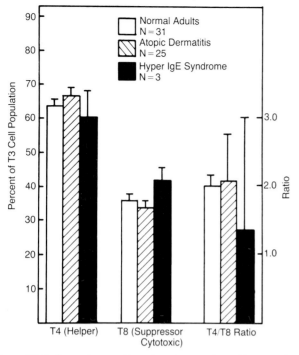

Figure 13–6. Percentages of lymphocytes reacting with monoclonal antibodies to T-cell surface antigens in patients with atopic dermatitis and with the hyper-IgE syndrome compared with normal controls. No differences were found between the three groups.

tients with the hyper-IgE syndrome. By contrast, lymphoproliferative responses to the antigens *Candida albicans* and tetanus toxoid have been absent or low. Because antigen-induced proliferation of blood lymphocytes is primarily a T-cell response, mixed leukocyte culture (MLC) studies were conducted in nine patients. Six of nine patients' T lymphocytes did not show proliferation in MLCs containing mononuclear cells (MNCs) from one or more genetically different family members. By contrast, T lymphocytes from five of the six patients who were unresponsive in intrafamilial MLC reactions proliferated vigorously when stimulated by unrelated subjects' MNCs. HLA-A and HLA-B locus typing done on nine of our patients and their first-degree relatives revealed no unusual antigens or antigen frequencies (Buckley and Sampson, 1981).

Regulatory T-Cell Studies

Because of the apparent abnormal regulation of IgE synthesis in such patients, we and others have searched for a regulatory T-cell defect. The inability of PWM and other polyclonal B-cell activators, such as *Staphylococcus Cowan 1* organisms to stimulate the production of IgE by human blood B cells in vitro severely limited studies of human IgE regulation for more than a decade (Claassen et al., 1990a, 1990b, 1992). Research on the control of human IgE production has been greatly advanced by the demonstration that both recombinant human IL-4 and IL-13 induce blood B cells to produce nanogram quantities of IgE when an effective second signal is provided (see earlier). During our initial studies of IL-4–induced human IgE synthesis, however, we found that a wide range of recombinant human IL-4 concentrations did not increase MNC IgE synthesis over baseline when cultured in tissue culture medium RPMI 1640 (Claassen et al., 1990a, 1990b, 1992).

We did observe that Iscove's modified Dulbecco's medium (containing human transferrin, bovine insulin, serum albumin, oleic, palmitic, and linoleic acids, and 10% fetal calf serum) supported the synthesis of nanogram quantities of IgE induced by small concentrations (2.5 to 5 ng/ml) of IL-4 (Claassen et al., 1990a, 1990b), thus providing a reproducibly positive in vitro system for assessing human IgE synthesis. Using this system, we found that B cells from hyper-IgE patients were relatively refractory to stimulation with IL-4 in vitro (Table 13–7); this suggested that they may have already been stimulated with excessive endogenous IL-4 in vivo (Claassen et al., 1991). It has been difficult to prove, however, that patients with the hyper-IgE syndrome produce excessive IL-4, because IL-4 cannot be measured in body fluids as a result of its short half-life.

Del Prete and associates (1989) reported defective IFN-γ and tumor necrosis factor–α (TNF-α) production by T cells from four patients with the hyper-IgE syndrome stimulated with mitogens in vitro. Paganelli and coworkers (1991) reported severely reduced or undetectable IFN-γ in supernatants of MNCs from five hyper-IgE patients after stimulation with mitogens or phorbol esters and calcium ionophores. Del Prete and colleagues (1989) found that the precursor frequency of T cells able to produce IFN-γ and TNF-α is markedly

Table 13–7. IL-4–Induced IgE Synthesis by Unfractionated MNC, T-Cell–Enriched and B-Cell–Enriched Subpopulations, and Recombinations in Hyper-IgE Syndrome, Atopic Eczema, and Normal Subjects*

Cells	Medium			IL-4 (10 ng/ml)		
	Hyper-IgE	Atopic	Nonatopic	Hyper-IgE	Atopic	Nonatopic
MNC	1.3	0	0.14	8.5	73.1	78.9
B	0	0	0	1.8	22.2	18.9
T	0	0	0.2	0	0	1.6
B plus hyper-IgE T	1.5	2.5	0.11	5.1	15.5	51.1
B plus atopic T	2.0	0.67	0.95	4.3	84.3	12.4
B plus nonatopic T	0	0.57	0	4.0	53.1	89.3

*Data area nanograms per milliliter of IgE in culture supernatants; MNC = mononuclear cells; IL = interleukin.
From Claassen JL, Levine AD, Schiff SE, Buckley RH. Mononuclear cells from patients with the hyper-IgE syndrome produce little IgE when stimulated with recombinant interleukin 4 in vitro. J Allergy Clin Immunol 88:713–721, 1991.

reduced when compared with controls but that the precursor frequency of T cells producing IL-4 is normal. Neither Vercelli and associates (1990) nor our studies (unpublished) found deficient IFN-γ production by T cells in patients with hyper-IgE.

Thus, there is as yet no clearly defined T-cell abnormality in the hyper-IgE syndrome. If such a deficiency is found, it is likely to be one of T_H1 cells or cytokines. However, abnormal IgE regulation does not explain the infection susceptibility of these patients because equally high levels of IgE are found in many patients with atopic dermatitis who have no susceptibility to abscess formation (Fiser and Buckley, 1979; Sampson and Buckley, 1981).

Chemotactic Studies

The defective polymorphonuclear (PMN) chemotaxis reported in some cases of hyper-IgE syndrome was suggested to be the basis for the patients' infection susceptibility (Hill and Quie, 1974). Such chemotactic abnormalities, however, are highly variable and infrequent. Indeed, Rebuck skin window studies in our first two patients showed normal PMN influx. Fluids from sites of infection in these patients contained numerous PMNs, and a brisk PMN leukocytosis occurs in the presence of infection. Only three of nine of our patients showed consistent depression of either PMN or mononuclear chemotaxis (one of each type and one with both) (Buckley and Sampson, 1981). In most patients with defective chemotaxis, repeated studies were normal. We found no correlation among chemotactic defects, medications, or the presence or absence of infection. The inconstancy of PMN chemotactic defects in this syndrome makes it highly unlikely that they are the basis of the extreme infection susceptibility seen in these patients.

Complement and Phagocytic Studies

Serum hemolytic complement activity has been normal in all patients tested. Our first two patients had normal levels of all nine complement components. Their sera were capable of generating C5a chemotactic factor normally.

PMN phagocytosis, metabolism, and killing have been normal in our patients and in studies of others. Because the clinical history in the hyper-IgE syndrome resembles that in CGD, phagocytic functional studies are often among the first tests performed. The granulocytes have normal phagocytic mechanisms, bacterial killing, and oxidative metabolism; the normal oxidative metabolism is indicated by normal nitroblue tetrazolium dye reduction and chemiluminescence tests.

Histologic sections of lymph nodes, spleen, and lung cysts obtained at surgery often demonstrate a striking tissue eosinophilia. This was particularly notable in the spleen of a boy who underwent splenectomy following trauma and in the wall of a giant lung cyst excised from another patient (Buckley and Sampson, 1981). Thus, it is possible that eosinophils or their products, such as eosinophil major basic protein, play a role in

the observed tissue destruction leading to formation of pneumatoceles. Normal thymic architecture, including that of Hassall's corpuscles, was observed at the postmortem examination of one patient.

A summary of the major immunologic features of hyper-IgE cases is presented in Table 13–8.

Treatment

Because the primary defect in the hyper-IgE syndrome is unknown, no definitive therapy is available. The most successful treatment is lifelong, continuous antistaphylococcal antibiotic therapy to prevent staphylococcal infections (Buckley, 1983). If pneumatoceles persist for more than 6 months, surgical excision should be strongly considered because the cysts may enlarge and compress adjacent normal lung, become infected with other organisms, or predispose to fungus ball formation. Although cutaneous abscesses are unusual in patients receiving antistaphylococcal antibiotics regularly, their occurrence may necessitate incision and drainage.

Although immunostimulants (e.g., transfer factor, levamisole) had been used in some patients prior to their referral to our institution, none experienced any clinical benefit; indeed, deterioration sometimes occurred because of antibiotic discontinuance or delay of surgery. Levamisole was inferior to placebo in a controlled study in hyper-IgE patients (Donabedian et al., 1982).

Based on the observation by Coffman and Carty (1986) that IFN-γ inhibits murine IL-4–induced IgE synthesis and on confirmation of these findings in humans (Pene et al. 1988), King and colleagues (1989) administered recombinant human IFN-γ to five patients with the hyper-IgE syndrome in an open clinical trial in doses of 0.05 and 0.1 mg/M^2 three times weekly for 2 and 6 weeks, respectively. There was a decline in the serum IgE level in two of five patients on the higher dose. Although no adverse effects were noted, there was no obvious clinical benefit.

Prognosis

If the hyper-IgE syndrome is recognized early in life and the child is kept on chronic antistaphylococcal

Table 13–8. Major Immunologic Features of 22 Patients with Hyper-IgE Syndrome

1. Markedly elevated IgE levels; IgD levels also elevated in a majority; other immunoglobulins may be elevated but are usually normal.
2. Positive immediate wheal-and-flare responses to a variety of food, inhalant, bacterial, and fungal antigens.
3. Marked eosinophilia in blood and sputum.
4. Impaired anamnestic (IgG) antibody responses and poor responses to neoantigens.
5. Depressed cell-mediated immunity to ubiquitous antigens in vivo in half and to specific antigens in vitro in a majority. Responses to mitogens are normal, as are percentages of CD4 and CD8 lymphocyte subpopulations.
6. Abnormal intrafamilial mixed leukocyte responses.
7. Decreased proportion of CD45RO+ CD3+ T cells.
8. Highly variable chemotactic abnormalities (not present in most).
9. Impaired IgE production in response to IL-4 in vitro.

antibiotic therapy, the prognosis is good. Several patients have reached maturity, indicating that the defect is compatible with prolonged survival. If the diagnosis is delayed, chronically infected giant pneumatoceles may develop and lung infections with agents other than staphylococci, such as *H. influenzae, Candida,* and *Aspergillus,* may occur. Putrid pyogenic secondary infections may develop within persistent pneumatoceles, and aspergilloma formation with severe hemoptysis may occur. The latter can lead to sudden death. In one of our patients, Hodgkin's disease developed at age 19. In another patient, Burkitt's lymphoma developed at age 7 (Gorin et al., 1989); these are the only known cases of malignancy in this syndrome.

GRAFT-VERSUS-HOST DISEASE

Elevated serum IgE concentrations have been noted during graft-versus-host disease (GVHD) in patients receiving allogeneic bone marrow transplants (Saryan et al., 1983; Sindel et al., 1984; Abedi et al., 1989). T-cell (as well as B-cell) function is known to be depressed for varying periods of time post-transplantation; this is associated with T-cell subset imbalances. Following allogeneic bone marrow transplantation, there is often a prolonged period of immunodeficiency because of the development of GVHD—even after cells of erythroid and myeloid lineage are fully functional. During this period, patients may experience allergic reactions to antibiotics (Lakin et al., 1975) or dietary antigens (Sindel et al., 1984), even if they were not allergic prior to transplantation. These findings suggest that GVHD is accompanied by a deficiency of T cells and/or cytokines important in down-regulating IgE synthesis.

ACQUIRED IMMUNODEFICIENCY SYNDROME

Patients with the acquired immunodeficiency syndrome (AIDS) usually have polyclonal hyperimmunoglobulinemia and depressed T-cell function, and they often have IgE-mediated hypersensitivities to sulfamethoxazole and other drugs (Gordin et al., 1984). Soon after the discovery of AIDS, patients with AIDS were reported to have a high frequency of allergic reactions. Studies by Maggi and coworkers (1987) demonstrated that T-cell clones derived from residual CD4[+] blood T cells from stage IV AIDS patients exhibited reduced production of IL-2 and IFN-γ and increased helper activity for IgG and IgE synthesis.

Romagnani and associates (1989, 1994) subsequently showed increased IL-4 production and decreased IFN-γ production by T cells from patients with late-stage AIDS when compared with T cells from normal controls. The explanation for the selective survival of CD4[+] T cells with this functional capacity in AIDS patients is unknown, but it has been postulated that a switch from T_H1 to T_H2 dominance results in human immunodeficiency virus (HIV) progression (Clerici and Shearer, 1993) (see Chapter 18).

References

Abedi MR, Backman L, Persson U, Ringden O. Serum IgE levels after bone marrow transplantation. Bone Marrow Transplant 4:255–260, 1989.

Ammann AJ, Cain WA, Ishizaka K, Hong R, Good RA. Immunoglobulin E deficiency in ataxia telangiectasia. N Engl J Med 281:469–472, 1969.

Ammann AJ, Hong R. Selective IgA deficiency: presentation of 30 cases and a review of the literature. Medicine 50:223–236, 1971.

Anwar ARE, Smithers SK, Kay AB. Killing of schistosomula of *Schistosoma mansoni* coated with antibody and/or complement by human leukocytes in vitro: requirement for complement in preferential killing by eosinophils. J Immunol 122:628–637, 1979.

Aversa G, Punnonen J, Cocks BG, de Waal Malefyt R, Vega F, Zurawski SM, Zurawski G, De Vries JE. An interleukin 4 (IL-4) mutant protein inhibits both IL-4 or IL-13–induced human immunoglobulin G4 (IgG4) and IgE synthesis and B cell proliferation: support for a common component shared by IL-4 and IL-13 receptors. J Exp Med 178:2213–2218, 1993.

Bazaral M, Hamburger RN. Standardization and stability of immunoglobulin E (IgE). J Allerg Clin Immunol 49:189–191, 1972.

Berg T, Johansson SGO. Immunoglobulin levels during childhood, with special regard to IgE. Acta Paediatr Scand 58:513–524, 1969.

Berger M, Kirkpatrick CH, Goldsmith PK, Gallin JI. IgE antibodies to *Staphylococcus aureus* and *Candida albicans* in patients with the syndrome of hyperimmunoglobulin E and recurrent infections. J Immunol 125:2437–2443, 1980.

Berglund G, Finnstrom O, Johansson SGO, Moller KL. Wiskott-Aldrich syndrome: a study of 6 cases with determination of the immunoglobulins A, D, G, M and ND. Acta Paediatr Scand 57:89–97, 1968.

Bergstedt-Lindqvist S, Moon H, Persson R, Moller G, Heusser C, Severinson E. Interleukin 4 instructs uncommitted B lymphocytes to switch to IgG1 and IgE. Eur J Immunol 18:1073, 1988.

Blum R, Geller G, Fish LA. Recurrent severe staphylococcal infections, eczematoid rash, extreme elevations of IgE, eosinophilia, and divergent chemotactic responses in two generations. J Pediatr 90:607–609, 1997.

Buckley RH. Clinical and immunologic features of selective IgA deficiency. In Bergsma D, Good RA, Finstad J, Paul NW, eds. Immunodeficiency in Man and Animals. Sinauer Associates, Stamford, Conn., 1975, pp. 134–142.

Buckley RH. The hyper-IgE syndrome. In Fauci AS, Lichtenstein L, eds. Current Therapy in Allergy and Immunology. Philadelphia, BC. Decker, 1983, pp. 304–306.

Buckley RH, Dees SC. The correlation of milk precipitins with IgA deficiency. N Engl J Med 281:465–469, 1969.

Buckley RH, Fiscus SA. Serum IgD and IgE concentrations in immunodeficiency disease. J Clin Invest 55:157–165, 1975.

Buckley RH, Sampson HA. The hyperimmunoglobulinemia E syndrome. In Franklin EC, ed. Clinical Immunology Update. New York, Elsevier North-Holland, 1981, pp. 147–167.

Buckley RH, Schiff SE, Hayward AR. Reduced frequency of CD45RO[+] T lymphocytes in blood of hyper IgE syndrome patients. J Allergy Clin Immunol 87:313, 1991.

Buckley RH, Schiff SE, Sampson HA, Schiff RI, Markert ML, Knutsen AP, Hershfield MS, Huang AT, Mickey GH, Ward FE. Development of immunity in human severe primary T cell deficiency following haploidentical bone marrow stem cell transplantation. J Immunol 136:2398–2407, 1986.

Buckley RH, Wray BB, Belmaker EZ. Extreme hyperimmunoglobulinemia E and undue susceptibility to infection. Pediatrics 49:59–70, 1972.

Burks AW, Sampson HA, Buckley RH. Anaphylactic reactions after gamma globulin administration in patients with hypogammaglobulinemia. N Engl J Med 314:560–564, 1986.

Butterworth AE, Wasson DL, Gleich GJ. Damage to schistosomula of *Schistosoma mansoni* induced directly by eosinophil major basic protein. J Immunol 122:221–229, 1979.

Capron M, Bozin H, Joseph M, Capron A. Evidence for IgE-dependent cytotoxicity by rat eosinophils. J Immunol 126:1764–1768, 1981.

Capron M, Rousseaux J, Mazingue C. Rat mast cell-eosinophil interaction in antibody-dependent eosinophil cytotoxicity to *Schistosoma mansoni* schistosomula. J Immunol 121:2518–2525, 1978.

Church JA, Frenkel LD, Wright DG, Bellanti JA. T lymphocyte dysfunction, hyperimmunoglobulinemia E, recurrent bacterial infections, and defective neutrophil chemotaxis in a Negro child. J Pediatr 88:982–985, 1976.

Claassen JL, Levine AD, Buckley RH. A cell culture system that enhances mononuclear cell IgE synthesis induced by recombinant human interleukin-4. J Immunol Methods 126:213–222, 1990a.

Claassen JL, Levine AD, Buckley RH. Recombinant human IL-4 induces IgE and IgG synthesis by normal and atopic donor mononuclear cells: similar dose response, time course, requirement for T cells, and effect of pokeweed mitogen. J Immunol 144:2123–2130, 1990b.

Claassen JL, Levine AD, Buckley RH. Mechanism of pokeweed mitogen inhibition of recombinant IL-4-induced human IgE synthesis. Cell Immunol 140:357–369, 1992.

Claassen JL, Levine AD, Schiff SE, Buckley RH. Mononuclear cells from patients with the hyper-IgE syndrome produce little IgE when stimulated with recombinant interleukin 4 in vitro. J Allergy Clin Immunol 88:713–721, 1991.

Clark RA, Root RK, Kimball HR, Kirkpatrick CH. Defective neutrophil chemotaxis and cellular immunity in a child with recurrent infections. Ann Intern Med 78:515–519, 1973.

Clerici M, Shearer GM. A $T_H1 \rightarrow T_H2$ switch is a critical step in the etiology of HIV infection. Immunol Today 14:107–111, 1993.

Coffman RL, Carty J. A T cell activity that enhances polyclonal IgE production and its inhibition by interferon-γ. J Immunol 136:949–954, 1986.

Davis SD, Schaller J, Wedgwood RJ. Job's syndrome. Recurrent, "cold," staphylococcal abscesses. Lancet 2:1013–1015, 1966.

De Saint-Basile G, Le Deist F, de Vallartay J, Cerf-Bensussan N, Journet O, Brousse N, Griscelli C, Fischer A. Restricted heterogeneity of T lymphocytes in combined immunodeficiency with hypereosinophilia (Omenn's syndrome). J Clin Invest 87:1352–1359, 1991.

De Vries JE, Punnonen J, Cocks BG, de Wall Malefyt R, Aversa G. Regulation of the human IgE responses by IL-4 and IL-13. Res Immunol 144:597–601, 1993.

Del Prete G, Tiri A, Maggi E, De Carli M, Macchia D, Parronchi P, Rossi ME, Pietrogrande MC, Ricci M, Romagnani S. Defective in vitro production of gamma interferon and tumor necrosis factor alpha by circulating T cells from patients with the hyperimmunoglobulin E syndrome. J Clin Invest 84:1830–1835, 1989.

Dessein AJ, Parker WL, James SL, David JR. IgE antibody and resistance to infection: I. Selective suppression of the IgE antibody response in rats diminishes the resistance and the eosinophil response to *Trichinella spiralis* infection. J Exp Med 153:423–436, 1981.

Donabedian H, Alling DW, Gallin JI. Levamisole is inferior to placebo in the hyperimmunoglobulin E recurrent infection (Job's) syndrome. N Engl J Med 307:290–292, 1982.

Donabedian H, Gallin JI. The hyperimmunoglobulin E recurrent infection (Job's) syndrome. Medicine 62:195–208, 1983.

Dreskin SC, Goldsmith PK, Gallin JI. Immunoglobulins in the hyperimmunoglobulin E and recurrent infection (Job's) syndrome. J Clin Invest 75:26–34, 1985.

Epstein LB, Ammann AJ. Evaluation of T lymphocyte effector function in immunodeficiency diseases: abnormality in mitogen-stimulated interferon production in patients with selective IgA deficiency. J Immunol 112:617–626, 1974.

Fiser PM, Buckley RH. Human IgE biosynthesis in vitro: studies with atopic and normal blood mononuclear cells and subpopulations. J Immunol 123:1788–1794, 1979.

Gascan H, Gauchat J, Aversa G, Vlasselaer PV, De Vries JE. Anti-CD40 monoclonal antibodies or CD4+ T cell clones and IL-4 induce IgG4 and IgE switching in purified human B cells via different signaling pathways. J Immunol 147:8–13, 1991.

Geha RS, Leung DYM. Hyperimmunoglobulin E syndrome. Immunodefic Rev 1:155–172, 1989.

Geha RS, Reinherz E, Leung D, McKee JT, Schlossman S, Rosen FS. Deficiency of suppressor T cells in the hyperimmunoglobulin E syndrome. J Clin Invest 68:783–791, 1981.

Gordin FM, Simon GL, Wofsy CB, Mills J. Adverse reactions to trimethoprim-sulfamethoxazole in patients with the acquired immunodeficiency syndrome. Ann Intern Med 100:495–499, 1984.

Gorin LJ, Jeha SC, Sullivan MP, Rosenblatt HM, Shearer WT.

Burkitt's lymphoma developing in a 7-year-old boy with hyper IgE syndrome. J Allergy Clin Immunol 83:5–10, 1989.

Hill HR, Quie PG. Raised serum IgE levels and defective neutrophil chemotaxis in three children with eczema and recurrent bacterial infections. Lancet 1:183–187, 1974.

Hill HR, Quie PG, Pabst HF, Ochs HD, Clark RA, Klebanoff SJ, Wedgwood RJ. Defect in neutrophil granulocyte chemotaxis in Job's syndrome of recurrent "cold" staphylococcal abscesses. Lancet 2:617–619, 1974.

Huntley CC, Dees SC. Eczema associated with thrombocytopenic purpura and purulent otitis media. Pediatrics 19:351–361, 1957.

Huntley CC, Thorpe DP, Lyerly AD, Kelsey WM. Rheumatoid arthritis with IgA deficiency. Am J Dis Child 113:411–418, 1967.

Iio A, Strober W, Broder S, Polmar SH, Waldmann TA: The metabolism of IgE in patients with immunodeficiency states and neoplastic conditions. J Clin Invest 59:743–755, 1977.

Ishizaka K, Ishizaka T. Identification of IgE-antibodies as a carrier of reaginic activity. J Immunol 99:1187–1192, 1967.

Ishizaka K, Ishizaka T, Hornbrook MM. Physiochemical properties of reaginic antibody: V. Correlation of reaginic activity with E-globulin antibody. J Immunol 97:840–853, 1966.

Josephs SH, Buckley RH. Serum IgD concentrations in normal infants, children and adults and in patients with elevated serum IgE. J Pediatr 96:417–420, 1979.

Juhlin L, Michaelson G. A new syndrome characterized by absence of eosinophils and basophils. Lancet 1:1233–1235, 1977.

Kikkawa Y, Kamimura K, Hamajima T. Thymic alymphoplasia with hyper-IgE globulinemia. Pediatrics 51:690–696, 1973.

King CL, Gallin JI, Malech HL, Abramson SL, Nutman TB. Regulation of immunoglobulin production in hyperimmunoglobulin E recurrent infection syndrome by interferon. Proc Natl Acad Sci U S A 86:10085–10089, 1989.

Kirchner SG, Sivit CJ, Wright PF. Hyperimmunoglobulinemia E syndrome: association with osteoporosis and recurrent fractures. Radiology 156:362, 1985.

Lakin JD, Strong DM, Sell KW. Polymyxin B reactions, IgE antibody and T cell deficiency: immunochemical studies in a patient after bone marrow transplantation. Ann Intern Med 83:204, 1975.

Leung DYM, Ambrosino DM, Arbeit RD, Newton JL, Geha RS. Impaired antibody responses in the hyperimmunoglobulin E syndrome. J Allergy Clin Immunol 81:1082–1087, 1988.

Leung DYM, Key L, Steinberg JJ, Young MD, Von Deck M, Wilkinson R, Geha RA. Increased in vitro bone resorption by monocytes in the hyperimmunoglobulin E syndrome. J Immunol 140:84–88, 1988.

Levy DA, Chen J. Healthy IgE-deficient person. N Engl J Med 283:541–542, 1970.

Lischner HW, Huff DS. T cell deficiency in DiGeorge syndrome. In Bergsma D, Good RA, Finstad J, Paul NW, eds. Immununodeficiency in Man and Animals. Sunderland, Mass., Sinauer Associates, 1975, pp. 16–21.

Luqman M, Johnson P, Trowbridge I, Bottomly K. Differential expression of the alternatively spliced exons of murine CD45 in T_H1 and T_H2 cloned lines. Eur J Immunol 21:17–22, 1991.

Maggi E, Macchia D, Parronchi P, Mazzetti M, Ravina A, Milo D, Romagnani S. Reduced production of interleukin-2 and interferon gamma and enhanced helper activity for IgG synthesis by cloned CD4+ T cells from patients with AIDS. Eur J Immunol 17:1685–1690, 1987.

Mann HB, Whitney DR. On a test of whether one of two random variables is stochastically larger than the other. Ann Math Stat 18:50–60, 1947.

McKenzie AMJ, Culpepper JA, de Waal Malefyt R, Briere F, Punnonen J, Aversa G, Sato A, Dang W, Cocks BG, Memon S, De Vries JE, Bancherau J, Zurawski G. Interleukin-13, a novel T cell derived cytokine that regulates monocyte and B cell function. Proc Natl Acad Sci U S A 90:3735–3739, 1993.

Melamed I, Cohen A, Roifman CM. Expansion of CD3+ CD4− CD8− T cell population expression high levels of IL-5 in Omenn's syndrome. Clin Exp Immunol 95:14–21, 1994.

Merten DF, Buckley RH, Pratt PC, Effmann EL, Grossman H. The hyperimmunoglobulinemia E syndrome: radiographic observations. Radiology 132:71–78, 1979.

Molina IJ, Sancho J, Terhorst C, Rosen FS, Remold-O'Donnell E. T cells of patients with the Wiskott-Aldrich syndrome have a restricted defect in proliferative responses. J Immunol 151:4383–4390, 1993.

Mosmann TR, Coffman RL. T$_H$1 and T$_H$2 cells: different patterns of lymphokine secretion lead to different functional properties. Ann Rev Immunol 7:145–173, 1989.

Motala C, Potter PC, Weinberg EG, Malherbe D, and Hughes J. Anti–*Staphylococcus aureus* specific IgE in atopic dermatitis. J Allergy Clin Immunol 78:583–589, 1986.

Nezelof C. Thymic dysplasia with normal immunoglobulins and immunologic deficiency: pure alymphocytosis. In Bergsma D, ed. Immunologic Deficiency Diseases in Man. New York, National Foundation–March of Dimes, 1968, pp. 104–115.

Okumura K, Tada T. Regulation of homocytotropic antibody formation in the rat: III. Effect of thymectomy and splenectomy. J Immunol 106:1019–1026, 1971.

Paganelli R, Scala E, Capobianchi MR, Fanales-Belasio E, D'Offizi G, Fiorilli M, Aiuti F. Selective deficiency of interferon-gamma production in the hyper IgE syndrome: relationship to in vitro IgE synthesis. Clin Exp Immunol 84:28–33, 1991.

Paul WE, Ohara J. B cell stimulatory factor-1/interleukin 4. Ann Rev Immunol 5:429–459, 1987.

Pene J, Rousset F, Briere F, Chretien I, Bonnefoy J, Spits H, Yokota T, Arai N, Arai K, Banchereau J, De Vries JE. IgE production by normal human lymphocytes is induced by interleukin 4 and suppressed by interferons γ and α and prostaglandin E$_2$. Proc Natl Acad Sci U S A 85:6880–6884, 1988.

Polmar SH, Waldmann TA, Balestra ST, Jost MC, Terry WD. Immunoglobulin E in immunologic deficiency diseases: I. Relation of IgE and IgA to respiratory tract disease in isolated IgE deficiency. J Clin Invest 51:326–330, 1972a.

Polmar SH, Waldmann TA, Terry WD. IgE in immunodeficiency. Am J Pathol 69:499, 1972b.

Punnonen J, Aversa G, Cocks BG, McKenzie ANJ, Menon S, Zurawski G, de Waal Malefyt R, De Vries JE. Interleukin 13 induces interleukin 4-independent IgG4 and IgE synthesis and CD23 expression by human B cells. Proc Natl Acad Sci U S A 90:3730–3734, 1993.

Romagnani S. Lymphokine production by human T cells in disease. Ann Rev Immunol 12:227–257, 1994.

Romagnani S, Maggi E, Del Prete GF, Tiri A, Macchia D, Parronchi P, Biswas P, Ricci M. T cells and T cell factors active in human IgE synthesis. In Pichler W, Stadler BM, Dahinden C, Pecound AR, Frei PC, Schneider C, de Weck AL. eds. Progress in Allergy and Clinical Immunobiology. Montreux, Switzerland, Hogrefe & Huber, 1989, pp. 138–144.

Sampson HA, Buckley RH. Human IgE synthesis in vitro: a reassessment. J Immunol 127:829–834, 1981.

Saryan JA, Rappeport J, Leung DYM, Parkman R, Geha RS. Regulation of human immunoglobulin E synthesis in acute graft versus host disease. J Clin Invest 71:556–564, 1983.

Schandene L, Ferster A, Mascart-Lemone F, Crusiaux A, Gerard C, Marchant A, Lybin M, Velu T, Sariban E, Goldman M. T helper type 2-like cells and therapeutic effects of interferon gamma in combined immunodeficiency with hypereosinophilia (Omenn's syndrome). Eur J Immunol 23:56–60, 1993.

Schmitt C, Ballet JJ. Serum IgE and IgG antibodies to tetanus toxoid and candidin in immunodeficient children with the hyper IgE syndrome. J Clin Immunol 3:178–183, 1983.

Schopfer K, Baerlocher K, Price P, Krech U, Quie PG, Douglas SD. Staphylococcal IgE antibodies, hyperimmunoglobulinemia E and *Staphylococcus aureus* infections. N Engl J Med 300:835–838, 1979.

Schwartz DP, Buckley RH. Serum IgE concentrations and skin reactivity to anti-IgE antibody in IgA deficient patients. N Engl J Med 284:513–517, 1971.

Sheerin KA, Buckley RH. Antibody responses to protein, polysaccha-ride, and φX 174 antigens in the hyperimmunoglobulinemia E (hyper IgE) syndrome. J Allergy Clin Immunol 87:803–811, 1991.

Simon HU, Higgins EA, Demetriou M, Datti A, Siminovitch KA, Dennis JW. Defective expression of CD23 and autocrine growth-stimulation in Epstein-Barr virus (EBV)–transformed B cells from patients with Wiskott-Aldrich syndrome (WAS). Clin Exp Immunol 91:43–49, 1993.

Sindel LJ, Buckley RH, Schiff SE, Ward FE, Mickey GH, Huang AT, Naspitz C, Koren H. Severe combined immunodeficiency with natural killer cell predominance: abrogation of graft-versus-host disease and immunologic reconstitution with HLA-identical bone marrow cells. J Allergy Clin Immunol 73:829–836, 1984.

Snyderman R, Rogers E, Buckley RH. Abnormalities of leukotaxis in atopic dermatitis. J Allergy Clin Immunol 60:121–126, 1977.

Soderberg-Warner M, Rice-Mendoza CA, Mendoza GR, Stiehm ER. Neutrophil and T lymphocyte characteristics of two patients with the hyper IgE syndrome. Pediatr Res 17:820–824, 1983.

Spriggs MK, Fanslow WC, Armitage RJ, Belmont J. The biology of the human ligand for CD40. J Clin Immunol 13:373–380, 1993.

Tada T, Ishizaka K. Distribution of E-forming cells in lymphoid tissues of the human and monkey. J Immunol 104:377–387, 1970.

Thyphronitis G, Tsokos GC, June CH, Levine AD, Finkelman FD. IgE secretion by Epstein-Barr virus–infected purified human B lymphocytes is stimulated by interleukin 4 and suppressed by interferon-γ. Proc Natl Acad Sci U S A 86:5580–5584, 1989.

Van der Giessen M, Reerink-Brongers EE, Veen TA. Quantitation of Ig classes and IgG subclasses in sera of patients with a variety of immunoglobulin deficiencies and their relatives. Clin Immunol Immunopathol 5:388–398, 1976.

Van Scoy RE, Hill HR, Ritts RE, Quie PG. Familial neutrophil chemotaxis defect, recurrent bacterial infections, mucocutaneous candidiasis, and hyperimmunoglobulinemia E. Ann Intern Med 82:766–771, 1975.

Veith MC, Butterworth AE. Enhancement of human eosinophil-mediated killing of *Schistosoma mansoni* larvae by mononuclear cell products in vitro. J Exp Med 157:1828–1843, 1983.

Vercelli D, Jabara HH, Cunningham-Rundles C, Abrams JS, Lewis DB, Meyer J, Schneider LC, Leung DYM, Geha RS. Regulation of immunoglobulin (Ig)E synthesis in the hyper IgE syndrome. J Clin Invest 85:1–6, 1990.

Vyas GN, Fudenberg HH. Immunobiology of human IgA: a serologic and immunogenetic study of immunization to IgA in transfusion and pregnancy. Clin Genet 1:45–64, 1974.

Vyas GN, Perkins HA, Fudenberg HH. Anaphylactoid tranfusion reactions associated with anti-IgA. Lancet 2:312–315, 1968.

Waldmann TA, Polmar SH, Balestra ST. Immunoglobulin E in immunologic deficiency diseases: II. Serum IgE concentration of patients with acquired hypogammaglobulinemia, myotonic dystrophy, intestinal lymphangiectasia and Wiskott-Aldrich syndrome. J Immunol 109:304–310, 1972.

Walsh GA, Richards KL, Douglas SD, Blumenthal MN. Immunoglobulin E anti–*Staphylococcus aureus* antibodies in atopic patients. J Clin Microbiol 13:1046–1048, 1981.

Weston WL, Humbert JR, August CS, Harnett I, Mass MF, Dean PB, Hagan IM. A hyperimmunoglobulin E syndrome with normal chemotaxis in vitro and defective leukotaxis in vivo. J Allergy Clin Immunol 59:112–119, 1977.

Wu CY, Sarfati M, Heusser C, Fournier S, Rubio-Trujillo M, Peleman R, Delespesse G. Glucocorticoids increase the synthesis of immunoglobulin E by interleukin 4-stimulated human lymphocytes. J Clin Invest 87:870–877, 1991.

Zhang K, Clark EA, Saxon A. CD40 stimulation provides an IFN-γ–independent and IL-4–dependent differentiation signal directly to human B cells for IgE production. J Immunol 146:1836–1842, 1991.

Chapter 14

Disorders of the IgA System

Charlotte Cunningham-Rundles

IgA IMMUNOGLOBULIN: OVERVIEW

IgA, the second most abundant immunoglobulin in human serum, has a chemical structure similar to that of IgG, but it is catabolized about five times faster (half-life, 3 to 6 days) (see Chapter 3). Although there are substantial amounts of IgA in serum, most of the IgA-producing B cells are in the mucosa of the sinopulmonary, genital, and gastrointestinal tracts. These cells produce secretory IgA, the most abundant immunoglobulin in human secretions. Based on the number of IgA-secreting plasma cells and its rapid rate of catabolism, it is estimated that 80% of the human B-cell system produces IgA (Mestecky and McGhee, 1987).

The secretory IgA present in human breast milk provides powerful protection to the infant against diarrhea and neonatal septicemia (Victoria et al., 1987; Ashraf et al., 1991). Almost all microbes that infect the mucosal surfaces stimulate the local secretion of IgA antibodies. The biologic importance of the secretory IgA system is underscored by the fact that most of the 40,000 children under the age of 5 years who die worldwide every day have contracted mucosal infections of either the gastrointestinal or respiratory tract (Hanson and Brandtzaeg, 1993).

Despite the fact that secretory IgA is so important in mucosal immunity, selective IgA deficiency is the most common primary immunodeficiency, but in most cases it is asymptomatic. The reasons for this are unknown, but presumably immunologic compensation provides complete restitution. Alternatively, IgA deficiency alone may not predispose to disease, but additional abnormalities in symptomatic individuals may be present.

One example is IgG2 subclass deficiency, which is occasionally linked to IgA deficiency (Oxelius et al., 1981) (see later, Selective IgA Subclass Deficiency).

This combination leads to recurrent infections, and in some cases to chronic pulmonary disease (Björkander et al., 1985). Some IgA-deficient individuals have a reduced antibody response to immunizations (even with normal IgG and IgM levels) (De Graeff et al, 1983), and others have an aberrant IgG subclass response to bacterial polysaccharide vaccines (Hammerström et al., 1985a). Another immunologic abnormality in some IgA-deficient individuals is the presence of one or more inactive C4 genes, the significance of which is unknown.

This chapter reviews the physiologic role of IgA, disorders of IgA regulation, the frequency and causes of IgA deficiency, the diseases associated with its absence, and the management of IgA deficiency.

HISTORICAL ASPECTS

Serum IgA was first identified by Grabar and Williams (1953) and was later isolated and characterized by Heremans (1974). IgA was soon found to be the main immunoglobulin in human milk by Hanson (1959) and by Gugler and Von Muralt (1959), and in saliva by Chodirker and Tomasi (1963). The importance of IgA in the intestinal tract was first noted by Crabbé and colleagues (1965), who reported a preponderance of IgA-producing cells in the human gut mucosa.

It was initially assumed that serum and secretory IgA were structurally identical, but in 1961 Hanson reported that secretory IgA had an extra antigenic epitope. By 1965, this extra determinant was identified as an additional chain, first known as a "transport" or "secretory" piece and now called *secretory component* (Tomasi, 1992). IgA in secretions is dimeric and, like the other polymeric immunoglobulin, IgM, contains a J chain.

More than 20 years ago, Brandtzaeg (1973, 1974) proposed a common epithelial mechanism for transporting IgA and IgM into mucosal secretions. The secretory component was proposed as the plausible epithelial cell surface receptor for both dimeric IgA and pentameric IgM. This foreshadowed molecular studies that showed that the secretory component is actually the extracellular portion of the polymeric immunoglobulin receptor (Mostov et al., 1984; Mostov and Deitcher, 1986).

STRUCTURE OF IgA

The structure of serum IgA is similar to that of IgG. It has two heavy and two light chains, arranged in a Y-shaped configuration. There are two antigen-binding sites at the ends of the arms and one cell-binding region called the *Fc portion* (Fig. 14–1). Human IgA occurs in two isotypes (subclasses), IgA1 and IgA2 (Fig. 14–1), which differ primarily by the length of the hinge region. IgA1 has an additional 13 amino acids in this portion, rendering IgA1 more susceptible to the action of bacterial proteases (Plaut, 1983). IgA2 exists in two allotypic (genetic) variants, IgA2m(1) and IgA2m(2) (Van Loghem et al., 1973) (see later, Selective IgA Subclass Deficiency), which differ in the points of attachment between heavy and light chains.

IgA1 is the predominant subclass in serum, and IgA2 is the predominant subclass in secretions. Serum IgA (both IgA1 and IgA2) is monomeric (containing two heavy chains and two light chains). Secretory IgA is dimeric (i.e., two IgA monomers) and is joined by

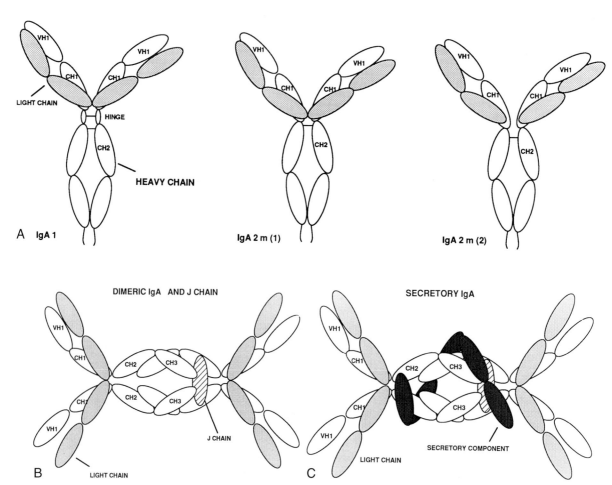

Figure 14–1. Theoretical models of IgA. *A,* IgA in serum is monomeric, containing two heavy and two light chains. IgA1 has an extended hinge region as compared with IgA2. For the IgA2m(1) allotype, the terminal cysteines of the light chains are disulfide-bonded; for IgA1 and IgA2m(2), they are linked to the heavy chain. *B,* Dimeric IgA is secreted by plasma cells lining the mucosal surfaces. The Fc regions are shown overlapped, with the J chain attached to the CH3 terminal cysteines of one pair of heavy chains. *C,* This model of secretory IgA, the final secreted form of IgA, is dimeric and includes the J chain and the secretory component (the secreted portion of the polymeric immunoglobulin receptor). The fifth "domain" of the secretory component is shown, disulfide-linked to the CH2 region of one of the IgA monomers (location still not established). (Adapted from Kerr MA: The structure and function of human IgA. J Biochem 271:285–296, 1990.)

the J chain and the 80-kD secretory component (Fig. 14–1).

FUNCTION OF IgA

IgA is the most prevalent immunoglobulin in exocrine secretions and represents the predominant class of antibodies produced by plasma cells of the sinopulmonary, gastrointestinal, and genitourinary tracts (Tomasi and Bienenstock, 1968; Mestecky and McGhee, 1987). External antigens contacting the mucosa stimulate the secretion of IgA antibodies. Secretory IgA combines with antigen at these surfaces to prevent mucosal penetration and exclude foreign antigens from entering the body. Secretory IgA antibodies can neutralize viruses, bind toxins, agglutinate bacteria, prevent bacteria from binding to cells, and bind to various food antigens. Thus, IgA is of crucial importance in preventing infectious agents from penetrating mucosal surfaces (Tomasi and Bienenstock, 1968; Arnold et al., 1977; Hanson, 1983; Mestecky and McGhee, 1987).

Table 14–1 summarizes some of the known binding activities of secretory IgA.

Two other roles for IgA in mucosal immunity have been identified. Dimeric IgA secreted by plasma cells is selectively transported to the lumen through the epithelial cell by the polymeric immunoglobulin receptor in a process known as *transcytosis*. Cleavage of this receptor releases the secretory component, and secretory IgA is discharged into the mucosal gland lumen. Dimeric IgA transiting through epithelial cells in this way may impede the replication of intracellular viruses (Mazanec et al., 1992). IgA can also complex with antigens that have penetrated the lamina propria and transport them across epithelial cells to facilitate antigen exclusion (Kaetzel et al., 1991).

Although secretory IgA has many known functions, the role of serum IgA is less certain. Plasma cells producing serum IgA are located predominantly in the bone marrow and to a lesser extent in the spleen (Mestecky and McGhee, 1987). The role of the abundant serum IgA antibodies to microbial and food antigens in the systemic immune response is uncertain (Mestecky and McGhee, 1987).

One clue to understanding the function of serum IgA may be the presence of receptors for the Fc portion of IgA on monocytes and granulocytes (Kerr, 1990; Monteiro et al., 1990). This receptor ($Fc\alpha R$), a glycosylated protein of 50 to 70 kD, can bind IgA1 or IgA2 monomers or even secretory IgA. Receptor-bound IgA antibodies can activate both granulocytes and monocytes and may initiate phagocytosis of bacteria and fungi. The $Fc\alpha R$ may play a role in the catabolism of IgA antibodies and in the clearance of IgA immune complexes from the circulation. Because IgA in the serum does not fix complement by the classical pathway, although it can do so by the alternative pathway (Russell and Mansa, 1989; Kerr, 1990), it has been suggested that it acts as a "discrete housekeeper," in which foreign antigens are bound by IgA into complexes and removed by the phagocytic system, but with little or no resultant inflammation (Conley and Delacroix, 1987).

Another biologic function is suggested by a biochemical feature of serum IgA, the presence of free cysteine residues located near the tip of the carboxy terminus of the Fc portion. These cysteines can complex IgA to other serum proteins, principally albumin, alpha$_1$-antitrypsin, and the heterogeneously charged (HC) protein. Both the heterogeneously charged protein and alpha$_1$-antitrypsin are leukocyte inhibitors. Thus, these complexes, as well as other IgA complexes, may inhibit neutrophil chemotaxis and exert a subtle immune control mechanism (Kerr, 1990). Other proteins binding to serum IgA include *fibronectin* and *lactoferrin* (Kerr, 1990).

IgA NEPHROPATHY AND HENOCH-SCHÖNLEIN PURPURA

Both IgA nephropathy and Henoch-Schönlein (anaphylactoid) purpura (HSP) are associated with either overproduction or abnormal deposition of IgA in the skin and kidneys. IgA nephropathy is a common cause of glomerulonephritis and renal failure and is associated with the deposition of IgA-containing immune complexes in the kidney (Clarkson et al., 1988) (see Chapter 25). The antigens involved are as yet unknown, despite the number of studies done to identify them. IgA-containing immune complexes are the only distinguishing feature of this disease, but IgA mesangial deposits also occur in other diseases. In IgA nephropathy, serum IgA is elevated in 50% of cases. Complement component levels are often elevated, and circulating IgA complexes are often found. IgA1 is the predominant subclass of IgA deposited in the kidney and is accompanied by variable amounts of IgG and C3 (Conley et al., 1980). Because the J chain is often identified, these deposits may be polymeric, but secretory component has not routinely been found in these

Table 14–1. Specific Secretory IgA Antibody Reactivity in Human Colostrum and Milk

Bacteria	Coxsackievirus
Escherichia coli O, K antigens, enterotoxin	Respiratory syncytial virus
	Cytomegalovirus
Salmonella	Influenza A virus
Shigella	Arboviruses—Semliki forest,
Vibrio cholerae	Ross river, Japanese B,
Bacteroides fragilis	dengue
Streptococcus	Parainfluenza, rhinovirus
Bordetella pertussis	
Clostridium diphtheriae, C. tetani	**Fungi**
Streptococcus mutans	*Candida albicans*
Neisseria gonorrhoeae	
Campylobacter	**Protozoa**
	Giardia
Viruses	
Rotavirus	**Other**
Poliovirus 1, 2, 3	Milk proteins
Echovirus	Soy lectin
	Peanut lectin
	Wheat gluten, gliadin

Modified from Cunningham-Rundles C. IgA deficiency. Immunol Allergy Clin North Am 8:435–450, 1988.

deposits (Komatsu et al., 1983). Some patients have increased numbers of circulating lymphocytes bearing IgA Fc receptors (Sakai et al., 1979).

Although Henoch-Schönlein purpura is historically older than IgA nephropathy, from a pathologic and immunologic point of view the two diseases are similar. Although Schönlein first reported the association of purpura and arthritis in 1837 and Henoch recognized the gastrointestinal and renal components in 1874, the first clinical description of HSP is attributed to Heberden (Clarkson et al., 1988) (see Chapter 24). Unlike IgA nephropathy, which has few characteristic clinical symptoms, Henoch-Schönlein purpura is usually manifested by a distinct rash and gastrointestinal and joint manifestations. A glomerular component is present in many cases and is responsible for most of the 1% to 3% mortality (Clarkson et al., 1988).

Clinical features are predominantly the result of a systemic leukocytoclastic vasculitis affecting the skin, joints, and intestinal tract. The specific agent of injury appears to be immune complexes, resulting in complement activation and neutrophil infiltration. The pathologic hallmark of the disease is the tissue deposition of IgA-containing immune complexes; deposits of IgA, C3, and (less often) IgG and IgM are found in the blood vessels and skin lesions.

Although Henoch-Schönlein purpura has been described in a subject with IgA deficiency (Martini et al., 1985), it is possible that IgA is not essential to this disease. Perhaps the IgA helps to recruit other immunologic mediators.

SELECTIVE IgA DEFICIENCY

Frequency

Serum IgA deficiency was first described in children with ataxia-telangiectasia (Thieffry et al., 1961), but soon IgA deficiency was identified in other patients and even in normal subjects (West et al., 1962).

Following the original report (West et al., 1962), many investigators studied the frequency of IgA deficiency in various populations. Its prevalence has ranged from 1/223 to 1/1000 in community populations from different countries (Bachmann, 1965; Grundbacher, 1972; Cassidy and Nordby, 1975) and from 1/400 to 1/3000 among healthy blood donors (Natvig et al., 1971; Frommel et al., 1973; Koistinen, 1975). These varying results may be the result of population differences, with the Finns having the highest frequency of IgA deficiency.

One difference in these studies is the serum IgA level used to establish a diagnosis of IgA deficiency. Some authors use 10 mg/dl or lower (Buckley and Dees, 1969); others use a level of 5 mg/dl or lower, as suggested by Hong and Ammann (1989). For our purposes here, we define selective IgA deficiency as a level of 5 mg/dl or lower.

Some studies have investigated the prevalence of IgA deficiency in predominantly male blood donors or in Rh-negative women. Although there are no apparent sex differences in the occurrence of IgA deficiency in healthy persons (Bachmann, 1965; Koistinen, 1975), male IgA-deficient individuals are more prevalent in hospitalized groups (Buckley, 1975). Buckley (1975) suggested that IgA deficiency may be less common in blacks than in whites. A correlated observation is that IgA deficiency is much less prevalent in Japanese blood donors (Kanoh et al., 1986) than in white donors; similarly, the incidence in Malaysians is low (Yadav and Iyngkaran, 1979).

IgA deficiency may be familial (see later, Patterns of Inheritance), but several studies have noted a higher frequency of mother-to-child inheritance of IgA deficiency than of father-to-child inheritance (Koistinen, 1976; Oen et al., 1982). One explanation is the transplacental passage of anti-IgA antibodies, which can result in IgA deficiency in the infant. Petty and colleagues (1985) studied the offspring of IgA-deficient mothers. Of these 27 children, 12 had IgA levels more than 1 standard deviation (SD) below normal, and 7 had levels more than 2 SDs below normal. Of the 7 with the lowest IgA levels, 5 had mothers who had anti-IgA antibodies during gestation.

In vitro studies have indicated that heterologous anti-human IgA can suppress mitogen-induced IgA synthesis by human B lymphocytes and that human anti-IgA suppresses the development of human IgA plaque-forming cells (Warrington et al., 1981, 1982; Hammarström et al., 1983). Two IgA-deficient mothers with circulating anti-IgA antibodies gave birth to four children with IgA deficiency (De Laat et al., 1991). In three of these children, anti-IgA antibodies developed before puberty. In all four, in vitro studies showed an IgA B-cell defect combined with excess IgA-specific T-suppressor function. These data suggest a means whereby IgA deficiency can be perpetuated among a population with a high prevalence of IgA deficiency.

IgA Deficiency in Healthy Subjects

Because secretory IgA is important in protecting mucous surfaces, it is a mystery why most IgA-deficient subjects remain healthy. For example, an early report described IgA deficiency in two healthy young physicians (Rockey et al., 1964). This lack of disease in IgA deficiency is usually attributed to a compensatory increase in IgM in the secretions (Brandtzaeg et al., 1986). In IgA-deficient individuals, there may be an increase in secretory IgM (IgM attached to secretory component) in the saliva and other intestinal fluids and in IgM-bearing plasma cells in the gastrointestinal mucosa. Similarly, the colostrum of IgA-deficient subjects has been shown to contain abundant amounts of IgM (Barros et al., 1985). The saliva of IgA-deficient individuals contains biologically active IgM antibody, such as secretory IgM to *Streptococcus mutans* (Arnold et al., 1977).

Although secretory IgM is functionally active, it may not confer mucosal protection equivalent to that of secretory IgA. Indeed, IgA-deficient blood donors harbor poliovirus longer after oral vaccination than normal subjects do (Savilahti et al., 1988). Additionally, secretory IgA is subject to rapid degradation in the intestinal lumen (Richman and Brown, 1977). Norhagen and associates (1989) also questioned the view that IgM can compensate for IgA deficiency in the secretions, and they could not relate salivary IgM levels to health or frequency of illness in 63 IgA-deficient subjects. Conversely, Mellander and colleagues (1986) found that infections are more common in IgA-deficient individuals with low or absent secretory IgM.

Nilssen and coworkers (1993) have shown that oral cholera-vaccinated, IgA-deficient individuals preferentially activate intestinal IgG-producing cells rather than IgM. The response to this vaccination (which in normal subjects produces a predominantly IgA response) was not significantly different for healthy, asymptomatic IgA-deficient individuals. These data suggest that there is still much to be learned about the immune compensations that occur in the healthy IgA-deficient subject.

Another reason some IgA-deficient individuals might remain healthy is that secretory IgA is produced in normal amounts. Up to 3% of IgA-deficient individuals have normal levels of secretory IgA (Hazenberg et al., 1968; Swanson et al., 1968; Ammann and Hong, 1971b) and possess normal numbers of IgA-bearing plasma cells in the intestine.

Association of IgA Deficiency with Specific Disorders

Despite the fact that most IgA-deficient subjects are not ill, IgA deficiency has been associated with an astonishing number of specific disorders (Ammann and Hong, 1970, 1971b; Hanson, 1983; Burks and Steele, 1986; Cunningham-Rundles, 1990; Strober and Sneller, 1991; Schaffer et al., 1991). A partial list is given in Table 14–2.

Sinopulmonary Infections

Recurrent sinopulmonary infection is the most frequent illness associated with selective IgA deficiency. Indeed, these infections often represent the reason why quantitative immunoglobulin levels are first obtained and the diagnosis established. The frequency of these infections in IgA-deficient subjects varies considerably. Most infections are caused by minor bacterial pathogens or, in the absence of exact bacteriologic diagnosis, various viral agents. Sinopulmonary infections are more likely to occur in IgA-deficient individuals who have IgG2 subclass deficiency, but they also occur in IgA-deficient individuals without a second known defect.

One group found that infections may be more common in IgA-deficient individuals with low or absent levels of secretory IgM (Mellander et al., 1986), although another group, studying a larger group of IgA-deficient subjects, did not find salivary IgM levels to be increased in healthy subjects or depressed in the more frequently infected individuals (Norhagen et al., 1989). Brandtzaeg and colleagues (1986) have suggested that some IgA-deficient patients with frequent infections

Table 14–2. Diseases/Conditions Associated with Selective IgA Deficiency

1. Allergic disorders (Ammann and Hong, 1971; Buckley 1975; Burgio et al., 1980; Baker et al., 1976; Collins-Williams et al., 1972; Burks and Steele, 1986)
2. Recurrent infections (Ammann and Hong, 1971b; Baker et al., 1976; Burgio et al., 1980)
3. Familial history of hypogammaglobulinemia (Fudenberg et al., 1962; Nell et al., 1972; Wollheim et al., 1964)
4. Malignancy (Ammann and Hong, 1971b; Kersey et al., 1988; Budman et al., 1978; Cunningham-Rundles et al., 1980; Spector et al., 1978)
5. Familial history of pulmonary fibrosis (Kirkpatrick and Ruth, 1966)
6. Chronic *Candida* granuloma (Claman et al., 1966; Fulginiti et al., 1966)
7. Mental retardation and seizures (Levin et al., 1963; Vassella et al., 1968; Haddow et al., 1970)
8. Mental retardation and cirrhosis (West et al., 1962)
9. Congenital sensory neuropathy (Haddow et al., 1970; Levin et al., 1963; Vassella et al., 1968)
10. Chronic nephritis (West et al., 1962)
11. Fatal varicella (Hobbs, 1968)
12. Chronic granulomatous disease (Douglas et al., 1969; Gerba et al., 1982)
13. Cystic fibrosis (Ammann and Hong, 1971b)
14. Endocrinopathy (Levin et al., 1963)
15. Hypersplenism and thrombocytopenia (Hobbs, 1968)
16. Pancreatitis (Penny et al., 1971)
17. Sarcoidosis (Claman et al., 1966; Sharma and Chandor, 1972)
18. Pernicious anemia (Odgers and Wangel, 1968)
19. Epilepsy (Fontana et al., 1978a, 1978b)
20. Gastrointestinal disease (see Table 14–3)
21. Autoimmune disease (see Table 14–4)
22. Chromosomal abnormalities (see Table 14–5)

have increased IgD B cells, rather than increased IgM B cells in the nasal mucosa.

There have been reports of chronic serious lung disease in patients with selective IgA deficiency, including cases of recurrent pneumonia, chronic obstructive lung disease, chronic bronchitis, bronchiectasis (Webb and Condemi, 1974; Hong and Ammann, 1989; Burks and Steele, 1986), and pulmonary hemosiderosis (Krieger and Brough, 1967). As noted, those with combined IgA and IgG2 deficiency are more likely to have severe, chronic respiratory infections (Björkander et al., 1985).

Allergy

Buckley and Dees (1969) first suggested that IgA deficiency and allergy are associated. Even in blood bank donors in whom IgA deficiency was discovered accidentally, allergy is more common (20%) than in healthy blood donors (10%) (Kaufman and Hobbs, 1970). IgE levels are often increased in IgA deficiency (Kanok et al., 1978). The most common allergic disorders reported in IgA-deficient individuals are allergic conjunctivitis, rhinitis, urticaria, atopic eczema, and bronchial asthma (Ammann and Hong, 1971b; Burks and Steele, 1986; Plebani et al., 1987). Many clinicians believe that IgA-deficient subjects with asthma have more refractory disease; perhaps their susceptibility to secondary respiratory infections aggravates the associated inflammation.

Food allergy may be more common in IgA-deficient

patients. In one study, a reduced IgA response to luminal antigens and a lack of IgM compensation was noted in the mucosa of atopic children (Sloper et al., 1981); delayed development of IgA in the intestinal tract of infants and young children has also been associated with atopy (Taylor et al., 1973).

Gastrointestinal Disease

Patients with IgA deficiency have an increased frequency of gastrointestinal diseases (Table 14–3). The best known association is infection with *Giardia lamblia*. Presumably, the lack of secretory IgA permits the attachment and proliferation of these protozoa on the intestinal epithelium (Zinneman and Kaplan, 1975). If giardiasis occurs in IgA deficiency, malabsorption resulting from flattened villi, often accompanied by nodular lymphoid hyperplasia, may develop. Diagnosis warrants multiple stool analyses and an examination of the duodenal fluid. Relapses after treatment with metronidazole or quinacrine hydrochloride are fairly common.

Nodular lymphoid hyperplasia and malabsorption also occur in IgA deficiency, but malabsorption can be present without nodular lymphoid hyperplasia (Jacobson and de Shazo, 1979). Severe diarrhea in association with IgA deficiency and lymphoid hyperplasia or malabsorption may be difficult to treat. Dramatic improvement has been reported after infusions of fresh plasma (Gryboski et al., 1967). Lactose intolerance appears to be increased in patients with IgA deficiency (Dubois et al., 1970).

Patients with celiac disease have a high incidence of IgA deficiency; approximately 1 of every 200 patients with celiac disease has IgA deficiency (Crabbé and Heremans, 1966, 1967; Hanson, 1983; Savilahti et al., 1984). This association is unique because gluten enteropathy is not associated with other primary immunodeficiencies. It is possible that there is increased absorption of wheat antigens because of the absence of secretory IgA. Indeed, secretory IgA can bind to wheat gluten and gliadin. Intestinal biopsy specimens of patients with coexisting IgA deficiency and celiac disease are similar to those of patients with celiac disease alone, and their responses to a gluten-free diet are also similar (Mann et al., 1970; Klemola, 1988).

Table 14–3. Gastrointestinal Diseases Associated with IgA Deficiency

Giardiasis	Regional enteritis
Nonspecific gastroenteritis	Total villous atrophy in the
Allergic disorders	presence of antiepithelial cell
Malabsorption	antibody
Celiac disease	Achlorhydria
Pancreatic insufficiency	Henoch-Schönlein syndrome
Nodular hepatitis	Cholelithiasis
Primary biliary cirrhosis	Gastrointestinal lymphoma
Pernicious anemia	Adenocarcinoma of stomach
Lactose intolerance	Nodular lymphoid hyperplasia
Ulcerative colitis	

Autoimmune Gastrointestinal Diseases

Associations between IgA deficiency and autoimmune intestinal diseases have been reported, including chronic hepatitis (Benbassat et al., 1973), biliary cirrhosis (James et al., 1986), and pernicious anemia (Odgers and Wangel, 1968). In these cases, autoantibodies to the relevant target organ are not uncommon. It is less clear whether the anti–basement membrane antibodies found in the sera of IgA-deficient individuals play a role in tissue damage; however, in one study, 3 of 31 patients with IgA deficiency and celiac disease had such an antibody (Ammann and Hong, 1971c). In another case, a serum antibody to the gastrointestinal epithelial cells was found in association with total villous atrophy and malabsorption (McCarthy et al., 1978).

Ulcerative colitis and regional enteritis are also associated with IgA deficiency; again, their therapeutic response is similar to that of non–IgA-deficient patients. One report described an IgA-deficient patient who had both ulcerative colitis and gluten-sensitive enteropathy (Falchuk and Falchuk, 1975).

Food allergy is a common clinical feature of IgA deficiency. This may represent another example of the abnormal processing of antigen at the mucosal surface. It has been suggested that there may be an increase in infantile atopy in IgA infants with delayed IgA maturation (Taylor et al., 1973). Similarly, another study showed a reduced IgA response and a lack of IgM compensation in the intestinal mucosa of atopic children (Sloper et al., 1981).

An unusual syndrome of malabsorption, IgA deficiency, diabetes mellitus, and a common HLA haplotype (HLA-B8 and DRw3) was reported in three persons in a kindred of 43 individuals (Van Thiel et al., 1977). Although some of these family members were healthy, there were multiple medical problems in others, including Graves' disease, vitiligo, rheumatic fever, multiple sclerosis, and hypocomplementemia. Henoch-Schönlein purpura has been described in IgA deficiency (Martini et al., 1985). Cholelithiasis has been described in several children with selective IgA deficiency (Danon et al., 1983).

Gastrointestinal Pathology

Several studies on the pathology and immunology of the gastrointestinal tract in IgA deficiency have been conducted. The main immunologic difference between the IgA-deficient and the normal intestinal tract is the substitution of IgM-secreting plasma cells for IgA-secreting cells (McClelland et al., 1979; Plebani et al., 1983; Klemola, 1988), even though there are some IgA-bearing B cells in the peripheral blood of IgA-deficient subjects (Scotta et al., 1982). This difference is evident in both healthy and ill IgA-deficient subjects. When nodular lymphoid hyperplasia develops, the nodules contain a proliferation of IgM plasma cells. This is in contrast with the lymphoid nodules of hypogammaglobulinemic patients, which contain a reduced number of plasma cells generally and an expanded population of immature B lymphocytes (Asherson and Webster, 1980).

Another gastrointestinal abnormality in IgA deficiency involves the intraepithelial lymphocytes in the intestinal tract. The lamina propria of the normal intestinal mucosa contains many T lymphocytes, but IgA-deficient individuals have an increased number of these cells (Kwitko et al., 1982). In both normal and IgA-deficient subjects, these cells express CD8, the T-suppressor cell phenotype. These CD8 cells may serve to limit local antibody production, cytokine secretion, or both. In agreement with this, there are increased CD8 cells in the epithelium following gluten challenge of both IgA-deficient and non–IgA-deficient celiac patients (Klemola, 1988). This implies that a sensitizing antigen stimulates the appearance of suppressor T lymphocytes.

Nonimmunologic abnormalities of the mucosal architecture may also be present. In one study, goblet cells were reportedly increased in the nasal mucosa in IgA deficiency (Karlson et al., 1985) but in another report were not present in increased amounts in the intestinal tract (Klemola, 1988).

Ultrastructural abnormalities of the gastrointestinal surface epithelium have been reported in IgA deficiency, including areas of missing glycocalyx and enterocytes with "frayed" microvilli (Giorgi et al., 1986). These abnormalities were found in the absence of associated disease and were thought to be characteristic of "normal" IgA-deficient individuals. The lesions described may permit the absorption of antigens from the intestinal lumen, even in the presence of compensatory mechanisms. IgA-deficient patients fed polyethylene glycol polymers have an abnormally large urinary excretion of high-molecular-weight polymers, indicating excess gastrointestinal absorption of high-molecular-weight substances (Cunningham-Rundles et al., 1988). Because polyethylene glycol is immunologically inert, this supports the hypothesis that structural gastrointestinal lesions are present in IgA deficiency.

Neurologic Disease

There have been a number of reported cases of selective IgA deficiency and mental retardation (West et al., 1962; Levin et al., 1963; Haddow et al., 1970). This is of interest because retardation also occurs in patients with ataxia-telangiectasia, most of whom have IgA deficiency (Aguilar et al., 1968). Ataxia-telangiectasia is a complex disorder, however, with several degenerative and demyelinating changes that are not clearly related to IgA deficiency.

The relationship of IgA deficiency to neurologic disease is complicated by the fact that anticonvulsant therapy can, for unknown reasons, reduce serum IgA levels. Hydantoin (Dilantin) has been implicated most often (Sorrell et al., 1971; Ruff et al., 1987), but sodium valproate can also reduce the serum IgA level (Joubert et al., 1977). In epileptics treated with hydantoin who were found to be IgA-deficient, the most prevalent HLA haplotypes were HLA-A1, HLA-A2, and HLA-B8 (Shakir et al., 1978). Serum IgA levels, however, are also sometimes low in untreated epileptic patients. Autoantibodies to muscle and brain nicotinic acetylcho-line receptors were found in three epileptics with IgA deficiency (Fontana et al., 1976, 1978).

Autoimmunity

Several autoimmune diseases are associated with selective IgA deficiency. Based on extensive reviews (Ammann and Hong, 1970, 1971b; Hong and Ammann, 1989; Cunningham-Rundles et al., 1981) autoimmunity may represent the most common association with IgA deficiency (Table 14–4). The most frequent of these conditions are juvenile rheumatoid arthritis, adult rheumatoid arthritis, and systemic lupus erythematosus.

The sera of IgA-deficient subjects often contain autoantibodies, even in the absence of autoimmune illness. Antibodies against thyroglobulin, thyroid microsomal antigens, basement membrane, smooth muscle cells, pancreatic cells, nuclear proteins, cardiolipin, human collagen, and adrenal cells have been identified (Ammann and Hong, 1970, 1971b; Ablin, 1972; Wells et al., 1973; Cunningham-Rundles et al., 1981; Pascual-Salcedo et al., 1988).

Cunningham-Rundles and colleagues (1981) found that IgA-deficient patients with high titers of antibodies to cow's milk are also more likely to have other autoantibodies. They suggested that IgA-deficient subjects with anti-food antibodies have enhanced gastrointestinal antigen absorption and that food-derived antigens could cross-react with internal tissue antigens. The sera of IgA-deficient individuals contain antibodies to a bovine mucoprotein of the fat globule membrane formed

Table 14–4. Autoimmune Diseases Associated with Selective IgA Deficiency

1. Rheumatoid arthritis (Bluestone et al., 1970; Cassidy et al., 1971)
2. Systemic lupus erythematosus (Ammann and Hong, 1970; Cassidy et al., 1969; Claman et al., 1966, 1970; Smith et al., 1970)
3. Thyroiditis (Ammann and Hong, 1970; 1971b; Cassidy et al., 1969a, 1969b; Goldberg et al., 1968)
4. Still's disease (Cassidy et al., 1968, 1969a, 1969b, 1973; Cassidy and Nordby, 1975; Bluestone et al., 1970)
5. Transfusion reactions (Miller et al., 1970; Schmidt et al., 1969; Vyas et al., 1968; Vyas and Fudenberg, 1969)
6. Pernicious anemia (Hobbs, 1968; Odgers and Wangel, 1968; Soothill et al., 1968; Ginsberg and Mullinax, 1970; Stricker and Linker, 1982)
7. Pulmonary hemosiderosis (Krieger and Brough, 1967; Ammann and Hong, 1970, 1971)
8. Myasthenia gravis (Liblau et al., 1992)
9. Vitiligo (Torrela et al., 1992)
10. Lupoid hepatitis (Claman et al., 1966)
11. Dermatomyositis (Cassidy et al., 1969b; Claman et al., 1970)
12. Coombs' positive hemolytic anemia (Heinz and Boyer, 1963; Hobbs, 1968; Sandler and Zlotnick, 1976)
13. Idiopathic Addison's disease (Francois et al., 1967)
14. Sjögren's syndrome (Claman et al., 1966; Hobbs, 1968)
15. Cerebral vasculitis (Ammann and Hong, 1970)
16. Idiopathic thrombocytopenia purpura (Claman et al., 1966)
17. Regional enteritis (Claman et al., 1970)
18. Ulcerative colitis (Claman et al., 1970)
19. Diabetes mellitus (Smith et al., 1970)
20. 21-Hydroxylase deficiency (Cobain et al., 1985)

by the mammary gland (Butler and Oskvig, 1974) and anti-chicken ovalbumin (Pudiffin et al., 1979), lending weight to this notion. Sera with high levels of immune complexes may potentially stimulate autoantibody production and even autoimmune disease (Cassidy et al., 1969a, 1969b; Ammann and Hong, 1970; Kornstadt and Nordhagen, 1974; Cunningham-Rundles et al., 1981) (see later, Milk Antibodies).

Anti-IgA Antibodies

A significant proportion of IgA-deficient individuals have serum anti-IgA antibodies. In the author's experience, this seems to be the only feature of IgA deficiency that is universally recalled. Blood or blood products given to IgA-deficient individuals with high titers of anti-IgA antibodies can lead to severe, even fatal, transfusion reactions; such reactions are rare, however, despite the high frequency of IgA deficiency in hospitalized patients not screened for anti-IgA antibodies prior to blood transfusions.

Anti-IgA antibodies can be directed to IgA1 (most commonly), IgA2, or the allotypic variant A2m(1) or A2m(2). These antibodies occur with a reported frequency of 9.6% to 44% in IgA-deficient subjects (Strober et al., 1968; Koistinen et al., 1977; Van Munster et al., 1978; Björkander et al., 1987). Anti-IgA antibodies are more common in IgA-deficient individuals with undetectable IgA but may occasionally occur when the IgA level is 10 mg/dl or higher. Ferreira and associates (1988) found that 39% of their IgA-deficient patients had anti-IgA antibodies; 22% of those in the antibody-positive group had IgA levels between 1.1 and 5 mg/dl, and the remaining 78% had IgA levels lower than 1.1 mg/dl.

Anti-IgA antibodies are usually of the IgG1 class, are more closely associated with the presence of HLA-DR3 (Hammerström et al., 1986), and are more common in IgA-deficient subjects who are also IgG2-deficient (Ferreira et al., 1988; Cunningham-Rundles et al., 1993). Because IgA-deficient and IgG2-deficient individuals often have poor antibody responses and may require immunoglobulin treatment (Oxelius et al., 1981), they are at particular risk for infusion reactions during immunoglobulin treatment.

IgA-Related Infusion Reactions

In the past, most IgA-related infusion reactions occurred following blood transfusions (Vyas and Fudenberg, 1969; Vyas et al., 1968; Schmidt et al., 1969; Leikola and Vyas, 1971); with the increased use of intravenous immunoglobulin (IVIG), however, more reactions now result from IVIG infusions. IVIGs contain varying amounts of IgA, but IgA-depleted preparations are available and are usually well tolerated, even in patients with high titers of anti-IgA antibodies (Cunningham-Rundles et al., 1993).

Malignancy

Carcinoma (particularly adenocarcinoma of the stomach) and lymphoma (usually of B-cell origin) are also associated with IgA deficiency (Kersey et al., 1988). Often the lymphomas are extranodal and involve the jejunum. Whether nodular lymphoid hyperplasia leads to lymphoma is not known. In general, IgA deficiency is more common than expected in cancer patients; in one cancer hospital, 12 of 4210 patients had selective IgA deficiency, an incidence of 1 in 342 (0.3%). One patient had gastric cancer and another had primary hepatoma (Cunningham-Rundles et al., 1980). Ten other cancers did not involve the gastrointestinal tract.

Other reported cancers in selective IgA deficiency include carcinoma of the stomach and colon, ovarian cancer, lymphosarcoma, melanoma, immunoblastic lymphoadenopathy, and thymoma (Kersey et al., 1988). One case of multiple neoplasms in an adolescent IgA-deficient child involving the thymus, scalp, hand, eyes, colon, and brain has been reported. This child had an IgA-deficient sibling who died of lymphosarcoma (Hamoudi et al., 1974).

Transient IgA Deficiency

Occasionally, IgA deficiency undergoes spontaneous remission (Blum et al., 1982). Petty and coworkers (1973) gave fresh-frozen plasma repeatedly to an IgA-deficient child with rheumatoid arthritis, resulting in permanent normalization of the serum IgA level. In a few such instances of transient IgA deficiency with recovery, the original IgA level was lower than 5 mg/dl; in most such cases, however, the IgA level is between 5 and 30 mg/dl (i.e., partial IgA deficiency) (Plebani et al., 1986). In this cohort of IgA-deficient subjects, half of those who had partial deficiency underwent spontaneous resolution, whereas none with an IgA level lower than 5 mg/dl experienced spontaneous recovery (Plebani et al., 1986). Resolution of IgA deficiency is much more common in children under 5 years of age (Joller et al., 1981), presumably the result of a delayed maturation of the IgA system.

Acquired IgA Deficiency

IgA deficiency many follow drug therapy or viral infection. Penicillamine (Proesman et al., 1976), sulfasalazine (Leickly and Buckley, 1986), hydantoin (Seager et al., 1975), cyclosporine (Murphy et al., 1993), gold (Johns et al., 1978), fenclofenac (Farr et al., 1985), sodium valproate (Joubert et al., 1977), and captopril (Hammarström et al., 1991) can produce a usually reversible IgA deficiency. On the other hand, congenital rubella and Epstein-Barr virus infections may result in persistent IgA deficiency (Saulsbury, 1989; Soothill et al., 1966).

A unique case of acquired IgA deficiency was reported by Hammarström and colleagues (1985b). They noted that an IgA-deficient bone marrow transplant donor transferred the deficiency to the recipient, who had previously had normal IgA levels.

Partial IgA Deficiency

Many patients have a serum IgA level lower than expected for age (i.e., <2 SDs from the mean, but above

5 mg/dl), a condition termed "partial" IgA deficiency. This is more common in children, presumably because of the immaturity of the IgA system. As noted earlier, such patients are more likely to undergo spontaneous remission than patients with an IgA level lower than 5 mg/dl. Many patients with partial IgA deficiency have normal levels of salivary IgA and are generally healthy. Partial IgA deficiency can be the result of deletions of genes controlling either the α1 or α2 chains, a condition termed *selective IgA1* (or *IgA2*) *subclass deficiency.*

Selective IgA Subclass Deficiency

In rare cases, IgA1 or IgA2 deficiency has been identified as a result of gene deletions on chromosome 14. Sometimes the α1 gene is deleted along with other heavy-chain genes (Olsson et al., 1991) (Fig. 14–2). The first case of selective IgA subclass deficiency was identified in an inbred Tunisian Berber family. The propositus was a healthy, 75-year-old woman with absent serum IgA1, IgG1, IgG2, and IgG4; increased IgG3, IgA2, and IgM; and normal IgE. The gene deletions included three IgG subclass genes, γ1, γ2, and γ4, and the pseudo-ε and α1 genes (Lefranc et al., 1982). Two brothers and one sister of the propositus were apparently heterozygous for this defect. Presumably, the good health of the index case was due to increased serum IgG3 and IgM levels and the presence of IgA2.

A similar, unrelated, Tunisian family was described by Lefranc and colleagues (1983). In this family, a 45-year-old Tunisian man whose only medical condition was a chronic cough had deleted genes for IgG1, IgG2, IgG4, and IgA1. Two other family members had two different chromosomal deletions, one a small deletion of the α1 gene and the other a larger deletion involving the γ1, γ2, γ4, and α1 genes.

Migone and associates (1984) and Carbonara and Demarchi (1986) reported additional families in whom similar deletions were found. Deletion of the α2 gene occurs less commonly than deletions involving α1 genes, but in one case, the α2 gene was deleted in conjunction with the pseudo-ε, γ2, γ4, and ε genes (Bottaro et al., 1989).

From these studies, it appears that there may be instability of a region of chromosome 14, with a potential "hot" recombination region being present between the γ2 and the switch α2 loci (Migone et al., 1984; Chaabani et al., 1985). Presumably, because of the location of this hot spot, no individuals have been both IgA1-deficient and IgA2-deficient.

To ascertain the frequency of such heavy-chain gene deletions, Carbonara and Demarchi (1986) studied 5000 normal Italian blood donors and found two subjects who lacked IgG2, IgG4, IgE, and IgA1. Although gene deletion is probably a rare cause of IgA1 deficiency, the data suggest that if the frequency of homozygous deletions were as high as that identified by this study (1/5000), the actual gene frequency might be of the order of 1/70.

Selective absence of IgA2 has been reported in a mother and daughter (Van Loghem et al., 1983). The mother had a low level of IgA1 and antibodies to IgA2, and the daughter had a normal IgA1 level. Both had normal IgG subclass levels. The molecular defect is not known.

Pathogenesis

T-cell abnormalities have been sought in IgA deficiency because a T-cell regulatory abnormality seems likely. In athymic or thymectomized animals, T cells are involved in B-cell differentiation into IgA-secreting plasma cells (McGhee et al., 1989). Neonatal thymectomy leads to IgA deficiency (Benveniste et al., 1969; Perey et al., 1970). The thymically impaired nude mouse is IgA-deficient (Pritchard et al., 1973). A reversible T-cell influence might explain why IgA deficiency can resolve spontaneously after exposure to certain drugs. Despite these reasons for suspecting a T-cell defect in IgA deficiency, few IgA-deficient patients seem to have identifiable defects using current analytical methods (see later, Cytogenetics).

3'- V – D – J – μ – δ – γ3 – γ1 – ψε1 – α1 – ψγ1 – γ2 – γ4 – ε – α2 – 3'

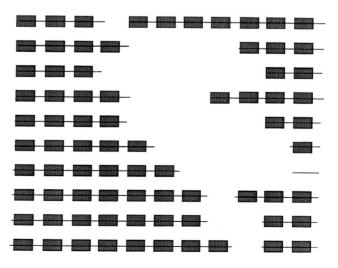

Figure 14–2. Immunoglobulin heavy-chain genes. The human immunoglobulin heavy-chain genes are grouped on chromosome 14 in the order shown. Deletions of certain genes can occur because of homologous recombination; the known deletion haplotypes are shown as gaps in the sequence. The α1 and α2 genes are not deleted together; IgA deficiency has not arisen by such deletions, but IgA2 or IgA1 deficiency is the result. (Adapted from Olsson PG, Hofker MH, Walter MA, et al. Ig H chain variable and C region genes in common variable immunodeficiency. J Immunol 147:2540–2546, 1991.)

Studies have shown that IgA deficiency is associated with certain major histocompatibility complex (MHC) haplotypes (see later, IgA Deficiency and the MHC). This suggests that the inheritance of a certain gene in the MHC area of chromosome 6 confers susceptibility to IgA deficiency. A gene of this sort may potentially activate IgA B-cell maturation.

Genetics

Patterns of Inheritance

In most cases, IgA deficiency appears to be inherited in a sporadic fashion. Many familial cases, however, have been described (Fudenberg et al., 1962; Kirkpatrick and Ruth, 1966; Goldberg et al., 1968; Huntley and Stephenson, 1968; Natvig et al., 1971; Tomkin et al., 1971; Nell et al., 1972; Beerman and Holm, 1974; Koistinen, 1976; Oen et al., 1982). Modes of inheritance reported include autosomal recessive (Van Loghem, 1974; Koistinen, 1976), multifactorial (Grundbacher, 1972; Nell et al., 1972; Buckley, 1975), and autosomal dominant with variable (Stocker et al., 1968; Vassallo et al., 1970) or incomplete expression (Cleland and Bell, 1978).

How often are relatives of IgA-deficient subjects also IgA-deficient? Oen and colleagues (1982) studied relatives of 60 IgA-deficient donors. In 48 families, no additional IgA-deficient members were discovered. In 21 of these families, all first-degree relatives of at least two consecutive generations were studied. For the remaining 12 families, IgA deficiency was found in three generations in one family, in two generations in six families, and in one generation in five families. Thus, among first-degree relatives of affected blood donors, the prevalence of IgA deficiency was 7.5%, a 38-fold increase over that of unrelated donors. As noted earlier, IgA deficiency is more common in the children of IgA-deficient women than in the offspring of IgA-deficient men (Petty et al., 1985).

IgA deficiency is also not uncommon in family members of patients with common variable immunodeficiency (CVI). Several families have shown IgA deficiency in the first generation, hypogammaglobulinemia in the second generation, and IgA deficiency in the third generation (Wollheim et al., 1964; Rosner et al., 1978; Ashman et al., 1992). This suggests that IgA deficiency and common variable immunodeficiency are genetically related diseases.

Cytogenetics

IgA deficiency has been reported in children with chromosomal abnormalities, particularly those involving chromosome 18 (Table 14–5). Ring chromosome 18 and deletion of the short, or long arm of chromosome 18 have been described. These patients have other congenital defects, such as facial, ear, and hand abnormalities; growth retardation; muscular hypotonia; and mental retardation. The 18q− syndrome (long-arm deletion) is a predictable syndrome of mental retardation, short stature, hypotonia, and facial and hand abnormalities (Werteleki and Gerald, 1971; Wilson et al., 1979). To discern which area of the long arm leads to these abnormalities when deleted, Wilson and associates (1979) studied patients with overlapping areas of deletions. The consistently deleted band was 18q21.3, but only two of these patients were IgA-deficient.

About half of patients with the 18p− syndrome and ring chromosome 18 are IgA-deficient (Lewkonia et al., 1980.) How these abnormalities lead to IgA deficiency is not well understood because no particular area of chromosome 18 is consistently abnormal or deleted.

IgA deficiency occurring in other chromosome abnormalities include a Turner syndrome variant with an Xq isochromosome (Silver et al., 1973; Choudat et al., 1979), IgE deficiency with multibranched chromosomes 1, 9, and 16 (Tiepolo et al., 1979), and Klinefelter's syndrome (Tsung and Ajlouni, 1978). IgA deficiency has been associated with the rare 20-nail dystrophy (Leong et al., 1982) and with alpha$_1$-antitrypsin deficiency (Casterline et al., 1978; Ostergaard, 1982). This latter association is of particular interest because alpha$_1$-antitrypsin is encoded near the α chain of IgA on chromosome 14 (Cox et al., 1982).

Most IgA-deficient individuals without physical or mental deficiencies, however, have no chromosome abnormalities. Herrmann and associates (1982) found no chromosome abnormalities in 70 IgA-deficient blood donors and in 10 symptomatic IgA deficient patients. Taalman and coworkers (1987) reported that 2 of 17 of the IgA-deficient children studied had chromosome abnormalities, but both children had pronounced physical and mental abnormalities.

IgA Deficiency and the Major Histocompatibility Complex

An association between IgA deficiency and certain HLA types of the MHC has been reported. In diabetes mellitus and concomitant IgA deficiency, HLA-B8 frequency was significantly increased (Van Thiel et al., 1977; Smith et al., 1978; Perez-Jimenez et al., 1981; Lakhanpal et al., 1988). Juvenile-onset diabetes mellitus itself, however, is associated with HLA-B8 (and HLA-DR3), and therefore a relationship between HLA-B8 and IgA deficiency may be secondary to this disease association. Similarly, there is an increased frequency of HLA-A1 and HLA-B8 in patients with autoimmune disorders and IgA deficiency (Ambrus et al., 1977), but again, this may result from the HLA-B8–autoimmunity association. In one study of IgA-deficient patients with recurrent upper respiratory tract infections, no association with HLA-B8 was found (Seignalet et al., 1978). In a group of IgA-deficient patients with epilepsy, a striking association with HLA-A2 was identified (Fontana et al., 1978).

Hammarström and Smith (1983) studied 21 unrelated healthy IgA-deficient Swedish blood donors and noted a significant increase in HLA-A1 ($P > .05$), HLA-B8 ($P > .01$), and HLA-DR3 ($P > .001$). This same group found no HLA-B8 predominance in selective

Table 14–5. Chromosome Abnormalities in Selective IgA Deficiency

Chromosome or Syndrome Involved	Associated Features	Reference
Chromosome 18		
18p –	Retardation and multiple anomalies	Ruvalcaba and Thuline (1969)
18p –	Multiple anomalies	Ogata et al. (1977)
18p –	Growth hormone deficiency	Leisti et al. (1973)
18q –	Multiple anomalies	Feingold et al. (1969)
18q –	Cleft palate, mental and growth retardation	Lewkonia et al. (1980)
18q –	Hypothyroidism	Faed et al. (1972)
18q –	—	Steward et al. (1970)
18q –	Dysmorphic features, pernicious anemia	Stricker and Linker (1982)
18q22 –	—	Wilson et al. (1979)
18q + mosaic	Retardation, multiple dysmorphic features	Lewkonia et al. (1980)
Ring 18	Multiple dysmorphic features, retardation	Finley et al. (1969)
Ring 18/18p	Short stature, hypotonia, facial abnormalities	Taalman et al. (1987)
Ring 18, trisomy 21		Burgio et al. (1980)
17–18p –, 21–22q	Two primary cancers	Goh et al. (1976)
Ring 22	Microcephaly, large, low-set ears, epicanthal fold, syndactyly of toes, unstable gait, mental retardation	Taalman et al. (1987)
Turner's syndrome	Changes of Turner's syndrome	Silver et al. (1973)
Xq isochromosome		Choudat et al. (1979)
Branched chromosomes 1, 9, and 16 (lymphocytes only)	IgE deficiency, recurrent pulmonary infections, neurologic degeneration	Tiepolo et al. (1979)
Polymorphic chromosome changes	—	Muñoz-López et al. (1977)
Klinefelter's syndrome	Changes of Klinefelter's syndrome	Tsung and Ajlouni (1978)
Karyotype instability with multiple 7/14 and 7/7 rearrangements	Microcephaly, growth retardation	Hustinx et al. (1979)

IgA-deficient patients with respiratory tract infections (Hammerström et al., 1984). In another Scandinavian study, 14 of 32 (44%) unrelated healthy IgA-deficient blood donors had HLA-A1 and HLA-B8, as compared with 25% in the healthy general population (Jersild et al., 1983). In a study of 23,782 healthy American blood donors, 67 IgA-deficient individuals were identified; HLA typing in 36 indicated a significant association with both HLA-A1, HLA-29, HLA-B8, and HLA-B14 (Strothman et al., 1986).

Wilton and colleagues (1985) studied HLA types in 17 individuals from 13 Australian families with complete or partial IgA deficiency (IgA levels, <30 mg/dl). They also studied DR antigens and complement components C4a, C4b, and Bf. Their report noted an increased frequency of HLA-A1, HLA-B8, and HLA-DR3; in addition, of the 29 independent haplotypes observed in the IgA-deficient subjects, 22 included deletions, duplications, or a defective C4 or 21-hydroxylase locus. The investigators suggested that there may be a gene regulating serum IgA concentration in the MHC region of chromosome 6 and that associations with three main extended haplotypes explained most previously reported HLA-IgA deficiency associations (Table 14–6). A survey of 150 other individuals with at least one of these haplotypes revealed only two who were IgA-deficient, which suggested recessive inheritance, with penetrance determined by another factor that was not linked to the MHC (Wilton et al., 1985). The HLA-B14, C4A2, C4B1/2, BfS haplotype (which also carries a C4B duplication) is itself associated with 21-hydroxylase IgA deficiencies (Cobain et al., 1985).

The MHC class III genes encoding complement components C2, C4A, and C4B and 21-hydroxylase have also been studied in patients with IgA deficiency or CVI. Twelve of 19 patients with CVI (63%) and 9 of 16 with IgA deficiency (56%) had rare C2, C4A, or 21-hydroxylase A deletions, compared with 5 of 34 (14%) in healthy individuals (Schaffer et al., 1989, 1991). Olerup and associates (1990, 1992) implicated the amino acid at codon 57 of the HLA-DQ-β chain in susceptibility to IgA deficiency. The *protective allele* had aspartic acid at position 57, whereas the *susceptibility allele* had an alanine or valine at this position. Despite these findings, other factors in addition to the genetic constituent must be involved; for example, several pairs of discordant twins have been reported, but only one of each set had IgA deficiency (Huntley and Stephenson, 1968; Lewkonia et al., 1976).

Laboratory Findings

Milk Antibodies

A common feature of IgA deficiency is the occurrence of increased levels of serum antibodies to cow's

Table 14–6. Histocompatibility Supratypes with IgA Deficiency

	Class I		Class III			Class II	
A1 Cw7	B8	C4AQO	C4B1	Bfs	DR3	
—	Bw65(14)	C4A2	C4B1/s	Bfs	DR1	DQW1
—	Bw57(17)	C4A6	C4B1	Bfs	—	

Data from Wilton et al., 1985; Schaffer et al., 1991; Olerup et al., 1992.

milk proteins and other proteins of Bovidae origin (cow, sheep, and goat) (Lopez and Hyslop, 1968; Buckley and Dees, 1969; Ammann and Hong, 1971a; Huntley et al., 1971). When these antibodies are in high titer, they can be visualized by the double-diffusion procedure in agar gels and are known as *milk precipitins* (Fig. 14–3) (Buckley and Dees, 1969). Up to 50% of IgA-deficient individuals have precipitins to cow's milk (Tomasi and Katz, 1971; Cunningham-Rundles et al., 1978, 1979a). The antibody appears to be directed against bovine IgM, a component of cow's milk (Tomasi and Katz, 1971). Most IgA-deficient individuals have IgG1 and IgG4 antibodies directed to ovalbumin and β-lactoglobulin and IgG1, IgG2, IgG3, and IgG4 (IgG1 > IgG2 > IgG3 > IgG4) antibodies to casein, bovine IgM, and gliadin, a component of wheat gluten (Husby et al., 1992).

The presence in IgA-deficient serum of large amounts of IgG milk antibodies directed to bovine IgM, and that cross-react with sheep and goat IgM, can cause confusion when such sera are examined for IgA deficiency if the IgA antiserum used is produced in these species. A false-positive result in radial immunodiffusion or in nephelometry can occur, leading to the interpretation of normal or increased IgA levels (Leikola and Vyas, 1971; Ammann and Hong, 1971a). This problem is not entirely solved by switching to rabbit antiserum because the sera of IgA-deficient subjects

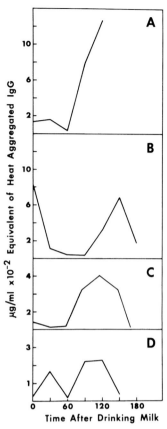

Figure 14–4. Immune complexes in IgA deficiency. Four IgA-deficient subjects (A–D) were given 100 ml of cow's milk to drink. Before and at 30-minute intervals after milk ingestion, the amount of circulating immune complex was measured in the serum using the Raji cell radioimmunoassay. (Adapted from Cunningham-Rundles C, Brandeis WE, Good RA, et al. Bovine antigens and the formation of circulating immune complexes in selective IgA deficiency. J Clin Invest 64:270–272, 1979. Copyright permission of The American Society for Clinical Investigation.)

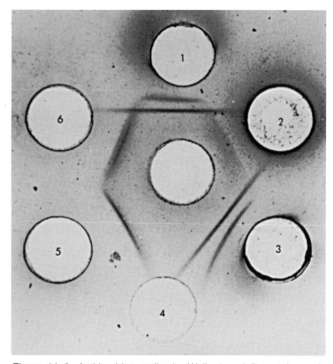

Figure 14–3. Anti-bovidae antibody. Wells 1 and 3 contain cow's milk, well 2 contains goat serum, well 4 contains horse serum, well 5 contains sheep serum, and well 6 contains cow serum. The center well is filled with serum from a patient with selective IgA deficiency. A precipitin line showing identity is seen between cow, sheep, and goat sera and cow's milk but not with horse serum. An additional precipitin line is seen with cow's milk, which is not present in cow, sheep, or goat serum.

may contain antibodies directed to rabbit IgM (Truedsson et al., 1982).

Immune Complexes

In IgA deficiency, the gastrointestinal tract is sufficiently leaky so that in most IgA-deficient individuals, circulating immune complexes develop in their serum 15 to 60 minutes after drinking a glass of milk (Fig. 14–4) (Cunningham-Rundles et al., 1978, 1979a, 1979b). The antigens identified in these immune complexes are bovine milk protein antigens (Cunningham-Rundles, 1981). These immune complexes are apparently benign, because renal disease, vasculitis, and arthritis are not common in IgA deficiency. Arthralgia, autoimmune disease, and neurologic disease, however, are common in IgA-deficient patients with high titers of immune complexes (Cunningham-Rundles et al., 1981).

Other Humoral Abnormalities

Other immunologic abnormalities in some IgA-deficient subjects include increased levels of serum IgG,

IgM, and/or IgE (but not IgD) (Ammann and Hong, 1971b; Buckley and Fiscus, 1975; Plebani et al., 1983). Other studies have demonstrated the presence of low-molecular-weight serum IgM (monomeric IgM instead of pentameric IgM) (Kwitko et al., 1982), increased J-chain–positive IgG B cells following stimulation with pokeweed mitogen (Yasuda et al., 1981), and a common cross-reactive idiotype on certain antibodies (Cunningham-Rundles and Feng, 1988).

An associated IgA2 deficiency or IgG2 and IgG4 deficiency may occur (Oxelius et al., 1981). The frequency of the IgA-IgG2 dual deficiency may differ in ethnic groups; Oxelius and coworkers (1981) found that 7 out of 37 (19%) IgA-deficient Swedish patients were IgG2-deficient, whereas Cunningham-Rundles and colleagues (1983), using the same methods, found that 3 out of 39 (8%) IgA-deficient American patients were IgG2-deficient.

IgA B Cells

A fundamental defect in IgA deficiency is the failure of IgA-bearing B lymphocytes to mature into IgA-secreting plasma cells. Examination of the α heavy-chain genes and their switch regions have shown no abnormalities in the few patients examined (Hammarström et al., 1985c). There are decreased (but not absent) numbers of IgA-bearing B cells in the peripheral circulation in these patients (Lawton et al., 1972), and they possess an immature phenotype—that is, IgA-bearing B cells that are also positive for IgM and IgD (Conley and Cooper, 1981). There is a paucity of IgA-bearing gastrointestinal plasma cells (Crabbé and Heremans, 1967).

This failure of terminal B-cell differentiation has been attributed to several factors:

1. Inadequate or defective T-helper cells (King et al., 1979).

2. The presence of IgA-specific T-cell suppressors (Waldmann et al., 1976; Atwater and Tomasi, 1978; Schwartz, 1980).

3. An intrinsic B-cell defect (Cassidy et al., 1979; Inoue et al., 1984).

4. The presence of maternal anti-IgA antibodies that suppress fetal IgA development (Petty et al., 1985).

T-Cell Abnormalities

Other than the regulatory abnormalities just postulated, T-cell immunity generally appears to be normal in IgA deficiency. Natural killer cells are also normal (Stannegard et al., 1983). Inconsistent cellular abnormalities that have been reported include reduced B-cell expression of IgA Fc receptors (Adachi et al., 1983), low serum thymic factor (Iwata et al., 1981), decreased lymphoproliferative responses to phytohemagglutinin on limiting dilution (Cowan et al., 1980), and reduced interferon-γ production following phytohemagglutinin stimulation (Epstein and Ammann, 1974).

Levitt and Cooper (1981) studied in vitro plasma cell differentiation in a family in whom three members were IgA-deficient. Two healthy IgA-deficient family members had subtle cellular abnormalities of B and T lymphocytes, whereas lymphocytes of the symptomatic IgA-deficient child had decreased in vitro production of all immunoglobulin classes. Following clinical improvement and plasma infusions from her healthy, nonimmunodeficient father, the child's in vitro lymphocyte culture results became similar to those of her healthy IgA-deficient brother and sister. These data suggest that the mechanisms for IgA deficiency in a given family are inherited.

Pathology

The pathologic findings in selective IgA deficiency depend on the associated diseases, if any. For patients with malabsorption, blunting of villi on jejunal biopsy occurs in patients with selective IgA deficiency and celiac disease. In the few patients studied, lymph node biopsy specimens reveal normal follicle formation and intact thymic-dependent and thymic-independent areas (Hobbs, 1968). As discussed, intestinal biopsy specimens usually reveal abundant plasma cells, mostly secreting IgM (Crabbé et al., 1965; Ammann and Hong, 1971c). A small number of IgA-containing plasma cells (usually IgA2) may be found (Andre et al., 1978).

A few autopsy reports are available. Krieger and Brough (1967) reported an unusual case with pulmonary hemosiderosis, bronchiectasis, and portal fibrosis of the liver. Detailed information was not given on the thymus, although the gland was present. Generalized hypertrophy of the lymph nodes was present along with loss of normal architecture and diminution of the follicles.

In a case of reticulum cell sarcoma and selective IgA deficiency, the autopsy showed massive lymphomatous infiltration of organs (Clinicopathologic Conference, 1962). Lymph node architecture was obliterated, but the thymus morphology was not presented. A patient with selective IgA deficiency and squamous cell carcinoma of the lung demonstrated massive infiltration of lymph nodes and other organs with metastatic tumor cells (Ammann and Hong, 1971b). The patient also had had celiac disease that had responded to a gluten-free diet; at autopsy, the intestinal villi appeared normal.

Immunologic attrition may occur in some individuals with selective IgA deficiency (Clinicopathologic Conference, 1962; Krieger and Brough, 1967; Case Records, 1971, 1975). Immunologic function may be normal during the greater part of the individual's life; with time, however, evidence of waning antibody-mediated and cell-mediated immunity may develop (Hong and Ammann, 1989). Whether this is associated with IgA deficiency or with the attendant illnesses is not known.

Evaluation

When IgA deficiency is identified in a healthy person with no significant medical history, no further evaluation is needed. More commonly, quantitative immunoglobulins are measured because a clinical problem that is difficult to manage has surfaced. In these cases, especially when infection has been present, it is useful to obtain IgG subclass levels. A combined IgA-IgG2 subclass–deficient patient may have a normal IgG level because of the elevation of other IgG subclasses and a history of serious or even life-threatening illness. Such patients may not respond to vaccination with pneumococcal polysaccharide. For these patients, intravenous immunoglobulin (IVIG) is sometimes indicated, but anti-IgA antibodies are common in these patients. Thus, assays for anti-IgA antibodies should be completed prior to IVIG therapy; if antibodies are present, IVIG should be given with trepidation and then under close supervision with premedication. An IgA-depleted IVIG preparation, such as Gammagard, should be used (Ferreira et al., 1988; Cunningham-Rundles et al., 1993).

In IgA-deficient patients with serious or persistent infections, with or without IgG2 subclass deficiency, the antibody responses to polysaccharide antigen (pneumonoccal or meningococcal vaccine) should be tested. Such tests are performed by obtaining a base line serum titer, immunizing, and obtaining a postvaccination serum titer 1 month later. The paired sera should be tested simultaneously to enhance the reliability of the results. Children under 2 years of age have poor responses to polysaccharide vaccines, and testing before age 2 is therefore not useful for these analyses.

Some IgA-deficient patients have persistent allergic symptoms. An allergic evaluation, including skin and/or radioallergosorbent testing, may be indicated.

IgA deficiency can be induced by various drugs (see earlier, Acquired IgA Deficiency). In IgA-deficient patients taking such a drug, a substitute drug (e.g., phenobarbital for phenytoin) can be given for 3 to 6 months and the IgA level redetermined. Sometimes, drug-induced IgA depression is not reversible.

Serum immunoglobulin studies on family members to ascertain the inheritance pattern, although of scientific interest, is not generally indicated. Determining immunoglobulin levels is recommended, however, for symptomatic family members. Similarly, HLA typing in patients or their families, except for research purposes, is not indicated. IgA-deficient patients with certain HLA types are no more likely to have specific medical problems (with the exception that HLA-DR3 IgA-deficient subjects have a higher incidence of anti-IgA antibodies) (Hammerström et al., 1984).

Quantitation of IgA1 and IgA2 levels in the partially IgA-deficient patient is difficult and expensive and not especially informative. In one report, IgA-deficient children (ages 3 to 10 years) had variable IgA1 and IgA2 levels, with both subclasses present in all children studied (Conley et al., 1983).

Although there is an association between IgA deficiency and autoimmune disease, the likelihood of an autoimmune disease developing in an individual IgA-deficient patient is probably low. Thus, extensive screening for autoantibodies is not indicated in the asymptomatic IgA-deficient patient.

Whether anti-IgA antibodies should be determined in all IgA-deficient patients is debatable. Although IgA antibodies can produce serious anaphylactic reactions if blood or blood products (including IVIG) are infused, the likelihood of such a reaction, if no known medical problems exist, is low. If an infusion of blood or blood products is anticipated, screening for IgA antibodies should be carried out. Tests for anti-IgA antibodies are not widely available but can be done in several commercial laboratories.

Management

There is no specific treatment for IgA deficiency because there are no drugs that activate IgA-producing B cells. Theoretically, an infusion of serum IgA or IgA-containing plasma can correct the serum IgA deficiency, but there is little or no transfer of infused IgA into the secretions (Stiehm et al., 1966; Butler et al., 1967). Nonetheless, there have been claims of the successful use of IgA-rich immunoglobulin preparations given intravenously (Blatrix et al., 1977; Skrede et al., 1977) or orally (Eibl et al., 1988). Human colostrum, rich in secretory IgA, has been given orally to a few immunodeficient patients with gastrointestinal disorders (Eibl et al., 1988).

Intermittent or continuous prophylactic antibiotics may be helpful in patients with recurrent respiratory tract infections, particularly those with chronic asthma, bronchitis, or sinusitis.

Associated diseases in IgA deficiency are treated conventionally using standard therapies and the results are equally as successful as those in nonimmunodeficient patients. For example, patients with systemic lupus erythematosus and selective IgA deficiency respond favorably to immunosuppressive treatment. An insufficient number of cases of selective IgA deficiency with associated diseases have been observed to predict their long-term prognosis. IgA-deficient asthmatic patients appear to be more resistant to standard antiasthma therapy, possibly because of their propensity to develop superimposed infections.

For the IgA-deficient individual with concomitant IgG2 subclass deficiency, or impaired antibody responses to bacterial or vaccine antigens, immunoglobulin replacement may be warranted, especially when lung damage is present or recurrent infections are prominent. IVIG in the usual therapeutic doses (300–400 mg/kg body weight, every 3 to 4 weeks) is indicated, using a product low in IgA (e.g., Gammagard SD) to decrease the risk of sensitization.

Transfusions with blood containing IgA may sensitize the selective IgA-deficient patient or may cause an anaphylactic reaction in a sensitized patient with anti-IgA antibodies (Vyas et al., 1968; Schmidt et al., 1969). Thus, patients with selective IgA deficiency who require blood transfusions should be given blood from an IgA-deficient donor or saline-washed erythrocytes. The use of autologous erythrocytes, gathered prior to elective sugery, is also indicated.

IgA-deficient patients, particularly those with anti-IgA antibodies, should wear a Medic-Alert bracelet.*

---

*For more information, the Medic-Alert Foundation can be reached at (415) 541-0900.

The diagnosis, a warning about blood transfusion, and the physician's name are inscribed.

Lactose intolerance is not uncommon in IgA deficiency, and milk should be avoided in lactose-intolerant, IgA-deficient patients. IgA-deficient subjects with milk precipitins probably should also avoid milk, although there is no clear association with disease. In one child who was given a bone marrow transplant for severe combined immunodeficiency, chronic graft-versus-host disease and IgA deficiency developed. His serum had high levels of circulating immune complexes containing milk protein, and ovine casein was detected in his skin. Exclusion of milk from the diet resulted in a precipitous drop of serum immune complex levels, with clinical improvement (Cunningham-Rundles et al., 1981).

Prognosis

Selective IgA deficiency is the mildest form of permanent primary immunodeficiency. In most cases, there are no significant medical problems and the prognosis is excellent. When IgA deficiency is associated with another illness, the prognosis is that of this illness (e.g., lupus erythematosus, juvenile rheumatoid arthritis). Insufficient data are available to determine whether early onset of associated disease is correlated with increased morbidity or mortality.

Selective IgA deficiency in an apparently healthy child, however, should not generate complacency. A reasonable initial search and a periodic review for diseases associated with selective IgA deficiency (see Tables 14–1 and 14–2) should be carried out.

As noted, a few patients with selective IgA deficiency, particularly young children with low but detectable levels of IgA, may recover spontaneously, although this is unusual (Blum et al., 1982).

References

Ablin RJ. Anti-tissue IgG antibodies and deficiency of IgA. Vox Sang 23:371–375, 1972.

Adachi M, Yodoi J, Masuda T, Takatsuki K, Uchino H. Altered expression of lymphocyte Fc receptor in selective IgA deficiency and IgA nephropathy. J Immunol 131:1246–1251, 1983.

Aguilar MM, Kamoshita S, Landing BH, Border E, Sedgwick RP. Pathological observations in ataxia-telangiectasia: report of five cases. J Neuropathol Exp Neurol 27:659–676, 1968.

Ambrus M, Hernadi E, Bajtai G. Prevalence of HLA-A1 and HLA-B8 antigens in selective IgA deficiency. Clin Immunol Immunopathol 7:311–314, 1977.

Ammann AJ, Hong R. Selective IgA deficiency and autoimmunity. Clin Exp Immunol 7:833–838, 1970.

Ammann AJ, Hong R. Anti-antisera antibody as a cause of double precipitin rings in immunoglobulin quantitation and its relation to milk precipitins. J Immunol 106:567–569, 1971a.

Ammann AJ, Hong R. Selective IgA deficiency: presentation of 30 cases and a review of the literature. Medicine 60:223–236, 1971b.

Ammann AJ, Hong R. Unique antibody to basement membrane in patients with selective IgA deficiency and celiac disease. Lancet 1:1264–1267, 1971c.

Andre C, Andre F, Fargier MC. Distribution of IgA1 and IgA2 plasma cells in various normal human tissues and in the jejunum of plasma IgA deficient patients. Clin Exp Immunol 33:327–331, 1978.

Arnold RR, Cole MF, Prince S, McGhee J. Secretory IgM antibodies

to *Streptococcus mutans* in subjects with selective IgA deficiency. Clin Immunol Immunopathol 8:475–486, 1977.

Asherson GL, Webster ADB. Gastrointestinal tract in hypogammaglobulinemia. In Asherson GL, Webster ADB, eds. Diagnosis and Treatment of Immunodeficiency Diseases. Oxford, Blackwell Scientific, 1980, pp. 61–77.

Ashman RF, Schaffer FM, Kemp JD, Yokoyama WM, Zhu ZB, Cooper MD, Volanakis JE. Genetic and immunologic analysis of a family containing five patients with common variable immune deficiency or selective IgA deficiency. J Clin Immunol 12:406–414, 1992.

Ashraf RN, Jalil F, Zaman S, Karlberg S, Khan SR, Lindblad BS, Hanson LÅ. Breast feeding and protection against neonatal sepsis in a high risk population. Arch Dis Child 66:488–490, 1991.

Atwater JS, Tomasi TB. Suppressor cells and IgA deficiency. Clin Immunol Immunopathol 9:379–382, 1978.

Bachmann R. Studies on the serum gamma A-globulin level. III. The frequency of A-gamma-A-globulinemia. Scand J Clin Lab Invest 17:316–320, 1965.

Barros MD, Porto MHO, Leser PG, Greemach AS, Carniero-Sampaio MMS. Study of colostrum of a patient with selective IgA deficiency. Allergol Immunopathol (Madr) 13:331–334, 1985.

Baker J, Hong R, Dick E, Reed C. Asthma, IgA deficiency, and respiratory infections. J Allergy Clin Immunol 58:713–716, 1976.

Beerman B, Holm G. Familial IgA defect. Scand J Haematol 12:307–311, 1974.

Benbassat J, Keren L, Zlotnic A. Hepatitis in selective IgA deficiency. Br Med J 4:762–763, 1973.

Benveniste J, Lespinats G, Salomon JC. Study of immunoglobulins in axenic mice thymectomized at birth. Proc Soc Exp Biol Med 130:936–940, 1969.

Björkander J, Bake B, Oxelius VA, Hanson LA. Impaired lung function in patients with IgA deficiency and low levels of IgG2 or IgG3. N Engl J Med 313:720–724, 1985.

Björkander J, Hammarström L, Smith CI, Buckley RH, Cunningham-Rundles C, Hanson LA. Immunoglobulin prophylaxis in patients with antibody deficiency syndromes and anti-IgA antibodies. J Clin Immunol 7:8–15, 1987.

Blatrix G, Thebault J, Steinbuch M. Propriétés et indications d'une nouvelle préparation d'immunoglobulines (IgGAM) enrichie en IgA et IgM. Rev Fr Transfus Immunohematol 20:419–426, 1977.

Bluestone R, Goldberg LS, Katz RM, Marchesano JM, Calabro JJ. Juvenile rheumatoid arthritis: a serologic survey of 200 consecutive patients. J Pediatr 77:98–102, 1970.

Blum PM, Stiehm ER, Hong R. Spontaneous recovery of selective IgA deficiency: additional case report and review. Clin Pediatr 21:77–80, 1982.

Bottaro A, de Marchi M, de Lange GG, Carbonara AO. Human Ig markers. Exp Clin Immunogenet 6:55–59, 1989.

Brandtzaeg P. Two types of IgA immunocytes in man. Nature New Biol 243:142–143, 1973.

Brandtzaeg P. Presence of J chains in human immunocytes containing various immunoglobulin classes. Nature 252:418–420, 1974.

Brandtzaeg P, Karlsson G, Hansson G, Petruson B, Björkander J, Hanson LÅ. The clinical condition of IgA-deficient patients is related to the proportion of IgD- and IgM-producing cells in their nasal mucosa. Clin Exp Immunol 67:626–636, 1986.

Buckley RH. Clinical and immunologic features of selective IgA deficiency. Birth Defects 11:134–141, 1975.

Buckley RH, Dees SC. Correlation of milk precipitins with IgA deficiency. N Engl J Med 281:465–469, 1969.

Buckley RH, Fiscus SA. Serum IgD and IgE concentrations in immunodeficiency diseases. J Clin Invest 55:157–161, 1975.

Budman DR, Koziner B, Cunningham-Rundles C, Filippa D, Good RA. IgA deficiency associated with angioimmunoblastic lymphadenopathy. N Engl J Med 298:1204, 1978.

Burgio GR, Duse M, Monafo V, Ascione A, Nespoli L. Selective IgA deficiency: clinical and immunological evaluation of 50 pediatric patients. J Pediatr 133:101–106, 1980.

Burks AW Jr, Steele RW. Selective IgA deficiency. Ann Allergy 57:3–13, 1986.

Butler JE, Oskvig R. Cancer, autoimmunity and IgA deficiency, related by a common antigen-antibody system. Nature 249:830–833, 1974.

Butler WT, Rosen R, Waldmann TA. The mechanism of appearance of immunoglobulin A in nasal secretion in man. J Clin Invest 46:1883–1887, 1967.

Carbonara AO, Demarchi M. Ig isotype deficiency caused by gene deletions. Monogr Allergy 20:13–17, 1986.

Case records of the Massachusetts General Hospital. N Engl J Med 284:39–47, 1971.

Case records of the Massachusetts General Hospital. N Engl J Med 284:39–47, 1975.

Cassidy JT, Burt A. Isolated IgA deficiency in juvenile rheumatoid arthritis (abstract). Arthritis Rheum 10:272, 1967.

Cassidy JT, Burt A, Petty R, Sullivan D. Selective IgA deficiency and autoimmunity (letter). N Engl J Med 284:985, 1971.

Cassidy JT, Burt A, Petty R, Sullivan D. Selective IgA deficiency in connective tissue diseases (letter). N Engl J Med 280:275, 1969a.

Cassidy JT, Nordby GL. Human serum immunoglobulin concentrations: prevalence of immunoglobulin deficiencies. J Allergy Clin Immunol 55:35–48, 1975.

Cassidy JT, Oldham G, Platts-Mills TAE. Functional assessment of a B cell defect in patients with selective IgA deficiency. Clin Exp Immunol 35:296–299, 1979.

Cassidy JT, Petty R, Burt A, Sullivan D. Anti-IgA antibodies in patients with selective IgA deficiency and connective tissue diseases (abstract). Clin Res 17:351, 1969b.

Cassidy JT, Petty RE, Sullivan DB. Abnormalities in the distribution of serum immunoglobulin concentration in juvenile rheumatoid arthritis. Clin Invest 52:1931–1936, 1973.

Casterline CL, Evans R, Battista VC, Talamo RC. IgA deficiency and Pi ZZ-antitrypsin deficiency. Chest 73:885–886, 1978.

Chaabani H, Bech-Hansen TN, Cox DW. A multigene deletion within the immunoglobulin heavy chain region. Am J Hum Genet 37:1164–1171, 1985.

Chodirker WB, Tomasi TB. Gammaglobulins: quantitative relationships in human serum and nonvascular fluids. Science 142:1080–1081, 1963.

Choudat D, Taillemite JL, Hirsch-Marie H, Choubrac P. Lebas FX. Relation entre isochromosome Xq et deficit serique en immunoglobuline A. Nouv Presse Med 8:2419–2420, 1979.

Claman HN, Hartley TF, Merrill D. Hypogammaglobulinemia, primary and secondary: immunoglobulin levels (gamma-G, gamma-A, gamma-M) in one hundred and twenty-five patients. J Allergy 38:215–225, 1966.

Claman HN, Merrill DA, Peakman D, Robinson A. Isolated severe gamma-A deficiency: immunoglobulin levels, clinical disorders, and chromosome studies. J Lab Clin Med 75:307–315, 1970.

Clarkson AR, Woodroffe AJ, Aaronson I. IgA nephropathy and Henoch-Schönlein purpura. In Schrier RW, Gottschalk CW, eds. Diseases of the Kidney, 4th ed. Boston, Little, Brown, 1988, pp. 2061–2083.

Cleland LG, Bell DA. The occurrence of systemic lupus erythematosus in two kindreds in association with selective IgA deficiency. J Rheumatol 5:288–293, 1978.

Clinicopathologic Conference. Rademacher's disease. Am J Med 32:80–95, 1962.

Cobain TJ, Stuckey MS, McCluskey J, Wilton A, Gedeon A, Garlepp MJ, Christiansen FT, Dawkins RL. The coexistence of IgA deficiency and 21-hydroxylase deficiency marked by specific supratypes. Ann N Y Acad Sci 458:76–84, 1985.

Collins-Williams C, Kokubu HL, Lamenza C, Nizami R, Chuiu AW, Lewis-McKinley C, Comerford TA, Varga EA. Incidence of isolated deficiency of IgA in the serum of Canadian children. Ann Allergy 30:11–16, 1972.

Conley ME, Arbetter A, Douglas SD. Serum levels of IgA1 and IgA2 in children and in patients with IgA deficiency. Mol Immunol 20:977–981, 1983.

Conley ME, Delacroix DL. Intravascular and mucosal immunoglobulin A: two separate but related systems of immune defence? Ann Intern Med 106:892–899, 1987.

Conley ME, Cooper MD. Immature IgA B cells in IgA-deficient patients. N Engl J Med 305:495–497, 1981.

Conley ME, Cooper MD, Michael AF. Selective deposition of immunoglobulin A in immunoglobulin A nephropathy, anaphylactoid purpura, nephritis and systemic lupus erythematosus. J Clin Invest 66:1432–1436, 1980.

Cowan MJ, Fujiwara P, Ammann AJ. Cellular immune defect in selective IgA deficiency using a microculture method for PHA

stimulation and limiting dilution. Clin Immunol Immunopathol 17:595–605, 1980.

Cox DW, Markovic VD, Teshima IE. Genes for immunoglobulin heavy chains and for alpha-1-antitrypsin are localized to specific regions of chromosome 14q. Nature 297:428–430, 1982.

Crabbé PA, Carbonara AO, Heremans JF. The normal human intestinal mucosa as a major source of plasma cells containing gamma-A immunoglobulin. Lab Invest 14:235–248, 1965.

Crabbé PA, Heremans JF. Lack of gamma A-immunoglobulin in serum of patients with steatorrhea. Gut 7:119–125, 1966.

Crabbé PA, Heremans JF. Selective IgA deficiency with steatorrhea. A new syndrome. Am J Med 42:319–326, 1967.

Cunningham-Rundles C. The identification of antigens in circulating immune complexes by an enzyme-linked immunosorbent assay: detection of bovine k-casein IgG complexes in human sera. Eur J Immunol 11:504–509, 1981.

Cunningham-Rundles C. IgA deficiency. Immunol Allergy Clin North Am 8:435–440, 1988.

Cunningham-Rundles C. Genetic aspects of immunoglobulin A deficiency. Adv Hum Genet 19:234–265, 1990.

Cunningham-Rundles C, Feng ZK. Analysis of a common inheritable idiotype in IgA-deficient sera using monoclonal antibodies. J Immunol 140:3880–3886, 1988.

Cunningham-Rundles C, Brandeis W, Good RA, Day NK. Milk precipitins, circulating immune complexes and IgA deficiency. Proc Natl Acad Sci U S A 75:3387–3389, 1978.

Cunningham-Rundles C, Brandeis WE, Good RA, Day NK. Bovine antigens and the formation of circulating immune complexes in selective IgA deficiency. J Clin Invest 64:270–272, 1979a.

Cunningham-Rundles C, Brandeis WE, Safai B, O'Reilly R, Day NK, Good RA. Selective IgA deficiency and circulating immune complexes containing bovine proteins in a child with chronic graft vs. host disease. Am J Med 67:883–889, 1979b.

Cunningham-Rundles C, Pudifin DJ, Armstrong D, Good RA. Selective IgA deficiency and neoplasia. Vox Sang 38:61–67, 1980.

Cunningham-Rundles C, Brandeis WE, Pudifin DJ, Day NK, Good RA. Autoimmunity in selective IgA deficiency: relationship to anti-bovine protein antibodies, circulating immune complexes and clinical disease. Clin Exp Immunol 45:299–304, 1981.

Cunningham-Rundles C, Oxelius VA, Good RA. IgG2 and IgG3 subclass deficiencies in selective IgA deficiency in the United States. Birth Defects 19:173–176, 1983.

Cunningham-Rundles C, Magnusson KE, Lindblad BS. Abnormal gastrointestinal absorption of polyethylene glycol in common variable immunodeficiency (abstract). Clin Res 36:65, 1988.

Cunningham-Rundles C, Zhou Z, Mankarious S, Courter S. Long-term use of IgA depleted intravenous immunoglobulin in immunodeficient subjects with anti-IgA antibodies. J Clin Immunol 13:272–278, 1993.

Danon YL, Dinari G, Garty BZ, Horodniceanu C, Nitzan M, Grunebaum M. Cholelithiasis in children with immunoglobulin A deficiency: a new gastroenterologic syndrome. J Pediatr Gastroenterol Nutr 2:663–666, 1983.

De Graeff PA, The TH, van Munster PJ, Out TA, Vossen JM, Zegers BJM. The primary immune response in patients with selective IgA deficiency. Clin Exp Immunol 54:778–784, 1983.

De Laat PCJ, Weemaes CMR, Bakkeren JAJM, van den Brandt FCA, van Lith TGPM, de Graaf R, van Munster PJJ, Stoelinga GBA. Familial selective IgA deficiency with circulating anti-IgA antibodies: a distinct group of patients? Clin Immunol Immunopathol 58:92–101, 1991.

Douglas SD, Davis WC, Fudenberg HH. Granulocytopathies: pleomorphism of neutrophil dysfunction. Am J Med 46:901–909, 1969.

Dubois RS, Roy CC, Fulginiti VA, Merrill DA, Murray RL. Disaccharidase deficiency in children with immunologic deficits. J Pediatr 76:377–385, 1970.

Eibl MM, Wolf HM, Furnkranz H, Rosenkranz A. Prevention of necrotizing enterocolitis in low-birth weight infants by IgA-IgG feeding. N Engl J Med 318:1–7, 1988.

Epstein LB, Ammann AJ. Evaluation of T lymphocyte effector function in immunodeficiency diseases: abnormalities in mitogen-stimulated interferon in patients with selective IgA deficiency. J Immunol 112:617–622, 1974.

Faed MJ, Whyle R, Patterson CR, McCathic M, Robertson J. Deletion of the long arm of chromosome 18 (46, XX, 18q⁻) associated with absence of IgA and hypothyroidism in an adult. J Med Genet 9:102–105, 1972.

Falchuk KR, Falchuk ZM. Selective immunoglobulin A deficiency ulcerative colitis and gluten-sensitive enteropathy—a unique association. Gastroenterology 69:503–506, 1975.

Farr M, Struthers GR, Scott DGI, Bacon PA. Fendofenac-induced selective IgA deficiency in rheumatoid arthritis. J Rheumatol 24:367–369, 1985.

Feingold M, Schwartz RS, Atkins L, Anderson R, Bartsocas CS, Page DL, Littlefield JW. IgA and partial deletion of chromosome 18. Am J Dis Child 117:129–136, 1969.

Ferreira A, Garcia-Rodriguez MC, Lopez-Trascasa M, Pascual-Salcedo D, Fontan G. Anti-IgA antibodies in selective IgA deficiency and in primary immunodeficient patients treated with gammaglobulin. Clin Immunol Immunopathol 47:199–207, 1988.

Finley SC, Finley WH, Uchida IA, Noto TA, Roddam RF. IgA absence associated with ring-18 chromosome. Lancet 1:1095–1096, 1968.

Fontana A, Grob PJ, Sauter R, Joller H. IgA deficiency, epilepsy and hydantoin medication. Lancet 2:228–231, 1976.

Fontana A, Joller H, Skvaril F, Grob P. Immunological abnormalities and HLA antigen frequencies in IgA-deficient patients with epilepsy. J Neurol Neurosurg Psychiatry 41:593–597, 1978.

Francois R, Rosenberg D, Bertrand J, Manuel Y, Reade P, Guibaud P. Deficit dissocie en immunoglobulins et insuffisance surrenalienne: association possible d'une carence immunitaire et d'une affection autoimmune. Ann Pediatr (Paris) 43:2778–2782, 1967.

Frommel D, Moullec J, Lambin P, Fine JM. Selective IgA deficiency: frequency among 15,200 French blood donors. Vox Sang 25:513–518, 1973.

Fudenberg H, German JL, Kunkel HG. The occurrence of rheumatoid factor and other abnormalities in families of patients with agammaglobulinemia. Arthritis Rheum 5:565–588, 1962.

Fulginiti VA, Sieber OF, Claman HN, Merrill MA. Serum immunoglobulin measurement during the first year of life and in immunoglobulin deficiency states. J Pediatr 68:723–730, 1966.

Gerba WM, Miller DR, Pahwa S, Cunningham-Rundles C, Gupta S. Chronic granulomatous disease and selective IgA deficiency. Am J Pediatr Hematol Oncol 4:155–160, 1982.

Ginsberg A, Mullinax F. Pernicious anemia and monoclonal gammopathy in a patient with IgA deficiency. Am J Med 48:787–791, 1970.

Giorgi PL, Catassi C, Sbarbati A, Bearzi I, Cinti S. Ultrastructural findings in the jejunal mucosa of children with IgA deficiency. J Pediatr Gastroenterol Nutr 5:892–898, 1986.

Goh KO, Reddy MM, Webb DR. Cancer in a familial IgA deficiency patient: abnormal chromosomes and B lymphocytes. Oncology 33:237–240, 1976.

Goldberg LS, Barnett EV, Fudenberg HH. Selective absence of IgA: a family study. J Lab Clin Med 72:204–209, 1968.

Grabar P, Williams CA. Méthode permettant d'étude conjugée des propriétés electrophorétique et immunochemiques d'un milange de protein: application au serum sanguin. Biochem Biophys Acta 10:193–194, 1953.

Grundbacher FJ. Genetic aspects of selective immunoglobulin A deficiency. J Med Genet 9:344–347, 1972.

Gugler E, Von Muralt G. Über immunoelectrophoretische untersuchurgen an Frauenmilchproteinen. Schweiz Med Wochenschr 89:925–929, 1959.

Gryboski JD, Self TW, Clemett A, Herskovic T. Selective IgA deficiency and intestinal nodular lymphoid hyperplasia correction of diarrhea with antibiotics and plasma. Pediatrics 42:833–837, 1967.

Haddow JE, Shapiro SR, Gall DG. Congenital sensory neuropathy in siblings. Pediatrics 45:651–655, 1970.

Hammarström L, Axelsson V, Bjorkander J, Hanson LA, Moller E, Smith CIE. HLA antigens in selective IgA deficiency. Tissue Antigens 24:35–39, 1984.

Hammarström L, Persson MAA, Smith CIE. Anti-IgA in selective IgA deficiency. In vitro effects and Ig subclass patterns of human anti-IgA. Scand J Immunol 18:509–513, 1983.

Hammarström L, Persson MAA, Smith CIE. Immunoglobulin subclass distribution of human anti-carbohydrate antibodies: aberrant pattern in IgA-deficient donors. Immunology 54:821–826, 1985a.

Hammarström L, Ringden O, Lonngvist B, Smith CIE, Wiebe T. Transfer of IgA deficiency to a bone marrow grafted patient with aplastic anemia. Lancet 1:778–781, 1985b.

Hammarström L, Carlsson B, Smith CIE, Wallin J, Wieslander L. Detection of IgA heavy chain constant region genes in IgA deficient donors: evidence against gene deletions. Clin Exp Immunol 60:661–664, 1985c.

Hammarström L, Smith CIE. HLA-A, B, C, and DR antigens in immunoglobulin A deficiency. Tissue Antigens 21:75–79, 1983.

Hammarström L, Smith CI, Berg CI. Captopril-induced IgA deficiency. Lancet 1:436, 1991.

Hamoudi AB, Ertel I, Newton WA, Reiner CB, Chatworthy HW. Multiple neoplasms in an adolescent child associated with IgA deficiency. Cancer 33:1134–1144, 1974.

Hanson LÅ. Comparative analysis of human milk and blood plasma by means of diffusion in gel methods. Experientia 15:473–474, 1959.

Hanson LÅ. Comparative immunological studies of immunoglobulins of human milk and serum. Int Arch Allergy Appl Immunol 18:241–267, 1961.

Hanson LÅ. Selective IgA-deficiency. In Chandra RK, ed. Primary and Secondary Immunodeficiency Disorders. New York, Churchill Livingstone, 1983, pp. 62–84.

Hanson LÅ, Brandtzaeg P. The discovery of the secretory IgA and mucosal immune system. Immunol Today 14:416–417, 1993.

Hazenberg BP, Hoedemaeker PJ, Nieuwenhuis P, Mandema E. Source of IgA in jejunal secretions. In Peeters H, ed. Protides of the Biological Fluids: Proceedings of the Sixteenth Colloquium. Oxford, Pergamon Press, 1968, pp. 491–497.

Heinz CF, Boyer JT. Dysgammaglobulinemia in the adult manifested as autoimmune hemolytic anemia. N Engl J Med 269:1329–1335, 1963.

Heremans JF. Immunoglobulin A. In Sela M, ed. The Antigens, Vol. II. London, Academic Press, 1974, pp. 365–522.

Herrmann RP, Chipper L, Bell S. Chromosome studies in healthy blood donors with IgA deficiency. Clin Genet 22:231–233, 1982.

Hobbs JR. Immune imbalance in dysgammaglobulinemia type IV. Lancet 1:110–114, 1968.

Hong R, Ammann RJ. Disorders of the IgA system. In Stiehm ER, ed. Immunologic Disorders of Infants and Children, 3rd ed. Philadelphia, WB Saunders, 1989, pp. 329–342.

Huntley CC, Robbins JB, Lyerly AD, Buckley RH. Characterization of precipitating antibodies to ruminant serum and milk proteins in humans with selective IgA deficiency. N Engl J Med 284:7–10, 1971.

Huntley CC, Stephenson RL. IgA deficiency: family studies. N C Med J 29:326–335, 1968.

Husby S, Oxelius VA, Svehag SE. IgG subclass antibodies to dietary antigens in IgA deficiency: quantitation and correlation with serum IgG subclass levels. Clin Immunol Immunopathol 62:83–90, 1992.

Hustinx TWJ, Scheres JMJC, Weemaes CMR, ter Haar BGA, Janssen AH. Karyotype instability with multiple 7/14 and 7/7 rearrangements. Hum Genet 49:199–208, 1979.

Inoue T, Okubo H, Kudo J, Ikuta T, Hachimine K, Shibata R, Yoshinari D, Fukada K, Ranase T. Selective IgA deficiency: analysis of Ig production in vitro. J Clin Immunol 4:235–241, 1984.

Iwata T, Incefy GS, Cunningham-Rundles S, Cunningham-Rundles C, Smithwick E, Geller N, O'Reilly R, Good RA. Circulating thymic hormone activity in patients with primary and secondary immunodeficiency diseases. Am J Med 71:385–394, 1981.

Jacobson KW, de Shazo RD. Selective immunoglobulin A deficiency associated with nodular lymphoid hyperplasia. J Allergy Clin Immunol 64:516–521, 1979.

James SP, Jones EA, Schafer DF, Hoofnagle JH, Varma RR, Strober W. Selective immunoglobulin A deficiency associated with primary biliary cirrhosis in a family with liver disease. Gastroenterology 90:283–288, 1986.

Jersild C, Staub-Nielsen L, Svegaard A. HLA and IgA deficiency in blood donors. Tissue Antigens 21:80, 1983.

Johns P, Felix-Davies DD, Hawkins CF, Macintosh P, Shadford MF, Stanworth DR, Thompson RA, Williamson N. IgA deficiency in patients with rheumatoid arthritis with D-penicillamine or gold (abstract). Ann Rheum Dis 37:289, 1978.

Joller PW, Buehler AK, Hitzig WH. Transitory and persistent IgA deficiency: reevaluation of 19 pediatric patients once found to be IgA deficient. J Clin Lab Immunol 6:97–101, 1981.

Joubert PH, Aucamp AK, Potgieter GM, Verster F. Epilepsy and IgA deficiency: the effect of sodium valproate. South Afr Med J 52:642–644, 1977.

Kaetzel CS, Robinson JK, Chintalacharuvu KR, Vaerman JP, Lamm ME. The polymeric immunoglobulin receptor (secretory component) mediates transport of immune complexes across epithelial cells: a local defense function for IgA. Proc Natl Acad Sci U S A 88:8796–8800, 1991.

Kanoh T, Mizumoto T, Yasuda N, Koya M, Ohno Y, Uchino H, Yoshimura K, Ohkubo Y, Yamaguchi H. Selective IgA deficiency in Japanese blood donors: frequency and statistical analysis. Vox Sang 50:81–86, 1986.

Kanok JM, Steinberg P, Cassidy JT, Petty RE, Bayne NK. Serum IgE levels in patients with selective IgA deficiency. Ann Allergy 41:220–228, 1978.

Karlson G, Hanson HA, Petruson B, Björkander J. Goblet cell number in the nasal mucosa relates to cell-mediated immunity in patients with selective antibody deficiency syndromes. Int Arch Allergy Appl Immunol 78:86–91, 1985.

Kaufman HS, Hobbs JR. Immunoglobulin deficiencies in an atopic population. Lancet 2:1061–1063, 1970.

Kerr MA. The structure and function of human IgA. J Biochem 271:285–296, 1990.

Kersey JH, Shapiro RS, Filipovich AH. Relationship of immunodeficiency to lymphoid malignancy. Pediatr Infect Dis J (Suppl) 7:S10–S12, 1988.

King MA, Wells JV, Nelson DS. IgA synthesis by peripheral blood mononuclear cells from normal and selectively IgA-deficient subjects. Clin Exp Immunol 38:306–310, 1979.

Kirkpatrick CH, Ruth WE. Chronic pulmonary disease and immunologic deficiency. Am J Med 41:427–432, 1966.

Klemola T. Immunohistochemical findings in the intestine of IgA-deficient persons. J Pediatr Gastroenterol Nutr 7:537–543, 1988.

Koistinen J. Familial clustering of selective IgA deficiency. Vox Sang 30:181–190, 1976.

Koistinen J. Selective IgA deficiency in blood donors. Vox Sang 29:192–202, 1975.

Koistinen J, Cardenas RM, Fudenberg HH. Anti-IgA antibodies of limited specificity in healthy IgA-deficient subjects. J Immunogenet 4:295–299, 1977.

Komatsu N, Nagura HH, Watanabe K, Nomoto Y, Kobayashi K. Mesangial deposition of J chain–linked polymeric IgA in IgA nephropathy. Nephron 33:61–64, 1983.

Kornstadt L, Nordhagen R. Immune deficiency and autoimmunity. Int Arch Allergy Appl Immunol 47:942–945, 1974.

Krieger I, Brough JA. Gamma-A deficiency and hypochromic anemia due to defective iron mobilization. N Engl J Med 269:886–894, 1967.

Kwitko AO, Roberts-Thomas PJ, Shearman DJC. Low molecular weight IgM in selective IgA deficiency. Clin Exp Immunol 50:198–202, 1982.

Lakhanpal S, O'Duffy JD, Homburg HA, Moore SB. Evidence for linkage of IgA deficiency with the major histocompatibility complex. Mayo Clin Proc 63:461–465, 1988.

Lawton AR, Royal SA, Self KS, Cooper MD. IgA determinants on B lymphocytes in patients with deficiency of circulating IgA. J Lab Clin Med 80:26–33, 1972.

Lefranc MP, Lefranc G, De Lange G, Out TA, van Denbroek PJ, van Nieuwkoop J, Radl J, Helal AM, Chabaani H, van Loghem E, Rabbits TH. Instability of the human immunoglobulin heavy chain constant region locus indicated by different inherited chromosomal deletions. Mol Biol Med 1:207–217, 1983.

Lefranc MP, Lefranc G, Rabbits TM. Inherited deletion of immunoglobulin heavy chain region genes in normal human individuals. Nature 300:760–762, 1982.

Leickly FE, Buckley RH. Development of IgA and IgG2 subclass deficiency after sulfasalazine therapy. J Pediatr 108:481–482, 1986.

Leikola J, Vyas GN. Human antibodies to ruminant IgM concealing the absence of IgA in man. J Lab Clin Med 77:629–638, 1971.

Leisti J, Leisti S, Perheentupa J, Savilahti E, Aula P. Absence of IgA and growth hormone deficiency associated with a short arm deletion of chromosome 18. Arch Dis Child 48:320–322, 1973.

Leong AB, Gange RW, O'Connor RD. Twenty nail dystrophy associated with selective IgA deficiency. J Pediatr 100:418–419, 1982.

Levin WC, Ritzmann SE, Haggard ME, Gregory RF, Reinarz JA. Selective a-beta-2A globulinemia (abstract). Clin Res 11:294, 1963.

Levitt D, Cooper MD. Immunoregulatory defects in a family with selective IgA deficiency. J Pediatr 98:52–58, 1981.

Lewkonia RM, Gairdner D, Doe WF. IgA deficiency in one of identical twins. Br Med J 1:311–313, 1976.

Lewkonia RM, Lin CC, Haslam RHA. Selective IgA deficiency with 18q+ and 18q− karyotypic anomalies. J Med Genet 17:453–456, 1980.

Liblau R, Fischer AM, Shapiro DE, Morel E, Bach JF. The frequency of selective IgA deficiency in myasthenia gravis. Neurology 42:516–518, 1992.

Lopez M, Hyslop E. Precipitating antibody to Bovidae serum proteins in dysgammaglobulinemic sera (abstract). Fed Proc 27:684, 1968.

Mann JG, Brown WR, Kern F. The subtle and variable clinical expressions of gluten-induced enteropathy (adult celiac disease, nontropical sprue): an analysis of twenty-one consecutive cases. Am J Med 48:357–366, 1970.

Martini A, Raveli A, Notarangelo LD, Burgio VL, Plebani A. Henoch-Schönlein syndrome and selective IgA deficiency. Arch Dis Child 60:160–162, 1985.

Mazanec MB, Kaetzel CS, Lamm ME, Fletcher D, Nedrud JG. Intracellular neutralization of virus by immunoglobulin A antibodies. Proc Natl Acad Sci U S A 89:6901–6905, 1992.

McCarthy DM, Katz SI, Gazzel L, Waldmann TA, Nelson DL, Strober W. Selective IgA deficiency associated with total villous atrophy of the small intestine and an organ-specific anti-epithelial cell antibody. J Immunol 120:932–938, 1978.

McClelland DBL, Shearman DJ, Van Furth R. Synthesis of immunoglobulin and secretory components by gastrointestinal mucosa in patients with hypogammaglobulinemia or IgA deficiency. Clin Exp Immunol 25:103–109, 1979.

McGhee JR, Mestecky J, Elson CO, Kiyono H. Regulation of IgA synthesis and immune response by T cells and interleukins. J Clin Immunol 9:175–199, 1989.

Mellander L, Björkander J, Carlson B, Hanson LA. Secretory antibodies in IgA-deficient and immunosuppressed individuals. J Clin Immunol 6:284–291, 1986.

Mestecky J, McGhee JR. Immunoglobulin A (IgA): molecular and cellular interactions involved in IgA biosynthesis and immune response. Adv Immunol 40:153–245, 1987.

Migone N, Olivero S, De Lange G, Delacroix DL, Altruda F, Silengo L, Demarchi M, Carbona AO. Multiple gene deletions within the human immunoglobulin heavy chain cluster. Proc Natl Acad Sci U S A 81:5811–5815, 1984.

Miller WV, Holland PV, Sugarbaker E, Strober W, Waldman TA. Anaphylactic reactions to IgA: a difficult transfusion problem. Am J Clin Pathol 54:618–624, 1970.

Monteiro RC, Kubagawa H, Cooper MD. Cellular distribution, regulation, and biochemical nature of an Fc alpha receptor in humans. J Exp Med 171:597–613, 1990.

Mostov KE, Deitcher DL. Polymeric immunoglobulin receptor expressed in MDCK cells transcytoses IgA. Cell 46:613–621, 1986.

Mostov KE, Friedlander M, Blobel G. The receptor for transepithelial transport of IgA and IgM contains multiple immunoglobulin-like domains. Nature 308:37–43, 1984.

Muñoz-López F, Ballesta-Martinez F, Martin-Mateos MA. Selective IgA deficiency. Immunologic and cytogenetic studies. Allergol Immunopathol (Madr) 5:671–675, 1977.

Murphy EA, Morris AJ, Walker E, Lee FD, Sturrock RD. Cyclosporine A induced colitis and acquired selective IgA deficiency in a patient with juvenile chronic arthritis. J Rheumatol 20:1397–1398, 1993.

Natvig JB, Harboe M, Fausa O, Tveit A. Family studies in individuals with selective absence of A-globulin. Clin Exp Immunol 8:229–236, 1971.

Nell PA, Ammann AJ, Hong R, Stiehm ER. Familial selective IgA deficiency. Pediatrics 49:71–79, 1972.

Nilssen DE, Friman V, Theman K, Björkander J, Kilarder A, Holmgren J, Hanson LÅ, Brandtzaeg P. B cell activation in duodenal mucosa after oral cholera vaccination in IgA-deficient subjects with or without IgG subclass deficiency. Scand J Immunol 38:201–208, 1993.

Norhagen GE, Enaptrom PE, Hammerstrom L, Söder PÖ, Smith CIE. Immunoglobulin levels in saliva in individuals with selective IgA deficiency. Compensatory IgM secretion and its correlation with HLA and susceptibility to infections. J Clin Immunol 9:279–286, 1989.

Odgers RJ, Wangel AG. Abnormalities in IgA-containing mononuclear cells in the gastric lesions of pernicious anemia. Lancet 2:846–849, 1968.

Oen K, Petty RE, Schroeder ML. Immunoglobulin A deficiency in genetic studies. Tissue Antigens 19:174–182, 1982.

Ogata K, Iinuma K, Kamimura K, Morinaga R, Kato J. A case report of a presumptive +i(18p) associated with serum IgA deficiency. Clin Genet 11:184–188, 1977.

Olerup O, Smith CIE, Hammarström L. Different amino acids at position 57 of the HLA-DQ-beta chain associated with susceptibility and resistance to IgA deficiency. Nature 347:289–290, 1990.

Olerup O, Smith CIE, Björkander J, Hammarström L. Shared HLA class II-associated genetic susceptibility and resistance, related to the HLA-DQB1 gene, in IgA deficiency and common variable immunodeficiency. Proc Natl Acad Sci U S A 89:10653–10657, 1992.

Olsson PG, Hofker MH, Walter MA, Smith S, Hammarström L, Smith CIE, Cox DW. Ig H chain variable and C region genes in common variable immunodeficiency. J Immunol 147:2540–2546, 1991.

Ostergaard PA. Combined IgA and alpha-1-antitrypsin deficiency in a boy with severe respiratory tract infections and asthma. Eur J Pediatr 138:83–85, 1982.

Oxelius VA, Laurell AB, Linquist B, Golebiowska H, Axelsson U, Björkander J, Hanson LA. IgG subclasses in selective IgA deficiency. N Engl J Med 304:1476–1477, 1981.

Pascual-Salcedo D, Rodriguez MCG, Trascasa ML, Fontana G. Anticardiolipin antibodies in patients with primary immunodeficiency disease. Ann Rheum Dis 47:410–413, 1988.

Penny R, Thompson RG, Polmar SH, Schulz RB. Pancreatitis malabsorption and IgA deficiency in a child with diabetes. J Pediatr 78:512–516, 1971.

Perey DYE, Frommel D, Hong R, Good RA. The mammalian homologue of the avian bursa of Fabricius. Lab Invest 22:212–227, 1970.

Perez-Jiminez F, Lopez PB, Tallo EP, Guzman JR, Molina JS, Perez-Perez JA. Selective IgA deficiency and the HLA-B8 antigen. Arch Intern Med 141:509–510, 1981.

Petty RE, Cassidy JT, Sullivan DB. Reversal of selective IgA deficiency in a child with juvenile rheumatoid arthritis after plasma transfusions. Pediatrics 51:44–48, 1973.

Petty RE, Sherry DD, Johannson J. Anti-IgA antibodies in pregnancy. N Engl J Med 313:1620–1625, 1985.

Plaut AG. The IgA1 proteases of pathogenic bacteria. Ann Rev Microbiol 37:603–622, 1983.

Plebani A, Mira E, Mevio E, Monafo V, Notarangelo LD, Avanzini A, Ugazio AG. IgM and IgD concentrations in the serum and secretions of children with selective IgA deficiency. Clin Exp Immunol 53:689–696, 1983.

Plebani A, Monafo V, Ugazio AG, Monti MA, Avanzini P, Massimi P, Burgio GR. Comparison of the frequency of atopic disease in children with severe and partial IgA deficiency. Int Arch Allergy Appl Immunol 82:485–486, 1987.

Plebani A, Ugazio AG, Monafo V, Burgio GR. Clinical heterogeneity and reversibility of selective immunoglobulin A deficiency in 80 children. Lancet 1:829–831, 1986.

Pritchard H, Riddaway J, Micklem HS. Immune response in congenitally thymus-less mice: II. Quantitative studies of serum immunoglobulins, the antibody response to sheep red blood cells and the effectiveness of thymus allografting. Clin Exp Immunol 13:125–138, 1973.

Proesman W, Jaeken J, Eeckels R. D-Penicillamine-induced IgA deficiency in Wilson's disease. Lancet 1:804–805, 1976.

Pudifin DJ, Cunningham-Rundles C, Good RA. Circulating antibodies to chicken ovalbumin in IgA-deficient subjects (abstract). Fed Proc 38:5263, 1979.

Richman LK, Brown WR. Immunochemical characterization of IgM in intestinal fluids. J Immunol 199:1515–1521, 1977.

Rockey JH, Hanson LÅ, Heremans JF, Kunkel HG. Beta-2A-agammaglobulinemia in two healthy men. J Lab Clin Med 63:205–212, 1964.

Rosner R, Vallejo V, Khan FA, Wessely Z, Gunwald HW, Calas C. Hypogammaglobulinemia and selective immunoglobulin A deficiency: double consanguinity in family. N Y State J Med 78:1459–1461, 1978.

Ruff ME, Pincus LG, Sampson HA. Phenytoin-induced IgA depression. Am J Dis Child 141:858–859, 1987.

Russell MW, Mansa B. Complement fixing properties of human IgA antibodies. Scand J Immunol 30:175–183, 1989.

Ruvalcaba RHA, Thuline HC. IgA absence associated with short arm deletion of chromosome No. 18. J Pediatr 74:964–965, 1969.

Sakai H, Nomoto Y, Arimori S, Komori K, Inouye H, Tsuji K. Increase of IgA-bearing peripheral blood lymphocytes in families of patients with IgA nephropathy. Am J Clin Pathol 72:452–456, 1979.

Sandler SC, Zlotnick A. IgA deficiency and autoimmune hemolytic disease. Arch Intern Med 136:93–94, 1976.

Saulsbury FT. Selective IgA deficiency temporally associated with Epstein-Barr virus infection. J Pediatr 115:268–271, 1989.

Savilahti E, Eskola J, Koskimies S. IgA deficiency in coeliac disease. In Griscelli C, Vossen J, eds. Progress in Immunodeficiency Research and Therapy. Amsterdam, Elsevier Science, 1984, pp. 257–259.

Savilahti E, Klemola T, Carlsson B, Mellander L, Stenvile M, Hovi T. Inadequacy of mucosal IgM antibodies in selective IgA deficiency: excretion of attenuated polio viruses is prolonged. J Clin Immunol 8:89–94, 1988.

Schaffer FM, Palermos J, Zhou ZB, Barger BO, Cooper MD, Volanakis JE. Individuals with IgA deficiency and common variable immunodeficiency share polymorphisms of major histocompatibility complex class III genes. Proc Natl Acad Sci U S A 86:8015–8019, 1989.

Schaffer FM, Monteiro RC, Volanakis JE, Cooper MD. IgA deficiency. Immunodefic Rev 3:15–44, 1991.

Schmidt AP, Taswell HF, Gleich GJ. Anaphylactic tranfusion reaction associated with anti-IgA antibody. N Engl J Med 280:188–193, 1969.

Schwartz SA. Heavy chain-specific suppression of immunoglobulin synthesis and secretion by lymphocytes from patients with selective IgA deficiency. J Immunol 124:2034–2038, 1980.

Scotta MS, Maggiore G, DeGiacomo C, Martini A, Burgio VL, Ugazio AG. IgA-containing plasma cells in the intestinal mucosa of children with selective IgA deficiency. J Clin Lab Immunol 9:173–175, 1982.

Seager J, Jamison DL, Wilson J, Hayward AR, Soothill JF. IgA deficiency, epilepsy and phenytoin treatment. Lancet 2:632–635, 1975.

Seignalet J, Michael FB, Guendon R, Thomas R, Robinet-Levy M, Lapinski H. HLA et dificit en IgA. Rev Fr Transfus Immunohematol 21:753–761, 1978.

Shakir RA, Behan PO, Dick H, Lambie DG. Metabolism of immunoglobulin A, lymphocyte function, and histocompatibility antigens in patients on anticonvulsants. J Neurol Neurosurg Psychiatry 41:307–311, 1978.

Sharma OP, Chandor SM. IgA deficiency in sarcoidosis. Am Rev Respir Dis 106:600–603, 1972.

Silver HKB, Shuster J, Gold P, Hawkins D, Freedman SO. Endocrinopathy and IgA deficiency. Clin Immunol Immunopathol 1:212–219, 1973.

Skrede S, Winther FO, Munthe E, Nordoy A. Transitory IgA-deficiency, persistent IgE-deficiency and recurrent respiratory tract infectious disease after splenectomy. Arch Otorhinolaryngol 217:423–429, 1977.

Sloper KS, Brook CGD, Kingston D, Pearson JR, Shiner M. Eczema and atopy in early childhood: low IgA plasma cell counts in the jejunal mucosa. Arch Dis Child 56:939–943, 1981.

Smith CK, Cassidy JT, Bole GG. Type I dysgammaglobulinemia, systemic lupus erythematosus and lymphoma. Am J Med 48:113–119, 1970.

Smith WI, Rabin BS, Huelimantel A, Van Thiel DH, Drash A. Immunopathology of juvenile-onset diabetes mellitus I: IgA deficiency and juvenile diabetes. Diabetes 27:1092–1099, 1978.

Soothill JF, Hayes K, Dudgeon JA. The immunoglobulins in congenital rubella. Lancet 2:1385–1388, 1966.

Soothill JF, Hill LE, Rowe DS. A quantitative study of the immunoglobulins in the antibody deficiency syndrome. In Bergsma D, Good RA, eds. Immunologic Deficiency Diseases in Man. National Foundation–Birth Defects: Original Article Series. Vol. 4, No. 1. Baltimore, Williams & Wilkins, 1968, pp. 71–81.

Sorrell TC, Forbes IJ, Burness FR, Rischbieth RHC. Depression of immunological function in patients treated with phenytoin sodium (sodium diphenylhydantoin). Lancet 2:1233–1235, 1971.

Spector BD, Perry GS, Good RA, Kersey JH. Immunodeficiency diseases and malignancy. In Twomey J, Good RA, eds. The Immunopathology of Lymphocyte Reticular Neoplasms. New York, Plenum, 1978, pp. 203–222.

Stannegard O, Björkander J, Hanson LÅ, Hermodsson S. Natural killer cells in common variable immunodeficiency and selective IgA deficiency. Clin Immunol Immunopathol 25:325–334, 1983.

Stewart JM, Go S, Ellis E, Robinson A. Absent IgA and deletions of chromosome 18. J Med Genet 7:11–19, 1970.

Stiehm ER, Vaerman J-P, Fudenberg HH. Plasma infusions in immunologic deficiency states: metabolic and therapeutic studies. Blood 28:918–937, 1966.

Stobo JD, Tomasi TB. A low molecular weight immunoglobulin antigenically related to 19S IgM. J Clin Invest 46:1329–1337, 1967.

Stocker F, Ammann P, Rossi E. Selective gamma-A-globulin deficiency, with dominant autosomal inheritance in a Swiss family. Arch Dis Child 43:585–588, 1968.

Stricker RB, Linker CA. Pernicious anemia, 18q deletion syndrome and IgA deficiency. JAMA 248:1359–1360, 1982.

Strober W, Weckner RD, Barlow MH, McFarlin DW, Waldmann TA. Immunoglobulin metabolism in ataxia-telangiectasia. J Clin Invest 47:1905–1908, 1968.

Strober W, Sneller MC. IgA deficiency. Ann Allergy 66:363–375, 1991.

Strothman R, White MB, Testin J, Chen SN, Ball MS. HLA and IgA deficiency in blood donors. Hum Immunol 16:289–294, 1986.

Swanson V, Dyce B, Citron P, Roulea C, Feinstein D, Haverback BJ. Absence of IgA in serum with presence of IgA-containing cells in the intestinal tract (abstract). Clin Res 16:119, 1968.

Taalman RDFM, Weemaes CMR, Hustinx TWJ, Scheres JMJC, Clement JME, Stoelinga GBA. Chromosome studies in IgA-deficient patients. Clin Genet 32:81–87, 1987.

Taylor B, Norman AP, Orgel HA, Stokes CR, Turner MW, Soothill JF. Transient IgA deficiency and pathogenesis of infantile atopy. Lancet 2:111–113, 1973.

Thieffry S, Arthuis M, Aicardi J, Lyon G. L'ataxie-telangiectasie (7 observations personnelles). Rev Neurol (Paris) 105:390–405, 1961.

Tiepolo L, Maraschio P, Gimeli G, Cuoco C, Gargani GF, Romano C. Multibranched chromosomes 1, 9, and 16 in a patient with combined IgA and IgE deficiency. Hum Genet 51:127–137, 1979.

Tomasi TB. The discovery of secretory IgA and the mucosal immune system. Immunol Today 13:416–418, 1992.

Tomasi TB, Bienenstock J. Secretory immunoglobulins. Adv Immunol 9:1–96, 1968.

Tomasi TB Jr, Katz L. Human antibodies against bovine immunoglobulin M in IgA-deficient sera. Clin Exp Immunol 9:3–10, 1971.

Tomkin GH, Mawhinney H, Nevin NC. Isolated absence of IgA with autosomal dominant inheritance. Lancet 2:124–125, 1971.

Torrelo A, Espana A, Balsa J, Ledo A. Vitiligo and polyglandular autoimmune syndrome with selective IgA deficiency. Int J Dermatol 31:343–344, 1992.

Truedsson L, Axelsson U, Laurell AB. Frequent occurrence of anti-rabbit IgM in IgA deficiency. Acta Pathol Microbiol Scand 90:315–316, 1982.

Tsung SH, Ajlouni K. Immune competence in patients with Klinefelter syndrome. Am J Med Sci 275:311–317, 1978.

Van Loghem E. Familial occurrence of isolated IgA deficiency associated with antibodies to IgA: evidence against a structural gene defect. Eur J Immunol 4:57–61, 1974.

Van Loghem E, Wang AC, Shuster J. A new genetic marker of human immunoglobulin determined by an allele at the alpha 2 locus. Vox Sang 24:481–490, 1973.

Van Loghem E, Zegers BJM, Bast EJE, Kater L. Selective deficiency of immunoglobulin A2. J Clin Invest 72:1918–1923, 1983.

Van Munster PJJ, Nadorp JHSM, Schuurman HJ. Human antibodies to immunoglobulin A (IgA). A radioimmunological method for differentiation between anti-IgA antibodies and IgA in the serum of IgA deficient individuals. J Immunol Methods 22:233–237, 1978.

Van Thiel DH, Smith WI, Rabin BS, Fisher SE, Lester R. A syndrome of immunoglobulin A deficiency, diabetes mellitus, malabsorption, and a common HLA haplotype: immunologic and genetic studies of forty-three family members. Ann Intern Med 86:10–19, 1977.

Vassallo CL, Zawadzki ZA, Simons JR. Recurrent respiratory infections in a family with immunoglobulin A deficiency. Am Rev Respir Dis 101:245–246, 1970.

Vassella F, Emrich HM, Kraus-Ruppert R, Aufdemaur F, Tonz O. Congenital sensory neuropathy in anhidrosis. Arch Dis Child 43:124–128, 1968.

Victoria CG, Smith PG, Vaughan JP, Nobre LC, Lombardi C, Teixeira AMB, Fuchs SMC, Moreira LB, Gigante LP, Barros FC. Evidence for protection by breast-feeding against infant deaths from infectious diseases in Brazil. Lancet 2:319–322, 1987.

Vyas GN, Fudenberg HH. Immunogenetic study of Am(1), the first allotype of human IgA. Clin Res 17:469, 1969.

Vyas GN, Perkins HA, Fudenberg HH. Anaphylactoid transfusion reactions associated with anti-IgA. Lancet 2:312–315, 1968.

Waldmann TA, Broder S, Krakauer R, Durm M, Meade B, Goldman C. Defect in IgA secretion and in IgA-specific suppressor cells in patients with selective IgA deficiency. Trans Assoc Am Physicians 89:219–224, 1976.

Warrington RJ, Sauder PJ, Rutherford WJ. Suppression of mitogen-induced human immunoglobulin (Ig)-A synthesis by heterologous antibody in IgA. Clin Immunol Immunopathol 19:372–382, 1981.

Warrington RS, Rutherford WJ, Sauder PJ, Bees WCH. Homologous antibody to human immunoglobulin (Ig)-A suppresses in vitro mitogen-induced IgA synthesis. Clin Immunol Immunopathol 23:698–704, 1982.

Webb RD, Condemi JJ. Selective immunoglobulin A deficiency and chronic obstructive lung disease: a family study. Ann Intern Med 80:618–621, 1974.

Wells JV, Michaeli D, Fudenberg HH. Antibodies to human collagen in subjects with selective IgA deficiency. Clin Exp Immunol 13:203–208, 1973.

Werteleki W, Gerald PS. Clinical chromosomal studies of the 18q− syndrome. J Pediatr 78:44–51, 1971.

West CD, Hong R, Holland NH. Immunoglobulin levels from the newborn period to adulthood and in immunoglobulin deficiency states. J Clin Invest 41:2054–2064, 1962.

Wilson MG, Towner JW, Forsman L, Siris E. Syndromes associated with the deletion of the long arm of chromosome 18. Am J Med Genet 8:155–174, 1979.

Wilton AN, Cobain TJ, Dawkins RL. Family studies of IgA deficiency. Immunogenetics 21:333–342, 1985.

Wollheim FA, Belfrage S, Coster C, Lindholm H. Primary "acquired" hypogammaglobulinemia: clinical and genetic aspects of nine cases. Acta Med Scand 176:18–23, 1964.

Yadav M, Iyngkaran N. Low incidence of selective IgA deficiency in normal Malaysians. Med J Malaysia 34:145–148, 1979.

Yasuda N, Kanoh T, Uchino H. J chain synthesis in lymphocytes from patients with selective IgA deficiency. Clin Exp Immunol 46:142–148, 1981.

Zinneman HH, Kaplan AP. The association of giardiasis with reduced intestinal secretory immunoglobulin A. Dig Dis Sci 125:207–213, 1975.

Chapter 15

Disorders of the Polymorphonuclear Phagocytic System

Paul G. Quie, Elaine L. Mills, Robert L. Roberts,
and Francisco J. D. Noya

INTRODUCTION

Phagocytic Function

Circulating polymorphonuclear leukocytes (PMNs), including neutrophils, eosinophils, and basophils, reach maturity in the bone marrow, circulate in the blood for a short time, and enter tissue spaces by diapedesis through capillary walls (see Chapter 5). The primary functions of neutrophils, the most abundant of these leukocytes, are engulfment and killing of microbes. Adequate numbers of neutrophils are necessary for normal host defense, a fact appreciated by clinicians for many years, because neutropenia as a consequence of congenital defects, malignancy, or chemotherapy results in increased susceptibility to severe, recurrent bacterial infections and a poor response to antibiotic therapy.

Patients with adequate numbers but deficient function of phagocytic leukocytes have been recognized. Functional activities include adherence, migration, phagocytosis, secretion, respiratory burst, and intracellular killing. Patients with congenital neutrophil dysfunction have characteristic clinical syndromes and are, indeed, models of understanding the contribution of neutrophils to inflammation and host defense (Malech and Gallin, 1987; Lehrer et al., 1988; Mills and Noya, 1993). The most common lesions in patients with deficient numbers or defective function of neutrophils are soft tissue inflammation and abscesses; common pathogens include *Staphylococcus aureus*, *Pseudomonas*, *Serratia* and other Enterobacteriaccae, *Aspergillus*, and *Candida*.

Laboratory Assessment of Phagocyte Activity

Numbers of circulating phagocytic cells (neutrophils, eosinophils, and monocytes) are easily determined by routine techniques in all hematology laboratories, and morphology is satisfactorily determined by standard staining techniques and electron microscopy. Functional evaluation of phagocytic cells, however, is not routinely performed in hospital laboratories but is available at most medical centers (see Chapter 9).

Neutrophil adherence is measured by passing blood over columns filled with nylon fibers (MacGregor et al., 1974). The percentage of cells sticking to nylon correlates well with adherence to endothelial cell monolayers (MacGregor et al., 1967). Congenital adhesion disorders are confirmed by flow cytometric analysis using monoclonal antibodies specific for adhesion molecules expressed on the cell surface (Arnaout et al., 1990).

Locomotion of neutrophils or monocytes is determined by measuring the distance moved during random motion (chemokinesis). Directional migration, that is, chemotaxis, may be measured by distance traveled through cellulose acetate filters in a Boyden chamber or by the "under agarose" method in response to a variety of chemoattractants. Phagocytic cells and attractants or buffer are placed in separate wells, cut in agarose, and incubated at 37°C. Numbers, patterns, and distance of cell migration on the plastic or glass surface under the agarose are recorded (Nelson et al., 1975).

Phagocytosis by neutrophils can be assessed by determining leukocyte-associated radioactivity after incubation with radiolabeled bacteria (Peterson et al., 1977) or visually by counting the number of particles—that is, yeast, oil red O, or latex beads—engulfed by the phagocyte.

Evaluation of intracellular killing of a variety of microbial species by neutrophils (Quie et al., 1967) is available in selected medical centers. The kinetics of intracellular killing can also be assessed.

The oxidative metabolic response of neutrophils during phagocytosis is determined by measuring superoxide generation directly or indirectly using either the nitroblue tetrazolium (NBT) dye reduction test or the chemiluminescence assay (Mills et al., 1980). The addition of luminol or lucigenin, which becomes electronically excited in the presence of oxidizing factors,

amplifies and increases the sensitivity of the chemiluminescence assay of superoxide generation (Stevens et al., 1978).

Flow cytometry studies are valuable for evaluating abnormalities in neutrophil adherence, phagocytosis, oxidative metabolism, and changes in intracellular calcium (Metcalf et al., 1986). Other laboratory tests of value in phagocytic disorders are discussed in Chapter 9.

DISORDERS OF LEUKOCYTE QUANTITY

Granulocytopenia (Neutropenia)

Neutropenia (defined as circulating neutrophils less than 500/mm³) is a frequent neutrophil disorder, leading to susceptibility to multiple exogenous and endogenous bacterial and fungal organisms. Neutropenia is common to a heterogeneous group of disorders resulting from decreased production or release of mature neutrophils from the bone marrow. It can be either congenital or secondary to infections such as parvovirus, drugs, toxins, neoplasia, antineutrophil antibodies, autoimmune disorders, or other acquired conditions. Neonatal neutropenia occurs in 50% of infants whose mothers have hypertension during pregnancy; this is due to transiently reduced neutrophil production (Koenig and Christensen, 1989). Neutropenia as a consequence of aplastic anemia (the most common cause of severe neutropenia) places patients at especially grave risk for severe infections because there is no reserve of circulating phagocytic monocytes. Common sites of infection are skin and mucous membranes, lungs, liver, and blood (Curnutte and Boxer, 1993). The most frequent infections are those caused by normal endogenous flora; thus polymicrobial infections are not uncommon. Neutropenia does not increase susceptibility to infection with viruses or parasites.

Acute bacteremic infections in children with severe granulocytopenia necessitate maximum intravenous therapeutic doses of a combination of β-lactam and aminoglycoside antibiotics, which should be continued until patients are afebrile. A continuing febrile course and persistent granulocytopenia are features of fungal superinfection, which often dictates empirical amphotericin B therapy (Newman et al., 1980).

Congenital Neutropenia

Patients with congenital neutropenia (Kostmann's syndrome) have persistent, severe absolute neutropenia and maturation arrest of myelopoiesis at the promyelocyte or myelocyte stage in the bone marrow (Kostmann, 1956). Typically, patients are well in early infancy but during the first few months of life experience recurrent pneumonia, otitis media, gingivitis and perineal or urinary tract infections. Until recently 50% of patients died as a result of infection before 1 year of age and only 30% survived more than 5 years (Alter, 1993). However, treatment with recombinant growth factors has improved this prognosis (Welte et al., 1990; Glasser et al., 1991; Dale et al., 1993). Progenitor cells of most patients with congenital neutropenia have the capacity for normal proliferation and differentiation to mature myeloid cells, although pharmacologic concentrations of growth factors may be required because of inability of the receptors for growth factor on the progenitor cells to transduce activation (Guba et al., 1994). Patients respond dramatically to recombinant human granulocyte colony-stimulating factor (rhG-CSF) with significant increases in blood neutrophils (Hammond et al., 1989).

Cyclic Neutropenia

Patients with cyclic neutropenia have regular cyclic fluctuations (usually every 21 days but with a range of 14 to 36 days) in the number of blood neutrophils, with periods of severe neutropenia (<200 cells/mm³), lasting 3 to 10 days, alternating with periods of normal neutrophil counts. The cycle length is usually constant in individual patients. Other leukocytes may also oscillate in cycles of the same length, although not necessarily in phase with neutrophils. For example, monocytosis and eosinophilia may coincide with the nadir of the neutrophil cycle, whereas fluctuation of platelets and reticulocytes may occur in phase with fluctuation of neutrophils.

Evaluation of the bone marrow reveals cyclic oscillations of hematopoietic progenitors. A paucity of mature neutrophils is observed during the nadir, whereas normal numbers of mature neutrophils are present in the bone marrow when peripheral counts are normal (Hammond et al., 1989). Bone marrow myeloid progenitors are present in high concentrations, and highest levels coincide with peripheral blood neutropenia. The defect in this disorder may be the inability of the myeloid precursor cells to respond to physiologic concentrations of G-CSF (Hammond et al., 1992).

Cyclic neutropenia is often familial, and genetic transmission may be autosomal dominant with variable expression (Dale and Hammond, 1988) or X-linked when associated with the hyper-immunoglobulin M syndrome (see Chapter 11).

Clinical signs and symptoms during periods of neutropenia include fever, malaise, periodontitis, mucosal ulcers, impetigo, sore throat, and lymph node enlargement, which resolve as the neutrophil count returns to normal. Although many patients live full lives, with a gradual amelioration of symptoms and less noticeable cycles, 10% of patients experience frequent serious infectious complications.

Therapy with recombinant human G-CSF increases neutrophil counts throughout the cycle, decreases duration of neutropenia, and shortens the length of the cycle from 21 to 14 days on average. Therapy with hematopoietic growth factors (e.g., G-CSF) can significantly ameliorate both the intermittent neutropenia of this disorder and its clinical consequences (Hanada et al., 1990).

Glycogen Storage Disease Type 1b

Glycogen storage disease (GSD) type 1b is characterized by glucose-6-phosphatase deficiency, hepato-

splenomegaly, fasting hypoglycemia, and lactic acidosis but normal latent glucose-6-phosphatase activity in the liver. Unlike patients with glycogen storage disease type 1a, these patients characteristically have neutropenia, functional neutrophil abnormalities, and recurrent infections such as pneumonia, stomatitis, and septicemia (Beaudet et al., 1980). Defects of locomotion and chemotaxis (Anderson et al., 1981b), oxidative metabolism, and bacterial killing have been described and attributed to the metabolic defects of the hexose monophosphate shunt (Seger et al., 1984) and of anaerobic glycolysis (Di Rocco et al., 1984). This disorder is also discussed in Chapters 16 and 19.

Acquired Neutropenias

Drug therapy is a frequent cause of neutropenia. Nitrogen mustard and chlorambucil have a direct cytolytic effect on neutrophils, causing these cells to disappear 7 to 10 days after therapy is begun. Azathioprine and 6-mercaptopurine affect the metabolism of neutrophils and result in cyclic variation in the numbers of circulating cells. Neutropenia develops in certain patients receiving phenothiazine; this is dependent on the duration of therapy as well as unknown host factors. Although severe aplasia of the bone marrow may be present, recovery is usually complete when the drug is discontinued. Sulfonamides, methicillin, and cephaloridine may also produce transient neutropenia. Neutropenia in human immunodeficiency virus–infected patients may be a consequence of antiviral therapy, notably with zidovudine (Balis et al., 1989), although impaired myelopoiesis caused by the virus is the major cause and may be a presenting finding in children (Doweiko, 1993).

The neutropenia observed in certain patients with rheumatoid arthritis, cirrhosis, lupus erythematosus, and malaria is believed to be due to abnormal cytophilic immunoglobulinemia, resulting in trapping of granulocytes in the spleen (Finch, 1972). Felty's syndrome, the triad of rheumatoid arthritis, splenomegaly, and neutropenia, previously required splenectomy to treat the neutropenia, but now growth factors (granulocyte-macrophage colony-stimulating factor [GM-CSF] and G-CSF) may be used (Kaiser et al., 1992). Immune-mediated neutropenia may occur in the neonate as a result of maternal antineutrophil antibodies or in older children as a result of neutrophil autoantibodies.

Myelokathexis

Myelokathexis is a rare form of severe congenital neutropenia characterized by persistent neutropenia, recurrent infections, and peculiar morphology of the polymorphonuclear leukocyte in the bone marrow (Zuelzer, 1964; O'Regan et al., 1977). Absolute PMN counts are usually less than 1000 cells/mm³ but transient leukocytosis occurs with acute infections. Bone marrow examination reveals an increased number of granulocytes at all stages of differentiation and an increased percentage of segmented mature forms. Most PMNs are hypersegmented with thin chromatin filaments connecting the nuclear lobes. The nuclei are often pyknotic and the cytoplasm vacuolated, suggestive of a degenerative process. Kinetic studies using radiolabeled granulocytes show that PMNs have an excessively short survival time in the blood and are impaired in their delivery from the bone marrow (Krill et al., 1964).

The basic defect in myelokathexis (*kathexis*, Greek for "holding fast") is thought to be an impaired mechanism of release of PMNs from the bone marrow (O'Regan et al., 1977). Administration of granulocyte colony stimulating factor (GM-CSF or G-CSF) to patients with myelokathexis has led to rapid mobilization of bone marrow PMNs and fewer abnormal-appearing myeloid cells (Ganser et al., 1989; Weston et al., 1991). Although patients improved clinically after normalization of the PMN count, neutrophil chemotaxis, superoxide production, and expression of the FcRγIII receptor (CD16) were all decreased compared with normal control values.

Wetzler and coworkers (1990) described a family in which two sisters had neutropenia and features of myelokathexis as just described. These patients also had moderate hypogammaglobulinemia, decreased numbers of B cells, and increased percentage of natural killer (NK) cells. In addition to recurrent respiratory infections, they both had multiple verrucae vulgaris on their hands and cervical papillomatosis. It was proposed that this constellation of warts, hypogammaglobulinemia, infections, and myelokathexis be called "WHIM syndrome." Mentzer and coworkers (1977) had previously described a father and daughter with similar clinical features. The cause of this syndrome is unclear, but it appears that both myeloid and lymphoid regulatory mechanisms are affected.

DISORDERS OF GRANULOCYTE MOVEMENT

Neutrophil Chemotaxis

Prompt accumulation of phagocytic cells in tissues invaded by bacteria is essential for preventing infectious lesions. Miles and associates (1957) provided graphic experimental evidence for this by demonstrating that delay of migration of neutrophil leukocytes for as little as 2 hours enabled bacteria to produce severe lesions by as much as 10,000-fold. These experimental observations are supported by clinical evidence for patients with defective leukotaxis who have recurrent severe infections. Disorders of chemotaxis may be primary or secondary to circulating inhibitory factors or to defective generation of intrinsic chemotactic factors (primarily complement components).

Leukocyte Adhesion Defect Type 1

Leukocyte adhesion defect (LAD) type 1 is an autosomal recessive hereditary disorder of neutrophils characterized by recurrent, life-threatening bacterial infections, impaired pus formation and wound healing, and a wide array of functional abnormalities of lymphocytes as well as neutrophils and monocytes. (See Chapter 16 for further discussion.)

Absence or deficient expression of the adhesion molecules CD11 and CD18 on the surface of neutrophils and other leukocytes results in defective cellular adherence (Anderson et al., 1984b; Fischer et al., 1988). Because most leukocyte adhesive functions are dependent on the expression and function of the leukocyte-specific heterodimers CD11a/CD18, CD11b/CD18, and CD11c/CD18, adhesion of leukocytes to endothelial, epithelial, and target cells; phagocytosis of foreign particles; and secretory activity of leukocytes associated with attachment to surfaces are compromised. Neutrophils do not accumulate at extravascular inflammatory sites, despite marked peripheral blood leukocytosis, because neutrophils do not adhere to and traverse the capillary endothelium in response to chemotactic stimuli.

Clinical Manifestations

Two clinical phenotypes have been identified: patients with severe life-threatening infections and those with moderate chronic periodontitis and less severe infections (Anderson and Springer, 1987). Patients with severe infections have undetectable CD11/CD18 glycoproteins on leukocyte surfaces; patients with less severe infections have diminished (3% to 10% of normal) CD11/CD18 glycoprotein on the surface of their neutrophils.

Patients with LAD have recurrent necrotic and indolent infections of soft tissues, primarily skin, mucous membranes, and intestinal tract (Anderson and Springer, 1987). Superficial lesions begin as small, erythematous, nonpurulent nodules that may progress to large ulcers and cellulitis without pus. Healing occurs slowly, often leaving dysplastic scars. During the neonatal period, septicemia or extension of the infection into the abdominal cavity may occur as a complication of omphalitis and separation of the umbilical cord may be delayed for 21 days or longer (Abramson et al., 1981). Later in childhood, gingivitis and periodontitis are a constant feature, often leading to gingival proliferation and severe loss of alveolar bone and teeth. Facial or deep neck cellulitis and facial nerve palsy may occur as complications. Recurrent otitis, sinusitis, and pneumonia are common. Perirectal abscess and cellulitis occur frequently and may progress to peritonitis and septicemia. Appendicitis, necrotizing enterocolitis, intestinal ulceration, bacterial tracheitis, *Candida* esophagitis, and erosive gastritis have also been reported (Anderson et al., 1985).

A wide spectrum of gram-positive and gram-negative bacteria are isolated from the infectious lesions of LAD patients; however, the most common pathogens are *S. aureus*, enterobacteria, *Pseudomonas* species, and *Candida albicans*. LAD patients are not abnormally susceptible to viral infections, and no untoward effects of live viral vaccines have been reported (Fischer et al., 1988).

Diagnosis

Extreme neutrophilia, especially during infections, is a constant feature and hallmark of LAD. Neutrophilia (>15,000 cells/mm³) is a common feature of LAD; this is due to diminished margination of the circulating neutrophils with enrichment of cells in the mainstream of the blood vessel. Absence of neutrophilia (especially in the newborn who is otherwise well but has delayed umbilical cord detachment) generally rules out the diagnosis of LAD.

Tests of neutrophil function in LAD patients reveal profound defects in adhesion-dependent functions such as adherence to glass or plastic surfaces, spreading, chemotaxis, aggregation, CR3-dependent binding, and phagocytosis of iC3b-coated particles. A deficient respiratory burst is triggered by particulate phagocytosis (Todd and Fryer, 1988). Conversely, adhesion-independent functions, such as intracellular microbicidal activity, and the respiratory burst and degranulation mediated by soluble stimuli are normal. Serum immunoglobulin levels, antibody responses, and delayed hypersensitivity reactions are normal but NK cytotoxicity (but not numbers) and T-cell cytotoxicity may be depressed in vitro.

The diagnosis of LAD is confirmed by flow cytometric analysis of peripheral blood PMNs using monoclonal antibodies for CD11 or CD18 (Arnaout, 1993).

Pathogenesis

The genetic basis of LAD is a variety of mutations within the common β (CD18) subunit gene of the leukocyte function–associated antigen 1 (LFA-1), Mac-1, and p150,95 glycoproteins (Kishimoto et al., 1987; Dimanche-Bortrel et al., 1988; Rodriguez et al., 1993), which is located on chromosome 21 (Corbi et al., 1988). The genes for the three CD11 α-subunits, which form a cluster in the short arm of chromosome 16 (Marlin et al., 1986), are normal. The defects in the β-subunit gene result in absence, insufficient quantity, or abnormal structure of the CD18 subunit precursor. In all patients, the CD18 subunit gene appears to be without gross deletions but there is a failure of the β (CD18) precursor to associate with the α-subunit precursor in the endoplasmic reticulum. This leads to decreased or absent expression of the αβ heterodimer on the cell surface or in intracellular granules (Springer et al., 1984; Lisowska-Grospierre et al., 1986; Corbi et al., 1988).

The diversity of the gene defects has led to the identification of five subtypes of LAD-1 (I to V), whose classification is based on the level of CD18 messenger ribonucleic acid (MRNA), on the size and levels of the CD18 protein precursor, and the resulting phenotype (Kishimoto et al., 1987). Patients with type I LAD-1 produce no β-subunit messenger RNA, have no CD18 precursor, and have a severe clinical phenotype; type II LAD-1 patients have a low level of mRNA, a trace of protein precursor, and a moderate clinical phenotype; type III LAD-1 patients have normal levels of mRNA, an aberrantly small protein precursor, and a moderate

clinical phenotype. It seems that low levels of β-subunit produced in types II and III LAD-1 are sufficient to allow the expression of approximately 3% to 10% of the normal amount of mature αβ complexes on leukocyte surfaces and a moderate clinical phenotype. Patients with type IV LAD-1 have normal levels of mRNA, an aberrantly large protein precursor, and a severe clinical phenotype; type V LAD-1 patients have normal levels of mRNA, a normal size of protein precursor, and a moderate or severe clinical phenotype. The expression of two clinical phenotypes in type V LAD-1 suggests that there are several distinct mutations within this group. Heterozygotes who are clinically unaffected have approximately half-normal amounts of CD11/CD18 subunits on the surfaces of their neutrophils and lymphocytes (Anderson et al., 1985).

Treatment

Patients with LAD require early and aggressive treatment of infections with appropriate antibiotics. Successful bone marrow transplantation has been reported in several LAD patients (LeDeist et al., 1989), and gene therapy has been proposed for these patients (Kraus et al., 1991).

Leukocyte Adhesion Defect Type 2

Two patients have been described with absence of neutrophil receptors (sialyl-Lewis X or CD15s) for E-selectin (CD62E), the adhesive molecule expressed on the surface of activated endothelial cells (Etzioni et al., 1992). The selectin adhesive molecules mediate the initial rolling motion of neutrophils and monocytes over endothelium at sites of inflammation (Bevilacqua and Nelson, 1993). The two unrelated boys with this defect had recurrent bacterial infections, periodontitis, and neutrophilia, as do patients with LAD type 1, but were also mentally retarded and had distinctive facies. These LAD type 2 patients had a normal density of CD11/CD18 on their leukocytes that could be increased with activation, unlike the LAD type 1 patients. Their neutrophils performed poorly in chemotaxis assays but had normal chemiluminescence responses. The authors suggest that these patients may have a defect in fucosylation that might account for the defect in their adhesive proteins and the abnormal Bombay blood phenotype that was also reported.

In vivo studies were performed on one of the original LAD II patients by Price et al. (1994). Chemotaxis of both neutrophils and monocytes was severely impaired (<6% of normal) as assessed by Rebuck's skin window and skin chamber techniques. Kinetic studies showed a reduced autologous neutrophil half-life of 3.2 hours (normal 7 hours) and an eightfold increase of the neutrophil turnover rate. The patient had a normal antibody response to bacteriophage φX174, indicating that T cell–B cell cooperation was normal.

HYPERIMMUNOGLOBULIN E SYNDROME (JOB'S SYNDROME)

The Biblical medical eponym *Job's syndrome* originated with the 1966 report of two fair-skinned, red-haired girls with severe eczema-like skin lesions, recurrent pulmonary and liver infections, and multiple cutaneous abscesses (Davis et al., 1966). Cultures of the abscesses invariably grew *S. aureus*, and the abscesses were referred to as "cold" because of the lack of local inflammation.

Bannatyne and coworkers (1969) suggested that Job's syndrome was a variant of chronic granulomatous disease (CGD), but this was later found to be incorrect inasmuch as their leukocytes could kill staphylococci normally (White et al., 1969; Pabst et al., 1971).

In 1972, Buckley and coworkers described two male patients with similar features of chronic dermatitis and recurrent infections. These patients had high levels of serum immunoglobulin E (IgE), as did the patients of Pabst and coworkers (1971). In 1974, Hill and Quie reported three patients with Job's syndrome with high IgG levels and a neutrophil chemotactic defect. Many patients of both sexes and various racial groups with the triad of severe eczematoid dermatitis, recurrent infections, and high levels of IgE have been reported (Clark et al., 1973; Van Scoy et al., 1975). The term hyperimmunoglobulin E (HIE) or hyper-IgE syndrome is now most widely used for referring to this disease entity. This syndrome is discussed in detail in Chapter 13.

Inheritance

Eight instances of familial occurrence of the hyper-IgE syndrome were noted in the 21 patients studied by Buckley and Sampson (1981). Both males and females were affected, and the authors suggested an autosomal dominant form of inheritance with incomplete penetrance. There is one report of a mother and daughter with hyper-IgE (Dreskin and Gallin, 1987). An association with particular human leukocyte antigen haplotypes has been suggested, but only a small number of patients have been studied (Jacobs and Norman, 1977). Therefore, the tendency for the development of the hyper-IgE syndrome may be genetically determined.

Clinical Manifestations

The clinical features of 43 patients with hyper-IgE syndrome in three medical centers have been reported (Buckley and Sampson, 1981; Donabedian and Gallin, 1983a; Leung and Geha, 1988). All patients had dermatitis and onset of infections in early childhood. The serum IgE levels ranged from 2150 to 90,000 IU/ml with a mean IgE level over 20,000 IU/ml.

Unlike patients with atopic dermatitis, patients with hyper-IgE syndrome do not usually experience allergy (Buckley and Sampson, 1981; Donabedian and Gallin, 1983a; Leung and Geha, 1988).

Eczematoid rashes are present in all patients with hyper-IgE syndrome. The rash is often papular and pruritic but may also be pustular and lichenified. The face and areas behind the ears are often involved, and flexural or extensor surfaces of limbs may be affected. Skin biopsy reveals dermal edema and infiltration of mast cells, eosinophils, and monocytes. The severity of the rash does not vary seasonally, and it is not provoked by allergens; these features distinguish hyper-IgE syndrome from atopic dermatitis.

Coarse facial features occur in the majority of patients and include a broad nasal bridge, prominent nose, and irregularly proportioned cheeks and jaw. These facial features may be noted in children but become more prominent in adults. The mechanism underlying these aberrations is not known.

Polyarticular arthritis of the wrists, metacarpal-phalangeal, and interphalangeal joints was reported in two patients (Donabedian and Gallin, 1983a). Osteoporosis with recurrent bone fractures is another noninfectious complication. Brestel and coworkers (1982) described a 9-year-old girl with hyper-IgE syndrome and osteogenesis imperfecta tarda with repeated long-bone fractures. Leung and Geha (1988) determined (by photon absorptiometry) the bone density of six patients with hyper-IgE syndrome and found that it was significantly decreased compared with that of age-matched controls. Isolated blood monocytes from these patients were noted to resorb bone actively, suggesting that activation of macrophages including osteoclasts might contribute to the osteopenia of hyper-IgE syndrome.

Recurrent pneumonia in patients with hyper-IgE syndrome often leads to pneumatoceles and empyema (Merten et al., 1979; Lui and Inculet, 1990; Shamberger et al., 1992). *S. aureus* and *C. albicans* are common pathogens but other organisms, including pneumococci, group A streptococcus, *Pseudomonas aeruginosa*, and *Haemophilus influenzae*, may be recovered (Stone and Wheeler, 1990).

Abscesses in patients with hyper-IgE syndrome may be mistaken for a tumor or cyst because of induration, persistence, and lack of warmth. These "cold" abscesses contain large volumes of pus and may be obstructive.

Botryomycosis, an unusual bacterial infection characterized by the formation of hard nodules containing bacterial and eosinophilic granules, has been reported in two patients with hyper-IgE syndrome (Buescher et al., 1988; Bulengo-Ransby et al., 1993). Botryomycosis has been reported in several patients with acquired immunodeficiency syndrome (AIDS) suggesting that abnormalities in immunoregulation may predispose to development of these lesions.

Chronic otitis media, otitis externa, and mastoiditis frequently occur in patients with hyper-IgE syndrome. Osteomyelitis occurs, but it is usually in spatial association with an overlying cellulitis or nearby abscess (Andrich et al., 1993).

Laboratory Findings

An extremely elevated serum level of IgE, often 20,000 IU/ml or greater, is typical of hyper-IgE syndrome. IgE elevations may occur early in infancy in these patients. Dreskin and Gallin (1987) followed IgE levels in a child with the syndrome whose serum IgE level was 160 IU/ml at age 5 months and rose to 5350 IU/ml at 2 years. Kamei and Honig (1988) described a child with the syndrome whose IgE level was 98 IU/ml at 8 months of age and rapidly increased to 10,000 IU/ml by 11 months of age.

Most patients with hyper-IgE syndrome have a mild to moderate eosinophilia. Buckley and Sampson (1981) reported eosinophil counts of 55% to 60% of the total white blood cell (WBC) count in infants with HIE, and Leung and Geha (1988) found eosinophil counts of 40% to 50%. Total WBC counts may be normal or markedly elevated, depending on the presence of acute infections. Patients with hyper-IgE syndrome may suffer from anemia secondary to chronic disease. The erythrocyte sedimentation rate is usually elevated, particularly during exacerbation of their disease. Histamine is an important mediator in IgE-induced allergic reactions, but urinary histamine levels are not correlated with increased incidence of infection or IgE levels (Dreskin et al., 1987).

A high percentage of the IgE in these patients is directed to *S. aureus*, and detection of high levels of anti–*S. aureus* IgE has been used to specifically confirm the diagnosis of hyper-IgE syndrome. Dreskin and colleagues (1985) reported that patients with HIE had markedly elevated levels of anti–*S. aureus* IgE compared with patients with atopic dermatitis or chronic granulomatous disease. They also found that the anti–*S. aureus* IgM but not IgG was elevated and that anti–*S. aureus* IgA was decreased. The infant with hyper-IgE syndrome reported by Kamei and Honig (1988) had anti–*S. aureus* IgE detected at 8 weeks of age (32% of total) that increased to 53% of the total IgE at 8 months of age. Lavoie and coworkers (1989) also reported that anti–*S. aureus* IgE could be detected in infants with hyper-IgE syndrome. However, determination of anti–*S. aureus* IgE requires a special technique and is not routinely available. Dreskin and coworkers (1987) also reported that the catabolism of IgE is slower in hyper-IgE syndrome patients, which also contributes to the serum elevations.

Immunologic Abnormalities

Several studies have shown that neutrophils from patients with hyper-IgE syndrome are defective in chemotaxis and that the presence of cold abscesses may be related to delay of inflammatory cells reaching the site of the infection (Hill and Quie, 1974). Defects in chemotaxis, however, has not been found in all patients, and repeated testing of the same patient's cells may not consistently demonstrate the defect.

The serum contains elevated levels of IgG anti-IgE that may circulate as free antibody or may form high-molecular-mass (>900 kD) complexes with IgE (Quinti et al., 1986). These IgG anti-IgE immune complexes are not unique to hyper-IgE syndrome and may also occur in asthma, allergic rhinitis, and atopic dermatitis.

The IgG-IgE complexes inhibit neutrophil chemotaxis and may be responsible for the chemotactic defect in hyper-IgE syndrome.

Donabedian and Gallin (1982) reported that mononuclear cells from patients with hyper-IgE syndrome produced a soluble factor in vitro that inhibited both neutrophil and monocyte chemotaxis. This inhibition was later shown to be produced by normal mononuclear cells when exposed to heat-killed staphylococci. The inhibitor is a protein with a molecular mass of 35 to 40 kD (Donabedian and Gallin, 1983a). The spontaneous production of this inhibitor is variable but correlates with the chemotactic defect in patients with hyper-IgE syndrome.

Buckley and Sampson (1981) found that all 21 of their hyper-IgE syndrome patients had low titers to diphtheria and tetanus and only 2 of 12 had a normal anamnestic response after a booster immunization with these antigens. Antibody response to capsular polysaccharide of *H. influenzae* was also deficient, and most had IgG2 subclass deficiency (Leung and Geha, 1988). However, IgG4 subclass may be elevated in both hyper-IgE syndrome and severe atopic dermatitis (Reinhold et al., 1988; Ishizaka et al., 1990).

Anergy to *Candida* and streptokinase-streptodornase was noted in half of the patients of Buckley and Sampson (1981). All nine of the hyper-IgE patients studied by Leung and Geha (1988) were anergic to *C. albicans* and tetanus toxoid. Patients with hyper-IgE syndrome have normal lymphoproliferative responses to mitogens, such as phytohemagglutinin, but respond poorly to soluble antigens such as *Candida* and tetanus toxoid (Soderberg-Warner et al., 1983).

Patients with hyper-IgE syndrome may have a deficiency of suppressor T lymphocytes (Katona et al., 1980). Geha and coworkers (1981) also found decreased numbers of CD8 suppressor T cells but normal numbers of CD4 helper T cells. B lymphocytes from hyper-IgE patients may spontaneously synthesize IgE in vitro, and this can be suppressed by the addition of normal CD8 lymphocytes (Kraemer et al., 1982). (See also discussion in Chapter 13.)

Mononuclear cells isolated from hyper-IgE patients were reported by Paganelli and coworkers (1991) to have defective production of interferon-γ (IFN-γ), an inhibitor of IgE production, suggesting that abnormalities in cytokine production may play a role in this disease (Geha, 1992).

Treatment

The most important therapeutic approach is prompt diagnosis and treatment of infectious complications. The lack of an inflammatory response in patients may mask the seriousness of the infection; delay of treatment may result in complications such as airway obstruction by peritonsillar abscesses and pneumatocele formation following pneumonia.

Prophylactic oral antibiotics benefit most patients with hyper-IgE syndrome. Dicloxacillin, trimethoprim-sulfamethoxazole, and other agents effective against staphylococci are used in therapeutic doses (Hattori et al., 1993). Deep-seated or extensive abscesses usually warrant intravenous antibiotics. Specimens for culture should be obtained, because these patients are susceptible to infections with many other bacteria in addition to *S. aureus*. Fungal infections are also common, and appropriate potassium hydroxide preparations should be completed and specimens for fungal cultures should be obtained. Surgical treatment is often required for drainage of abscesses, chest tube placement, and lobectomy or pneumonectomy.

The dermatitis in patients with hyper-IgE syndrome is often severe and may be the source of infection, physical discomfort, and psychologic distress. Topical steroids are useful for controlling the eczematoid dermatitis; oral steroids are sometimes necessary for severe exacerbations. A topical antifungal medication, such as clotrimazole, may be helpful. Oral candidiasis may be treated with nystatin suspension or clotrimazole troches. Antihistamines, such as hydroxyzine or diphenhydramine, help to control pruritus.

Plasmapheresis has been used in hyper-IgE patients unresponsive to conventional therapy. There was a decrease in the severity of the eczematoid rash and normalization of chemotactic and lymphocyte proliferative responses (Ishikawa et al., 1982). Leung and Geha (1988) recommended five treatments in a 10-day period, followed by weekly plasmapheresis to maintain the beneficial effects. They also recommended intravenous immunoglobulin (IVIG) after plasmapheresis to reduce the frequency of serious infections. Clinical trials using IVIG in the treatment of hyper-IgE syndrome indicate that it is effective in treating the severe eczema in these patients and in reducing IgE production (Kimata, 1995).

Levamisole, ascorbic acid, cimetidine, and transfer factor have also been used in treatment on the basis of their ability to improve the in vitro chemotaxis of neutrophils; however, results have been dubious. Levamisole was tested in a double-blind, placebo-controlled study; those receiving the drug were found to have more infections than those given the placebo (Donabedian et al., 1982). IFN-γ improves the chemotaxis of neutrophils from hyper-IgE syndrome patients in vitro and decreases IgE serum levels (Jeppson et al., 1991), but its clinical effectiveness is unproven.

Prognosis

The prognosis for a near-normal life span is favorable for patients diagnosed early and followed up carefully. When diagnosis is delayed bronchiectasis or pneumatoceles may develop and lead to severe pulmonary complications.

Hodgkin's disease and other lymphomas (Burkitt's and histiocytic) have been reported in four patients with hyper-IgE syndrome under 20 years of age (Gorin et al., 1989). The association between the development of a lymphoid neoplasm and other forms of immunodeficiency is well established and may be due to defective tumor surveillance by the patient's abnormal immune system.

LEUKOTACTIC DISORDERS

Leukotactic Disorders with Dermatologic Abnormalities

An association exists between abnormalities of the skin, recurrent infections, and abnormal leukotaxis. Phagocytic cells have a capacity for rapid locomotion that allows them to rapidly localize and kill invading bacteria. It is not surprising that the skin and mucous membranes are particularly vulnerable to lesions as a consequence of deficient neutrophil chemotaxis (Quie et al., 1991). Pincus and colleagues (1975) described a 4-year-old child with ichthyosis, severe subcutaneous abscesses infected with staphylococci and gram-negative bacteria, and abnormal PMN chemotaxis. Dahl and associates (1976) described a child with incontinentia pigmenti with depressed PMN chemotaxis and severe recurrent infections. The frequent infections may be secondary to an abnormal epithelial barrier as well as to the defective leukocyte chemotaxis.

Shwachman Syndrome

Abnormal neutrophil chemotaxis was found in 13 of 14 patients with Shwachman syndrome (Aggett et al., 1979). These patients have pancreatic insufficiency, malabsorption, dyschrondroplasia, eczema, and marked susceptibility to recurrent infections (Mortureux et al., 1992). Parents of children with Shwachman syndrome also have depressed neutrophil chemotaxis, and because this syndrome is inherited as a recessive characteristic, abnormal granulocyte chemotaxis may be a primary defect, although intermittent neutropenia is also often present.

Diabetes Mellitus

Neutrophil chemotaxis in diabetic persons is moderately depressed (Mowat and Baum, 1971; Hill et al., 1983). However, there is no correlation between the leukotactic defect and the age of the patient, degree of control, or serum concentrations of glucose cholesterol, triglycerides, or creatinine. Incubation of diabetic leukocytes with insulin in a glucose-containing medium returns their chemotactic responsiveness to normal. Hyperglycemic sera inhibits killing of *Candida albicans* by neutrophils from diabetic patients but not with normal neutrophils (Wilson and Reeves, 1986).

Molenaar and coworkers (1976) reported that leukotaxis was defective in 52 first-degree relatives of patients with diabetes; the relatives all had normal blood glucose levels. Thus, depressed granulocyte chemotaxis may be a primary abnormality in diabetes, not secondary to insulin therapy or metabolic abnormalities.

Hill and colleagues (1983) demonstrated that peripheral blood monocytes as well as neutrophils from patients with diabetes mellitus exhibit depressed chemotaxis. This topic is discussed in Chapter 19.

Metabolic Storage Diseases

Mannosidosis is a storage disease characterized by mental deficiency and recurrent infections resulting from a congenital deficiency of acidic α-D-mannosidase, leading to the accumulation of mannose within cells, including circulating leukocytes (see Chapter 19). A patient with this enzymatic disorder was shown to have defective neutrophil chemotaxis and delayed bacterial phagocytosis, abnormalities proposed to be secondary to accumulated mannose (Desnick et al., 1976). Chemotactic effects also occur in Gaucher's disease, a deficiency of the lysosomal enzyme glucocerebrosidase, and intravenous enzyme replacement has been reported to correct this defect (Zimran et al., 1993).

Transient Leukotactic Disorders

Disorders of leukotaxis may be transient when secondary to another disorder. Anderson and associates (1974) found a marked depression of granulocyte chemotaxis and random migration in 35 children with measles. Leukotactic function returned to normal approximately 10 days after onset of measles, with resolution of the rash and clinical improvement.

Hill and associates (1976) observed depressed leukocyte chemotactic responsiveness in four patients with allergic rhinitis and severe staphylococcal furunculosis. Neutrophil chemotaxis was normal when the patients were well but became abnormal when allergic symptoms developed, at which point staphylococcal abscesses appeared.

Depressed neutrophil chemotaxis was noted in bone marrow transplant recipients, especially during graft-versus-host reactions or when the patient was receiving antithymocyte globulin, and patients with defective neutrophil chemotaxis had more severe bacterial infections (Zimmerli et al., 1991). Severe impairment of neutrophil chemotaxis has been reported in patients with cancer receiving high doses of interleukin-2, which might account for the frequent episodes of bacterial sepsis in these patients (Klempner et al., 1990).

McCall and coworkers (1971) found depressed granulocyte chemotactic responsiveness in 22 patients with severe bacterial infections. However, Hill and coworkers (1974a) reported neutrophil chemotaxis responsiveness to be increased rather than depressed in patients with bacterial infections. In contrast to a 30% mortality rate in the patients of McCall and colleagues (1971), Hill's patients experienced no mortality and responded well to antibiotics. Thus, increased chemotactic responsiveness appears to be an early response to infection, but chemotaxis may become depressed in severe infection.

Protein-Calorie Malnutrition

Children with severe protein-calorie malnutrition have delayed chemotactic responsiveness (Schopfer and Douglas, 1976). They have greatly increased susceptibility to bacterial, fungal, and viral infections and a paucity of leukocytes in lesions despite the presence of pyogenic microorganisms. Because these children also exhibit decreased antibody production, decreased cell-mediated immunity, low levels of complement components, and defective intraleukocyte killing of

bacteria and fungi, the role of chemotactic defects in their susceptibility to infection is difficult to assess (see Chapter 19).

Tuftsin Deficiency

Tuftsin deficiency is a congenital familial disorder (or a disorder acquired as a result of splenectomy) characterized by increased susceptibility to infection and defective granulocyte phagocytosis (Constantopoulos et al., 1972, 1973; Constantopoulos, 1983). Tuftsin is a tetrapeptide (threonyl-lysyl-prolyl-arginine) synthesized by the spleen in the form of a cytophilic gamma globulin termed *leukokinin*. Leukokinin binds to granulocytes and is cleaved by the granulocyte enzyme leukokinase to form tuftsin. Tuftsin, in turn, enhances the phagocytic ability of the granulocytes and monocytes (Najjar and Constantopoulos, 1972) and may also stimulate procoagulant activity in monocytes and macrophages (Kornberg et al., 1990). Symptoms of hereditary tuftsin deficiency include respiratory infections (bronchitis, pneumonia, bronchiectasis), enlarged and fluctuant lymph nodes, and seborrheic skin rashes. The usual organisms are *Pneumococcus*, *S. aureus*, and *Candida*. Immunoglobulins, complement, and NBT reduction are normal, but serum tuftsin activity is markedly deficient.

Secondary tuftsin deficiency occurs after splenectomy or splenic infiltration (e.g., Hodgkin's disease) or infarction (e.g., sickle cell disease) (Najjar, 1975). The granulocytes of patients with myelofibrosis and leukemia fail to show phagocytic stimulation even with saturating amounts of tuftsin (Constantopoulos et al., 1973). Few new reports of tuftsin deficiency have been reported, in part because of the difficulty in performing the tuftsin assay.

Localized Juvenile Periodontitis

Localized juvenile periodontitis (LJP) is usually diagnosed in adolescents 11 to 13 years of age, and its incidence in the United States is estimated at 0.1% although it may be much higher in some ethnic groups (Nisengard et al., 1994). Often there is little gingival inflammation on inspection, but radiographs reveal a characteristic pattern of marked, localized, alveolar bone loss that rapidly leads to tooth loss if untreated. The disease may progress to generalized juvenile periodontitis with more generalized alveolar bone loss in older adolescents.

Specimens of the gram-negative anaerobic bacterium *Actinobacillus actinomycetemcomitans* can be obtained from culture from the gingiva of 97% of patients with LJP, and most patients have antibodies in the serum and crevicular fluid to this organism. Tetracycline suppresses growth of *A. actinomycetemcomitans* and is the treatment of choice for these patients, although surgery may also be required. Antibiotics are not effective in generalized juvenile periodontitis, as different bacteria including *Porphyromonas (Bacteroides) gingivalis* are associated with this form of disease (Adair, 1992).

Peripheral blood neutrophils from patients with LJP

exhibit decreased chemotactic responsiveness that appears to be due to a defect in the chemotactic receptors on the neutrophil (Van Dyke, 1985; Perez et al., 1991). Siblings of patients with LJP also exhibit a chemotactic defect in their neutrophils, although they do not show clinical signs of LJP; this suggests that the tendency to acquire LJP is genetic but that microbial factors, such as leukotoxins produced by bacteria, also play a role.

Papillon-Lefèvre Syndrome

The Papillon-Lefèvre syndrome is a rare form of periodontitis affecting pre-pubertal children associated with palmer-plantar hyperkeratosis (Coccia et al., 1966). Gingival bleeding on brushing the teeth is noted by age 2, complete loss of all primary teeth usually occurs by 4 years, and loss of all permanent teeth occurs by age 16. This disease has an autosomal recessive pattern of inheritance, and a defect in neutrophil chemotaxis is suspected (Burgett, 1993).

Rapidly Progressive Periodontitis

Rapidly progressive periodontitis (RPP) usually occurs in late adolescence to about 35 years of age. In the active phase of the disease, patients experience gingival bleeding and inflammation with severe alveolar bone loss. The anaerobe *P. gingivalis* is frequently recovered from the gingiva of patients with rapidly progressive periodontitis, although other bacteria, including spirochetes, may also be isolated (Riviere et al., 1991).

Secretory products of *P. gingivalis* inhibit neutrophil chemotaxis and phagocytosis (Odell and Wu, 1992), which may contribute to the chemotactic defects reported in some of these patients. Furthermore, more than 90% of patients with adult onset of progressive periodontitis are smokers (Haber and Kent, 1992), and the function of oral PMNs is compromised by soluble factors in tobacco and tobacco smoke (Kenney et al., 1977; MacFarlane et al., 1992).

Acute Necrotizing Ulcerative Gingivitis

The acute necrotizing ulcerative form of gingivitis has a rapid onset and presents with painful, ulcerative gingival lesions. It usually occurs at times of great physical or psychologic stress and is often found in young military personnel under battle conditions and college students at examination time. Treatment consists of proper plaque control and débridement and sometimes antibiotics (Nisengard et al., 1994).

Microscopic examination of the gingiva reveals bacteria, primarily *Prevotella intermedia* and an intermediate-sized spirochete, neutrophils, and necrotic tissue (Riviere et al., 1991). Defects in neutrophil chemotaxis and phagocytosis have been reported in patients with this disease (Cogen et al., 1983).

Newborn Infants

All newborn infants have depressed neutrophil chemotactic responsiveness, which may be related to decreased neutrophil membrane deformability (Miller, 1975); this may lead to the decreased ability of newborns to localize infections (see Chapter 10). Neonatal neutrophils also have impaired adherence and fluidity, resulting in delayed accumulation at inflammatory sites (Anderson et al., 1981a, 1990). The cellular basis for defective locomotion of neutrophils from neonates may be related to abnormality of microtubule assembly and, therefore, deformability (Anderson et al., 1984a).

Actin is a major component of microfilaments, necessary for all motion. Monomeric G-actin is rapidly polymerized to filamentous F-actin when the neutrophil is activated. Harris and coworkers (1992) reported that the F-actin content of neutrophils from normal newborns was significantly decreased compared with that of normal adults after stimulation with chemotactic peptide, which may also explain the defects in chemotaxis in newborns. Decreased mobilization of the adhesion glycoprotein CD11b/CD18 (Mac-1) from the neutrophil granules to the cell surface may also depress the response to inflammatory stimuli (Jones et al., 1990).

Actin Dysfunction

Disorders of actin polymerization may account for defective chemotaxis of neutrophils outside the neonatal period. In 1974, Boxer and colleagues described a male infant with recurrent bacterial infections whose neutrophils contained normal amounts of actin protein, but the actin polymerization in the patient's cells was decreased compared with that of normal individuals. The parents of this patient were studied several years later (Southwick et al., 1988), and the F-actin (polymerized) content of their stimulated neutrophils was about half-normal; this suggested this the disorder was recessively inherited. Other cases of aberrant actin polymerization associated with defective neutrophil chemotaxis and recurrent infections have been reported (Coates et al., 1991; Jung, 1991; Howard et al., 1994); a recessive pattern of inheritance has also been suggested in these patients.

Burns

Decreased chemotaxis of neutrophils has also been noted in patients with large thermal burns (Grogan and Miller, 1973). In studies using guinea pigs, neutrophil chemotaxis was greatly depressed immediately after the burn injury (induced under anesthesia) and normalized by 7 to 10 days (Bjornson and Somers, 1993). Hasslen and coworkers (1992) examined neutrophils from patients with major thermal injuries (second-degree to third-degree burns over more than 40% of the body) and found that the content of polymerized actin (F-actin) was increased in their cells, which may make the cells less deformable and inhibit chemotaxis. Davis and coworkers (1980) found that peripheral blood neutrophils from burn patients (>35% burn on average) had discharged their specific granule contents and the degranulation correlated with decreased chemotaxis. This disorder is also discussed in Chapter 19.

CHRONIC GRANULOMATOUS DISEASE

Chronic granulomatous disease (CGD) is a genetic syndrome characterized by susceptibility to recurrent severe infections and is associated with dysfunctional NADPH oxidase and defective microbicidal function of phagocytic cells but normal B-cell and T-cell function (Dinauer and Orkin, 1992; Quie, 1993). At least eight genetic subtypes are now recognized, with one X-linked subtype accounting for the majority of the cases (Cornutte, 1993).

Historical Aspects

Two years after Bruton's first description of agammaglobulinemia (Bruton, 1952), Janeway and colleagues (1954) described five children with recurrent, severe, life-threatening *Staphylococcus, Proteus,* or *Pseudomonas* infections with increased levels of serum gamma globulin. Four patients with similar clinical manifestations were extensively investigated by Good and colleagues in Minnesota and reported by Berendes (1957) and Bridges (1959) and their coworkers. All were male children with hepatosplenomegaly, suppurative lymphadenitis, pyogenic skin lesions, severe pulmonary disease, and hypergammaglobulinemia. Specific antibody responses were normal and the increased gamma globulin concentrations were appropriate to the severity of their infections. The severity and progressive nature of the infectious process were believed to be a consequence of a "generalized disease of the reticuloendothelial system." Early death of all patients in spite of heroic treatment efforts prompted Bridges and coworkers (1959) to call this syndrome a "fatal granulomatous disease of childhood."

Johnston and McMurry (1967) described five boys and reviewed 23 previously reported patients with a clinical syndrome of hepatosplenomegaly, recurrent suppurative infections, and hypergammaglobulinemia. All of the patients were boys, and 16 had a brother or brothers with a similar constellation of clinical findings, which strongly suggested X-linked transmission of the syndrome. Johnston and McMurry proposed that the syndrome be called *chronic familial granulomatosis.* Quie and coworkers (1967) reported defective intracellular bacterial killing by neutrophils. The term "chronic granulomatous disease" has been used since then to describe this syndrome.

Quie et al. (1967) and Holmes et al. (1967) first noted that CGD granulocytes ingested bacteria normally but did not kill them (Fig. 15–1). Ordinarily, the engulfment process in phagocytic cells is associated with a burst of respiratory oxidative activity, increased oxygen consumption, and a shift to glucose metabolism via the hexose monophosphate shunt (see Chapter 5). In the resting state, only 1% of glucose is metabolized by the hexose monophospate shunt, but during phagocytosis as much as 10% of glucose is oxidized by this route. Phagocytosis also stimulates lipid turnover as new membranes are formed during degranulation and phagocytic particle engulfment.

Phagocytic cells from patients with CGD did not re-

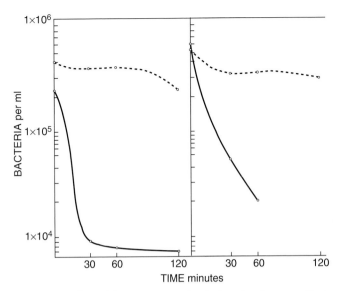

Figure 15–1. Bacterial assay comparing leukocytes from a patient with chronic granulomatous disease and a normal person. There was rapid killing of greater than 99% of bacteria incubated with normal leukocytes during 2 hours (solid line). There was essentially no killing of either staphylococci *(left)* or *Serratia (right)* by the leukocytes of the patient *(dashed line).* (Redrawn from Quie PG, Kaplan EL, Laxdal T, Dossett J. Phagocyte abnormalities. In Kagan BM, Stiehm ER, eds. Immunologic Incompetence. Chicago, Year Book Medical, 1971.)

spond with the expected oxidative respiratory burst during phagocytosis, and this abnormal response to membrane stimulation was associated with defective intracellular killing of catalase-positive microbial species.

Clinical Manifestations

The overall clinical findings of CGD are summarized in Table 15–1. The prognosis has improved with more vigilant care and use of antibiotics, IFN-γ, and bone marrow transplantation.

Infections

Most patients with CGD have at least one unusual or severe infection during the first year of life, and more than 80% are identified with unusual susceptibility to serious infections before their second birthday (Johnston and Newman, 1977). Diagnosis of CGD, however, may be delayed until adolescence or adulthood; the oldest reported individual with CGD was diagnosed in the sixth decade of life (Schapiro et al., 1991).

Patients with CGD usually manifest a typical response to infection with fever, an appropriate localized inflammatory response, leukocytosis, and an elevated erythrocyte sedimentation rate. Incomplete resolution of the inflammatory response results in granulomatous lesions characterized by collections of phagocytes and giant cells often containing pigmented lipid material.

The areas of the body primarily involved in CGD are those that receive constant challenge from bacteria, such as the skin, lungs, and perianal tissue (Fig. 15–2).

Table 15–1. Clinical Findings in 28 Cases
of Granulomatous Disease

Finding	Fraction of Patients Involved
Marked lymphadenopathy	28/28
Hepatomegaly	27/27
Pneumonitis	27/27
Onset by age 2	25/25
Suppuration of nodes	27/28
Splenomegaly	26/27
Dermatitis	25/26
Onset by age 1	22/25
Death by age 7	18/23
Persistent rhinitis	14/25
Death from pneumonitis	10/19
Conjunctivitis	12/24
Onset with lymphadenitis	9/22
Onset with dermatitis	9/22
Ulcerative stomatitis	10/25
Perianal abscess	9/25
Persistent diarrhea	8/24
Osteomyelitis	7/25

From Johnston RB Jr, McMurray JS. Chronic familial granulomatosis: report of five cases and review of the literature. Am J Dis Child 114:370–378, 1967. Copyright 1967, American Medical Association.

The onset of illness is usually in the first few months of life but may be delayed. The earliest lesions are typically eczematoid reactions of the skin around the ears and nose. These progress to purulent dermatitis and enlarged local lymph nodes. With recurrences, tissue necrosis, granuloma formation, and suppurative adenopathy occur.

Abscess formation is the hallmark of CGD and may occur in any organ of the body, particularly in the liver, spleen, lungs, and bones (Quie, 1969). Brain abscesses resulting from *Aspergillus* species are often fatal, although pneumonia caused by *Aspergillus* is much more common (Cohen et al., 1981).

Infections of the genitourinary tract are common (Aliabadi et al., 1989; Walther et al., 1992). Cutaneous infections may result in persistent drainage, prolonged healing, and residual scarring. Surprisingly, septicemia and meningitis are uncommon.

Osteomyelitis may develop at multiple sites even

during antibiotic therapy, but complete healing of all affected bones occurs (Wolfson et al., 1969). The small bones of the hands and feet are common sites (Forrest et al., 1988). Although bone enlargement and destruction occur, there is minimal sclerosis, presumably because of the granulomatous cellular response. The bacteria recovered from the bones are similar to those recovered from lymph nodes or organ abscesses.

Although an infectious pathogen is not isolated in each febrile episode in CGD patients, most infections are caused by a relatively limited spectrum of catalase-positive microbes; the most common are *S. aureus, Serratia marcescens, Escherichia coli, Pseudomonas,* and *Aspergillus* species (Lazarus and Neu, 1975) (Fig. 15–3). Catalase-negative microbes, such as streptococci, are killed normally by CGD neutrophils because microbial hydrogen peroxide, which is concentrated in phagocytic vacuoles, contributes to microbial "suicide." Catalase-positive microbes, in contrast, inactivate peroxide and thus persist within CGD neutrophils and form a nidus for chronic inflammation and granuloma formation.

Unusual organisms, such as *Chromobacterium violaceum,* and *Legionella* species, have also been isolated from CGD patients (Macher et al., 1982; Peerless et al., 1985; Ephros et al., 1989). The bacille Calmette-Guérin strain of *Mycobacterium bovinum* has been isolated from CGD lymph nodes and lungs of patients immunized with bacille Calmette-Guérin. Atypical mycobacteria and *Nocardia* species have also been isolated from a patient with CGD (Seger et al., 1984).

Pulmonary Disorders

Pulmonary disorders occur in nearly all children with CGD and include recurrent pneumonia, hilar lymphadenopathy, empyema, and lung abscesses. Because antibiotic treatment does not result in rapid clearing,

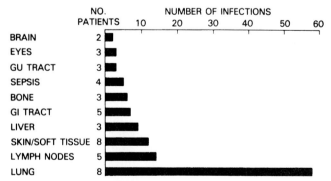

Figure 15–2. Sites of 119 infections in 14 patients with chronic granulomatous disease followed for 150 patient-years. GU = genitourinary; GI = gastrointestinal. (Reproduced with permission from Gallin JI, Buescher ES, Seligmann BE, Nath J, Gaither TE, Katz P. Recent advances in chronic granulomatous disease. Ann Intern Med 99:657–674, 1983.)

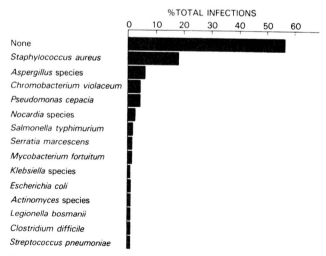

Figure 15–3. Organisms causing 119 major febrile episodes (necessitating treatment with intravenous antibiotic drugs) in 14 patients with chronic granulomatous disease followed for 150 patient-years. (Reproduced with permission from Gallin JI, Buescher ES, Seligmann BE, Nath J, Gaither TE, Katz P. Recent advances in chronic granulomatous disease. Ann Intern Med 99:657–674, 1983.)

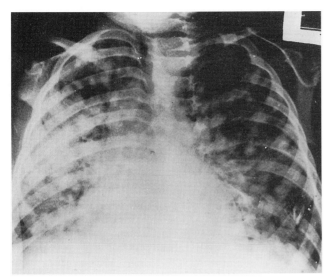

Figure 15–4. Chest roentgenogram of a patient with chronic granulomatous disease. Respiration was severely compromised, and death occurred 7 days after this chest film was taken. (From Quie PG. Clinical manifestations of chronic granulomatous disease of childhood. In Williams RC Jr, Fudenberg HH, eds. Phagocytic Mechanisms in Health and Disease. New York, Intercontinental Medical Book, 1972.)

lung infiltrates persist for weeks or months (Fig. 15–4). The chest radiograph may show reticulonodular densities, which represent areas of granuloma (Fig. 15–5). In certain patients, areas of bronchopneumonia resolve into discrete areas of consolidation termed *encapsulating*

pneumonia; these areas are considered distinctive and diagnostic of CGD (Wolfson et al., 1968).

Gastrointestinal Disorders

Mucous membrane complications include ulcerative stomatitis, gingivitis, persistent rhinitis, and conjunctivitis (Cohen et al., 1985). Diarrhea is relatively common and enteritis, and colitis may be indistinguishable from Crohn's disease (Ament and Ochs, 1973; Fisher et al., 1987). Ament and Ochs (1973) also described perianal fistulas, vitamin B_{12} malabsorption, and steatorrhea. Rectal and jejunal biopsy specimens of seven of nine patients disclosed the presence of histiocytes. One child presented with ascites and bilateral inguinal hernias (Subramian et al., 1974).

Obstructive Lesions

A fairly common manifestation of CGD—intestinal obstruction associated with gastric antral narrowing—was first described by Griscom and coworkers (1974). Biopsy specimens revealed sterile noncaseating granulomas with histiocytic and round cell infiltration. The obstruction may lead to vomiting, delayed gastric emptying, and malnutrition. Clinical benefits have been noted with corticosteroid therapy (Chin et al., 1987).

Similar obstructive lesions associated with diffuse granulomatous lesions have been observed in the esophagus, intestine, and ureters (Harris and Boles, 1973; Gallin et al., 1983).

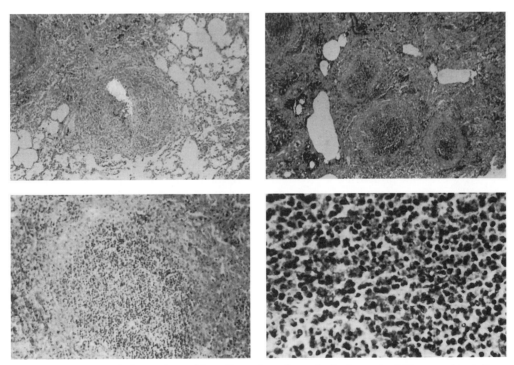

Figure 15–5. Histologic sections of lung tissue from the patient whose chest film was shown in Figure 15–4. Note granulomas throughout the lung parenchyma, which consist primarily of mononuclear cells. (From Quie PG. Clinical manifestations of chronic granulomatous disease of childhood. In Williams RC Jr, Fudenberg HH, eds. Phagocytic Mechanisms in Health and Disease. New York, Intercontinental Medical Book, 1972.)

Growth

Patients with CGD are generally shorter in stature than their parents or normal siblings. Serious and prolonged infections may account for some of this growth failure; however, when Payne and associates (1983) reviewed clinical information for 14 patients with CGD, most were short (approximately in the third percentile) by age 2 years. Several of the patients had relative freedom from serious infection until this age. Short stature in these patients persisted throughout childhood and adolescence in spite of catch-up growth during extended asymptomatic periods.

The short stature may be secondary to chronic infection, but gastrointestinal tract abnormalities and malnutrition may also contribute. The short stature may also be a genetic feature of CGD, reflecting membrane defects in cells other than the hematopoietic system.

Collagen Disease

Both systemic and discoid lupus erythematosus have been reported in patients with X-linked or autosomal recessive CGD (Manzi et al., 1991). Juvenile rheumatoid arthritis with highly positive rheumatoid factor has been reported in a girl with autosomal recessive (p47 cytosolic factor–deficient) CGD (Lee and Yap, 1994). Many mothers of boys with X-linked CGD have been reported to have discoid lupus, recurrent aphthous ulcers, or both, but without serologic evidence of lupus, such as antinuclear antibodies (Kragballe et al., 1981). A female carrier of documented X-linked cytochrome–positive CGD has been reported with discoid lupus and recurrent aphthous ulcers (Yeaman et al., 1992).

Pathogenesis

As noted earlier, the hallmark of CGD is a failure of the NADPH oxidase of phagocytic cells to generate superoxide and other reactive oxygen species (Segal, 1989; Babior, 1991) that participate in intracellular killing of ingested microorganisms. The four structural components of NADPH oxidase in resting cells are the two subunits of the plasma membrane cytochrome b_{558}, a 91-kD and a 22-kD protein called gp91-phox and p22-phox, and the two cytosolic proteins, a 47-kD and a 67-kD protein called p47-phox and p67-phox (gp designates glycoprotein; p, protein; and phox, phagocytic oxidase). Microbial attachment to receptors on the phagocytic cell surface or other appropriate stimuli cause assembly of these components in the plasma membrane and activation of NADPH oxidase. Defects in any of these four components result in loss of enzymatic activity and expression of CGD.

Genetic Types

Chronic granulomatous disease is inherited as either an X-linked or an autosomal recessive disorder. The gene for the gp91-phox subunit of cytochrome b_{558} is located on the short arm of the X chromosome (Dinauer et al., 1987) and mutations in this gene account

for all cases of X-linked CGD. Designated X91, this is the most common type of the disease and is responsible for almost 60% of all CGD patients (Segal et al., 1983; Roos et al., 1992; Curnutte, 1993) (Table 15–2).

In rare circumstances, patients have mutations in the p22-phox gene in the long arm of chromosome 16 that inactivate the p22-phox subunit of cytochrome b_{558} and lead to an autosomal recessive form of CGD; A22 CGD accounts for about 5% of all CGD patients. However, most CGD patients with autosomal recessive inheritance have a defect in one of the two cytosolic components of the NADPH oxidase, p47-phox or p67-phox (Nunoi et al., 1988). Mutations in the p47-phox gene on the long arm of chromosome 7 and mutations in the p67-phox gene on the long arm of chromosome 31 lead to A47 and A67 CGD, respectively, and together account for 38% of all patients with CGD (Curnutte et al., 1988; Clark et al., 1989; Roos, 1994).

Most cases of X-linked CGD have a grossly intact gp91-phox on Southern blot analysis, but the protein product is absent and cytochrome b_{558} is completely missing on the outer membrane of phagocytic cells. In X-linked gp91-phox CGD as well as autosomal p22-phox CGD, both subunits of cytochrome b_{558} are usually missing, indicating that single subunits lack the stability of the combined subunits of the heterodimer (Verhoeven et al., 1988; Roos, 1994). Intact neutrophils of X91 CGD patients with total absence of protein produce no superoxide and do not reduce NBT. Intermediate levels of cytochrome b_{558} and superoxide production are found in heterozygotic female carriers, and NBT scores are approximately 50% of normal. In the few cases in which mutations in gp91-phox lead to normal levels of nonfunctional cytochrome b_{558}, phagocytic cells produce no superoxide and do not reduce NBT.

In variant forms of CGD, levels of gp91-phox and p22-phox protein are diminished and oxidase activity is low but usually measurable (Roos, 1994). In some variant forms, the NADPH oxidase activity is between 5% and 25% of normal and the quantity of superoxide produced and NBT reduced is proportional to the level of measurable cytochrome b_{558} (Roos, 1994). In a rare variant with very low levels of cytochrome b_{558} and an abnormal oxidase (2% to 5% of normal), neutrophils produce minimal quantities of superoxide and have weakly positive NBT scores (Curnutte et al., 1988).

Table 15–2. Genetic Defects and Chromosome Locations of Types of Chronic Granulomatous Disease (CGD)

Chromosome	Gene Product	Type	Frequency in CGD Patients (%)
X	gp91-phox	X91	57
16	p22-phox	A22	5
7	p47-phox	A27	33
1	p67-phox	A67	5

From Curnutte JT. Classification of chronic granulomatous disease. Hematol Oncol Clin North Am Imm 2:241–252, 1988; Curnutte JT. Presentation, Western Society for Pediatric Research, February 7–9, 1994; and Roos D. The genetic basis of chronic granulomatous disease. Immunol Rev 138:121–157, 1994.

Gene Defects

The mutations leading to X-linked CGD (X91) are extremely heterogeneous in nature, and more than 40 mutations have been found in 46 families studied by various investigators and reported by Roos (1994). When large deletions occur on the distal short arm of the X chromosome, other genes may be affected. McLeod's hemolytic anemia, Duchenne's muscular dystrophy, and X-linked retinitis pigmentosa have been associated with CGD (Baehner et al., 1986; Orkin, 1989).

In all but one patient described with A22 CGD, the gene is intact but the protein product is lacking and cytochrome b_{558} is completely missing. All A22 CGD patients lack NADPH oxidase activity, including a patient with normal levels of nonfunctional cytochrome b_{558}. As with X91 CGD, the mutations leading to A22 CGD are heterogenous in nature (Dinauer et al., 1990; Babior, 1991; Roos, 1994).

In contrast to the great heterogeneity of mutations in X91 and A22 CGD, only a few different mutations are known to cause A47 and A67 CGD (Roos, 1994). Neutrophils from all patients analyzed had normal mRNA for p47-phox and p67-phox but no detectable protein and absent NBT reduction or superoxide production when stimulated (Curnutte et al., 1988; Lomax et al., 1989; Leto et al., 1990; Casimir et al., 1991; Chanock et al., 1991; Roos, 1994).

Clinical Correlates with Genetic Types

A difference in severity of infectious lesions has been observed in CGD patients with different inheritance patterns. Weening and colleagues (1985a) compared clinical severity in seven CGD patients with X-linked inheritance (absence of gp91-phox) and five patients with autosomal recessive inheritance (absence of p47-phox). Although no significant differences in site of infections or etiology of infections were noted, CGD patients with X-linked inheritance were hospitalized twice as frequently and onset of infections occurred at an earlier age than in patients with autosomal recessive CGD.

Diagnosis

Oxidase Activity

The defining defect of CGD is the failure of neutrophils to react with increased NADPH oxidase activity upon appropriate stimulation. The oxidase activity is usually measured by superoxide generation (by reduction of ferricytochrome c) but can be measured by oxygen consumption or production of hydrogen peroxide. Flow cytometric methods have been introduced to diagnose CGD (Roesler et al., 1991).

Nitroblue Tetrazolium Dye Test and Chemiluminescence

The NBT dye reduction assay is an excellent screening test for CGD, because superoxide generated by the respiratory burst in normal cells reduces the soluble yellow NBT dye to formazan, a deep blue insoluble pigment. Neutrophils from CGD patients generate little or no superoxide, and the NBT test is negative; that is, neutrophils from CGD patients do not contain formazan because NBT remains soluble and colorless in the absence of superoxide. Female carriers of CGD are chimeric and both NBT-positive and NBT-negative cells are observed. The NBT slide test is sensitive and specific for diagnosis of CGD and for identifying the carrier state of X-linked CGD in females (Baehner and Nathan, 1968).

A chemiluminescence assay is a sensitive but less specific indicator of superoxide generation. The assay is a useful screening test for CGD because neutrophils from CGD patients generate essentially no chemiluminescence and intermediate values are found in female carriers of X-linked CGD (Mills et al., 1980).

These assays, however, may fail to detect the X-linked origin of the disease in some families because about one third of all X-linked defects arise from new mutations in germline cells (Roos, 1994). Furthermore, the carrier state may be obscured in carriers of gp91-phox deficiency with extreme lyonization toward the normal phenotype. Conversely, extreme lyonization toward the abnormal phenotype may result in CGD in a female and point away from the X-linked nature of the disease.

Definition of Genetic Types

To differentiate the types of CGD, Western blot analysis of neutrophil lysates with antibodies against gp91-phox, p22-phox, p47-phox, and p67-phox detects the presence of these constitutive proteins of NADPH oxidase. In patients with A47 or A67 CGD, the relevant protein is absent. In the case of either A22 or X91 CGD, both subunits of cytochrome b_{558} are usually undetectable, and the distinction between these two forms can usually be made by NBT slide testing of family members. Detection of a female carrier identifies the disease as X-linked and points to a defect in the gp91-phox gene (Roos, 1994).

When both subunits of cytochrome b_{558} are detectable, the cell-free oxidase system may point to a defect in cytochrome b_{558}. In the cell-free oxidase assay, neutrophil cell membranes are combined with neutrophil cytosol in the presence of activating agents and cofactors. In CGD patients, absent or very reduced oxidase activity is detected by this assay. Membranes from normal neutrophils restore NADPH oxidase function in CGD patients with absent gp91-phox or absent p22-phox. Cytosol from normal neutrophils restores the NADPH oxidase response in CGD patients with p47-phox or p67-phox deficiency (Clark et al., 1989). Carriers of autosomal types of CGD have no detectable abnormalities in any assays of NADPH oxidase activity, but superoxide production has been shown to be significantly lower than normal in carriers of A67 CGD (de Boer et al., 1994) and in carriers of A47 CGD (Verhoeven et al., 1988).

Prenatal Diagnosis

Before the availability of molecular biology techniques, prenatal diagnosis of CGD depended on obtaining umbilical cord phagocytes at fetoscopy for measurement of oxidase activity (Newburger et al., 1979). Currently, fetal DNA obtained by chronic villus biopsy or amniocentesis can be analyzed for specific gene defects by Southern blot analysis, polymerase chain reaction, and restriction fragment length polymorphism analysis to provide a more definitive prenatal diagnosis of CGD (Orkin, 1989; de Boer et al., 1992; Roos, 1994).

Treatment

Antibiotic Therapy

The primary aim of therapy for patients with CGD is prevention and cure of infectious lesions. The skin is a frequent portal of entry, and efforts to improve skin hygiene are effective. Prophylaxis with trimethoprim-sulfamethoxazole or other antibiotics is now the rule (Margolis et al., 1990). Itraconazole has been used to treat aspergillosis, and a double-blind trial is under way using oral itraconazole prophylactically to prevent fungal infections (Spencer et al., 1994). Infectious lesions develop in CGD patients despite prophylactic antibiotics and adjunctive therapies and require vigorous diagnostic measures as well as aggressive early antimicrobial therapy (Mouy et al., 1989; Pogrebniak et al., 1993).

Treatment of Obstructive Lesions

A frequent complication of CGD is obstruction of the gastrointestinal or genitourinary tract by granulomas. The gastric outlet is often the site of obstruction in the gastrointestinal tract, and this may be the first clinical manifestation of CGD (Dickerman et al., 1986). Many patients respond to more intense antibiotic therapy, but steroids are often required and usually bring relief within a few days. Granulomas may also occur anywhere in the genitourinary tract from the kidney to the urethra and may be associated with dysuria. These lesions also respond to a combination of antibiotic and oral steroid therapy (Chin et al., 1987; Southwick and van der Meer, 1988). Surgery must be considered in the treatment of certain obstructions in CGD patients, but postoperative complications are frequent. Salazosulfapyridine has been used for gastric outlet obstructions in addition to steroids (Stopyrowa et al., 1989).

Leukocyte Transfusions

Leukocyte transfusions may contribute to successful control of life-threatening infection processes (McCullough et al., 1969; Raubitschek et al., 1973; Yomtovian et al., 1981; Gallin et al., 1983). A 16-year-old girl with CGD and multiple hepatic abscesses was treated with a combination of interferon-γ and intralesional granulocyte infusions and experienced complete recovery (Lekstrom-Himes et al., 1994).

Interferon-γ

A randomized double-blind study of a recombinant human IFN-γ has shown that this well-tolerated treatment reduced the frequency and severity of infectious episodes (International Chronic Granulomatous Disease Cooperative Study Group, 1991). IFN-γ treatment of CGD patients with detectable but deficient levels of cytochrome b_{558} (i.e., variant CGD patients) had demonstrated increased NADPH oxidase activity (Ezekowitz et al., 1988) and prompted a placebo-controlled study of IFN-γ in 128 CGD patients with different inheritance patterns.

An impressive clinical benefit was observed in CGD patients receiving IFN-γ compared with those receiving placebo. Of CGD patients receiving IFN-γ, 77% were infection free after 12 months. Only 30% of CGD patients in the placebo group were free of serious infections for 12 months. The difference in infection rates was significant ($P = .0001$) (International Chronic Granulomatous Disease Cooperative Study Group, 1991). The infections that did occur in IFN-γ–treated CGD patients were less severe, requiring fewer days of hospitalization and parenteral antibiotic treatment. Individual patients with pre-existing pulmonary nodules and gastrointestinal nodules improved after IFN-γ treatment. The most frequent reactions to IFN-γ injections were flu-like symptoms, headache, myalgia, and mild fever, usually effectively prevented by acetaminophen.

No difference in NADPH oxidative response, bacterial killing, or cytochrome b_{558} was noted between the placebo and the IFN-γ recipients. Other unidentified biologic responses to IFN-γ may contribute to enhanced resistance in patients treated with this recombinant cytokine (Klebanoff et al., 1992; Malmvall and Follin, 1993). The minimal toxicity and significant clinical effectiveness have led to a standard recommendation of recombinant human IFN-γ, 50 μ/m² body surface, administered subcutaneously three times each week (International Chronic Granulomatous Disease Cooperative Study Group, 1991) for CGD patients of all ages and inheritance patterns.

Transfusions and Kell's Blood Group

Anemia may be present in patients with CGD as a result of constant severe infections, and whole-blood transfusions may be required. The frequent occurrence of Ko erythrocytes in CGD is a potential transfusion hazard (Giblett et al., 1971). This is a rare null Kell phenotype linked to the X chromosome that is not uncommon in CGD patients (Marsh et al., 1975). As a result of previous transfusions with Kell-positive erythrocytes, antibodies to Kell antigens may develop that cause subsequent transfusion reactions with all but Ko cells. Thus, Kell phenotyping should be done for all patients with CGD; if Ko is present, transfusion is best avoided or Ko erythrocytes used.

Bone Marrow Transplantation

Bone marrow transplantation has been accomplished in patients with CGD. One patient (a 2½-year-old boy) was given 5.5×10^6 nucleated marrow cells from a human leukocyte antigen–identical, unrelated female donor 4 days after receiving cyclophosphamide (Forfoozanfar et al., 1977). Evidence of successful engraftment of donor granulocyte precursors included clinical improvement over 3 years, 12% circulating NBT-positive cells, and neutrophils with female nuclear clubs. This offers an approach to the cure of CGD as well as other phagocytic defects (Rappeport et al., 1982; Hobbs et al., 1992).

Gene Therapy

Chronic granulomatous disease is an ideal candidate disease for gene therapy because the biochemical defect is known and the involved genes have been cloned (Royer-Pokora et al., 1986; Dinauer et al., 1987; Leto et al., 1990; Volpp and Lin, 1993). Moreover, hematopoietic progenitor cells, the therapeutic target for gene therapy for CGD, have been receptive for CGD gene transfer. Hematopoietic progenitor cells from A47 CGD patients have been transfected with a retroviral vector containing p47-phox complementary DNA (cDNA), and NADPH oxidase activity was corrected when these cells were differentiated in vitro to mature neutrophils and monocytes (Sekhsar et al., 1993). Similarly, transduction of progenitor cells corrected the gp91-phox and p22-phox CGD oxidase defect to 2.5% and 4.9% of normal superoxide production, respectively, in nine patients (Li et al., 1994). These studies provide the basis for gene therapy for both X-linked and autosomal forms of CGD.

Prognosis

Susceptibility to serious bacterial and fungal infection is still the hallmark of CGD; however, the quality of life of CGD patients has dramatically improved during the past three decades. Knowledge of decreased effectiveness of host defenses prompted antimicrobial prophylaxis and early aggressive treatment of infection. Indeed, patients diagnosed during the 1960s and 1970s are now adults and are productively involved in their communities (Quie, 1993). IFN-γ therapy has further decreased the frequency of infections requiring hospitalization or intravenous antibiotics, and CGD patients receiving IFN-γ appear to respond more appropriately to antibacterial and antifungal therapy when infections do occur (Quie, 1995, personal observation). Correction of the specific functional defect in CGD phagocytic cells by genetic engineering is a realistic expectation and may soon provide CGD patients with normal host defenses.

ENZYME DEFECTS

Myeloperoxidase Deficiency

Using a benzidine staining method for leukocyte myeloperoxidase, Graham (1920) observed that leukocytes from patients with severe infections were mark-edly depleted in cytoplasmic myeloperoxidase. Several additional families have been described with complete absence of myeloperoxidase (Grignaschi et al., 1963; Undritz, 1966; Lehrer and Cline, 1969). Most of these patients suffered chronic *C. albicans* infections; their leukocytes are incapable of killing intracellular *C. albicans* (Lehrer and Cline, 1969). Granulocytes lacking myeloperoxidase are incapable of killing *C. albicans*. Five patients with myeloperoxidase deficiency have been reported with severe *C. albicans* infections. Three of these patients also had diabetes mellitus (Parry et al., 1981; Weber et al., 1987).

Davis and colleagues (1971) described an adult male with myeloperoxidase leukemia, candidiasis, and pneumonia, with a presumed acquired myeloperoxidase deficiency. Peripheral and bone marrow leukocytes showed no myeloperoxidase activity. In addition, a partial leukocyte bactericidal deficiency was present. After 60 minutes of incubation, few bacteria had been killed by the patients' leukocytes whereas more than 90% had been killed by normal leukocytes. However, after 4 hours of incubation, the patient's leukocytes killed nearly 90% of the bacteria. A supernormal respiratory burst may provide normal host defense (Nauseef, 1988).

Myeloperoxidase deficiency may be quite common, and most patients with this disorder do not suffer unusually severe infections. Automated differential white blood cell counters that identify granulocytes by myeloperoxidase content have been used for screening; granulocyte myeloperoxidase deficiency may occur with an incidence of 1 in 4000 (Parry et al., 1981). The myeloperoxidase gene has been localized to chromosome 17 (Weil et al., 1987).

Eosinophil Peroxidase Deficiency

Both myeloperoxidase in neutrophils and eosinophil peroxidase catalyze the peroxidation reaction but these peroxidases are distinct gene products with different heme and protein moieties. Isolated eosinophil peroxidase deficiency was identified in five individuals by examination of 131,000 peripheral blood samples for routine automated analysis by flow cytometry with peroxidase staining (Zabacchi et al., 1992).

Although the numbers are limited, the subjects with eosinophil peroxidase deficiency did not display any clinical disorder attributable to this defect, as is the case for most individuals with myeloperoxidase deficiency. Eosinophil peroxidase deficiency was confirmed in these patients by lack of Sudan black staining, absent or very low peroxidase activity of their eosinophils, and lack of immunogold labeling of their eosinophils with anti–eosinophil peroxidase antibodies. The eosinophil specific granules were also smaller than granules in normal eosinophils, and the ratio of the granule core to the granule matrix was also greater in the deficient cells. Presentey (1984) studied another group of patients and confirmed these findings.

There have been other reports of eosinophil peroxidase deficiency, and it has been found to occur in a pair of identical twins (Hoffman and Tielens, 1987;

Lepelley et al., 1987; Lanza et al., 1988; Andres et al., 1993).

Glucose-6-Phosphate Dehydrogenase Deficiency

Cooper and coworkers (1972) described a white female with severe infections and complete absence of leukocyte glucose-6-phosphate dehydrogenase (G6PD) activity. Phagocytosis of particles by the patient's leukocytes was normal but was accompanied by minimal stimulation of hexose monophosphate shunt activity and less than 25% of normal H_2O_2 production. The patient's leukocytes were unable to kill intracellular bacteria. However, patients with G6PD levels that are 25% or more of normal usually have normal leukocyte bactericidal activity.

Baehner and associates (1971) showed that patients with absent G6PD had deficient cellular NADH and NADPH; furthermore, despite normal NADH and NADPH oxidase activity, there was little hexose monophosphate shunt activity or H_2O_2 produced. Accordingly, NBT dye cannot be reduced. G6PD–deficient leukocytes do not kill *S. aureus*, *E. coli*, or *Serratia* but do kill *Streptococcus faecalis* normally, suggesting a leukocyte bactericidal deficiency similar to that in CGD. Thus, normal quantities of reduced pyridine nucleotides (NADH and NADPH), as well as oxygen and oxidase activity, may be necessary for normal hexose monophosphate shunt and bactericidal activity (Gray et al., 1973).

Glutathione Reductase Deficiency

Glutathione is an important intracellular antioxidant in leukocytes and also plays a role in many regulatory functions in the cell (Roos et al., 1979). Three children from a consanguineous marriage were discovered to have reduced (10% to 15% of normal) levels of glutathione reductase. Hemolytic crises resulting from the ingestion of fava beans and premature cataracts developed. When granulocytes were incubated with bacteria, the respiratory burst stopped abruptly after 5 minutes and no more superoxide or hydrogen peroxide was produced. Intracellular killing of *S. aureus* was normal, suggesting that an initial respiratory burst is adequate for intracellular killing of bacteria. Susceptibility to infection was not increased.

Glutathione Synthase Deficiency

Several patients with deficient glutathione synthase have been identified. These patients have low reduced glutathione in erythrocytes and granulocytes (Mohler et al., 1970). During phagocytosis, increased hydrogen peroxide production is associated with abnormal degranulation and microtubule disruption. Intracellular killing of *S. aureus* is impaired. Therapy with vitamin E has resulted in granulocyte metabolic response and normal bactericidal activity (Boxer et al., 1979). Ascorbate and *N*-acetylcysteine have also been used to treat this disorder and resulted in a fourfold to sixfold increase in glutathione in patients' lymphocytes and plasma (Jain et al., 1994).

OTHER PHAGOCYTIC DISORDERS

Human Immunodeficiency Virus Infection

Neutrophil and monocyte dysfunction has been described in human immunodeficiency virus (HIV)–infected children. A depressed oxygen burst with less superoxide and hydrogen peroxide during phagocytosis may contribute to increased susceptibility to bacterial and fungal infections in HIV-infected patients (Chen et al., 1993). Patients with HIV infection also have lower plasma and intracellular levels of glutathione, which may make them susceptible to injury by oxygen intermediates.

Chédiak-Higashi Syndrome

The Chédiak-Higashi syndrome (CHS) is an autosomal recessive disorder characterized by recurrent pyogenic infections, partial oculocutaneous albinism, a progressive neuropathy, and giant cytoplasmic granules in many cells, particularly peripheral blood leukocytes (Barak and Nir, 1987). Other granule-containing cells, including lymphocytes, platelets, Schwann cells, melanocytes, renal tubule epithelium, gastric mucosa, pancreas, and thyroid cells, also contain abnormally large lysosomal granules (Blume and Wolff, 1972). This disorder is also discussed in Chapter 16.

Clinical Manifestations

Patients with CHS suffer from frequent and severe pyogenic infections but these are not as severe as in patients with CGD. Most patients with CHS undergo an "accelerated" phase, characterized by fever, jaundice, hepatosplenomegaly, lymphadenopathy, pancytopenia, and diffuse mononuclear cell infiltrates. This accelerated phase may begin in childhood or adulthood and may be either a form of neoplasia or an abnormal inflammatory response to a virus. A severe bleeding diathesis may contribute to a fatal outcome.

The diagnosis of CHS is relatively simple. The physical appearance of patients is characteristic as a result of partial oculocutaneous albinism, and the patient's leukocytes contain characteristic large cytoplasmic inclusions that are evident on a peripheral blood smear (Fig. 15–6).

Pathogenesis

Leukocytes from patients with Chédiak-Higashi syndrome are abnormal in several functional assays. Degranulation of the giant intracellular inclusions does not occur during phagocytosis. Abnormal capping and orientation of leukocytes in gradients of chemoattractants may be explained by the cytoskeletal abnormalities, which include disordered assembly of microtubules and abnormal tubulin tyrosinolation (Nath et al.,

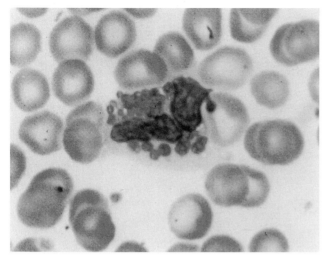

Figure 15–6. Giant granulocyte granules from a patient with the Chédiak-Higashi syndrome.

1982). Peripheral neutropenia is common and may be secondary to increased intramedullary destruction of granulocytes; the hypersplenism may result from the autophagocytic activity. On the basis of striking elevations of serum muramidase (lysozyme) activity and increased numbers of granulocytic precursors in the bone marrow, Blume and Wolff (1972) suggested an accelerated rate of granulocyte turnover.

Root and colleagues (1972) demonstrated defective bactericidal activity in CHS granulocytes. Neutrophils from two patients with CHS phagocytized *S. aureus* at normal rates, but intracellular bacterial killing of *S. aureus* was defective. Streptococci and pneumococci were also killed at a lower rate than normal. The characteristic cytoplasmic inclusions of CHS leukocytes remain intact during phagocytosis and, although seemingly incorporated into the phagocytic vacuole, do not discharge their contents into the vacuole. Resting CHS leukocytes have twice the normal hexose monophosphate shunt activity, as measured by oxidation of [^{14}C]-glucose, and a normal burst in oxygen consumption and increased H_2O_2 formation occur during phagocytosis.

The finding of a defect in intracellular killing despite normal hexose monophosphate shunt activity suggests that there may be two phases of intracellular killing. The initial phase may be dependent on lysosomal factors (which are compromised in CHS) and the latter phase on the respiratory oxidative response, which is essentially normal in CHS.

Defective natural killer (NK) function in patients with CHS has been described (Katz et al., 1982; Targan and Oseas, 1983). The NK cells are present in CHS patients but are functionally deficient because of refractoriness to activation stimuli, such as interferon. Prolonged incubation of NK cells from CHS patients results in activity similar to that of resting NK cells from normal individuals, suggesting that the molecules and structures involved in lytic activity are present but respond abnormally to stimuli. Bone marrow trans-

plantation corrected the NK defect in one patient (Virelizier et al., 1982).

Treatment

The management of Chédiak-Higashi syndrome warrants prompt attention to the patient's recurrent bacterial infections; prophylactic antibiotics should be considered. The outcome is usually fatal once the patient enters the accelerated phase, but successful treatment has been reported with a combination of steroids and cytotoxic agents (Harville et al., 1994). Ascorbic acid corrects some of the defects related to microtubule function of CHS in phagocytes in vitro, but its use in patients has not been conclusive, possibly because of the high concentrations of ascorbic acid required to replicate the in vitro studies (Gallin et al., 1979).

Likewise, IFN-γ treatment was not able to restore NK function in patients, although the cytokine is partially effective in vitro (Targan and Oseas, 1983). A series of 10 patients were treated with allogeneic bone marrow transplantation, with 7 alive and well up to 13 years after transplantation (Haddad et. al., 1995).

Specific Granule Deficiency

Specific granule deficiency is a rare autosomal recessive hereditary disorder characterized by susceptibility to recurrent and severe infections of the skin, mucous membranes, and lungs (Strauss et al., 1974; Boxer et al., 1982; Gallin et al., 1982; Ambruso et al., 1984; Curnutte and Boxer, 1993). Neutrophils of these patients have bilobed or kidney-shaped nuclei (resembling Pelger-Hüet cells) and absence of specific (secondary) neutrophil granules by electron microscopy. They lack specific granule factors such as lactoferrin and vitamin B$_{12}$–binding protein but have normal levels of lysozyme, β-glucuronidase, and myeloperoxidase, which are present in the azurophilic granules. The eosinophil-specific granule proteins (major basic protein, eosinophil cationic protein, and eosinophil-derived neurotoxin) are also lacking in these patients; however, eosinophil peroxidase can be detected (Rosenberg and Gallin, 1993).

Because specific granules are a source of receptors for chemoattractants and help to "up-regulate" neutrophil membrane receptor activity during stimulation (Gallin et al., 1982), chemotaxis is deficient in these patients. Because cytochrome b and flavoproteins necessary for the normal respiratory burst are located in specific granules (Borregaard et al., 1985), several abnormalities of neutrophil oxidative metabolism have been noted. These included high resting oxidase activity, diminished oxidative response to stimuli, and defective bactericidal activity. The importance of specific granule contents as modulators of inflammation, chemoattractants, and adhesiveness is demonstrated by patients with specific granule deficiency. There is associated susceptibility to infection, including recurrent skin abscesses and progressive pulmonary disease. Frequent etiologic agents are *S. aureus,* enteric bacilli, *P. aerugi-*

nosa, and *C. albicans.* Despite the recurrent infections, most patients survive when infections are treated promptly and aggressively.

Transcobalamin II Deficiency

A child with recurrent pyoderma, purulent rhinitis, tonsillitis, and bronchitis was found to be deficient in transcobalamin II (Seger et al., 1980). This defect was autosomally transmitted, but the anemia, immune defects, and pancytopenia were corrected by hydroxycobalamin. Transcobalamin is necessary for transport and conversion of vitamin B_{12} into coenzymes necessary for intracellular methylation reactions. Granulocytes from this child did not kill intracellular *S. aureus,* even though phagocytosis and degranulation were normal. Enzyme replacement via plasma transfusions resulted in normal bactericidal activity, which suggests that methylation reactions contribute to the respiratory burst of granulocytes. This disorder is also discussed in Chapter 11.

Neutrophil Dysfunction in Severe Infection

Leukocyte bactericidal deficiency is found in patients with serious acute infections who have had no prior history of increased susceptibility to infection. This may be a more frequent phenomenon than is presently realized. Tan and colleagues (1971) reported two adult males with serious infections whose leukocytes did not kill intracellular staphylococci. Other aspects of the immune response were normal. Abnormal bactericidal function of leukocytes in one patient with severe staphylococcal abscesses and in one with a severe postoperative wound infection with *E. coli* and *Bacteroides* was reported by Messner et al. (1973).

McCall and colleagues (1971) studied the function of toxic neutrophils of patients with severe infections. *Toxic* neutrophils were defined as cells with prominently stained azurophilic granules that may be due to abnormal maturation. Döhle bodies (light blue cytoplasmic inclusions representing aggregated endoplasmic reticulum) and cytoplasmic vacuoles were also present, and more than 90% of the neutrophils were judged toxic. It seems likely that the mechanism causing formation of toxic neutrophils also results in the chemotactic and bactericidal defects. Copeland and associates (1971), confirming a bactericidal defect against staphylococci but not gram-negative organisms in neutrophils from severely infected patients, suggested that abnormal release and activation of cellular proteolytic enzymes during severe infections may interfere with intraleukocyte bacterial mechanisms.

Another mechanism to account for defects of neutrophil function in bacterial infections is the release of bacterial toxins. *Staphylococcus epidermidis* organisms isolated from the blood of patients with clinically significant infections release a factor that inhibits neutrophil bactericidal activity (Noble et al., 1990). This virulence factor is not usually found in *S. epidermidis,* which is considered to be a contaminant. *Pseudomonas* proteases, staphylococcal membrane-damaging toxins, and *Bordetella pertussis* adenylate cyclase may severely impair neutrophil function (Krause and Lew, 1988).

References

Abramson JS, Mills EL, Sawyer MK, Regelmann WE, Nelson JD, Quie PQ. Recurrent infections and delayed separation of the umbilical cord in an infant with abnormal phagocytic cell locomotion and oxidative response during particle phagocytosis. J Pediatr 99:887–894, 1981.

Adair SM. Oral conditions. In McCarney ER, Kreipe RE, Orr DP, Comerci GD, eds. Textbook of Adolescent Medicine. Philadelphia, WB Saunders, 1992, pp. 291–297.

Aggett PJ, Harries JT, Harvery BM, Soothill JF. An inherited disorder of neutrophil mobility in Shwachman syndrome. J Pediatr 94:391–394, 1979.

Aliabadi H, Gonzalez R, Quie PG. Urinary tract disorders in patients with chronic granulomatous disease. N Engl J Med 321:706–708, 1989.

Al-Mohanna F, Parhar R, Kawaasi A, Ernst P, Sheth K, Harfi H, Al-Sediary S. Inhibition of neutrophil functions by human immunoglobulin E. J Allergy Clin Immunol 92:757–766, 1993.

Alter BP. The bone marrow failure syndromes. In Nathan DJ, Oski FA, eds. Hematology of Infancy and Childhood. Edition III. Philadelphia, WB Saunders, 1993, pp. 159–241.

Ambruso DR, Sasada M, Nishlyama H, Kubo A, Komiyama A, Allen RH. Defective bactericidal activity and absence of specific granules in neutrophils from a patient with recurrent bacterial infections. J Clin Immunol 4:23–30, 1984.

Ament ME, Ochs HD. Gastrointestinal manifestations of chronic granulomatous disease. N Engl J Med 288:382–387, 1973.

Anderson DC, Springer TA. Leukocyte adhesion deficiency: an inherited defect in the Mac-1, LFA-1 and p150,95 glycoproteins. Annu Rev Med 38:175–194, 1987.

Anderson DC, Hughes GJ, Smith CW. Abnormal mobility of neonatal polymorphonuclear leukocytes. Relationship to impaired redistribution of surface adhesion sites by chemotactic factor of colchicine. J Clin Invest 68:863–874, 1981a.

Anderson DC, Mace ML, Brinkley BR, Martin RR, Smith CW. Recurrent infection in glycogenesis type 1B: abnormal neutrophil mobility related to impaired redistribution of adhesion sites. J Infect Dis 143:447–459, 1981b.

Anderson DC, Hughes BJ, Wible LJ, Perry GJ, Smith CW, Brinkley BR. Impaired mobility of neonatal PMN leukocytes: relationship to abnormalities of cell orientation and assembly of microtubules in chemotactic gradients. J Leukoc Biol 35:1–15, 1984a.

Anderson DC, Schmalstieg FC, Arnaout AM, Kohl J, Tosi MF, Dana N, Buffone GJ, Hughes BJ, Brinkley BR, Dickey WD, Springer JS, Boyer LA, Hollerson JM, Smith CW. Abnormalities of polymorphonuclear leukocyte function associated with a heritable deficiency of high molecular weight surface glycoproteins (GP138): common relationship to diminished cell adherence. J Clin Invest 74:536–551, 1984b.

Anderson DC, Schmalstieg FC, Finegold MJ, Hughes BJ, Rothlein R, Miller LJ, Kohl S, Tosi MF, Jacobs RL, Waldrop TC, Goldman AS, Shearer WT, Springer TA. The severe and moderate phenotypes of heritable Mac-1, LFA-1 deficiency: their quantitative definition and relation to leukocyte dysfunction and clinical features. J Infect Dis 152:668–689, 1985.

Anderson DC, Rothlein R, Marlin SD, Krater SS, Smith CW. Impaired transendothelial migration by neonatal neutrophils: abnormalities of Mac-1 (CD11b/CD18)–dependent adherence reactions. Blood 76:2613–2621, 1990.

Anderson R, Sher R, Radson AR, Koornhof HJ. Defective chemotaxis in measles patients. S Afr Med J 48:1819–1820, 1974.

Andres MC, Hidalgo C, Balsa A, Fernandez de Castro M. Eosinophilia in rheumatoid arthritis marked by eosinophil peroxidase deficiency. Clin Lab Haematol 15:67–73, 1993.

Andrich MP, Chen CC, Gallin JI. Abnormal bone scintigraphy before clinical symptoms in a patient with defective phagocyte function. Clin Nucl Med 18:153–154, 1993.

Arnaout MA. Molecular basis for leukocyte adhesion deficiency. In Horton M, ed. Biochemistry of Macrophages and Related Cell Types. New York, Plenum, 1993, pp. 335–346.

Arnaout MA, Dana N, Gapta SK, Tenen DG, Fathallah DM. Point mutations impairing cell surface expression of the common β subunit (CD18) in a patient with leukocyte adhesion molecule (LEU-CAM) deficiency. J Clin Invest 85:977–981, 1990.

Babior BM. The respiratory burst oxidase and the molecular basis of chronic granulomatous disease. Am J Hematol 37:263–266, 1991.

Baehner RL, Nathan DG. Quantitative nitroblue tetrazolium test in chronic granulomatous disease. N Engl J Med 287:971–976, 1968.

Baehner RL, Johnston RB Jr, Nathan DG. Reduction of pyridine nucleotide (RPN) content in G-6-PD deficient granulocytes (PMN): an explanation for their defective bactericidal function (abstract). Prog Am Soc Clin Invest 13:4a, 1971.

Baehner RL, Kunkel LM, Monaco AP, Haines JL, Conneally PM, Palmer C, Heerema N, Orkin SH. DNA linkage of X-chromosome linked chronic granulomatous disease. Proc Natl Acad Sci U S A 83:3398–3401, 1986.

Balis FM, Pizzo PA, Murphy RF. The pharmacokinetics of zidovudine administered by continuous infusion in children. Ann Intern Med 110:279–285, 1989.

Bannatyne RM, Skowron PN, Weber JL. Job's syndrome—a variant of chronic granulomatous disease. J Pediatr 75:236–242, 1969.

Barak Y, Nir E. Chediak-Higashi syndrome. Am J Pediatr Hematol Oncol 9:42–55, 1987.

Beaudet AL, Anderson DC, Michels VV, Arion WJ, Lange AJ. Neutropenia and impaired neutrophil migration in type 1B glycogen storage disease. J Pediatr 97:906–910, 1980.

Berendes H, Bridges RA, Good RA. A fatal granulomatous disease of childhood. The clinical study of a new syndrome. Minn Med 40:309–312, 1957.

Bevilacqua MP, Nelson RM. Selectins. J Clin Invest 91:379–387, 1993.

Bjornson AB, Somers SD. Down-regulation of chemotaxis of polymorphonuclear leukocytes following thermal injury involves two distinct mechanisms. J Infect Dis 168:120–127, 1993.

Blume RS, Wolff SM. The Chediak-Higashi syndrome: studies in four patients and a review of the literature. Medicine (Baltimore) 51:247–280, 1972.

Borregaard N, Boxer LA, Smolen JE, Tauber AI. Anomalous neutrophil granule distribution in a patient with lactoferrin deficiency: pertinence to the respiratory burst. Am J Hematol 18:255–260, 1985.

Boxer LA, Hedley-Whyte ET, Stossel TP. Neutrophil actin dysfunction and abnormal neutrophil behavior. N Engl J Med 291:1093–1099, 1974.

Boxer LA, Oliver JM, Spielberg SP, Allen JM, Schulman JD. Protection of granulocytes by vitamin E in glutathione synthetase deficiency. N Engl J Med 301:901–904, 1979.

Boxer LA, Coats TD, Haak RA, Wolach JB, Hoffstein S, Baehner RL. Lactoferrin deficiency associated with altered granulocyte functions. N Engl J Med 307:404–410, 1982.

Brestel EP, Klingberg WG, Veltri RW, Dorn JS. Osteogenesis imperfecta tarda in a child with hyper-IgE syndrome. Am J Dis Child 136:774–776, 1982.

Bridges RA, Berendes H, Good RA. A fatal granulomatous disease of childhood. Am J Dis Child 97:387–408, 1959.

Bruton OC. Agammaglobulinemia. Pediatrics 9:722–728, 1952.

Buckley RH, Sampson HA. The hyperimmunoglobulinemia E syndrome. In Franklin EC, ed. Clinical Immunology Update. New York, Elsevier, 1981, pp. 148–167.

Buckley RH, Wray BB, Belmaker EZ. Extreme hyperimmunoglobulin E and undue susceptibility to infection. Pediatrics 49:59–70, 1972.

Buescher ES, Hebert A, Rapini RP. Staphylococcal botryomycosis in a patient with the hyperimmunoglobulin E–recurrent infection syndrome. Pediatr Infect Dis J 7:431–433, 1988.

Bulengo-Ransby SM, Headington JT, Cantu-Gonzalez G, Rasmussen JE. Staphylococcal botryomycosis and hyperimmunoglobulin E (Job's) syndrome in an infant. J Am Acad Dermatol 28:109–111, 1993.

Burgett F. Periodontal disease. In Regezi J, Sciubba J, eds. Oral Pathology. Philadelphia, WB Saunders, pp. 553–557, 1993.

Cappell MS, Manzione NC. Recurrent colonic histoplasmosis after standard therapy with amphotericin B in a patient with Job's syndrome. Am J Gastroenterol 86:119–120, 1991.

Casimir CM, Bu-Ghanim H, Rodaway AR, Bentley DL, Rowe P, Segal AW. Autosomal recessive chronic granulomatous disease caused by deletion at a dinucleotide repeat. Proc Natl Acad Sci U S A 88:2753–2757, 1991.

Chanock SJ, Barrett DM, Curnutte JT, Orkin SH. Gene structure of the cytosolic component, phox-47 and mutations in autosomal recessive chronic granulomatous disease. Blood 78:165a, 1991.

Chen TP, Roberts RL, Wu KW, Ank BJ, Stiehm ER. Decreased superoxide anion and hydrogen peroxide production by neutrophils and monocytes in HIV infected children and adults. Pediatr Res 34:544–550, 1993.

Chin TW, Stiehm ER, Falloon J, Gallin J. Corticosteroids in the treatment of obstructive lesions of chronic granulomatous disease. J Pediatr 111:349–352, 1987.

Clark RA, Root RK, Kimball HR, Kirkpatrick CH. Defective neutrophil chemotaxis and cellular immunity in a child with recurrent infections. Ann Intern Med 78:515–519, 1973.

Clark RA, Maleech HL, Gallin JI, Nunoi H, Volpp BD, Pearson DW, Nauseff WM, Curnutte JT. Genetic variants of chronic granulomatous disease: prevalence of deficiencies of two cytosolic components of the NADPH oxidase system. N Engl J Med 321:647–652, 1989.

Coates TD, Torkildson JC, Torres M, Church JA, Howard TH. An inherited defect of neutrophil motility and microfilamentous cytoskeleton associated with abnormalities in 47-kd and 89-kd proteins. Blood 78:1338–1346, 1991.

Coccia CT, McDonald RE, Mitchell DF. Papillon-Lefèvre syndrome: precocious periodontosis with palmar-plantar hyperatosis. J Periodontal 37:408–414, 1966.

Cogen RB, Stevens AW Jr, Cohen-Cole S, Kirks K, Freeman A. Leukocyte function in the etiology of acute necrotizing ulcerative gingivitis. J Periodontol 54:402–407, 1983.

Cohen MS, Isturiz RE, Malech HL, Root RK. Fungal infection in chronic granulomatous disease. Am J Med 71:59–66, 1981.

Cohen MS, Leong PA, Simpson DM. Phagocytic cells in periodontal defense. J Periodontol 56:611–617, 1985.

Constantopoulos A. Congenital tuftsin deficiency. Ann N Y Acad Sci 419:214–219, 1983.

Constantopoulos A, Najjar VA, Smith JW. Tuftsin deficiency: a new syndrome with defective phagocytosis. J Pediatr 80:564–572, 1972.

Constantopoulos A, Likhile V, Crosby WH, Najjar VA. Phagocytic activity of the leukemic cell and its response to the phagocytosis-stimulating tetrapeptide, tuftsin. Cancer Res 33:1230–1234, 1973.

Cooper MR, DeChatelet LR, McCall CE, LaVia MF, Spurr CL, Baehner RL. Complete deficiency of leukocyte glucose-6-phosphate dehydrogenase with defective bactericidal activity. J Clin Invest 51:769–778, 1972.

Copeland JL, Karrh LR, McCoy J, Guckian JC. Bactericidal activity of polymorphonuclear leukocytes from patients with severe bacterial infections. Texas Rep Biol Med 29:555–562, 1971.

Corbi AL, Larson RS, Kishimoto TK, Springer TA, Morton CC. Chromosomal location of the genes encoding the leukocyte adhesion receptors LFA-1, Mac-1, and p150,95. J Exp Med 167:1597–1607, 1988.

Curnutte JT. Chronic granulomatous disease: the solving of a clinical riddle at the molecular level. Clin Immunol Immunopathol 67:S2–S15, 1993.

Curnutte JT, Berkow RL, Roberts RL, Shurin SB, Scott PJ. Chronic granulomatous disease due to a defect in the cytosolic factor required for nicotinamide adenine dinucleotide phosphate oxidase activation. J Clin Invest 81:606–610, 1988.

Curnutte JT, Boxer LA. Disorders of granulopoiesis and granulocyte function. In Nathan DJ, Oski FA, eds. Hematology of Infancy and Childhood, 3rd ed. Philadelphia, WB Saunders, 1993, pp. 797–847.

Curnutte JT, Whitten DM, Babior BM. Defective superoxide production by granulocytes from patients with chronic granulomatous disease. N Engl J Med 290:593–597, 1977.

Dahl MV, Greene WH Jr, Quie PG. Infection, dermatitis, increased IgE, and impaired neutrophil chemotaxis. Arch Dermatol 112:1387–1390, 1976.

Dale DC, Bonilla MA, Davis MW, Nakanishi AM, Hammond WP, Kurtzberg J, Wang W, Jakubowski A, Winton E, Lalezari P, Robinson W, Glaspy JA, Emerson S, Gabrilove J, Vincent M, Boxer LA. A randomized controlled phase III trial of recombinant human granulocyte colony-stimulating factor (Filgrastim) for treatment of severe chronic neutropenia. Blood 81:2496–2502, 1993.

Dale DC, Hammond WP. Cyclic neutropenia: a clinical review. Blood Rev 2:178–185, 1988.

Dana N, Todd RF III, Pitt J, Springer TA, Arnaout MA. Deficiency of a surface membrane glycoprotein (Mo1) in man. Clin Invest 73:153–159, 1984.

Davis AT, Brunning RD, Quie PG. Polymorphonuclear leukocytes and myeloperoxidase deficiency in a patient with myelomonocytic leukemia. N Engl J Med 285:789–790, 1971.

Davis JM, Dineen P, Gallin JI. Neutrophil degranulation and abnormal chemotaxis after thermal injury. J Immunol 124:1467–1471, 1980.

Davis SD, Schaller J, Wedgwood RJ. Job's syndrome. Recurrent "cold" staphylococcal abscesses. Lancet 1:1013–1017, 1966.

de Boer M, de Klein A, Hossle JP, Seger R, Corbel L, Weening RS, Roos D. Cytochrome b₅₅₈–negative, autosomal recessive chronic granulomatous disease: two new mutations in the cytochrome b₅₅₈ light chain of the NADPH oxidase (p22-phox). Am J Hum Genet 51:1127–1135, 1992.

de Boer M, Hilarius-Stokman PM, Hossle J-P, Verhoeven AJ, Graf N, Kenney RT, Seger R, Roos D. Autosomal recessive chronic granulomatous disease with absence of the 67-kD cytosolic NADPH oxidase component: identification of mutation and detection of carriers. Blood 83:531–536, 1994.

Desnick RJ, Sharp HL, Grabowski GA, Brunning RD, Quie PG, Sung JH, Gorlin RJ, Ikonne JU. Mannosidosis: clinical, morphologic, immunologic and biochemical studies. Pediatr Res 10:985–996, 1976.

Dickerman JD, Collettii RB, Tampas JP. Gastric outlet obstruction in chronic granulomatous disease of childhood. Am J Dis Child 140:567–570, 1986.

Dimanche-Bortrel MT, Guyot A, De Sainte-Basile G, Fischer A, Griscelli C, Lisowska-Grospierre B. Heterogeneity in the molecular defect leading to the leukocyte adhesion deficiency. Eur J Immunol 18:1575–1579, 1988.

Dinauer MC, Orkin SH. Chronic granulomatous disease. Annu Rev Med 43:117–124, 1992.

Dinauer MC, Orkin SH, Brown R, Jesaitis AJ, Parkos CA. The glycoprotein encoded by the X-linked chronic granulomatous disease locus is a component of the neutrophil cytochrome b complex. Nature 327:717–720, 1987.

Dinauer MC, Pierce EA, Burns GAP, Curnutte JT, Orkin SH. Human neutrophil cytochrome b light chain (p22-phox). Gene structure chromosomal location, and mutations in cytochrome-negative autosomal recessive chronic granulomatous disease. J Clin Invest 86:1729–1737, 1990.

Di Rocco M, Borrone C, Dallegri F, Frumento G, Patrone F. Neutropenia and impaired neutrophil function in glycogenosis type Ib. J Inherited Metab Dis 7:151–154, 1984.

Donabedian H, Alling DW, Gallin JI. Levamisole is inferior to placebo in the hyperimmunoglobulin E recurrent-infection (Job's) syndrome. N Engl J Med 307:290–292, 1982.

Donabedian H, Gallin JI. Mononuclear cells from patients with the hyperimmunoglobulin E–recurrent infection sydrome produce an inhibitor of leukocyte chemotaxis. J Clin Invest 69:1155–1163, 1982.

Donabedian H, Gallin JI. The hyperimmunoglobulin E recurrent-infection (Job's) syndrome: a review of the NIH experience and the literature. Medicine (Baltimore) 62:195–208, 1983a.

Donabedian H, Gallin JI. Two inhibitors of neutrophil chemotaxis are produced by hyperimmunoglobulin E recurrent infection syndrome mononuclear cells exposed to heat killed staphylococci. Infect Immun 40:1030–1037, 1983b.

Doweiko JP. Management of the hematologic manifestations of HIV disease. Blood Rev 7:121–126, 1993.

Dreskin SC, Gallin JI. Evolution of the hyperimmunoglobulin E and recurrent infection (HIE, Job's) syndrome in a young girl. J Allergy Clin Immunol 80:746–751, 1987.

Dreskin SC, Goldsmith PK, Gallin GI. Immunoglobulins in the hyperimmunoglobulin E and recurrent infection (Job's) syndrome. J Clin Invest 75:26–34, 1985.

Dreskin SC, Goldsmith PK, Strober W, Zech LA, Gallin JI. Metabolism of immunoglobulin E in patients with markedly elevated serum immunoglobulin E levels. J Clin Invest 79:1764–1772, 1987.

Ephros M, Engelhard D, Maayan S, Bercovier H, Avital A, Yatsiv I. *Legionella gormanii* pneumonia in a child with chronic granulomatous disease. Pediatr Infect Dis J 8:726–727, 1989.

Etzioni A, Frydman M, Pollack S, Avidor I, Philips ML, Paulson JC,

Gershoni-Baruch R. Recurrent severe infections caused by a novel leukocyte adhesion deficiency. N Engl J Med 327:1789–1792, 1992.

Ezekowitz RAB. Chronic granulomatous disease: an update and a paradigm for the use of interferon-gamma as adjunct immunotherapy in infectious diseases. Curr Top Microbiol Immunol 181:283–292, 1992.

Ezekowitz RAB, Dinauer MC, Jaffe HS, Orkin SH, Newburger PE. Partial correction of the phagocytic defect in patients with X-linked chronic granulomatous disease by subcutaneous inferferon gamma. N Engl J Med 319:146–151, 1988.

Finch SC. Granulocyte disorders: benign quantitative abnormalities of granulocytes. In Williams WJ, Beutler E, Erslev AJ, eds. Hematology, Vol 1. New York, McGraw-Hill, 1972, pp. 628–654.

Fischer A, Lisowka-Cropierre B, Anderson DC, Springer RA. Leukocyte adhesion deficiency: molecular basis and functional consequences. Immunodefic Rev 1:39–54, 1988.

Fischer A, Trung PH, Descamps-Latscha B, Usowska-Grospierre B, Gerota I, Scheinmetzier C, Durandy A, Vierilizer JL, Griscelli G. Bone-marrow transplantation for inborn error of phagocytic cells associated with defective adherence, chemotaxis and oxidative response during opsonized particle phagocytosis. Lancet 2:473–476, 1983.

Fisher JE, Khan AR, Heitlinger L, Allen JE, Afshani E. Chronic granulomatous disease of childhood with acute ulcerative colitis: a unique association. Pediatr Pathol 7:91–96, 1987.

Foroozanfar N, Hobbs JR, Hugh-Jones K. Bone marrow transplant from an unrelated donor for chronic granulomatous disease. Lancet 1:210–213, 1977.

Forrest CB, Forehand JR, Axtell RA, Roberts RL, Johnston RB. Clinical features and current management of chronic granulomatous disease. Hematol Oncol Clin North Am 2:253–266, 1988.

Gallin JI, Buescher ES, Seligmann BE, Nath J, Gaither TE, Katz P. Recent advances in chronic granulomatous disease. Ann Intern Med 99:657–674, 1983.

Gallin JI, Ellin RJ, Hubert RT, Fauci AS, Kaliner MA, Wolff SM. Efficacy of ascorbic acid in Chédiak-Higashi syndrome (CHS): studies in humans and mice. Blood 53:226–234, 1979.

Gallin JI, Fletcher MP, Seligmann BE, Hoffsteins S, Cehrs K, Mounessa N. Human neutrophil specific granule deficiency: a model to assess the role of neutrophil-specific granules in the evolution of the inflammatory response. Blood 59:1317–1329, 1982.

Ganser A, Ottmann OG, Erdmann H, Schulz G, Hoelzer D. The effect of recombinant human granulocyte-macrophage colony-stimulating factor on neutropenia and related morbidity in chronic severe neutropenia. Ann Intern Med 111:887–892, 1989.

Geha RS. Regulation of IgE synthesis in humans. J Allergy Clin Immunol 90:143–150, 1992.

Geha RS, Reinherz E, Leung D, McKee KT, Schlossman S, Rosen FS. Deficiency of suppressor T cells in the hyperimmunoglobulin E syndrome. J Clin Invest 68:783–791, 1981.

Giblett ER, Klebanoff SJ, Pincus SH, Swanson J, Park BH, McCullough J. Kell phenotypes in chronic granulomatous disease: a potential transfusion hazard. Lancet 1:1235–1236, 1971.

Glasser L, Duncan BR, Corrigan JJ. Measurement of serum granulocyte colony-stimulating factor in a patient with congenital agranulocytosis (Kostmann's syndrome). Am J Dis Child 145:925–928, 1991.

Gorin LJ, Jeha SC, Sullivan MP, Rosenblatt HM, Shearer WT. Burkitt's lymphoma developing in a 7-year old boy with hyper-IgE syndrome. J Allergy Clin Immunol 83:5–10, 1989.

Graham GS. The neutrophil granules of the circulating blood in health and in disease—a preliminary report. NY J Med 20:46–55, 1920.

Gray GR, Stamatoyannopoulos G, Naiman GC, Kilman MR, Klebanoff SJ, Austin T, Yoshida A, Robinson GCF. Neutrophil dysfunction, chronic granulomatous disease and non-spherocytic haemolytic anemia caused by complete deficiency of glucose-6-phosphate dehydrogenase. Lancet 2:530–534, 1973.

Grignaschi VJ, Sperperato AM, Etcheverry MJ, Macario AJL. Un nuevo chadro citoquimico: negatividad espontanea de dos reaccionis de peroxidasas monocitos de dos hermonos. Rev Assoc Med Argent 77:218–221, 1963.

Griscom NT, Kirkpatrick JA Jr, Girdany BR, Berdon WE, Grand RJ, Mackie GG. Gastric antral narrowing in chronic granulomatous disease of childhood. Pediatrics 54:456–460, 1974.

Grogan JB, Miller RC. Impaired function of polymorphonuclear leukocytes in patients with burns and other trauma. Surg Gynecol Obstet 137:784–788, 1973.

Guba SC, Sartor CA, Hutchinson R, Boxer LA, Emerson SG. Granulocyte colony-stimulating factor (G-CSF) production and G-CSF receptor structure in patients with congenital neutropenia. Blood 83:1486–1492, 1994.

Haber J, Kent RI. Cigarette smoking in a periodontal practice. J Periodontol 63:100–106, 1992.

Haddad E, Le Deist F, Blanche S, Benkerrou M, Rohrlich P, Vilmer E, Griscelli C, Fischer A. Treatment of Chédiak-Higashi syndrome by allogenic bone marrow transplantation: report of 10 cases. Blood 85:3228–3333, 1995.

Hajjar FM. Neutrophils in the newborn: normal characteristics and quantitative disorders. Semin Perinatol 14:374–383, 1990.

Hammond WP, Chatta GS, Andrews RG, Dale DC. Abnormal responsiveness of granulocyte-committed progenitor cells in cyclic neutropenia. Blood 79:2536–2539, 1992.

Hammond WP, Price TH, Souza LM, Dale DC. Treatment of cyclic neutropenia with granulocyte colony-stimulating factor. N Engl J Med 320:1306–1311, 1989.

Hanada T, Ono I, Nagasawa T. Childhood cyclic neutropenia treated with recombinant human granulocyte colony-stimulating factor. Br J Haematol 75:135–137, 1990.

Harris BH, Boles ET. Intestinal lesions in chronic granulomatous disease in childhood. J Pediatr Surg 8:955–956, 1973.

Harris MC, Shalit M, Southwick FS. Diminished actin polymerization by neutrophils from newborn infants. Pediatr Res 33:27–31, 1992.

Harville TO, Williams LW, Graham ML. Successful treatment of Chédiak-Higashi syndrome with bone marrow transplantation (BMT). J Allergy Clin Immunol 93:276, 1994.

Hasslen SR, Ahrenholz DH, Solem LD, Nelson RD. Actin polymerization contributes to neutrophil chemotactic dysfunction following thermal injury. J Leukoc Biol 52:495–500, 1992.

Hattori K, Hasui M, Masuda K, Masuda M, Ogino H, Kobayashi Y. Successful trimethoprim-sulfamethoxazole therapy in a patient with hyperimmunoglobulin E syndrome. Acta Pediatr 82:324–326, 1993.

Hill HR, Quie PG. Raised serum IgE levels and defective neutrophil chemotaxis in three children with eczema and recurrent bacterial infections. Lancet 1:183–187, 1974.

Hill HR, Augustine NH, Rallison ML, Santos JI. Defective monocyte chemotactic responses in diabetes mellitus. J Clin Immunol 3:70–73, 1983.

Hill HR, Gerrard JM, Hogan NA, Quie PG. Hyperactivity of neutrophil leukotactic responses during active bacterial infection. J Clin Invest 53:996–1002, 1974a.

Hill HR, Ochs HD, Quie PG, Pabst HF, Klebanoff SJ, Wedgwood RJ. Effect in neutrophil granulocyte chemotaxis in Job's syndrome of recurrent "cold" staphylococcal abscesses. Lancet 2:617–619, 1974b.

Hill HR, Williams PB, Krueger GG, Janis B. Recurrent staphylococcal abscesses associated with defective neutrophil chemotaxis and allergic rhinitis. Ann Intern Med 85:39–43, 1976.

Hobbs JR, Monteil M, McCluskey DR, Jurges E, Eitumi M. Chronic granulomatous disease 100% corrected by displacement bone marrow transplantation from a volunteer unrelated donor. Eur J Pediatr 151:806–810, 1992.

Hoffman JJML, Tielens AGWM. Partial deficiency of eosinophil peroxidase. Blut 54:165–169, 1987.

Holmes B, Page AR, Good RA. Studies of the metabolic activity of leukocytes from patients with genetic abnormality of phagocytic function. J Clin Invest 46:1422–1432, 1967.

Howard T, Li Y, Torres M, Guerrero A, Coates T. The 47-kD protein increased in neutrophil actin dysfunction with 47 and 89 kD protein abnormalities is lymphocyte-specific protein. Blood 83:231–241,1994.

Howard TH, Watts RG. Actin polymerization and leukocyte function. Curr Opin Hematol 1:61–68, 1994.

International Chronic Granulomatous Disease Cooperative Study Group. A controlled trial of interferon gamma to prevent infection in chronic granulomatous disease. N Engl J Med 324:509–516, 1991.

Ishikawa I, Fukuda Y, Kitada H, Yuri T, Shinoda A, Hayakawa Y, Sawano K, Usui T. Plasma exchange in a patient with hyper-IgE syndrome. Ann Allergy 49:295–300, 1982.

Ishizaka A, Joh K, Shibata R, Wagatsuma Y, Nakanishi M, Tomizawa K, Kojima K. Regulation of IgE and IgG4 synthesis in patients with hyper IgE syndrome. Immunology 70:414–416, 1990.

Jacobs JC, Norman ME. A familial defect of neutrophil chemotaxis with asthma, eczema, and recurrent skin infections. Pediatr Res 11:732–736, 1977.

Jain A, Buist RM, Kennaway NG, Powell BR, Auld PAM, Martensson J. Effect of ascorbate or N-acetylcysteine treatment in a patient with hereditary glutathione synthetase deficiency. J Pediatr 124:229–233, 1994.

Janeway C, Craig J, Davidson M, Doroney W, Gitlin D, Sullivan JC. Hypergammaglobulinemia associated with severe recurrent and chronic nonspecific infection. Am J Dis Child 88:388–392, 1954.

Jeppson JD, Jaffe HS, Hill HR. Use of recombinant human interferon gamma to enhance neutrophil chemotactic responses in Job syndrome of hyperimmunoglobulinemia E and recurrent infections. J Pediatr 118:383–387, 1991.

Johnston RB Jr, McMurray JS. Chronic familial granulomatosis: report of five cases and review of the literature. Am J Dis Child 114:370–378, 1967.

Johnston RB, Newman SL. Chronic granulomatous disease. Pediatr Clin North Am 24:365–376, 1977.

Johnston RB Jr, Klemperer MR, Alper CA, Rosen FS. The enhancement of bacterial phagocytosis by serum. J Exp Med 129:1275–1290, 1969.

Jones DH, Schmalstieg FC, Dempsey K, Krater SS, Nannen DD, Smith CW, Anderson DC. Subcellular distribution and mobilization of Mac-1 (CD11b/CD18) in neonatal neutrophils. Blood 75:488–498, 1990.

Jung LKL. Association of aberrant F-actin formation with defective leukocyte chemotaxis and recurrent pyoderma. Clin Immunol Immunopathol 61:41–54, 1991.

Kaiser U, Kausmann M, Kolb G, Pfluger KH, Havemann K. Felty's syndrome: favorable response to granulocyte-macrophge colony-stimulating factor in the acute phase. Acta Haematol 87:190–194, 1992.

Kamei R, Honig PJ. Neonatal Job's syndrome featuring a vesicular eruption. Pediatr Dermatol 5:75–82, 1988.

Katona IM, Tata G, Scanlon RT, Bellanti JA. Hyper IgE syndrome: a disease with suppressor T cell deficiency. Ann Allergy 45:295–300, 1980.

Katz PA, Zaytoun A, Fauci A. Deficiency of active natural killer cells in the Chédiak-Higashi syndrome. Localization of the defect using a single cell assay. J Clin Invest 69:1231–1238, 1982.

Kenney EB, Kraal JH, Saxe SR, Jones J. The effect of cigarette smoke on oral polymorphonuclear leukocytes. J Periodont Res 12:227–234, 1977.

Kimata H. High-dose intravenous γ-globulin treatment for hyperimmunoglobulinemia E syndrome. J Allergy Clin Immunol 95:771–774, 1995.

Kishimoto TK, Hollander N, Roberts TM, Anderson DC, Springer TA. Heterogeneous mutations in the β subunit common to the LFA-1, Mac-1, and p150,95 glycoproteins cause leukocyte adhesion deficiency. Cell 50:193–202, 1987.

Klebanoff SJ, Olszowski S, Van Voorhis WC, Ledbetter JA, Waltersdorph AM, Schlechte KG. Effects of gamma-interferon on human neutrophils: protection from deterioration on storage. Blood 80:225–234, 1992.

Klempner MS, Noring R, Mier JW, Atkins MB. An acquired chemotactic defect in neutrophils from patients receiving interleukin-2 immunotherapy. N Engl J Med 322:959–965, 1990.

Koenig JL, Christensen RD. Incidence, neutrophil kinetics and natural history of neonatal neutropenia associated with maternal hypertension. N Engl J Med 321:557–562, 1989.

Kornberg A, Catane R, Peller S, Kaufman S, Fridkin M. Tuftsin induces tissue factor–like activity in human mononuclear cells and in monocyte cell lines. Blood 76:814–819, 1990.

Kostmann R. Infantile genetic agranulocytosis. Acta Paediatr Scand [Suppl.] 45:1–178, 1956.

Kraemer MJ, Ochs HD, Furukawa CT, Wedgwood RJ. In vitro studies of the hyper-IgE disorders: suppression of spontaneous IgE synthesis by allogeneic suppressor T lymphocytes. Clin Immunol Immunopathol 25:157–164, 1982.

Kragballe K, Borregaard N, Brandrup F, Koch C, Johansen KS. Relation of monocyte and neutrophil oxidative metabolism to skin and oral lesions in carriers of chronic granulomatous disease. Clin Exp Immunol 43:390–398, 1981.

Kraus JC, Mayo-Bond L, Rogers CE, Weber KL, Todd RF III, Wilson JM. An in vivo animal model of gene therapy for leukocyte adhesion deficiency. J Clin Invest 88:1412–1417, 1991.

Krause KH, Lew DP. Bacterial toxins and neutrophil activation. Semin Hematol 25:112–122, 1988.

Krill CE, Smith HD, Mauer AM. Chronic idiopathic granulocytopenias. N Engl J Med 270:973–979, 1964.

Lanza F, Castoldi GL, Masotti M. Eosinophil peroxidase deficiency detected by the Technicon H1 system. Blut 56:143–144, 1988.

Lavoie A, Rottem M, Grodofsky MP, Douglas SD. Anti-*Staphylococcus aureus* IgE antibodies for diagnosis of hyperimmunoglobulinemia E-recurrent infection syndrome in infancy. Am J Dis Child 143:1038–1041, 1989.

Lazarus GM, Neu HC. Agents responsible for infection in chronic granulomatous disease of childhood. J Pediatr 86:415–417, 1975.

LeDeist F, Blanche S, Keable S, Gaud C, Pham H, Descamp-Latscha B. Successful HLA nonidentical bone marrow transplantation in three patients with the leukocyte adhesion deficiency. Blood 74:512–516, 1989.

Lee BW, Yap HK. Polyarthritis resembling juvenile rheumatoid arthritis in a girl with chronic granulomatous disease. Arthritis Rheum 37:773–776, 1994.

Lehrer RI, Cline MJ. Leukocyte myeloperoxidase deficiency and disseminated candidiasis. The role of myeloperoxidase in resistance to *Candida* infection. J Clin Invest 48:1478–1488, 1969.

Lehrer RI, Ganz T, Selsted ME, Babior BM, Burnutte JT. Neutrophils and host defense. Ann Intern Med 109:127–142, 1988.

Lehrer RI, Hanifin J, Cline MJ. Defective bactericidal activity in myeloperoxidase-deficient human neutrophils. Nature 233:78–79, 1969.

Lekstrom-Himes JA, Holland SM, DeCarlo ES, Miller J, Leitman SF, Chang R, Baker AR, Gallin JI. Treatment with intralesional granulocyte instillations and interferon-γ for a patient with chronic granulomatous disease and multiple hepatic abscesses. Clin Infect Dis 19:770–773, 1994.

Lepelley P, Zandecki M, Paquet S, Lerche B, Estienne MH, Fenaux P, Torpier G, Cosson A. Total peroxidase deficiency in eosinophils: a report on twin sisters, one with a refractory anaemia. Eur J Haematol 39:77–81, 1987.

Leto TL, Lomax KJ, Volpp BD, Nunoi H, Sechler JMG, Nauseef WM, Clark RA, Gallin JI, Malech HL. Cloning of a 67-kD neutrophil oxidase factor with similarity to a non-catalytic region of p60$_{c-src}$. Science 248:727–729, 1990.

Leung DYM, Geha RS. Clinical and immunologic aspects of the hyperimmunoglobulin E syndrome. Hematol Oncol Clin North Am 2:81–100, 1988.

Li F, Linton GF, Sekhsaria S, Whiting-Theobald N, Katkin JP, Gallin JI. CD34$^+$ peripheral blood progenitors as a target for genetic correction of the two flavocytochrome b$_{558}$ defective forms of chronic granulomatous disease. Blood 84:53–58, 1994.

Lisowska-Grospierre B, Bohler MC, Fischer A, Mawas C, Springer TA, Griscelli C. Defective membrane expression of the LFA-1 complex may be secondary to the absence of the β chain in a child with recurrent bacterial infection. Eur J Immunol 16:205–208, 1986.

Lomax KR, Leto TL, Nunoi H, Gallin JI, Malech HL. Recombinant 47-kilodalton cytosol factor restores NADPH oxidase in chronic granulomatous disease. Science 245:409–412, 1989. (Erratum in Science 246:987, 1989.)

Loos H, Roos D, Weening R, Houwerzijl J. Familial deficiency of glutathione reductase in human blood cells. Blood 38:53–62, 1976.

Lui RC, Inculet RI. Job's syndrome: a rare cause of recurrent lung abscess in childhood. Ann Thorac Surg 50:992–994, 1990.

MacFarlane GD, Herzberg MC, Wolff LF, Hardie NA. Refractory periodontitis associated with abnormal polymorphonuclear leukocyte phagocytosis and cigarette smoking. J Periodontol 63:908–912, 1992.

MacGregor RR, Macarak EJ, Kefalides NA. Comparative adherence of granulocytes to endothelial monolayers and nylon fiber. J Clin Invest 61:69–78, 1967.

MacGregor RR, Spagnuolo PJ, Lentneh AZ. Inhibition of granulocyte adherence by ethanol, prednisone and aspirin measured with an assay system. N Engl J Med 291:642–646, 1974.

Macher AM, Casale TB, Fauci AL. Chronic granulomatous disease of

childhood and *Chromobacterium violaceum* infections in the southeastern United States. Ann Intern Med 97:51–55, 1982.

Malech HL, Gallin JI. Neutrophils in human diseases. N Engl J Med 317:687–694, 1987.

Malmvall BE, Follin P. Successful interferon-gamma therapy in a chronic granulomatous disease (CGD) patient suffering from *Staphylococcus aureus* hepatic abscess and invasive *Candida albicans* infection. Scand J Infect Dis 25:61–66, 1993.

Manzi S, Urbach AH, McCune AB, Altman HA, Kaplan SS, Medsger TA Jr, Ramsey-Goldman R. Systemic lupus erythematosus in a boy with chronic granulomatous disease: case report and review of the literature. Arthritis Rheum 34:101–105, 1991.

Margolis DM, Melnick DA, Alling DW, Gallin JI. Trimethoprimsulfamethoxazole prophylaxis in the management of chronic granulomatous disease. J Infect Dis 162:723–726, 1990.

Marlin SD, Morton CC, Anderson DC, Springer TA. LFA-1 immunodeficiency disease: definition of the genetic defect and chromosomal mapping of α and β subunits of the lymphocyte function-associated antigen 1 (LFA-1) by complementation in hybrid cells. J Exp Med 164:855–867, 1986.

Marsh WL, Uretsky SC, Douglas SD. Antigens of the Kell blood group system on neutrophils and monocytes: their relation to chronic granulomatous disease. J Pediatr 87:1117–1120, 1975.

McCall CE, Caves J, Cooper R, DeChatelet L. Functional characteristics of human toxic neutrophils. J Infect Dis 124:68–75, 1971.

McClain K, Estrov Z, Chen H, Mahoney DH. Chronic neutropenia of childhood: frequent association with parvovirus infection and correlations with bone marrow culture studies. Br J Haematol 85:57–62, 1993.

McCullough J, Benson S, Yunis EJ, Quie PG. Effect of blood bank storage on leukocyte function. Lancet 2:1333–1337, 1969.

Mentzer WC Jr, Johnston RB Jr, Baehner RL, Nathan DG. An unusual form of chronic neutropenia in a father and daughter with hypogammaglobulinemia. Br J Haematol 36:313–322, 1977.

Merten DF, Buckley RH, Pratt PC, Effman EL, Grossman H. Hyperimmunoglobulin E syndrome: radiographic observations. Radiology 132:71–78, 1979.

Messner RP, Reed WP, Palmer DL, Bolin RB, Davis AT, Quie PG. Transient defects in leukocytic intracellular bactericidal capacity. Clin Immunol Immunopathol 1:523–538, 1973.

Metcalf JS, Gallin JI, Nauseef WM, Root RK. Quantitation using radiolabeled ligands (binding). In Metcalf JS, Nauseef WM, Root RK, Gallin JI, eds. Laboratory Manual of Neutrophil Function. New York, Raven Press, 1986, pp. 80–86.

Miles AA, Miles EM, Burke J. The value and duration of defense reactions of the skin to the primary lodgement of bacteria. Br J Exp Pathol 38:79–96, 1957.

Miller ME. Developmental maturation of human neutrophil motility and its relationship to membrane deformability. In Ballanti JA, Dayton DH, eds. The Phagocytic Cell in Host Resistance. New York, Raven Press, 1975, pp. 295–307.

Mills EL, Noya FJD. Congenital neutrophil deficiencies. In Abramson JS, Wheeler JD, eds. The Neutrophil. New York, Oxford University Press, 1993, pp. 183–227.

Mills EL, Rhool KS, Quie PG. X-linked inheritance in females with chronic granulomatous disease. J Clin Invest 66:332–340, 1980.

Mohler DN, Majerus PW, Minnuch V, Hess CE, Garrick MD. Glutathione synthetase deficiency as a cause of hereditary hemolytic disease. N Engl J Med 283:1253–1257, 1970.

Molenaar DM, Palumbo PJ, Wilson WR, Ritts RE Jr. Leukocyte chemotaxis in diabetic patients with their nondiabetic first-degree relatives. Diabetes 25(Suppl. 2):880–883, 1976.

Mortureux P, Taïeb A, Bazeille JES, Hehunstre JP, Maleville J. Shwachman's syndrome: a case report. Pediatr Dermatol 9:57–61, 1992.

Mouy R, Fischer A, Vilmer E, Seger R, Griscelli C. Incidence, severity, and prevention of infections in chronic granulomatous disease. J Pediatr 114:550–560, 1989.

Mowat AG, Baum J. Chemotaxis of polymorphonuclear leukocytes from patients with diabetes mellitus. N Engl J Med 284:621–627, 1971.

Najjar VA. Defective phagocytosis due to deficiencies involving the tetrapeptide tuftsin. J Pediatr 87:1121–1124, 1975.

Najjar VA, Constantopoulos A. A new phagocytosis-stimulating tetrapeptide hormone, tuftsin, and its role in diseases. J Reticuloendothel Soc 12:197–215, 1972.

Nath J, Flavin M, Gallin JI. Tubulin tyrosinolation in human polymorphonuclear leukocytes: studies in normal subjects and in patients with the Chédiak-Higashi syndrome. J Cell Biol 95:519–526, 1982.

Nauseef WM. Myeloperoxidase deficiency. Hematol Oncol Clin North Am 2:135–159, 1988.

Nelson RD, Quie PG, Simmons RL. Chemotaxis under agarose: a new and simple method for measuring chemotaxis and spontaneous migration of human polymorphonuclear leukocytes and monocytes. J Immunol 115:1650–1656, 1975.

Newburger PE, Cohen HJ, Rothchild SB, Hobbins JC, Malawista SE, Mahoney MJ. Prenatal diagnosis of chronic granulomatous disease. N Engl J Med 300:178–181, 1979.

Newman KA, Schimpff SC, Wade JC. Antibiotic prophylaxis of infections for patients with granulocytopenia. In Verhoef J, Peterson PJ, Quie PG, eds. Infections in the Immunocompromised Host: Pathogenesis, Prevention and Therapy. Amsterdam, North-Holland Biomedical, 1980, pp. 187–190.

Nisengard RJ, Newman MG, Zambon JJ. Periodontal disease. In Nisengard RJ, Newman MG, eds. Oral Microbiology and Immunology, 2nd ed. Philadelphia, WB Saunders, 1994, pp. 360–384.

Noble MA, Grant SK, Hajen E. Characterization of a neutrophil-inhibitory factor from clinically significant *Staphylococcus epidermidis*. J Infect Dis 162:909–913, 1990.

Nunoi H, Rotrosen D, Gallin JI, Malech HL. Two forms of autosomal chronic granulomatous disease lack distinct neutrophil cytosol factors. Science 242:1298–1301, 1988.

Odell EW, Wu PJ. Susceptibility of *Porphyromonas gingivalis* and *P. asaccharolytica* to the non-oxidative killing mechanisms of human neutrophils. Arch Oral Biol 8:597–601, 1992.

O'Regan S, Newman AJ, Graham RC. 'Myelokathexis': Neutropenia with marrow hyperplasia. Am J Dis Child 131:655–658, 1977.

Orkin SH. Molecular genetics of chronic granulomatous disease. Annu Rev Immunol 7:277–357, 1989.

Pabst HF, Holmes B, Quie PG, Gewurz H, Rodey G, Good RA. Immunologic abnormalities in Job's syndrome (abstract). Proceeding of the Society for Pediatric Research, Atlantic City, NJ, 1971.

Paganelli R, Scala E, Capobianchi MR, Fanales-Belasio E, D'Offizi G, Fiorilli N, Aiuti F. Selective deficiency of interferon-gamma production in the hyper-IgE syndrome: relationship to in vitro IgE synthesis. Clin Exp Immunol 84:28–33, 1991.

Parry MF, Root RK, Metcalf JA, Belaney KK, Kaplow LS, Richar WJ. Myeloperoxidase deficiency. Ann Intern Med 95:293–301, 1981.

Payne NR, Hays NT, Regelmann WE, Sorenson M, Mills EL, Quie PG. Growth in patients with chronic granulomatous disease. J Pediatr 102:397–399, 1983.

Peerless AG, Liebhaber M, Anderson S, Lehrer RI, Stiehm ER. *Legionella* pneumonia in chronic granulomatous disease. J Pediatr 106:783–785, 1985.

Perez HD, Kelly E, Elfman F. Armitage G, Winkler J. Defective polymorphonuclear leukocyte formyl peptide receptor(s) in juvenile periodontitis. J Clin Invest 87:971–976, 1991.

Peterson PK, Verhof J, Schmeling D, Quie PG. Kinetics of phagocytosis and bacterial killing by human polymorphonuclear leukocytes and monocytes. J Infect Dis 136:502–509, 1977.

Pincus SH, Thomas IT, Clark RA, Ochs HD. Defective neutrophil chemotaxis with variant ichthyosis, hyperimmunoglobulinemia E, and recurrent infections. J Pediatr 87:908–911, 1975.

Pogrebniak HA, Gallin JI, Malech HL, Baker AR, Moskaluk CA, Travis WD, Pass HI. Surgical management of pulmonary infections in chronic granulomatous disease of childhood. Ann Thorac Surg 55:844–849, 1993.

Presentey B. Ultrastructure of human eosinophils genetically lacking peroxidase. Acta Haematol 71:334–340, 1984.

Price TH, Ochs HD, Gershoni-Baruch G, Harlan JM, Etzioni A. In vivo neutrophil and lymphocyte function studies in a patient with leukocyte adhesion deficiency type II. Blood 84:1635–1639, 1994.

Quie PG. Chronic granulomatous disease of childhood. Adv Pediatr 16:287–300, 1969.

Quie PG. Chronic granulomatous disease in childhood: a saga of discovery and understanding. Pediatr Infect Dis J 12:395–398, 1993.

Quie PG, Belani KK. Corticosteroids for chronic granulomatous disease. J Pediatr 111:393–394, 1987.

Quie PG, White JG, Holmes B, Good RA. In vitro bactericidal capacity of human polymorphonuclear leukocytes: diminished activity in chronic granulomatous disease of childhood. J Clin Invest 46:668–679, 1967.

Quie PG, Kaplan EL, Page AR, Gruskay FL, Malawista SE. Defective polymorphonuclear leukocyte function and chronic granulomatous disease in 2 female children. N Engl J Med 278:976–980, 1968.

Quie PG, Mills EL, Holmes B. Molecular events during phagocytosis by human neutrophils. Prog Hematol 10:193–210, 1977.

Quie PG, Muller SA, Goltz RW. Immunodeficiency and immunosuppression. In Orkin M, Maibach HI, Dahl MV, eds. Dermatology. Norwalk, Conn., Appleton & Lange, 1991, pp. 393–404.

Quinti I, Brozek C, Wood N, Geha RS, Leung DYM. Circulating IgG autoantibodies to IgE in atopic syndromes. J Allergy Clin Immunol 77:586–590, 1986.

Rappeport JM, Newburger PE, Goldblum RM, Goldman AS, Nathan DG, Parkman R. Allogeneic bone marrow transplantation for chronic granulomatous disease. J Pediatr 101:952–955, 1982.

Raubitschek AA, Levin AS, Stites DP, Shaw EB, Fudenberg HH. Normal granulocyte infusion therapy for aspergillosis in chronic granulomatous disease. Pediatrics 51:230–233, 1973.

Reinhold U, Pawelec G, Wehrmann W, Herold M, Wernet P, Kreysel HW. Immunoglobulin E and immunoglobulin G subclass distribution in vivo and relationship to in vitro generation of interferon-gamma and neopterin in patients with severe atopic dermatitis. Int Arch Allergy Appl Immunol 87:120–126, 1988.

Riviere GR, Wagoner MA, Baker-Zander SA, Weisz KS, Adams DF, Simonson L, Lukehart SA. Identification of spirochetes related to *Treponema pallidum* in necrotizing ulcerative gingivitis and chronic periodontitis. N Engl J Med 325:539–543, 1991.

Rodriguez CR, Nueda A, Grospuerre B, Sanchez-Madrid F, Fischer A. Springer TA, Corbi AL. Characterization of two new CD18 alleles causing severe leukocyte adhesion deficiency. Eur J Immunol 23:2792–2798, 1993.

Roesler J, Hecht M, Freihorst J, Lohmann-Matthes ML, Emmendorffer A. Diagnosis of chronic granulomatous disease and of its mode of inheritance by dihydrorhodamine 123 and flow microcytofluorometry. Eur J Pediatr 150:161–165, 1991.

Roos D. The respiratory burst of phagocytic leukocytes. Drug Invest 3:48–61, 1991.

Roos D. The genetic basis of chronic granulomatous disease. Immunol Rev 138:121–157, 1994.

Roos D, Weening RS, Voetman AA, van Schaik MLJ, Bot AAM, Meerhof LJ, Loos JA. Protection of phagocytic leukocytes by endogenous glutathione: studies in a family with glutathione reductase deficiency. Blood 53:851–866, 1979.

Roos D, de Boer M, Borregard N, Bjerrum OW, Valerius NH, Seger RA, Muhlbach T, Belohradsky BH, Weening RS. Chronic granulomatous disease with partial deficiency of cytochrome b_{558} and incomplete respiratory burst: variants of the X-linked, cytochrome b_{558}–negative form of the disease. J Leukoc Biol 51:164–171, 1992.

Root RK, Rosenthal AS, Balestra DJ. Abnormal bactericidal, metabolic and lysosomal functions of Chédiak-Higashi syndrome leukocytes. J Clin Invest 51:649–665, 1972.

Rosenberg HF, Gallin JI. Neutrophil-specific granule deficiency includes eosinophils. Blood 82:268–273, 1993.

Royer-Pokora B, Kunkel LM, Monaco AP, Goff SC, Newburger PE, Baehner RL, Cole FS, Curnutte JT, Orkin SH. Cloning the gene for an inherited human disorder—chronic granulomatous disease—on the basis of its chromosomal location. Nature 322:32–38, 1986.

Schapiro BL, Newburger PE, Klempner MS, Dinauer MC. Chronic granulomatous disease presenting in a 69-year-old man. N Engl J Med 325:1786–1790, 1991.

Schopfer K, Douglas SD. Neutrophil function in children with kwashiorkor. J Lab Clin Med 88:450–461, 1976.

Segal AW. The electron transport chain of the microbicidal oxidase of phagocytic cells and its involvement in the molecular pathology of chronic granulomatous disease. J Clin Invest 83:1785–1793, 1989.

Segal AW, Cross AR, Garcia RC, Borregaard N, Valerius NH, Soothill FF, Jone OTG. Absence of cytochrome b_{245} in chronic granulomatous disease: a multicenter European evaluation of its incidence and relevance. N Engl J Med 308:245–250, 1983.

Seger R. Inborn errors of oxygen-dependent microbial killing by neutrophils. In: Herausgegeben VP, Frick GA, eds. Advances in

Internal Medicine and Pediatrics. Berlin, Springer-Verlag, 1984, pp. 46–52.

Seger R, Galle J, Wildfeuer A, Frater-Schroder M, Linnell J, Hitzig WH. Impaired functions of lymphocytes and granulocytes in transcobalamin II deficiency and their response to treatment. In Seligmann M, Hitzig WH, eds. Primary Immunodeficiencies. Amsterdam, Elsevier/North Holland, 1980, pp. 353–362.

Seger R, Steinmann B, Tiefenauer L, Matsunaga T, Gitzelmann R. Glycogenosis 1B: Neutrophil microbicidal defects due to impaired hexose monophosphate shunt. Pediatr Res 18:297–299, 1984.

Sekhsar S, Gallin JI, Linton GF, Mallory RC, Malech HL. Peripheral blood progenitors as a target for genetic correction of p47-phox–deficient chronic granulomatous disease. Proc Natl Acad Sci U S A 90:7446–7450, 1993.

Shamberger RC, Wohl ME, Perez-Atayde A, Hendren WH. Pneumatocele complicating hyperimmunoglobulin E syndrome (Job's syndrome). Ann Thorac Surg 54:1206–1208, 1992.

Soderberg-Warner M, Rice-Mendoza A, Mendoza GR, Stiehm ER. Neutrophil and T lymphocyte characteristics of two patients with hyper-IgE syndrome. Pediatr Res 17:820–824, 1983.

Solberg CO. Enhanced susceptibility to infection. A new method for the evaluation of neutrophil granulocyte functions. Acta Pathol Microbiol Scand Sect 8 80:10–18, 1972.

Southwick FS, van der Meer JWM. Recurrent cystitis and bladder mass in two adults with chronic granulomatous disease. Ann Intern Med 109:118–121, 1988.

Southwick FS, Dabiri GA, Stossel TP. Neutrophil actin dysfunction is a genetic disorder associated with partial impairment of neutrophil actin assembly in three family members. J Clin Invest 82:1525–1531, 1988.

Spencer DA, John P, Ferryman SR, Weller PH, Darbyshire P. Successful treatment of invasive pulmonary aspergillosis in chronic granulomatous disease with orally administered itraconazole suspension. Am J Respir Crit Care Med 149:239–241, 1994.

Springer TA, Thompson WS, Miller LJ, Schmalstieg FC, Anderson DC. Inherited deficiency of the Mac-1, LFA-1, p150,95 glycoprotein family and its molecular basis. J Exp Med 160:1901–1918, 1984.

Stevens P, Winston DJ, Van Dyke K. In vitro circulation of opsonic and granulocyte function by luminol-dependent chemiluminescence: utility in patients with severe neutropenia and cellular deficiency states. Infect Immun 22:41–51, 1978.

Stone BD, Wheeler JG. Disseminated cryptococcal infection in a patient with hyperimmunoglobulinemia E syndrome. J Pediatr 117:92–95, 1990.

Stopyrowa J, Fyderek K, Sikorska B, Kowalczyk D, Zembala M. Chronic granulomatous disease of childhood: gastric manifestation and response to salazosulfapyridine therapy. Eur J Pediatr 149:28–30, 1989.

Strauss RG, Bove KE, Jones JR, Mauer AM, Fulginiti VA. An anomaly of neutrophil morphology with impaired function. N Engl J Med 290:478–484, 1974.

Subramaniam S, Tuman D, Rausen AR, Douglas SD. "Ascites" and inguinal hernias: unusual presentation for chronic granulomatous disease of childhood. Mt Sinai J Med 41:566–569, 1974.

Tan JS, Akabutu JJ, Mauer AM, Phair JP. Isolated neutrophil dysfunction in adults: a new entity (abstract). Prog Am Soc Clin Invest 90a:301, 1971.

Targan SR, Oseas R. The "lazy" NK cells of Chédiak-Higashi syndrome. J Immunol 130:2671–2674, 1983.

Todd RF III, Fryer DR. The CD11/CD18 leukocyte glycoprotein deficiency. Hematol Oncol Clin North Am 2:13–31, 1988.

Undritz VE. Die Aliws-Grignaschi-anomalies: der erblichkostitutionelle Peroxydasedefect der neutrophilen und monozyten. Blut 14:129–136, 1966.

Van Dyke TE. Role of the neutrophil in oral disease: receptor deficiency in leukocytes from patients with juvenile periodontitis. Rev Infect Dis 7:419–424, 1985.

Van Scoy RE, Hill HR, Ritts RE Jr, Quie PG. Familial neutrophil chemotaxis defect, recurrent bacterial infections, mucocutaneous candidiasis, and hyperimmunoglobulinemia E. Ann Intern Med 82:766–771, 1975.

Verhoeven AJ, van Schaik MLJ, Roos D, Weening RS. Detection of carriers of the autosomal form of chronic granulomatous disease. Blood 71:505–507, 1988.

Virelizier JL, Lagrue A, Durandy A, Arenzana F, Oury E, Griscelli C. Reversal of natural killer defect in Chédiak-Higashi syndrome after bone-marrow transplantation. N Engl J Med 306:1055–1056, 1982.

Volpp BD, Lin Y. In vitro molecular reconstitution of the respiratory burst in B lymphoblasts from p47-phox–deficient chronic granulomatous disease. J Clin Invest 91:201–207, 1993.

Walther MM, Malech H, Berman A, Choyke P, Venzon DJ, Linehan WM, Gallin JD. The urologic manifestations of chronic granulomatous disease. J Urol 147:1314–1318, 1992.

Weber ML, Abela A, de Repentigny L, Garel L, Lapointe N. Myeloperoxidase deficiency with extensive candidal osteomyelitis of the base of the skull. Pediatrics 80:876–879, 1987.

Weening RS. Continuous therapy with sulfamethoxazole-trimethoprim in patients with chronic granulomatous disease. J Pediatr 103:127–130, 1983.

Weening RS, Adriaansz LH, Weemaes CMR, Lutter R, Roos D. Clinical differences in chronic granulomatous disease in patients with cytochrome b–negative or cytochrome b–positive neutrophils. J Pediatr 107:102–104, 1985a.

Weening RS, Corbeel L, de Boer M, Lutter R, Van Zweiten R, Hamers MN, Roos D. Cytochrome b deficiency in an autosomal form of chronic granulomatous disease. A third form of chronic granulomatous disease recognized by monocyte hybridization. J Clin Invest 75:915–920, 1985b.

Weil SC, Rosner GL, Reid MS. cDNA cloning of human myeloperoxidase: decrease in myeloperoxidase mRNA upon induction of HL-60 cells. Proc Natl Acad Sci U S A 84:2157–2161, 1987.

Welte K, Zeidler C, Reiter A, Muller W, Odenwald E, Souza L, Riehm H. Differential effects of granulocyte-macrophage colony-stimulating factor in children with severe congenital neutropenia. Blood 75:1056–1063, 1990.

Weston B, Axtell RA, Todd RF, Vincent M, Balazovich KJ, Suchard SJ, Boxer LA. Clinical and biologic effects of granulocyte colony stimulating factor in the treatment of myelokathexis. J Pediatr 118:229–234, 1991.

Wetzler M, Talpaz M, Kleinerman ES, King A, Huh YO, Gutterman JU, Kurzrock R. A new familial immunodeficiency disorder characterized by severe neutropenia, a defective marrow release mechanism, and hypogammaglobulinemia. Am J Med 89:663–672, 1990.

White LR, Ianette A, Kaplan EL, Davis SD, Wedgwood RJ. Leukocyte in Job's syndrome (letter). Lancet 1:630, 1969.

Wilson CB, Ochs HD, Almquiest J, Dassel S, Mauseth R, Ochs WH. When is umbilical cord separation delayed? J Pediatr 107:292–293, 1985.

Wilson RM, Reeves WG. Neutrophil phagocytosis and killing in insulin-dependent diabetes. Clin Exp Immunol 63:478–484, 1986.

Windhorst DB, Page AR, Holmes B, Quie PG, Good RA. The pattern of genetic transmission of the leukocyte defect in fatal granulomatous disease of childhood. J Clin Invest 47:1026–1034, 1968.

Wolfson JJ, Kane WJ, Laxdal SD, Good RA, Quie PG. Bone findings in chronic granulomatous disease of childhood. A genetic abnormality of leukocyte function. J Bone Joint Surg [Am] 51:1573–1583, 1969.

Wolfson JJ, Quie PG, Laxdal S, Good RA. Roentgenologic manifestations in children with a genetic defect of polymorphonuclear leukocyte function: chronic granulomatous disease of childhood. Radiology 91:37–48, 1968.

Yeaman GR, Froebel K, Galea G, Ormerod A, Urbaniak SJ. Discoid lupus erythematosus in an X-linked cytochrome-positive carrier of chronic granulomatous disease. Br J Dermatol 126:60–65, 1992.

Yomtovian R, Abramson J, Quie PG. Granulocyte transfusion therapy in chronic granulomatous disease: report of a patient and review of the literature. Transfusion 21:739–743, 1981.

Zabacchi G, Soranzo MR, Menegazzi R, Vecchio M, Knowles A, Piccinini C, Spessotto P, Patriarca P. Eosinophil peroxidase deficiency: morphological and immunocyto-chemical studies of the eosinophil-specific granules. Blood 80:2903–2910, 1992.

Zimmerli W, Zarth A, Grathwohl A, Speck B. Neutrophil function and pyogenic infections in bone marrow transplant recipients. Blood 77:393–399, 1991.

Zimran A, Abrahmov A, Aker A, Matzner Y. Correction of neutrophil chemotaxis defect in patients with Gaucher disease by low-dose enzyme replacement therapy. Am J Hematol 43:69–71, 1993.

Zuelzer WW. Myelokathexis—a new form of chronic granulocytopenia. N Engl J Med 270:699–704, 1964.

Chapter 16

Disorders of the Mononuclear Phagocytic System

Naynesh R. Kamani and Steven D. Douglas

The monocyte, or mononuclear phagocyte (MNP), is the first cell to appear in phylogeny as a cell involved in host defense. The role of the mononuclear phagocyte in the coelomic cavity of marine invertebrates is as a scavenger for dead cells, microbes, and debris. With evolution, the mononuclear phagocyte assumed additional roles in the immune system as an antigen-presenting and -processing cell and as an important source of cytokines, complement components, and numerous enzymes. As a professional phagocyte, it ingests microorganisms and participates in the removal of apoptotic cells. These varied functions of the mononuclear phagocyte are discussed in greater detail in Chapter 6. Deficiencies in mononuclear phagocyte function can thus lead to diverse pathologic processes affecting host defense, tissue remodeling, metabolic storage diseases, and inflammatory conditions. Disorders of mononuclear phagocyte proliferation may affect circulating monocytes or any of a number of tissue macrophages. This chapter reviews the qualitative and quantitative defects affecting cells of the mononuclear phagocyte system.

The circulating monocyte arises in the bone marrow from the pluripotential hematopoietic stem cell. The two primary phagocytic cells in blood, monocytes and neutrophils, arise from a common committed progenitor represented by the granulocyte-macrophage colony-forming unit. With maturation, these progenitors are restricted to differentiation along those two cell lineages. The stage at which these progenitors become irreversibly committed to becoming monocytes is not known, but it is probably before the promonocyte stage. Monocytes circulate in the blood for short periods of time and then migrate to tissues, where they differentiate into tissue macrophages. The half-life of the circulating monocyte is estimated to be about 70 hours. In the tissues, in addition to their role as immunoregulatory and phagocytic cells, they assume functions unique to the tissues. Tissue macrophages include the hepatic Kupffer cell, the alveolar macrophage in the lungs, the osteoclast, the microglial cells in the brain, and the dermal Langerhans cell.

Studies of the mononuclear phagocyte in humans have lagged behind studies of lymphocytes and granulocytes because of the difficulty in isolating sufficient numbers of these cells for in vitro investigation. In peripheral blood, the monocyte is present in far lower numbers than lymphocytes or granulocytes. In addition, methods available for separating monocytes from other mononuclear leukocytes are generally inefficient. Techniques for isolating highly enriched monocyte populations are available but are often clinically impractical for use in infants and children, who require large blood volumes. The in vitro evaluation of different measures of monocyte function, such as chemotaxis, adhesion, and phagocytosis, is technically cumbersome. Techniques used to isolate monocytes may themselves induce functional changes (see Chapter 6). These factors as well as the lack of standardized assays for the evaluation of monocyte immunoregulatory function have led to problems in the laboratory studies of disorders affecting the mononuclear phagocyte system.

The tissue macrophage has been even more difficult to study than its circulating monocyte precursor. With the exception of the alveolar macrophage obtainable by bronchial washing and fetal monocyte/macrophages isolated from the placenta after delivery (Wilson et al., 1983), most tissue macrophages cannot be isolated for in vitro study. For this reason, the assessment of the tissue macrophage has been limited to gross and indirect functional evaluation (i.e., skin testing and clearance studies) and to morphologic and immunocytometric assessment.

Despite these technical problems, great progress has been made in understanding the function of the human mononuclear phagocyte system.

DISORDERS WITH AN ALTERATION IN MONOCYTE/MACROPHAGE NUMBER

Monocytosis

The life cycle of the blood monocyte is reviewed in Chapter 6. Normally, monocytes make up 1% to 9% of the total circulating leukocytes, with the absolute monocyte count ranging between 0 and 1200/mm³ in children. Monocyte counts decrease with age. In the newborn period, monocyte counts can reach 1900/mm³ (Weinberg et al., 1985). A monocyte count greater than 750/mm³ in childhood and exceeding 500/mm³ in adults is considered to be *monocytosis* (Miale, 1977; Oski and Naiman, 1982).

Monocytosis can occur in a wide variety of pathologic states, some of which are outlined in Table 16–1. In addition to the hematologic disorders that might be expected to be characterized by monocytosis, a large number of infectious, inflammatory, and immune disorders are associated with increased numbers of circulating monocytes. Collagen-vascular disease, inflammatory bowel disease, sarcoidosis, and infections such

Table 16–1. Disorders Associated with Monocytosis

Infections
  Bacterial: subacute bacterial endocarditis, syphilis, tuberculosis, acute bacterial infection
  Viral: cytomegalovirus

Inflammatory and granulomatous diseases
  Sarcoidosis
  Inflammatory bowel disease, sprue
  Collagen-vascular disease: systemic lupus erythematosus, periarteritis nodosa, rheumatoid arthritis

Hematologic disorders
  Hematologic malignancies: preleukemia, acute monocytic leukemia, chronic myelocytic leukemia, juvenile chronic myelocytic leukemia
  Lymphoid malignancies: lymphoma, multiple myeloma
  Other malignancies
  Polycythemia vera
  Hemolytic anemia, immune thrombocytopenic purpura, chronic neutropenias
  Postsplenectomy state

Miscellaneous
  Drug-related: chlorpromazine, ampicillin

Adapted from Lichtman MA. Monocyte and macrophage disorders: self limited proliferative responses. Monocytosis and monocytopenia. In Williams WJ, Beutler E, Ersler AJ, Lichtman MA, eds. Hematology, 4th ed. New York, McGraw-Hill, 1990, pp. 882–885.

as subacute bacterial endocarditis and tuberculosis have been principal causes. As would be expected, the administration of macrophage colony-stimulating factor (M-CSF) results in marked monocytosis, typically to 20% to 30% of the total white blood cell count (Bajorin et al., 1991). In some disorders, the monocytosis is reactive, for example, the "compensatory" monocytosis in children with cyclic neutropenia. Monocytosis may also be a harbinger of recovery from agranulocytosis. However, despite the monocytosis seen in these neutropenic states, acute or chronic bacterial infection frequently develops in some children, which suggests the need for polymorphonuclear neutrophils in early bacterial surveillance (Baehner and Johnston, 1972; Steigbigel et al., 1974).

When seen in association with benign conditions, monocytosis is not associated with any specific clinical manifestations. Monocytosis associated with malignancies (such as acute myelomonocytic leukemia), however, can be associated with tissue infiltration with serious consequences and release of procoagulant materials, which can lead to disseminated intravascular coagulation.

Monocytopenia

Isolated or primary monocytopenia does not occur, and even a reduction in peripheral monocyte count is an uncommon event. When it does occur, monocytopenia may be associated with abnormalities in monocyte-dependent immune functions.

Patients with aplastic anemia often have a marked monocytopenia and neutropenia. Monocyte-dependent lymphocyte proliferative responses (as in the mixed leukocyte culture [MLC] reaction and responses to specific antigens) are depressed in aplastic anemia

(Twomey et al., 1973). Monocyte-mediated, antibody-dependent cellular cytoxicity (MMADCC) is also deficient in the peripheral blood of patients with aplastic anemia (Poplack et al., 1976).

Monocytopenia is a characteristic feature of hairy cell leukemia (HCL), an uncommon lymphoproliferative disorder seen in older adults. It is characterized by massive splenomegaly, mild to moderate pancytopenia, vasculitis in a significant number of patients, and bone marrow replacement with atypical cells with prominent cytoplasmic projections termed "hairy cells" (Flandrin et al., 1984). Patients with HCL are prone to infections with a variety of organisms, including *Mycobacterium tuberculosis* and atypical mycobacteria, *Toxoplasma,* and *Legionella* (Golomb and Hanauer, 1981). In addition to monocytopenia, monocytes are absent from the spleen and monocyte migration in Rebuck's skin window preparations is either absent or markedly reduced. A variant form of HCL in which monocytopenia is not a feature has been described (Sainati et al., 1990).

Corticosteroids affect monocyte/macrophage function in several ways. Monocytopenia occurs after steroid administration, as does diminished monocyte/macrophage mobilization to areas of inflammation. In vitro, glucocorticoids impair a number of other monocyte/macrophage functions, including chemotactic responsiveness, phagocytic activity, microbicidal function, and macrophage processing and presentation of antigen (Gerrard et al., 1984). Glucocorticoids modulate the expression of monocyte and macrophage Fc receptors for immunoglobulin G (IgG) and inhibit the clearance of IgG-coated erythrocytes by splenic macrophages (Schreiber et al., 1992). These effects on mononuclear phagocyte function may contribute to the predisposition of patients treated with steroids to infections with fungi, mycobacteria, and other opportunistic organisms. Profound monocytopenia may occur in patients with acquired immunodeficiency syndrome (AIDS).

Transient monocytopenia has been noted between 2 and 4 hours after administration of tumor necrosis factor-α (TNF-α) and interferon-γ (IFN-γ) to patients with malignancies. Similarly, administration of M-CSF and granulocyte-macrophage colony-stimulating factor (GM-CSF) leads to transient monocytopenia within 15 minutes. This effect is most likely secondary to monocyte margination resulting from increased monocyte adherence to endothelium (Ulich et al., 1990; Aulitzky et al., 1991).

PROLIFERATIVE DISORDERS OF MONONUCLEAR PHAGOCYTES

Reactive Hyperplasia

Several illnesses are characterized by a profound hyperplasia of the mononuclear phagocyte system. These diseases are characterized clinically by hepatosplenomegaly and lymph node hypertrophy. Microscopic examination of the enlarged organs reveals macrophage hyperplasia and numerous multinucleated giant cells. These multinucleated giant cells occur in response to infection with certain intracellular agents (tuberculosis, leprosy, cryptococcosis), as a reaction in the presence of foreign chemicals (silicosis or berylliosis), in the presence of excessive hematopoietic cell destruction (hemolytic anemia or pulmonary hemosiderosis), or in a variety of granulomatous disorders (sarcoidosis, Wegener's granulomatosis) (Hassan et al., 1989).

Although these granulomatous diseases share common histologic and clinical features, each has distinct immunopathologic characteristics. For example, tuberculosis may be associated with macrophage activation. Delayed hypersensitivity reactions are demonstrable, and the macrophages manifest increased phagocytic and microbicidal activity (King et al., 1975). By contrast, in the other illnesses in which delayed hypersensitivity reactions are demonstrable, such as exposure to beryllium (Alekseeva, 1966), macrophages do not manifest increased microbial killing (Golde, 1975).

Further reactive hyperplasia may occur in the absence of delayed hypersensitivity reactions; for example, in disorders with excessive hemolysis and erythrophagocytosis, delayed hypersensitivity is absent, phagocytosis of bacteria is reduced, and the tumoricidal capacity of macrophages is defective (Gill et al., 1966; Weinberg and Hibbs, 1977). Studies of monocyte Fc receptor activity in patients with immune hemolytic anemias indicate an increase in the number of Fc receptor sites with restricted specificity for autologous immunoprotein–coated erythrocytes (Kay and Douglas, 1977).

The Histiocytosis Syndromes

Classification of the neoplastic disorders of the mononuclear phagocyte system is complicated by the fact that these disorders encompass a wide spectrum of cellular differentiation and proliferation. At one extreme is acute monocytic leukemia, an aggressive proliferative malignancy characterized by infiltration of the bone marrow with undifferentiated monoblasts; at the other end of the spectrum is the clinically benign eosinophilic granuloma (Table 16–2). A classification of the histiocytosis syndromes in children has been proposed based on the immunobiology of the mononuclear phagocyte and Langerhans cells (Writing Group of the Histiocyte Society, 1987; Broadbent et al., 1989).

Class I: Langerhans Cell Histiocytosis

The entity of Langerhans cell histiocytosis (LCH) includes a diverse group of clinical syndromes characterized by a proliferation of Langerhans cells that have distinctive pathologic and immunophenotypic features (Egeler and D'Angio, 1995). Birbeck's granules, rod-shaped cytoplasmic granules with expanded rounded ends, can be seen on electron microscopy and are pathognomonic for LCH. Langerhans cells have a distinctive immunophenotype: $S100^+$, $CD1^+$, $CD4^+$, $CD11c^+$, $CD14^+$, $CD15^+$, $CD30^-$, $CD45^-$, and vimentin$^+$ (McMillan et al., 1986). S100 protein, present in nor-

Table 16–2. The Histiocytosis Syndromes

Langerhans cell histiocytoses (class I)
  Eosinophilic granuloma
  Letterer-Siwe disease
  Hand-Schüller-Christian disease

Hemophagocytic syndromes (class II)
  Familial erythrophagocytic lymphohistiocytosis (FEL)
  Infection-associated hemophagocytic syndrome (IAHS)
  Sinus histiocytosis with massive lymphadenopathy
  X-linked lymphoproliferative syndrome (XLP)

Malignant histiocytosis syndromes (class III)
  Leukemias
    Acute myelocytic leukemia (AML)
    Chronic myelocytic leukemia (CML)
    Adult chronic myelocytic leukemia
    Juvenile chronic myelocytic leukemia
    Chronic myelomonocytic leukemia (CMML)
  Malignant histiocytosis
  True histiocytic lymphoma

mal Langerhans cells and LCH cells, is an acidic, calcium-binding neural specific protein that is also present in neurons, glial cells, and neuroectodermal tumor cells.

Langerhans cell histiocytosis occurs primarily in children and young adults. The clinical spectrum of LCH can extend from the localized entity of eosinophilic granuloma to a multisystem disease involving the bones, skin, liver, lymph nodes, lungs, spleen, eyes, ears, and bone marrow. Immunologic evaluations have revealed varying abnormalities of T-cell number and function. Some patients have a relative lack of suppressor $CD8^+$ T cells with a resultant increase in CD4/CD8 ratios.

Therapy is dependent on the extent of the disease. Patients with progressive multisystem disease may respond to chemotherapy with single or multiple agents (Ishii et al., 1992; Egeler et al., 1993). Successful allogeneic bone marrow transplantation has been performed in a few patients with chemotherapy-resistant progressive LCH (Ringden et al., 1987; Stoll et al., 1990; Greinix et al., 1992).

Class II: The Hemophagocytic Syndromes

The hemophagocytic syndromes encompass several benign proliferative disorders of the non-Langerhans–cell histiocytes. They include two disorders in which histiocytes proliferate after an infection. In two other disorders (familial erythrophagocytic lymphohistiocytosis and sinus histiocytosis with massive lymphadenopathy), the pathogenesis remains obscure, although immunoregulatory defects of the T cell may result in proliferation of these cells. These disorders are also discussed in Chapter 27.

Infection-Associated Hemophagocytic Syndrome

Infection-associated hemophagocytic syndrome (IAHS) is characterized by fever, generalized constitutional symptoms, hepatosplenomegaly, and generalized lymphadenopathy. It is most often associated with viral

infections. A similar hemophagocytic syndrome has been described in association with a number of gram-positive and gram-negative bacterial infections and fungal, mycobacterial, and rickettsial infections (Woda and Sullivan, 1993). The most severe cases of virus-associated hemophagocytic syndromes occur in immunosuppressed patients.

Laboratory findings include pancytopenia, abnormal liver function with elevated liver enzymes and triglycerides, and a rapidly developing coagulopathy. Histologic differentiation of benign hemophagocytic syndromes from malignant histiocytosis is made on the basis of the benign nature of the histiocytes in IAHS. Histologic features in the tissues are dependent on the stage of disease, with minimal histiocytic infiltration early on, followed by increasing proliferation with time. Erythrophagocytosis can be detected in bone marrow and in liver sinusoids but may not be seen in abundance.

Therapy is usually supportive. Immunosuppressive therapy may be deleterious and is not recommended. The prognosis for those who survive the coagulopathy is generally good (McClain et al., 1988).

Familial Erythrophagocytic Lymphohistiocytosis

Familial erythrophagocytic lymphohistiocytosis (FEL) is a rare condition seen in young children that involves the entire reticuloendothelial system. The age of onset is usually in the first few months of life. It is a familial disorder with an autosomal recessive mode of inheritance. It presents abruptly or insidiously with fever, hepatosplenomegaly, pancytopenia, and neurologic and hepatic manifestations, including a bleeding diathesis. Bone and skin lesions are not prominent, but spinal fluid pleocytosis and hypertriglyceridemia are characteristically present. Elevated levels of cerebrospinal fluid neopterin were observed in two children with FEL, suggestive of increased macrophage activation within the central nervous system. Levels returned to normal with the achievement of remission after cytotoxic therapy (Howells et al., 1990, 1992). Lesional cells are found in the bone marrow, spleen, liver, lymph nodes, and meninges and express varying degrees of hemophagocytosis.

Immunologic deficiency has been described in some cases, with defects in both humoral and cellular immune function (Ladisch et al., 1978). The pediatric patient has cutaneous anergy, depressed antibody responses, and a profound defect in monocyte-mediated antibody-dependent cellular cytotoxicity (ADCC). These immunologic defects are accompanied by a plasma factor that suppresses the responses of normal lymphocytes in culture and may reflect abnormal plasma lipid and ganglioside metabolism. Some of these children have been treated by repeated plasma exchange with complete but temporary clinical remission lasting several weeks and correction of the immunodeficiency (Ladisch et al., 1982, 1984; Wong et al., 1983).

Marked elevations in serum ferritin levels and levels of cytokines including interleukin-6 (IL-6), IFN-γ, and soluble IL-2 receptor occur in children with hemophagocytic syndromes including IAHS, FEL, and malignant histiocytosis (Esumi et al., 1989; Fujiwara et al., 1993). Because of overlapping clinical, laboratory, and pathologic features, it is sometimes difficult to distinguish between FEL and IAHS. Promising results have been achieved with the use of etoposide-containing cytotoxic therapeutic regimens in infants with FEL (Loy et al., 1991). An FEL-like hemophagocytic syndrome occurs in the accelerated phase of Chédiak-Higashi syndrome (Bejaoui et al., 1989).

X-Linked Lymphoproliferative Syndrome

The X-linked lymphoproliferative (XLP) syndrome is a disorder seen exclusively in males in which males carrying the XLP gene usually die after a primary Epstein-Barr virus (EBV) infection (see Chapters 12 and 27). At the time of death, patients demonstrate a diffuse proliferation of histiocytes similar to that seen in IAHS. EBV-induced infectious mononucleosis, which follows a benign course in the majority of children, results in a fatal illness in most children with XLP. In studies of families with XLP, affected male children have normal immunologic function before their encounter with EBV infection. The affected males who have survived EBV infection have developed a combined immunodeficiency with hypogammaglobulinemia and cellular immune dysfunction. Furthermore, B-cell non-Hodgkin's lymphomas develop in many patients. Genetic detection of XLP carriers and presymptomatic affected males is now possible using restriction fragment length polymorphism (RFLP) analysis at the *DXS42* and *DXS37* loci on the X chromosome (Skare et al., 1989). The XLP gene has been localized to Xq25 based on the detection of Xq25 deletions in three affected patients (Skare et al., 1993).

The histopathologic features of XLP evolve with time. Lymphoid depletion with histiocyte proliferation in the lymph node sinuses and splenic red pulp have been seen in autopsies. Treatment of the acute EBV infection with acyclovir has been tried unsuccessfully in several patients. Immunosuppressive therapy usually leads to the onset of fatal lymphoid malignancy. In the near future, prevention of EBV infection with antiviral agents, intravenous immunoglobulin, or vaccination may offer the best hope for these patients (Woda and Sullivan, 1993).

Sinus Histiocytosis with Massive Lymphadenopathy

First described by Rosai and Dorfman in 1972, sinus histiocytosis with massive lymphadenopathy (SHML) is seen most commonly in children in the second decade of life. It is characterized by a chronic, painless, massive cervical lymphadenopathy associated with low-grade fever, leukocytosis, increased erythrocyte sedimentation rate, and hypergammaglobulinemia. The course is benign, with lymphadenopathy persisting for several months and occasionally years (Rosai and Dorfman, 1972; Foucar and Foucar, 1990). Lymph node histology reveals complete effacement of lymph node architecture by benign-appearing histiocytes and lymphocytes with significant leukocytophagocytosis and some erythrophagocytosis (Fig. 16–1). The etiology

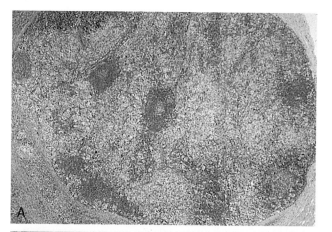
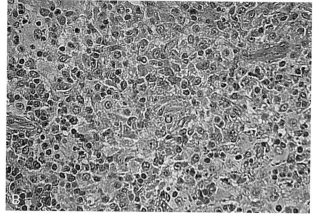

Figure 16–1. Sinus histiocytosis with massive lymphadenopathy (Rosai-Dorfman disease). *A.* Low-power view of lymph node showing almost total effacement of lymph node architecture. *B.* High-power view showing proliferation of sinusoidal histiocytes with leukophagocytosis.

of this syndrome remains undefined. In situ hybridization studies of tissues involved by SHML have revealed human herpesvirus-6 DNA in seven of nine involved tissues examined and EBV DNA in one of nine tissues (Levine et al., 1992). Effective therapy is unavailable, and immunosuppressive therapy should be discouraged because of the usually excellent long-term prognosis (Komp, 1990).

Class III: Malignant Histiocytosis Syndromes

This subgroup of the histiocytic disorders includes the overtly malignant proliferations of circulating monocytes and tissue macrophages or histiocytes. The term *mononuclear phagocyte and immunoregulatory effector system* (M-PIRE) has been suggested to consolidate the monocyte and free and fixed histiocytes into a single family of cells, all derived from a bone marrow stem cell (Foucar and Foucar, 1990; Ben-Ezra and Koo, 1993). Thus, malignancies of the M-PIRE system include malignant neoplasms of monocytes, macrophages, and dendritic and interdigitating reticulum cells. Because there are no distinctive clonal markers for histiocytes, a number of these malignancies have been mistakenly identified in the past as representing malignancies of T cells or vice versa.

Acute Monocytic Leukemia

Acute monocytic leukemia is a hematologic malignancy lumped under the heading of acute nonlymphocytic leukemia (ANLL) or French-American-British (FAB) class M5 in the FAB classification of ANLL. It constitutes the majority of cases of ANLL in children under age 2. A diagnosis of acute monocytic leukemia M5 can be made when the marrow has more than 30% blasts that are nonspecific esterase-positive and bear the cell surface marker CD14 (see Chapter 6). Acute monocytic leukemia carries a poor overall survival.

Malignant Histiocytosis

Malignant histiocytosis is a severe, systemic neoplastic disorder with a predilection for the entire reticuloendothelial system. The diagnosis is made on the basis of the discovery of atypical neoplastic histiocytes in any part of the reticuloendothelial system. Erythrophagocytosis may be present but is not diagnostic for this disorder. Morphologically, the cells are of varying sizes with irregularly contoured nuclei. Other features of mononuclear phagocytic cells can be discerned ultrastructurally. Cytochemically, the cells are of histiocytic origin. They are S100 negative and positive for CD4 and HLA-DR. A number of these neoplasms previously diagnosed as malignant histiocytosis would now be classified as malignant lymphoma. When malignant histiocytosis occurs as localized tumor nodules, it is classified as a *true histiocytic lymphoma.*

Secondary Histiocytoses

By virtue of their role as a scavenger of particulate material and organic debris, macrophages are involved in a variety of metabolic disorders characterized by abnormal accumulation of intracellular material. This material accumulates because of a defect of the enzymatic pathway necessary for degradation of the ingested material or excessive production of a cell product.

Lysosomal Storage Diseases

Lysosomes are acid hydrolase–containing membrane-bound organelles within the cytoplasm of cells throughout the body. They contain a number of different enzymes that are vital to the metabolism of several lipid, glycolipid, and glycosaminoglycan substrates. By a process called *exocytosis*, lysosomal enzymes are released into surrounding tissues and recognized by specific cell surface receptors found on adjoining cells via the terminal mannose-6-phosphate residue on the enzymes. The lysosome contents are ingested into surrounding cells via endocytosis after ligand-receptor interaction.

Lysosomal storage diseases result from specific deficiencies of individual lysosomal enzymes. Depending on the missing enzyme, substrates such as sphingolipids, glycogen, or mucopolysaccharide accumulate

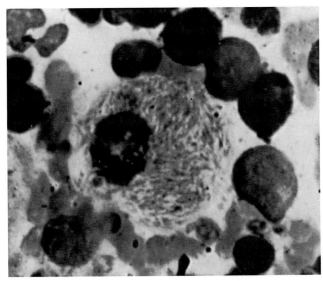

Figure 16–2. Gaucher cell. Accumulation of glucosylceramide within monocyte/macrophage in the bone marrow of a patient with Gaucher's disease due to deficiency of beta glucocerebrosidase activity. Note the large foamy-looking cell. (Courtesy of Dr. J. Peyser.)

within the lysosomes, eventually affecting other cellular functions and contributing to the specific disease phenotype. In lysosomal storage diseases, macrophages throughout the reticuloendothelial system are affected. These distended macrophages assume characteristic appearances in different lysosomal storage diseases. The Gaucher cell (Fig. 16–2) and the sea-blue histiocyte of Niemann-Pick disease represent some of these characteristic cells (Fig. 16–3). An exhaustive discussion of the various lysosomal storage disorders is beyond the scope of this chapter.

In in vitro experiments with fibroblasts from patients with Hurler's syndrome, Neufeld (1974) showed that cross-correction of "giant lysosomes" in abnormal α-1-iduronidase–deficient fibroblasts occurred when they were cocultured with normal fibroblasts. These results

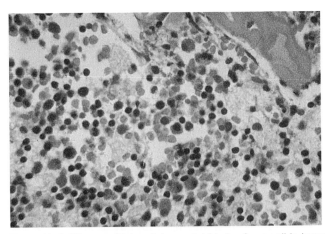

Figure 16–3. Niemann-Pick cell. Large lipid-laden foam cell in bone marrow of a patient with Niemann-Pick disease type A. Sphingomyelin accumulates in macrophages throughout the reticuloendothelial system and brain because of a deficiency of sphingomyelinase. (Courtesy of Dr. C. August.)

form the basis for the successful reversal of the consequences of substrate accumulation noted after allogeneic bone marrow transplantation (BMT) in a number of lysosomal storage disorders. Bone marrow transplants provide a source of enzymatically normal hematopoietic cells. The experience to date with bone marrow transplantation suggests that although existing neurologic abnormalities cannot be reversed, progressive neurologic deterioration can be arrested (Krivit et al., 1992).

For Gaucher's disease, which is the most prevalent lysosomal storage disorder, the use of mannose-terminated human glucocerebrosidase (alglucerase) via intravenous infusion has shown promise. After intravenous alglucerase, improvements are noted within 6 months with increased hemoglobin values and platelet counts, a reduction in liver and spleen size, and improvements in skeletal findings (Barton et al., 1991; Beutler et al., 1991; Fallet et al., 1992). Based on the promising results after allogeneic bone marrow transplantation, some of these diseases may respond to the infusion of autologous genetically corrected hematopoietic progenitors. Somatic cell gene therapy is being explored and offers the best hope for curing these disorders.

MONONUCLEAR PHAGOCYTE SECRETORY FUNCTIONS

Monocytes and macrophages make and secrete a wide variety of inflammatory substances. They are capable of producing essentially all of the complement components and of extensive production of prostaglandins. Research has focused on the mutual interaction between cytokines and monocyte/macrophages (i.e., on monocyte synthesis of cytokines and the effects of cytokines on these cells). These interactions are vital to normal homeostasis and immune and inflammatory responses.

Monokine Secretion

Monocytes synthesize interleukin-1α and -1β (IL-1α and IL-1β) and TNF-α. IL-1 plays a central role in a number of host responses to inflammation (see Chapter 6). Thus, a number of monocyte stimuli result in IL-1 secretion. Among the protean effects of IL-1 are the production of fever, increased synthesis of acute-phase reactants through a direct action on hepatocytes, the production of collagenase, an increase in prostaglandin synthesis, and increased adherence of both polymorphonuclear leukocytes and lymphocytes to endothelial cells.

TNF-α was originally described on the basis of its ability in vitro to lyse certain tumor cells. It plays a central role in the cachexia associated with metastatic malignancy. TNF-α may also play an etiologic role in endotoxic shock. Recombinant TNF-α administered intravenously leads to a clinical picture similar to that induced by endotoxin (Beutler and Cerami, 1986).

Human monocytes, in vitro, produce M-CSF, granulocyte colony-stimulating factor (G-CSF), and GM-CSF. A number of different agents and cytokines induce the formation of colony-stimulating factors (CSFs) by human monocytes. Lipopolysaccharide and numerous cytokines, including IL-3, IL-4, and IFN-γ, induce CSF synthesis by monocytes (Hamilton, 1993).

Under appropriate circumstances, IL-1α, IL-1β, TNF-α, and GM-CSF may lead to enhanced cytotoxicity and direct lysis of tumor cells. All of these compounds have been cloned and synthesized by recombinant technology; they are currently being assessed in therapeutic trials in the treatment of malignancy. G-CSF enhances granulocyte production. GM-CSF also enhances the production of monocytes. Both agents are being used to accelerate hematopoietic recovery after myelosuppressive or myeloablative chemotherapy.

Wound Healing

A number of polypeptide growth factors secreted by mononuclear phagocytes and lymphocytes play a central role in wound healing and matrix generation. These include IL-1, TNF-α, platelet-derived growth factor (PDGF), and transforming growth factor-β (TGF-β). Although mononuclear phagocytes are not the primary cellular source of TGF-β and PDGF, they synthesize and release these cytokines upon activation after the onset of an inflammatory response (Wahl, 1992). Both PDGF and TGF-β are instrumental in fibroblast proliferation and tissue repair, and their secretion is regulated in an autocrine or paracrine fashion. These cytokines play important roles in disease processes characterized by excessive matrix generation, such as fibrotic disorders of the skin, lungs, and liver (Czaja et al., 1989; Khalil et al., 1989; Kulozik et al., 1990). Increased TGF-β messenger ribonucleic acid (mRNA) and protein synthesis has been demonstrated in myelofibrosis (Terui et al., 1990) and in a number of collagen-vascular diseases (Connor et al., 1989; Peltonen et al., 1990).

The wound-healing (vulnerary) properties of both TGF-β and PDGF suggest a therapeutic role for these cytokines. Wound healing in experimental tissue repair models can be accelerated with local application of TGF-β (Mustoe et al., 1987) and PDGF (Pierce et al., 1991). Effects of TGF-β can be demonstrated in both normal and monocytopenic animals (Lynch et al., 1989). In contrast, effects of PDGF are macrophage-dependent and seen only in normal models of wound healing (Pierce et al., 1989). Antagonists of TGF-β, such as IL-4 and IFN-γ, may counteract the fibrosis induced by these cytokines in such disorders as hepatitis C (Castilla et al., 1991). Because of the overlapping effects of different cytokines in influencing the inflammatory response, quantitative or qualitative deficiencies in individual cytokines may not result in defects of wound healing.

Pulmonary Disease

Alveolar Macrophages

Human alveolar macrophages are the predominant cell type found within the alveolar air spaces and are usually located within the acellular lining that covers alveolar epithelium. They function as the first line of defense against all foreign particulate matter and inhaled microorganisms that are small enough to reach the alveoli. Besides its well-recognized phagocytic and microbicidal properties, the pulmonary alveolar macrophage (PAM) is important in immunoregulation and in the secretion of a number of soluble mediators of inflammation.

Studies of PAMs recovered during bronchoalveolar lavage in healthy adults provide the basis of most of our knowledge about human PAMs, although PAMs isolated from other species have also been investigated extensively. Approximately 10 million to 20 million cells are recovered in a typical lavage procedure from a healthy, nonsmoking adult. Over 90% of these cells are PAMs, and most of the remaining cells are lymphocytes. Morphologically, human PAMs are large mononuclear cells, usually 15 to 20 μm (10 to 50 μm) in diameter. The cell membrane of the PAM is convoluted, and many membrane-bound cytoplasmic inclusions represent primary lysosomes that contain a variety of hydrolytic enzymes.

Pulmonary alveolar macrophages play an important role in repair processes and ongoing tissue breakdown in the normal lung. Cathepsin D is important in the final breakdown of collagen, and fibronectin is important in the normal healing process. Inflammatory mediators, such as IFN-γ and lipopolysaccharide, actively but nonsynchronously modulate PAM cathepsin D and fibronectin activity (Rossman et al., 1990).

Pulmonary Emphysema

Connective tissues and their collagen and elastin constituents are fundamental to pulmonary structure and function. Small airway obstruction results when the supporting structures of the conducting airways are impaired by changes in elastin and collagen architecture. These changes lead to two general forms of disease: emphysematous and fibrotic disorders.

Emphysematous pulmonary changes occur when proteolytic enzymes (elastase) chronically released from activated normal macrophages cause a gradual loss of pulmonary elastin. These enzymes are released as a consequence of cell death or injury or by active secretion. For example, cigarette smoke stimulates the synthesis and secretion of elastolytic enzymes from PAMs, undoubtedly contributing to the link between smoking and emphysema.

The enzymatic activity of macrophage proteases is usually opposed by the 52-kD serum glycoprotein alpha$_1$-antitrypsin. The most common congenital deficiency of alpha$_1$-antitrypsin is the result of a point mutation (Glu^{342}→Lys^{342}). This leads to defective secretion of this critical antiprotease and the early onset of severe emphysema. Alveolar macrophages as well as the Kupffer cells of the liver synthesize alpha$_1$-antitrypsin. The local balance of proteases and antiproteases is essential to the maintenance of normal pulmonary structure and function (Mornex et al., 1986).

Pulmonary Fibrosis

A number of interstitial lung diseases, including idiopathic pulmonary fibrosis and asbestosis, are characterized by alveolar wall fibrosis with interstitial remodeling, an increase in the number of activated alveolar macrophages, and extracellular matrix accumulation. Alveolar macrophages from these patients demonstrate enhanced IL-1β and TNF-α release, suggesting that these monokines are important in the pathogenesis of fibrotic disorders of the lung (Rom et al., 1991; Zhang et al., 1993).

Liver Disease

A major source of tissue macrophages is the Kupffer cells of the liver. Accordingly, it might be anticipated that liver disease would result in abnormal MNP function. In fact, monocytes from patients with chronic liver disease express diminished chemotactic responsiveness, diminished phagocytic activity, and depressed bactericidal killing (Hassner et al., 1981; Holdstock et al., 1982).

As in the lung, Kupffer cell–derived cytokines may play an important role in the pathogenesis of hepatic fibrosis. Kupffer cell–conditioned medium induces a PDGF-mediated activation of hepatic lipocytes into proliferative cells, producing increased amounts of collagen (Friedman and Arthur, 1989).

DISORDERS OF MONONUCLEAR PHAGOCYTE CELL SURFACE RECEPTORS

Mononuclear phagocytes possess a variety of cell surface receptors that play vital roles in their effector and immunoregulatory functions during host defense. Genetic defects involving absence of some of these cell surface receptors have been described. These include leukocyte adhesion defects and the bare lymphocyte syndrome. A number of studies have uncovered abnormalities of receptor expression or function in diverse disorders of host defense, malignant conditions, and inflammatory diseases.

Integrins

Integrins are heterodimer glycoproteins made up of noncovalently linked α- and β-chains. The α-chain is the larger and more variable of the two subunits. Common β-subunits combine with unique α-subunits to create functionally distinct receptors. Members of the integrin family of adhesion receptors mediate cell-cell and cell-matrix interactions. The leukocyte integrins, or β_2 subfamily, are made up of three different α-chains, CD11a (leukocyte function–associated antigen-1 [LFA-1]), CD11b (Mo1 or Mac-1), and CD11c (p150,95), that associate with a single common 94-kD β-chain, CD18. The β-subunit amino acid sequence of the β_2 subfamily has homology with the β-subunit of the fibronectin receptor and glycoprotein IIb/IIIa (β_3) and the very-late-antigen β_1 integrins, very-late-antigen molecules (Hemler et al., 1986; Hynes, 1992).

Leukocyte Adhesion Defects

The leukocyte adhesion defect (LAD) syndrome type 1 is an autosomal recessive inherited disorder characterized by recurrent and life-threatening bacterial and fungal infections (see Chapter 15). Defective synthesis of the β-chain of LFA-1, Mac-1, and p150,95 receptors occurs in monocytes, granulocytes, and certain lymphocytes and is associated with impaired cell adhesion in a unique group of patients with recurrent infections (Marlin et al., 1986). These patients have recurrent bacterial infections, necrotic skin lesions, and delayed separation of the umbilical cord after birth. In addition, they experience severe gingivitis, periodontitis, and alveolar bone loss (Fig. 16–4), which lead to early loss of deciduous and permanent teeth (Anderson et al., 1986).

Clinically, two phenotypic presentations of LAD-1 are recognized. In the severe phenotype, there are no detectable α-β complexes on leukocytes. In the moderate phenotype (partial LAD-1), leukocytes express 1% to 10% Mac-1, p160,95, and LFA-1. The severity of clinical and laboratory manifestations parallels the degree of integrin expression. The hallmark of LAD-1 is absence of granulocytes at sites of infection in the presence of peripheral blood leukocytosis. This is secondary to defective neutrophil and monocyte adhesion to vascular endothelium. Rebuck's skin window tests in severely affected patients show no mobilization of neutrophils or monocytes. Adhesion-dependent chemotaxis and aggregation of monocytes and granulocytes in vitro are deficient. Other cell-cell adhesion–dependent functions of lymphocytes (lymphocyte proliferation, ADCC, and natural killer cell cytoxicity) are also abnormal.

Allogeneic bone marrow transplantation has successfully corrected the defect in LAD-1. Because these patients have hyperactive marrows, mixed but stable hematopoietic chimerism often results after marrow transplantation despite the use of conditioning regimens that would be considered myeloablative. Gene therapy with hematopoietic stem cells transfected with the normal β-subunit–encoding gene offers the best hope for cure for these patients.

A new leukocyte adhesion defect, LAD-2, has been described in two unrelated children of consanguineous parents (Etzioni et al., 1992) (see Chapter 15). These children had severe mental retardation, distinctive facies, short-limbed dwarfism, the Bombay (hh) erythrocyte phenotype, and recurrent bacterial infections including localized cellulitis without pus formation. The patients' neutrophils lacked the fucosylated sialyl-Lewis X carbohydrate structure, which serves as the ligand for E- and P-selectins involved in neutrophil recruitment. Both patients had leukocytosis and abnor-

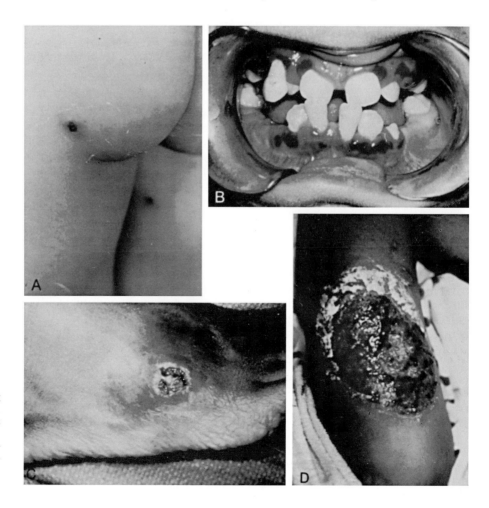

Figure 16–4. Ulcerative skin lesions *(A, C, D)* and periodontitis *(B)* in a patient with leukocyte adhesion defect type 1. Periodontitis leads to alveolar gum loss with early loss of the deciduous and permanent teeth. Because of the chemotactic defect, skin lesions are ulcerative and nonpurulent. (Courtesy of Dr. Donald C. Anderson.)

mal adhesion-dependent neutrophil functions despite having normal CD18 expression. Although the patients' monocytes were not studied, they most likely lacked this adhesion molecule ligand.

Glanzmann's Thrombasthenia

Patients with Glanzmann's thrombasthenia have defective expression of the integrin GPIIb/IIIa on platelets. This leads to a mild bleeding diathesis because platelets cannot aggregate on exposure to fibrin (Ruggeri et al., 1982). The expression of the leukocyte integrins Mac-1, LFA-1, and p150,95 is unaffected. Conversely, platelets of patients with LAD express GPIIb/IIIa normally (Pidard et al., 1987; Setiadi et al., 1991).

Familial Monocyte Dysfunction

A familial monocyte dysfunction syndrome has been described in a young adult male with recurrent febrile episodes and frequent oral and skin infections. The patient's monocytes showed markedly reduced expression of a number of cell surface receptors including HLA-DR antigens, C3b and Fc receptors for IgG, and cytoskeletal vimentin intermediate filaments. His monocytes also demonstrated impaired phagocytosis and antigen-presenting function. Similar monocyte abnormalities were demonstrable in a sister with a longstanding history of asthenia and a nephew who had frequent but mild respiratory infections (Prieto et al., 1990).

Histocompatibility Antigens

The histocompatibility (HLA) antigens present on many cells, including monocytes, play a critical role in a number of immune responses. Class I HLA antigens (HLA-A, -B, and -C antigens) are found on virtually all cells and exist on the surface as heterodimers of 44 and 12 kd. Class II HLA antigens (HLA-DP, -DQ, -DR antigens) are heterodimers of 29 and 34 kD. They have a restricted tissue distribution and are preferentially expressed on monocytes, B cells, and activated T cells (see Chapters 2 and 4). Class II antigens are also expressed on alveolar macrophages and other tissue macrophages. Alveolar macrophages express five times more DR antigens per unit surface area than do peripheral blood monocytes. However, the degree of expression of these antigens on monocyte/macrophages does not correlate with their ability to present antigen to lymphocytes (Moore et al., 1983). Cytotoxic T (CD8$^+$) cells recognize foreign antigen (e.g., viruses) in the context of class I antigens. Helper T cells (CD4$^+$) recognize foreign antigen in association with class II antigens on antigen-presenting cells.

Bare Lymphocyte Syndrome

Several families have been described in which class I antigens and associated β_2-microglobulin are poorly expressed, and a second group has been described in which class II expression is also severely defective (Schuurman et al., 1979; Lisowska-Grospierre et al., 1983; Touraine, 1984) (see Chapter 12). Patients with defective class I and/or defective class II expression characteristically have a severe primary immunodeficiency. Defective HLA antigen expression has been demonstrated on T cells, B cells, and macrophages, although the disorder is commonly referred to as the bare lymphocyte syndrome. Clinical manifestations include candidiasis, bacterial pneumonia, *Pneumocystis* pneumonia, severe diarrhea, septicemia, and an increased susceptibility to viral infections, including herpesvirus, coxsackievirus, and poliomyelitis (Touraine and Betuel, 1983; Griscelli et al., 1989).

Prenatal diagnosis in utero based on the defective expression of these molecules has been accomplished (Schuurman et al., 1985). In HLA class II deficiency, class II molecules cannot be induced on any cell type by IFN-γ. The class II molecule–encoding genes on chromosome 6 are normal. A defective gene for a regulatory DNA-binding protein, RF-X, that leads to absent HLA class II gene transcription appears to be responsible for this genetic defect.

Allogeneic bone marrow transplantation is the therapy of choice. Successful transplantation of human fetal liver stem cells into an affected fetus in utero has been reported (Touraine, 1992).

CD14

Antibodies that recognize the CD14 cluster define a 55-kD glycoprotein cell surface molecule that is localized to myeloid cells. It is anchored to the cell membrane by a phosphatidylinositol (PI) linkage mechanism. Anti-CD14 antibodies preferentially stain monocytes, but weak staining of granulocytes and B cells occurs. CD14 is a receptor for gram-negative bacteria, lipopolysaccharide (LPS), or LPS-coated particles. Monocytes can be activated by small amounts of LPS to secrete IL-6 in the presence of serum containing LPS-binding protein, a protein that enhances LPS-CD14 binding (Ziegler-Heitbrock and Ulevitch, 1993).

The most primitive myelomonocytic progenitors lack CD14; thus, CD14-positive acute monocytic leukemia and acute myelomonocytic leukemia cells represent more mature cells. The magnitude of CD14 expression by alveolar macrophages is a marker for disease activity in a number of inflammatory diseases, including sarcoidosis and extrinsic allergic alveolitis. CD14 can be released into cellular supernatants or plasma by protease digestion or by the actions of phospholipases on the glycosyl-phosphatidylinositol (GPI) anchor. This soluble CD14 (sCD14) is thought to be derived from the membrane glycoprotein, because sCD14 levels correlate with CD14 cell surface expression. Patients with sepsis have decreased levels of monocyte CD14 expression but increased circulating sCD14 levels. Because patients with paroxysmal nocturnal hemoglobinuria have a defect in the phosphatidylinositol-anchoring mechanism, monocytes from these patients have decreased to absent CD14 expression (Haziot et al., 1988).

Atherosclerosis

Macrophages possess scavenger receptors that mediate endocytosis of low-density lipoproteins and a wide range of other negatively charged macromolecules (Goldstein et al., 1985). At least two carboxyl terminally distinct types of receptor units have been described on human macrophages (Naito et al., 1992). Atherosclerotic plaques are characterized by an inflammatory cell infiltrate in which macrophages (foam cells) are a prominent component. Foam cells, believed to be derived from circulating blood monocytes that have migrated into the subendothelial intima, express both types of scavenger receptors. They have an augmented capacity for TNF-α and IL-1 secretion (Tipping and Hancock, 1993).

Endothelial cells in these atherosclerotic lesions are characterized by a marked increase in the expression of adhesion molecules endothelial leukocyte adhesion molecule-1 (ELAM-1) and intracellular adhesion molecule-1 (ICAM-1) compared with that in endothelium from noninflamed sites (van der Wal et al., 1992). These findings suggest that macrophage-derived cytokines modulate adhesion molecule expression on vascular endothelium and play an important role in the pathogenesis of atherosclerosis. Dietary supplementation with fish oil containing n-3 polyunsaturated fatty acids induces suppression of monocyte chemotaxis in healthy volunteers. This negative effect on monocyte migration into the intima may explain the beneficial effects of n-3 polyunsaturated fatty acids in atherosclerotic vascular disease (Schmidt et al., 1992).

Immunoglobulin (Fc) Receptors

Cells of the mononuclear phagocyte system have the capacity to identify and remove foreign organisms and antigens via cell surface receptors that recognize the Fc portion of several immunoglobulin classes. At least three biochemically distinct receptors that recognize the Fc domain of IgG antibody (Fcγ receptors) have now been described. These have been designated FcγRI, FcγRII, and FcγRIII (Table 16–3). FcγR molecules are membrane glycoproteins with molecular masses ranging from 40 to 72 kD (see Chapter 3). Each of them is present on human macrophages, but only FcγRI and FcγRII are found on fresh circulating monocytes (Schreiber et al., 1992).

Deficient FcR Function

Fcγ receptors mediate cell attachment and stimulate several signal transduction events. They are important for the clearance of immune complexes and for internalization of IgG-coated cells or microorganisms. Defective function of Fc receptors has been associated with certain HLA haplotypes (Lawley et al., 1981) and with susceptibility to autoimmune diseases (Salmon et al., 1984, 1986). In addition to promoting phagocytosis, the membrane Fc receptors on the mononuclear phagocyte are the receptors for a nonphagocytic form of cytotoxicity called antibody-dependent cellular cytotoxicity (ADCC). Monocyte-mediated ADCC is impaired in a variety of disorders, including AIDS, various malignancies, aplastic anemia, and familial erythrophagocytic lymphohistiocytosis (Ladisch et al., 1978).

Genetic polymorphism in the expression of Fc receptors for different classes of immunoglobulin on the mononuclear phagocyte may also contribute to defective clearance of opsonized particles (see Chapter 3). Initially, certain ethnic and family groups were described whose lymphocytes did not proliferate when stimulated with certain murine monoclonal antibodies to the mitogenic receptor on T lymphocytes, CD3 (e.g., OKT3 or Leu-4); this was dependent on the IgG subclass of the stimulating murine monoclonal antibody and whether the monocytes of the donor had the appropriate Fc receptor to bind that IgG subclass. Nonresponders to murine IgG1 antibodies (Leu-4) lack a 40-kD low-affinity Fc receptor on their monocytes; nonresponders to IgG2b murine antibodies (OKT3) lack a 77-kD receptor (Abo et al., 1984; Tax et al., 1984; Ceuppens et al., 1985).

Absence of functional FcγRI on phagocytic cells has been identified in four members of a single family whose monocytes were unable to support T-cell proliferation on stimulation with a murine anti-CD3 antibody of the mIgG2a subclass. These four individuals were healthy and had no increased susceptibility to infections, autoimmune disease, or circulating immune

Table 16–3. Human Immunoglobulin G Fc Receptors

Characteristic	FcRI	FcRII	FcRIII
Molecule	72 kD	40 kD	60 kD
CD designation	CD64	CD32	CD16
Affinity for IgG monomer	High	Low	Low
Sites/cell	$1-4 \times 10^4$	$3-6 \times 10^4$	$1-2 \times 10^5$
Cells	Monocytes, macrophages (cell line HL60, U937)	Monocytes, macrophages, neutrophils, eosinophils, platelets, B cells, cell lines HL60, K562, Daudi, Raji	Neutrophils, eosinophils, macrophages, NK, K, Tγ cells
Specificity, human IgG subclass	1 = 3 > 4; 2 none	1 = 3 > 2, 4	1
Monoclonal antibodies	32, 44.1, 22.2	IV-3, KU79	3G8, 4F7, VEP13, Leu-11a, Leu-11b, B73.1

Abbreviations: IgG = immunoglobulin G; K = killer; NK = natural killer.
Adapted from Anderson CL, Looney RJ. Human leukocyte IgG Fc receptors. Immunol Today 7:264–266, 1986.

complexes. Because of functionally intact FcγRII, their monocytes could bind aggregated human IgG and ingest IgG-coated particles (Ceuppens et al., 1988).

Uremia

Macrophage Fcγ receptor function is impaired in patients with end-stage renal disease (see Chapter 19). Patients with uremia demonstrate decreased in vivo clearance of IgG-coated autologous erythrocytes. In vitro, monocyte recognition of IgG-sensitized red blood cells via FcγRI was also decreased (Ruiz et al., 1990). These defects may partly explain the susceptibility of uremia patients to recurrent pyogenic infections. Macrophage Fcγ receptor function is decreased in patients with systemic lupus erythematosus, dermatitis herpetiformis, and Sjögren's syndrome (Boswell and Schur, 1989). In these diseases, the defect has been attributed to the occupation of Fcγ receptors by immune complexes (Frank et al., 1983; Kimberly and Ralph, 1983). The degree of binding of immune complexes to Fc receptors is dependent on the class and subclass of the antibody molecule involved and on the capacity of these complexes to fix complement, because complement receptors (C3bi) are important in the removal of immune complexes.

Congenital Asplenia

Asplenia syndrome is characterized by the presence of right atrial isomerism (two right atria), complex congenital cardiovascular malformations, and asplenia (Waldman et al., 1977) (see Chapter 19). These children are susceptible to overwhelming infections after corrective cardiac surgery. Fc receptor–mediated clearance of sensitized autologous erythrocytes is markedly impaired in children with the asplenia syndrome (Wang and Hsieh, 1991). Additional immunologic findings in these patients include impaired phagocytosis, subtle T-cell defects, and poor antibody responses to polysaccharide antigens (Biggar et al., 1981).

DISORDERS INVOLVING ABNORMAL MONOCYTE/MACROPHAGE MOTILITY

Macrophage motility is a critical element of the response to infection. As discussed in Chapter 6, mononuclear phagocyte movement can be either random or directed, depending on whether it occurs in the absence or presence of attracting stimuli. In vitro assessment of directed movement (chemotaxis) generally utilizes a chamber in which the movement of monocytes through a membrane in response to a chemotactic stimulus (e.g., C5a) is evaluated (Gallin and Wolff, 1976).

Mucocutaneous Candidiasis

Defective chemotaxis to both C5a and lymphocyte-derived chemotactic factor was observed in the monocytes of a patient with chronic mucocutaneous candidiasis (Snyderman et al., 1973) (see Chapter 12). This disorder, characterized by infection of cutaneous and mucosal surfaces with *Candida albicans,* has been associated with a variety of defects of cell-mediated immunity (Kirkpatrick, 1989; Oyefara et al., 1994).

Wiskott-Aldrich Syndrome

The Wiskott-Aldrich syndrome (WAS) is an X-linked immunodeficiency disorder characterized by recurrent infections and inability to respond to polysaccharide antigens (see Chapter 12). It is characterized by deficient or defective expression of the glycoprotein sialophorin (CD43) on the surface of T cells, monocytes, platelets, neutrophils, and some B cells. The WAS gene defect is expressed in each of these cell types, as suggested by the finding of a nonrandom pattern of X-chromosome inactivation in monocytes and T and B cells of female carriers (Greer et al., 1989). ICAM-1 serves as a ligand for CD43 and their interaction leads to antigen-specific T-cell activation (Rosenstein et al., 1991).

Patients have a variety of immune defects (Blaese et al., 1975), including a defect in a monocyte-mediated ADCC (Poplack et al., 1976), abnormal monocyte chemotaxis (Altman et al., 1974), and diminished spontaneous monocyte cytotoxic activity (Blaese et al., 1980). Fc receptor expression on the mononuclear phagocyte of these patients is normal. Monocytes manifest decreased responsiveness to C5a (Altman et al., 1974). The serum contains high levels of chemotactic activity and causes normal monocytes to manifest decreased chemotaxis.

Chédiak-Higashi Syndrome

Defective monocyte chemotaxis occurs in patients with the Chédiak-Higashi syndrome (see Chapter 15). This is an inherited disorder of humans and several animal species characterized by partial oculocutaneous albinism, neutropenia, and recurrent infections (Blume and Wolff, 1972). Gallin and associates (1975) reported defective monocyte chemotaxis in human, mink, and cattle Chédiak-Higashi cells. Their monocytes demonstrate abnormal chemotactic responsiveness to four different chemotactic stimuli:

- Nonactivated serum
- Endotoxin-activated serum
- Dialyzable transfer factor
- A kallikrein–plasminogen activator mixture

Random migration and microbicidal activity are also abnormal.

The pathognomonic feature of this syndrome is the presence of large lysosomal inclusions in all granule-forming cells, possibly resulting from failure of phagocytic degranulation (Fig. 16–5). It has been hypothesized that the decreased chemotaxis results from decreased cell distensibility secondary to the large intracellular lysosomal inclusions (Clark et al., 1972). Giant cytoplasmic granules along with normal-appearing Birbeck's granules have been demonstrated in

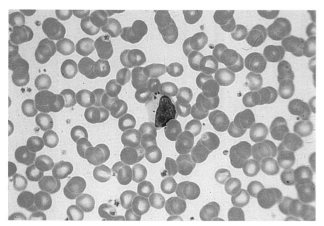

Figure 16–5. Chédiak-Higashi syndrome: mononuclear cell. Note the large cytoplasmic lysosomal granules.

the epidermal Langerhans cells of patients with Chédiak-Higashi syndrome. The underlying genetic defect has not been elucidated. Prenatal diagnosis has been accomplished by the demonstration of large lysosomes in amniotic fluid and chorionic villus cells (Diukman et al., 1992).

DISORDERS OF MICROBICIDAL ACTIVITY/OXIDATIVE METABOLISM

The mononuclear phagocyte plays a central role in host defense against many microorganisms, although the granulocyte is a more efficient microbicidal cell for most infectious agents. The production of reactive oxygen intermediates is critical for microbial killing, just as it is for the granulocyte. There are several organisms for which the mononuclear phagocyte plays a more pronounced microbicidal role than the granulocyte does. Macrophages activated by T-cell products, such as IFN-γ, are principally responsible for the elimination of many facultative intracellular microorganisms (e.g., *Listeria monocytogenes*). In cases of macrophage or T-cell immaturity or immunodeficiency, macrophage activation may be impaired and thus these organisms become established.

Selected Infections

Even with activation, the cells of the mononuclear phagocyte system may have trouble eliminating some microorganisms that have developed unique mechanisms for evading the microbicidal systems of the mononuclear phagocyte. *Toxoplasma gondii, M. tuberculosis, Chlamydia,* and *Legionella* have all become effective pathogens by inhibiting the fusion of the phagosome with the lysosome (Horowitz, 1983). Other organisms, such as *Leishmania* and *Mycobacterium lepraemurium,* do not inhibit fusion of phagosomes and lysosomes but can survive within the inhospitable environment of the phagolysosome. Still others, such as *Trypanosoma cruzi,* avoid the unfavorable milieu of the phagolysosome by remaining in the host cell cytoplasm.

Leprosy

The persistence of the infecting organism can have important secondary effects on the mononuclear phagocyte. Lepromatous leprosy in particular is characterized by several functional defects (Kaplan and Cohn, 1986). Macrophages that have ingested *Mycobacterium leprae* are refractory to activation by IFN-γ (Sibley and Krahenbuhl, 1987). Furthermore, there may be defective regulation of surface Fc receptor numbers, interference with normal macrophage T-cell interaction, and deficient IL-1 production (Birdi et al., 1980; Salgame et al., 1980; Watson et al., 1984; Mistry et al., 1985).

The mononuclear phagocyte may also contribute to the pathogenesis of certain infections. Intestinal bacteria may be spread throughout the body as passengers in mononuclear phagocytes (Wells et al., 1987). The monocyte/macrophage may play a central role in the dissemination of human immunodeficiency virus (HIV) in AIDS (see Chapter 18).

Chronic Granulomatous Disease

Chronic granulomatous disease (CGD) is an inherited group of disorders in which phagocytic cells (neutrophils, monocytes, and eosinophils) fail to activate one of their most potent microbicidal mechanisms—that of the respiratory burst (see Chapter 15). This results in an inability of patients' phagocytes to generate reactive oxygen radicals and kill certain microorganisms after their ingestion. Most patients with CGD suffer from recurrent bacterial and fungal infections. The defect in the respiratory burst resulting in defective microbicidal activity has been demonstrated in the monocytes from patients with CGD (Davis et al., 1968; Nathan et al., 1969; Weening et al., 1985). Chronic granulomatous disease can be caused by a defect in any one of the four subunits of reduced nicotinamide-adenine dinucleotide phosphate (NADPH) oxidase, the enzyme that catalyzes the oxidative burst. The disease may be inherited in an X-linked or autosomal recessive fashion (Curnutte, 1992).

IFN-γ treatment reduces the frequency of serious infections in patients with CGD (Ezekowitz et al., 1988; Sechler et al., 1988; International Chronic Granulomatous Disease Cooperative Study Group, 1991; Gallin, 1992). Although IFN-γ is a potent activator of monocytes and macrophages, its exact mechanism of action in CGD remains unknown (Woodman et al., 1992). Cytokines other than IFN-γ, including TNF-α, IL-1, IL-3, and IL-6, increase the defective respiratory burst in monocytes from children with CGD (Jendrossek et al., 1993).

Osteopetrosis

Malignant osteopetrosis is a fatal congenital bone disorder inherited in an autosomal recessive pattern. It is characterized by dense and sclerotic bones secondary to defective osteoclast function (Fig. 16–6). Osteoclasts are members of the mononuclear phagocyte family. Affected infants have cranial nerve palsies, deafness,

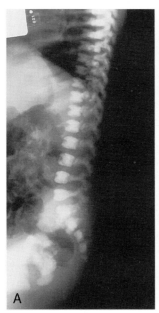
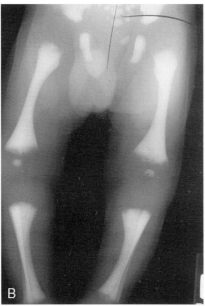

Figure 16–6. Osteopetrosis. *A*, X-rays of spine, thickening of vertebral end plates, diffuse osteosclerosis, and classic bone-within-bone (radiolucent insets in vertebral bodies) appearance. *B*, X-rays of long bones demonstrating diffusely sclerotic bone with poor definition of medullary canal.

and blindness and die within the first decade of life from infection or bleeding secondary to pancytopenia resulting from encroachment of marrow spaces by sclerotic bone. The precise molecular defect that causes osteopetrosis is unknown.

Most patients with osteopetrosis show no consistent abnormalities of humoral or cellular immunity; their peripheral blood monocytes have normal phagocytic activity and chemotactic responsiveness. The monocytes from one patient had defective adherence to glass surfaces, and monocytes from five other patients showed impaired bactericidal capacity (Reeves et al., 1979; Beard et al., 1986). Allogeneic bone marrow transplantation from unaffected histocompatible sibling donors has resulted in reversal of the hematopoietic consequences of bone encroachment, rapid remodeling of bone, and normalization of monocyte bactericidal capacity (Coccia et al., 1980; Sorell et al., 1981; Sieff et al., 1983).

Patients with osteopetrosis have increased numbers of osteoclasts demonstrable on bone biopsy (Shapiro et al., 1988). Evidence suggests that osteoclast-derived oxygen radicals are vital to normal bone resorption (Garrett et al., 1990; Ries et al., 1992). Because leukocyte superoxide production is defective in most osteopetrotic patients, Key and coworkers (1992) have used IFN-γ in these patients and showed enhancement of bone resorption and leukocyte function.

In the osteopetrotic (*op/op*) mouse, a defect in the macrophage-colony stimulating factor (M-CSF) gene results in absence of M-CSF activity and absence of or reduction in osteoclast numbers. Two studies have demonstrated normal serum levels of M-CSF in children with osteopetrosis (Orchard et al., 1992; Naffakh et al., 1993). Treatment of *op/op* mice with M-CSF results in normalization of osteoclast numbers and bone resorption. The mutant microphthalmic (*mi/mi*) mouse is a better animal model of human osteopetrosis because it has normal numbers of osteoclasts with de-

fective superoxide production. M-CSF alone or in combination with IFN-γ results in amelioration of osteopetrosis in the *mi/mi* mouse (Rodriguiz et al., 1993).

Severe osteoporosis with a propensity for repeated bone fractures has been seen in some patients with the hyper-IgE syndrome (see Chapter 13). An increase in in vitro bone resorption by monocytes activated via the cyclooxygenase pathway has been demonstrated in these patients and may contribute to their osteopenia (Leung et al., 1988).

Glycogen Storage Disease Type 1b

Glycogen storage disease (GSD) type 1b is characterized by hypoglycemia during fasting because of an inability to convert glucose-6-phosphate to glucose as a result of an inherited hepatic defect (see Chapters 15 and 19). It differs from GSD type 1a in that patients are prone to recurrent bacterial infections and are often neutropenic. Decreased chemiluminescence of one patient's monocytes in the presence of normal monocyte chemotaxis has been shown (Ueno et al., 1986). Studies of phagocyte function in three patients with GSD type 1b demonstrated markedly reduced respiratory burst activity in both neutrophils and monocytes. The phagocyte dysfunction was associated with decreased calcium mobilization in response to formylmethionyl-leucyl-phenylalanine (f-Met-Leu-Phe) along with defective intracellular stores of calcium (Kilpatrick et al., 1990). Recombinant GM-CSF may be useful in the short-term treatment of serious infections in patients with GSD type 1b (Hurst et al., 1993).

MONOCYTE/MACROPHAGE IMMUNOREGULATORY DYSFUNCTION

The cells of the mononuclear phagocyte system play a central role in specific immune responses through their functions of processing and presenting antigens, secreting cytokines (e.g., IL-1), and ultimately acting as effector cells in many T cell–dependent microbicidal processes (Unanue, 1981; Shevach, 1984). Monocytes and macrophages can serve as both helper and suppressor cells in in vitro assays of immune function. Although it is difficult to correlate in vitro abnormalities noted in tissue culture with clinical effects, some links seem clearly established.

Partial degradation of antigen (or antigen processing) is also critical in permitting immune responses. T cells require the presentation of antigen fragments in association with class II major histocompatibility complex (MHC) antigens on the MNP surface. In patients with the bare lymphocyte syndrome, lack of MHC antigens may lead to a diminished immunologic response. If proteolytic processes are inhibited (e.g., by chloroquine), large protein antigens cannot be degraded to peptide fragments and the immune response may be inhibited (Chesnut et al., 1982; Grey et al., 1982).

Eibl and colleagues (1982) have described one patient with common variable hypogammaglobulinemia in whom monocytes did not present antigen to lymphocytes. The mechanism of defective antigen presentation has not been elucidated.

MONOCYTE/MACROPHAGE DYSFUNCTION IN THE NEWBORN

The neonatal period is characterized by a state of relative immunodeficiency during which the infant is susceptible to a variety of infections that are uncommon in later life (see Chapter 10). The circulating monocyte count in newborn infants is significantly higher than that found in older children or adults. Functional differences between neonatal and adult macrophages play a significant role in this immunodeficiency in experimental animals. Newborn rats produce antibody poorly, are extraordinarily susceptible to lethal infections with *L. monocytogenes,* and are easily tolerized to soluble antigens. These abnormalities can all be corrected by the administration of macrophages, but not lymphocytes, from adult rats but not newborn rats (Blaese et al., 1979).

The phagocytic and bactericidal abilities of newborn monocytes are usually reported as normal, although their responses may be impaired if the cells are stressed by high ratios of challenging bacteria (Wilson and Haas, 1984). Ingestion or binding via Fc, complement, and mannosyl/fucosyl receptors and by receptors for unopsonized *Pseudomonas aeruginosa* is normal in cord blood monocyte–derived macrophages (Conly and Speert, 1991). The expression of Mac-1 on newborn monocytes is normal, but these cells fail to dramatically increase surface antigen density after exposure to ionophore or f-Met-Leu-Phe, as do adult MNPs. Another group of critical cell surface antigens, class II major histocompatibility (DR) antigens, is expressed to a significantly lower extent on cord blood monocytes than on adult monocytes (Stiehm et al., 1983).

The mononuclear phagocytes, particularly after activation by lymphokines such as IFN-γ, are the principal defense against intracellular pathogens, such as *T. gondii.* Cord blood and adult monocytes have a similar capacity to kill *T. gondii* in vitro when stimulated with exogenous IFN-γ (Wilson and Haas, 1984). However, newborn T cells are poor producers of IFN-γ, and thus newborns may have an increased susceptibility to infection as a secondary consequence (Bryson et al., 1980; Wilson, 1986). Cord blood mononuclear cells, unlike those from adults, do not produce IFN-γ in vitro when stimulated with endotoxin from *Salmonella typhimurium.* This functional immaturity can be corrected experimentally by using monocytes cultured for 2 weeks or by treatment with conditioned medium. Recombinant GM-CSF, M-CSF, or IFN-γ can partially enhance IFN-γ production by cord blood mononuclear cells (McKenzie et al., 1993).

Cord blood monocytes produce IL-1 normally (Glover et al., 1987), and they appear to process and present soluble antigens, such as tetanus toxoid, in a normal fashion to immune T cells (Mori and Hayward, 1984). Term neonatal cord blood monocytes secrete TNF-α normally, but preterm monocytes secrete significantly less TNF-α activity than term infant or adult monocytes do (Weatherstone and Rich, 1989; Bortolussi et al., 1992). Cord blood monocytes have normal ADCC and spontaneous toxicity mediated by the macrophage's mannosylfucosyl receptor (Blaese et al., 1979). Upon stimulation with phytohemagglutinin or phorbol myristate acetate, mononuclear cells from term neonates produced less granulocyte colony-stimulating factor (G-CSF) and IL-3 than adult cells. There was an associated reduction in their respective messenger RNA transcripts (Cairo et al., 1992). These data may partly explain the cytopenias seen in stressed neonates.

Delayed cutaneous hypersensitivity, a process dependent on intact mononuclear phagocyte function, is also deficient in newborns (Uhr et al., 1960). This is undoubtedly contributed to by impaired mononuclear phagocyte migration. Newborns demonstrate a delayed influx of mononuclear phagocyte in Rebuck's skin windows, and defective in vitro monocyte chemotaxis has also been reported (Klein et al., 1977). This defect, however, is not as pronounced as that of the neonatal granulocyte.

The results of some investigations may help to elucidate the mechanisms that underlie these monocyte functional defects in the newborn. IL-6, which is produced primarily by monocytes and macrophages, has a number of diverse stimulatory effects on B cells, T cells, and hematopoietic progenitors. In response to stimulation by IL-1, monocytes from term and preterm neonates produced less IL-6 than did monocytes from adults (Schibler et al., 1992). Interleukin-8 is a monokine that promotes neutrophil chemotaxis, adherence, C3bi binding, and superoxide generation. Term and preterm neonatal monocytes produced significantly lower amounts of IL-8 upon stimulation by IL-1 or TNF-α (Schibler et al., 1993). In both studies, monocytes from preterm neonates produced less IL-6 and IL-8 than did term neonatal monocytes.

The fetal monocyte/macrophage may serve as a

reservoir for human immunodeficiency virus type 1 (HIV-1). Cord blood monocyte–derived macrophages are capable of sustaining productive infection with monocytotropic strains of HIV-1. In vitro studies have shown that they are more susceptible to infection than adult monocyte/macrophages. They may thus play an important role in the pathogenesis of perinatally acquired HIV infection (Ho et al., 1992; Lioy et al., 1993).

MISCELLANEOUS DISORDERS

Human Immunodeficiency Virus Infection

Most of the observations regarding monocyte/macrophage function during HIV infection have been made on patients with late-stage HIV infection, that is, AIDS. Results of these studies have often been contradictory. Most studies reveal normal peripheral blood monocyte counts, although monocytopenia has also been reported. Monocytes from HIV-infected patients demonstrate normal expression of a number of monocyte cell surface receptors, including HLA determinants, CD4, CD11, CR3, CD14, and Fc receptors (Haas et al., 1987; Davidson et al., 1988). Disparate results showing aberrant expression of these receptors in HIV-infected patients can be partially explained by the fact that HIV envelope glycoproteins p41 and gp120 can induce phenotypic or functional changes (Wahl et al., 1989; Meltzer et al., 1990).

As with studies of phenotypic expression, investigations of monocyte function have shown variable findings. Depressed phagocytosis, IL-1 secretion, and microbicidal activity have all been described (Smith et al., 1984; Lane and Fauci, 1985; Poli et al., 1985), although in a number of other studies these monocyte functions have been normal. Bender and colleagues (1987) showed that impaired Fc and C3 mediate clearance by macrophages from HIV-infected patients. Tissue macrophages such as the dermal Langerhans' cells and lymph node follicular dendritic cells show marked degenerative and immunophenotypic changes. Unlike blood monocytes and other tissue macrophages, these cells have high levels of CD4 expression that may render them more susceptible to the effects of HIV. Macrophages are the major tissue reservoirs for HIV during all changes of infection and may aid in spreading infection to other tissues or individuals by playing a "Trojan horse" role. Because of their role as immunoregulatory cells, they may also control the rate of disease progression (Meltzer and Gendelman, 1992; Ho et al., 1994).

Whipple's Disease (Intestinal Lipodystrophy)

Whipple's disease is a rare disorder affecting predominantly middle-aged men. It is a chronic, systemic illness characterized by anemia, skin pigmentation, joint symptoms, weight loss, diarrhea, and malabsorption. The presence of characteristic periodic acid–Schiff (PAS)–positive material in the macrophages of the mucosa of the small bowel and other affected tissues is the major diagnostic feature. Bacillary bodies are found in the macrophages of involved tissues, and reports of successful antibiotic treatment indicate that the disease is an infectious disorder. The bacillus associated with Whipple's disease has been identified by a molecular genetic approach as a gram-positive actinomycete, tentatively named *Tropheryma whippelii* (Relman et al., 1992). There seems to be abundant evidence that these patients cannot mount an effective immune response to this organism, which leads to the massive accumulation of PAS-positive bacterial degradation products in the macrophages. PAS-positive macrophages continue to persist in biopsy specimens for months to years after therapy.

A unique form of macrophage dysfunction has been demonstrated in a patient with Whipple's disease (Bjerknes et al., 1985). His macrophages showed almost no intracellular degradation and elimination of *Escherichia coli, Staphylococcus pyogenes,* or zymosan particles over a prolonged period of observation. Monocyte phagocytosis and killing were normal, as was granulocyte intracellular degradation of bacterial or zymosan particles. Studies of the same patient (Bjerknes et al., 1988) 4 years after diagnosis continued to demonstrate significant impairment of intracellular degradation of zymosan particles, *E. coli* proteins, and *E. coli* DNA. These findings suggest a primary cellular immune defect in these patients. Morphologic changes similar to those seen in Whipple's disease have been noted in patients with AIDS and massive *Mycobacterium avium–intracellulare* infection.

Malacoplakia

Malacoplakia is a rare chronic granulomatous disorder of unknown etiology. It is characterized by the presence of submucosal aggregates of histiocytes that contain dense, lamellated calcium and iron-containing inclusion bodies known as Michaelis-Gutmann bodies. Malacoplakia is most frequently seen in immunosuppressed adults or those who are chronically infected. Rare cases in children have been reported (Charney et al., 1985). The genitourinary tract is primarily involved in about 75% of cases (Long and Althausen, 1989). Clinical manifestations of malacoplakia depend on the site of involvement. Malacoplakia of the lower urinary tract manifests with hematuria and bladder irritative symptoms. Renal parenchymal involvement often presents with fever and a flank mass.

The pathogenesis of malacoplakia is unknown. Electron microscopic evaluation of Michaelis-Gutmann bodies suggests that these bodies represent phagolysosomes containing incompletely digested engulfed bacteria. Decreased monocyte bactericidal activity against *E. coli* agonists has been demonstrated in some patients with malacoplakia (Abdou et al., 1977). Other studies of patients with biopsy-proven malacoplakia have failed to show similar defects in monocyte bactericidal activity (McClure, 1983). A primary or secondary monocyte/macrophage lysosomal defect leading to an inability to degrade phagocytosed microorganisms may be responsible in evoking a granulomatous inflammatory response to the bacterial debris.

References

Abdou NI, NaPombejara C, Sagawa A, Ragland C, Stechschulte DJ, Nilsson U, Gourley W, Wantanabe I, Lindsey NJ, Allen MS. Malakoplakia: evidence for monocyte lysosomal abnormality correctable by cholinergic agonist in vitro and in vivo. N Engl J Med 297:1413–1419, 1977.

Abo T, Tilden AB, Bolch CM, Kumangai K, Troup GM, Cooper MD. Ethnic differences in the lymphocyte proliferative response induced by a murine IgG1 antibody, Leu-4, to the T3 molecule. J Exp Med 160:303–309, 1984.

Alekseeva OG. Ability of beryllium compounds to cause allergy of the delayed type. Fed Proc 25 (Suppl.):T843–T845, 1966.

Altman LC, Snyderman R, Blaese RM. Abnormalities of chemotactic lymphokine synthesis and monocyte leukocyte chemotaxis in Wiskott-Aldrich syndrome. J Clin Invest 54:486–493, 1974.

Anderson CL, Looney RJ. Human leukocyte IgG Fc receptors. Immunol Today 7:264–266, 1986.

Anderson DC, Schmalstieg FC, Feingold MJ, Hughes BJ, Rothlein R, Miller LJ, Kohl S, Tosi MF, Jacobs RL, Woldrop TC, Goldman AS, Shearer WT, Springer TA. The severe and moderate phenotypes of heritable Mac-1/LFA-1 deficiency: their quantitative definition and relation to leukocyte dysfunction and clinical features. J Infect Dis 1952:668–689, 1986.

Aulitzky WE, Tilg H, Vogel W, Aulitzky W, Berger M, Gastl G, Herold M, Huber C. Acute hematologic effects of interferon alpha, interferon gamma, tumor necrosis factor alpha and interleukin 2. Ann Hematol 62:25–31, 1991.

Baehner RL, Johnston RB. Monocyte function in children with neutropenia and chronic infection. Blood 40:31–40, 1972.

Bajorin DF, Cheung NKV, Houghton AN. Macrophage colony-stimulating factor: biologic effects and potential applications for cancer therapy. Semin Hematol 28(Suppl.):42–48, 1991.

Barton NW, Brady RO, Dambrosia JM, Di-Bisceglie AM, Doppelt SH, Hill SC, Mankin HJ, Murray GJ, Parker RI, Argoff CE, Grewal RP, Yu K-T, and collaborators. Replacement therapy for inherited enzyme deficiency—macrophage-targeted glucocerebrosidase for Gaucher's disease. N Engl J Med 324:1464–1470, 1991.

Beard CJ, Key L, Newburger PE, Ezekowitz RA, Arceci R, Miller B, Proto P, Ryan T, Anast C, Simons ER. Neutrophil defect associated with malignant infantile osteopetrosis. J Lab Clin Med 198:498–505, 1986.

Bejaoui M, Veber F, Girault D, Guad C, Blanche S, Griscelli C, Fisher A. The accelerated phase of Chédiak-Higashi syndrome. Arch Fr Pediatr 46:733–736, 1989.

Bender BS, Bohnsack JF, Sourlis SH, Frank MM, Quinn TC. Demonstration of defective C3-receptor–mediated clearance by the reticuloendothelial system in patients with acquired immunodeficiency syndrome. J Clin Invest 79:715–720, 1987.

Ben-Ezra JM, Koo CH. Langerhans' cell histiocytosis and malignancies of the M-PIRE system. Am J Clin Pathol 99:464–471, 1993.

Beutler B, Cerami A. Cachexin and tumor necrosis factor as two sides of the same biological coin. Nature 320:584–588, 1986.

Beutler E, Kay A, Saven A, Garver P, Thurston D, Dawson A, Rosenbloom B. Enzyme replacement therapy for Gaucher disease. Blood 78:1183–1189, 1991.

Biggar WD, Ramirez RA, Rose V. Congenital asplenia: immunologic assessment and clinical review of eight surviving patients. Pediatrics 67:648–651, 1981.

Birdi TJ, Salgame PR, Mahadevan PR, Antia NH. Role of macrophages in defective cell mediated immunity of lepromatous leprosy: II. Macrophage and lymphocyte interactions. Int J Lepr Other Mycobact Dis 48:178–182, 1980.

Bjerknes R, Laerum OD, Odegaard S. Impaired bacterial degradation by monocytes and macrophages from a patient with treated Whipple's disease. Gastroenterology 89:1139–1146, 1985.

Bjerknes R, Odegaard S, Bjerkwig R, Borkje B, Laerum OD. Whipple's disease. Demonstration of a persisting monocyte and macrophage dysfunction. Scand J Gastroenterol 23:611–619, 1988.

Blaese RM, Strober W, Waldmann TA. Immunodeficiency in the Wiskott-Aldrich syndrome. In Bergsma D, Good RA, Finstad J, eds. Immunodeficiency in Man and Animals. Sunderland, MA, Sinauer Associates, 1975, pp. 250–254.

Blaese RM, Poplack DG, Muchmore AV. The mononuclear phagocyte system: role in expression of immunocompetence in neonatal and adult life. Pediatrics 64(Suppl.):820–822, 1979.

Blaese RM, Muchmore AV, Lawrence EC, Poplack DG. The cytolytic effector function of monocytes in immunodeficiency diseases. In Seligmann M, Hitzig W, eds. Primary Immunodeficiencies. Amsterdam, Elsevier, 1980, pp. 319–398.

Blume RS, Wolff SM. The Chédiak-Higashi syndrome: studies in four patients and a review of the literature. Medicine (Baltimore) 51:247–280, 1972.

Bortolussi R, Rajaraman K, Serushago B. Role of tumor necrosis factor-α and interferon-γ in newborn host defense against Listeria monocytogenes infection. Pediatr Res 32:460–464, 1992.

Boswell J, Schur PH. Monocyte function in systemic lupus erythematosus. Clin Immunol Immunopathol 52:271–278, 1989.

Broadbent V, Gadner H, Komp DM, Ladisch S. Histiocytosis syndromes in children: II. Approach to the clinical and laboratory evaluation of children with Langerhans cell histiocytosis. Clinical Writing Group of the Histiocyte Society. Med Pediatr Oncol 17:492–495, 1989.

Bryson YJ, Winter HS, Gard SE, Fisher TJ, Stiehm ER. Deficiency of immune interferon production by leukocytes of normal newborns. Cell Immunol 55:191–200, 1980.

Cairo MS, Suen Y, Knoppel E, Dana R, Park L, Clark S, van-de-Veu C, Sender L. Decreased G-CSF and IL-3 production and gene expression from mononuclear cells of newborn infants. Pediatr Res 31:574–578, 1992.

Castilla A, Prieto J, Fausto N. Transforming growth factors β1 and α in chronic liver disease. Effects of interferon alfa therapy. N Engl J Med 324:933–940, 1991.

Ceuppens JL, Bloemmen FJ, Van Wauwe JP. T-cell unresponsiveness to the mitogenic activity of OKT3 antibody results from a deficiency of monocyte Fc gamma receptors for murine IgG2a and inability to cross-link the T3Ti complex. J Immunol 135:3882–3886, 1985.

Ceuppens JL, Baroja ML, Vaeck FV, Anderson CL. Defect in the membrane expression of high affinity 72-kD Fc γ receptors on phagocytic cells in four healthy subjects. J Clin Invest 82:571–578, 1988.

Charney EB, Witzleben CL, Douglas SD, Kamani N, Kalichman MA. Medical management of bilateral renal malakoplakia. Arch Dis Child 60:254–256, 1985.

Chesnut RW, Colon SM, Grey HM. Requirements for the processing of antigens by antigen presenting B-cells. I. Functional comparison of B cell tumors and macrophages. J Immunol 129:2382–2388, 1982.

Clark RA, Kimball HR, Padgett GA. Granulocyte chemotaxis in the Chédiak-Higashi syndrome of mink. Blood 39:644–649, 1972.

Coccia PF, Krivit W, Cervenka J, Clawson C, Kersey JH, Kim T, Nesbit ME, Ramsey NKC, Warkentin PL, Teitelbaum SL, Kahn AJ, Brown DM. Successful bone marrow transplantation for infantile malignant osteopetrosis. N Engl J Med 302:701–708, 1980.

Conly ME, Speert DP. Human neonatal monocyte-derived macrophages and neutrophils exhibit normal nonopsonic and opsonic receptor–mediated phagocytosis and superoxide anion production. Biol Neonate 60:361–366, 1991.

Connor TB, Roberts AB, Sporn MB, Danielpour D, Dart LL, Michels RG, de Bustros S, Enger C, Kato H, Lansing M, Hayashi H, Glaser BM. Correlation of fibrosis and transforming growth factor-β type 2 levels in the eye. J Clin Invest 83:1661–1666, 1989.

Curnutte JT. Molecular basis of the autosomal recessive forms of chronic granulomatous disease. Immunodefic Rev 3:149–172, 1992.

Czaja MJ, Weiner FR, Flanders KC, Giambrone MA, Wind R, Biempica L, Zern MA. In vitro and in vivo association of transforming growth factor-β1 with hepatic fibrosis. J Cell Biol 108:2477–2482, 1989.

Davidson BL, Kline RL, Rowland J, Quinn TC. Surface markers of monocyte function and activation in AIDS. J Infect Dis 158:438–486, 1988.

Davis WC, Huber H, Douglas SD, Fudenberg HH. A defect in circulating mononuclear phagocytes in chronic granulomatous disease of childhood. J Immunol 101:1093–1095, 1968.

Diukman R, Tanigawara S, Cowan MJ, Golbus MS. Prenatal diagnosis of Chédiak-Higashi syndrome. Prenat Diagn 12:877–885, 1992.

Egeler RM, deKraker J, Voute PA. Cytosine-arabinoside, vincristine and prednisolone in the treatment of children with disseminated Langerhans cell histiocytosis with organ dysfunction: experience at a single institution. Med Pediatr Oncol 21:265–270, 1993.

Egeler RM, D'Angio GJ. Langerhans cell histiocytosis. J Pediatr 127: 1–11, 1995.

Eibl MM, Mannhalter JW, Zlabinger G, Mayr WR, Tilz GP, Ahmad R, Zielinski CC. Defective macrophage function in a patient with common variable immunodeficiency. N Engl J Med 307:803–806, 1982.

Esumi N, Ikushima S, Todo S, Imashuku S. Hyperferritinemia in malignant histiocytosis, virus-associated hemophagocytic syndrome and familial erythrophagocytic lymphohistiocytosis. A survey of pediatric cases. Acta Pediatr Scand 78:268–270, 1989.

Etzioni A, Frydman M, Pollack S, Avidor I, Phillips ML, Paulson JC, Gershoni-Baruch R. Recurrent severe infections caused by a novel leukocyte alhesion deficiency. N Engl J Med 327:1789–1792, 1992.

Ezekowitz RAB, Dinauer MC, Jaffe HS, Orkin SH, Newburger PE. Partial correction of phagocytic defect in patients with X-linked chronic granulomatous disease by subcutaneous interferon gamma. N Engl J Med 319:146–151, 1988.

Fallet S, Grace ME, Sibille A, Mendelson DS, Shapiro RS, Hermann G, Grabowski GA. Enzyme augmentation in moderate to life-threatening Gaucher disease. Pediatr Res 31:496–502, 1992.

Flandrin G, Sigaux F, Sebahoun G, Bouffette P. Hairy cell leukemia: clinical presentation and follow-up of 211 patients. Semin Oncol 11:458–471, 1984.

Foucar K, Foucar E. The mononuclear phagocyte and immunoregulatory effector (M-PIRE) system: evolving concepts. Semin Diagn Pathol 7:4–18, 1990.

Frank MM, Lawley TJ, Hamburger MI, Brown EJ. Immunoglobulin G Fc receptor–mediated clearance in autoimmune diseases. Ann Intern Med 98:206–218, 1983.

Friedman SL, Arthur MJ. Activation of cultured rat hepatic lipocytes by Kupffer cell conditioned medium. Direct enhancement of matrix synthesis and stimulation of cell proliferation via induction of platelet-derived growth factor receptors. J Clin Invest 84:1780–1785, 1989.

Fujiwara F, Hibi S, Imashuku S. Hypercytokinemia in hemophagocytic syndrome. Am J Pediatr Hematol Oncol 15:92–98, 1993.

Gallin JI. Interferon-gamma in the treatment of the chronic granulomatous diseases of childhood. Clin Immunol Immunopathol 61:S100–S105, 1992.

Gallin JI, Klimerman JA, Padgett GA, Wolff SM. Defective mononuclear chemotaxis in the Chédiak-Higashi syndrome of humans, mink and cattle. Blood 45:863–870, 1975.

Gallin JI, Wolff SM. Leukocyte chemotaxis: physiological considerations and abnormalities. Clin Haematol 4:567–607, 1976.

Garrett IR, Boyce BF, Oreffo ROC, Bonewald L, Poser J, Mundy GR. Oxygen-derived free radicals stimulate osteoclastic bone resorption in rodent bone in vitro and in vivo. J Clin Invest 85:632–639, 1990.

Gerrard TL, Cupps TR, Jurgensen CH, Fauci AS. Hydrocortisone-mediated inhibition of monocyte antigen presentation: dissociation of inhibitory effect and expression of DR antigens. Cell Immunol 85:330–339, 1984.

Gill FA, Kaye D, Hook EW. The influence of erythrophagocytosis on the interaction of macrophages and salmonella in vitro. J Exp Med 124:173–183, 1966.

Glover DM, Brownstein D, Burchett S, Larsen A, Wilson CB. Expression of HLA class II antigens and secretion of interleukin-1 by monocytes and macrophages from adults and neonates. Immunology 61:195–201, 1987.

Golde DW. Disorders of mononuclear phagocyte proliferation, maturation, and function. Clin Haematol 4:705–721, 1975.

Goldstein JL, Brown MS, Anderson RGW, Russel DW, Schneider WJ. Receptor-mediated endocytosis: concepts emerging from the LDL receptor system. Annu Rev Cell Biol 1:1–39, 1985.

Golomb HM, Hanauer SB. Infectious complications associated with hairy cell leukemia. J Infect Dis 143:639–643, 1981.

Greer WL, Wong PC, Peacocke M, Ip P, Rubin LA, Siminovitch KA. A marker for detection of the carrier state and identification of cell lineages expressing the gene defect. Genomics 4:60–67, 1989.

Greinix HT, Storb R, Sanders JE, Petersen FB. Marrow transplantation for treatment of multisystem progressive Langerhans cell histiocytosis. Bone Marrow Transplant 10:39–44, 1992.

Grey HM, Colon SM, Chesnut RW. Requirements for the processing of antigens by antigen presenting B-cells. II. Biochemical comparison of the fate of antigen B cell tumors and macrophages. J Immunol 129:2389–2395, 1982.

Griscelli C, Lisowska-Grospierre B, Mach B. Combined immunodeficiency with defective expression in MHC class II genes. Immunodefic Rev 1:135–153, 1989.

Haas JG, Reithmuller G, Ziegler-Heitbrock HWL. Monocyte phenotype and function in patients with acquired immunodeficiency syndrome (AIDS) and AIDS-related disorders. Scand J Immunol 26:371–379, 1987.

Hamilton J. Colony stimulating factors, cytokines and monocyte-macrophages—some controversies. Immunol Today 14:18–24, 1993.

Hassan NF, Kamani N, Meszaros MM, Douglas SD. Induction of multinucleated giant cell formation from human blood–derived monocytes by phorbol myristate acetate in in vitro culture. J Immunol 143:2179–2184, 1989.

Hassner A, Kletter Y, Shlag D, Yedvab M, Aronson M, Shibole S. Impaired monocyte function in liver cirrhosis. Br Med J [Clin Res] 282:1262–1263, 1981.

Haziot A, Chen S, Ferrero E, Low MG, Silber R, Goyert SM. The monocyte differentiation antigen, CD14, is anchored to the cell membrane by a phosphatidylinositol linkage. J Immunol 141:547–552, 1988.

Hemler ME, Huang C, Schwartz L. The VLA protein family. J Biol Chem 262:3300–3309, 1986.

Ho W, Lioy J, Song L, Cutilli JR, Polin RA, Douglas SD. Infection of cord blood monocyte–derived macrophages with human immunodeficiency virus type 1. J Virol 66:573–579, 1992.

Ho W, Cherukuri R, Douglas SD. The macrophage and HIV-1. In Zwilling BS, Eisenstein TK, eds. Macrophage-Pathogen Interactions. New York, Marcel Dekker, 1994, pp. 569–587.

Holdstock G, Leslie B, Hill S, Tanner A, Wright R. Monocyte function in cirrhosis. J Clin Pathol 35:972–979, 1982.

Horowitz MA. The Legionnaires' disease bacterium inhibits phagosome-lysosome fusion in human monocytes. J Exp Med 158:2108–2125, 1983.

Howells DW, Strobel S, Smith I, Levinsky RJ, Hyland K. Central nervous system involvement in the erythrophagocytic disorders of infancy: the role of cerebrospinal fluid neopterins in their differential diagnosis and clinical management. Pediatr Res 28:116–119, 1990.

Howells DW, Hyland K, Smith I, Strobel S. Tryptophan and serotonin metabolism in familial erythrophagocytic lymphohistiocytosis. J Inherited Metab Dis 15:891–897, 1992.

Hurst D, Kilpatrick L, Becker J, Lipani J, Kleman K, Perrine S, Douglas SD. Recombinant human GM-CSF treatment of neutropenia in glycogen storage disease 1b. Am J Pediatr Hematol Oncol 15:71–76, 1993.

Hynes RO. Integrins: versatility, modulation and signaling in cell adhesion. Cell 69:11–25, 1992.

International Chronic Granulomatous Disease Cooperative Study Group. A controlled trial of interferon gamma to prevent infection in chronic granulomatous disease. N Engl J Med 324:509–516, 1991.

Ishii E, Matsuzaki A, Okamura J, Inoue T, Kajiwara M, Uozumi T, Yoshida N, Miyazaki S, Miyake K, Matsumoto T, Tasaka H, Ueda K. Treatment of Langerhans cell histiocytosis in children with etoposide. Am J Clin Oncol 15:515–517, 1992.

Jendrossek V, Peters AMJ, Buth S, Liese J, Wintergerst U, Belohradsky BH, Gahr M. Improvement of superoxide production in monocytes from patients with chronic granulomatous disease by recombinant cytokines. Blood 81:2131–2136, 1993.

Kaplan G, Cohn ZA. The immunobiology of leprosy. Int Rev Exp Pathol 28:45–78, 1986.

Kay NE, Douglas SD. Monocyte-erythrocyte interaction in vitro in immune hemolytic anemias. Blood 50:889–897, 1977.

Key LL, Ries WL, Rodriguiz RM, Hatcher HC. Recombinant human interferon gamma therapy for osteopetrosis. J Pediatr 121:119–124, 1992.

Khalil N, Bereznay O, Sporn M, Greenberg AH. Macrophage production of transforming growth factor β and fibroblast collagen synthesis in chronic pulmonary inflammation. J Exp Med 170:727–737, 1989.

Kilpatrick L, Garty BA, Lundquist KF, Hunter K, Stanley CA, Baker L, Douglas SD, Korchak HM. Impaired metabolic function and signaling defects in phagocytic cells in glycogen storage disease type 1b. J Clin Invest 86:196–202, 1990.

Kimberly RP, Ralph P. Endocytosis by the mononuclear phagocyte system and autoimmune disease. Am J Med 74:481–493, 1983.

King GW, Bain G, LoBuglio AF. The effect of tuberculosis and neoplasia on human monocyte staphylocidal activity. Cell Immunol 16:389–395, 1975.

Kirkpatrick CH. Chronic mucocutaneous candidiasis. Eur J Clin Microbiol Infect Dis 8:448–456, 1989.

Klein RB, Fischer TJ, Gard SE, Biberstein M, Rich KC, Stiehm ER. Decreased mononuclear and polymorphonuclear chemotaxis in human newborns, infants, and young children. Pediatrics 60:467–472, 1977.

Komp DM. The treatment of sinus histiocytosis with massive lymphadenopathy (Rosai-Dorfman disease). Semin Diagn Pathol 7:83–86, 1990.

Krivit W, Shapiro E, Hoogerbrugge PM, Moser HW. State of the art review. Bone marrow transplantation treatment for storage disease. Keystone, January 23, 1992. Bone Marrow Transplant 10(Suppl. 1):87–96, 1992.

Kulozik M, Hogg A, Lankat-Buttgereit B, Krieg T. Colocalization of transforming growth factor β2 with α 1(I) procollagen mRNA in tissue sections of patients with systemic sclerosis. J Clin Invest 86:917–922, 1990.

Ladisch S, Poplack DG, Holiman B, Blaese RM. Immunodeficiency in familial erythrophagocytic lymphohistiocytosis. Lancet 1:581–583, 1978.

Ladisch S, Ho W, Matheson D, Pilkington R, Hertman G. Immunologic and clinical effects of repeated blood exchange in familial erythrophagocyte lymphohistiocytosis. Blood 60:814–821, 1982.

Ladisch S, Ulsh L, Gillard B, Wong C. Modulation of the immune response by gangliosides. Inhibition of adherent monocyte accessory function in vitro. J Clin Invest 74:2074–2081, 1984.

Lane HC, Fauci AS. Immunologic abnormalities in the acquired immunodeficiency syndrome. Annu Rev Immunol 3:477–500, 1985.

Lawley TJ, Hall RP, Fauci AS, Katz SI, Hamburger MI, Frank MM. Defective Fc receptor function associated with the HLA-B8/DRw 3 haplotype: studies in patients with dermatitis herpetiformis and normal subjects. N Engl J Med 304:185–192, 1981.

Leung DYM, Key L, Steinberg JJ, Young MC, VonDeck M, Wilkinson R, Geha RS. Increased in vitro bone resorption by monocytes in the hyperimmunoglobulin E syndrome. J Immunol 140:84–88, 1988.

Levine PH, Jahan N, Murari P, Manak M, Jaffe ES. Detection of human herpesvirus 6 in tissues involved by sinus histiocytosis with massive lymphadenopathy (Rosai-Dorfman disease). J Infect Dis 166:291–295, 1992.

Lichtman MA. Monocyte and macrophage disorders: self limited proliferative responses. Monocytosis and monocytopenia. In Williams WJ, Beutler E, Ersler AJ, Lichtman MA, eds. Hematology, 4th ed. New York, McGraw-Hill, 1990, pp. 882–885.

Lioy J, Ho W, Cutilli JA, Polin RA, Douglas SD. Thiol suppression of human immunodeficiency virus type 1 replication in primary cord blood monocyte–derived macrophages in vitro. J Clin Invest 91:495–498, 1993.

Lisowska-Grospierre B, Durandy A, Virilizier JL, Fischer A, Griscelli C. Combined immunodeficiency with defective expression of HLA: modulation of an abnormal HLA synthesis and functional studies. Birth Defects 19:87–91, 1983.

Long JP, Althausen AF. Malacoplakia: a 25-year experience with a review of the literature. J Urol 141:1328–1331, 1989.

Loy TS, Diaz-Arias AA, Perry MC. Familial erythrophagocytic lymphohistiocytosis. Semin Oncol 18:34–38, 1991.

Lynch SE, Colvin RB, Antoniades HN. Growth factors in wound healing. J Clin Invest 84:640–646, 1989.

Marlin SD, Morton CC, Anderson DC, Springer TA. LFA-1 immunodeficiency disease. J Exp Med 164:855–867, 1986.

McClain K, Gehrz R, Grierson H, Purtilo D, Filipovich A. Virus associated histiocytic proliferations in children. Frequent association with Epstein-Barr virus and congenital or acquired immunodeficiencies. Am J Pediatr Hematol Oncol 10:196–205, 1988.

McClure J. Malakoplakia. J Pathol 140:275–330, 1983.

McKenzie SM, Kline J, Douglas SD, Polin RA. Enhancement in vitro of the low interferon-γ production of leukocytes from human newborn infants. J Leukoc Biol 53:691–696, 1993.

McMillan EM, Humphrey GB, Stoneking L, Strauss LC, Civin CI, Abo T, Balch C. Analysis of histiocytosis X infiltrates with monoclonal antibodies directed against cells of histiocytic, lymphoid, and myeloid lineage. Clin Immunol Immunopathol 38:295–301, 1986.

Meltzer MS, Gendelman HE. Mononuclear phagocytes as targets, tissue reservoirs, and immunoregulatory cells in human immunodeficiency virus disease. Curr Top Microbiol Immunol 181:239–263, 1992.

Meltzer MS, Skillman DS, Gomatos PJ, Kalter DC, Gendelman HE. Role of mononuclear phagocytes in the pathogenesis of human immunodeficiency virus infection. Annu Rev Immunol 8:169–194, 1990.

Miale JB. Leukocytes. In Laboratory Medicine—Hematology, 3rd ed. St. Louis, CV Mosby, 1977, pp. 759–790.

Mistry NF, Birdi TJ, Mahadevan PR, Anita NH. *Mycobacterium leprae*–induced alterations in macrophage Fc receptor expression and monocyte-lymphocyte interaction in familial contacts of leprosy patients. Scand J Immunol 22:415–423, 1985.

Moore ME, Rossman MD, Schreiber AD, Douglas SD. DR framework antigens and 63D3 antigens on human peripheral blood monocytes and alveolar macrophages. Clin Immunol Immunopathol 29:119–128, 1983.

Mori M, Hayward AR. Persistence of Ia antigen and antigen presenting activity by cultured human monocytes. Clin Immunol Immunopathol 30:387–392, 1984.

Mornex JF, Chytil-Weir A, Martinet Y, Courtney M, LeCocq JP, Crystal RG. Expression of the alpha-1-antitrypsin gene in mononuclear phagocytes of normal and alpha-1-antitrypsin–deficient individuals. J Clin Invest 77:1952–1961, 1986.

Mustoe TA, Pierce GF, Thomason A, Gramates P, Sporn MB, Deuel TF. Transforming growth factor type beta induces accelerated healing of incisional wounds in rats. Science 237:1333–1336, 1987.

Naffakh N, Legall S, Danos O, Heard JM, Cournot G, Motoyoshi K, Vilmer E. Macrophage colony-stimulating factor: serum levels and cDNA structure in malignant osteopetrosis. Blood 81:2817–2818, 1993.

Naito M, Suzuki H, Mori T, Matsumoto A, Kodama T, Takahashi K. Coexpression of type I and type II human macrophage scavenger receptors in macrophages of various organs and foam cells in atherosclerotic lesions. Am J Pathol 141:591–599, 1992.

Nathan DC, Baehner RL, Weaver DK. Failure of nitroblue tetrazolium reduction in the phagocytic vacuoles of leucocytes in chronic granulomatous disease. J Clin Invest 48:1895–1904, 1969.

Neufeld EF. The biochemical basis for mucopolysaccharidoses and mucolipidoses. Prog Med Genet 10:81–101, 1974.

Orchard PJ, Dahl N, Aukerman SL, Blazar BR, Key LL. Circulating macrophage-stimulating factor is not reduced in malignant osteopetrosis. Exp Hematol 20:103–105, 1992.

Oski FA, Naiman JL. Normal blood values in the newborn period. In Hematologic Problems in the Newborn, 3rd ed. Philadelphia, WB Saunders, 1982, pp. 1–31.

Oyefara BI, Kim HC, Danziger RN, Carroll M, Greene JM, Douglas SD. Autoimmune hemolytic anemia in chronic mucocutaneous candidiasis. Clin Diagn Lab Immunol 1:38–43, 1994.

Peltonen J, Kahari L, Jaakkola S, Kahari VM, Varga J, Uitto J, Jimenez SA. Evaluation of transforming growth factor β and type 1 procollagen gene expression in fibrotic skin diseases by in situ hybridization. J Invest Dermatol 94:365–371, 1990.

Pidard D, Fischer A, Bouillot C, Le Deist F, Nurden AT. Inherited deficiencies can affect separately the platelet membrane glycoprotein IIb-IIIa complex and the leukocyte LFA-1, Mac-1, and p150,95 complexes (abstract). International Society for Thrombosis and Hemostasis, Bruxelles, 1987.

Pierce GF, Mustoe TA, Lingelbach J, Masakowski VR, Gramates P, Deuel TF. Transforming growth factor β reverses the glucocorticoid-induced wound-healing deficit in rats: possible regulation in macrophages by platelet-derived growth factor. Cell Biol 86:2229–2233, 1989.

Pierce GF, Mustoe TA, Altrock BW, Deuel TF, Thomason A. Role of platelet-derived growth factor in wound healing. J Cell Biochem 45:319–326, 1991.

Poli G, Bottazzi B, Acero R, Bersani L, Rossi V, Introna M, Lazzarin A, Galli M, Mantovani A. Monocyte function in intravenous drug abusers with lymphadenopathy syndrome and in patients with acquired immunodeficiency syndrome: selective impairment of chemotaxis. Clin Exp Immunol 62:136–142, 1985.

Poplack DG, Bonnard GD, Holiman BJ, Blaese RM. Monocyte mediated antibody dependent cellular cytotoxicity: a clinical test of monocyte function. Blood 48:809–816, 1976.

Prieto J, Subira ML, Castilla A, Civeira MP, Serrano M. Monocyte disorder causing cellular immunodeficiency: a family study. Clin Exp Immunol 79:1–6, 1990.

Reeves JD, August CS, Humbert JR, Weston WL. Host defense in infantile osteopetrosis. Pediatrics 65:202–206, 1979.

Relman DA, Schmidt TM, MacDermott RP, Falkow S. Identification of the uncultured bacillus of Whipple's disease. N Engl J Med 327:293–301, 1992.

Ries WL, Key LL, Rodriguiz RM. Nitroblue tetrazolium reduction and bone resorption by osteoclasts in vitro inhibited by a manganese-based superoxide dismutase mimic. J Bone Miner Res 7:931–939, 1992.

Ringden O, Ahstrom L, Lonnquist B, Baryd I, Svedmyr E, Gahrton G. Allogeneic bone marrow transplantation in a patient with chemotherapy-resistant progressive histiocytosis X. N Engl J Med 316:733–735, 1987.

Rodriguiz RM, Key LL, Ries WL. Combination macrophage-colony stimulating factor and interferon-γ administration ameliorates the osteopetrotic condition in microphthalmic (mi/mi) mice. Pediatr Res 33:384–389, 1993.

Rom WN, Travis WD, Brody AJ. Cellular and molecular basis of the asbestos-related diseases. Am Rev Respir Dis 143:408–422, 1991.

Rosai J, Dorfman RF. Sinus histiocytosis with massive lymphadenopathy: a pseudolymphomatous benign disorder. Cancer 30:1176–1188, 1972.

Rosenstein Y, Park JK, Hahn WC, Rosen FS, Bierer BE, Burakoff SJ. CD43, a molecule defective in Wiskott-Aldrich syndrome, binds ICAM-1. Nature 354:233–235, 1991.

Rossman MD, Maida BT, Douglas SD. Monocyte-derived macrophage and alveolar macrophage fibronectin production and cathepsin D activity. Cell Immunol 126:268–277, 1990.

Ruggeri ZM, Bader R, Demarco L. Glanzmann's thrombasthenia: deficient binding of von Willebrand factor to thrombin stimulated platelets. Proc Natl Acad Sci U S A 79:6038–6041, 1982.

Ruiz P, Gomez F, Schreiber AD. Impaired function of macrophage Fcγ receptors in end-stage renal disease. N Engl J Med 322:717–722, 1990.

Sainati L, Matules E, Mulligan S, de Oliveira MP, Rani S, Lampert IA, Catovsky D. A variant form of hairy cell leukemia resistant to γ-interferon: clinical and phenotypic characteristics of 17 patients. Blood 76:157–162, 1990.

Salgame PR, Birdi TJ, Mahadevan PR, Anita NH. Role of macrophages in defective cell mediated immunity in lepromatous leprosy. I. Factor(s) from macrophages affecting protein synthesis and lymphocyte transformation. Int J Lepr Other Mycobact Dis 48:172–177, 1980.

Salmon JE, Kimberly RP, Gibofsky A, Fotino M. Defective mononuclear phagocyte function in systemic lupus erythematosus: dissociation of Fc receptor–ligand binding and internalization. J Immunol 133:2525–2531, 1984.

Salmon JE, Kimberly RP, Gibofsky A, Fotino M. Altered phagocytosis by monocytes from HLA-DR2 and DR3-positive healthy adults is Fc-gamma-receptor specific. J Immunol 136:3625–3630, 1986.

Schibler KR, Liechty KW, White WL, Rothstein G, Christensen RD. Defective production of interleukin-6 by monocytes: a possible mechanism underlying several host defense deficiencies of neonates. Pediatr Res 31:18–21, 1992.

Schibler KR, Trautman MS, Liechty KW, White WL, Rothstein G, Christensen RD. Diminished transcription of IL-8 by monocytes from preterm neonates. J Leukoc Biol 63:399–406, 1993.

Schmidt EB, Varming K, Pederson JO, Lervang HH, Grunnet N, Jersild C, Dyerberg J. Long-term supplementation with n-3 fatty acids. II: Effect on neutrophil and monocyte chemotaxis. Scand J Clin Lab Invest 52:229–236, 1992.

Schreiber AD, Rossman MD, Levinson AI. The immunobiology of human Fc gamma receptors on hematopoietic cells and tissue macrophages. Clin Immunol Immunopathol 62:566–572, 1992.

Schuurman RKB, Van Rood JJ, Vossen JM, Schellekons P, Feltkamp-Vrom TH, Doyer TM, Grelig-Meyling F, Visser HKA. Failure of lymphocyte membrane HLA-A and B expression in two siblings with combined immunodeficiency. Clin Immunol Immunopathol 14:418–434, 1979.

Schuurman HJ, Huber J, Zegers BJM, Roord JJ. Placental diagnosis of the bare lymphocyte syndrome. N Engl J Med 313:757–758, 1985.

Sechler JM, Malech HL, White CJ, Gallin JI. Recombinant human interferon-gamma reconstitutes defective phagocyte function in patients with chronic granulomatous disease of childhood. Proc Natl Acad Sci U S A 85:4874–4878, 1988.

Setiadi H, Antoine C, Wautier JL. Normal expression of the adhesive structure Mo-1 on monocytes from patients with Glanzmann's thrombasthenia. J Mal Vasc 16:30–31, 1991.

Shapiro F, Key LL, Anast C. Variable osteoclast appearance in human infantile osteopetrosis. Calcif Tissue Int 43:67–76, 1988.

Shevach EM. Macrophages and other accessory cells. In Paul WE, ed. Fundamental Immunology, 2nd ed. New York, Raven Press, 1984, pp. 71–108.

Sibley LD, Krahenbuhl JL. Mycobacterium leprae–burdened macrophages are refractory to activation by gamma interferon. Infect Immun 55:446–450, 1987.

Sieff CA, Chessels JM, Levinsky RJ, Pritchard J, Rogers DW, Casey A, Muller K, Hall CM. Allogeneic bone marrow transplantation in infantile malignant osteopetrosis. Lancet 1:437–441, 1983.

Skare JC, Grierson HL, Sullivan JL, Nussbaum RL, Purtilo DT, Sylla BS, Lenoir GM, Reilly DS, White BN, Milunsky A. Linkage analysis of seven kindreds with the X-linked lymphoproliferative syndrome (XLP) confirms that the XLP locus is near DXS42 and DXS37. Hum Genet 82:354–358, 1989.

Skare J, Wu BL, Madan S, Pulijaal V, Purtilo D, Haber D, Nelson D, Sylla B, Grierson H, Nitowsky H, Glaser J, Wissink J, White B, Holden J, Houseman D, Lenoir GM, Wyandt H, Milunsky A. Characterization of three overlapping deletions causing X-linked lymphoproliferative disease. Genomics 16:254–255, 1993.

Smith PD, Ohura K, Masure H, Lane HC, Fauci AS, Wahl SM. Monocyte function in the acquired immune deficiency syndrome. Defective chemotaxis. J Clin Invest 74:2121–2128, 1984.

Snyderman R, Altman LC, Frankel A, Blaese RM. Defective mononuclear leucocyte chemotaxis: a previously unrecognized immune dysfunction. Ann Intern Med 78:509–513, 1973.

Sorell M, Kapoor N, Kirkpatrick D, Rosen JF, Chaganti RS, Lopes C, Dupont B, Pollack MS, Terrin BN, Harris MB, Vine D, Rose JS, Goossen C, Lane J, Good RA, O'Reilly RJ. Marrow transplantation for juvenile osteopetrosis. Am J Med 70:1280–1287, 1981.

Steigbigel RT, Lambert LH, Remington JS. Phagocytic and bactericidal properties of normal human monocytes. J Clin Invest 53:131–152, 1974.

Stiehm ER, Mann D, Newland C, Sztein MB, Steeg PS, Oppenheim JJ, Blaese RM. Deficient DR antigen expression on human neonatal monocytes: reversal with lymphokines. Birth Defects 19:295–298, 1983.

Stoll M, Freund M, Schmid H, Deicher H, Riehm H, Poliwada H, Link H. Allogeneic bone marrow transplantation for Langerhans cell histiocytosis. Cancer 66:284–288, 1990.

Tax WJM, Hermes FFM, Willems R, Copel JA, Koene RAP. Fc receptors for murine IgG-1 on human monocytes: polymorphism and role in antibody induced T-cell proliferation. J Immunol 133:1185–1189, 1984.

Terui T, Niitsu Y, Mahara K, Fujisaki Y, Urushizaki Y, Mogi Y, Kohgo Y, Watanabe N, Ogura M, Saito H. The production of transforming growth factor-β in acute megakaryoblastic leukemia and its possible implication in myelofibrosis. Blood 75:1540–1548, 1990.

Tipping PG, Hancock WW. Production of tumor necrosis factor and interleukin-1 by macrophages from human atheromatous plaques. Am J Pathol 142:1721–1728, 1993.

Touraine JL. The bare lymphocyte syndrome: report on the registry. Lancet 1:319–320, 1984.

Touraine JL. Rationale and results of in utero transplants of stem cells in humans. Bone Marrow Transplant 10(Suppl. 1):121–126, 1992.

Touraine JL, Betuel H. The blue lymphocyte syndrome: immunodeficiency resulting from the lack of expression of HLA antigens. Birth Defects: Original Article Series No. 3, 19:83–85, 1983.

Twomey JJ, Douglas CC, Sharkey O. The monocytopenia of aplastic anemia. Blood 41:187–195, 1973.

Ueno N, Tomita M, Ariga T, Ohkawa M, Nagano S, Takahashi Y, Arashima S, Matsumoto S. Impaired monocyte function in glycogen storage disease type 1b. Eur J Pediatr 145:312–314, 1986.

Uhr JW, Dancis J, Neumann CG. Delayed type hypersensitivity in premature neonatal humans. Nature 187:1130–1131, 1960.

Ulich TR, del Castillo J, Watson LR, Yin SM, Garnick MB. In vivo hematologic effects of recombinant human macrophage colony-stimulating factor. Blood 75:846–850, 1990.

Unanue ER. The regulatory role of macrophages in antigenic stimulation. Adv Immunol 31:1–125, 1981.

van der Wal AC, Das PK, Tigges AJ, Becker AE. Adhesion molecules on the endothelium and mononuclear cells in human atherosclerotic lesions. Am J Pathol 141:1427–1433, 1992.

Wahl SM. Transforming growth factor beta (TGF-β) in inflammation. A cause and a cure. J Clin Immunol 12:61–74, 1992.

Wahl SM, Allen JB, Gartner S, Orenstein JM, Popvic M, Chenoweth DE, Arthur LO, Farrar WL, Wahl LM. Human immunodeficiency virus-1 and its envelope glycoprotein down-regulate chemotactic ligand receptors and chemotactic function of peripheral blood monocytes. J Immunol 142:3553–3559, 1989.

Waldman JD, Rosenthal A, Smith AL, Shurin S, Nadas AS. Sepsis and congenital asplenia. J Pediatr 90:555–559, 1977.

Wang J, Hsieh K. Immunologic study of the asplenia syndrome. Ped Infect Dis J 10:819–822, 1991.

Watson S, Bullock W, Nelson K, Schauf V, Gelber R, Jacobson R. Interleukin 1 production by peripheral blood mononuclear cells from leprosy patients. Infect Immun 45:787–789, 1984.

Weatherstone KB, Rich EA. Tumor necrosis factor/cachectin and interleukin-1 secretion by cord blood monocytes from premature and term neonates. Pediatr Res 25:342–346, 1989.

Weening RS, Corbeel L, De Boer M, Lutter R, van Zwieten R, Hamers MN, Roos D. Cytochrome b deficiency in an autosomal form of chronic granulomatous disease recognized by monocyte hybridization. J Clin Invest 75:915–920, 1985.

Weinberg AG, Rosenfeld CR, Manroe BL, Browne R. Neonatal blood cell count in health and disease. II. Values for lymphocytes, monocytes, and eosinophils. J Pediatr 106:462–466, 1985.

Weinberg JB, Hibbs JB. Endocytosis of red blood cells or haemoglobin by activated macrophages inhibits their tumoricidal effect. Nature 269:245–247, 1977.

Wells CL, Maddaus MA, Simmons RL. Role of the macrophage in the translocation of intestinal bacteria. Arch Surg 122:48–53, 1987.

Wilson CB. Immunologic basis for increased susceptibility of the neonate to infection. J Pediatr 108:1–12, 1986.

Wilson CB, Haas JE. Cellular defenses against *Toxoplasma gondii* in newborns. J Clin Invest 73:1606–1616, 1984.

Wilson CB, Haas JE, Weaver WM. Isolation, purification and characteristics of mononuclear phagocytes from human placentas. J Immunol Methods 56:305–317, 1983.

Woda BA, Sullivan JL. Reactive histiocytic disorders. Am J Clin Pathol 99:459–463, 1993.

Wong CG, Ladisch S, Sweely CC. Hepatic ganglioside abnormalities in a patient with familial erythrophagocytic lymphohistiocytosis. Pediatr Res 17:413–417, 1983.

Woodman RC, Erickson RW, Rae J, Jaffe HS, Curnutte JT. Prolonged recombinant interferon-gamma therapy in chronic granulomatous disease: evidence against enhanced neutrophil oxidase activity. N Engl J Med 79:1558–1562, 1992.

Writing Group of the Histiocyte Society. Histiocytosis syndromes in children. Lancet 1:208–209, 1987.

Zhang Y, Lee TC, Guillemin B, Yu M, Rom WN. Enhanced IL-1β and tumor necrosis factor-α release and messenger RNA expression in macrophages from idiopathic pulmonary fibrosis or after asbestos exposure. J Immunol 150:4188–4196, 1993.

Ziegler-Heitbrock HWL, Ulevitch RJ. CD14: Cell surface receptor and differentiation marker. Immunol Today 14:121–125, 1993.

Chapter 17

Disorders of the Complement System

Richard B. Johnston, Jr.

Knowledge of the biology and biochemistry of the complement system has grown rapidly (see Chapter 7). A great deal is now known about the relationships between structure and function of the complement proteins. On the basis of this current knowledge, no better example exists in nature of the exquisitely sensitive interplay that occurs between biochemical reactions and their control mechanisms, nor do better examples exist of how an imbalance in such an interaction can lead to disease. In the complement system, an imbalance occurs when an individual is born without one of the 31 proteins that compose the system in its broadest context. (As presently understood, the system consists of 20 well-defined plasma constituents, five cell membrane regulatory proteins, and seven membrane receptors that permit expression of the biologic activity of the system. One membrane protein serves as both regulator and receptor.) An acquired, partial deficiency of one or more of these proteins can occur commonly, secondary either to increased consumption of the system or to decreased synthesis. In all but the mildest cases, the complement deficiency creates a potential for disease that warrants diagnosis. Although cure is not possible, proper management in most instances can prevent serious consequences.

Genetic deficiencies of the complement system include those of plasma components, plasma control proteins, and serosal control protein.

GENETIC DEFICIENCIES OF PLASMA COMPONENTS

Primary deficiency of serum complement in humans was first reported in 1960 (Alper and Rosen, 1984; Figueroa and Densen, 1991; Silverstein, 1960). Congenital deficiencies of all 11 complement component proteins of the classical pathway, factor D of the alternative pathway, and five control proteins have now been described (Table 17–1).* There are two major categories of clinical findings associated with any of these deficiencies in humans, collagen-vascular disease and a predisposition to infection.

---

*Several animal strains are also known to lack a complement component: C4-deficient and C2-deficient guinea pigs (Bitter-Suermann et al., 1981; Ellman et al., 1971), C5-deficient rats (Arroyave et al., 1977), C3-deficient dogs (Winkelstein et al., 1982; Quezado et al., 1994), C5-deficient mice (Cinader et al., 1964; Wetzel et al., 1990), C6-deficient rabbits (Rother et al., 1966), and C8-deficient rabbits (Komatsu et al., 1985).

Most of the inherited deficiencies of complement components that have been described in humans are the result of decreased protein synthesis resulting from the inheritance of two nonfunctioning (null) genes. Individuals who are heterozygous for deficiency of a component possess one normal gene and one null gene and have approximately half-normal levels of the deficient component. This pattern of inheritance has been termed *autosomal codominant*. Deficiencies of C1rs, C4, C2, C3, C5, C6, C7, C8, and C9 all appear to be inherited in this manner, as is C1q dysfunction. Deficiencies of the control proteins factors I, H, and D are probably also inherited as codominant traits. An incomplete deficiency of C4 (2% to 5% of normal levels) has been inherited in one family as an autosomal dominant trait (Muir et al., 1984). Properdin deficiency is inherited as an X-linked trait. C1 INH deficiency has dominant inheritance, but 10% of propositi are apparently spontaneous mutants. (For reviews of genetic deficiencies, see Colten and Rosen, 1992; Figueroa and Densen, 1991; Kölble and Reid, 1993; Ross and Densen, 1984; Tedesco et al., 1993; Würzner et al., 1992.)

C1q Deficiency

Primary selective deficiency of C1q has been described in several patients (Berkel et al., 1979, 1981; Fiqueroa and Densen, 1991; Leyva-Cobián et al., 1981; Loos et al., 1980; Minta et al., 1982; Nishino et al., 1981; Steinsson et al., 1983; Uenaka et al., 1982; Wara

Table 17–1. Genetic Deficiencies of Plasma Complement Components and Associated Clinical Findings

Deficient Component†	Infection*			Collagen-Vascular Disease*		
	Common‡	*Less Common*	*Occasional*	*Common*	*Less Common*	*Occasional*
C1q			Pneumococcal B/M, other pyogenic	SLE	GN	DV/DLE
C1r		Other pyogenic	Pneumococcal B/M, DGI	SLE		GN
C1rs		Other pyogenic		SLE		
C4		Other pyogenic		SLE	Other CVD	GN
C2		Other pyogenic, pneumococcal B/M, meningococcal M			SLE, GN, DV/DLE, other CVD	
C3	Other pyogenic	Pneumococcal B/M, meningococcal M			GN, DV/DLE	SLE, other CVD
C5	Meningococcal M	DGI	Other pyogenic			SLE, GN
C6	Meningococcal M	DGI	Other pyogenic			SLE, GN, other CVD
C7	Meningococcal M		DGI, other pyogenic			SLE, other CVD
C8	Meningococcal M	DGI	Other pyogenic			SLE, GN
C9		Meningococcal M				
Factor D			DGI, meningococcal M			

*A finding was reported as common if it occurred in 50% or more of reported cases, less common if reported in about 5% to 50% of cases, and occasional if present in one or two cases or <5% of the more frequent deficiencies.

†No genetic complete deficiency of factor B has been reported to date.

‡B/M = bacteremia or meningitis; DGI = disseminated gonococcal infection; DV/DLE = dermal vasculitis or typical discoid lupus erythematosus; GN = glomerulonephritis in various forms, often membranoproliferative; M= meningitis; other CVD = other collagen-vascular diseases (almost all possible diagnoses have been reported); other pyogenic = serious deep or systemic infection caused by or typically caused by a pyogenic bacterium (abscess, osteomyelitis, pneumonia, bacteremia other than pneumococcal, meningitis other than meningococcal or pneumococcal, cellulitis, myopericarditis, and peritonitis); SLE = typical systemic lupus erythematosus or an SLE-like syndrome without characteristic serologic findings.

Modified from Johnston RB Jr. J Pediatr Infect Dis 12:933–941, 1993. Data from Figueroa JE, Densen P. Clin Microbiol Rev 4:359–395, 1991; and Ross SC, Densen P. Medicine 63:243–273, 1984.

et al., 1975). Most have had systemic lupus erythematosus (SLE), an SLE-like syndrome without typical SLE serology, a chronic rash that has shown an underlying vasculitis on biopsy, or membranoproliferative glomerulonephritis (MPGN). One man was well until he developed SLE at 37 years of age (Nishino et al., 1981). Three C1q-deficient children suffered from infections, including meningitis, recurrent septicemia, recurrent otitis media, pyoderma, pneumonia, stomatitis, and persistent moniliasis of the oral cavity and nails (Berkel et al., 1979, 1981). Two of these children died from meningitis-septicemia. C1q has usually been completely absent by both hemolytic and immunochemical assays. C1q deficiency can occur in families; however, obligate heterozygotes do not have half-normal levels, and the inheritance pattern is not yet clear. The whole-complement hemolytic titer, or CH_{50}, measured as the capacity of serum to induce lysis of antibody-coated sheep red blood cells, is completely absent in C1q-deficient sera. In fact, a zero (or near-zero) CH_{50} value is found with deficiency of each of the classical pathway components except C9.

Four additional families have been reported in whom the sera lacked functional C1q activity but contained an antigenically altered C1q protein (Chapuis et al., 1982; Hannema et al., 1984; Kölble and Reid, 1993; Thompson et al., 1980). Four of the affected individuals in these families had glomerulonephritis, a lupus-like syndrome, or both; two have been completely healthy. In one of the families, the parents had both normal and abnormal C1q protein in the sera (Thompson et al., 1980), suggesting that the patients had inherited one abnormal codominant trait from each parent. Functional C1 levels and whole-complement titers have been normal in the obligate heterozygous carriers who have been studied. C1q is encoded by three genes in a 24-kb stretch of the short arm of chromosome 1.

C1rs Deficiency

Complete deficiency of C1r has been reported in several families (Day and Good, 1980; Kölble and Reid, 1993; Lee et al., 1978; Loos and Heinz, 1986; Moncada et al., 1972; Pickering et al., 1971; Rich et al., 1979). Almost all affected individuals have had some sort of collagen-vascular disease, especially chronic glomerulonephritis by clinical diagnosis, MPGN when a kidney biopsy specimen was obtained, SLE, or a syndrome of clinical findings resembling SLE but without positive titers for antinuclear antibody or other serologic abnormalities seen with typical lupus. This same spectrum has been seen with deficiencies of the other early-acting components of the classical pathway (C1, C4, and C2). That is, some patients have had typical SLE, and others have had a syndrome with the clinical manifestations of lupus but few, if any, serologic abnormalities. For the sake of simplicity, this spectrum has been grouped as simply "SLE" in Table 17–1. A few patients have had severe infections; one infant with C1r deficiency had pneumonia, empyema, cervical and hepatic abscesses, and pneumococcal bacteremia (Garty et al., 1987). The genes for C1r and C1s are closely linked on

the terminal portion of the short arm of chromosome 12, and deficiency of C1r appears to be invariably associated with partial deficiency of C1s.

C1s Deficiency

To date, only two individuals have been reported to have isolated C1s deficiency. One had typical SLE (Pondman et al., 1968), and the other had disseminated gonococcocal infection (Ellison et al., 1987). The molecular basis for deficiency of C1r/C1s or for C1s alone is not presently understood.

C4 Deficiency

The first report of congenital absence of C4 was of an 18-year-old girl who presented with an SLE-like syndrome (Hauptmann et al., 1974). Most of the cases reported subsequently have also had an SLE syndrome or typical SLE, in some cases with severe glomerulonephritis (reviewed in Ross and Densen, 1984; Figueroa and Densen, 1991). Most of the patients have been children or adolescents. Henoch-Schönlein purpura, glomerulonephritis, and Sjögren's syndrome have been diagnosed in individual cases (Ross and Densen, 1984). Infections have occurred on occasion, usually superimposed on severe SLE (Jackson et al., 1979; Tappeiner et al., 1982). One young boy with C4 deficiency had an abnormal antibody response to injected antigens and depressed lymphoproliferative responses to mitogens or foreign cells (Jackson et al., 1979). He later died of cytomegalovirus pneumonia. The abnormal lymphocyte functions shown in this boy may be related to the fact that the two genes that direct the synthesis of C4, C4A and C4B, are located on the short arm of chromosome 6 in an alignment of six genes related to the immune response and host defense. From centomer toward telomer, these are HLA-DR, C4B, C4A, factor B, C2, and HLA-B. Linkage disequilibrium within this array of genes is common, and certain extended haplotypes, including a null C4 gene, appear to be more commonly associated with a variety of disorders that may reflect abnormalities of immunologic regulation (Colten and Rosen, 1992; McLean and Winkelstein, 1984). A decrease in antibody response also has been found in C4-deficient guinea pigs (Ellman et al., 1971).

Muir et al. (1984) described a patient with hereditary incomplete C4 deficiency determined by a gene not linked to the HLA system.

C4B is hemolytically four times more active than C4A, and persons whose C4 is composed only of the C4A isotype (about 3% of the general population) have an increased risk of serious pyogenic bacterial infections (reviewed in Fasano et al., 1990; Bishof et al., 1990). Failure of C4B expression has been shown to result usually from mutations that cause the C4B gene to transcribe a molecule with the properties of C4A. Complete deficiency of C4A results from gene deletions, stop codons, or other mutations that lead to failure of transcription (Barba et al., 1993; Colten and Rosen, 1992).

C2 Deficiency

The most frequent complement deficiency reported has been deficiency of C2. It has been estimated that the prevalence of this condition is from 1 in 10,000 to 1 in 28,000 people and that the abnormal gene occurs in 1.2% of the population (Glass et al., 1976; Rynes et al., 1982). The first two clearly identified cases were healthy immunologists (Klemperer et al., 1967); however, since then, the disorder has been found in association with a variety of collagen-vascular diseases as well as in normal subjects. SLE has been most common, but discoid lupus, MPGN, Henoch-Schönlein purpura, rheumatoid arthritis, dermatomyositis, Crohn's disease, and idiopathic thrombocytopenic purpura have all been reported in patients with C2 deficiency (Figueroa and Densen, 1991; Ross and Densen, 1984). Common variable immunodeficiency was associated with C2 deficiency in one individual (Seligmann et al., 1979).

Two types of C2 deficiency are recognized (Johnson et al., 1992b). In type I C2 deficiency, the synthesis of C2 cannot be detected although the C2 mRNA content is normal; serum C2 is undetectable. This defect in C2 synthesis results from a 28-base pair deletion in the gene (Johnson et al., 1992a). In over 90% of C2-deficient kindreds, this defect is associated with the haplotype HLA-B18, DR2 (Kölble and Reid, 1993; Truedsson et al., 1993). In type II C2 deficiency, C2 builds up inside the cell but is not secreted normally; serum C2 levels are 0.5% to 4% of normal (Johnson et al., 1992b). The molecular basis for this defect is not understood.

In most of the early reported cases, patients showed no definite predisposition to infection. It is now clear, however, that there is a definite risk in C2-deficient individuals of sustaining a serious bacteremic infection, especially with the pneumococcus, but also with meningococci, *Haemophilus influenzae*, enteric bacteria, and staphylococci (Borzy et al., 1984; Day et al., 1973; Figueroa and Densen, 1991; Glovsky et al., 1976; Hyatt et al., 1981; Leggiadro et al., 1983; Newman et al., 1978; Ross and Densen, 1984; Sampson et al., 1982; Thong et al., 1980). Most of these patients were young children, but one was a girl who had pneumococcal meningitis at 4 years of age and *H. influenzae* arthritis, pneumonia, and bacteremia at 16 years of age. She had been completely healthy in the 12 years between the two episodes of infection (Hyatt et al., 1981). Another child had no serious infections until he had meningococcemia at 16 years of age (Leggiadro et al., 1983). These cases suggest that C2 deficiency should be considered in any patient, after the first two years of life, who has pneumococcal bacteremia, no matter how healthy he or she has been previously.

It is not clear why a few patients with C2 deficiency suffer recurrent bacteremic illnesses and why most have no trouble with infections at all. Antibody response has been normal to the extent it has been studied. Presumably, the alternative pathway should fix C3 to the invading organism well enough to permit efficient opsonization and phagocytic clearance in most cases. Factor B, however, can be moderately reduced in individuals with C2 deficiency and, of eight patients with recurrent infection that were studied, three had clearly abnormal alternative pathway function (Hyatt et al., 1981; Newman et al., 1978). On the other hand, alternative pathway activity was normal in five of these patients; thus, failure of the back-up opsonization system seems unlikely as a general explanation for the infections that occur in C2-deficient individuals.

It is also not clear why there is a tendency for collagen-vascular disease to develop in patients with deficiency of C2 or the other early-acting components of the classical pathway. There are at least four possibilities:

1. It is possible that the association is artifactual—that it results from the preferential screening of patients with collagen-vascular disease for an underlying complement abnormality. This appears not to be the case; for example, C2 deficiency was significantly more common among 545 patients from a rheumatology clinic than it was among samples of over 10,000 normal blood donors (Glass et al., 1976).

2. A complement deficiency could make it difficult for individuals to clear a putative infectious agent adequately. The disease state, then, could begin with direct tissue injury by the agent or through the formation of immune complexes. Because infectious agents have never been proven to cause collagen-vascular disease, this possibility remains speculative. Perhaps related, however, are studies with a *Mycoplasma pulmonis*–induced chronic arthritis in mice, which has been used as a model for rheumatoid arthritis. In this model, chronic arthritis is significantly greater in C5-deficient mice than in normal mice (Keystone et al., 1978).

3. A third possibility is suggested by the observations that complement increases the solubility of immune complexes through the covalent binding of C3 fragments and that complement is essential for the normal removal of immune complexes from the circulation through binding to complement receptor (CR1) on erythrocytes and transport to the mononuclear phagocyte system (reviewed in Davies et al., 1993; Schifferli et al., 1985). Sera deficient in early classical pathway components lack the normal ability to prevent aggregation of complexes at the time of the antigen-antibody reaction and to support normal clearance, particularly by the spleen (Davies et al., 1993; Schifferli et al., 1985). It seems likely that this abnormality contributes to the high incidence of collagen-vascular disease in individuals in whom C1q, C1r, C1s, C4, C2, or C3 is absent.

4. If the genes controlling C2, C4, and factor B synthesis, which are located between the genes for the class I and II MHC (major histocompatibility complex), are closely linked to the MHC, the complement deficiencies may only be markers for defects or for tissue phenotypes encoded within this complex that could lead to the autoimmune state. To date, it does not appear that the MHC class II genes linked to the C2 null gene (pseudogene) of type I deficiency play any role in determining the different clinical consequences of C2 deficiency (Truedsson et al., 1993).

C3 Deficiency

Because both pathways converge to cleave and activate C3, there is no way to compensate for absence of this protein. Without C3, opsonization of most pyogenic bacteria is inefficient and the chemotactic fragment from C5 is not generated effectively. One would expect trouble from organisms that must be well opsonized to be cleared, and this has been the case: congenital absence of C3 has been associated with recurrent, severe pyogenic infections such as pneumococcal pneumonia and meningococcal meningitis (Ross and Densen, 1984). In most of these patients, the clinical picture in regard to the type and severity of infections has been identical to that seen in hypogammaglobulinemia.

Increased susceptibility to infection, however, has not been present in all C3-deficient individuals, and the reason for this is not clear. There are some data to suggest that, at least for neutrophils, IgG is the major opsonin and C3 serves to increase the extent of binding rather than ingestion (Newman and Johnston, 1979). For some organisms, however, C3 may not be an essential opsonin. Thus, on exposure to a small inoculum of a pathogen, or to a pathogen that could be well opsonized without C3, some patients may do well if sufficient antibody is present.

Several individuals with C3 deficiency have had MPGN, SLE, or dermal vasculitis (Ross and Densen, 1984). The molecular basis for C3 deficiency appears to be heterogeneous, and serum levels vary from undetectable to about 3% of normal (Colten and Rosen, 1992).

C5 Deficiency

The first individual described with congenital deficiency of C5 had SLE at 11 years of age (Rosenfeld et al., 1976b). She had frequent skin infections and subcutaneous abcesses both before and after the diagnosis of SLE. Serum was markedly deficient in generating chemotactic activity, and normal activity was restored by the addition of C5 (Rosenfeld et al., 1976a), supporting the role of C5a as the primary chemoattractant in serum. Deficient chemotaxis was considered to be a plausible explanation for her frequent and subcutaneous skin infections. In none of the almost 30 additional cases that have been reported have the patients suffered frequent cutaneous infections (Figueroa and Densen, 1991; Ross and Densen, 1984; Weinstein et al., 1983), nor have they experienced collagen-vascular disease. Rather, most have had meningococcal meningitis at least once and four have had disseminated gonococcal infection (see Table 17–1).

The genetic abnormalities responsible for deficiency of C5, C6, C7, C8, and C9 have not yet been fully defined, although molecular defects have been determined in a few individuals.

Deficiency of C6, C7, C8, or C9

The same high incidence of neisserial infections and the frequent occurrence of collagen-vascular disease that have been seen with C5 deficiency exist also in patients with deficiency of C6, C7, or C8. Of 238 patients described with deficiency of one of these three components (Adams et al., 1983; Burdash et al., 1983; Ellison et al., 1983; Figueroa and Densen, 1991; Liston, 1983; Merino et al., 1983; Ross and Densen, 1984; Strate et al., 1983; Weinstein et al., 1983; Zimran et al., 1984), 151 (63%) have had at least one serious neisserial infection (140 meningococcal, nine disseminated gonococcal, two both), and 13 have had a collagen-vascular syndrome. These numbers should not be taken too literally, because the presence of disease led to the complement study, but the emphasis on predisposition to neisserial infections, especially meningococcal, seems valid. The reason for this predisposition is not clear, but its occurrence suggests a dependence on complement-mediated bacteriolysis for host defense against neisserial species (Nicholson and Lepow, 1979; Vogler et al., 1979). The collagen-vascular syndromes seen in these patients include discoid lupus, sclerodactyly, Sjögren's syndrome, nephritis, rheumatoid arthritis, and ankylosing spondylitis, in addition to SLE (Figueroa and Densen, 1991; Ross and Densen, 1984).

C6 and C7 are encoded on chromosome 5q and share similar structures. Four patients have been reported to be deficient in both C6 and C7 (Lachmann et al., 1978; Würzner et al., 1992).

The C8 molecule consists of three chains (α, β, and γ) linked as two subunits (α-γ and β). The two subunits are under the control of separate genes. Two major forms of C8 deficiency have been described, corresponding to the subunit structure of the molecule (Tedesco et al., 1983, 1993). About 90% of reported cases have been whites with β deficiency; 10% have been nonwhites with α-γ deficiency (Tedesco et al., 1993). The clinical picture has been equivalent with all types of deficiency.

In contrast to deficiency of any of the other ten components or subcomponents of the classical pathway, deficiency of C9 does not result in a zero hemolytic complement titer but in a titer of one third to one half normal. Gram-negative bacteria also can be lysed to some extent with C9-deficient sera (Harriman et al., 1981; Pramoonjago et al., 1992). This result confirms previous work with purified components showing that the C5b678 complex can lyse cells, although at a slower rate than with the entire "membrane attack complex," which also contains C9. Meningococcal meningitis has occurred in about one third of the reported cases; three cases have had SLE (Figueroa and Densen, 1991). C9 deficiency is particularly common in Japan, where it is reported to occur in about 0.1% of the general population (Tedesco et al., 1993).

A collation of the results of seven studies suggests that about 14% of patients presenting with sporadic meningococcal disease might be expected to have a defect in C5, C6, C7, C8, or C9 (Tedesco et al., 1993). The frequency of underlying complement deficiency (any component) increases to almost one third in individuals with more than one episode of meningococcal disease.

Factor D Deficiency

Identical twin sisters had isolated deficiency of factor D activity of the alternative pathway. The deficiency was partial (6% to 12% of normal) but persistent. Both sisters had recurrent sinusitis and bronchitis; one also had bronchiectasis. Hemolytic complement activity in the serum was normal, but alternative pathway activity was markedly deficient (Kluin-Nelemans et al., 1984). A third patient, who had no detectable serum factor D protein, had disseminated gonococcal infection twice and meningococcal meningitis once. Serum hemolytic complement activity was reduced but not absent; alternative pathway activity was undetectable. His mother and sister had approximately half-normal levels of alternative pathway activity and factor D protein in their sera (Hiemstra et al., 1989).

Heterozygous Deficiency of Complement Component

Glass and coworkers (1976) first suggested that the heterozygous deficiency of C2 (possession of one null allele) is associated with an increased incidence of rheumatologic disease. This suggestion was raised by the finding that the prevalence of heterozygous C2 deficiency is much higher in patients with SLE or juvenile rheumatoid arthritis than in a large number of normal blood donors. A similar suggestion has been raised in regard to heterozygous deficiency of C4. Individuals carrying a null allele for one of the two loci for C4 (C4A or C4B) may have an increased incidence of SLE, discoid lupus, or urticaria/angioedema (Agnello et al., 1983; Fielder et al., 1983; Ripoche et al., 1983). Partial deficiency of several different complement components (C2, factor B, C3, C6, C7, and C8) was found on analysis of sera from 44 patients with MPGN (Coleman et al., 1983). These deficiencies could not be ascribed to complement consumption or to the nephrotic syndrome, and in some cases they were present in

family members. Three individuals from two large families apparently carrying one silent gene for factor H also had chronic renal disease (vasculitis-nephritis syndrome or IgA nephropathy) (Wyatt et al., 1982). A possible relationship between nephritis and certain polymorphic variants of complement proteins has been proposed (McLean and Winkelstein, 1984). Thus, it is possible that suboptimal functioning of the complement system may in itself predispose to nephritis.

GENETIC DEFICIENCIES OF PLASMA CONTROL PROTEINS

Several control proteins modulate activity of the complement system. Their importance to the system has been emphasized by the striking clinical problems that result from their absence (Table 17–2). Two of these deficiencies, hereditary angioedema and factor I deficiency, are classical experiments of nature that provide considerable insight into the delicate balance between activation and regulation of the system.

Hereditary Angioedema

Hereditary angioedema results when an individual is born without the ability to synthesize normally functioning C1 inhibitor. In about 85% of affected patients, the concentration of inhibitor is reduced to 5% to 30% of normal (type I); in the other 15%, the serum contains normal or elevated concentrations of an immunologically cross-reacting but nonfunctional protein (type II) (Rosen et al., 1965). Both forms of the disease are transmitted as autosomal dominant traits, and the two cannot be distinguished clinically. About 10% of propositi are apparently spontaneous mutants. In type I disease, the defective mutant mRNA or protein (or both) appear to inhibit translation of normal C1 INH (Kramer et al., 1993). The mutation in the type II form occurs most commonly in the Arg at the critical reactive center of the inhibitor (Colten and Rosen, 1992).

Table 17–2. Genetic Deficiencies of Plasma Complement Control Proteins and Associated Clinical Findings

Deficient Protein†	Infection*			Collagen-Vascular Disease*		
	Common‡	Less Common	Occasional	Common	Less Common	Occasional
C1 INH	Hereditary angioedema					
Factor I	Other pyogenic, meningococcal M	Pneumococcal B/M				
Factor H		Meningococcal B/M	Other pyogenic		GN	SLE
Properdin		Meningococcal M	Pneumococcal B/M, other pyogenic		DV/DLE	
C4 binding protein						Other CVD

*A finding was reported as common if it occurred in 50% or more of reported cases, less common if reported in about 5% to 50% of cases, and occasional if present in one or two cases or <5% of the more frequent deficiencies.

†No genetic deficiency of the plasma control proteins C1q inhibitor, S protein, SP-40, histidine-rich glycoprotein, or anaphylatoxin inactivator has been reported to date.

‡B/M = bacteremia or meningitis; C1 INH = C1 inhibitor; DV/DLE = dermal vasculitis or typical discoid lupus erythematosus; GN = glomerulonephritis in various forms, often membranoproliferative; M = meningitis; other CVD = other collagen-vascular diseases; other pyogenic = serious deep or systemic infection caused by or typically caused by a pyogenic bacterium; SLE = systemic lupus erythematosus.

Modified from Johnston RB Jr. J Pediatr Infect Dis 12:933–941, 1993. Data from Figueroa JE, Densen P. Clin MIcrobiol Rev 4:359–395, 1991; and Ross SC, Densen P. Medicine 63:243–273, 1984.

In the absence of C1 inhibitor (C1 INH) function, the activation of C1 leads to uncontrolled C̄1s activity with breakdown of C4 and C2 and release of a vasoactive peptide, or kinin, from C2 (Frank, 1982; Donaldson, 1983; Gigli, 1983; Strang et al., 1988). Bradykinin is also generated during an attack (Schapira et al., 1983), presumably because C1 inhibitor also controls activity of the kallikrein system through which bradykinin is formed. Episodic, localized, typically nonpitting edema results from the vasodilatory effects of the kinins at the level of the postcapillary venule. The mechanism by which C1 is activated in these individuals is not known.

Clinical Features

Swelling of the affected part occurs rapidly, without associated urticaria, itching, discoloration, or redness, and usually without severe pain (Fig. 17–1). Intense abdominal cramping can occur, however, from swelling of the intestinal wall. Concurrent subcutaneous edema is often absent, and patients have been subjected to abdominal surgery or psychiatric examination before the proper diagnosis was made. Laryngeal edema can be fatal. Attacks last 2 or 3 days, then gradually abate. They may occur at sites of trauma, after vigorous exercise, with menses, or with emotional stress. Attacks can begin in the first 2 years of life but are usually not severe until late childhood or adolescence (Donaldson and Rosen, 1966; Frank et al., 1976; Gigli, 1983). SLE has been described in patients with congenital hereditary angioedema (Donaldson et al., 1977; Kohler et al., 1974).

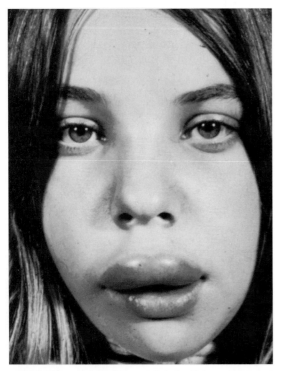

Figure 17–1. Edema of the lip associated with hereditary angioneurotic edema.

Diagnosis

During an attack of hereditary angioedema, marked depression of C4 and C2 significantly reduces the total hemolytic complement titer. In contrast to the pattern in SLE or other immune complex diseases, in hereditary angioedema, C4 is characteristically low, even between attacks, and C3 is normal. Concentrations of C1 INH can be determined with antibody, but a false-normal result can be anticipated in about 15 percent of cases. Because C1 acts as an esterase, the specific diagnosis can be made by showing increased capability of patients' sera to hydrolyze synthetic esters. When complement is activated in normal serum with aggregated IgG, C1 INH binds to C1r, reducing its antigenicity; hereditary angioedema can be diagnosed by showing persistence of C1r antigen after complement (C1) activation (Ziccardi and Cooper, 1980).

Treatment

The treatment of hereditary angioedema starts with the avoidance of precipitating factors, usually trauma. Fresh plasma transfusions have been used prophylactically when trauma is unavoidable (e.g., with surgery or dental work), but this carries the potential risk from infusion of the substrate for the uncontrolled (or partially controlled), activated enzyme, namely, C4 and C2. The infusion of purified C1 inhibitor has been effective in aborting acute attacks (Gadek et al., 1980) and in long-term prophylaxis (Bork and Witzke, 1989), but this material is available only for experimental use. The semisynthetic androgen danazol, which has minimal virilizing activity, has proved useful in preventing acute episodes (Agostoni et al., 1980; Gelfand et al., 1976; Gigli, 1983; Hosea et al., 1980). The clinical improvement noted with danazol is associated with increased serum levels of normal C1 inhibitor in both forms of the disease (Frank, 1982). The mechanism by which this increase is achieved is as yet unknown.

Because of its androgenic effects, danazol is not approved or recommended for use in children. Two children with severe disease, however, ages 5 and 9, have been treated with danazol, without apparent adverse effects (Tappeiner et al., 1979; Barakat and Castaldo, 1993). Fortunately, the attacks in most children with the disease are considerably less severe than those in adults. Epinephrine, at a dose of about 0.01 ml/kg, can reduce swelling; antihistamines rarely do. Corticosteroids have not been found to be helpful. Epsilon-aminocaproic acid (EACA), an inhibitor of plasminogen activation, can be effective as a prophylactic agent. The adult dosage of 7 to 8 g daily should be scaled down for the child and kept as low as possible because side effects of EACA, especially myopathy, can be severe. The preoperative administration of EACA can prevent postoperative edema (Gigli, 1983). One injection of meperidine (Demerol) may reduce the pain of an abdominal attack. Tracheostomy should be performed without hesitation in patients with laryngeal obstruction.

Factor I Deficiency

Deficiency of factor I (formerly called C3b inactivator) was one of the first complement abnormalities to be elucidated. The first report in 1970 described the original case as having a deficiency of C3 resulting from its hypercatabolism (Alper et al., 1970a). This is, of course, precisely the case because (as described in Chapter 7), unless the C$\overline{3bBb}$ enzyme is dismantled, it continues to cleave C3 to C3b. Levels of uncleaved C3 in the serum have ranged from undetectable to about 15% of normal (Barrett and Boyle, 1984; reviewed in Figueroa and Densen, 1991; Ross and Densen, 1984; Teisner et al., 1984). Factor B is also decreased because it is consumed in the process. C3b can easily be detected on the surface of red cells, confirming the presence of unchecked activation of the alternative pathway in the circulation. Intravenous infusion of plasma or purified factor I induces a prompt rise in serum C3 concentration and in C3-dependent functions such as opsonization (Alper et al., 1970b; Barrett and Boyle, 1984). Plasma infusions carry the risk of anaphylaxis (Wahn et al., 1984) because fresh C3 in plasma is cleaved, releasing C3a.

These patients suffer the same severe infections seen in individuals with C3 deficiency—namely, recurrent skin infections, pneumonia, septicemia, and meningitis caused by pyogenic bacteria. The defect is inherited as an autosomal codominant trait, in that both parents have about half-normal levels of factor I.

Factor H Deficiency

The effects of factor H deficiency on the complement system are similar to those of factor I deficiency. Without the assistance of factor H in the dismantling of the alternative pathway C3 convertase, C$\overline{3bBb}$, there is increased cleavage of C3 in vivo so that C3 and factor B levels are markedly reduced. Systemic pyogenic bacterial infections have been common, especially those caused by meningococci (Figueroa and Densen, 1991). Glomerulonephritis, especially MPGN, has occurred in almost 50% of cases. Total hemolytic complement activity and alternative pathway activity have been low or undetectable in all patients tested.

Properdin Deficiency

Complete deficiency of properdin has been described in maternally related males from several families (Densen et al., 1985; Figueroa and Densen, 1991; Sjöholm et al., 1982; Sjöholm and Nilsson, 1985; Späth et al., 1985). The disorder is inherited as an X-linked trait; the gene is on the short arm of the X chromosome. About half of patients have had a serious pyogenic bacterial infection, most often meningococcal meningitis or meningococcemia. One quarter of reported cases have not had serious illness (Figueroa and Densen, 1991).

In contrast to the situation with deficiency of factor I or factor H, in which serum hemolytic complement activity is markedly decreased because of C3 deficiency, the classical pathway hemolytic titers have been normal in the properdin-deficient sera. Functions of the alternative pathway, however, including opsonization, have been markedly reduced, presumably because the C3 convertase that is generated is inactivated too rapidly to function efficiently. Meningococci isolated from one patient with meningococcemia were lysed poorly in patient serum until properdin was added. Immunization of the patient with meningococcal vaccine permitted normal meningococcal killing by his serum, indicating that induction of efficient classical pathway activity could circumvent deficient alternative pathway killing of that strain (Densen et al., 1987).

Deficiency of C4 Binding Protein (C4bp)

Three members of a single family were reported to have partial deficiency (about 25% of normal adult values) of serum C4bp as detected by radial immunodiffusion using specific antibody (Trapp et al., 1987). One had atypical Behçet's disease and recurrent angioedema; the other two were healthy. The in vitro conversion of serum C3 in response to classical pathway activation was accelerated in the patients' sera, as shown previously for C4bp-depleted serum.

DEFICIENCY OF SEROSAL COMPLEMENT CONTROL PROTEIN: C5a/IL-8 INHIBITOR (Familial Mediterranean Fever)

There is strong evidence to indicate that serosal fluids contain yet another complement control protein and that a genetic defect in this protein results in disease. In particular, peritoneal and synovial fluids from individuals with familial Mediterranean fever (FMF) lack a serine protease that normally destroys the chemotactic activity of C5a (Ayesh et al., 1990; Matzner et al., 1990; Matzner and Brzezinski, 1984). This C5a inhibitor can also inactivate interleukin-8 (IL-8), a second important chemotactic factor for neutrophils (Ayesh et al., 1993). Patients with FMF suffer recurrent episodes of fever in association with painful inflammation of the joints and pleural and peritoneal cavities. Thus, it appears that C5a, IL-8, or both are generated at serosal surfaces under normal conditions and that serosal fluids contain an inhibitor of these chemotactic agents that serves to prevent the inflammatory response that would otherwise ensue.

DEFICIENCY OF CELL MEMBRANE REGULATORY PROTEINS

Deficiencies in cell membrane regulatory proteins include C3b receptor deficiency, paroxysmal nocturnal hemoglobinuria, and leukocyte adhesion defect type I.

C3b Receptor (CR1) Deficiency

The receptor for C3b (complement receptor 1, CR1) on cell surface membranes assists in the disruption of

C4b-bearing or C3b-bearing immune complexes that the cell encounters in the plasma or on the surface of adjacent cells (Ross and Medof, 1985). The average number of CR1 per erythrocyte is small (mean, <2,000/cell) compared with that of circulating neutrophils, monocytes, or B lymphocytes (21,000 to 148,000/cell) (Cornacoff et al., 1983). Because of the much higher number of circulating erythrocytes than leukocytes, however, most of the CR1 in the circulation resides on erythrocytes. Erythrocytes play an important role in clearing immune complexes from the circulation, and this capability appears to depend on their expression of the CR1 receptor (Cornacoff et al., 1983). Thus, a reduction in the number of CR1 exhibited on erythrocytes could impair the disposal of circulating immune complexes and accelerate the development of tissue injury.

Patients with SLE and some of their asymptomatic family members have reduced numbers of CR1 on erythrocytes, which appears to be inherited as an autosomal codominant trait (Minota et al., 1984; Wilson et al., 1982). This deficiency could increase the individual's risk of developing immune complex disease and thereby contribute to the pathogenesis of SLE. In agreement with this concept, a primate model has shown a protective role of higher levels of erythrocyte CR1 against immune complex–mediated glomerulonephritis (Hebert et al., 1991a). The congenital nature of the CR1 deficiency in SLE is difficult to detect because in SLE a secondary deficiency can be caused by accelerated catabolism of CR1 in association with complement activation at the cell surface (Pascual et al., 1993; Ross et al., 1985) or by autoantibody to CR1 (Wilson et al., 1985). Renal glomerular epithelial cells (podocytes) normally secrete a CR1 in the urine that can bind C3b-coated erythrocytes; CR1 antigen is lost from podocytes and the secretion of urinary CR1 is decreased in SLE with severe proliferative nephritis (Pascual et al., 1994).

Paroxysmal Nocturnal Hemoglobinuria

Membrane-bound complement control proteins serve to protect host cells, especially erythrocytes, against complement lysis that might otherwise occur when complement is activated by physiologic or inflammatory conditions. That is, a small amount of C3b can be deposited on erythrocyte membranes under normal physiologic conditions or in an area of inflammation. This C3b can trigger activation of the alternative pathway if left unopposed. Similarly, the terminal complement components, as a membrane attack complex, can attach to bystander cells in an area of inflammation. Three of the membrane complement control proteins—CR1, membrane cofactor protein, and decay accelerating factor (DAF, CD55)—prevent the formation of the full C3-cleaving enzyme, $C\overline{3bBb}$, that is triggered by C3b deposition. The other two, membrane inhibitor of reactive lysis (MIRL, CD59) and C8 binding protein (C8bp, homologous restriction factor), prevent the full development of the membrane

attack complex that creates the hole (Lachmann, 1991).

Paroxysmal nocturnal hemoglobinuria (PNH) is a hemolytic anemia that occurs when DAF, CD59, and C8bp are not expressed on the erythrocyte surface (Rosse, 1990). The condition is acquired as a somatic mutation in a hematopoietic stem cell; granulocytes, monocytes, lymphocytes, and platelets share the defective expression of these three (and other) membrane proteins. This abnormality is caused by a mutation in the PIG-A gene on the X chromosome, whose product is required for the normal synthesis of a glycosyl-phosphatidylinositol molecule that anchors at least 40 proteins to the cell membrane, including DAF, CD59, and C8bp (Bessler et al., 1994a, 1994b; Miyata et al., 1994).

One patient with genetic isolated CD59 deficiency had a mild PNH-like disease in spite of the normal expression of membrane DAF (Yamashina et al., 1990). One part of the DAF molecule is an antigenic epitope that is identified as the Cromer blood group. Rare individuals who are Cromer-negative (known as the Inab phenotype) lack erythrocyte DAF, but in contrast to the individual with CD59 deficiency, isolated DAF deficiency has not resulted in hemolytic anemia (Holguin et al., 1992).

Because of the potent capability of CR1 to regulate complement activation through either pathway, a soluble form of the molecule (sCR1) is being studied as a possible means of suppressing inflammation. Impressive reductions have been reported in inflammatory end points in animal models of various conditions, including myocardial infarction, rejection of tissue grafts, ischemia-reperfusion injury, burns, immune complex vasculitis, and adult respiratory distress syndrome (reviewed in Johnston, 1993; Tomlinson, 1993). Human recombinant soluble DAF, which lacks the glycophospholipid anchor of the native molecule, appears to have similar properties (Moran et al., 1992).

DEFECTS OF CELL MEMBRANE RECEPTORS FOR COMPLEMENT PROTEINS

Plasma membranes of inflammatory leukocytes express at least eight receptors for complement components or their products (Ghebrehiwet et al., 1994; Johnston, 1993). These receptors permit expression of the biologic activity of the complement system but do not influence complement activation (with the exception of CR1, which serves both functions; see earlier). CR1 and CR3 on phagocytes promote the uptake of C3-coated microorganisms in vitro and presumably in vivo. CR3 plays an additional critical role in allowing phagocytes to migrate out of the blood stream into sites of inflammation.

Deficient surface expression of the entire CR3 molecule presents as leukocyte adhesion defect type I, a syndrome of recurrent infections beneath the skin and in the mouth (see Chapters 14 and 15).

An isolated patient has also been described with a presumably genetic defect only in the iC3b binding epitope on CR3 (Witte et al., 1993). He had SLE and defective phagocytosis of C3-opsonized bacteria in vitro but no history of recurrent infections.

SECONDARY COMPLEMENT DISORDERS ASSOCIATED WITH INCREASED ACTIVATION

A large number of conditions exists in which partial deficiency of one or more complement components has been caused by an underlying disease process that leads to consumption of complement, decreased synthesis, or (rarely) both (Table 17–3). In many of these conditions, activation of complement is an integral component of the pathogenesis of the disease state (Eichenfield and Johnston, 1989).

Secondary complement disorders characterized by increased activation and consumption of complement are described next.

Chronic Hypocomplementemic Nephritis with Autoantibody to Complement Proteins

Depression of serum complement is a common feature of many types of acute nephritis (Hebert et al., 1991b). In these acute disorders, complement levels return to normal as the nephritis subsides. In some patients, however, particularly those with membrano-proliferative glomerulonephritis, low complement levels, especially low C3, persist (Gotoff et al., 1965; West et al., 1965). In 1969, a factor was described in some of these patients that accelerated the cleavage of C3 in serum (Spitzer et al., 1969). The factor was termed *C3 nephritic factor* (see Chapter 25). It was subsequently

---

Table 17–3. Secondary Disorders of Complement

DISORDERS CAUSED PRIMARILY BY ACTIVATION AND CONSUMPTION
  Chronic hypocomplementemic nephritis with autoantibody to
    complement proteins
  Partial lipodystrophy
  Hypocomplementemic nephritis with inhibitor to factor H
  Immune complex diseases
  Infection
  Thermal injury
  Adult respiratory distress syndrome
  Postperfusion, dialysis, and leukapheresis syndromes
  Acute pancreatitis
  Atheroembolic disease
  Reaction to radiographic contrast media
  Sickle cell disease, β thalassemia major, and splenectomy
  C1 inhibitor deficiency with B-cell lymphoproliferative disorder or
    autoantibody
  Hypocomplementemic vasculitis syndrome
  Porphyria
DEFICIENCIES CAUSED PRIMARILY BY DECREASED SYNTHESIS OR INCREASED
  CATABOLISM
  The newborn state
  Malnutrition and anorexia nervosa
  Liver cirrhosis
  Hepatic failure
  Reye syndrome
  Increased C1q catabolism with hypogammaglobulinemia
  Nephrotic syndrome
DECREASED ALTERNATIVE PATHWAY FUNCTION ASSOCIATED WITH
  HYPOGAMMAGLOBULINEMIA

---

found that the activity of this factor also requires factor B and factor D and thus appears to act through the alternative pathway. This nephritic factor of the alternative pathway has been identified as an autoantibody to the alternative pathway C3 convertase, $\overline{C3bBb}$ (Davis et al., 1977; Kim et al., 1978), which acts to stabilize the enzyme and allow the persistent cleavage of C3 through suppression of the decay-promoting activity of factor H.

A nephritic factor that binds to the classical pathway convertase, $\overline{C4b2a}$, has been described in patients with acute postinfectious glomerulonephritis or SLE. This factor is also an autoantibody of the IgG class that markedly prolongs the half-life of the convertase (Halbwachs et al., 1980). Autoantibodies to other new antigens formed during complement activation can be detected commonly in patients with various types of MPGN (Strife et al., 1990).

The mechanism by which nephritic factor is formed as an autoantibody is uncertain (Spitzer et al., 1990). The significance of nephritic factor–mediated hypocomplementemia is clear, however. First, by permitting prolonged activation of the complement system it may enhance tissue injury. Second, if the process is severe enough, C3 can be markedly decreased, which increases the host's susceptibility to infection. Pyogenic infections, including meningitis, have occurred in these patients when the C3 level has been reduced to below about 10% of normal (Edwards et al., 1983a; Thompson et al., 1983; Wahn et al., 1987).

Partial Lipodystrophy

Nephritic factor has been demonstrated in patients with partial lipodystrophy who have not had nephritis. In this disorder, there is loss of fat from the face and upper body which is often acute and follows a viral infection. Of the 21 individuals with partial lipodystrophy reviewed in one study, 17 had depressed levels of C3 with normal levels of C4 and C2. Most of these 17 patients had detectable nephritic factor, and although 10 were clinically well, 7 had overt nephritis, especially MPGN (Sissons et al., 1976). The relationship can be explained by the observation that adipocytes can produce C3, factor D, and factor B and can activate the alternative pathway (Choy et al., 1992). The addition of sera containing nephritic factor to adipocytes induces their lysis (Mathieson et al., 1993).

Hypocomplementemic Nephritis with Inhibitor of Factor H

The importance of factor H in restraining the uncontrolled conversion of C3 has been illustrated by an experiment of nature. Meri and colleagues (1992) described a patient who had a circulating monoclonal dimer of immunoglobulin light chains that reacted directly with factor H. When added to normal serum, the patient's serum induced almost complete consumption of the normal C3. The patient had hypocomplementemic MPGN, emphasizing the important role that complement can play in the pathogenesis of renal injury.

Immune Complex Diseases

Immune complexes can induce the consumption of complement components. Activation generally occurs through the fixation of C1q to antibody and thus primarily involves the classical pathway. Circulating immune complexes are a common feature of autoimmune diseases, with SLE being the prototype. Complement fixation to these complexes potentiates their clearance from the circulation. This can result in tissue deposition, most notably in the kidney and skin (common sites of injury in these disorders), and the degree of complement depletion often parallels disease activity. Complement abnormalities are most pronounced in patients with SLE who have active renal disease (Schur, 1975). In these patients, serum levels of C1q, C4, C2, and C3 are decreased. Decreased levels of factor B have also been observed. C1q, C4, and C3 can be frequently detected in the kidney by immunofluorescence; the deposition of late-acting components can also be seen (Biesecker et al., 1982). Evidence for complex-induced complement activation in rheumatoid arthritis has also been presented (Miller et al., 1986; Nydegger et al., 1977).

Immune complex formation and hypocomplementemia have been observed in a variety of other conditions, including subacute bacterial endocarditis, infected ventriculojugular shunts, infectious mononucleosis, acute viral hepatitis and hepatitis B, Felty's syndrome, serum sickness, primary biliary cirrhosis, and lepromatous leprosy (Alpert et al., 1971; Breedveld et al., 1987; Dobrin et al., 1975; Jones et al., 1979; reviewed in Lachmann and Peters, 1982; Lawley et al., 1984; Perrin et al., 1973). Nephritis or arthritis may develop in these infections as a result of immune complex deposition and complement activation. Circulating immune complexes and decreased C3 have also been reported in both dermatitis herpetiformis and celiac disease (Mohammed et al., 1976).

Infection

In addition to the consumption of early complement components by microbial agents that have interacted with antibody, infections can activate complement in the absence of demonstrable immune complex formation. In patients with gram-negative bacteremia and shock, the bacteria, endotoxin, or both initiate direct activation of the alternative pathway and consumption of C3 (Fearon et al., 1975; Kalter et al., 1985). Gram-negative bacteremia without shock can activate the complement system, but component levels may not be seriously depleted (Fearon et al., 1975; Kalter et al., 1985; Palestine and Klemperer, 1976). Activation of the alternative pathway and complement depletion can be associated with cryptococcal septicemia (Macher et al., 1978), pneumococcal pneumonia (Reed et al., 1976), acquired immunodeficiency syndrome (Tausk et al., 1986), or typhoid fever (Mayes et al., 1984).

Certain viruses can activate the alternative pathway in vitro (McSharry et al., 1981), and complement activation appears to play a role in the pathogenesis of the viral-induced syndromes of dengue hemorrhagic shock (Bokisch et al., 1973) and Argentine hemorrhagic fever (de Bracco et al., 1978). Substantial decreases in C1, C4, and C2 have been found in association with malarial paroxysms (Neva et al., 1974). Studies with an animal model suggest that complement depletion secondary to a localized infection may predispose to infection elsewhere (White et al., 1986).

Microorganisms have evolved various means of countering the antimicrobial effects of the complement system, and one consists of destroying the chemotactic capability of C5a. Group A *Streptococcus pyogenes* (reviewed in O'Connor et al., 1991) and group B streptococci (Hill et al., 1988; Bohnsack et al., 1991) express a surface peptidase that cleaves and inactivates C5a. This peptidase activity could be involved in the pathogenesis of impetigo and in the poor inflammatory response characteristic of localized group B streptococcal infection.

Thermal Injury and Adult Respiratory Distress Syndrome

Thermal burns can induce massive activation of the complement system, especially the alternative pathway, within a few hours after injury (reviewed in Gelfand et al., 1982; Davis et al., 1987). Generation of C3a and C5a occurs, which stimulates neutrophils to aggregate and become sequestered in the lung (Hammerschmidt et al., 1980; Till and Ward, 1986). These events probably play an important part in the development of adult respiratory distress syndrome after burn injury (Till and Ward, 1986). The released C3a and C5a may also induce neutrophil degranulation and depress neutrophil chemotaxis (Davis et al., 1980). These effects and depressed opsonization resulting from complement deficiency undoubtedly contribute to the severe predisposition to infection that exists after burn injury (Gelfand et al., 1982). Studies support complement activation and pulmonary granulocyte entrapment as having a pathogenic role in adult respiratory distress syndrome that results from insults other than burns, including sepsis and severe trauma (Hallgreen et al., 1987; Hammerschmidt et al., 1980; Hammerschmidt, 1986; Sprung et al., 1986; Zilow et al., 1986, 1990).

Postperfusion, Dialysis, and Leukapheresis Syndromes

The use of pump-oxygenator systems in open heart surgery has been associated with a systemic inflammation-like reaction characterized by increased capillary permeability, accumulation of interstitial fluid, fever, and profound dysfunction of the lungs, kidneys, and central nervous system. This reaction has been termed *postperfusion syndrome*. A similar syndrome can occur in individuals undergoing renal dialysis with cellophane membrane dialyzers or in patients subjected to nylon fiber filtration leukapheresis. In each of these situations, complement is activated by the procedure and complement-derived products, especially the anaphylatoxin C3a, can be detected in plasma (Chenowith et al., 1981; Hakim et al., 1984; Hammerschmidt et al., 1978; Nusbacher et al., 1978; Salama et al., 1988). Leukopenia and hemolysis are common, and the membrane attack complex (C5b~9) can be identified in the membranes of lysed erythrocytes (Salama et al., 1988).

Acute Pancreatitis, Atheroembolic Disease, and Reaction to Radiographic Contrast Media

In some patients with acute pancreatitis, respiratory distress syndrome develops. Profound complement activation can accompany pancreatitis, and complement split products have been implicated in the development of pulmonary sequelae (reviewed in Horn et al., 1980). Atheroembolic disease can be associated with hypocomplementemia (Cosio et al., 1985), perhaps because of the activity of enzymes of the coagulation system. The intravenous injection of iodinated radiographic contrast medium can induce a rapid and significant cleavage of C3, perhaps through the alternative pathway, which could explain at least some of the reactions that occur in 5% to 8% of individuals who undergo this procedure (Arroyave and Tan, 1977; Kolb et al., 1978; Von Zabern et al., 1983). Nonionic contrast media can inactivate C2 and activate the alternative pathway by interfering with factors I and H (Von Zabern et al., 1984).

Sickle Cell Disease, β Thalassemia Major, and Splenectomy

Sera from some patients with sickle cell disease have been found to opsonize pneumococci normally through the antibody-dependent classical pathway but abnormally through the alternative pathway (Johnston et al., 1973; Winkelstein and Drachman, 1968), and 10% to 25% of individuals with splenectomy, sickle cell disease, or β thalassemia major have normal classical pathway activity but defective alternative pathway activity as measured by the hemolysis of rabbit erythrocytes (Corry et al., 1979, 1981). Levels of C3 can be decreased in patients' sera (DeCeulaer et al., 1986). Other studies have suggested that the complement deficiency of sickle cell disease is the result of activation of complement within the circulation (Chudwin et al., 1985; DeCeulaer et al., 1981; Larcher et al., 1982; reviewed in Wilson, 1983; Wang et al., 1993). Hemoglobin (DeCeulaer et al., 1981; Wilson, 1983) was proposed as an activating stimulus, but it is now clear that membranes serve that role (Poskitt et al., 1973; Wang et al., 1993). The deoxygenation of erythrocytes from patients with sickle cell disease alters their membrane to increase the exposure of phosphatidyl ethanolamine and phosphatidyl serine on the outer leaflet. Erythrocytes altered in this way activate the alternative pathway, consuming its constituents and fixing C3 onto the membrane surface (Wang et al., 1993). The cause of the alternative pathway abnormality in β thalassemia or after splenectomy is not known.

C1 Inhibitor Deficiency with B-Cell Lymphoproliferative Disorder or Autoantibody

Acquired C1 INH deficiency has been detected in a small percentage of patients with B-cell lymphoproliferative disorders, including B-cell lymphosarcoma, chronic lymphocytic leukemia, macroglobulinemia, multiple myeloma, and cryoglobulinemia (Sheffer et al., 1985). The condition presents as late-onset recurrent angioedema; it can be differentiated from hereditary angioedema by the presence of markedly decreased levels of C1q, in addition to decreased C1 INH and C4. Because some patients have had a malignant B-cell clone that produces IgA, which cannot fix complement, it has seemed unlikely that the monoclonal immunoglobulin present on the surface of the neoplastic B cells and secreted into the serum is responsible for the consumption of C1 and C1 INH. Four patients have been identified, however, who had circulating anti-idiotypic antibody to the monoclonal immunoglobulin expressed by their malignancy (Geha et al., 1985). The interaction between the anti-idiotypic antibody and the patient's monoclonal immunoglobulin, then, might be responsible for the increased consumption of C1q and the consequent consumption of C1 INH. Individuals with acquired angioedema but no malignancy may have an autoantibody to normal C1 INH that blocks its function (reviewed in Mandle et al., 1994).

Hypocomplementemic Vasculitis Syndrome

A syndrome has been described in both adults and children of recurrent urticaria and angioedema, vasculitis with deposition of immunoglobulin and complement in the vessel wall, and depression of C1 through C5, especially C1q, but normal levels of C1 INH (reviewed in Marder et al., 1984; Waldo et al., 1985). About half the patients have had mild nephritis, often MPGN. The syndrome cannot be attributed to circulating immune complexes, and its pathogenesis is presently obscure. Corticosteroid treatment has been effective in some cases (Geha and Akl, 1976).

Porphyria

In patients with erythropoietic protoporphyria or porphyria cutanea tarda, exposure of the skin to light of certain wave lengths activates complement, generating C5-derived chemotactic activity and reduced levels of serum C3 and C5 (Lim et al., 1984). Phototoxicity is associated histologically with lysis of capillary endothelial cells, mast cell degranulation, and the appearance of neutrophils in the dermis (Lim et al., 1981), all changes that can result from complement activation.

SECONDARY COMPLEMENT DISORDERS ASSOCIATED WITH DECREASED SYNTHESIS OR INCREASED CATABOLISM

Some secondary complement disorders may result from the decreased synthesis or increased catabolism of complement.

The Newborn

Cord serum was reported to show subnormal complement activity in 1927 (Nattan-Larrier et al., 1927). All studies published since then have confirmed this finding, although the extent of the reported abnormality has varied. In earlier studies, comparisons were made with maternal values; however, it was subsequently appreciated that complement levels are elevated during normal pregnancy. Even when normal adult values are used as standards, though, the newborn state is the most common condition associated with complement deficiency (reviewed in Johnston et al., 1979). Activity of the classical pathway, measured as total hemolytic complement (CH_{50}), has been found to be 57% to 90% as high in term infants as in normal adults; the overall mean for 119 infants (seven studies) was 74% of the mean for adults (Johnston et al., 1979; Norman et al., 1975; Notarangelo et al., 1984; Sawyer et al., 1971; Shapiro et al., 1981; Strunk et al., 1979; Tannous et al., 1982). Values in preterm babies were even lower (58% of adult levels) (Notarangelo et al., 1984; Sawyer et al., 1971; Strunk et al., 1979; Geelen et al., 1990; Miyano et al., 1987).

The alternative pathway has been more abnormal (56% of adult mean, 85 term babies) (Adamkin et al., 1978; Johnston et al., 1979; Notarangelo et al., 1984; Shapiro et al., 1981; Strunk et al., 1979). Preterm babies had only slightly lower values (Notarangelo et al., 1984; Strunk et al., 1979). Values in babies small for gestational age were equivalent in both pathways to those in term infants (Notarangelo et al., 1984; Shapiro et al., 1981). All individual components of either pathway that have been measured have been mildly to moderately decreased (Johnston et al., 1979; Lassiter et al., 1992b; Zach and Hostetter, 1989).

In the studies that reported the percentage of babies with values significantly lower than those of normal adults, about half of babies at term had clearly subnormal activity of the classical pathway, measured by CH_{50} (Johnston et al., 1979) or by opsonization of a group B streptococcus (Edwards et al., 1983b). About 75% of term babies had clearly subnormal activity of the alternative pathway by hemolytic assay (lysis of rabbit erythrocytes) (Edwards et al., 1983b; Johnston et al., 1979); about one third of babies had decreased alternative pathway opsonization of pneumococci, endotoxin, or *Escherichia coli* (Johnston et al., 1979; Mills et al., 1979; Stossel et al., 1973). Complement-dependent bacteriolysis (Lassiter et al., 1992a) and opsonization of pneumococci (Geelen et al., 1990) have been reported to be normal in newborns (see Chapter 10).

The data that are available suggest that complement component levels reach the adult range by 3 to 6 months of age, with the exception of C1q and properdin, which can be low until the child is 12 to 18 months of age (Davis et al., 1979; Fireman et al., 1969).

However the data are analyzed, the newborn infant displays a deficiency in complement function relative to a normal adult. The degree of deficiency is such that it probably would not predispose a normal adult to infection. It seems likely, however, that the deficiency of multiple components and of both pathways found in neonates, especially in conjunction with the decreased phagocyte function known to exist in this population, does increase their likelihood of serious infection. In the presence of high levels of transferred maternal antibody, the relatively mild deficiency of classical pathway function might not be detrimental. In the absence of such antibody, however, the alternative pathway probably would offer inadequate protection against a large inoculum of microorganisms in a majority of newborn infants (Zilow et al., 1993). With this configuration of abnormalities, infections caused by extracellular bacteria would be predicted and, in fact, these organisms are particularly troublesome to the neonate. These considerations, though, remain to be proven.

Malnutrition and Anorexia Nervosa

In patients with malnutrition or anorexia nervosa, there may be significant depletion of components and decreased functional activity of complement (reviewed in Keusch et al., 1984; Kim and Michael, 1975; Sirisinha et al., 1977; Suskind et al., 1976). Both classical and alternative pathways can be deficient (see Chapter 19). Although the synthesis of components is depressed in these conditions, sera from some patients with malnutrition also appear to contain immune complexes and endotoxin, which could accelerate depletion (Klein et al., 1977; Suskind et al., 1976).

Liver Cirrhosis, Hepatic Failure, and Reye Syndrome

Severe chronic cirrhosis of the liver or fulminant hepatic failure can result in decreased complement levels, especially decreased C3 (Larcher et al., 1983, 1985; Le Prévost et al., 1975; Petz, 1971). Decreased synthesis of C3 has been documented in some patients. Individuals with Reye syndrome can have marked deficiency of complement components (Marder et al., 1981; Pickering et al., 1979). Some of these patients have circulating immune complexes, and deficiency may be due, at least in part, to activation and consumption. In the majority, however, low levels, at least of C3, might be better explained by decreased synthesis of the control proteins factors H and I, with consequent consumption of C3 (Marder et al., 1981).

Increased C1q Catabolism Associated with Hypogammaglobulinemia

In patients with hypogammaglobulinemia, there is a variable decrease in serum concentrations of C1q that is proportional to the decrease in IgG (reviewed by Atkinson et al., 1978; Kohler and Müller-Eberhard, 1972). The deficiency can be corrected by infusion of IgG, in agreement with the concept that weak, reversible interactions between C1q and IgG protect C1q from hypercatabolism.

Nephrotic Syndrome

Children with nephrotic syndrome are at increased risk for serious bacterial infection (see Chapters 19 and 25). Serum levels of C3, C4, and properdin have been slightly decreased or normal in these children; but factor B has been commonly deficient, and this deficiency has been associated with defective opsonization of *Escherichia coli* or zymosan (McLean et al., 1977; Anderson et al., 1979). In one study, there was a highly positive correlation ($r = .8$) between serum factor B and serum albumin concentrations, suggesting that factor B (molecular weight, 100 kD) was being lost in the urine (McLean et al., 1977). Similarly, factor D (molecular weight, 25 kD) normally is reabsorbed in the proximal tubule, and tubular dysfunction leads to renal losses (Kölble and Reid, 1993).

ALTERNATIVE PATHWAY DYSFUNCTION WITH HYPOGAMMAGLOBULINEMIA

The alternative complement pathway can be activated in the absence of specific antibody by a variety of surfaces that provide a microenvironment in which the alternative pathway C3 convertase is relatively protected against inactivation. A large body of experimental data has indicated that antibody to the surface can enhance alternative pathway activation (reviewed in Fries et al., 1984; Ratnoff et al., 1983). Sera from patients with hypogammaglobulinemia function defectively in the alternative pathway (Corry et al., 1979; Polhill et al., 1978a), and this defect disappears when the patient is given immunoglobulin replacement therapy (Polhill et al., 1978a).

DIAGNOSIS OF COMPLEMENT DISORDERS

The techniques available for study of the complement system have been described in detail in Chapter 7. It should only be emphasized that testing for total hemolytic complement (CH_{50}) serves as a useful screening procedure for most of the complement disorders (see Chapter 9). This assay depends on the ability of all nine components of the classical pathway to interact and lyse antibody-coated sheep erythrocytes. The dilution of serum that lyses 50% of the cells determines the end point, or CH_{50} value. This value is 0 (or essentially so) in deficiencies of C1 through C8. As noted, a deficiency of C9 results in a CH_{50} value 30% to 50% of normal. Values in the acquired deficiencies vary with the severity of the underlying disorder.

Deficiency of the serum control proteins factor I or factor H permits consumption of C3, with partial reduc-

tion in the CH_{50} value. The CH_{50} assay, however, is not able to detect deficiency of factors B or D or properdin. Alternative pathway activity can be measured with a hemolytic assay that depends on the capability of rabbit erythrocytes to serve as both an activating (permissive) surface and a target of alternative pathway activity (see Chapter 7; Polhill et al., 1978b).

The indications for studying complement activity (i.e., for obtaining a serum CH_{50} value as a screening test) are presented in Table 17–4. The bases for these indications have been discussed here in detail. The indications given are conservative, and the list may be expanded in the future. Table 17–4 illustrates why the hemolytic complement assay should be available as a screening test to every physician.

MANAGEMENT OF COMPLEMENT DISORDERS

Treatment of the acquired disorders of the complement systems depends on control of the underlying disease. Specific therapy for the hereditary deficiencies of complement does not presently exist. Careful management, however, could make a major impact on the health and survival of the patient. For example, knowledge that an individual has a genetic deficiency of a complement component can alert the physician to the threat of a rapidly developing systemic bacterial infection. If the physician knows that a complement component, especially C2, C3, C5, C6, C7, C8, properdin, factor H, or factor I, is absent in a patient, cultures can be obtained more vigorously and fever of unknown origin treated more quickly with antibiotics. An antipneumococcal drug might be included in the case of C2 deficiency, or an antineisserial drug might be used in the case of deficiency of a late-acting component or properdin. Long-term penicillin therapy might be considered when meningococcal disease is endemic and for patients with a history of previous severe infections (Potter et al., 1990).

The patient and close household contacts should be

Table 17–4. Indications for Studying Complement Activity*

DEFINITE INDICATIONS
  Systemic lupus erythematosus (SLE)
  Recurrent pyogenic infections
  Second episode of bacteremia at any age
  Second episode of meningococcal meningitis or gonococcal arthritis
  Chronic nephritis, especially membranoproliferative glomerulonephritis
  Recurrent angioedema without urticaria
  Partial lipodystrophy
PROBABLE INDICATIONS
  Nonepidemic meningococcal meningitis in an adolescent or young adult
  Disseminated gonococcal infection
  Pneumococcal bacteremia after infancy
  Other chronic immune complex disease or vasculitis syndrome
  Recurrent angioedema with urticaria

*The list is conservative, and additional indications may exist in individual patients.

immunized with vaccines for pneumococci, *Haemophilus influenzae,* and *Neisseria meningitidis.* High titers of specific antibody might opsonize these organisms well enough to prevent dissemination of at least small numbers of invading organisms, and immunization of household members could decrease infections and, perhaps, the nasopharyngeal carriage of these bacteria in people with whom the patient has regular contact. In the case of a defect in C1, C4, or C2, increased antibody can facilitate fixation of C3 through the alternative pathway (Polhill et al., 1978a). In the case of properdin deficiency, the presence of specific antibody facilitates efficient activation of the classical pathway by meningococci; bacteriolysis occurs rapidly, circumventing a need for the alternative pathway and properdin (Figueroa and Densen, 1991).

Knowing that deficiency of an early-acting component exists can alert the physician to the possible development of collagen-vascular disease, which could permit earlier diagnosis. Hemizygous carriers of C2 deficiency could be sought, because they appear to have an increased likelihood of having a rheumatic disease. Other family members should be studied in the case of any genetic complement deficiency, and genetic counseling can be offered as indicated.

References

Adamkin D, Stitzel A, Urmson J, Farnett ML, Post E, Spitzer R. Activity of the alternative pathway of complement in the newborn infant. J Pediatr 93:604–608, 1978.

Adams EM, Hustead S, Rubin P, Wagner R, Gewurz A, Graziano FM. Absence of the seventh component of complement in a patient with chronic meningococcemia presenting as vasculitis. Ann Intern Med 99:35–38, 1983.

Agnello V, Gell J, Tye MJ. Partial genetic deficiency of the C4 component of complement in discoid lupus erythematosus and urticaria/angioedema. J Am Acad Dermatol 9:894–898, 1983.

Agostoni A, Cicardi M, Martignoni C, Bergamaschini L, Marasini B. Danazol and stanozolol in long-term prophylactic treatment of hereditary angioedema. J Allergy Clin Immunol 65:75–79, 1980.

Alper CA, Abramson N, Johnston RB Jr, Jandl JH, Rosen FS. Increased susceptibility to infection associated with abnormalities of complement-mediated functions and of the third component of complement (C3). N Engl J Med 282:350–354, 1970a.

Alper CA, Abramson N, Johnston RB Jr, Jandl JH, Rosen FS. Studies in vivo and in vitro on an abnormality in the metabolism of C3 in a patient with increased susceptibility to infection. J Clin Invest 49:1975–1985, 1970b.

Alper CA, Rosen FS. Inherited deficiencies of complement proteins in man. Springer Semin Immunopathol 7:251–261, 1984.

Alpert E, Isselbacher KJ, Schur PH. The pathogenesis of arthritis associated with viral hepatitis: complement-component studies. N Engl J Med 285:185–189, 1971.

Anderson DC, York TL, Rose G, Smith CW. Assessment of serum factor B, serum opsonins, granulocyte chemotaxis, and infection in nephrotic syndrome of children. J Infect Dis 140:1–11, 1979.

Arroyave CM, Levy RM, Johnson JS. Genetic deficiency of the fourth component of complement (C4) in Wistar rats. Immunology 33:453–459, 1977.

Arroyave CM, Tan EM. Mechanism of complement activation by radiographic contrast media. Clin Exp Immunol 29:89–94, 1977.

Atkinson JP, Fisher RI, Reinhardt R, Frank MM. Reduced concentrations of the first component of complement in hypogammaglobulinemia: correction by infusion of γ-globulin. Clin Immunol Immunopathol 9:350–355, 1978.

Ayesh SK, Ferne M, Flechner I, Babior BM, Matzner Y. Partial characterization of a C5a-inhibitor in peritoneal fluid. J Immunol 144:3066–3070, 1990.

Ayesh SK, Azar Y, Babior BM, Matzner Y. Inactivation of interleukin-8 by C5a-inactivating protease from serosal fluid. Blood 81:1424–1427, 1993.

Barakat A, Castaldo AJ. Hereditary angioedema: danazol therapy in a 5-year-old child (letter). Am J Dis Child 147:931–932, 1993.

Barba G, Rittner C, Schneider PM. Genetic basis of human complement C4A deficiency: detection of a point mutation leading to nonexpression. J Clin Invest 91:1681–1686, 1993.

Barrett DJ, Boyle MDP. Restoration of complement function in vivo by plasma infusion in factor I (C3b inactivator) deficiency. J Pediatr 104:76–81, 1984.

Berkel AI, Loos M, Sanal Ö, Ersoy F, Yegin O. Selective complete C1q deficiency: report of two new cases. Immunol Lett 2:263–267, 1981.

Berkel AI, Loos M, Sanal Ö, Mauff G, Güngen Y, Örs Ü, Ersoy F, Yegin O. Clinical and immunological studies in a case of selective complete C1q deficiency. Clin Exp Immunol 38:52–63, 1979.

Bessler M, Mason P, Hillmen P, Luzzatto L. Somatic mutations and cellular selection in paroxysmal nocturnal haemoglobinuria. Lancet 343:951–953, 1994a.

Bessler M, Mason PJ, Hillmen P, Miyata T, Yamada N, Takeda J, Luzzatto L, Kinoshita T. Paroxysmal nocturnal haemoglobinuria (PNH) is caused by somatic mutations in the PIG-A gene. EMBO J 13:110–117, 1994b.

Biesecker G, Lavin L, Ziskind M, Koffler D. Cutaneous localization of the membrane attack complex in discoid and systemic lupus erythematosus. N Engl J Med 306:264–270, 1982.

Bishof NA, Welch TR, Beischel LS. C4B deficiency: a risk factor for bacteremia with encapsulated organisms. J Infect Dis 162:248–250, 1990.

Bitter-Suermann D, Hoffmann T, Burger R, Hadding U. Linkage of total deficiency of the second component (C2) of the complement system and of genetic C2-polymorphism to the major histocompatibility complex of the guinea pig. J Immunol 127:608–612, 1981.

Bohnsack JF, Zhou X, Williams PA, Cleary PP, Parker CJ, Hill HR. Purification of the proteinase from Group B streptococci that inactivates human C5a. Biochim Biophys Acta 1079:222–228, 1991.

Bokisch VA, Top FH, Russell PK, Dixon FJ, Müller-Eberhard HJ. The potential pathogenic role of complement in dengue hemorrhagic shock syndrome. N Engl J Med 289:996–1000, 1973.

Bork K, Witzke G. Long-term prophylaxis with C1-inhibitor (C1 INH) concentrate in patients with recurrent angioedema caused by hereditary and acquired C1-inhibitor deficiency. J Allergy Clin Immunol 83:677–682, 1989.

Borzy MS, Wolff L, Gewurz A, Buist NRM, Lovrein E. Recurrent sepsis with deficiencies of C2 and galactokinase. Am J Dis Childh 138:186–191, 1984.

Breedveld FC, Fibbe WE, Hermans J, Van der Meer JW, Cats A. Factors influencing the incidence of infections in Felty's syndrome. Arch Intern Med 147:915–920, 1987.

Burdash NM, Blackburn BB, Farrar WE Jr. Meningococcal meningitis and complement (C6) deficiency. J S C Med Assoc 79:440–441, 1983.

Chapuis RM, Hauptmann G, Grosshans E, Isliker H. Structural and functional studies in C1q deficiency. J Immunol 129:1509–1512, 1982.

Chenowith DE, Cooper SW, Hugli TE, Stewart RW, Blackstone EH, Kirklin JW. Complement activation during cardiopulmonary bypass: evidence for generation of C3a and C5a anaphylatoxins. N Engl J Med 304:497–508, 1981.

Choy LN, Rosen BS, Spiegelman BA. Adipsin and an endogenous pathway of complement from adipose cells. J Biol Chem 267:12736–12741, 1992.

Chudwin DS, Korenblit AD, Kingzette M, Artrip S, Rao S. Increased activation of the alternative complement pathway in sickle cell disease. Clin Immunol Immunopathol 37:93–97, 1985.

Cinader B, Dubiski S, Wardlaw AC. Distribution, inheritance, and properties of an antigen, MUBI, and its relation to hemolytic complement. J Exp Med 120:897–924, 1964.

Coleman TH, Forristal J, Kosaka T, West CD. Inherited complement component deficiencies in membranoproliferative glomerulonephritis. Kidney Int 24:681–690, 1983.

Colten HR, Rosen FS. Complement deficiencies. Annu Rev Immunol 10:809–834, 1992.

Cornacoff JB, Hebert LA, Smead WL, VanAman ME, Birmingham

DJ, Waxman FJ. Primate erythrocyte-immune complex clearing mechanism. J Clin Invest 71:236–247, 1983.

Corry JM, Marshall WC, Guthrie LA, Peerless AG, Johnston RB Jr. Deficient activity of the alternative pathway of complement in β thalassemia major. Am J Dis Childh 135:529–531, 1981.

Corry JM, Polhill RB Jr, Edmonds SR, Johnston RB Jr. Activity of the alternative complement pathway after splenectomy: comparison to activity in sickle cell disease and hypogammaglobulinemia. J Pediatr 95:964–969, 1979.

Cosio FG, Zager RA, Sharma HM. Atheroembolic renal disease causes hypocomplementaemia. Lancet 2:118–121, 1985.

Davies KA, Erlendsson K, Beynon HLC, Peters AM, Steinsson K, Valdimarsson H, Walport MJ. Splenic uptake of immune complexes in man is complement-dependent. J Immunol 151:3866–3873, 1993.

Davis AE III, Arnaout MA, Alper CA, Rosen FS. Transfer of C3 nephritic factor from mother to fetus: is C3 nephritic factor IgG? N Engl J Med 297:144–145, 1977.

Davis CA, Vallota EH, Forristal J. Serum complement levels in infancy: age related changes. Pediatr Res 13:1043–1046, 1979.

Davis CF, Moore FD, Rodrick ML, Fearon DT, Mannick JA. Neutrophil activation after burn injury: contributions of the classic complement pathway and of endotoxin. Surgery 102:477–484, 1987.

Davis JM, Dineen P, Gallin JI. Neutrophil degranulation and abnormal chemotaxis after thermal injury. J Immunol 124:1467–1471, 1980.

Day NK, Geiger H, McLean R, Michael A, Good RA. C2 deficiency: development of lupus erythematosus. J Clin Invest 52:1601–1607, 1973.

Day NK, Good RA. The complement system in human disease. In Grieco MH, ed. Infections in the Abnormal Host. New York, Yorke Medical Books, 1980, pp. 38–67.

de Bracco MME, Rimoldi MT, Cossio PM, Rabinovich A, Maiztegui JI, Carballal G, Arana RM. Argentine hemorrhagic fever: alterations of the complement system and anti-Junin–virus humoral response. N Engl J Med 299:216–221, 1978.

DeCeulaer K, Wilson WA, Morgan AG, Serjeant GR. Plasma haemoglobin and complement activation in sickle cell disease. J Clin Lab Immunol 6:57–60, 1981.

DeCeulaer K, Forbes M, Maude GH, Pagliccua A, Serjeant GR. Complement and immunoglobulin levels in early childhood in homozygous sickle cell disease. J Clin Immunol 21:37–41, 1986.

Densen P, Weiler J, Griffiss M, Hoffmann LG. Familial properdin deficiency and fatal meningococcemia. N Engl J Med 316:922–926, 1987.

Dobrin RS, Day NK, Quie PG, Moore HL, Vernier RL, Michael AF, Fish AJ. The role of complement, immunoglobulin and bacterial antigen in coagulase-negative staphylococcal shunt nephritis. Am J Med 59:660–673, 1975.

Donaldson VH. The challenge of hereditary angioneurotic edema. N Engl J Med 308:1094–1095, 1983.

Donaldson VH, Rosen FS. Hereditary angioneurotic edema: a clinical survey. Pediatrics 37:1017–1027, 1966.

Donaldson VH, Hess EV, McAdams AJ. Lupus erythematosus–like disease in three unrelated women with hereditary angioneurotic edema. Ann Intern Med 86:312–313, 1977.

Edwards KM, Alford R, Gewurz H, Mold C. Recurrent bacterial infections associated with C3 nephritic factor and hypocomplementemia. N Engl J Med 308:1138–1141, 1983a.

Edwards MS, Buffone GJ, Fuselier PA, Weeks JL, Baker CJ. Deficient classical complement pathway activity in newborn sera. Pediatr Res 17:685–688, 1983b.

Eichenfield LF, Johnston RB Jr. Secondary disorders of the complement system. Am J Dis Child 143:595–602, 1989.

Ellison RT, Curd JG, Kohler PF, Reller LB, Judson FN. Underlying complement deficiency in a patient with disseminated gonococcal infection. Sex Transm Dis 14:201–204, 1987.

Ellison RT III, Kohler PF, Curd JG, Judson FN, Reller LB. Prevalence of congenital or acquired complement deficiency in patients with sporadic meningococcal disease. N Engl J Med 308:913–916, 1983.

Ellman L, Green I, Judge F, Frank MM. In vivo studies in C4-deficient guinea pigs. J Exp Med 134:162–175, 1971.

Fasano MB, Densen P, McLean RH, Winkelstein JA. Prevalence of homozygous C4B deficiency in patients with deficiencies of terminal complement components and meningococcemia. J Infect Dis 162:1220–1221, 1990.

Fearon DT, Ruddy S, Schur PH, McCabe WR. Activation of the properdin pathway of complement in patients with gram-negative bacteremia. N Engl J Med 292:937–940, 1975.

Fielder AHL, Walport MJ, Batchelor JR, Rynes RI, Black CM, Dodi IA, Hughes GRV. Family study of the major histocompatibility complex in patients with systemic lupus erythematosus: importance of null alleles of C4A and C4B in determining disease susceptibility. Br Med J 286:425–428, 1983.

Figueroa JE, Densen P. Infectious diseases associated with complement deficiencies. Clin Microbiol Rev 4:359–395, 1991.

Fireman P, Zuchowski DA, Taylor PM. Development of human complement system. J Immunol 103:25–31, 1969.

Frank MM. The C1 esterase inhibitor and hereditary angioedema. J Clin Immunol 2:65–68, 1982.

Frank MM, Gelfand JA, Atkinson JP. Hereditary angioedema: the clinical syndrome and its management. Ann Intern Med 84:580–593, 1976.

Fries LF, Gaither TA, Hammer CH, Frank MM. C3b covalently bound to IgG demonstrates a reduced rate of inactivation by factors H and I. J Exp Med 160:1640–1655, 1984.

Gadek JE, Hosea SW, Gelfand JA, Santaella M, Wickerhauser M, Triantaphyllopoulos DC, Frank MM. Replacement therapy in hereditary angioedema: successful treatment of acute episodes of angioedema with partly purified C1 inhibitor. N Engl J Med 302:542–546, 1980.

Garty BZ, Conley ME, Douglas SD, Kolski GB. Recurrent infections and staphylococcal liver abscess in a child with C1r deficiency. J Allergy Clin Immunol 80:631–635, 1987.

Geelen SPM, Fleer A, Bezemer AC, Gerards LJ, Rijkers GT, Verhoef J. Deficiencies in opsonic defense to pneumococci in the human newborn despite adequate levels of complement and specific IgG antibodies. Pediatr Res 27:514–518, 1990.

Geha RS, Akl KF. Skin lesions, angioedema, eosinophilia, and hypocomplementemia. J Pediatr 89:724–727, 1976.

Geha RS, Quinti I, Austen KF, Cicardi M, Sheffer A, Rosen FS. Acquired C1-inhibitor deficiency associated with anti-idiotypic antibody to monoclonal immunoglobulins. N Engl J Med 312:534–540, 1985.

Gelfand JA, Donelan M, Hawiger A, Burke JF. Alternative complement pathway activation increases mortality in a model of burn injury in mice. J Clin Invest 70:1170–1176, 1982.

Gelfand JA, Sherins RJ, Alling DW, Frank MM. Treatment of hereditary angioedema with danazol: reversal of clinical and biochemical abnormalities. N Engl J Med 295:1444–1448, 1976.

Ghebrehiwet B, Lim BL, Peerschke EIB, Willis AC, Reid KBM. Isolation, cDNA cloning, and overexpression of a 33-kD cell surface glycoprotein that binds to the globular "heads" of C1q. J Exp Med 179:1809–1821, 1994.

Gigli I. Hereditary angioneurotic edema (hereditary angioedema). In Franklin EC, ed. Clinical Immunology Update: Reviews for Physicians. New York, Elsevier, 1983, pp. 317–335.

Glass D, Raum D, Gibson D, Stillman JS, Schur PH. Inherited deficiency of the second component of complement: rheumatic disease associations. J Clin Invest 58:853–861, 1976.

Glovsky MM, Opelz G, Terasaki PI. Genetic, opsonic, and bactericidal studies in a C2 deficient family. Clin Res 24:327A, 1976.

Gotoff SP, Fellers FX, Vawter GF, Janeway CA, Rosen FS. The beta$_{1c}$ globulin in childhood nephrotic syndrome: laboratory diagnosis of progressive glomerulonephritis. N Engl J Med 273:524–529, 1965.

Hakim RM, Breillat J, Lazarus JM, Port FK. Complement activation and hypersensitivity reactions to dialysis membranes. N Engl J Med 311:878–882, 1984.

Halbwachs L, Leveillé M, Lesavre P, Wattel S, Leibowitch J. Nephritic factor of the classical pathway of complement: immunoglobulin G autoantibody directed against the classical pathway C3 convertase enzyme. J Clin Invest 65:1249–1256, 1980.

Hallgreen R, Samuelsson T, Modig J. Complement activation and increased alveolar capillary permeability after major surgery and in adult respiratory distress syndrome. Crit Care Med 15:189–193, 1987.

Hammerschmidt DE. Clinical utility of complement anaphylatoxin assays. Complement 3:166–176, 1986.

Hammerschmidt DE, Craddock PR, McCullough J, Kronenberg RS, Dalmasso AP, Jacob HS. Complement activation and pulmonary leukostasis during nylon fiber filtration leukapheresis. Blood 51:721–730, 1978.

Hammerschmidt DE, Weaver LJ, Hudson LD, Craddock PR, Jacob HS. Association of complement activation and elevated plasma-C5a with adult respiratory distress syndrome: pathophysiological relevance and possible prognostic value. Lancet 1:947–949, 1980.

Hannema AJ, Kluin-Nelemans JC, Hack CE, Eerenberg-Belmer AJM, Mallée C, van Helden HPT. SLE-like syndrome and functional deficiency of C1q in members of a large family. Clin Exp Immunol 55:106–114, 1984.

Harriman GR, Esser AF, Podack RR, Wunderlich AC, Braude AI, Lint TF, Curd JG. The role of C9 in complement-mediated killing of *Neisseria*. J Immunol 127:2386–2390, 1981.

Hauptmann G, Grosshans E, Heid LE. Lupus érythematéux aigus et déficits héréditaires en complément: a propos d'un cas par déficit complet en C4. Ann Dermatol Syphilgr 101:479–496, 1974.

Hebert LA, Cosio FG, Birmingham DJ, Mahan JD, Sharma HM, Smead WL, Goel R. Experimental immune complex-mediated glomerulonephritis in the nonhuman primate. Kidney Int 39:44–56, 1991a.

Hebert LA, Cosio FG, Neff JC. Diagnostic significance of hypocomplementemia. Kidney Int 39:811–821, 1991b.

Hiemstra PS, Langeler E, Compier B, Keepers Y, Leijh PCJ, van den Barselaar MT, Overbosch D, Daha MR. Complete and partial deficiencies of complement factor D in a Dutch family. J Clin Invest 84:1957–1961, 1989.

Hill HR, Bohnsack JF, Morris EZ, Augustine NH, Parker CJ, Cleary PP, Wu JT. Group B streptococci inhibit the chemotactic activity of the fifth component of complement. J Immunol 141:3551–3556, 1988.

Holguin MH, Martin CB, Bernshaw NJ, Parker CJ. Analysis of the effects of activation of the alternative pathway of complement on erythrocytes with an isolated deficiency of decay accelerating factor. J Immunol 148:498–502, 1992.

Horn JK, Ranson JHC, Goldstein IM, Weissler J, Curatola D, Taylor R, Perez HD. Evidence of complement catabolism in experimental acute pancreatitis. Am J Pathol 101:205–216, 1980.

Hosea SW, Santaella ML, Brown EJ, Berger M, Katusha K, Frank MM. Long-term therapy of hereditary angioedema with danazol. Ann Intern Med 93:809–812, 1980.

Hyatt AC, Altenburger KM, Johnston RB Jr, Winkelstein JA. Increased susceptibility to severe pyogenic infections in patients with an inherited deficiency of the second component of complement. J Pediatr 98:417–419, 1981.

Jackson CG, Ochs HD, Wedgwood RJ. Immune response of a patient with deficiency of the fourth component of complement and systemic lupus erythematosus. N Engl J Med 300:1124–1129, 1979.

Johnson CA, Densen P, Hurford RK Jr, Colten HR, Wetsel RA. Type I human complement C2 deficiency: a 28-base pair gene deletion causes skipping of exon 6 during RNA splicing. J Biol Chem 267:9347–9353, 1992a.

Johnson CA, Densen P, Wetsel RA, Cole FS, Goeken NE, Colten HR. Molecular heterogeneity of C2 deficiency. N Engl J Med 326:871–874, 1992b.

Johnston RB Jr. The complement system in host defense and inflammation: the cutting edges of a double-edged sword. Pediatr Infect Dis J 12:933–941, 1993.

Johnston RB Jr, Altenburger KM, Atkinson AW Jr, Curry RH. Complement in the newborn infant. Pediatrics 64(Suppl.):781–786, 1979.

Johnston RB Jr, Newman SL, Struth AG. An abnormality of the alternate pathway of complement activation in sickle-cell disease. N Engl J Med 288:803–808, 1973.

Jones EA, Frank MM, Jaffe CJ, Vierling JM. Primary biliary cirrhosis and the complement system. Ann Intern Med 90:72–84, 1979.

Kalter ES, Daha MR, ten Cate JW, Verhoef J, Bouma BN. Activation of inhibition of Hageman factor–dependent pathways and the complement system in uncomplicated bacteremia or bacterial shock. J Infect Dis 151:1019–1027, 1985.

Keusch GT, Torun B, Johnston RB Jr, Urrutia JJ. Impairment of hemolytic complement activation by both classical and alternative pathways in serum from patients with kwashiorkor. J Pediatr 105:434–436, 1984.

Keystone E, Taylor-Robinson D, Pope C, Taylor G, Furr P. Effect of inherited deficiency of the fifth component of complement on arthritis induced in mice by *Mycoplasma pulmonis*. Arthritis Rheum 21:792–797, 1978.

Kim Y, Michael AF. Hypocomplementemia in anorexia nervosa. J Pediatr 87:582–585, 1975.

Kim Y, Shvil Y, Michael AF. Hypocomplementemia in a newborn infant caused by placental transfer of C3 nephritic factor. J Pediatr 92:88–90, 1978.

Klein K, Suskind RM, Kulapongs P, Mertz G, Olson RE. Endotoxemia, a possible cause of decreased complement activity in malnourished Thai children. In Suskind RM, ed. Malnutrition and the Immune Response. New York, Raven Press, 1977, pp. 321–328.

Klemperer MR, Austen F, Rosen FS. Hereditary deficiency of the second component of complement (C'2) in man: further observations of a second kindred. J Immunol 98:72–78, 1967.

Kluin-Nelemans HC, van Velzen-Blad H, van Helden HPT, Daha MR. Functional deficiency of complement factor D in a monozygous twin. Clin Exp Immunol 58:724–730, 1984.

Kohler PF, Müller-Eberhard HJ. Metabolism of human C1q: studies in hypogammaglobulinemia, myeloma, and systemic lupus erythematosus. J Clin Invest 51:868–875, 1972.

Kohler PF, Percy J, Campion WM, Smyth CJ. Hereditary angioedema and "familial" lupus erythematosus in identical twin boys. Am J Med 56:406–411, 1974.

Kolb WP, Lang JH, Lasser EC. Nonimmunologic complement activation in normal human serum induced by radiographic contrast media. J Immunol 121:1232–1238, 1978.

Kölble K, Reid KBM. Genetic deficiencies of the complement system and association with disease—early components. Int Rev Immunol 10:17–36, 1993.

Komatsu M, Yamamoto KI, Kawashima T, Migita S. Genetic deficiency of the α-γ-subunit of the eighth complement component in the rabbit. J Immunol 134:2607–2609, 1985.

Kramer J, Rosen FS, Colten HR, Rajczy K, Strunk RC. Transinhibition of C1 inhibitor synthesis in type I hereditary angioneurotic edema. J Clin Invest 91:1258–1262, 1993.

Lachmann PJ. The control of homologous lysis. Immunol Today 12:312–315, 1991.

Lachmann PJ, Hobart MJ, Woo P. Combined genetic deficiency of C6 and C7 in man. Clin Exp Immunol 33:193–203, 1978.

Lachmann PJ, Peters DK. Complement. In Lachmann PJ, Peters DK, eds. Clinical Aspects of Immunology, 4th ed. Oxford, Blackwell, 1982, pp. 18–49.

Larcher VF, Manolaki N, Vegnente A, Vergani D, Mowat AP. Spontaneous bacterial peritonitis in children with chronic liver disease: clinical features and etiologic factors. J Pediatr 106:907–912, 1985.

Larcher VF, Wyke RJ, Davis LR, Stroud CE, Williams R. Defective yeast opsonisation and functional deficiency of complement in sickle cell disease. Arch Dis Child 57:343–346, 1982.

Larcher VF, Wycke RJ, Vergani D, Mowat AP, Williams R. Yeast opsonisation and complement in children with liver disease: analysis of 69 cases. Pediatr Res 17:296–300, 1983.

Lassiter HA, Tanner JE, Miller RD. Inefficient bacteriolysis of *Escherichia coli* by serum from human neonates. J Infect Dis 165:290–298, 1992a.

Lassiter HA, Watson SW, Seifring ML, Tanner JE. Complement factor 9 deficiency in serum of human neonates. J Infect Dis 166:53–57, 1992b.

Lawley TJ, Bielory L, Gascon P, Yancey KB, Young NS, Frank MM. A prospective clinical and immunologic analysis of patients with serum sickness. N Engl J Med 311:1407–1413, 1984.

Le Prévost C, Frommel D, Dupuy J-M. Complement studies in alpha-1 antitrypsin deficiency in children. J Pediatr 87:571–573, 1975.

Lee SL, Wallace SL, Barone R, Blum L, Chase PH. Familial deficiency of two subunits of the first component of complement. Arthritis Rheum 21:958–967, 1978.

Leggiadro RJ, Warren AB, Swift AJ, Winkelstein JR. Meningococcemia in genetically determined deficiency of the second component of complement. J Infect Dis 148:941, 1983.

Leyva-Cobián F, Moneo I, Mampaso F, Sánchez-Bayle M, Ecija JL, Bootello A. Familial C1q deficiency associated with renal and cutaneous disease. Clin Exp Immunol 44:173–180, 1981.

Lim HW, Perez HD, Poh-Fitzpatrick M, Goldstein IM, Gigli I. Generation of chemotactic activity in serum from patients with erythropoietic protoporphyria and porphyria cutanea tarda. N Engl J Med 304:212–216, 1981.

Lim HW, Poh-Fitzpatrick MB, Gigli I. Activation of the complement system in patients with porphyrias after irradiation in vivo. J Clin Invest 74:1961–1965, 1984.

Liston TE. Relapsing *Neisseria meningitidis* infection associated with C8 deficiency. Clin Pediatr (Phila) 22:605–607, 1983.

Loos M, Heinz H. Component deficiencies. I. The first component, C1q, C1r, C1s. Prog Allergy 39:212–231, 1986.

Loos M, Laurell AB, Sjöholm AG, Mårtensson U, Berkel I. Immunochemical and functional analyses of a complete C1q deficiency in man: evidence that C1r and C1s are in the native form, and that they reassociate with purified C1q to form macromolecular C1. J Immunol 124:59–63, 1980.

Macher AM, Bennett JE, Gadek JE, Frank MM. Complement depletion in cryptococcal sepsis. J Immunol 120:1686–1690, 1978.

Mandle R, Baron C, Roux E, Sundel R, Gelfand J, Aulak K, Davis AE III, Rosen FS, Bing DH. Acquired C1 inhibitor deficiency as a result of an autoantibody to the reactive center region of C1 inhibitor. J Immunol 152:4680–4685, 1994.

Marder HK, Strife CF, Forristal J, Partin J, Partin J. Hypocomplementemia in Reye syndrome: relationship to disease stage, circulating immune complexes, and C3b amplification loop protein synthesis. Pediatr Res 15:362–365, 1981.

Marder RJ, Potempa LA, Jones JV, Toriumi D, Schmid FR, Gewurz H. Assay, purification and further characterization of 7S C1q-precipitins (C1q-p) in hypocomplementemic vasculitis, urticaria syndrome and systemic lupus erythematosus. Acta Pathol Microbiol Immunol Scand (Suppl.) 284:25–34, 1984.

Mathieson PW, Würzner R, Oliveira DBG, Lachmann PJ, Peters DK. Complement-mediated adipocyte lysis by nephritic factor sera. J Exp Med 177:1827–1831, 1993.

Matzner Y, Brzezinski A. C5a-inhibitor deficiency in peritoneal fluids from patients with familial Mediterranean fever. N Engl J Med 311:287–290, 1984.

Matzner Y, Ayesh SK, Hochner-Celniker D, Ackerman Z, Ferne M. Proposed mechanism of the inflammatory attacks in familial Mediterranean fever. Arch Intern Med 150:1289–1291, 1990.

Mayes JT, Schreiber RD, Cooper NR. Development and application of an enzyme-linked immunosorbent assay for the quantitation of alternative complement pathway activation in human serum. J Clin Invest 73:160–170, 1984.

McLean RH, Forsgren A, Björkstén B, Kim Y, Quie PG, Michael AF. Decreased serum factor B concentration associated with decreased opsonization of *Escherichia coli* in the idiopathic nephrotic syndrome. Pediatr Res 11:910–916, 1977.

McLean RH, Winkelstein JA. Genetically determined variation in the complement system: relationship to disease. J Pediatr 105:179–188, 1984.

McSharry JJ, Pickering RJ, Caliguiri LA. Activation of the alternative complement pathway by enveloped viruses containing limited amounts of sialic acid. Virology 114:507–515, 1981.

Meri S, Koistinen V, Miettinen A, Törnroth T, Seppälä IJT. Activation of the alternative pathway of complement by monoclonal λ light chains in membranoproliferative glomerulonephritis. J Exp Med 175:939–950, 1992.

Merino J, Rodriquez-Valverde V, Lamelas JA, Riestra JL, Casanueva B. Prevalence of deficits of complement components in patients with recurrent meningococcal infections. J Infect Dis 148:331, 1983.

Miller JJ III, Olds LC, Silverman ED, Milgrom H, Curd JG. Different patterns of C3 and C4 activation in the varied types of juvenile arthritis. Pediatr Res 20:1332–1337, 1986.

Mills EL, Björkstén B, Quie PG. Deficient alternative complement pathway activity in newborn sera. Pediatr Res 13:1341–1344, 1979.

Minota S, Terai C, Nojima Y, Takano K, Takai E, Miyakawa Y, Takaku F. Low C3b receptor reactivity on erythrocytes from patients with systemic lupus erythematosus detected by immune adherence hemagglutination and radioimmunoassays with monoclonal antibody. Arthritis Rheum 27:1329–1335, 1984.

Minta JO, Winkler CJ, Biggar WD, Greenberg M. A selective and complete absence of C1q in a patient with vasculitis and nephritis. Clin Immunol Immunopathol 22:225–237, 1982.

Miyano A, Nakayama M, Fujita T, Kitajima H, Imai S, Shimizu A. Complement activation in fetuses: assessment by the levels of complement components and split products in cord blood. Diagn Clin Immunol 5:86–90, 1987.

Miyata T, Yamada N, Iida Y, Nishimura J, Takeda J, Kitani T, Kinoshita T. Abnormalities of PIG-A transcripts in granulocytes from patients with paroxysmal nocturnal hemoglobinuria. N Engl J Med 330:249–255, 1994.

Mohammed I, Holborow EJ, Fry L, Thompson BR, Hoffbrand AV, Stewart JS. Multiple immune complexes and hypocomplementaemia in dermatitis herpetiformis and coeliac disease. Lancet 2:487–490, 1976.

Moncada B, Day NKB, Good RA, Windhorst DB. Lupus erythematosus–like syndrome with a familial defect of complement. N Engl J Med 286:689–693, 1972.

Moran P, Beasley H, Gorrell A, Martin E, Gribling P, Fuchs H, Gillett N, Burton LE, Caras IW. Human recombinant soluble decay accelerating factor inhibits complement activation in vitro and in vivo. J Immunol 149:1736–1743, 1992.

Muir WA, Hedrick S, Alper CA, Ratnoff OD, Schacter B, Wisnieski JJ. Inherited incomplete deficiency of the fourth component of complement (C4) determined by a gene not linked to human histocompatibility leukocyte antigens. J Clin Invest 74:1509–1514, 1984.

Nattan-Larrier L, Lépine P, May J. Dosage comparatif de l'alexine dans le sang de la mère et dans le sang de l'enfant au moment de la naissance. C R Soc Biol (Paris) 97:671–672, 1927.

Neva FA, Howard WA, Glew RH, Krotoski WA, Gam AA, Collins WE, Atkinson JP, Frank MM. Relationship of serum complement levels to events of the malarial paroxysm. J Clin Invest 54:451–460, 1974.

Newman SL, Johnston RB Jr. Role of binding through C3b and IgG in polymorphonuclear neutrophil function: studies with trypsin-generated C3b. J Immunol 123:1839–1846, 1979.

Newman SL, Vogler LB, Feigin RD, Johnston RB Jr. Recurrent septicemia associated with congenital deficiency of C2 and partial deficiency of factor B and the alternative complement pathway. N Engl J Med 299:290–292, 1978.

Nicholson A, Lepow IH. Host defense against *Neisseria meningitidis* requires a complement-dependent bactericidal activity. Science 205:298–299, 1979.

Nicholson-Weller A, March JP, Rosenfeld SI, Austen KF. Affected erythrocytes of patients with paroxysmal nocturnal hemoglobinuria are deficient in the complement regulatory protein, decay accelerating factor. Proc Natl Acad Sci (U S A) 80:5066–5070, 1983.

Nishino H, Shibuya K, Nishida Y, Mushimoto M. Lupus erythematosus-like syndrome with selective complete deficiency of C1q. Ann Intern Med 95:322–324, 1981.

Norman ME, Gall EP, Taylor A, Laster L, Nilsson UR. Serum complement profiles in infants and children. J Pediatr 87:912–916, 1975.

Notarangelo LD, Chirico G, Chiara A, Columbo A, Rondini G, Plebani A, Martini A, Ugazio AG. Activity of classical and alternative pathways of complement in preterm and small for gestational age infants. Pediatr Res 18:281–285, 1984.

Nusbacher J, Rosenfeld SI, MacPherson JL, Thiem PA, Leddy JP. Nylon fiber leukapheresis: associated complement component changes and granulocytopenia. Blood 51:359–365, 1978.

Nydegger UE, Zubler RH, Gabay R, Joliat G, Karagevrekis C, Lambert PH, Miescher PA. Circulating complement breakdown products in patients in rheumatoid arthritis: correlation between plasma C3d, circulating immune complexes, and clinical activity. J Clin Invest 59:862–868, 1977.

O'Connor SP, Darip D, Fraley K, Nelson CM, Kaplan EL, Cleary PP. The human antibody response to streptococcal C5a peptidase. J Infect Dis 163:109–116, 1991.

Palestine AG, Klemperer MR. In vivo activation of properdin factor B in normotensive bacteremic individuals. J Immunol 117:703–705, 1976.

Pangburn MK, Schreiber RD, Müller-Eberhard HJ. Deficiency of an erythrocyte membrane protein with complement regulatory activity in paroxysmal nocturnal hemoglobinuria. Proc Natl Acad Sci (U S A) 80:5430–5434, 1983.

Parker CJ, Weidmer T, Sims PJ, Rosse WF, Characterization of the complement sensitivity of paroxysmal nocturnal hemoglobinuria erythrocytes. J Clin Invest 75:2074–2084, 1985.

Pascual M, Duchosal MA, Steiger G, Giostra E, Pechère A, Paccaud J-P, Danielsson C, Schifferli JA. Circulating soluble CR1 (CD35): serum levels in diseases and evidence for its release by human leukocytes. J Immunol 151:1702–1711, 1993.

Pascual M, Steiger G, Sadallah S, Paccaud J-P, Carpentier J-L, James

R, Schifferli J-A. Identification of membrane-bound CR1 (CD35) in human urine: evidence for its release by glomerular podocytes. J Exp Med 179:889–899, 1994.

Perrin LH, Lambert PH, Nydegger UE, Miescher PA. Quantitation of C3PA (properdin factor B) and other complement components in diseases associated with a low C3 level. Clin Immunol Immunopathol 2:16–27, 1973.

Petz LD. Variable mechanisms for low serum-complement in liver disease. Lancet 2:1033–1034, 1971.

Pickering RJ, Michael AE Jr, Herdman RC, Good RA, Gewurz H. The complement system in chronic glomerulonephritis: three newly associated aberrations. J Pediatr 78:30–43, 1971.

Pickering RJ, Urizar RE, Hanson PA, Laffin RJ. Abnormalities of the complement system in Reye syndrome. J Pediatr 94:218–222, 1979.

Polhill RB Jr, Newman SL, Pruitt KM, Johnston RB Jr. Kinetic assessment of alternative complement pathway activity in a hemolytic system. II. Influence of antibody on alternative pathway activation. J Immunol 121:371–376, 1978a.

Polhill RB Jr, Pruitt KM, Johnston RB Jr. Kinetic assessment of alternative complement pathway activity in a hemolytic system. I. Experimental and mathematical analyses. J Immunol 121:363–370, 1978b.

Pondman KW, Stoop JW, Cormane RH, Hannema AJ. Abnormal C'1 in a patient with systemic lupus erythematosus. J Immunol 101:811, 1968.

Poskitt TR, Fortwengler HP Jr, Lunskis BJ. Activation of the alternate complement pathway by autologous red cell stroma. J Exp Med 138:715–722, 1973.

Potter PC, Frasch CE, van der Sande WJM, Cooper RC, Patel Y, Orren A. Prophylaxis against *Neisseria meningitidis* infections and antibody responses in patients with deficiency of the sixth component of complement. J Infect Dis 161:932–937, 1990.

Pramoonjago P, Kinoshita T, Hong K, Takatakozono Y, Kozono H, Inagi R, Inoue K. Bactericidal activity of C9-deficient human serum. J Immunol 148:837–843, 1992.

Quezado ZMN, Hoffman WD, Winkelstein JA, Yatsiv I, Koev CA, Cork LC, Elin RJ, Eichacker PQ, Natanson C. The third component of complement protects against *Escherichia coli* endotoxin-induced shock and multiple organ failure. J Exp Med 179:569–578, 1994.

Ratnoff WD, Fearon DT, Austen KF. The role of antibody in the activation of the alternative complement pathway. Springer Semin Immunopathol 6:361–371, 1983.

Reed WP, Davidson MS, Williams RC Jr. Complement system in pneumococcal infections. Infect Immun 13:1120–1125, 1976.

Rich KC Jr, Hurley J, Gewurz H. Inborn C1r deficiency with a mild lupus-like syndrome. Clin Immunol Immunopathol 13:77–84, 1979.

Ripoche J, Fontaine M, Godin M, Hauptmann G, Goetz J. Partial deficiency of the fourth component of human complement (C4) and autoantibody directed against C4 in a patient with SLE. Ann Immunol (Paris) 134D:233–245, 1983.

Rosen FS, Charache P, Pensky J, Donaldson V. Hereditary angioneurotic edema: two genetic variants. Science 148:957–958, 1965.

Rosenfeld SI, Baum J, Steigbigel RT, Leddy JP. Hereditary deficiency of the fifth component of complement in man. II. Biological properties of C5-deficient human serum. J Clin Invest 57:1635–1643, 1976a.

Rosenfeld SL, Kelly ME, Leddy JP. Hereditary deficiency of the fifth component of complement in man. I. Clinical, immunochemical, and family studies. J Clin Invest 57:1626–1634, 1976b.

Ross GD, Medof ME. Membrane complement receptors specific for bound fragments of C3. Adv Immunol 37:217–267, 1985.

Ross GD, Yount WJ, Walport MJ, Winfield JB, Parker CJ, Fuller CR, Taylor RP, Myones BL, Lachmann PJ. Disease-associated loss of erythrocyte complement receptors (CR₁, C3b receptors) in patients with systemic lupus erythematosus and other diseases involving autoantibodies and/or complement activation. J Immunol 135:2005–2014, 1985.

Ross SC, Densen P. Complement deficiency states and infection: epidemiology, pathogenesis and consequences of neisserial and other infections in an immune deficiency. Medicine 63:243–273, 1984.

Rosse WF. Phosphatidylinositol-linked proteins and paroxysmal nocturnal hemoglobinuria. Blood 75:1595–1601, 1990.

Rother K, Rother U, Müller-Eberhard HJ, Nilsson UR. Deficiency of the sixth component of complement in rabbits with an inherited complement defect. J Exp Med 124:773–785, 1966.

Rynes RI, Britten AFH, Pickering RJ. Deficiency of the second complement component: association with the HLA haplotype A10, B18 in a normal population. Ann Rheum Dis 41:93–96, 1982.

Salama A, Hugo F, Heinrich D, Höge R, Müller R, Kiefel V, Mueller-Eckhardt C, Bhakdi S. Deposition of terminal C5b-9 complement complexes on erythrocytes and leukocytes during cardiopulmonary bypass. N Engl J Med 318:408–414, 1988.

Sampson HA, Walchner AM, Baker PJ. Recurrent pyogenic infections in individuals with absence of the second component of complement. J Clin Invest 2:39–45, 1982.

Sawyer MK, Forman ML, Kuplic LS, Stiehm ER. Developmental aspects of the human complement system. Biol Neonate 19:148–162, 1971.

Schapira M, Silver LD, Scott CF, Schmaier AH, Prograis LJ Jr, Curd JG, Colman RW. Prekallikrein activation and high-molecular-weight kininogen consumption in hereditary angioedema. N Engl J Med 308:1050–1054, 1983.

Schifferli JA, Steiger G, Hauptmann G, Spaeth PJ, Sjöholm AG. Formation of soluble immune complexes by complement in sera of patients with various hypocomplementemic states: differences between inhibition of immune precipitation and solubilization. J Clin Invest 76:2127–2133, 1985.

Schur PH. Complement in lupus. Clin Rheum Dis 1:519–543, 1975.

Seligmann M, Brouet JC, Sasportes M. Hereditary C2 deficiency associated with common variable immunodeficiency. Ann Intern Med 91:216–217, 1979.

Shapiro R, Beatty DW, Woods DL, Malan AF. Serum complement and immunoglobulin values in small-for-gestational-age infants. J Pediatr 99:139–141, 1981.

Sheffer AL, Austen KF, Rosen FS, Fearon DT. Acquired deficiency of the inhibitor of the first component of complement: report of five additional cases with commentary on the syndrome. J Allergy Clin Immunol 75:640–646, 1985.

Silverstein AM. Essential hypocomplementemia: report of a case. Blood 16:1338–1341, 1960.

Sirisinha S, Suskind RM, Edelman R, Kulapongs P, Olson RE. The complement system in protein-calorie malnutrition—a review. In Suskind RM, ed. Malnutrition and the Immune Response. New York, Raven Press, 1977, pp. 309–320.

Sissons JGP, West RJ, Fallows J, Williams DG, Boucher BJ, Amos N, Peters DK. The complement abnormalities of lipodystrophy. N Engl J Med 294:461–465, 1976.

Sjöholm AG, Nilsson LÅ. Properdin deficiency in a secondary Swedish family: absence of clinical manifestations. Complement 2:73, 1985.

Sjöholm AG, Braconier JH, Söderström C. Properdin deficiency in a family with fulminant meningococcal infections. Clin Exp Immunol 50:291–297, 1982.

Späth PJ, Misiano G, Schaad UB, Rohner R, Scherz R, Uring-Lambert B, Hauptmann G, Butler R. Association of heterozygous C4A and complete factor P deficient conditions. Complement 2:74, 1985.

Spitzer RE, Vallota EH, Forristal J, Sudora E, Stitzel A, Davis NC, West CD. Serum C'3 lytic system in patients with glomerulonephritis. Science 164:436–437, 1969.

Spitzer RE, Stitzel AE, Tsokos GC. Evidence that production of autoantibody to the alternative pathway C3 convertase is a normal physiologic event. J Pediatr 116:S103–S108, 1990.

Sprung CL, Schultz DR, Marcial E, Caralis PV, Gelbard MA, Arnold PI, Long WM. Complement activation in septic shock patients. Crit Care Med 14:525–528, 1986.

Steinsson K, McLean RH, Merrow M, Rothfield NF, Weinstein A. Selective complete C1q deficiency associated with systemic lupus erythematosus. J Rheumatol 10:590–594, 1983.

Stossel TP, Alper CA, Rosen FS. Opsonic activity in the newborn: role of properdin. Pediatrics 52:134–137, 1973.

Strang CJ, Cholin S, Spragg J, Davis AE, Schneeberger EE, Donaldson VH, Rosen FS. Angioedema induced by a peptide derived from complement component C2. J Exp Med 168:1685–1698, 1988.

Strate M, Olsen H, Teisner B, Brandslund I. Normal bacterial capacity against *Neisseria meningitidis* in serum from a patient with a hemolytically inactive complement factor 8 (C8). Acta Pathol Microbiol Immunol Scand (B) 91:431–434, 1983.

Strife CF, Prada AL, Clardy CW, Jackson E, Forristal J. Autoantibody to complement neoantigens in membranoproliferative glomerulonephritis. J Pediatr 116:S98–S102, 1990.

Strunk RC, Fenton LJ, Gaines JA. Alternative pathway of complement activation in full term and premature infants. Pediatr Res 13:641–643, 1979.

Suskind R, Edelman R, Kulapongs P, Pariyanonda A, Sirisinha S. Complement activity in children with protein-calorie malnutrition. Am J Clin Nutr 29:1089–1092, 1976.

Tannous R, Spitzer RE, Clarke WR, Goplerud CP, Cavender-Zylich N. Decreased chemotactic activity in activated newborn plasma: role of higher chemotactic factor inactivator activity and lower complement levels. J Lab Clin Med 99:331–341, 1982.

Tappeiner G, Hintner H, Glatzl J, Wolff K. Hereditary angio-oedema: treatment with danazol. Br J Dermatol 100:207–212, 1979.

Tappeiner G, Hintner H, Scholz S, Albert E, Linert J, Wolff K. Systemic lupus erythematosus in hereditary deficiency of the fourth component of complement. J Am Acad Dermatol 7:66–79, 1982.

Tausk FA, McCutchan JA, Spechko P, Schrieber RD, Gigli I. Altered erythrocyte C3b receptor expression, immune complexes and complement activation in homosexual men in varying risk groups for acquired immune deficiency syndrome. J Clin Invest 78:977–982, 1986.

Tedesco F, Densen P, Villa MA, Petersen BH, Sirchia G. Two types of dysfunctional eighth component of complement (C8) molecules in C8 deficiency in man: reconstitution of normal C8 from the mixture of two abnormal C8 molecules. J Clin Invest 71:183–191, 1983.

Tedesco F, Nürnberger W, Perissutti S. Inherited deficiencies of the terminal complement components. Int Rev Immunol 10:51–64, 1993.

Teisner B, Brandslund I, Folkersen J, Rasmussen JM, Poulson LO, Svehag SE. Factor I deficiency and C3 nephritic factor: immunochemical findings and association with *Neisseria meningitidis* infection in two patients. Scand J Immunol 20:291–297, 1984.

Thompson RA, Haeney M, Reid KBM, Davies JG, White RHR, Cameron AH. A genetic defect of the C1q subcomponent of complement associated with childhood (immune complex) nephritis. N Engl J Med 30:22–24, 1980.

Thompson RA, Yap PL, Brettle RB, Dunmow RE, Chapel H. Meningococcal meningitis associated with persistent hypocomplementaemia due to circulating C3 nephrotic factor. Clin Exp Immunol 52:153–156, 1983.

Thong YH, Simpson DA, Müller-Eberhard HJ. Homozygous deficiency of the second component of complement presenting with recurrent bacterial meningitis. Arch Dis Child 55:471–473, 1980.

Till GO, Ward PA. Systemic complement activation and acute lung injury. Fed Proc 45:13–18, 1986.

Tomlinson S. Complement defense mechanisms. Curr Opin Immunol 5:83–89, 1993.

Trapp RG, Fletcher M, Forristal J, West CD. C4 binding protein deficiency in a patient with atypical Behcet's disease. J Rheumatol 14:135–138, 1987.

Truedsson L, Alper CA, Awdeh ZL, Johansen P, Sjöholm AG, Sturfelt G. Characterization of type I complement C2 deficiency MHC haplotypes: strong conservation of the complotype/HLA-B-region and absence of disease association due to linked class II genes. J Immunol 151:5856–5863, 1993.

Uenaka A, Akimoto T, Aoki T, Tsuyuguchi I, Nagaki K. A complete selective C1q deficiency in a patient with discoid lupus erythematosus (DLE). Clin Exp Immunol 48:353–358, 1982.

Vogler LB, Newman SL, Stroud RM, Johnston RB Jr. Recurrent meningococcal meningitis with absence of the sixth component of complement: an evaluation of underlying immunologic mechanisms. Pediatrics 64:465–467, 1979.

Von Zabern I, Przykleuk H, Vogt W, Sachsenheimer W. Effect of radiographic contrast media on complement components C3 and C4: generation of C3b-like C3 and C4b-like C4. Int J Immunopharmacol 5:503–514, 1983.

Von Zabern I, Przykleuk H, Nolte R, Vogt W. Effect of metrizamide, a nonionic radiographic contrast agent, on human serum complement: comparison with ionic contrast media. Int Arch Allergy Appl Immunol 73:321–329, 1984.

Wahn V, Göbel U, Day NK. Restoration of complement function by plasma infusion in factor I (C3b inactivator) deficiency. J Pediatr 105:673, 1984.

Wahn V, Müller W, Rieger C, Rother U. Persistently circulating C3 nephritic factor (C3 NeF)–stabilized alternative pathway C3 convertase (C3 CoF) in serum of an 11-year-old girl with meningococcal septicemia: simultaneous occurrence with free C3 NeF. Pediatr Res 22:123–129, 1987.

Waldo FB, Leist PA, Strife CF, Forristal J, West CD. Atypical hypocomplementemic vasculitis syndrome in a child. J Pediatr 106:745–750, 1985.

Wang RH, Phillips G Jr, Medof ME, Mold C. Activation of the alternative complement pathway by exposure of phosphatidylethanolamine and phosphatidylserine on erythrocytes from sickle cell disease patients. J Clin Invest 92:1326–1335, 1993.

Wara DW, Reiter EO, Doyle NE, Gewurz H, Ammann AJ. Persistent C1q deficiency in a patient with a systemic lupus erythematosus-like syndrome. J Pediatr 86:743–745, 1975.

Weinstein MP, Gocke DJ, Gewurz A. Complement deficiency and sporadic meningococcal disease. N Engl J Med 309:615, 1983.

West CD, McAdams AJ, McConville JM, Davis NC, Holland NH. Hypocomplementemic and normocomplementemic persistent (chronic) glomerulonephritis; clinical and pathologic characteristics. J Pediatr 67:1089–1112, 1965.

Wetzel RA, Fleischer DT, Haviland DL. Deficiency of the murine fifth complement component (C5): a two base pair gene deletion in a 5' exon. J Biol Chem 265:2435–2440, 1990.

White JC, Nelson S, Winkelstein JA, Booth FVM, Jakab GJ. Impairment of antibacterial defense mechanisms of the lung by extrapulmonary infection. J Infect Dis 153:202–208, 1986.

Wilson JG, Jack RM, Wong WW, Schur PH, Fearon DT. Autoantibody to the C3b/C4b receptor and absence of this receptor from erythrocytes of a patient with systemic lupus erythematosus. J Clin Invest 76:182–190, 1985.

Wilson JG, Wong WW, Schur PH, Fearon DT. Mode of inheritance of decreased C3b receptors on erythrocytes of patients with systemic lupus erythematosus. N Engl J Med 307:981–986, 1982.

Wilson WA. Nature of complement deficiency in sickle cell disease. Arch Dis Child 58:235–236, 1983.

Winkelstein JA, Drachman RH. Deficiency of pneumococcal serum opsonizing activity in sickle-cell disease. N Engl J Med 279:459–466, 1968.

Winkelstein JA, Johnson JP, Swift AJ, Ferry F, Yolken R, Cork LC. Genetically determined deficiency of the third component of complement in the dog: *in vitro* studies on the complement system and complement-mediated serum activities. J Immunol 129:2598–2602, 1982.

Witte T, Dumoulin F-L, Gessner JE, Schubert J, Götze O, Neumann C, Todd RF III, Deicher H, Schmidt RE. Defect of a complement receptor 3 epitope in a patient with systemic lupus erythematosus. J Clin Invest 92:1181–1187, 1993.

Würzner R, Orren A, Lachmann PJ. Inherited deficiencies of the terminal components of human complement. Immunodefic Rev 3:123–147, 1992.

Wyatt RJ, Julian BA, Weinstein A, Rothfield NF, McLean RH. Partial H (β1H) deficiency and glomerulonephritis in two families. J Clin Immunol 2:110–117, 1982.

Yamashina M, Ueda E, Kinoshita T, Takami T, Ojima A, Ono H, Tanaka H, Kindi N, Orii T, Okada N, Okasa H, Inoue K, Kitani T. Inherited complete deficiency of 20-kilodalton homologous restriction factor (CD59) as a cause of paroxysmal nocturnal hemoglobinuria. N Engl J Med 323:1184–1189, 1990.

Zach TL, Hostetter MK. Biochemical abnormalities of the third component of complement in neonates. Pediatr Res 26:116–120, 1989.

Ziccardi RJ, Cooper NR. Development of an immunochemical test to assess C1 inactivator function in human serum and its use for the diagnosis of hereditary angioedema. Clin Immunol Immunopathol 15:465–471, 1980.

Zilow G, Geiger U, Kirschfin M, Rother U, Joka T. C3a as a prognostic indicator for the development of adult respiratory distress syndrome (ARDS) in polytrauma patients. Immunobiology 173:475, 1986.

Zilow G, Sturm JA, Rother U, Kirschfink M. Complement activation and the prognostic value of C3a in patients at risk of adult respiratory distress syndrome. Clin Exp Immunol 79:151–157, 1990.

Zilow G, Zilow EP, Burger R, Linderkamp O. Complement activation in newborn infants with early onset infection. Pediatr Res 34:199–203, 1993.

Zimran A, Kuperman O, Shemesh O, Hershko C. Recurrent *Neisseria meningitidis* bacteremia: association with deficiency of the eighth component of complement (C8) in a Sephardic Jewish family. Arch Intern Med 144:1481–1482, 1984.

Chapter 18

Pediatric Human Immunodeficiency Virus Infection

Gareth Tudor-Williams and Philip A. Pizzo

The first reports of an acquired immunodeficiency syndrome (AIDS) in children possibly caused by a transmissible agent appeared in 1982 (Centers for Disease Control [CDC], 1982; Ammann et al., 1983). The intervening years have seen more than 1000 reports that relate specifically to human immunodeficiency virus type 1 (HIV-1) infection in children. Women and children now constitute the fastest growing groups of newly infected individuals in the United States. As a result of HIV-1 infection, pediatricians throughout the world are increasingly required to recognize and treat children with profoundly impaired immunity. Unlike families of children with other life-threatening diseases, the parents of HIV-infected children are also frequently infected, ill, and face discrimination rather than support from their communities. The care of such children therefore involves a comprehensive, multidisciplinary approach.

Although at this time there are no cures for HIV disease, many advances are being made. This chapter provides an overview of the current state of understanding of the disease, selected clinical issues, and approaches to the management of HIV-1 infected children.

EPIDEMIOLOGY

Worldwide, more than 2.5 million people were estimated to have had AIDS by mid-1993, a 20% increase over the previous year. Thirteen million adults and at least 1 million children were thought to be infected; 8 million of these infections had occurred in sub-Saharan Africa (Quinn, 1994). The spread of HIV-1 throughout the world has varied from region to region by a few years, but there are now no countries free of the virus (National Commission on AIDS, 1993). In the United States, this is reflected by the rapid spread of disease into rural communities. The annual incidence of reported new cases per 100,000 inhabitants more than doubled in 25 states, including Arkansas, the Dakotas, Iowa, Minnesota, Nebraska, South Carolina, Wisconsin, and Wyoming, in the year ending June 1993 compared with the previous year (CDC, 1993c).

HIV-1 infection became the leading cause of death among young men (aged 25 to 44 years) in 64 cities and of young women in 9 cities in 1990 (Selik et al., 1993). By the same year, in New York State, AIDS was the leading cause of death in Hispanic children under 4 years of age (CDC, 1991b). Worldwide, infant and child mortality rates will increase as much as 30% above previously projected rates as a direct consequence of perinatal HIV infection (Quinn, 1994).

Mode of Transmission

There has been a shift toward heterosexual acquisition of HIV-1 in developed countries, and this has always been the dominant mode of transmission in developing countries. In the United States, heterosexual contact eclipsed drug abuse as an HIV risk factor for the first time in 1992 (CDC, 1993e). Women now represent 5 of every 11 newly infected adults worldwide (Merson, 1993). In children, the screening of donors for blood and blood products has almost completely eliminated this source of infection.

Vertical transmission (from infected mothers to their infants) will account for almost all new cases in young children in the future. In addition, a small proportion of children may be infected as the result of child sexual abuse (Gutman et al., 1991). Projecting the numbers of new, vertically acquired cases is difficult, because the numbers of HIV infected women in their childbearing years continues to increase while estimates of the transmission rate vary. In 1991, it was estimated that there would be 1800 new cases of HIV-infected children in the United States, based on projections of 6000 infected mothers delivering per year, with a transmission rate of 30% (Gwinn et al., 1991).

The finding that zidovudine (AZT) could significantly reduce the rate of mother-to-child transmission when administered to HIV-infected women during pregnancy and delivery, and for the first 6 weeks of life to their offspring, promises to reduce the numbers of HIV-infected children in countries where this therapy is available and is broadly administered (CDC, 1994a). Unfortunately, it is unlikely to reduce the transmission rates in developing countries where most of these children will be born, because it is improbable that such treatment will soon be available or safely administered in these countries.

Several large studies have confirmed the extremely low risk of transmission through casual interactions among household contacts (Friedland et al., 1986; Mann et al., 1986; Simonds and Chanock, 1993). There has been one well-documented description of transmission from a child with AIDS to an unrelated 2-year-old in the same household. The authors concluded that the mode of transmission was an unrecognized exposure of the 2-year-old's mucous membranes or excoriated skin to blood from nosebleeds or a laceration of the child with AIDS (Fitzgibbon et al., 1993). A second report described transmission between siblings with hemophilia. The brothers could not recall sharing equipment for infusions of factor VIII, but the potential for a needle stick transmission in this setting is high (CDC, 1993b). An earlier, brief report of suspected household transmission between young children, possibly by biting, was not supported by genotypic analysis (Wahn et al., 1986). Rogers and colleagues (1990) documented lack of HIV transmission in seven individuals known to have bitten HIV-infected children.

There have been no reports of transmission in out-of-home child care settings or in school. Only one case of HIV transmission attributed to sports has been reported worldwide to date (Torre et al., 1990). This involved a collision of heads during a soccer match, with copious bleeding from both players. Other modes of transmission for the person who became infected however, could not be definitively excluded. Adolescents are at risk from unprotected sexual intercourse or the use of contaminated needles. The magnitude of this risk is underscored by the fact that 20% of people developing AIDS in the United States are aged 20 to 29 years. Given the prolonged incubation period, it is clear that a substantial proportion acquired their infection as teenagers (Gayle and D'Angelo, 1991).

Orphans

The implications of HIV infection affecting both children and their parents are far-reaching. For example, it is estimated that by the end of the century, 10 million children under 15 years of age may be orphaned as a result of the premature death of their parents (Quinn, 1994).

Demographics

Demographically, minority groups in the United States are disproportionally affected, with 54% of cases occurring in black, non-Hispanic children and 24% in Hispanics. The annual rate per 100,000 people is 7.4 and 2.0, respectively, compared to 0.4 in white, non-Hispanic children (CDC, 1993e). Males and females are equally represented among children under 5 years, although 62% of older children are male because of blood product acquired disease in hemophiliacs prior to the introduction of screening.*

PATHOGENESIS

Current and future strategies for therapeutic intervention require a clear understanding of the pathogenesis of HIV-1 infection in children. It can be assumed that the viral life cycle is essentially the same in children and adults, but much remains to be learned regarding the influence of growth and cellular differentiation, which are an integral part of the pediatric host, on viral replication and pathogenesis. These influences may help explain some of the differences in the course of disease noted between adults and children.

Molecular and Cellular Biology

Considerations of molecular and cellular biology involve an understanding of viral structure, life cycle, cellular tropism, and regulation of gene expression.

Structure

HIV-1 is a member of the Lentivirinae subfamily of retroviruses. The distinguishing feature of all retroviruses is their ability to transcribe genetic material in a reverse direction, from RNA into DNA. The HIV-1 virion comprises a bullet-shaped, electron–dense nucleocapsid that contains the genomic RNA, surrounded by an envelope (Fig. 18–1) (Greene, 1991; Haseltine, 1991; Bryant and Ratner, 1992; Stevenson et al.,

---

*Epidemiologic information is updated quarterly by the Centers for Disease Control (CDC). The HIV/AIDS surveillance report can be obtained by writing to CDC, OD/OPS/MASO, 1/B49, Mailstop A-22, Atlanta, GA 30333.

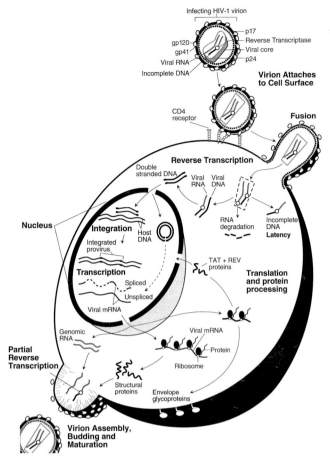

Figure 18–1. Life cycle of the human immunodeficiency virus type 1.

scriptase (p66, p51), integrase (p31), and protease (p10) and a cellular-derived transfer RNA molecule, tRNALys, required for the initiation of reverse transcription. Evidence has suggested that the process of reverse transcription is initiated at the time of assembly or shortly thereafter, and partial reverse transcripts of viral DNA may also be identifiable in the virion (Trono, 1992). The restricted pool of deoxynucleoside triphosphates and other substrates within the virion probably limits the extent of reverse transcription that can occur extracellularly.

Life Cycle, Cellular Tropism, and Regulation of Gene Expression

As shown in Figure 18–1, the life cycle begins with the attachment of the virion to a target cell. The CD4 differentiation antigen of T lymphocytes and macrophages serves as the principal cell surface receptor for HIV-1 (Dalgleish et al., 1984; Klatzmann et al., 1984; Gartner et al., 1986; Ho et al., 1986). Physiologically, the CD4 receptor stabilizes the interaction between major histocompatibility complex (MHC) class II molecules on an antigen-presenting cell and the T-cell receptor reactive with the MHC class II peptide complex. Binding of virions to the T cell involves the interaction of specific conformational domains of gp120 with the CD4 molecule (Lasky et al., 1987).

The binding affinity appears to vary among HIV isolates, with lower affinities observed for primary isolates than for laboratory-adapted viruses (Ivey-Hoyle et al., 1991; Daar et al., 1990). This may explain in part the disappointing results of clinical trials using soluble CD4 as a decoy to block viral binding to CD4+ cells, although other mechanisms are also implicated (Brighty et al., 1991).

Conformational alterations in the binding epitopes of gp120 are crucial determinants of the cellular tropism of HIV-1 variants (York-Higgins et al., 1990; Cheng-Meyer et al., 1991). Cordonnier and colleagues (1989) showed that a single amino acid substitution in a highly conserved domain of gp120 abrogated the ability of a cloned virus to infect monocytes, although it was still able to infect T-cell lines. Chesebro and associates (1992) have defined critical amino acids in the third variable region (V3 loop) as determinants of macrophage tropism.

Following binding to the target cell surface, evidence has suggested that the virus gains entry by simple fusion of the two membranes (Stein et al., 1987; Dimitrov et al., 1991). Alternatively, virus may be transmitted from one infected cell directly to another uninfected cell by cell fusion in a process that can result in syncytia formation in vitro (Sodroski et al., 1986). Clinical isolates of HIV-1 vary in their ability to induce syncytia in donor peripheral blood mononuclear cells (PBMCs) (Tersmette et al., 1988). Syncytium-inducing (SI) variants tend to be recovered from patients later in the course of disease, whereas non–syncytium-inducing (NSI) isolates can be detected throughout HIV-1 infection.

In a prospective study of 225 asymptomatic men,

1992). The components of the virion are assigned numbers based on their molecular weights (in kilodaltons) and migration on Western blots. The genomic organization is illustrated in Figure 18–2.

The envelope consists of a lipid bilayer derived from the host cell plasma membrane during virus budding. Under high-resolution electron microscopy, the virion is seen as a sphere with 72 external knobs projecting from the surface. The knobs are formed by trimers or tetramers of two glycoproteins; gp120 (the surface glycoprotein) is anchored noncovalently to gp41 (the transmembrane protein). A variety of additional host proteins, including class I and class II histocompatibility antigens, may be incorporated into the viral envelope as the virions bud (Gelderblom et al., 1987).

The core contains the duplex single-stranded RNA genome bound to nucleic acid binding proteins p9 and p7. Surrounding this nucleoid core is the cylindric or bullet-shaped capsid formed by the p24 core antigen protein. It has been recommended that this should more accurately be renamed p25 (CA) protein but, because p24 is widely used in the clinical literature, we shall use p24 throughout this review (Leis et al., 1988). Lining the inside of the viral envelope with its amino terminal inserted into the membrane is the p17 matrix protein.

In addition to these structural proteins, the mature virion also packages the viral enzymes reverse tran-

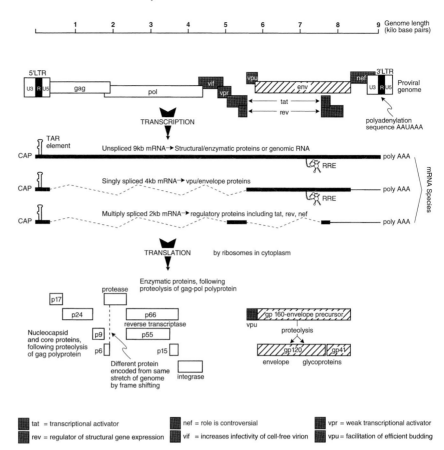

Figure 18–2. Genomic organization of HIV-1, transcription of spliced (2- and 4-kb) and full-length (9-kb) messenger RNA species, and translation of structural, enzymatic, and regulatory proteins. RRE = rev responsive element; TAR = transactivation response element.

71% of those with SI variants progressed to AIDS within 30 months, compared with 16% of men with NSI variants. This biologic phenotype has not yet been fully defined at a molecular level, and its precise role in pathogenesis in vivo remains speculative. It appears to be a useful independent marker, however, for disease progression in adults (Koot et al., 1993). The infectivity of HIV-1 during cell-to-cell transmission has been shown to be more rapid and 10^2 to 10^3 times greater than the infectivity of cell-free virus stocks (Sato et al., 1992; Dimitrov et al., 1993b). Cell fusion appears to be mediated by the transmembrane protein gp41, which contains a fusogenic domain resembling that of the F proteins of the paramyxoviruses (Richardson and Choppin, 1983; Kowalski et al., 1987).

Other mechanisms for virus entry must also exist because certain cells, such as fetal brain cells, glial cells, and colorectal cells, which do not express detectable CD4 on their surface, have been shown to be infectable by HIV-1 (Takeda et al., 1988). Alternative host glycoproteins, such as Fc receptors, may play a role in viral binding, although gp41 is still thought to be involved in fusion and entry.

Following fusion, the virion capsid is released into the host cell cytoplasm and uncoating occurs. *Reverse transcription* then proceeds in a complex series of steps involving the sequential creation of a partial, "strong stop" complementary DNA (cDNA) strand, degradation of the RNA component of the RNA-DNA duplex, and "jumping" of the cDNA from the 5' to the 3' end of the same or the second RNA strand to enable completion of

the cDNA (Varmus and Swanstrom, 1991). The process is catalyzed by the pol gene product of HIV-1, reverse transcriptase (RT) (see Fig. 18–2). In its active form, the enzyme is a dimer of two proteins, p51 and p66; the smaller component is a truncated derivative of p66. It acts as an RNA-dependent DNA polymerase to produce a minus-strand DNA copy of the RNA template. It then functions as a DNA-dependent DNA polymerase to make the plus-strand DNA from the minus-strand DNA template. The carboxy terminal end of p66 includes the RNase H domain, which degrades viral RNA following reverse transcription. Retroviruses without a functional RNase H enzyme can only generate short DNA fragments that remain hybridized to viral RNA and are nonreplicating (Tanese et al., 1991). Reverse transcription (RT) yields a double-stranded DNA replica of the RNA genome, with additional flanking sequences called long terminal repeats (LTRs) in place of the short terminal repeats of the RNA genome.

Unlike cellular polymerases, HIV-1 RT is error-prone and lacks a "proofreading" mechanism. One base per 1.7 to 4.0 kb is estimated to be mis-incorporated (Takeuchi et al., 1988; Bebenek et al., 1989; Hubner et al., 1992). Because the genome is approximately 9 kb, this may produce several mis-incorporations per replication cycle and accounts for the rapid mutation rates observed in vivo. Some mutations may be lethal to the virus, but others may confer significant biologic advantage and result in selection of that strain or *quasispecies* within the host (Meyerhans et al., 1989). Under different selection pressures of humoral and cellular responses and different antiretroviral therapies, this process may result in a heterogeneous population of viruses or "swarm" in infected individuals.

The double-stranded proviral DNA is translocated into the nucleus and integrated into the host chromosomal DNA by another pol gene-encoded enzyme, integrase. Integration depends on the state of activation of the host cell. In quiescent T lymphocytes, substantial amounts of unintegrated HIV DNA have been demonstrated that retained the capacity to integrate after in vitro activation of the cells (Stevenson et al., 1990).

Bukrinsky and colleagues (1991) found that lymphocytes from asymptomatic HIV-infected individuals contained a higher ratio of unintegrated to integrated proviral DNA compared with lymphocytes from AIDS patients. The implication of these findings is that there may be potentially large inducible pools of proviral DNA in asymptomatic patients. Studies have revealed that integration is not essential for virus replication in macrophages, although transcription off the unintegrated circularized DNA is less efficient (see Fig. 18–1) (Cara et al., 1993). Other studies, however, have suggested that unintegrated viral DNA does not persist for prolonged periods if the cells remain unstimulated (Zack et al., 1990).

The integrated proviral DNA functions like a host cell gene, providing a formidable obstacle to the eradication of HIV from infected individuals. Transcription is dependent initially on interactions between cellular transcription factors and the HIV promoter sequences in the 5'-LTR. Cellular transcription factors include the constitutively expressed Sp1 protein and the inducible nuclear factor kappa B (NFκB), which normally regulates the expression of T-cell genes involved in cell growth following activation. NF-κB can be induced by a variety of cytokines, such as tumor necrosis factor alpha (TNF-α), and interleukin-1 (IL-1) (Osborn et al., 1989; Duh et al., 1989), or by gene products of viruses, such as human T-cell leukemia virus type 1 (HTLV-1) and human herpes viruses such as herpes simplex virus (HSV) or human herpes virus 6 (HHV-6) (Siekevitz et al., 1987; Mosca et al., 1987; Ensoli et al., 1989; Heng et al., 1994) and JC virus (Gendelman et al., 1986). Other upstream regulatory sequences are being characterized that regulate LTR-driven gene expression in certain cells at different stages of differentiation (Zeichner et al., 1992). These may play an important role in the pathogenesis of perinatally acquired HIV disease.

The formation of a transcription complex on the 5'-LTR initiates a low level of transcription of viral messenger RNA (mRNA) by the host enzyme RNA polymerase II (Fig. 18–3A and B). The early mRNA transcripts are multiply spliced, resulting in the synthesis of the HIV-1 regulatory proteins tat, rev, and nef. In studies of the kinetics of expression, these mRNAs can be detected within 8 to 12 hours of infection of cell lines in vitro (Klotman et al., 1991). The tat protein is a potent transactivator, increasing transcription from the HIV LTR by as much as two orders of magnitude (Fisher et al., 1986). The protein binds to the *transacti-*

vation response element (TAR) at the 5' end of all HIV mRNAs (see Fig. 18–2 and 18–3B). It is thereby brought into close proximity with the transcription start site of the proviral DNA. In conjunction with the cellular proteins of the transcription complex, tat increases the rate of transcription initiation and allows elongation to take place (Laspia et al., 1989).

The resulting increased production of multiply spliced mRNA leads to higher levels of translation of the rev protein (Fig. 18–3C). This also acts in the nucleus, binding to the rev response element (RRE), which is a segment of RNA in the env region, with a complex secondary structure. It appears that in the absence of rev all mRNAs containing the RRE are held up in the nucleus to be spliced or degraded. Following binding with rev, export into the cytoplasm can occur, and production of structural and enzymatic proteins proceeds (Fig. 18–3D) (Cullen and Greene, 1989). The roles of the auxiliary proteins are indicated in Figure 18–2 (Cullen and Greene, 1990). The precise function of the nef protein in HIV-1 is controversial, but it is required for the maintenance of high virus loads and clinical disease progression in rhesus monkeys with simian immunodeficiency virus (SIV) infection (Kestler et al., 1991). In addition, down-regulation of CD4 receptor expression is a widely accepted role of the nef protein (Inoue et al., 1993; Anderson et al., 1993).

As depicted in Figure 18–2, the viral core structural proteins are encoded by the gag (*g*roup-specific *a*nti*g*en) gene and the enzymatic proteins by the pol (*pol*ymerase) gene via a gag-pol fusion protein. The ribosomes slip back by one nucleotide (ribosomal frameshifting) during translation with 5% to 10% efficiency, thereby gaining access to the pol open reading frame (Jacks et al., 1988). This mechanism ensures that a much higher ratio of gag-to-pol proteins is produced. The polyproteins are modified post-translationally by the attachment of a myristyl group onto their shared amino terminal glycine. Myristoylation appears to be required for intracellular transport to the cell membrane (Bryant and Ratner, 1990). During the final stages of virion assembly, the polyproteins are cleaved into functional proteins by the viral protease enzyme (Fitzgerald and Springer, 1991). Proteolysis of the gag proteins results in self-assembly of the virion nucleocapsid, with a predisposition for budding from the host cell.

Translation of the envelope precursor gp160 occurs in the rough endoplasmic reticulum. The protein is promptly glycosylated and is cleaved by cellular proteases in the Golgi complex into its components, gp120 and gp 41, which are inserted across the host cytoplasmic membrane (Willey et al., 1988). Full-length genomic RNA is packaged into the assembling virion through interactions with a conserved zinc finger sequence of the p9 gag protein (Gorelick et al., 1990). The host cell membrane, replete with gp120 anchored by gp41 and incidental host cell surface proteins, forms the viral envelope for the infectious, mature virion. A new round of infection can now occur, either by direct interaction during budding of the envelope glycoproteins with a neighboring CD4+ cell or by the release of mature virions to infect distant cells.

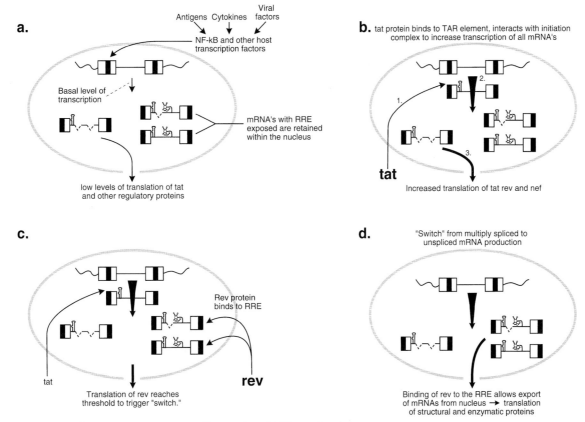

Figure 18–3. Function of tat and rev proteins in self-regulation of HIV-1 replication.

a, Host-transcription factors, influenced by a variety of signals, bind to the 5'-LTR. A low level of transcription is initiated. The 9- and 4-kb mRNAs are retained in the nucleus because of the presence of the unbound rev response element (RRE). Only the multiply spliced 2-kb mRNA lacking an RRE can move out to the ribosomes in the cytoplasm, resulting in low levels of transcription of the regulatory proteins only.

b, The tat protein is an extremely potent transactivator: 1, low concentrations of tat bind to the TAR element and interact with the initiation complex; 2, this results in increased transcription of all mRNAs; 3, at this stage, the 9- and 4-kb mRNAs are still retained in the nucleus—only the 2-kb messages can be exported, resulting selectively in increased translation of the regulatory proteins.

c, The rev protein reaches a threshold concentration, binding in a multimeric fashion to the RRE and thereby enabling export of all mRNAs from the nucleus.

d, As a result of rev binding, production of HIV-1 proteins is effectively switched from purely regulatory to all structural and enzymatic proteins also.

Ovals = nuclear membrane; LTR = long terminal repeat; mRNA = messenger RNA; TAR = *trans*activation response element.

Immunopathogenesis

Immunopathogenetic considerations include the course of the infection, mechanisms of CD4 depletion, interactions with cellular and humoral immune systems, and host genetic factors.

Course of HIV Infection

Immunopathologic studies in adults have revealed a common pattern of events following acute infection, although great individual variation has been noted (Levy, 1993 [more than 1300 references]; Fauci, 1993; Weiss, 1993). In children, there are many gaps in our knowledge, but in broad terms a similar pattern is discernible. Acute infection by cell-associated or cell-free virus may occur parenterally (e.g., via a break in the integrity of the placental barrier) or across a mucosal surface (e.g., by ingestion of contaminated maternal blood during delivery) (Sato, 1992).

Within 3 to 6 weeks, an acute mononucleosis-like illness is experienced by 50% to 70% of adults (Tindall and Cooper, 1991). The equivalent clinical manifestations of primary infection are not as evident in infants. This may be due to the timing of perinatal transmission (see later), differences in transmitted viral burden or phenotype, or immaturities of the host immune response. Additionally, infants of infected mothers generally have pre-existing (maternally derived) HIV-specific antibodies, unlike acute infection occurring outside the perinatal period, which may attenuate the acute syndrome.

The acute illness is associated with high levels of viremia and wide dissemination of the virus, particularly to lymphoid tissue but also to other organs, including the central nervous system. In adults, an abrupt drop in CD4$^+$ lymphocyte counts in the peripheral blood is observed (Daar et al., 1991). Within 1 to 12 weeks, antiviral immune responses develop and coincide with a dramatic decrease in circulating viral burden. Cellular immune responses in the form of cytotoxic T lymphocytes (CTLs) appear before a humoral antibody response (Safrit et al., 1993). Trapping of virus-antibody-complement immune complexes on the cytoplasmic processes of follicular dendritic cells (FDCs) in lymph nodes may contribute to the removal of virus from the circulation (Fox et al., 1991).

With the decrease in circulating virus, a partial recovery of CD4+ lymphocyte counts is seen although not usually back to pre-illness baseline levels. In infants, it is difficult to document such a pattern because CD4+ lymphocyte counts in "normal" (i.e., uninfected) infants are much higher during the first 2 years of life, falling to adult levels by the time a child is 6 years of age (European Collaborative Study, 1992; McKinney and Wilfert, 1992).

A clinically asymptomatic period follows primary infection, which may last for many years in adults. In children, there appears to be a subset with more rapid disease progression (see later, Perinatal Transmission), and a second group that may follow a pattern of clinical latency, which is generally shorter than that seen in adult disease (Blanche et al., 1989, 1990; Scott et al., 1989; Tovo et al., 1992; Byers et al., 1993). Recently, a child with putatively perinatally acquired HIV infection has been reported to have cleared his infection (Bryson et al., 1995). This report is provocative but additional confirmation is necessary to support its conclusions.

It is becoming clear, however, that there is no period of viral latency, and throughout the course of infection progressive destruction of CD4+ T cells and of the FDC network in lymph nodes is taking place (Vago et al., 1989; Michael et al., 1992; Pantaleo et al., 1993a). Figure 18–4 shows a section of a lymph node from a relatively asymptomatic 2-year-old with a CD4 count of 2965 (36%). In situ hybridization of HIV-1 RNA reveals an abundance of virus localized to the germinal centers. Dual in situ and immunohistochemical staining reveals a pattern consistent with the attachment

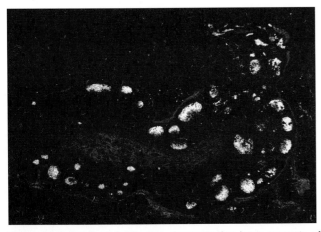

Figure 18–4. In situ hybridization demonstrating large amounts of HIV-1 RNA in the germinal centers of a lymph node from a 3-year-old boy with well-preserved CD4+ count (36%; absolute count, 2695 cells/mm³). (1.3× darkfield view using antisense probes that bind HIV-1 RNA. The gray reticulin stain reveals an orderly distribution of reticulin around the node, without extensive fibrosis in the tissue. The white grains represent hybridization signals using ³⁵S-labeled RNA antisense probes.) (Courtesy of Dr. Cecil Fox.)

of immune-complexed virions to the surface of the interlacing processes of the FDC. The amount of virus in the lymphoid tissue may not be directly reflected by measurements of circulating viral burden or by the degree of immune impairment. The final breakdown of the germinal centers and FDC architecture and the profound impairment of HIV-specific host defenses result in a recurrence of high levels of viremia and depletion of virus trapped in lymphoid tissue.

Late-stage disease in both adults and children is marked by a precipitous decline in CD4+ lymphocyte counts and by the risk of opportunistic infections, neoplasms, and death.

Mechanisms of CD4 Depletion

The central event in the course of HIV disease appears to be the development of functional abnormalities and progressive destruction of the CD4+ lymphocyte population. Numerous theories about how this occurs have been proposed, and it seems probable that both direct and indirect mechanisms are involved. Direct killing may occur because of the accumulation of unintegrated viral DNA, inhibition of cellular protein synthesis, or disruption during budding and release of virions (Garry, 1989). Studies demonstrating much higher levels of virus in peripheral blood mononuclear cells than were previously detectable support the role of direct cell killing in cytopathicity (Bagasra et al., 1992; Embretson et al., 1993; Patterson et al., 1993; Piatak et al., 1993b).

Numerous indirect mechanisms have been postulated. Syncytia formation, in which infected cells fuse with neighboring uninfected CD4+ cells, can be demonstrated in vitro. This capability correlates with cytopathicity and with disease progression (see earlier, Life Cycle), but has only rarely been observed in vivo (Lifson et al., 1986).

The host's immune response may destroy virus-infected cells, principally by HIV-specific cytotoxic T cells and also by antibody-dependent cell-mediated cytotoxicity (ADCC) in conjunction with natural killer (NK) cells (Walker et al., 1987).

The virus may trigger autoimmune destruction through the molecular mimicry of cellular antigens. For example, gp120 and gp41 glycoproteins share some structural homology with regions of the MHC class II molecules. Anti-HIV envelope antibodies may therefore cross-react with the patient's class II molecules, and there are limited data from patients supporting this in vivo (Golding et al., 1989). Such an alloreaction has been likened to a chronic graft-versus-host type disease, opening up possible novel approaches to therapy (Habeshaw et al., 1992).

The role of HIV proteins as superantigens remains speculative (Imberti et al., 1991). It is possible that such superantigens might activate a subset of T cells bearing particular variable beta (V$_\beta$) regions, resulting in greater viral replication and direct cell killing of those cells (Pantaleo et al., 1993b).

A number of researchers has proposed that HIV infection leads to early priming of lymphocytes to undergo *apoptosis* (programmed cell death) on further stimulation (Groux et al., 1992; Banda et al., 1992; Cohen, 1993). A major fraction of such lymphocytes, however, has been shown to be CD8$^+$ cells (Meyaard et al., 1992). The relative contribution of apoptosis to the loss of CD4$^+$ lymphocytes in vivo awaits clarification. In infants and children, dysregulation of this mechanism could be of considerable importance because thymic apoptosis of autoreactive T-cell clones is occurring naturally at a high rate (Jenkinson et al., 1989; Economides et al., 1993).

The thymus is an important target organ in the immunopathogenesis of HIV-1 disease. Pathologic studies of the thymus in children at autopsy reveal extensive involvement, with thymitis and precocious involution. Thymic epithelial cells around Hassall's corpuscles are the major target of injury, as judged by immunofluorescent studies using anti-HIV IgG probes (Joshi and Oleske, 1985).

Interactions With Cellular and Humoral Immune Systems

CD4$^+$ Lymphocytes

In addition to the numerical destruction of CD4$^+$ lymphocytes described earlier, functional abnormalities have been noted (Miedema et al., 1988; Clerici et al., 1989). A progressive series of defects in T-helper (T$_H$) function with advancing disease has been identified, as measured in vitro by interleukin-2 (IL-2) production from PBMCs. Initially, a loss of response to recall antigens (influenza A or tetanus toxoid), followed by a loss of response to HLA alloantigens and finally to phytohemagglutinin (PHA), has been reported both in adults and children (Clerici et al., 1989; Roilides et al., 1991a). The defects may be mediated by HIV envelope proteins (Chanh et al., 1988; Diamond et al., 1988) and have been shown to be partially reversible with antiretroviral therapy (Clerici et al., 1992b). Improved function was associated with a lower incidence of infections (Clerici et al., 1992c). Some caution is required in interpreting the pediatric data because it is difficult to distinguish HIV-induced suppression of T$_H$ function from the absence of T$_H$ function resulting from the lack of maturation or immunologic priming (Shearer and Clerici, 1993).

There is accumulating evidence based on IL-2/IL-4 production by PBMCs in vitro that a switch in T-lymphocyte clonal maturation patterns occurs during disease progression, from T-helper 1 (T$_H$1) to T-helper 2 (T$_H$2) patterns (Clerici et al., 1993a). T$_H$1 clones promote cell-mediated effector responses via the production of the cytokines IL-2, IL-12, and inteferon-gamma (IFN-γ). T$_H$2 clones produce IL-4, IL-5, IL-6, and IL-10, which lead to B-cell activation and hypergammaglobulinemia and down-regulate the immunoprotective T$_H$1 cellular immunity (Clerici and Shearer, 1993). This change in cytokine profile is predictive of a decline in CD4$^+$ lymphocyte counts and disease progression and death (Lucey et al., 1991; Viganó, et al., 1995).

There is much interest in attempting to reverse this switch by the administration of T$_H$1-type cytokines (Fauci, 1993). Infusions of IL-2 for 5 days every 8 weeks are being administered to HIV-infected adults with CD4$^+$ lymphocyte counts over 200 cells/mm^3 at the National Institute of Allergy and Infectious Diseases. Preliminary data have shown significant improvements in CD4$^+$ counts in about half of the recipients. Side effects are common, and increases in plasma HIV viral titers (by branched chain DNA measurements) have been noted after each infusion. IL-12 has been shown to restore defective T$_H$1-type cell-mediated responses in vitro (Clerici et al., 1993b).

Critical subsets of CD4$^+$ lymphocytes may be preferentially infected by HIV, and this may be obscured when total CD4$^+$ percentages and absolute counts are monitored. Multiparameter flow cytometric analysis was used to identify activation and differentiation antigens on CD4$^+$ and CD8$^+$ cells from 67 HIV-infected children and matched uninfected controls (Plaeger-Marshall et al., 1993). CD4$^+$/CD45RA$^+$ (naive) subset cells were significantly lower in the infected children. A unique and dominant function of this subset in cord blood is the suppression of immunoglobulin production (Clement et al., 1990). Disproportionate loss of these cells may be a factor in the polyclonal B-cell stimulation and hypergammaglobulinemia associated with pediatric HIV infection. The CD29$^+$/CD45RO$^+$ (memory) subset, which provides helper functions and participates in responses to recall antigens, may also be reduced, potentially contributing to early functional defects (Brunell, 1993). Identification of specific subset deficiencies may provide prognostic information as well as potential therapeutic options by supplying mediators secreted by the deficient subsets.

CD8$^+$ Lymphocytes

Two separate CD8$^+$ cell-mediated responses to HIV infection have been described (Levy, 1993). The first is the classical CTL response, which is HLA-dependent (MHC class I restricted) and requires cell-to-cell contact. The second is mediated by a novel lymphokine released by CD8$^+$ cells, which suppresses HIV replication in CD4$^+$ lymphocytes.

Cytotoxic T cells are present in high number in asymptomatic adults but decrease, particularly in functional activity, with disease progression (Hoffenbach et al., 1989). The CTL can kill cells expressing a wide variety of HIV peptides, including reverse transcription, envelope, core, vif, and nef protein derivatives (Nixon et al., 1992). The peptides expressed in the grooves of the MHC class I molecules, however, are usually derived from cytoplasmic proteins. In HIV-infected cells, envelope proteins are formed close to the cell surface and are rapidly transferred across the cell membrane. These would have to be misdirected intracellularly to be processed into CTL-inducing target peptides. Physiologically therefore, dominant CTL responses are directed to peptides derived from gag, pol, and regulatory proteins.

Several studies have detected CTL responses in acute infection before the appearance of neutralizing antibody (Clerici et al., 1991; Levy, 1993; Safrit et al.,

1993). In one of these studies, Safrit and colleagues (1993) demonstrated that the CTL response is temporally associated with a decline in circulating viral load, before a humoral response has developed. The role of CTL in chronic HIV disease is less clear. Disease progression with increasing levels of HIV-infected cells takes place in the presence of these CD8$^+$ cells. There is some evidence that HIV genotypic variants that can escape recognition by CTL, CTL *escape mutants,* may emerge over time (Phillips et al., 1991).

The ability of CD8$^+$ lymphocytes to suppress HIV replication has been demonstrated in vitro using PBMCs from asymptomatic individuals (Walker et al., 1991). In the presence of CD8$^+$ cells, the cultures did not yield HIV. When CD8$^+$ cells were removed by panning, virus production from the CD4$^+$ lymphocytes remaining in culture was detected. Replacement of CD8$^+$ cells at low levels suppressed viral replication without direct killing of virus-infected cells. CD8$^+$ cells separated from the CD4$^+$ cells by a 0.4-μm filter and supernatants from CD8$^+$ cell cultures were found to mediate this inhibition, although cell-to-cell contact was more efficient (Mackewicz and Levy, 1992). Suppression of replication appears to occur at or before mRNA transcription, but the precise mechanism and the soluble factor(s) responsible for inhibition have yet to be characterized.

In children with vertically acquired infection, HIV-specific CTL responses have been deficient (Luzuriaga et al., 1993). In a detailed study of three infants who were probably infected intrapartum, Luzuriaga and colleagues found a peak of circulating virus titers between 3 and 16 weeks of age. The titers declined in the absence of a CTL response or broadly neutralizing antibody response and without antiretroviral therapy. CTL responses remained undetectable throughout the reported follow-up period to 23 months of age. This was despite an early expansion of the CD8$^+$/DR$^+$ subset of activated T cells and intact CTL responses in mixed lymphocyte cultures. In a study of four symptomatic children, Plaeger-Marshall and colleagues (1992) showed that CD8-mediated viral inhibition is attenuated or absent.

Buseyne and associates (1993) detected specific CTL activity to at least one of four HIV target proteins in 24 of 25 perinatally infected children and in none of four seroreverting infants. Responses were weaker than in adults and diminished as children became symptomatic. The mean age of the infected children studied was 51 months (range, 3 to 168), and the authors conceded that there may be some selection bias for better immune function compared with the other pediatric cohorts mentioned. The one child with rapid disease progression who died at 7 months had undetectable CTL responses to gag proteins on the one occasion he was tested. The authors made the point that intrauterine infection could result in the presence of HIV antigens in the thymus at the time of T-cell differentiation and produce tolerance, which may contribute to the more rapid disease progression in these children compared with children infected intrapartum.

In the study by Plaeger-Marshall and coworkers (1992), CD8$^+$ cell percentages were significantly higher in HIV-infected children compared with controls. This was attributable to subsets that were CD45RA$^-$, CD38$^+$, CD57$^+$, or HLA-DR$^+$, confirming an earlier report that noted increased expression of the CD45RO antigen on CD8$^+$ T cells (Froebel et al., 1991). CD45RA is lost (and the CD45RO isoform is expressed) when CD8 cells become effectors of cytotoxicity (Yamashita and Clement, 1989). The increase in this subset may therefore reflect a specific CTL response, consistent with the increased HLA-DR$^+$ subset. Both of these, however, may result from nonspecific immune activation associated with HIV infection.

HIV-specific CTL activities have been reported in seroreverting infants of HIV-infected mothers (Rowland-Jones et al., 1993; Cheynier et al., 1992). Helper T-cell reactivity measured by IL-2 release from PBMCs in response to envelope peptides has been detected in exposed but uninfected high-risk individuals, although CTL assays were not performed in this study (Clerici et al., 1992a). Unusually high frequencies of HIV-specific CTL responses to envelope proteins have been found in normal, uninfected subjects. Whether these observations are the result of cross-reactivity with certain cellular proteins or whether they represent triumphs of cellular immunity in controlling and possibly clearing virus remains controversial.

Cytotoxic Natural Killer Cells and Antibody-Dependent Cellular Cytotoxicity (ADCC)

As with the CTL responses, natural killer (NK) cell activity has been found to be defective with advancing HIV disease (Cai et al., 1990). In this study, the decrease in NK cell activity did not correlate with altered numbers of CD16$^+$ (NK) lymphocytes. Defective triggering by NK cells of NK cytotoxic factor production by target cells and abnormalities of tubulin distribution have been identified (Bonavida et al., 1986; Sirianni et al., 1988). The cytokines IL-2 and IL-12 enhance NK function in vitro, providing an additional rationale for the use of such immunomodulators in HIV-infected individuals (Rook et al., 1983; Chehimi et al., 1992) (see earlier, CD4$^+$ Lymphocytes).

NK cells are mediators of antibody-dependent cellular cytotoxicity. IgG1 isotype antibodies to specific domains of gp41 or gp120 bind to antigen on the surface of infected cells. Effector NK cells attach by Fc receptors to the antibody-antigen complexes, and the target cells are killed by a cytotoxic process mediated by cytokines such as *perforins* (Yagita et al., 1992). Theoretically, this non-MHC restricted killing of virus-infected cells might be helpful in preventing perinatal transmission, but studies to date have not shown any relationship between ADCC in mothers or their infants and subsequent infection status of the child (Broliden et al., 1993). A significantly higher frequency of ADCC was seen in asymptomatic HIV-infected children than in those with AIDS. This is presumably due to declining NK function because anti-gp120 antibody levels do not drop significantly with disease progression, and the passive administration of antibodies does not affect ADCC (Wong et al., 1993).

Neutralizing Antibody

The viral proteins, believed to be primarily involved in antibody neutralization, have been localized to the envelope gp120 and the external portion of gp41 (Levy, 1993). The principal neutralizing domain (PND) is located at the crown of the third variable region (V3 loop) in the N-terminal portion of gp120 (Broliden et al., 1991). The PND is a linear epitope conserved among many strains. Immunization with this region of gp120 over time induces antibodies that neutralize a large number of HIV-1 strains that share this envelope domain (Berman et al., 1992). In addition, the V3 region contains conformational epitopes that can be better recognized by immune sera if the envelope is glycosylated (Steimer et al., 1991).

HIV-1 infected individuals do not consistently have strong neutralizing antibodies to their autologous virus strain. This may reflect escape by the virus from the humoral immune response (McKeating et al., 1989). Interestingly, HIV-1 sera can neutralize HIV-1 but not HIV-2 strains, yet HIV-2 sera may neutralize some HIV-1 strains (Weiss et al., 1988).

The clinical relevance of the humoral immune response remains uncertain. Neutralizing antibodies do not prevent cell-to-cell infection, and their effect in controlling viral spread following infection is not clear. In a study of 58 HIV-infected children, however, Robert-Guroff and colleagues (1993) found that low titers of neutralizing antibodies to HIV-1$_{MN}$ are associated with an increased frequency of major clinical events during the follow-up period. No such correlates were found with levels of binding antibody to V3 epitopes, which suggests that the neutralization involves conformational epitopes.

The evidence for the role of maternal antibodies in preventing perinatal transmission is controversial (see later, Perinatal Transmission).

Antibody-Dependent Enhancement

In dengue virus infection, and in other retroviral diseases, such as caprine and equine lentivirus infections, antibodies that enhance viral replication in vivo have been identified that correlate with increased morbidity and mortality (Kliks et al., 1989; McGuire et al., 1986; Issel et al., 1992). Factors in fresh human serum from HIV-infected individuals have been described that caused increased syncytial formation in MT2 cells at dilutions of sera from 1:4 to 1:64 (Robinson et al., 1988). A possible explanation for enhancement in HIV infection is that infectious virus complexed to non-neutralizing antibody may be brought into closer proximity to CD4 receptors by the antibody binding to Fc or by complement receptors on the lymphocyte. The role of the CD4 receptor is not clear because the phenomenon occurs in the presence of CD4 (Leu-3a) antibodies in macrophages (Homsy et al., 1988). In this situation, virus may fuse directly with the cell membrane after the antibody-virus complex binds to the cell receptors. HIV strain variation, in which certain sera neutralize one HIV strain yet enhance cytopathicity of another, has been described. The clinical rele-

vance of antibody-dependent enhancement is controversial (Montefiori et al., 1991; Shadduck et al., 1991), but it raises some concerns regarding active or passive immunization in the treatment of HIV disease.

Neutrophils and Monocytes

Bactericidal activity of neutrophils against *Staphylococcus aureus* in vitro was defective in 8 of 12 children with asymptomatic infection and in 8 of 9 children with symptomatic HIV disease (Roilides et al., 1990). This defect was partially corrected by granulocyte-macrophage colony-stimulating factor (GM-CSF), but this cytokine is detrimental in patients with HIV infection when administered without concomitant antiretroviral therapy (Pluda et al., 1990b).

Decreased phagocytosis and bactericidal activity of monocytes from adults with AIDS-related complex, but not from asymptomatic individuals, was also noted in one study (Szkaradkiewicz, 1992). In contrast, Nottet and colleagues (1993) found no differences in macrophage phagocytic function when healthy donor macrophages were infected in vitro with HIV-1. Peripheral blood monocytes are not very susceptible to HIV infection and need to undergo differentiation into macrophages in the tissues. Chronically infected tissue macrophages are thought to be a major reservoir for the production and spread of HIV in the host (Levy, 1993).

Host Genetic Factors

Some intriguing preliminary observations have been made regarding host genetic factors that may play a role in protection from infection and delaying disease progression. Up to three log differences in end-point titrations were noted in experiments comparing the susceptibility of peripheral blood leukocytes from 12 healthy donors to HIV isolates (Williams and Cloyd, 1991). Some familial segregation was noted among donors, but no relation with human leukocyte antigen (HLA) polymorphism could be demonstrated. Intriguing information from a study of prostitutes in Nairobi, Kenya, indicates that seroconversion did not occur in a small subgroup of women, despite frequent exposure. The genetic, immunologic, or behavioral reasons for this are being investigated; preliminary data have revealed that MHC class 1 alleles Aw28 and Bw70 are associated with a decreased risk of seroconversion whereas Aw19 is associated with an increased risk (Plummer et al., 1993).

In a study of heterosexual partners of HIV-positive drug users and infants of HIV-infected mothers, HLA antigens B52 and B44 were associated with "resistance" to infection but B51 was associated with HIV "susceptibility" (Fabio et al., 1992). The HLA-DR11 phenotype was significantly more common than expected among HIV+ individuals transmitting infection in this cohort. In studies of rapid versus slow disease progression, HLA-B35 has been associated with a significantly faster rate (Sahmoud et al., 1993; Itescu and Winchester, 1992). Other HLA haplotypes were associated with more rapid declines in CD4+ counts in the Multicenter AIDS Cohort (Kaslow et al., 1990).

Analyses of long term survivors is currently being undertaken to determine whether any particular HLA haplotype confers an advantage.

CLINICAL CONSIDERATIONS

Clinical issues include perinatal transmission and complications of HIV infection.

Perinatal Transmission

Perinatal transmission encompasses the transmission of virus from an infected mother to her child prenatally (intrauterine transmission), during delivery (intrapartum), or following delivery through breast-feeding (postpartum). Table 18–1 outlines some evidence for transmission at each stage. In the literature on HIV, the term "perinatal" is used synonymously with *vertical*, to describe mother-infant transmission.

Timing and Rate of Transmission

Most infants born to infected mothers are themselves uninfected. Published transmission rates in untreated mother-infant pairs varied from 13% in the European Collaborative Study to about 40% in Africa (Gwinn et al., 1991; Hoff et al., 1988; Goedert et al., 1989; European Collaborative Study, 1991; Blanche et al., 1989; Ryder et al., 1989). The reasons for such geographic

Table 18–1. Evidence for Three Routes of HIV-1 Perinatal Transmission

Route of Transmission	References
Intrauterine (Rubella Model)	
Virus detected in aborted fetuses as early as 8 weeks of gestation	Courgnaud et al., 1991
	Sprecher et al., 1986
	Mano and Chermann, 1987
	Jovaisas et al., 1985
Placental trophoblasts and Hofbauer cells can be infected in vitro and in vivo	Lewis et al., 1990
	Douglas et al., 1991
	Maury et al., 1989
Virus isolated from amniotic fluid	Mundy et al., 1987
Chorioamnionitis associated with increased transmission	Ryder et al., 1989
Molecular analysis of transmitted virus	Mulder-Kampinga et al., 1993
Intrapartum (Hepatitis B Model)	
Discordant twin studies	Goedert et al., 1991
	Young and Nelson, 1990
Lack of detectable virus in a proportion of infected children within first 48 hours of birth	De Rossi et al., 1992
	Krivine et al., 1992
	Bryson et al., 1993a
Bimodal pattern of disease postnatally	Blanche et al., 1989, 1990
	Scott et al., 1989
	Tovo et al., 1992
	Byers et al., 1993
Postpartum (HTLV-1 Model)	
Virus can be cultured from breast milk	Thiry et al., 1985
	Davis, 1991
Mothers infected postnatally can transmit virus to breast-fed infants	Stiehm and Vink, 1991
	Hira et al., 1990
	Zeigler et al., 1985
Transmission by wet nurse	Colebunders et al., 1988

variation have yet to be identified definitively. Higher levels of maternal viremia, lower CD4 counts, and more advanced maternal disease have been associated with increased risk of transmission in some cohorts (Ryder et al., 1989; Boue et al., 1990; D'Arminio Monforte et al., 1991; Tibaldi et al., 1993; Boyer et al., 1994) but not in others (Tovo et al., 1991; Papaevangelou et al., 1992). Most transmitting mothers in the United States, however, are asymptomatic at delivery (Scott et al., 1985). Intrapartum events that increase fetal exposure to maternal blood, such as amniocentesis, placenta previa, abruptio placentae, fetal scalp monitoring, episiotomy, and second-degree tears, are associated with an increased risk of transmission (Boyer et al., 1994).

Some selection of maternal viral quasi-species may occur, with preliminary evidence for preferential transmission of non-SI variants and certain gp120 glycosylation motifs (Wolinsky et al., 1992; Mo et al., 1993). In contrast, Lamers and colleagues (1994) found that sequences in samples obtained from two infants within 4 weeks of birth displayed greater genetic variation than maternal samples. The influence of viral genotype and phenotype is a focus of much research. Viruses with a rapid-high replicative capacity do not appear to be transmitted more readily than those with a slow-low phenotype (Scarlatti et al., 1993).

The rate of disease progression in infants has been linked to the severity of disease in the mother at the time of delivery, but whether this is the result of a larger viral inoculum, earlier intrauterine transmission, or transmission of other pathogens that might influence disease progression is not clear (Blanche et al., 1994).

Maternal immune factors are equally controversial. High titer antibodies to certain epitopes of gp120 of HIV-1 laboratory isolates were initially associated with lower transmission rates (Rossi et al., 1989; Goedert et al., 1989), but this has not been confirmed in subsequent studies (Halsey et al., 1992). Preliminary data suggested that higher maternal neutralizing antibody titers to autologous HIV isolates may correlate with decreased transmission (Bryson et al., 1993b; Scarlatti et al., 1993). A phase III study of passive immunization of mothers (and of babies within 12 hours of birth) with human immune globulin containing high titers of antibody to HIV structural proteins (HIVIG) is under way (AIDS Clinical Trial Group [ACTG] study 185).

Any theories regarding vertical transmission have to explain the well-documented discordance of transmission from one pregnancy to the next and between twins. A multinational study of 100 sets of twins born to seropositive mothers demonstrated that transmission is more common to the first-born twin ($p = .004$) (Goedert et al., 1991). Fifty percent of vaginally delivered and 38% of cesarean section–delivered first-born twins were infected, as opposed to 19% of second-born twins delivered by either route. Confounding variables, such as increased monitoring of the first twin with scalp electrodes, were excluded. The first-born twin has more prolonged exposure to cervical and vaginal secretions, which have been shown to harbor infectious virus (Vogt et al., 1987; Pomerantz et al., 1988).

Intrapartum transmission is presumed to occur across the infant's mucous membranes, principally in the oropharynx and possibly in the esophagus and stomach. In support of this mechanism, four out of four healthy Rhesus monkeys inoculated orally at birth with cell-free simian immunodeficiency virus (SIV), equivalent to 5 ml of viremic plasma, became infected (Baba et al., 1994). Field studies are being conducted to test whether cleansing of the birth canal during labor can reduce the risk of transmission. Successful interventions to reduce perinatal infection, particularly in parts of the world where antiretroviral therapy is not yet an option, are likely to require a more precise understanding of the mechanisms and timing of transmission.

A placebo-controlled study in the United States of zidovudine given to mothers during pregnancy and delivery and to their infants postnatally has demonstrated a highly significant reduction in transmission, from 25.5% to 8.3% (see later, Treatment; CDC, 1994b; Connor et al.,1994). This is clearly of great importance for the management of women who can be identified as infected early enough in pregnancy. It does not, however, clarify the issue of timing of transmission because treatment was started in the second trimester and extended throughout the perinatal period.

In Utero Versus Intrapartum Transmission

With the advent of highly sensitive techniques for detecting virus in the peripheral circulation of the infant, it is becoming possible to define the predominant route more accurately. A consensus opinion from the Pediatric Virology Committee of the AIDS Clinical Trials Group defined an infant infected in utero as one in whom virus could be cultured or HIV-1 genome detected by polymerase chain reaction (PCR) from blood within 48 hours of birth (Bryson et al., 1992). A child infected intrapartum would have negative results within the first 48 hours, becoming positive from day 7 to day 90. Breast-fed infants are excluded from this category. This is a reasonable working definition, although it does not exclude the possibility that infants are becoming infected in utero but only develop detectable viremia postnatally as viral replication is up-regulated following immune stimulation. Large prospective studies using this definition are in progress. The existing evidence for transmission at each stage of the perinatal period is summarized in Table 18–1. Using the above criteria, preliminary estimates indicate that in the absence of breast-feeding, 50% to 70% of transmission occurs around the time of delivery (Boyer et al., 1994).

As mentioned, a bimodal pattern of disease progression has been observed in perinatally infected children (Blanche et al., 1989, 1990; Scott et al., 1989; Tovo et al., 1992; Byers et al., 1993). One explanation for this is that children infected in utero may have dissemination of virus to organs such as the thymus at a critical stage of development (Uittenbogaart et al., 1993). This

may result in early and profound impairment of cellular and humoral immunity, with more rapid disease progression. Consistent with this are reports that infants who have detectable virus by culture, PCR, or p24 antigen levels within the first week of life are at increased risk for rapid disease progression (Burgard et al., 1992; Krivine et al., 1992; Bryson et al., 1993a; Levine et al., 1993). Early reports of an embryopathy associated with HIV disease, suggesting first-trimester transmission, have not been confirmed (Marion et al., 1986; Iosub et al., 1987).

Despite several studies documenting the presence of HIV-1 in the breast milk of seropositive mothers, the additional risk of infection by this route rather than in utero or intrapartum appears to be around 15% to 20% (Thiry et al., 1985; Davis, 1991; Dunn et al., 1992; Ruff et al., 1992). The risk may be higher if the mother's primary infection occurs in the perinatal period, consistent with wide dissemination of virus and a lack of protective secretory IgA at the time of acute infection (Van De Perre et al., 1991; Stiehm and Vink, 1991). Ryder and colleagues did not find a statistically significant difference in infection rates of breast-fed as opposed to bottle-fed infants in Zaire. In this setting, however, bottle feeding was associated with a higher morbidity (Ryder et al., 1991).

Mathematical modeling has demonstrated that the benefits of breast-feeding can outweigh the risks of transmission in countries in which safe water supplies and maintenance of sterility of bottle feeding equipment cannot be guaranteed (Lederman, 1992). The World Health Organization (WHO) (1992) encourages breast-feeding in countries "where infectious diseases and malnutrition are the main causes of infant deaths and the infant mortality rate is high." In the United States, the United Kingdom, and other countries with relatively safe alternatives to breast-feeding, bottle feeding is strongly encouraged (Brierley et al., 1988).

Diagnosis

The diagnosis of HIV infection is normally established in adults by serologic tests for HIV-specific IgG antibodies, which become detectable within 4 to 24 weeks of initial infection (Horsburgh et al., 1989). Several licensed enzyme-linked immunosorbent assays (ELISAs) are available, and the results can be confirmed by Western blot (Consortium for Retrovirus Serology Standardization, 1988). The Western blot allows a profile of antibody reactivity to the range of HIV-1 proteins to be assessed. Antibodies to the envelope glycoproteins gp160, gp120, and gp41 tend to persist, whereas those to the gag proteins may be lost with advancing disease. This loss of reactivity has prognostic significance in children (Walter et al., 1990). Hypogammaglobulinemia may result in false-negative test results by ELISA or Western blot (Rogers et al., 1991).

For perinatally infected infants, these tests are of no diagnostic value beyond confirming the serologic status of the mother. Almost 100% of infants of infected mothers acquire IgG antibodies to HIV transplacentally. These passively acquired antibodies gradually wane, with a median time to disappearance of 10 months, although up to 2% of uninfected infants have detectable antibodies at 18 months (European Collaborative Study, 1991; Blanche et al., 1989). Positive ELISA and Western blots are therefore only diagnostic of infection in children over the age of 18 months.

The current approach to establishing the diagnosis in infants is to use tests that directly detect the virus or its components (Table 18–2) (Husson et al., 1990; Rogers et al., 1991; Tudor-Williams, 1991; Consensus Report, 1992). The three most widely accepted methods are

- Virus culture
- Detection of proviral genome by PCR
- Detection of serum p24 antigen by ELISA

Virus can be cultured from plasma, PBMCs, or whole blood in qualitative or quantitative assays (Jackson et al., 1988; Ho et al., 1989; Coombs et al., 1989; Alimenti et al., 1992). The requirement for Biosafety Level 2 or 3 facilities, and the lengthy, labor-intensive nature of these assays, makes them expensive and limits their availability. Culture of the virus is essential, however, if one wants to perform additional studies, such as phenotypic assays and neutralizing studies against autologous viral isolates.

Polymerase chain reaction techniques have become increasingly automated and are at the point of being licensed by the Food and Drug Administration for diagnostic use. Proviral DNA extracted from PBMC or whole blood (including dried blood spots on filter papers) can be amplified (Cassol et al., 1992). By the use of a reverse transcription step prior to amplification

(RT-PCR), virion RNA from plasma or the various species of mRNA in cells or whole blood can be detected. For diagnostic purposes, the DNA PCR method is more straightforward; for research purposes, increasingly reliable methods of quantitative RNA PCR are being studied (Piatak et al., 1993a; Mulder et al., 1994). PCR is more rapid than culture and provides a similar degree of sensitivity and specificity, approaching 100% by 2 to 3 months of age (Consensus Report, 1992). Quality assurance procedures for rapidly detecting contamination and false-positive results in a PCR laboratory are mandatory. Careful selection of primers in highly conserved regions of the genome are important because genotypic variation can affect the efficiency of amplification (Candotti et al., 1991).

The sensitivity of p24 antigen detection has been considerably enhanced by the use of immune complex disruption/dissociation (ICD p24) techniques (Bollinger et al. 1992). Both in vivo and in vitro lysis of virions release p24 antigen, which is immediately complexed with antibody. Acid hydrolysis of such complexes frees the p24 antigen to bind with the test reagent. Preliminary results in the neonatal period are promising (Walter et al., 1993; Chandwani et al., 1993). In one study, however, 2 of 22 cord blood samples from seroreverting infants tested falsely positive just above the cutoff value. When a second serum sample was used, all 29 children evaluated in the first 3 weeks of life were correctly assigned (Miles et al., 1993).

Despite the sensitivity of culture, PCR and, to a marginally lesser extent, ICD p24 antigen assays, between 50 and 70% of children who subsequently prove to be infected have negative results in the first few days of life (Krivine et al., 1992). This suggests peripartum transmission with extremely low or absent circulating viral burden initially (see earlier). The need for follow-up samples to confirm an initial positive result or establish a negative diagnosis is apparent.

Several tests have been developed that demonstrate evidence of infection less directly. In vitro antibody production (IVAP) and enzyme-linked immunospot (Elispot) methodologies detect the presence of B cells that secrete specific HIV antibodies in vitro (Pahwa et al., 1989; Nesheim et al., 1992). These methods have low sensitivity and specificity in the first 3 months of life and have not become widely used. Detection of IgA-specific antibodies (which do not cross the placenta) offers promise, although they cannot usually be detected earlier than 2 months of age (Martin et al., 1991; Landesman et al., 1991). The assays in development are in ELISA format, are much less costly than PCR or culture, and may prove useful as an additional screening test. HIV-infected cells can be detected by flow cytometry; fluorescent anti-p24 antibody probes that bind with intracellular p24 antigen in lymphocytes may be a potentially sensitive diagnostic technique (Ohlsson-Wilhelm et al., 1990; Connelly et al., 1992).

Prenatal diagnosis has been attempted in a limited number of women—for example, those undergoing cordocentesis for clinical indications (Cullen et al., 1992). HIV has also been cultured from amniotic fluid (Mundy et al., 1987). Any invasive procedures in the

Table 18–2. CDC 1994 Revised Diagnostic Classification System for HIV Infection in Children Younger Than 13 Years Old

Confirmed HIV Infection
1. In a child < 18 months of age who is known to be HIV-seropositive or born to an HIV-infected mother—positive results by any of the following HIV detection tests on two separate samples (excluding cord blood):
   a. HIV virus culture
   b. HIV polymerase chain reaction (PCR)
   c. HIV antigen (p24) (FDA-licensed assay) *or*
   d. Diagnosis of AIDS based on the 1987 AIDS case definition
2. In a child > 18 months of age:
   a. HIV antibody-positive by repeatedly reactive EIA and confirmatory test, *or*
   b. Any of the criteria in (1) above

Exposed Infection Status
A child who does not meet the criteria above but who is
   a. HIV-seropositive by EIA and confirmatory test (< 18 months old at the time of test) *or*
   b. Born to an HIV-infected mother, infant's antibody status unknown

Seroreverter
A child born to an HIV-infected mother has seroreverted (SR) and is assumed uninfected when
   a. He or she has been documented HIV antibody-negative (two or more negative ELISA tests after 6 months of age) *and*
   b. Has no other laboratory evidence of infection (has not had two positive viral detections tests, described above) *and*
   c. Has not had any clinical condition listed in category C (see Table 18–3)

Abbreviation: FDA = Food and Drug Administration.

prenatal period, however, run the risk of carrying maternal blood to the infant and causing infections.

Clinical and indirect laboratory parameters may also indicate HIV infection. A new classification system (see later) for pediatric HIV disease has been developed (Table 18–3) (CDC, 1994b). The onset of category C symptoms is diagnostic, but category A symptoms have poor specificity (Mayers et al., 1991). Persistent oral candidiasis and parotitis were found to be highly discriminatory for HIV infection in the European collabo-

rative study, whereas lymphadenopathy, hepatosplenomegaly, eczema, fever, rhinitis, otitis, and non–gram-negative pneumonias were not (European Collaborative Study, 1991). Low CD4 counts and percentages, taking into account the age-dependent normal range, were suggestive but not diagnostic (Erkeller-Yuksel et al., 1992; McKinney and Wilfert, 1992). Hypergammaglobulinemia is a frequent finding by 3 months of age but is of poor positive predictive value, because many uninfected infants of infected

Table 18–3. CDC 1994 Revised Classification System for HIV Infection in Children Less Than 13 Years Old

Category N: No Symptoms
Child has no signs or symptoms that are believed to be the result of HIV infection and/or are indicative of immunologic deficits attributable to HIV infection, or has only one of the conditions listed in category A, below

Category A: Mildly Symptomatic
Two or more of the conditions listed below occurring in an HIV-infected or exposed child; conditions listed in categories B and C must not have occurred:
- Lymphadenopathy (≥0.5 cm at ≥ two sites; bilateral = one site)
- Hepatomegaly
- Splenomegaly
- Dermatitis
- Parotitis
- Recurrent or persistent upper respiratory tract infections, including sinusitis or otitis media (four or more episodes in a 12-month period)

Category B: Moderately Symptomatic
Symptomatic conditions occurring in a child that are not included among conditions listed in clinical category C and that are attributed to HIV infection and/or are indicative of immunologic deficits attributable to HIV infection

Examples of conditions in clinical category B include, *but are not limited to*
- Anemia, <8 g/dl, or neutropenia, <1000/mm^3, or thrombocytopenia, <100,000/mm^3
- Bacterial meningitis, pneumonia, or sepsis (single episode)
- Candidiasis, oropharyngeal (thrush), persistent in child > 6 months of age
- Cardiomyopathy
- Diarrhea, recurrent or chronic
- Hepatitis
- Herpes stomatitis, recurrent (≤ two episodes within 1 year)
- Herpes zoster (shingles) involving at least two distinct episodes or more than one dermatome
- Leiomyosarcoma
- Lymphoid interstitial pneumonia or pulmonary lymphoid hyperplasia complex (LIP/PLH)
- Nephropathy
- Nocardiosis
- Persistent fever > 1 month
- Varicella (persistent or complicated primary chickenpox)

Category C: Severely Symptomatic
Any condition listed in the 1987 surveillance case definition for AIDS, *with the exception of LIP*. The conditions in clinical category C are strongly associated with severe immunodeficiency, occur frequently in HIV-infected individuals, and cause serious morbidity or mortality:
- Serious bacterial infections, multiple or recurrent (any combination of at least two culture-proven infections within a 2-year period of the following types: septicemia, pneumonia, meningitis, bone or joint infection, or abcess of an internal organ or body cavity; excludes otitis media, superficial skin or mucosal abcesses, and indwelling catheter related infections).

Category C: Severely Symptomatic *Continued*
- Candidiasis, esophageal
- Candidiasis, pulmonary (bronchi, trachea, lungs)
- Cytomegalovirus disease with onset of symptoms at age > 1 month (other than liver, spleen, or nodes)
- Cytomegalovirus retinitis
- Cryptococcosis
- Cryptosporidiosis or isosporiasis with diarrhea persisting 1 month
- Coccidioidomycosis, disseminated (at site other than or in addition to lungs or cervical or hilar lymph nodes)
- Encephalopathy (at least one of the following progressive findings present at least 2 months: (1) failure to attain or loss of developmental milestones or loss of intellectual ability verified by standard developmental scale or neuropsychologic tests; (2) impaired brain growth (acquired microcephaly or brain atrophy demonstrated on serial CT or MRI); (3) acquired symmetric motor deficit manifested by two or more of the following—paresis, pathologic reflexes, ataxia, gait disturbance)
- Herpes simplex virus infection causing a mucocutaneous ulcer that persists longer than 1 month, or bronchitis, pneumonitis, or esophagitis for any duration affecting a child older than 1 month of age
- Histoplasmosis, disseminated (at site other than or in addition to lungs or cervical or hilar lymph nodes)
- Kaposi's sarcoma
- Lymphoma, primary in brain
- Lymphoma, small, noncleaved cell (Burkitt's), or immunoblastic or large-cell lymphoma of B-cell or unknown immunologic phenotype
- *Mycobacterium tuberculosis,* disseminated or extrapulmonary
- *Mycobacterium,* other species or unidentified species, disseminated or extrapulmonary
- *Mycobacterium avium* complex or *M. kansasii,* disseminated (at site other than or in addition to lungs, skin, or cervical or hilar lymph nodes)
- *Pneumocystis carinii* pneumonia
- Progressive multifocal leukoencephalopathy
- Toxoplasmosis of the brain with onset at age > 1 month
- Wasting syndrome: persistent weight loss—>10% of baseline, or an infant who crosses two percentile lines or is below the fifth percentile and falling away from curve—that is unresponsive to oral alimentation

mothers have high levels of passively acquired IgG (Kline et al., 1993). By 6 months of age, however, hypergammaglobulinemia was found to be a useful indicator and was positive in 77% of infected and 3% of uninfected children (European Collaborative Study, 1991). β_2-microglobulin and neoterin levels are non-specific indicators of infection that may have greater value in monitoring disease progression than in establishing a diagnosis (Chan et al., 1990; Ellaurie and Rubinstein, 1990; Ellaurie et al., 1992; Siller et al., 1993).

The differential diagnosis of HIV infection in symptomatic infants and children includes the primary combined immunodeficiency disorders, other congenital infections (e.g., toxoplasmosis, syphilis, parvovirus B19, listeriosis), and the extensive list of causes of failure to thrive. A careful history that includes maternal risk factors may suggest HIV exposure. Initial laboratory tests, including an immunoglobulin profile and lymphocyte subsets using age-adjusted standards, may indicate a cellular or humoral immune abnormality. Direct tests for the presence of HIV, as outlined earlier, should be done prior to an extensive workup for rare primary immunodeficiency diseases.

Classification Systems

Classification systems have been developed for children 13 years old and younger, but there are differences in HIV infection in children compared with adults.

HIV Infection in Children Under 13 Years of Age

The 1987 classification system proposed by the CDC (1987) was revised in 1994 to reflect the spectrum of clinical and immune abnormalities (CDC, 1994b).

The clinical categories are outlined in Table 18–3; the signs and symptoms should be HIV-related. For example, hepatitis is ascribed to category B only when other causes of hepatitis, such as other viral infections or drug toxicities, have been excluded. Category C conditions include all those listed in the 1987 surveillance case definition for AIDS, except for lymphocytic interstitial pneumonitis (LIP). Several studies have indicated that LIP is not associated with shortened survival (Blanche et al., 1990; Tovo et al., 1992). LIP and any category C conditions, however, are reportable to state and local health departments as AIDS.

Table 18–4 shows the new classification grid, and the CD4 absolute count and percentage axes are shown in Table 18–5. Children are categorized according to two CD4 counts and are not reclassified to a higher level if the counts subsequently improve. Clinically and epidemiologically, the classification grid allows greater precision in describing and staging children with HIV infection.

This classification system requires systematic laboratory testing of children, both to establish the diagnosis and to monitor immune parameters. In addition, there are geographic variations in clinical manifestations of AIDS, such as severe diarrheal disease and measles in sub-Saharan Africa, which make this classification less appropriate. A clinical case definition for AIDS was published by WHO (1986). Subsequent field evaluation demonstrated 90% specificity but only 35% sensitivity and positive predictive value (Lepage et al., 1989). Proposals for a revision are being considered (Belec et al., 1992).

For adolescents, the revised classification system published by the CDC in 1993 should be used (CDC, 1993a). This includes an expansion of the surveillance case definition for AIDS to include all HIV-infected persons with CD4 counts lower than 200/mm³ or less than 14% and patients with pulmonary tuberculosis, recurrent pneumonia, or invasive cervical cancer.

Comparison of HIV Infection in Adults and Children

The proposed new classification of clinical conditions for children with HIV contains much overlap with the current classification for adults and adolescents. A number of important differences, however, have become apparent.

The most important difference is that disease progression may be more rapid in children. Disease progression has a bimodal distribution (see earlier), but even for the children in the later peak, the period of latency is reduced compared to that of adults (Tovo et al., 1992; Byers et al., 1993). The long-term survivors who did not develop *Pneumocystis carinii* pneumonia had a median survival of 8.4 years.

In infants, the subtle initial symptoms must be distinguished from problems associated with prematurity, intrauterine drug exposure, or congenital infections other than HIV. It is unusual to detect a mononucleosis-like illness described in adults with acute HIV infection. The incidence of encephalopathy is higher in children, ranging from 30% to 90% with advancing disease (European Collaborative Study, 1990). Failure

Table 18–4. CDC 1994 Classification Grid for HIV Infection in Children
Less Than 13 Years Old*

Immunologic (CD4⁺ T-Cell) Categories	Clinical Categories			
	No Symptoms (N)	Mild Symptoms (A)	Moderate Symptoms (B)	Severe Symptoms (C)
1. No evidence of suppression	N1	A1	B1	C1
2. Evidence of moderate suppression	N2	A2	B2	C2
3. Severe suppression	N3	A3	B3	C3

*Children whose HIV infection status is not confirmed are classified using the above grid with a letter E (exposed) placed in front of the classification (e.g., EN2).

Table 18–5. CDC 1994 CD4$^+$ T-Lymphocyte Categories for HIV-Infected
Children Younger Than 13 Years of Age

Absolute CD4 Count and Percentage Categories	Age		
	<12 Months	1–5 Years	6–12 Years
1. No evidence of immunosuppression	>1500 ≥25%	≥1000 ≥25%	≥500 ≥25%
2. Evidence of moderate immunosuppression	750–1499 15–24%	500–749 15–24%	200–499 15–24%
3. Severe immunosuppression	<750 <15%	<500 <15%	<200 <15%

to thrive, in particular the failure of normal linear growth, is considered a specific manifestation of pediatric HIV infection (Working Group on Antiretroviral Therapy: National Pediatric HIV Resource Center, 1993; McKinney et al., 1993). Recurrent bacterial infections, particularly with polysaccharide encapsulated bacteria, are more common, reflecting the immaturity of the humoral immune system. Toxoplasmosis and cryptococcosis are less common in children. LIP has been seen almost exclusively in the pediatric population. Malignancies, in particular Kaposi's sarcoma, are less commonly found in children.

COMPLICATIONS

Complications of pediatric HIV infection can be of two major types, organic-specific and infectious.

Organic-specific complications include LIP, central nervous system problems, growth and endocrine dysfunction, nutritional and gastrointestinal problems, hematologic manifestations, and malignancies.

Lymphocytic Interstitial Pneumonitis

LIP is a chronic lung disorder of uncertain cause that affects up to 40% to 50% of vertically HIV-infected children (Connor et al., 1991b). It is less common in older children and hemophiliacs. The disorder is characterized by a diffuse, interstitial, reticulonodular infiltrate on plain x-ray (Fig. 18–5). If it is associated with larger nodules and hilar or mediastinal lymphadenopathy, it is referred to as pulmonary lymphoid hyperplasia (PLH), which appears to represent one end of the continuum of this process (Joshi et al., 1990). Clinically, there is a wide spectrum of severity, from an asymptomatic individual in whom LIP is a purely radiologic diagnosis to someone with severely compromised exercise tolerance and oxygen dependency.

A presumptive diagnosis may be made on the basis of suggestive x-ray changes that persist for months, are unresponsive to antimicrobial therapy, and are not the result of other specific infectious pathogens. *P. carinii* pneumonia can coexist with LIP, and any new onset of oxygen dependency should prompt an induced sputum examination and consideration of bronchoscopy to

look for pneumocysts or trophozoites. A definitive diagnosis of LIP is made by lung biopsy, although this is rarely necessary. Characteristic findings are a diffuse lymphoid infiltration of the alveolar septa and peribronchiolar areas, with varying degrees of lymphoid aggregation that may show organization into early germinal centers. Both Epstein-Barr virus (EBV) DNA and HIV RNA have been identified by *in situ* hybridization in biopsy specimens from children with LIP (Andiman et al., 1985; Joshi et al., 1987; Katz et al., 1992). The precise etiologic role of either and why LIP is less frequently seen in adults are unclear. The fact that children may be experiencing a primary infection with EBV may be relevant. Other viral agents causing primary infections in childhood, such as HHV-6, may play a role in the pathogenesis of LIP.

LIP may remit spontaneously. Treatment for LIP is only indicated in the presence of hypoxemia and shortness of breath. High-dose oral steroids are used for at least 6 weeks to suppress the lymphocytic proliferation. Symptoms frequently return on weaning steroids, and the lowest maintenance dose must be sought for each individual.

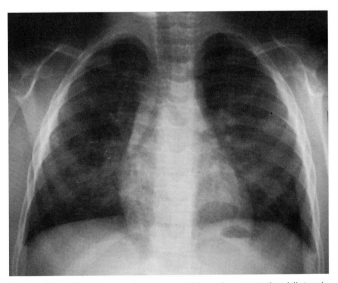

Figure 18–5. Chest x-ray of a 4-year-old boy demonstrating bilateral perihilar infiltrates of mild to moderate lymphoid interstitial pneumonitis (LIP). (Courtesy of Dr. Irwin Feuerstein.)

Central Nervous System Problems

Neurologic problems occur frequently in symptomatic HIV-infected children; estimates vary from 31% to 89% in different series (European Collaborative Study, 1990; Belman, 1992). Of 131 children that were followed at the National Cancer Institute until death, 86 (66%) had neurodevelopmental evidence of encephalopathy at some stage of their disease. Lower CD4 percentages and positive p24 antigen levels are significantly associated with the presence of CNS abnormalities.

Only macrophage-tropic strains of HIV gain entry into the central nervous system, which suggests that infected peripheral blood macrophages are the "Trojan horses" that carry HIV across the blood-brain barrier (Levy, 1993). HIV can be identified in the microglia (CNS macrophages) and, to a lesser extent, in astrocytes. Neurons are not directly infected, and several mechanisms for neuronal cell damage have been proposed. HIV proteins, in particular gp120 and possibly tat, may be toxic to neuroglial cells. *In vivo* support for this has been demonstrated in a transgenic mouse model, in which the expression of gp120 alone correlated with reactive astrocytosis, microglial activation and clustering, and neuronal dendritic vacuolization (Toggas et al., 1994). Activated macrophages may produce toxic factors such as TNF-α, which has been implicated in demyelination (Epstein and Gendelman, 1993). Metabolic products, such as quinolinic acid, can mediate neuronal toxicity by binding to postsynaptic N-methyl-D-aspartate (NMDA) receptors, causing toxic calcium influx. One study in HIV-infected children has shown a significant relation between cerebrospinal fluid (CSF), quinolinic acid levels, and encephalopathy (Brouwers et al., 1993). Nitric oxide, in conjunction with superoxide anion, is believed to be a mediator of neuronal damage following NMDA receptor stimulation (Dawson et al., 1993). Arachidonic acid metabolites, such as leukotrienes and prostaglandins, may cause toxicity by different mechanisms (Lipton, 1994; Epstein and Gendelman, 1993). Until the pathogenesis of CNS damage is more clearly understood, reducing the virus burden using agents that penetrate the CNS is the most logical approach to intervention.

HIV encephalopathy is rarely evident at birth, but it may present in infancy with such signs as delayed acquisition of a social smile, poor head control, or truncal hypotonia. Subsequently progressive motor abnormalities, such as spastic diplegia and oral motor dysfunction, become apparent (European Collaborative Study, 1990; Civitello, 1991; Belman, 1992). Expressive language is frequently more affected than receptive language. The course varies from "static" (with acquisition of developmental milestones at a slower rate than normal) to "progressive," (with overt loss of previously acquired skills). Acquired microcephaly resulting from cerebral atrophy may be noted. Seizures are unusual in the absence of other complications because HIV infection is predominately a disease of white matter (Civitello, 1991). Cerebrovascular disease resulting in strokes can occur (Park et al., 1990). Giant

aneurysms in the circle of Willis have also been described (Lang et al., 1992; Husson et al., 1992).

Computed tomography (CT) scans can demonstrate ventricular enlargement and cortical atrophy (Fig. 18–6) or cerebral calcification, which is seen particularly in the basal ganglia in association with HIV infection (Fig. 18–7) (DeCarli et al., 1993). DeCarli and colleagues found that calcification is a hallmark of vertically acquired HIV infection and is rare in children with transfusion-acquired disease, even if the transfusion was administered in the neonatal period. Of the children with vertically acquired disease, 33% had calcifications, and all of these patients were encephalopathic. Possibly, cerebral calcification is a surrogate marker of intrauterine transmission. Cerebellar atrophy was noted in 12% of scans from this series of symptomatic children. Abnormalities on CT scan were significantly associated with declines in neuropsychologic function. In addition, we have found a significant relation between the presence of CT scan abnormalities and declining CD4 percentages.

Magnetic resonance imaging (MRI) techniques are better than CT scans at delineating white matter abnormalities (Fig. 18–8) (Kauffman et al., 1992).

Early reports suggested that PCR detection of HIV DNA of the cerebrospinal fluid is a marker for CNS involvement in adults (Shaunak et al., 1990). A subse-

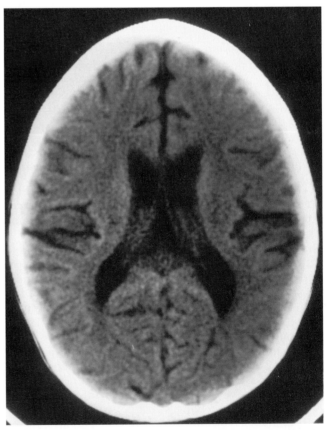

Figure 18–6. Cranial CT scan of an 8-year-old girl with perinatally acquired HIV-1 infection, demonstrating enlargement of the ventricles and widening of the sulci because of cerebral atrophy. This may be partially reversible with zidovudine therapy. (Courtesy of Dr. Nicholas Patronas.)

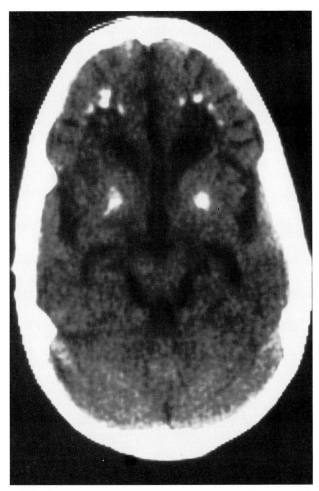

Figure 18–7. Cranial CT scan showing typical distribution of basal ganglia and frontal periventricular calcification. This is a hallmark of perinatally acquired HIV-1 infection (see text). Marked cerebral atrophy is also present. (Courtesy of Dr. Nicholas Patronas.)

and radiologic findings have been associated with zidovudine therapy, particularly when given as a continuous infusion (Pizzo et al., 1988; Brouwers et al., 1990). Improvements in encephalopathic symptoms have been noted anecdotally with corticosteroid treatments (Stiehm et al., 1992). The rapidity with which steroids can induce improvements in a subset of patients suggests that they reverse some toxic effect on the CNS rather than inhibiting primary infection. Modulation of proinflammatory cytokines is a possible mechanism.

Growth and Endocrine Dysfunction

Growth failure is a common finding, and the cause is multifactorial. In one retrospective analysis of 170 children born to infected mothers, the 62 HIV-infected children had significantly decreased linear growth and weight gain by the age of 4 months compared with uninfected controls (McKinney et al., 1993). These decreases were proportional, so that weight for height measurements were normal and the children did not appear wasted. Several studies have shown that growth failure is a specific marker of HIV disease progression (Brettler et al., 1990; McKinney et al., 1991; Tovo et al., 1992).

Growth failure may be a result of inadequate nutri-

quent study, however, found that HIV-1 sequences could be amplified from CSF in 80% of patients, independent of clinical stage or neurologic symptoms (Chiodi et al., 1992). As a supplemental marker for HIV-related neurologic disease, CSF quinolinic acid determinations may be more useful than PCR.

Pathologic findings post mortem include cerebral atrophy, calcification, focal necrosis, gliosis, reactive astrocytosis, vascular lesions, and inflammatory infiltrates, including multinucleated giant cells. Ultrastructural studies and in situ hybridization have demonstrated HIV to be present in these giant cells (Epstein et al., 1988b; Kure et al., 1991).

Spinal cord disease resulting from HIV-induced vacuolar myelopathy is well described in adults but infrequently seen in children (Sharer et al., 1990). We have found evidence of cytomegalovirus (CMV) in the cervical spine and nerve roots of one child associated with a painful radiculomyelopathy.

Therapeutically, the only currently licensed antiretroviral agent that penetrates the blood-brain barrier significantly is zidovudine. Striking improvements in motor abnormalities, neurophysiologic functioning,

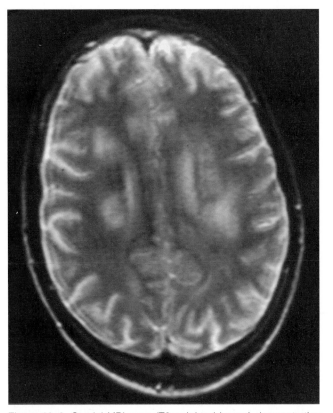

Figure 18–8. Cranial MRI scan (T2-weighted image) demonstrating extensive periventricular white matter changes consistent with HIV-1 leukomalacia. Cytomegalovirus may cause a similar appearance, but usually shows greater evidence of subependymal involvement. Periventricular multifocal leukomalacia, associated with JC virus infection, is usually subcortical initially, with finger-like projections to the surface of the gray matter, and may be more diffuse and patchy. (Courtesy of Dr. Nicholas Patronas.)

tional intake, caused by suppressed appetite, oropharyngeal pathology, or neurologic disease (see other topics). HIV enteropathy or pathogenic bacterial colonization of the small intestine may result in malabsorption (Miller et al., 1991). The metabolic requirements of HIV-infected children may be increased, and wasting may be the result of dysregulation of cytokines following immune activation (Matsuyama et al., 1991; Grunfeld et al., 1992).

Large systematic studies of endocrine abnormalities at different stages of HIV disease are lacking. In one series of nine children with growth failure, there was one case of primary hypothyroidism, six cases of deficient nocturnal thyroid-stimulating hormone (TSH) increase, and one child with growth hormone deficiency (Laue et al., 1990). End-organ resistance may contribute to growth failure; in vitro resistance to growth hormone, insulin-like growth factor-1 (IGF-1), and insulin has been demonstrated in erythroid progenitor cells from HIV-infected children (Geffner et al., 1993). Of 124 children at various stages of HIV disease, we have noted an elevated TSH level in 35 (28%). The prevalence is increased as CD4$^+$ counts fall—42% of children with <200 CD4$^+$ cells/mm^3 had an elevated TSH level. The thyroid-binding globulin level is frequently elevated (74% of 73 patients tested). These data suggest that compensated hypothyroidism is a frequent enough finding to merit annual testing of thyroxine and TSH in symptomatic children.

We have observed three cases of adrenal insufficiency associated with severe salt craving requiring therapy with fludrocortisone acetate. CMV infection of the adrenal gland is a recognized complication of HIV infection (Bleiweiss et al., 1986), but without invasive studies this diagnosis can only be presumptive. In the absence of other evidence of CMV end-organ infection, we do not treat children with adrenal insufficiency with anti-CMV drugs.

In view of the documented efficacy of promoting anabolism in catabolic states and data demonstrating improvements in immune parameters in immunodeficient animal models, we have started a trial of growth hormone or IGF-1 as adjunctive therapy in HIV-infected children with growth failure (see later, Treatment: Immune Modulators).

Nutritional and Gastrointestinal Complications

As discussed, the cause of wasting in HIV-infected children varies. Infections of the gastrointestinal tract frequently contribute. *Candida albicans* and HSV are the most common causes of oropharyngeal pathology (Smith et al., 1993). Since children with esophagitis may not complain of dysphagia, a barium swallow is indicated in children with loss of appetite and weight loss. Infectious pathogens that have been associated with diarrhea in HIV-infected children include *Cryptosporidia, Mycobacterium avium–intracellulare* (MAI), *Microsporidium, Salmonella,* and *Shigella* (Pickering and Cleary, 1991). HIV infection of enterochromaffin cells in the intestinal mucosa may dysregulate motility, and

cytokines released by macrophages in the lamina propria may promote secretory diarrhea (Matsuyama et al., 1991). Disaccharide intolerance caused by lactase deficiency has been documented and may improve with dietary manipulation (Yolken et al., 1991). The role of specific nutrient deficiencies has not been systematically reported, although selenium deficiency was documented in 61% of 23 children with wasting (Miller et al., 1993) and in 37% of 22 other symptomatic children (Mantero-Atienza et al., 1992).

Fluctuating elevations of hepatic transaminases are a frequent finding and can be a diagnostic challenge. Infectious causes other than HIV should be investigated, in particular the hepatitis viruses, CMV, EBV, and *M. avium-intracellulare* (see later). Cryptosporidial infection of the biliary tree is described in adults, and we have seen this at autopsy in one child (Margulis et al., 1986). Many drugs that HIV-infected children receive may be implicated, especially the rifamycins and antifungal azoles. Ceftriaxone and other antibiotics are implicated in biliary sludging (Zinberg et al., 1991).

Pancreatitis was an uncommon finding in children prior to the AIDS era. It can result from opportunistic infections, such as CMV, or, more commonly, as a side effect of therapy, in particular as a dose-dependent toxicity of dideoxyinosine (ddI) (Miller et al., 1992; Butler et al., 1993). The precise mechanism is not well understood (Underwood and Frye, 1993).

Therapeutic interventions for growth failure must be individualized after a thorough diagnostic evaluation. In the absence of specific infections or endocrine complications that can be treated, we use a combination of appetite stimulants, enteral supplements and, if necessary, parenteral feeding to counteract wasting. Studies of early nutritional intervention in HIV-infected infants are in progress to test whether the early onset of growth failure can be ameliorated.

Hematologic Manifestations

All three cell lines from the bone marrow can be affected by HIV infection, although evidence for direct infection of bone marrow precursors is scant (Scadden et al., 1989; Molina et al., 1990). HIV can infect human bone marrow stromal fibroblasts, which are important sources of trophic and inhibitory regulators of hematopoietic progenitors (Scadden et al., 1990). Disruption of the bone marrow microenvironment may explain many of the effects of HIV on hematopoiesis.

The most common hematologic abnormality is anemia which, depending on definition, stage of disease, and concomitant myelosuppressive drug exposure, is seen in up to 94% of children (Pizzo et al., 1988; Ellaurie et al., 1990; Butler et al., 1991). Severe anemia has been shown to be an indicator for disease progression in some series (Ellaurie et al., 1990; Tovo et al., 1992). Pure red cell aplasia has been occasionally described as resulting from human parvovirus B19 infections (Frickhofen et al., 1990; Parmentier et al., 1992).

Neutropenia (variously defined as an absolute neutrophil count of less than 500 to 1500) is also common and is the major dose-limiting toxicity to zidovudine therapy in infants. Side effects of therapy are the most common cause of neutropenia, but opportunistic infections with CMV and *M. avium-intracellulare* may be implicated.

Thrombocytopenia may be the presenting complaint of HIV infection (Rigaud et al., 1992). It may be the result of direct effects of HIV or of opportunistic infections of the bone marrow, autoimmune destruction, sequestration in the spleen, antiretroviral medication or, rarely, an artifact caused by platelet clumping in EDTA-anticoagulated samples (Wong et al., 1993).

Bone marrow aspirates and biopsies in HIV-infected children typically show evidence of maturational arrest of each cell line. The cell lines may be differentially affected. Dyserythropoiesis with megaloblastic changes and nucleated red blood cells, dysmegakaryopoiesis, and left-shifting of the leukocyte precursors may be found.

A variety of coagulopathies have been described. Vitamin K deficiency is not uncommon and is an easily corrected coagulopathy. Lupus-like anticoagulants have been noted to cause a prolongation of the activated partial thromboplastin time that is not corrected by the addition of normal plasma (Scadden et al., 1989). Disseminated intravascular coagulation (DIC) may complicate fulminant infections but does not appear more common in HIV-infected children. We have seen a DIC-like picture in some children treated with G-CSF, but the mechanism of this is not fully elucidated.

Malignancies

Immunodeficiency is known to be associated with an increased risk of pediatric malignancy (Penn, 1988; Groopman and Broder, 1989). In adults with HIV, the risk of Kaposi's sarcoma is estimated to be 20,000 times greater than in the general population, although among transmission groups homosexual and bisexual men are disproportionately affected (Beral et al., 1990). Non-Hodgkin's lymphoma is about 60 times more common in AIDS patients than in the general United States population (Pluda et al., 1990a; Beral et al., 1991).

In children, the anticipated increased incidence of non-Hodgkin's lymphoma has yet to materialize, although it is an uncommon tumor in the general population under 19 years of age. The cumulative number of children under the age of 13 years in whom a malignancy was the AIDS-defining illness was 99 (as of December 1993). This represented 2% of the total 5210 children with AIDS. Of these, 25 had Kaposi's sarcoma, 39 had Burkitt's lymphoma (which is not normally associated with immunosuppression), 20 had an immunoblastic lymphoma, and 15 had primary CNS lymphoma. Grouping the lymphomas together yields a 360-fold increased risk of observed to expected cases in the AIDS group 0 to 19 years old. In addition, an increased incidence of leiomyomas and leiomyosarcomas, which have also not previously been associated with immunodeficiency, has been reported (Mueller et al., 1992a).

Of the more than 350 HIV-infected children evaluated at the Pediatric Branch of the National Cancer Institute, we have seen two non-Hodgkin's lymphomas of the central nervous system (both related to vessels). In addition, we have diagnosed three Ki-1[+] large cell anaplastic lymphomas, one nasopharyngeal Burkitt's lymphoma, one large cell pulmonary lymphoma (a second tumor in a hemophiliac who had a complete remission of the nasopharyngeal Burkitt's, listed earlier), one mucosa-associated lymphoid tumor, one leiomyosarcoma of the liver, and three leiomyomas diagnosed incidentally at post mortem.

We have had some encouraging preliminary results in obtaining remission in HIV-associated high-grade lymphomas using a dose-intensive three-cycle regimen of cyclophosphamide and methotrexate intravenously and cytarabine and methotrexate intrathecally. Figure 18–9 shows gallium scans of a 3-year-old boy with a high-grade B-cell lymphoma before and after two cycles of chemotherapy. Clinically, it can be impossible to differentiate between an EBV-driven polyclonal immunoproliferative disorder or lymphoma, and biopsy is essential in children presenting with new or asymmetric regional lymphadenopathy.

Recurrent Bacterial Infections

Infectious complications include recurrent bacterial, mycobacterial, viral, protozoal, and fungal infections.

Recurrent, serious bacterial infections are a hallmark of the B-cell defect in HIV-infected children, which may often manifest itself before evidence of a T-cell deficiency. If central venous catheter–associated infections are excluded, the most common bacterial pathogens are the polysaccharide encapsulated organisms, particularly *Streptococcus pneumoniae* (Krasinski et al., 1988; Roilides et al., 1991b). Excluding otitis media, among 204 infectious episodes in the larger series (reported by Roilides) of 105 HIV-infected children, soft tissue infections were most frequent (34%), followed by bacteremias, pneumonia, and sinusitis. Late onset group B streptococcal disease as late as 5 months of age has been described (Di John et al., 1990). An increasing incidence of *Pseudomonas* infections has been reported (Roilides et al., 1992). These were most commonly associated with central venous catheters, especially if a *Pseudomonas* species other than *P. aeruginosa* was isolated. Only 4 of the 13 bacteremic children in this series were neutropenic. Of the catheter-related infections, 65% were cured without removal of the line.

Several case reports have noted that *Bordetella pertussis* may present in older children and adults with HIV infection, despite complete prior immunizations (Adamson et al., 1989; Nordmann et al., 1992). Nasopharyngeal carriage may be extremely prolonged, despite erythromycin therapy. Impaired antibody responses to bacterial toxoids have been documented in HIV-infected children (Borkowsky et al., 1992). It has been hypothesized that cell-mediated immunity may be re-

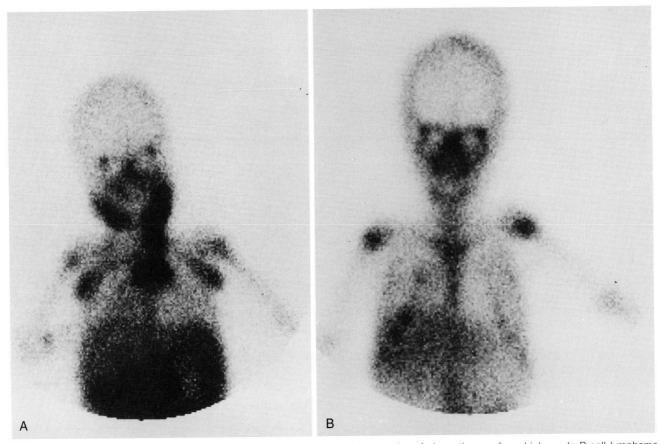

Figure 18–9. Gallium images of a 3-year-old boy, before (*A*) and after (*B*) two cycles of chemotherapy for a high-grade B-cell lymphoma. (Images were obtained with a General Electric starport gamma camera using a medium energy collimator after the administration of approximately 2 mCi of gallium-67 citrate. The pretreatment image obtained 120 hours after administration of the tracer shows abnormally increased uptake throughout the left side of the neck and in the superior mediastinum and both axillae. A follow-up scan 7 weeks later after completion of two cycles of therapy shows no abnormal uptake in the neck or axillae.) (Courtesy of Dr. Steven Falen.)

quired to eliminate an intracellular phase of *B. pertussis* (Doebbeling et al., 1990).

Mycobacterial Infections

Mycobacterial infections are of increasing concern. *M. avium–intracellulare* has been found in almost one in five children with advanced disease (CD4, <50 cells/mm³) (Lewis et al., 1992). Typical presentation includes recurrent fevers, night sweats, abdominal pain and bloating, and weight loss. A diagnosis of systemic infection requires culture of the organisms from blood, because stool and respiratory isolates may only represent colonization. However, in most prospectively studied adults with such colonization, bacteremia eventually develops (Chin et al., 1994).

Current therapy consists of at least three agents, which usually include a macrolide antibiotic (clarithromycin or azithromycin) plus ethambutal and rifampin. The safety and toxicity of prophylactic rifabutin in children with CD4 counts lower than 100 are being assessed. Efficacy studies in adults with less than 75 CD4 cells/mm³ indicate that rifabutin can halve the incidence of *M. avium–intracellulare* infection during the course of treatment (Nightingale et al., 1993).

Mycobacterium tuberculosis is an emerging problem,

and the identification of strains multiply resistant to isoniazid, rifampin, and other drugs in Miami and New York poses a serious threat to patients and their caregivers (Khouri et al., 1992; Starke et al., 1992; Fischl et al., 1992; Beck-Sague et al., 1992). Diagnosis is confounded by anergy in HIV-infected children. Gastric lavage was more sensitive than bronchoalveolar lavage in one series of 20 children (Abadco and Steiner, 1992).

Guidelines for therapy have been reviewed by the Advisory Council for the Elimination of Tuberculosis (CDC, 1993d). Several studies have shown some benefit of isoniazid as prophylaxis against tuberculosis in HIV-infected adults who have positive tuberculin skin tests or in anergic individuals at high risk (Pape et al., 1993). Isoniazid prophylaxis has been recommended for all HIV-infected children who are household or day care contacts with active TB. If the contact has mycobacteria with multiple drug resistance, the choice of drug must be individually tailored (Working Group on Antiretroviral Therapy, 1993).

Viral Infections

HIV-infected children are at substantially greater risk for serious morbidity and mortality from a wide variety of viral pathogens. Of the herpes group, primary varicella can be associated with visceral dissemination (Jura et al., 1989) and encephalitis (Silliman et al., 1993). Subsequent varicella zoster virus (VZV) infection may recur with increasing frequency as the underlying immunodeficiency progresses, although it is seen at all stages of disease. Lesions may be atypical, with hyperkeratosis and increased pigmentation or hypopigmentation without obvious vesiculation (Pahwa et al., 1988; Leibovitz et al., 1992). They are usually painful. Chronic suppressive therapy with acyclovir or foscarnet may be required, but the development of drug resistance is a problem (Pahwa et al., 1988; Jacobson et al., 1990). The role of BV-araU, a bromovinyl uracil derivative with promising in vitro activity against VZV, is being explored in this setting (Hiraoka et al., 1991).

Herpes simplex virus has been associated with severe herpetic gingivostomatitis, esophagitis, and chronic labial infections (Hanson and Kaplan, 1990). Oral acyclovir may be useful for preventing frequent occurrences of severe mucocutaneous HSV infections (Working Group on Antiretroviral Therapy, 1993).

Cytomegalovirus (CMV) may cause retinitis, pneumonitis, enterocolitis, hepatitis and, more rarely, esophagitis, pancreatitis, or adrenal insufficiency (Hanson and Kaplan, 1990). It may be necessary to treat retinitis with a combination of ganciclovir and foscarnet in children who relapse on ganciclovir alone (Butler et al., 1992a). Retinal implants with slow-release formulations of ganciclovir are being used in adults with some promise. It may be possible to use this approach in children older than 6 years of age.

Epstein-Barr virus is implicated in the cause of LIP and also in the polyclonal lymphoproliferative disorder, which may be difficult to distinguish from lymphoma (see earlier, Malignancies). Interactions between HHV-6 and HHV-7 in this population are largely unknown, although seroepidemiologic studies suggest that most children seroconvert by age 2 or 3 years (Pruksananonda et al., 1992; Clark et al., 1993a). *In vitro,* individual CD4 cells can be coinfected with HHV-6 and HIV, and HHV-6 transactivates the HIV LTR through interactions with NF-κB (Ensoli et al., 1989; Lusso and Gallo, 1994). Studies are in progress to assess the role of HHV-6 in disease progression in HIV-infected children.

Respiratory pathogens, particularly respiratory syncytial virus (RSV), parainfluenza III, and adenoviruses may cause severe and even fatal pneumonitis and may also be shed for prolonged periods, creating a significant dilemma in terms of patient isolation policies. *P. carinii* pneumonia may be complicated by superinfection with any of these respiratory pathogens and carries a poor prognosis.

Measles is associated with a high incidence of pneumonitis and occasionally encephalitis (Kaplan et al., 1992). The case fatality rate of measles pneumonitis is estimated to be between 33% and 45%, although this may be an overestimate based on series of hospitalized patients. The clinical presentation is frequently atypical, and rash is absent in about 30% of cases. Treatment options are limited, enhancing the need for widespread preventative vaccination in the community.

Hepatitis viruses A, B, and C may be more fulminant, and the B and C forms in particular can result in a chronic aggressive or frequently relapsing course (Martin et al., 1989; Bodsworth et al., 1991).

Protozoal and Fungal Infections

It is appropriate to discuss protozoal and fungal infections together, because one of the most significant opportunistic pathogens, *P. carinii,* has features of both groups. Morphologically, and in terms of treatment, *P. carinii* resembles a protozoon, but at a biochemical and molecular level it has features of a fungus (Masur, 1992).

Pneumocystis carinii *Infection*

Early in the HIV epidemic, *P. carinii* was noted to be a cause of pulmonary disease in young children with HIV despite apparently high CD4 counts (Rubinstein et al., 1986). *P. carinii* pneumonia was the AIDS indicator disease in 38% of 3471 reported pediatric AIDS cases through 1991. An early and frequently fatal peak is observed in infants around the age of 6 months who are presumably experiencing their primary infection.

Scott and colleagues (1989) reported a median survival time of 1 month from the onset of *P. carinii* pneumonia in a natural history study of HIV-infected children. The presenting features were tachypnea (88%), dyspnea (88%), cough (86%), and fever (79%) in the series of 27 cases reported by Connor and associates (1991a). The presentation may be insidious over a week rather than acute. Hypoxemia is the hallmark of the disease. Radiologically, *P. carinii* pneumonia can present as a spectrum with almost no infiltrates to frank consolidation.

The diagnosis can frequently be established by sputum induction but, if this is negative and clinical suspicion is high, bronchoalveolar lavage is indicated (Ognibene et al., 1989). Open lung biopsy is rarely necessary.

Therapy should take into account which prophylactic regimen (if any) the child has broken through. The drug of choice for treatment remains trimethoprim/sulfamethoxazole-(TMP/SMX), and only a documented serious allergic response (angioneurotic edema, for example) should prompt alternative therapy. Based on data from adult studies, adjunctive steroids are used for any child with an arterial oxygen pressure lower than 70 mm Hg (National Institutes of Health/University of California Expert Panel, 1990). Intravenous pentamidine may be used in patients who have broken through TMP/SMX prophylaxis, but careful monitoring for hypoglycemia, pancreatitis, and dysrhythmias is mandatory. Atovaquone is a hydroxynaphthoquinone with activity against both *P. carinii* and *Toxoplasma gondii* (see later). It can only be given orally, and the bioavailability of the initial tablet preparation was erratic. Absorption was improved twofold to threefold if it was taken with fat-containing meals, which many individuals with advanced HIV disease could not tolerate. A new microparticle suspension is currently in phase I studies in adults and children.

Prophylaxis for *P. carinii* pneumonia is a constantly

evolving field (CDC 1991a, 1995). It is currently rec-ommended that all children with severe immunosup-pression as defined by $CD4^+$ lymphocyte counts receive prophylaxis. In addition, all perinatally exposed infants and proven HIV-infected infants younger than 1 year of age should receive prophylaxis through 12 months of age (CDC, 1995). Any child with a history of *P. carinii* pneumonia, regardless of CD4 count, should receive secondary prophylaxis.

The drug of choice in both situations is TMP/SMX (150 mg TMP/m²/day, two divided doses on 3 consecu-tive days/week). Alternative regimens include aerosol-ized pentamidine for children old enough to comply with nebulized treatment, dapsone (2 mg/kg/day), or intravenous pentamidine. Breakthroughs have been reported with all four regimens but are least frequent with TMP/SMX and most frequent with intravenous pentamidine (Mueller et al., 1991).

Other Protozoal and Fungal Infections

Toxoplasma gondii infections have been the subject of several case reports but the prevalence is much lower in children than in adults (Miller and Remington, 1991). From the literature on adults, chronic sup-pressive therapy with daily pyrimethamine-sulfadia-zine and folinic acid is recommended following treat-ment for active ocular or CNS toxoplasmosis (Working Group on Antiretroviral Therapy, 1993). Cryptospori-dial infection may cause intractable diarrhea in some children, and there are few effective therapies (Curry et al., 1991). Complications include ascending infection of the biliary tree and pancreatitis. The role of *Isospora* and *Microsporidia* is not well documented in children, but *Giardia lamblia* has been implicated as a cause of chronic diarrhea and malabsorption (Smith et al., 1992).

Of the fungal pathogens, *Candida albicans* is the most prevalent. Recurrent oropharyngeal candidiasis was seen in 71% of 123 deceased patients whom we fol-lowed throughout their symptomatic disease stage. *Candida* esophagitis was diagnosed in 24%, usually on clinical and radiologic evidence. Disseminated candidi-asis or fungemias are rare, except in patients with chronic indwelling intravenous devices (Walsh et al., 1993). *Torulopsis glabrata* and other candidal species may cause fungemia in association with such catheters. For persistent or recurrent mucocutaneous candidiasis, chronic suppressive therapy is frequently required. If topical treatment with clotrimazole fails, oral ketocona-zole or fluconazole is used. Resistance and break-through infections occur that may require parenteral therapy with amphotericin B (Working Group on Anti-retroviral Therapy: National Pediatric HIV Resource Center, 1993).

Cryptococcus neoformans is less prevalent in pediatric patients than in adults but can cause meningitis, with an insidious onset of malaise and altered mental status in older children (Ting et al., 1991). Chronic sup-pressive therapy with oral fluconazole is required fol-lowing initial treatment with amphotericin B and 5-flucytosine (Working Group on Antiretroviral Ther-apy, 1993).

Histoplasmosis presenting with fever, cough, pulmo-nary interstitial infiltrates, and sometimes dissemina-tion to the CNS is seen particularly in endemic areas of the midwestern United States (Hanson and Kaplan, 1990). Pulmonary aspergillosis is an occasional compli-cation that in our experience has been unusual in HIV-infected children, unless they have profound, persistent neutropenia (Walsh et al., 1993). Anecdotally, we have found *Aspergillus fumigatus* at post mortem in nodules on the heart valves in a child with pulmonary aspergil-losis.

TREATMENT

Treatment strategies for HIV disease are constantly evolving as our understanding of the immunopatho-genesis grows and as improved therapies are devel-oped. Because currently recommended standards of care may have been modified by the time this chapter is in print, this discussion is limited to the broad princi-ples of treatment and a review of published clinical studies to date.

Table 18–6 summarizes the main components of therapy with some examples that are in use or are being evaluated in clinical trials.

Antiretroviral Therapy

The central role of the virus in the immunopatho-genesis of HIV disease is becoming increasingly clear as more sensitive detection methods delineate the abun-dance of virus in the circulation and lymphoid organs at all stages of disease (Bagasra et al., 1992; Embretson et al., 1993; Pantaleo et al., 1993a; Piatak et al., 1993b). If antiretroviral agents were developed that could com-pletely prevent viral replication, it would be rational to use these at the earliest possible stage of disease. In adults and adolescents, this would be at the time of acute infection, with the aim of reducing the initial burst of viremia and limiting the seeding of virus to the lymphoid organs, brain, and other sites. In infants, it would similarly be at the earliest stage of infection, which includes the perinatal period to diminish trans-mission or as soon as infection is confirmed postnatally. The agents that are available cannot switch off viral replication completely, allowing subpopulations of vi-rus to evolve and mutate into potentially resistant or more pathogenic strains. Long-term therapy is neces-sary, requiring physicians to balance carefully the po-tential benefits of early intervention against the side effects, cost, and selection of more resistant quasispe-cies associated with each drug.

Reverse Transcriptase Inhibitors

Antiretroviral agents are generally targeted to spe-cific steps in the viral life cycle. Of these targets, the virus-encoded reverse transcriptase enzyme has been the most exploited to date. Being an RNA-dependent and DNA-dependent DNA polymerase, it could be an-ticipated that nucleoside analogs might provide suitable substrates for the enzyme. Both purine (adenosine and

Table 18–6. Components of Therapy for HIV-Infected Children with Selected Examples

Treatment Category	Examples

Antiretroviral therapy: Aimed at molecular targets of HIV-1 life cycle (see Figs. 18–1 and 18–2); both single agents and combinations are being studied	Reverse transcription:
	  Nucleoside analogs (AZT, ddI, ddC, 3TC, d4T)
	  Non-nucleoside RT inhibitors (nevirapine, BHAP compounds)
	Protease (e.g., KN1-272, Ro 31-8959)
	Transcription (antisense oligonucleotides)
	Translation (α-glucosidase-1 inhibitor)
	Budding (IFN-α)

Immune modulators	Interleukin-2 and other cytokines TNF-α blockers (pentoxyphylline, thalidomide) Antioxidants (N-acetylcysteine, procysteine) Therapeutic vaccines (gp120, gp160) Growth factors (rhGH, rhIGF-1) HIV antibodies (HIVIG, immune plasma)
Prophylactic measures	Intravenous immunoglobulin *Pneumocystis carinii* pneumonia prophylaxis *Mycobacterium avium–intracellulare* prophylaxis Immunizations (routine, influenza) For contacts of tuberculosis, varicella zoster virus, measles
Chronic suppressive therapy	*Candida* species therapy Cytomegalovirus therapy Varicella zoster virus therapy Herpes zoster virus therapy Toxoplasmosis therapy Cryptococcosis therapy
Supportive therapy	Psychosocial support Nutritional intervention Pain management

guanosine and their precursor inosine) and pyrimidine (thymidine and cytidine) nucleoside analogs have been identified that have potent activity against a wide range of retroviruses.

Each drug requires intracellular anabolic phosphorylation by cellular kinases to form the active triphosphate. The rate of phosphorylation depends on the state of activation of the host cell; zidovudine is more efficiently phosphorylated in phytohemagglutin (PHA)-stimulated PBMC, as opposed to ddI and dideoxycytidine (ddC), which are metabolized to their triphosphate forms fivefold to 15-fold more efficiently in resting PBMCs (Gao et al., 1993). This is of possible relevance in the perinatal period, because neonates have a lower proportion of activated lymphocytes (Erkeller-Yuksel et al., 1992). All active anti-HIV analogs lack the 3′-hydroxyl moiety on the deoxyribose ring so that no phosphodiester link can be formed with the next nucleotide, resulting in chain termination. Such analogs act as competitive inhibitors and chain terminators, with inhibition constants ranging from 0.005 to 0.2 μM (Yarchoan et al., 1989). Mammalian DNA polymerase-α is more selective than the HIV reverse transcriptase and is inhibited only by 100- to 230- μM concentrations of these agents. Inhibition constants for mitochondrial DNA polymerase γ, however, are in the range of 0.016 to 0.4 μM, which has been implicated in some of the toxicities of these compounds, particularly zidovudine-associated myopathy (Chariot et al., 1993).

Zidovudine (ZDV, AZT)

Zidovudine (3′-azido-2′,3′-dideoxythymidine; azidothymidine; ZDV, AZT) prolongs the short-term survival

of adults with advanced HIV-1 disease (Fischl et al., 1987) and delays the development of AIDS-defining conditions in symptomatic and asymptomatic adults with CD4 counts below 500 cells/mm³ (Fischl et al., 1990; Volberding et al., 1990; Graham et al., 1992). Optimism from these initial studies, however, has been tempered by data from the Veterans Affairs Cooperative Study and the European Concorde Study (Hamilton et al., 1992; Aboulker and Swart, 1993).

In summary, it appears that disease progression occurs in 12 to 18 months in patients with more advanced disease (CD4 counts lower than 200 cells/mm³) at the time of initiation of monotherapy. In asymptomatic individuals with counts above 200 cells/mm³, drug failure is seen after 2 to 3 years of treatment (Saag, 1994). Within this framework, there is considerable individual variation.

The most compelling evidence to date for the efficacy of zidovudine as an antiretroviral agent is provided by the ACTG 076 trial to diminish perinatal transmission (CDC, 1994a; Connor et al., 1994). This was a placebo-controlled study of zidovudine given to mothers antepartum and intrapartum and to infants for 6 weeks after birth. At an interim analysis of 364 evaluable infants in February 1994, the estimated rate of transmission was 25.5% in the placebo recipients (n = 184) and 8.3% in the zidovudine-treated group (n = 180).

In children with symptomatic disease, uncontrolled clinical trials have demonstrated improvements in clinical, neurodevelopmental, and virologic parameters with zidovudine therapy (Pizzo et al., 1988; McKinney et al., 1990, 1991; Brouwers et al. 1990). Pharmacokinetic studies demonstrated good oral bioavailability

(65%) and reasonable levels in the cerebrospinal fluid (24% of serum levels) (Balis et al., 1989a,b) The plasma half-life was only 1 hour in children older than 12 months but was considerably prolonged in neonates (14 hours after maternal ingestion in one study) (Chavanet et al., 1989; Watts et al., 1991).

The optimal dose of zidovudine monotherapy is yet to be defined. Recommendations are as follows: 0 to 2 weeks of age, 2 mg/kg/dose every 6 hours; 2 to 4 weeks of age, 3 mg/kg/dose every 6 hours; 4 weeks to 13 years of age, 180 mg/m²/dose every 6 hours (Working Group on Antiretroviral Therapy, 1993). For children temporarily unable to take oral medication, zidovudine can be given intravenously at two thirds of the oral dose. The higher incidence of neurologic disease in children has prompted the use of comparatively high doses.

Data from a trial of over 400 minimally symptomatic children comparing the 90- with the 180-mg/m²/dose (ACTG study 128), however, have shown no difference in neurologic or other clinical end points. The lower dose may therefore become the recommended initial dose for children with no pre-existing neurologic disease. One noncomparative study using a 100-mg/m²/dose (or less) every 6 hours failed to show any neurodevelopmental improvements in 60 symptomatic children over 6 to 12 months of follow-up (Blanche et al., 1991). In view of the short plasma half-life, the Pediatric Branch of the National Cancer Institute has been investigating the delivery of zidovudine by continuous intravenous infusion. Twenty-two of 38 evaluable children who had progressive encephalopathy on intermittent oral zidovudine (480 to 720 mg/m²/day) have shown significant neurodevelopmental gains on continuous infusion at 360 to 480 mg/m²/day total dose.

The primary toxicities are anemia (30% to 40% of symptomatic children) and neutropenia. These may occur at any stage during treatment but are more frequent in children with more advanced disease. Dose reduction (to no lower than 75 mg/m²/dose) is indicated. Neutropenia may be ameliorated with granulocyte colony-stimulating factor (G:CSF), which has to be titrated for each child (Mueller et al., 1992b). Many children respond to 1 µg/kg/day subcutaneously but a minority require doses as high as 20 µg/kg/day. We have observed a coagulopathy with decreased platelets, fibrinogen, and a prolonged PTT in three children on higher doses of G-CSF. The mechanism for this disseminated intravascular coagulation-like picture is under investigation. Erythropoietin may be considered for transfusion-dependent anemia, despite dose reduction, but the response is less predictable than with G-CSF for neutropenia. We use an initial subcutaneous or intravenous dose of 150 units/kg three times per week. This can be increased incrementally every 8 weeks to a maximum of 1500 units/kg/dose. Neither G-CSF nor erythropoietin have yet been approved by the Food and Drug Administration for this indication. Zidovudine was approved in 1990 for use in children older than 3 months.

Zidovudine monotherapy can no longer be recommended as initial therapy, inasmuch as ACTG study 152 indicated in February 1995 that it was less effective and more toxic than didanosine or the combination of didanosine and zidovudine.

Didanosine (ddI)

Didanosine (2',3'-dideoxyinosine; ddI) is metabolized intracellularly to its active form, 2',3'-dideoxyadenosine triphosphate (Lambert et al., 1990). This has a long intracellular half-life of more than 12 hours, and ddI itself has a longer plasma half-life than zidovudine, allowing 8 to 12-hour dosing. The oral bioavailability is highly variable (about 19%) and, because ddI is acid-labile, the drug must be taken with antacid (Balis et al., 1992). Penetration of the blood-brain barrier is poor.

ACTG study 116A compared ddI to zidovudine as first-line therapy for adults with advanced HIV disease. No difference in disease progression was found, but the survival trends favored zidovudine (relative risk, 1.4) (Sande et al., 1993). Adults who had tolerated zidovudine for at least 16 weeks (median, 14 months) reached study morbidity and mortality end points less frequently if they were switched to 500 mg/day of ddI rather than continuing on zidovudine (ACTG studies 116B/117) (Kahn et al., 1992). In a randomized study of 312 adults with disease progression on zidovudine, switching to ddI was associated with fewer new AIDS-defining events or deaths after 2 years of follow-up (Spruance et al., 1994). The benefit was most apparent among those with a CD4 count above 100 cells/mm³ at entry.

Studies of ddI in children were initiated concurrently with the adult studies. In the phase I/II trial, 43 children with symptomatic HIV-1 infection received escalating doses from 60 to 540 mg/m²/day in three divided doses. Median CD4 counts increased from 218 to 327 cells/mm³, and p24 antigen levels declined during the first 24 weeks (Butler et al., 1991). As in adults, bone marrow suppression was not observed, but pancreatitis was observed in two patients on higher doses (360 mg/m²/day or more), and peripheral atrophy of the retinal pigment epithelium occurred in three children. In 1991, the data from this study contributed to the simultaneous licensing of ddI for adults and children, an historic event in the history of the FDA. We have subsequently followed over 100 children on ddI monotherapy. In summary, ddI appears to have a more sustained positive impact on CD4 counts than zidovudine but, because of its poor penetrance of the CSF, it is not the drug of choice for children with evidence of HIV encephalopathy.

DdI is nonmyelosuppressive but may be associated with pancreatitis in 5 to 7% of recipients. This complication appears to be more frequent if ddI is given concurrently with intravenous pentamidine. Six of 6000 adults receiving ddI under the expanded access program died with acute pancreatitis (Yarchoan et al., 1991). Retinal depigmentation is non–sight-threatening, and we do not stop treatment with ddI on this basis alone (Whitcup et al., 1992). Peripheral neuropathy is an uncommon toxicity in children, although it is well recognized in adults (Lambert et al., 1990). Despite the recognized problems with oral bioavailability, it is not our practice to monitor levels on all children. Ensuring optimal antacid treatment prior to each dose is crucial; children on less than 20 ml of the commercial liquid formulation need additional antacid.

The interim analysis of a large randomized trial (ACTG study 152) comparing ddI or zidovudine monotherapy with a combination of the two as first-line therapy for symptomatic children was terminated in February 1995, when the zidovudine monotherapy arm was found to be less active and more toxic than ddI monotherapy and/or the combination arm. Another study (ACTG 144) is comparing 100 versus 300 mg/m²/day of ddI for children progressing on or intolerant to zidovudine.

Zalcitibine (ddC)

Like zidovudine, zalcitibine (2',3'-dideoxycytidine; ddC) is a pyrimidine nucleoside analog and is about 10 times more potent in vitro than zidovudine on a molar basis (Yarchoan et al., 1991). Despite the in vitro data, a study of 635 adults with CD4 counts lower than 200/mm³ (ACTG 114) demonstrated that both mortality and disease progression are significantly more frequent on ddC compared with zidovudine monotherapy (Remick et al., 1993). Moderate to severe peripheral neuropathy was observed in 23% of the ddC recipients versus 6% in the zidovudine group. In addition, oral ulcers and rash were common toxicities. Granulocytopenia (10%) and anemia (6%) occurred, although at a lower frequency than with zidovudine. Pancreatitis is an uncommon toxicity. Subsequently, ddI or ddC monotherapy has been compared in 467 adults who had disease progression or were intolerant to zidovudine (Abrams et al., 1994). The median CD4 count was lower than 50 cells/mm³ at entry. After 16 months median follow-up, there were 100 deaths in the ddI arm and 88 in the ddC arm, yielding an adjusted relative risk of 0.63 in favor of ddC. Disease progression was not significantly different, and adverse events were common in both groups. Because the study did not include a placebo arm, it is not possible to determine whether either drug was better than no treatment in patients with advanced disease. It appears, however, that ddC is equivalent to ddI in this context.

Data in children are limited. Pharmacokinetic studies demonstrated a short plasma half-life (0.8 hour), with 54% oral bioavailability (Pizzo et al., 1990). Penetration of the blood-brain barrier is poor. During 8 weeks of ddC monotherapy in this dose escalation pilot study, improvements in CD4 counts and p24 antigen were observed in most of the children. Mouth sores occurred in 9 of 15 patients, however, and a rash was noted in 3 of 6 patients at the higher dose level (0.04 mg/kg every 6 hours). Subsequently, an alternating schedule of zidovudine for 3 weeks and of ddC for 1 week was well tolerated, with less myelosuppression than when zidovudine was administered alone (Pizzo et al., 1990). An ACTG protocol 138 is comparing two doses of ddC (0.01 versus 0.005 mg/kg every 8 hours) in 170 children who have progressed on or are intolerant of zidovudine.

3-Thiacytidine (3-TC)

The negative enantiomer of 2'-deoxy-3'-thiacytidine (3-TC) has been given to more than 100 children, most of whom have had disease progression or toxicity to zidovudine or ddI. Of those with disease progression (n = 68), the median number of weeks of prior therapy with nucleoside analogs was 166; thus, this represents a heavily pretreated cohort. Median bioavailability was 25% to 52%, and the plasma half-life was 2.25 hours, allowing twice-daily dosing. An optimal nonmyelosuppressive pediatric dose appears to be 4 to 8 mg/kg/day. The drug has been well tolerated and is associated with weight gain and improvements in energy levels and appetite in a majority of children. Immune complex dissociation (ICD) of p24 antigen levels and serum viremia by RNA PCR were significantly decreased at weeks 4 and 12. ICD of p24 remained significantly lower at week 24 and serum RNA PCR levels showed sustained improvement at 24 weeks. CD4 percentages were stable at week 24 for both previously treated and untreated patients. A marginal decline (10 cells/mm³) was noted in absolute CD4 counts at week 24 in the pretreated group. Four children (6% of the study cohort), all with advanced HIV disease and other potential risk factors, have had pancreatitis while on 3-TC. Two children have experienced behavioral changes, with marked hyperactivity.

Stavudine (d4T)

Stavudine (2',3'-didehydro-3'-deoxythymidine; d4T) has shown promising short-term antiviral activity, as judged by surrogate markers, but it may be more myelosuppressive than 3-TC (Yarchoan et al., 1991). An efficacy trial comparing zidovudine alone versus a combination of zidovudine and d4T has opened for children over 6 months of age (ACTG 240).

Non-Nucleoside Reverse Transcriptase Inhibitors

Several structurally distinct groups of compounds have been identified that specifically inhibit HIV-1 reverse transcriptase at sites remote from the nucleoside binding domains. These include nevirapine (BI-RG-587), pyridinone (L-697,639), TIBO (R-82913), HEPT, and BHAP (U-87201). All have high antiviral potency in vitro and have been shown to be synergistic with nucleoside analogs. They do not require intracellular metabolism and have low cellular toxicity. Pharmacokinetic profiles are encouraging, with good bioavailability. They are equally active against zidovudine-sensitive or zidovudine-resistant isolates. Their "Achilles heel" has been the rapid emergence of resistant HIV strains when they are given as single agents, both in vitro and in vivo (Richman, 1993). For this reason, they are likely to be of most benefit when used in combination with the nucleoside analogs. One of these agents, nevirapine, has completed phase I testing in children (ACTG 165). Skin rashes have been the most prominent adverse effects, and these are less frequent if the drug is started at a low dose. Several combination studies with zidovudine and/or ddI are in progress.

HIV-1 Resistance to Reverse Transcriptase Inhibitors

The chronic, persistent nature of HIV-1 disease, with substantial levels of virus replication at all stages and a naturally high mutation rate caused by the error-prone nature of the reverse transcriptase, make it predictable that drug-resistant mutants will emerge under the selective pressure of prolonged treatment. The *pol* gene codon mutations that result in amino acid substitutions associated with resistance to several of the reverse transcriptase inhibitors in current use are listed in Table 18–7. Site-directed mutagenesis experiments with construction of recombinant infectious HIV-1 clones containing specific resistance mutations have enabled the contribution of different codon changes to be evaluated (St. Clair et al., 1991).

Partial resistance to zidovudine is conferred by one to three mutations, whereas four to five mutations are required to produce a highly zidovudine-resistant virus (Kellam et al., 1992). Relatively low level resistance to ddI is conferred by the amino acid substitution at codon 74 (St. Clair et al., 1991). In contrast, 1000-fold reduction in sensitivity to 3-TC is associated with the substitution at codon 184 (Tisdale et al., 1993). Through conformational changes adjacent to the nucleoside binding sites, certain mutations that confer resistance to one nucleoside analog (e.g., codon 74 to ddI, or 181 to 3-TC) increase susceptibility to other nucleoside analogs (such as zidovudine) to which the virus has already developed resistance mutations (St. Clair et al., 1991; Tisdale et al., 1993).

It has been hypothesized that multiple mutations required to escape triple RT inhibitor combinations might result in nonviable viruses, the "convergent combination therapy" concept (Chow et al., 1993b). Subsequent reports demonstrated that HIV-1 was capable of developing multidrug-resistant variants in vitro, with growth kinetics similar to that of wild-type viruses (Chow et al., 1993a; Emini et al., 1993; Larder et al., 1993). It seems likely that such selection can occur in vivo also. The possibility that combination therapy may delay the development of resistance, however, is under investigation.

Risk factors for the development of zidovudine resistance include low $CD4^+$ counts, a positive p24 antigen by standard ELISA, the presence of a syncitium-inducing phenotype, and a high plasma viral load at initia-

tion of therapy (Richman et al., 1990; Mayers et al., 1993). The clinical relevance of drug resistance is the subject of continued controversy (Richman, 1993). Drug resistance develops gradually, and mixtures of viruses with different resistance phenotypes may coexist. Clinical end points may not be the immediate result of increases in viral replication but simply an opportunistic consequence of immunosuppression. Proving that drug resistance causes disease progression is confounded by covariables such as virus burden, syncytium-inducing phenotype, and impaired host defenses. Surrogate markers for disease progression have been shown to deteriorate following the rapid emergence of resistance to the non-nucleoside reverse transcriptase inhibitors, nevirapine, and L-697,661 (Richman, 1992).

Two studies in children have demonstrated a highly significant relation between zidovudine resistance and disease progression, but these do not prove causality for the reasons discussed earlier (Tudor-Williams et al., 1992; Ogino et al., 1993). Ogino and colleagues (1993) documented improvements in growth following a change of retroviral therapy. This has been noted anecdotally in adults also and tends to support the argument that zidovudine drug resistance plays a role in disease progression.

High-level resistance to ddI occurs less readily in adults (Reichman et al., 1993) and has not been documented during prolonged therapy in children (Husson et al., 1993; Dimitrov et al., 1993a). Husson and associates (1993) noted the ddI resistance mutation at codon 74 in six of seven post-therapy isolates at a median of 66 weeks' treatment. This was associated with only a threefold reduction in sensitivity to ddI but up to an 11-fold cross-resistance to ddC. The fact that ddI is more active in resting cells in which viral replication is slower may be an explanation for the slower emergence of high-level resistance (Gao et al., 1993). Given the lower levels of phenotypic resistance to ddI, it will be even more difficult to demonstrate clinical correlates of resistance than with zidovudine.

Combination Regimens

As with other infectious diseases (particularly those caused by mycobacteria) and various malignancies, in the absence of curative monotherapy, combinations of the most active agents are undergoing evaluation. Drugs with additive or synergistic antiviral activity, lack of cross-resistance, and nonoverlapping toxicities are potential candidates. These theoretical benefits are well illustrated by zidovudine and ddI (Husson et al., 1994). In addition, zidovudine appears to be more effective for treating the central nervous system, whereas ddI has a more sustained impact on maintenance of the immune system. The potential for unexpected additive toxicities must be considered, however, and such adverse events may be more likely with increasing numbers of drugs used together.

Pilot studies of various different dose combinations of zidovudine and ddI in children (Husson et al., 1994) and in adults (Collier et al., 1993; Yarchoan et al., 1994) have been published. These relatively short-term

Table 18–7. Recognized HIV-1 *pol* Gene Mutations Associated With Resistance to Specific Reverse Transcriptase Inhibitors

Reverse Transcriptase Inhibitor	*pol* Gene Codon Mutations Associated with Resistance
Zidovudine	41, 67, 70, 215, 219
ddI	74, 135
ddC	69 (74)
3-TC	184
Non-nucleoside RTIs	98–108, 181–190

Abbreviations: ddI, dideoxyinosine; ddC, dideoxycytidine; 3-TC = 2'-deoxy-3-thiacytidine; RTIs = reverse transcriptase inhibitors.

pilot studies demonstrated that zidovudine and ddI in combination are well tolerated, with no evidence of enhanced toxicities. Clinical and laboratory improvements were consistently noted in patients naive to therapy but were less apparent in children who had received prior zidovudine treatment (median, 18 months). On the basis of these, phase III trials of combination therapy compared to monotherapy with one or other agent are in progress in over 800 children (ACTG protocol 152). In addition, a phase II study of zidovudine plus d4T, zidovudine plus IFN-α, and small pilot studies of triple combination therapy with zidovudine, ddI, and either nevirapine or 3-TC are underway. In Europe, a phase II study comparing zidovudine with zidovudine plus ddC in symptomatic children is in progress (PENTA 3, the Pediatric European Network for Treatment of AIDS).

Protease Inhibitors

Of the other identified molecular targets, the HIV-1 protease is the most promising. A variety of compounds have been designed containing nonhydrolyzable moieties that mimic the putative transition state of the protease-catalyzed reaction (Mimoto et al., 1991; Kageyama et al., 1993) or as symmetric inhibitors designed rationally on the basis of crystallographic resolution of the enzyme structure (Erickson et al., 1990; Roberts et al., 1990). Only preliminary data are available in children, because the lead compounds have had poor bioavailability in pediatric formulations. However, appropriate formulations will permit initiation of additional pediatric studies by mid-1995. Rapid development of resistance also appears to be a problem with this class of agents, which suggests that they may be more useful in combination with reverse transcriptase inhibitors than as single agents.

Institution of Antiretroviral Therapy

As the results of clinical trials become available, and as newer agents are evaluated, the indications for starting treatment are likely to change. To improve the outlook for HIV-infected children, as many as possible should receive treatment as part of carefully designed clinical trials. For these reasons, it is recommended that the decision to start antiretroviral therapy be made in consultation with a physician experienced in managing children with HIV (Working Group on Antiretroviral Therapy, 1993).*

A multidisciplinary Working Group convened in Washington, DC, in September 1992 to develop current consensus guidelines, and their recommendations were published in June 1993 (Working Group on Antiretroviral Therapy, 1993). No major studies (apart from

the ACTG 076 trial) have been published since then that substantially alter the recommendations. In children with an established diagnosis of HIV infection, treatment should be started if they are moderately or severely symptomatic (see Table 18–3) or have evidence of "significant" immunodeficiency.

The thresholds for starting *P. carinii* pneumonia prophylaxis include children with severe immunosuppression and known or presumed HIV-infected infants less than 1 year of age (category 3, Table 18–5; also see earlier, Protozoal and Fungal Infections). To diminish the risk of opportunistic infections for as long as possible, it has been recommended that antiretroviral therapy should be started at absolute CD4 counts of 250 cells/mm^3 above these thresholds. For children over age 6, the threshold for *P. carinii* pneumonia prophylaxis is 200 cells/mm^3 and antiretroviral agents may be initiated if the counts fall below 500 cells/mm^3 (Working Group on Antiretroviral Therapy: National Pediatric HIV Resource Center, 1993). Didanosine alone, or in combination with zidovudine, is recommended as initial therapy.

Indications for alternative therapy include intolerance or clinical disease progression. The most widely accepted sign of disease progression that is believed to be attributable to HIV disease itself is growth failure or neurodevelopmental deterioration. Each is clearly defined, with suggested schedules for monitoring CNS function, in the recommendations of the Working Group.

Laboratory Markers

The most extensively used surrogate marker for determining response to therapy and disease progression has been the measurement of CD4$^+$ T lymphocytes in the peripheral blood. Recommendations for standardization of flow cytometric methods have been widely adopted (CDC, 1992). It is important to recognize that there may be considerable intrapatient daily fluctuations in absolute CD4$^+$ cell numbers. The absolute count is derived by multiplying the CD4% by the total lymphocyte count, which can be influenced by such factors as intercurrent infections and drug treatment. It has been shown in a cohort of uninfected infants of infected mothers that the CD4% fluctuates significantly less than absolute counts (Raszka et al., 1994). Because of the fluctuations, changes in classification of disease state or in therapy should be based on two observations. In addition, the confounding effect of age, with declining counts through the first 4 to 6 years of life, requires an adjustment to allow prospective data to be analyzed. One method is to convert counts into standard deviation *(z)** scores using formula based on data from the European Collaborative Study (1992). This report contained smoothed centile curves for lymphocyte subsets for children younger than 4 years. Similar

---

*Information about clinical trials in the United States is available by calling 800-TRIALSA for ACTG studies or 301-402-1387 for the Pediatric Branch of the National Cancer Institute. In Europe, the Pediatric European Network for Treatment of AIDS (PENTA) studies are being coordinated through the Medical Research Council HIV Clinical Trials Centre (Great Britain, telephone, 0171-380-9991 or -9993).

*A *z* score of −1.0 means that the child's CD4% or absolute count is 1 SD below the mean for age. A *z* score of 0 would mean the child's counts are equal to the mean for age. Because the *z* score is derived from age-adjusted data, it can be useful for longitudinal studies of individual children, bearing in mind the caveats noted.

curves are being prepared on combined North American and European data, which may be more widely applicable.

Improvements in CD4 counts have been used in many pediatric studies as an indicator of antiretroviral efficacy (Pizzo et al., 1988; Butler et al., 1991; McKinney et al., 1991; Husson et al., 1994). Indeed, these data were an important part of the licensing of ddI by the FDA. As a prognostic marker, a CD4 count below 500 cells/mm³ was strongly correlated with disease progression in untreated children (Duliege et al., 1992). In a cohort of 147 children, the risk of death was significantly associated with very low CD4⁺ counts (equivalent to lower than 50 cells/mm³ in adults) (Butler et al., 1992b). It is recognized, however, that CD4 counts are an incomplete surrogate marker for disease progression in adults (Choi et al., 1993; Aboulker and Swart, 1993). Many centers caring for HIV-1 infected children have reported patients surviving for 5 years or more with lower than 5% CD4⁺ lymphocytes. A low CD4 count, therefore, should not be a reason for therapeutic nihilism (Butler et al., 1992b).

Measurement of p24 antigen, particularly using immune complex dissociation (ICD p24), has utility in early diagnosis (see earlier, Establishing the Diagnosis), and has also been widely used as a surrogate marker of antiretroviral efficacy in short-term trials (McKinney et al., 1991; Butler et al., 1991; Husson et al., 1994). In some adult studies, p24 antigen has been shown to be a useful marker for disease progression (Rinaldo et al., 1989; MacDonell et al., 1990). In most multivariate analyses, however, p24 antigen by standard ELISA has not been a good independent predictor of AIDS (Fahey et al., 1990; Fernandez-Cruz et al., 1990). In one cohort of 54 children, persistence of p24 antigenemia was associated with both clinical deterioration and death (Epstein et al., 1988a). Butler and colleagues, however, found that for children receiving antiretroviral therapy, p24 antigen levels did not predict survival (Butler et al., 1992b). ICD p24 antigen levels may well prove to be more useful than standard ELISA for detecting antiretroviral activity in short-term trials, because a greater proportion of patients can be predicted to be positive initially. Preliminary data have suggested that trends in ICD p24 antigen may correlate with disease progression in a cohort of children on ddI (Tudor-Williams et al., 1993). For a given individual, however, the variation in patterns is so great that it has not been possible to define criteria that strongly predict poor outcome in the next 6 months or year.

Quantitative culture methods for both plasma, PBMCs, and whole blood have been developed (Ho et al., 1989; Coombs et al., 1989; Alimenti et al., 1991) and may be useful to demonstrate antiviral efficacy (Husson et al., 1994), but these methods are, highly labor-intensive and expensive. They are therefore not widely available for the long-term monitoring of cohorts of children, but this will change with the wider availability of commercial assays.

Quantitative DNA, and particularly RNA PCR, methods offer more rapid, sensitive, and reproducible ways to measure viral load (Mulder et al., 1994; Aoki et al., 1992; Piatak et al., 1993a). Branched DNA signal amplification is a novel non-PCR assay that uses a sandwich nucleic acid hybridization method (Cao et al., 1993). It appears to be slightly less sensitive than PCR, but does not require the purchase of a thermal cycler. Both this and several PCR applications have been formatted for 96-well microplates with nonisotopic methods of detection to enable them to be used with routine laboratory equipment. These offer a more direct measurement of HIV virus burden than p24 antigen, but a significant proportion of detectable RNA has been shown to be from noninfectious (defective or neutralized) particles (Piatak et al., 1993b). The utility of these newer techniques in predicting disease progression or death will take some time to establish.

Immune Modulators

Paradoxically, although HIV infection primarily results in immune deficiency, the immunopathogenesis also involves chronic immune activation (Habeshaw et al., 1992; Fauci, 1993). In children this is manifested, for example, by nonspecific B-cell activation with hypergammaglobulinemia, lymphadenopathy, increased expression of T-cell activation antigens, and elevated serum neopterin and β_2-microglobulin levels (European Collaborative Study, 1991; Siller et al., 1993). The consequences of activation in CD4+ infected cells are up-regulation of reverse transcription, integration, transcription, and viral replication, and possibly increased apoptotic cell death, particularly in the microenvironment of the lymph nodes (Fauci, 1993).

Agents that may selectively block aspects of immune activation are under evaluation. Little data are available from pediatric cohorts. Pentoxyphylline, an inhibitor of TNF-α production, has been shown under certain in vitro conditions to inhibit HIV-1 replication (Fazely et al., 1991). However, clinical studies in adults were unimpressive and pediatric studies have not been pursued. Thalidomide selectively inhibits TNF-α production from PBMCs induced by lipopolysaccharide. It also induces a switch from T_H2 to T_H1 responses (see earlier, Interactions with the Cellular Immune System). Similarly, intriguing in vitro data suggesting that IL-12 may restore T_H1-type cell-mediated responses are being investigated (Clerici et al., 1993b). A trial in adults using intermittent infusions of IL-2 has shown promising early effects on CD4⁺ lymphocyte counts, but each infusion is associated with an abrupt rise in plasma viremia (Fauci, 1993; Kovacs et al., 1995). Such therapeutic interventions need to be used in conjunction with optimal antiretroviral therapy.

Intracellular levels of glutathione are low in the leukocytes of adults with HIV infection (Buhl et al., 1989). Glutathione is the main scavenger of intracellular reactive oxygen species. Depletion of glutathione allows greatly enhanced in vitro production of HIV in response to cytokine stimulation such as that by TNF-α (Roederer et al., 1990). Glutathione itself does not cross cell membranes. N-acetylcysteine increases intracellular glutathione synthesis and has been used clinically to treat acetaminophen liver toxicity, which is thought to be mediated by production of reactive oxygen species. N-acetylcysteine has been shown to suppress HIV replication in chronically infected cells and to block the up-regulation of HIV by cytokines (Kalebic et al., 1991; Roederer et al., 1990). In clinical trials, however, the bioavailability of N-acetylcysteine was poor, and there was little evidence of clinical benefit (Walker et al., 1993). Other thiol-related drugs such as procysteine are being investigated in adults.

IFN-α has antiviral activity by interfering with the release of mature virions, but also stimulates natural killer cells and expression of class I and II antigens on cell membranes (Ammann, 1993). Synergism with zidovudine in vitro has been demonstrated, but it has been more difficult to demonstrate convincing synergism in clinical trials. Adults with Kaposi's sarcoma have response rates of 30% to 50%. We have used rIFN-α-2b in conjunction with continuous infusion zidovudine in a child with HIV encephalopathy and aneurysms of the circle of Willis. The white matter changes improved considerably, but the aneurysms continued to enlarge. We have also used rIFN-α for Ki-1$^+$ lymphomas and children with EBV-driven polyclonal lymphadenopathy. Experience is too limited to draw definite conclusions, but the treatment has been generally well tolerated. A phase I study in combination with zidovudine in HIV-infected children is nearing completion at present (ACTG 153).

Postinfection therapy with a variety of HIV-vaccines is under evaluation in adults, pregnant women, and children. The rationale is to stimulate humoral and CTL responses using selected envelope glycoproteins or whole, inactivated virus lacking the surface glycoproteins. Much controversy exists regarding optimal epitopes for inclusion in vaccines for different geographic locations, adjuvants, and appropriate methods for monitoring responses. There are concerns that immune stimulation under some circumstances could be harmful by inducing enhancing antibodies or by nonspecific up-regulation of HIV replication (Levy, 1993). Preliminary data from the Department of Defense recombinant gp160 and gp120 trials, and with an inactivated vaccine, have shown stability of CD4$^+$ lymphocytes, increased proliferative resonses to the envelope glycoproteins used as immunogens, and no apparent increases in viral burden. Long-term follow-up is required to assess clinical benefit.

Passive immunotherapy using plasma from HIV-infected donors with high titers of anti-HIV antibodies provided no discernible clinical or laboratory benefit in a randomized study of 63 adults with advanced disease (Jacobson et al., 1993). Two other controlled studies, however, showed some clinical promise (Levy et al., 1994; Vittecoq et al., 1995).

Growth hormone and its active intermediate, insulin-like growth factor-1 (IGF-1), have been found to increase proliferative responses of lymphocytes or cell lines of lymphocytic origin, to restore thymic atrophy in diabetic and hypophysectomized rats, and to replenish the rodent analogs of CD4$^+$ lymphocytes (Binz et al., 1990; Geffner et al., 1990; Gjerset et al., 1990; Petersen et al., 1990). Growth hormone also accelerates peripheral T-cell reconstitution after bone marrow transplantation in severe combined immunodeficient mice (Murphy et al., 1992). In BALB/c mice, IGF-1 increased CD4$^+$ T lymphocytes and splenic B cells, both numerically and in functional assays (Clark et al., 1993b). In addition to positive effects on the immune system, IGF-1 in conjunction with growth hormone promotes anabolism, with reversal of negative nitrogen balance, increases in muscle mass, and stimulation of longitudinal bone growth (Ammann, 1993). Using an in vitro erythroid progenitor cell colony-formation assay, Geffner and colleagues (1993) have shown that more advanced HIV-1 infection in children is associated with resistance to the growth-promoting effects of IGF-1 and growth hormone.

A pilot study of growth hormone and IGF-1 is being conducted at the Pediatric Branch of the National Cancer Institute to assess the effect on immune function and growth in HIV-infected children. There are in vitro data to show that the growth factors may increase viral replication, but this can be completely suppressed by the use of either zidovudine or ddI. We are treating the children with a combination of both antiretroviral agents.

Prophylactic Measures

Prophylactic measures include the use of intravenous immunoglobulin and active and passive immunizations.

Intravenous Immunoglobulin

A double-blind study of 372 HIV-1 infected children compared human intravenous immune globulin (IVIG; 400 mg/kg) every 28 days with placebo (0.1% albumin), over a median length of follow-up of 17 months. A reduction of bacterial infections and hospitalizations was observed for those children with CD4$^+$ counts above 200 cells/mm^3 at entry (Mofenson et al., 1992). Subsequent age-adjusted CD4$^+$ slope analysis demonstrated a slowing of CD4$^+$ count decline by 13.5 cells/month in the IVIG recipients (Mofenson et al., 1993). The benefits, however, were not observed in children receiving trimethoprim-sulfamethoxazole for *P. carinii* pneumonia prophylaxis and were not found in another study of children with lower CD4$^+$ counts (Spector et al., 1993). The consensus of the Working Group was that children with significant recurrent bacterial infections, hypogammaglobulinemia, or documented poor functional antibody development may be candidates for IVIG 400 mg/kg every 28 days (Working Group on Antiretroviral Therapy, 1993). Higher doses may be useful in children with thrombocytopenia (0.5 to 1.0 g/kg/dose for 3 to 5 days).

Active and Passive Immunization

Most childhood immunizations are currently recommended. Inactivated poliovirus vaccine should be substituted for oral polio vaccine, even after seroreversion, to prevent spread to immunodeficient family members (Working Group on Antiretroviral Therapy, 1993).

The new varicella vaccine is not recommended until further studies are completed. Pneumococcal vaccine is recommended at age 2 years, and influenza vaccine is recommended annually in symptomatic children (although the data supporting efficacy of the latter are lacking in this population). Bacille Calmette-Guérin (BCG) is a subject of controversy; the current recommendation is not to give BCG in the United States, but WHO recommends that it be given to asymptomatic children in areas of high prevalence (Khouri et al., 1992).

Passive immunization is recommended for susceptible children with symptomatic HIV infection who are in contact with measles or varicella zoster. Children receiving IVIG are considered susceptible if the last dose was given more than 2 weeks prior to exposure. In some urban areas where measles outbreaks are frequent, antibody responses in HIV-infected children should be checked after measles-mumps-rubella (MMR) vaccination. If the response has been poor, a second dose of MMR should be given. If the child fails to respond to a second dose, regular IVIG prophylaxis should be considered. Children with a documented past history of varicella or recurrent zoster need not be treated with varicella zoster immune globulin (VZIG). If a susceptible child is re-exposed more than 2 weeks after VZIG, however, another dose is recommended. The administration of VZIG may prolong the incubation period to 28 days, so clinic visits should be postponed for this period.

Prophylaxis for *P. carinii* pneumonia, *M. avium–intracellulare,* and tuberculosis and chronic suppressive therapy for specific infectious complications of HIV infection are mentioned earlier; see Infectious Complications.

Supportive Therapy

Caring for a child with HIV infection imposes a heavy burden for any caregiver. In the context of perinatal transmission, this is frequently compounded by illness in the parent, social isolation, and feelings of guilt. An effective multidisciplinary team needs to determine the major concerns for each caregiver. These may be emotional, financial, or legal (e.g., regarding schooling). Caregivers may need more information about HIV, help informing the child or siblings about the diagnosis, advice about treatment for themselves, or help with substance abuse problems. Without addressing these issues, the child is unlikely to receive optimal care. A social worker and primary nurse are assigned to each family attending our clinic. The team includes psychologists, dietitians, clergy, teachers, occupational and physical therapists, and recreation therapists. Formal and informal group support is provided for both children and their caregivers. Involvement of appropriate community-based supportive services, from early intervention programs to hospice services, may be required. Ideally, care for all infected and affected family members should be coordinated in one facility. This requires close collaboration among pediatricians, adult physicians, obstetricians-gynecologists, and their affiliated teams.

Medical supportive care includes teaching parents to be alert for subtle signs of new illness and to seek help promptly. Fevers need to be evaluated carefully, with early intervention for treatable bacterial or opportunistic infections. Creative and aggressive attention to pain management is important. Pain is frequently associated with procedures, but also arises, for example, from infectious complications, side effects of drugs, or spasticity associated with central nervous system involvement. Nutritional monitoring and dietary intervention should begin early, because malnutrition may enhance immunodeficiency (Beisel et al., 1981). Iron, vitamin, and other micronutrient deficiencies should be considered. Providing sufficient calories and protein to maintain linear growth and weight gain is frequently difficult. A variety of calorically dense formulas and supplements should be available to find one that the child can tolerate. Dietary advice should be sensitive to the family's ethnic and cultural constraints. Appetite stimulants, such as cyproheptadine (Periactin), dronabinol (Marinol), and megestrol acetate, (Megace) are worth considering but rarely improve caloric intake more than 10% to 20%. If oral intake remains inadequate, tube feeding may be necessary. Gastrostomy sites, may heal poorly and leak, however, and nasogastric tubes may exacerbate sinusitis and upper airway infection. Parenteral nutrition may therefore become necessary.

FUTURE CONSIDERATIONS

Numerous refinements of existing antiretroviral therapies in various combinations can be expected over the next few years. The role of new therapeutic strategies, particularly the use of immunomodulating therapies, and of gene therapy approaches that were beyond our scope here, offer cause for continuing optimism for better control of established HIV infection. Such advances depend on gaining increased insights into both viral pathogenesis and host defenses in this disease. Validation of the new techniques for monitoring viral burden as surrogate markers for drug efficacy can perhaps enable more rapid identification of useful treatment strategies. Much work is being done to improve both the diagnostic and therapeutic options for the opportunistic infections associated with immunosuppressed hosts. Lessons learned from HIV-infected individuals may help in the care of children undergoing cancer chemotherapy, and vice versa. Multidisciplinary approaches should continue to focus on ways to improve the quality of lives that may be extended by medical advances. More family-based care facilities can help in this regard.

The prevention of perinatal transmission is of the highest priority. The results of the ACTG 076 study will provide a major impetus to develop less complicated but equally effective interventions that may be useful worldwide. Targeted prevention, however, can only be achieved if HIV-infected mothers can be identified prenatally. Success in this arena requires a concerted effort by health professionals, community organizations, and public health planners.

References

Abadco DL, Steiner P. Gastric lavage is better than bronchoalveolar lavage for isolation of *Mycobacterium tuberculosis* in childhood pulmonary tuberculosis. Pediatr Infect Dis J 11:735–738, 1992.

Aboulker JP, Swart AM. Preliminary analysis of the Concorde trial. Concorde Coordinating Committee (letter). Lancet 341:889–890, 1993.

Abrams D, Goldman A, Launer C, Korvick J, Neaton J, Crane L, Grodesky M, Wakefield S, Muth K, Kornegay S, Cohn D, Harris A, Luskin-Hawk R, Markowitz N, Sampson J, Thompson M, Deyton L. A comparative trial of didanosine or zalcitabine after treatment with zidovudine in patients with human immunodeficiency virus infection. N Engl J Med 330:657–662, 1994.

Adamson PC, Wu TC, Meade BD, Rubin M, Manclark CR, Pizzo PA. Pertussis in a previously immunized child with human immunodeficiency virus infection. J Pediatr 115:589–592, 1989.

Alimenti A, Luzuriaga K, Stechenberg B, Sullivan JL. Quantitation of human immunodeficiency virus in vertically infected infants and children. J Pediatr 119:225–229, 1991.

Alimenti A, O'Neill M, Sullivan JL, Luzuriaga K. Diagnosis of vertical human immunodeficiency virus type 1 by whole blood culture. J Infect Dis 166:1146–1148, 1992.

Ammann A. The clinical evaluation of cytokines and immunomodulators in HIV infection. Ann N Y Acad Sci 693:178–185, 1993.

Ammann AJ, Cowan MJ, Wara DW, Weintrub P, Dritz S, Goldman H, Perkins HA. Acquired immunodeficiency in an infant: possible transmission by means of blood products. Lancet 1:956–958, 1983.

Anderson S, Shugars DC, Swanstrom R, Garcia JV. Nef from primary isolates of human immunodeficiency virus type 1 suppresses surface CD4 expression in human and mouse T cells. J Virol 67:4923–4931, 1993.

Andiman WA, Martin K, Rubinstein A, Pahwa S, Eastman R, Katz BZ, Pitt J, Miller G. Opportunistic lymphoproliferations associated with Epstein-Barr viral DNA in infants and children with AIDS. Lancet 2:1390–1393, 1985.

Aoki SS, Yarchoan R, Kageyama S, Hoekzema DT, Pluda JM, Wyvill KM, Broder S, Mitsuya H. Plasma HIV-1 viremia in HIV-1 infected individuals assessed by polymerase chain reaction. AIDS Res Hum Retroviruses 8:1263–1270, 1992.

Baba T, Koch J, Mittler E, Greene M, Wyand M, Penninck D, Ruprecht R. Mucosal infection of neonatal Rhesus monkeys with cell-free SIV. AIDS Res Hum Retroviruses 10:351–357, 1994.

Bagasra O, Hauptman SP, Lischner HW, Sachs M, Pomerantz RJ. Detection of human immunodeficiency virus type 1 provirus in mononuclear cells by in situ polymerase chain reaction. N Engl J Med 326:1385–1391, 1992.

Balis FM, Pizzo PA, Eddy J, Wilfert C, McKinney R, Scott G, Murphy RF, Jarosinski PF, Falloon J, Poplack DG. Pharmacokinetics of zidovudine administered intravenously and orally in children with human immunodeficiency virus infection. J Pediatr 114:880–884, 1989a.

Balis FM, Pizzo PA, Murphy RF, Eddy J, Jarosinski PF, Falloon J, Broder S, Poplack DG. The pharmacokinetics of zidovudine administered by continuous infusion in children. Ann Intern Med 110:279–285, 1989b.

Balis FM, Pizzo PA, Butler KM, Hawkins ME, Brouwers P, Husson RN, Jacobsen F, Blaney SM, Gress J, Jarosinski P, Poplack DG. Clinical pharmacology of 2′,3′-dideoxyinosine in human immunodeficiency virus-infected children. J Infect Dis 165:99–104, 1992.

Banda NK, Bernier J, Kurahara DK, Kurrle R, Haigwood N, Sekaly RP, Finkel TH. Crosslinking CD4 by human immunodeficiency virus gp120 primes T cells for activation-induced apoptosis. J Exp Med 176:1099–1106, 1992.

Bebenek K, Abbotts J, Roberts J, Wilson S, Kunkel T. Specificity and mechanism of error-prone replication by human immunodeficiency virus-1 reverse transcriptase. J Biol Chem 264:16948–16956, 1989.

Beck-Sague C, Dooley SW, Hutton MD, Otten J, Breeden A, Crawford JT, Pitchenik AE, Woodley C, Cauthen G, Jarvis WR. Hospital outbreak of multidrug-resistant Mycobacterium tuberculosis infec-tions: factors in transmission to staff and HIV-infected patients. JAMA 268:1280–1286, 1992.

Beisel WR, Edelman R, Nauss K, Suskind RM. Single nutrient effects on immunological functions. JAMA 254:52–58, 1981.

Belec L, Mbopi Keou F, Georges A. A case for the revision of the WHO clinical definition for African AIDS. AIDS 6:880–881, 1992.

Belman AL. Acquired immunodeficiency syndrome and the child's central nervous system. Pediatr Clin North Am 39:691–714, 1992.

Beral V, Peterman TA, Berkelman RL, Jaffe HW. Kaposi's sarcoma among persons with AIDS: a sexually transmitted infection? Lancet 335:123–128, 1990.

Beral V, Peterman T, Berkelman R, Jaffe H. AIDS-associated non-Hodgkin's lymphoma. Lancet 337:805–809, 1991.

Berman PW, Matthews TJ, Riddle L, Champe M, Hobbs MR, Nakamura GR, Mercer J, Eastman DJ, Lucas C, Langlois AJ. Neutralization of multiple laboratory and clinical isolates of human immunodeficiency virus type 1 (HIV-1) by antisera raised against gp120 from the MN isolate of HIV-1. J Virol 66:4464–4469, 1992.

Binz K, Joller P, Froesch P, Binz H, Zapf J, Froesch ER. Repopulation of the atrophied thymus in diabetic rats by insulin-like growth factor I. Proc Natl Acad Sci U S A 87:3690–3694, 1990.

Blanche S, Rouzioux C, Guihard Moscato M-L, Veber F, Mayaux M-J, Jacomet C, Tricoire J, De Ville A, Vial M, Firtion G, De Crepy A, Douard D, Robin M, Courpotin C, Ciraru-Vigneron N, Le Deist F, Griscelli C. A prospective study of infants born to women seropositive for human immunodeficiency virus type 1. HIV Infection in Newborns French Collaborative Study Group. N Engl J Med 320:1643–1648, 1989.

Blanche S, Tardieu M, Duliege A-M, Rouzioux C, Le Deist F, Fukunaga K, Caniglia M, Jacomet C, Messiah A, Griscelli C. Longitudinal study of 94 symptomatic infants with perinatally acquired human immunodeficiency virus infection. Am J Dis Child 144:1210–1215, 1990.

Blanche S, Duliege A-M, Navarette MS, Tardieu M, Debre M, Rouzioux C, Seldrup J, Kouzan S, Griscelli C. Low-dose zidovudine in children with an human immunodeficiency virus type 1 infection acquired in the perinatal period. Pediatrics 88:364–370, 1991.

Blanche S, Mayaux MJ, Rouzioux C, Teglas JP, Firtion G, Monpoux F, Ciraru VN, Meier F, Tricoire J, Courpotin C, Vilmer E, Griscelli C, Delfraissy J-F, French Pediatric HIV Infection Study Group. Relation of the course of HIV infection in children to the severity of the disease in their mothers at delivery. N Engl J Med 330:308–312, 1994.

Bleiweiss IJ, Pervez NK, Hammer GS, Dikman SH. Cytomegalovirus-induced adrenal insufficiency and associated renal cell carcinoma in AIDS. Mt Sinai J Med 53:676–679, 1986.

Bodsworth NJ, Cooper DA, Donovan B. The influence of human immunodeficiency virus type 1 infection on the development of the hepatitis B virus carrier state. J Infect Dis 163:1138–1140, 1991.

Bollinger RC, Kline RL, Francis HL, Moss MW, Bartlett JG, Quinn TC. Acid dissociation increases the sensitivity of p24 antigen detection for the evaluation of antiviral therapy and disease progression in asymptomatic human immunodeficiency virus–infected persons. J Infect Dis 165:913–916, 1992.

Bonavida B, Katz J, Gottlieb M. Mechanism of defective NK cell activity in patients with acquired immunodeficiency syndrome (AIDS) and AIDS-related complex: I. Defective trigger on NK cells for NKCF production by target cells, and partial restoration by IL 2. J Immunol 137:1157–1163, 1986.

Borkowsky W, Rigaud M, Krasinski K, Moore T, Lawrence R, Pollack H. Cell-mediated and humoral immune responses in children infected with human immunodeficiency virus during the first four years of life. J Pediatr 120:371–375, 1992.

Boue F, Pons JC, Keros L, Chambrin V, Papiernik E, Henrion R, Delfraissy JF. Risk for HIV 1 perinatal transmission varies with the mother's stage of HIV infection. Int Conf AIDS 6:1990.

Boyer P, Dillon M, Navaie M, Deveikis A, Keller M, O'Rourke S, Bryson Y. Factors predictive of maternal-fetal transmission of HIV-1. JAMA 271:1925–1930, 1994.

Brettler DB, Forsberg A, Bolivar E, Brewster F, Sullivan J. Growth failure as a prognostic indicator for progression to acquired immunodeficiency syndrome in children with hemophilia. J Pediatr 117:584–588, 1990.

Brierley J, Roth C, Warwick C. Breast-feeding and HIV infection. Lancet 1:1346, 1988.

Brighty D, Rosenberg M, Chen I, Ivey-Hoyle M. Envelope proteins from clinical isolates of HIV-1 that are refractory to neutralization by soluble CD4 possess high affinity for the CD4 receptor. Proc Natl Acad Sci U S A 88:7802–7805, 1991.

Broliden K, Sievers E, Tovo PA, Moschese V, Scarlatti G, Broliden PA, Fundaro C, Rossi P. Antibody-dependent cellular cytotoxicity and neutralizing activity in sera of HIV-1-infected mothers and their children. Clin Exp Immunol 93:56–64, 1993.

Broliden PA, Makitalo B, Akerblom L, Rosen J, Broliden K, Utter G, Jondal M, Norrby E, Wahren B. Identification of amino acids in the V3 region of gp120 critical for virus neutralization by human HIV-1–specific antibodies. Immunology 73:371–376, 1991.

Brouwers P, Moss H, Wolters P, Eddy J, Balis F, Poplack DG, Pizzo PA. Effect of continuous-infusion zidovudine therapy on neuro-psychologic functioning in children with symptomatic human immunodeficiency virus infection. J Pediatr 117:980–985, 1990.

Brouwers P, Heyes MP, Moss HA, Wolters PL, Poplack DG, Markey SP, Pizzo PA. Quinolinic acid in the cerebrospinal fluid of children with symptomatic human immunodeficiency virus type 1 disease: relationships to clinical status and therapeutic response. J Infect Dis 168:1380–1386, 1993.

Brunell P. Antibody in human immunodeficiency virus infection. Ann N Y Acad Sci 693:9–13, 1993.

Bryant M, Ratner L. Myristoylation-dependent replication and assembly of human immunodeficiency virus I. Proc Natl Acad Sci U S A 87:523–527, 1990.

Bryant M, Ratner L. Biology and molecular biology of human immunodeficiency virus. Pediatr Infect Dis J 11:390–400, 1992.

Bryson Y, Luzuriaga K, Sullivan J, Wara D. Proposed definition for in utero versus intrapartum transmission of HIV-1. N Engl J Med 327:1246–1247, 1992.

Bryson Y, Dillon M, Garratty E, Dickover R, Keller M, Deveikis A. The role of timing of HIV maternal-fetal transmission (in utero vs. intrapartum) and HIV phenotype on onset of symptoms in vertically infected infants. Int Conf AIDS 9:c10–c12, 1993a.

Bryson Y, Lehman D, Garratty E, Dickover R, Plaeger-Marshall S, O'Rourke S. The role of maternal autologous neutralizing antibody in prevention of maternal fetal HIV-1 transmission (abstract). J Cell Biochem S17E:95, 1993b.

Bryson YJ, Pang S, Wei LS, Dickover R, Diagne A, Chen IS. Clearance of HIV infection in a perinatally infected infant. N Engl J Med 332:833–838, 1995.

Buhl R, Holroyd K, Mastrangeli A, Cantin AM, Jaffe HA, Wells FB, Saltini C, Crystal RG. Systemic glutathione deficiency in symptom-free HIV-seropositive individuals. Lancet 2:1294–1298, 1989.

Bukrinsky M, Stanwick T, Dempsey M, Stevenson M. Quiescent T lymphocytes as an inducible virus reservoir in HIV-1 infection. Science 254:423–427, 1991.

Burgard M, Mayaux MJ, Blanche S, Ferroni A, Guihard MM, Allemon MC, Ciraru VN, Firtion G, Floch C, Guillot F, EL, Vial M, Griscelli C, Rouzioux C, HIV Infection in Newborns French Collaborative Study Group. The use of viral culture and p24 antigen testing to diagnose human immunodeficiency virus infection in neonates. N Engl J Med 327:1192–1197, 1992.

Buseyne F, Blanche S, Schmitt D, Griscelli C, Riviere Y. Detection of HIV-specific cell-mediated cytotoxicity in the peripheral blood from infected children. J Immunol 150:3569–3581, 1993.

Butler KM, Husson RN, Balis FM, Brouwers P, Eddy J, El-Amin D, Gress J, Hawkins M, Jarosinski P, Moss H, Poplack D, Santacroce S, Venzon D, Wiener L, Wolters P, Pizzo PA. Dideoxyinosine in children with symptomatic human immunodeficiency virus infection. N Engl J Med 324:137–144, 1991.

Butler KM, De Smet MD, RNH, Mueller B, Manjunath K, Montrella K, Lovato G, Jarosinski P, Nussenblatt RB, Pizzo PA. Treatment of aggressive cytomegalovirus retinitis with ganciclovir in combination with foscarnet in a child infected with human immunodeficiency virus. J Pediatr 120:483–486, 1992a.

Butler KM, Husson RN, Lewis LL, Mueller BU, Marshall D, Venzon D, Pizzo PA. CD4 status and p24 antigenemia: are they useful predictors of survival in pediatric antiretroviral recipients? Am J Dis Childh 146:932–936, 1992b.

Butler KM, Venzon D, Henry N, Husson RN, Mueller BU, Balis FM, Jacobsen F, Lewis LL, Pizzo PA. Pancreatitis in human immunodeficiency virus–infected children receiving dideoxyinosine. Pediatrics 91:747–751, 1993.

Byers B, Caldwell B, Oxytoby M. Pediatric Spectrum of Disease Project. Survival of children with perinatal HIV-infection: evidence for two distinct populations. Presented at the Ninth International Conference on AIDS, Berlin, 1993.

Cai Q, Huang XL, Rappocciolo G, Rinaldo CJ. Natural killer cell responses in homosexual men with early HIV infection. J AIDS 3:669–676, 1990.

Candotti D, Jung M, Kerouedan D, Rosenheim M, Gentilini M, M'Pele P, Huraux J. Genetic variability affects the detection of HIV by polymerase chain reaction. AIDS 5:1003–1007, 1991.

Cao Y, Kokka R, Kern D, Urdea M, Wu Y, Ho DD. Comparison of quantitative bDNA technique with end-point-dilution culture, p24 antigen assay, and RT-PCR quantitation of HIV-1 in plasma. Int Conf AIDS 9:A32–0794, 1993.

Cara A, Guarnaccia F, Gallo R, Reitz M, Lori F. Different replication of HIV-1 integrase defective mutant in PBL and macrophages. Presented at the Annual Meeting of the Laboratory of Tumor Cell Biology, Bethesda, Md., 1993.

Cassol SA, Lapointe N, Salas T, Hankins C, Arella M, Fauvel M, Delage G, Boucher M, Samson J, Charest J. Diagnosis of vertical HIV-1 transmission using the polymerase chain reaction and dried blood spot specimens. J AIDS 5:113–119, 1992.

CDC [Centers for Disease Control]. Unexplained immunodeficiency and opportunistic infections in infants—New York, New Jersey, California. MMWR 31:665–667, 1982.

CDC [Centers for Disease Control]. Classification system for human immunodeficiency virus (HIV) infection in children under 13 years of age. MMWR 36:225–236, 1987.

CDC [Centers for Disease Control]. Guidelines for prophylaxis against *Pneumocystis carinii* pneumonia for children with human immunodeficiency virus infection/exposure. MMWR 40:1–13, 1991a.

CDC [Centers for Disease Control]. Mortality attributable to HIV infection/AIDS—United States, 1981–1990. MMWR 40:41–44, 1991b.

CDC [Centers for Disease Control]. Guidelines for the performance of CD4 + T-cell determinations in persons with human immunodeficiency virus infection. MMWR 41:1–17, 1992.

CDC [Centers for Disease Control]. 1993 revised classification system for HIV infection and expanded surveillance case definition for AIDS among adolescents and adults. MMWR 41:1–19, 1993a.

CDC [Centers for Disease Control]. HIV transmission between two adolescent brothers with hemophilia. MMWR 42:948–951, 1993b.

CDC [Centers for Disease Control]. HIV/AIDS Surveillance Report 5:1–19, 1993c.

CDC [Centers for Disease Control]. Initial therapy for tuberculosis in the era of multidrug resistance: recommendations of the Advisory Council for the Elimination of Tuberculosis. MMWR 42:1–8, 1993d.

CDC [Centers for Disease Control]. Update: Acquired immunodeficiency syndrome—United States, 1992. MMWR 42:547–557, 1993e.

CDC [Centers for Disease Control]. Zidovudine for the prevention of HIV transmission from mother to infant. MMWR 43:285–287, 1994a.

CDC [Centers for Disease Control]. Revised classification system for human immunodeficiency virus infection in children less than 13 years of age. MMWR 43:1–12, 1994b.

CDC [Centers for Disease Control]. 1995 Revised guidelines for prophylaxis against *Pneumocystis carinii* pneumonia for children infected with or perinatally exposed to human immunodeficiency virus. MMWR 44:1–11, 1995.

Chan MM, Campos JM, Josephs S, Rifai N. β$_2$-microglobulin and neopterin: predictive markers for human immunodeficiency virus type 1 infection in children? J Clin Microbiol 28:2215–2219, 1990.

Chandwani S, Moore T, Kaul A, Krasinski K, Borkowsky W. Early diagnosis of human immunodeficiency virus type 1-infected infants by plasma p24 antigen assay after immune complex disruption. Pediatr Infect Dis J 12:96–97, 1993.

Chanh T, Kennedy R, Kanda P. Synthetic peptides homologous to HIV transmembrane glycoprotein suppress normal human lymphocyte blastogenic response. Cell Immunol 111:77–86, 1988.

Chariot P, Benbrik E, Schaeffer A, Gherardi R. Tubular aggregates and partial cytochrome c oxidase deficiency in skeletal muscle of patients with AIDS treated with zidovudine. Acta Neuropathol (Berl) 85:431–436, 1993.

Chavanet P, Diquet B, Waldner A. Perinatal pharmacokinetics of zidovudine. N Engl J Med 321:1548–1549, 1989.

Chehimi J, Starr SE, Frank I, Rengaraju M, Jackson SJ, Llanes C, Kobayashi M, Perussia B, Young D, Nickbarg E. Natural killer (NK) cell stimulatory factor increases the cytotoxic activity of NK cells from both healthy donors and human immunodeficiency virus-infected patients. J Exp Med 175:789–796, 1992.

Cheng-Meyer C, Shiodo T, Levy J. Host range, replicative, and cytopathic properties of human immunodeficiency virus type 1 are determined by very few amino acid changes in Tat and gp120. J Virol 65:6931–6941, 1991.

Chesebro B, Wehrly K, Nishio J, Perryman S. Macrophage-tropic human immunodeficiency virus isolates from different patients exhibit unusual V3 envelope sequence homogeneity in comparison with T-cell-tropic isolates: definition of critical amino acids involved in cell tropism. J Virol 66:6547–6554, 1992.

Cheynier R, Langlade DP, Marescot MR, Blanche S, Blondin G, Wain HS, Griscelli C, Vilmer E, Plata F. Cytotoxic T lymphocyte responses in the peripheral blood of children born to human immunodeficiency virus-1–infected mothers. Eur J Immunol 22:2211–2217, 1992.

Chin DP, Hopewell PC, Yajko DM, Vittinghoff E, Horsburgh CJ, Hadley WK, Stone EN, Nassos PS, Ostroff SM, Jacobson MA. Mycobacterium avium complex in the respiratory or gastrointestinal tract and the risk of *M. avium* complex bacteremia in patients with human immunodeficiency virus infection. J Infect Dis 169:289–295, 1994.

Chiodi F, Keys B, Albert J, Hagberg L, Lundeberg J, Uhlen M, Fenyo EM, Norkrans G. Human immunodeficiency virus type 1 is present in the cerebrospinal fluid of a majority of infected individuals. J Clin Microbiol 30:1768–1771, 1992.

Choi S, Lagakos SW, Schooley RT, Volberding PA. CD4+ lymphocytes are an incomplete surrogate marker for clinical progression in persons with asymptomatic HIV infection taking zidovudine. Ann Intern Med 118:674–680, 1993.

Chow YK, Hirsch MS, Kaplan JC, D'Aquila RT. HIV-1 error revealed (letter). Nature 364:679–793, 1993a.

Chow YK, Hirsch MS, Merrill DP, Bechtel LJ, Eron JJ, Kaplan JC, D'Aquila RT. Use of evolutionary limitations of HIV-1 multidrug resistance to optimize therapy [see erratum in Nature 364:679, 737, 1993]. Nature 361:650–654, 1993b.

Civitello L. Neurological complications of HIV infection in children. Pediatr Neurosurg 17:104–112, 1991.

Clark DA, Freeland ML, Mackie LK, Jarrett RF, Onions DE. Prevalence of antibody to human herpesvirus 7 by age (letter). J Infect Dis 168:251–252, 1993a.

Clark R, Strasser J, McCabe S, Robbins K, Jardieu P. Insulin-like growth factor-1 stimulation of lymphopoiesis. J Clin Invest 92:540–548, 1993b.

Clement LT, Vink PE, Bradley GE. Novel immunoregulatory functions of phenotypically distinct subpopulations of CD4+ cells in the human neonate. J Immunol 145:102–108, 1990.

Clerici M, Shearer G. A Th1-Th2 switch is a critical step in the etiology of HIV infection. Immunol Today 14:107–111, 1993.

Clerici M, Stocks N, Zajac R, Boswell R, Lucey D, Via C, Shearer G. Detection of three distinct patterns of T helper cell dysfunction in asymptomatic, human immunodeficiency virus-seropositive patients. J Clin Invest 84:1892–1899, 1989.

Clerici M, Lucey DR, Zajac RA, Boswell RN, Gebel HM, Takahashi H, Berzofsky JA, Shearer GM. Detection of cytotoxic T lymphocytes specific for synthetic peptides of gp160 in HIV-seropositive individuals. J Immunol 146:2214–2219, 1991.

Clerici M, Giorgi JV, Chou CC, Gudeman VK, Zack JA, Gupta P, Ho HN, Nishanian PG, Berzofsky JA, Shearer GM. Cell-mediated immune response to human immunodeficiency virus (HIV) type 1 in seronegative homosexual men with recent sexual exposure to HIV-1. J Infect Dis 165:1012–1019, 1992a.

Clerici M, Landay AL, Kessler HA, Phair JP, Venzon DJ, Hendrix CW, Lucey DR, Shearer GM. Reconstitution of long-term T helper cell function after zidovudine therapy in human immunodeficiency virus–infected patients. J Infect Dis 166:723–730, 1992b.

Clerici M, Roilides E, Butler K, DePalma L, Venzon D, Shearer G, Pizzo P. Changes in T-helper function in human immunodeficiency virus-infected children during didanosine therapy as a measure of antiretroviral activity. Blood 80:2196–2202, 1992c.

Clerici M, Hakim F, Venzon D, Blatt S, Hendrix C, Wynn T, Shearer G. Changes in interleukin-2 and interleukin-4 production in asymptomatic, human immunodeficiency virus-seropositive individuals. J Clin Invest 91:759–765, 1993a.

Clerici M, Lucey D, Berzofsky J, Pinto L, Wynn T, Blatt S, Dolan M, Hendrix C, Wolf S, Shearer G. Restoration of HIV-specific cell-mediated immune responses by interleukin-12 in vitro. Science 262:1721–1724, 1993b.

Cohen J. Apoptosis: physiological cell death. J Lab Clin Med 124:761–765, 1994.

Colebunders R, Kapita B, Nekwei W, Bahwe Y, Lebughe I, Oxtoby M, Ryder R. Breastfeeding and transmission of HIV. Lancet 2:1487, 1988.

Collier AC, Coombs RW, Fischl MA, Skolnik PR, Northfelt D, Boutin P, Hooper CJ, Kaplan LD, Volberding PA, Davis LG, Henrard D, Weller S, Corey L. Combination therapy with zidovudine and didanosine compared with zidovudine alone in HIV-1 infection. Ann Intern Med 119:786–793, 1993.

Connelly M, McSharry J, Rao P. A simple and rapid flow cytometric method for the detection of HIV infected cells and their immunophenotype. Presented at the International Conference on AIDS, Florence, Italy, 1992.

Connor E, Bagarazzi M, McSherry G, Holland B, Boland M, Denny T, Oleske J. Clinical and laboratory correlates of *Pneumocystis carinii* pneumonia in children infected with HIV. JAMA 265:1693–1697, 1991a.

Connor E, Marquis J, Oleske J. Lymphoid interstitial pneumonitis. In Pizzo PA, Wilfert CM, eds. The Challenge of HIV Infection in Infants, Children, and Adolescents. Baltimore, Williams & Wilkins, 1991b, pp. 343–354.

Connor EM, Sperling RS, Gelber R, Kiselev P, Scott G, O'Sullivan MJ, VanDyke R, Bey M, Shearer W, Jacobson RL, Jimenez E, O'Neil E, Bazin B, Delfraissy JF, Culnane M, Coombs R, Elkins M, Moye J, Stratton P, Balsley J, for the Pediatric AIDS Clinical Trials Group Protocol 076 Study Group. Reduction of maternal-infant transmission of human immunodeficiency virus type I with zidovudine treatment. N Engl J Med 331:1173–1180, 1994.

Consensus Report. Early diagnosis of HIV infection in infants. J AIDS 5:1169–1178, 1992.

Consortium for Retrovirus Serology Standardization. Serological diagnosis of human immunodeficiency virus infection by Western blot testing. JAMA 260:674–679, 1988.

Coombs RW, Collier AC, Allain J-P, Nikora B, Leuther M, Gjerset GF, Corey L. Plasma viremia in human immunodeficiency virus infection. N Engl J Med 321:1626–1631, 1989.

Cordonnier A, Montagnier L, Emerman M. Single amino-acid changes in HIV envelope affect viral tropism and receptor binding. Nature 340:571–574, 1989.

Courgnaud V, Laure F, Brossard A, Bignozzi C, Goudeau A, Barin F, Brechot C. Frequent and early in utero HIV-1 infection. AIDS Res Hum Retroviruses 7:337–341, 1991.

Cullen B, Greene W. Regulatory pathways governing HIV-1 replication. Cell 58:423–426, 1989.

Cullen B, Greene W. Functions of the auxiliary gene products of the human immunodeficiency virus type 1. Virology 178:1–5, 1990.

Cullen M, Viscarello R, Paryani S, Sanchez-Ramos L. Prenatal diagnosis of HIV infection: the use of cordocentesis, polymerase chain reaction, and p24 antigen assay. Am J Obstet Gynecol 166:386, 1992.

Curry A, Turner AJ, Lucas S. Opportunistic infections in human immunodeficiency virus disease: review highlighting diagnostic and therapeutic aspects. J Clin Pathol 44:182–193, 1991.

Daar E, Li X, Moudgil T, Ho D. High concentrations of recombinant soluble CD4 are required to neutralize primary human immunodeficiency virus type 1 isolates. Proc Natl Acad Sci U S A 87:6574–6578, 1990.

Daar ES, Moudgil T, Meyer RD, Ho DD. Transient high levels of viremia in patients with primary human immunodeficiency virus type 1 infection. N Engl J Med 324:961–964, 1991.

Dalgleish A, Beverley P, Clapham P, Crawford D, Greaves M, Weiss R. The CD4 (T4) antigen is an essential component of the receptor for the AIDS virus. Nature 312:763–767, 1984.

D'Arminio Monforte A, Ravizza M, Muggiasca ML, Novati R, Bini T, Tornaghi R, Zuccotti GV, Cavalli G, Musicco M, Giovannini M. HIV-infected pregnant women: possible predictors of vertical transmission. Int Conf AIDS 7:1991.

Davis MK. Human milk and HIV infection: epidemiologic and laboratory data. In Symposium on Immunology of Milk and the Neonate. New York, Plenum Press, 1991, pp. 271–280.

Dawson VL, Dawson TM, Uhl GR, Snyder SH. Human immunodeficiency virus type 1 coat protein neurotoxicity mediated by nitric oxide in primary cortical cultures. Proc Natl Acad Sci U S A 90:3256–3259, 1993.

DeCarli C, Civitello LA, Brouwers P, Pizzo PA. The prevalence of computed tomographic abnormalities of the cerebrum in 100 consecutive children symptomatic with the human immune deficiency virus. Ann Neurol 34:198–205, 1993.

De Rossi A, Ometto L, Mammano F, Zanotto C, Giaquinto C, Chieco-Bianchi L. Vertical transmission of HIV-1: lack of detectable virus in peripheral blood cells of infected children at birth. AIDS 6:1117–1120, 1992.

Di John D, Krasinski K, Lawrence R, Borkowsky W, Johnson JP, Schieken LS, Rennels MB. Very late onset of group B streptococcal disease in infants infected with the human immunodeficiency virus. Pediatr Infect Dis J 9:925–928, 1990.

Diamond D, Sleckman B, Gregory T, Lasky L, Greenstein J, Burakoff S. Inhibition of CD4+ T cell function by the HIV envelope protein, gp120. J Immunol 141:3715–3717, 1988.

Dimitrov D, Golding H, Blumenthal R. Initial steps in HIV-1 envelope glycoprotein mediated cell fusion monitored by a new assay based on redistribution of fluorescence markers. AIDS Res Hum Retroviruses 7:799–805, 1991.

Dimitrov DH, Hollinger FB, Baker CJ, Kline MW, Doyle M, Bremer JW, Shearer WT. Study of human immunodeficiency virus resistance to 2'-3'-dideoxyinosine and zidovudine in sequential isolates from pediatric patients on long-term therapy. J Infect Dis 167:818–823, 1993a.

Dimitrov D, Willey R, Sato H, Chang L-J, Blumenthal R, Martin M. Quantitation of human immunodeficiency virus type 1 infection kinetics. J Virol 67:2182–2190, 1993b.

Doebbeling BN, Feilmeier ML, Herwaldt LA. Pertussis in an adult man infected with the human immunodeficiency virus. J Infect Dis 161:1296–1298, 1990.

Douglas GC, Fry GN, Thirkill T, Holmes E, Hakim H, Jennings M, King BF. Cell-mediated infection of human placental trophoblast with HIV in vitro. AIDS Res Hum Retroviruses 7:735–740, 1991.

Duh E, Maury E, Folks T, Fauci A, Rabson A. Tumor necrosis factor alpha activates human immunodeficiency virus type 1 through induction of nuclear factor binding to the NF-kappa B sites in the long terminal repeat. Proc Natl Acad Sci U S A 86:5974–5978, 1989.

Duliege AM, Messiah A, Blanche S, Tardieu M, Griscelli C, Spira A. Natural history of human immunodeficiency virus type 1 infection in children: prognostic value of laboratory tests on the bimodal progression of the disease. Pediatr Infect Dis J 11:630–635, 1992.

Dunn D, Newell M, Ades E, Peckham C. Risk of human immunodeficiency virus type 1 transmission through breastfeeding. Lancet 340:585–588, 1992.

Economides A, Anisman D, Schmid I, Zack J, Hays E, Uittenbogaart C. Apoptosis in human HIV-1 infected thymocytes (abstract). J Cell Biochem S17E:62, 1993.

Ellaurie M, Rubinstein A. Beta-2-microglobulin concentrations in pediatric human immunodeficiency virus infection. Pediatr Infect Dis J 9:807–809, 1990.

Ellaurie M, Burns ER, Rubinstein A. Hematologic manifestations in pediatric HIV infection: severe anemia as a prognostic factor. Am J Pediatr Hematol Oncol 12:449–453, 1990.

Ellaurie M, Calvelli T, Rubinstein A. Neopterin concentrations in pediatric human immunodeficiency virus infection as predictor of disease activity. Pediatr Infect Dis J 11:286–289, 1992.

Embretson J, Zupancic M, Ribas JL, Burke A, Racz P, Tenner RK, Haase AT. Massive covert infection of helper T lymphocytes and macrophages by HIV during the incubation period of AIDS. Nature 362:359–362, 1993.

Emini EA, Graham DJ, Gotlib L, Condra JH, Byrnes VW, Schleif WA. HIV and multidrug resistance (letter). Nature 364:679, 1993.

Ensoli B, Lusso P, Schachter F, Josephs S, Rappaport J, Negro F, Gallo R, Wong-Staal F. Human herpes virus-6 increases HIV-1 expression in co-infected T cells via nuclear factors binding to the HIV-1 enhancer. EMBO J 8:3019–3027, 1989.

Epstein LG, Gendelman HE. Human immunodeficiency virus type 1 infection of the nervous system: pathogenetic mechanisms. Ann Neurol 33:429–436, 1993.

Epstein LG, Boucher CA, Morrison SH, Connor EM, Oleske JM, Lange JM, van der Noordaa J, Bakker M, Dekker J, Scherpbier H, van den Berg H, Boer K, Goudsmit M. Persistent human immunodeficiency virus type 1 antigenemia in children correlates with disease progression. Pediatrics 82:919–924, 1988a.

Epstein LG, Sharer LR, Goudsmit J. Neurological and neuropathological features of human immunodeficiency virus infection in children. Ann Neurol 23(Suppl):S19–S23, 1988b.

Erickson J, Neidhart DJ, VanDrie J, Kempf DJ, Wang XC, Norbeck DW, Plattner JJ, Rittenhouse JW, Turon M, Wideburg N. Design, activity, and 2.8 A crystal structure of a C2 symmetric inhibitor complexed to HIV-1 protease. Science 249:527–533, 1990.

Erkeller-Yuksel FM, Deneys V, Hannet I, Hulstaert F, Hamilton C, Mackinnon H, Turner Stokes L, Munhyeshuli V, Vanlangendonck F, De Bruyere M, Bach BA, Lydyard PM. Age-related changes in human blood lymphocyte subpopulations. J Pediatr 120:216–222, 1992.

European Collaborative Study. Neurologic signs in young children with human immunodeficiency virus infection. Pediatr Infect Dis J 9:402–406, 1990.

European Collaborative Study. Children born to women with HIV-1 infection: natural history and risk of transmission. Lancet 337:253–260, 1991.

European Collaborative Study. Age-related standards for T lymphocyte subsets based on uninfected children born to human immunodeficiency virus 1–infected mothers. Pediatr Infect Dis J 11:1018–1026, 1992.

Fabio G, Scorza R, Lazzarin A, Marchini M, Zarantonello M, D'Arminio A, Marchisio P, Plebani A, Luzzati R, Costigliola P. HLA-associated susceptibility to HIV-1 infection. Clin Exp Immunol 87:20–23, 1992.

Fahey JL, Taylor JMG, Detels R, Hofmann B, Melmed R, Nishanian P, Giorgi JV. The prognostic value of cellular and serologic markers in infection with human immunodeficiency virus type 1. N Engl J Med 322:166–172, 1990.

Fauci A. Multifactorial nature of human immunodeficiency virus disease: implications for therapy. Science 262:1011–1018, 1993.

Fazely F, Dezube BJ, Allen RJ, Pardee AB, Ruprecht RM. Pentoxifylline (Trental) decreases the replication of the human immunodeficiency virus type 1 in human peripheral blood mononuclear cells and in cultured T cells. Blood 77:1653–1656, 1991.

Fernandez-Cruz E, Desco M, Garcia MM, Longo N, Gonzalez B, Zabay JM. Immunological and serological markers predictive of progression to AIDS in a cohort of HIV-infected drug users. AIDS 4:987–994, 1990.

Fischl MA, Richman DD, Grieco MH, Gottlieb MS, Volberding PA, Laskin OL, Leedom JM, Groopman JE, Mildvan D, Schooley RT, Jackson GG, Durack DT, King D, Group TACW. The efficacy of azidothymidine (AZT) in the treatment of patients with AIDS and AIDS-related complex. N Engl J Med 317:185–191, 1987.

Fischl MA, Richman DD, Hansen N, Collier AC, Carey JT, Para MF, Hardy WD, Dolin R, Powderly WG, Allan JD, Wong B, Merigan TC, McAuliffe VJ, Hyslop NE, Rhame FS, Balfour HH, Spector SA, Volberding P, Pettinelli C, Anderson J, Group TACT. The safety and efficacy of zidovudine (AZT) in the treatment of subjects with mildly symptomatic human immunodeficiency virus type 1 (HIV) infection. Ann Intern Med 112:727–737, 1990.

Fischl MA, Uttamchandani RB, Daikos GL, Poblete RB, Moreno JN, Reyes RR, Boota AM, Thompson LM, Cleary TJ, Lai S. An outbreak of tuberculosis caused by multiple-drug-resistant tubercle bacilli among patients with HIV infection. Ann Intern Med 117:177–183, 1992.

Fisher A, Feinberg M, Josephs S, Harper M, Marsell L, Reyes G, Gonda M, Aldovini A, Debouk C, Gallo R, Wong-Staal F. The trans-activator gene of HTLV-III is essential for virus replication. Nature 320:367–371, 1986.

Fitzgerald P, Springer J. Structure and function of retroviral proteases. Annu Rev Biophys Biophys Chem 20:299–320, 1991.

Fitzgibbon J, Gaur S, Frenkel L, Laraque F, Edlin B, Dubin D. Transmission from one child to another of human immunodeficiency virus type 1 with a zidovudine-resistance mutation. N Engl J Med 329:1835–1841, 1993.

Fox CH, Tenner-Racz K, Racz P, Firpo A, Pizzo PA, Fauci AS.

Lymphoid germinal centers are reservoirs of human immunodeficiency virus type 1 RNA. J Infect Dis 164:1051–1057, 1991.

Frickhofen N, Abkowitz JL, Safford M, Berry JM, Antunez-de-Mayolo J, Astrow A, Cohen R, Halperin I, King L, Mintzer D, Cohen B, Young NS. Persistent B19 parvovirus infection in patients infected with human immunodeficiency virus type 1 (HIV-1): a treatable cause of anemia in AIDS. Ann Intern Med 113:926–933, 1990.

Friedland GH, Saltzman BR, Rogers MF, Kahl PA, Lesser ML, Mayers MM, Klein RS. Lack of transmission of HTLV-III/LAV infection to household contacts of patients with AIDS or AIDS-related complex with oral candidiasis. N Engl J Med 314:344–339, 1986.

Froebel KS, Doherty KV, Whitelaw JA, Hague RA, Mok JY, Bird AG. Increased expression of the CD45RO (memory) antigen on T cells in HIV-infected children. AIDS 5:97–99, 1991.

Gao WY, Shirasaka T, Johns DG, Broder S, Mitsuya H. Differential phosphorylation of azidothymidine, dideoxycytidine, and dideoxyinosine in resting and activated peripheral blood mononuclear cells. J Clin Invest 91:2326–2333, 1993.

Garry R. Potential mechanisms for the cytopathic properties of HIV. AIDS 3:683–694, 1989.

Gartner S, Markovits P, Markovitz D, Kaplan M, Gallo R, Popovic M. The role of mononuclear phagocytes in HTLV-III/LAV infection. Science 233:215–219, 1986.

Gayle H, D'Angelo L. Epidemiology of acquired immunodeficiency syndrome and human immunodeficiency virus infection in adolescents. J Pediatr Infect Dis 10:322–328, 1991.

Geffner ME, Bersch N, Lippe BM, Rosenfeld RG, Hintz RL, Golde DW. Growth hormone mediates the growth of T-lymphoblast cell lines via locally generated insulin-like growth factor-I. J Clin Endocrinol Metab 71:464–469, 1990.

Geffner ME, Yeh DY, Landaw EM, Scott ML, Stiehm ER, Bryson YJ, Israele V. In vitro insulin-like growth factor-I, growth hormone, and insulin resistance occurs in symptomatic human immunodeficiency virus-1-infected children. Pediatr Res 34:66–72, 1993.

Gelderblom H, Hausmann E, Ozel M, Pauli G, Koch M. Fine structure of human immunodeficiency virus (HIV) and immunolocalization of structural proteins. Virology 156:171–176, 1987.

Gendelman H, Phelps W, Feigenbaum L, Ostrove J, Adachi A, Howley P, Khoury G, Ginsberg H, Martin M. Trans-activation of the human immunodeficiency virus long terminal repeat sequence by DNA viruses. Proc Natl Acad Sci U S A 83:9759–9763, 1986.

Gjerset RA, Yeargin J, Volkman SK, Vila V, Arya J, Haas M. Insulin-like growth factor-I supports proliferation of autocrine thymic lymphoma cells with a pre-T cell phenotype. J Immunol 145:3497–3501, 1990.

Goedert JJ, Drummond JE, Minkoff HL, Stevens R, Blattner WA, Landesman SH, Mendez H, Robert-Guroff M, Holman S, Rubinstein A, Willoughby A. Mother-to-infant transmission of human immunodeficiency virus type 1: association with prematurity or low anti-gp120. Lancet 2:1351–1354, 1989.

Goedert JJ, Duliege A, Amos C, Felton S, Biggar R. The International Registry of HIV-exposed twins. High risk of HIV-1 infection for first-born twins. Lancet 338:1471–1475, 1991.

Golding H, Shearer G, Hillman K, Lucas P, Manischewitz J, Zajac R, Clerici M, Gress R, Boswell R, Golding B. Common epitope in human immunodeficiency virus (HIV) I-GP41 and HLA class II elicits immunosuppressive autoantibodies capable of contributing to immune dysfunction in HIV I-infected individuals. J Clin Invest 83:1430–1435, 1989.

Gorelick R, Nigida S, Bess J, Arthur L, Henderson L, Rein A. Noninfectious human immunodeficiency virus type 1 mutants deficient in genomic RNA. J Virol 64:3207–3211, 1990.

Graham NMH, Zeger SL, Park LP, Vermund SH, Detels R, Rinaldo CR, Phair JP. The effects on survival of early treatment of human immunodeficiency virus infection. N Engl J Med 326:1037–1042, 1992.

Greene WC. The molecular biology of human immunodeficiency virus type 1 infection. N Engl J Med 324:308–317, 1991.

Groopman JE, Broder S. Cancers in AIDS and other immunodeficiency states. In DeVita VT, Hilman S, Rosenberg S, eds. Cancer: Principles and Practice of Oncology. Philadelphia, JB Lippincott, 1989, pp. 1953–1970.

Groux H, Torpier G, Monte D, Mouton Y, Capron A, Ameisen J-C. Activation-induced death by apoptosis in CD4+ T cells from human immunodeficiency virus-infected asymptomatic individuals. J Exp Med 175:331–340, 1992.

Grunfeld C, Pang M, Shimuzu L, Shigenga JK, Jensen P, Feingold KR. Resting energy expenditure, caloric intake and short-term weight change in human immunodeficiency virus infection and the acquired immunodeficiency syndrome. Am J Clin Nutr 55:455–460, 1992.

Gutman LT, St. Claire KK, Weedy C, Herman-Giddens ME, Lane BA, Niemeyer JG, McKinney RE. Human immunodeficiency virus transmission by child sexual abuse. Am J Dis Child 145:137–141, 1991.

Gwinn M, Pappaioanou M, George J, Hannon W, Wasser S, Redus M, Hoff R, Grady G, Willoughby A, Novello A, Peterson L, Dondero T, Curran J. Prevalence of HIV infection in childbearing women in the United States: surveillance using newborn blood samples. JAMA 265:1704–1708, 1991.

Habeshaw J, Hounsell E, Dalgleish A. Does the HIV envelope induce a chronic graft-versus-host-like disease? Immunol Today 13:207–210, 1992.

Halsey N, Markham R, Wahren B, Boulos R, Rossi P, Wigzell H. Lack of association between maternal antibodies to V3 loop peptides and maternal-infant transmission. J AIDS 5:153–157, 1992.

Hamilton JD, Hartigan PM, Simberkoff MS, Day PL, Diamond GR, Dickinson GM, Drusano GL, Egorin MJ, George WL, Gordin FM, Hawkes CA, Jensen PC, Klimas NG, Labriola AM, Lahart CJ, O'Brien WA, Oster CN, Weinhold KJ, Wray NP, Zolla-Pazner SB, the Veterans Affairs Cooperative Study Group on AIDS Treatment. A controlled trial of early versus late treatment with zidovudine in symptomatic human immunodeficiency virus infection: results of the Veterans Affairs Cooperative Study. N Engl J Med 326:437–443, 1992.

Hanson I, Kaplan S. Opportunistic infections. Semin Pediatr Infect Dis 1:31–39, 1990.

Haseltine W. Molecular biology of the human immunodeficiency virus type 1. FASEB J 5:2349–2360, 1991.

Heng MC, Heng SY, Allen SG. Co-infection and synergy of human immunodeficiency virus-1 and herpes simplex virus-1. Lancet 343:255–258, 1994.

Hira SK, Mangrola UG, Mwale C, Chintu C, Tembo G, Brady WE, Perine PL. Apparent vertical transmission of human immunodeficiency virus type 1 by breast-feeding in Zambia. J Pediatr 117:421–424, 1990.

Hiraoka A, Masaoka T, Nagai K, Horiuchi A, Kanamaru A, Niimura M, Hamada T, Takahashi M. Clinical effect of BV-araU on varicella-zoster virus infection in immunocompromised patients with haematological malignancies. J Antimicrob Chemother 27:361–367, 1991.

Ho D, Rota T, Hirsch M. Infection of monocyte/macrophages by human T lymphotropic viruses type III. J Clin Invest 77:1712–1715, 1986.

Ho DD, Moudgil T, Alam M. Quantitation of human immunodeficiency virus type 1 in the blood of infected persons. N Engl J Med 321:1621–1625, 1989.

Hoff R, Berardi VP, Weiblen BJ, Mahoney-Trout L, Mitchell ML, Grady GF. Seroprevalence of human immunodeficiency virus among childbearing women. Estimation by testing samples of blood from newborns. N Engl J Med 318:525–530, 1988.

Hoffenbach A, Langlade DP, Dadaglio G, Vilmer E, Michel F, Mayaud C, Autran B, Plata F. Unusually high frequencies of HIV-specific cytotoxic T lymphocytes in humans. J Immunol 142:452–462, 1989.

Homsy J, Tateno M, Levy J. Antibody-dependent enhancement of HIV infection. Lancet 1:1285–1286, 1988.

Horsburgh CJ, Ou CY, Jason J, Holmberg SD, Longini IJ, Schable C, Mayer KH, Lifson AR, Schochetman G, Ward JW. Duration of human immunodeficiency virus infection before detection of antibody. Lancet 2:637–640, 1989.

Hubner A, Kruhoffer M, Grosse F, Krauss G. Fidelity of human immunodeficiency virus type 1 reverse transcriptase in copying natural RNA. J Mol Biol 223:595–600, 1992.

Husson RN, Comeau AM, Hoff R. Diagnosis of human immunodeficiency virus infection in infants and children. Pediatrics 86:1–10, 1990.

Husson RN, Saini R, Lewis LL, Butler KM, Patronas N, Pizzo PA. Cerebral artery aneurysms in children infected with human immunodeficiency virus. J Pediatr 121:927–930, 1992.

Husson RN, Shirasaka T, Butler KM, Pizzo PA, Mitsuya H. High-level resistance to zidovudine but not to zalcitabine or didanosine in human immunodeficiency virus from children receiving antiretroviral therapy. J Pediatr 123:9–16, 1993.

Husson R, Mueller B, Farley M, Woods L, Kovacs A, Goldsmith J, Ono R, Lewis L, Balis F, Brouwers P, Avramis V, Church J, Butler K, Rasheed S, Jarosinski P, Venzon D, Pizzo P. Zidovudine and didanosine combination therapy in children with human immunodeficiency virus infection. Pediatrics 93:316–322, 1994.

Imberti L, Sottini A, Bettinardi A, Puoti M, Primi D. Selective depletion of T cells that bear specific T cell receptor V-beta sequences. Science 254:860–862, 1991.

Inoue M, Koga Y, Djordjijevic D, Fukuma T, Reddy EP, Yokoyama MM, Sagawa K. Down-regulation of CD4 molecules by the expression of Nef: a quantitative analysis of CD4 antigens on the cell surfaces. Int Immunol 5:1067–1073, 1993.

Iosub S, Bamji M, Stone RK, Gromisch DS, Wasserman E. More on human immunodeficiency virus embryopathy. Pediatrics 80:512–516, 1987.

Issel CJ, Horohov DW, Lea DF, Adams WJ, Hagius SD, McManus JM, Allison AC, Montelaro RC. Efficacy of inactivated whole-virus and subunit vaccines in preventing infection and disease caused by equine infectious anemia virus. J Virol 66:3398–3408, 1992.

Itescu S, Winchester R. Diffuse infiltrative lymphocytosis syndrome: a disorder occurring in human immunodeficiency virus-1 infection that may present as a sicca syndrome. Rheum Dis Clin North Am 18:683–697, 1992.

Ivey-Hoyle M, Culp J, Caikin M, Hellmig B, Matthews T. Envelope glycoproteins from biologically diverse isolates of human immunodeficiency viruses have widely different affinities for CD4. Proc Natl Acad Sci U S A 88:7802–7805, 1991.

Jacks T, Power M, Masiarz F, Luciw P, Barr P, Varmus H. Characterization of ribosomal frameshifting in HIV-1 *gag-pol* expression. Nature 331:280–283, 1988.

Jackson J, Coombs R, Sannerud K, Rhame F, Balfour H. Rapid and sensitive viral culture method for human immunodeficiency virus type 1. J Clin Microbiol 26:1416–1418, 1988.

Jacobson JM, Colman N, Ostrow NA, Simson RW, Tomesch D, Marlin L, Rao M, Mills JL, Clemens J, Prince AM. Passive immunotherapy in the treatment of advanced human immunodeficiency virus infection [see published erratum appears in J Infect Dis 168:802, 1993]. J Infect Dis 168:298–305, 1993.

Jacobson MA, Berger TG, Fikrig S, Becherer P, Moohr JW, Stanat SC, Biron KK. Acyclovir-resistant varicella zoster virus infection after chronic oral acyclovir therapy in patients with the acquired immunodeficiency syndrome (AIDS). Ann Intern Med 112:187–191, 1990.

Jenkinson E, Kingston R, Smith C, Williams G, Owen J. Antigen-induced apoptosis in developing T cells: a mechanism for negative selection of the T cell receptor repertoire. Eur J Immunol 19:2175–2177, 1989.

Joshi VV, Oleske JM. Pathologic appraisal of the thymus gland in acquired immunodeficiency syndrome in children. A study of four cases and a review of the literature. Arch Pathol Lab Med 109:142–146, 1985.

Joshi VV, Kauffman S, Oleske JM, Fikrig S, Denny T, Gadol C, Lee E. Polyclonal polymorphic B-cell lymphoproliferative disorder with prominent pulmonary involvement in children with acquired immune deficiency syndrome. Cancer 59:1455–1462, 1987.

Joshi VV, Oleske JM, Connor EM. Morphologic findings in children with acquired immune deficiency syndrome: pathogenesis and clinical implications. In Childhood AIDS. Hemisphere Publishing, 1990, pp. 155–165.

Jovaisas E, Koch M, Schafer A, Stauber M, Lowenthal D. LAV/HTLV-III in 20-week fetus. Lancet 2:1129, 1985.

Jura E, Chadwick EG, Josephs SH, Steinberg SP, Yogev R, Gershon AA, Krasinski KM, Borkowsky W. Varicella-zoster virus infections in children infected with human immunodeficiency virus. Pediatr Infect Dis J 8:586–590, 1989.

Kageyama S, Mimoto T, Murakawa Y, Nomizu M, Ford HJ, Shirasaka T, Gulnik S, Erickson J, Takada K, Hayashi H. In vitro anti-human immunodeficiency virus (HIV) activities of transition state mimetic HIV protease inhibitors containing allophenylnorstatine. Antimicrob Agents Chemother 37:810–817, 1993.

Kahn JO, Lagakos SW, Richman DD, Cross A, Pettinelli C, Liou S-H,

Brown M, Volberding PA, Crumpacker CS, Beall G, Sacks HS, Merigan TC, Beltangady M, Smaldone L, Dolin R, the NIAID AIDS Clinical Trials Group. A controlled trial comparing zidovudine with didanosine in human immunodeficiency virus infection. N Engl J Med 327:581–587, 1992.

Kalebic T, Kinter A, Poli G, Anderson ME, Meister A, Fauci AS. Suppression of human immunodeficiency virus expression in chronically infected monocytic cells by glutathione, glutathione ester, and N-acetylcysteine. Proc Natl Acad Sci U S A 88:986–990, 1991.

Kaplan LJ, Daum RS, Smaron M, McCarthy CA. Severe measles in immunocompromised patients. JAMA 267:1237–1241, 1992.

Kaslow RA, Duquesnoy R, VanRaden M, Kingsley L, Marrari M, Friedman H, Su S, Saah AJ, Detels R, Phair J. A1, Cw7, B8, DR3 HLA antigen combination associated with rapid decline of T-helper lymphocytes in HIV-1 infection: a report from the Multicenter AIDS Cohort Study. Lancet 335:927–930, 1990.

Katz B, Berkman A, Shapiro E. Serologic evidence of active Epstein-Barr virus infection in Epstein-Barr virus-associated lymphoproliferative disorders of children with acquired immunodeficiency syndrome. J Pediatr 120:228–232, 1992.

Kauffman WM, Sivit CJ, Fitz CR, Rakusan TA, Herzog K, Chandra RS. CT and MR evaluation of intracranial involvement in pediatric HIV infection: a clinical-imaging correlation. Am J Neuroradiol 13:949–957, 1992.

Kellam P, Boucher CA, Larder BA. Fifth mutation in human immunodeficiency virus type 1 reverse transcriptase contributes to the development of high-level resistance to zidovudine. Proc Natl Acad Sci U S A 89:1934–1938, 1992.

Kestler HW, Ringler DJ, Mori K, Panicali DL, Sehgal PK, Daniel MD, Desrosiers RC. Importance of the nef gene for maintenance of high virus loads and for the development of AIDS. Cell 65:651–662, 1991.

Khouri YF, Mastrucci MT, Hutto C, Mitchell CD, Scott GB. Mycobacterium tuberculosis in children with human immunodeficiency virus type 1 infection. Pediatr Infect Dis J 11:950–955, 1992.

Klatzmann D, Champagne E, Chamaret S, Gruest J, Guetard D, Hercend T, Gluckman J-C, Montagnier L. T-lymphocyte T4 behaves as the receptor for human retrovirus LAV. Nature 312:767–768, 1984.

Kliks SC, Nisalak A, Brandt WE, Wahl L, Burke DS. Antibody-dependent enhancement of dengue virus growth in human monocytes as a risk factor for dengue hemorrhagic fever. Am J Trop Med Hyg 40:444–451, 1989.

Kline M, Hollinger F, Rosenblatt H, Bohannon B, Kozinetz C, Shearer W. Sensitivity, specificity and predictive value of physical examination, culture and other laboratory studies in the diagnosis during early infancy of vertically acquired human immunodeficiency virus infection. Pediatr Infect Dis J 12:33–36, 1993.

Klotman ME, Kim S, Buchbinder A, DeRossi A, Baltimore D, Wong-Staal F. Kinetics of expression of multiply spliced RNA in early human immunodeficiency virus type 1 infection of lymphocytes and monocytes. Proc Natl Acad Sci U S A 88:5011–5015, 1991.

Koot M, Keet I, Vos A, De Goede R, Roos M, Coutinho R, Miedema F, Schellekens P, Tersmette M. Prognostic value of syncytium-inducing phenotype for rate of CD4+ cell depletion and progression to AIDS. Ann Intern Med 118:681–688, 1993.

Kovacs JA, Baseler M, Dewar RJ, Vogel S, Davey RT, Falloon J, Polis MA, Walker RE, Stevens R, Salman NP, Metcalf JA, Masur H, Lane HC. Increases in CD4 T lymphocytes with intermittent courses of Interleukin-2 in patients with human immunodeficiency virus infection: a preliminary study. N Engl J Med 332:567–575, 1995.

Kowalski M, Potz J, Basiripour L, Dorfman T, Goh W, Terwilliger E, Dayton A, Rosen C, Haseltine W, Sodroski J. Functional regions of the envelope glycoprotein of human immunodeficiency virus type 1. Science 237:1351–1355, 1987.

Krasinski K, Borkowsky W, Bonk S, Lawrence R, Chandwani S. Bacterial infections in human immunodeficiency virus–infected children. Pediatr Infect Dis J 7:323–328, 1988.

Krivine A, Firtion G, Cao L, Francoual C, Henrion R, Lebon P. HIV replication during the first weeks of life. Lancet 339:1187–1189, 1992.

Kure K, Llena JF, Lyman WD, Soeiro R, Weidenheim KM, Hirano A, Dickson DW. Human immunodeficiency virus–1 infection of the nervous system: an autopsy study of 268 adult, pediatric, and fetal brains. Hum Pathol 22:700–710, 1991.

Lambert JS, Seidlin M, Reichman RC, Plank CS, Laverty M, Morse GD, Knupp C, McLaren C, Pettinelli C, Valentine FT, Dolin R. 2′,3′-dideoxyinosine (ddI) in patients with the acquired immunodeficiency syndrome or AIDS-related complex. N Engl J Med 322:1333–1340, 1990.

Lamers SL, Sleasman JW, She JX, Barrie KA, Pomeroy SM, Barrett DJ, Goodenow MM. Persistence of multiple maternal genotypes of human immunodeficiency virus type I in infants infected by vertical transmission. J Clin Invest 93:380–390, 1994.

Landesman S, Weiblen B, Mendez H, Willoughby A, Goedert J, Rubinstein A, Minkoff H, Moroso G, Hoff R. Clinical utility of HIV-IgA immunoblot assay in the early diagnosis of perinatal HIV infection. JAMA 266:3443–3446, 1991.

Lang C, Jacobi G, Kreuz W, Hacker H, Herrmmann G, Keul H-G, Thomas E. Rapid development of giant aneurysm at the base of the brain in an 8-year-old boy with perinatal HIV infection. Acta Histochem (Suppl.) 42:S83–S90, 1992.

Larder BA, Kellam P, Kemp SD. Convergent combination therapy can select viable multidrug-resistant HIV-1 in vitro. Nature 365:451–453, 1993.

Lasky L, Nakamura G, Smith D, Fennie C, Shimasaki C, Patzer E, Berman P, Gregory T, Capon D. Delineation of a region of the human immunodeficiency virus type 1 gp120 glycoprotein critical for interaction with the CD4 receptor. Cell 50:975–985, 1987.

Laspia M, Rice A, Mathews M. HIV-1 *tat* protein increases transcriptional initiation and stabilizes elongation. Cell 59:283–292, 1989.

Laue L, Pizzo PA, Butler K, Cutler GB. Growth and neuroendocrine dysfunction in children with acquired immunodeficiency syndrome. J Pediatr 117:541–545, 1990.

Lederman S. Estimating infant mortality from human immunodeficiency virus and other causes in breast-feeding and bottle-feeding populations. Pediatrics 89:290–296, 1992.

Leibovitz E, Kaul A, Rigaud M, Bebenroth D, Krasinski K, Borkowsky W. Chronic varicella zoster in a child infected with human immunodeficiency virus: case report and review of the literature. Cutis 49:27–31, 1992.

Leis J, Baltimore D, Bishop J, Coffin J, Fleissner E, Goff S, Oroszlan S, Robinson H, Skalka A, Temin H, Vogt V. Standardized and simplified nomenclature for preoteins common to all retroviruses. J Virol 62:1808–1809, 1988.

Lepage P, van de Perre P, Dabis F, Commenges D, Orbinski J, Hitimana D, Bazubagira A, van Goethem C, Allen S, Butzler J. Evaluation and simplification of the World Health Organization clinical case definition for paediatric AIDS. AIDS 3:221–225, 1989.

Levine M, Denamur E, Simon F, De Crepy A, Blot P, Vilmer E. Conversion of HIV viral markers during the first months of life in HIV infected children born to seropositive mothers. Presented at the Ninth International Conference on AIDS, Berlin, June 6–11, 1993.

Levy J. Pathogenesis of human immunodeficiency virus infection. Microbiol Rev 57:183–289, 1993.

Levy J, Youvan Y, Lee ML, the Passive Hyperimmune Therapy Study Group. Passive hyperimmune plasma therapy in the treatment of acquired immunodeficiency syndrome: results of a 12-month multicenter double-blind controlled trial. Blood 84:2130–2135, 1994.

Lewis LL, Butler KM, Husson RN, Mueller BU, Fowler CL, Steinberg SM, Pizzo PA. Defining the population of human immunodeficiency virus-infected children at risk for *Mycobacterium avium-intracellulare infection*. J Pediatr 121:677–683, 1992.

Lewis SH, Reynolds-Kohler C, Fox HE, Nelson JA. HIV-1 in trophoblastic and villous Hofbauer cells, and haematological precursors in eight-week fetuses. Lancet 335:565–568, 1990.

Lifson J, Reyes G, McGrath M, Stein B, Engleman E. AIDS retrovirus induced cytopathology: giant cell formation and involvement of CD4 antigen. Science 232:1123–1127, 1986.

Lipton S. HIV displays its coat of arms. Nature 367:113–114, 1994.

Lucey DR, Melcher GP, Hendrix CW, Zajac RA, Goetz DW, Butzin CA, Clerici M, Warner RD, Abbadessa S, Hall K, Shearer G. Human immunodeficiency virus infection in the US Air Force: seroconversions, clinical staging, and assessment of a T helper cell functional assay to predict change in CD4+ T cell counts. J Infect Dis 164:631–637, 1991.

Lusso P, Gallo R. Human herpesvirus 6 in AIDS. Lancet 343:555–556, 1994.

Luzuriaga K, McQuilken P, Alimenti A, Somasundaran M, Hesselton R, Sullivan JL. Early viremia and immune responses in vertical human immunodeficiency virus type 1 infection. J Infect Dis 167:1008–1013, 1993.

MacDonell KB, Chmiel JS, Poggensee L, Wu S, Phair JP. Predicting progression to AIDS: combined usefulness of CD4 lymphocyte counts and p24 antigenemia. Am J Med 89:706–712, 1990.

Mackewicz C, Levy JA. CD8+ cell anti-HIV activity: nonlytic suppression of virus replication. AIDS Res Hum Retroviruses 8:1039–1050, 1992.

Mann JM, Quinn TC, Francis H, Nzilambi N, Bosenge N, Bila K, McCormick JB, Ruti K, Asila PK, Curran JW. Prevalence of HTLV-III/LAV in household contacts of patients with confirmed AIDS and controls in Kinshasa, Zaire. JAMA 256:721–724, 1986.

Mano H, Chermann J-C. Fetal human immunodeficiency virus type 1 infection of different organs in the second trimester. AIDS Res Human Retroviruses 7:83–88, 1987.

Mantero-Atienza E, Indacochea F, Cabrejos C, Sotomayor MC, Fletcher MA, Sauberlich HE, Shor PG, Baum MK. Selenium deficiency associated with HIV-1 infection in children. Int Conf AIDS 8:7336, 1992.

Margulis SJ, Honig CL, Soave R, Govoni AF, Mouradian JA, Jacobson IM. Biliary tract obstruction in the acquired immunodeficiency syndrome. Ann Intern Med 105:207–210, 1986.

Marion RW, Wiznia AA, Hutcheon RG, Rubinstein A. Human T-cell lymphotropic virus type III (HTLV-III) embryopathy. Am J Dis Child 140:638–640, 1986.

Martin NL, Levy JA, Legg H, Weintrub PS, Cowan MJ, Wara DW. Detection of infection with human immunodeficiency virus (HIV) type 1 in infants by an anti-HIV immunoglobulin A assay using recombinant proteins. J Pediatr 118:354–358, 1991.

Martin P, Di BA, Kassianides C, Lisker MM, Hoofnagle JH. Rapidly progressive non-A, non-B hepatitis in patients with human immunodeficiency virus infection. Gastroenterology 97:1559–1561, 1989.

Masur H. Prevention and treatment of Pneumocystis pneumonia [see erratum in N Engl J Med 328:1136, 1993]. N Engl J Med 327:1853–1860, 1992.

Matsuyama T, Kobayashi N, Yamamoto N. Cytokines and HIV infection: is AIDS a tumor necrosis factor disease? AIDS 5:1405–1417, 1991.

Maury W, Potts B, Rabson A. HIV-1 infection of first trimester and term human placental tissue: a possible mode of maternal-fetal transmission. J Infect Dis 160:583–588, 1989.

Mayers D, Wagner K, Chung R, Lane J, Vahey M, White F, Ruiz N, Hicks C, Weislow O, Gardner L, Burke D. Zidovudine (AZT) resistance is temporally associated with clinical failure in patients on AZT therapy. Presented at the First National Conference on Human Retroviruses, Washington, DC, American Society for Microbiology, 1993.

Mayers M, Davenny K, Schoenbaum E, Feingold A, Selwyn P, Robertson V, Ou C-Y, Rogers M, Naccarato M. A prospective study of infants of human immunodeficiency virus seropositive and seronegative women with a history of intravenous drug use or of intravenous drug-using sex partners in the Bronx. Pediatrics 88:1248–1256, 1991.

McGuire TC, Adams DS, Johnson GC, Klevjer AP, Barbee DD, Gorham JR. Acute arthritis in caprine arthritis-encephalitis virus challenge exposure of vaccinated or persistently infected goats. Am J Vet Res 47:537–540, 1986.

McKeating JA, Gow J, Goudsmit J, Pearl LH, Mulder C, Weiss RA. Characterization of HIV-1 neutralization escape mutants. AIDS 3:777–784, 1989.

McKinney R, Wilfert C. Lymphocyte subsets in children younger than 2 years old: normal values in a population at risk for human immunodeficiency virus infection and diagnostic and prognostic application to infected children. Pediatr Infect Dis J 11:639–644, 1992.

McKinney RE, Pizzo PA, Scott GB, Parks WP, Maha MA, Nusinoff-Lehrmann S, Riggs M, Eddy J, Lane BA, Eppes SC, Wilfert CM, the Pediatric Zidovudine Phase I Study Group. Safety and tolerance of intermittent intravenous and oral zidovudine therapy in human immunodeficiency virus-infected pediatric patients. J Pediatr 116:640–647, 1990.

McKinney RE, Maha MA, Connor EM, Feinberg J, Scott GB, Wulfsohn M, McIntosh K, Borkowsky W, Modlin JF, Weintrub P, O'Donnell K, Gelber RD, Knowlton-Rogers G, Nusinoff-Lehrman S, Wilfert CM, Group TPOS. A multicenter trial of oral zidovudine in children with advanced human immunodeficiency virus disease. N Engl J Med 324:1018–1025, 1991.

McKinney R, Robertson W, Duke Pediatric AIDS Clinical Trials Unit. Effect of human immunodeficiency virus infection on the growth of young children. J Pediatr 123:579–582, 1993.

Merson M. The HIV pandemic: global spread and global response. Presented at the Ninth International Conference on AIDS, Berlin, June 6–11, 1993.

Meyaard L, Otto S, Jonker R, Mijnster M, Keet R, Miedema F. Programmed death of T cells in HIV-1 infection. Science 257:217–219, 1992.

Meyerhans A, Cheynier R, Albert J, Seth M, Kwok S, Sninsky J, Morfeldt-Manson L, Asjo B, Wain-Hobson S. Temporal fluctuations in HIV quasispecies in vivo are not reflected by sequential HIV isolations. Cell 58:901–910, 1989.

Michael N, Vahey M, Burke D, Redfield R. Viral DNA and mRNA expression correlate with the stage of human immunodeficiency virus (HIV) type 1 infection in humans: evidence for viral replication in all stages of HIV disease. J Virol 66:310–316, 1992.

Miedema F, Petit A, Terpstra F, Schattenkerk J, deWolf F, Al B, Roos M, Lange J, Danner S, Goudsmit J, Schellekens P. Immunological abnormalities in human immunodeficiency virus (HIV) infected asymptomatic homosexual men. HIV infects the immune system before CD4+ T helper depletion occurs. J Clin Invest 82:1908–1914, 1988.

Miles S, Balden E, Magpantay L, Wei L, Leiblein A, Hofheinz D, Toedter G, Stiehm E, Bryson Y. Rapid serologic testing with immune-complex–dissociated HIV p24 antigen for early detection of HIV infection in neonates. N Engl J Med 328:297–302, 1993.

Miller MJ, Remington JS. Toxoplasmosis in infants and children with HIV infection or AIDS. In Pizzo PA, Wilfert CM, eds. Pediatric AIDS. Baltimore, Williams & Wilkins, 1991, pp. 299–307.

Miller TL, Orav EJ, Martin SR, Cooper ER, McIntosh K, Winter HS. Malnutrition and carbohydrate malabsorption in children with vertically transmitted human immunodeficiency virus 1 infection. Gastroenterology 100:1296–1302, 1991.

Miller TL, Winter HS, Luginbuhl LM, Orav EJ, McIntosh K. Pancreatitis in pediatric human immunodeficiency virus infection. J Pediatr 120:223–227, 1992.

Miller T, Orav E, McIntosh K, Lipshultz S. Is selenium deficiency clinically significant in pediatric HIV infection? Presented at the Ninth International Conference on AIDS, Berlin, June 6–11, 1993.

Mimoto T, Imai J, Tanaka S, Hattori N, Takahashi O, Kisanuki S, Nagano Y, Shintani M, Hayashi H, Sakikawa H. Rational design and synthesis of a novel class of active site-targeted HIV protease inhibitors containing a hydroxymethylcarbonyl isostere: use of phenylnorstatine or allophenylnorstatine as a transition-state mimic. Chem Pharmacol Bull (Tokyo) 39:2465–2467, 1991.

Mo H, Zhu T, Cao Y, Gu G, Koup R, Borkowsky W, Ho D. Genotype and phenotype characteristics of the HIV-1 transmitted from mother to infant (abstract). J Cell Biochem S17E: 98, 1993.

Mofenson LM, Moye JJ, Bethel J, Hirschhorn R, Jordan C, Nugent R. Prophylactic intravenous immunoglobulin in HIV-infected children with CD4+ counts of 0.20 × 10(9)/L or more: effect on viral, opportunistic, and bacterial infections. The National Institute of Child Health and Human Development Intravenous Immunoglobulin Clinical Trial Study Group. JAMA 268:483–488, 1992.

Mofenson LM, Bethel J, Moye JJ, Flyer P, Nugent R. Effect of intravenous immunoglobulin (IVIG) on CD4+ lymphocyte decline in HIV-infected children in a clinical trial of IVIG infection prophylaxis: The National Institute of Child Health and Human Development Intravenous Immunoglobulin Clinical Trial Study Group. J AIDS 6:1103–1113, 1993.

Molina JM, Scadden DT, Sakaguchi M, Fuller B, Woon A, Groopman JE. Lack of evidence for infection of or effect on growth of hematopoietic progenitor cells after in vivo or in vitro exposure to human immunodeficiency virus. Blood 76:2476–2482, 1990.

Montefiori DC, Lefkowitz LJ, Keller RE, Holmberg V, Sandstrom E, Phair JP. Absence of a clinical correlation for complement-mediated, infection-enhancing antibodies in plasma or sera from HIV-1-infected individuals: Multicenter AIDS Cohort Study Group. AIDS 5:513–517, 1991.

Mosca J, Bednarik D, Raj N, Rosen C, Sodroski J, Haseltine W, Pitha P. Herpes simplex virus type-1 can reactivate transcription of latent human immunodeficiency virus. Nature 325:67–70, 1987.

Mueller BU, Butler KM, Husson RN, Pizzo PA. Pneumocystis carinii pneumonia despite prophylaxis in children with human immunodeficiency virus infection. J Pediatr 119:992–994, 1991.

Mueller BU, Butler KM, Feuerstein IM, Higham MC, Husson RN, Manjunath K, Montrella KA, Pizzo PA. Smooth muscle tumors in children with human immunodeficiency virus infection. Pediatrics 90:460–463, 1992a.

Mueller BU, Jacobsen F, Butler KM, Husson RN, Lewis LL, Pizzo PA. Combination treatment with azidothymidine and granulocyte colony-stimulating factor in children with human immunodeficiency virus infection. J Pediatr 121:797–802, 1992b.

Mulder J, McKinney N, Christopherson C, Sninsky J, Greenfield L, Kwok S. Rapid and simple PCR assay for quantitation of human immunodeficiency virus type 1 RNA in plasma: application to acute retroviral infection. J Clin Microbiol 32:292–300, 1994.

Mulder-Kampinga G, Kuiken C, Dekker J, Scherpbier H, Boer K, Goudsmit J. Genomic human immunodeficiency virus type 1 RNA variation in mother and child following intra-uterine virus transmission. J Gen Virol 74:1747–1756, 1993.

Mundy D, Schinazi R, Gerber A, Nahmias A, Randall HJ. Human immunodeficiency virus from amniotic fluid. Lancet 2:459–460, 1987.

Murphy WJ, Durum SK, Longo DL. Human growth hormone promotes engraftment of murine or human T cells in severe combined immunodeficient mice. Proc Natl Acad Sci U S A 89:4481–4485, 1992.

National Commission on AIDS. AIDS: An Expanding Tragedy. Washington, DC, National Commission on AIDS, 1993.

National Institutes of Health/University of California Expert Panel. Consensus statement on the use of corticosteroids as adjunctive therapy for Pneumocystis pneumonia in the acquired immunodeficiency syndrome. N Engl J Med 323:1500–1504, 1990.

Nesheim S, Lee F, Sawyer M, Jones D, Lindsay M, Slade B, Shaffer N, Holmes R, Ashby R, Grimes V. Diagnosis of human immunodeficiency virus infection by enzyme-linked immunospot assays in a prospectively followed cohort of infants of human immunodeficiency virus-seropositive women. Pediatr Infect Dis J 11:635–639, 1992.

Nightingale SD, Cameron DW, Gordin FM, Sullam PM, Cohn DL, Chaisson RE, Eron LJ, Sparti PD, Bihari B, Kaufman DL. Two controlled trials of rifabutin prophylaxis against Mycobacterium avium complex infection in AIDS. N Engl J Med 329:828–833, 1993.

Nixon DF, Broliden K, Ogg G, Broliden PA. Cellular and humoral antigenic epitopes in HIV and SIV (editorial). Immunology 76:515–534, 1992.

Nordmann P, Francois B, Menozzi FD, Commare MC, Barois A. Whooping cough associated with Bordatella parapertussis in a human immunodeficiency virus-infected child. Pediatr Infect Dis J 11:248, 1992.

Nottet HS, deGraff L, de Vas NM, Bakker LJ, van Strijp JA, Visser MR, Verhoef J. Phagocytic function of monocyte-derived macrophages is not affected by human immunodeficiency virus type 1 infection. J Infect Dis 168:84–91, 1993.

Ogino MT, Dankner WM, Spector SA. Development and significance of zidovudine resistance in children infected with human immunodeficiency virus. J Pediatr 123:1–8, 1993.

Ognibene FP, Gill VJ, Pizzo PA, Kovacs JA, Godwin C, Suffredini AF, Shelhamer JH, Parrillo JE, Masur H. Induced sputum to diagnose Pneumocystis carinii pneumonia in immunosuppressed pediatric patients. J Pediatr 115:430–433, 1989.

Ohlsson-Wilhelm B, Cory J, Kessler H, Eyster M, Rapp F, Landay A. Circulating human immunodeficiency virus (HIV) p24 antigen-positive lymphocytes: a flow cytometric measure of HIV infection. J Infect Dis 162:1018–1024, 1990.

Osborn L, Kunkel S, Nabel G. Tumor necrosis factor alpha and interleukin 1 stimulate the human immunodeficiency virus enhancer by activation of the nuclear factor kappa B. Proc Natl Acad Sci U S A 86:2336–2340, 1989.

Pahwa S, Biron K, Lim W, Swenson P, Kaplan MH, Sadick N, Pahwa R. Continuous varicella-zoster infection associated with acyclovir resistance in a child with AIDS. JAMA 260:2879–2882, 1988.

Pahwa S, Chirmule N, Leombruno C, Lim W, Harper R, Bhalla R, Pahwa R, Nelson R, Good R. *In vitro* synthesis of human immunodeficiency virus-specific antibodies in peripheral blood lymphocytes of infants. Proc Natl Acad Sci U S A 86:7532–7536, 1989.

Pantaleo G, Graziosi C, Demarest J, Butini L, Montroni M, Fox C, Orenstein J, Kotler D, Fauci A. HIV infection is active and progressive in lymphoid tissue during the clinically latent stage of disease. Nature 362:292–293, 1993a.

Pantaleo G, Graziosi C, Fauci A. The immunopathogenesis of human immunodeficiency virus infection. N Engl J Med 328:327–335, 1993b.

Papaevangelou V, Moore T, Nagaraj V, Krasinski K, Borkowsky W. Lack of predictive value of maternal human immunodeficiency virus p24 antigen for transmission of infection to their children. Pediatr Infect Dis J 11:851–855, 1992.

Pape JW, Jean SS, Ho JL, Hafner A, Johnson WJ. Effect of isoniazid prophylaxis on incidence of active tuberculosis and progression of HIV infection. Lancet 342:268–272, 1993.

Park YD, Belman AL, Kim T-S, Kure K, Llena JF, Lantos G, Bernstein G, Dickson DW. Stroke in pediatric acquired immunodeficiency syndrome. Ann Neurol 28:303–311, 1990.

Parmentier L, Boucary D, Salmon D. Pure red cell aplasia in an HIV-infected patient. AIDS 6:234–235, 1992.

Patterson BK, Till M, Otto P, Goolsby C, Furtado MR, McBride LJ, Wolinsky SM. Detection of HIV-1 DNA and messenger RNA in individual cells by PCR-driven in situ hybridization and flow cytometry. Science 260:976–979, 1993.

Penn I. Tumors of the immunocompromised patient. Annu Rev Med 39:63–73, 1988.

Petersen BH, Rapaport R, Henry DP, Huseman C, Moore WV. Effect of treatment with biosynthetic human growth hormone (GH) on peripheral blood lymphocyte populations and function in growth hormone-deficient children. J Clin Endocrinol Metab 70:1756–1760, 1990.

Phillips RE, Rowland JS, Nixon DF, Gotch FM, Edwards JP, Ogunlesi AO, Elvin JG, Rothbard JA, Bangham CR, Rizza CR, McMichael AJ. Human immunodeficiency virus genetic variation that can escape cytotoxic T cell recognition. Nature 354:453–459, 1991.

Piatak M, Luk K-C, Williams B, Lifson J. Quantitative competitive polymerase chain reaction for accurate quantitation of HIV DNA and RNA species. BioTechniques 14:70–80, 1993a.

Piatak MJ, Saag MS, Yang LC, Clark SJ, Kappes JC, Luk KC, Hahn BH, Shaw GM, Lifson JD. High levels of HIV-1 in plasma during all stages of infection determined by competitive PCR. Science 259:1749–1754, 1993b.

Pickering L, Cleary K. Problems of the digestive tract. In Pizzo PA, Wilfert CM, eds. Pediatric AIDS. Baltimore, Williams & Wilkins, 1991, pp. 384–397.

Pizzo PA, Eddy J, Falloon J, Balis FM, Murphy RF, Moss H, Wolters P, Brouwers P, Jarosinski P, Rubin M, Broder S, Yarchoan R, Brunetti A, Maha M, Nusinoff-Lehrman S, Poplack DG. Effect of continuous intravenous infusion of zidovudine (AZT) in children with symptomatic HIV infection. N Engl J Med 319:889–896, 1988.

Pizzo PA, Butler K, Balis F, Brouwers E, Hawkins M, Eddy J, Einloth M, Falloon J, Husson R, Jarosinski P, Meer J, Moss H, Poplack DG, Santacroce S, Wiener L, Wolters P. Dideoxycytidine alone and in an alternating schedule with zidovudine in children with symptomatic human immunodeficiency virus infection. J Pediatr 117:799–808, 1990.

Plaeger-Marshall S, Hausner MA, Isacescu V, Giorgi JV. CD8 T-cell-mediated inhibition of HIV replication in HIV infected adults and children. AIDS Res Hum Retroviruses 8:1375–1376, 1992.

Plaeger-Marshall S, Hultin P, Bertolli J, O'Rourke S, Kobayashi R, Kobayashi AL, Giorgi JV, Bryson Y, Stiehm ER. Activation and differentiation antigens on T cells of healthy, at-risk, and HIV-infected children. J AIDS 6:984–993, 1993.

Pluda JM, Yarchoan R, Jaffe ES, Feuerstein IM, Solomon D, Steinberg SM, Wyvill KM, Raubitschek A, Katz D, Broder S. Development of non-Hodgkin lymphoma in a cohort of patients with severe human immunodeficiency virus (HIV) infection on long-term antiretroviral therapy. Ann Intern Med 113:276–282, 1990a.

Pluda JM, Yarchoan R, Smith PD, McAtee N, Shay LE, Oette D, Maha M, Wahl SM, Myers CE, Broder S. Subcutaneous recombinant granulocyte-macrophage colony-stimulating factor used as a single agent and in an alternating regimen with azidothymidine in leuko-

penic patients with severe human immunodeficiency virus infection. Blood 76:463–472, 1990b.

Plummer FA, Fowke K, Nagelkerke NJ, Simonsen JN, Bwayo J, Ngugi E. Evidence of resistance to HIV among continuously exposed prostitutes in Nairobi, Kenya. Int Conf AIDS 9:a07–3, 1993.

Pomerantz RJ, de la Monte S, Donegan SP, Rota TR, Vogt MW, Craven DE, Hirsch MS. Human immunodeficiency virus (HIV) infection of the uterine cervix. Ann Intern Med 108:321–327, 1988.

Pruksananonda P, Hall CB, Insel RA, McIntyre K, Pellett PE, Long CE, Schnabel KC, Pincus PH, Stamey FR, Dambaugh TR, Stewart JA. Primary human herpesvirus 6 infection in young children. N Engl J Med 326:1445–1450, 1992.

Quinn T. Population migration and the spread of types 1 and 2 human immunodeficiency viruses. Proc Natl Acad Sci U S A 91:2407–2414, 1994.

Raszka WJ, Meyer GA, Waecker NJ, Ascher DP, Moriarty RA, Fischer GW, Robb ML. Variability of serial absolute and percent CD4+ lymphocyte counts in healthy children born to human immunodeficiency virus 1–infected parents. Pediatr Infect Dis J 13:70–71, 1994.

Reichman RC, Tejani N, Lambert JL, Strussenberg J, Bonnez W, Blumberg B, Epstein L, Dolin R. Didanosine (ddI) and zidovudine (ZDV) susceptibilities of human immunodeficiency virus (HIV) isolates from long-term recipients of ddI. Antiviral Res 20:267–277, 1993.

Remick S, Follansbee S, Olson R, Pollard R, Reiter W, Salgo M. Safety and tolerance of zalcitabine (ddC, HIVID) in a double-blind, comparative trial (ACTG 114; N3300). Int Conf AIDS 9:b26–2115, 1993.

Richardson C, Choppin P. Oligopeptides that specifically inhibit membrane fusion by paramyxoviruses: studies on the site of action. Virology 131:518–532, 1983.

Richman DD. Loss of nevirapine activity associated with the emergence of resistance in clinical trials. The ACTG 164/168 Study Team. Int Conf AIDS 8:3576, 1992.

Richman D. HIV drug resistance. Annu Rev Pharmacol Toxicol 32:149–164, 1993.

Richman DD, Grimes JM, Lagakos SW. Effect of stage of disease and drug dose on zidovudine susceptibilities of isolates of human immunodeficiency virus. J AIDS 3:743–746, 1990.

Rigaud M, Leibovitz E, Sin Quee C, Kaul A, Nardi M, Pollack H, Lawrence R, DiJohn D, Krasinski K, Karpatkin M, Borkowsky W. Thrombocytopenia in children infected with human immunodeficiency virus: long-term follow-up and therapeutic considerations. J AIDS 5:450–455, 1992.

Rinaldo C, Kingsley L, Neumann J, Reed D, Gupta P, Lyter D. Association of human immunodeficiency virus (HIV) p24 antigenemia with decrease in CD4+ lymphocytes and onset of AIDS during the early phase of HIV infection. J Clin Microbiol 27:880–884, 1989.

Robert-Guroff M, Roilides E, Muldoon R, Venzon D, Husson R, Marshall D, Gallo RC, Pizzo PA. Human immunodeficiency virus (HIV) type 1 strain MN neutralizing antibody in HIV-infected children: correlation with clinical status and prognostic value. J Infect Dis 167:538–546, 1993.

Roberts NA, Martin JA, Kinchington D, Broadhurst AV, Craig JC, Duncan IB, Galpin SA, Handa BK, Kay J, Krohn A. Rational design of peptide-based HIV proteinase inhibitors. Science 248:358–361, 1990.

Robinson WJ, Montefiori DC, Mitchell WM. Antibody-dependent enhancement of human immunodeficiency virus type 1 infection. Lancet 1:790–794, 1988.

Roederer M, Staal FJT, Raju PA, Ela SW, Herzenberg LA, Herzenberg LA. Cytokine-stimulated human immunodeficiency virus replication is inhibited by N-acetyl-L-cysteine. Proc Natl Acad Sci U S A 87:4884–4888, 1990.

Rogers M, Ou C-Y, Kilbourne B, Schochetman G. Advances and problems in the diagnosis of human immunodeficiency virus infection in infants. Pediatr Infect Dis J 10:523–531, 1991.

Rogers M, White C, Sanders R, Schable C, Ksell T, Wasserman R, Bellanti J, Peters S, Wray B. Lack of transmission of human immunodeficiency virus from infected children to their household contacts. Pediatrics 85:210–214, 1990.

Roilides E, Mertins S, Eddy J, Walsh TJ, Pizzo PA, Rubin M. Impairment of neutrophil chemotactic and bactericidal function in children infected with human immunodeficiency virus type 1 and partial reversal after in vitro exposure to granulocyte-macrophage colony-stimulating factor. J Pediatr 117:531–540, 1990.

Roilides E, Clerici M, DePalma L, Rubin M, Pizzo PA, Shearer GM. T helper cell responses in children infected with human immunodeficiency virus type 1. J Pediatr 118:724–730, 1991a.

Roilides E, Marshall D, Venzon D, Butler K, Husson R, Pizzo PA. Bacterial infections in human immunodeficiency virus type 1–infected children: the impact of central venous catheters and antiretroviral agents. Pediatr Infect Dis J 10:813–819, 1991b.

Roilides E, Butler KM, Husson RN, Mueller BU, Lewis LL, Pizzo PA. *Pseudomonas* infections in children with human immunodeficiency virus infection. Pediatr Infect Dis J 11:547–553, 1992.

Rook AH, Masur H, Lane HC, Frederick W, Kasahara T, Macher AM, Djeu JY, Manischewitz JF, Jackson L, Fauci AS, Quinnan GJ. Interleukin-2 enhances the depressed natural killer and cytomegalovirus-specific cytotoxic activities of lymphocytes from patients with the acquired immune deficiency syndrome. J Clin Invest 72:398–403, 1983.

Rossi P, Moschese V, Broliden PA, Fundaro C, Quinti I, Plebani A, Giaquinto C, Tovo PA, Ljunggren K, Rosen J. Presence of maternal antibodies to human immunodeficiency virus 1 envelope glycoprotein gp120 epitopes correlates with the uninfected status of children born to seropositive mothers. Proc Natl Acad Sci U S A 86:8055–8058, 1989.

Rowland-Jones S, Nixon DF, Aldhous MC, Gotch F, Ariyoshi K, Hallam N, Kroll JS, Froebel K, McMichael A. HIV-specific cytotoxic T-cell activity in an HIV-exposed but uninfected infant. Lancet 341:860–861, 1993.

Rubinstein A, Morecki R, Silverman B, Charytan M, Krieger BZ, Andiman W, Ziprkowski MN, Goldman H. Pulmonary disease in children with acquired immune deficiency syndrome and AIDS-related complex. J Pediatr 108:498–503, 1986.

Ruff AJ, Halsey NA, Coberly J, Boulos R. Breast-feeding and maternal-infant transmission of human immunodeficiency virus type 1. J Pediatr 121:325–329, 1992.

Ryder RW, Nsa W, Hassig SE, Behets F, Rayfield M, Ekungola B, Nelson AM, Mulenda U, Francis H, Mwandagalirwa K, Davachi F, Rogers M, Nzilambi N, Greenberg A, Mann J, Quinn TC, Piot P, Curran JW. Perinatal transmission of the human immunodeficiency virus type 1 to infants of seropositive women in Zaire. N Engl J Med 320:1637–1642, 1989.

Ryder RW, Manzila T, Baende E, Kabagabo U, Behets F, Batter V, Paquot E, Binyingo E, Heyward WL. Evidence from Zaire that breast-feeding by HIV-1-seropositive mothers is not a major route for perinatal HIV-1 transmission but does decrease morbidity. AIDS 5:709–714, 1991.

Saag M. What to do when zidovudine fails. N Engl J Med 330:706–707, 1994.

Safrit J, Cao Y, Andrews C, Ho D, Koup R. Role of cytotoxic T lymphocytes in acute HIV-1 infection. Presented at the International Conference on AIDS, Berlin, June 6–11, 1993.

Sahmoud T, Laurian Y, Gazengel C, Sultan Y, Gautreau C, Costagliola D. Progression to AIDS in French haemophiliacs: association with HLA-B35. AIDS 7:497–500, 1993.

Sánde MA, Carpenter CC, Cobbs CG, Holmes KK, Sanford JP. Antiretroviral therapy for adult HIV-infected patients. Recommendations from a state-of-the-art conference. National Institute of Allergy and Infectious Diseases State-of-the-Art Panel on Anti-Retroviral Therapy for Adult HIV-Infected Patients. JAMA 270:2583–2589, 1993.

Sato H, Ornstein J, Dimitrov D, Martin M. Cell-to-cell spread of HIV-1 occurs within minutes and may not involve the participation of virus particles. Virology 186:712–724, 1992.

Scadden DT, Zon LI, Groopman JE. Pathophysiology and management of HIV-associated hematologic disorders. Blood 74:1455–1463, 1989.

Scadden DT, Zeira M, Woon A, Wang Z, Schieve L, Ikeuchi K, Lim B, Groopman JE. Human immunodeficiency virus infection of human bone marrow stromal fibroblasts. Blood 76:317–322, 1990.

Scarlatti G, Leitner T, Hodara V, Halapi E, Rossi P, Albert J, Fenyo E. Neutralizing antibodies and viral characteristics in mother-to-child transmission of HIV-1. AIDS 7:S45–S48, 1993.

Scott GB, Fischl MA, Klimas N, Fletcher MA, Dickinson GM, Levine RS, Parks WP. Mothers of infants with the acquired immunodeficiency syndrome. Evidence for both symptomatic and asymptomatic carriers. JAMA 253:363–366, 1985.

Scott GB, Hutto C, Makuch RW, Mastrucci MT, O'Connor T, Mitchell CD, Trapido EJ, Parks WP. Survival in children with perinatally acquired human immunodeficiency virus type 1 infection. N Engl J Med 321:1791–1796, 1989.

Selik R, Chu S, Buehler J. HIV infection as leading cause of death among young adults in US cities and States. JAMA 269:2991–2994, 1993.

Shadduck PP, Weinberg JB, Haney AF, Bartlett JA, Langlois AJ, Bolognesi DP, Matthews TJ. Lack of enhancing effect of human anti-human immunodeficiency virus type 1 (HIV-1) antibody on HIV-1 infection of human blood monocytes and peritoneal macrophages. J Virol 65:4309–4316, 1991.

Sharer LR, Dowling PC, Michaels J, Cook SD, Menonna J, Blumberg BM, Epstein LG. Spinal cord disease in children with HIV-1 infection: a combined molecular biological and neuropathological study. Neuropathol Appl Neurobiol 16:317–331, 1990.

Shaunak S, Albright RE, Klotman ME, Henry SC, Bartlett JA, Hamilton JD. Amplification of HIV-1 provirus from cerebrospinal fluid and its correlation with neurologic disease. J Infect Dis 161:1068–1072, 1990.

Shearer G, Clerici M. Abnormalities of immune regulation in human immunodeficiency virus infection. Pediatr Res 33:S71–S74, 1993.

Siekevitz M, Josephs S, Dukovich M, Peffer N, Wong-Staal F, Greene W. Activation of the HIV-1 LTR by T cell mitogens and the transactivator protein of HTLV-1. Science 238:1575–1578, 1987.

Siller L, Martin N, Kostuchenko P, Beckett L, Rautonen J, Cheng S, Wara DW. Serum levels of soluble CD8, neopterin, beta 2-microglobulin and p24 antigen as indicators of disease progression in children with AIDS on zidovudine therapy. AIDS 7:369–373, 1993.

Silliman CC, Tedder D, Ogle JW, Simon J, Kleinschmidt D, Masters B, Manco JM, Levin MJ. Unsuspected varicella-zoster virus encephalitis in a child with acquired immunodeficiency syndrome. J Pediatr 123:418–422, 1993.

Simonds R, Chanock S. Medical issues related to caring for human immunodeficiency virus-infected children in and out of the home. Pediatr Infect Dis J 12:845–852, 1993.

Sirianni MC, Soddu S, Malorni W, Arancia G, Aiuti F. Mechanism of defective natural killer cell activity in patients with AIDS is associated with defective distribution of tubulin [see erratum in J Immunol 141:1709, 1988]. J Immunol 140:2565–2568, 1988.

Smith PD, Quinn TC, Strober W, Janoff EN, Masur H. Gastrointestinal infections in AIDS. Ann Intern Med 116:63–77, 1992.

Smith PD, Eisner MS, Manischewitz JF, Gill VJ, Masur H, Fox CF. Esophageal disease in AIDS is associated with pathologic processes rather than mucosal human immunodeficiency virus type 1. J Infect Dis 167:547–552, 1993.

Sodroski J, Goh W, Rosen C, Campbell K, Haseltine W. Role of the HTLV-III/LAV envelope in syncytium formation and cytopathicity. Nature 322:470–474, 1986.

Spector S, Gelber RD, Connor EM, Wara D, McGrath N, Balsley JS, Pediatric AIDS Clinical Trials Group, NICHD Pediatric HIV Centers. Results of a Double-Blind Placebo-Controlled Trial to Evaluate Intravenous Gammaglobulin in Children With Symptomatic HIV Infection Receiving Zidovudine: ACTG 051. Washington, DC, American Society of Pediatrics/Society for Pediatric Research, 1993.

Sprecher S, Soumenkoff G, Puissant F, Degueldre M. Vertical transmission of HIV in 15-week fetus. Lancet 2:288, 1986.

Spruance S, Pavia A, Peterson D, Berry A, Pollard R, Patterson T, Frank I, Remick S, Thompson M, MacArthur R, Morey G, Ramirez-Ronda C, Bernstein B, Sweet D, Crane L, Peterson E, Pachucki C, Green S, Brand J, Rios A, Dunkle L, Smaldone L. Didanosine compared with continuation of zidovudine in HIV-infected patients with signs of clinical deterioration while receiving zidovudine. Ann Intern Med 120:360–368, 1994.

St. Clair MH, Martin JL, Tudor-Williams G, Bach MC, Vavro CL, King DM, Kellam P, Kemp SD, Larder BA. Resistance to ddI and sensitivity to AZT induced by a mutation in HIV-1 reverse transcriptase. Science 253:1557–1559, 1991.

Starke JR, Jacobs RF, Jereb J. Resurgence of tuberculosis in children. J Pediatr 120:839–855, 1992.

Steimer KS, Scandella CJ, Skiles PV, Haigwood NL. Neutralization of divergent HIV-1 isolates by conformation-dependent human antibodies to Gp120. Science 254:105–108, 1991.

Stein B, Gowda S, Lifson J, Penhallow R, Bensch K, Engleman E. pH-independent HIV entry into CD4-positive cells via virus envelope fusion to the plasma membrane. Cell 49:659–668, 1987.

Stevenson M, Stanwick T, Dempsey M, Lamonica C. HIV-1 replication is controlled at the level of T cell activation and proviral integration. EMBO J 9:1551–1560, 1990.

Stevenson M, Bukrinsky M, Haggerty S. HIV-1 replication and potential targets for intervention. AIDS Res Hum Retroviruses 8:107–117, 1992.

Stiehm ER, Vink P. Transmission of human immunodeficiency virus infection by breast-feeding. J Pediatr 118:410–412, 1991.

Stiehm ER, Bryson YJ, Frenkel LM, Szelc CM, Gillespie S, Williams ME, Watkins ME. Prednisone improves human immunodeficiency virus encephalopathy in children. Pediatr Infect Dis J 11:49–50, 1992.

Szkaradkiewicz A. Phagocytosis and microbicidal capacity of human monocytes in the course of HIV infection. Immunol Lett 33:145–150, 1992.

Takeda A, Tuazon C, Ennis F. Antibody-enhanced infection by HIV-1 via Fc receptor-mediated entry. Science 242:580–583, 1988.

Takeuchi Y, Nagumo T, Hoshino H. Low fidelity of cell-free DNA synthesis by reverse transcriptase of human immunodeficiency virus. J Virol 62:3900–3902, 1988.

Tanese N, Telesnitsky A, Goff S. Abortive reverse transcription by mutants of moloney murine leukemia virus deficient in the reverse transcriptase-associated RNase H function. J Virol 65:4387–4397, 1991.

Tersmette M, De Goede R, Al B, Winkel I, Gruters R, Cuypers H, Huisman H, Miedema F. Differential syncytium-inducing capacity of human immunodeficiency virus isolates: frequent detection of syncytium-inducing isolates in patients with acquired immunodeficiency syndrome (AIDS) and AIDS-related complex. J Virol 62:2026–2032, 1988.

Thiry L, Sprecher G, Goldberger S, Jonckheer T, Levy J, Van de Perre P, Henrivaux P, Le Clerc J, Clumeck N. Isolation of AIDS virus from cell-free breast milk of three healthy virus carriers (letter). Lancet 2:891–892, 1985.

Tibaldi C, Tovo PA, Ziarati N, Palomba E, Salassa B, Sciandra M, D'Ambrosio R, Ponti A, Sinicco A. Asymptomatic women at high risk of vertical HIV-1 transmission to their fetuses. Br J Obstet Gynaecol 100:334–337, 1993.

Tindall B, Cooper D. Primary HIV infection: host responses and intervention strategies. AIDS 5:1–14, 1991.

Ting SF, Glader BE, Prober CG. Cryptococcus infection in a nine-year-old child with hemophilia and the acquired immunodeficiency syndrome. Pediatr Infect Dis J 10:76–77, 1991.

Tisdale M, Kemp SD, Parry NR, Larder BA. Rapid in vitro selection of human immunodeficiency virus type 1 resistant to 3′-thiacytidine inhibitors due to a mutation in the YMDD region of reverse transcriptase. Proc Natl Acad Sci U S A 90:5653–5656, 1993.

Toggas S, Masliah E, Rockenstein E, Rall G, Abraham C, Mucke L. Central nervous system damage produced by expression of the HIV-1 coat protein gp120 in transgenic mice. Nature 367:188–193, 1994.

Torre D, Sampietro C, Ferraro G, Zeroli C, Speranza F. Transmission of HIV-1 infection via sports injury. Lancet 335:1105, 1990.

Tovo PA, Palomba E, Gabiano C, Galli L, de Martino M. Human immunodeficiency virus type 1 (HIV-1) seroconversion during pregnancy does not increase the risk of perinatal transmission. Br J Obstet Gynaecol 98:940–942, 1991.

Tovo PA, De Martino M, Gabiano C, Cappello N, D'Elia R, Loy A, Plebani A, Zuccotti GV, Dallacasa P, Ferraris G, Caselli D, Fundaro C, D'Argenio P, Galli L, Principi N, Stegagno M, Ruga E, Palomba E. Prognostic factors and survival in children with perinatal HIV-1 infection. Lancet 339:1249–1253, 1992.

Trono D. Partial reverse transcripts in virions from human immunodeficiency and murine leukemia viruses. J Virol 66:4893–4900, 1992.

Tudor-Williams G. Early diagnosis of vertically acquired HIV-1 infection. AIDS 5:103–105, 1991.

Tudor-Williams G, St. Clair MH, McKinney RE, Maha M, Walter E, Santacroce S, Mintz M, O'Donnell K, Rudoll T, Vavro CL, Connor EM, Wilfert CM. HIV-1 sensitivity to zidovudine and clinical outcome in children. Lancet 339:15–19, 1992.

Tudor-Williams G, Mueller B, Stocker V, Venzon D, Marshall D, Brouwers P, Butler K, Pizzo P. Serum p24 antigen levels and disease progression in HIV-1 infected children (abstract). J Cell Biochem S17E:100, 1993.

Uittenbogaart C, Anisman D, Schmid I, Hays E, Aldrovandi G, Zack J. Role of HIV infection of thymocytes in the pathogenesis of pediatric AIDS (abstract). J Cell Biochem S17E: 94, 1993.

Underwood T, Frye C. Drug-induced pancreatitis. Clin Pharm 12:440–448, 1993.

Vago L, Antonacci M, Cristina S, Parravicini C, Lazzarin A, Moroni M, Negri C, Uberti-Foppa C, Musicco M, Costanzi G. Morphogenesis, evolution and prognostic significance of lymphatic tissue lesions in HIV infection. Appl Pathol 7:298–309, 1989.

Van De Perre P, Simonon A, Msellati P, Hitimana D-G, Vaira D, Bazubagira A, Van Goethem C, Stevens AM, Karita E, Sondag-Thuli D, Dabis F, Lepage P. Postnatal transmission of human immunodeficiency virus type 1 from mother to infant. N Engl J Med 325:593–598, 1991.

Varmus H, Swanstrom R. Replication of Retroviruses. RNA Tumor Viruses. Cold Spring Harbor, NY, Cold Spring Harbor Laboratory, 1991, pp. 369–512.

Viganó A, Principi N, Villa ML, Riva C, Crupi L, Trabattoni D, Shearer GM, Clereci M. Immunologic characterization of children vertically infected with human immunodeficiency virus, with slow or rapid disease progression. J Pediatr 126:368–374, 1995.

Vittecoq D, Chevret S, Morandjoubert L, Heshmati F, Audat F, Bary M, Dusautoir T, Bismuth A, Viard JP, Barré-Sinoussi B, Bach JF, and Lefrère JJ. Passive Immunotherapy in AIDS—a double-blind randomized study based on transfusions of plasma rich in anti-human immunodeficiency virus I antibodies vs. transfusions of seronegative plasma. Proc Natl Acad Sci U S A 92:1195–1199, 1995.

Vogt MW, Witt DJ, Craven DE, Byington R, Crawford DF, Hutchinson MS, Schooley RT, Hirsch MS. Isolation patterns of the human immunodeficiency virus from cervical secretions during the menstrual cycle of women at risk for the acquired immunodeficiency syndrome. Ann Intern Med 106:380–382, 1987.

Volberding PA, Lagakos SW, Koch MA, Pettinelli C, Myers MW, Booth DK, Balfour HH, Reichman RC, Bartlett JA, Hirsch HH, Murphy RL, Hardy D, Soeiro R, Fischl MA, Bartlett JG, Merigan TC, Hyslop NE, Richman DD, Valentine FT, Corey L. Zidovudine in asymptomatic human immunodeficiency virus infection. N Engl J Med 322:941–949, 1990.

Wahn V, Kramer H, Voit T, Bruster H, Scrampical B, Scheid A. Horizontal transmission of HIV infection between two siblings. Lancet 2:694, 1986.

Walker B, Chakrabarti S, Moss B, Paradis T, Flynn T, Durno A, Blumberg R, Kaplan J, Hirsch M, Schooley R. HIV-specific cytotoxic T lymphocytes in seropositive individuals. Nature 328:345–348, 1987.

Walker CM, Thomson HG, Hsueh FC, Erickson AL, Pan LZ, Levy JA. CD8+ T cells from HIV-1-infected individuals inhibit acute infection by human and primate immunodeficiency viruses. Cell Immunol 137:420–428, 1991.

Walker R, Lane H, Boenning C, Polis M, Kovacs J, Falloon J, Davey R, Masur H, Fauci A. The safety, pharmacokinetics, and antiviral activity of n-acetylcysteine in HIV-infected individuals. Am Rev Respir Dis (Suppl.) 147:A1004, 1993.

Walsh T, Gonzalez C, Roilides E, Mueller B, Ali N, Lewis L, Whitcomb T, Marshall D, Pizzo P. Fungemia complicating pediatric HIV infection. Presented at the First National Conference on Retroviruses and Related Infections, American Society of Microbiology, Washington, DC, 1993.

Walter EB, McKinney RE, Lane BA, Weinhold KJ, Wilfert CM. Interpretation of Western blots of specimens from children infected with human immunodeficiency virus type 1: implications for prognosis and diagnosis. J Pediatr 117:255–258, 1990.

Walter E, Weinhold K, Wilfert C. Enhanced p24 antigen detection in sera from human immunodeficiency virus-infected children. Pediatr Infect Dis J 12:94–96, 1993.

Watts DH, Brown ZA, Tartaglione T, Burchett SK, Opheim K, Coombs R, Corey L. Pharmacokinetic disposition of zidovudine during pregnancy. J Infect Dis 163:226–232, 1991.

Weiss R. How does HIV cause AIDS? Science 260:1273–1279, 1993.

Weiss RA, Clapham PR, Weber JN, Whitby D, Tedder RS, O'Connor T, Chamaret S, Montagnier L. HIV-2 antisera cross-neutralize HIV-1. AIDS 2:95–100, 1988.

Whitcup S, Butler K, Pizzo P, Nussenblatt R. Retinal lesions in children treated with dideoxyinosine. N Engl J Med 326:1226–1227, 1992.

Willey R, Bonifacino J, Potts B, Martin M, Klausner R. Biosynthesis, cleavage, and degradation of the human immunodeficiency virus 1 envelope glyoprotein gp160. Proc Natl Acad Sci U S A 85:9580–9584, 1988.

Williams LM, Cloyd MW. Polymorphic human gene(s) determines differential susceptibility of CD4 lymphocytes to infection by certain HIV-1 isolates. Virology 184:723–728, 1991.

Wolinsky SM, Wike CM, Korber BT, Hutto C, Parks WP, Rosenblum LL, Kunstman KJ, Furtado MR, Munoz JL. Selective transmission of human immunodeficiency virus type-1 variants from mothers to infants. Science 255:1134–1137, 1992.

Wong VK, Gillette SG, Roth MJ, Miles S, Stiehm ER. Plasma immunotherapy in a child with acquired immunodeficiency syndrome. Pediatr Infect Dis J 12:947–951, 1993.

Working Group on Antiretroviral Therapy: National Pediatric HIV Resource Center. Antiretroviral therapy and medical management of the human immunodeficiency virus-infected child. Pediatr Infect Dis J 12:513–522, 1993.

WHO [World Health Organization]. Acquired immunodeficiency syndrome (AIDS): provisional WHO clinical case definition for AIDS. Wkly Epidemiol Rec 61:72–73, 1986.

WHO [World Health Organization]. Consensus statement from the WHO/Unicef consultation on HIV transmission and breast-feeding. Wkly Epidemiol Rec 67:177–179, 1992.

Yagita H, Nakata M, Kawasaki A, Shinkai Y, Okumura K. Role of perforin in lymphocyte-mediated cytolysis. Adv Immunol 51:215–242, 1992.

Yamashita N, Clement LT. Phenotypic characterization of the post-thymic differentiation of human alloantigen-specific CD8+ cytotoxic T lymphocytes. J Immunol 143:1518–1523, 1989.

Yarchoan R, Mitsuya H, Myers CE, Broder S. Clinical pharmacology of 3'-azido-2',3'-dideoxythymidine (zidovudine) and related dideoxynucleosides [see erratum in N Engl J Med 322:280, 1990]. N Engl J Med 321:726–738, 1989.

Yarchoan R, Pluda JM, Perno CF, Mitsuya H, Broder S. Anti-retroviral therapy of human immunodeficiency virus infection: current strategies and challenges for the future [see erratum in Blood 78:3330, 1991]. Blood 78:859–884, 1991.

Yarchoan R, Lietzau JA, Nguyen BY, Brawley OW, Pluda JM, Saville MW, Wyvill KM, Steinberg SM, Agbaria R, Mitsuya H, Broder S. A randomized pilot study of alternating or simultaneous zidovudine and didanosine therapy in patients with symptomatic human immunodeficiency virus infection. J Infect Dis 169:9–17, 1994.

Yolken RH, Hart W, Oung I, Shiff C, Greenson J, Perman JA. Gastrointestinal dysfunction and disaccharide intolerance in children infected with human immunodeficiency virus. J Pediatr 118:359–363, 1991.

York-Higgins D, Cheng-Mayer C, Bauer D, Levy J, Dina D. Human immunodeficiency virus type 1 cellular host range, replication, and cytopathicity are linked to envelope region of the viral genome. J Virol 64:4016–4020, 1990.

Young KY, Nelson RP. Discordant human immunodeficiency virus infection in dizygotic twins detected by polymerase chain reaction. Pediatr Infect Dis J 9:454–456, 1990.

Zack J, Arrigo S, Weitsman S, Go A, Haislip A, Chen I. HIV-1 entry into quiescent primary lymphocytes: molecular analysis reveals a labile, latent viral structure. Cell 61:213–222, 1990.

Zeichner S, Hirka G, Andrews P, Alwine J. Differentiation-dependent human immunodeficiency virus long terminal repeat regulatory elements active in human teratocarcinoma cells. J Virol 66:2268–2273, 1992.

Ziegler J, Cooper D, Gold J, Johnston R. Postnatal transmission of AIDS-associated retrovirus from mother to infant. Lancet 1:896–898, 1985.

Zinberg J, Chernaik R, Coman E, Rosenblatt R, Brandt LJ. Reversible symptomatic biliary obstruction associated with ceftriaxone pseudolithiasis. Am J Gastroenterol 86:1251–1254, 1991.

Chapter 19

The Secondary Immunodeficiencies

Eric T. Sandberg, Mark W. Kline,
and William T. Shearer

The immunologically intact individual may develop alterations in immune function as a result of exogenous factors such as infections, drugs, malnutrition, surgery, or immaturity. These secondary immunodeficiencies are considerably more common in clinical practice than are the primary immunodeficiencies. Secondary immunodeficiencies can result in abnormalities of humoral immunity (in nephrosis), cellular immunity (in viral infections), phagocytosis (in aplastic anemia), or even opsonic function (in sickle cell disease). The study of these secondary immune defects can provide theoretical insight into normal functions. Furthermore, practical case management of the primary disorder may be strongly influenced by an understanding of the resulting immune dysfunction. Abnormal immune function may be an early clue to a specific diagnosis (e.g., neutropenia in the hypoglycemic neonate with glycogenosis type 1b). Marked hypergammaglobulinemia in an infant may cause one to suspect human immunodeficiency virus (HIV) infection involving both the infant and the mother.

Findings such as recurrent infection, infection with unusual organisms, or poor response to therapy suggest an immune deficit. An overall classification of secondary immunodeficiency is outlined in Table 19–1. These secondary effects may occur in diverse settings, such as hereditary, metabolic, and infectious disease. Iatrogenic causes include chemotherapy, radiation therapy, and surgery. Two of the most common secondary immunodeficiencies, those associated with neonatal immaturity and HIV infection, are covered in Chapters 10 and 18.

HEREDITARY DISEASES

Chromosomal Abnormalities

Down Syndrome

Impaired immune competence of patients with Down syndrome (trisomy 21) is clinically manifested by three major findings: increased susceptibility to infection, a high risk of developing malignancy, and a high frequency of autoantibodies (Ugazio et al., 1990). Early reports emphasized the increased morbidity of Down syndrome patients resulting from respiratory and gastrointestinal infections (Siegel, 1948). The availability of antimicrobials has markedly reduced the risk

Table 19–1. The Secondary Immunodeficiencies

I. *Premature and newborn infant*
II. *Acquired immunodeficiency syndrome*
III. *Hereditary diseases*
   A. Chromosomal abnormalities
   B. Chromosome instability syndromes
   C. Enzyme deficiencies
   D. Hemoglobinopathies
   E. Myotonic dystrophy
   F. Congenital asplenia
   G. Skeletal dysplasias
IV. *Specific organ system dysfunction*
   A. Diabetes mellitus
   B. Protein-losing enteropathy
   C. Nephrotic syndrome
   D. Uremia
V. *Nutritional deficiency*
   A. Protein-calorie malnutrition
   B. Iron deficiency
   C. Vitamin A deficiency
VI. *Immunosuppressive agents*
   A. Radiation
   B. Antibodies
   C. Glucocorticosteroids
   D. Cyclosporine
   E. Cytotoxic drugs
   F. Anti-convulsant drugs
VII. *Infectious diseases*
   A. Bacterial infection
   B. Fungal infection
   C. Viral infection
   D. Parasitic infection
VIII. *Infiltrative and hematologic diseases*
   A. Histiocytosis
   B. Sarcoidosis
   C. Lymphoid malignancy
   D. Leukemia
   E. Hodgkin's disease
   F. Lymphoproliferative disease
   G. Agranulocytosis and aplastic anemia
IX. *Surgery and trauma*
   A. Burns
   B. Splenectomy
   C. Head injury

of early mortality for Down syndrome patients, yet pneumonia and other respiratory diseases continue to be a major cause of death (Oster et al., 1975). One striking finding linked to their predisposition to infection is a high carrier rate of hepatitis B (e.g., HBsAg-positive) (Sutnick et al., 1972; Hollingsworth et al., 1974). Since many of these patients live in institutional settings, it is unclear if this reflects an increased risk of exposure or inefficient biologic processing of the hepatitis B virus. In one study, immunization with hepatitis B vaccine led to expected seroconversion rates and antibody titers (Troisi et al., 1985). Although hepatitis B immunization is advisable, proof of disease protection is lacking. Other studies suggest that trisomic patients have abnormal IgG subclass response (Avanzini et al., 1988) and a poor response to intradermal hepatitis B vaccine (Ahman et al., 1993) (see Chapter 11).

The high risk of malignancy in Down syndrome is most striking for childhood leukemia, including both acute lymphoblastic leukemia (ALL) and acute non-lymphoblastic leukemia (ANLL) (Schuler et al., 1972; Robison and Neglia, 1987). For individuals younger than 3 years old, acute megakaryoblastic leukemia, a

form of ANLL, is as much as 400 times more prevalent in children with Down syndrome as it is in normal children (Iselius et al., 1990). Patients with normal somatic karyotypes who have ALL or ANLL often exhibit an extra copy of chromosome 21 in their leukemic cell lines (Heim and Mitelman, 1987). This information supports the possibility that the susceptibility of Down syndrome patients to leukemia may be a direct result of the extra copy of an unidentified gene locus on chromosome 21 (Rowley, 1981).

The frequent presence of autoantibodies, often antithyroid antibodies, suggests a defect in immune regulation in Down syndrome patients (Burgio et al., 1965; Levo and Green, 1977; Ugazio et al., 1977). Although clinical correlates of these autoantibodies are limited, Cutler and coworkers (1986) showed an increased frequency of hypothyroidism in young children with Down syndrome. The presence of IgA antibodies to gluten has been associated with lower body weight in adults with Down syndrome (Kanavin et al., 1988). The combination of hyperthyroidism, hypoparathyroidism, and alopecia areata offers further support to the association of autoimmunity and Down syndrome (DuVivier and Munro, 1975; Ruch et al., 1985; Blumberg and AvRuskin, 1987).

Humoral immunity in Down syndrome has been extensively studied. Circulating B cell numbers are normal (Reiser et al., 1976). Immunoglobulin levels vary depending on age with low IgG levels in infants and high levels in children older than 5 years (Burgio and Ugazio, 1978). IgM levels are decreased, most prominently after childhood. The data concerning specific antibody responses are diverse. Antibody responses to ϕX174 phage (Lopez et al., 1975), influenza vaccine (Gordon et al., 1971; Philip et al., 1986), and pneumococcal vaccine (Nurmi et al., 1982) are low. Responses to tetanus immunization have been reported to be normal (Hawkes et al., 1978) or low (Griffiths and Sylvester, 1967; Philip et al., 1986). Thus, minor defects in the humoral response of Down syndrome patients occur, but no major defects of the B cell compartment exist.

By contrast, cell-mediated immunity is profoundly abnormal in Down syndrome. A long-standing observation is the high percentage of circulating natural killer (NK) cells (Maccario et al., 1984). NK cells from Down syndrome patients coexpress CD3 and CD8 (Abo et al., 1982), suggesting that these cells may not be synonymous with CD16$^+$ NK cells. However, despite increased numbers of NK cells (Cossarizza et al., 1990; Murphy and Epstein, 1992), NK cell activity (Montagna et al., 1988) (Fig. 19–1) and antibody-dependent cellular cytotoxicity are impaired in Down syndrome (Nair and Schwartz, 1984). Although numbers of circulating total T cells (CD3$^+$) are generally normal, the ratio of CD4$^+$ to CD8$^+$ cells is decreased in Down syndrome (Burgio et al., 1983; Philip et al., 1986). In addition, the proportion of cells expressing the $\alpha\beta$ chains of the T cell receptor is decreased in Down syndrome peripheral blood while the proportion of cells expressing the $\gamma\delta$ chains is increased (Murphy and Epstein, 1992). This suggests the possibility that $\alpha\beta$ T

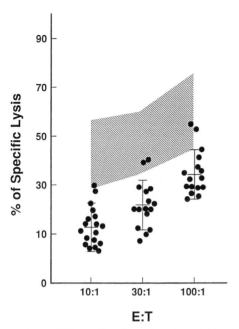

Figure 19–1. Natural killer cell activity of peripheral blood mononuclear cells from 16 subjects with Down syndrome using three different effector-to-target ratios, 10:1, 30:1, and 100:1. Vertical bars represent the mean ± 1 SD of patient samples. The shaded area represents the mean ± 1 SD of the age-matched karyotypically normal controls. (From Montagna D, Maccario R, Ugazio AG, et al. Cell-mediated cytotoxicity in Down syndrome: impairment of allogeneic mixed lymphocyte reaction, NK and NK-like activities. Eur J Pediatr 148:53–57, 1988. Courtesy of Springer-Verlag.)

cells, which are dependent on the thymus for maturation, may not emigrate efficiently from the Down syndrome thymus gland. The additional finding that Down syndrome peripheral blood has a decreased proportion of CD45R[+], CD4[+] naive cells also supports this hypothesis (Murphy and Epstein, 1992).

Studies of lymphocyte proliferative responses have yielded varying results. In vitro responses to phytohemagglutinin (PHA) and tuberculin were normal in some studies (Hayakawa et al., 1968; Fowler et al., 1973; Philip et al., 1986) but diminished in others (Agarwal et al., 1970; Rigas et al., 1970). However, the in vitro proliferation, interleukin (IL)-2 production, and antibody responses to influenza and tetanus antigen have been shown to be decreased in Down syndrome (Philip et al., 1986). Bertotto and colleagues (1987) found that T-cell proliferation to anti-CD3 antibody is diminished. Delayed hypersensitivity responses are reported as normal (Hollingsworth et al., 1974) or decreased (Mellman et al., 1970).

It has been postulated that the immunodeficiency of Down syndrome, particularly the T cell defect, is related to the severe anatomic abnormalities present in the thymus gland (Benda and Strassman, 1965; Levin et al., 1979). Marked depletion of cortical thymocytes, poor corticomedullary demarcation, and enlarged Hassall's corpuscles are present. There is evidence that these anatomic abnormalities in the thymus gland occur as early as 18 weeks of fetal gestation and are accompanied by abnormalities in the spleen (Insoft et

al., 1993, 1994). Alterations in thymocyte subpopulations in patients with Down syndrome suggest abnormal maturation of T cells in the thymus gland (Larocca et al., 1988).

Abnormalities in the expression and response to cytokines and inflammatory adhesion molecules have been implicated in the thymic abnormalities in Down syndrome (Murphy et al., 1992a, 1992b, 1993). In brief, messenger RNA (mRNA) for interferon-γ and tumor necrosis factor (TNF) is overexpressed in Down syndrome thymus glands. Additionally, thymocyte proliferation is more sensitively inhibited by these cytokines than in normal controls. This cytokine dysregulation is accompanied by overexpression of CD18 leukocyte integrins and their ligand, ICAM-1, molecules that are implicated in thymocyte maturation. In light of the role of ICAM-1 in thymocyte depletion (Carlow et al., 1992), these observations may explain the anatomic depletion of cortical thymocytes.

Phagocytic dysfunction is well documented in Down syndrome. Impaired chemotaxis, both of neutrophils and monocytes (Khan et al., 1975; Barroeta et al., 1983), phagocytosis (Rosner et al., 1973), quantitative nitroblue tetrazolium (NBT) dye reduction, and bacterial killing (Kretschmer et al., 1974; Seger et al., 1976) have been reported in children with Down syndrome.

The hypothesis that the extra chromosome 21 in Down syndrome leads to a gene dosage effect causing immunodeficiency has been advanced. Best documented is the finding that the activity of superoxide-dismutase 1 (SOD-1), located on chromosome 21, is 150% of controls (Baeteman et al., 1984). Conversion of leukocyte superoxide, a key component of cell killing, to hydrogen peroxide by excessive SOD-1 might contribute to a susceptibility to catalase-positive bacteria and fungi. The location of CD18 on chromosome 21 may explain an increased expression of CD18 leukocyte integrins in the thymus, as discussed previously. Likewise, the cloning of the interferon-γ response element on chromosome 21 (Soh et al., 1994) suggests that the increased sensitivity of trisomic thymocytes to interferon-γ may be a result of an extra copy of chromosome 21.

Therapeutic options for patients with Down syndrome are limited. As discussed previously, routine immunizations should include hepatitis B vaccine. Dietary supplementation with zinc has often been suggested, but a well-controlled 6-month trial showed no immunologic benefit (Lockitch et al., 1989). The value of thymic hormones or intravenous immunoglobulin is unproven.

ICF Syndrome

The complex of *i*mmunodeficiency, *c*entromeric instability, and *f*acial anomalies has been called the ICF syndrome (Maraschio et al., 1989). This rare autosomal disorder brings patients to medical attention during the first year of life with severe recurrent respiratory infections. Four of 15 reported patients died as a result of severe infections (Smeets et al., 1994). Characterization of the immunodeficiency in this disorder remains incomplete. Serum immunoglobulin levels are generally low, and some patients demonstrate agammaglobulinemia. The number of B cells is usually normal, and T cell numbers may be either reduced or normal. NK cell activity may be impaired (Fasth et al., 1990).

Diagnosis of ICF syndrome requires cytogenetic evaluation of cultured peripheral lymphocytes. Studies reveal structural abnormalities of the heterochromatic regions of chromosomes 1 and 16. Similar findings are seen less frequently with chromosome 9. These changes are rarely found in cells from other tissues, such as fibroblasts or bone marrow cells. ICF is distinct from the chromosome instability syndromes (see below). The chromosomal abnormalities in ICF are limited to specific chromosomal regions, compared with the diverse locations of points of breakage found in the chromosomal instability syndromes. Although both groups of patients exhibit immunodeficiency and autosomal recessive inheritance, patients with ICF syndrome have no hypersensitivity to ionizing radiation, nor do they have an increased incidence of malignancies. The facial anomalies seen in ICF syndrome are characterized by epicanthal folds, hypertelorism, a flat nasal bridge, and macroglossia (Gimelli et al., 1993).

Other Chromosomal Abnormalities

Another striking association of chromosomal abnormality and immunodeficiency occurs with deletions of chromosome 22q11 and DiGeorge anomaly (Driscoll et al., 1992). See Chapter 12. A related phenotype was noted in a child with deletion of 10p that presented with congenital heart disease, hypoparathyroidism, and an imbalance of immunoregulatory T cells (Greenberg et al., 1986). Two other rare secondary immunodeficiencies associated with chromosomal abnormalities include a female patient with a deletion of Xp11-p22 who exhibited humoral and cellular deficits (Nurmi et al., 1981) and a female infant with a deletion of chromosome 5p (*cri-du-chat* syndrome), cardiovascular defects, shortened forearms, and syndactyly of fingers in association with thymic dysplasia and lymphocyte-depleted lymph nodes (Taylor and Josifek, 1981).

Abnormalities of chromosome 18 have been associated with immunoglobulin deficiencies (see Chapter 14). Studies by Feingold and Schwartz (1968) and Finley and associates (1968) reported the first patients with IgA deficiency and a ring-18 chromosome. IgA deficiency may be associated with deletions of the short arm of chromosome 18 (Ruvalcaba and Thuline, 1969). However, patients with ring-18 chromosomes may have normal immunoglobulins (Richards and Hobbs, 1968); ring-18 chromosomes have been associated with an IgM paraproteinemia and normal IgA levels (Jensen et al., 1969). Studies in infants with trisomy 18 as well as in other chromosomal abnormalities suggest disturbances in phagocytosis (Seger et al., 1976).

A common entity, Turner syndrome, (45XO) is associated with a variety of immune abnormalities. An increased incidence of respiratory infections has been noted. Decreases in serum immunoglobulin levels are commonly noted (Jensen et al., 1976; Lorini et al.,

1983). Cases with combined humoral and cell-mediated defects have been reported (Donti et al., 1989; Robson and Potter, 1990).

Chromosome Instability Syndromes

Several syndromes with a predisposition toward chromosomal breakage are associated with an increased risk of malignancy and immunodeficiency (Table 19–2). Cultured cells from these patients are hypersensitive to ionizing radiation and demonstrate a high frequency of chromosomal aberrations. *Ataxia-telangiectasia*, the most common of these disorders, includes prominent defects in cellular and humoral immunity and is discussed in Chapter 12.

Bloom's syndrome is a rare autosomal recessive disorder characterized by growth retardation, sunlight sensitivity, and a strong predisposition to malignancy. These children present during infancy and childhood with respiratory and gastrointestinal infections caused by a variety of microorganisms (Hutteroth et al., 1975). There is an increased risk of chronic lung disease in adults (German and Passarge, 1989). Limited immunologic studies in Bloom's syndrome have disclosed low serum IgG levels (Weemaes et al., 1979), decreased NK activity (Ueno et al., 1985), and impaired lymphocytic proliferative responses to mitogens. Etzioni and colleagues (1989) demonstrated defective regulatory T-cell function for IgG synthesis. Kondo and colleagues (1992) documented an increase in serum IgG levels over time in two patients.

Another chromosomal instability syndrome, *Fanconi's anemia*, also predisposes to infection. In a series of 25 children with Fanconi's anemia, 10 died of confirmed or suspected infections (Rogers et al., 1989). Single-case reports have described selective IgA deficiency (Standen et al., 1989) and impaired T-cell function (Pedersen et al., 1977).

A more recently described chromosomal instability syndrome is the *Nijmegen breakage syndrome*, characterized by microcephaly, mental retardation, *café-au-lait* spots, and immunodeficiency (Weemaes et al., 1981) (see Chapter 12). A defect in the primary and secondary antibody response to vaccination has been noted (Weemaes et al., 1984). Hypogammaglobulinemia and an impaired proliferative response of T cells can be severe in some patients (Taalman et al., 1989). Nijmegen breakage syndrome may have considerable overlap with the less well-defined *Seemanova's syndrome* (Taalman et al., 1989), which is manifested by microcephaly, normal intelligence, "bird"-like facies, immune abnormalities, and an increased risk of lymphoreticular malignancies (Seemanova et al., 1985).

Table 19–2. Chromosome Instability Syndromes with Immunodeficiency

Ataxia-telangiectasia
Bloom's syndrome
Fanconi's anemia
Nijmegen breakage syndrome
Seemanova's syndrome

Evidence of impaired immune function in Seemanova syndrome includes hypogammaglobulinemia and decreased mitogen proliferation (Seemanova et al., 1985; Seyschab et al., 1992).

Enzyme Deficiencies

Glycogen Storage Disease Type 1b

In glycogen storage disease (GSD), inherited hepatic enzyme defects prevent the conversion of glucose-6-phosphate to glucose, resulting in fasting hypoglycemia (see Chapters 15 and 16). An absence of glucose-6-phosphatase occurs in type 1a, and an absence of glucose-6-phosphate translocase occurs in type 1b. Clinically, the two syndromes are similar with the notable exception of the presence of neutropenia and increased risk of infection in GSD type 1b (Lange et al., 1980). A summary of 21 GSD type 1b patients showed that 15 had moderate to severe infections (Ambruso et al., 1985). The most common infections were recurrent otitis, pneumonia, and skin infections. Bacterial infections predominated; the most common agents were *Staphylococcus aureus*, group A *Streptococcus*, and *Escherichia coli*. In light of the neutrophil's key role in protection of the oral cavity (Van Dyke et al., 1985), it is not surprising that 8 of 21 patients had recurrent oral or anal mucosal ulcers or both (Ambruso et al., 1985).

In the largest published study of the immune dysfunction in GSD type 1b, Ambruso and associates (1985) found that 14 of 16 patients demonstrated abnormal bone marrow morphology, notably myeloid hyperplasia and maturational arrest. Despite normal white blood cell counts, nearly all patients demonstrated neutropenia at some point. Neutrophil chemotaxis was decreased in 14 of 15 patients. Others have reported abnormal respiratory burst activity of both neutrophils and monocytes (Kilpatrick et al., 1990). As shown in Figure 19–2, the respiratory burst, as assessed by superoxide anion generation, is reduced in GSD type 1b neutrophils compared with cells of normal controls and GSD type 1a patients. No defect in neutrophil degranulation was noted.

Glycoprotein Storage Diseases

Genetic errors of glycoprotein metabolism involve faulty catabolism of the oligosaccharide side chain of glycoproteins. They are considered a subset of the lysosomal storage diseases. Although these disorders are rare, the initial presentation may include recurrent infections.

Mannosidosis results from a deficiency of the acidic α–D-mannosidase. The predominant clinical features, psychomotor retardation and coarse facies, are accompanied by frequent respiratory and ear infections, particularly in infancy (Chester et al., 1982). Desnick and colleagues (1976) studied the in vitro responses of patients' leukocytes and found impaired chemotactic responsiveness and decreased bacterial phagocytosis. T-cell responsiveness to phytohemagglutinin (PHA) and concanavalin A was also severely impaired. The exact

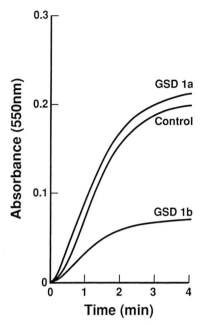

Figure 19–2. Superoxide anion generation in neutrophils from control, glycogen storage disease (GSD) 1a and GSD 1b patients stimulated with 10^{-7} M f-Met-Leu-Phe. (From Kilpatrick L, Garty BZ, Lundquist KF, et al. Impaired metabolic function and signaling defects in phagocytic cells in glycogen storage disease type 1b. J Clin Invest 86:196–202, 1990. Copyright permission of the American Society for Clinical Investigation.)

biochemical basis for these defects is not known, but the partially degraded oligosaccharides, glycopeptides, and glycoproteins with α-mannoside residues may interfere with normal ligand-receptor binding of the plasma membrane.

Another glycoprotein disorder, *aspartyglucosaminuria*, is the most common recessively inherited lysosomal storage disorder in the Finnish population. Although adult patients demonstrate marked psychomotor abnormalities, an early clinical feature is recurrent respiratory and ear infections. As noted for mannosidosis, this susceptibility usually diminishes after 6 years of age (Arvio et al., 1993) but may persist into adulthood. Indeed, Aula and coworkers (1982), in a review of 138 patients, reported that among patients who died after age 25, many had purulent infections of the lung or brain.

Still another glycoprotein storage disease, *fucosidosis*, results from a deficiency of the enzyme α-fucosidase. Recurrent sinus and pulmonary infections are common (Willems et al., 1991). Rubin and colleagues (1991) reported a 6-year-old affected girl with recurrent infections; routine immunologic studies were normal, but the trachea mucus was thinner than normal. They speculated that impaired mucus glycoprotein assembly or secretion was responsible for the abnormal mucus and her increased susceptibility to infection.

Galactosemia

Galactosemia is a heterogeneous group of inborn errors of galactose metabolism. The most common form is a deficiency of galactose-1-phosphate uridyl transferase. In treated patients, no predilection toward infection is present. However, there is an extremely high death rate in untreated neonates caused by *E. coli* sepsis (Levy et al., 1977). The period of greatest risk is from the end of the first week of life through the second week. The explanation for the selective propensity to *E. coli* infection is unknown, but Litchfield and Wells (1978) suggest that galactosemic neutrophils have reduced bactericidal activity. Published studies of neutrophil function in these patients are lacking.

Because of this risk of fulminant sepsis, it is important to identify galactosemia among neonates with jaundice. With widespread neonatal screening, many infants with galactosemia are detected before developing infectious complications. In the case of a neonate with a positive reaction to screening for galactosemia, an immediate clinical evaluation is required. If signs of disease such as jaundice, hepatomegaly, or poor feeding are present, the use of prophylactic antibiotics should be considered until bacterial cultures can be examined and metabolic stabilization with a specialized diet has been accomplished.

Sickle Cell Disease

Sickle cell disease (SCD) is the most common lethal autosomal recessive condition among African populations. Most of these patients have hemoglobin SS, leading to the most severe form of the disease. Individuals with sickle cell trait (hemoglobin AS) are partially protected from *Plasmodium falciparum* malaria. In geographic areas where *P. falciparum* is an important contributor to mortality, as much as 30% of the population has sickle cell trait, and as many as 2% of newborns have SS disease (Fleming et al., 1979). In Africa, with its high infant mortality, survival of children with sickle cell disease in the first year of life is not appreciably less than that of their unaffected peers. However, by age 5 years, only 2% of children with SCD are still alive (Molineaux et al., 1979). The relatively good survival in the first year of life is partially accounted for by the continued synthesis of fetal hemoglobin during this period. The value of improved care in a nonmalarial environment is proved by a survival rate of nearly 75% in a large Jamaican SS cohort followed to 19 years of age (Serjeant and Serjeant, 1993).

In the United States, increased mortality is also evident, largely because of a high incidence of meningitis and septicemia (Powars, 1975; Overturf et al., 1977). In areas without endemic malaria, *Streptococcus pneumoniae* (pneumococcus) is the most common pathogen (Kabins and Lerner, 1970; Seeler et al., 1972); the relative risk of pneumococcal meningitis for children with SCD is 500-fold that of the unaffected population (Barrett-Connor, 1971). *Haemophilus influenzae* type b, also poses a threat for the patient with SCD. Powars and colleagues (1983) found that the relative risk of *H. influenzae* septicemia in these children younger than the age of 9 years is fourfold that of normal children. The risk of infection in SCD variants, such as hemoglobin SC disease is higher than normal but much less than that in SS disease (Serjeant and Serjeant, 1993).

Septicemia with gram-negative enteric organisms is more common in the second decade, when pneumococcal infection becomes less prevalent (Overturf et al., 1977). *Salmonella* infections are frequently associated with osteomyelitis (Hook et al., 1957; Engh et al., 1971). The immune response to most organisms is normal in children with SCD. Of particular relevance is their normal response to parvovirus B19, an important cause of transient aplastic crisis. Rao and colleagues (1992) found a positive antibody response with clearance of the virus in eight patients with acute parvovirus B19 infection associated with an aplastic crisis.

Tissue hypoxia and functional inactivation of the reticuloendothelial system caused by chronic hemolysis may contribute to the increased susceptibility to infection. Focal vascular impairment with tissue necrosis may provide a nidus of entry through the mucosa for enteric infections such as *Salmonella*.

Splenic Function

The role of the spleen in host defense is discussed later in the text on splenectomy. Although the progressive fibrosis and shrinkage of the spleen in patients with sickle cell disease is well known, the occurrence of splenic hypofunction in the presence of splenomegaly was identified by Pearson and coworkers (1969) using technetium scanning. In some children with SCD transfusions of normal red blood cells reversed the functional asplenia (Pearson et al., 1970). The splenic hypofunction has been attributed to sluggish blood flow in the spleen, sickling of the red blood cells, increased blood viscosity, obstruction of vessels, infarction, and fibrosis (Usami et al., 1975). Falter and coworkers (1973) demonstrated that the release of factor VIII after epinephrine infusion was compromised in children with SCD with abnormal splenic uptake of technetium, providing another indicator of splenic insufficiency; this correlated with susceptibility to severe bacterial infections. An increased percentage (>5%) of pocked erythrocytes has also been used as an indicator of poor splenic function (Holroyde et al., 1969; Pearson et al., 1979).

Humoral Factors

Evans and Reindorf (1968) found normal levels of serum immunoglobulins in 24 children and 15 adults with SCD. Gavrilis and colleagues (1974) reported low IgM concentrations associated with the absence of splenic function, but this was not confirmed (Sullivan et al., 1978).

A normal antibody response was noted following subcutaneous immunization with *Salmonella* vaccines (Robbins and Pearson, 1965), but patients with SCD responded less well to intravenous immunization (Schwartz and Pearson, 1972). Ammann and associates (1977) found a normal response to an octavalent pneumococcal polysaccharide vaccine in children with SCD older than 2 years.

Winkelstein and Drachman (1968) showed that sera from patients with SCD had a deficiency of heat-labile opsonic activity against the pneumococcus; Johnston and associates (1973) and Corry and colleagues (1979) reported that the opsonic defect was in the alternative complement pathway (see Chapter 17). The deficient factor has not been identified. CH_{50}, C3PA, properdin, C3, and C3 inactivator activity are normal (Johnston et al., 1975; Strauss et al., 1977). A deficiency of properdin factor B in the serum of patients with SCD has been reported (Wilson et al., 1976).

Management

Early identification of patients with SCD through newborn screening improves clinical management. Immunization with polyvalent pneumococcal polysaccharide vaccine is effective in children older than 2 years (Ammann et al., 1977). Although equivalent studies are lacking for the quadravalent meningococcal vaccine and influenza vaccine, both are recommended for patients with SCD (American Academy of Pediatrics, 1994). Prophylactic antibiotics also are of value. Daily oral antibiotic therapy reduced pneumococcal septicemia in patients by 84% (Gaston et al., 1986). Thus, antibiotic prophylaxis should be initiated before 4 months of age, before fetal hemoglobin synthesis comes to a stop, and probably should be continued throughout childhood. Many centers use the same management guidelines for all SCD variants.

Myotonic Dystrophy

Myotonic dystrophy is a progressive muscular disorder inherited in an autosomal dominant manner and characterized by weakness, wasting, and myotonia, particularly of the facial, neck, and distal muscles. Immunoglobulin levels are often decreased secondary to a shortened IgG half-life (Zinneman and Rotstein, 1956). Wochner and associates (1966) also studied serum protein metabolism of patients with myotonic dystrophy and found a unique hypercatabolism of IgG. These patients had a mean IgG concentration of 700 mg/dl with a half-life of 11.4 days; in controls, the mean was 22.9 days. Serum concentrations and catabolic rates of IgA, IgM, and albumin were normal. IgG isolated from a patient with myotonic dystrophy had a normal survival in controls. Synthetic rates of IgG were normal. Thus, the metabolic abnormality is specific for IgG but the mechanism is obscure.

Congenital Asplenia

Congenital absence of the spleen occurs most frequently in the context of complex congenital cardiovascular anomalies and less often in association with structural abnormalities of the gastrointestinal and genitourinary tracts (Ivemark, 1955; Ruttenburg et al., 1964; Van Mierop et al., 1972; Rose et al., 1975) (see Chapter 16). From an embryologic viewpoint, asplenia is the most dramatic consequence of bilateral right-sidedness, resulting from a primary defect in morphogenesis. Prognosis is primarily determined by the severity of the cardiovascular defects. However, for patients

with isolated asplenia or those undergoing successful cardiovascular surgery, the continuing threat of overwhelming infection is substantial. A diagnosis of asplenia should be entertained in all children with congenital heart disease or recurrent sepsis. The peripheral blood smear demonstrates Howell-Jolly bodies; these are present in both functional and anatomic asplenia. Definitive diagnosis of congenital asplenia is best achieved by radionuclide scan.

Infants with congenital asplenia have a high mortality rate. In one series, infants with asplenia and cardiac defects had an 85% mortality rate; most died in the first month of life from their heart disease (Waldman et al., 1977). In infants surviving longer than a month, death from sepsis was more frequent than death from cardiac causes. Death from sepsis occurred in two of seven patients with isolated asplenia. Gram-negative organisms were the most frequent cause of sepsis in asplenic infants younger than 6 months of age and *Haemophilus* and pneumococcus were the most frequent causes in older children (Waldman et al., 1977).

The susceptility to infection associated with asplenia has been attributed to the absence of the phagocytic function of the spleen. Wang and Hsieh (1991) showed a decreased clearance of sensitized autologous erythrocytes in asplenic patients. Additionally, a subtle T-cell defect was suggested by an impaired proliferative response to mitogens and a decreased CD4:CD8 ratio. Biggar et al. (1981) described a deficient antibody response to pneumococcal vaccine in children with congenital asplenia.

Asplenia is a component of multiple genetic syndromes (Table 19–3). Asplenia with congenital heart disease is the most frequent combination. Hurwitz and Caskey (1982) identified 32 cases of asplenia with congenital heart disease in a review of 21 years of autopsies at a large children's hospital. Familial asplenia is not uncommon and may be a subset of a developmental defect that includes polysplenia (Niikawa et al., 1983). Both autosomal dominant and autosomal recessive inheritance have been suggested (Niikawa et al., 1983; Gillis et al., 1992). Crawfurd (1978) described two siblings with asplenia, polycystic kidneys, and enlarged cystic pancreas. Asplenia has also been reported in association with microgastria and limb reduction defects (Lueder et al., 1989). Stormorken and colleagues (1985) reported an association of bleeding tendency, extreme miosis, and asplenia in a six-generation

Table 19–3. Syndromes Associated with Congenital Asplenia

Asplenia with congenital heart disease
  (Ivemark's syndrome)
Familial asplenia
Asplenia with cystic liver, kidney, and pancreas
Asplenia with microgastria and limb reduction defects
Thrombocytopenia, asplenia, and miosis
  (Stormorken's syndrome)
Distinctive facies, mental retardation, short stature, and
  cryptorchidism (Smith-Fineman-Myers syndrome)
Caudal deficiency and asplenia

family. Ades and colleagues (1991) reported two brothers with Smith-Fineman-Myers syndrome, one of whom had asplenia. Asplenia has also been associated with caudal deficiency (Fullana et al., 1986).

Treatment of children with congenital asplenia must take into consideration their age, associated medical conditions, and geographic location. Immunization with *H. influenzae* type b, pneumococcal, and meningococcal vaccines is recommended. Travel to areas where malaria or babesiosis is common is unwise. Continuous antimicrobial prophylaxis should be considered for all asplenic children, especially for those younger than 5 years of age (American Academy of Pediatrics, 1994). Additional antibiotics should be started promptly in febrile illness.

Skeletal Dysplasias

Skeletal abnormalities are noted in both primary and secondary immunodeficiency. As discussed in Chapter 13, patients with the *hyper-IgE syndrome* may demonstrate osteoporosis. Patients with *adenosine deaminase (ADA) deficiency* often exhibit bony rib abnormalities (Chapter 12). *Omenn syndrome* and ADA deficiency have been associated with short-limbed dwarfism (Schofer et al., 1991; MacDermot et al., 1991). Chronic illness may nonspecifically limit skeletal growth and immune competence in tandem. However, some studies suggest a relationship between growth and immunity, particularly in the roles of IL-1 and IL-6 in bone growth and immune development (Horowitz, 1993). Common cellular progenitors give rise to both monocytes and osteoclasts.

Schimke and associates (1974) described a child with short stature, renal dysfunction, and impaired cellular immunity. Spranger and coworkers (1991) summarized five similar patients and called the disorder *Schimke's immuno-osseous dysplasia*. These patients all had recurrent infections and intermittent lymphopenia, usually by the end of the third year of life. An increased proportion of CD4+ CD8+ (double-positive) cells were present in the circulation, suggesting a defect in intrathymic T-cell maturation. These findings imply that renal disease was secondary to immune complex deposition triggered by their frequent infections.

Short stature, hair abnormalities, and immunodeficiency are noted in cartilage-hair hypoplasia (see Chapter 12). van der Burgt and colleagues (1991) described seven patients with *cartilage-hair hypoplasia* and variable cellular immune deficits. Lymphopenia, an inverted CD4:CD8 ratio, and decreased lymphocyte proliferation were noted in some patients. Defects in humoral immunity are rare. The increased risk of infections present in children may abate in adults. Severe varicella may occur. Bone marrow transplantation corrects immune abnormalities but does not restore growth potential (Hong, 1989).

Excessive growth may also be associated with secondary immunodeficiency. The *Marshall-Smith syndrome*, characterized by accelerated skeletal maturation, failure to thrive, and dysmorphic features, is associated with frequent respiratory infections (Johnson et al.,

1983). In part, this may be due to structural abnormalities, but the presence of decreased numbers of T cells and an absence of suppressor T cells suggest an intrinsic immune abnormality. *Weaver's syndrome*, also characterized by skeletal overgrowth, has been associated with recurrent infections (Ramos-Arroyo et al., 1991).

SPECIFIC ORGAN SYSTEM DYSFUNCTION

Diabetes Mellitus

Primary immunologic dysfunction in patients with diabetes mellitus is suggested by the observation that insulin-dependent diabetic children have a genetically determined predisposition to autoimmune disease, particularly thyroid dysfunction (Farid, 1988). Many studies have focused on HLA haplotypes that are associated with diabetes. Inheritance of HLA antigens DR3 and DR4 contributes to the susceptibility to diabetes. Immunologic markers, such as islet cell antibodies and insulin autoantibodies, also have predictive value in the development of diabetes (see Chapter 26).

Less detail exists regarding the effect of diabetes on the immune system. Although most measures of humoral and cell-mediated immunity are normal in patients with diabetes mellitus, there is considerable debate regarding their increased susceptibility to infection (Bagdade, 1976). Adults may be predisposed to bacterial and fungal infections, particularly of the skin and urinary tract (Kass, 1960). The frequency of vaginal yeast infections is increased in women with diabetes. Diabetic vasculopathy may contribute to the increased susceptibility to infection in adults with long-standing disease. Children with diabetes do not appear to have an increased incidence of infection (Miller and Baker, 1972).

Defects in the inflammatory response have been described in both children and adults with diabetes mellitus (see Chapter 15). Mobilization of polymorphonuclear leukocytes (PMNs) is reduced in Rebuck's windows (Brayton et al., 1970) as well as in vitro (Mowat and Baum, 1971). Miller and Baker (1972) found impaired polymorphonuclear leukocyte (PMN) chemotaxis and reduced serum chemotactic factors in children with diabetes. Their finding of normal phagocytosis of yeast particles contrasts with the results of Serlenga and colleagues (1993) who noted an impairment of phagocytosis. Hill and associates (1974b) reported impaired leukotaxis and normal nitroblue tetrazolium (NBT) dye reduction by neutrophils of patients with juvenile diabetes mellitus. Correction of the chemotactic defect with insulin has been demonstrated (Mowat and Baum, 1971; Miller and Baker, 1972; Hill et al., 1974b). Bybee and Rogers (1964) found normal phagocytes in leukocytes from non-acidotic diabetic patients but noted that ketoacidosis suppressed ingestion of staphylococci. In well-controlled diabetic patients, neutrophils did not increase their bactericidal activity in response to infection to the same degree as neutrophils from controls (Repine et al., 1980). Increased natural killer cell activity has been noted (Sensi et al., 1981), but this change may be part of the prediabetic profile that predisposes the child to autoimmune disease.

Abnormal phagocytosis and bactericidal activity were reported in patients with ketoacidosis and mild diabetes (Bagdade et al., 1974). Tan and associates (1975) have demonstrated impaired intracellular killing as well as a phagocytic defect in some diabetics in a nonketoacidotic state. Similar studies have been performed on leukocytes from diabetic children (Dziatkowiak et al., 1982). These observations are consistent with the hypothesis that alterations in energy metabolism affect chemotaxis and phagocytosis.

Protein-Losing Enteropathy

Excessive gastrointestinal (GI) protein loss may cause hypoproteinemia in a number of disorders (Table 19–4) (see Chapters 12 and 23). All proteins appear to be lost into the intestinal tract at the same rate, regardless of molecular size (Waldmann and Schwab, 1965; Waldmann, 1966). However, reduction in the serum concentration of proteins varies, since synthetic rates dif-

Table 19–4. Diseases Associated with Protein-Losing Enteropathy

Intestinal Surface Abnormalities
Acute transient exudative gastroenteropathy
Allergic gastroenteropathy
Angioneurotic edema
Gastrocolic fistula
Giant hypertrophy of the gastric mucosa
   (Ménétrier's disease)
Gluten-induced enteropathy
Neoplasms
Regional enteritis
Ulcerative colitis

Cardiac
Atrial septal defect
Constrictive pericarditis
Familial cardiomyopathy
Thrombosis of inferior vena cava
Tricuspid insufficiency

Infection
Acquired immunodeficiency syndrome
Hookworm
Mycoplasma pneumoniae
Shigella dysenteriae
Strongyloides
Tropical sprue
Tuberculosis
Whipple's disease

Vasculitic Syndromes
Systemic lupus erythematosus
Henoch-Schönlein purpura
Churg-Strauss syndrome

Other
Aminopterin administration
Hirschsprung's disease
Intestinal lymphangiectasia
Pancreatitis
Postgastrectomy syndrome
Protein-calorie malnutrition

fer. Levels of albumin and immunoglobulin are the most markedly depressed. IgM, ceruloplasmin, and transferrin concentrations are mildly depressed, but α_2-macroglobulin and fibrinogen levels are usually normal (Jarnum and Petersen, 1961; Waldmann, 1966). Although significant hypogammaglobulinemia may be present, antibody responses are normal (Ulstrom et al., 1956, 1957; Waldmann, 1966) and increased susceptibility to infection is unusual. Reductions in the concentrations of all three major immunoglobulins are associated with normal or increased synthetic rates and increased fractional catabolic rates.

Etiology

Protein loss occurs most commonly in patients with gastrointestinal surface abnormalities, such as regional enteritis, ulcerative colitis (Schwartz and Jarnum, 1959; Steinfeld et al., 1960), sprue (Parkins, 1960; London et al., 1961), and celiac disease (Rotem and Czerniak, 1964). Milk allergy has been incriminated as a cause of protein-losing enteropathy in infants (Waldmann et al., 1967). Edema, hypoalbuminemia, and hypogammaglobulinemia were associated with growth retardation, iron deficiency anemia, and eosinophilia. In three patients studied, there was significant improvement noted on a milk-free diet and a return of symptoms when milk was reintroduced. Transient hypoproteinemia and edema have followed gastroenteritis in a few children (Degnan, 1957; Waldmann et al., 1961; Pitman et al., 1964; Herskovic et al., 1968).

Gastrointestinal protein loss also may occur as the result of lymphatic obstruction. The concurrent loss of lymphocytes into the intestinal tract and subsequent lymphopenia distinguish this mechanism of protein loss from the enteropathy caused by surface abnormalities. Direct obstruction of the intestinal lymphatics may occur in entities such as intestinal lymphangiectasia, neoplasia, and regional enteritis. Indirect lymphatic obstruction occurs as the result of the effects of high venous pressures on lymphatic flow as seen in patients with congestive heart failure, especially in those with constrictive pericarditis. A few cases of constrictive pericarditis in children have been reported (Davidson et al., 1961; Plauth et al., 1964; Nelson et al., 1975). Patients with other causes of congestive heart failure, such as congenital heart disease and rheumatic fever, have been found to have excessive gastrointestinal protein losses (Waldmann, 1966).

Several vasculitic conditions, including systemic lupus erythematosus (SLE) (Pelletier et al., 1992), Henoch-Schönlein purpura (Kobayashi et al., 1991), and Churg-Strauss syndrome (Malaval et al., 1993), have been described as causes of gastrointestinal protein loss. Intestinal protein loss in SLE most likely occurs as the result of increased microvascular permeability (Perednia and Curosh, 1990).

Serum Protein Metabolism

In 1956, Ulstrom and coworkers reported four infants with edema, anemia, and marked irritability without signs of hepatic or renal disease. Marked hypoproteinemia was present with a uniform reduction of albumin and all globulins. Despite the inability to demonstrate gamma globulin by Tiselius' apparatus or paper electrophoresis, the authors found that the two infants had normal isohemagglutinin levels and had anitoxin titers following diphtheria and tetanus immunization. *H. influenzae* agglutinins were demonstrated in one of the infants. Turnover studies indicated increased degradation of protein; however, the origin and site of destruction were not apparent (Ulstrom et al., 1957).

Sturgeon and Brubaker (1956) noted similar cases, stressing hypocupremia as part of a multiple deficiency syndrome. After Citrin and coworkers (1957) demonstrated the loss of albumin into the stomach of a patient with hypertrophic gastritis, Gordon (1959) found increased fecal excretion of ^{131}I polyvinylpyrolidone (PVP) in patients with idiopathic hypercatabolic hypoproteinemia and called the condition *exudative enteropathy*. Schwartz and Jarnum (1959) immediately confirmed Gordon's findings.

Waldmann and coworkers (1961) studied 20 patients with hypoproteinemia and edema using ^{131}I albumin and ^{131}I PVP. Gastrointestinal symptoms were not always present. Eighteen had a normal to increased rate of synthesis of albumin with increased fecal loss. Twelve of the 15 patients examined had intestinal lymphangiectasia. Dilated lymphatic channels with a thickening of the elastica interna and muscular layers of the media were characteristic findings. Chylous effusions were present in four patients. Jarnum and Peterson (1961) suggested that the transport of protein and lymph into the lumen of the gut and the peritoneal cavity was due to increased pressure in the lymphatic vessels.

Chylous ascites, sometimes in association with peripheral lymphedema, has frequently been reported with hypoproteinemia (Rosen et al., 1962). Pomeranz and Waldmann (1963) demonstrated systemic lymphatic abnormalities by lymphangiography in four patients with intestinal lymphangiectasia, including one child with congenital chylous ascites.

Immunologic Abnormalities

Lymphopenia has been reported in patients with intestinal lymphangiectasia and protein-losing enteropathy associated with regional enteritis, Whipple's disease, and constrictive pericarditis (Strober et al., 1967). Normal lymphocyte counts were reported in protein-losing enteropathies associated with sprue, gluten enteropathy, allergic enteropathy, and variable agammaglobulinemia. The lymphopenic enteropathies appear to be secondary to structural abnormalities of the lymphatic channels—for example, intestinal lymphangiectasia (Strober et al., 1967; Weiden et al., 1972). Diminished skin test responses to purified protein derivative (PPD), mumps, *Trichophyton,* and *Candida albicans*; negative reactions to dinitrochlorobenzene; and prolonged skin allograft retention were related to lymphopenia. Although immunoglobulin levels were depressed (IgG of 450 ± 210 mg/dl; IgA of 110 ± 30 mg/dl; IgM of

70 ± 20 mg/dl), the antibody response of five patients to tularemia antigen was normal. Three of five patients responded to a single injection of 100 μg of Vi antigen, but the overall response was significantly lower than that in controls. Despite these defects in cell-mediated and humoral immunity, significant infections occurred in only two children under 10 years; furunculosis, pneumonia, and peritonitis associated with severe debilitation developed.

In a child with intestinal lymphangiectasia with lymphopenia and impaired cutaneous delayed hypersensitivity, the lymphocyte response to PHA was normal, suggesting a quantitative defect of lymphocyte function (McGuigan et al., 1968). Weiden and colleagues (1972) found impaired lymphocyte responses to mitogens, antigens, and allogeneic cells in patients with intestinal lymphangiectasia. Lymphocytes from chylous effusions were normal, suggesting GI loss of recirculating long-lived lymphocytes.

Illustrative examples of gastrointestinal anomalies producing combined immunodeficiency were reported by Fawcett and associates (1986), who described severe B-cell and T-cell defects in two children originally thought to have food allergy. These children suffered from a malrotation of the small intestine and a cavernous hemangioma of the midjejunum, respectively. Following surgical correction there was gradual restoration of both B-cell and T-cell immunity (Figs. 19–3 and 19–4). In addition to the normalization of serum IgG and mitogen reactivity, the number of T lymphocytes and the inverted CD4:CD8 ratios became normal. These two cases emphasize the importance of a careful immune evaluation in children with diarrhea when a food allergy is suspected.

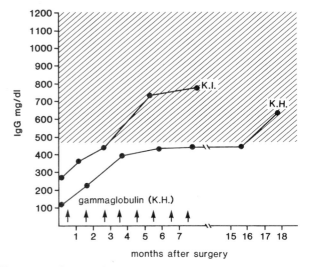

Figure 19–3. Serum IgG concentrations in two patients with anatomic intestinal abnormalities corrected by surgery. Patient K. H. had a malrotation of the small bowel, and patient K. I. had a cavernous hemangioma of the mid-jejunum. Patient K. H. received intravenous gamma globulin replacement therapy for several months until IgG levels were self-sustained. The shaded area represents the 95% confidence range for age-matched controls. (From Fawcett WA IV, Ferry GD, Gorin LJ, et al. Immunodeficiency secondary to structural intestinal defects. Malrotation of the small bowel and cavernous hemangioma of the jejunum. Am J Dis Child 140:169–172, 1986.)

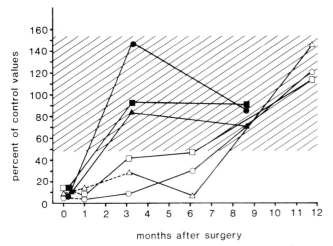

Figure 19–4. Reactivity of peripheral blood lymphocytes to mitogens in patient K. H. *(open symbols)* and patient K. I. *(closed symbols)* after corrective surgery. PHA = squares; conconavalin A (ConA) = circles; PWM (pokeweed mitogen) = triangles. The values are given in terms of percentage of normal values, and the shaded area represents the 95% confidence normal range. (From Fawcett WA IV, Ferry GD, Gorin LJ, et al. Immunodeficiency secondary to structural intestinal defects. Malrotation of the small bowel and cavernous hemangioma of the jejunum. Am J Dis Child 140:169–172, 1986. Copyright 1986, American Medical Association.)

Treatment

Treatment of protein-losing enteropathy depends on the identification of the underlying disorder. In localized lesions of the gastrointestinal tract, surgical resection may provide complete remission. Remissions have followed surgery for giant hypertrophy of the gastric mucosa, congenital jejunal stenosis, Hirschsprung's disease, localized intestinal lymphangiectasia, constrictive pericarditis, and intra-atrial septal defects (Waldmann 1966). However, most of the diseases producing protein-losing enteropathy are too diffuse for surgical therapy. No specific treatment is necessary for the acute transient enteropathies. Allergic gastroenteropathy has been treated successfully with a milk-free diet (Waldmann et al., 1967). Gluten-free diets have been beneficial in patients with celiac disease and nontropical sprue. Diffuse intestinal lymphangiectasia has been more difficult to manage. A low-fat diet with replacement of long-chain triglycerides by medium-chain triglycerides has led to improvement in a few patients (Jeffries et al., 1964; Amirhakimi et al., 1969; Holt, 1964; McGuigan et al., 1968). Corticosteroids have not been of value in treating intestinal lymphangiectasia. Corticosteroids and some of the cytotoxic drugs have been effective in regional enteritis and ulcerative colitis.

Nephrotic Syndrome

Volhard and Fahr (1914) first reported pneumococcal peritonitis as a fatal complication of the nephrotic syndrome. Subsequently, other pneumococcal infections were noted in the nephrotic syndrome; this suggests a unique susceptibility not found in other patients with edema (e.g., congestive heart failure, malnutri-

tion). The infections often develop in patients who are nasopharyngeal carriers of the involved pneumococcus (MacLeod and Farr, 1937).

Group A streptococci, staphylococci, and *Haemophilus influenzae* type b follow pneumococci as etiologic agents of infections in the nephrotic syndrome. With the advent of antibiotics and the successful treatment of edema with corticosteroids, bacterial infections, particularly skin infections, are much less common. Pneumococcal peritonitis (Rubin et al., 1975; Gorensek et al., 1988) and systemic infection with enteric organisms (Wilfert and Katz, 1968; Krensky et al., 1982) still occur.

Hypoproteinemia develops in patients with nephrotic syndrome because of proteinuria. Barandun and colleagues (1960) have shown that in some children there is additional protein loss through the GI tract. The characteristic serum electrophoretic pattern reveals decreases in the albumin, β globulin, and γ globulin fractions with elevations of α_2 globulin (Bongiovanni and Wolman, 1949). Metabolic studies in patients with the nephrotic syndrome indicate that synthetic and catabolic rates of many proteins are increased (Kelley et al., 1950). The IgG synthetic rate is generally normal (Al-Bander et al., 1992). Barth and coworkers (1964) reported a normal IgM catabolic rate. Of the serum immunoglobulins, the greatest depletion affects the smallest species, IgG. Giangiacomo and coworkers (1975) found elevated IgM levels in the idiopathic nephrotic syndrome, but this was not confirmed (Ingelfinger et al., 1976). Serum IgG and IgA values may remain low during periods of remission (Giangiacomo et al., 1975). IgE concentrations may be increased (Groshong et al., 1973) (see Chapter 25).

Children with the nephrotic syndrome have an impaired antibody response to pneumococci (Hodes, 1952) and pneumococcal polysaccharide (Hodges, 1954). Kunin and coworkers (1959) found a normal antibody response to influenza virus vaccine in such children. The differences in the reported antibody responses to viral and bacterial products may be related to the severity of the disease as well as the immunogen.

Complement levels are elevated in the nephrotic syndrome, except for patients with immune complex glomerulonephritis (Pickering et al., 1970). Properdin factor B (C3 proactivator) may be decreased (Michael et al., 1973).

Neutrophil function was abnormal in a study of 18 children with nephrotic syndrome (Anderson et al., 1979). Children with nephrotic syndrome in relapse demonstrated neutrophil chemotactic scores that were significantly depressed compared with those in children with disease in remission or in controls. Opsonic activity of the serum, C3 deposition on activated zymosan particles, and serum factor B concentration were all significantly abnormal in patients in relapse, and correlation was made with systemic bacterial infections.

Significant improvement in prognosis came first with the availability of antimicrobial agents and then with corticosteroids (Leutscher and Deming, 1950; Saxena and Crawford, 1965; Arneil and Lam, 1966). However, steroids may mask the response to infection or potentiate certain viral infections such as varicella zoster. The steroid dose should be lowered if the child contracts such an infection. Passive immunization is indicated (see Chapter 29) if a susceptible child is exposed to measles or varicella. Cytotoxic drugs, including nitrogen mustard, cyclophosphamide, and azathioprine, that are used in steroid-resistant nephrotic syndrome also decrease host resistance.

Uremia

Chronic renal failure produces uremia and often necessitates treatment with hemodialysis. Both uremia and hemodialysis treatment adversely affect immune responses (Goldblum and Reed, 1980) (see Chapter 16). Hemodialysis often requires a link between the dialysis machine and the intravascular compartment for 10 to 15 hours a week. The combination of frequent needlesticks and increased carriage of cutaneous staphylococci predisposes hemodialysis patients to infections of the vascular access site. Bacterial contamination of dialysis equipment has been linked to sepsis (Curtis et al., 1967). Even when organisms cannot pass through the dialysis membrane, their bacteria-derived products, such as endotoxin, may pass into the blood stream and produce sepsis-like symptoms in patients (Hindman et al., 1975). In addition, the interaction of serum and hemodialysis equipment may interfere with complement function. The hemodialysis membrane activates the alternative pathway to generate C5 cleavage products. These C5 fragments can affect neutrophil adherence to endothelial surfaces or to other neutrophils. The changes in neutrophils may account for the peripheral leukopenia and the pulmonary leukostasis temporally associated with the hemodialysis procedure (reviewed in Goldblum and Reed, 1980).

Immune function is also compromised by the metabolic derangements accompanying uremia. In general, the duration and severity of the uremic state, rather than the underlying cause of renal failure, determine the extent of immune alterations. The glomerular filtration rate must be reduced to less than 25% of normal before immune dysfunction becomes detectable (Byron et al., 1976). Uremia impairs the integrity of mucocutaneous barriers. Associated dermatologic problems include dryness, pruritis, and excoriation (Young et al., 1973). The intestinal mucosa may be compromised by the ulcerative defects that occur in chronic renal failure.

Uremia increases susceptibility to infections of the lung, skin, urinary tract, and gastrointestinal tract (Montgomerie et al., 1968). Mailloux and colleagues (1991) followed 222 uremic patients on dialysis over a 16-year period and reported that infection was the leading cause of death, although the death rate from infection dropped from 44% in the first four years of the study to 22% in the last four years. Infections in uremic subjects also result in considerable morbidity necessitating frequent hospitalization (Lowrie et al., 1973). *S. aureus,* mycobacteria, and hepatitis B virus are common pathogens in uremic patients (Szmuness et al., 1974; Bradley et al., 1987; Garcia-Leoni et al., 1990).

Cellular Immunity

Impaired cell-mediated immunity is the predominant defect in uremia. Lymphopenia with decreased CD3, CD4, and CD8 cells is reported (Raska et al., 1983; Kurz et al., 1986). The thymus is hypocellular and shows fatty infiltration and cystic degeneration (Wilson et al., 1965). The lymph nodes have a decreased number of secondary follicles (Black and de Chabon, 1964). Marked decrease occurs in cutaneous delayed hypersensitivity to a wide variety of antigens (Kirkpatrick et al., 1964). There are diminished lymphocyte proliferative responses (Huber et al., 1969; Raska et al., 1983). Johnston and Slavin (1976) successfully transferred tuberculin sensitivity with cells from a uremic donor to a non-uremic recipient but not to a uremic recipient. They concluded that intrinsic lymphocyte activity was intact in uremia but functional immunosuppressive factors were present in the plasma.

A dramatic example of altered cell-mediated immunity in uremia was noted during some of the early human renal allografts. Hume and colleagues (1955) found good survival of kidney allografts from unrelated donors transplanted to uremic patients compared with survival of kidney allografts in non-uremic dogs and astutely suggested that uremic recipients were not fully immunocompetent. These observations were confirmed by studies that showed prolonged survival of skin allografts in uremic subjects (Dammin et al., 1957). Later studies showed that lymphocytes from uremic donors were unable to mount a normal graft-versus-host reaction (Bridges et al., 1964; Carpenter et al., 1966).

Humoral Immunity

Humoral immunity is less severely compromised in uremic subjects than is cellular immunity. Immunoglobulin levels (Dammin et al., 1957) are generally normal. Numbers of circulating B cells may be reduced in the uremic patient, but this deficiency is improved by maintenance hemodialysis (Hoy et al., 1978). Yet, high rates of infection and abnormal antibody formation to pneumococcal polysaccharide antigens (Goldblum and Reed, 1980), influenza virus (Pabico et al., 1974), and hepatitis B vaccine (Stevens et al., 1984) suggest subtle humoral immunodeficiency. Raskova and colleagues (1987) showed impaired B-cell activation in vitro to both T cell–dependent and T cell–independent antigens.

Neutrophil Dysfunction

Early studies of neutrophil function in uremia were normal (Brayton et al., 1970; Quie, 1972; Abrutyn et al., 1977), but subsequent studies have described defective chemotaxis (Lewis and Van Epps, 1987), phagocytosis (Alexiewicz et al., 1991), and oxidative metabolism (Lewis, 1991). Metabolic disturbances present in renal failure, such as iron overload, zinc deficiency, secondary hyperparathyroidism, and circulating plasma factors, may account for the functional abnormalities of neutrophils (Haag-Weber and Horl, 1993) (see Chapter 16).

In sum, multiple facets of the immune system are impaired in uremic patients. Secondary metabolic derangements aggravate these responses. Special vaccine protocols (e.g., high-dose hepititis B vaccine) and aggressive clinical management of potential infectious episodes can minimize morbidity and mortality.

NUTRITIONAL DEFICIENCIES

Protein-Calorie Malnutrition

Malnutrition refers to an inadequacy of nutrients that is sufficient to interfere with normal physiologic function. Inadequate nutrition adversely affects many aspects of immune function (Kuvibidila et al., 1993), and it is the most common cause of secondary immunodeficiency in the world. The deficiencies are usually multiple and involve varying degrees of caloric and protein deprivation.

Protein-calorie malnutrition (PCM) has been separated into two clinical extremes: *marasmus*, an insufficiency of all food; and *kwashiorkor*, a deficiency of protein in a diet usually high in calories. Protein-calorie malnutrition is a serious problem in most developing countries (e.g., India and some nations in Latin America and Africa). Economic and cultural considerations, such as premature weaning, are major causes of malnutrition. The age at which malnutrition occurs is important, and early deprivation leads to severe impairment of immunologic function. The severity of malnutrition, as assessed by arm circumference measurements, accurately predicts the risk of death (Alam et al., 1989). Severe malnutrition may also occur with gastrointestinal, hepatic, renal, or cardiopulmonary diseases and malignancies.

Marasmus generally occurs early in infancy. The patients are grossly underweight and wasted, but edema and skin and hair changes are absent. Kwashiorkor, more common during the second year of life, is characterized by growth retardation, dermatitis, edema, moon facies, hepatomegaly, abnormal hair, apathy, and misery. There is overlap between the two syndromes, and malnutrition of lesser severity is even more common. Serum albumin levels are markedly depressed in kwashiorkor and slightly depressed in marasmus. Decreased concentrations of cholesterol, lipase, amylase, and esterase are characteristic of kwashiorkor. The infants are infrequently anemic, with low transferrin levels. Kwashiorkor patients at autopsy show thymic and lymphoid fatty infiltration and atrophy (Smythe et al., 1971). Often there is an associated zinc deficiency, which by itself can produce T-cell abnormalities (Chandra, 1980b).

Malnutrition markedly increases susceptibility to infection, resulting in increased morbidity and mortality from many infectious diseases. Nearly 50% of malnourished children requiring hospital admission are infected. Bacterial infections are frequent (Smythe and Campbell, 1959; Phillips and Wharton, 1968), particularly pneumonia. Although the specific etiology of pneumonia is often difficult to establish, tuberculous, *Pneumocystis carinii*, and staphylococcal pneumonias are not uncommon. Gram-negative infections of the blood and gastrointestinal and urinary tracts are common.

Measles causes a particularly high mortality in these patients; the rash may be absent, and giant cell pneumonia is common (Smythe et al., 1971). Herpes infections are often severe (Templeton, 1970), and the prevalence of hepatitis B antigenemia is high (Suskind et al., 1973). Many children have fungal and parasitic infections, including *P. carinii* (Hughes et al., 1974).

The interplay between malnutrition and infection results in a vicious circle. Each episode of infection increases the need for calories and protein and at the same time causes anorexia; both of these aggravate the nutritional deficiency, making the patient even more susceptible to infection.

Nonspecific Immune Factors

Several factors, including anatomic barriers, phagocytosis, lysozyme, interferon, and hormones, are involved in nonspecific host defense, but in malnutrition few have been completely characterized. Many of these factors are adversely affected (Neumann et al., 1975), and some, such as localized defects of the mucous membranes, may be critical in the pathogenesis of respiratory, gastrointestinal, and urinary tract infections.

Several defects of PMN function have been described in protein-calorie malnutrition (see Chapter 15). Studies of chemotaxis have produced conflicting results, perhaps influenced by different degrees of malnutrition or the presence of infection (Schopfer and Douglas, 1976b; Douglas and Schopfer, 1976). Engulfment and opsonic activity are normal (Seth and Chandra, 1972; Douglas and Schopfer, 1974; Keusch et al., 1977), but bactericidal and candidicidal activity are diminished. Reduced incorporation of radioactive iodine (^{131}I) into trichloroacetic acid (TCA)–precipitable proteins by phagocytizing PMNs from children with kwashiorkor suggests impairment of the myeloperoxidase–H_2O_2–iodide killing system (Douglas and Schopfer, 1976); however, myeloperoxidase activity was reported as normal, and the leukocyte defects may be secondary to the high incidence of infections (Schopfer and Douglas, 1976b). The defects in phagocytosis, when present, are mild, and their contribution to infection is subtle.

Anderson and investigators (1983), studying 37 malnourished American black and Hispanic inner city infants, detected diminished migration of neutrophils in response to bacterial chemotactic factor and decreased adherence of neutrophils to surfaces and particles. Moreover, these abnormalities were corrected with restoration of adequate nutrition.

Decreased levels of a number of complement components were found, except for C4 in patients with PCM (Sirisinha et al., 1973) (see Chapter 17). Anticomplementary activity was present in 25% of their sera.

Children with kwashiorkor and those with infection had more frequent and more severe disorders.

The skin and mucous membranes act as an initial barrier to potential pathogens. Dietary deficiencies may compromise the integrity of these surfaces. Lack of vitamin A may lead to metaplastic hyperkeratosis. Riboflavin and pyridoxine deficiency may result in dermatitis, cheilitis, or angular stomatitis. Protein deficiency predisposes to skin and mucosal atrophy. Malnutrition may also influence cellular components of this first line of defense. Lymphocytes and plasma cells in the interstitial space are reduced. Migration of lymphoblasts from the mesentery is also affected (Chandra and Wadhwa, 1989).

Humoral Immunity

Serum immunoglobulin concentrations are normal or elevated in infants with protein-calorie malnutrition (Keet and Thom, 1969; Rosen et al., 1971; Smythe et al., 1971; Neumann et al., 1975; Chandra, 1977). During infection, γ globulin synthesis is increased, and the preferential utilization of protein precursors restricts the synthesis of albumin and exacerbates the clinical manifestations of kwashiorkor (Cohen and Hansen, 1962). Although serum IgA values are often elevated, there is a mild but significant decrease in secretory IgA (Sirisinha et al., 1975; Reddy et al., 1976) (see Chapter 8). Isohemagglutinin titers are normal (Kahn et al., 1957). Antibody responses to typhoid vaccine (Pretorius and de Villiers, 1962), keyhole-limpet hemocyanin (KLH), and pneumococcal polysaccharide (Neumann et al., 1975) were reported as normal. However, antibody responses to diphtheria toxoid (Scrimshaw and Behar, 1961) and yellow fever vaccine (Brown and Katz, 1966) are impaired.

The most striking abnormality of the B-cell system is the high levels of serum IgE (Table 19–5). Although intestinal parasitism may contribute to these high levels, neither this nor the occurrence of allergy explains the abnormality (Stiehm, 1980). A likely explanation is that nutritional deprivation affects immunoregulatory subsets of T cells and leads to overproduction of IgE.

Red blood cells from infants with PCM appear to be agglutinated by antisera to serum complement components and immunoglobulins (Smythe et al., 1971). These autoimmune phenomena may be related to concurrent infections.

Thymic Alterations

Smythe and coworkers (1971) reported varying degrees of lymph node germinal center depletion in malnourished infants. Malnourished patients also have thymic atrophy and depletion of paracortical cells in peripheral lymphoid tissue (Vint, 1937; Smythe et al., 1971; Schonland, 1972). Morphologic changes of the thymus in malnutrition are summarized by Dourov (1986). Thymic atrophy and fibrotic changes are common, usually involving the cortex earlier than the medulla. Although many tissues such as liver, kidney, and heart may undergo atrophy during malnutrition,

Table 19–5. Serum IgE Levels in Malnourished Children

	IgE Level (IU/ml)*	
Author	Malnourished (± 1 SD)	Controls (± 1 SD)
Johansson et al. (1968)		
Ethiopian children		
With parasites	4400 ± 4150†	
Without parasites	860 ± 1190†	160 ± 116
Neumann et al. (1975)		
Ghanaian children	1489 ± 410†	829 ± 244
Purtilo et al. (1976)		
Brazilian children		
With parasites	1636	2593
Without parasites		129
Suskind et al. (1976)		
Thai children	16/25 had levels > 1000 IU/ml	1/11 had levels > 1000 IU/ml
Chandra (1977)		
Indian children		
With infection	360 ± 110†	56 ± 37
With parasites	2865 ± 581	3410 ± 736
Without infection or parasites	427 ± 129†	36 ± 21

*Values represent the IgE level (IU/ml) ± 1 SD.
†Significantly increased.
From Stiehm ER. Humoral immunity in malnutrition. Fed Proc 39:3093–3097, 1980.

thymic atrophy is distinguished by a greater loss of cells than a decrease in cell size. Also, in contrast to other tissues, thymic tissue does not show the capacity to regenerate readily when proper diet is restored. These findings are not limited to malnutrition but are found in a variety of chronic debilitating diseases.

Cellular Immunity

Impairment of cell-mediated immunity is the most common immunologic abnormality in protein-calorie malnutrition (Edelman, 1973; McMurray, 1984). Lymphopenia occurs in about 25% of the children dying from malnutrition (Smythe et al., 1971). Tuberculin tests may be negative in PCM in the presence of active tuberculosis or following bacille Calmette-Guérin (BCG) vaccination (Harland and Brown, 1965). Cutaneous delayed hypersensitivity reactions to other antigens are also impaired (Ferguson et al., 1974; Neumann et al., 1975). Delayed hypersensitivity reactions following dinitrochlorobenzene (DNCB) sensitization were absent in 70% of infants with PCM (Smythe et al., 1971). Transfer of cutaneous reactions to tuberculin was accomplished in children with PCM using lysates of leukocytes from a strongly positive donor, indicating that the capacity for recruitment of nonsensitive cells in the delayed hypersensitivity reaction was normal (Brown and Katz, 1967). However, Walker and others (1975) could not show any difference in the response to transfer factor of children with PCM and controls.

The absolute number of T cells is diminished in PCM (Chandra, 1974; Ferguson et al., 1974; Schopfer and Douglas, 1976a). Imbalances in immunoregulatory subsets of T cells have been observed in malnutrition

(Chandra, 1980a). In some studies, the in vitro lymphocyte response to PHA has been normal (Ferguson et al., 1974; Schlesinger and Stekel, 1974), although severely malnourished infants may have an impaired response (Chandra, 1974; Neumann et al., 1975; Schopfer and Douglas, 1976a). Pokeweed mitogen appears to produce a normal or increased lymphocyte response (Schopfer and Douglas, 1976a).

Iron Deficiency

Iron deficiency is common among children throughout the world, including the United States. The relationship between iron status and immunity has been debated for more than half a century (MacKay, 1928). Although numerous studies have evaluated diverse immunologic parameters in the presence of iron deficiency, methodologic concerns cloud the interpretations. The issue is further complicated by the varying biologic responses to iron conditions in infecting organisms: for example, the increased virulence of *E. coli* in the presence of added iron (Sussman, 1974) and enhanced tetanus toxin elaboration in the presence of iron deprivation (Masawe and Msazumuhire, 1973). Critical reviews provide a reasoned perspective (Dallman, 1987; Dhur et al., 1989).

The fundamental unanswered question is whether the incidence of infections is increased in the presence of iron deficiency or supplementation. A common methodologic approach is to study a population with a high prevalence of iron deficiency in which one group receives iron supplementation and a control group does not. In two large studies, one in Chile (Heresi et al., 1985) and the other in India (Damodaran et al., 1979), no difference was found in morbidity between children receiving iron supplements and a control group. In contrast, Cantwell (1972), studying children with severe iron deficiency, found a slight decrease in hospitalizations in an iron-treated group compared with controls.

Other studies have measured immunologic abnormalities in iron deficiency. Humoral immunity is generally intact. Serum immunoglobulins and salivary IgA are normal (Chandra and Saraya, 1975; MacDougall et al., 1975). The same authors found normal total hemolytic complement (CH_{50}). A subsequent study noted a decrease in the CH_{50} levels when iron deficiency was severe (Jagadeesan and Reddy, 1983). Several studies report decreased T-cell numbers and impaired cutaneous delayed hypersensitivity, consistent with impaired cell mediated immunity (Chandra and Saraya, 1975; MacDougall et al., 1975; Krantman et al., 1982). Impaired lymphocyte proliferation has been noted by several groups (Joynson et al., 1972; Chandra and Saraya, 1975; MacDougall et al., 1975) but not by others (e.g., Kulapongs et al., 1974). Variations in laboratory techniques and the state of nutrition may account for these discrepancies.

Impaired bactericidal activity of neutrophils in iron-deficient patients is reversible after iron supplementation (Chandra, 1973; Yetgin et al., 1979; Walter et al., 1986). Conflicting evidence exists for a defect in phagocytic function as assessed by hexose monophosphate shunt activity and myeloperoxidase activity (reviewed in Dhur et al., 1989).

Vitamin A Deficiency

Deficiency of vitamin A (retinol and its derivatives) has long been appreciated as a significant factor in the increased severity of infection seen in the malnourished host (Bloch, 1924). Neonates have low stores of vitamin A, largely because of poor placental transport, and children younger than 5 years of age are at greatest risk of vitamin A deficiency (reviewed by Rumore, 1993). Although isolated vitamin A deficiency is rare, it is often seen in populations at risk for PCM. Many reports have demonstrated an important impact of therapeutic and supplemental vitamin A on the health of children. Meta-analysis of published studies found a 30% reduction in all-cause mortality (Glasziou and Mackerras, 1993). A significant reduction was noted for treatment of hospitalized patients and in community-based supplementation studies (Fawzi et al., 1993). Rahmathullah and colleagues (1990) noted the greatest reduction in mortality in children younger than 3 years of age. In contrast, Stansfield and associates (1993) found an increased prevalence of childhood morbidity during a trial of megadose vitamin A supplementation. Their study was criticized for a low follow-up rate and for a failure to assess the duration or severity of the morbidity (Semba and Hussey, 1993).

Of the infectious diseases for which vitamin A status is thought to be important, the relationship with measles has been investigated most extensively. As mentioned previously, measles remains a devastating disease in populations at high risk for malnutrition. Infections in general, and measles in particular, induce depression of serum vitamin A levels (Arroyave and Calcano, 1979; Arrieta et al., 1992). Treatment of severe measles with vitamin A dramatically improves morbidity and mortality (Hussey and Klein, 1990). Coutsoudis and colleagues (1992) found that vitamin A treatment of measles allows a more rapid reversal of the infection-induced lymphopenia. They also noted an increase in measles IgG antibody concentrations in the treated patients.

An understanding of the effects of vitamin A that determine resistance to infection and may contribute to increased survival has been delineated in part. Many authors have emphasized the role of vitamin A in augmenting nonspecific immunity through maintenance of the physical and biologic integrity of epithelial tissue (Olson, 1972; Chandra, 1988). Semba and associates (1993) found altered lymphocyte profiles in children with clinical evidence of vitamin A deficiency. They noted that affected children have lower CD4:CD8 ratios, lower proportions of CD4 naive T cells, and higher proportions of CD8[+], CD45RO[+] T cells and that these abnormalities reversed with vitamin A supplementation. An important role for vitamin A in B-cell lymphopoiesis was demonstrated by Buck and associates (1990). Decreased natural killer cell activity has been shown in animal models of vitamin A deficiency (Nauss and Newberne, 1985; Bowman et al., 1990).

Vitamin A deficiency also impairs the humoral immune response (reviewed by Ross, 1992). Semba and colleagues (1992) reported improved tetanus toxoid titers in children at risk for malnutrition who were given vitamin A supplementation 2 weeks prior to vaccination. Their results contrast with those of Brown and associates (1980), who gave a dose of vitamin A concurrently with immunization and found no detectable difference in tetanus titers. Animal studies support the concept that primary antibody response is impaired in vitamin A deficiency (Lavasa et al., 1988; Pasatiempo et al., 1990).

In addition to vitamin A's anti-infective properties, some studies have emphasized a broader interaction of vitamin A and the immune system. Specifically, vitamin A may reduce the risk of cancer, particularly that of epithelial origin (Ziegler et al., 1986). In experimental models, vitamin A enhances rejection of certain immunogenic tumors consistent with a role in immunosurveillance (Malkovsky et al., 1983). The identification of a family of nuclear receptors for retinoic acid in diverse tissues has led to many studies of the function of vitamin A in gene regulation (Petkovich, 1992).

IMMUNOSUPPRESSIVE AGENTS

Immunosuppressive agents may be classified as:

- *Physical* (radiation, thoracic duct drainage)
- *Biologic* (anti–lymphocyte globulin, anti–T cell antibody)
- *Chemical* (corticosteroids, alkylating agents, and inhibitors of protein or nucleic acid synthesis)

Anti-inflammatory and cytotoxic drugs are widely used in children for a variety of disorders. Their effects on host defense are mostly derived from studies done on experimental animals with considerable variation as to species, dosage, route, timing, and type of response studied. Their effects in humans are derived from a few studies in normal individuals and are complicated by immunologic alterations present in the underlying disease. In general, antimetabolites inhibit cell proliferation and are most effective when given at the peak of this cell proliferation. Unlike anti-inflammatory agents, drugs that inhibit dividing cells generally do not affect chemotaxis or phagocytosis. Radiation and cytotoxic drugs do not affect the uptake of colloid by the reticuloendothelial system but do block its phagocytic function (Benaceraf et al., 1959).

Radiation

The injurious effect of ionizing radiation on immunity is well demonstrated by increased susceptibility to infections and tumors in irradiated experimental animals (United Nations Scientific Committee on the Effects of Atomic Radiation, 1972). Specific immune responses are primarily affected, although nonspecific factors, such as macrophage and granulocyte function,

may also be altered. Phagocytosis is relatively radioresistant, whereas antigen processing by macrophages is easily impaired by low-dose radiation. The effect on the antibody response depends on antigen dose, frequency of administration, rate, and temporal relationship of irradiation to antigen administration. Although the lag phase may be shortened or lengthened, the antibody response is generally radioresistant.

By contrast, cell-mediated immunity is significantly impaired by radiation. Children with acute lymphocytic leukemia who receive prophylactic craniospinal irradiation have lymphopenia and impaired lymphocyte responses to PHA for more than a year after treatment (Campbell et al., 1973; Petrini et al., 1983). In patients with Hodgkin's disease, T-cell lymphocytopenia and B-cell lymphocytosis persisted for over a year along with impaired in vitro lymphocyte responses to mitogens and antigens persisting for 10 years in some patients (Fuks et al., 1976; Kaplan et al., 1983).

Two studies in patients with intractable rheumatoid arthritis given fractionated total lymphoid irradiation (2000 to 3000 rad) are particularly revealing for their description of the alterations in immunoregulatory T cells (Kotzin et al., 1981; Trentham et al., 1981). Irradiation produced lymphocytopenia, especially among T-helper cells (Table 19–6). Along with a decrease in lymphocyte reactivity to mitogens and antigens, there was a fourfold reduction in the ability of pokeweed mitogen (PWM)–stimulated lymphocytes to secrete IgM and IgG, which was attributable to functional suppressor T lymphocytes (Kotzin et al., 1981). There is evidence suggesting that changes in T-cell subsets depend on the amount of radiation as well as the target area (Uh et al., 1994). Another factor that may influence the CD4:CD8 ratio is the emergence of CD8$^+$ natural killer cells following radiotherapy for Hodgkin's disease (Macklis et al., 1992).

Therapeutic Antibodies

Anti-Lymphocyte Globulin

Anti-lymphocyte globulin (ALG) or anti-thymocyte globulin (ATG) is the purified, concentrated, and sterile γ globulin fraction of animal (usually equine) antiserum specific for human lymphocytes or thymocytes, respectively. A commercial preparation, ATGAM, is available.

ALG is used primarily to inhibit allograft rejection. Because its distribution is largely intravascular, it acts predominantly on circulating lymphocytes; however, the normal recirculation of lymphocytes leads to depletion in lymphoid organs. Immune responses mediated by recirculating long-lived lymphocytes are suppressed by ALG. Thymic-dependent antibody responses are inhibited by ALG given before but not after antigen (Berenbaum, 1979). Secondary antibody responses are generally unaffected (Lance et al., 1973).

ALG abrogates or reduces cutaneous delayed hypersensitivity reactions in previously sensitized individuals (Revillard and Brochier, 1971). Survival of grafts is prolonged, independent of histocompatibility differ-

Table 19–6. Analysis of Lymphocyte Subsets in 11 Patients with Rheumatoid Arthritis Before and After
Total Lymphoid Irradiation

Cell Feature	Controls	Patients	
		Before Therapy	After Therapy
Absolute lymphocyte count (No./mm³)	2038 ± 73*	1621 ± 133	573 ± 84
Percent CD3⁺ cells (absolute No./mm³)	75 ± 2.3 (1520 ± 49)	63 ± 4.6 (922 ± 110)	49 ± 5.2 (345 ± 61)
Percent CD8⁺ cells (absolute No./mm³)	23 ± 2.9 (469 ± 59)	18 ± 2.6 (246 ± 30)	27 ± 3.6 (182 ± 35)
Percent CD4⁺ cells (absolute No./mm³)	43 ± 3.4 (870 ± 69)	46 ± 4.4 (680 ± 85)	23 ± 3.5 (152 ± 31)
Helper:suppressor ratio CD4⁺:CD8⁺	1.72 ± 0.9	2.22 ± 0.1	0.76 ± .23

*Results expressed as the means ± standard errors.
Modified from Kotzin BL, Strober S, Engleman EG, et al. Treatment of intractable rheumatoid arthritis with total lymphoid irradiation. Reprinted with permission from The New England Journal of Medicine 305: 969–976, 1981.

ences (Simmons et al., 1971; Najarian and Simmons, 1971). Responses to vaccines are inhibited in a minority of individuals, and pre-existing antibody titers are unaffected (Pirofsky et al., 1972). In vitro, lymphocytes show an increase in spontaneous DNA synthesis whereas the response to tuberculin is suppressed (Melli et al., 1968).

In addition to its use in organ transplantation, ATG has been shown to be of benefit in diseases, such as aplastic anemia, that are believed to be mediated by suppressive lymphocytes (Champlin et al., 1983). The beneficial effects of ATG in a girl with agranulocytosis have been reported (Chudwin et al., 1983). In contrast to the use of monoclonal antibodies for immunosuppression (see later), ALG poses a slight risk for malignant transformation, particularly for post-transplantation lymphoproliferative disease (Dresdale et al., 1993).

Monoclonal Antibodies Directed Against T Cells

Monoclonal antibodies to a variety of T-cell surface antigens have been used clinically, as an immunosuppressive agent in organ transplantation (Cosimi et al., 1981), as a reagent to deplete mature T cells from histoincompatible bone marrow before administration to congenitally immunodeficient individuals (Reinherz et al., 1982), and in the treatment of acute graft-versus-host disease seen after bone marrow transplantation (Martin et al., 1984; Shearer et al., 1985). The prototype of this group is OKT3, a commercially available mouse monoclonal antibody directed against the epsilon chain of the T-cell receptor. Administration of OKT3 results in profound lymphopenia (Chatenoud et al., 1982). The antibody causes the release of cytokines with resultant fever, gastrointestinal distress, and, rarely, pulmonary edema (Thistlethwaite et al., 1987).

Because conventional immunosuppression of patients who have received transplants results in an increased incidence of solid tumors, lymphomas, and lymphoproliferative disease (Penn, 1981), it is not surprising that use of OKT3 also is associated with an increased incidence of malignancies (Swinnen et al., 1990). New monoclonals, such as anti-CD4, may prove to be useful in conferring long-term tolerance with less toxicity (Cosimi et al., 1990). The use of "humanized" monoclonal anti–T cell antibodies (Woodle et al., 1992)

and toxin-conjugated anti–T cell antibodies (Vitetta et al., 1993) may permit more selective targeting of immunosuppression and, consequently, less nonspecific immune suppression. Nonetheless, the removal of target T cells causes at least a temporary state of immune dysfunction.

Glucocorticoids

Corticosteroids and adrenocorticotropic hormone (ACTH) depress resistance to a wide variety of bacterial, viral, protozoal, and fungal agents (Dale and Petersdorf, 1973). Steroids have many effects on cells, from cytoplasmic binding to inhibition of synthesis of carbohydrate, proteins, and nucleic acids, and, ultimately, cell death (Baxter et al., 1971; Berenbaum, 1979). The biochemical action of corticosteroids on lymphoid cells is not perfectly clear but may relate, at least in part, to the well-defined effects of steroid hormones on eukaryotic cells (O'Malley, 1984), involving steroid-receptor binding to the cell membrane and transplantation of the complex to the cell nucleus. Within the cell nucleus, interaction with DNA occurs through binding of the receptor-steroid complex to 5' flanking regions of target genes, resulting in alteration of transcription (Gronemeyer, 1992). There is variability in susceptibility of different species, and humans are relatively more resistant to the effects of corticosteroids than are a number of animal species (Claman, 1972).

The mechanism of action of glucocorticoids is mediated in part by lipocortins, which inhibit phospholipase A_2, arachidonic acid metabolites, and IL-1 (Lew et al., 1988). The ensuing anti-inflammatory effects are diverse. It has long been appreciated that leukocyte trafficking is also disturbed. Corticosteroids suppress the accumulation of leukocytes at the site of inflammation (Perper et al., 1974); this is partially due to reduced granulocyte adherence to vascular epithelium (Ebert and Barclay, 1952; Fauci et al., 1976). Corticosteroids also block the reticuloendothelial cell clearance of opsonized and non-opsonized particles (Vernon-Roberts, 1972). Corticosteroids cause lymphocytopenia and monocytopenia (Fauci and Dale, 1975), presumably as a result of redistribution of the recirculating lymphocyte and monocyte pools and delaying release of bone marrow monocyte precursors (Fauci et al., 1976).

A prominent lytic effect on lymphocytes has been

well described. Haynes and Fauci (1978) determined that intravenous corticosteroids produced a sudden, but transient, decrease in normal T-helper lymphocytes whereas T-suppressor lymphocytes were unaffected. Silverman and coworkers (1984) documented a transient panlymphopenia occurring 5 hours after high-dose intravenous methylprednisolone in nine children with rheumatic diseases. T-helper cells were much more depressed than were T-suppressor cells. Bactericidal and fungicidal activity of monocytes is reduced (Rinehart et al., 1975), whereas granulocyte function is probably not significantly altered (Fauci et al., 1976).

Large doses of corticosteroids decrease levels of serum immunoglobulins (Butler and Rossen, 1973) and complement components (Atkinson and Frank, 1973). Corticosteroids in moderately low doses do not affect antibody synthesis in humans (Tuchinda et al., 1972). When the effects of single doses of oral prednisone (60 mg) were compared with those of 5 days of oral prednisone (20 mg every 6 hours), there was a greatly prolonged period (60 hours) of depressed pokeweed mitogen–driven immunoglobulin synthesis as measured by an in vitro plaque-forming assay in the volunteers who were treated for 5 days when contrasted to that of the volunteers receiving a single dose (5 hours) (Cupps et al., 1984). Ten hours after completion of the 5-day treatment, isolated blood cells revealed an enrichment in T-suppressor (CD8$^+$) cells that coincided with a depressed synthesis of immunoglobulin by B cells in vitro.

Cutaneous delayed hypersensitivity responses are suppressed by corticosteroids, but lymphocytes from steroid-treated donors transfer the response, suggesting that inflammatory effector cells, primarily macrophages, are inhibited (Weston et al., 1973; Fauci et al., 1976). In patients on alternate-day prednisone therapy, lymphocyte numbers and in vitro responses return to normal on the off-day of therapy and delayed hypersensitivity reactions remain intact (Fauci and Dale, 1975). Renal transplant rejection is blocked by large doses of corticosteroids (Bell et al., 1971).

In vitro studies of lymphocytes from humans treated with corticosteroids indicate that responses to antigens are more easily suppressed than responses to mitogens (Fauci and Dale, 1975; Fauci et al., 1976). A block of T-cell activation is central to the resulting immunosuppression. Interleukin-2 (IL-2) synthesis is inhibited both at the transcription level and through decreased messenger RNA stability (Boumpas et al., 1991). Balow and Rosenthal (1973) showed that corticosteroids suppress the reaction between migration inhibitory factor (MIF) and macrophages rather than MIF synthesis, adding to the evidence that the major effect of corticosteroids is not on lymphocyte function but on effector cells that express cellular immunity. In patients on alternate-day prednisone therapy, lymphocyte numbers and in vitro responses return to normal on the day-off therapy and delayed hypersensitivity reactions remain intact (Fauci and Dale, 1975).

In summary, the main anti-inflammatory actions of corticosteroids result from effects on the function and distribution of the nonspecific cellular effectors of inflammation such as macrophages, monocytes, and granulocytes. These effects include:

- Decreased production of proinflammatory cytokines (IL-1, IL-6, and tumor necrosis factor [TNF])
- Inhibition of arachidonic acid metabolism and production of the prostaglandins and leukotrienes
- Inhibition of platelet activating factor production by the elaboration of lipocortin, which inhibits phospholipase A$_2$
- Blunting of the response of effector cells, such as macrophages and monocytes, to the enhancing effects of interferon-γ and MIF produced by lymphoid cells

In addition, significant inhibition of the expression of class II MHC antigens and intercellular adhesion molecules modulates accumulation of phagocytic inflammatory effectors and the distribution of lymphoid elements (Boumpas et al., 1993).

Cyclosporine

Cyclosporine is the prototype of a powerful class of drugs that confer immunosuppression by inhibiting intracellular signaling of T cells (Kahan, 1989). FK506 and rapamycin are additional drugs within the same group (Sigal and Dumont, 1992). These differ from glucocorticoids and cytotoxic drugs by their increased immunologic specificity. Cyclosporine binds intracellularly to a cyclophilin, which allows subsequent interaction with calcineurin, a calcium-calmodulin–dependent phosphatase. Inhibition of calcineurin results in inhibition of IL-2 production through an interaction with the IL-2 promoter (O'Keefe et al., 1992). This results in reversible inhibition of T cell–mediated alloimmune and autoimmune responses.

Cyclosporine has played a significant role in the development of successful organ transplantation. Patients receiving kidney, liver, heart, and lung transplants have all benefited from its use (Kahan, 1989). Several autoimmune conditions are ameliorated by cyclosporine, including uveitis, psoriasis, and insulin-dependent diabetes (Nussenblatt et al., 1983; Ellis et al., 1986; Bougneres et al., 1988). Because of the specificity of cyclosporine, the broad spectrum of infections seen in most immunosuppression regimens is avoided. The use of cyclosporine in solid organ transplantation has reduced the incidence of acute bacterial and fungal infections without altering the risk of viral infection (Canadian Multicentre Transplant Study Group, 1986; Showstack et al., 1989). Although there is a relative sparing of B-cell function, inhibition of antibody responses to some T cell–independent antigens occurs (O'Garra et al., 1986). Macrophage function, including antigen presentation, phagocytosis, and cytotoxicity, is unaffected (Esa et al., 1988; Granelli-Piperno et al., 1988).

The most common toxicity of cyclosporine is renal dysfunction and hypertension. Bone marrow suppression that complicates the use of many other immunosuppressive agents is notably absent. As with other therapies that interfere with T-lymphocyte function, the risk of lymphoproliferative disorders is increased. Malatack and colleagues (1991) described 12 children with lymphoproliferative disease related to administration of cyclosporine following liver transplantation. Five of these patients died. Tumors developed as early as 10 weeks and as late as 7 years after transplantation.

Cockburn and Krupp (1989) reported a 28 times higher prevalence of lymphomas in organ transplant recipients treated with cyclosporine compared with a 34- to 59-fold increased risk in patients receiving conventional immunosuppressive therapy. Their data suggested that the latency period for the development of lymphoproliferative disorders is shorter for cyclosporine-treated patients compared with patients receiving conventional therapy. In addition, the occurrence of other malignancies was increased in patients receiving cyclosporine. The most frequently noted neoplasms involved the skin, with a disproportionate percentage being Kaposi's sarcoma.

Cytotoxic Drugs

Cyclophosphamide

The alkylating agent cyclophosphamide cross-links complementary DNA strands, effectively inhibiting cell replication. In addition, in large doses it has a direct lympholytic effect. In experimental animals, cyclophosphamide decreases anti-DNA titers in New Zealand black/New Zealand white (NZB/NZW) mice, decreases small lymphocytes (immunologic memory cells) in NZB mice, inhibits new and ongoing antibody synthesis, suppresses skin graft rejection in animals, and suppresses graft-versus-host disease in mice (reviewed in Bunch and O'Duffy, 1980; Kovarsky, 1983). In humans, cyclophosphamide results in decreased immunoglobulin production, decreased B cell and T cell function, and inhibited T-suppressor cell function. In children with minimal-change nephrotic syndrome who were given 2.5 mg/kg/day of cyclophosphamide for 8 weeks, a lymphopenia was produced, particularly among the helper (CD4$^+$) T cells (Feehally et al., 1984). These changes in CD4$^+$ cells were believed to be due not to the disease process itself but to the drug therapy with cyclophosphamide.

Cyclophosphamide is most effective during the early phases of the immune response. It also has anti-inflammatory effects (Stevens and Willoughby, 1969). In guinea pigs, there is evidence for a restricted effect on B cells (Turk and Poulter, 1972); in humans, there is effective suppression of T cells as evidenced by prolongation of graft survival (Starzl et al., 1971). Large doses (3.5 to 9 mg/kg/day) effectively suppress antibody response (Santos et al., 1971), and lower doses prevent cutaneous delayed hypersensitivity (Townes et al., 1976). Massive doses suppress bone marrow rejection in patients with leukemia (Santos et al., 1971). Alepa and colleagues (1970) reported inhibition of in vitro lymphocyte responses to PHA and pokeweed mitogen (PWM). Clinical application of cyclophosphamide is limited by the severe toxicity, which can manifest as granulocytopenia and hemorrhagic cystitis (Kovarsky, 1983).

Methotrexate

Methotrexate binds to folic reductase, blocking recycling of folic acid derivatives and thereby affecting DNA synthesis in late S phase (Jolivet et al., 1983). There is little or no action on resting cells. It also has potent anti-inflammatory properties, such as inhibiting the response to histamine (Currey, 1971). The effect of methotrexate on antibody response varies with the dose and frequency of administration (Berenbaum, 1979). Methotrexate does not particularly suppress delayed hypersensitivity reactions (Santos et al., 1964).

Purine Antagonists

The purine analogs *azathioprine* and *6-mercaptopurine* (an azathioprine metabolite) block both the *de novo* and salvage pathways of purine synthesis resulting in impairment of DNA and RNA synthesis (Chan et al., 1987). Any immune response that is dependent on cell proliferation may be inhibited, depending on the dose of drug and timing of the administration of antigen (Schwartz, 1965). In addition to specific immune responses, the inflammatory response may be suppressed (Page et al., 1964). The primary antibody response is more easily inhibited than the secondary response (Maibach and Epstein, 1965; Hersh et al., 1965). IgG antibody is more easily inhibited than IgM (Swanson and Schwartz, 1967). Induction of delayed hypersensitivity is inhibited or delayed (Swanson and Schwartz, 1967), whereas reactions in previously sensitized individuals are usually unaffected (Hersh et al., 1965; Maibach and Epstein, 1965). Allograft rejection is variably suppressed, depending on the organ grafted and histocompatibility differences (Starzl et al., 1967). Abdou and others (1973) reported depression of the in vitro lymphocyte response to PWM but not to PHA in patients receiving 2.5 to 4 mg/kg of azathioprine.

Anticonvulsant Drugs

Anticonvulsant drugs, principally *phenytoin* (Dilantin), produce several untoward effects on the immune system, resulting in serum sickness (Josephs et al., 1980); lymphocytotoxic antibodies (Ooi et al., 1977); selective and reversible (off-drug) IgA deficiency (Gilhus and Aarli, 1981) (see Chapter 14); and transient hypogammaglobulinemia, decreased antibody formation, and abnormal suppressor cell activity (Dosch et al., 1982). In addition, reversible cases of agranulocytosis (Sharafuddin et al., 1991) and IgG subclass deficiency (Ishizaka et al., 1992) have been reported.

Guerra and coworkers (1986) reported a healthy 28-year-old man who had been given phenytoin for convulsions secondary to head trauma. Serum sickness developed, followed by permanent hypogammaglobulinemia, deficiency of functional antibodies, and paucity of B lymphocytes. In addition, recurrent respiratory infections, indistinguishable from common variable immunodeficiency, occurred.

Despite these documented changes, some authors caution against routine immune surveillance in asymptomatic patients on phenytoin (Burks et al., 1989). From the scattered case reports, these phenytoin effects seem to represent true drug hypersensitivity, occurring only in individuals whose immune systems are predisposed to react to the drug. From the prospective study of 118 patients (Bardana et al., 1983) with epilepsy, it seems that even prior to treatment with phenytoin, patients with idiopathic epilepsy showed an increased incidence of low serum IgA concentration (13.5% below lowest normal value versus 2.5% for controls). After treatment for 18 months, this percentage increased to 33% (versus 4% for controls). Thus, patients with idiopathic convulsive disorders may be predisposed to immunologic disturbances. This syndrome is also discussed in Chapters 11 and 14.

INFECTIOUS DISEASES

Bacterial Infections

Contradictory reports on PMN function in patients with bacterial infection reflect variations in host, type and stage of infection, treatment, and methodology. Increased migration into Rebuck's windows (Perillie et al., 1962) and increased chemotaxis in vitro (Hill et al., 1974a) are contrasted with decreased chemotaxis in other studies (Mowat and Baum, 1971; McCall et al., 1971). Reticuloendothelial clearance of ^{131}I-aggregated albumin may be increased, decreased, or normal in patients with severe infections (Wagner et al., 1963). Phagocytosis may be normal (Weinstein and Young, 1976) or depressed (McCall et al., 1971). Some patients may show a slight but significant transient impairment of bactericidal function (Copeland et al., 1971; McCall et al., 1971; Solberg and Hellum, 1972). Results will depend upon the test organism (Messner et al., 1973; Weinstein and Young, 1976) and may reflect antiphagocytic surface determinants (Howard and Glynn, 1971). In some studies, deficiencies of opsonins appear to play a role (Weinstein and Young, 1976) (see Chapter 15).

Selected bacteria can induce specific immune function abnormalities. For example, lipoarabinomannan (LAM), a mycobacterial cell wall component, can suppress in vitro T-cell proliferative responses to mitogens and antigens in patients with leprosy and in healthy individuals (Kaplan et al., 1987). Furthermore, LAM inhibits antigen-induced proliferation of CD4$^+$ T-cell clones specific for influenza virus (Moreno et al., 1988).

The immunosuppressive effects of LAM may be mediated by CD8$^+$ suppressor T cells (Mehra et al., 1982, 1984; Kaplan et al., 1987). However, modulation of lymphokine function also has been implicated. Decreased levels of circulating IL-2 and interferon-γ have been reported in patients with lepromatous leprosy (Nogueira et al., 1983; Makonkawkeyoon et al., 1990). In one study, LAM exhibited a down-regulatory effect on mitogen-induced accumulation of mRNAs for IL-2, IL-3, granulocyte-macrophage colony–stimulating factor (GM-CSF), and IL-2α receptor (Chujor et al., 1992).

Given the ability of mycobacteria to survive within host macrophages, it is likely that the effects of LAM include impairment of macrophage activation, antigen processing, and mycobacterial killing.

Superantigens are proteins made by microorganisms that bind specifically to class II major histocompatibility complex (MHC) molecules (Schlievert, 1993) and activate T cells directly (see Chapters 2 and 4). The best characterized superantigens are those belonging to the family of pyrogenic toxins produced by *S. aureus* and the group A streptococci, including staphylococcal toxic shock syndrome toxin-1, the staphylococcal enterotoxins, and streptococcal pyrogenic exotoxins. Superantigens stimulate polyclonal proliferation of all T cells bearing particular β-chain variable regions, with resultant massive lymphokine secretion and eventual cell death. Several systemic illnesses, including toxic shock syndrome, toxic shock-like syndrome, and scarlet fever, result from host effects of these superantigens.

Superantigens can induce nonresponsiveness in murine T cells either by clonal deletion (White et al., 1989) or functional inactivation (Rammensee et al., 1989). Experimental evidence suggests that *S. aureus* enterotoxins that are able to stimulate lymphoproliferation can also induce antigen-specific nonresponsiveness in human CD4$^+$ T cells (O'Hehir and Lamb, 1990). A decrease in specific mitogen-activated V-β chain–containing T-cell numbers has been described in animals after administration of staphylococcal enterotoxins (MacDonald et al., 1991). A decrease in circulating immune cells as well as depletion of immune cells from the spleen and lymph nodes has been observed in some humans with toxic shock syndrome or toxic shock-like syndrome (Larkin et al., 1982; Jackson et al., 1991). Interaction between pyrogenic toxins and endotoxin has been implicated in the pathogenesis of this immune cell lethality (Leonard and Schlievert, 1992).

Fungal Infections

Like certain bacteria, fungi have been implicated as a cause of immunosuppression in animals and humans. Administration of killed *C. albicans* to mice results in transient depression of T-cell mitogen responses (Rivas and Rogers, 1983). In addition, animals given killed *Candida* or a polysaccharide extract of *Candida* develop increased susceptibility to infection with *Mycobacterium tuberculosis* (Mankiewicz et al., 1959; Mankiewicz and Liivak, 1960). Chronic mucocutaneous candidiasis has been associated with depressed delayed hypersensitivity responses; amphotericin B therapy may result in restoration of immune responsiveness (Paterson et al., 1971). Other fungal infections, including disseminated histoplasmosis, also have been associated with T cell immunosuppression (Nickerson et al., 1981).

Parasitic Infections

Parasitism is an important cause of immune response abnormalities in individuals in developing countries. Patients with malaria develop impaired humoral immune function with poor antibody responses to tetanus toxoid (Greenwood et al., 1972), *Salmonella typhi* (Greenwood et al., 1972), pneumococcal vaccine (McBride et al., 1977), and meningococcal vaccine (Williamson and Greenwood, 1978). The severity of the immune defect correlates with the degree of parasitism. Cell-mediated immunity, as reflected by cutaneous delayed hypersensitivity and reactivity to T cell mitogens, appears to be normal.

T-suppressor cells, which decrease lymphocyte responses to mitogens and schistosome antigens, have been observed in human splenic tissue obtained from patients with *Schistosoma mansoni* infection (Ellner et al., 1980). Adult schistosomes evade destruction by sensitized lymphocytes and antibodies directed against molecules expressed on the exterior surface of the intestinal epithelium of the parasite, despite intimate association of antigens and immune effectors within the host's vascular system. Virtually no inflammation is observed around viable adult parasites. This may be accomplished by masking parasite antigens by absorption of host molecules (Allison et al., 1974).

Infection with *Trypanosoma cruzi* (the cause of Chagas' disease) has been associated with production of molecules on the parasite's surface that block complement activation (Rimoldi et al., 1988). *Trypanosoma brucei gambiense* (the cause of African trypanosomiasis) infection has been linked to depression of both humoral and cellular immune responses. Finally, patients infected with certain filarial nematodes, including *Wuchereria bancrofti* and *Onchocerca volvulus*, have depressed lymphocyte proliferative responses to soluble parasite antigens, associated with an inability to produce IL-1, IL-2, and interferon-γ (Nutman et al., 1987; Elkhalifa et al., 1991; Soboslay et al., 1992). Treatment of onchocerciasis with ivermectin may reverse this immunosuppression (Soboslay et al., 1992).

Viral Infections

HIV Infection

Human immunodeficiency virus (HIV), the best known example of a virus capable of causing immunosuppression, is discussed in detail in Chapter 18.

Measles

Historically, measles provided the first evidence of virus-induced immunosuppression. It was observed early in the century that the tuberculin skin response was temporarily blunted during the course of natural measles (von Pirquit, 1908). It is now known that measles can infect a variety of immune cells, including monocytes, T cells, and B cells, and can suppress NK cell activity, immunoglobulin synthesis, and antigen-mediated T-cell proliferation (Casali et al., 1984; McChesney et al., 1986; Griffin et al., 1990; Leopardi et al., 1993). The result of this immune suppression is an increased risk of infection with other organisms. The immune suppression of measles generally is transient but may persist in some individuals with severe disease.

Influenza

Epidemiologic studies indicate that there is an increased risk of systemic and pulmonary bacterial infections during influenza epidemics (Mills, 1984). Similarly, the incidence of bacterial otitis media is increased markedly by concomitant infection with several respiratory viruses, including respiratory syncytial virus, influenza, and adenovirus (Henderson et al., 1982). Acute influenza produces transient lymphopenia, primarily affecting T cells. Immune abnormalities include diminished lymphocyte proliferation (Lewis et al., 1986; del Gobbo et al., 1989), increased NK cell activity caused by interferon production (Ennis et al., 1981), and generation of suppressor lymphocytes that inhibit IL-2 production (del Gobbo et al., 1990). In addition, influenza infection causes secretion of IL-1 and TNF (Vacheron et al., 1990), and expansion of the subpopulation of circulating T cells (Carding, 1990).

Adenovirus Infection

Adenovirus infection has been associated with a deficiency in the production of and the response to IL-2 (Berencsi et al., 1991) as well as an overall diminution in host response attributable to effects on macrophage function (Berencsi et al., 1985). One adenovirus-produced protein inhibits the cellular actions of interferons (Mathews and Shenk, 1991), and another binds MHC class I antigens and prevents cytotoxicity by CD8+ lymphocytes (Wold and Gooding, 1991).

Herpes Infections

Infection with herpesviruses can result in significant immunosuppression. Simultaneous infection with multiple herpesviruses or a herpesvirus and a disparate organism has been reported, including cytomegalovirus and herpes simplex virus infection (Weiss et al., 1987), cytomegalovirus and *P. carinii* pneumonia (Pahwa et al., 1983) and Epstein-Barr virus and disseminated *C. albicans* infection (Gudnason et al., 1990). In addition, an epidemiologic association has been noted between herpesvirus infections and opportunistic infections (Schooley et al., 1983).

Epstein-Barr Virus

The immunologic changes that occur in association with Epstein-Barr virus infection are complex. In vitro T-cell anergy occurs during acute infectious mononucleosis, possibly as a result of T cell receptor–specific impairment (Perez-Blas et al., 1992). T-cell regulatory changes and secreted IL-10 (Burdin et al., 1993) lead to polyclonal expansion of B cells and enhanced immunoglobulin production. Cells transformed by Epstein-Barr virus also secrete a homolog of IL-10 that acts as an inhibitory cytokine (Hsu et al., 1990). An increased number of phenotypic NK cells has been reported in individuals with infectious mononucleosis, but NK function is decreased (Williams et al., 1989). The immunologic alterations induced by Epstein-Barr virus usually are transient but, rarely, can lead to long-term immune dysregulation and clinical sequelae (Joncas et al., 1989) (see Chapter 27).

Cytomegalovirus

Cytomegalovirus induces immune suppression through productive infection of monocytes (Carney and Hirsch, 1981; Weinshenker et al., 1988). Cytomegalovirus induces an inhibitor of IL-1 that may account for most of the immune-suppressive effects (Rodgers et al., 1985). As a consequence, infected monocytes are less able to present antigens, such as tetanus toxoid and *C. albicans* to autologous lymphocytes (Buchmeier and Cooper, 1989). Carriers of cytomegalovirus have elevated numbers of circulating NK cells with suppressor activity (Gratama et al., 1989). Some infants with congenital cytomegalovirus infection have a long-term defect in cell-mediated immunity with impaired lymphocyte proliferation (Pass et al., 1983).

Herpes Simplex 1 and 2

Numerous studies document immune suppression after infection with herpes simplex 1 or 2. After selective infection of T-helper cells, the T-suppressor cell population is expanded (Whittum et al., 1984), resulting in impaired lymphocyte proliferation and decreased antibody production. In addition, herpes simplex glycoproteins can inhibit complement-mediated cytolysis (Harris et al., 1990) and bind the Fc portion of IgG, preventing Fc-mediated phagocytosis (Bell et al., 1990). Individuals who suffer recurrent herpes simplex lesions may have a number of immunologic abnormalities, including lymphopenia, impaired neutrophil phagocytosis, and exaggerated suppressor lymphocyte activity (Doutlik et al., 1989). It is hypothesized that heightened suppressor activity may inhibit normal cell-mediated immunity and allow frequent lesion recurrences (Vestey et al., 1989).

Human Herpesvirus 6

A newly identified herpesvirus, human herpesvirus 6, is capable of direct infection of NK cells (Lusso et al., 1993), possibly leading to immune suppression. Furthermore, the virus can cause up-regulation of the CD4 molecule on CD8+ lymphocytes, theoretically rendering the individual more susceptible to HIV infection (Lusso et al., 1991). Additional studies are needed to define the role of this virus in producing immune suppression.

INFILTRATIVE AND HEMATOLOGIC DISEASES

Langerhans Cell Histiocytosis

Abt and Denholz (1936) described a syndrome based on cases reported by Letterer and Siwe characterized by hepatosplenomegaly, generalized lymphadenopathy, hemorrhagic cutaneous manifestations, anemia, and bone changes occurring in infancy. Subsequently, investigators linked histiocytosis X, Hand-Schüller-Christian disease, eosinophilic granuloma of bone, Letterer-Siwe disease, and self-healing reticulohistiocytosis as a spectrum of histiocytic syndromes (Favara, 1991). Histiocytosis with diffuse involvement of the reticuloendothelial system (RES) occurs predominantly in infants and is usually progressively fatal, whereas focal histiocytosis of bone or soft tissue is usually a benign self-limited process (Newton and Hamoudi, 1973; Lahey, 1975). Despite the clinical heterogeneity of these syndromes, the uniformity of the pathologic features in all forms of this disease strongly suggests a common basis.

The lesions consist of histiocytes that resemble the dendritic antigen-presenting Langerhans' cell of the skin and other organs. Some studies indicate that Langerhans' cell histiocytosis is a clonal proliferative disease with highly variable biologic behavior (Willman et al., 1994) rather than a reactive process (Komp, 1987). The hypothesis that the clonal proliferation seen in histiocytosis is driven by viral infection is not supported by DNA studies (McClain et al., 1994). Histiocytosis is also discussed in Chapters 16 and 27.

Leikin and associates (1973) measured immunoglobulins, delayed cutaneous hypersensitivity, and in vitro lymphocyte responses to mitogens and allogeneic cells in six infants with Letterer-Siwe disease. Despite secondary abnormalities of the thymus and lymphoid tissues at autopsy, most immunologic studies were essentially normal. Subsequently, 14 children with histiocytosis were studied before initiation of therapy (Martin-Mateos et al., 1991). Patients with early disease demonstrated slightly elevated serum immunoglobulin levels and decreased CD8+ lymphocytes. Children with advanced disease showed hypogammaglobulinemia and lymphopenia. Maennle and colleagues (1991) reported three children with sinus histiocytosis. Immune abnormalities of hypogammaglobulinemia, decreased lymphocyte proliferation, and cutaneous anergy correlated with a history of recurrent infections. An excellent review is available (Egeler and D'Angio, 1995).

Omenn Syndrome

By contrast, several infants with some features of Letterer-Siwe disease whose immunologic function has been markedly or variably defective have been described (Omenn, 1965; Barth et al., 1972; Cederbaum et al., 1974; Ochs et al., 1974) (see Chapter 12). A diagnosis of combined immunodeficiency has been established at autopsy in some of these children. A chronic maternal-fetal graft-versus-host reaction has been postulated to explain the phenomenon (Cederbaum et al., 1974). Thus, all infants presenting with the clinical syndrome of histiocytosis require careful histologic, immunologic, and genetic investigation.

Immunologic studies of more than 100 members of the original kindred with this autosomal recessive syndrome revealed that two affected children had abnormalities of T cell subsets; similarly, many unaffected family members, including obligate heterozygotes, had decreased CD4 (helper) and increased CD8 (suppressor) lymphocytes (Karol et al., 1983). It is thought that Omenn syndrome represents a variant form of severe combined immunodeficiency diseases (SCID) in which immature lymphocytes fail to completely differentiate into mature T cells and B cells. Bone marrow transplantation is often curative (Gomez et al., 1995).

Sarcoidosis

Sarcoidosis is a chronic, multisystem, granulomatous disorder that most commonly affects young adults. Although essentially all organs of the body may be affected by sarcoidosis, the lungs are most commonly involved and account for the most morbidity and mortality (Thomas and Hunninghake, 1987). Although the cause of sarcoidosis is unknown, the host immune response clearly plays a major role in the pathogenesis. Sarcoidosis demonstrates a dichotomy of heightened immune activity at sites of disease activity and impaired responses elsewhere (Hunninghake et al., 1979). The diagnosis rests on characteristic clinical and radiologic findings combined with histologic evidence of noncaseating epithelioid cell granulomas in more than one organ. In the past, a positive Kveim-Siltzbach skin test has been used for diagnosis, but possible contamination of antigen by infectious viral particles has limited its usefulness.

Since sarcoidosis in children is relatively uncommon (McGovern and Merritt, 1956; Jasper and Denny, 1968; Waldman and Stiehm, 1977; Pattishall and Kendig, 1990), immunologic studies are largely limited to adult subjects. Immunologic characterization of the disease includes lymphocytic activation within the lungs (Hunninghake and Crystal, 1981) and depressed cellular immunity in peripheral blood lymphocytes (Pasquali et al., 1985). Despite these aberrations, patients with sarcoidosis generally do not show an increased susceptibility to infection. Pascual and colleagues (1973) found elevated serum lysozyme levels in sarcoidosis that correlated with disease activity. Macrophages are the likely source of the lysozyme. Serum angiotensin-converting enzyme level is elevated in 60% of patients with sarcoidosis, but it also is elevated in many other disorders (Bascom and Johns, 1986).

Etiology

A number of agents have been isolated from sarcoid tissue in the search for the cause, but these findings have not been reproducible (Mitchell and Scadding, 1974). Mitchell and Rees (1969) reported the transfer of granulomatous reactions from human sarcoid tissue to mice. These results have been reproduced by some (Taub and Siltzbach, 1972; Mitchell and Rees, 1976) but not by others (Iwai and Takahashi, 1976). Although viruses, particularly of the herpes group, have been a prime suspect based on sero-epidemiologic evidence (Byrne et al., 1973), conclusive support for a viral etiology is lacking (Steplewski, 1976). Siltzbach (1976) has suggested that the transfer experiments are also consistent with transmission by lymphokines or lymphocyte activation.

Of the many etiologic factors that have been considered, mycobacterial infections have received the greatest amount of attention. However, attempts to fulfill Koch's postulates have failed (Bowman et al., 1972).

A further possibility is that both mycobacterial and viral infection may interact to produce sarcoidosis. James and Neville (1977) suggested that a virus-induced T-cell defect combined with an exposure to mycobacteria might produce sarcoidosis.

Genetic factors that contribute to the pathogenesis of sarcoidosis have been suggested by the marked differences between the prevalence of sarcoidosis in black and white Americans. Blacks are affected eight times more frequently than whites, and disease in blacks can be more severe (Johns et al., 1976). The genetic influence of MHC loci is suggested by studies that show an association of specific manifestations of sarcoidosis with particular MHC antigens. For example, erythema nodosum and arthritis are noted frequently in patients with human leukocyte antigen (HLA)-B8 (James and Neville, 1977; Guyatt et al., 1982), and uveitis is noted in those with HLA-B27 (Scharf and Zonis, 1980).

A potential role of environmental factors in the pathogenesis of sarcoidosis is indicated by the similar clinical and pathologic characteristics of berylliosis and sarcoidosis (Thomas and Hunninghake, 1987). The mechanisms by which beryllium induces granuloma formation are not known. It is thought that beryllium binds to endogenous proteins to render them immunogenic. The possibility that beryllium may persist for long periods of time could explain the chronic nature of immune activation.

B and T Lymphocytes

The absolute number of circulating lymphocytes is usually decreased in patients with sarcoidosis (Hedfors et al., 1974; Ramachandar et al., 1975; Tannenbaum et al., 1976). Hedfors and coworkers (1974) report a modest but significant deficiency of T cells as measured by E rosettes, an observation confirmed in other laboratories (Kalden et al., 1976; Veien et al., 1976). Daniele and Rowlands (1976) have demonstrated antibodies to T lymphocytes in the sera of 9 of 15 patients with sarcoidosis. Circulating B cells as identified by surface membrane immunoglobulin, erythrocyte antibody (EA), or erythrocyte antibody and complement (EAC) rosettes are normal (Kalden et al., 1976; Hedfors, 1976) or increased (Hedfors, 1975; Fernandez et al., 1976). Kataria and colleagues (1976) found increased numbers of lymphocytes with surface membrane immunoglobulin but normal numbers of EAC rosette-forming lymphocytes.

Humoral Immunity

Serum immunoglobulin levels may be normal in sarcoidosis, but IgG is increased in about half the patients (Blasi and Olivieri, 1974; James et al., 1975). Other deviations in immunoglobulins are not uncommon (Celikoglu et al., 1971). Buckley and associates (1966) reported significant elevations of IgA and IgG but not of IgM or C3 in a series of 16 patients with active sarcoidosis. Low levels of IgD (Buckley and Trayer, 1972) and high levels of IgE (Bergmann et al., 1972) have been recorded. The variability does not consistently reflect disease activity or staging (James et al., 1975), but ethnicity may affect results, since IgA and IgG have been reported to be higher in normal black patients (Goldstein et al., 1969). Levels of secretory immunoglobulins in patients with pulmonary sarcoidosis are similar to those in other bronchopulmonary diseases (Blasi and Olivieri, 1974).

With the exception of the failure to form antibody to mycobacteriophage (Mankiewicz, 1967), patients with sarcoidosis generally exhibit normal or accentuated antibody responses. Carnes and Raffel (1949) reported that complement-fixing antibodies to mycobacterial antigens were comparable in patients with sarcoidosis and tuberculin-positive controls. Using the Middlebrook-Dubos test for antibody to mycobacteria, Flemming and others (1951) found a normal response in patients with sarcoidosis. The antibody response to typhoid and pertussis vaccines (Sones and Israel, 1954) and tetanus toxoid (Greenwood et al., 1958) is essentially normal in sarcoidosis, although the primary response to tetanus toxoid is diminished. Quinn and colleagues (1955) reported normal titers of mumps antibody in patients with sarcoidosis. Sones and Israel (1954) found normal immediate wheal-and-flare reactions and normal Prausnitz-Küstner responses.

The presence of high titers of antibody to Epstein-Barr virus has been noted (Hirshaut et al., 1970; Hedfors, 1975), but the lack of difference in titers in acute and chronic sarcoidosis argues against Epstein-Barr virus as the causative agent (James et al., 1975). Increased antibody titers to other members of the herpes group (Wahren et al., 1971) and other viruses (Byrne et al., 1973) have also been recorded. The frequency of autoantibodies to gastric, thyroid, mitochondrial, and nucleic acid antigens was increased in one study (Veien et al., 1976) and normal in another (James et al., 1975). Hedfors and Norberg (1974) used a platelet aggregation assay to demonstrate immune complexes in 6 of 26 patients with sarcoidosis. Other investigators have less commonly found immune complexes (Agnello et al., 1970).

Serum complement, reflecting an acute phase reaction, may be increased in active sarcoidosis (Buckley et al., 1966) but CH_{50}, C2, and C4 levels are generally normal in subacute and chronic cases (Simececk et al., 1971; Scheffer et al., 1971).

Cutaneous Delayed Hypersensitivity

Decreased cutaneous delayed hypersensitivity reactions to tuberculin were first observed by Jadassohn in 1914 and Schaumann in 1917, a period in which most adults tested had positive tuberculin reactions. These results with tuberculin and purified protein derivative (PPD) have been confirmed, although the percentage of nonreactors has varied (Citron, 1957; Sones and Israel, 1954). In the pediatric age group, 14 of 86 patients had positive tuberculin test results (Jasper and Denny, 1968). Citron (1957) and Siltzbach (1969) have shown that increasing the test strength of tuberculin from 10 to 100 tuberculin units (TU) significantly increased the number of reactors. The depression of de-

layed hypersensitivity reactions appears to be an acquired defect, since the conversion from a positive to a negative test in newly acquired sarcoidosis and a return of reactivity with remission have been observed (Nitter, 1953; Sommer, 1964; Israel and Sones, 1967).

Israel and Sones (1966, 1967) noted that tuberculin anergy persisted in most patients with sarcoidosis during remission; furthermore, only 1 of 12 patients given BCG remained tuberculin-positive after 12 weeks. Israel and Sones (1966), using a BCG vaccine that converted 95% of controls, reported a low degree of reactivity in patients with sarcoidosis and noted three patients in whom conversion had not occurred with BCG prior to the development of their disease. This suggested that the immunologic defect might be the basis for the disease.

However, more extensive data obtained in a BCG and vole bacillus vaccination study in Britain indicated no preceding impairment of delayed hypersensitivity in sarcoidosis. Sutherland and associates (1965) found that the incidence of intrathoracic sarcoidosis was similar in vaccinated subjects and tuberculin-negative or tuberculin-positive unvaccinated controls. They concluded that the incidence of sarcoidosis (1.49/10,000) was not related to the level of previous tuberculin sensitivity but that tuberculin sensitivity tended to be depressed in sarcoidosis at and shortly after the onset of disease.

In other studies, the loss of tuberculin reactivity is relative, since the addition of cortisone to the antigen and the use of depot tuberculin increase the number of reactors (Pyke and Scadding, 1952). Patients with sarcoidosis also have a decreased response to mumps, coccidioidin, *Trichophyton,* and pertussis (Friou, 1952; Sones and Israel, 1954), indicating a broad spectrum of impairment of cutaneous delayed hypersensitivity reactions. Epstein and Mayock (1957) found that patients with sarcoidosis had normal contact sensitivity to the potent allergen pentadecyl catechol of poison ivy. However, a diminished response was observed with the less potent chemical sensitizers dinitrochlorobenzene (DNCB) and paranitrosodimethyl aniline.

Skin allograft rejection was normal in five patients with sarcoidosis (Snyder, 1964). In this study, skin tests to PPD, histoplasmin, blastomycin, and coccidioidin were negative, but all patients rejected their grafts by day 14. Lymphocytes from patients with sarcoidosis produce smaller graft-versus-host reactions in immunosuppressed rats (Topilsky et al., 1972).

Further insight into the immunologic defect in sarcoidosis comes from experiments on the transfer of delayed hypersensitivity reactions with viable leukocytes (Urbach et al., 1952; Sones and Israel, 1954) or transfer factor (Lawrence and Zweiman, 1968). In patients with sarcoidosis who receive leukocytes from tuberculin-sensitive donors, a positive skin test result develops, excluding a cutaneous abnormality and suggesting that the defect is in the leukocyte. In five of seven patients with sarcoidosis, transfer factor conferred a transient local immunity but systemic transfer was observed in only two of the five. Horsmanheimo and Virolainen (1976) reported transfer of systemic tuberculin sensitivity with transfer factor in six of eight patients with sarcoidosis.

In Vitro Cell-Mediated Immunity

Hirschhorn and coworkers (1964) showed that peripheral blood leukocytes from patients with sarcoidosis had an impaired response to PHA. Buckley and associates (1966) found a significantly decreased response to PHA in sick patients with sarcoidosis, whereas the lymphocytic response from patients in remission was normal. Normal responses to PHA were reported (Girard et al., 1971; Fernandez et al., 1976; Hedfors, 1976), whereas other studies indicated some impairment (Siltzbach et al., 1970; Topilsky et al., 1972; Kataria et al., 1973). Impaired responses to concanavalin A were reported by Hedfors (1976) but were normal in other studies (Girard et al., 1971). Hedfors (1975) and Horsmanheimo (1974) have reported an impaired lymphocyte response to PPD in patients with sarcoidosis, but other patients with stage I disease or extrapulmonary manifestations had normal in vitro responses (Kalden et al., 1976). Belcher and colleagues (1974) and Mangi and associates (1974) demonstrated a serum inhibitor that reduced the in vitro response of normal lymphocytes to PHA, *Candida,* and mumps. Several investigators have reported increased thymidine incorporation by unstimulated lymphocytes in culture. Fernandez and colleagues (1976) suggested that increased spontaneous DNA synthesis might be due to replicating B cells.

Originally, Kveim preparations stimulated blast transformation of lymphocytes from patients with sarcoidosis (Hirschhorn et al., 1964; Schweiger and Mandi, 1967), but studies with thymidine incorporation were negative (Siltzbach et al., 1970; Izumi et al., 1973). However, Zweiman and Israel (1976) reported positive proliferative responses in 14 of 45 patients with variation caused by the source of Kveim material. There was no correlation with in vivo Kveim reactivity, clinical stage, or lymphocyte response to other antigens in vitro. Inhibition of leukocyte migration with Kveim material has yielded conflicting results (Brostoff and Walker, 1971; Becker et al., 1972; Topilsky et al., 1972; Williams et al., 1972; Zweiman and Israel, 1976).

Immunoregulation

Hunninghake and Crystal (1981) have demonstrated an imbalance of local immunoregulatory T lymphocytes in patients with active sarcoidosis (i.e., those with high-intensity alveolitis). Their findings demonstrated a relative excess of T-helper lymphocytes (CD4[+]) in lung (obtained by bronchoalveolar lavage). Thus, the CD4:CD8 ratio of lung cells was high (10.8:1 versus 1.8:1 for control), and the CD4[+] cell population was shown to secrete a monocyte chemotactic factor that stimulated granuloma formation and polyclonal B-cell activation. In addition, the CD4:CD8 ratio of lymphocytes in the peripheral blood of patients was low (0.81 versus 1.9 for control). T cells obtained from lungs of patients with active disease spontaneously replicate in

tissue culture and release IL-2, which further stimulates T-cell replication (Pinkston et al., 1983; Hunninghake et al., 1983). An increased expression of the IL-2 receptor on pulmonary lymphocytes also supports the concept that the accumulation of lymphocytes in the lung may be due in part to in situ proliferation (Muller-Quernheim et al., 1989). T cells also secrete factors that produce a local polyclonal activation of B cells, resulting in large amounts of immunoglobulin in fluid surrounding lung tissue. These imbalances of immunoregulatory subsets of lymphocytes in lung and blood were thought to explain the excess production of immunoglobulins in the lung (Hunninghake et al., 1979; Lawrence et al., 1980) and the defective antibody and immunoglobulin production of blood lymphocytes (Katz and Fauci, 1978; Lawrence et al., 1982). A role for suppressor monocytes in peripheral blood has also been demonstrated (Goodwin et al., 1979; Lawrence et al., 1982).

In addition to the expansion of the number of T cells in the lung tissue of patients with sarcoidosis, there is a dramatic increase in the number of tissue macrophages known to secrete fibronectin, growth factors, and IL-1 (Hunninghake, 1984). Crystal and associates (1984), having reviewed the role of macrophages and immunoregulatory subsets of lymphocytes in sarcoidosis, suggested that the alveolar macrophage plays a central role in stimulating T-cell replication.

Lymphoid Malignancies

Infections

Infections are common complications in patients with lymphoid malignancies. In one large series, Bodey and Hersh (1969) reported that 79% of deaths in acute leukemia were due to infection. In a more recent study, Fernbach (1984) found an infection incidence of 86% in autopsied cases of children with acute leukemia. Deaths resulted from infection in 45% of children with lymphoma. In Hodgkin's disease, infection is responsible for death in 20% to 60% of patients. Most infections in Hodgkin's disease occur during the terminal period, when the patient's condition has become refractory to therapy.

Fever is a common sign in Hodgkin's disease, and several studies have sought to distinguish the intrinsic fever of Hodgkin's disease from the fever of a complicating infection (Boggs and Frei, 1960). The majority of febrile episodes occurring at the time of diagnosis were a result of the disease. The characteristics of the fever in infection or in Hodgkin's disease were similar. Murchison-Pel-Ebstein fever was rare. Fever was more common in patients in stage III or IV than in stage I or II, and the fever of infection was more common as the disease progressed. Fever at diagnosis was associated with a poorer prognosis.

By contrast, more than 70% of the febrile episodes in patients with acute leukemia were caused by infection (Bodey, 1966a; Freireich et al., 1970). Raab and others (1960) identified infection as the cause of fever in 102 of 149 episodes of fever in 55 patients with acute leukemia. Fever was more likely to be a result of infection when it appeared late, beyond the mean duration of survival. There were no characteristics of the fever of infection that could differentiate it from fever caused by underlying disease.

Organisms Implicated

Pneumonia and septicemia are the most frequent infections, and multiple infections are not unusual. The major causes of septicemia in children with lymphoid malignancies are *Pseudomonas, E. coli, Klebsiella-Enterobacter,* and *S. aureus.* The common pyogenic organisms, *Streptococcus pneumoniae* and *H. influenzae,* are also incriminated, particularly in the splenectomized patient with Hodgkin's disease. The sites of origin of septicemia are usually the respiratory tract, the gastrointestinal tract, or the skin. Although *S. aureus* septicemia has become more amenable to treatment, the fatality rate for patients with *Pseudomonas* infections is high.

When less common bacterial agents, such as *Listeria monocytogenes, Bacteroides, Serratia marcescens,* and clostridial species cause infections in patients with leukemia and lymphoma, a marked impairment of host resistance is suggested. Although tuberculosis was often associated with Hodgkin's disease in the past, it is now much less common (Silver, 1963). Lowther (1959) found the incidence of tuberculosis in patients with acute leukemia no higher than in the general population. Local and disseminated fungal infections caused by *Candida* species, *Cryptococcus neoformans, Nocardia* species, *Histoplasma capsulatum, Aspergillus* species, and *Mucor* species are being observed with increasing frequency in patients with lymphoid malignancies. Bodey (1966b) noted 161 fungal infections in 454 patients with acute myelogenous leukemia and in some patients with acute lymphoblastic leukemia.

Immune Avoidance

Although the interaction of malignancy with the immune system is appreciated clinically by the increased risk of infection, the compromised immune function also may facilitate progression of the cancer. The concept of tumor cell escape from T-cell surveillance has been best delineated for Epstein-Barr virus (EBV) and associated Burkitt's lymphoma (BL). A down-regulation of several EBV proteins in BL tumor cells may permit their evasion from normal immune surveillance (Rowe et al., 1987). Additionally, down-regulation of cellular adhesion molecules that facilitate lymphocyte-tumor interactions may contribute to this escape (Gregory et al., 1988). The absence of cell adhesion markers in other lymphomas suggests cancer spread by immune avoidance may be a common mechanism of cancer spread (Medeiros et al., 1989). Defective immunosurveillance may be restored by immunotherapy. Kwak and colleagues (1992) immunized B-cell lymphoma patients with immunoglobulin derived from their own tumor cells, which had been conjugated to a protein carrier, and noted a specific immunologic response to the therapy.

Leukemia

Although the increased susceptibility to infection in patients with acute leukemia can often be related to decreased numbers of circulating mature neutrophils, infections may occur when the leukocyte count is normal or high, suggesting other factors. Local leukocyte mobilization is markedly decreased in acute leukemias (Senn and Jungi, 1975). Granulocyte clearance is normal in acute lymphoblastic leukemia but impaired in acute myelocytic leukemia. Reticuloendothelial clearance rates are prolonged in some patients with acute leukemia (Groch et al., 1965).

B-Cell and T-Cell Function

In contrast to patients with lymphomas, patients with acute leukemia generally have normal antibody and cell-mediated immunity until they receive excessive chemotherapy or reach a terminal state. Kiran and Gross (1969) reported normal initial levels of IgG with a significant temporary fall associated with chemotherapy. IgG levels below 350 mg/dl were common in the preterminal stage of the disease. McKelvey and Carbone (1965) reported normal IgG and IgM values and slightly diminished IgA values. B-lymphocyte counts and serum immunoglobulin levels were followed in a cohort of 14 children who completed therapy for acute lymphoblastic leukemia (Alanko et al., 1992). The number of B cells normalized within 1 month, and serum immunoglobulins returned to normal within 6 months after cessation of therapy in most patients. The antibody responses of patients with acute leukemia appear to be intact (Larson and Tomlinson, 1953; Silver et al., 1960; Heath et al., 1964; Libansky, 1965). Delayed hypersensitivity responses are generally normal (Lamb et al., 1962). T-cell and B-cell enumeration in acute lymphocytic leukemia is distorted by the increased number of leukemic cells lacking either marker (Hitzig et al., 1976). The in vitro lymphocyte response to mitogens may be suppressed by massive chemotherapy (Hersh and Oppenheim, 1965) but is usually normal in children in remission receiving conventional therapy (Borella and Webster, 1971).

In a hypogammaglobulinemic child with acute lymphocytic leukemia, Broder and colleagues (1981) demonstrated a T-prosuppressor leukemic lymphocyte that could be induced on interaction with normal T and B cells to differentiate into a normal T-suppressor cell with the CD3 antigen and the CD25 (IL-2 receptor) antigen. In chronic lymphocytic leukemia, the accompanying hypogammaglobulinemia is secondary to a paucity of normal, immunoglobulin-secreting cells and to an intrinsic B-cell defect rather than to excess T-suppressor cells or deficient T-cell help (Fernandez et al., 1983).

Hodgkin's Disease

Hodgkin's disease was the first lymphoma to be associated with abnormalities of the immune response. In some cases, the immunologic defects may be related to the clinical stage of the disease and the histologic type (Lukes and Butler, 1966; Lukes et al., 1966) (see Chapter 27). The four histologic expressions of Hodgkin's disease are lymphocytic predominance, nodular sclerosis, mixed cellularity, and lymphocytic depletion. Lymphocytic depletion is associated with a greater impairment of immunologic function and a poorer prognosis. Hodgkin's disease may be clinically classified according to its anatomic distribution and systemic symptoms. This clinical staging correlates with immunologic status and ultimate prognosis.

Phagocytic Function

Leukocytosis is present in more than 50% of patients with Hodgkin's disease, despite the presence of lymphopenia as the disease progresses (Aisenberg, 1965a). Phagocytic function of the reticuloendothelial system, measured by clearance of ^{125}I-labeled aggregated human serum albumin, is normal or enhanced (Sheagren et al., 1967). Blood granulocyte clearance is decreased in patients in stages III and IV, but neutrophil mobilization is normal (Senn and Jungi, 1975).

The bactericidal capacity of mononuclear phagocytes is normal in Hodgkin's disease (Steigbigel et al., 1976). Leukocyte chemotaxis is abnormal, apparently associated with excessive levels of chemotactic factor inactivator (Ward and Berenberg, 1974). Perez-Soler and colleagues (1985) found impaired superoxide production in monocytes from patients with active disease compared with patients in remission and normal controls.

B and T Cells

Lymphocyte depletion of lymphoid tissue is well recognized in Hodgkin's disease (Lukes and Butler, 1966) and may be associated with peripheral leukopenia (Young et al., 1972; Eltringham and Kaplan, 1973). Studies of T and B lymphocytes in Hodgkin's disease show decreased percentages of T cells when using E rosetting (Andersen, 1974; Bobrove et al., 1975) but normal percentages when using specific anti–T cell sera (Chin et al., 1973; Bobrove et al., 1975). Absolute numbers of T cells are generally reduced in patients with lymphopenia. The finding of reduced numbers of B cells is not infrequent and is associated with low T-cell levels (Bobrove et al., 1975).

In Vivo Cell-Mediated Immunity

Defects of cell-mediated immunity are often seen in patients with Hodgkin's disease. In earlier decades, when most adults had positive tuberculin test findings, many patients with Hodgkin's disease had negative tuberculin results despite a history of tuberculosis or tuberculosis proved at autopsy. Schier and coworkers (1956) showed that tuberculin negativity was part of a generalized cutaneous anergy; in a control group 71% responded to PPD, 90% to mumps, 92% to *C. albicans*, and 66% to *Trichophyton*; in Hodgkin's disease, the response rates to the same antigens were 23%, 14%,

19%, and 16%, respectively. Others have also noted anergy in Hodgkin's disease, even in patients who were asymptomatic or in good condition (Sokal and Primikirios, 1961; Lamb et al., 1962).

In contrast, patients with other lymphomas or leukemia do not show a loss of cutaneous delayed hypersensitivity reactivity until the disease is far advanced. Lamb and colleagues (1962) found anergy in only 3 of 208 controls, 3 of 25 patients with leukemia, and 1 of 20 patients with other lymphomas; all were in good condition. In advanced disease, 5 of 10 patients with leukemia and 13 of 21 patients with other lymphomas were anergic.

In general, approximately one half the patients with Hodgkin's disease do not react to any antigens; of those with reactions, positive tests are fewer and of diminished intensity. The anergic state is relative, since increasing the concentration of the antigen may increase the number of positive reactions. The tuberculin reaction in advanced Hodgkin's disease may be delayed (Morgenfeld and Bonchil, 1968); a negative reaction at 48 hours may become positive in 5 to 7 days. Conversion from tuberculin positivity to negativity has been noted with the development of the disease, and reconversion to tuberculin positivity has been reported with remissions. Thus, the anergy of Hodgkin's disease may occur early in the disease when the patient is asymptomatic or in good clinical condition, in contrast to the relatively late appearance of anergy in seriously debilitated patients with leukemia, carcinoma, or non-Hodgkin's lymphoma.

In order to distinguish the anergic patient from those not exposed to antigen, Aisenberg (1962) attempted to sensitize 37 patients with Hodgkin's disease to DNCB. All 25 patients with active Hodgkin's disease were anergic, whereas 12 patients with disease quiescent for more than 2 years became sensitized. Brown and coworkers (1967) were able to sensitize 35 of 50 patients to DNCB; the reactors tended to have localized disease and normal lymphocyte counts. Sokal and Aungst (1969) found that patients with advanced Hodgkin's disease who showed positive tuberculin skin test findings after BCG vaccination had a longer survival than those who remained anergic.

Prolonged allograft survival was reported in more than half the patients with Hodgkin's disease (Kelly et al., 1960; Miller, 1962). Although the ability to reject grafts is impaired, it is difficult to pinpoint the effect of chemotherapy.

Attempts to transfer delayed hypersensitivity to patients with Hodgkin's disease who have normal leukocytes or transfer factor have been almost uniformly unsuccessful (Fazio and Calciati, 1962; Good et al., 1962; Muftuoglu and Balkuv, 1967). Chase (1966), discussing the mechanism of inactivation of donor cells by patients with Hodgkin's disease, suggests that nonantibody plasma factors may alter the immunocompetent cells. Insufficient numbers of functional lymphocytes in the recipient may also be responsible. These abnormal lymphocyte transfer reactions in Hodgkin's disease reflect impaired cell-mediated immunity (Aisenberg, 1965b). By contrast, an abnormally prolonged reaction by normal lymphocytes in some patients may be ascribed to delayed rejection. Depressed reactivity of Hodgkin's lymphocytes in normal recipients suggests an impaired graft-versus-host capability.

In Vitro Cell-Mediated Immunity

Hersh and Oppenheim (1965) reported decreased in vitro transformation of lymphocytes in response to PHA in Hodgkin's disease. Less transformation was seen in anergic patients than in those with positive skin tests. In three cases, plasma factors contributed to the impaired PHA response. Similar findings were reported by Trubowitz and coworkers (1966) and by Aisenberg (1965c). Brown and coworkers (1967) found that the PHA response in Hodgkin's disease was related to clinical staging and histology. Jackson and associates (1970) also found a reduced lymphocyte response in patients with systemic symptoms and advanced disease; most patients with stage I disease showed normal responses.

Han and Sokal (1970) and Winkelstein and others (1974) reported considerable variability of in vitro lymphocyte responses to PHA in active Hodgkin's disease. Although the mean response was significantly lower than that of the controls, half the patients had normal responses. A few patients in remission exhibited a diminished PHA response. Chemotherapy diminished the response in some cases. Patients with nodular sclerosing disease had normal PHA responses. In general, a diminished PHA response is correlated with advanced disease, systemic symptoms, lymphopenia, cutaneous anergy, and radiation therapy. Because PHA is such a strong lymphocyte stimulator, the response to it may remain positive when the patient is nonreactive to weaker antigenic stimuli.

Gotoff and others (1973) demonstrated impaired synthesis of a lymphokine, macrophage aggregation factor, by lymphocytes from patients with Hodgkin's disease. Subnormal mixed leukocyte culture reactions of Hodgkin's lymphocytes suggest a relative excess of suppressor lymphocytes (Twomey et al., 1975).

Monocyte-related immunosuppression may be present in Hodgkin's disease, resulting in an increased number of bacterial and fungal infections (Coker et al., 1983).

Removal of glass-adherent cells from mononuclear cells of patients with Hodgkin's disease resulted in increased PHA responsiveness (Sibbitt et al., 1978). Increased prostaglandin E_2 (PGE_2) production by monocytes from patients, and reversal of their suppressive activity by indomethacin has been documented (Goodwin et al., 1977; Passwell et al., 1983). Another cause of suppression includes circulating plasma factors. Pui and colleagues (1989) showed that increased serum levels of soluble CD8 was associated with aggressive clinical disease and suggested that this correlated with suppressor T cell activity. Although the understanding of immune suppression remains incomplete, these studies establish Hodgkin's disease as an immunoregulatory disorder.

Humoral Immunity

Serum immunoglobulins are usually normal in Hodgkin's disease (Ultmann et al., 1966; Goldman and Hobbs, 1967). Both hypergammaglobulinemias and hypogammaglobulinemias may be seen in about 10% of patients; the latter is associated with advanced disease. There are no consistent changes in specific immunoglobulin levels. The secondary antibody response is usually normal, but many patients have an impaired primary response (Schier et al., 1956; Barr and Fairley, 1961). Saslaw and colleagues (1961) reported that in only 15 of 37 patients with Hodgkin's disease, agglutinins developed following tularemia vaccination; in controls, agglutinins developed in 45 of 48 patients. Aisenberg and Leskowitz (1963) found a normal antibody response to pneumococcal polysaccharide in 15 of 19 Hodgkin's patients, all of whom were anergic to DNCB. The four patients who did not form antibody had widely disseminated advanced disease and died within 6 months.

Total serum complement is either normal or elevated in most patients with Hodgkin's disease (Schier et al., 1956; Rottino and Levy, 1959).

Lymphoproliferative Disease in Transplant Recipients

Transplantation of human tissue or organs is a lifesaving therapy for many patients with congenital or acquired disorders such as malignancy. Potent immunosuppression must generally be utilized to achieve and maintain successful engraftment. Transplantation to both immunologically normal and immunologically deficient humans is attended by the predictable development of continually proliferating B lymphocytes known as lymphoproliferative disease. The suppression of cell-mediated immunity that allows successful transplantation also permits proliferation of transformed B lymphocytes (see Chapter 27).

Pathophysiology

With rare exceptions (Garcia et al., 1987), Epstein-Barr virus infection has been implicated as the causative agent of post-transplantation lymphoproliferative disease. The sequence of pathophysiology has recently been reviewed (Malatack et al., 1991). EBV infects B cells through a cell-specific complement receptor (CD21) on the B-cell surface. The normal immune response controls the infection by development of EBV-specific cytotoxic T cells directed against infected B cells (Klein, 1975). Without these cytotoxic T cells, the EBV-induced B-cell proliferation continues. Initial proliferation is polyclonal and can be reversed if the normal immune response is restored. Indeed, a decreased dose of immunosuppressive drugs may allow sufficient restoration of the immune system to halt progression of the lymphoproliferation without compromising graft survival tissue. Unimpeded progression of the disease may lead to a monoclonal malignant lymphoma that requires surgical excision even if immune dysfunction can be reversed.

Three clinical phases of progression have been described (Malatack et al., 1991). The initial phase consists of lymphatic hyperplasia in the otherwise symptom-free patient. Progression to a systemic phase is associated with clinical disorders including pancreatitis, meningoencephalitis, and pneumonitis. Whether these symptoms are a direct result of EBV infection or from other opportunistic infection remains unresolved. Further advancement of the disease may result in a lymphoma-like disease indistinguishable from that of a non-Hodgkin's lymphoma.

Pathologic classification of these lymphoproliferative tumors emphasizes the progressive nature of the disease (Nalesnik et al., 1988). Polymorphic tumors consist of lymphoid cells in various stages of differentiation. Monomorphic tumors contain lymphocytes in the same stage of differentiation. Monomorphic lymphoid cells are further classified by clonality using immunocytochemical staining or genetic analysis of gene rearrangements. Polyclonal tumors have an intermediate ratio of kappa to lambda light chains, whereas monoclonal tumors express a skewed ratio with either kappa or lambda light chains in great excess.

Risk in Transplantation

The incidence of lymphomas in immunosuppressed transplant recipients is 100-fold higher than in the general population (Penn, 1981). One multicenter study examined more than 45,000 kidney transplant recipients and found a 40-fold increase in non-Hodgkin's lymphoma during the first post-transplant year (Opelz and Henderson, 1993). A similar risk occurs for heart and liver transplant recipients (Krikorian et al., 1978; Okano et al., 1988). Schubach and colleagues (1982) reported the development of monoclonal immunoblastic cell populations in donor cells following allogeneic bone marrow transplantation for leukemia.

Immunodeficiency and immunosuppression are predisposing conditions for the development of malignancy, especially EBV-associated B-cell lymphomas. The case of a 12-year-old immunodeficient patient, David, maintained in gnotobiotic isolation for his entire life span, has been particularly enlightening (Shearer et al., 1985; Rosenblatt et al., 1987). Subsequent to haploidentical bone marrow transplantation using sibling bone marrow treated with monoclonal anti–T cell antibody, multiple tumors developed in various organs as a result of EBV-stimulated host B-cell proliferations of diverse clonal origins. The B-cell proliferations were shown to contain the EBV genome and either oligoclonal or monoclonal rearrangements of immunoglobulin genes. These findings suggested that EBV initiated an evolution of polyclonal activation of B cells to oligoclonal B-cell proliferations and, finally, to monoclonal B-cell lymphoma.

Other Lymphomas

Immunologic defects have also been described in lymphosarcoma and reticulum cell sarcoma. Immuno-globulin levels may be normal, elevated, or low. Miller (1962) found that 60% of patients with lymphosarcoma had normal immunoglobulin levels, 25% had elevated levels, and 15% had hypogammaglobulinemia. In reticulum cell sarcoma, the figures were 11%, 24%, and 65%, respectively. Antibody responses are usually impaired (Barr and Fairley, 1961; Saslaw et al., 1961; Heath et al., 1964), and delayed hypersensitivity is depressed (Sokal and Primikirios, 1961; Lamb et al., 1962; Hersh and Irvin, 1969). The greatest impairment is found in diffuse lymphoma, particularly in those cases with histiocytic features (Jones et al., 1977). The in vitro lymphocytic response to PHA is also impaired (Hersh and Irvin, 1969). Leukocyte mobilization and granulocyte clearance rates are normal (Senn and Jungi, 1975).

Certain lymphoreticular malignancies are characterized by the presence of B, T, or monocytic markers on their cell surfaces (Hansen and Good, 1974). Chronic lymphocytic leukemia is predominantly a B-cell malignancy (Grey et al., 1971); acute lymphoblastic leukemia (ALL) is most often a T-cell or null cell disease (Gajl-Peczalska et al., 1974). Many lymphomas in children are of T-cell origin (Kaplan et al., 1974; Gajl-Peczalska et al., 1975); in contrast, lymphomas in adults are usually derived from B cells (Aisenberg and Bloch, 1972).

Agranulocytosis and Aplastic Anemia

Bone marrow failure may affect one or more cellular elements. The term aplastic anemia should be restricted to disorders of the red cell series but often implies pancytopenia. A congenital form of aplastic anemia, *Fanconi's anemia,* was discussed earlier (see Chromosome Instability Syndromes). Acquired forms of aplastic anemia have been linked epidemiologically to a recent history of hepatitis, a history of autoimmune disease, and the previous use of various drugs (Baumelou et al., 1993) (see Chapter 27). The immunologic deficiency is determined by the cell line affected, usually the granulocyte. Monocytopenia has been noted in aplastic anemia (Twomey et al., 1973).

The risk of major bacterial infections is primarily related to the absolute granulocyte count. Children with chronic neutropenia generally have infections involving the skin, mucous membranes, and lungs, usually caused by *S. aureus* or enteric organisms (Pincus et al., 1976).

Acquired aplastic anemia has been associated with hypogammaglobulinemia, thymoma, and other immunologic abnormalities in adults (Jeunet and Good, 1968; Morley and Forbes, 1974). Brookfield and Singh (1974) have described hypogammaglobulinemia in an infant with congenital hypoplastic anemia. Neutropenia has been reported in dysgammaglobulinemia (Rieger et al., 1974) and in certain forms of cellular immunodeficiency (Lux et al., 1970).

Laboratory Findings

Foon and coworkers (1984), studying 16 young male patients with hepatitis-associated aplastic anemia, documented significant reductions in circulating T cells, mitogen reactivity of T cells, in vivo response to skin-test antigens, and low serum IgG and IgM levels. Cines and colleagues (1982) studied 16 patients with neutropenia of uncertain etiology. They discovered that the majority had underlying immunologic disturbances, such as immune thrombocytopenia and autoimmune hemolytic anemia. Suppressor lymphocytes may play a role in certain forms of aplastic anemia, including *Blackfan-Diamond syndrome*; these lymphocytes are capable of suppressing erythroid colony formation of normal bone marrow cells in vitro (Hoffman et al., 1977).

Treatment

Management of neutropenic states includes attempts to reverse the primary defect and prevention and treatment of infectious complications. Neutropenia has been corrected with plasma infusions (Rieger et al., 1974; Pachman et al., 1975), leukocyte transfusions (Vallejos et al., 1975), and bone marrow transplantation (see Chapter 32). Lithium has been shown to increase the number of circulating neutrophils in selected patients (Gerner et al., 1981).

Supportive therapeutic measures are directed at the complications of the disease (Freireich et al., 1970). Hemorrhage caused by thrombocytopenia may be managed by platelet transfusions. In leukopenia, acute leukemia, aplastic anemia, and lymphomas, the granulocyte count often predicts susceptibility to infection. Patients with fewer than 400 granulocytes/mm³ are at higher risk, and those with granulocyte counts of 400 to 800/mm³ are at moderate risk. Prompt recognition of infection, with confirmation by appropriate cultures, provides the basis for control. In acute leukemia, in which more than 70% of febrile episodes are associated with infection, antimicrobial therapy should be started immediately after culture specimens are obtained. Selection of an antimicrobial agent depends on the severity of the infection, the probable location of the infection, and the prior response to antibiotics. Broad-spectrum antibiotics are used until the organism is identified and sensitivity patterns are determined (see Chapter 31).

Prevention of infection by strict environmental protection is being tested in some centers. Life-island isolation units provide a barrier between the patient and the environment, and the endogenous flora may be suppressed with oral nonabsorbable and topical antibiotics (Freireich et al., 1970; Schimpff et al., 1975). Laminar air-flow units in hospital rooms provide a more natural setting and control transport of organisms.

However, many infections in patients with depressed resistance are endogenous and are almost impossible to prevent, short of favorably altering host resistance. Transfusion of granulocytes in large numbers raises circulating blood levels for short periods of time (half-life ~6 hours).

During remission of leukemia, there does not appear to be increased susceptibility to bacterial infection and normal childhood activity should be maintained. Live virus vaccines are contraindicated in patients with leukemia and lymphomas and in those receiving immunosuppressive drugs or radiation therapy. Progressive vaccinia (Davidson and Hayhoe, 1962) and other complications of live vaccines may occur.

A major advance in the treatment of agranulocytosis has been the use of biologic substances that stimulate hematopoiesis. Recombinant human granulocyte colony-stimulating factor (rhG-CSF) has proved effective in congenital agranulocytosis (Bonilla et al., 1989) and cyclic neutropenia (Hammond et al., 1989). Absolute neutrophil counts rise dramatically, and the number of infections decreases.

SURGERY AND TRAUMA

Burns

Thermal burns are a major cause of acquired immunodeficiency. Children younger than 5 years of age are the most prone to thermal injury. Although most burns in this age group are caused by scalds, most of the fatal injuries result from flame burns (Finkelstein et al., 1992). Wartime injuries have become increasingly more likely to be associated with burns (Sparkes, 1993). Septicemia is a common complication of burn patients surviving the initial period of shock (see Chapter 31). The major causes are *Pseudomonas*, *Proteus*, streptococci, and *S. aureus* (Rabin et al., 1961a; Kefalides et al., 1964; Balch, 1968). Tetanus and other clostridial infections may also occur. Patients with burns are also susceptible to viral infections such as generalized herpes simplex and varicella (Foley et al., 1970). The burned area is a site for viral proliferation, much like that of eczematoid skin for vaccinia and varicella infection. Fungal infections have also been reported (Rabin et al., 1961b; Foley, 1969; Nash et al., 1971; Law et al., 1972).

Inflammatory Changes

With thermal injury to the integument, the primary defense against bacterial invasion is compromised. Local changes at the site of thermal injury include arteriolar constriction, which impairs blood flow, dilation of venules and venous stasis, formation of microthrombi, and sloughing of endothelial cells (Branemark et al., 1968). These changes lead to impaired margination of PMNs and interference with phagocytosis (Knisely, 1968). Depression of reticuloendothelial function occurs following severe burns (McRipley and Garrison, 1965; Smith and Goldman, 1972). Blood bactericidal activity is normal or elevated, but phagocytic function is diminished (Alexander et al., 1966; Balch, 1968; Rittenbury and Hanback, 1967; Alexander and Wixson, 1970). Abnormal neutrophil function precedes the onset of sepsis (Alexander and Meakins, 1972) (see Chapter 15).

Humoral Immunity

Serum immunoglobulin levels fall during the first few days after thermal injury and gradually return to normal after several weeks (Kefalides et al., 1964; Barr, 1965; Alexander et al., 1966). Arturson and coworkers (1969) found all five immunoglobulins decreased in serum, with the lowest levels occurring 2 days after the burn. Normal levels of IgM and IgD were regained at the end of the first week and of IgA, IgG, and IgE during the second week. IgG levels were diminished in 40 burn patients studied by Munster and Hoagland (1969), but no significant change was noted in IgA and IgM levels. Kohn and Cort (1969) also found that IgG was the major immunoglobulin affected. Daniels and colleagues (1974a) showed that immunoglobulin changes in burned children were similar to those in burned adults, with decreases of IgG confined to the first week. The most extensive decreases occurred in the youngest age group.

Deficiencies in complement components C3 and C4 have also been recorded (Daniels et al., 1974b) (see Chapter 17). Björnson and Alexander (1974) reported decreased serum opsonic activity in patients with extensive burns, which were related to alterations in the alternate complement pathway.

Fox and Lowbury (1953) found high titers of agglutinins to *Pseudomonas pyocyanea* in patients with burns who were colonized with *Pseudomonas*. Normal controls and burned patients who were not colonized with *Pseudomonas* also had serum agglutinins. Antibodies to staphylococcal polysaccharide and α-hemolysin develop in burn patients colonized with *S. aureus* (Jones and Lowbury, 1963). However, the titers varied and tended to be lower in patients with severe burns who died. Alexander and Moncrief (1966) found a brisk anamnestic response to tetanus toxoid but an impaired primary response to xenogeneic erythrocytes. The primary response to bacterial antigens was normal. Burn patients show an increased incidence of circulating autoantibodies, mainly directed against skin antigens (Leguit et al., 1973). Immunosuppressive serum factors were discovered in the blood of burn patients, as measured by effects upon in vitro lymphocyte proliferation, but the in vivo significance of these polypeptide factors is not known (Alexander et al., 1978; Ninnemann et al., 1982).

Cellular Immunity

Following thermal injury, there is an initial lymphopenia (Sakai et al., 1974) and depletion of lymphocytes in all lymphoid tissue (Baker, 1945). Lymphocyte counts return to normal within the first week. Several studies indicate that T-cell function is reduced following thermal injury. Delayed hypersensitivity skin reactions are depressed in patients with extensive (30%) burns (Casson et al., 1966). Grafts of allogeneic skin have prolonged survival on a burn patient (Jackson, 1954; Alexander and Moncrief, 1966; Chambler and Batchelor, 1969). In experimental animals, thermal injury depresses the response to tuberculin (Rapaport et al., 1968), depletes thoracic duct lymphocytes (Casson et al., 1968), and prolongs allograft survival (Rapaport et al., 1964). Both the stimulatory capacity and the responsiveness of lymphocytes from burn patients

are markedly impaired in mixed leukocyte cultures for at least 3 weeks (Leguit et al., 1973; Sakai et al., 1974). There is little effect on the lymphocyte response to PHA (Daniels et al., 1971; Mahler and Batchelor, 1971). Munster (1984) suggested that suppressor T-cell proliferation might contribute to the immune dysfunction. An increased serum concentration of IL-2 receptor (CD25) in the post-burn period may indicate early T-cell activation and refractoriness to further immune stimulation (Teodorczyk-Injeyan et al., 1991).

Treatment

Three major tenets of care must be considered in the treatment of a burn patient to minimize the risk of secondary infection: nutrition, débridement, and antibiotics (see Chapter 31).

Proper nutritional support decreases the risk of infection and improves survival. The benefit of high-calorie diets with protein supplements has been demonstrated in children (Alexander et al., 1980).

Burned tissue may release factors that impede normal immune function. Prompt excision of devitalized tissue in burned children decreases mortality (Tompkins et al., 1988).

Penicillin prophylaxis against β-hemolytic streptococcal infection is used in some burn centers (Altemeier and MacMillan, 1968). Gamma globulin prophylaxis is advocated by certain investigators (Kefalides et al., 1964; Altemeier and MacMillan, 1968). Silver nitrate (Monafo and Moyer, 1965), sulfamylon (Moncrief et al., 1966), silver sulfadiazine (Fox, 1968), and gentamicin (Altemeier and MacMillan, 1968; Stone and Whitehead, 1970) have been widely used for topical prophylaxis. Silver nitrate (0.5% solution) is a nontoxic antiseptic agent that decreases bacterial colonization. Its disadvantages are mainly due to secondary electrolyte derangements and its staining characteristics. Sulfamylon acetate is a safe chemotherapeutic agent that suppresses bacterial colonization. Occasional sensitivity reactions have been noted, and infections with resistant staphylococci have appeared late in the postburn period. Gentamicin sulfate ointment (0.1%) is a safe and effective local antibiotic that is rarely associated with resistance.

Kefalides and colleagues (1964) found that prophylactic antibiotic combinations of polymyxin B and tetracycline, colistin and penicillin, and polymyxin B and chloramphenicol did not prevent colonization of burned areas with *S. aureus* and *Pseudomonas aeruginosa*. In burns of from 10% to 30% of the body surface, plasma or γ globulin reduced mortality by 50% compared with saline and albumin therapy. In children younger than 6 years, *Pseudomonas* antibody titers were low, supporting the argument for passive immunization. Active immunization with specific strains of *Pseudomonas* may protect burn patients from septicemia (Wesley et al., 1974). However, infection with resistant strains remains a significant clinical problem. High-titer *Pseudomonas* intravenous immunoglobulin (Ps-IVIG) therapy may offer enhanced protection to the immune-compromised burn patient (Shirani et al., 1984).

Splenectomy

The association of splenectomy with increased susceptibility to infection was first noted by Morris and Bullock in 1919 but did not achieve wide appreciation until King and Schumacker in 1952 reported severe infection in five infants who had undergone splenectomy for spherocytosis. Since then, many reports have shown an increased risk of infection after splenectomy (Table 19–7). This risk of infection and the accompanying mortality are influenced strongly by the underlying disease. Singer (1973) noted that the increased risk of infection after splenectomy was three times greater for idiopathic thrombocytopenia or spherocytosis than for trauma. In children requiring splenectomy for Hodgkin's disease, severe bacterial infections developed in 10% (Chilcote et al., 1976). In a review of 12,000 published cases, Holdsworth and colleagues (1991) confirmed that young children and infants have an increased risk of infection independent of the reason for splenectomy but suggested that no increased risk of infection exists in otherwise healthy splenectomized adults.

The infections may occur any time from a few weeks to decades from the time of surgery, but they are more common in the first two years. Infants are at higher risk. The infections are usually of rapid onset and are fatal in approximately 50% of cases. The etiologic agent is primarily pneumococcal, but meningococci, *E. coli, H. influenzae,* staphylococci, and *Streptococcus pyogenes* are also responsible. Splenectomy also predisposes to malaria (Coatney, 1968), babesiosis (Western et al., 1970), and viral infections (Smith et al., 1957; Forward and Ashmore, 1960; Diamond, 1969). The risk of babesiosis infection in splenectomized adults was emphasized in a review of 22 cases, 6 of which resulted in death (Rosner et al., 1984).

Pathogenesis

The spleen is a major organ in the reticuloendothelial system and with the liver plays a dominant role in the clearance of microorganisms from the blood stream (Saba, 1970). The spleen is aided by the presence of specific (antibody) and nonspecific (complement) opsonins. The spleen also plays an important role in antibody synthesis (Ellis and Smith, 1966). The relative importance of the spleen as an organ of clearance and antibody synthesis varies, depending on genetic factors, age, immune status of the host and the type, route, and dose of the organism. The spleen's role in mounting an immune response is particularly important in young, nonimmunized patients with bacteremia.

In early studies of splenectomized children, immunoelectrophoretic patterns were normal (Broberger et al., 1960), but in subsequent reports IgM levels were decreased (Schumacher, 1970; Claret et al., 1975) or normal (Sullivan et al., 1978). Wang and colleagues (1988) found that in vitro IgM synthesis by PWM-stimulated patient cells was decreased. Diminished properdin levels were noted by Carlisle and Saslaw (1959), but Winkelstein and Lambert (1975) found normal levels of C3, C5, and properdin factor B as well as normal pneumococcal opsonizing activity in 24 splenectomized children. Defective alternative complement pathway activity was found in 10% of splenectomized patients and 16% of patients having functional asplenia on the basis of sickle cell disease (Corry et al., 1979).

A deficiency of tuftsin, a phagocytosis-promoting tetrapeptide derivative of IgG produced by the spleen, has been noted (Constantopoulos et al., 1972) (see Chapter 15).

A number of studies have reported a normal antibody response following subcutaneous or intramuscular injection of antigen in splenectomized patients (McFadzean and Tsang, 1956; Saslaw et al., 1959; Ammann et al., 1977; Sullivan et al., 1978). In contrast, the immune response to intravenously administered antigens is impaired in splenectomized animals (Rowley, 1981) and humans (Sullivan et al., 1978). Similarly, Hosea and coworkers (1981b) demonstrated a defective antibody response to a polyvalent (14 serotypes) pneumococcal vaccine in splenectomized patients.

Shinefield and associates (1966) demonstrated increased susceptibility to pneumococcal infection in a pathogen-free strain of mice undergoing splenectomy. Following intravenous injection of small numbers of organisms, multiplication of pneumococci occurred in a higher proportion in splenectomized mice and at a more rapid rate. Although no decrease in the clearance of carbon particles or pneumococci was found, high concentrations of pneumococci were present in the spleens of normal mice. This suggests that the spleen protects by removing and killing small but critical numbers of circulating pneumococci. Studies of the clearance of ^{123}I-labeled pneumococci in rabbits (Schulkind et al., 1967) showed that the spleen was more efficient than the liver in clearing microorganisms, particularly in the nonimmune animal.

Hosea and associates (1981a) showed that the macrophages of the reticuloendothelial system in the splenectomized subject require increased amounts of spe-

Table 19–7. Pediatric Mortality Rate in Postsplenectomy Sepsis

Disease	Eraklis et al. (1972)			Walker et al. (1976)			Holdsworth et al. (1991)		
	Patients	*Deaths*	*%*	*Patients*	*Deaths*	*%*	*Patients*	*Deaths*	*%*
Trauma	342	3	0.9	389	1	0.3	883	9	1.0
Congenital hemolytic anemia	394	2	0.5	201	4	2.0	707	13	1.8
Idiopathic thrombocytopenia	262	7	2.7	109	3	2.8	384	6	1.6
Thalassemia	45	2	4.4				168	9	5.4

cific antibody to produce intravascular clearance of opsonized particles. Ellis and Smith (1966) postulated that the spleen of the nonimmune host rapidly synthesizes opsonizing antibody in addition to serving as a phagocytic organ. The splenectomized host may be incapable of producing an immediate antibody response early in the course of bacteremia or may be unable to limit multiplication of circulating bacteria. Immunoregulatory imbalance may play a role in the poor immune response of splenectomized patients, particularly a lack of T-cell help (Amsbaugh et al., 1978; Drew et al., 1984). Splenosis, the regrowth of splenic tissue unattached to the splenic artery, did not reverse these immunologic abnormalities (Drew et al., 1984).

Treatment

Splenectomy is usually indicated for children with hereditary spherocytosis, but it is preferable to delay the operation until after infancy (Diamond, 1969). In patients with idiopathic thrombocytopenic purpura, splenectomy is indicated when medical management fails to control bleeding. Traumatic rupture and primary splenic tumor are usually treated by splenectomy, but medical management is possible (Aronson et al., 1977). Subtotal splenectomy should also be considered (De Boer and Downie, 1971). The use of splenic implants requires further study.

Medical therapy of the splenectomized patient includes the use of antibiotics promptly for febrile episodes. Travel to areas of endemic malaria or babesiosis should be discouraged or done with an appreciation of the potential consequences. Because many bacterial pathogens in asplenic individuals are sensitive to oral antibiotics, daily oral prophylaxis is often recommended (American Academy of Pediatrics, 1994). Postsplenectomy patients older than 2 years of age should receive pneumococcal and meningococcal vaccines, in addition to their routine vaccinations. In a retrospective analysis of pneumococcal infection in Denmark, Konradsen and Henrichsen (1991) suggested that the use of these vaccines and prompt use of penicillin for fever in postsplenectomized children was efficacious in preventing severe infections.

Head Injury

Impaired immune responses after major blunt trauma in adults may increase the risk of secondary infection (Munster, 1984). More than 75% of all non-neurologic deaths following nonthermal trauma in adults is attributable to infection (Baker et al., 1980). Abnormal immune parameters following blunt trauma in adults include impaired delayed cutaneous hypersensitivity (Meakins et al., 1978), decreased lymphocyte proliferation to mitogens (O'Mahony et al., 1984), and decreased T-cell numbers, particularly CD4$^+$ cells (Faist et al., 1986). Studies in children are less extensive despite the fact that nearly half of all deaths in children older than 1 year are due to accidents (Gratz, 1979).

Wilson and colleagues (1989) studied antibody responses in 10 children who had suffered blunt trauma. Although secondary responses to diphtheria and tetanus were normal, the primary response to a neoantigen, bacteriophage φX174, was markedly abnormal in all but one child. The same group (Wilson et al., 1991) studied cutaneous delayed hypersensitivity in children receiving intensive care for major head trauma. Approximately half of the patients were anergic to a panel of seven antigens. Proven infection was three times more common in the anergic group than in patients with at least one positive skin test. The number of peripheral B cells also was decreased. T cells, monocytes, and granulocytes were not affected. Gooding and colleagues (1993) examined the value of intravenous immunoglobulin in a similar population of children after head injury but found no therapeutic benefit.

References

Abdou NI, Zweiman B, Casella SR. Effects of azathioprine therapy on bone marrow–dependent and thymus-dependent cells in man. Clin Exp Immunol 13:55–64, 1973.

Abo T, Cooper MD, Balch CM. Characterization of HNK-1$^+$ (Leu-7) human lymphocytes. I. Two distinct phenotypes of human NK cells with different cytotoxic capability. J Immunol 129:1752–1757, 1982.

Abrutyn E, Solomons NW, St Clair L, MacGregor RR, Root RK. Granulocyte function in patients with chronic renal failure: surface adherence, phagocytosis, and bactericidal activity in vitro. J Infect Dis 135:1–8, 1977.

Abt A, Denholz EJ. Letterer-Siwe's disease. Am J Dis Child 51:499–522, 1936.

Ades LC, Kerr B, Turner G, Wise G. Smith-Fineman-Myers syndrome in two brothers. Am J Med Genet 40:467–470, 1991.

Agarwal SS, Blumberg BS, Gerstley BJ, London WT, Sutnick AI, Loeb LA. DNA polymerase activity as an index of lymphocyte stimulation: studies in Down's syndrome. J Clin Invest 49:161–169, 1970.

Agnello V, Winchester RJ, Kunkel HG. Precipitin reactions of the C1q component of complement with aggregated gamma-globulin and immune complexes in gel diffusion. Immunol 19:909–919, 1970.

Ahman L, Back E, Bensch K, Olcen P. Non-efficacy of low-dose intradermal vaccination against hepatitis B in Down's syndrome. Scand J Infect Dis 25:16–23, 1993.

Aisenberg AC. Studies on delayed hypersensitivity in Hodgkin's disease. J Clin Invest 41:1964–1970, 1962.

Aisenberg AC. Lymphopenia in Hodgkin's disease. J Clin Invest 251:1037–1042, 1965a.

Aisenberg AC. Studies of lymphocyte transfer reactions in Hodgkin's disease. J Clin Invest 44:555–564, 1965b.

Aisenberg AC. Quantitative estimation of the reactivity of normal and Hodgkin's disease lymphocytes with thymidine-2-C^{14}. Nature 205:1233–1235, 1965c.

Aisenberg AC, Bloch KJ. Immunoglobulins on the surface of neoplastic lymphocytes. N Engl J Med 287:272–276, 1972.

Aisenberg AC, Leskowitz S. Antibody formation in Hodgkin's disease. N Engl J Med 268:1269–1272, 1963.

Alam N, Wojtyniak B, Rahaman MM. Anthropometric indicators and risk of death. Am J Clin Nutr 49:884–888, 1989.

Alanko S, Pelliniemi TT, Salmi TT. Recovery of blood B-lymphocytes and serum immunoglobulins after chemotherapy for childhood acute lymphoblastic leukemia. Cancer 69:1481–1486, 1992.

Al-Bander HA, Martin VI, Kaysen GA. Plasma IgG pool is not defended from urinary loss in nephrotic syndrome. Am J Physiol 262:F333–F337, 1992.

Alepa FP, Zvaifler NJ, Sliwinski AJ. Immunologic effects of cyclophosphamide treatment in rheumatoid arthritis. Arthritis Rheum 13:754–760, 1970.

Alexander JW, Brown W, Mason AD Jr, Moncrief JA. The influence of infection upon serum protein changes in severe burns. J Trauma 6:780–789, 1966.

Alexander JW, MacMillan BG, Stinnett JD, Ogle CK, Bozian RC, Fischer JE, Oakes JB, Morris MJ, Krummel R. Beneficial effects of aggressive protein feeding in severely burned children. Ann Surg 192:505–517, 1980.

Alexander JW, Meakins JL. A physiological basis for the development of opportunistic infections in man. Ann Surg 176:273–287, 1972.

Alexander JW, Moncrief JA. Alterations of the immune response following severe thermal injury. Arch Surg 93:75–83, 1966.

Alexander JW, Ogle CK, Stinnett JD, MacMillan BG. A sequential, prospective analysis of immunologic abnormalities and infection following severe thermal injury. Ann Surg 188:809–816, 1978.

Alexander JW, Wixson D. Neutrophil dysfunction and sepsis in burn injury. Surg Gynecol Obstet 130:431–438, 1970.

Alexiewicz JM, Smogorzewski M, Fadda GZ, Massry SG. Impaired phagocytosis in dialysis patients: studies on mechanisms. Am J Nephrol 11:102–111, 1991.

Allison AC, Andrade ZA, Brunner KT, Butterworth AE, Capron A, Cohen S, Colley DG, Coombs RRA, David JR, Davis A, Hoffman DB, Hopwood BEC, Houba V, Jordan P, Lambert PH, Mahmoud AAF, Sher A, Smithers SR, Sturrock RF, Torrigiani G, Warren KS, Webbe G, Weigle WO. Immunology of schistosomiasis. Bull WHO 51:553–595, 1974.

Altemeier WA, MacMillan BG. Comparative studies of topical silver nitrate. Sulfamylon and gentamicin. Ann N Y Acad Sci 150:966–979, 1968.

Ambruso DR, McCabe ER, Anderson D, Beaudet A, Ballas LM, Brandt IK, Brown B, Coleman R, Dunger DB, Falletta JM, Friedman HS, Haymond MW, Keating JP, Kinney TR, Leonard JV, Mahoney DH, Matalon R, Roe TF, Simmons P, Slonim AE. Infectious and bleeding complications in patients with glycogenosis Ib. Am J Dis Child 139:691–697, 1985.

American Academy of Pediatrics. Immunization in special clinical circumstances. In Peter G, ed. 1994 Red Book: Report of the Committee on Infectious Diseases. Elk Grove Village, Ill., American Academy of Pediatrics, 1994, pp. 57–58.

Amirhakimi GH, Samloff IM, Bryson MF, Forbes GB. Intestinal lymphangiectasia. Metabolic studies. Am J Dis Child 117:178–185, 1969.

Ammann AJ, Addiego J, Wara DW, Lubin B, Smith WB, Mentzer WC. Polyvalent pneumococcal-polysaccharide immunization of patients with sickle-cell anemia and patients with splenectomy. N Engl J Med 297:897–900, 1977.

Amsbaugh DF, Prescott B, Baker PJ. Effect of splenectomy on the expression of regulatory T cell activity. J Immunol 121:1483–1485, 1978.

Andersen E. Depletion of thymus-dependent lymphocytes in Hodgkin's disease. Scand J Haematol 12:263–269, 1974.

Anderson DC, Krishna GS, Hughes BJ, Mace ML, Mintz AA, Smith CW, Nichols BL. Impaired polymorphonuclear leukocyte motility in malnourished infants: relationship to functional abnormalities of cell adherence. J Lab Clin Med 101:881–895, 1983.

Anderson DC, York TL, Rose G, Smith CW. Assessment of serum factor B, serum opsonins, granulocyte chemotaxis, and infection in nephrotic syndrome of children. J Infect Dis 140:1–11, 1979.

Arneil GC, Lam CN. Long-term assessment of steroid therapy in childhood nephrosis. Lancet 2:819–821, 1966.

Aronson DZ, Scherz AW, Einhorn AH, Becker JM, Schneider KM. Nonoperative management of splenic trauma in children: a report of six consecutive cases. Pediatrics 60:482–485, 1977.

Arrieta AC, Zaleska M, Stutman HR, Marks MI. Vitamin A levels in children with measles in Long Beach, California. J Pediatr 121:75–78, 1992.

Arroyave G, Calcano M. Descenso de los niveles sericos de retinol y su proteina de enlace (RBP) durante las infecciones. Arch Latinoam Nutr 29:233–260, 1979.

Arturson G, Hogman CF, Johansson SG, Killander J. Changes in immunoglobulin levels in severely burned patients. Lancet 1:546–548, 1969.

Arvio M, Autio S, Louhiala P. Early clinical symptoms and incidence of aspartylglucosaminuria in Finland. Acta Paediatr 82:587–589, 1993.

Atkinson JP, Frank MM. Effect of cortisone therapy on serum complement components. J Immunol 111:1061–1066, 1973.

Aula P, Autio S, Raivio KO, Rapola J. Aspartylglucosaminuria. In Durand P, O'Brien JS, eds. Genetic Errors of Glycoprotein Metabolism. Milan, edi-ermes, 1982, pp. 123–143.

Avanzini MA, Soderstrom T, Wahl M, Plebani A, Burgio GR, Hanson LA. IgG subclass deficiency in patients with Down's syndrome and aberrant hepatitis B vaccine response. Scand J Immunol 28:465–470, 1988.

Baeteman MA, Mattei MG, Baret A, Mattei JF. Immunoreactive copper-zinc superoxide-dismutase (SOD-1) in mosaic trisomy 21 and normal subjects. Acta Paediatr Scand 73:341–344, 1984.

Bagdade JD. Infection in diabetes, predisposing factors. Postgrad Med 59:160–164, 1976.

Bagdade JD, Root RK, Bulger RJ. Impaired leukocyte function in patients with poorly controlled diabetes. Diabetes 23:9–15, 1974.

Baker CC, Oppenheimer L, Stephens B, Lewis FR, Trunkey DD. Epidemiology of trauma deaths. Am J Surg 140:144–150, 1980.

Baker RD. The internal lesion in burns with special reference to the liver and to splenic nodules. Am J Pathol 21:717–733, 1945.

Balch HH. Septicemia in burned patients. Ann N Y Acad Sci 150:991–1000, 1968.

Balow JE, Rosenthal AS. Glucocorticoid suppression of macrophage migration inhibitory factor. J Exp Med 137:1031–1041, 1973.

Barandun S, Aebersold J, Bianchi R, Kluthe R, Muralt GV, Poretti G, Riva G. "Protein diarrhoe": Zugleich ein Beitrag zur Frage der sogenannten essentiellen Hypoproteinamie. Schweiz Med Wschr 90:1458–1467, 1960.

Bardana EJ Jr, Gabourel JD, Davies GH, Craig S. Effects of phenytoin on man's immunity. Evaluation of changes in serum immunoglobulins, complement, and antinuclear antibody. Am J Med 74:289–296, 1983.

Barr M, Fairley GH. Circulating antibodies in reticuloses. Lancet 1:1305–1310, 1961.

Barr S. Serum and plasma proteins in thermally injured patients treated with plasma, its admixture with albumin or serum alone. Ann Surg 161:112–126, 1965.

Barrett-Connor E. Bacterial infection and sickle cell anemia. An analysis of 250 infections in 166 patients and a review of the literature. Medicine 50:97–112, 1971.

Barroeta O, Nungaray L, Lopez-Osuna M, Armendares S, Salamanca F, Kretschmer RR. Defective monocyte chemotaxis in children with Down's syndrome. Pediatr Res 17:292–295, 1983.

Barth WF, Vergara GG, Khurana SK, Lowman JT, Beckwith JB. Rapidly fatal familial histiocytosis associated with eosinophilia and primary immunological deficiency. Lancet 2:503–506, 1972.

Barth WF, Wochner RD, Waldmann TA, Fahey JL. Metabolism of human gamma macroglobulins. J Clin Invest 43:1036–1048, 1964.

Bascom R, Johns CJ. The natural history and management of sarcoidosis. Adv Intern Med 31:213–241, 1986.

Baumelou E, Guiguet M, Mary JY. Epidemiology of aplastic anemia in France: a case-control study. I. Medical history and medication use. The French Cooperative Group for Epidemiological Study of Aplastic Anemia. Blood 81:1471–1478, 1993.

Baxter JD, Harris AW, Tomkins GM, Cohn M. Glucocorticoid receptors in lymphoma cells in culture: relationship to glucocorticoid killing activity. Science 171:189–191, 1971.

Becker FW, Krull P, Deicher H, Kalden JR. Leucocyte-migration test in sarcoidosis. Lancet 1:120–123, 1972.

Belcher RW, Carney JF, Nankervis GA. Effect of sera from patients with sarcoidosis on in vitro lymphocyte response. Int Arch Allergy Appl Immunol 46:183–190, 1974.

Bell PR, Briggs JD, Calman KC, Paton AM, Wood RF, Macpherson SG, Kyle K. Reversal of acute clinical and experimental organ rejection using large doses of intravenous prednisolone. Lancet 1:876–880, 1971.

Bell S, Cranage M, Borysiewicz L, Minson T. Induction of immunoglobulin G Fc receptors by recombinant vaccinia viruses expressing glycoproteins E and I of herpes simplex virus type 1. J Virol 64:2181–2186, 1990.

Benaceraf B, Kivy-Rosenberg E, Sebestyen MM, Zweifach BW. The effect of high doses of x-irradiation on the phagocytic, proliferative and metabolic properties of the RES. J Exp Med 110:49–64, 1959.

Benda DE, Strassman GS. The thymus in mongolism. J Ment Defic Res 9:109–120, 1965.

Berenbaum MC. Time-dependence and selectivity of immunosuppressive agents. Immunology 36:355–365, 1979.

Berencsi K, Bakay M, Beladi I. The role of macrophages in adenovirus-induced immunosuppression in mice. Acta Virol 29:61–65, 1985.

Berencsi K, Bakay M, Beladi I. Impaired interleukin-2 production by spleen cells from mice infected with human adenovirus. Acta Virol 35:350–356, 1991.

Bergmann KC, Zaumseil I, Lachmann B. IgE Konzentrationen im Serum von Patienten mit Sarkoidose und Lungentuberkulose. Dtsch Gesundheitsw 27:1774–1775, 1972.

Bertotto A, Arcangeli C, Crupi S, Marinelli I, Gerli R, Vaccaro R. T cell response to anti-CD3 antibody in Down's syndrome. Arch Dis Child 62:1148–1151, 1987.

Biggar WD, Ramirez RA, Rose V. Congenital asplenia: immunologic assessment and a clinical review of eight surviving patients. Pediatrics 67:548–551, 1981.

Björnson AB, Alexander JW. Alterations of serum opsonins in patients with severe thermal injury. J Lab Clin Med 83:372–382, 1974.

Black MM, de Chabon A. Reactivity of lymph nodes in azotaemic patients. Am J Clin Pathol 41:503–508, 1964.

Blasi A, Olivieri D. Immunoglobulins in serum and bronchial secretions in pulmonary sarcoidosis. In Proceedings of the Sixth International Conference on Sarcoidosis. Tokyo, Tokyo University Press, 1974, pp. 204–207.

Bloch CE. Blindness and other diseases in children arising from deficient nutrition (lack of fat-soluble A factor). Am J Dis Child 27:139–148, 1924.

Blumberg D, AvRuskin T. Down's syndrome, autoimmune hyperthyroidism, and hypoparathyroidism: a unique triad. Am J Dis Child 141:1149, 1987.

Bobrove AM, Fuks Z, Strober S, Kaplan HS. Quantitation of T and B lymphocytes and cellular immune function in Hodgkin's disease. Cancer 36:169–179, 1975.

Bodey GP. Infectious complications of acute leukemia. Med Times 94:1076–1085, 1966a.

Bodey GP. Fungal infections complicating acute leukemia. J Chronic Dis 19:667–687, 1966b.

Bodey GP, Hersh EM. The problem of infection in children with malignant disease. In Neoplasia in Childhood. Anderson Hospital. Chicago, Year Book Medical Publishers 1969, pp. 135–154.

Boggs DR, Frei E. Clinical studies of fever and infection in cancer. Cancer 13:1240–1253, 1960.

Bongiovanni AM, Wolman IJ. Plasma protein fractionation in pediatrics: a review of its present status. Am J Med Sci 218:700–714, 1949.

Bonilla MA, Gillio AP, Ruggeiro M, Kernan NA, Brochstein JA, Abboud M, Fumagalli L, Vincent M, Gabrilove JL, Welte K, Souza LM, O'Reilly RJ. Effects of recombinant human granulocyte colony–stimulating factor on neutropenia in patients with congenital agranulocytosis. N Engl J Med 320:1574–1580, 1989.

Borella L, Webster RG. The immunosuppressive effects of long-term combination chemotherapy in children with acute leukemia in remission. Cancer Res 31:420–426, 1971.

Bougneres PF, Carel JC, Castano L, Boitard C, Gardin JP, Landais P, Hors J, Mihatsch MJ, Paillard M, Chaussain JL, Bach JF. Factors associated with early remission of type I diabetes in children treated with cyclosporine. N Engl J Med 318:663–670, 1988.

Boumpas DT, Anastassiou ED, Older SA, Tsokos GC, Nelson DL, Balow JE. Dexamethasone inhibits human interleukin 2 but not interleukin 2 receptor gene expression in vitro at the level of nuclear transcription. J Clin Invest 87:1739–1747, 1991.

Boumpas DT, Chrousos GP, Wilder RL, Cupps TR, Balow JE. Glucocorticoid therapy for immune-mediated diseases: basic and clinical correlates. Ann Intern Med 119:1198–1208, 1993.

Bowman BU, Amos WT, Geer JC. Failure to produce experimental sarcoidosis in guinea pigs with *Mycobacterium tuberculosis* and mycobacteriophage DS6A. Am Rev Respir Dis 105:85–94, 1972.

Bowman TA, Goonewardene IM, Pasatiempo AM, Ross AC, Taylor CE. Vitamin A deficiency decreases natural killer cell activity and interferon production in rats. J Nutr 120:1264–1273, 1990.

Bradley JR, Evans DB, Calne RY. Long-term survival in haemodialysis patients. Lancet 1:295–296, 1987.

Branemark PI, Breine U, Joshi M, Urbaschek B. Part I. Pathophysiology of thermal burns. Microvascular pathophysiology of burned tissue. Ann N Y Acad Sci 150:474–494, 1968.

Brayton RG, Stokes PE, Schwartz MS, Louria DB. Effect of alcohol and various diseases on leukocyte mobilization, phagocytosis and intracellular bacterial killing. N Engl J Med 282:123–128, 1970.

Bridges JM, Nelson SD, McGeown MG. Evaluation of lymphocyte transfer test in normal and uremic subjects. Lancet 1:581–584, 1964.

Broberger O, Gyulai F, Hirschfeldt J. Splenectomy in childhood. Acta Paediatr 49:679–689, 1960.

Broder S, Uchiyama T, Muul LM, Goldman C, Sharrow S, Poplack DG, Waldmann TA. Activation of leukemic pro-suppressor cells to become suppressor-effector cells. Influence of cooperating normal T cells. N Engl J Med 304:1382–1387, 1981.

Brookfield EG, Singh P. Congenital hypoplastic anemia associated with hypogammaglobulinemia. J Pediatr 85:529–531, 1974.

Brostoff J, Walker JG. Leucocyte migration inhibition with Kveim antigen in Crohn's disease. Clin Exp Immunol 9:707–711, 1971.

Brown KH, Rajan MM, Chakraborty J, Aziz KM. Failure of a large dose of vitamin A to enhance the antibody response to tetanus toxoid in children. Am J Clin Nutr 33:212–217, 1980.

Brown RE, Katz M. Failure of antibody production to yellow fever vaccine in children with kwashiorkor. Trop Geogr Med 18:125–128, 1966.

Brown RE, Katz M. Passive transfer of delayed hypersensitivity reaction to tuberculin in children with protein calorie malnutrition. J Pediatr 70:126–128, 1967.

Brown RS, Haynes HA, Foley HT, Godwin HA, Berard CW, Carbone PP. Hodgkin's disease. Immunologic, clinical, and histologic features of 50 untreated patients. Ann Intern Med 67:291–302, 1967.

Buchmeier NA, Cooper NR. Suppression of monocyte functions by human cytomegalovirus. Immunol 66:278–283, 1989.

Buck J, Ritter G, Dannecker L, Katta V, Cohen SL, Chait BT, Hammerling U. Retinol is essential for growth of activated human B cells. J Exp Med 171:1613–1624, 1990.

Buckley CE, Trayer HR. Serum IgD concentrations in sarcoidosis and tuberculosis. Clin Exp Immunol 10:257–265, 1972.

Buckley CE III, Nagaya H, Sieker HO. Altered immunologic activity in sarcoidosis. Ann Intern Med 64:508–520, 1966.

Bunch TW, O'Duffy JD. Disease-modifying drugs for progressive rheumatoid arthritis. Mayo Clin Proc 55:161–179, 1980.

Burdin N, Peronne C, Banchereau J, Rousset F. Epstein-Barr virus transformation induces B lymphocytes to produce human interleukin 10. J Exp Med 177:295–304, 1993.

Burgio GR, Severi F, Rossoni R, Vaccaro R. Mongolism and thyroid autoimmunity. Lancet 1:166–167, 1965.

Burgio GR, Ugazio AG. Immunity in Down's syndrome. Eur J Pediatr 127:293–294, 1978.

Burgio GR, Ugazio A, Nespoli L, Maccario R. Down syndrome: a model of immunodeficiency. Birth Defects 19:325–327, 1983.

Burks AW, Charlton R, Casey P, Poindexter A, Steele R. Immune function in patients treated with phenytoin. J Child Neurol 4:25–29, 1989.

Butler WT, Rossen RD. Effects of corticosteroids on immunity in man. I. Decreased serum IgG concentration caused by 3 or 5 days of high doses of methylprednisolone. J Clin Invest 52:2629–2640, 1973.

Bybee JD, Rogers DE. The phagocytic activity of polymorphonuclear leukocytes obtained from patients with diabetes mellitus. J Lab Clin Med 64:1–13, 1964.

Byrne EB, Evans AS, Fouts DW, Israel HL. A seroepidemiological study of Epstein-Barr virus and other viral antigens in sarcoidosis. Am J Epidemiol 97:355–363, 1973.

Byron PR, Mallick NP, Taylor G. Immune potential in human uraemia. 1. Relationship of glomerular filtration rate to depression of immune potential. J Clin Pathol 29:765–769, 1976.

Campbell AC, Hersey P, MacLennan IC, Kay HE, Pike MC. Immunosuppressive consequences of radiotherapy and chemotherapy in patients with acute lymphoblastic leukaemia. Br Med J 2:385–388, 1973.

Canadian Multicentre Transplant Study Group. A randomized clinical trial of cyclosporine in cadaveric renal transplantation. Analysis at three years. N Engl J Med 314:1219–1225, 1986.

Cantwell RJ. Iron deficiency anemia of infancy: some clinical principles illustrated by the response of Maori infants to neonatal parenteral iron administration. Clin Pediatr 11:443–449, 1972.

Carding SR. A role for gamma/delta T cells in the primary immune response to influenza virus. Res Immunology 141:603–606, 1990.

Carlisle HN, Saslaw S. Properdin levels in splenectomized persons. Proc Soc Exp Biol Med 102:150–154, 1959.

Carlow DA, Van Oers NSC, Teh SJ, Teh HS. Deletion of antigen-specific immature thymocytes by dendritic cells requires LFA-1/ICAM interactions. J Immunol 148:1595–1603, 1992.

Carnes WH, Raffel S. A comparison of sarcoidosis and tuberculosis with respect to complement fixation with antigens derived from the tubercle bacillus. Bull Johns Hopkins Hosp 85:204–220, 1949.

Carney WP, Hirsch MS. Mechanisms of immunosuppression in cytomegalovirus mononucleosis. II. Virus-monocyte interactions. J Infect Dis 144:47–54, 1981.

Carpenter CB, Glassock RJ, Gleason R, Corson JM, Merrill JP. The application of the normal lymphocyte transfer reaction to histocompatibility testing in man. J Clin Invest 45:1452–1466, 1966.

Casali P, Rice GP, Oldstone MB. Viruses disrupt functions of human lymphocytes. Effects of measles virus and influenza virus on lymphocyte-mediated killing and antibody production. J Exp Med 159:1322–1337, 1984.

Casson PR, Gesner BM, Converse JM, Rapaport FT. Immunosuppressive sequelae of thermal injury. Surg Forum 19:509–511, 1968.

Casson P, Solowey AC, Converse JM, Rapaport FT. Delayed hypersensitivity status of burned patients. Surg Forum 17:268–270, 1966.

Cederbaum SD, Niwayama G, Stiehm ER, Neerhout RC, Ammann AJ, Berman W Jr. Combined immunodeficiency presenting as the Letterer-Siwe syndrome. J Pediatr 85:466–471, 1974.

Celikoglu S, Vieria LO, Siltzbach LE. Serum immunoglobulin levels in sarcoidosis. In Levinsky L, Macholda F, eds. Proceedings of the Fifth International Conference on Sarcoidosis: XIVth Scientific Conference of the Medical Faculty of Charles University, Prague 1969. Prague, Universita Karlova, 1971, pp. 168–170.

Chambler K, Batchelor JR. Influence of defined incompatibilities and area of burn on skin-homograft survival in burned subjects. Lancet 1:16–18, 1969.

Champlin R, Ho W, Gale RP. Antithymocyte globulin treatment in patients with aplastic anemia: a prospective randomized trial. N Engl J Med 308:113–118, 1983.

Chan GL, Canafax DM, Johnson CA. The therapeutic use of azathioprine in renal transplantation. Pharmacotherapy 7:165–177, 1987.

Chandra RK. Reduced bactericidal capacity of polymorphs in iron deficiency. Arch Dis Child 48:864–866, 1973.

Chandra RK. Rosette-forming T lymphocytes and cell-mediated immunity in malnutrition. Br Med J 3:608–609, 1974.

Chandra RK. Immunoglobulins and antibody response in malnutrition—a review. In Suskind R, ed. Malnutrition and the Immune Response. New York, Raven Press, 1977, pp. 155–168.

Chandra RK. Cell-mediated immunity in nutritional imbalance. Fed Proc 39:3088–3092, 1980a.

Chandra RK. Nutritional deficiency, immune responses, and infectious illness. Fed Proc 39:3086–3087, 1980b.

Chandra RK. Increased bacterial binding to respiratory epithelial cells in vitamin A deficiency. BMJ 297:834–835, 1988.

Chandra RK, Saraya AK. Impaired immunocompetence associated with iron deficiency. J Pediatr 86:899–902, 1975.

Chandra RK, Wadhwa M. Nutritional modulation of intestinal mucosal immunity. Immunol Invest 18:119–126, 1989.

Chase MW. Delayed-type hypersensitivity and the immunology of Hodgkin's disease with a parallel examination of sarcoidosis. Cancer Res 26:1097–1120, 1966.

Chatenoud L, Baudrihaye MF, Kreis H, Goldstein G, Schindler J, Bach JF. Human in vivo antigenic modulation induced by the anti-T cell OKT3 monoclonal antibody. Eur J Immunol 12:979–982, 1982.

Chester MA, Lundblad A, Ockerman P, Autio S. Mannosidosis. In Durand P, O'Brien JS, eds. Genetic Errors of Glycoprotein Metabolism. Milan, Edi-ermes, 1982, pp. 89–115.

Chilcote RR, Baehner RL, Hammond D. Septicemia and meningitis in children splenectomized for Hodgkin's disease. N Engl J Med 295:798–800, 1976.

Chin AH, Saiki JH, Trujillo JM, Williams RC Jr. Peripheral blood T- and B-lymphocytes in patients with lymphoma and acute leukemia. Clin Immunol Immunopathol 1:499–510, 1973.

Chudwin DS, Cowan MJ, Greenberg PL, Wara DW, Ammann AJ. Response of agranulocytosis to prolonged antithymocyte globulin therapy. J Pediatr 103:223–227, 1983.

Chujor CS, Kuhn B, Schwerer B, Bernheimer H, Levis WR. Specific inhibition of mRNA accumulation for lymphokines in human T cell line Jurkat by mycobacterial lipoarabinomannan antigen. Clin Exp Immunol 87:398–403, 1992.

Cines DB, Passero F, Guerry D IV, Bina M, Dusak B, Schreiber AD. Granulocyte-associated IgG in neutropenic disorders. Blood 59:124–132, 1982.

Citrin Y, Sterling K, Halsted JA. The mechanism of hypoproteinemia associated with giant hypertrophy of the gastric mucosa. N Engl J Med 257:906–912, 1957.

Citron KM. Skin tests in sarcoidosis. Tubercle 38:33–41, 1957.

Claman HN. Corticosteroids and lymphoid cells. N Engl J Med 287:388–397, 1972.

Claret I, Morales L, Montaner A. Immunological studies in the post-splenectomy syndrome. J Pediatr Surg 10:59–64, 1975.

Coatney GR. Simian malarias in man: facts, implications, and predictions. Am J Trop Med Hyg 17:147–155, 1968.

Cockburn IT, Krupp P. The risk of neoplasms in patients treated with cyclosporine A. J Autoimmun 2:723–731, 1989.

Cohen S, Hansen JDL. Metabolism of albumin and gamma globulin in kwashiorkor. Clin Sci 23:351–359, 1962.

Coker DD, Morris DM, Coleman JJ, Schimpff SC, Wiernik PH, Elias EG. Infection among 210 patients with surgically staged Hodgkin's disease. Am J Med 75:97–109, 1983.

Constantopoulos A, Najjar VA, Smith JW. Tuftsin deficiency: a new syndrome with defective phagocytosis. J Pediatr 80:564–572, 1972.

Copeland JL, Karrh LR, McCoy J, Guckian JC. Bactericidal activity of polymorphonuclear leukocytes from patients with severe bacterial infections. Tex Rep Biol Med 29:555–562, 1971.

Corry JM, Polhill RB Jr, Edmonds SR, Johnston RB Jr. Activity of the alternative complement pathway after splenectomy: comparison to activity in sickle cell disease and hypogammaglobulinemia. J Pediatr 95:964–969, 1979.

Cosimi AB, Colvin RB, Burton RC, Rubin RH, Goldstein G, Kung PC, Hansen WP, Delmonico FL, Russell PS. Use of monoclonal antibodies to T-cell subsets for immunologic monitoring and treatment in recipients of renal allografts. N Engl J Med 305:308–314, 1981.

Cosimi AB, Delmonico FL, Wright JK, Wee SL, Preffer FI, Jolliffe LK, Colvin RB. Prolonged survival of nonhuman primate renal allograft recipients treated only with anti-CD4 monoclonal antibody. Surgery 108:406–413, 1990.

Cossarizza A, Monti D, Montagnani G, Ortolani C, Masi M, Zannotti M, Franceschi C. Precocious aging of the immune system in Down syndrome: alteration of B lymphocytes, T-lymphocyte subsets, and cells with natural killer markers. Am J Med Genet Suppl 7:213–218, 1990.

Coutsoudis A, Kiepiela P, Coovadia HM, Broughton M. Vitamin A supplementation enhances specific IgG antibody levels and total lymphocyte numbers while improving morbidity in measles. Pediatr Infect Dis J 11:203–209, 1992.

Crawford MD. Renal dysplasia and asplenia in two sibs. Clin Genet 14:338–344, 1978.

Crystal RG, Bitterman PB, Rennard SI, Hance AJ, Keogh BA. Interstitial lung diseases of unknown cause. Disorders characterized by chronic inflammation of the lower respiratory tract. N Engl J Med 310:235–244, 1984.

Cupps TR, Edgar LC, Thomas CA, Fauci AS. Multiple mechanisms of B cell immunoregulation in man after administration of in vivo corticosteroids. J Immunol 132:170–175, 1984.

Currey HL. A comparison of immunosuppressive and anti-inflammatory agents in the rat. Clin Exp Immunol 9:879–887, 1971.

Curtis JR, Wing AJ, Coleman JC. Bacillus cereus bacteraemia: a complication of intermittent haemodialysis. Lancet 1:136–138, 1967.

Cutler AT, Benezra-Obeiter R, Brink SJ. Thyroid function in young children with Down syndrome. Am J Dis Child 140:479–483, 1986.

Dale DC, Petersdorf RG. Corticosteroids and infectious diseases. Med Clin North Am 57:1277–1287, 1973.

Dallman PR. Iron deficiency and the immune response. Am J Clin Nutr 46:329–334, 1987.

Dammin GJ, Couch NP, Murray JE. Prolonged survival of skin homografts in uremic patients. Ann N Y Acad Sci 64:967–976, 1957.

Damodaran M, Naidu AN, Sarma KV. Anaemia and morbidity in rural preschool children. Indian J Med Res 69:448–456, 1979.

Daniele RP, Rowlands DT. Antibodies to T cells in sarcoidosis. Ann N Y Acad Sci 278:88–100, 1976.

Daniels JC, Larson DL, Abston S, Ritzmann SE. Serum protein profiles in thermal burns. I. Serum electrophoretic patterns, immunoglobulins, and transport proteins. J Trauma 14:137–152, 1974a.

Daniels JC, Larson DL, Abston S, Ritzmann SE. Serum protein profiles in thermal burns. II. Protease inhibitors, complement factors, and c-reactive protein. J Trauma 14:153–162, 1974b.

Daniels JC, Sakai H, Cobb EK, Lewis SR, Larson DL, Ritzmann SE. Evaluation of lymphocyte reactivity studies in patients with thermal burns. J Trauma 11:595–601, 1971.

Davidson E, Hayhoe FGJ. Prolonged generalized vaccinia complicating acute leukemia. Br Med J 2:1298–1299, 1962.

Davidson JD, Waldmann TA, Goodman DS, Gordon JRS. Protein-losing gastroenteropathy in congestive heart failure. Lancet 1:899–902, 1961.

De Boer J, Downie HG. Partial splenectomy in dogs: an experimental tool for studies of the spleen. Can J Physiol Pharmacol 49:1110–1112, 1971.

Degnan TJ. Idiopathic hypoproteinemia. J Pediatr 51:448–452, 1957.

del Gobbo V, Balestra E, Marini S, Villani N, Calio R. Influenza virus infection reduces cellular immunity functions. Adv Exp Med Biol 257:247–254, 1989.

del Gobbo V, Villani N, Marini S, Balestra E, Calio R. Suppressor cells induced by influenza virus inhibit interleukin-2 production in mice. Immunol 69:454–459, 1990.

Desnick RJ, Sharp HL, Grabowski GA, Brunning RD, Quie PG, Sung JH, Gorlin RJ, Ikonne JU. Mannosidosis: clinical, morphologic, immunologic, and biochemical studies. Pediatr Res 10:985–996, 1976.

Dhur A, Galan P, Hercberg S. Iron status, immune capacity and resistance to infections. Comp Biochem Physiol 94A:11–19, 1989.

Diamond LK. Splenectomy in childhood and the hazard of overwhelming infection. Pediatrics 43:886–889, 1969.

Donti E, Nicoletti I, Venti G, Filipponi P, Gerli R, Spinozzi F, Cernetti C, Rambotti P. X-ring Turner's syndrome with combined immunodeficiency and selective gonadotropin defect. J Endocrinol Invest 12:257–263, 1989.

Dosch HM, Jason J, Gelfand EW. Transient antibody deficiency and abnormal T-suppressor cells induced by phenytoin. N Engl J Med 306:406–409, 1982.

Douglas SD, Schopfer K. Phagocyte function in protein-calorie malnutrition. Clin Exp Immunol 17:121–128, 1974.

Douglas SD, Schopfer K. Analytical review: host defense mechanisms in protein-energy malnutrition. Clin Immunol Immunopathol 5:1–5, 1976.

Dourov N. Thymic atrophy and immune deficiency in malnutrition. Curr Top Pathol 75:127–150, 1986.

Doutlik S, Kutinova L, Benda R, Kaminkova J, Krcmar M, Votruba T, Suchankova A, Vonka V, Vacek Z. Some immunological characteristics of subjects suffering from frequent herpes simplex virus recrudescences. Acta Virol 33:435–446, 1989.

Dresdale AR, Lutz S, Drost C, Levine TB, Fenn N, Paone G, del Busto R, Silverman NA. Prospective evaluation of malignant neoplasms in cardiac transplant recipients uniformly treated with prophylactic antilymphocyte globulin. J Thorac Cardiovas Surg 106:1202–1207, 1993.

Drew PA, Kiroff GK, Ferrante A, Cohen RC. Alterations in immunoglobulin synthesis by peripheral blood mononuclear cells from splenectomized patients with and without splenic regrowth. J Immunol 132:191–196, 1984.

Driscoll DA, Budarf ML, Emanuel BS. A genetic etiology for DiGeorge syndrome: consistent deletions and microdeletions of 22q11. Am J Hum Genet 50:924–933, 1992.

DuVivier A, Munro DD. Alopecia areata, autoimmunity, and Down's syndrome. Br Med J 1:191–192, 1975.

Dziatkowiak H, Kowalska M, Denys A. Phagocytic and bactericidal activity of granulocytes in diabetic children. Diabetes 31:1041–1043, 1982.

Ebert RH, Barclay WR. Changes in connective tissue reaction induced by cortisone. Ann Intern Med 37:506–518, 1952.

Edelman R. Cutaneous hypersensitivity in protein-calorie malnutrition. Lancet 1:1244–1245, 1973.

Egeler RM, D'Angio GJ. Langerhans cell histiocytosis. J Pediatr 127:1–11, 1995.

Elkhalifa MY, Ghalib HW, Dafa'Alla T, Williams JF. Suppression of human lymphocyte responses to specific and non-specific stimuli in human onchocerciasis. Clin Exp Immunol 86:433–439, 1991.

Ellis CN, Gorsulowsky DC, Hamilton TA, Billings JK, Brown MD, Headington JT, Cooper KD, Baadsgaard O, Duell EA, Annesley TM, Turcotte JG, Voorhees JJ. Cyclosporine improves psoriasis in a double-blind study. JAMA 256:3110–3116, 1986.

Ellis EF, Smith RT. The role of the spleen in immunity. With special reference to the post-splenectomy problem in infants. Pediatrics 37:111–119, 1966.

Ellner JJ, Olds GR, Kamel R, Osman GS, el Kholy A, Mahmoud AA. Suppression splenic T lymphocytes in human hepatosplenic schistosomiasis mansoni. J Immunol 125:308–312, 1980.

Eltringham JR, Kaplan HS. Impaired delayed hypersensitivity responses in 154 patients with untreated Hodgkin's disease. Natl Cancer Inst Monogr 36:107–115, 1973.

Engh CA, Hughes JL, Abrams RC, Bowerman JW. Osteomyelitis in the patient with sickle-cell disease. J Bone Joint Surg 53:1–15, 1971.

Ennis FA, Meager A, Beare AS, Qi Y, Riley D, Schwarz G, Schild GC, Rook AH. Interferon induction and increased natural killer cell activity in influenza infections in man. Lancet 2:891–893, 1981.

Epstein WL, Mayock RL. Induction of allergic contact dermatitis in patients with sarcoidosis. Proc Soc Exp Biol Med 96:786–787, 1957.

Eraklis AJ, Filler RM. Splenectomy in childhood: a review of 1413 cases. J Pediat Surg 7:382–388, 1972.

Esa AH, Paxman DG, Noga SJ, Hess AD. Sensitivity of monocyte subpopulations to cyclosporine. Arachidonate metabolism and in vitro antigen presentation. Transplant Proc 20:80–86, 1988.

Etzioni A, Lahat N, Benderly A, Katz R, Pollack S. Humoral and cellular immune dysfunction in a patient with Bloom's syndrome and recurrent infections. J Clin Lab Immunol 28:151–154, 1989.

Evans HE, Reindorf C. Serum immunoglobulin levels in sickle cell disease and thalassemia major. Am J Dis Child 116:586–590, 1968.

Faist E, Kupper TS, Baker CC, Chaudry IH, Dwyer J, Baue AE. Depression of cellular immunity after major injury: its association with posttraumatic complications and its reversal with immunomodulation. Arch Surg 121:1000–1005, 1986.

Falter ML, Robinson MG, Kim OS, Go SC, Taubkin SP. Splenic function and infection in sickle cell anemia. Acta Haematol 50:154–161, 1973.

Farid NR. Immunologic aspects of diabetes mellitus. In Chandra RK, ed. Nutrition and Immunology. New York, Alan R. Liss, 1988, pp. 269–313.

Fasth A, Forestier E, Holmberg E, Holmgren G, Nordenson I, Soderstrom T, Wahlstrom J. Fragility of the centromeric region of chromosome 1 associated with combined immunodeficiency in siblings: a recessively inherited entity? Acta Paediatr Scand 79:605–612, 1990.

Fauci AS, Dale DC. Alternate-day prednisone therapy and human lymphocyte subpopulations. J Clin Invest 55:22–32, 1975.

Fauci AS, Dale DC, Balow JE. Glucocorticosteroid therapy: mechanisms of action and clinical considerations. Ann Intern Med 84:304–315, 1976.

Favara BE. Langerhans' cell histiocytosis pathobiology and pathogenesis. Semin Oncol 18:3–7, 1991.

Fawcett WA IV, Ferry GD, Gorin LJ, Rosenblatt HM, Brown BS, Shearer WT. Immunodeficiency secondary to structural intestinal defects: malrotation of the small bowel and cavernous hemangioma of the jejunum. Am J Dis Child 140:169–172, 1986.

Fawzi WW, Chalmers TC, Herrera MG, Mosteller F. Vitamin A supplementation and child mortality. A meta-analysis. JAMA 269:898–903, 1993.

Fazio M, Calciati A. Transporto degli anticorpi di Tipo tubercolinico ritardato nel linfogranuloma. Minerva Med 53:2394–2397, 1962.

Feehally J, Beattie TJ, Brenchley PE, Coupes BM, Houston IB, Mallick NP, Postlethwaite RJ. Modulation of cellular immune function by cyclophosphamide in children with minimal change nephropathy. N Engl J Med 310:415–420, 1984.

Feingold M, Schwartz RS. IgA and partial deletions of chromosome 18. Lancet 2:1086, 1968.

Ferguson AC, Lawlor GJ Jr, Neumann CG, Oh W, Stiehm ER. Decreased rosette-forming lymphocytes in malnutrition and intrauterine growth retardation. J Pediatr 85:717–723, 1974.

Fernandez B, Press P, Girard JP. Distribution and function of T- and B-cell subpopulations in sarcoidosis. Ann N Y Acad Sci 278:80–87, 1976.

Fernandez LA, MacSween JM, Langley GR. Immunoglobulin secretory function of B cells from untreated patients with chronic lymphocytic leukemia and hypogammaglobulinemia: role of T cells. Blood 62:767–774, 1983.

Fernbach DJ. Natural history of acute leukemia. In Sutow WW, Fernbach DJ, Vietti TJ, eds. Clinical Pediatric Oncology. St. Louis, C. V. Mosby, 1984, pp. 332–377.

Finkelstein JL, Schwartz SB, Madden MR, Marano MA, Goodwin CW. Pediatric burns: an overview. Pediatr Clin North Am 39:1145–1163, 1992.

Finley SC, Finley WH, Noto TA, Uchida IA, Roddam RF. IgA absence associated with a ring-18 chromosome. Lancet 1:1095–1096, 1968.

Fleming AF, Storey J, Molineaux L, Iroko EA, Attai ED. Abnormal haemoglobins in the Sudan savanna of Nigeria: I. Prevalence of haemoglobins and relationships between sickle cell trait, malaria and survival. Ann Trop Med Parasitol 73:161–172, 1979.

Flemming JW, Runyon EH, Cummings MM. An evaluation of the hemagglutination test for tuberculosis. Am J Med 10:704–710, 1951.

Foley FD. The burn autopsy. Fatal complications of burns. Am J Clin Pathol 52:1–13, 1969.

Foley FD, Greenawald KA, Nash G, Pruitt BA Jr. Herpesvirus infection in burned patients. N Engl J Med 282:652–656, 1970.

Foon KA, Mitsuyasu RT, Schroff RW, McIntyre RE, Champlin R, Gale RP. Immunologic defects in young male patients with hepatitis-associated aplastic anemia. Ann Intern Med 100:657–662, 1984.

Forward AD, Ashmore PG. Infection following splenectomy in infants and children. Can J Surg 3:229–233, 1960.

Fowler I, Hollingsworth DR, Traurig H. Response to stimulation in vitro of lymphocytes from patients with Down's syndrome. Proc Soc Exp Biol Med 144:475–477, 1973.

Fox CL Jr. Silver sulfadiazine—a new topical therapy for *Pseudomonas* in burns: therapy of *Pseudomonas* infection in burns. Arch Surg 96:184–188, 1968.

Fox JE, Lowbury EJL. Immunity to *Pseudomonas pyocyanea* in man. J Pathol Bacteriol 65:519–531, 1953.

Freireich EJ, Bodey GP, DeJongh DS, Curtis JE, Hersh EM. Supportive therapeutic measures for patients under treatment for leukemia or lymphoma. In Leukemia-Lymphoma. Anderson Hospital. Chicago, Year Book Medical Publishers, 1970, pp. 275–284.

Friou GJ. A study of the cutaneous reactions to oidiomycin, trichophytin, and mumps skin test antigens in patients with sarcoidosis. Yale J Biol Med 24:533–539, 1952.

Fuks Z, Strober S, Bobrove AM, Sasazuki T, McMichael A, Kaplan HS. Long-term effects of radiation of T and B lymphocytes in peripheral blood of patients with Hodgkin's disease. J Clin Invest 58:803–814, 1976.

Fullana A, Garcia-Frias E, Martinez-Frias ML, Razquin S, Quero J. Caudal deficiency and asplenia anomalies in sibs. Am J Med Genet Suppl 2:23–29, 1986.

Gajl-Peczalska KJ, Bloomfield CD, Coccia PF, Sosin H, Brunning RD, Kersey JH. B and T cell lymphomas: analysis of blood and lymph nodes in 87 patients. Am J Med 59:674–685, 1975.

Gajl-Peczalska KJ, Zusman J, Kersey JH, Nesbit ME. B lymphocytes in acute lymphoblastic leukemia: the effects of radiation and chemotherapy. Fed Proc 33:610, 1974.

Garcia CR, Brown NA, Schreck R, Stiehm ER, Hudnall SD. B-cell lymphoma in severe combined immunodeficiency not associated with the Epstein-Barr virus. Cancer 60:2941–2947, 1987.

Garcia-Leoni ME, Martin-Scapa C, Rodeno P, Valderrabano F, Moreno S, Bouza E. High incidence of tuberculosis in renal patients. Eur J Clin Microbiol Infect Dis 9:283–285, 1990.

Gaston MH, Verter JI, Woods G, Pegelow C, Kelleher J, Presbury G, Zarkowsky H, Vichinsky E, Iyer R, Lobel JS, Diamond S, Holbrook CT, Gill FM, Ritchey K, Falletta J. Prophylaxis with oral penicillin in children with sickle cell anemia: a randomized trial. N Engl J Med 314:1593–1599, 1986.

Gavrilis P, Rothenberg SP, Guy R. Correlation of low serum IgM levels with absence of functional splenic tissue in sickle cell disease syndromes. Am J Med 57:542–545, 1974.

German J, Passarge E. Bloom's syndrome. XII. Report from the Registry for 1987. Clin Genet 35:57–69, 1989.

Gerner RH, Wolff SM, Fauci AS, Aduan RP. Lithium carbonate for recurrent fever and neutropenia. JAMA 246:1584–1586, 1981.

Giangiacomo J, Cleary TG, Cole BR, Hoffsten P, Robson AM. Serum immunoglobulins in the nephrotic syndrome: a possible cause of minimal-change nephrotic syndrome. N Engl J Med 293:8–12, 1975.

Gilhus NE, Aarli JA. The reversibility of phenytoin-induced IgA deficiency. J Neurol 226:53–61, 1981.

Gillis J, Harvey J, Isaacs D, Freelander M, Wyeth B. Familial asplenia. Arch Dis Child 67:665–666, 1992.

Gimelli G, Varone P, Pezzolo A, Lerone M, Pistoia V. ICF syndrome with variable expression in sibs. J Med Genet 30:429–432, 1993.

Girard JP, Poupon MF, Press P. Culture of peripheral blood lymphocytes from sarcoidosis: response to mitogenic factor. Int Arch Allergy Appl Immunol 41:604–619, 1971.

Glasziou PP, Mackerras DE. Vitamin A supplementation in infectious diseases: a meta-analysis. Br Med J 306:366–370, 1993.

Goldblum SE, Reed WP. Host defenses and immunologic alterations associated with chronic hemodialysis. Ann Intern Med 93:597–613, 1980.

Goldman JM, Hobbs JR. The immunoglobulins in Hodgkin's disease. Immunol 13:421–431, 1967.

Goldstein RA, Israel HL, Rawnsley HM. Effect of race and stage of disease on the serum immunoglobulins in sarcoidosis. JAMA 208:1153–1155, 1969.

Gomez L, Le Deist F, Blanche S, Cavazzano-Calvo M, Griscelli C, Fischer A. Treatment of Omenn syndrome by bone marrow transplantation. J Pediatr 127:76–81, 1995.

Good RA, Kelly WD, Rotstein J, Varco RL. Immunological deficiency diseases: agammaglobulinemia, hypogammaglobulinemia, Hodgkin's disease and sarcoidosis. Prog Allergy 6:187–319, 1962.

Gooding AM, Bastian JF, Peterson BM, Wilson NW. Safety and efficacy of intravenous immunoglobulin prophylaxis in pediatric head trauma patients: a double-blind controlled trial. J Crit Care 8:212–216, 1993.

Goodwin JS, DeHoratius R, Israel H, Peake GT, Messner RP. Suppressor cell function in sarcoidosis. Ann Intern Med 90:169–173, 1979.

Goodwin JS, Messner RP, Bankhurst AD, Peake GT, Saiki JH, Williams RC Jr. Prostaglandin-producing suppressor cells in Hodgkin's disease. N Engl J Med 297:963–968, 1977.

Gordon MC, Sinha SK, Carlson SD. Antibody responses to influenza vaccine in patients with Down's syndrome. Am J Ment Defic 75:391–399, 1971.

Gordon RS. Exudative enteropathy. Abnormal permeability of the gastrointestinal tract demonstrable with labelled polyvinylpyrolidone. Lancet 1:325–326, 1959.

Gorensek MJ, Lebel MH, Nelson JD. Peritonitis in children with nephrotic syndrome. Pediatrics 81:849–856, 1988.

Gotoff SP, Lolekha S, Lopata M, Kopp J, Kopp RL, Malecki TJ. The macrophage aggregation assay for cell-mediated immunity in man: studies of patients with Hodgkin's disease and sarcoidosis. J Lab Clin Med 82:682–691, 1973.

Granelli-Piperno A, Keane M, Steinman RM. Evidence that cyclosporine inhibits cell-mediated immunity primarily at the level of the T lymphocyte rather than the accessory cell. Transplantation 46:53S–60S, 1988.

Gratama JW, Langelaar RA, Oosterveer MA, van der Linden JA, den Ouden Noordermeer A, Naipal AM, Visser JW, de Gast GC, Tanke HJ. Phenotypic study of CD4$^+$ and CD8$^+$ lymphocyte subsets in relation to cytomegalovirus carrier status and its correlate with pokeweed mitogen–induced B lymphocyte differentiation. Clin Exp Immunol 77:245–251, 1989.

Gratz RR. Accidental injury in childhood: a literature review on pediatric trauma. J Trauma 19:551–555, 1979.

Greenberg F, Valdes C, Rosenblatt HM, Kirkland JL, Ledbetter DH. Hypoparathyroidism and T cell immune defect in a patient with 10p deletion syndrome. J Pediatr 109:489–492, 1986.

Greenwood BM, Bradley-Moore AM, Bryceson AD, Palit A. Immunosuppression in children with malaria. Lancet 1:169–172, 1972.

Greenwood R, Smellie H, Barr M, Cunliffe AC. Circulating antibodies in sarcoidosis. Br Med J 1:1388–1391, 1958.

Gregory CD, Murray RJ, Edwards CF, Rickinson AB. Downregulation of cell adhesion molecules LFA-3 and ICAM-1 in Epstein-Barr virus–positive Burkitt's lymphoma underlies tumor cell escape from virus-specific T cell surveillance. J Exp Med 167:1811–1824, 1988.

Grey HM, Rabellino E, Pirofsky B. Immunoglobulins on the surface of lymphocytes. IV. Distribution in hypogammaglobulinemia, cellular immune deficiency, and chronic lymphatic leukemia. J Clin Invest 50:2368–2375, 1971.

Griffin DE, Ward BJ, Jauregui E, Johnson RT, Vaisberg A. Natural killer cell activity during measles. Clin Exp Immunol 81:218–224, 1990.

Griffiths AW, Sylvester PE. Mongols and non-mongols compared in their response to active tetanus immunisation. J Ment Defic Res 11:263–266, 1967.

Groch GS, Perillie PE, Finch SC. Reticuloendothelial phagocytic function in patients with leukemia and multiple myeloma. Blood 26:489–499, 1965.

Gronemeyer H. Control of transcription activation by steroid hormone receptors. FASEB J 6:2524–2529, 1992.

Groshong T, Mendelson L, Mendoza S, Bazaral M, Hamburger R, Tune B. Serum IgE in patients with minimal-change nephrotic syndrome. J Pediatr 83:767–771, 1973.

Gudnason T, Potter C, Sharp H, Quie PG. Disseminated *Candida albicans* infection in a patient with Epstein-Barr virus infection. Clin Pediatr 29:583–586, 1990.

Guerra IC, Fawcett WA IV, Redmon AH, Lawrence EC, Rosenblatt HM, Shearer WT. Permanent intrinsic B cell immunodeficiency caused by phenytoin hypersensitivity. J Allergy Clin Immunol 77:603–607, 1986.

Guyatt GH, Bensen WG, Stolmon LP, Fagnilli L, Singal DP. HLA-B8 and erythema nodosum. Can Med Assoc J 127:1005–1006, 1982.

Haag-Weber M, Horl WH. Uremia and infection: mechanisms of impaired cellular host defense. Nephron 63:125–131, 1993.

Hammond WP, Price TH, Souza LM, Dale DC. Treatment of cyclic neutropenia with granulocyte colony–stimulating factor. N Engl J Med 320:1306–1311, 1989.

Han T, Sokal JE. Lymphocyte response to phytohemagglutinin in Hodgkin's disease. Am J Med 48:728–734, 1970.

Hansen JA, Good RA. Malignant disease of the lymphoid system in immunological perspective. Hum Pathol 5:567–599, 1974.

Harland PSEG, Brown RE. Tuberculin sensitivity following BCG vaccination in undernourished children. East Afr Med J 42:233–238, 1965.

Harris SL, Frank I, Yee A, Cohen GH, Eisenberg RJ, Friedman HM. Glycoprotein C of herpes simplex virus type 1 prevents complement-mediated cell lysis and virus neutralization. J Infect Dis 162:331–337, 1990.

Hawkes RA, Boughton CR, Schroeter DR. The antibody response of institutionalized Down's syndrome patients to seven microbial antigens. Clin Exp Immunol 31:298–304, 1978.

Hayakawa H, Matsui I, Higurashi M, Kobayashi N. Hyperblastic response to dilute PHA in Down's syndrome. Lancet 1:95–96, 1968.

Haynes BF, Fauci AS. The differential effect of in vivo hydrocortisone on the kinetics of subpopulations of human peripheral blood thymus-derived lymphocytes. J Clin Invest 61:703–707, 1978.

Heath RB, Fairley GH, Malpas JS. Production of antibodies against viruses in leukemia and related diseases. Br J Haematol 10:365–370, 1964.

Hedfors E. Immunological aspects of sarcoidosis. Scand J Respir Dis 56:1–19, 1975.

Hedfors E. Characterization of peripheral blood lymphocytes in sarcoidosis. Ann NY Acad Sci 278:101–107, 1976.

Hedfors E, Holm G, Pettersson D. Lymphocyte subpopulations in sarcoidosis. Clin Exp Immunol 17:219–226, 1974.

Hedfors E, Norberg R. Evidence for circulating immune complexes in sarcoidosis. Clin Exp Immunol 16:493–496, 1974.

Heim S, Mitelman F. Cancer Cytogenetics. New York, Alan R. Liss, 1987, pp. 94, 162.

Henderson FW, Collier AM, Sanyal MA, Watkins JM, Fairclough DL, Clyde WA Jr, Denny FW. A longitudinal study of respiratory viruses and bacteria in the etiology of acute otitis media with effusion. N Engl J Med 306:1377–1383, 1982.

Heresi G, Olivaress M, Pizzaro F, Cayazao M, Hertrampf E, Walter T, Stekel A. Effect of iron fortification on infant morbidity. In XIII International Congress of Nutrition, Brighton, England, 1985. London, Libbey, 1986, p. 129.

Hersh EM, Carbone PP, Wong EP, Freireich EJ. Inhibition of the primary immune response in man by antimetabolites. Cancer Res 25:997–1001, 1965.

Hersh EM, Irvin WS. Blastogenic responses of lymphocytes from patients with untreated and treated lymphomas. Lymphology 2:150–160, 1969.

Hersh EM, Oppenheim JJ. Impaired in vitro lymphocyte transformation in Hodgkin's disease. N Engl J Med 273:1006–1012, 1965.

Herskovic T, Spiro HM, Gryboski JD. Acute transient gastrointestinal protein loss. Pediatrics 41:818–821, 1968.

Hill HR, Gerrard JM, Hogan NA, Quie PG. Hyperactivity of neutrophil leukotactic responses during active bacterial infection. J Clin Invest 53:996–1002, 1974a.

Hill HR, Sauls HS, Dettloff JL, Quie PG. Impaired leukotactic responsiveness in patients with juvenile diabetes mellitus. Clin Immunol Immunopathol 2:395–403, 1974b.

Hindman SH, Favero MS, Carson LA, Petersen NJ, Schonberger LB, Solano JT. Pyogenic reactions during haemodialysis caused by extramural endotoxin. Lancet 2:732–734, 1975.

Hirschhorn K, Schreibman RR, Bach FH, Siltzbach LE. In vitro studies of lymphocytes from patients with sarcoidosis and lymphoproliferative diseases. Lancet 2:842–843, 1964.

Hirshaut Y, Glade P, Vieria BD, Ainbender E, Dvorak B, Siltzbach LE. Sarcoidosis, another disease associated with serologic evidence for herpes-like virus infection. N Engl J Med 283:502–506, 1970.

Hitzig WH, Pluss HJ, Joller P, Pilgrim U, Tacier-Eugster A, Jakob M. Studies on the immune status of children with acute lymphocytic leukaemia. I. Early phase before and after first remission. Clin Exp Immunol 26:403–413, 1976.

Hodes H (quoted by Janeway CA). In Metcoff J, ed. Proceedings of the Fourth Annual Conference on the Nephrotic Syndrome. New York, National Kidney Disease Foundation, 1952, p. 46.

Hodges R. In Metcoff J, ed. Proceedings of the Sixth Annual Conference on the Nephrotic Syndrome. Cleveland, National Kidney Disease Foundation, 1954, pp. 265–271.

Hoffman R, Zanjani ED, Lutton JD, Zalusky R, Wasserman LR. Suppression of erythroid-colony formation by lymphocytes from patients with aplastic anemia. N Engl J Med 296:10–13, 1977.

Holdsworth RJ, Irving AD, Cuschieri A. Postsplenectomy sepsis and its mortality rate: actual versus perceived risks. Br J Surg 78:1031–1038, 1991.

Hollingsworth DR, Hollingsworth JW, Roeckel I, McKean HE, Holland N. Immunologic reactions and Australia antigenemia in Down's syndrome. J Chronic Dis 27:483–490, 1974.

Holroyde CP, Oski FA, Gardner FH. The "pocked" erythrocyte. Red-cell surface alterations in reticuloendothelial immaturity of the neonate. N Engl J Med 281:516–520, 1969.

Holt PR. Dietary treatment of protein loss in intestinal lymphangiectasia: the effect of eliminating dietary long-chain triglycerides on albumin metabolism in this condition. Pediatrics 34:629–635, 1964.

Hong R. Associations of the skeletal and immune systems. Am J Med Genet 34:55–59, 1989.

Hook EW, Campbell GC, Weens HS, Cooper GR. *Salmonella* osteomyelitis in patients with sickle cell anemia. N Engl J Med 257:403–407, 1957.

Horowitz MC. Cytokines and estrogen in bone: anti-osteoporotic effects. Science 260:626–627, 1993.

Horsmanheimo M. Lymphocyte transforming factor in sarcoidosis. Cell Immunol 10:338–343, 1974.

Horsmanheimo M, Virolainen M. Transfer of tuberculin sensitivity by transfer factor in sarcoidosis. Clin Immunol Immunopathol 6:231–237, 1976.

Hosea SW, Brown EJ, Hamburger MI, Frank MM. Opsonic requirements for intravascular clearance after splenectomy. N Engl J Med 304:245–250, 1981a.

Hosea SW, Burch CG, Brown EJ, Berg RA, Frank MM. Impaired immune response of splenectomised patients to polyvalent pneumococcal vaccine. Lancet 1:804–807, 1981b.

Howard CJ, Glynn AA. The virulence for mice of strains of *Escherichia coli* related to the effects of K antigens on their resistance to phagocytosis and killing by complement. Immunol 20:767–777, 1971.

Hoy WE, Cestero RV, Freeman RB. Deficiency of T and B lymphocytes in uremic subjects and partial improvement with maintenance hemodialysis. Nephron 20:182–188, 1978.

Hsu DH, de Waal Malefyt R, Fiorentino DF, Dang MN, Vieira P, de Vries J, Spits H, Mosmann TR, Moore KW. Expression of interleukin-10 activity by Epstein-Barr virus protein BCRF1. Science 250:830–832, 1990.

Huber H, Pastner D, Dittrich P, Braunsteiner H. In vitro reactivity of human lymphocytes in uraemia—a comparison with the impairment of delayed hypersensitivity. Clin Exp Immunol 5:75–82, 1969.

Hughes WT, Price RA, Sisko F, Havron WS, Kafatos AG, Schonland M, Smythe PM. Protein-calorie malnutrition. A host determinant for *Pneumocystis carinii* infection. Am J Dis Child 128:44–52, 1974.

Hume DM, Merrill JP, Miller BS, Thorn GW. Experiences with renal homotransplantation in the human: report of nine cases. J Clin Invest 34:327–332, 1955.

Hunninghake GW. Release of interleukin-1 by alveolar macrophages of patients with active pulmonary sarcoidosis. Am Rev Respir Dis 129:569–572, 1984.

Hunninghake GW, Bedell GN, Zavala DC, Monick M, Brady M. Role of interleukin-2 release by lung T-cells in active pulmonary sarcoidosis. Am Rev Respir Dis 128:634–638, 1983.

Hunninghake GW, Crystal RG. Pulmonary sarcoidosis: a disorder mediated by excess helper T–lymphocyte activity at sites of disease activity. N Engl J Med 305:429–434, 1981.

Hunninghake GW, Gadek JE, Kawanami O, Ferrans VJ, Crystal RG. Inflammatory and immune processes in the human lung in health and disease: evaluation by bronchoalveolar lavage. Am J Pathol 97:149–206, 1979.

Hurwitz RC, Caskey CT. Ivemark syndrome in siblings. Clin Genet 22:7–11, 1982.

Hussey GD, Klein M. A randomized, controlled trial of vitamin A in children with severe measles. N Engl J Med 323:160–164, 1990.

Hutteroth TH, Litwin SD, German J. Abnormal immune responses of Bloom's syndrome lymphocytes in vitro. J Clin Invest 56:1–7, 1975.

Ingelfinger JR, Link DA, Davis AE, Grupe WE. Serum immunoglobulins in idiopathic minimal change nephrotic syndrome. N Engl J Med 294:50–51, 1976.

Insoft RM, Murphy M, Popek EJ, Pike-Nobile L, Epstein LB. Overexpression of IFN-gamma, TNF and ICAM-1 in fetal and postnatal Down syndrome thymus. J Interferon Res 13:S160, 1993.

Insoft RM, Murphy M, Popek EJ, Pike-Nobile L, Epstein LB. Abnormalities in the fetal and postnatal spleen in Down syndrome: implications for deficient immune function. Pediatr Res 35:13A, 1994.

Iselius L, Jacobs P, Morton N. Leukaemia and transient leukaemia in Down syndrome. Hum Genet 85:477–485, 1990.

Ishizaka A, Nakanishi M, Kasahara E, Mizutani K, Sakiyama Y, Matsumoto S. Phenytoin-induced IgG2 and IgG4 deficiencies in a patient with epilepsy. Acta Paediatr 81:646–648, 1992.

Israel H, Sones M. A study of bacillus Calmette-Guérin vaccination and the Kveim reaction. Ann Intern Med 64:87–91, 1966.

Israel HL, Sones M. The tuberculin reaction in patients recovered from sarcoidosis. In Turiaf J, Chabot J, eds. La Sarcoidose, Paris, Masson, 1967, pp. 295–298.

Ivemark BI. Implications of agenesis of the spleen on the pathogenesis of conotruncus anomalies in childhood: analysis of the heart malformations in spleen agenesis syndrome with fourteen new cases. Acta Paediatr 44(Suppl.):1–110, 1955.

Iwai K, Takahashi S. Transmissibility of sarcoid-specific granulomas in the footpads of mice. Ann NY Acad Sci 278:249–259, 1976.

Izumi T, Nilsson BS, Ripe E. In vitro lymphocyte reactivity to different Kveim preparations in patients with sarcoidosis. Scand J Respir Dis 54:123–127, 1973.

Jackson D. A clinical study of the use of skin homografts for burns. Br J Plast Surg 7:26–43, 1954.

Jackson MA, Burry VF, Olson LC. Multisystem group A beta-streptococcal disease in children. Rev Infect Dis 13:783–788, 1991.

Jackson SM, Garrett JV, Craig AW. Lymphocyte transformation changes during the clinical course of Hodgkin's disease. Cancer 25:843–850, 1970.

Jadassohn J. Sie tuberkulide. Arch Dermatol Syph 119:10–83, 1914.

Jagadeesan V, Reddy V. Complement system in iron deficiency anemia. Experientia 39:146, 1983.

James DG, Neville E. Pathobiology of sarcoidosis. Pathobiol Annu 7:31–61, 1977.

James DG, Neville E, Walker A. Immunology of sarcoidosis. Am J Med 59:388–394, 1975.

Jarnum S, Petersen VP. Protein-losing eneropathy. Lancet 1:417–421, 1961.

Jasper PL, Denny FW. Sarcoidosis in children. With special emphasis on the natural history and treatment. J Pediatr 73:499–512, 1968.

Jeffries GH, Chapman A, Sleisenger MH. Low-fat diet in intestinal lymphangiectasia: its effect on albumin metabolism. N Engl J Med 270:761–766, 1964.

Jensen K, Christensen KR, Jacobsen P, Nielsen J, Friedrich U, Tsuboi T. Ring chromosome 18 and gamma-M-globulin abnormality. Lancet 2:497–498, 1969.

Jensen K, Petersen PH, Nielsen EL, Dahl G, Nielsen J. Serum immunoglobulin M, G, and A concentration levels in Turner's syndrome compared with normal women and men. Hum Genet 31:329–334, 1976.

Jeunet FS, Good RA. Thymoma, immunologic deficiencies, and hematologic abnormalities. Birth Defects 4:192–206, 1968.

Johns CJ, Macgregor MI, Zachary JB, Ball WC. Extended experience in the long-term corticosteroid treatment of pulmonary sarcoidosis. Ann NY Acad Sci 278:722–731, 1976.

Johnson JP, Carey JC, Glassy FJ, Paglieroni T, Lipson MH. Marshall-Smith syndrome: two case reports and a review of pulmonary manifestations. Pediatrics 71:219–223, 1983.

Johnston MF, Slavin RG. Mechanism of inhibition of adoptive transfer of tuberculin sensitivity in acute uremia. J Lab Clin Med 87:457–461, 1976.

Johnston RB Jr, Newman SL, Struth AG. An abnormality of the alternate pathway of complement activation in sickle-cell disease. N Engl J Med 288:803–808, 1973.

Johnston RB Jr, Newman SL, Struth AG. Increased susceptibility to infection in sickle cell disease: defects of opsonization and of splenic function. In Bergsma D, Good RA, eds. Immunodeficiency in Man and Animals. Stamford, Conn., Sinauer Associates, 1975, pp. 322–327.

Jolivet J, Cowan KH, Curt GA, Clendeninn NJ, Chabner BA. The pharmacology and clinical use of methotrexate. N Engl J Med 309:1094–1104, 1983.

Joncas J, Monczak Y, Ghibu F, Alfieri C, Bonin A, Ahronheim G, Rivard G. Brief report: killer cell defect and persistent immunological abnormalities in two patients with chronic active Epstein-Barr virus infection. J Med Virol 28:110–117, 1989.

Jones RJ, Lowbury EJL. Staphylococcal antibodies in burned patients. Br J Exp Pathol 44:575–585, 1963.

Jones SE, Griffith K, Dombrowski P, Gaines JA. Immunodeficiency in patients with non-Hodgkin lymphomas. Blood 49:335–344, 1977.

Josephs SH, Rothman SJ, Buckley RH. Phenytoin hypersensitivity. J Allergy Clin Immunol 66:166–172, 1980.

Joynson DH, Walker DM, Jacobs A, Dolby AE. Defect of cell-mediated immunity in patients with iron-deficiency anaemia. Lancet 2:1058–1059, 1972.

Kabins SA, Lerner C. Fulminant pneumococcemia and sickle cell anemia. JAMA 211:467–471, 1970.

Kahan BD. Cyclosporine. N Engl J Med 321:1725–1738, 1989.

Kahn E, Stein H, Zoutendyk A. Isohemagglutinins and immunity in malnutrition. Am J Clin Nutr 5:70–71, 1957.

Kalden JR, Peter HH, Lohmann E, Schedel J, Diehl V, Vallee D. Estimation of T- and K-cell activity in the peripheral blood of sarcoidosis patients. Ann NY Acad Sci 278:52–68, 1976.

Kanavin O, Scott H, Fausa O, Ek J, Gaarder PI, Brandtzaeg P. Immunological studies of patients with Down's syndrome: measurements of autoantibodies and serum antibodies to dietary antigens in relation to zinc levels. Acta Med Scand 224:473–477, 1988.

Kaplan G, Gandhi RR, Weinstein DE, Levis WR, Patarroyo ME, Brennan PJ, Cohn ZA. *Mycobacterium leprae* antigen–induced suppression of T cell proliferation in vitro. J Immunol 138:3028–3034, 1987.

Kaplan HS, Hoppe RS, Strober S. Selective immunosuppressive effects of total lymphoid irradiation. In Chandra RK, ed. Primary and Secondary Immunodeficiency Disorders. New York, Churchill Livingstone, 1983, pp. 272–279.

Kaplan J, Mastrangelo R, Peterson WD Jr. Childhood lymphoblastic lymphoma, a cancer of thymus-derived lymphocytes. Cancer Res 34:521–525, 1974.

Karol RA, Eng J, Cooper JB, Dennison DK, Sawyer MK, Lawrence EC, Marcus DM, Shearer WT. Imbalances in subsets of T lymphocytes in an inbred pedigree with Omenn's syndrome. Clin Immunol Immunopathol 27:412–427, 1983.

Kass EH. Hormones and host resistance to infection. Bacteriol Rev 24:177–195, 1960.

Kataria YP, LoBuglio AF, Bromberg PA, Hurtubise PE. Sarcoid lymphocytes: B- and T-cell quantitation. Ann NY Acad Sci 278:69–79, 1976.

Kataria YP, Sagone AL, LoBuglio AG, Bromberg PA. In vitro observations on sarcoid lymphocytes and their correlation with cutaneous anergy and clinical severity of disease. Am Rev Respir Dis 108:767–776, 1973.

Katz P, Fauci AS. Inhibition of polyclonal B–cell activation by suppressor monocytes in patients with sarcoidosis. Clin Exp Immunol 32:554–562, 1978.

Keet MP, Thom H. Serum immunoglobulins in kwashiorkor. Arch Dis Child 44:600–603, 1969.

Kefalides NA, Arana JA, Bazan A, Velarde N, Rosenthal SM. Evaluation of antibiotic prophylaxis and gamma globulin, plasma, albumin and saline-solution therapy in severe burns. Ann Surg 159:496–506, 1964.

Kelley VC, Ziegler MR, Doeden D, McQuarrie L. Labeled methionine as an indicator of protein formation in children with lipoid nephrosis. Proc Soc Exp Biol Med 75:153–155, 1950.

Kelly WD, Lamb DL, Varco RL, Good RA. Investigation of Hodgkin's disease with respect to problems of homotransplantation. Ann NY Acad Sci 87:187–202, 1960.

Keusch GR, Urrutia JJ, Fernandez R, Guerrero O, Casteneda G. Humoral and cellular aspects of intracellular bacterial killing in Guatemalan children with protein-calorie malnutrition. In Suskind R, ed. Malnutrition and the Immune Response. New York, Raven Press, 1977, pp. 245–252.

Khan AJ, Evans HE, Glass L, Skin YH, Almonte D. Defective neutrophil chemotaxis in patients with Down syndrome. J Pediatr 87:87–89, 1975.

Kilpatrick L, Garty BZ, Lundquist KF, Hunter K, Stanley CA, Baker L, Douglas SD, Korchak HM. Impaired metabolic function and signaling defects in phagocytic cells in glycogen storage disease type 1b. J Clin Invest 86:196–202, 1990.

King H, Shumacker HB. Susceptibility to infection after splenectomy. Ann Surg 136:239–242, 1952.

Kiran O, Gross S. The G-immunoglobulins in acute leukemia in children: hematologic and immunologic relationships. Blood 33:198–206, 1969.

Kirkpatrick CH, Wilson WEC, Talmage DW. Immunologic studies in human organ transplantation: I. Observation and characterization of suppressed cutaneous reactivity in uremia. J Exp Med 119:727–742, 1964.

Klein G. The Epstein-Barr virus and neoplasia. N Engl J Med 293:1353–1357, 1975.

Knisely MH. Enforced postponement of selective phagocytosis following burn: a contribution to the biophysics of disease. Ann NY Acad Sci 150:510–527, 1968.

Kobayashi K, Manaka K, Ebihara Y, Funazu Y, Ueno M, Funazu K, Mizuno Y, Takeuchi M, Serizawa H, Miura S. A case of Schönlein-Henoch purpura complicated with protein-losing enteropathy and hyperamylasemia. Nippon Shokakibyo Gakkai Zasshi 88:2171–2176, 1991.

Kohn J, Cort DF. Immunoglobulins in burned patients. Lancet 1:836–837, 1969.

Komp DM. Langerhans cell histiocytosis. N Engl J Med 316:747–748, 1987.

Kondo N, Motoyoshi F, Mori S, Kuwabara N, Orii T, German J. Long-term study of the immunodeficiency of Bloom's syndrome. Acta Paediatr 81:86–90, 1992.

Konradsen HB, Henrichsen J. Pneumococcal infections in splenectomized children are preventable. Acta Paediatr Scand 80:423–427, 1991.

Kotzin BL, Strober S, Engleman EG, Calin A, Hoppe RT, Kansas GS, Terrell CP, Kaplan HS. Treatment of intractable rheumatoid arthritis with total lymphoid irradiation. N Engl J Med 305:969–976, 1981.

Kovarsky J. Clinical pharmacology and toxicology of cyclophosphamide: emphasis on use in rheumatic diseases. Semin Arthritis Rheum 12:359–372, 1983.

Krantman HJ, Young SR, Ank BJ, O'Donnell CM, Rachelefsky GS, Stiehm ER. Immune function in pure iron deficiency. Am J Dis Child 136:840–844, 1982.

Krensky AM, Ingelfinger JR, Grupe WE. Peritonitis in childhood nephrotic syndrome: 1970–1980. Am J Dis Child 136:732–736, 1982.

Kretschmer RR, Lopez-Osuna M, de la Rosa L, Armendares S. Leukocyte function in Down's syndrome. Quantitative NBT reduction and bactericidal capacity. Clin Immunol Immunopathol 2:449–455, 1974.

Krikorian JG, Anderson JL, Bieber CP, Penn I, Stinson EB. Malignant neoplasms following cardiac transplantation. JAMA 240:639–643, 1978.

Kulapongs P, Vithayasai V, Suskind R, Olson RE. Cell-mediated immunity and phagocytosis and killing function in children with severe iron-deficiency anaemia. Lancet 2:689–691, 1974.

Kunin CM, Schwartz R, Yaffe S, Knapp J, Fellers FX, Janeway CA, Finland M. Antibody response to influenza virus vaccine in children with nephrosis: effect of cortisone. Pediatrics 23:54–62, 1959.

Kurz P, Kohler H, Meuer S, Hutteroth T, Meyer zum Buschenfelde KH. Impaired cellular immune response in chronic renal failure: evidence for a T cell defect. Kidney Int 29:1209–1214, 1986.

Kuvibidila S, Yu L, Ode D, Warrier RP. The immune response in protein-energy malnutrition and single-nutrient deficiencies. In Klurfeld DM, ed. Nutrition and Immunology. New York, Plenum Press, 1993, pp. 121–155.

Kwak LW, Campbell MJ, Czerwinski DK, Hart S, Miller RA, Levy R. Induction of immune responses in patients with B-cell lymphoma against the surface-immunoglobulin idiotype expressed by their tumors. N Engl J Med 327:1209–1215, 1992.

Lahey E. Histiocytosis X—an analysis of prognostic factors. J Pediatr 87:184–189, 1975.

Lamb D, Pilney F, Kelly WD, Good RA. A comparative study of the incidence of anergy in patients with carcinoma, leukemia, Hodgkin's disease and other lymphomas. J Immunol 89:555–558, 1962.

Lance EM, Medawar PB, Taub RN. Antilymphocyte serum. Adv Immunol 17:1–92, 1973.

Lange AJ, Arion WJ, Beaudet AL. Type Ib glycogen storage disease is caused by a defect in the glucose-6-phosphate translocase of the microsomal glucose-6-phosphatase system. J Biol Chem 255:8381–8384, 1980.

Larkin SM, Williams DN, Osterholm MT, Tofte RW, Posalaky Z. Toxic shock syndrome: clinical, laboratory, and pathological findings in nine fetal cases. Ann Intern Med 96:858–864, 1982.

Larocca LM, Piantelli M, Valitutti S, Castellino F, Maggiano N, Musiani P. Alterations in thymocyte subpopulations in Down's syndrome (trisomy 21). Clin Immunol Immunopathol 49:175–186, 1988.

Larson DL, Tomlinson LJ. Quantitative antibody studies in man. III. Antibody response in leukemia and other malignant lymphomas. J Clin Invest 32:317–321, 1953.

Lavasa S, Kumar L, Chakravarti RN, Kumar M. Early humoral immune response in vitamin A deficiency—an experimental study. Indian J Exp Biol 26:431–435, 1988.

Law EJ, Kim OJ, Stieritz DD, MacMillan BG. Experience with systemic candidiasis in the burned patient. J Trauma 12:543–552, 1972.

Lawrence EC, Martin RR, Blaese RM, Teague RB, Awe RJ, Wilson RK, Deaton WJ, Bloom K, Greenberg SD, Stevens PM. Increased bronchoalveolar IgG-secreting cells in interstitial lung diseases. N Engl J Med 302:1186–1188, 1980.

Lawrence EC, Theodore BJ, Teague RB, Gottlieb MS. Defective immunoglobulin secretion in response to pokeweed mitogen in sarcoidosis. Clin Exp Immunol 49:96–104, 1982.

Lawrence HS, Zweiman B. Transfer factor deficiency response—a mechanism of anergy in Boeck's sarcoid. Trans Assoc Am Physicians 81:240–248, 1968.

Leguit P Jr, Feltkamp TE, Van Rossum A, Van Loghem E, Eijsvoogel VP. Immunological studies in burn patients: 3. Autoimmune phenomena. Int Arch Allergy Appl Immunol 45:392–404, 1973.

Leikin S, Puruganan G, Frankel A, Steerman R, Chandra R. Immunologic parameters in histocytosis-X. Cancer 32:796–802, 1973.

Leonard BAB, Schlievert PM. Immune cell lethality induced by streptococcal pyrogenic exotoxin A and endotoxin. Infect Immun 60:3747–3755, 1992.

Leopardi R, Ilonen J, Mattila L, Salmi AA. Effect of measles virus infection on MHC class II expression and antigen presentation in human monocytes. Cell Immunol 147:388–396, 1993.

Leutscher JA Jr, Deming QB. Treatment of nephrosis with cortisone. J Clin Invest 29:1576–1587, 1950.

Levin S, Schlesinger M, Handzel Z, Hahn T, Altman Y, Czernobilsky B, Boss J. Thymic deficiency in Down's syndrome. Pediatics 63:80–87, 1979.

Levo Y, Green P. Down's syndrome and autoimmunity. Am J Med Sci 273:95–99, 1977.

Levy HL, Sepe SJ, Shih VE, Vawter GF, Klein JO. Sepsis due to *Escherichia coli* in neonates with galactosemia. N Engl J Med 297:823–825, 1977.

Lew W, Oppenheim JJ, Matsushima K. Analysis of the suppression of IL-1 alpha and IL-1 beta production in human peripheral blood mononuclear adherent cells by a glucocorticoid hormone. J Immunol 140:1895–1902, 1988.

Lewis DE, Gilbert BE, Knight V. Influenza virus infection induces functional alterations in peripheral blood lymphocytes. J Immunol 137:3777–3781, 1986.

Lewis SL. C5a receptors on neutrophils and monocytes from chronic dialysis patients. In Horl WH, Schollmeyer PJ, eds. New Aspects of Human Polymorphonuclear Leukocytes. New York, Plenum Press, 1991, pp. 167–181.

Lewis SL, Van Epps DE. Neutrophil and monocyte alterations in chronic dialysis patients. Am J Kidney Dis 9:381–395, 1987.

Libansky J. Study of immunologic reactivity in haemoblastosis: circulating antibody formation as a response to antigenic stimulus in leukemia, malignant lymphoma, myeloma, and myelofibrosis. Blood 25:169–178, 1965.

Litchfield WJ, Wells WW. Effect of galactose on free radical reactions of polymorphonuclear leukocytes. Arch Biochem Biophys 188:26–30, 1978.

Lockitch G, Puterman M, Godolphin W, Sheps S, Tingle AJ, Quigley G. Infection and immunity in Down syndrome: a trial of long-term low oral doses of zinc. J Pediatr 114:781–787, 1989.

London DR, Bamforth J, Creamer B. Steatorrhea presenting with gastrointestinal protein loss. Lancet 2:18–19, 1961.

Lopez V, Ochs HD, Thuline HC, Davis SD, Wedgwood RJ. Defective antibody response to bacteriophage φX174 in Down syndrome. J Pediatr 86:207–211, 1975.

Lorini R, Ugazio AG, Cammareri V, Larizza D, Castellazzi AM, Brugo MA, Serevi F. Immunoglobulin levels, T-cell markers, mitogen responsiveness and thymic hormone activity in Turner's syndrome. Thymus 5:61–66, 1983.

Lowrie EG, Lazarus JM, Mocelin AJ, Bailey GL, Hampers CL, Wilson RE, Merrill JP. Survival of patients undergoing chronic hemodialysis and renal transplantation. N Engl J Med 288:863–867, 1973.

Lowther CP. Leukemia and tuberculosis. Ann Intern Med 51:52–56, 1959.

Lueder GT, Fitz James A, Dowton SB. Congenital microgastria and hypoplastic upper limb anomalies. Am J Med Genet 32:368–370, 1989.

Lukes RJ, Butler JJ. The pathology and nomenclature of Hodgkin's disease. Cancer Res 26:1063–1081, 1966.

Lukes RJ, Craver LF, Hall TC, Rappaport H, Ruben P. Report of the nomenclature committee. Cancer Res 26:1311, 1966.

Lusso P, De Maria A, Malnati M, Lori F, DeRocco SE, Baseler M, Gallo RC. Induction of CD4 and susceptibility to HIV-1 infection in human CD8$^+$ T lymphocytes by human herpesvirus 6. Nature 349:533–535, 1991.

Lusso P, Malnati MS, Garzino Demo A, Crowley RW, Long EO, Gallo RC. Infection of natural killer cells by human herpesvirus 6. Nature 362:458–462, 1993.

Lux SE, Johnston RB Jr, August CS, Say B, Penchaszadeh VB, Rosen FS, McKusick VA. Chronic neutropenia and abnormal cellular immunity in cartilage-hair hypoplasia. N Engl J Med 282:231–236, 1970.

Maccario R, Ugazio AG, Nespoli L, Alberini C, Montagna D, Porta F, Bonetti F, Burgio GR. Lymphocyte subpopulations in Down's syndrome: high percentage of circulating HNK-1$^+$, Leu 2a$^+$ cells. Clin Exp Immunol 57:220–226, 1984.

MacDermot KD, Winter RM, Wigglesworth JS, Strobel S. Short stature/short limb skeletal dysplasia with severe combined immunodeficiency and bowing of the femora: report of two patients and review. J Med Genet 28:10–17, 1991.

MacDonald HR, Baschieri S, Lees RK. Clonal expansion precedes anergy and death of V$_\beta$8$^+$ peripheral T cells responding to staphylococcal enterotoxin B in vivo. Eur J Immunol 21:1963–1966, 1991.

MacDougall LG, Anderson R, McNab GM, Katz J. The immune response in iron-deficient children: impaired cellular defense mechanisms with altered humoral components. J Pediatr 86:833–843, 1975.

MacKay HM. Anaemia in infancy: its prevalence and prevention. Arch Dis Child 3:117–124, 1928.

Macklis RM, Mauch PM, Burakoff SJ, Smith BR. Lymphoid irradiation results in long-term increases in natural killer cells in patients treated for Hodgkin's disease. Cancer 69:778–783, 1992.

MacLeod CM, Farr LE. Relation of the carrier state to pneumococcal peritonitis in young children with the nephrotic syndrome. Proc Soc Exp Biol Med 37:556–558, 1937.

Maennle DL, Grierson HL, Gnarra DG, Weisenburger DD. Sinus histiocytosis with massive lymphadenopathy: a spectrum of disease associated with immune dysfunction. Pediatr Pathol 11:399–412, 1991.

Mahler D, Batchelor JR. Phytohaemagglutinin transformation of lymphocytes in burned patients. Transplantation 12:409–411, 1971.

Maibach HI, Epstein WL. Immunologic responses of healthy volunteers receiving azathioprine (Imuran). Int Arch Allergy 27:102–109, 1965.

Mailloux LU, Bellucci AG, Wilkes BM, Napolitano B, Mossey RT, Lesser M, Bluestone PA. Mortality in dialysis patients: analysis of the causes of death. Am J Kidney Dis 18:326–335, 1991.

Makonkawkeyoon S, Kasinrerk W, Supajatura V, Hirunpetcharat C, Vithayasai V. Immunologic defects in leprosy patients: II. Interleukin 1, interleukin 2, and interferon production in leprosy patients. Int J Lepr Other Mycobact Dis 58:311–318, 1990.

Malatack JF, Gartner JC Jr, Urbach AH, Zitelli BJ. Orthotopic liver transplantation, Epstein-Barr virus, cyclosporine, and lymphoproliferative disease: a growing concern. J Pediatr 118:667–675, 1991.

Malaval T, Li V, Jang G, Martins-Ramos J, Mezin P, Fournet J, Hostein J. Churg-Strauss syndrome with rectal localization and exudative enteropathy. Gastroenterol Clin Biol 17:386–390, 1993.

Malkovsky M, Edwards AJ, Hunt R, Palmer L, Medawar PB. T-cell–mediated enhancement of host-versus-graft reactivity in mice fed a diet enriched in vitamin A acetate. Nature 302:338–340, 1983.

Mangi RJ, Dwyer JM, Kantor FS. The effect of plasma upon lymphocyte response in vitro: demonstration of a humoral inhibitor in patients with sarcoidosis. Clin Exp Immunol 18:519–528, 1974.

Mankiewicz E. Le role des mycobacteries lysogenes dans l'etiologie de la sarcoidose. In Turiaf J, Chabot J, eds. La Sarcoidose. Paris, Masson, 1967, pp. 487–495.

Mankiewicz E, Liivak M. Effect of *Candida albicans* on the evolution of experimental tuberculosis. Nature 187:250–251, 1960.

Mankiewicz E, Stackiewicz E, Livak M. A polysaccharide isolated from *Candida albicans* as a growth-promoting factor for tuberculosis. Can J Microbiol 5:261–267, 1959.

Maraschio P, Tupler R, Dainotti E, Piantanida M, Cazzola G, Tiepolo L. Differential expression of the ICF (immunodeficiency, centromeric heterochromatin, facial anomalies) mutation in lymphocytes and fibroblasts. J Med Genet 26:452–456, 1989.

Martin-Mateos MA, Munoz-Lopez F, Monferrer R, Cruz M. Immunological findings in 14 cases of Langerhans cells histiocytosis. J Invest Allergy Clin Immunol 1:308–314, 1991.

Martin PJ, Shulman HM, Schubach WH, Hansen JA, Fefer A, Miller G, Thomas ED. Fatal Epstein-Barr virus–associated proliferation of donor B cells after treatment of acute graft-versus-host disease with a murine anti-T-cell antibody. Ann Intern Med 101:310–315, 1984.

Masawe AE, Msazumuhire H. Growth of bacteria in vitro in blood from patients with severe iron deficiency anemia and from patients with sickle cell anemia. Am J Clin Pathol 59:706–711, 1973.

Mathews MB, Shenk T. Adenovirus virus–associated RNA and translation control. J Virol 65:5657–5662, 1991.

McBride JS, Micklem HS, Ure JM. Immunosuppression in murine malaria: I. Response to type III pneumococcal polysaccharide. Immunol 32:635–644, 1977.

McCall CE, Caves J, Cooper R, DeChatlet L. Functional characteristics of human toxic neutrophils. J Infect Dis 124:68–75, 1971.

McChesney MB, Fujinami RS, Lampert PW, Oldstone MB. Viruses disrupt functions of human lymphocytes: II. Measles virus suppresses antibody production by acting on B lymphocytes. J Exp Med 163:1331–1336, 1986.

McClain K, Jin H, Gresik V, Favara B. Langerhans cell histiocytosis: lack of a viral etiology. Am J Hematol 47:16–20, 1994.

McFadzean AJS, Tsang KC. Antibody formation in cryptogenic splenomegaly: II. Response to antigen injected subcutaneously. Trans R Soc Trop Med Hyg 50:438–441, 1956.

McGovern JP, Merritt DH. Sarcoidosis in childhood. Adv Pediatr 8:97–135, 1956.

McGuigan JE, Purkerson ML, Trudeau WL, Peterson ML. Studies of the immunologic defects associated with intestinal lymphangiectasia, with some observations on dietary control of chylous ascites. Ann Intern Med 68:398–404, 1968.

McKelvey E, Carbone PP. Serum immune globulin concentrations in acute leukemia during intensive chemotherapy. Cancer 18:1291–1296, 1965.

McMurray DN. Cell-mediated immunity in nutritional deficiency. Prog Food Nutr Sci 8:193–228, 1984.

McRipley RJ, Garrison DW. Effect of burns in rats on defense mechanisms against *Pseudomonas aeruginosa*. J Infect Dis 115:159–170, 1965.

Meakins JL, McLean AP, Kelly R, Bubenik O, Pietsch JB, MacLean LD. Delayed hypersensitivity and neutrophil chemotaxis: effect of trauma. J Trauma 18:240–247, 1978.

Medeiros LJ, Weiss LM, Picker LJ, Clayberger C, Horning SJ, Krensky AM, Warnke RA. Expression of LFA-1 in non-Hodgkin's lymphoma. Cancer 63:255–259, 1989.

Mehra V, Brennan PJ, Rada E, Convit J, Bloom BR. Lymphocyte suppression in leprosy induced by unique *M. leprae* glycolipid. Nature 308:194–196, 1984.

Mehra V, Convit J, Rubinstein A, Bloom BR. Activated suppressor T cells in leprosy. J Immunol 129:1946–1951, 1982.

Melli G, Mazzei D, Rugarli C, Ortolani C, Bazzi C. Blastosis during anti-lymphocyte–globulin treatment. Lancet 2:975, 1968.

Mellman WJ, Younkin LH, Baker D. Abnormal lymphocyte function in trisomy 21. Ann NY Acad Sci 171:537–542, 1970.

Messner RP, Reed WP, Palmer DL, Bolin RB, Davis AT, Quie PG. A transient defect in leukocytic bactericidal capacity. Clin Immunol Immunopathol 1:523–532, 1973.

Michael AF, McLean RH, Roy LP, Westberg NG, Hoyer JR, Fish AJ, Vernier RL. Immunologic aspects of the nephrotic syndrome. Kidney Int 3:105–115, 1973.

Miller DG. Patterns of immunological deficiency in lymphomas and leukemias. Ann Intern Med 57:703–716, 1962.

Miller ME, Baker L. Leukocyte functions in juvenile diabetes mellitus: humoral and cellular aspects. J Pediatr 81:979–982, 1972.

Mills EL. Viral infections predisposing to bacterial infections. Annu Rev Med 35:469–479, 1984.

Mitchell DN, Rees RJ. A transmissible agent from sarcoid tissue. Lancet 2:81–84, 1969.

Mitchell DN, Rees RJW. The nature and physical characteristics of a transmissible agent from human sarcoid tissue. Ann NY Acad Sci 278:233–248, 1976.

Mitchell DN, Scadding JG. Sarcoidosis. Am Rev Respir Dis 110:774–802, 1974.

Molineaux L, Fleming AF, Cornille Brogger R, Kagan I, Storey J. Abnormal haemoglobins in the Sudan savanna of Nigeria: III. Malaria, immunoglobulins and antimalarial antibodies in sickle cell disease. Ann Trop Med Parasitol 73:301–310, 1979.

Monafo WW, Moyer LS. Effectiveness of dilute aqueous silver nitrate in the treatment of major burns. Arch Surg 91:200–210, 1965.

Moncrief JA, Lindberg RB, Switzer WE, Pruitt BA Jr. The use of a topical sulfonamide in the control of burn wound sepsis. J Trauma 6:407–419, 1966.

Montagna D, Maccario R, Ugazio AG, Nespoli L, Pedroni E, Faggiano P, Burgio GR. Cell-mediated cytotoxicity in Down syndrome: impairment of allogeneic mixed lymphocyte reaction, NK, and NK-like activities. Eur J Pediatr 148:53–57, 1988.

Montgomerie JZ, Kalmanson GM, Guze LB. Renal failure and infection. Medicine 47:1–32, 1968.

Moreno C, Mehlert A, Lamb J. The inhibitory effects of mycobacterial lipoarabinomannan and polysaccharides upon polyclonal and monoclonal human T cell proliferation. Clin Exp Immunol 74:206–210, 1988.

Morganfeld MD, Bonchil G. Tuberculin reactions in Hodgkin's disease. N Engl J Med 278:565, 1968.

Morley A, Forbes I. Impairment of immunological function in aplastic anaemia. Aust NZ J Med 4:53–57, 1974.

Morris DH, Bullock FD. The importance of the spleen in resistance to infection. Ann Surg 70:513–521, 1919.

Mowat AG, Baum J. Polymorphonuclear leucocyte chemotaxis in patients with bacterial infections. Br Med J 3:617–619, 1971.

Muftuoglu AU, Balkuv S. Passive transfer of tuberculin sensitivity to patients with Hodgkin's disease. N Engl J Med 277:126–129, 1967.

Muller-Quernheim J, Kronke M, Strausz J, Schykowski M, Ferlinz R. Interleukin-2 receptor gene expression by bronchoalveolar lavage lymphocytes in pulmonary sarcoidosis. Am Rev Respir Dis 140:82–88, 1989.

Munster AM. Immunologic response of trauma and burns: an overview. Am J Med 76:142–145, 1984.

Munster AM, Hoagland HC. Serum immunoglobulin patterns after burns. Surg Forum 20:76–77, 1969.

Murphy M, Epstein LB. Down syndrome (DS) peripheral blood contains phenotypically mature CD3$^+$ TCR alpha, beta$^+$ cells but abnormal proportions of TCR alpha, beta$^+$, TCR gamma, delta$^+$ and CD4$^+$ CD45RA$^+$ cells: evidence for an inefficient release of mature T cells by the DS thymus. Clin Immunol Immunopathol 62:245–251, 1992.

Murphy M, Friend DS, Pike-Nobile L, Epstein LB. Tumor necrosis factor-alpha and IFN-gamma expression in human thymus: localization and overexpression in Down syndrome (trisomy 21). J Immunol 149:2506–2512, 1992.

Murphy M, Hyun W, Hunte B, Levine AD, Epstein LB. A role for tumor necrosis factor-alpha and interferon-gamma in the regulation of interleukin-4–induced human thymocyte proliferation in vitro: heightened sensitivity in the Down syndrome (trisomy 21) thymus. Pediatr Res 32:269–276, 1992b.

Murphy M, Insoft RM, Pike-Nobile L, Derbin KS, Epstein LB. Overexpression of LFA-1 and ICAM-1 in Down syndrome thymus. J Immunol 150:5696–5703, 1993.

Nair MP, Schwartz SA. Association of decreased T-cell-mediated natural cytotoxicity and interferon production in Down's syndrome. Clin Immunol Immunopathol 33:412–424, 1984.

Najarian JS, Simmons RL. The clinical use of antilymphocyte globulin. N Engl J Med 285:158–166, 1971.

Nalesnik MA, Jaffe R, Starzl TE, Demetris AJ, Porter K, Burnham JA, Makowka L, Ho M, Locker J. The pathology of posttransplant lymphoproliferative disorders occurring in the setting of cyclosporine A–prednisone immunosuppression. Am J Pathol 133:173–192, 1988.

Nash G, Foley FD, Goodwin MN Jr, Bruck HM, Greenwald KA, Pruitt BA Jr. Fungal–burn wound infection. JAMA 215:1664–1666, 1971.

Nauss KM, Newberne PM. Local and regional immune function of vitamin A–deficient rats with ocular herpes simplex virus (HSV) infections. J Nutr 115:1316–1324, 1985.

Nelson DL, Blaese RM, Strober W, Bruce R, Waldmann TA. Constrictive pericarditis, intestinal lymphangiectasia, and reversible immunologic deficiency. J Pediatr 86:548–554, 1975.

Neumann CG, Lawlor CJ Jr, Stiehm ER, Swenseid ME, Newton C, Herbert J, Ammann AJ, Jacob M. Immunologic responses in malnourished children. Am J Clin Nutr 28:89–104, 1975.

Newton WA Jr, Hamoudi AB. Histiocytosis: a histologic classification with clinical correlation. Perspect Pediatr Pathol 1:251–283, 1973.

Nickerson DA, Havens RA, Bullock WE. Immunoregulation in disseminated histoplasmosis: characterization of splenic suppressor cell populations. Cell Immunol 60:287–297, 1981.

Niikawa N, Kohsaka S, Mizumoto M, Hamada I, Kajii T. Familial clustering of situs inversus totalis, and asplenia and polysplenia syndromes. Am J Med Genet 16:43–47, 1983.

Ninnemann JL, Condie JT, Davis SE, Crockett RA. Isolation immunosuppressive serum components following thermal injury. J Trauma 22:837–844, 1982.

Nitter L. Changes in the chest roentgenogram in Boeck's sarcoid of the lungs. Acta Radiol 105(Suppl.):7–202, 1953.

Nogueira N, Kaplan G, Levy E, Sarno EN, Kushner P. Defective interferon production in leprosy: reversal with antigen and interleukin 2. J Exp Med 158:2165–2170, 1983.

Nurmi T, Leinonen M, Haiva VM, Tiilikainen A, Kouvalainen K. Antibody response to pneumococcal vaccine in patients with trisomy-21 (Down's syndrome). Clin Exp Immunol 48:485–490, 1982.

Nurmi T, Uhari M, Linna SL, Herva R, Tiilikainen A, Kouvalainen

K. Immunodeficiency associated with a deletion in the short arm of the X-chromosome. Clin Exp Immunol 45:107–112, 1981.

Nussenblatt RB, Palestine AG, Chan CC. Cyclosporin A therapy in the treatment of intraocular inflammatory disease resistant to systemic corticosteroids and cytotoxic agents. Am J Ophthalmol 96:275–282, 1983.

Nutman TB, Kumaraswami V, Ottesen EA. Parasite-specific anergy in human filariasis: insights after analysis of parasite antigen-driven lymphokine production. J Clin Invest 79:1516–1523, 1987.

Ochs HD, Davis SD, Mickelson E, Lerner KG, Wedgwood RJ. Combined immunodeficiency and reticuloendotheliosis with eosinophilia. J Pediatr 85:463–465, 1974.

O'Garra A, Warren DJ, Holman M, Popham AM, Sanderson CJ, Klaus GG. Effects of cyclosporine on responses of murine B cells to T cell–derived lymphokines. J Immunol 137:2220–2224, 1986.

O'Hehir RE, Lamb JR. Induction of specific clonal anergy in human T lymphocytes by *Staphylococcus aureus* enterotoxins. Proc Natl Acad Sci USA 87:8884–8888, 1990.

Okano M, Thiele GM, Davis JR, Grierson HL, Purtilo DT. Epstein-Barr virus and human diseases: recent advances in diagnosis. Clin Microbiol Rev 1:300–312, 1988.

O'Keefe SJ, Tamura J, Kincaid RL, Tocci MJ, O'Neill EA. FK-506- and CsA-sensitive activation of the interleukin-2 promoter by calcineurin. Nature 357:692–694, 1992.

Olson JA. The biological role of vitamin A in maintaining epithelial tissues. Isr J Med Sci 8:1170–1178, 1972.

O'Mahony JB, Palder SB, Wood JJ, McIrvine A, Rodrick ML, Demling RH, Mannick JA. Depression of cellular immunity after multiple trauma in the absence of sepsis. J Trauma 24:869–875, 1984.

O'Malley BW. Steroid hormone action in eucaryotic cells. J Clin Invest 74:307–312, 1984.

Omenn G. Familial reticuloendotheliosis with eosinophilia. N Engl J Med 273:427–432, 1965.

Ooi BS, Kant KS, Hanenson IB, Pesce AJ, Pollak VE. Lymphocytotoxins in epileptic patients receiving phenytoin. Clin Exp Immunol 30:56–61, 1977.

Opelz G, Henderson R. Incidence of non-Hodgkin lymphoma in kidney and heart transplant recipients. Lancet 342:1514–1516, 1993.

Oster J, Mikkelsen M, Nielsen A. Mortality and life-table in Down's syndrome. Acta Paediatr Scand 64:322–326, 1975.

Overturf GD, Powars D, Baraff LJ. Bacterial meningitis and septicemia in sickle cell disease. Am J Dis Child 131:784–787, 1977.

Pabico RC, Douglas RG, Betts RF, McKenna BA, Freeman RB. Influenza vaccination of patients with glomerular diseases: effects on creatinine clearance, urinary protein excretion, and antibody response. Ann Intern Med 81:171–177, 1974.

Pachman LM, Schwartz AD, Barron R, Golde DW. Chronic neutropenia: response to plasma with high colony-stimulating activity. J Pediatr 87:713–719, 1975.

Page AR, Condie RM, Good RA. Suppression of plasma cell hepatitis with 6-mercaptopurine. Am J Med 36:200–214, 1964.

Pahwa S, Kirkpatrick D, Ching C, Lopez C, Pahwa R, Smithwick E, O'Reilly R, August C, Pasquariello P, Good RA. Persistent cytomegalovirus infection: association with profound immunodeficiency and treatment with interferon. Clin Immunol Immunopathol 28:77–89, 1983.

Parkins RA. Protein-losing enteropathy in the sprue syndrome. Lancet 2:1366–1368, 1960.

Pasatiempo AM, Kinoshita M, Taylor CE, Ross AC. Antibody production in vitamin A-depleted rats is impaired after immunization with bacterial polysaccharide or protein antigens. FASEB J 4:2518–2527, 1990.

Pascual RS, Gee JB, Finch SC. Usefulness of serum lysozyme measurement in diagnosis and evaluation of sarcoidosis. N Engl J Med 289:1074–1076, 1973.

Pasquali JL, Godin D, Urlacher A, Pelletier A, Pauli G, Storck D. Abnormalities of in vitro responses to polyclonal activation of peripheral blood lymphocytes in patients with active sarcoidosis. Eur J Clin Invest 15:82–88, 1985.

Pass RF, Stagno S, Britt WJ, Alford CA. Specific cell-mediated immunity and the natural history of congenital infection with cytomegalovirus. J Infect Dis 148:953–961, 1983.

Passwell J, Levanon M, Davidsohn J, Ramot B. Monocyte PGE2 secretion in Hodgkin's disease and its relation to decreased cellular immunity. Clin Exp Immunol 51:61–68, 1983.

Paterson PY, Semo R, Blumenschein G, Swelstad J. Mucocutaneous candidiasis, anergy and a plasma inhibitor of cellular immunity: reversal after amphotericin B therapy. Clin Exp Immunol 9:595–602, 1971.

Pattishall EN, Kendig EL. Sarcoidosis. In Chernick V, ed. Kendig's Disorders of the Respiratory Tract in Children. Philadelphia, WB Saunders, 1990, pp. 769–780.

Pearson HA, Cornelius EA, Schwartz AD, Zelson JH, Wolfson SL, Spencer RP. Transfusion-reversible functional asplenia in young children with sickle-cell anemia. N Engl J Med 283:334–337, 1970.

Pearson HA, McIntosh S, Ritchey AK, Lobel JS, Rooks Y, Johnston D. Developmental aspects of splenic function in sickle cell diseases. Blood 53:358–365, 1979.

Pearson HA, Spencer RP, Cornelius EA. Functional asplenia in sickle-cell anemia. N Engl J Med 281:923–926, 1969.

Pedersen FK, Hertz H, Lundsteen C, Platz P, Thomsen M. Indication of primary immune deficiency in Fanconi's anemia. Acta Paediatr Scand 66:745–751, 1977.

Pelletier S, Ekert P, Landi B, Coutellier A, Bletry O, Herson S. Exudative enteropathy in disseminated lupus erythematosus. Ann Gastroenterol Hepatol 28:259–262, 1992.

Penn I. The price of immunotherapy. Curr Probl Surg 18:681–751, 1981.

Perednia DA, Curosh NA. Lupus-associated protein-losing enteropathy. Arch Intern Med 150:1806–1810, 1990.

Perez-Blas M, Regueiro JR, Ruiz-Contreras JR, Arnaiz-Villena A. T lymphocyte anergy during acute infectious mononucleosis is restricted to the clonotypic receptor activation pathway. Clin Exp Immunol 89:83–88, 1992.

Perez-Soler R, Lopez-Berestein G, Cabanillas F, McLaughlin P, Hersh EM. Superoxide anion (O-2) production by peripheral blood monocytes in Hodgkin's disease and malignant lymphoma. J Clin Oncol 3:641–645, 1985.

Perillie PE, Nolan JP, Finch SC. Studies of the resistance to infection in diabetes mellitus: local exudative cellular response. J Lab Clin Med 59:1008–1015, 1962.

Perper RJ, Sanda M, Chinea G, Oronsky AL. Leukocyte chemotaxis in vivo. I. Description of a model of cell accumulation using adoptively transferred ^{51}Cr-labeled cells. J Lab Clin Med 84:378–393, 1974.

Petkovich M. Regulation of gene expression by vitamin A: the role of nuclear retinoic acid receptors. Annu Rev Nutr 12:443–471, 1992.

Petrini B, Wasserman J, Rotstein S, Blomgren H. Radiotherapy and persistent reduction of peripheral T cells. J Clin Lab Immunol 11:159–160, 1983.

Philip R, Berger AC, McManus NH, Warner NH, Peacock MA, Epstein LB. Abnormalities of the in vitro cellular and humoral responses to tetanus and influenza antigens with concomitant numerical alterations in lymphocyte subsets in Down syndrome (trisomy 21). J Immunol 136:1661–1667, 1986.

Phillips I, Wharton B. Acute bacterial infection in kwashiorkor and marasmus. Br Med J 1:407–409, 1968.

Pickering RJ, Herdman RC, Michael AF, Vernier RL, Gewurz H, Fish AJ, Good RA. Chronic glomerulonephritis associated with low serum complement activity (chronic hypocomplementemic glomerulonephritis). Medicine 49:207–226, 1970.

Pincus SH, Boxer LA, Stossel TP. Chronic neutropenia in childhood: analysis of 16 cases and a review of the literature. Am J Med 61:849–861, 1976.

Pinkston P, Bitterman PB, Crystal RG. Spontaneous release of interleukin-2 by lung T lymphocytes in active pulmonary sarcoidosis. N Engl J Med 308:793–800, 1983.

Pirofsky B, Beaulieu R, August A. Immunologic effects of antithymocyte antisera in the human. In Seiler FR, Schwick HG, eds. ALG Therapy and Standardization Workshop. Marburg, Behringwerke AG, 1972, pp. 237–242.

Pitman FE, Harris RC, Barker HG. Transient edema and hypoproteinemia. Am J Dis Child 108:189–197, 1964.

Plauth WH Jr, Waldmann TA, Wochner RD, Braunwald NS, Braunwald E. Protein-losing enteropathy secondary to constrictive pericarditis in childhood. Pediatrics 34:636–648, 1964.

Pomerantz M, Waldmann TA. Systemic lymphatic abnormalities associated with gastrointestinal protein loss secondary to intestinal lymphangiectasia. Gastroenterology 45:703–711, 1963.

Powars D, Overturf G, Turner E. Is there an increased risk of *Hae-*

mophilus influenzae septicemia in children with sickle cell anemia? Pediatrics 71:927–931, 1983.

Powars DR. Natural history of sickle cell disease—the first ten years. Semin Hematol 12:267–285, 1975.

Pretorius PJ, de Villiers LS. Antibody response in children with protein malnutrition. Am J Clin Nutr 10:379–383, 1962.

Pui CH, Ip SH, Thompson E, Dodge RK, Brown M, Wilimas J, Carrabis S, Kung P, Berard CW, Crist WM. Increased serum CD8 antigen level in childhood Hodgkin's disease relates to advanced stage and poor treatment outcome. Blood 73:209–213, 1989.

Pyke DA, Scadding JG. Effect of cortisone upon skin sensitivity to tuberculin in sarcoidosis. Br Med J 2:1126–1128, 1952.

Quie PG. Disorders of phagocyte function. Curr Probl Pediatr 2:3–53, 1972.

Quinn EL, Bunch DC, Yagle EM. The mumps skin test and complement fixation test as a diagnostic aid in sarcoidosis. J Invest Dermatol 24:595–598, 1955.

Raab SO, Hoeprich PD, Wintrobe MM, Cartwright GE. The clinical significance of fever in acute leukemia. Blood 16:1609–1628, 1960.

Rabin ER, Graby CD, Vogel JEH. Fatal *Pseudomonas* infection in burned patients: a clinical, bacteriologic and anatomic study. N Engl J Med 265:1225–1231, 1961a.

Rabin ER, Lundberg GD, Mitchell ET. Mucormycosis in severely burned patients. N Engl J Med 264:1286–1289, 1961b.

Rahmathullah L, Underwood BA, Thulasiraj RD, Milton RC, Ramaswamy K, Rahmathullah R, Babu G. Reduced mortality among children in southern India receiving a small weekly dose of vitamin A. N Engl J Med 323:929–935, 1990.

Ramachandar K, Douglas SD, Siltzbach LE, Taub RN. Peripheral blood lymphocyte subpopulations in sarcoidosis. Cell Immunol 16:422–426, 1975.

Rammensee HG, Kroschewski R, Frangoulis B. Clonal anergy induced in mature V-beta 6[+] T lymphocytes on immunizing Mls-1b mice with Mls-1a expressing cells. Nature 339:541–544, 1989.

Ramos-Arroyo MA, Weaver DD, Banks ER. Weaver syndrome: a case without early overgrowth and review of the literature. Pediatrics 88:1106–1111, 1991.

Rao SP, Miller ST, Cohen BJ. Transient aplastic crisis in patients with sickle cell disease: B19 parvovirus studies during a 7-year period. Am J Dis Child 146:1328–1330, 1992.

Rapaport FT, Converse JM, Horn L, Ballantyne DL, Mulholland JH. Altered reactivity to skin homografts in severe thermal injury. Ann Surg 159:390–395, 1964.

Rapaport FT, Milgrom F, Kano K, Gesner B, Solowey AC, Casson P, Silverman HI, Converse JM. Immunologic sequelae of thermal injury. Ann NY Acad Sci 150:1004–1008, 1968.

Raska K Jr, Raskova J, Shea SM, Frankel RM, Wood RH, Lifter J, Ghobrial I, Eisinger RP, Homer L. T cell subsets and cellular immunity in end-stage renal disease. Am J Med 75:734–740, 1983.

Raskova J, Ghobrial I, Czerwinski DK, Shea SM, Eisinger RP, Raska K Jr. B-cell activation and immunoregulation in end-stage renal disease patients receiving hemodialysis. Arch Intern Med 147:89–93, 1987.

Reddy V, Raghuramulu N, Bhaskaram C. Secretory IgA in protein-calorie malnutrition. Arch Dis Child 51:871–874, 1976.

Reinherz EL, Geha R, Rappeport JM, Wilson M, Penta AC, Hussey RE, Fitzgerald KA, Daley JF, Levine H, Rosen FS, Schlossman SF. Reconstitution after transplantation with T-lymphocyte–depleted HLA haplotype-mismatched bone marrow for severe combined immunodeficiency. Proc Natl Acad Sci U S A 79:6047–6051, 1982.

Reiser K, Whitcomb C, Robinson K, MacKenzie MR. T and B lymphocytes in patients with Down's syndrome. Am J Ment Defic 80:613–619, 1976.

Repine JE, Clawson CC, Goetz FC. Bactericidal function of neutrophils from patients with acute bacterial infections and from diabetics. J Infect Dis 142:869–875, 1980.

Revillard JP, Brochier J. Selective deficiency of cell-mediated immunity in humans treated with antilymphocytes globulins. Transplant Proc 3:725–729, 1971.

Richards BW, Hobbs JR. IgA and ring-18 chromosome. Lancet 1:1426–1427, 1968.

Rieger CH, Moohr JW, Rothberg RM. Correction of neutropenia associated with dysgammaglobulinemia. Pediatrics 54:508–511, 1974.

Rigas DA, Elsasser P, Hecht T. Impaired in vitro response of circulat-

ing lymphocytes to phytohemagglutinin in Down's syndrome: dose- and time-response curves and relation to cellular immunity. Int Arch Allergy Appl Immunol 39:587–608, 1970.

Rimoldi MT, Sher A, Heiny S, Lituchy A, Hammer CH, Joiner K. Developmentally regulated expression by *Trypanosoma cruzi* of molecules that accelerate the decay of complement C3 convertases. Proc Natl Acad Sci U S A 85:193–197, 1988.

Rinehart JJ, Sagone AL, Balcerzak SP, Ackerman GA, LoBuglio AF. Effects of corticosteroid therapy on human monocyte function. N Engl J Med 292:236–241, 1975.

Rittenbury MS, Hanback LD. Phagocytic depression in thermal injuries. J Trauma 7:523–540, 1967.

Rivas V, Rogers TJ. Studies on the cellular nature of *Candida albicans*–induced suppression. J Immunol 130:376–379, 1983.

Robbins JB, Pearson HA. Normal response of sickle cell anemia patients to immunization with *Salmonella* vaccines. J Pediatr 66:877–882, 1965.

Robison LL, Neglia JP. Epidemiology of Down syndrome and childhood acute leukemia. In McCoy E, Epstein C, eds. Oncology and Immunology of Down Syndrome. New York, Alan R. Liss, 1987, pp. 19–32.

Robson SC, Potter PC. Common variable immunodeficiency in association with Turner's syndrome. J Clin Lab Immunol 32:143–146, 1990.

Rodgers BC, Scott DM, Mundin J, Sissons JG. Monocyte-derived inhibitor of interleukin 1 induced by human cytomegalovirus. J Virol 55:527–532, 1985.

Rogers PC, Desai F, Karabus CD, Hartley PS, Fisher RM. Presentation and outcome of 25 cases of Fanconi's anemia. Am J Pediatr Hematol Oncol 11:141–145, 1989.

Rose V, Izukawa T, Moes CAF. Syndromes of asplenia and polysplenia: a review of cardiac and non-cardiac malformations in 60 cases with special reference to diagnosis and prognosis. Br Heart J 37:840–852, 1975.

Rosen EU, Geefhuysen J, Ipp T. Immunoglobulin levels in protein calorie malnutrition. South Afr Med J 45:980–982, 1971.

Rosen FS, Smith DH, Earle JR, Janeway CA, Gitlin D. The etiology of hypoproteinemia in a patient with congenital chylous ascites. Pediatrics 30:696–706, 1962.

Rosenblatt HM, Lewis DE, Sklar J, Cleary ML, Parikh N, Galili N, Ritz J, Shearer WT. Epstein-Barr virus-transformed B-cell line (DV-1) derived from bone marrow of a patient with severe combined immunodeficiency and immunoblastic lymphoma. Pediatr Res 21:331–337, 1987.

Rosner F, Kozinn PJ, Jervis GA. Leukocyte function and serum immunoglobulins in Down's syndrome. N Y State J Med 73:672–675, 1973.

Rosner F, Zarrabi MH, Benach JL, Habicht GS. Babesiosis in splenectomized adults. Review of 22 reported cases. Am J Med 76:696–701, 1984.

Ross AC. Vitamin A status: relationship to immunity and the antibody response. Proc Soc Exp Biol Med 200:303–320, 1992.

Rotem Y, Czerniak P. Gastrointestinal protein leakage in celiac disease as studied by labeled PVP. Am J Dis Child 107:58–66, 1964.

Rottino A, Levy AL. Behavior of total serum complement in Hodgkin's disease and other malignant lymphomas. Blood 14:246–254, 1959.

Rowe M, Rowe DT, Gregory CD, Young LS, Farrell PJ, Rupani H, Rickinson AB. Differences in B cell growth phenotype reflect novel patterns of Epstein-Barr virus latent gene expression in Burkitt's lymphoma cells. EMBO J 6:2743–2751, 1987.

Rowley JD. Down syndrome and acute leukaemia: increased risk may be due to trisomy 21. Lancet 2:1020–1022, 1981.

Rubin BK, MacLeod PM, Sturgess J, King M. Recurrent respiratory infections in a child with fucosidosis: is the mucus too thin for effective transport? Pediatr Pulmonol 10:304–309, 1991.

Rubin HM, Blau EB, Michaels RH. Hemophilus and pneumococcal peritonitis in children with the nephrotic syndrome. Pediatrics 56:598–601, 1975.

Ruch W, Schurmann K, Gordon P, Burgin-Wolff A, Girard J. Coexistent coeliac disease, Graves' disease and diabetes mellitus type 1 in a patient with Down syndrome. Eur J Pediatr 144:89–90, 1985.

Rumore MM. Vitamin A as an immunomodulating agent. Clin Pharm 12:506–514, 1993.

Ruttenburg HD, Neufield HN, Lucas RV Jr. Syndrome of congenital cardiac disease with asplenia: distinction from other forms of congenital cyanotic cardiac disease. Am J Cardiol 13:387–406, 1964.

Ruvalcaba RH, Thuline HC. IgA absence associated with short arm deletion of chromosome no. 18. J Pediatr 74:964–965, 1969.

Saba TM. Physiology and physiopathology of the reticuloendothelial system. Arch Intern Med 126:1031–1052, 1970.

Sakai H, Daniels JC, Beathard GA, Lewis SR, Lynch JB, Ritzmann SE. Mixed lymphocyte culture reaction in patients with acute thermal burns. J Trauma 14:53–57, 1974.

Santos GW, Owens AH, Sensenbrenner LL. Effects of selected cytotoxic agents on antibody production in man. Ann NY Acad Sci 114:404–423, 1964.

Santos GW, Sensenbrenner LL, Burke PJ, Colvin M, Owens AH Jr, Bias WB, Slavin RE. Marrow transplantation in man following cyclophosphamide. Transplant Proc 3:400–404, 1971.

Saslaw S, Arlisle HD, Bouroncle B. Antibody response in hematologic patients. Proc Soc Exp Biol Med 106:654–656, 1961.

Saslaw S, Bouroncle BA, Wall RL, Doan CA. Studies on antibody response in splenectomized persons. N Engl J Med 261:120–125, 1959.

Saxena KM, Crawford JD. The treatment of nephrosis. N Engl J Med 272:522–526, 1965.

Scharf Y, Zonis S. Histocompatibility antigens (HLA) and uveitis. Surv Ophthalmol 24:220–228, 1980.

Schaumann J. Études sur le lupus pernio et ses rapports avec les sarcoides et la tuberculose. Ann Dermatol Syph (Paris) 6:357–373, 1916.

Scheffer AL, Ruddy S, Israel HL. Serum complement levels in sarcoidosis. In Levinsky L, Macholda F, eds. Proceedings of the Fifth International Conference on Sarcoidosis: XIVth Scientific Conference of the Medical Faculty of Charles University, Prague, 1969. Prague, Universita Karlova, 1971, pp. 195–197.

Schier WW, Roth A, Ostroff G, Schrift MH. Hodgkin's disease and immunity. Am J Med 20:94–99, 1956.

Schimke RN, Horton WA, King CR, Martin NL. Chondroitin-6-sulfate mucopolysaccharidosis in conjunction with lymphopenia, defective cellular immunity and the nephrotic syndrome. Birth Defects 10:258–266, 1974.

Schimpff SC, Greene WH, Young VM, Fortner CL, Cusack N, Block JB, Wiernik PH. Infection prevention in acute nonlymphocytic leukemia: laminar air flow room reverse isolation with oral, nonabsorbable antibiotic prophylaxis. Ann Intern Med 82:351–358, 1975.

Schlesinger L, Stekel A. Impaired cellular immunity in marasmic infants. Am J Clin Nutr 27:615–620, 1974.

Schlievert PM. Role of superantigens in human disease. J Infect Dis 167:997–1002, 1993.

Schofer O, Blaha I, Mannhardt W, Zepp F, Stallmach T, Spranger J. Omenn phenotype with short-limbed dwarfism. J Pediatr 118:86–89, 1991.

Schonland M. Depression of immunity in protein-calorie malnutrition: a post-mortem study. J Trop Pediatr Environ Child Health 18:217–224, 1972.

Schooley RT, Hirsch MS, Colvin RB, Cosimi AB, Tolkoff Rubin NE, McCluskey RT, Burton RC, Russell PS, Herrin JT, Delmonico FL, Giorgi JV, Henle W, Rubin RH. Association of herpesvirus infections with T-lymphocyte–subset alterations, glomerulopathy, and opportunistic infections after renal transplantation. N Engl J Med 308:307–313, 1983.

Schopfer K, Douglas SD. In vitro studies of lymphocytes from children with kwashiorkor. Clin Immunol Immunopathol 5:21–30, 1976a.

Schopfer K, Douglas SD. Neutrophil function in children with kwashiorkor. J Lab Clin Med 88:450–461, 1976b.

Schubach WH, Hackman R, Neiman PE, Miller G, Thomas ED. A monoclonal immunoblastic sarcoma in donor cells bearing Epstein-Barr virus genomes following allogeneic marrow grafting for acute lymphoblastic leukemia. Blood 60:180–187, 1982.

Schuler D, Dobos M, Fekete G, Machay T, Nemeskéri A. Down's syndrome and malignancy. Acta Paediatr Acad Sci Hung 13:245–252, 1972.

Schulkind ML, Ellis EF, Smith RT. Effect of antibody upon clearance of ^{125}I-labeled pneumococci by the spleen and liver. Pediatr Res 1:178–184, 1967.

Schumacher MJ. Serum immunoglobulin and transferrin levels after childhood splenectomy. Arch Dis Child 45:114–117, 1970.

Schwartz AD, Pearson HA. Impaired antibody response to intravenous immunization in sickle cell anemia. Pediatr Res 6:145–149, 1972.

Schwartz M, Jarnum S. Gastrointestinal protein loss in idiopathic (hypercatabolic) proteinemia. Lancet 1:327–328, 1959.

Schwartz RS. Immunosuppressive drugs. Prog Allergy 9:246–289, 1965.

Schweiger O, Mandi L. Effect of Kveim substance on the respiration of circulating leukocytes of patients suffering from pulmonary sarcoidosis or other lung disease. Am Rev Respir Dis 96:1064–1066, 1967.

Scrimshaw NS, Behar M. Protein malnutrition in young children. Science 133:2039–2047, 1961.

Seeler RA, Metzger W, Mufson MA. *Diplococcus pneumoniae* infections in children with sickle cell anemia. Am J Dis Child 123:8–10, 1972.

Seemanova E, Passarge E, Beneskova D, Houstek J, Kasal P, Sevcikova M. Familial microcephaly with normal intelligence, immunodeficiency, and risk for lymphoreticular malignancies: a new autosomal recessive disorder. Am J Med Genet 20:639–648, 1985.

Seger R, Wildfeuer A, Buchinger G, Romen W, Catty D, Dybas L, Haferkamp O, Stroder J. Defects in granulocyte function in various chromosome abnormalities (Down's-, Edwards'-, cri-du-chat syndrome). Klin Wochenschr 54:177–183, 1976.

Semba R, Hussey G. Vitamin A supplementation and childhood morbidity. Lancet 342:1176, 1993.

Semba RD, Muhilal, Scott AL, Natadisastra G, Wirasasmita S, Mele L, Ridwan E, West KP Jr, Sommer A. Depressed immune response to tetanus in children with vitamin A deficiency. J Nutr 122:101–107, 1992.

Semba RD, Muhilal, Ward BJ, Griffin DE, Scott AL, Natadisastra G, West KP Jr, Sommer A. Abnormal T-cell subset proportions in vitamin A–deficient children. Lancet 341:5–8, 1993.

Senn HJ, Jungi WF. Neutrophil migration in health and disease. Semin Hematol 12:27–45, 1975.

Sensi M, Pozzilli P, Gorsuch AN, Bottazzo GF, Cudworth AG. Increased killer cell activity in insulin-dependent (type 1) diabetes mellitus. Diabetologia 20:106–109, 1981.

Serjeant GR, Serjeant BE. Management of sickle cell disease: lessons from the Jamaican Cohort Study. Blood Rev 7:137–145, 1993.

Serlenga E, Garofalo AR, DePergola G, Ventura MT, Tortorella C, Antonaci S. Polymorphonuclear cell–mediated phagocytosis and superoxide anion release in insulin-dependent diabetes mellitus. Cytobios 74:189–195, 1993.

Seth V, Chandra RK. Opsonic activity, phagocytosis, and bactericidal capacity of polymorphs in undernutrition. Arch Dis Child 47:282–284, 1972.

Seyschab H, Schindler D, Friedl R, Barbi G, Boltshauser E, Fryns JP, Hanefeld F, Korinthenberg R, Krageloh Mann I, Scheres JM, Schinzel A, Seemanova E, Tommerup N, Hoehn H. Simultaneous measurement, using flow cytometry, of radiosensitivity and defective mitogen response in ataxia-telangiectasia and related syndromes. Eur J Pediatr 151:756–760, 1992.

Sharafuddin MJ, Spanheimer RG, McClune GL. Phenytoin-induced agranulocytosis: a nonimmunologic idiosyncratic reaction? Acta Haematol 86:212–213, 1991.

Sheagren JN, Block JB, Wolff SM. Reticuloendothelial system phagocytic function in patients with Hodgkin's disease. J Clin Invest 46:855–862, 1967.

Shearer WT, Finegold MJ, Guerra IC, Rosenblatt HM, Lewis DE, Pollack MS, Taber LH, Sumaya CV, Grumet FC, Cleary ML, Warnke R, Sklar J. Epstein-Barr virus–associated B-cell proliferations of diverse clonal origins after bone marrow transplantation in a 12-year-old patient with severe combined immunodeficiency. N Engl J Med 312:1151–1159, 1985.

Shinefield HR, Steinberg CR, Kaye D. Effect of splenectomy on the susceptibility of mice inoculated with *Diplococcus pneumoniae*. J Exp Med 123:777–794, 1966.

Shirani KZ, Vaughan GM, McManus AT, Amy BW, McManus WF, Pruitt BA Jr, Mason AD Jr. Replacement therapy with modified immunoglobulin G in burn patients: preliminary kinetic studies. Am J Med 76:175–180, 1984.

Showstack J, Katz P, Amend W, Bernstein L, Lipton H, O'Leary M, Bindman A, Salvatierra O. The effect of cyclosporine on the use of hospital resources for kidney transplantation. N Engl J Med 321:1086–1092, 1989.

Sibbitt WL Jr, Bankhurst AD, Williams RC Jr. Studies of cell subpopulations mediating mitogen hyporesponsiveness in patients with Hodgkin's disease. J Clin Invest 61:55–63, 1978.

Siegel M. Susceptibility of mongoloids to infection: I. Incidence of pneumonia, influenza A and *Shigella dysenteriae* (Sonne). Am J Hyg 48:53–62, 1948.

Sigal NH, Dumont FJ. Cyclosporin A, FK-506, and rapamycin: pharmacologic probes of lymphocyte signal transduction. Annu Rev Immunol 10:519–560, 1992.

Siltzbach LE. Etiology of sarcoidosis. Practitioner 202:613–618, 1969.

Siltzbach LE. Discussion of sarcoidosis. Ann N Y Acad Sci 278:247–248, 1976.

Siltzbach LE, Glade PR, Hurschaut Y, Veira LOBP, Celikoglu IS, Hirschhorn K. In vitro stimulation of peripheral lymphocytes in sarcoidosis. In Levinsky L, Macholda F, eds. Proceedings of the Fifth International Conference on Sarcoidosis: XIVth Scientific Conference of the Medical Faculty of Charles University, Prague, 1969. Prague, Universita Karlova, 1971, pp. 217–224.

Silver RT. Infections, fever and host resistance in neoplastic diseases. J Chronic Dis 16:677–701, 1963.

Silver RT, Utz JP, Fahey J, Freireich EJ. Antibody response in patients with acute leukemia. J Lab Clin Med 56:634–643, 1960.

Silverman ED, Myones BL, Miller JJ III: Lymphocyte subpopulation alterations induced by intravenous megadose pulse methylprednisolone. J Rheumatol 11:287–290, 1984.

Simececk C, Zavagal V, Sach J, Kulich V. Serum proteins and serum complement in sarcoidosis. In Levinsky L, Macholda F, eds. Proceedings of the Fifth International Conference on Sarcoidosis: XIVth Scientific Conference of the Medical Faculty of Charles University, Prague, 1969. Prague, Universita Karlova, 1971, pp. 188–194.

Simmons RL, Moberg AW, Gewurz H, Soll R, Najarian JS. Immunosuppression by anti–human lymphocyte globulin: correlation of human and animal assay systems with clinical results. Transplant Proc 3:745–748, 1971.

Singer DB. Postsplenectomy sepsis. In Rosenberg HS, Bolande RP, eds. Perspectives in Pediatric Pathology. Chicago, Year Book Medical Publishers, 1973, pp. 285–311.

Sirisinha S, Edelman R, Suskind R, Charupatana C, Olson RE. Complement and C3-proactivator levels in children with protein-calorie malnutrition and effect of dietary treatment. Lancet 1:1016–1020, 1973.

Sirisinha S, Suskind R, Edelman R, Asvapaka C, Olson RE. Secretory and serum IgA in children with protein-calorie malnutrition. Pediatrics 55:166–170, 1975.

Smeets DF, Moog U, Weemaes CM, Vaes-Peeters G, Merkx GF, Niehof JP, Hamers G. ICF syndrome: a new case and review of the literature. Hum Genet 94:240–246, 1994.

Smith CH, Erlandson M, Schulman I, Stern G. Hazard of severe infections in splenectomized infants and children. Am J Med 22:390–404, 1957.

Smith CW, Goldman AS. Selective effects of thermal injury on mouse peritoneal macrophages. Infect Immun 5:938–941, 1972.

Smythe PM, Brereton Stiles GG, Grace HJ, Mafoyane A, Schonland M, Coovadia HM, Loening WE, Parent MA, Vos GH. Thymolymphatic deficiency and depression of cell-mediated immunity in protein-calorie malnutrition. Lancet 2:939–943, 1971.

Smythe PM, Campbell JAH. The significance of the bacteremia of kwashiorkor. South Afr Med J 33:777, 1959.

Snyder GB. The fate of skin homografts in patients with sarcoidosis. Bull Johns Hopkins Hosp 115:81–91, 1964.

Soboslay PT, Dreweck CM, Hoffmann WH, Luder CGK, Heuschkel C, Gorgen H, Banla M, Schulz-Key H. Ivermectin-facilitated immunity in onchocerciasis: reversal of lymphocytopenia, cellular anergy and deficient cytokine production after single treatment. Clin Exp Immunol 89:407–413, 1992.

Soh J, Donnelly RJ, Kotenko S, Mariano TM, Cook JR, Wang N, Emanuel S, Schwartz B, Miki T, Pestka S. Identification and sequence of an accessory factor required for activation of the human interferon gamma receptor. Cell 76:793–802, 1994.

Sokal JE, Aungst CW. Response to BCG vaccination and survival in advanced Hodgkin's disease. Cancer 24:128–134, 1969.

Sokal JE, Primikirios N. The delayed skin test response in Hodgkin's disease and lymphosarcoma. Effect of disease activity. Cancer 14:597–607, 1961.

Solberg CO, Hellum KB. Neutrophil granulocyte function in bacterial infections. Lancet 2:727–730, 1972.

Sommer E. Primary and secondary anergy in sarcoidosis. Acta Med Scand (Suppl.) 425:195–197, 1964.

Sones M, Israel HL. Altered immunologic reactions in sarcoidosis. Ann Intern Med 40:260–268, 1954.

Sparkes BG. Mechanisms of immune failure in burn injury. Vaccine 11:504–510, 1993.

Spranger J, Hinkel GK, Stoss H, Thoenes W, Wargowski D, Zepp F. Schimke immuno-osseous dysplasia: a newly recognized multisystem disease. J Pediatr 119:64–72, 1991.

Standen GR, Hughes IA, Geddes AD, Jones BM, Wardrop CA. Myelodysplastic syndrome with trisomy 8 in an adolescent with Fanconi anaemia and selective IgA deficiency. Am J Hematol 31:280–283, 1989.

Stansfield SK, Pierre Louis M, Lerebours G, Augustin A. Vitamin A supplementation and increased prevalence of childhood diarrhoea and acute respiratory infections. Lancet 342:578–582, 1993.

Starzl TE, Marchioro TL, Porter KA, Iwasaki Y, Cerilli GJ. The use of heterologous antilymphoid agents in canine renal and liver homotransplantation and in human renal homotransplantation. Surg Gynecol Obstet 124:301–308, 1967.

Starzl TE, Putnam CW, Halgrimson CG, Schroter GT, Martineau G, Launois B, Corman JL, Penn I, Booth AS Jr, Groth CG, Porter KA. Cyclophosphamide and whole organ transplantation in human beings. Surg Gynecol Obstet 133:981–991, 1971.

Steigbigel RT, Lambert LH Jr, Remington JS. Polymorphonuclear leukocyte, monocyte, and macrophage bactericidal function in patients with Hodgkin's disease. J Lab Clin Med 88:54–62, 1976.

Steinfeld JL, Davidson JD, Gordon JRS, Greene FE. The mechanism of hypoproteinemia in patients with regional enteritis and ulcerative colitis. Am J Med 29:405–415, 1960.

Steplewski Z. The search for viruses in sarcoidosis. Ann N Y Acad Sci 278:260–263, 1976.

Stevens CE, Alter HJ, Taylor PE, Zang EA, Harley EJ, Szmuness W. Hepatitis B vaccine in patients receiving hemodialysis: immunogenicity and efficacy. N Engl J Med 311:496–501, 1984.

Stevens JE, Willoughby DA. The anti-inflammatory effect of some immunosuppressive agents. J Pathol 97:367–373, 1969.

Stiehm ER. Humoral immunity in malnutrition. Fed Proc 39:3093–3097, 1980.

Stone HH, Whitehead JB. The management of *Pseudomonas* infections in severely burned patients. Med J Aust (Suppl) 1:6–10, 1970.

Stormorken H, Sjaastad O, Langslet A, Sulg I, Egge K, Diderichsen J. A new syndrome: thrombocytopathia, muscle fatigue, asplenia, miosis, migraine, dyslexia and ichthyosis. Clin Genet 28:367–374, 1985.

Strauss RG, Ashbrock T, Forristal J, West CD. Alternative pathway of complement in sickle cell disease. Pediatr Res 11:285–289, 1977.

Strober W, Wochner RD, Carbone PP, Waldmann TA. Intestinal lymphangiectasia: a protein-losing enteropathy with hypogammaglobulinemia, lymphocytopenia and impaired homograft rejection. J Clin Invest 46:1643–1656, 1967.

Sturgeon P, Brubaker C. Copper deficiency in infants: a syndrome characterized by hypocupremia, iron deficiency anemia, and hypoproteinemia. Am J Dis Child 92:254–265, 1956.

Sullivan JL, Ochs HD, Schiffman G, Hammerschlag MR, Miser J, Vichinsky E, Wedgwood RJ. Immune response after splenectomy. Lancet 1:178–181, 1978.

Suskind RM, Olson LC, Olson RE. Protein calorie malnutrition and infection with hepatitis-associated antigen. Pediatrics 51:525–530, 1973.

Sussman M. Iron and infection. In Jacobs A, Worwood M, eds. Biochemistry and Medicine. New York, Academic Press, 1974, pp. 649–679.

Sutherland I, Mitchell DN, D'Arcy Hart P. Incidence of intrathoracic sarcoidosis among young adults participating in a trial of tuberculosis vaccines. Br Med J 2:497–503, 1965.

Sutnick AI, London WT, Blumberg BS, Gerstley BJ. Persistent anicteric hepatitis with Australia antigen in patients with Down's syndrome. Am J Clin Pathol 57:2–12, 1972.

Swanson MA, Schwartz RS. Immunosuppressive therapy: the relation between clinical response and immunologic competence. N Engl J Med 277:163–170, 1967.

Swinnen LJ, Costanzo-Nordin MR, Fisher SG, O'Sullivan EJ, Johnson MR, Heroux AL, Dizikes GJ, Pifarre R, Fisher RI. Increased incidence of lymphoproliferative disorder after immunosuppression with the monoclonal antibody OKT3 in cardiac-transplant recipients. N Engl J Med 323:1723–1728, 1990.

Szmuness W, Prince AM, Grady GF, Mann MK, Levine RW, Friedman EA, Jacobs MJ, Josephson A, Ribot S, Shapiro FL, Stenzel KH, Suki WN, Vyas G. Hepatitis B infection. A point-prevalence study in 15 US hemodialysis centers. JAMA 227:901–906, 1974.

Taalman RD, Hustinx TW, Weemaes CM, Seemanova E, Schmidt A, Passarge E, Scheres JM. Further delineation of the Nijmegen breakage syndrome. Am J Med Genet 32:425–431, 1989.

Tan JS, Anderson JL, Watanakunakorn C, Phair JP. Neutrophil dysfunction in diabetes mellitus. J Lab Clin Med 85:26–33, 1975.

Tannenbaum H, Pinkus GS, Schur PH. Immunological characterization of subpopulations of mononuclear cells in tissue and peripheral blood from patients with sarcoidosis. Clin Immunol Immunopathol 5:133–141, 1976.

Taub RN, Siltzbach LE. Induction of granulomas in mice by injection of human sarcoid and ileitis homogenates. In Iwai K, Hosoda Y, eds. Proceedings of the Sixth International Conferences on Sarcoidosis. Tokyo, 1972. Baltimore, University Park Press, 1974, pp. 20–21.

Taylor MJ, Josifek K. Multiple congenital anomalies, thymic dysplasia, severe congenital heart disease, and oligosyndactyly with a deletion of the short arm of chromosome 5. Am J Hum Genet 9:5–11, 1981.

Templeton AC. Generalized herpes simplex in malnourished children. J Clin Pathol 23:24–30, 1970.

Teodorczyk-Injeyan JA, Sparkes BG, Mills GB, Peters WJ. Immunosuppression follows systemic T lymphocyte activation in the burn patient. Clin Exp Immunol 85:515–518, 1991.

Thistlethwaite JR Jr, Gaber AO, Haag BW, Aronson AJ, Broelsch CE, Stuart JK, Stuart FP. OKT3 treatment of steroid-resistant renal allograft rejection. Transplantation 43:176–184, 1987.

Thomas PD, Hunninghake GW. Current concepts of the pathogenesis of sarcoidosis. Am Rev Respir Dis 135:747–760, 1987.

Tompkins RG, Remensnyder JP, Burke JF, Tompkins DM, Hilton JF, Schoenfeld DA, Behringer GE, Bondoc CC, Briggs SE, Quinby WC Jr. Significant reductions in mortality for children with burn injuries through the use of prompt eschar excision. Ann Surg 208:577–585, 1988.

Topilsky M, Siltzbach LE, Williams M, Glade PR. Lymphocyte response in sarcoidosis. Lancet 1:117–120, 1972.

Townes AS, Sowa JM, Shulman LE. Controlled trial of cyclophosphamide in rheumatoid arthritis. Arthritis Rheum 19:563–573, 1976.

Trentham DE, Belli JA, Anderson RJ, Buckley JA, Goetzl EJ, David JR, Austen KF. Clinical and immunologic effects of fractionated total lymphoid irradiation in refractory rheumatoid arthritis. N Engl J Med 305:976–982, 1981.

Troisi CL, Heiberg DA, Hollinger FB. Normal immune response to hepatitis B vaccine in patients with Down's syndrome: a basis for immunization guidelines. JAMA 254:3196–3199, 1985.

Trubowitz S, Masek B, Del Rosario A. Lymphocyte response to phytohemagglutinin in Hodgkin's disease, lymphatic leukemia and lymphosarcoma. Cancer 19:2019–2023, 1966.

Tuchinda M, Newcomb RW, DeVald BL. Effect of prednisone treatment on the human immune response to keyhole limpet hemocyanin. Int Arch Allergy Appl Immunol 42:533–544, 1972.

Turk JL, Poulter LW. Selective depletion of lymphoid tissue by cyclophosphamide. Clin Exp Immunol 10:285–296, 1972.

Twomey JJ, Douglass CC, Morris SM. Inability of leukocytes to stimulate mixed leukocyte reactions. J Natl Cancer Inst 51:345–351, 1973.

Twomey JJ, Laughter AH, Farrow S, Douglass CC. Hodgkin's disease: an immunodepleting and immunosuppressive disorder. J Clin Invest 56:467–475, 1975.

Ueno Y, Miyawaki T, Seki H, Hara K, Sato T, Taniguchi N, Takahashi H, Kondo N. Impaired natural killer cell activity in Bloom's syndrome could be restored by human recombinant IL-2 in vitro. Clin Immunol Immunopathol 35:226–233, 1985.

Ugazio AG, Jayakar SD, Marcioni AF, Duse M, Monafo V, Pasquali F, Burgio GR. Immunodeficiency in Down's syndrome: relationship between presence of human thyroglobulin antibodies and HBsAg carrier status. Eur J Pediatr 126:139–146, 1977.

Ugazio AG, Maccario R, Notarangelo LD, Burgio GR. Immunology of

Down syndrome: a review. Am J Med Genet 7(Suppl.):204–212, 1990.

Uh S, Lee SM, Kim HT, Chung Y, Kim YH, Park C, Huh SJ, Lee HB. The effect of radiation therapy on immune function in patients with squamous cell lung carcinoma. Chest 105:132–137, 1994.

Ulstrom RA, Smith NJ, Heimlich E. Transient dysproteinemia in infants, a new syndrome. Am J Dis Child 92:219–253, 1956.

Ulstrom RA, Smith NJ, Nakamura K, Heimlich E. Transient dysproteinemia in infants: II. Studies of protein metabolism using amino acid isotopes. Am J Dis Child 93:536–547, 1957.

Ultmann JE, Cunningham JK, Gellhorn A. The clinical picture of Hodgkin's disease. Cancer Res 26:1047–1062, 1966.

United Nations Scientific Committee on the Effects of Atomic Radiation. Ionizing Radiation: Levels and Effect. New York, United Nations, 1972.

Urbach F, Sones M, Israel HL. Passive transfer of tuberculin sensitivity to patients with sarcoidosis. N Engl J Med 247:794–797, 1952.

Usami S, Chien S, Scholtz PM, Bertles JF. Effect of deoxygenation on blood rheology in sickle cell disease. Microvas Res 9:324–334, 1975.

Vacheron F, Rudent A, Perin S, Labarre C, Quero AM, Guenounou M. Production of interleukin 1 and tumour necrosis factor activities in bronchoalveolar washings following infection of mice by influenza virus. J Gen Virol 71:477–479, 1990.

Vallejos C, McCredie KB, Bodey GP, Hester JP, Freireich EJ. White blood cell transfusions for control of infections in neutropenic patients. Transfusion 15:28–33, 1975.

van der Burgt I, Haraldsson A, Oosterwijk JC, van Essen AJ, Weemaes C, Hamel B. Cartilage hair hypoplasia, metaphyseal chondrodysplasia type McKusick: description of seven patients and review of the literature. Am J Med Genet 41:371–380, 1991.

Van Dyke TE, Levine MJ, Genco RJ. Neutrophil function and oral disease. J Oral Pathol 14:95–120, 1985.

Van Mierop LHS, Gessner IH, Schiebler GL. Asplenia and polysplenia syndrome. Birth Defects 8:74–82, 1972.

Veien NK, Hardt F, Bendixen G, Ringsted J, Brodthagen H, Faber V, Genner J, Heckscher T, Svejgaard A, Freisleben S, Sorensen S, Wanstrup J, Wiik A. Immunological studies in sarcoidosis: a comparison of disease activity and various immunological parameters. Ann N Y Acad Sci 278:47–51, 1976.

Vernon-Roberts B. The Macrophage. Cambridge, England, Cambridge University Press, 1972, p. 92.

Vestey JP, Norval M, Howie S, Maingay J, Neill WA. Variation in lymphoproliferative responses during recrudescent orofacial herpes simplex virus infections. Clin Exp Immunol 77:384–390, 1989.

Vint FW. Post-mortem findings in the natives of Kenya. East Afr Med J 13:332–340, 1937.

Vitetta ES, Thorpe PE, Uhr JW. Immunotoxins: magic bullets or misguided missiles? Immunol Today 14:252–259, 1993.

Volhard F, Fahr T. Die Brightsche Nierenkrankheit: Klinik, Pathologie und Atlas. Berlin, Springer, 1914.

von Pirquit C. Das verhalten der kutanen Tuberkulinreaktion während der Masern. Deutsche Med Wchnschr 34:1297–1300, 1908.

Wagner HN Jr, Iho M, Horwich RB. Studies of the reticuloendothelial system (RES). II. Changes in the phagocytic capacity of the RES in patients with certain infections. J Clin Invest 42:427–434, 1963.

Wahren B, Carlens E, Espmark A, Lundbeck H, Lofgren S, Madar E, Henle G, Henle W. Antibodies to various herpesviruses in sera from patients with sarcoidosis. J Natl Cancer Inst 47:747–755, 1971.

Waldman DJ, Stiehm ER. Cutaneous sarcoidosis of childhood. J Pediatr 91:271–273, 1977.

Waldman JD, Rosenthal A, Smith AL, Shurin S, Nadas AS. Sepsis and congenital asplenia. J Pediatr 90:555–559, 1977.

Waldmann TA. Protein-losing enteropathy. Gastroenterology 50:422–443, 1966.

Waldmann TA, Schwab PJ. IgC (7S gamma globulin) metabolism in hypogammaglobulinemia: studies in patients with defective gamma globulin synthesis, gastrointestinal protein loss, or both. J Clin Invest 44:1523–1533, 1965.

Waldmann TA, Steinfeld JL, Dutcher TF, Davidson JD, Gordon RS Jr. The role of the gastrointestinal system in "idiopathic hypoproteinemia." Gastroenterology 41:197–207, 1961.

Waldmann TA, Wochner RD, Laster L, Gordon RS Jr. Allergic gastroenteropathy: a cause of excessive gastrointestinal protein loss. N Engl J Med 276:762–769, 1967.

Walker AM, Garcia R, Pate P, Mata LJ, David JR. Transfer factor in the immune deficiency of protein-calorie malnutrition: a controlled study with 32 cases. Cell Immunol 15:372–381, 1975.

Walker W. Splenectomy in childhood: a review in England and Wales,1960–4. Br J Surg 63:36–43, 1976.

Walter T, Arredondo S, Arevalo M, Stekel A. Effect of iron therapy on phagocytosis and bactericidal activity in neutrophils of iron-deficient infants. Am J Clin Nutr 44:877–882, 1986.

Wang JK, Hsieh KH. Immunologic study of the asplenia syndrome. Pediatr Infect Dis J 10:819–822, 1991.

Wang WC, Herrod HG, Valenski WR, Wyatt RJ. Lymphocyte and complement abnormalities in splenectomized patients with hematologic disorders. Am J Hematol 28:239–245, 1988.

Ward PA, Berenberg JL. Defective regulation of inflammatory mediators in Hodgkin's disease: supernormal levels of chemotactic-factor inactivator. N Engl J Med 290:76–80, 1974.

Weemaes CM, Bakkeren JA, ter Haar BG, Hustinx TW, van Munster PJ. Immune responses in four patients with Bloom syndrome. Clin Immunol Immunopathol 12:12–19, 1979.

Weemaes CM, Hustinx TW, Scheres JM, van Munster PJ, Bakkeren JA, Taalman RD. A new chromosomal instability disorder: the Nijmegen breakage syndrome. Acta Paediatr Scand 70:557–564, 1981.

Weemaes CM, The TH, van Munster PJ, Bakkeren JA. Antibody responses in vivo in chromosome instability syndromes with immunodeficiency. Clin Exp Immunol 57:529–534, 1984.

Weiden PL, Blaese RM, Strober W, Block JB, Waldmann TA. Impaired lymphocyte transformation in intestinal lymphangiectasia: evidence for at least two functionally distinct lymphocyte populations in man. J Clin Invest 51:1319–1325, 1972.

Weinshenker BG, Wilton S, Rice GP. Phorbol ester–induced differentiation permits productive human cytomegalovirus infection in a monocytic cell line. J Immunol 140:1625–1631, 1988.

Weinstein RJ, Young LS. Neutrophil function in gram-negative rod bacteremia: the interaction between phagocytic cells, infecting organisms, and humoral factors. J Clin Invest 58:190–199, 1976.

Weiss RL, Colby TV, Spruance SL, Salmon VC, Hammond ME. Simultaneous cytomegalovirus and herpes simplex virus pneumonia. Arch Pathol Lab Med 111:242–245, 1987.

Wesley J, Fisher A, Fisher MW. Immunization against *Pseudomonas* in infection after thermal injury. J Infect Dis (Suppl.) 130:S152–S158, 1974.

Western KA, Benson GD, Gleason NN, Healy GR, Schultz MG. Babesiosis in a Massachusetts resident. N Engl J Med 283:854–856, 1970.

Weston WL, Claman HN, Krueger GG. Site of action of cortisol in cellular immunity. J Immunol 110:880–883, 1973.

White J, Herman A, Pullen AM, Kubo R, Kappler JW, Marrack P. The V-beta–specific superantigen staphylococcal enterotoxin B: stimulation of mature T cells and clonal deletion in neonatal mice. Cell 56:27–35, 1989.

Whittum JA, Niederkorn JY, McCulley JP, Streilein JW. Role of suppressor T cells in herpes simplex virus–induced immune deviation. J Virol 51:556–558, 1984.

Wilfert CM, Katz SL. Etiology of bacterial sepsis in nephrotic children 1963–1967. Pediatrics 42:840–843, 1968.

Willems PJ, Gatti R, Darby JK, Romeo G, Durand P, Dumon JE, O'Brien JS. Fucosidosis revisited: a review of 77 patients. Am J Med Genet 38:111–131, 1991.

Williams ML, Loughran TP Jr, Kidd PG, Starkebaum GA. Polyclonal proliferation of activated suppressor/cytotoxic T cells with transient depression of natural killer cell function in acute infectious mononucleosis. Clin Exp Immunol 77:71–76, 1989.

Williams WJ, Pioli E, Jones DJ, Dighero M. The Kmif (Kveim-induced macrophage migration inhibition factor) test in sarcoidosis. J Clin Pathol 25:951–954, 1972.

Williamson WA, Greenwood BM. Impairment of the immune response to vaccination after acute malaria. Lancet 1:1328–1329, 1978.

Willman CL, Busque L, Griffith BB, Favara BE, McClain KL, Duncan MH, Gilliland DG. Langerhans'-cell histiocytosis (histiocytosis X)—a clonal proliferative disease. N Engl J Med 331:154–160, 1994.

Wilson NW, Gooding A, Peterson B, Bastian JF. Anergy in pediatric head trauma patients. Am J Dis Child 145:326–329, 1991.

Wilson NW, Ochs HD, Peterson B, Hamburger RN, Bastian JF. Abnormal primary antibody responses in pediatric trauma patients. J Pediatr 115:424–427, 1989.

Wilson WA, Hughes GR, Lachmann PJ. Deficiency of factor B of the complement system in sickle cell anaemia. Br Med J 1:367–369, 1976.

Wilson WEC, Kirkpatrick CH, Talmage DW. Suppression of immunologic responsiveness in uremia. Ann Intern Med 62:1–14, 1965.

Winkelstein JA, Drachman RH. Deficiency of pneumococcal serum opsonizing activity in sickle-cell disease. N Engl J Med 279:459–466, 1968.

Winkelstein JA, Lambert GH, Swift A. Pneumococcal serum opsonizing activity in splenectomized children. J Pediatr 87:430–433, 1975.

Winkelstein JA, Mikulla JM, Sartiano GP, Ellis LD. Cellular immunity in Hodgkin's disease: comparison of cutaneous reactivity and lymphoproliferative responses to phytohemagglutinin. Cancer 34:549–553, 1974.

Wochner RD, Drews G, Strober W, Waldmann TA. Accelerated breakdown of immunoglobulin G (IgG) in myotonic dystrophy: a hereditary error of immunoglobulin catabolism. J Clin Invest 45:321–329, 1966.

Wold WS, Gooding LR. Region E3 of adenovirus: a cassette of genes involved in host immunosurveillance and virus-cell interactions. Virology 184:1–8, 1991.

Woodle ES, Thistlethwaite JR, Jolliffe LK, Zivin RA, Collins A, Adair JR, Bodmer M, Athwal D, Alegre ML, Bluestone JA. Humanized OKT3 antibodies: successful transfer of immune modulating properties and idiotype expression. J Immunol 148:2756–2763, 1992.

Yetgin S, Altay C, Ciliv G, Laleli Y. Myeloperoxidase activity and bactericidal function of PMN in iron deficiency. Acta Haematol 61:10–14, 1979.

Young AW Jr, Sweeney EW, David DS, Cheigh J, Hochgelerenl EL, Sakai S, Stenzel KH, Rubin AL. Dermatologic evaluation of pruritus in patients on hemodialysis. N Y State J Med 73:2670–2674, 1973.

Young RC, Corder MP, Haynes HA, DeVita VT. Delayed hypersensitivity in Hodgkin's disease. A study of 103 untreated patients. Am J Med 52:63–72, 1972.

Ziegler RG, Mason TJ, Stemhagen A, Hoover R, Schoenberg JB, Gridley G, Virgo PW, Fraumeni JF Jr. Carotenoid intake, vegetables, and the risk of lung cancer among white men in New Jersey. Am J Epidemiol 123:1080–1093, 1986.

Zinneman HH, Rotstein J. A study of gamma globulins in dystonia myotonica. J Lab Clin Med 47:907–916, 1956.

Zweiman B, Israel HL. Comparative in vitro reactivities of leukocytes from sarcoids and normals to different Kveim preparations. Ann N Y Acad Sci 278:700–710, 1976.

PART III

IMMUNOLOGIC ASPECTS OF PEDIATRIC ILLNESSES

Chapter 20

Allergic Disorders

David S. Pearlman and C. Warren Bierman

Since the discovery in the late 1800s of specific immune substances in the blood and their connection with the development of specific immunity, antiserum has been used to modify the course of many diseases. Most of the antiserum used was prepared from the horse, a good antibody producer and a source of large amounts of serum. Horse antiserum, however, often caused a curious illness apparently unrelated to the disease for which the serum was employed. In 1905, Clemens von Pirquet and Bela Schick, observing that individuals with horse "serum sickness" developed precipitating antibodies to horse serum proteins, suggested for the first time that antibodies not only could prevent disease but also could cause disease as well.

That the development of antibodies could alter subsequent responsiveness in an unfavorable fashion was a concept of great significance, and the term *allergy* (which means changed activity) was coined by von Pirquet in 1906 to designate such a state of altered reactivity, regardless of whether it was beneficial or detrimental to the host. The clinically opposite states of *hyposensitivity* (as in acquired specific resistance to measles) and *hypersensitivity* (as in the untoward reactivity to horse serum proteins) were both thought to be based on fundamentally similar mechanisms, namely antigen-antibody interaction.

Through the years, however, allergy has assumed a different meaning and refers now to the unfavorable consequences of immune reactivity. Immune mechanisms may result in undesirable clinical manifestations with characteristic patterns. It is often erroneously assumed, however, that clinical manifestations typical of allergic reactions necessarily have an immune basis.

The term *allergy* is used here to refer to a clinical event or disorder mediated specifically by an immune reaction in which the consequence of this reaction is detrimental to the host. *Allergic disorders* are considered to include those constellations of clinical symptoms and signs that commonly, but not exclusively, are the ultimate manifestations of antigen-antibody interactions. Allergic disorders may be triggered or aggravated by various mechanisms, both immune and nonimmune.

Allergic reactivity, both in the sense in which it was used by von Pirquet and in the sense of its current usage, is present in all normal subjects. Transfusion reactions caused by administering mismatched blood, dermatitis induced by contact with the leaves from the poison ivy plant, and the rejection of a transplanted kidney are undesirable manifestations of allergic reactivity that occur in normal subjects. Other forms of allergic reactivity are not shared by all. Hay fever, allergic asthma, and allergic infantile eczema are found in a minority of the population, and these cannot be readily induced in individuals not predisposed to their development. Although an association between these disorders and *skin-sensitizing (reaginic) antibody,* identified more recently as immunoglobulin E (IgE) antibody, was recognized long ago, the basis for the development of these disorders is poorly understood. The term *atopy* ("strange disease") still applies to these dis-

orders in the same sense as it was first used by Coca and Cooke in 1923.

CLASSIFICATION OF ALLERGIC REACTIONS

The manifestations of allergic reactions are based on the nature of the allergen involved, the route of contact with the allergen, the biologic properties of the antibodies present, and the vulnerability of various tissues to the effects of antigen-antibody interaction. These manifestations can involve a variety of immune mechanisms, some defined only recently.

Classically, allergic reactions have been divided into two general categories: *immediate hypersensitivity* and *delayed-type hypersensitivity* (DTH), also called *cell-mediated immunity* (CMI). This classification is based on (1) the time interval between allergen contact and the appearance of clinical manifestations and (2) dependence either on humoral antibody (immediate hypersensitivity) or on cell-mediated immune reactions (delayed-type hypersensitivity). In addition, "late" reactions, which sometimes occur a few hours after immediate reactions, are mediated by the same humoral (IgE) antibody responsible for the immediate reaction. Another classification of clinical allergic reactions based on the different mechanisms by which immune reactions may initiate tissue damage was proposed by Gell and Coombs (1968). According to this classification, immune tissue injury is divided into four types of reactions:

Type I (anaphylactic) reactions: Now known to be mediated by IgE antibody. Examples of type I reactions include allergic urticaria and angioedema, systemic *anaphylaxis** (so-called allergic shock), hay fever, and allergic asthma.

Type II (cytotoxic) reactions: Caused by antibody attaching to and harming a cell or tissue. Examples include transfusion reactions caused by antibody reactive with formed elements of the blood, ABO hemolytic disease of the newborn, and autoimmune hemolytic anemia.

Type III (toxic immune complexes) reactions: Caused by the deposition of immune microprecipitates in or around blood vessels. Examples include lesions seen in the serum sickness syndrome, glomerulonephritis, and connective tissue disorders such as systemic lupus erythematosus.

Type IV (delayed-type hypersensitivity) reactions: Caused by the interaction between antigen and specifically sen-

---

*Anaphylaxis was first described in 1902 by Portier and Richet, who observed that the injection of a relatively harmless amount of sea anemone toxin into dogs rendered these animals unusually sensitive to toxin injected many days later. The degree of hypersensitivity was so great that a subsequent injection was followed by the sudden and violent death of the animal. The term anaphylaxis ("against protection") was applied to this heightened and untoward responsiveness in the belief that the first injections of toxin used up some natural protective substance in the body, leaving the animals sensitive to the toxin's effects. An immunologic interpretation was later applied to this phenomenon, but the term has been used for a variety of allergic reactions mediated by various serum antibodies.

sitized T, or thymus-derived, lymphoid cells. Examples include tuberculin reactions, contact dermatitis, and the rejection of foreign tissue.

These classifications do not take into account the profound interrelationships between the various types of immune tissue injury and other immune and related nonimmune types of injury, such as that occurring through activation of the alternative complement pathway. In addition, many (probably most) allergic manifestations involve more than one immune mechanism. However, any attempt to provide a classification of allergic mechanisms necessarily suffers from oversimplification and from the incompleteness of current immunologic information.

ANTIBODIES OF ALLERGIC REACTIVITY

Even before the recognition of the role of antibodies in allergic reactions, considerable diversity in antibody function was recognized. Such antibody can cause precipitation, agglutination, opsonization, lysis, and antigen neutralization, indicating the heterogeneity of antibody molecules. Prausnitz and Küstner (1921) demonstrated that the serum from an individual who was clinically sensitive to fish (Küstner) contained a substance that could sensitize the skin of a nonsensitive individual (Prausnitz), so that a local anaphylactic reaction occurred if fish antigen was injected at the site of serum transfer. This skin-sensitizing substance was recognized as a special kind of antibody present in people with atopic disorders and was termed *atopic reagin*, or *reaginic antibody.*

We now recognize several classes of antibodies, all of which help to protect the host from the deleterious effects of infectious agents and other foreign antigens. However, these antibodies may also result in detrimental reactions through immune mechanisms identical to those operative in host defense.

Immunoglobulin E Antibodies

Antibody of the IgE class fulfills all the criteria for reaginic or skin-sensitizing antibody and is mainly, but not necessarily exclusively, responsible for such antibody activity (Ishizaka and Ishizaka, 1967). IgE antibodies usually mediate type I reactions and are the antibodies implicated in allergic rhinitis, allergic asthma, and some cases of atopic dermatitis. They are also involved in anaphylactic and allergic urticarial reactions and in "late" allergic responses, occurring 4 to 8 hours after contact with allergen (Kaliner, 1984). These late responses are believed to be especially important in the pathogenesis of end-organ hyperresponsiveness to various stimuli and nonimmune stimuli in asthma and perhaps other atopic allergic disorders. The IgE-mediated late-phase response appears to be associated with cellular infiltration including T cells, eosinophils, polymorphonuclear leukocytes (PMNs) to a lesser extent, and other cells, all of which probably play an important role in promoting long-lasting obstruction and airway hyperirritability.

IgE antibody is an efficient liberator of histamine and other pharmacologic substances (mediators) responsible for the clinical manifestations of allergic reactions (see Mediator Activation and Release). The mediator-releasing ability of IgE antibody is related to its unusual affinity for tissue mast cells and blood basophils, the cells from which many of these mediators emanate.

The production of skin-sensitizing antibody was initially thought to be an abnormal phenomenon limited to atopic individuals, but IgE (and presumably IgE antibody) is present in most individuals, although generally at a lower concentration than in atopic subjects. Furthermore, IgE antibody can be induced by appropriate stimulation in most persons. Certain people are particularly disposed to produce this kind of antibody.

IgE levels and the formation of IgE antibody appear to be under the influence of at least two separate genetic control mechanisms: one concerned with the ability to mount an IgE antibody response to a specific antigen and another that controls basal IgE levels (Huang and Marsh, 1993). IgE levels tend to be high in atopic disorders, especially in atopic dermatitis, but they may also be normal or low even in the presence of large quantities of specific IgE antibodies to various antigens (see also Chapters 3 and 13).

Other Antibody Classes

Immunoglobulin G (IgG) and immunoglobulin M (IgM) antibodies can mediate type II and type III reactions, such as autoimmune hemolytic anemia, poststreptococcal and lupus nephritis, and serum sickness. Antibodies of these classes may also contribute to the development of autoallergic disorders of solid tissues. Aggregated IgG can induce anaphylactic shock if given intravenously and liberates vasoactive agents if it is injected into the skin. Certain IgG antibodies may exhibit reagin-like activity, promoting type I allergic reactions in a manner similar to that of IgE (Parish, 1970). Specifically, there is evidence that IgG4 may possess reagin-like activity (Stanworth and Smith, 1973). In addition, IgM and IgG antibodies can liberate vasoactive agents through the activation of the complement system (see Chemical Mediators of Allergic Reactions later), and their participation sometimes results in urticaria, angioedema, allergic rhinitis, and allergic asthma. IgM has also been implicated in the pathogenesis of an acquired form of cold urticaria (Wanderer et al., 1971).

Delayed-type hypersensitivity (DTH) results in allergic contact dermatitis to poison ivy and various chemicals and plays an important role in certain autoallergic disorders of solid tissues. An experimental allergic rhinitis resembling IgE-mediated allergic rhinitis can be produced via a DTH mechanism.

Cooperative Effects of Antibodies in Allergic Reactions

The normal humoral response to antigenic stimulation is the formation of antibodies of many immunoglobulin classes with different biologic activities. Thus, sensitized individuals tend to produce a spectrum of antibodies to a specific antigen, and subsequent antigenic contact results in a mixture of immune reactions. Allergic manifestations, in other words, are generally the result of the combined effects of several immune reactions. For example, in serum sickness, antibodies of the IgE, IgM, and IgG classes may occur. IgE antibodies (and perhaps IgG and IgM antibodies through complement activation) are responsible for the urticarial component of the syndrome; IgG and IgM antibodies (and possibly IgE and immunoglobulin A [IgA]) participate in the vasculitis of serum sickness (Cochrane, 1971).

Patients with hypersensitivity diseases of the lung (Fink, 1993) may exhibit a biphasic response to inhalation of the offending allergen, the first phase beginning rapidly after allergen inhalation and the second occurring hours later. IgE antibodies produce the early phase of the reaction, and precipitating IgG and IgM antibodies may be at least partly responsible for the later phase. Evidence is accumulating in addition for the participation of DTH. There may be a cooperative dependence among these different kinds of immune reactions, with the IgE-mediated reaction being required before immune complex damage can occur.

Inhibitory Effects of Antibodies on Allergic Reactions

Antibody of one type may interfere with the biologic effects of other immune reactions. Interference with antibody formation, with antigen-antibody interaction, and with cellular immune reactions is well documented. Circulating antibody, for instance, may inhibit the DTH-mediated rejection of foreign grafts, mainly by neutralizing tumor antigens and rendering them unavailable for reaction with specifically sensitized lymphoid cells (immune enhancement). Immunotherapy with ragweed in individuals with asthma and hay fever results in the production of circulating IgG antibodies, which, compared with the IgE antibodies causing the disorder, are relatively inefficient in causing mediator release on contact with antigen. IgG antibodies mixed with IgE antibodies of the same specificity block the ability of the IgE antibodies to induce mediator release from skin or peripheral blood leukocytes, when mixed with the appropriate antigen, by competing with the IgE antibodies for antigen. The production of this so-called blocking antibody may account in part for the amelioration of allergic symptoms seen after immunotherapy.

With the exception of IgE, which is frequently elevated in atopic disorders, there are no consistent abnormalities of immunoglobulins in allergic disorders (Pearlman, 1969). In individuals with primary immunodeficiencies the incidence of true allergic reactions is extremely low, as would be expected. In certain immunodeficiencies, however, clinical phenomena often considered to be of allergic origin are sometimes noted. An eczematoid eruption resembling atopic dermatitis is seen in children with X-linked agammaglobulinemia and the Wiskott-Aldrich syndrome. High IgE levels have been recorded in the Wiskott-Aldrich syndrome and thymic aplasia, but in most immunodeficient states IgE production is deficient (McLaughlan et al., 1974). Connective tissue diseases, such as rheumatoid arthritis, are noted in congenital and acquired agammaglobulinemia. In these disorders, there is a deficit of some immune reactants but not others. Various allergic manifestations seem to occur in subjects with mild to moderate deficiencies in immunoglobulin levels. These allergic manifestations may result from an unbalanced immune system or from microorganisms not held in check by the deficient immune system (Pearlman, 1971).

ALLERGENS

All antigens are potential allergens, and the number implicated in allergic reactions is legion. Allergenicity depends to a large extent on the nature of the antigen involved; some antigens act regularly as allergens, whereas others do so only occasionally. The quantity, route, and form of antigen exposure influence the degree of allergenicity. In addition, host factors are important: differences occur on both an individual and a racial level and are genetically determined (Marsh, 1975; Orgel, 1975).

Because allergic reactivity depends on antigen exposure and on antibody formation, it is not surprising that allergic reactions are less common in infants than in older subjects. Allergic sensitization in utero appears to occur, but this is rare, primarily because of the relative protection against antigenic stimulation afforded the fetus.

"Passive" allergic sensitization does occur in the sense that transplacental IgG antibody is responsible for ABO and Rh hemolytic disease of the newborn, but IgE antibodies associated with allergic asthma or hay fever are not transmitted to the fetus. Passive sensitization may conceivably occur through breast feeding, but this sensitization would probably exert its greatest effects in the gastrointestinal tract. Rapid postnatal sensitization can occur, and allergic reactions in the first month have been recorded. Early milk sensitivity can be caused by milk given to newborns in the nursery.

Food Allergens

The relative importance of various kinds of allergens depends on a person's age. Food antigens are encountered early in life and are important allergens in infancy. Cow's milk, presented to the infant in huge quantities, is the chief offender (1 quart of milk per day for a 6-month-old child is the equivalent of 8 to 10 quarts a day for an average adult). Wheat, corn, egg, soy and other legumes, and nuts are also offenders of some frequency. Increased gastrointestinal absorption of incompletely digested protein may also be a factor in food allergies in early life. Fish, seafood, strawberries, nuts, beef, white potatoes, and pork are other common food allergens in older subjects. Food hypersensitivity may be lost with time, although severe food sensitivity to certain allergens, such as peanuts, is frequently not lost.

Because the symptoms of food allergy are often poorly defined and since diagnosis is difficult, there is a tendency to consider food allergy as an entity separate from other kinds of allergic reactivity. However, there is no reason to believe that allergic responses to foods differ from those to other antigens. Signs and symptoms of food-induced allergic reactions may include local or systemic urticaria and angioedema, atopic dermatitis (Sampson, 1984), other erythematous skin eruptions, gastrointestinal disturbances, asthma, rhinitis, and, in highly sensitive individuals, anaphylactic shock (Metcalfe, 1984). Symptoms may be provoked not only by ingestion but also by inhalation. The response to ingestion of an offending food may be immediate or delayed for hours; the latter event results in a diagnostic dilemma.

The delay in the appearance of symptoms after the ingestion of a food may be related to:

- The time it takes for digestive processes to alter the ingested food to a form to which the person has become sensitized
- Non-IgE immune reactions (Metcalfe, 1984)
- Reactions mediated by nonimmune mechanisms

Other Allergens

Several kinds of antigens, in addition to food, are encountered early in life. Among these are infectious agents; there is a strong association between viral respiratory infections and an asthma-like respiratory disorder beginning in infancy. IgE antibody to the etiologic viral agent has been demonstrated in many such children (Welliver et al., 1981). It is not clear, however, that these "allergic" manifestations are induced by an immune response to the invading organisms.

Other allergens encountered early include common inhalants present in the home, such as animal (especially cat) allergens, house dust mites, insects (in particular, cockroaches in inner city areas), and molds. House dust mites have been implicated as the prevalent allergenic ingredient of house dust in most countries. Concentrations of house mites are significantly greater in moist climates. Their clinical importance is correspondingly greater in areas where humidity tends to stay above 50% for prolonged periods. Animal allergens from domestic or farm animals may result in sensitization in early childhood. Anaphylactic reactions to stinging insects, such as bees, wasps, hornets, and fire ants, usually occur in later childhood or in adult life after sensitization by previous stings. Exposure to pollens and seasonal molds sufficient to induce sensitization to cause major problems usually requires a few years. Antibiotics and other drugs assume increasing importance as potential allergens with repeated usage.

Incomplete Allergens

Most allergens both sensitize and induce allergic reactions. Some low-molecular-weight substances, however, are incomplete allergens (*haptens*) in their original state and must be attached to a suitable carrier before they can sensitize or induce an allergic reaction. Chemical contactants, which are responsible for allergic contact dermatitis, and drugs are examples of such haptenic allergens. Because conjugation to a carrier substance is necessary for sensitization, the degree to which a given chemical or drug can react with skin or other body tissues is an important determinant of potential allergenicity. Some drugs that cannot participate in such a reaction themselves nevertheless give rise to highly reactive metabolic derivatives, which act as potent inducers of allergic reactions. Penicillin is a good example, although the native molecule is not totally devoid of reactivity (see Penicillin Reactions). Because there is variation from one individual to another in the metabolic pathways of various drugs, it is conceivable that these differences may affect individual susceptibility to sensitization.

Much cross-antigenicity exists in nature, and, similarly, there are many examples of cross-allergenicity. Cross-reactivity is based on structural similarities between different molecules (*epitopes*) and is greatest among antigens that have similar biologic backgrounds. For example, individuals sensitized to one breed of dog are often reactive to various breeds of dogs, sensitivity to Kentucky bluegrass pollen is often associated with sensitivity to other grass pollens, and sensitivity to benzylpenicillin is often associated with sensitivity to ampicillin or other penicillin derivatives. Sensitivity is probably strongest to the sensitizing allergen (antibodies react more strongly with the antigen that induced sensitivity than with cross-reactive antigens). Cross-reactive antigens also exhibit individual antigenic peculiarities; it is possible to develop sensitivity to one breed of dog yet be relatively unreactive to another, or to react to one grass but not another.

CHEMICAL MEDIATORS OF ALLERGIC REACTIONS

Mast Cells and Basophils

Two classical effector cells are involved in the allergic inflammatory reaction. It is through the mast cell and basophil that the combination of antigen and antibody induces the allergic response.

Mast cells are more prevalent than basophils. They are found in connective tissues, particularly near small blood vessels, nerves, and glandular ducts, and are associated with lymphoid tissues. The skin and gastrointestinal mucosa are among the organ systems rich in mast cells (Metcalfe, 1983). The basophil is the circulating blood-borne counterpart of the mast cell.

Mast cells and basophils share many features. Both contain preformed mediators, such as histamine; both have surface high affinity receptors for IgE, and mediator activation and release of both cells appear to be modulated by cyclic adenosine monophosphate (cAMP) levels. Both cell types have many granules in their cytoplasm that contain chemical mediators of inflammation. When stimulated, they degranulate and release these mediators.

There are also distinct differences between basophils and mast cells. Basophils are formed in bone marrow and appear to be derivatives of promyelocytes. Mast cells leave bone marrow as progenitors and complete their maturation in peripheral tissues. They differ in morphology, size, granular size, and content of mediators. Mast cells appear to generate quantities of arachidonic acid metabolites that are an order of magnitude greater than those produced by basophils.

There are two major types of mast cells in humans: (1) the mucosal mast cell (MC_T) and (2) the connective tissue mast cell (MC_{TC}) (Irani and Schwartz, 1990).

The morphologic changes that mast cells and basophils undergo during degranulation differ. Basophil degranulation results from fusion of individual granules to cell membrane with extrusion of the granule. Mast cell granules fuse intracellularly to form chains of connected granules that are released into the intracellular space through newly formed channels to the cell membrane (Schleimer et al., 1983).

Mediators released by mast cells and basophils are of two types:

1. Preformed mediators include histamine, neutrophil chemotactic factor, various inflammatory proteases, and heparin.
2. Newly formed mediators include arachidonic acid metabolites (prostaglandins and slow-reacting substance of anaphylaxis, or SRS-A), platelet activating factor (PAF), and others.

Mediator Activation and Release

Release of mediators from basophils and mast cells can be caused by various stimuli, such as specific antigen, anaphylatoxins, lymphokines, and some neuropeptides. Also, mediator release is enhanced by many substances, such as the interferons, platelet factors, adenosine, prostaglandin D_2, 5-hydroxy-6,8,11,14-eicosatetraenoic acid (5-HETE), and 5-hydroperoxy-6,8,11,14-eicosatetraenoic acid (5-HPETE).

IgE antibody–dependent mediator release has been well studied, and the events in this process identified to date are outlined briefly here (Kaliner and Austen, 1975). The process begins with the interaction between antibody attached to mediator cells (mast cells or basophils) and antigen. When two or more antibody molecules are bridged on the surface of the mediator cell through such interactions, a membrane-associated serine proesterase is activated, presumably through a strategic perturbation of the cell membrane. The activated esterase plays an important, although undefined, role in the early phase of the process of mediator activation and release. Calcium ion flux is also an essential step in the early phase of the process, with a subsequent energy-dependent and calcium ion–dependent step involved both in mediator generation and in the release phase of preformed or activated mediators. The entire process leaves the mediator cell viable and free to replenish its mediator stores.

By this process, at least four mediators are activated or released more or less concomitantly: histamine, SRS-A, PAF, and eosinophil chemotactic factor of anaphylaxis (ECF-A). Other substances, such as *kallikreins* involved in kinin generation and *neutrophil chemotactic factors,* may be released as well; secondarily, activation of other mediators, such as *kinins* and *prostaglandins,* occurs.

The processes of mediator generation and release are influenced strongly by intracellular levels of the cyclic nucleotides cAMP and cyclic guanosine monophosphate (cGMP) and, therefore, by agents that alter cellular levels of these nucleotides. Increases in cAMP levels decrease mediator production and release, whereas decreases in cAMP levels and increases in cGMP levels augment mediator generation and release. Thus, adrenergic agents (through beta-adrenergic receptor activation), prostaglandins (through activation of nonadrenergic receptors, which generate cAMP production), and methylxanthines (which may act on adenosine receptors) diminish mediator activation and release. Cholinergic and adrenergic agents, acting through alpha-receptor stimulation, enhance the process of mediator generation or release through depression of cAMP levels or augmentation of cGMP production. Histamine also inhibits its own release, possibly through enhancement of cAMP levels.

There are extensive interrelationships between the activation, release, and degradation of the chemical mediators (Austen and Orange, 1975). The release or activation of various *primary mediators* from mediator cells not only results in alterations in blood flow, vascular permeability, or contraction of some smooth muscles but also is instrumental in activating other mediators, such as plasma kinins. Some primary mediators also attract to the area of the reaction PMNs, eosinophils, and other cells. These cells may elaborate a variety of *secondary mediators* on their own that, in the case of PMNs, can mediate further tissue damage or, in the case of eosinophils, can result in prostaglandin generation and the elaboration of various other agents capable of inhibiting mediator generation or release. Eosinophils may also induce direct tissue damage by releasing toxins, including a highly toxic basic protein, eosinophil cationic protein, eosinophil peroxidase, arylsulfatase B, β-glucuronidase, eosinophil collagenase, and the enzyme phenol oxidase (Gleich et al., 1992).

Histamine

Histamine is present in human skin, intestinal mucosa, heart, and lungs in large amounts, and it has been identified in brain tissue and nerve endings (Grzanna and Schultz, 1982). Histamine appears to be important in homeostasis. Its actions range from local and systemic cardiovascular effects to regulating the microcirculation, mediating gastric secretion, and perhaps acting as a neurotransmitter in the central nervous system.

In the allergic reaction, histamine is released from basophils and mast cells. Histamine acts to dilate small blood vessels, increase capillary and venular permeability, contract bronchial and other smooth muscle, and stimulate mucous glands and ganglionic neurons (Pipcorn et al., 1988).

Along with certain proteases, histamine is a key pharmacologic mediator of pruritus. Some of its actions, especially the bronchoconstricting effects, may be mediated in part through activation of cholinergic mechanisms (Gold, 1973). Histamine is the mediator of the *triple response of Lewis:*

- Erythema from dilation of small blood vessels
- The development of a central wheal from increased capillary permeability
- Secondary erythema from peripheral dilatation of surrounding blood vessels induced by an axon reflex mechanism

Histamine is also responsible for many wheal-and-flare reactions (urticaria, or hives) induced by immune and nonimmune mechanisms. Interaction between antigen and IgE antibody is an especially effective means by which histamine is liberated from its intercellular storage sites, and histamine is thought to play an important role in allergic disorders in which IgE antibody is involved, such as allergic rhinitis.

Histamine release can also be initiated by non-IgE immune pathways. Reaginic IgG antibodies may mediate wheal-and-flare reactions, and IgG and IgM antibodies complexed with antigen can liberate histamine indirectly through activation of certain complement components (discussed later). Histamine release can occur nonimmunologically by heat or cold injury and after exposure to basic amines, surface-active agents, certain drugs (e.g., polymyxin B or codeine), and various foods (e.g., strawberries, nuts, or eggs) (Paton, 1957; Beall, 1964).

Histamine activates at least three specific receptors: H_1, H_2, and H_3. The effects of this stimulation are noted in Table 20–1. In addition, histamine acts through H_3 receptor activation to inhibit its own liberation from mediator cells. Histamine does not appear to play a great role in asthma; however, it does participate in mediating symptoms of rhinitis.

Much of the histamine is made within the cells that store it through decarboxylation of histidine. A large population of cells associated with the vasculature,

other than mast cells, appears to manufacture but not store histamine. Histamine turnover in these cells is rapid, and the rate of histamine formation can be altered by a variety of stimuli. This so-called *induced histamine* in conjunction with catecholamines and corticosteroids may affect the regulation of the microcirculation (Schayer, 1963). The rate of histamine formation is increased in anaphylaxis, at least in animals; this suggests that histamine may perpetuate such reactions.

Metabolites of Arachidonic Acid

Metabolites of arachidonic acid are released by mast cells and other cell types involved in the immediate allergic response. These metabolites are all products of either the cyclooxygenase or the lipoxygenase pathway (Stenson and Parker, 1983).

Cyclooxygenase products exert their effects in both the cells in which they are synthesized and neighboring cells but generally do not affect more remote parts of the body because of their rapid degradation in vivo. They appear to act through specific receptors.

The lipoxygenase pathway leads to the formation of monohydroxy and dihydroxy fatty acids and leukotrienes. These fatty acids and leukotriene-B_4 (LTB_4) are chemotactic agents, whereas LTC_4, LTD_4, and LTE_4 are bronchoconstrictors (constituting SRS-A).

There are significant differences between cyclooxygenase and lipoxygenase pathways. Cyclooxygenase is found in every cell, whereas lipoxygenase appears to be present in only a few cell types, including neutrophils, platelets, macrophages, and cells of the skin and testis. Cyclooxygenases from different tissues appear to be identical, but lipoxygenases differ from cell type to cell type. Cyclooxygenases are not calcium-dependent, whereas lipoxygenases are.

Arachidonic acid metabolites are not stored in mast cells but are synthesized as a result of a specific stimulus. Such stimuli appear to be specific for each cell: thrombin in platelets, chemotactic peptides in neutrophils, and IgE in mast cells. Histamine released by stimulated mast cells may contribute to activation of arachidonate metabolism. Table 20–2 summarizes the major arachidonate metabolites and their biologic effects.

Table 20–1. Effect of Histamine on Tissues with Various Receptors

H_1 Receptors	H_2 Receptors	H_1 and H_2 Receptors	H_3 Receptors
Bronchoconstriction	↑ Gastric acid secretion	Vasodilation	Modulate cholinergic and sensory nerves
↑ Vascular permeability	↑ Pepsin secretion	Flushing	
Contraction gastrointestinal muscle	↑ cAMP levels	Headache	Inhibit mast cell histamine release
↑ cAMP levels	↓ Lymphocyte toxicity	Tachycardia	
Prostaglandin generation	↑ Chemotaxis	Hypotension	
↑ Chemotaxis	↑ Chemokinesis	Wheal-flare reaction	
↓ Chemokinesis	↓ Histamine release		

Abbreviations: cAMP = cyclic adenosine monophosphate.
Modified from Marquardt DL. Histamine. Clin Rev Allergy 1:343–351, 1983.

Table 20–2. Chemical Mediators of Allergic Reactions from Arachidonate Metabolites

Compound	Source	Biologic Effects
Cyclooxygenase Pathway		
PGD_2	Mast cells	↑ PMN chemokinesis, bronchoconstriction
PGE_2	Macrophages and mast cells	↑ cAMP, induces fever and vascular permeability, bronchodilation
$PGF_{2\alpha}$	Macrophages and mast cells	Stimulates guanylate cyclase, bronchoconstriction
TXA_2	Platelets, macrophages, and mast cells	Block's PGE-induced cAMP production
PGI_2	Vascular endothelium, macrophages, and mast cells	↑ Vascular permeability, ↑ chemokinesis, may bronchodilate or constrict (depending on concentration)
Lipoxygenase Pathway		
5-HETE	PMNs and mast cells	PMN chemotaxis, ↑ histamine release
LTB_4	PMNs and macrophages	PMN chemotaxis, bronchoconstriction
$LTVC_4$	PMNs and macrophages, mast cells	Potent bronchoconstrictor, ↑ microvascular permeability
LTD_4	PMNs and others	Very potent bronchoconstrictor, ↑ microvascular tone and permeability
LTE_4	PMNs and others	Very potent bronchodilator

Abbreviations: PGD_2 = prostaglandin D_2; TXA_2 = thromboxane A_2; 5-HETE = 5-hydroxy-6,8,11,14-eicosatetraenoic acid; LTB_4 = leukotriene B_4; PMN = polymorphonuclear leukocyte; cAMP = cyclic adenosine monophosphate.
Modified from Stenson WF, Parker CW. Metabolites of arachidonic acid. Clin Rev Allergy 1:369–384, 1983.

Arachidonic acid metabolites play a significant role in inflammation. Mast cells form large amounts of prostaglandin D_2 (PGD_2), which causes central and peripheral airways to contract, inhibits platelet aggregation, and is chemotactic. PGD_2 potentiates the bronchoconstrictor response to both histamine and methacholine in asthmatics (Fuller et al., 1986) via thromboxane receptors. A thromboxane synthase inhibitor has been found to inhibit bronchial hyperresponsiveness in subjects with asthma (Fujimura et al., 1986). Lipoxygenase products are mediators in anaphylaxis and asthma. In the rhesus monkey model, bronchial challenge induces arachidonate metabolites, and the results are increased pulmonary resistance, increased respiratory rate, and decreased dynamic compliance.

Platelet Activating Factor

Platelet activating factor (PAF) is an endogenously formed phospholipid with potent toxic actions. It was so named because it was considered responsible for the in vivo platelet activation occurring during anaphylaxis and acute serum sickness (Benveniste et al., 1976). Its structure was characterized in 1979 by Demopoulos et al. PAF is associated with human mast cells and possibly basophils as well as eosinophils, neutrophils, and platelets.

PAF is produced and secreted when cells are stimulated by a variety of means, including specific antigen and anti-IgE antibody. Its formation and secretion are Ca^{2+}-dependent and possibly modulated by cAMP. In human blood, plasma, or serum, PAF is activated in seconds by an acetyl hydrolase, possibly from PMNs (O'Flaherty and Wykle, 1983). Although PAF may cause increased bronchial responsiveness, it can cause a sustained increase in pulmonary resistance and compliance lasting from days to weeks (Cuss et al., 1986).

The mechanism of action of PAF is not totally clear. PMNs and platelets have receptor sites and, within seconds of PAF challenge, take up intracellular Ca^{2+}. PAF appears to induce metabolism and release of arachidonic acid metabolites. In human PMNs, LTB_4

may be a mediator of the platelet aggregation response to PAF. PAF may be involved in human anaphylaxis (O'Flaherty et al., 1981) and in other inflammatory diseases, such as the acute stage of systemic lupus erythematosus, endotoxemia, extensive bodily injury, and adult respiratory distress syndrome (O'Flaherty and Wykle, 1983).

Chemotactic Factors

When mast cells are stimulated by an intradermal injection of antigen and serial biopsy specimens are examined, a consistent cellular response pattern is seen. Neutrophils infiltrate the site within 20 minutes and persist for up to 2 hours, followed by the appearance of eosinophils over the next 2 to 4 hours. In at least 40% of allergic subjects, a second skin response of induration and edema develops, peaking at 6 to 8 hours after the injection and lasting up to 12 hours. This can be increased to 100% if the concentration of the antigen employed for skin testing is increased (Frew and Kay, 1988).

A biopsy specimen of this late reaction shows a mixed infiltrate of eosinophils, neutrophils, basophils, monocytes, and lymphocytes. These cellular infiltrates result from a variety of chemotactic factors, all induced by human mast cell stimulation (Bierman et al., 1991).

Neutrophil Chemotactic Factors

Factors released after mast cell stimulation include the following:

- High-molecular-weight neutrophil chemotactic factor (NCF)
- Arachidonic acid metabolites of the lipoxygenase and cyclooxygenase pathways (see previous topic)
- Eosinophilic chemotactic factors (although preferential for eosinophils, they also attract PMNs)
- Inflammatory factor of anaphylaxis (IF-A), which is preformed in mast cell granules

Neutrophil chemotactic factor is the only specific neutrophil chemotactic mediator that has been identified in humans during mast cell–mediated reactions, and it has been demonstrated after both antigen and exercise challenge (Lee and O'Hickey, 1989). However, the other factors identified are potent in vitro chemotactic stimuli for human PMNs (Atkins and Wasserman, 1983).

Eosinophil Chemotactic Factors

Chemotactic factors for eosinophils were the first mast cell chemotactic factors identified. Eosinophil chemotactic factor of anaphylaxis, a low-molecular-weight tetrapeptide found preformed in human mast cell granules, is weakly chemoattractive for eosinophils. Other low-molecular-weight factors, especially PAF, that attract human eosinophils preferentially and deactivate their further movement have been identified. Higher-molecular-weight eosinophil chemotactic compounds have been recovered from the blood of patients with physical urticarias. Histamine also modulates eosinophil chemotaxis. At low concentrations, it augments eosinophil responsiveness (H_1 effect); at high concentrations, it inhibits migration (H_2 effect).

Lymphocyte Chemotactic Factors

Two lymphocyte chemotactic factors have been found after rat mast cell stimulation—one with a molecular mass of 12,000 daltons and specific for T lymphocytes, the other with a molecular mass less than 2000 daltons and specific for B lymphocytes. Whether there is a counterpart of these factors in humans is not clear.

OTHER FACTORS INFLUENCING ALLERGIC REACTIVITY

Kinins

Plasma kinins constitute a group of physiologically active peptides with powerful inflammatory activities (Wilhelm, 1971). Kinins cause vasodilatation, increase capillary permeability, cause nonvascular smooth muscle to contract, generate pain, and promote leukocyte immigration. Various kinins are found throughout the animal kingdom and are responsible for some of the inflammatory actions induced by venoms of insects and other animals.

Two kinins have been identified in human plasma: a nonapeptide (bradykinin, so named because it induces slower contraction of guinea pig ileum than histamine) and a less potent decapeptide (kallidin, identical to bradykinin except for an extra amino acid, lysine). A third kinin, methionyl-lysyl-bradykinin, has been isolated from human urine and also appears to play a role in inflammation.

Generation of kinin activity is complex, involving the sequential activities of a number of enzymes, which, in turn, are activated by various mechanisms. Active kinin is formed by proteolytic cleavage of inactive plasma or tissue substrates as a last step of the reaction. Enzymes capable of generating kinin activity are found in basophils and PMNs and are liberated by IgE and other immune mechanisms. Kinin inactivation occurs rapidly as a result of plasma or tissue proteinases.

There is an extensive interrelationship between kallikrein activation, kinin formation, and kinin inactivation on the one hand and the activities of various components of the complement and clotting systems on the other (Kaplan and Austen, 1975). Kinins have been implicated in anaphylactic shock, asthma, and other allergic disorders (Christiansen et al., 1987). Although increased kinin activity occurs in these disorders, the degree to which kinin activity contributes to their production is not yet clear.

Complement

Treatment of fresh serum with immune aggregates led to the discovery of a factor that causes vasodilatation, increased capillary permeability, and contraction of smooth muscles. This substance, termed anaphylatoxin, was thought to be involved in the mediation of anaphylactic reactions. More recently, it has been demonstrated that C5a, a product of the complement system, is an anaphylatoxin. The similarity between the actions noted for anaphylatoxin and those of histamine is readily apparent, and the activity of these anaphylatoxins seems, in fact, to be mediated through the liberation of histamine.

Anaphylatoxins may promote urticaria or serum sickness and may participate in so-called atopic disorders. Plasminogen, carried by eosinophils, when activated to plasmin, can generate biologically active complement components. Chemotactic factors associated with the complement system activated by immune reactions induce tissue damage by attracting PMNs and other cells that secondarily liberate tissue-damaging substances. C2 kinin may increase capillary permeability, and immunologically activated complement is capable of activating Hageman factor, which, in turn, affects bradykinin activation (Vogt, 1974). The role of complement in the pathogenesis of hereditary angioneurotic edema is discussed in Chapter 17. There is no evidence that allergic factors are involved in that disorder.

Lymphocytes

T lymphocytes participate in reactions directly involving antigen. After antigen activation, CD4 T lymphocytes elaborate lymphokines that are proinflammatory proteins. The CD4 cells perform the following functions (Corrigan and Kay, 1993):

1. Increase the production of granulocytes from precursors.
2. Prolong their survival in tissues.
3. Promote direct chemotaxis and the synthesis of adhesion molecules.
4. Prime granulocytes for response.
5. Activate B lymphocytes to produce specific antibodies.

CD4 T lymphocytes are thus involved in production of lymphokines and antibodies. Their exact role in asthma and allergic inflammation is currently being studied.

Interleukins

T lymphocytes can be subdivided into T_H2 and T_H1 cells based on the pattern of secreted lymphokines. T_H1 cells produce interleukin-2 (IL-2), interferon-γ (IFN-γ), and tumor necrosis factor-β (TNF-β), and T_H2 cells secrete IL-4, IL-5, and IL-6. Both cells secrete IL-3, TNF-α, and granulocyte-macrophage colony-stimulating factor (GM-CSF) (Mosmann and Coffman, 1989). The interleukins are protein mediators by which one cell communicates with another. Their functions, the cells that produce them, and the cells that respond are shown in Table 20–3, which presents the first 13 interleukins. Nineteen interleukins have now been described, but they have not all been fully characterized. (See Appendix 2.)

Cell Adhesion Molecules

Adhesion molecules play an important role in cell recruitment. Adhesion molecules include intracellular adhesion molecule-1 (ICAM-1), endothelial leukocyte adhesion molecule–1 (ELAM-1), and vascular cell ad-hesion molecule–1 (VCAM-1). In addition, the integrins are a large supergene family that includes leukocyte adhesion molecule on lymphocytes, granulocytes, and macrophages (LEUCAM). These agents are important in the recruitment and activation of eosinophils, neutrophils, and platelets in asthma and other allergic diseases and usually act together with interleukins to carry out their function.

Other Mediators

Among other mediators, acetylcholine and the catecholamines should be considered important in modulating the allergic reaction. Acetylcholine is found mainly within the synaptic vesicles of the central and peripheral nervous systems. It can induce vasodilatation and contraction of bronchial smooth muscle and stimulate secretory glands, such as tracheal and bronchial mucous glands.

The catecholamines (epinephrine and norepinephrine) are pharmacologic antagonists of many of the previously discussed mediators. They may act to oppose the actions of these mediators as well as modulate their activation and release.

In sum, many chemical mediators are activated or released by immune reactions. These mediators amplify the effects of antigen-antibody interaction. The kind of mediator released depends on the specific immune

Table 20–3. Role of Interleukins in Atopic Disease*

Interleukin	Function*	Producing Cells†	Responding Cells‡
IL-1	Leukocyte activation	Macrophages and other cells	Leukocytes
IL-2	Eosinophil activation, stimulates B cell growth and antibody secretion	T cells	Eosinophils, B cells, T cells
IL-3	Maintenance of mast cells and eosinophils in airway	Mast cells, CD4 T_H1 cells	Mast cells, eosinophils
IL-4	Cofactor for IgE synthesis, induces B cell proliferation and IgE gene transcription	CD4 T_H2 cells	B cells (not yet switched)
IL-5	Differentiates mature lymphocytes, prolongs survival of eosinophils, promotes eosinophil adhesion to vascular endothelium, primes eosinophils for activation	CD4 T cells, mast cells, B cells	Eosinophils, lymphocytes
IL-6	Stimulates IgE synthesis in B cells already making IgE	Fibroblasts, alveolar macrophages, blood mononuclear cells	CD4 T_H2 cells, immunoglobulin-producing B cells
IL-7	Promotes growth of pre-B and pre-T cells	Stromal cells	Pre-B cells, pre-T cells
IL-8	Attracts and activates neutrophils, stimulates lymphocyte chemotaxis	Alveolar macrophages, monocytes	Neutrophils, lymphocytes
IL-9	Stimulates mast cells, erythroid maturation	T cells	Mast cells, erythroid precursors
IL-10	Inhibits cytokine synthesis, cofactor for mast cell proliferation	T cells, B cells, macrophages	Mast cells
IL-11	Megakaryocyte and plasma cell growth factor	Stromal cells	Megakaryocytes, plasma cells
IL-12	Regulates IFN-γ (with IL-3)	B cells	T cells
IL-13	Activates monocytes, induces proliferation of B cells (action similar to IL-4 but weaker)	T cells	Monocytes, B cells

Abbreviations: IL = interleukin; IgE = immunoglobulin E; IFN-γ = interferon-γ.
*May require prior priming by another cell.
†These interleukins may be produced by many cells including epithelial cells. Those listed have been studied.
‡Many other cells may respond. Listed are the cells that have been studied.

mechanism involved. Several mediators may be released by one immune mechanism; more than one mechanism can result in the release of a given mediator. Chemical mediators may be released by nonimmune mechanisms as well, which in turn may result in manifestations indistinguishable from true allergic reactions.

The relative contribution of these mediators to the pathogenesis of allergic disorders may vary from one disorder to another and probably within a given disorder from time to time. Furthermore, drug therapy used in allergic disorders may alter (perhaps at times unfavorably) the relative contribution of chemical mediators in inducing a particular disorder.

DIAGNOSIS OF ALLERGIC DISEASE

The diagnosis of allergic disorders is basically a clinical one, although laboratory findings may aid in the diagnosis. A thorough history and physical examination are indispensable, not only in defining relevant symptoms and signs but also in excluding other disorders that may masquerade as allergy. Moreover, findings (such as urticaria) often associated with allergic reactions may represent manifestations of underlying systemic nonallergic disease. Because allergic reactions may affect any tissue or organ system, the manifestations of allergic reactions are legion. Commonly, allergic manifestations are referable to the route by which allergenic contact is made, so abnormalities of the skin, mucous membranes, and respiratory and gastrointestinal tracts are encountered frequently. Certain manifestations, such as urticaria, conjunctivitis, rhinitis, and paroxysmal wheezing, occur so frequently with allergic reactions that they are mistakenly assumed to be necessarily a result of allergy. However, allergic manifestations can be caused by nonimmune (nonallergic) mechanisms.

Because allergy, by definition, is induced by contact with allergens, correlation should be sought between allergic symptoms and the time (year, month, day, or even hour) and location (work, home, room, or neighbor's or relative's house) of their occurrence. The examiner should obtain a family history because an allergic predisposition is often familial. A history of a previous atopic disorder should be sought because multiple manifestations of atopic allergy in the same individual are common. Understanding the nature of and response to medication can also be a diagnostic aid.

Some allergens that are ordinarily well tolerated may provoke symptoms when the patient is having difficulty with another allergen. The patient sometimes behaves as if one allergic reaction has primed his or her tissues for reactivity to another. In certain instances, cross-antigenicity between the weak, ordinarily well-tolerated allergen and other potent seasonal allergens may exist, and a simple additive effect is present. In other instances, there is no apparent antigenic relationship and the effect appears to be nonspecific. This priming phenomenon has been reproduced experimentally (Connell, 1968).

Immunoglobulin E Skin Tests

Skin testing with suspected allergens is an extremely useful procedure in the diagnosis of allergy. The kind of local allergic reaction sought must be representative of the type of allergic tissue damage responsible for the disorder in question. In atopic disorders and other reactions caused by IgE-mediated mechanisms, such as drug allergies, skin-sensitizing antibodies to suspected allergens are involved. In testing for evidence of IgE antibody, one introduces the allergen into the skin by pricking or puncturing the epidermis or by inoculating the allergen intradermally. The end point of the reaction is the development of a local wheal and flare (hive), which usually reaches its peak within 15 to 20 minutes and subsides shortly thereafter.

Scratch and puncture tests are less sensitive than intradermal tests and therefore are safer, particularly for highly sensitive individuals. A scratch or puncture test should be performed first; intradermal tests can follow nonreactive scratch or puncture tests. Although large reactions are more likely to be significant than small reactions, the size of the reaction does not always correlate with the intensity of symptoms.

Skin tests are merely correlative, and a positive test indicates only that reaginic antibody is present. (Even this must be qualified because some allergen extracts can release histamine by nonimmune mechanisms.) The correlation between a positive skin test and clinical reactivity is high for inhalants and pollens but poorer for food allergens. The possibility exists that the food antigens used for testing differ in form from the digested food that induces the clinical reaction. In some instances, local production of antibody may be sufficient to cause allergic symptoms but inadequate to sensitize peripheral tissues, so that antibody cannot be demonstrated by skin or serologic tests (Huggins and Brostoff, 1975).

Because atopic individuals have more IgE antibody than normal individuals, multiple positive skin tests support the diagnosis of atopy. Skin testing is occasionally performed in infants, but it is more valuable after infancy. Skin testing is a potentially dangerous procedure that must be performed cautiously. Appropriate drugs and equipment for the treatment of severe allergic reactions should always be at hand.

When direct skin testing has not been feasible, such as in patients with extensive dermatitis, passive transfer tests had been used before the acquired immunodeficiency syndrome (AIDS) epidemic. Serum from the individual was injected into the skin of a nonsensitive recipient, and allergen was injected into the site of transfer after a suitable latent period (usually 2 hours). Such tests (also called *PK tests* after Prausnitz and Küstner) have been replaced by serologic tests (see In Vitro Tests). Skin testing on mucosal surfaces, especially the conjunctiva, appears to offer little advantage over conventional skin testing.

In Vitro Tests

Several in vitro tests have been introduced to diagnose allergic sensitization. The proliferative response of peripheral blood lymphocytes to antigens in culture has been claimed by some to be useful in identifying sensitivity to drug, food, and pollen antigens, but the proliferative response to an antigen represents an index of previous experience with that antigen, and its value as a diagnostic aid in clinical allergy is doubtful.

Antigen-induced degranulation of basophilic leukocytes from sensitized individuals or degranulation of human basophils or rat mast cells passively sensitized with serum from sensitized individuals has been used to test for IgE-mediated reactivity to drugs and other allergens. The sensitivity of peripheral blood leukocytes to antigen-induced histamine release has also been used as an index of severity of clinical sensitivity, and some correlation has been established between in vitro leukocyte sensitivity and intensity of clinical symptoms (Lichtenstein et al., 1968). In addition, there is a general (but imperfect) relationship between clinical improvement after immunotherapy and decreased in vitro sensitivity to the antigen (Sadan et al., 1969). None of these tests, however, has proved helpful in general as a practical diagnostic procedure.

Serologic Tests

Radioallergoabsorbent Test

The measurement of IgE serum antibody has also been made possible through immunoassays. The best known and most widely employed is the radioallergosorbent test (RAST) (Yunginger and Gleich, 1975). In this test, antigen is coupled to some insoluble material, and the coupled allergen is then exposed to antiserum containing IgE antibody. Radiolabeled anti-IgE antibody is then allowed to react with the antigen-antibody complexes, which may contain IgE antibody; the amount of IgE antibody present is calculated on the basis of the radioactivity (anti-IgE antibody) that has reacted with the immune complexes. RAST correlates well with skin testing.

Variations of RAST using radiolabeling or enzyme-linked immunoassays (ELISAs) are now numerous but are based on similar principles. The main advantages of serologic over allergy skin tests are their safety and the fact that they are not influenced by medications and can be used to detect antibody in patients with dermatoses or other conditions that preclude skin testing. However, compared with skin tests, they tend to be less sensitive and more expensive and provide the same amount of information or less.

Radioimmunosorbent Test

IgE levels are measured by test procedures somewhat similar to those used for detecting specific IgE antibody. One such test is a variation of the RAST called the radioimmunosorbent test (RIST). In this test, serum IgE serves as the antigen and competes with a known amount of radiolabeled IgE for anti-IgE. The displacement of radiolabeled IgE by IgE in the serum is a measure of the amount of serum IgE present.

Variations on the RIST, such as the double radioim-munoassay (RIA), the paper radioimmunosorbent test (PRIST), which is more sensitive than RIST for measuring IgE, and the enzyme-linked immunosorbent assays (ELISAs), are also available. The finding of an elevated IgE level in an individual with a suspected allergic diathesis is evidence in favor of such a suspicion. However, normal or even low IgE levels occur sufficiently often in allergic disorders mediated by IgE antibody that IgE levels are only infrequently a helpful diagnostic tool. Normal IgE levels are given in Chapter 9.

Patch Tests for Contact Dermatitis

In contact dermatitis in which the underlying allergic mechanism is caused by cell-mediated immunity, skin testing is performed by applying the suspected allergen superficially to the skin of the affected individual under a patch (patch test). The patch is left in place for 24 to 48 hours or removed earlier if burning or itching develops; the skin is examined 24 to 48 hours thereafter for a local reaction typical of contact dermatitis. Patch testing should not be done when extensive dermatitis is present because the local application of allergen may result in exacerbation of the dermatitis.

Provocative Tests

Provocative tests are sometimes used to identify a suspected allergen. Patch testing for contact dermatitis is a provocative test in the sense that both the route of allergen contact and the site of the reaction mimic the clinical situation. Provocation by inhalation or ingestion of pollens, foods, and other allergens is a useful diagnostic procedure, but the danger of producing a severe allergic reaction must be kept in mind, particularly when the clinical reaction has been pronounced.

Provocative tests are most valuable in patients with a food allergy. Elimination of suspected foods from the diet and subsequent challenge with each of the foods are especially useful in identifying moderate or mild food allergy. In severe food hypersensitivity, an association between allergic reactivity and the inciting food has most likely been made already by the patient or the patient's parents. When challenging with food, it should be eliminated from the diet for at least 1 week. Elimination may result in relief of symptoms, if the particular food is the sole or chief allergen involved. The food should then be added to the diet for at least 4 days before the challenge can be considered negative.

A diagnosis of food-induced asthma can be made only with a double-blind placebo-controlled food challenge (DBPCFC) after strict elimination of suspected food allergens. A positive reaction occurs within minutes to 2 hours of ingestion, and the reaction may range from signs and symptoms of rhinoconjunctivitis to significant falls in the forced expiratory volume in 1 second (FEV_1) or peak expiratory flow rate (PEFR) (Sampson et al., 1989). Provocation of gastrointestinal symptoms by a given substance does not establish an allergic mechanism of the reaction. For example, intolerance of milk may result from lactase deficiency rather than from milk allergy.

Eosinophilia

Eosinophilia in the blood or mucous secretions is common in various allergic disorders, particularly in atopic disorders, and its presence is used as circumstantial evidence of an allergic reaction. Nasal eosinophilia occurring in clumps is so common in allergic rhinitis that it is almost diagnostic. Eosinophilia may disappear, however, during asymptomatic periods or when infection supervenes. Nasal eosinophilia is a frequent finding in nonallergic infants under 3 months of age and thus cannot be used as a diagnostic aid in early infancy.

Because chemotactic factors that attract eosinophils can be activated by nonimmune as well as allergic stimuli, eosinophil accumulation can be seen in nonallergic inflammatory conditions. This, in fact, was found in a small population of children and adults (nonallergic rhinitis with eosinophilia [NARES syndrome]) in whom the incidence of idiosyncratic reaction to aspirin appears to be increased (Pearlman, 1984b). The presence of eosinophilia in respiratory secretions seems to be more a reflection of mast cell mediator release than the specific cause of an inflammatory response, but it also suggests that drugs useful for allergic reactions (e.g., corticosteroids) are likely to be of therapeutic benefit.

Controversial Diagnostic and Therapeutic Techniques

A variety of techniques of unproven value are employed by some practitioners for diagnosis and therapy of allergic disorders. These include intracutaneous and sublingual provocative tests, some kinds of intracutaneous end-point titration, leukocytotoxic tests, and sublingual desensitization. Although an occasional patient may benefit from these procedures, no scientific validation of these techniques as a general diagnostic or therapeutic approach has been forthcoming. An additional complicating issue is the fact that many practitioners using these techniques consider any adverse clinical reaction to a foreign substance as an ''allergy'' to that substance. At this time, these procedures, at best, can be considered controversial (Terr, 1993).

PRINCIPLES OF ALLERGIC THERAPY

Despite the wide range of clinical manifestations of allergic reactions, the pathogenesis of such reactions is fundamentally similar, based on an initial immune event that serves to release or activate pharmacologic intermediates, which, in turn, induce reversible tissue changes. This basic pathogenesis permits some generalization in the therapeutic approach to various allergic disorders. The specifics of therapy may vary with the type, severity, and location of the allergic tissue damage involved.

The principles of allergic therapy include the prevention or modification of the initiating immune reaction and the reversal by drugs of the tissue changes produced by the chemical mediators of allergic reactions (Pearlman, 1975). These principles are considered in the order of their importance, namely:

- Allergen avoidance
- Drug therapy
- Immunotherapy (also referred to as *hyposensitization* and *desensitization*)

Allergen Avoidance

Allergen avoidance is the mainstay of therapy for all allergic disorders and the most effective means of preventing allergic reactions. In many instances, identification of allergens is difficult, and even when they are identified, avoidance may be impossible. Because clinical reactivity is proportional to the degree of allergen exposure, any reduction in contact with offensive allergens can be beneficial.

Atopic individuals often become sensitized to household materials ordinarily considered innocuous, such as house mites, animals (especially cats), molds, and plant products used in the stuffing of furniture and toys. Control of exposure to these substances is important and feasible. Because atopic individuals commonly become sensitized to these substances, limitation of environmental exposure to these substances should also be done prophylactically. The degree of environmental manipulation warranted depends on the intensity of symptoms and is largely a matter of compromise and common sense. Particular emphasis is placed on environmental control of the child's bedroom (Buckley and Pearlman, 1988).

Individuals sensitive to one allergen must be warned against contact with closely related allergens, such as ampicillin and other penicillins in benzyl penicillin hypersensitivity. Because nonimmunogenic irritants may aggravate allergic disorders (for example, cigarette smoke in asthma or wool in atopic dermatitis), they should be avoided.

Infants fed diets restricted in the amounts of cow products, egg, wheat, and chicken during the first 9 months of life experience less allergic rhinitis and asthma than those fed diets unrestricted in these foods (Johnstone and Dutton, 1966). Other studies have suggested that restriction of cow's milk in the first few months of life either diminishes or delays the likelihood of atopic dermatitis and other allergic disorders. However, there are as many studies that refute these findings. In the absence of proof, it seems wise to institute dietary restrictions of these foods for the first 6 months of life only in children with unusually strong family histories of atopic disease.

Drug Therapy

Allergic reactions can often be reversed or ameliorated by drug therapy. The judicious use of drugs has reduced the morbidity and discomfort of various allergic disorders remarkably, and they can be lifesaving.

The main drugs used in allergic disorders (Weinberger and Hendeles, 1988) include:

- Adrenergic agents
- Methylxanthines
- Antihistamines
- Expectorants
- Cromolyn sodium
- Adrenal glucocorticosteroids

Antibiotics are considered briefly here because of their frequent use as adjuncts in the treatment of allergic disease.

Adrenergic Agents

The manifestations of allergic reactions can be traced to variable combinations of vasodilatation, edema, smooth muscle spasm, stimulation of mucus secretion, and tissue damage induced by chemical mediators of allergic reactions and the resulting infiltration of inflammatory cells. The catecolamines, epinephrine and norepinephrine, are physiologic antagonists of the actions of various chemical mediators implicated in allergic reactions; these adrenergic agents are among the most effective antiallergic drugs. The effectiveness of adrenergic agents depends on their ability to constrict blood vessels, minimize edema, and dilate contracted smooth muscle tissue. In addition, catecholamines have been shown to inhibit IgE-mediated antigen-induced mediator release. Although certain adrenergic drugs such as epinephrine possess all of these properties, others have only certain actions.

The activities of adrenergic agents depend on their abilities to interact with specific cell-associated (usually membrane-associated) proteins termed alpha- and beta-receptors. In general, alpha-receptor activation leads to excitatory responses (e.g., vasoconstriction), whereas beta-receptor activation results in relaxation (e.g. bronchodilatation). Thus, phenylephrine, a predominantly alpha-receptor agonist, is a potent vasoconstrictor used in allergic rhinitis; it does not dilate bronchial smooth muscle tissue. Isoproterenol, predominantly a beta-receptor agonist, is an extremely effective bronchodilator, but it has essentially no vasoconstrictor properties. Ephedrine is similar to epinephrine, with both alpha- and beta-receptor activators, and exhibits the combined activities of phenylephrine and isoproterenol. Although less potent than epinephrine, it can be given orally.

Beta$_1$- and Beta$_2$-Receptors

There are at least two subpopulations of beta receptors: beta$_1$ and beta$_2$. Beta$_1$-receptor activation increases cardiac rate and contraction, relaxes intestinal smooth muscle, and stimulates lipolysis; beta$_2$-receptor activation causes bronchodilatation and vascular and uterine muscle relaxation but stimulates skeletal muscle and induces glycogenolysis. Various drugs with predominant beta$_2$-receptor activating properties are now available for use, particularly for asthma therapy (Bierman, 1983).

Beta$_2$-Agonists

New, relatively specific beta$_2$-receptor agonists available in North America include albuterol (salbutamol), bitolterol, pirbuterol, and terbutaline. Salmeterol, a similar drug with a longer duration of action (12 hours for salmeterol versus 5 hours for albuterol), has been approved for twice daily maintenance therapy in children 12 years and older and in adults. *It is recommended that it be used when needed in addition to, not instead of, maintenance anti-inflammatory therapy and should not be used for aute asthma treatment.* Short-acting adrenergic drugs are especially useful in inhalant form for the treatment of acute and chronic asthma.

Although these agents are most effective when inhaled from metered-dose inhalers, some are available by the oral route, both in syrup form and as tablets (albuterol, terbutaline, metaproterenol). When given orally, both albuterol and terbutaline produce bronchodilation that peaks after 2 hours and may last 4 to 8 hours (Wolfe et al., 1985). When the agent is administered subcutaneously, the bronchodilation response is observed in 5 minutes and may persist up to 3 to 4 hours. Administration by inhalation produced a rapid reaction with 75% of maximal effect achieved within 5 minutes and peak activity in 30 to 90 minutes (Spector and Garza-Gomez, 1977).

Because of the multiplicity, rapidity, and potency of its actions, epinephrine is the most useful drug in the treatment of anaphylactic reactions. Adrenergic agents are not always effective in allergic disorders and may have undesirable effects. For example, in several studies, the chronic routine use of short-acting β$_2$-agents without concomitant anti-inflammatory agents has been associated with a mild increase in bronchial hyperresponsiveness and evidence of asthma deterioration (Position Statement, 1992). In severe asthma, epinephrine may not reverse bronchial obstruction, and excessive use of some aerosolized adrenergic drugs can increase bronchial obstruction temporarily. The latter phenomenon may sometimes be caused by sensitivity to the metabisulfite used as an antioxidant in solution of adrenergic drugs. As a result, it has been removed from many of these solutions.

Methylxanthines

The methylxanthines, theophylline and its ethylenediamine derivative aminophylline, are potent drugs used in asthma. Their most important action is dilation of bronchial smooth muscle. Methylxanthines also inhibit antigen-induced mediator release. Overdosage with these drugs in children and adolescents makes the drugs less desirable than they were in the past when they were the most effective agents available for chronic asthma. Manifestations of toxicity include nausea and vomiting, hematemesis, palpitations, dizziness, headache, convulsions, excessive thirst, hypotension, and death. Abdominal pain resulting from gastric irritation, with or without nausea, is also common and may be caused by the drug or the vehicle in which it is formulated. It is important to recognize, however, that this can be a central nervous system (CNS) effect, related to drug blood level, and that toxic gastrointestinal symptoms can result from theophylline given by rectum or parenterally.

Peak blood theophylline levels of less than 15 μg/ml are considered relatively safe; in severe asthma, blood theophylline levels between 5 and 15 μg/ml are probably optimal (Weinberger and Hendeles, 1988). However, because of the variability in blood levels, caused in part by the influence of food ingestion in relation to timing of oral drug administration for some preparations and the effects of certain drugs and viral infections on drug metabolism, it is recommended that blood levels be kept toward the lower end of the so-called optimal therapeutic range on a chronic basis. In addition, some individuals are unusually sensitive to the CNS effects of methylxanthines, and blood levels significantly less than 20 μg/ml (and probably less than 10 μg/ml) do not preclude the occurrence of undesirable obvious or subtle side effects. Moreover, subtle behavior changes, sleep disturbances, and learning difficulties have been recognized with increased frequency in some children receiving "ideal" therapeutic doses of theophylline compounds.

The absorption of these compounds varies according to the route of administration. Oral doses given every 8 to 12 hours are preferred for chronic administration. Absorption is generally good. Aminophylline used intravenously in severe asthma may be effective, even after epinephrine resistance. However, intravenous aminophylline is used less commonly in patients with acute severe asthma because of the effectiveness of improved β_2-agonist aerosol solutions, and controversy whether its addition to β_2-therapy gives sufficient benefit in the face of risk for increasing adverse effects.

Methylxanthines are not given intramuscularly because of their tendency to cause extreme irritation. Prolonged use of proper dosages of methylxanthines is usually well tolerated. Dosage for chronic oral use or for intravenous use in acute severe asthma should be governed by assaying blood levels of the drug and clinical assessment for possible side effects.

Antihistamines

Antihistamines are a varied group of compounds that act as competitive antagonists of histamine activity (Pearlman, 1976). Some actions of histamine are blocked well by conventional antihistamines, but others, such as stimulation of gastric secretions, are not. Three histamine receptors have been identified: H_1, H_2, and H_3.

H_1 receptors are present in the nose, eyes, and skin, and their activation is responsible for the itching of eczema and hives and for the major symptoms of hay fever and perennial rhinitis. They play only a secondary role in asthma.

H_2 receptor activation is responsible for the histamine-induced gastric acid secretion, and H_2 receptor antagonists, such as cimetidine and ranitidine, are useful in the therapy of syndromes of gastric acid hypersecretion. Although H_2 receptors probably play some role in histamine-induced vascular responses, the use of H_2 antagonists in the treatment of allergic disorders at this time is experimental. H_2 antagonists, however, are recommended in conjunction with H_1 antagonists in the treatment of anaphylaxis (see Anaphylactic Reactions).

H_3 receptors appear to be located primarily in the brain and lung, but their exact function is unknown.

Conventional *first-generation antihistamines* (H_1 antagonists) are divided structurally into at least five groups. When one antihistamine is ineffective or side effects are encountered, it is common practice to select another from a different group, although the scientific basis for this practice is lacking. The antihistamine groups and representative examples of each group are as follows:

1. Ethylenediamines—tripelennamine (Pyribenzamine).
2. Ethanolamines—diphenhydramine (Benadryl).
3. Alkylamines—chlorpheniramine (Chlor-Trimeton).
4. Piperazines—hydroxyzine (Atarax, Vistaril).
5. Phenothiazines—promethazine (Phenergan).

Antihistamines with antiserotonin activity, such as cyproheptadine (Periactin), are of special value in the treatment of some cases of cold urticaria.

There is a structural similarity between some antihistamines and biogenic amines, such as acetylcholine; some of the side effects of antihistamines are related to their ability to act as competitive antagonists of biogenic amines. Thus, an atropine-like drying of the mouth may be encountered. Drowsiness is probably the most common side effect of antihistamines; it varies with the antihistamine involved and individual susceptibility to this effect. The older first-generation H_1 antagonists may significantly impair CNS function even in the absence of apparent sedation.

Second-generation H_1 antihistamines with little CNS penetration and few or no CNS side effects, such as sedation, are now available (e.g., terfenadine [Seldane], astemizole [Hismanal], loratadine [Claritin]). Others should be available shortly. Some have cardiac side effects (terfenadine and astemizole) when administered to patients with hepatic disease, possibly with macrolide antibiotics (such as erythromycin) or antifungal agents (such as ketoconazole).

Antihistamines are readily absorbed when given orally, the usual route of administration. They can also be given intramuscularly or intravenously for more rapid effect. Intravenous infusion must be done slowly, because rapid infusion may produce hypotension.

Because the therapeutic effectiveness of antihistamines depends on successful competition with histamine at histamine receptors, the timing of administration of an antihistamine has an important bearing on its ability to inhibit an allergic response. The presence of antihistamine at receptor sites before histamine liberation is more advantageous than the arrival of antihistamine after histamine has begun to exert its effect.

Clinically, the administration of antihistamines before the anticipated onset of paroxysmal sneezing (as may occur each morning with hay fever) is more beneficial than administration of the drug after symptoms have already begun. Although most antihistamines have an 8- to 24-hour duration of action, astemizole is an exception. A short course of astemizole results in long-acting antihistamine activity in the skin and mucous membranes because its active metabolite, desmethyl astemizole, has a half-life of 9.5 days. For this reason it may have to be discontinued for 6 weeks before diagnostic challenge or skin testing with histamine or antigen (Simons and Simons, 1991).

Corticosteroids

Systemic Corticosteroids

Adrenal glucocorticoids ("steroids") are used in all forms of allergic disorders, but their effectiveness varies from one allergic disorder to another. Adrenal glucocorticoids are most effective in controlling delayed-type hypersensitivity reactions, such as contact dermatitis, but they are also invaluable in the management of severe asthma. Their effectiveness in urticarial disorders is less impressive. The undesirable side effects associated with the administration of systemic steroids are well known (Lieberman et al., 1972); therefore, long-term therapy is reserved for severe asthma or other disease unresponsive to other treatment. Short-term systemic therapy is used in acute asthma, severe hay fever, and self-limited disorders, such as contact dermatitis and serum sickness.

Because of the relatively slow onset of action of glucocorticosteroids (several hours to several days), even when given intravenously, these agents are never the drug of choice in acute allergic reactions. When used in the treatment of acute asthma or other allergic reactions, high doses (for example, 1 mg of methylprednisolone per kilogram of body weight given intravenously every 6 hours) are used until the desired effect is achieved. When given for short periods of time (less than a week), steroids may be discontinued abruptly, even when used in high doses. With more prolonged steroid use or in individuals who have received long-term steroid therapy within the previous few months, the dose should be tapered gradually.

When long-term steroid therapy is necessary, an alternate-day regimen may achieve sufficient therapeutic effect with fewer side effects and less adrenal suppression. Alternate-day therapy is used only with short-acting steroids, such as prednisone, prednisolone, and methylprednisolone. The steroid is given orally, in one dose, in the early morning (before 8 A.M.) every second day. Daily steroid therapy is first used to achieve the desired therapeutic effect, and then alternate-day therapy is begun using two to three times the daily dose. For chronic therapy of respiratory disorders, corticosteroid use by topical aerosol may be employed in place of alternate-day systemic therapy (discussed later). Adrenocorticotropic hormone (ACTH) offers no advantage over glucocorticoids and is not recommended.

Topical Corticosteroids

Topical steroids are extremely effective in controlling allergic dermatitis. Although the chronic use of topical steroids is not usually associated with severe side effects, extensive and frequent topical application, especially of the potent fluorinated steroid preparations, may lead to systemic absorption with adrenal suppression and to skin atrophy.

Aerosolized Corticosteroids

Topical inhalational steroids (beclomethasone dipropionate, triamcinolone acetonide, flunisolide), which are inactivated rapidly by the liver, are useful in the treatment of chronic severe asthma and rhinitis (Godfrey, 1975). In high dosage, sufficient blood levels of active drug can be achieved to cause adrenal suppression; at standard doses, this rarely occurs.

Short-term studies of aerosolized steroids have demonstrated efficacy and safety in both steroid-dependent and non–steroid-dependent children. Their use is associated with decreased need for other medications, including oral corticosteroids. They improve symptom scores, improve pulmonary function, and may decrease bronchial hyperreactivity.

Most steroid-dependent children can be weaned from oral steroids, although they often continue to need them for acute exacerbations.

Aerosolized steroids, in doses recommended by the manufacturer for use in children, have resulted in slower growth rates in some studies. The significance of this is not clear at present (Tinkelman et al., 1993). They have not interfered with the hypothalamic-pituitary-adrenal axis as determined by normal diurnal serum cortisol levels or responses to ACTH and intravenous metyrapone. However, impaired pituitary-adrenal reserves may exist in previously steroid-dependent children for as long as a year after discontinuation of oral steroids, and aerosolized steroids in usually nonsuppressive dosages may prolong adrenal suppression in already suppressed individuals. Thus, during periods of stress and exacerbations of asthma, systemic corticosteroids should be added.

The effectiveness of inhaled steroids is related to effectiveness of delivery. Up to 80% of steroids with some delivery systems are delivered to the nasopharynx. Spacer units aid in the production of smaller particles so that more of the drug is delivered to the lung (Toogood, 1990). This technique also reduces such side effects as candidiasis and hoarseness. Despite positive cultures, clinical *Candida* infections are infrequent, respond well to oral nystatin, and do not require discontinuation of aerosolized drug. Local effects of aerosolized steroids on the bronchial mucous membranes, such as local atrophy and impaired resistance to infection, are theoretical and have not been seen in bronchial biopsy specimens from patients who have used them for years.

Initial dosages used should be at the higher end of dosages recommended by the manufacturer in order to achieve control as rapidly as possible. In order to facilitate inhalation of aerosolized drug, a short-term increase in oral steroid dosage (3 to 5 days) to improve pulmonary function may be in order at onset of therapy. Because full benefit from an aerosolized drug may not be reached for weeks, it is wise to be conservative in attempting to reduce systemic steroids during this period. One rule of thumb in attempting to reduce alternate-day steroids is to decrease the oral dosage by 2.5 mg/wk, assuming maintenance of clinical stability.

After a patient is controlled with aerosolized steroid and is no longer taking oral steroids, an attempt should be made to lower the dose of aerosolized drug gradually to the lowest dose necessary for control, while maintaining other nonsteroidal antiasthmatic drugs.

Indications for the use of aerosolized steroids include the following:

1. Children with chronic severe asthma dependent on systemic steroid therapy.

2. Children with chronic severe asthma not requiring continuous systemic daily around-the-clock nonsteroid medications with poor control of symptoms.

3. Children not responding to an 8-week trial of cromolyn sodium or nedocromil sodium.

Aerosolized steroids are not indicated or are not useful in:

1. Status asthmaticus, in which airway penetration is prevented by severe bronchospasm.

2. Infrequent asthma, characterized by normal interval periods; this is better treated by aggressive bronchodilator therapy, immunotherapy as appropriate, and occasional short courses of systemic steroids.

3. Exercise-induced asthma.

4. The young asthmatic patient who cannot properly inhale aerosols, even with spacer devices.

Cromolyn Sodium and Nedocromil Sodium

Cromolyn sodium (disodium cromoglycate, Intal) is used in the treatment of asthma as a ''preventative'' (Falliers, 1975). It differs from other antiallergic agents in having no direct action on target cells, although inhibition of cyclic nucleotide phosphodiesterase by the drug and some effect on calcium transport have been documented. Cromolyn acts locally on the respiratory mucosa presumably by blocking the release or activation of certain chemical mediators, principally those from mast cells. Cromolyn is supplied in a metered-dose inhaler (1 mg per activation) and in a 20-mg ampule for aerosol administration. Cromolyn should initially be given four times a day, but in some children asthma control can be maintained on a twice-a-day schedule (anecdotal).

About 20 years after the introduction of cromolyn, nedocromil was introduced. Nedocromil is a drug that appears to have a mechanism of action similar to that of cromolyn (Eady, 1986). It is also available in a metered-dose inhaler at a concentration of 1.75 mg per activation. Clinical studies have shown that both drugs are effective in allergic asthma, exercise-induced asthma, and asthma induced by a variety of irritants. Both drugs prevent the immediate and late reactions to inhaled antigens and reduce the nonspecific increase of hyperresponsiveness after late reactions.

Nedocromil and cromolyn both produce greater inhibition of histamine release from bronchoalveolar mast cells if the drugs are preincubated with cells than if they are added after the stimulus. Cromolyn inhibits the ability of eosinophils to kill complement-coated *Schistosoma* organisms and to express complement C3b and Fcγ receptors. Nedocromil inhibits the release of proteins from eosinophil granules and leukotriene C_4 (LTC_4) formation by eosinophils. The two drugs differ in their effect on eosinophil chemotaxis; cromolyn inhibits zymosan-induced chemotaxis but nedocromil does not (Bruijnzeel et al., 1990), whereas nedocromil inhibits eosinophilic chemotaxis but cromolyn does not.

In humans, exercise-induced asthma is inhibited by cromolyn and nedocromil. Furthermore, nedocromil is more effective than cromolyn in inhibiting bronchoconstriction caused by sulfur dioxide and in inhibiting cough. The mechanism of action of these two agents is not clear, but they may work through neurophysiologic mechanisms (Foreman and Pearce, 1993).

Expectorants

Expectorants such as glyceryl guaiacolate and iodides are used in asthma to liquefy mucus. Few patients respond to iodides. There is little evidence to support the effectiveness of glyceryl guaiacolate or iodides in most patients. Long-term use of iodides can result in goiter, gastric irritation, salivary gland inflammation, skin eruptions, and acne in adolescents and adults. The long-term use of glyceryl guaiacolate is apparently without side effects. However, the best way to promote mucus removal is by adequate hydration, so oral (with or without inhalational) fluids are an essential part of expectorant therapy.

Anticholinergic Drugs

Acetylcholine is the neurohumoral transmitter of all preganglionic autonomic neurons, of all postganglionic neurons, and of somatic efferent fibers to skeletal muscle (Weiner, 1980). These impulses can be blocked by atropine, other belladonna alkaloids, and synthetic analogs.

Because airways are constricted by the vagal nerve, atropine in the human induces bronchodilation. In the asthmatic, the onset of action is later than that with sympathomimetic bronchodilators; it peaks at 30 to 60 minutes and persists for 4 to 6 hours. Ipratropium bromide (Atrovent), a synthetic analog, is the only member of this group approved by the Food and Drug Administration for metered-dose inhaler use at present. It acts locally and is poorly absorbed into the systemic circulation. Hence, its use is associated with minimal occurrence of mouth dryness, cough, headache, dizziness, or eye abnormalities as compared with use of atropine (Davis et al., 1984).

Anticholinergic agents induce bronchodilation almost as effectively as β_2-bronchodilators but they take longer to work and last longer. There is some evidence that when administered with sympathomimetic agents their effects are additive, but they are not as useful as β_2-adrenergic agents administered by themselves. Their effect on exercise is variable and their major use at present may be in adults with chronic obstructive pulmonary disease.

Antibiotics

Allergic disorders frequently mimic infection. Because infection and respiratory allergic disorders frequently coexist, antibiotics are often used in allergic disorders. Viral agents are the major culprits in acute exacerbations of asthma; bacterial agents are rarely the problem. However, both otitis media and sinusitis are common in allergic children and may exacerbate asthma. When they are present, antibiotic therapy may be needed. Further coagulase-positive staphylococcal infections occur frequently in atopic dermatitis for which systemic therapy is necessary. Because "allergic" children may become sensitized to antibiotics more readily, it is important to minimize their indiscriminate use. Topical antibiotics are especially likely to sensitize; the only antibiotics applied to the skin should be those not used systemically (e.g., bacitracin).

Combination Drugs

Several drugs are marketed in combination form for therapy of asthma, allergic rhinitis, and other allergic drug reactions. Vasoconstrictor-antihistamine combinations are rational but combination asthma drugs containing ephedrine, aminophylline, or theophylline and a sedative (e.g., Tedral or Marax) have been superseded by more effective agents and their use should be discouraged.

Immunotherapy (Hyposensitization, Desensitization, Injection Therapy)

The observation that repeated injections of an allergen into a sensitive patient result in decreased sensitivity to the same allergen was made more than 80 years ago; injection therapy for allergic disorders has been used ever since. Its effectiveness has been the subject of much controversy, but various studies have provided evidence for its value in pollinosis, in house dust mite sensitivity, and in Hymenoptera sensitivity for the treatment of upper and lower respiratory tract allergen. Its effectiveness in mold hypersensitivity remains to be established clearly. Hyposensitization to animal (especially cat) allergens is effective if the appropriate allergens (not necessarily danders) are used. Hyposensitization with bacterial vaccines has no proven value (Lieberman and Patterson, 1974; Norman, 1980; Lichtenstein, et al., 1984). Although total elimination of symptoms may follow injection therapy, more commonly only partial benefit occurs, and in some instances there is little benefit. Injection therapy is used primarily in respiratory allergic disorders mediated by IgE antibody and severe allergic reactions to Hymenoptera insect stings.

The rationale for injection therapy was based initially on the presumption that grass and other allergens were toxins. Repeated injections of small but increasing amounts of antigen were given to induce immunity to the "toxin," as had been demonstrated for other toxins, such as cholera toxin. Although there are many theories to explain the rationale for injection therapy, its use was mainly empirical, based on its safety and apparent effectiveness. Subsequent controlled trials have clearly demonstrated the effectiveness of immunotherapy (Van Metre et al., 1982). Therapy is begun using small doses of antigen, which do not provoke clinical symptoms (or much antibody response). Increased quantities of antigen are injected at frequent intervals initially; later, when larger and more immunogenic doses are reached, injections are given at greater intervals.*

Indications for Immunotherapy

Because injection therapy is directed toward specific allergens, it should be instituted only after specific allergens have been identified. Injection therapy is used only for allergens that cannot be avoided. Since injection therapy for allergic rhinitis may prevent asthma (Johnstone, 1960), some believe that injection therapy is indicated in all instances in which unavoidable allergens can be identified. This position also makes sense theoretically because allergic mechanisms have been implicated in inducing nonspecific bronchial hyperreactivity, believed to be important in chronic asthma (Cockroft, 1983; Kaliner, 1984). Nevertheless, others (including the authors) believe that the use of such therapy should be based on the severity of the symptoms and inability to provide satisfactory control with environmental and drug therapy.

Injection therapy is indicated for Hymenoptera allergy in children only when systemic and potentially life-threatening symptoms have occurred. Injection of specific venoms of the Hymenoptera insects (not whole-body extracts except for fire ants) induces adequate protection.

Oral hyposensitization of food-sensitive individuals has been attempted with limited success. This treatment is not indicated if the food can be avoided, but it

---

*There may be more than one way to increase clinical tolerance to an allergen. For example, in an individual sensitive to a given drug that cannot be avoided, extremely small amounts of the drug are given subcutaneously, and the dose is gradually increased every 20 to 30 minutes until a therapeutic concentration is reached. The therapeutic concentration of the drug is then maintained for the duration of therapy. Production and maintenance of antigen excess and reduction of mediator stores by repeated injections of antigen may explain the effectiveness of this kind of desensitization. This may also account for the increasing tolerance to parenteral antigen early in the course of injection treatment in atopic disorders. Another goal of injection therapy in atopic disorders and insect allergy is to form "blocking" antibodies, which can block the release of histamine and other chemical mediators by combining with the antigen, thereby preventing its combination with reaginic antibody. IgE antibody titers to the antigen tend to fall with long-term injection therapy, suggesting that a form of immunologic tolerance may develop. Inhibition of IgE antibody formation by enhancement of suppressor T-cell activity has also been suggested as a mechanism by which injection therapy operates. Antibody-independent inhibition of cellular mediator release (cellular desensitization) also occurs in some patients.

can be considered in severe food hypersensitivity when accidental ingestion may occur.

Procedure for Immunotherapy

Despite minor variations, the basic procedure for all injection therapy is similar. Injections of the allergen extract are given subcutaneously in progressively increasing doses small enough not to provoke a clinical response. The usual initial dose is 0.05 mL of a 1:100,000 dilution or greater. When some form of intradermal skin test end-point titration is done, the patient usually tolerates a dose that is equal to 0.1 mL of the end-point dilution that initiates skin reaction (Van Metre et al., 1982).

New methods for standardization of allergens are being used; the new standard in the United States will be the BAU (biological allergen unit), but to date only a few antigens have been standardized.

Injections are repeated every 3 to 7 days (occasionally at shorter intervals), and the dose of extract is increased approximately 50% each time until a peak or maintenance dose is reached. The peak dose is the highest concentration of extract tolerated without a systemic or severe local reaction or, in the absence of any reaction, the highest concentration of allergen extract available. This peak dose is administered throughout the year—initially weekly but gradually every 2 to 4 weeks. During the symptomatic period of the year, a return to weekly injections at the same or lower doses may be advisable. To perform preseasonal hyposensitization, injections are begun a few weeks before the allergy season, so that the peak dose is reached just before the time when symptoms occur. The injections are then stopped abruptly until the following season.

Large local reactions or systemic reactions are indications for reduction of subsequent dosage. Selection of too large a starting dose and increasing doses too rapidly are common causes of reactions. Because most severe reactions occur within 30 minutes after injections, all patients should remain under close observation for at least this period of time. Severe allergic reactions including anaphylactic shock may occur after allergy injections, and physicians using such therapy should be prepared to deal with them immediately (see Anaphylactic Reactions, following).

Various different techniques for preparing modified allergen to reduce reactions have been tried. To date only alum-precipitated and alum-pyridine extracts are available in the United States. Efficacy of this preparation has been shown for grass antigens and not for ragweed (FDA Panel Report on Allergenic Extracts, 1985).

The effectiveness of injection therapy is related to the total dose of antigen used (Franklin and Lowell, 1967; Lichtenstein et al., 1968). Because many patients appear to be sensitive to a large number of allergens, it is common to treat such patients with many antigens. Because of limitations on the volume of antigen extract used, the concentration of each allergen may be relatively small, even at peak or maintenance doses. In view of the relationship between allergen dose and the effectiveness of therapy, it may be important to minimize the number of different allergens used so that therapeutic concentrations of the most problematic antigens can be reached.

The duration of injection therapy is determined by its effectiveness. Therapy may be discontinued if it has produced the desired relief for at least two consecutive years. Because of a tendency for clinical sensitivity to recur after injection therapy has been discontinued, many prefer to continue therapy. Benefit may not be apparent in the first year of therapy, and a trial of less than 2 years cannot be considered adequate.

ANAPHYLACTIC REACTIONS

Many allergic reactions are life-threatening (Sheffer, 1985). These can occur with extreme rapidity and immediate treatment is critical. Death is most commonly from asphyxia (airway obstruction resulting from laryngeal edema or severe bronchospasm) and/or cardiovascular collapse (anaphylactic shock) resulting from transudation of fluid from the intravascular space. Signs and symptoms include pallor, weakness, pruritus, erythema, urticaria, dyspnea, wheezing, cyanosis, nausea, vomiting, diarrhea, abdominal cramps, palpitations, cardiac arrhythmias, frothy sputum with pulmonary edema, hypotension, and localized or generalized edema. A tingling sensation may herald the reaction, and the patient may complain of feeling odd or faint. With edema of the upper airway, the patient may complain of a "thick" throat before any respiratory impairment is perceived. On the other hand, the reaction may produce cardiovascular collapse so rapidly that there are no warning symptoms or signs.

Etiology

Severe anaphylactic reactions are often caused by injection of drugs (especially penicillin) or biologics (foreign serum, intravenous immune globulin), by hyposensitization therapy with allergenic extracts, or by skin testing in extremely sensitive individuals. Severe allergic reactions can also be provoked by ingestion of food allergens (especially fish, milk, peanuts, other nuts, and shellfish) or, in inordinately sensitive individuals, by inhalation of allergens (foods, pollens, animal danders). In addition, severe allergy to insect stings, most notably by bees, hornets, wasps, yellow jackets (insects of the order Hymenoptera), or fire ants, can cause anaphylaxis. Anaphylaxis can also result from the use of radiocontrast media or the use of latex in procedures for patients with spina bifida (Kelly et al., 1991). Anaphylaxis may also occur with exercise in some subjects or after ingestion of specific food followed by exercise in others.

Diagnosis

Diagnosis depends on the nature of the clinical reaction and on establishing a relationship between a possible offensive substance and the reaction. An association between substances eaten, inhaled, injected, or touched and the symptoms observed should be regarded as highly suggestive and a causal relationship assumed until the relationship can be investigated. Skin testing with suspected allergens is sometimes useful, but it should be performed with caution, beginning with extremely low concentrations of the suspected allergens. In the case of drugs or foreign sera, for example, it is advisable to begin with at least a thousandfold dilution of the material and to start with a scratch or prick test rather than an intradermal test. As soon as an obvious reaction occurs, the allergen should be wiped from the skin.

When skin tests are used to identify the cause of a severe allergic reaction, it must be remembered that a positive skin reaction may occur without severe hypersensitivity and that a negative skin reaction does not completely exclude the possibility that the material in question plays a role in the reaction investigated. Negative reactions may occur:

1. If the testing material is in a form different from that which provoked the reaction in the first place (some foods and antibiotics).

2. If testing is performed too soon after the reaction during a transient anergic period ("refractory period").

3. If testing is performed too long after the original reaction (years or possibly months), so that the level of IgE antibody has waned. The latter occurs frequently in penicillin hypersensitivity.

4. If anaphylaxis is caused by non-IgE antibody such as immune complex or complement-mediated agents, by modulators of arachidonic acid metabolism, or by direct histamine-releasing agents.

Because of the possible occurrence of a refractory period, testing should be deferred for 1 month after a systemic reaction.

Treatment

Treatment of severe allergic reactions begins with the immediate intramuscular injection of 0.2 to 0.5 ml (0.01 ml/kg) of 1:1000 aqueous epinephrine. This may be repeated at 20-minute intervals if necessary. If the material that provoked the reaction was injected into an extremity, a tourniquet should be placed proximal to the site of injection to retard absorption. If the material was injected intradermally or subcutaneously, infiltration of the injection site with 0.2 ml of aqueous epinephrine and application of ice may slow absorption. Diphenhydramine (Benadryl), 1 mg/kg up to 50 mg, should be given intravenously, slowly over a 5- to 10-minute period, or intramuscularly. An H_2 antihistamine, cimetidine (300 mg), should be infused intravenously over a 5- to 10-minute period as well. Parenteral or oral antihistamines may be repeated every 4 to 6 hours as necessary.

Oxygen by mask should be administered while an intravenous infusion of 5% dextrose in water is started to provide a route for subsequent fluid, colloid, or drug therapy. An adequate airway should be ensured. An intubation and tracheostomy set should be available nearby, and appropriate surgical or anesthesiology personnel should be notified. In addition to fluids, plasma may be required to maintain an appropriate blood volume. Maintenance of adequate blood pressure may require pressor agents. A cardiac monitor should be in place, because anaphylaxis may lead to decreased coronary blood flow.

The value of adrenal steroids in acute severe allergic reactions is unclear, because the onset of their therapeutic effects requires several hours. However, in acute reactions not immediately responsive to epinephrine and antihistamine therapy, they should be given. Methylprednisolone or equivalent given intravenously in large doses (1 to 2 mg/kg body weight every 6 hours) is recommended. After symptoms diminish, adequate control can be maintained with oral antihistamines alone or in combination with ephedrine. Late complications of anaphylaxis include occlusion of the airway, hypotension, cardiac arrhythmias, hypoxic seizures, and metabolic acidosis. For therapy of these conditions a hospital intensive care unit and blood gas laboratory are essential.

Prevention

Subsequent avoidance of the inciting allergens is imperative. Sensitive individuals should be told of possible hidden sources of allergens. Individuals sensitive to an antibiotic should be warned against the subsequent use of a structurally related antibiotic. In severe insect hypersensitivity, hyposensitization should be instituted, preferably by a physician with experience in hyposensitization therapy. In children, hyposensitization is indicated if a reaction has involved respiratory or cardiovascular symptoms, but otherwise it may not be warranted (Schuberth et al., 1983). Immunizations should be kept up to date in order to minimize the necessity for using foreign antisera.

Exercise-Induced Anaphylaxis

This syndrome of pruritus, urticaria, angioedema, wheezing, and hypotension after exercise was first described by Sheffer and Austen in 1980. Histologic changes consist of mast cell degranulation after exercise challenge (Sheffer et al., 1985). One half to two thirds of the patients are atopic. This syndrome has also been noted in patients who exercise after ingesting specific foods (shellfish or celery) or in some who exercise within 2 hours of eating any food.

Therapy has been unsatisfactory because reactions do not occur after each exercise episode. Recommendations for treatment include avoidance of exercise for 2 hours after eating and that patients carry epinephrine and an antihistamine with them when they exercise.

Anaphylaxis Caused by Latex

Latex has been shown to cause immediate reactions, including anaphylaxis, as well as delayed reactions. Three groups appear to be at especially high risk: children with meningomyelocele or genitourinary abnormalities (generally who require multiple surgeries), workers exposed to latex in industry, and health-care workers. There is as yet no standard screening procedure for diagnoses. Accordingly, procedures for all patients with spina bifida should be performed in an environment free of latex, as should any medical procedure for patients with a positive history. Latex-free gloves are available, but latex-free condoms are not available at present.

Skin testing has not been standardized, but antigen extracted from latex gloves or latex extract may be the best available diagnostic substance. However, one should be careful in testing these patients because anaphylaxis has been induced by epicutaneous tests in very sensitive patients (Committee Report, 1993).

ATOPIC ALLERGIC DISORDERS

Allergic reactivity is a normal phenomenon that plays a potentially beneficial role in the body's defense against infection and oncogenesis. Allergic reactions can be elicited in all normal subjects and are an undesirable concomitant of this protective response. Certain kinds of allergic responsiveness, such as allergic rhinitis, asthma, and atopic dermatitis, occur only in a segment of the population genetically predisposed to their development. Coca and Cooke (1923) applied the term "atopic" to these disorders and to the individuals in whom they occur. Atopic individuals often have high levels of skin-sensitizing antibody and tissue and blood eosinophilia. Also, individuals with one disorder often develop other atopic manifestations.

Pathogenesis

Immunologic explanations for the pathogenesis of these disorders are based on the presence of skin-sensitizing IgE antibody. Although atopic individuals seem to respond better to antigens encountered by mucosal surfaces and tend to have higher levels of IgE antibodies, normal subjects also synthesize these antibodies. Furthermore, IgE antibody may not be important in all atopic states, including in some cases of asthma and atopic dermatitis.

Immunologic theories do not entirely explain the role of nonimmune stimuli (irritants, psychologic factors, exercise, chemicals) or the end-organ hypersensitivity to chemical mediators that occurs in these disorders. For example, in nearly all asthmatics with chronic symptoms, bronchial obstruction can be produced by small amounts of acetylcholine, histamine, kinins, prostaglandins, or leukotrienes that do not produce changes in normal individuals (Szentivanyi, 1968; Boushey et al., 1980). On the other hand, IgE antibody has been implicated not only in triggering symptoms of asthma and other atopic disorders but also in causing end-organ hyperresponsiveness (Cockroft et al., 1977).

Pharmacologic theories of atopic allergy suggest abnormal production or metabolism of chemical mediators or their physiologic antagonists or an imbalanced

nervous system. Autonomic disturbances in allergic patients led years ago to the speculation that the atopic abnormality was caused by vagotonia, a relative hyperfunction of the cholinergic component of the autonomic nervous system.

Szentivanyi (1968) proposed that the underlying abnormality in asthma, and perhaps in other atopic disorders, is a relative deficiency in beta-adrenergic receptor function. This hypothesis helped to refocus attention on pharmacologic and metabolic abnormalities present in atopic individuals. Evidence forthcoming from numerous laboratories has indicated various abnormalities in chemical mediator responses of the autonomic nervous system at cellular and subcellular levels in patients with atopic disorders. Whatever the explanation for these abnormalities, the immune aberrations associated with atopic disorders do not appear to be the entire basis for the development of such disorders (Pearlman, 1984a).

Allergic Rhinitis

Allergic rhinitis is the most common atopic disorder. Two forms are recognized:

- *Perennial* rhinitis, in which symptoms are present throughout the year
- *Seasonal* rhinitis ("hay fever"), in which symptoms are confined to a certain characteristic portion of the year, usually spring, summer, and/or fall

Many individuals have both forms, with seasonal exacerbations on top of perennial rhinitis.

Allergic rhinitis can begin at any age and has been reported in early infancy. More commonly, it begins in later infancy or early childhood, usually as perennial allergic rhinitis. Seasonal allergic rhinitis may occur early in life but usually occurs later than perennial rhinitis. Allergic rhinitis is basically a wheal and erythema reaction of the nasal mucosa mediated by IgE antibody. Histamine is a principal mediator of the reaction, but other mediators also play an important role. A late-phase reaction to allergen also occurs, similar to that in allergic asthma. A large proportion of individuals with allergic rhinitis exhibit bronchial hyperreactivity to chemical mediators.

Clinical Manifestations

Perennial allergic rhinitis generally presents with nasal stuffiness, with or without serous nasal discharge. There may be sniffling, varying from occasional to extremely repetitive, accompanied by nose wrinkling and nose rubbing. A characteristic form of the latter is the allergic salute, accomplished by pressing the undersurface of the nose upward by the palm of the hand. The chronicity of symptoms presumably reflects the nature of the inciting allergenic agents, namely, allergens to which there is continuous exposure, for example, from house dust mites and domestic animals. Symptoms may be of the same intensity year-round, but often they are worse in the winter, perhaps because of increased exposure to indoor allergens at that time of year. Seasonal allergens present in the air for a limited time, including pollens and molds, may contribute. Foods occasionally cause perennial or seasonal rhinitis.

Hay fever symptoms are similar, but nasal itching, paroxysmal sneezing, and serous nasal discharge tend to be more prominent and manifestations of eye involvement are more likely. Symptoms are commonly most pronounced in the early morning or late evening and can include excess tearing; itching of the eyes, palate, pharynx, face, or ears; headache; paranasal sinus and eustachian tube involvement; and fatigue. Anosmia and epistaxis may also occur.

Symptoms are usually more intense in older adolescents or adults than in younger children, but the severity of symptoms is not necessarily correlated with age. Symptoms also tend to be more prominent later in the problematic pollen season, a phenomenon probably related to the "priming" effect of repeated allergen exposure increasing general nasal mucous membrane sensitivity (Connell, 1968).

Physical findings usually include mucosal hyperemia and edema; the surface may glisten because of superficial watery secretion. Physical findings are related to the severity and chronicity of the process and can be highly variable. In severe rhinitis, the nasal mucosa appears pale and swollen ("boggy"), sometimes with a bluish coloration. Polypoid changes in the mucosa may cause complete obstruction of the nares or sinuses. There may be conjunctival injection and increased lacrimation, and the eyelid mucosa may assume a cobblestone appearance. Patients with allergic rhinitis often exhibit a distinctive facial appearance, with flattening of the malar eminences and infraorbital cyanosis; this results in dark circles ("allergic shiners") under the eyes, which may be demarcated by skin pleats, extending from under the eye to the epicanthal fold ("allergic pleats"). Excessive upward rubbing of the nose can result in a transverse crease over the end of the cartilaginous portion of the nose ("allergic crease"). Pharyngeal lymphoid follicles may be prominent, and enlargement of adenoids, tonsils, and cervical nodes may occur.

Diagnosis

Diagnosis of allergic rhinitis is based on the history and physical findings just described. Nasal eosinophilia is a characteristic finding that supports the diagnosis, but it is not necessarily present or consistent and may be influenced by disease activity, concurrent infection, or medication use. The presence of more than 15 eosinophils per 100 cells or of clumps of eosinophils suggests allergic rhinitis. Testing for pollen, mold, and other inhalant allergens can be helpful in determining the offending allergens for avoidance and immunotherapy if necessary. Testing for food allergens is generally not of value in rhinitis.

Perennial allergic rhinitis should be differentiated from *vasomotor rhinitis,* a nonallergic, noninfectious condition with a similar constellation of symptoms. Although nasal eosinophilia and IgE antibody are not present, one form of nonallergenic rhinitis with nasal

eosinophilia has been identified in children and adults (Jacobs et al., 1981). Rhinitis caused by viral infections or chronic use of topical medications and other causes of nasal obstruction must be considered in the differential diagnosis (Pearlman, 1984b). *Vernal conjunctivitis,* a distressing disorder of unknown (but possibly allergic) etiology, occurs in the spring and summer.

Complications

Sinusitis, often asymptomatic, is a more common complication of allergic rhinitis than is generally appreciated. There may be no specific signs of the disease, and its presence may not be appreciated unless x-ray films of the sinuses are taken.

Serous otitis media occurs frequently in children with allergic rhinitis (Kraemer et al., 1983), but it also commonly occurs in the absence of allergic disease. The middle ear may be the site of an allergic reaction, or nasal obstruction may block the eustachian tube with secondary involvement of the middle ear (Bluestone, 1983). The chief symptom of serous otitis media is hearing loss, usually mild and often undetected, particularly because of the age group most commonly affected (3 to 8 years old). Hearing loss can be severe and lead to learning disorders and psychologic disturbances. Other symptoms may include a feeling of fullness in the head or in the ears, "popping" sounds in the ear, and low-pitched tinnitus. Physical findings variably include thickened, dull, and relatively immobile tympanic membranes, a fluid level in the middle ear with or without air bubbles, and distorted or absent tympanic membrane landmarks. The ears may also appear completely normal.

Nasal polyps are generally nonallergic in origin, and when they occur in children, cystic fibrosis must be ruled out (see Pearlman, 1984b).

Treatment

The best treatment for allergic rhinitis is avoidance of allergens. Antihistamines, alone or in conjunction with vasoconstrictor drugs, often afford relief of symptoms, particularly in seasonal allergic rhinitis. Cromolyn sodium (Nasalcrom) can also be used topically by itself or in conjunction with antihistamines.

With eye involvement, topical vasoconstrictors are helpful, as are short-term topical steroids in more resistant cases. Simple standard aqueous eye lubricants may be helpful.

With severe debilitating rhinitis, short-term systemic steroid therapy can be considered. Beclomethasone dipropionate (Vancenase, Beconase), flunisolide (Nasalide), and triamcinolone acetonide (Nasacort) are effective topical steroid preparations with little systemic effect in recommended dosages; they tend to be effective in ameliorating nasal symptoms and can be used with other therapy or alone.

If symptoms are severe and/or prolonged and offending allergens are identified, immunotherapy may be indicated. Asymptomatic sinusitis with mild radiographic changes (mucosal thickening of less than 5 mm) is often left untreated. In more severe sinusitis, however, antibiotic therapy must be used until resolution of inflammation, which may require weeks of therapy. Maximizing nasal and sinus ostia patency by use of decongestants and topical steroids is recommended, although there are few data concerning their efficacy in improving resolution of disease.

Treatment of polyps is difficult; polyps removed surgically tend to recur. Nasal polyps and severe aspirin idiosyncracy are often associated; if so, aspirin and certain other compounds should be avoided (Samter and Beers, 1968). Other nonallergic associations with polyposis, such as cystic fibrosis and infection, should be excluded.

Serous otitis media is treated with an antihistamine-vasoconstrictor combination to promote adequate drainage of fluid from the middle ear (although efficacy has also not been proved), and a 7-day course of oral steroids with or without antibiotics may be helpful. Antibiotics are sometimes also used. Myringotomy, with implantation of a small plastic tube to promote adequate ventilation, or adenoidectomy may be necessary.

Course

The course of allergic rhinitis is variable. Mild rhinitis may disappear spontaneously, but severe rhinitis tends to persist. Severe long-standing allergic rhinitis in a young child may result in alteration of facial development, with an elongated facies and dental malocclusion. Serous otitis media may occasionally result in permanent hearing loss.

Atopic Dermatitis (Eczema)

Atopic dermatitis is a chronic dermatosis characterized by erythema, papules, vesiculation, oozing, crusting, and intense itching (see Chapter 21). It commonly begins in early infancy ("infantile eczema") but may develop at any age. Its inclusion as an atopic disorder is based chiefly on its association with asthma and allergic rhinitis and the common occurrence of skin-sensitizing (IgE) antibodies in this disorder. A family history of atopic disease is observed in most individuals with atopic dermatitis, and patients with atopic dermatitis are at greatly increased risk for development of allergic rhinitis and asthma. In addition to the presence of IgE antibodies to a variety of allergens, IgE levels are high (generally higher than in other atopic disorders) in about 80% of patients and eosinophilia is common.

In some instances, primarily in preschool children, food or inhalant allergens aggravate the dermatitis, and their avoidance leads to amelioration of symptoms (Sampson, 1983). In older children and adults, patch testing with environmental allergens may produce eczema-like contact reactions (Adinoff et al., 1988).

Treatment with immunotherapy may benefit patients with inhalant sensitivity. When a specific allergen causes exacerbations of this disorder, it is generally not the only or dominant etiologic factor. In most cases, it is difficult to identify a specific allergen, in fact,

and in some patients IgE antibodies are not demonstrable.

The immediate wheal-and-flare skin lesion associated with the action of skin-sensitizing antibody is not typical of the skin changes in atopic dermatitis, although the late-phase reaction may be. Abnormalities in T-cell regulation and cytokine production may be related to elevated serum IgE and the rash of atopic dermatitis (Leung, 1992). Products elaborated by eosinophils may play an important role in the pathogenesis of disease (Sampson, 1992).

The histopathologic picture depends on the stage of the disease and includes secondary changes that occur as a result of infection or scratching. The multiple nonimmune factors that aggravate the disease, such as temperature changes, sweating, contact with detergents and soaps, local or systemic infection, and friction caused by rubbing and scratching, suggest a multifactorial etiology. Thus, an allergic reaction may be just one of the multiple events that play a role in this disorder.

Etiology

Individuals with atopic dermatitis have itchy skin, suggesting that the underlying basis of atopic dermatitis is a constitutional predisposition to the development of pruritus (Rostenberg and Solomon, 1971). The itching leads to scratching, skin trauma, and the chronic changes characteristic of this disorder. Thus, the trauma caused by scratching plays a major role in the pathogenesis of atopic dermatitis, although it is not essential to the development of dermatologic lesions. Unusual responsiveness to skin stroking (*white dermographism*) and to the injection of acetylcholine (a "delayed branch" reaction instead of erythema) has been described. Biochemical abnormalities, such as a high norepinephrine content and an abnormal surface lipid composition, have also been reported in the skin of patients with atopic dermatitis (Sulzberger and Frick, 1971).

IgE-mediated tissue injury and tissue injury mediated by other immune mechanisms play a role in atopic dermatitis, but immune mechanisms do not appear to be the entire basis of this disorder. On the other hand, the association between skin eruptions that resemble atopic dermatitis and immunodeficiencies is striking, suggesting the possibility of some cause-and-effect relationship (Pearlman, 1971).

Clinical Manifestations

The infantile form of eczema begins typically at about 2 to 3 months of age as an erythematous eruption with small papules and vesicles. This leads to fissuring of the skin with oozing and crusting of the lesions. Early in the disease and in mild cases, the lesions may have a dry and scaly appearance. The head and neck, forehead, cheeks, and creases behind the ears are most commonly involved in infancy, although involvement of the trunk and the extremities (more commonly on the extensor surfaces) does occur. Involvement of the antecubital and popliteal areas is less common; these are the characteristic locations in the older child. Itching is prominent and leads to scratching and excoriation. Secondary skin infection often occurs.

With chronicity of the dermatitis, thickening (lichenification) of the skin in the affected areas occurs, particularly in the antecubital and popliteal areas and the wrists. Many individuals with atopic dermatitis have ichthyosis and dry, scaly skin in unaffected areas. Scarring rarely occurs, but skin pigmentation in the involved areas may be increased or decreased. The course is marked by exacerbations and remissions.

Atopic dermatitis may be confused with seborrheic dermatitis, contact dermatitis, candidiasis, and histiocytosis X (Kahn, 1975). The distinction between seborrheic dermatitis and atopic dermatitis may be especially difficult in some cases, and the two may coexist. Seborrhea in infancy tends to involve the scalp, forehead, and ears; is not pruritic; and occurs in plaques of yellowish greasy scales. Eczematous eruptions that resemble atopic dermatitis are also seen in patients with Wiskott-Aldrich syndrome, ataxia-telangiectasia, phenylketonuria, and X-linked agammaglobulinemia. An eczematoid eruption has been reported in the hyper-IgE syndrome of recurrent furunculosis and markedly elevated IgE (Buckley et al., 1972) and in Job's syndrome (Hill et al., 1974).

The diagnosis of atopic dermatitis is based on the character and distribution of lesions, aided by a strong family or personal history of atopy. Skin testing often reveals a number of positive reactions to foods and inhalant allergens, but, as noted, these are not necessarily etiologic factors. With foods, a general rule is that a positive skin test suggests the possibility of etiologic involvement, and a negative skin test virtually rules it out (Sampson, 1983).

Treatment

For patients with atopic dermatitis, good general skin care with vigorous specific local treatment is the most important aspect of therapy. Avoiding ingestion, inhalation, or contact with suspected allergens, minimizing contact with irritants (soap, detergents, or rough clothing, such as wool), and ensuring proper hydration of the skin are essential elements of therapy.

Patients should avoid excessive bathing, and they can add lubricants (Alpha-Keri, Lubath, Domol) to the bath halfway through the bath or use them after bathing. Oils should be added to the bath water only after allowing the skin to be hydrated; adding the oil halfway through the bath is usually satisfactory. Superfatted soaps may be used (Lowila, Dove, Basis, Neutrogena) but should be thoroughly rinsed from the skin. In wet climates, an alternative regimen using Cetaphil in place of soap and water and avoiding water altogether can be useful.

Patients should thoroughly rinse their clothes after each wash to eliminate any residual detergent. Antihistamines can relieve itching, but sedative doses may be required. Fingernails should be kept short to minimize trauma caused by scratching. Lightweight socks or mittens may be used to cover the hands while the infant sleeps. During the acute weeping stage of dermatitis, cool soaks with Burow's solution or plain water applied for 15- or 20-minute intervals every 3 to 4 hours relieves itching and promotes drying of the lesions.

Steroid creams are extremely valuable in diminishing the inflammatory reaction, but they should not be applied to weeping or infected skin. The fluorinated steroid preparations are particularly potent. Topical steroids should be applied frequently and liberally until dermatitis is controlled. (However, significant systemic absorption of steroids from the more potent steroid preparations can occur with topical use when they are applied frequently, especially when used over large areas of dermatitis.) Chronic use of topical steroids can lead to skin atrophy. Less potent topical steroids (e.g., hydrocortisone) should be used on the face and, if possible, when topical steroids are employed for prolonged periods, reserving the more potent preparations for flares of eczema. With chronic and lichenified lesions, steroid ointments may be used instead of creams. In severe atopic dermatitis, a short course (several days) of systemic steroid therapy may be necessary.

Coal tar preparations are also useful in chronic dermatitis. Because of their photosensitizing properties, they should be used cautiously if the patient has extensive contact with sunlight. The incorporation of 10% urea in steroid preparations can increase skin hydration but can be irritating. Secondary skin infection should be treated with systemic antibiotics. Group A beta-hemolytic streptococcal and hemolytic staphylococcal infections require systemic antibiotic therapy. Immunotherapy is rarely indicated in the treatment of atopic dermatitis.

Course

Although atopic dermatitis is rarely associated with permanent physical scarring, disfigurement resulting from active atopic dermatitis, particularly in older children and adolescents, may result in severe psychologic problems. The development of keratoconus and cataracts is a rare complication of protracted atopic dermatitis. Skin infections with *Herpesvirus hominis* (eczema herpeticum) can be severe. Close contact with an individual with herpes simplex must be avoided. Malnutrition resulting from an inadequate diet caused by excessive dietary restrictions must be avoided.

The course is variable; atopic dermatitis may disappear by ages 3 to 5 or persist indefinitely. It may also develop for the first time during any part of childhood or adult life.

Bronchial Asthma

Asthma is a largely reversible obstructive pulmonary disorder in which allergic reactions often play an important role. Although allergic reactions frequently induce asthma, the underlying problem is not necessarily of immune origin (Pearlman, 1989).

Pathogenesis

A striking characteristic of almost all patients with chronic symptomatic asthma is a "nonspecific" bronchial hyperresponsiveness to acetylcholine and other chemical mediators that regulate airway resistance or are components of the inflammatory response (Boushey et al., 1980). Asthma can be provoked by a large variety of factors, such as allergic reactions, irritants, exercise, chemicals, drugs, infection, and emotional factors. All these factors, allergic and nonallergic, cause the release of mediators or activation of an irritant mechanism that, especially in a hypersensitive bronchial tree, leads to bronchial obstruction.

Bronchial hypersensitivity is such an important feature of chronic asthma that the term "reactive airway disorder" has come into use in recognition of its importance in this condition. However, "nonspecific" airway hyperreactivity does not appear to be a necessary component of asthma (Pearlman, 1989). All hyperreactivity is specific ultimately, and various combinations of specific hyperreactivity are observed when bronchial responses to different challenges are measured.

IgE antibody plays a major role in allergic asthma because of its inordinate propensity to liberate chemical mediators. Moreover, it has been implicated in inducing bronchial hyperreactivity (Cockroft et al., 1977), perhaps through its ability to induce late-phase inflammatory responses (Lam et al., 1983). Various kinds of immune tissue injury may result in mediator release and undoubtedly play a role in asthma.

Epidemiology

The onset of asthma may occur at any age, but approximately half of all asthma patients experience their first symptoms during childhood. At least 8% of all children are affected by asthma, usually within the first 6 years of life and often in infancy (Gergen et al., 1988). More school is missed as a result of asthma than because of any other chronic illness. Asthma is a grossly underdiagnosed and undertreated childhood disorder (Speight et al., 1983). This applies to all ages, in fact, a point of concern that led to the development of national and international guidelines for the recognition and treatment of asthma (National Asthma Education Program [NAEP], 1991; International Consensus Report on Diagnosis and Treatment of Asthma, 1992).

Clinical Manifestations

The clinical hallmarks of asthma are episodic wheezing, dyspnea, and cough. In some children, however, wheezing may never be overt, and evidence of pulmonary obstruction may be elicited only by careful auscultation or pulmonary function testing. Moreover, significant air flow limitation can occur in the absence of any detectable wheezing. Wheezing, therefore, is a common but not necessary indicator of airway obstruction. Prolonged cough, with or without overt wheezing, is a common presentation of asthma in early life.

Between paroxysms of wheezing, the patient is often asymptomatic. In severe chronic asthma, symptoms of pulmonary obstruction may be constant, with superimposed episodes of greater airway obstruction. The degree of pulmonary obstruction varies from one patient

to the next and from one attack to the next, ranging from mild attacks that abate spontaneously to severe episodes unresponsive to heroic therapy, leading to death resulting from respiratory failure.

Asthma attacks may occur at any time, sometimes within minutes of contact with a known precipitating factor but often without obvious cause. Asthma tends to be more severe at night, possibly related to the fall in endogenous corticosteroid and catecholamine secretions at this time. In addition, there is an increased bronchial sensitivity to chemical mediators at night, and airway resistance increases in the recumbent position.

Airway obstruction is caused by a combination of mucosal edema; contraction of bronchial smooth muscle; the production of thick, tenacious bronchial mucus; and an inflammatory response characterized by accumulation of eosinophils, T lymphocytes, macrophages, and other cells. Although most prominent in chronic symptomatic asthma, *inflammation* has been identified even in mild asymptomatic asthma leading to a generally accepted notion that inflammation is the underlying pathologic basis of asthma, and control of inflammation is the critical therapeutic issue for asthma therapy.

Asthma early in life is frequently associated with viral respiratory infection (certain viruses, especially the respiratory syncytial virus, are special offenders) and in infancy may present as bronchiolitis. Recurrent bronchiolitis is a clue that a child may have asthma. Other viral respiratory infections also trigger asthmatic attacks, particularly in early childhood (Pattemore et al., 1992). Bacterial respiratory infections rarely provoke or aggravate asthma (McIntosh et al., 1973). When asthma occurs only with infections, the term asthmatic bronchitis or wheezy bronchitis is often used.

Except for the absence of evidence of allergy, the characteristics of the various asthma-like syndromes including asthmatic bronchitis are indistinguishable, and all are considered to be forms of asthma (Williams and McNicol, 1969). As the child gets older, allergens, initially perennial inhalants (animal allergens, house dust mites, or molds) and later seasonal allergens, tend to provoke symptoms. However, inhalant allergens can play an important role in asthma even in infancy. Foods sometimes provoke asthma, especially in infancy.

Precipitating Factors in Asthma

In addition to respiratory infections and specific allergens, various irritants (smoke, cold air, air pollutants, or odors), emotional factors, changes in temperature and humidity, cough, chemicals, and exercise all can trigger or aggravate asthma. Exercise-induced asthma can be a major problem (Spector, 1992). Exercise tolerance in children with inadequately controlled asthma is diminished and can limit normal childhood functioning to the point that the child may be reoriented to an unnecessarily sedentary existence. Strenuous exercise (especially running and bicycling) can precipitate severe asthma even in asthmatics with normal pulmonary functions at rest and, occasionally, is the only known precipitant of asthma in a child.

Acetylsalicylic acid (ASA), known to precipitate asthma by nonallergic mechanisms in adults, has also been shown to do so in childhood. Metabisulfite, an antioxidant in some drugs, including bronchodilator preparations, and employed as a greening agent on foods, may also induce asthma.

The role that each of the various possible precipitating factors plays in an individual child with asthma varies considerably. In some patients, no initiating or aggravating factors can be identified. Because exposure to one asthmogenic stimulus can heighten bronchial hyperreactivity, which can change from time to time, some factors may appear to be problematic during certain periods but well tolerated during others (Cockroft, 1983).

Asthma that occurs without an allergic response to exogenous allergens has been termed intrinsic asthma, implying that such individuals are responding to intrinsic allergens (such as normal respiratory bacterial flora) or to other internal factors. Asthma triggered by exogenous environmental allergens was thus termed extrinsic asthma. The concept from which these terms arose is probably incorrect, and the terms tend to be more confusing than helpful.

Physical Examination

Physical findings depend on the degree of pulmonary obstruction, so that between attacks the physical examination may be normal. Edelson and Rebuck (1985) have extensively reviewed the clinical assessment of asthma.

The earliest sign of airway obstruction is a prolonged expiratory phase of respiration; expiratory wheezes may also be heard on forced expiration, often before the child is symptomatic. With increasing airway obstruction, air exchange diminishes, the respiratory rate increases, breathing becomes labored, and expiratory and inspiratory wheezes and rhonchi become prominent.

A hacking cough may be present, but the child often attempts to suppress the cough. (On the other hand, persistent night cough or other episodic or chronic cough may be the main clinical manifestation of asthma.) Accessory respiratory muscles are used and supraclavicular, suprasternal, and intercostal retractions may be seen. The child often raises the shoulders as respiration becomes more labored. Hyperinflation of the chest occurs, with increased anteroposterior chest diameter, hyperresonance to percussion, more distant heart sounds, and limitation of diaphragmatic excursion. The child is often pale, but with increased severity of asthma, circumoral cyanosis results. Wheezing may decrease in intensity with a decrease in bronchial air exchange. With further progression, there may be signs of respiratory failure, generalized cyanosis, pulsus paradoxus, cardiac arrhythmia or standstill, and vascular collapse.

With long-standing asthma, a barrel chest or pigeon-breast deformity may be noted. Clubbing is rare, even in chronic severe asthma, and should suggest an alternative diagnosis.

Laboratory Findings

X-Rays

Radiographic findings may be normal between attacks, although there is often evidence of bronchial thickening. With airway obstruction, hyperinflation with depression of the diaphragm and peribronchial densities may be seen. Atelectasis and patchy pneumonic densities are common in asthma, especially in very young patients. These features are often diagnosed as pneumonitis, implying infection, although other evidence of infection may be lacking. Segmental atelectasis or atelectasis of an entire lobe, particularly the right middle lobe, may be seen.

Asymptomatic pneumothorax is an infrequent finding, with or without mediastinal emphysema. If the latter is present, there may be associated subcutaneous emphysema, observed radiographically and clinically.

With hyperinflation, the heart may appear small, and the pulmonary artery may be prominent.

Pulmonary Function

During an acute asthmatic attack, pulmonary function tests indicate increased airway resistance with airflow obstruction and air trapping (McFadden, 1975, 1980). The forced expiratory volume in 1 second (FEV_1), maximum midexpiratory flow (MMEF), and peak expiratory flow rate (PEFR) all are decreased, and the residual volume (RV), functional residual capacity (FRC), and total lung capacity (TLC) are increased. The vital capacity (VC) may be decreased or normal. Lung compliance and specific airway conductance (sGaw) are diminished, and there is a defect in elastic recoil. Ventilation tends to be grossly uneven, with a profound ventilation-perfusion imbalance, which is largely responsible for the hypoxemia commonly observed. Diffusing capacity is normal or, in chronic severe asthma, may be increased along with an increase in total lung capacity.

Characteristically, some reversal of these abnormalities in response to bronchodilator therapy is demonstrable, and, between attacks, pulmonary functions may be normal. However, residual significant pulmonary function abnormalities occur for many days after an acute episode, even when symptoms have abated, indicating the chronicity of so-called acute asthma (McFadden, 1975). Moreover, airway obstruction in the absence of overt wheezing is common in individuals with chronic asthma, even during asymptomatic periods (Levison et al., 1974).

Measurement of pulmonary functions to determine peak flow and/or FEV_1 is extremely helpful for documenting the amount of air-flow limitation and is an important adjunct to physical signs in assessing degree of asthma, acutely and chronically. Many patients do not perceive air-flow limitation until FEV_1 decreases to 50% of normal or less.

Blood Gas Values

Blood gas determinations are important in assessing the severity and response to treatment. Hypoxemia is an early finding and is virtually always present in acute asthmatic attacks. Hypercapnia, even with profound hypoxemia, is not usually seen except in severe attacks. In fact, because of the hyperventilation that usually occurs with bronchoconstriction, hypocapnia is more common. Indeed, a normal $Paco_2$ in the presence of hyperventilation implies carbon dioxide retention and is cause for great concern. A normal blood pH is usually maintained, although there may be a mild, compensated metabolic acidosis, or, with hyperventilation, a mild respiratory alkalosis.

With respiratory failure, profound respiratory acidosis may occur. With long-standing asthma, the hemoglobin and hematocrit may be elevated. These may also be increased during an acute asthmatic attack as a result of dehydration resulting from poor fluid intake and excessive respiratory water loss.

Diagnosis

The diagnosis of asthma is based on the historical and physical features previously described, but it can be aided by demonstrating a reversal of airway obstruction with bronchodilator therapy. Particularly in chronic severe asthma, the pulmonary function abnormalities may not always be completely reversible, however. In patients with questionable histories and normal pulmonary function, the demonstration of bronchial obstruction by an exercise test can be diagnostic.

Bronchoconstriction induced by the inhalation of low concentrations of methacholine chloride (Mecholyl) or histamine is also used as a diagnostic test but must be employed with extreme caution and only by those experienced in its use. A negative test result does not rule out asthma, however, particularly if the test is performed during a quiescent phase.

Blood and sputum eosinophilia is often present irrespective of the implication of allergic factors. The sputum may contain Charcot-Leyden crystals and Curschmann's spirals.

Differential Diagnosis

Asthma must be differentiated from other causes of airway obstruction. Upper airway obstruction caused by infection, tumors, or anomalies of the nose, nasopharynx, or larynx and dysfunction of the vocal cords may present with wheezing; with upper airway obstruction, in contrast to asthma, inspiratory wheezing with little expiratory wheezing is common. Lower airway obstruction with expiratory wheezing may occur with cystic fibrosis; a foreign body in the trachea, bronchi, or esophagus; compression of the bronchus by enlarged lymph nodes (infection, neoplasia); vascular abnormalities (aortic ring, anomalous pulmonary vessels); or other congenital anomalies such as bronchogenic cyst (Ellis, 1993). Because asthma is common, the possibility that nonasthmatic causes of airway obstruction (especially foreign body and cystic fibrosis) may coexist with asthma should be kept in mind.

Treatment of Chronic Asthma

Goals

Goals of asthma therapy are to achieve normal functioning without adverse effects of therapy. Specifically, these goals are to:

- Prevent troublesome daytime and nighttime symptoms
- Gain the ability to exercise normally, including competitive sports
- Prevent exacerbations of asthma
- Maintain normal or as near-normal lung functions as possible while avoiding undesirable effects of asthma medications and other forms of therapy

Treatment of asthma consists of reducing exposure to known or suspected allergens and irritants and using bronchodilators, anti-inflammatory and "preventive" drugs, and immunotherapy for unavoidable clinically significant allergens. The importance of inflammation in asthma has led to the formulation of therapeutic guidelines that emphasize the use of anti-inflammation therapy early in asthma as the underpinning for all patients with asthma who require chronic treatment (all but "mild" asthma, somewhat arbitrarily defined as asthma with short-lived symptoms up to twice a week with nocturnal symptoms less than twice a month) (National Asthma Education Program [NAEP], 1991). Although anti-inflammatory drugs such as cromolyn sodium, nedocromil sodium, and topical and systemic steroids, constitute important treatment options, the most "potent" anti-inflammatory modality potentially is avoidance of allergens and other irritating agents when possible. Immunotherapy may also play an important role in preventing or ameliorating inflammation (Pearlman, 1989).

The potentially serious nature of asthma justifies rigorous environmental control of asthmogenic factors in the child's home. In unusual circumstances (for example, a child in contact with farm animals to which there is marked sensitivity), a move to a different home or area is advisable. A move to another part of the country is rarely recommended because of the economic and other hardships imposed by such a move and the frequency with which sensitization to allergens indigenous to the new area occurs.

Home Monitoring

When feasible, home assessment of peak flow in children with moderate or severe asthma is strongly recommended as part of the treatment plan to facilitate self-assessment and continued self-care. A scheme of three color zones, green, yellow, and red, has been proposed (National Asthma Education Program, 1991) based on percentage of the patient's normal or best peak flow (or, when that is unknown, the "predicted" normal, which is the average for a normal population):

- Red zone, less than 50% peak flow, which does not increase after use of a bronchodilator

- Yellow zone, 50% to 80% of normal
- Green zone, more than 80% of normal

Acute and chronic pharmacotherapeutic needs are based on consideration of not only symptoms but also lung functions according to these zones. A sustained decrease in peak flows into the red zone, for example, calls for consideration of systemic steroids (Table 20–4).

Severity Guidelines

Categorization of asthma as mild, moderate, or severe is necessarily somewhat arbitrary, because there can be much variability in asthma, between asthmatics and within a single asthma patient. Frequency and intensity of symptoms, lability of asthma, and severity and chronicity of obstruction are all important issues in characterizing asthma severity, but they occur in various combinations and can change from time to time in a given patient during the natural course of the disease. Nevertheless, the classification of severity and recommendations for pharmacotherapy published by the NAEP are adopted for consideration here (see Table 20–4).

Pharmacotherapy

In general, beta$_2$-agonists taken by inhalation are drugs of first choice for relieving acute episodes of asthma. They are used on an as-needed basis, ordi-narily up to every 4 hours; in severe asthmatic episodes, however, they are used more frequently on a temporary basis. For chronic asthma, they may be used routinely three to four times a day in addition to other pharmacotherapy; in our opinion, however, short-acting beta$_2$-agonists ordinarily are best prescribed on an as-needed basis, using the patient's need for frequent use of beta$_2$-agonists as a sign that asthma is not under adequate control and the treatment regimen is not adequate.

All patients with more than mild asthma (see Table 20–4) should receive routine "anti-inflammatory" agents. Inhaled cromolyn sodium is recommended for younger children (especially preschool and perhaps preadolescent children) before considering inhaled corticosteroids, but the latter can be utilized at any age when control of chronic symptoms is necessary. Whether theophylline has clinically significant anti-inflammatory actions is an unsettled issue. It is generally accepted that short-acting (4 to 6 hours) beta$_2$-agonists do not have an anti-inflammatory activity.

Exercise-induced bronchospasm (or asthma) may be prevented by giving medicine before exercise. Cromolyn sodium, nedocromil sodium, and/or adrenergic drugs such as albuterol or terbutaline, administered by inhalation 10 minutes before exercise, are particularly useful. Asthmatic children should be strongly encouraged to participate in normal athletic activities to the

---

Table 20–4. Classification and General Management of Asthma in Children

Mild asthma	Treatment
Brief episodes up to twice a week Asymptomatic between episodes Brief if any exercise-related symptoms Little (less than twice a month) or no nocturnal symptoms FEV$_1$ or peak flow at least 80% of "normal"*	Inhaled beta$_2$-agonist every 4 to 6 hours as needed. (For very young children unable to cooperate adequately, an oral beta$_2$ agent can be used.) Inhaled beta$_2$-agonist, cromolyn sodium, or both 10 to 15 minutes before exercise if needed as a preventative
Moderate asthma	Treatment
Episodes greater than twice a week Episodes last for hours to days Emergency care, if necessary, infrequent FEV$_1$ or peak flow 60% to 80% of normal (without medication)	Inhaled beta$_2$-agonist as necessary. (If needed more than three or four times a day, increase dose of current other daily medication or add another class of medication.) "Anti-inflammatory" agents routinely. This may be cromolyn sodium or nedocromil sodium or inhaled corticosteroids. (A trial of nonsteroidal anti-inflammatory agents is encouraged first at youngest ages.) Theophylline and/or long-acting beta$_2$-agonist can be added to or used in place of the above agents, but are not considered anti-inflammatory
Severe asthma	Treatment
Symptoms more or less continuous in the absence of medication Frequent asthma exacerbations Frequent nocturnal symptoms Activity generally limited Periodic emergency treatment; occasional hospitalization Any life-threatening episodes FEV$_1$ or peak flow less than 60% without medication	Inhaled beta$_2$-agonist as necessary. Routine inhaled corticosteroid Cromolyn sodium or nedocromil sodium, theophylline, and/or long-acting beta$_2$-agents may be used as steroid-sparing or for added control of nocturnal or other symptoms Consideration of oral corticosteroids QOD if possible at lowest dose if other therapy not adequate

Once control is established, pharmacotherapy is reduced to the lowest amount necessary to maintain control. This may (and often does) mean increasing routine and/or as-necessary medications periodically to control mild to moderate increases in symptoms and periodic aggressive therapy including short "bursts" of systemic steroids to control moderate to severe exacerbations.

*Defined as the best function achievable for the child or, until that is established, the "predicted" (average) value for a normal population.
Abbreviation: FEV$_1$ = forced expiratory volume in 1 second.
Adapted from National Asthma Education Program. Expert Panel Report. Guidelines for the Diagnosis and Management of Asthma. Bethesda, Md., National Heart, Lung, and Blood Institute publication 91-3042, National Institutes of Health, 1991, and from the International Consensus Report on Diagnosis and Treatment of Asthma. Bethesda, Md., National Heart, Lung, and Blood Institute publication 92-3091, National Institutes of Health, 1992.

extent that they can; restrictions on physical activity because of rare or occasional wheezing should be avoided.

Short courses (5 to 10 days) of systemic steroids should be instituted early in the treatment of acute severe asthma poorly responsive to nonsteroid drugs. When used, steroids should be given in a dosage sufficient to achieve adequate control of symptoms and employed for as brief a period as possible. If long-term use is necessary in chronic severe asthma when topical therapy is not adequate, alternate-day therapy with prednisone or methylprednisolone given in the morning should be prescribed. The lowest dose necessary to maintain control should be employed, and periodic attempts to decrease and, if possible, eliminate steroid therapy should be made.

Antihistamines generally are not effective in asthma, although they may be beneficial in relieving upper respiratory symptoms that aggravate asthma. In an occasional patient, asthma appears to be aggravated by antihistamines. Although there are theoretical objections to the use of antihistamines in asthma because of their potential drying effect on mucus, this effect, if it occurs, is probably minimal and there is no general contraindication to the use of antihistamines for allergic rhinitis in an asthmatic individual.

Immunotherapy should be considered if allergy to unavoidable allergens significantly aggravates the asthma.

Treatment of Acute Asthma

Adrenergic Agents

Adrenergic agents are the drugs of first choice in the treatment of acute asthma. The administration of beta-adrenergic drugs by inhalation is preferred (e.g., albuterol, bitolterol mesylate [Tornalate], pirbuterol, and terbutaline). This generally is as effective as the parenteral route, is associated with fewer side effects, and can be repeated every 20 to 30 minutes initially in the absence of any systemic side effects. Nebulization through a compressed-air device or driven by pressurized oxygen is a particularly effective means of delivering medication. Albuterol (0.15 mg/kg per dose up to 5 mg) is recommended. Hand-held metered-dose inhalers can also be effective. Spacer devices into which an adrenergic agent can be sprayed can facilitate effective inhalation of the agent in children, including very young patients who are unable to coordinate inhalational maneuvers with drug activation.

As an alternative for children too small or too ill to cooperate for effective administration by inhalation, even by compressed air–driven nebulization by mask, parenteral adrenergic drugs may be used. Epinephrine (1:1000 aqueous solution, 0.2 to 0.3 ml given subcutaneously) is the parenteral drug of choice for rapid relief of asthmatic paroxysms. It may be repeated at 20-minute intervals for a total of three doses. As a preferred alternative, a single injection of sustained-release epinephrine (Sus-Phrine, 1:200, 0.05 to 0.15 ml) can be used and is likely to be as effective as repeated use of aqueous epinephrine, with fewer side effects. Terbutaline (Bricanyl), 0.01 mg/kg up to 0.25 mg (0.25 ml), may also be used for two doses instead of epinephrine.

Caution: In severe asthma with acidosis and profound hypoxemia, epinephrine and other adrenergic agents may cause cardiac arrhythmias and cardiac arrest. Relative or apparently complete lack of responsiveness to epinephrine ("epinephrine fastness") or other agents may be caused by acidosis, bronchial obstruction by thick mucous plugs, pneumothorax, or simply severe asthma.

The distress of asthma is probably caused more by the discomfort of increased airway resistance than the perception of hypoxemia. Drugs that decrease airway resistance and relieve discomfort do not necessarily lessen hypoxemia. Subjective improvement in asthma, therefore, is not a reliable guide to tissue oxygenation. (Increased use of accessory respiratory muscles or retractions indicates severe pulmonary obstruction. Pulsus paradoxus may occur with extreme obstruction.)

Because of ventilation-perfusion imbalance that characteristically occurs in asthma, the asthmatic patient has hypoxemia but can usually eliminate carbon dioxide adequately. In fact, asthmatics tend to hyperventilate and decrease carbon dioxide below normal. An elevated or even normal Pa_{CO_2} in the presence of hyperpnea is an ominous sign.

Hypercapnia tends to occur when the FEV_1 decreases to about 20% to 30% of normal (Georg, 1981). In severely ill patients, there is no substitute for oximetry or for periodic determination of arterial blood gases. If this is not feasible, it is best to assume that the patient is hypoxemic and needs oxygen. Excessively high concentrations of oxygen (approaching 100%) should be avoided because they may lead to atelectasis and, rarely, may inhibit respiratory drive.

Intravenous Fluids

An intravenous infusion may be needed to ensure hydration and as a route for drug administration. Patients with severe asthma are often dehydrated. Fluid and caloric intake is characteristically decreased, and fluid losses, particularly from the respiratory tract, are increased. Adequate hydration is necessary for liquefaction of inspissated bronchial mucus. At the same time, overhydration must be avoided; a large fluid intake in the presence of a marked negative intrathoracic pressure that occurs in severe asthma may promote pulmonary edema. When urinary output is established, potassium should be added, particularly for patients receiving steroids. For patients with possible cardiovascular or renal insufficiency, fluid therapy should be more conservative.

Initially, only intravenous fluids are given. When oral fluids are tolerated, clear liquids only should be given as long as the patient has moderate or severe respiratory distress.

Correction of Acidosis

If the patient is in severe distress, administer sodium bicarbonate, 2 mEq/kg body weight, intravenously without delay over a 10-minute period. Further correct the pH to 7.3, using the following formula:

$$\text{mEq sodium bicarbonate} = \text{base deficit} \times 0.3 \times \text{body weight (kg)}$$

If the patient is not in extreme difficulty, determine the pH first and correct as necessary to pH 7.3 using the preceding formula. The effect of bicarbonate therapy can be assessed within minutes, and additional bicarbonate can then be given if indicated. Arterial or venous (not capillary) blood must be used for pH determinations. There is often a (compensated) metabolic acidosis in children with severe asthma. The inclusion of 5% dextrose in intravenous fluids lessens ketosis and helps maintain a normal blood pH.

Aminophylline (Theophylline)

The added effectiveness of theophylline when optimal doses of beta-agonists are used in acute asthma is an unsettled issue. Some studies indicate benefit, and at least as many indicate no therapeutic benefit with the disadvantage of increasing side effects. The authors do not recommend adding theophylline in general. If it is used, it is important to be aware that the amount of aminophylline tolerated or needed varies considerably from individual to individual because of individual variability in its metabolism. Ideally, aminophylline is administered by constant infusion, but it can also be given over a 20-minute period every 4 to 6 hours.

Theophylline blood levels should be measured and therapy aimed at achieving a theophylline level of more than 10 but less than 20 μg/ml (1 to 2 mg/dl) of serum. Before choosing an aminophylline dose, it is important to ascertain that the patient has not already had an excessive amount of theophylline, what other conditions the patient has, or what other medications the patient is receiving that may interfere with theophylline metabolism. Theophylline given by the oral route should not generally be relied upon in severe asthma.

Corticosteroids

Corticosteroids should be administered promptly in all instances of severe asthma (status asthmaticus) nonresponsive to adrenergic agents. Steroids are generally indicated for all patients deemed sick enough to require emergency admission to the hospital. Steroids should also be given in acute severe asthmatic attacks to patients who are already receiving oral or inhaled steroids.

High doses of steroids are employed for severe asthma. Methylprednisolone should be given intravenously using a dose of 1 to 2 mg per kg body weight in 20-minute infusions every 4 to 6 hours until the patient obtains relief. The dose can then be reduced. It is usually unnecessary to use high doses for more than 24 to 48 hours. Adrenocorticosteroids are administered ordinarily for 5 to 10 days. Because the onset of steroid action is delayed several hours, steroids cannot be relied upon to provide immediate reversal of bronchial obstruction. They may facilitate the action of adrenergic agents in a shorter period, however. The usefulness of inhaled steroids in the treatment of acute severe asthma is unproven.

Antibiotics

If there is evidence of bacterial infection or if there is a question of bacterial infection in life-threatening asthma, antibiotics should be used. Antibiotics are used frequently in asthma when no clear indication of infection exists; their excessive use has been partly responsible for the frequent sensitization of allergic patients to penicillin and other antibiotic and chemotherapeutic agents. One should remember these principles:

1. Asthma is frequently accompanied by patchy atelectasis, which is often misinterpreted as bronchopneumonia on x-ray study.
2. Leukocytosis of 15,000 cells/μl or even higher may be seen in severe asthma in the absence of demonstrable bacterial infection, particularly after epinephrine administration; it is not an indication *per se* for antibiotic therapy.
3. Sinusitis may precipitate asthma and, if present, should be treated with antibiotics.

Sedation

Sedatives to relieve anxiety have been grossly misused in asthma and have been responsible for the death of some asthmatics. Psychologic factors are undoubtedly significant in asthma and may in some instances precipitate or aggravate an asthmatic attack. Patients with asthma have good reason to be anxious; however, anxiety is usually secondary to hypoxemia rather than the cause of it.

Sedatives that depress the respiratory center, such as barbiturates, are contraindicated in asthma. Tranquilizers, particularly members of the phenothiazine group (e.g., chlorpromazine), should not be used because they depress respiration and bronchial reflexes, especially in the presence of hypoxemia. They also exert multiple effects on the central nervous system. The combination of adrenergic agents and phenothiazines may precipitate profound hypotension.

Expectoration

Plugging of large and small airways by thick, tenacious mucus is a characteristic and important component of the obstructive process in asthma; thus mucus removal is an essential aspect of therapy. Children with asthma rapidly learn that expectoration of mucus is difficult, and coughing is an uncomfortable and often futile exercise, best avoided if possible. Removal of mucus is facilitated by periodic stimulation of coughing and by systemic and local hydration through humidification to liquefy secretions.

Postural drainage is effective in promoting productive coughing and can be used every 2 to 4 hours according to the patient's tolerance. Postural drainage is not a useful procedure if the patient has significant bronchospasm and may even aggravate bronchospasm. Aerosolized adrenergic bronchodilators should be used before postural drainage.

Intravenous Beta-Adrenergic Therapy

Intravenous isoproterenol has been used successfully as an alternative to mechanical ventilation. The criteria for respiratory failure are those summarized by Rachelefsky (1979). Intravenous albuterol and terbutaline (Bohn et al., 1983; Van Renterghem et al., 1987) have also been used. Before such therapy or mechanical ventilation is considered, specialists who are experts in the treatment of severe asthma in children and the use of these therapeutic modalities should be involved in the patient's care.

Mechanical Ventilatory Assistance

Respiratory failure should be considered to be present when three or more of the following criteria are present:

1. Severe inspiratory retractions.
2. Barely audible inspiratory breath sounds.
3. Minimal thoracic movement with hyperinflation.
4. Depressed level of consciousness with decreased response to painful stimuli.
5. Cyanosis in 40% inspired oxygen.

In addition, the presence of a $Paco_2$ greater than 45 mm Hg and a rate of rise greater than 5 mm Hg/hour are indications for mechanical ventilatory assistance.

Other Diagnostic and Therapeutic Procedures

The following principles apply:

1. Blood gas and pH values should be monitored. Although patients survive most asthmatic attacks without benefit of blood gas monitoring, the severity of asthma and response to therapy are extremely difficult to judge on clinical grounds alone, even in the most experienced hands. Close monitoring of arterial blood gases and pH in a severely ill asthmatic patient may prove to be lifesaving. Alternatively, venous (not capillary) blood can be used for pH determinations and, if necessary, as an index of $Paco_2$.

2. A chest radiograph should be considered to exclude infection, pneumothorax, and large airway mucus plugging if the episode is severe or the response to therapy poor. Sinus radiographs should be considered.

3. Atropine sulfate, 1.0 to 2.0 mg by inhalation, or ipratropium (Atrovent), two to four inhalations, can be tried alone or with adrenergic drugs, every 4 to 8 hours. (This is not approved by the Food and Drug Administration for children under 12 years of age.)

4. As the patient improves, do not wean from therapy too rapidly.

5. Permit the patient to rest as much as possible.

6. The best treatment of severe asthmatic attacks is prevention. Treat asthma early and adequately. Identify and remove environmental allergens and irritants.

Complications

Asthma rarely results in bronchiectasis or emphysema. When these do occur, intercurrent lung infection or other chronic lung disease is probably responsible. However, atelectasis, pneumothorax, and bacterial respiratory infection may be complications of or associated with acute asthma.

Atelectasis ordinarily resolves spontaneously, even after many weeks of collapse. Asthma may result in chest deformity and, occasionally, short stature. Sudden death of unknown causes has also been reported in asthmatic children. Complications of long-term steroid therapy are many and include cushingoid appearance and growth retardation (Lieberman et al., 1972; Reimer et al., 1975). Improper use of other medications may result in aggravation of asthma and severe toxic reactions to the drugs themselves, including death (frequently caused by overuse of sedatives).

Although the complications of drug overuse must always be kept in mind, it is important to recognize the serious effects of inadequate pharmacologic therapy as well. Most deaths of patients with asthma are due to inadequate recognition and delayed or inadequate therapy by patients, parents, and physicians.

Pulmonary hypersensitivity to *Aspergillus* antigens can result in allergic bronchopulmonary aspergillosis (Kabalin and Greenberger, in press). The disease is more common in Great Britain than in the United States. The disease has features of immune involvement of IgE-mediated mechanisms as well as type II and type IV (Gell and Coombs, 1968) mechanisms. The source of the antigen is intrinsic, because the organism grows within the bronchial mucus. Systemic invasion by the organism does not occur. The tissue reaction may result in bronchiectasis of the proximal, medium-sized bronchi, usually with little involvement of the distal airways.

Clinically, the disorder may result in symptoms identical to those of other pneumonitic syndromes, but, in addition, wheezing with other evidence of bronchial obstruction is the rule. Cough with expectoration of thick, often brownish mucous plugs containing viable mycelia is noted. Eosinophilia of blood and sputum is common and often intense. Serum IgE levels usually are elevated, sometimes markedly.

Prognosis

It is commonly stated that children outgrow asthma, but more often it is the pediatrician rather than the asthma that a child outgrows (Levison et al., 1974; Pearlman, 1989). Most asthmatic children improve significantly by adulthood, usually at puberty, and some appear to become asthma-free for the remainder of their lives. In long-term follow-up studies, however, fewer than a third of all asthmatic children remain asymptomatic, even after a prolonged symptom-free interval (Ryssing, 1959), and there is increasing evidence that abnormalities in pulmonary function may persist in many individuals for years after the last asthmatic episode (Levison et al., 1974). Moreover, many asymptomatic adults who do not smoke but have a history of chronic or frequent asthma in childhood exhibit a significant degree of irreversible pulmonary obstruction. Asthmatic children subject to passive smoking at home may be at particularly increased risk (Woolcock et al., 1979). Thus, asthma is a chronic pulmonary disorder in which the tip of the pathologic iceberg may be visible only some of the time.

NON-ATOPIC ALLERGIC DISORDERS

Serum Sickness

At one time serum sickness was caused chiefly by the administration of horse antisera. With the increased use of antibiotics and the decreased use of animal antisera, however, the etiology of this disorder has been altered. Drugs, particularly penicillin, are now the leading causes of this disorder, although the use of horse-derived antilymphocyte globulin in transplantation procedures has also been associated with the development of serum sickness (Lawley et al., 1985). Nearly any foreign substance can cause this syndrome, the likelihood being related to the immunogenicity of the substance, the route of administration, and the amount of antigen given. Thus, drugs, insect bites or stings, vaccines, hyposensitization extracts, and perhaps foods may also cause serum sickness.

Etiology

Serum sickness is mainly a toxic immune complex disorder resulting from the deposition of circulating antigen-antibody aggregates in the blood vessels. The antigens are unrelated to the tissues in which they are deposited, and the tissues injured are thus innocent bystanders. Increased permeability of the vessels as a result of activation or release of vasoactive amines is necessary for localization of the complexes. There is experimental evidence that this is mediated by IgE antibody (Cochrane, 1971). Localized complement-fixing complexes (with IgG or IgM antibody) activate chemotactic factors, which attract neutrophil leukocytes, which are in turn responsible for a necrotizing vasculitis (Cochrane and Dixon, 1968; Lawley et al., 1985).

Any tissue may be affected, but the deposition of complexes in large arteries and kidney, joint, and heart tissues is especially common. The amount, molecular size, and duration in the circulation affect the severity and course of the illness. High concentrations of immune complexes present for a brief period ordinarily induce transient lesions that heal completely. Low levels of immune complexes for a longer duration may result in permanent lesions. The latter occur most frequently in collagen-vascular disorders, such as systemic lupus erythematosus.

Clinical Manifestations

Serum sickness appears clinically from 1 to 3 weeks, most commonly 7 to 10 days, after initial exposure to the sensitizing antigen. There is a shorter latent period (1 to 5 days) if sensitization has occurred previously. Skin rashes are common features of the syndrome, occurring in over 90% of the cases. They are usually urticarial but may also be maculopapular or take other forms. Itching is common and may precede the onset of the rash. Tender lymphadenopathy may appear initially in the drainage area of the injection site. Polyarthralgias occur in half the cases and joint effusions may develop, but overt arthritis is rare. Peripheral neuritis, especially of the brachial plexus, has been reported occasionally and may take the form of the Guillain-Barré syndrome.

Occasionally, central nervous system involvement may occur. Mild to moderate fever is frequently present. Headache, malaise, nausea and vomiting, and abdominal pain are common. Acute life-threatening allergic reactions, such as laryngeal edema, severe asthma, and anaphylactic shock, can occur and seem to be more common in individuals with atopic disorders.

Laboratory Findings

The blood count discloses an initial leukocytosis followed by leukopenia, the latter caused primarily by neutropenia. Eosinophilia may occur late in the disease, particularly during the recovery phase. Atypical lymphocytes and plasma cells may be observed in smears of peripheral blood. Examination of the urine may reveal albuminuria, hyaline casts, and a few red blood cells. Complement levels, characteristically low in the active phase of experimental acute serum sickness, are generally normal in human disease.

Diagnosis and Treatment

Diagnosis rests on the presence of the characteristic signs and symptoms, in addition to a history of exposure to a sensitizing substance at an appropriate preceding time. Treatment depends on the nature and severity of symptoms encountered. Aqueous epinephrine (1:1000) is the initial treatment for laryngeal edema, wheezing, and anaphylactic shock, as discussed elsewhere (see Anaphylactic Reactions).

Antihistamines are of use in controlling urticaria and itching. Ephedrine may also be used to control urticaria. Glucocorticoids may be helpful in controlling severe manifestations. These can be given for a few days and then stopped, thus avoiding the problems associated with long-term steroid use. Acetylsalicylic acid (ASA) is used to control joint symptoms. Serum sickness usually lasts only a few days, during which time elimination of the antigen from the body is occurring. If the disorder is prolonged, constant or repeated exposure to the inciting antigen may be taking place.

Course

The prognosis for patients with serum sickness is excellent, and complete recovery ensues in almost all instances. Serum sickness may recur if there is re-exposure to the same antigens; subsequent reactions may be more severe than the original one. In most cases of acute serum sickness, the causative antigen can be identified and avoided. Up-to-date immunizations are especially important for individuals with horse or horse serum sensitivity. Fortunately, except as noted for transplantation procedures, antisera derived from animals have largely been replaced by antisera of human origin. If there is a suggestive history of reactivity to a serum or drug and there is a need to use the serum or drug, skin testing should be done before its use. A negative skin reaction does not necessarily rule out the possibility of a systemic reaction, however.

Urticaria

Urticaria (hives) is a skin eruption commonly associated with allergic reactions and characterized by raised itchy wheals surrounded by erythema. The disorder is usually transient, and the eruption lasts a few minutes to several hours. The acute form is experienced eventually by about one of every four individuals and may occur at any age. Chronic urticaria (lasting or recurring for 6 weeks or more) is much less common and occurs more frequently in adults than in children. Urticaria is thought to occur more often in atopic individuals, but this is not well documented.

Pathology

The initial response in urticaria is erythema caused by dilation of small blood vessels in the dermis. Increased capillary permeability and transudation of fluid occurs, resulting in local edema, which appears as a pale swelling (the wheal). Secondary arteriolar dilatation around the edematous area (the flare) then occurs, by an axon reflex mechanism. Pruritus may precede the development of the erythema or wheals. The wheals vary in size from tiny swellings visible only on close examination to the confluent involvement of a large area of the body.

When the reaction occurs in the subcutaneous or submucosal tissues, it tends to be more diffuse and less erythematous. It may also be unaccompanied by itching, probably because of absence of the nerve receptors in subepidermal tissue. The term angioneurotic edema *(angioedema)* refers to this reaction in the deeper dermal and subcutaneous tissue. Urticaria and angioedema can occur together, or either may occur alone. Both are due to the same pathophysiology, but urticaria involves the superficial vessels whereas angioedema affects the deeper cutaneous blood vessels.

All of the features of an urticarial reaction can be reproduced locally by the injection of histamine into the skin, and histamine is thought to be the chief mediator of urticarial reactions (Kaplan et al., 1975). Kinins, acetylcholine, proteases, and other mediators may also be involved. Allergic mechanisms may cause urticaria or angioedema, but they are not the sole cause. The nonimmune release of histamine and other mediators by drugs, chemicals, physical factors, and psychogenic factors may initiate an urticarial reaction. Often, the cause of the reaction cannot be identified, especially in chronic urticaria, in which an etiologic agent is identified in fewer than half the cases.

Many patients with chronic urticaria appear to have autoantibodies to their activated high affinity receptors on skin mast cells and react with a wheal and flare to intradermal injection of autologous serum (Hide et al., 1993). Whatever the cause of chronic urticaria, once the condition arises, there appears to be a lower threshold for itch, wheal, and erythema formation, and various physical factors, such as pressure as well as some drugs (e.g., ASA), appear to precipitate or intensify the urticaria secondarily (Warin and Champion, 1974).

Etiology

Foods are among the chief etiologic agents; eggs, milk, wheat, shellfish, berries, cheese, nuts, and citrus fruits are the principal offenders. Drugs are common causes of urticaria, and ASA and penicillin are among the leading drug offenders. Several drugs induce allergic photosensitivity, which in turn causes urticaria (Epstein, 1972).

Infection with pyogenic bacteria and, less frequently, with viral or fungal agents may be associated with urticaria. Parasitic infestations, especially with roundworms or protozoa, can also cause urticaria. Injectable biologicals (vaccines, foreign antisera, allergenic extracts), contactants (animal saliva, chemicals, topical drugs), and inhalants (pollen, molds, house dust mites, animal emanations) may induce urticaria. Insect stings or bites cause local urticaria, but with severe hypersensitivity generalized urticaria can occur. Scabies infestation may be associated with various forms of eruption including urticaria.

Insects, particularly fleas, may cause a peculiar form of urticaria known as papular urticaria. In this disorder, lesions characteristically occur in crops on the extremities, particularly on extensor surfaces. The eruption begins as a wheal and erythema but progresses to the development of papules, the form in which the physician first sees the disorder.

Urticaria may be a manifestation of systemic disease, such as carcinoma, lymphoma or leukemia, systemic lupus erythematosus, periarteritis nodosa, rheumatoid arthritis, dermatomyositis, or liver disease, especially hepatitis or obstructive jaundice. Emotional stimuli may induce or intensify urticarial or angioedematous reactions and pruritus, but chronic urticaria is probably rarely (if ever) solely psychologic in origin. A hereditary abnormality of the complement system (hereditary angioneurotic edema) results in angioedema (see Chapter 17).

Physical factors, such as heat, cold, light, and pressure, have been implicated in the production of urticaria and other skin reactions; this reaction to physical factors is termed *physical allergy.* The role of allergic mechanisms in hypersensitivity to physical factors remains to be clarified. In some instances, sensitivity to the physical agent has been transferred to nonsensitive individuals by serum. Immunoglobulins may play a pathogenic role in some forms of cold-induced urticaria (Wanderer et al., 1971). A rare familial form of cold-induced urticaria presents with an erythematous maculopapular eruption associated with a burning rather than pruritic sensation (though pruritus can occur) and may be accompanied by fever and leukocytosis. Heat-induced (cholinergic) urticaria may be a particular problem in adolescence. (See Baer and Harber [1971] for a detailed consideration of hypersensitivities to physical factors; see Mathews [1980] and Warin and Champion [1974] for reviews of urticaria in general.)

Diagnosis

The diagnosis of urticaria and angioedema depends primarily on the appearance of the eruption. Angioedema usually affects the lips and eyelids and, to a lesser extent, the tongue and genitalia, but other parts of the body may also be affected. If it affects the larynx, it can be life-threatening. Rarely, angioneurotic edema may be confused with edema secondary to cardiac disease, renal disease, or myxedema. Urticaria may be a component of erythema multiforme and must be differentiated from urticaria pigmentosa.

Identification of causative factors rests mainly on a history of contact with a known or suspected sensitizing substance. Skin testing may be used as an aid in implicating possible allergens, but it is rarely diagnostic. Elimination diets and provocative tests with suspected offenders may be helpful, but the latter should not be done if symptoms are severe. Parasitic infestation or other infections should be excluded.

Treatment

The most effective treatment is avoidance of the substance responsible for the reaction. ASA-containing products should be avoided. When foods or drugs are identified as problems, the patient should be informed of hidden sources of these substances. Infections and parasitic infestations should be treated. Protective clothing, sunscreen preparations, and limitation of exposure to cold or sunlight are important in cold or solar urticaria.

Various drugs help to control urticaria and angioedema; their use in severe reactions may be lifesaving. Epinephrine is the most potent and the drug of choice in controlling life-threatening angioedema and severe urticaria. The use of aqueous epinephrine results in rapid reversal of symptoms. Its short duration of action may be prolonged by using a long-acting preparation such as Sus-Phrine.

Antihistamines, hydroxyzine, and diphenhydramine, for example, are also valuable in acute urticaria; they are less successful in chronic urticaria. In chronic urticaria not controlled by classic H_1 antihistamines (hydroxyzine is the first choice), H_2 antihistamines (cimetidine or ranitidine) can be added. Oral ephedrine may be used with antihistamines if the latter do not control symptoms by themselves. Cyproheptadine is especially effective in some patients with cold urticaria.

Adrenal steroids are not particularly useful in acute urticaria, and their effectiveness in chronic urticaria is not well documented. However, their effectiveness in some patients with urticaria is striking, and in resistant chronic urticaria a therapeutic trial with steroids may be justified. Treatment of subjects with autoimmune urticaria who do not respond to antihistamines and

steroids is experimental. The use of cyclosporine at a dose of 2.5 mg/kg appears to help about half of these patients (Barlow et al., 1993).

Urticaria and angioedema (except hereditary angioedema) are ordinarily more bothersome than serious and are usually transient problems. Occasionally, urticaria recurs over a period of months or years, but even in most of these individuals it eventually disappears.

Hypersensitivity Pneumonitis

Hypersensitivity pneumonitis (HP), or *extrinsic allergic alveolitis*, is a pulmonary and constitutional illness that results from hypersensitivity to a variety of inhaled allergens (Table 20–5). Although HP is multicausal, the clinical, immunologic, and pathophysiologic findings are similar regardless of the etiology. This disorder is also discussed in Chapter 22.

Historical Aspects

Hypersensitivity pneumonitis was first reported in 1713 by Ramazani, who described a pneumonia-like illness in individuals working with shell grains that were not properly dried before storage. The classical description of farmer's lung disease was published in 1932 (Campbell, 1932); however, only since 1941 has a reaction to other organic dusts has been noted, and this entity has become well known. Most of the studies of this disease are related to adults who have been exposed to various etiologic agents in their job. More cases are now being recognized in children as a result of their hobbies, exposure to home humidifying systems, and even inhaled medications.

Clinical Manifestations

Hypersensitivity pneumonitis can occur as an acute, intermittent, systemic, and respiratory illness or as an insidious chronic progressive pulmonary disease. In the acute form, symptoms consist of chills, fever, malaise, cough, and dyspnea. Symptoms or signs are frequently mistaken for those of infectious pneumonitis. Acute reactions may resolve within 12 to 18 hours after contact but may occasionally persist for several days unless terminated by corticosteroid therapy.

In the insidious form, prolonged and continued exposure to the offending dust may result in coughing and dyspnea, which may progress without the cycle of exacerbation and alleviation seen in the acute form. Symptoms may consist of dyspnea on exertion, anorexia, weight loss, and fatigue, often without fever. Positive physical findings may be limited to fine basilar rales and, rarely, clubbing of the fingers. In children, the insidious form is marked by dramatic weight loss, thought by some to be related to malabsorption and steatorrhea associated with duodenal reaction to swallowing the causative antigen.

Laboratory Findings

In the acute form of hypersensitivity pneumonitis, the patient may have leukocytosis, a count as high as

Table 20–5. Causes of Hypersensitivity Pneumonitis (HP)

Antigen	Name	Mode of Exposure
Thermophilic antigen		
Actinomyces	Farmer's lung	Moldy hay
	Bagassosis	Moldy sugarcane
	Fog fever	Cattle
	Mushroom lung	Moldy compost
	Humidifier lung (some cases)	Air conditioning, humidifiers
Other fungal antigens		
Aspergillus clavatus	Cheese washer's lung	Moldy cheese
Penicillium casei	Cheese worker's lung	Cheese mold
Merulius lacrymans	Dry rot HP	Moldy moist wood
Aspergilllus sp.	Malt worker's lung	Moldy malt and barley dust
Cryptostroma corticale	Maple bark lung	Moldy maple bark
Mucor stolonifer	Paprika slicer's lung	Moldy paprika pods
Pullularia	Sauna taker's disease	Contaminated water
Pullularia/graphium	Sequoiosis	Moldy redwood dust
Cephalosporium	Sewer water HP	Sewer water home flood
Penicillium frequentans	Suberosis	Moldy cork
Other antigens		
Avian serum proteins	Bird breeder's disease	Bird droppings (parrot, parakeet, dove, pigeon)
Streptomyces albus	Dirt HP	Processed dirt
Duck proteins	Duck fever	Feathers
Chicken proteins	Plucker's lung	Chicken processing
Gerbil proteins	Gerbil lung	Gerbil excreta
Amebae	Humidifier fever	Contaminated water
Toluene diisocyanate	TDI disease	Plastics industry
Bovine and porcine proteins	Pituitary snuff disease	Pituitary powder
Porcine proteins	Pancreatic powder lung	Enzyme replacement in cystic fibrosis
Pyrethrum	Pyrethrum HP	Insecticide
Rat serum proteins	Rat lung	Rat excreta
Turkey proteins	Turkey handler's lung	Turkey droppings
Unknown antigens	Coffee worker's lung	Coffee dust
	Coptic lung	Cloth wrappings of mummies
	Grain measurer's lung	Cereal grains
	Tap water disease	Contaminated tap water
	Tea grower's lung	Tea leaves
	Thatched roof lung	Thatch or contaminants
	Tobacco grower's lung	Tobacco leaves
	Air conditioner lung (some cases)	Air conditioning or humidification systems
	Wood dust disease	Sawdust

Abbreviations: TDI = toluene diisocyanate.
Modified from Schatz M, Patterson R. Hypersensitivity pneumonitis—general considerations. Clin Rev Allergy 1:451–467, 1983.

25,000 cells/μl, with a predominance of polymorphonuclear leukocytes (PMNs) with or without eosinophilia. The chest radiograph shows a diffuse interstitial infiltrate with fine reticular densities, multiple small nodules, and patchy infiltrates at the lung bases. In the chronic form, diffuse interstitial fibrosis with coarsening of the bronchovascular markings and contraction of lung tissue is seen. Hyperinflation is uncommon in adults but may occur in children.

Pulmonary function tests in general show restrictive impairment of pulmonary function with reduced forced vital capacity (FVC) but a normal FEV_1/FVC ratio. Increased stiffness of the lung with decreased compliance in the chronic phase of the disease may be accompanied by alveolar capillary blockage with reduced gas transfer and diminished carbon monoxide diffusion. Functional residual capacity and total lung capacity are low. Arterial blood gases reveal diminished arterial partial pressure of oxygen (Pa_{O_2}), decreased oxygen saturation, and diminished arterial partial pressure of carbon dioxide (Pa_{CO_2}). FEV_1 and other flow rates are usually normal unless the patient has significant bronchiolitis or superimposed asthma, much more common in children than in adults.

Skin testing with a suspected antigen may result in an Arthus-type skin reaction with a maximum reaction appearing at 24 to 48 hours. Serum precipitating antibodies to the suspected antigens are frequently found by gel diffusion but are not diagnostic because they may occur in the absence of the disease. Patients with farmer's lung disease, for instance, have been found to have a broad immune response with elevated specific antibodies to a variety of respiratory viruses and *Mycoplasma*, which may indicate either wide antigenic exposure or unknown peculiarities in host responsiveness. Serum complement has been reported to be decreased in asymptomatic individuals but normal in symptomatic patients with pigeon breeder's disease who underwent inhalation challenge with pigeon antigens. Peripheral blood lymphocytes from patients with hypersensitivity pneumonitis undergo proliferation and release macrophage migration inhibition factor when cultured in vitro with appropriate fungal or avian antigens. In contrast, lymphocytes from asymptomatic individuals do not react in this manner, even though they may have serum precipitating antibodies to these antigens.

Diagnosis and Treatment

A diagnosis of hypersensitivity pneumonitis is based on the history and physical and laboratory findings. A provocative natural or laboratory challenge with a suspected antigen may be necessary. Treatment consists of eliminating the antigen from the patient's environment, which may necessitate changing one's job or home location. In patients with severe involvement, corticosteroids may be needed for several months until pulmonary function is stable.

Syndromes of Pulmonary Eosinophilia

Pulmonary infiltrations associated with blood or pulmonary eosinophilia or both and presumed therefore to be caused by allergic reactions have been described (Lecks and Kravis, 1969; Liebow and Carrington, 1969; Rosenow, 1972). (See Chapter 22.) Pulmonary infiltration with eosinophilia (PIE) includes a heterogeneous group of reactions, including bronchial asthma, collagen-vascular disease, and idiopathic PIE syndromes. In general, these syndromes are clinically mild and transient. Unusual reactions to drugs (especially nitrofurantoin, sulfonamides, and penicillin), pollens, and roundworms (for example, *Ascaris*) may result in densities on chest radiographs, eosinophilia, and cough (this is often termed Löffler's syndrome).

Physical Features

Physical findings are minimal and may consist of only a few crepitant rales. Lung biopsy reveals patchy bronchopneumonic foci with small areas of alveolar exudate containing many eosinophils. The syndrome usually lasts no more than 3 or 4 weeks; occasionally it is more prolonged.

Treatment and Prognosis

Treatment consists of limiting exposure to the offending antigen, but adrenal steroids are useful in severe forms of eosinophilic pneumonitis.

The prognosis is generally excellent and pulmonary residua are uncommon. In some instances, the problem can be prolonged; however, and especially in tropical eosinophilia caused by infestation with filariae, progression to granuloma formation and pulmonary fibrosis occurs (McNanty and Nutman, 1993). (See Chapter 22.)

Contact Dermatitis

Allergic contact dermatitis is an inflammatory response of the skin based on delayed-type hypersensitivity mechanisms, resulting from contact between the skin and sensitizing allergen (see Chapter 21). The skin serves both as the site of reaction and as the route by which sensitization occurs. The reaction is usually confined to the area exposed directly to the allergen. Because sensitization is generalized, regardless of the particular location of the skin in which sensitization occurred, subsequent contact with any skin area results in a reaction. Moreover, in sensitized individuals, dermatitis can be induced systemically by ingestion of the allergen (Baer and Leider, 1949).

In mild reactions, erythema with papulation is observed. In more severe reactions, vesiculation with denudation and weeping is observed. In acute reactions, there is a sharp demarcation between involved and uninvolved skin. In chronic reactions, the skin is erythematous, thickened, and scaly, with a poor demarcation between involved and uninvolved skin. Pruritus is characteristic and often intense.

In a previously sensitized individual, contact with the allergen usually leads to a response within 24 to 48 hours, occasionally within 12 hours after exposure. The course of the reaction depends on the degree of sensitization and the intensity and duration of the reexposure. A mild or moderate reaction to a single exposure may subside completely within a few days, whereas a severe reaction may last 2 to 3 weeks. With continued allergen exposure, a reaction may last indefinitely.

Sensitization may develop as early as 7 to 10 days after contact with an allergen or only after repeated contact for weeks or years. The ease with which sensitization develops varies according to the nature of the contactant involved. Some substances, such as oleoresins and *Rhus* antigens from poison ivy or oak, are potent sensitizers effective in most individuals; others are weak and sensitize only a few individuals. After sensitization occurs, it lasts indefinitely, although the degree may diminish with time in the absence of further allergen contact. The capacity to develop contact sensitivity occurs in fetal life, increases in infancy, stabilizes in childhood, and wanes in late adult life.

ADVERSE DRUG REACTIONS

Allergic reactions or pseudoallergic reactions to drugs represent some 3% to 25% of overall adverse drug reactions (Mathews, 1984). Drug *allergy* refers to adverse drug reactions that are immunologically mediated; *pseudoallergic* reactions denote reactions that simulate drug allergy in their manifestation but are not initiated by a demonstrable drug-derived antigen and an antibody or sensitized cells. Numerous agents in addition to IgE can induce mast cells and basophils to release mediators, resulting in reactions ranging from urticaria to generalized systemic reactions. Table 20–6 classifies allergic and pseudoallergic drug reactions.

The management of adverse drug reactions involve early recognition and appropriate therapy. Life-threatening reactions, such as acute systemic anaphylaxis, must be recognized and treated promptly. The most common cause of drug-induced anaphylaxis is penicillin, although a variety of other antibiotics, certain egg-based vaccines (measles-mumps-rubella and in-

Table 20–6. Allergic and Pseudoallergic Drug Reactions

Anaphylaxis
Cutaneous: urticaria, angioedema, contact dermatitis, photodermatitis, purpura, exfoliative dermatitis, maculopapular eruptions, Stevens-Johnson syndrome, erythema nodosum
Respiratory: asthma, hypersensitivity pneumonitis, rhinosinusitis, pulmonary infiltrates with eosinophilia
Hematologic: thrombocytopenia, agranulocytosis, hemolytic anemia
Hypersensitivity vasculitis and serum sickness
Liver disease: hepatitis granulomas
Renal disease
Drug-induced systemic lupus erythematosus
Other: drug fever, lymphadenopathy, eosinophilia

Modified from Mathews KP. Clinical spectrum of allergic and pseudoallergic drug reactions. J Allergy Clin Immunol 74:558–566, 1984.

fluenza), and other protein-containing drugs can lead to IgE sensitization. The management of anaphylaxis has been reviewed earlier (see Anaphylactic Reactions).

Serum sickness–like reactions to a new drug, by contrast, usually occur 7 to 10 days, or later, after the initiation of drug therapy. If the agent has been used previously, a serum sickness–like reaction may occur within hours to days after readministration of the drug. Although penicillin is the most common cause, cefaclor and sulfonamides can also induce serum sickness–like reactions. Other drug reactions—such as rash, destruction of formed elements of the blood, drug fever, vasculitis, and specific organ involvement (e.g., liver, kidney, and lungs)—must be suspected and differentiated from a manifestation of the underlying disease.

Therapy for drug reactions involves:

1. Stopping the drug.
2. Suppressing unpleasant symptoms (e.g., with antihistamines for pruritus or urticaria and topical steroids for contact dermatitis).
3. Counteracting the reaction (e.g., with systemic corticosteroids for generalized exfoliative dermatitis or Coombs-positive hemolytic anemia).
4. Medical supportive measures (e.g., dialysis for acute renal shutdown until kidney function returns).

Confirmation by laboratory tests depends on the type of reaction and the organ system(s) involved. Skin tests are useful for IgE-mediated reactions, such as for predicting penicillin allergy (discussed later), and allergy to egg-based vaccines and other protein-containing drugs. Skin testing is not useful for predicting allergic reactions to other antibiotics or other non–protein-containing drugs. Other laboratory tests include a complete blood count, total eosinophil count, a Coombs' test for a patient with anemia, or an antinuclear antibody test for a patient who is taking a drug known to induce systemic lupus erythematosus. Patch testing may be useful in identifying the cause of a contact dermatitis, but it must be done with great caution because it can exacerbate a healing contact dermatitis. When a drug must be used for which there is no substitute, cautious readministration may be the only method of determining drug allergy or tolerance. If such a challenge is to be undertaken, the patient and family must first be informed of the risk involved and then the test carried out in a setting with appropriate emergency equipment to treat severe adverse reactions. If a trial test proves negative, the physician should still use great caution in proceeding with therapy.

With an established history of drug allergy, avoidance of all substances that may cross-react with the offending drug is essential. The patient and the patient's family must be informed of the type of reaction to expect, other substances that may cross-react with the drug, and the risk of re-exposure. The patient should also be given identification, such as a Medic Alert bracelet, so that others will be alerted to the problem in an emergency bracelet.* The patient's medical records should be labeled prominently with the drug to which the patient is allergic.

Penicillin Reactions

Penicillin and its semisynthetic derivatives remain the drugs of choice in many pediatric infections because of their wide margin of safety, even in high dosages. The actual incidence of allergic reactions in children is unknown, although in adults it appears to be between 1% and 2% (Adkinson, 1984).

Classification

Penicillin reactions can be classified as acute explosive or anaphylactic, occurring minutes after penicillin administration; accelerated reactions, manifested primarily by urticaria and occurring hours after administration; and late-onset reactions, occurring days to weeks after therapy. Late-onset reactions may range from serum sickness–like reactions to drug fever or eosinophilia. Most of the semisynthetic penicillins produce reactions similar to those to penicillin. The two exceptions appear to be ampicillin and amoxicillin, which can induce nonimmune maculopapular rashes, and methicillin, which can induce toxic renal damage.

Diagnosis

Penicillin allergy can be predicted by skin testing of penicillin and its major and minor breakdown products. Penicillin is degraded primarily (95%) to the penicilloyl moiety, the so-called major determinant, and a minor amount is degraded to benzyl penilloate and benzyl penicilloate, to so-called minor determinants. The major determinant is available for skin testing as a synthetic hapten, penicilloyl-polylysine. However, the minor determinants, which are the main causes of acute anaphylaxis, are not yet commercially available, although clinical trials leading to their marketing are under way. A positive skin test reaction to penicillin or the major or minor determinants suggests that the patient may have a clinical reaction if given penicillin. Negative tests indicate that a penicillin reaction is un-

---

*Medic Alert Foundation, P.O. Box 1009, Turlock, CA 95380.

likely. Ampicillin or amoxicillin allergy may be associated with a delayed skin test reaction to these drugs, which correlates with clinical reaction to challenge (Bierman et al., 1972).

There appears to be a small but significant likelihood of cross-reactivity between penicillins and cephalosporins. Therefore, patients with penicillin allergy should be given cephalosporins with caution.

Radiocontrast Media Reactions

Radiocontrast media (RCM) can be associated with anaphylactoid (allergic-like) reactions (urticaria, wheezing, dyspnea, hypotension, or shock) or vasomotor reactions (nausea, vomiting, flushing, or warmth). Occasional fatalities have occurred. Although statistics are not available for the frequency of such reactions in pediatrics, approximately 1.6% of adults who receive intravenous infusions of radiocontrast media may experience reactions that require emergency treatment. The incidence of reactions in patients who have had an initial reaction range from 36% to 60%. Infusions of radiocontrast media can cause rises in plasma histamine and complement and kinin activation. The mechanism of reaction is not clear but may involve complement activation.

In patients who have had prior reactions, administration of prednisone at 12 hours, 7 hours, and 1 hour before the procedure along with 50 mg of diphenhydramine and 25 mg of ephedrine 1 hour before the procedure has reduced the reaction rate to 3% (Greenberger and Patterson, 1991). Results of skin testing do not predict the patient at risk for a reaction.

Aspirin and Nonsteroidal Anti-Inflammatory Drug Reactions

Urticaria or angioedema in reaction to acetylsalicylic acid (ASA) and related nonsteroidal anti-inflammatory drugs (NSAIDs) has long been known. ASA and NSAID hypersensitivity manifested as bronchospasm (sometimes extremely severe) has also been reported, usually in adults but more recently in children. A triad of nasal polyposis, severe ASA-induced bronchospasm, and rhinitis with sinusitis is recognized. The cause of this ASA hypersensitivity is unknown, but it does not appear to be of immune (allergic) origin (Samter and Beers, 1968; Samter, 1973).

Various hypotheses have been advanced to explain the mechanism of ASA and NSAID hypersensitivity:

1. Cyclooxygenase blockade with diversion of arachidonate into the lipogenase pathway.
2. Mast cell discharge through a non-IgE mechanism.
3. Complement consumption with formation of C3a.
4. Activation of the complement system with formation of kinins.
5. A biochemical abnormality of connective tissue.
6. ASA-induced alteration of immunoglobulins.

There are two main forms of ASA hypersensitivity:

- Rhinitis with urticaria and/or angioedema, associated with nasal polyposis in a minority of these patients
- Bronchospasm associated with nasal polyposis in approximately 30% to 40% of the patients in some series (Stevenson, 1984)

In the bronchospastic form, ASA-induced rhinitis and/or urticaria or angioedema may also occur. Characteristically, at least in older children and adults, females are affected more commonly than males, and there is little association with allergic disorders (Falliers, 1973; Stevenson and Mathison, 1985).

In the bronchospastic form, the onsets of ASA sensitivity and nonallergic asthma tend to coincide, usually occurring in late childhood or adulthood, in contrast to the generally earlier onset of allergic asthma. Tartrazine (FD&C Yellow Dye No. 5) sensitivity may also be associated with ASA hypersensitivity, but the reported incidence has varied from less than 5% to more than 80% of ASA-sensitive patients.

Patients can be desensitized with ASA and NSAIDs. Such desensitization may improve the associated rhinosinusitis but does not alter bronchial hyperreactivity. To maintain this desensitized state, the patient must take ASA or NSAIDs daily. Otherwise, full sensitivity returns in 7 days (Manning and Stevenson, 1991).

Reactions to Food and Drug Additives

Sulfites are widely used as food and drug preservatives and antioxidants in drugs. Six patients with asthma had severe life-threatening reactions after restaurant meals and were subsequently shown to have asthma by double-blind challenge with potassium metabisulfite (Stevenson and Simon, 1981). Since then, acute asthma has been documented with bronchodilator solutions, epinephrine, local anesthetics, corticosteroids, antibiotics, analgesics, and eyedrops that contain sulfites (Simon, 1984). Preliminary studies suggest that these reactions may be mediated through the mast cell (Sprenger et al., 1989).

References

Adinoff AD, Tellez P, Clark RAF. Atopic dermatitis and aeroallergen contact sensitivity. J Allergy Clin Immunol 81:736–742, 1988.

Adkinson NF Jr. Risk factors for drug allergy. J Allergy Clin Immunol 74:567–572, 1984.

Atkins PC, Wasserman SI. Chemotactic mediators. Clin Rev Allergy 1:358–395, 1983.

Austen KF, Orange RP. Bronchial asthma: the possible role of chemical mediators of immediate hypersensitivity in the pathogenesis of subacute chronic disease. Am Rev Respir Dis 112:423–436, 1975.

Baer RL, Harber LC. Reactions to light, heat, and trauma. In Samter M, ed. Immunological Diseases, 2nd ed. Boston, Little, Brown, 1971, pp. 973–984.

Baer RL, Ledier M. The effects of feeding certified food azo dyes in paraphenylenediamine-hypersensitive subjects. J Invest Dermatol 13:223–232, 1949.

Barlow RJ, Black AK, Greaves MW. Treatment of severe chronic urticaria with cyclosporin A. Eur J Dermatol 3:273–275, 1993.

Beall GN. Urticaria: a review of laboratory and clinical observations. Medicine (Baltimore) 43:131–151, 1964.

Benveniste J, Egido J, Gutierrec-Millet V. Evidence for the involvement of the IgE basophil system in acute serum sickness. Clin Exp Immunol 26:449–454, 1976.

Bierman CW. Adrenergic drugs. Clin Rev Allergy 1:87–104, 1983.

Bierman CW, Pierson WE, Zeitz SJ, Hoffman LS, VanArsdel PP Jr. Reaction associated with ampicillin allergy. JAMA 220:1098–1100, 1972.

Bierman CW, Maxwell D, Rytina E, Emanuel MB, Lee TH. Effect of H_1 receptor blockade on late cutaneous reactions to antigen: a double-blind controlled study. J Allergy Clin Immunol 87:1013–1019, 1991.

Bluestone CD. Eustachian tube dysfunction: physiology, pathophysiology, and role of allergy in pathogenesis of otitis media. J Allergy Clin Immunol 72:242–251, 1983.

Bohn D, Kalloghlian A, Jenkins J. Intravenous salbutamol in the treatment of status asthmaticus in children. Crit Care Med 12:392–396, 1983.

Boushey HA, Holtzman MJ, Sheller JR, Adele JA. Bronchial hyperreactivity. Am Rev Respir Dis 121:389–413, 1980.

Bruijnzeel PL, Warringa RA, Kok PT, Kreukniet J. Inhibition of neutrophil and eosinophil induced chemotaxis by nedocromil sodium and sodium cromoglycate. Br J Pharmacol 99:798–802, 1990.

Buckley JM, Pearlman DS. Controlling the environment. In Bierman CW, Pearlman DS, eds. Allergic Diseases from Infancy to Childhood, 2nd ed. Philadelphia, WB Saunders, 1988, pp. 239–252.

Buckley RH, Wray BB, Belmaker EZ. Extreme hyperimmunoglobulinemia E and undue susceptibility to infection. Pediatrics 49:59–70, 1972.

Campbell JM. Acute symptoms following work with hay. Br Med J 2:1143–1144, 1932.

Christiansen SC, Proud D, Cochrane CG. Detection of tissue kallikrein in the bronchoalveolar lavage fluid of asthmatic subjects. J Clin Invest 79:188–197, 1987.

Coca AF, Cooke RA. On the classification of the phenomena of hypersensitiveness. J Immunol 8:163–182, 1923.

Cochrane CG. Mechanisms involved in the deposition of immune complexes in tissues. J Exp Med 134:75–89, 1971.

Cochrane CG, Dixon FJ. Cell and tissue damage through antigen-antibody complexes. In Miescher PA, Müller-Eberhard HJ, eds. Textbook of Immunopathology. New York, Grune & Stratton, 1968, pp. 94–110.

Cockroft, DW. Mechanism of perennial allergic asthma. Lancet 2:253–255, 1983.

Cockroft DW, Ruffin RE, Dolovich J, Hargreave FE. Allergen-induced increase in non-allergic bronchial reactivity. Clin Allergy 7:503–513, 1977.

Committee Report. Task Force on Allergic Reactions to Latex. J Allergy Clin Immunol 92:16–18, 1993.

Connell JT. Quantitative intranasal pollen challenge. II. Effect of daily pollen challenge, environmental pollen exposure, and placebo challenge on the nasal membrane. J Allergy 41:123–139, 1968.

Corrigan CA, Kay AB. Lymphocytes. In Middleton E Jr, Reed CE, Ellis EF, et al, eds. Allergy, Principles and Practice, 4th ed. St. Louis, CV Mosby, 1993, pp. 206–211.

Cuss FM, Dixon CM, Barnes PJ. Effects of inhaled platelet activating factor on bronchial responsiveness in man. Lancet 2:189–192, 1986.

Davis A, Vickerson F, Worsley G, Mindorff C, Kazim F, Levison H. Determination of dose-response relationship for nebulized ipratropium in asthmatic children. J Pediatr 105:1002–1005, 1984.

Demopoulos CA, Pinkard RN, Hanahan DJ: Platelet-activating factor: evidence for 1-O-alkyl-2-acetyl-sn-glyceryl-3-phosphorylcholine as the active component. J Biol Chem 254:935–939, 1979.

Eady RP. Pharmacology of nedocromil sodium. Eur J Respir Dis 69(Suppl. 147):112–119, 1986.

Edelson JD, Rebuck AS. The clinical assessment of asthma. Arch Intern Med 145:321–323, 1985.

Ellis EF. Asthma in infancy and childhood. In Middleton RJ, Reed CE, Ellis EF, et al, eds. Allergy, Principles and Practice, 4th ed. St. Louis, CV Mosby, 1993, pp. 1225–1262.

Epstein JH. Photoallergy. Arch Dermatol 106:741–748, 1972.

Falliers CJ. Aspirin and subtypes of asthma: risk factor analysis. J Allergy Clin Immunol 52:141–147, 1973.

Falliers CJ. Cromolyn sodium (disodium cromoglycate) prophylaxis (review). Pediatr Clin North Am 22:141–146, 1975.

FDA Panel Report on Allergenic Extracts. Fed Reg 50:3082, 1985.

Fink JN. Hypersensitivity pneumonitis. In Middleton RJ, Reed CE, Ellis EF, et al., eds. Allergy, Principles and Practice, 4th ed. St. Louis, CV Mosby, 1993, pp. 1415–1431.

Foreman JC, Pearce FL. Cromolyn and nedocromil. In Middleton E Jr, Reed CE, Ellis EF, et al., eds. Allergy, Principles and Practice, 4th ed. St. Louis, Mosby–Year Book, 1993, pp. 926–940.

Franklin W, Lowell FC. Comparison of two dosages of ragweed extract in the treatment of pollenosis. JAMA 201:915–917, 1967.

Frew AJ, Kay AB. The relationship between infiltrating $CD4^+$ lymphocytes, activated eosinophils and the magnitude of the allergen-induced late phase cutaneous reaction. J Immunol 141:4158–4164, 1988.

Fujimura M, Sasaki F, Nakatsumi Y, Takahashi Y, Hifumi S, Taga K, Mifune J, Tanaka T, Matsuda T. Effects of thromboxane synthetase inhibitor (OKY-046) and a lypoxygenase inhibitor (AA-861) on bronchial responsiveness to acetylcholine in asthmatic subjects. Thorax 41:955–959, 1986.

Fuller RW, Dixon CM, Dollery CT, Barnes PJ. Prostaglandin D_2 potentiates airway responses to histamine and methacholine. Am Rev Respir Dis 133:252–254, 1986.

Gell PGH, Coombs RRA. Clinical Aspects of Immunology, 2nd ed. Philadelphia, FA Davis, 1968.

Georg J. The treatment of status asthmaticus. Allergy 36:219–232, 1981.

Gergen PJ, Mullally DI, Evans R III. National survey of prevalence of asthma among children in the United States, 1976 to 1980. Pediatrics 81:1–7, 1988.

Gleich GJ, Adolphson CR, Leiferman RL. Eosinophils. In Gallin JI, Goldstein IM, Snyderman R, eds. Inflammation: Basic Principles and Clinical Correlates. New York, Raven, 1992, pp. 663–700.

Godfrey S. The place of a new aerosol steroid, beclomethasone dipropionate, in the management of childhood asthma. Pediatr Clin North Am 22:147–155, 1975.

Gold WM. Vagally mediated reflex bronchoconstriction in allergic asthma. Chest 63(Suppl.):11S, 1973.

Greenberger PA, Patterson R. The prevention of immediate generalized reactions to radiocontrast media in high risk patients. J Allergy Clin Immunol 87:867–872, 1991.

Grzanna R, Schultz LD. The contribution of mast cells to the histamine content of the central nervous system: a regional analysis. Life Sci 30:1959–1964, 1982.

Hide M, Francis DM, Grattan CE, Hakimi J, Kochan JP, Greaves MW. Autoantibodies against the high-affinity IgE receptor as a cause of histamine release in chronic urticaria. N Engl J Med 328:1599–1604, 1993.

Hill HR, Ochs HD, Quie PG, Clark RA, Pabst HF, Klebanoff SJ, Wedgwood RJ. Defect in neutrophil granulocyte chemotaxis in Job's syndrome of recurrent "cold" staphylococcal abscesses. Lancet 42:617–619, 1974.

Huang SK, Marsh DG. Immunogenesis of allergic diseases. In Middleton E Jr, Reed CE, Ellis EF, Adkinson NF Jr, Yunginger JW, Busse WW, eds. Allergy: Principles and Practice, 4th ed. St. Louis, CV Mosby, 1993, pp. 60–72.

Huggins KG, Brostoff J. Local production of specific IgE antibodies in allergic rhinitis patients with negative skin tests. Lancet 2:148–150, 1975.

International Consensus Report on Diagnosis and Treatment of Asthma. Bethesda, Md., National Heart, Lung, and Blood Institute publication 92-3091, National Institutes of Health, 1992.

Irani AA, Schwartz LB. Neutral proteases as indicators of human mast cell heterogeneity. Monogr Allergy 27:146–162, 1990.

Ishizaka K, Ishizaka I. Identification of IgE antibodies as a carrier of reaginic activity. J Immunol 99:1187–1198, 1967.

Jacobs RL, Freedman PM, Boswell RN. Nonallergic rhinitis with eosinophilia (NARES syndrome). J Allergy Clin Immunol 67:253–262, 1981.

Johnstone DE. Comparative value of hyposensitization and symptomatic therapy in pollenosis in children. NY J Med 60:1448–1451, 1960.

Johnstone DE, Dutton AM. Dietary prophylaxis of allergic disease in children. N Engl J Med 274:715–719, 1966.

Kabalin CS, Greenberger PA. Allergic bronchopulmonary aspergillosis. In Bierman CW, Pearlman DS, Busse WW, Shapiro GC, eds. Allergy, Clinical Immunology and Asthma. Management in Infants, Children and Adults, 3rd ed. Philadelphia, WB Saunders (in press).

Kahn G. Eczematoid eruptions in children. Pediatr Clin North Am 22:203–215, 1975.

Kaliner M, Austen KF. Immunologic release of chemical mediators from human tissues. Annu Rev Pharmacol 15:177–189, 1975.

Kaliner MA. Hypotheses on the contribution of late phase allergic responses to the understanding and treatment of allergic diseases. J Allergy Clin Immunol 73:311–315, 1984.

Kaplan AP, Austen KF. Activation and control mechanisms of Hageman factor–dependent pathways of coagulation, fibrinolysis, and kinin generation and their contribution to the inflammatory response. J Allergy Clin Immunol 56:491–506, 1975.

Kaplan AP, Gray L, Shaff RE, Horakova Z, Beaven MA. In vivo studies in mediator release in cold urticaria and cholinergic urticaria. J Allergy Clin Immunol 55:394–402, 1975.

Kelly K, Sitlock M, Davis JP. Anaphylactic reactions during general anesthesia among pediatric patients. United States, January 1990–1991. MMWR 40:437–443, 1991.

Kraemer MJ, Richardson MA, Weiss NS, Furukawa CT, Shapiro GG, Pierson WE, Bierman OW. Risk factors for persistent middle ear effusions. Recurrent otitis, nasal congestion, atopy and cigarette smoke. JAMA 249:1022–1025, 1983.

Lam S, Tan F, Chan H, Chan-Yeung M. Relationship between types of asthmatic reaction, nonspecific bronchial reactivity, and specific IgE antibodies in patients with red cedar asthma. J Allergy Clin Immunol 72:134–139, 1983.

Lawley TJ, Bielory L, Gascon P, Yancey KB, Young NS, Frank MM. A prospective clinical and immunological analysis of patients with serum sickness. N Engl J Med 311:1407–1413, 1985.

Lecks HI, Kravis LP. The allergist and the eosinophil. Pediatr Clin North Am 16:125–148, 1969.

Lee TH, O'Hickey SP. Exercise-induced asthma and late phase reactions. Eur Respir J 2:195–197, 1989.

Leung DYM. Immunopathology of atopic dermatitis. Springer Semin Immunopathol 13:427–440, 1992.

Levison H, Collins-Williams C, Bryan AC, Reilly BJ, Orange RP. Asthma: current concepts. Pediatr Clin North Am 21:957–965, 1974.

Lichtenstein LM, Norman PS, Winkenwerder WL. Clinical and in vitro studies on the role of immunotherapy in ragweed hay fever. Am J Med 44:514–524, 1968.

Lichtenstein LM, Valentine MD, Norman PS. A re-evaluation of immunotherapy for asthma (editorial). Am Rev Respir Dis 129:657–659, 1984.

Lieberman P, Patterson P, Kunske R. Complications of long-term steroid therapy for asthma. J Allergy Clin Immunol 49:329–336, 1972.

Lieberman P, Patterson R. Immunotherapy for atopic disease. Adv Intern Med 19:391–411, 1974.

Liebow AA, Carrington CB. The eosinophilic pneumonias. Medicine (Baltimore) 48:257–285, 1969.

Manning ME, Stevenson DD. Aspirin sensitivity: a distressing reaction that is now often treatable. Postgrad Med 90:227–233, 1991.

Marquardt DL. Histamine. Clin Rev Allergy 1:343–351, 1983.

Marsh DG. Allergens and the genetics of allergy. In Sela M, ed. The Antigens. Vol. 3. New York, Academic Press, 1975, pp. 271–359.

Mathews KP. Management of urticaria and angioedema. J Allergy Clin Immunol 66:347–357, 1980.

Mathews KP. Clinical spectrum of allergic and pseudoallergic drug reactions. J Allergy Clin Immunol 74:558–566, 1984.

McFadden ER Jr. The chronicity of acute attacks of asthma—mechanical and therapeutic implications. J Allergy Clin Immunol 56:18–26, 1975.

McFadden ER Jr. Asthma: pathophysiology. Semin Respir Med 1:297–303, 1980.

McIntosh K, Ellis EF, Hoffman LS, Lybass TB, Eller JJ, Fulginiti VA. The association of viral and bacterial respiratory infections with exacerbations of wheezing in young asthmatic children. J Pediatr 82:578–590, 1973.

McLaughlan P, Stanworth DR, Webster ADB, Asherson GL. Serum IgE in immune deficiency disorders. Clin Exp Immunol 16:375–381, 1974.

McNanty S, Nutman TB. Eosinophilia and eosinophil-related disorder. In Middleton E Jr, Reed CE, Ellis EF, et al, eds. Allergy,

Principles and Practice, 4th ed. St. Louis, CV Mosby, 1993, pp. 1081–1085.

Metcalfe DD. Effector cell heterogeneity in immediate hypersensitivity reactions. Clin Rev Allergy 1:311–325, 1983.

Metcalfe DD. Food hypersensitivity. J Allergy Clin Immunol 73:749–762, 1984.

Mosmann TR, Coffman RL: T$_H$1 and T$_H$2 cells: different patterns of lymphokine secretion lead to different functional properties. Ann Rev Immunol 7:145–152, 1989.

National Asthma Education Program (NAEP). Expert Panel Report. Guidelines for the Diagnosis and Management of Asthma. Bethesda, Md., National Heart, Lung, and Blood Institute publication 91-3042, National Institutes of Health, 1991.

Norman PS. An overview of immunotherapy: implications for the future. J Allergy Clin Immunol 65:87–96, 1980.

O'Flaherty JT, Hammett MJ, Shewmake TB, Wykle RL, Love SH, McCall CE, Thomas MJ. Evidence for 5,12-dihydroxy-6,8,10,14-eicosatetraenoate as a mediator of human neutrophil aggregation. Biochem Biophys Res Commun 103:552–558, 1981.

O'Flaherty JT, Wykle RL. Biology and biochemistry of platelet activating factor. Clin Rev Allergy 1:353–367, 1983.

Orgel HA. Genetic and developmental aspects of IgE. Pediatr Clin North Am 22:17–32, 1975.

Parish WE. Short-term anaphylactic IgG antibodies in human sera. Lancet 2:591–592, 1970.

Paton WDM. Histamine release by compounds of simple chemical structure. Pharmacol Rev 9:269–328, 1957.

Pattemore PK, Johnston SL, Bardin PG. Viruses as precipitants of asthma symptoms. I. Epidemiology. Clin Exp Allergy 22:325–336, 1992.

Pearlman DS. Immunoglobulins and allergic disease. Pediatr Clin North Am 16:109–123, 1969.

Pearlman DS. Immunologic basis of allergic disease. In Kagan BM, Stiehm ER, eds. Immunologic Incompetence. Chicago, Year Book Medical, 1971, pp. 345–355.

Pearlman DS. Rationale for therapy of allergic disorders. Pediatr Clin North Am 22:101–110, 1975.

Pearlman DS. Antihistamines: pharmacology and clinical use. Drugs 12:258–273, 1976.

Pearlman DS. Bronchial asthma. A perspective from childhood to adulthood. Am J Dis Child 138:459–466, 1984a.

Pearlman DS. Chronic rhinitis in children. Clin Rev Allergy 2:197–211, 1984b.

Pearlman DS. Bronchial asthma: a perspective from childhood through adulthood—update. Pediatr Asthma Allergy Immunol 3:191–205, 1989.

Pipcorn U, Karlsson G, Enerback L. Cellular response of the human allergic nasal mucosa to natural allergy exposure. J Allergy Clin Immunol 82:1046–1054, 1988.

Portier P, Richet C. De l'action anaphylactique de certaines venins. C R Soc Biol (Paris) 54:170–172, 1902.

Position Statement. Inhaled β$_2$-adrenergic agonists in asthma. American Academy of Allergy and Immunology Committee on Drugs. News & Notes 2):11–13, 1991.

Prausnitz C, Küstner H. Studien über überempfindlichkeit. Zentralbl Bakteriol Abt 1 Orig 86:160–169, 1921.

Rachelefsky GS. New drugs in the treatment of asthma. Pediatr Update 1:303–328, 1979.

Ramazani: De morbis artificim Distriba, 1713. Chicago, University of Chicago Press, 1930.

Reimer LG, Morris HG, Ellis EF. Growth of asthmatic children during treatment with alternate day steroids. J Allergy Clin Immunol 55:224–231, 1975.

Rosenow EC III. The spectrum of drug-induced pulmonary disease. Ann Intern Med 77:977–991, 1972.

Rostenberg A Jr, Solomon LM. Atopic dermatitis and infantile eczema. In Samter M, ed. Immunological Diseases. Boston, Little, Brown, 1971, pp. 920–935.

Ryssing E. Continued follow-up investigation concerning the fate of 298 asthmatic children. Acta Paediatr 48:255–260, 1959.

Sadan N, Rhyne MB, Mellits ED, Goldstein EO, Levy DA, Lichtenstein LM. Immunotherapy of pollenosis in children. N Engl J Med 280:623–627, 1969.

Sampson HA. Role of immediate food hypersensitivity in the pathogenesis of atopic dermatitis. J Allergy Clin Immunol 71:473–480, 1983.

Sampson HA. Immunologically mediated adverse reactions to foods:

role of T cells and cutaneous reactions. Ann Allergy 53:472–475, 1984.

Sampson HA. Atopic dermatitis. Ann Allergy 69:469–479, 1992.

Sampson HA, Broadbent KR, Bernhisel-Broadbent J. Spontaneous release of histamine from basophils and histamine-releasing factor in patients with atopic dermatitis and food allergy. N Engl J Med 321:229–232, 1989.

Samter M. Intolerance to aspirin. Hosp Pract 8(12):85–90, 1973.

Samter M, Beers RR Jr. Intolerance to aspirin. Clinical studies and consideration of pathogenesis. Ann Intern Med 68:975–983, 1968.

Schayer RW. Induced synthesis of histamine, microcirculatory regulation and the mechanism of action of the adrenal glucocorticoid hormones. Prog Allergy 7:187–212, 1963.

Schleimer RP, MacGlashan DW Jr, Schulman ES, Peters SP, Adams GK III, Adkinson NF Jr, Lichtenstein LM. Human mast cells and basophils—structure, function, pharmacology and biochemistry. Clin Rev Allergy 1:327–341, 1983.

Schuberth, KC, Lichtenstein LM, Kagey-Sobotka A, Szklo M, Kwiterouich KA, Valentine MD. Epidemiologic study of insect allergy in children. 2. Effect of accidental stings on allergic children. J Pediatr 102:361–365, 1983.

Sheffer AL. Anaphylaxis. J Allergy Clin Immunol 75:227–233, 1985.

Sheffer AL, Austen KF. Exercise induced anaphylaxis. J Allergy Clin Immunol 66:106–111, 1980.

Sheffer AL, Fonferko EB, Murphy GF, Austen KF. Ultrastructural changes of cutaneous mast cells (MC) in response to defined stimuli of the physical allergy class. J Allergy Clin Immunol 75:114, 1985.

Simon RA. Adverse reactions to drug additives. J Allergy Clin Immunol 74:623–630, 1984.

Simons FER, Simons KJ. Pharmacokinetic optimization of histamine H_1 receptor antagonist therapy. Clin Pharmacokinet 21:372–393, 1991.

Spector SL. Exercise-induced bronchospasm: mechanisms and management. J Respir Dis 13(Suppl.):S7–S13, 1992.

Spector SL, Garza-Gomez MG. Dose-response effects of albuterol aerosol compared with isoproterenol and placebo aerosols. J Allergy Clin Immunol 59:280–286, 1977.

Speight ANP, Lee DA, Hey EN. Underdiagnosis and undertreatment of asthma in childhood. Br Med J 286:1253–1256, 1983.

Sprenger, JD, Altman LC, Marshall SG, Pierson WE, Koenig JQ. Studies of neutrophil chemotactic factor of anaphylaxis in metabisulfite sensitivity. Ann Allergy 62:117–121, 1989.

Stanworth DR, Smith AK. Inhibition of reagin-mediated PCA reactions in baboons by the human IgG-4 sub-class. Clin Allergy 3:37–41, 1973.

Stenson WF, Parker CW. Metabolites of arachidonic acid. Clin Rev Allergy 1:369–384, 1983.

Stevenson DD. Diagnosis, prevention and treatment of adverse reactions to aspirin and non-steroidal anti-inflammatory drugs. J Allergy Clin Immunol 74:617–622, 1984.

Stevenson DD, Simon RA. Sensitivity to ingested metabisulfites in asthma subjects. J Allergy Clin Immunol 68:26–32, 1981.

Stevenson DD, Mathison DA. Aspirin sensitivity in asthmatics. When may this drug be safe? Postgrad Med 78:111–113, 116–119, 1985.

Sulzberger MB, Frick OL. Atopic dermatitis. In Fitzpatrick TB et al., eds. Dermatology in General Medicine. New York, McGraw-Hill, 1971, pp. 680–696.

Szentivanyi A. The beta adrenergic theory of the atopic abnormality in bronchial asthma. J Allergy 42:203–232, 1968.

Terr AI. Unconventional theories and unproven methods in allergy. In Middleton E Jr, Reed CE, Ellis EF, et al, eds. Allergy, Principles and Practice, 4th ed. St. Louis, CV Mosby, 1993, pp. 1767–1793.

Tinkelman DG, Reed CE, Nelson HS, Offord KP. Aerosol beclomethasone dipropionate compared with theophylline as primary treatment of chronic mild to moderately severe asthma in children. Pediatrics 92:64–77, 1993.

Toogood JH. Complications of topical steroid therapy for asthma. Am Rev Respir Dis 141:S89–S96, 1990.

Van Metre TE Jr, Adkinson NF Jr, Amodio FJ, Kagey-Sobotka A, Lichtenstein LM, Mardiney MR Jr, Norman PS, Rosenberg GL. A comparison of immunotherapy schedules for injection treatment of ragweed pollen hay fever. J Allergy Clin Immunol 69:181–193, 1982.

Van Renterghem D, Lamont H, Elinck W, Pauwels R, Van der Straeten M. Intravenous versus nebulized terbutaline in patients with acute severe asthma: a double-blind randomized study. Ann Allergy 59:313–316, 1987.

Vogt W. Activation, activities and pharmacologically active products of complement. Pharmacol Rev 26:125–169, 1974.

von Pirquet G. Allergie. Muench Med Wochenschr 53:1457, 1906.

von Pirquet CF, Schick B. Die Serumkrankenheit. Vienna, Verlag Franz Deuticke, 1905. (Schick B, trans. Baltimore, Williams & Wilkins, 1951.)

Wanderer A, Maseli R, Ellis EF, Ishizaka K. Immunologic characterization of serum factors responsible for cold urticaria. J Allergy 48:13–22, 1971.

Warin RP, Champion RH. Urticaria. Philadelphia, WB Saunders, 1974.

Weinberger M, Hendeles L. Pharmacologic management. In Bierman CW, Pearlman DS, eds. Allergic Diseases from Infancy to Childhood, 2nd ed. Philadelphia, WB Saunders, 1988, pp. 253–258.

Weiner N. Atropine, scopolamine, and related antimuscarinic drugs. In Gilman AG, Goodman LS, Gilman A, eds. The Pharmacologic Basis of Therapeutics, 6th ed. New York, Macmillan, 1980, pp. 120–137.

Welliver RC, Wong DT, Sun M, Middleton E Jr, Vaughan RS, Ogra PL. The development of respiratory virus–specific IgE and the release of histamine in nasopharyngeal secretions after infection. N Engl J Med 305:841–846, 1981.

Wilhelm DL. Kinins in human disease. Annu Rev Med 22:63–84, 1971.

Williams HB, McNicol KN. Prevalence, natural history and relationship of wheezy bronchitis and asthma in children: an epidemiological study. Br Med J 2:321–325, 1969.

Wolfe JD, Yamate M, Biedermann AA, Chu TJ. Comparison of the acute cardiopulmonary effects of oral albuterol, metaproterenol and terbutaline in asthmatics. JAMA 253:2068–2072, 1985.

Woolcock AJ, Leeder SR, Peat JK, Blackburn CRB. The influence of lower respiratory illness in infancy and childhood and subsequent cigarette smoking on lung function in Sydney school children. Am Rev Respir Dis 120:5–14, 1979.

Yunginger JW, Gleich GJ. The impact of the discovery of IgE on the practice of allergy. Pediatr Clin North Am 22:3–15, 1975.

Chapter 21

Dermatologic Disorders

Lynne Morrison and Jon M. Hanifin

The entities discussed in this chapter are diverse and include:

1. Autoimmune disorders such as immunologically mediated blistering skin diseases and lupus erythematosus (LE).

2. Reactive erythemas, which are cutaneous reactions secondary to a variety of antigenic stimuli.

3. Figurate erythemas such as erythema multiforme (EM), a morphologically defined group of reactive lesions with an annular appearance.

4. Henoch-Schönlein purpura (HSP).

5. Hypersensitivity dermatitis, including both atopic and allergic contact dermatitis.

6. Psoriasis.

The skin manifestations of primary immunodeficiency diseases are discussed in chapters dealing with those disorders. Although cutaneous lupus is discussed here, skin manifestations of other collagen-vascular diseases are covered elsewhere. By far the most common of the diseases covered in this chapter is atopic dermatitis. Henoch-Schönlein purpura and erythema multiforme minor are fairly common but are not seen with the frequency of atopic dermatitis, and the remaining diseases are considered uncommon to rare.

Because of the diversity of this group of skin disorders, there are no unifying historical or laboratory features that suggest a diagnosis of an immunologically mediated disease. The diagnosis frequently rests on recognition of the individual morphologic features of the various dermatoses as well as histologic findings. In the immunologically mediated blistering skin diseases, immunohistology is essential in establishing a correct diagnosis.

Again, because of the wide range of entities considered here, the therapies vary widely and can range from simple observation in neonatal lupus with only skin findings or mild Henoch-Schönlein purpura to systemic corticosteroids in bullous diseases.

In general, many of the diseases discussed here are cutaneous reactions to an inciting allergen, and identification and elimination of the allergen are of prime importance. This consideration applies to allergic contact dermatitis, reactive erythemas such as erythema multiforme, figurate erythemas, and Henoch-Schönlein purpura. Avoidance of exacerbating environmental agents is of great importance in managing atopic dermatitis. Therapeutic control of the skin eruption often involves but is not limited to topical corticosteroids. Therapy for psoriasis includes ultraviolet light, topical corticosteroids, tar, topical calcipotriol, and anthralin. Systemic therapy is generally required for the bullous diseases. Both dermatitis herpetiformis and linear immunoglobulin A (IgA)/bullous dermatosis are treated with dapsone, and pemphigus and bullous pemphigoid are most often treated with systemic corticosteroids. Dapsone and tetracycline (in appropriately aged children) are alternatives to corticosteroids in bullous pemphigoid.

IMMUNOBULLOUS DISEASES

Dermatitis Herpetiformis

Dermatitis herpetiformis (DH) is an intensely pruritic, chronic, papulovesicular eruption with a characteristic distribution involving extensor surfaces. Histologically, it is characterized by subepidermal blister formation with infiltration of neutrophils in the papillary tips. Because the clinical and histologic findings can overlap those of other immunologically mediated blistering diseases, direct immunofluorescence (IF) studies of perilesional skin are most reliable for diagnosing dermatitis herpetiformis (Zone, 1991; McCord and Hall, 1993). The characteristic direct immunofluorescence features of dermatitis herpetiformis demonstrate granular deposition of IgA in the papillary tips or continuously beneath the basement membrane zone.

The disease usually occurs between the third and fifth decades, but cases of juvenile dermatitis herpetiformis have been reported. The exact prevalence in the pediatric age group is hard to determine, because the disease was confused with linear IgA/bullous dermatosis until direct immunofluorescence studies were routinely performed in these patients. Some authors consider that juvenile dermatitis herpetiformis is rare.

History

The initial description of dermatitis herpetiformis is generally attributed to Dr. Louis Duhring in 1884. Over the next 80 years, the clinical description was refined, the histopathologic features were described, systemic ingestion of iodide was found to exacerbate the eruption, and a favorable response to sulfapyridine was noted. An association with gluten-sensitive enteropathy was first described by Marks and colleagues in 1966, and gluten sensitivity is now thought to play a role in the pathogenesis of dermatitis herpetiformis. In 1971 Cormane and Gianetti recognized the presence of immunoglobulins in the skin, suggesting an immune pathogenesis. Since then, the granular deposition of IgA in the papillary tips has become the diagnostic hallmark of dermatitis herpetiformis and a focus of investigation. A strong association with human leukocyte antigen B8 (HLA-B8), HLA-DR3, and HLA-DQ2 was recognized in the mid-1970s, indicating a genetic basis for an immune disorder (McCord and Hall, 1993).

Clinical Features

Dermatitis herpetiformis in children occurs most frequently between 2 and 7 years of age. The cutaneous eruption in children is similar to that in adults, with red papules or papulovesicles and an intense burning or stinging itch that leads to rapid excoriation of lesions. The lesions are often grouped and distributed symmetrically over extensor areas including elbows, knees, buttocks, upper back, posterior neck, and scalp (Fig. 21–1). Small hemorrhagic papules and vesicles of the palms and soles are present in the majority of patients (Rabinowitz and Esterly, 1993). Mucous membrane involvement rarely occurs.

Gluten-sensitive enteropathy has been found in 75% to 90% of children with dermatitis herpetiformis (Zone, 1991; Rabinowitz and Esterly, 1993). Signs of malabsorption are not usually present in children with the disease, but some may have chronic diarrhea and anemia. A gluten-free diet can induce remission of both the gastrointestinal and cutaneous lesions.

Pathogenesis

The strong association between gluten ingestion and the skin eruptions suggests an as yet obscure patho-

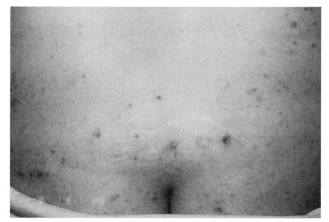

Figure 21–1. Excoriated lesions with typical extensor distribution in a patient with dermatitis herpetiformis. Although the primary lesions are vesicopapules, the patient may present with excoriated lesions because of the intense pruritus.

genic relationship with the intestinal abnormality. Gluten may act as an antigen that stimulates circulating or local IgA antibodies, which bind to the skin as cross-reacting antibodies or as immune complexes. Alternatively, a gluten-induced intestinal defect may allow passage of other dietary antigens that initiate the development of circulating IgA antibodies, which subsequently bind to the skin (Zone, 1991, 1993).

Diagnosis

Clinical and routine histologic features overlap those of other immunologically mediated vesicobullous dermatoses such as linear IgA/bullous dermatosis, bullous pemphigoid, or epidermolysis bullosa acquisita. Accurate diagnosis necessitates direct immunofluorescence studies of biopsy specimens, which show granular deposition of IgA in dermal papillary tips (Fig. 21–2). The biopsy specimen for immunofluorescence must be from perilesional skin of typically affected areas.

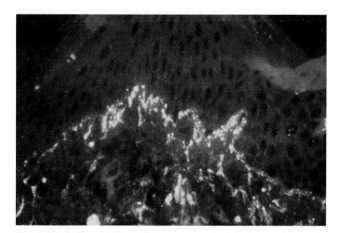

Figure 21–2. Direct immunofluorescence of a biopsy specimen of a patient with dermatitis herpetiformis showing the characteristic granular deposition of IgA in the dermal papillary tips.

Treatment and Prognosis

Institution of a gluten-free diet can lead to complete control of skin disease and reversal of intestinal abnormalities. This treatment requires strict adherence and patience, because 1 to 2 years of a gluten-free diet may be needed to obtain control (Zone, 1991; Rabinowitz and Esterly, 1993).

Alternatively, dapsone at a dose of 1.5 to 2 mg/kg/day is effective and usually controls the symptoms and eruption within a few days of beginning therapy (Rabinowitz and Esterly, 1993). A combination of dapsone and a gluten-free diet may be used with either a decrease in or discontinuance of the dapsone as the dietary regimen takes effect. Side effects of dapsone include a dose-related hemolytic anemia, methemoglobinemia, and rare idiosyncratic effects including agranulocytosis, neuropathy, and toxic hepatitis.

Typically, dermatitis herpetiformis in the adult population is a lifelong disease with treatment-free remissions occurring in under 1% of patients. Although the long-term prognosis for children is not clear, it is best to consider juvenile DH a lifelong disease.

Linear IgA/Bullous Dermatosis of Childhood

Linear IgA/bullous dermatosis (LABD), also known as *chronic bullous disease of childhood*, is a blistering cutaneous eruption that usually presents in preschool children. It is self-limited but lasts several years. The characteristic finding is the linear deposition of IgA along the basement membrane by immunofluorescence studies of perilesional skin (Marsden, 1990). The exact incidence and prevalence of LABD are not known because of its rarity. Cases are reported in both black and white children and the frequency is the same in females and males.

History

LABD was initially considered a variant of dermatitis herpetiformis because of shared histologic features. However, it has now been clearly differentiated from the latter, based on the linear IgA deposition in immunofluorescence studies, absence of gluten-sensitive enteropathy, and HLA typing differences (McCord and Hall, 1993; Smith and Zone, 1993).

Clinical Features

Patients have large, tense bullae, which may be clear or hemorrhagic. The bullae can arise on either normal skin or pre-existing urticarial lesions. Sites of predilection are the lower abdomen, genital area, and buttocks, as well as the face and scalp. Other characteristic features include clustering of blisters and annular configurations of blisters encircling a crusted healing lesion, referred to as a "crown of jewels" or "rosette" (McCord and Hall, 1993; Rabinowitz and Esterly, 1993). The eruption may be mildly to markedly pruritic (Fig. 21–3).

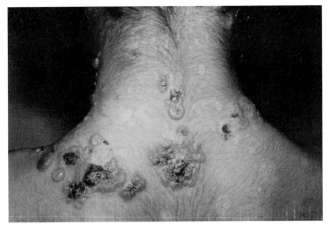

Figure 21–3. Tense blisters with an annular configuration in a patient with linear IgA/bullous dermatosis.

Mucous membrane involvement is relatively common, in contrast to the situation in dermatitis herpetiformis. Oral and ocular lesions are noted in a significant number of patients, and conjunctival scarring has been identified. Patients do not have an associated gluten-sensitive enteropathy, in contrast to those with childhood dermatitis herpetiformis. Some, but not all, studies suggest that there may be an increased frequency of HLA-B8 in these patients, but there is no increased frequency of HLA-R3 and HLA-DQ2 as there is in dermatitis herpetiformis (McCord and Hall, 1993; Rabinowitz and Esterly, 1993).

Pathogenesis

LABD is thought to be an autoimmune process mediated by IgA autoantibodies directed against a basement membrane antigen of skin. Immunoelectron microscopy reveals two patterns of IgA deposition: one with immunoglobulin deposition in the sub–lamina densa and the other with deposition of immunoglobulin within the lamina lucida (Rabinowitz and Esterly, 1993; Smith and Zone, 1993). There are no clinical differences related to the two immunoelectron microscopic findings. It was originally proposed that LABD was simply bullous pemphigoid mediated by IgA rather than an immunoglobulin G (IgG) antibody to the bullous pemphigoid antigen. However, the IgA autoantibody from patients with the lamina lucida type of LABD reacts with a 97-kD antigen that is different from the 180- and 230-kD bullous pemphigoid antigen.

Diagnosis

Clinically, LABD has a heterogeneous presentation and may be confused with other immunologically mediated blistering skin diseases such as bullous pemphigoid or dermatitis herpetiformis. Occasionally, when mucous membrane changes predominate, the disease can resemble cicatricial pemphigoid. Histology shows a subepidermal blister with a neutrophilic infiltrate, often indistinguishable from findings in dermatitis herpetiformis. Direct immunofluorescence studies are diagnostic and the most reliable means of establishing a diagnosis (Marsden, 1990; Rabinowitz and Esterly, 1993; Smith and Zone, 1993). The characteristic finding is linear deposition of IgA along the basement membrane zone of perilesional skin. In addition, a circulating IgA anti–basement membrane zone antibody is present in serum from 31% to 72% of patients.

Treatment and Prognosis

Patients usually respond to dapsone in doses of 1.5 to 2.0 mg/kg/day. If improvement is not satisfactory, addition of either sulfapyridine or small amounts of systemic corticosteroids may be helpful. Topical steroids are generally ineffective. Topical antipruritics or systemic antihistamines may provide symptomatic relief. LABD is a self-limited disease, usually resolving after 2 to 3 years.

Other Rare Bullous Diseases

Pemphigus Vulgaris

There are three immunobullous diseases that usually occur in adults but occasionally are seen in children. Pemphigus vulgaris (PV) is a serious chronic, intraepidermal bullous dermatosis with autoantibodies directed against antigens on the surface of epidermal cells. It affects both the mucosa and skin, producing flaccid blisters that may be limited in extent or generalized with large areas of denuded skin. Patients with active pemphigus vulgaris typically have a positive Nikolsky sign (i.e., generation of a blister by displacement of perilesional skin by friction). Patients with widespread disease are subject to fluid and electrolyte imbalances, are susceptible to cutaneous and systemic infection, and often require inpatient management. The presentation in children does not differ significantly from that in adults; however, diagnosis in children has been delayed for months to years because the index of suspicion is low for pemphigus in a young child. Pemphigus vulgaris should be included in the differential diagnosis in children with chronic mucous membrane erosions.

Biopsy specimens of oral or cutaneous bullae or erosions characteristically show suprabasilar acantholysis, a diagnostic pathologic finding in pemphigus. Direct immunofluorescence shows deposition of both IgG and C3 in the epidermal intercellular spaces. Furthermore, circulating autoantibodies are detected in the majority of patients.

Management of the disease depends on the degree of severity. Mild localized lesions may respond to topical corticosteroids; however, more severe disease necessitates the use of systemic corticosteroids.

Bullous Pemphigoid

Bullous pemphigoid (BP) is an autoimmune bullous disorder characterized by tense subepidermal blisters and typically occurs in the elderly population. Childhood cases are rare, but the disorder has been reported in infants 2 months of age. Most childhood cases occur before 8 years of age. Bullous pemphigoid is manifest as tense blisters arising either on an urticarial base or on normal skin. The blisters heal without scarring. Clinical features of the disease are similar in adults and children. Mucous membrane lesions are more common in children. Lesions of the palms and soles may occur in children less than 1 year of age (Rabinowitz and Esterly, 1993). Histologically, subepidermal blister formation with a dermal inflammatory infiltrate heavily mixed with eosinophils is seen. Direct immunofluorescence shows linear deposition of IgG and C3 on the basement membrane. As with pemphigus, systemic corticosteroids are often necessary. Sulfones, such as dapsone and sulfapyridine, are alternatives.

Epidermolysis Bullosa Acquisita

Epidermolysis bullosa acquisita (EBA) is another subepidermal blistering disease that usually occurs in adults. However, several well-documented cases in children have been reported (Rabinowitz and Esterly, 1993). Cases beginning in children as young as 3 months of age have been noted.

Epidermolysis bullosa acquisita, like pemphigus and bullous pemphigoid, is an autoimmune disorder thought to be mediated by antibodies to type VII collagen. The cutaneous eruption classically presents as noninflammatory blistering with skin fragility. The blisters and erosions, which are usually localized to acral and extensor surfaces, heal with atrophic scarring and milia. Nail dystrophy and scarring alopecia may also occur. The similarity of epidermolysis bullosa acquisita to inherited epidermolysis bullosa accounts for its name.

Affected children, like affected adults, are found by routine histologic examination to have subepidermal blister formation with a dermal inflammatory infiltrate significantly mixed with neutrophils. Direct immunofluorescence shows linear deposition of IgG along the basement membrane, as found in bullous pemphigoid; indirect immunofluorescence on salt split-skin substrates can help differentiate the two diseases.

Epidermolysis bullosa acquisita in adults is generally refractory to therapy. In contrast, the childhood disease responds fairly well to the combination of prednisone and dapsone (Rabinowitz and Esterly, 1993). The prognosis for these children is not known.

LUPUS ERYTHEMATOSUS

Cutaneous Lupus Erythematosus

The cutaneous manifestations of lupus erythematosus (LE) can be classified clinically into various forms, including (1) acute cutaneous lupus; (2) chronic cutaneous lupus, also referred to as discoid LE; (3) subacute cutaneous LE; and (4) neonatal LE (Rothfield, 1993). Acute cutaneous lupus is similar in adults and children and is associated with active systemic lupus. The systemic manifestations usually overshadow the cutaneous changes. The most characteristic feature is the facial butterfly erythema; however, similar changes may extend to the upper extremities and trunk. These changes are typically transient and improve as the systemic disease is brought under control (see Chapter 24).

The most common form of chronic cutaneous lupus erythematosus is discoid lupus erythematosus (DLE). Other variants include lupus panniculitis and hypertrophic discoid lupus erythematosus. The cutaneous findings in children and adults are similar (Hurwitz, 1981). Red papules and plaques with scaling and prominent follicular hyperkeratosis occur. The lesions expand and heal with central scarring and pigmentary change and, when present in the scalp, can lead to permanent alopecia. They are mostly distributed over the face, scalp, and ears. Discoid lupus erythematosus can be confused with polymorphous light eruption, lymphocytic infiltrate of Jessner, rosacea, sarcoid, granuloma faciale, and lichen planus. A cutaneous biopsy is helpful in establishing the diagnosis.

Chronic cutaneous lupus can occur as an isolated manifestation of lupus erythematosus or as one feature of the systemic disease. Only 5% of adults with discoid lupus develop systemic disease, whereas in children there is a greater tendency for systemic involvement (George and Tunnessen, 1993). Other features unique to childhood discoid lupus erythematosus are lack of female preponderance and lower incidence of photosensitivity.

Subacute cutaneous lupus erythematosus (SCLE) is a recently recognized entity that presents as either papulosquamous or annular lesions with a prominent photodistribution (Lee, 1993). The lesions, in contrast to those in discoid lupus, do not scar. Most patients with subacute cutaneous lupus have relatively mild systemic involvement, and the skin disease is the greatest problem.

Neonatal Lupus Erythematosus

Neonatal lupus erythematosus (NLE) is an uncommon autoimmune disease occurring in the neonatal period in which the major findings are nonscarring skin lesions and congenital heart block (see Chapter 24). Mothers of infants with neonatal lupus usually have anti–Ro/SS-A autoantibodies that cross the placenta into the infant and contribute to the pathogenesis of the disease (Watson and Provost, 1987).

History

McCuistion and Schoch (1954) first reported lupus erythematosus in a newborn and hypothesized that a maternal factor passing transplacentally caused the eruption. In the early 1980s, Weston and colleagues (1982) identified the anti–Ro/SS-A autoantibody as a serologic marker of neonatal lupus erythematosus. Subsequently, it was recognized that many infants with congenital heart block had anti–Ro/SS-A autoantibodies.

Clinical Manifestations

About half of the infants with neonatal lupus erythematosus have cutaneous lesions and half have congenital heart block, but rarely do the two occur together. Liver disease and thrombocytopenia with petechiae or purpura are uncommon features. Liver disease and thrombocytopenia are generally not present at birth but develop a few weeks after birth and resolve within a few more weeks.

The cutaneous lesions are scaling, erythematous plaques and patches that lack the follicular plugging of discoid lupus erythematosus. They resolve without scarring or atrophy but may show residual hypopigmentation. The lesions are most often distributed over the face and scalp, particularly in periorbital and forehead areas, and are commonly exacerbated by sunlight. Less often, they occur in photoprotected areas such as the diaper area. Lesions are transient, typically appearing several weeks after birth or, less often, at birth, and resolve by 6 months of age (McCuistion and Schoch, 1954). Postinflammatory hypopigmentation may take months to resolve, and, occasionally, persistent telangiectasias have been observed.

Complete heart block in neonatal lupus erythematosus begins during gestation as early as the sixteenth week (Watson and Provost, 1987; Lee, 1993). Although other cardiac problems are not usually present, patent ductus arteriosus has been reported in a few cases. Suspicion of heart block might arise during a routine obstetric examination with detection of a slow fetal heart rate. Diagnosis of heart block can be confirmed by fetal ultrasonography. The heart block is due to fibrosis and calcification of the conduction system that involves the atrioventricular node and also affects the sinoatrial node in some cases. Because the pathologic change is fibrosis, the heart block is generally permanent.

Pathogenesis

Several observations support the hypothesis that anti–Ro/SS-A autoantibodies are involved in the pathogenesis of neonatal lupus erythematosus (Lee, 1993). First, these autoantibodies are regularly present in the serum of mothers of babies with neonatal lupus. Second, these IgG autoantibodies can pass through the placenta and into the child's serum. Third, the infant's skin lesions begin to resolve as the maternal autoantibodies diminish and disappear. Furthermore, IgG antibodies have been shown to be present in neonatal lupus lesions. Particulate deposits of IgG have been demonstrated in the epidermis in skin lesions and in the conduction system in myocardium of affected cardiac tissue. A similar pattern was demonstrated in human skin grafted to immunodeficient mice after passive transfer of both serum from mothers of infants with neonatal lupus and purified Ro autoantibodies, suggesting that the particulate deposits of IgG are due to anti–Ro/SS-A autoantibodies.

It is not clear why some infants develop skin disease and others present only with cardiac disease. The antibody specificities in these two groups are not significantly different. Genetic factors may play a role in the disease. The mothers of infants with neonatal lupus have an increased incidence of HLA-B8 and HLA-DR3 antigens. Sex steroids may be important because cutaneous lesions of neonatal lupus erythematosus occur three times more commonly in female than in male infants. Of interest, there is no sexual predilection for the heart block.

Sun exposure may potentiate or initiate the skin lesions but is not essential, because they occur in photoprotected areas and at birth.

Diagnosis

Clinical findings, serologic findings, skin biopsy results, and cardiac evaluation are all important in establishing a diagnosis of neonatal lupus erythematosus. If a diagnosis of neonatal lupus is suspected, the sera of mother and infant should be evaluated for autoantibodies. In about 95% of the cases, anti–Ro/SS-A autoantibodies are detected (Watson and Provost, 1987; Lee, 1993). Anti–La/SS-B antibodies are also present in many patients. A few patients with only anti–U$_1$-RNP autoantibodies have been reported. Characteristic clinical findings in association with the presence of either anti–Ro/SS-A, anti–La/SS-B, or anti–U$_1$-RNP antibodies strongly suggest the diagnosis of neonatal lupus erythematosus.

A skin biopsy showing vacuolar changes along the epidermal junction with sparse lymphohistiocytic infiltrate can confirm the diagnosis. Immunofluorescence studies show particulate deposition of IgG in epidermal cells.

During gestation, a slow heart rate may be detected on routine obstetric examination and confirmed by ultrasonography and postnatal electrocardiography. Blood and liver tests should also be done.

Treatment and Prognosis

Management of skin disease includes protection from and avoidance of sun exposure and nonfluorinated low-potency topical steroids. Because the skin changes are transient and nonscarring, more aggressive treatment is not indicated.

Treatment of cardiac disease may not be necessary but, if indicated, consists of pacemaker implantation. Systemic steroids can be considered when heart failure ensues.

The skin lesions generally heal by 6 months of age without scarring or atrophy, although persistent telangiectasias have been noted in some patients. Pigmentary change may take months to resolve. Despite a markedly decreased heart rate, about half the infants with heart block related to neonatal lupus erythematosus do not need treatment, and the other half require pacemaker placement. A small number fail to respond to pacemaker placement, presumably because of myocardial disease.

Children with congenital heart block who survive infancy generally have a good prognosis regardless of organ system involvement. Rarely, some children develop cardiac rhythm disturbances or congestive heart failure during later childhood. The long-term outlook is unknown, but there are occasional reports of connective tissue disease arising in adulthood.

About half the mothers of infants with neonatal lupus are asymptomatic at the time of delivery. However, at 5 years after delivery, 86% of the mothers had either symptoms of Sjögren's disease (Lee, 1993) or a diagnosis of systemic lupus erythematosus or subacute cutaneous lupus erythematosus.

REACTIVE ERYTHEMAS

The reactive erythemas are a diverse group of cutaneous immunologic disorders representing varied host reactions to various antigenic stimuli. In some cases, the different patterns may occur together or occur at different times in the chronology of the process, suggesting that some of these conditions have similar causes or pathogenic mechanisms. Many of the disorders are associated with urticaria. Also, although certain of the reactive erythemas are associated with certain drugs (e.g., erythema multiforme with sulfonamides), with specific inflammatory diseases (e.g., erythema marginatum with rheumatic fever), or with infections (e.g., erythema chronicum migrans with Lyme disease), the physician should realize that virtually any of the reaction patterns may be triggered by any antigen.

Erythema Multiforme and Stevens-Johnson Syndrome

Erythema multiforme (EM) is an acute, self-limited mucocutaneous eruption, occurring as a cutaneous response to a variety of triggering agents. The disease is usefully classified into two forms: erythema multiforme minor and erythema multiforme major, including the Stevens-Johnson syndrome (Huff, 1991). Erythema multiforme minor affects primarily cutaneous surfaces, especially acral areas, with limited mucous membrane involvement. Erythema multiforme major is the more severe form, with evolution of lesions to bullae, extensive mucosal erosions, and marked constitutional symptoms.

History

Although the cutaneous eruptions of erythema multiforme have been recognized for centuries, von Hebra in 1866 first used the term and recognized the multiform rash as it evolved from papules to target lesions. Subsequently, patients with severe mucosal involvement and skin changes similar to those of erythema multiforme minor were reported by Stevens and Johnson in 1922. This is now considered as a more severe variant of erythema multiforme and is commonly referred to as the Stevens-Johnson syndrome.

Clinical Manifestations

Erythema multiforme minor most often occurs in young adults, but approximately 20% of cases occur in children, usually in preteen or adolescent age groups. The disease is rare in infants. The course and evolution of lesions in children are similar to those in adults. Erythema multiforme minor is relatively common, slightly more frequent in males, and without a racial predilection. Recurrent episodes are common, occurring in about half of cases. Seasonal outbreaks are common (Huff, 1993).

Stevens-Johnson syndrome is much less common than erythema multiforme minor. One survey of hospitalized patients found an annual incidence of 1 to 10 cases per million. In contrast to erythema multiforme minor, erythema multiforme major occurs at any age but is more likely to occur in the pediatric population, particularly in the second decade (Huff, 1993).

A clinical prodrome is absent in most patients with erythema multiforme minor. The primary lesions begin as red macules, which rapidly evolve into papules that may itch or burn. These may extend to form small plaques that clear centrally to produce annular lesions. The plaques may develop central duskiness surrounded by concentric zones of red to pink, producing the target or iris lesion, the hallmark of erythema multiforme. Lesions are typically distributed symmetrically and most prominently over the distal extremities. In erythema multiforme minor, the mucosal changes are limited to the mouth and present as discrete erosions with erythematous borders, often accompanied by cervical lymphadenopathy (Fritsch and Elias, 1993; Huff, 1993).

Erythema multiforme major is commonly preceded by fever, headache, and malaise. Mucous membrane and skin lesions begin abruptly, and cutaneous lesions may initially resemble those of erythema multiforme minor but evolve quickly into large areas of tender erythema and blisters. The blisters usually break, leaving extensive, denuded, tender erosions involving from 10% to 90% of the body surface. Mucosal involvement is generally severe and usually involves at least two sites. The majority of patients have oral, mucosal, lip, and eye lesions. Mucosal changes include bullae that rupture to leave painful erosions, swelling, and hemorrhagic crusting. Ocular lesions are painful and manifest as erythema, erosions, and purulent conjunctivitis (Fritsch and Elias, 1993; Huff, 1993).

Pathogenesis

For years it has been postulated that erythema multiforme is a hypersensitivity reaction to a variety of precipitating factors. The association between preceding herpes simplex virus (HSV) infection and erythema multiforme is well established, and HSV infection is probably the most common precipitating cause of erythema multiforme minor (Huff, 1993). The HSV-associated reaction typically occurs between 3 and 21 days after an episode of HSV infection and often recurs. Other factors associated with outbreaks of erythema multiforme include infectious mononucleosis, tuberculosis, histoplasmosis, coccidioidomycosis, *Yersinia* infections, vaccinia, and x-ray therapy.

Immunocytochemical studies indicate that the dermal infiltrate in erythema multiforme consists primarily of T lymphocytes, with both helper and suppressor subsets present. Keratinocytes may express class II histocompatibility antigens, which they do not do constitutively. This suggests that lymphocyte-produced interferon-γ (IFN-γ) has activated the keratinocytes. This information, together with the finding of HSV antigens and nucleic acids in keratinocytes of the lesions, suggests that a cellular immune response to HSV antigens within the epidermis is responsible for the final lesion production in erythema multiforme.

The best-documented precipitating factors of the Stevens-Johnson syndrome are drugs, mycoplasma infections, and HSV infections (Fritsch and Elias, 1993). Drugs commonly involved include sulfonamides, anticonvulsants, and nonsteroidal anti-inflammatory agents. Similar to the hypothesis put forth for erythema multiforme minor, it has been proposed that an antigen from either a drug or an infectious agent localizes at the mucocutaneous site of the eruption and a cell-mediated immune response causes the tissue damage.

Diagnosis

Proposed criteria for the diagnosis of erythema multiforme minor (Huff, 1993) include:

- A self-limited illness not lasting more than 4 weeks
- Fixed discrete lesions lasting at least 7 days
- Some lesions with characteristic features of target lesions
- Minimal or no mucosal involvement
- Compatible histology

Atypical urticaria is most frequently confused with erythema multiforme, but urticaria is much more transient and is histologically distinct.

The Stevens-Johnson syndrome with severe mucous membrane involvement can resemble other immunologically mediated blistering diseases such as pemphigus vulgaris, bullous pemphigoid, and paraneoplastic pemphigus. Direct immunofluorescence studies of biopsy specimens are important in differentiating these conditions.

There is overlap between erythema multiforme major and toxic epidermal necrolysis and some feel that the latter is a more severe form of EM major. Acute severe graft-versus-host disease can also resemble Stevens-Johnson syndrome. History and routine histology can usually distinguish these two entities.

Treatment

Episodes of erythema multiforme minor can be so mild that only symptomatic treatment is necessary. It is important to identify and eliminate potential precipitating factors. In recurrent cases secondary to HSV infection, prophylactic acyclovir prevents most episodes of recurrent HSV and erythema multiforme (Huff,

1993). There is no good evidence that systemic steroids are of value in treating this condition.

Erythema multiforme major can be associated with severe complications, including sepsis, fluid and electrolyte imbalances, and pneumonia. Consideration of care in a burn unit is appropriate for those having large denuded areas of the skin. Careful attention to regular cultures of skin erosions, mouth, blood, and sputum is important, as is meticulous fluid and electrolyte balance monitoring. Ophthalmologic consultation should be sought promptly to prevent ocular complications.

It is essential to discontinue any potential causative medications or treat underlying infections. Although some authors have suggested early use of systemic corticosteroids while new lesions are still evolving, there have been no controlled studies of the use of systemic steroids in the treatment of Stevens-Johnson syndrome (Eichenfield and Honig, 1991). Studies have shown that management of pediatric patients with meticulous wound care, careful fluid and electrolyte therapy, good ophthalmologic care, and avoidance of systemic corticosteroids can lead to good outcomes (Prendiville et al., 1989). Systemic corticosteroids in patients with extensive skin erosions can increase the risk of infection and prolong the hospital stay.

Prognosis

Erythema multiforme minor typically has a course of 1 to 4 weeks and resolves without sequelae. About half the patients have recurrent episodes, often associated with HSV infections. Erythema multiforme major has a more prolonged course, lasting 3 to 4 weeks. Mucosal erosions may heal with scarring, including ocular scarring. Scarring can lead to esophageal and anal strictures and vaginal or urethral stenosis. Skin lesions usually heal without sequelae; however, permanent loss of nails may occur.

Figurate Erythemas

The figurate erythemas are a poorly defined, descriptive group of erythematous lesions caused by reaction to unknown antigens that have in common a lymphocytic inflammatory infiltrate around vessels in the upper and middle dermis. Most of the lesions are annular (but occasionally irregular or gyrate), multiple, chronic, and remitting. As with chronic urticaria, a cause is seldom identified, but patients should be assessed for an antigenic source for the reactive lesions. Infections, drugs, autoimmune diseases, and malignancies have all been associated with cases of figurate erythemas.

Erythema Annulare Centrifugum

Erythema annulare centrifugum (EAC) is the most common of the figurate erythemas. The appearance can vary considerably depending on the acuteness and intensity of the process, the depth of blood vessels affected, and the degree of involvement of the epidermis. The lesions range from the initial and transient pink indurated papules to annules with central clearing and often a trailing collarette of scale. This latter appearance can resemble that of tinea, which is easily ruled out with potassium hydroxide (KOH) examination. The rings are multiple, sometimes generalized, sometimes clustered over only one area. Erythema annulare centrifugum may appear at any age, including the newborn period (Fried et al., 1957). Lesions are usually chronic or recurring and may continue for years. They can be quite dynamic, enlarging over days to weeks and then fading while others appear. Itching is variable but is seldom severe.

The etiology is obscure, but reactions to fungal infections are probably the most common associations. The immunologic nature of these lesions can occasionally be demonstrated when intradermal trichophytin antigen reproduces the process, which results in an enlarging annular lesion that can continue for weeks (Champion, 1992). *Candida* infections, ingestion of blue cheese, carcinomas, lymphomas, drugs, and a variety of bacterial and viral infections have been reported in association with erythema annulare centrifugum (Troy and Goetz, 1991).

Differential diagnosis includes, in addition to dermatophytosis, granuloma annulare, mycosis fungoides, sarcoid, lupus erythematosus, and leprosy.

Management is aimed primarily at eliminating the suspected antigen. Topical corticosteroids can reduce the inflammation of the superficial and scaly lesions. Prednisone controls the process but is rarely justified for such benign and minimally symptomatic lesions.

Erythema Marginatum

Erythema marginatum, classically associated with rheumatic fever, consists of superficial, macular or urticarial erythemas in rings or ring segments that may coalesce into a polycyclic or reticular pattern (see Chapter 24). Typically, lesions are evanescent, appearing for a few hours in the afternoon, expanding rapidly, clearing centrally, and then fading, although some may last 2 to 3 days. Erythema marginatum occurs in 10% to 18% of patients with rheumatic fever and is considered to be specific (it is part of the Jones criteria for rheumatic fever), although we have seen morphologically similar lesions associated with hepatitis B.

Erythema Chronicum Migrans

This annular erythema centered on the tick bite inoculation of *Borrelia burgdorferi* can be the cutaneous prodrome to Lyme disease (see Chapter 24). It differs from erythema annulare centrifugum in usually being solitary and retains a central papulation at the bite site. Lesions usually occur on the extremities or trunk 4 to 20 days after the bite (Schachner and Hansen, 1988) and usually persist for 1 to 2 months. Treatment with penicillin, tetracycline, or amoxicillin may prevent the later development of Lyme disease, although the value of prophylaxis remains controversial (Shapiro et al., 1992).

HENOCH-SCHÖNLEIN PURPURA

Henoch-Schönlein purpura (HSP) (also termed *anaphylactoid purpura*, or Henoch-Schönlein vasculitis) is an illness affecting skin, joints, the gastrointestinal tract, the kidneys, and, in rare instances, the central nervous system and other organs subject to hemorrhage (Allen et al., 1960; Hall, 1991; Jones and Callen, 1991). The condition can occur at any age but is more common in children, usually between 2 and 12 years of age. Symptoms typically appear suddenly and subside over 3 to 4 weeks, although they may recur in about 50% of patients and rarely persist or recur for years. This disorder is also discussed in Chapters 22, 24, and 25.

The cutaneous manifestation of Henoch-Schönlein purpura is purpuric, usually palpable and symmetrically arrayed over the buttocks and lower extremities. Lesions can appear in any site, and the earliest may be urticarial or petechial, evolving within hours to the typical palpable purpura. These gradually darken, flatten, and fade, usually within 2 weeks, leaving transient brownish pigmentation. Although skin lesions appear at some point in 100% of patients, the presenting complaint is cutaneous in only about 60% and skin lesions may occur weeks after arthritic or gastrointestinal symptoms. In other cases, purpuric eruptions may be the only manifestation. In some patients, soft tissue swelling may occur over the head or extremities and be quite painful. This edema is more common in younger children and is distinct from the joint manifestations that occur in up to 85% of children. The latter are limited to arthralgias and sometimes periarticular swelling. True inflammatory arthritis is uncommon, self-limited, and leaves no joint damage.

Gastrointestinal symptoms occur in 70% to 95% of patients and include abdominal pain and vomiting (Jones and Callen, 1991). Evidence of gastrointestinal hemorrhage ranging from guaiac-positive stools to melena is seen in about 70% of cases. Occasional severe and even fatal manifestations such as hemorrhage and intussusception occur. It is important to consider Henoch-Schönlein purpura in any case of unexplained abdominal pain. Of the patients reported by Allen and colleagues (1960), 15% had severe pain before the development of purpura and many required laparotomy.

Renal disease occurs in about 30% of children (Crumb, 1976), usually in the first month (see Chapter 25). This is usually transient microscopic hematuria or proteinuria, but glomerulonephritis and renal failure occur. Of the 131 children studied by Allen and colleagues (1960), 6 developed severe renal disease and 2 died. In addition, 40% of those with acute renal disease had late renal findings not present initially. Thus, all patients with Henoch-Schönlein purpura should have periodic urinalysis for 2 years after onset.

Pathology

Skin biopsy specimens show changes typical of leukocytoclastic vasculitis with perivascular neutrophilic infiltrate, erythrocyte extravasation, and nuclear debris. In some cases epidermal necrosis and bulla formation are seen. Renal histopathology is highly variable, ranging from mild glomerular changes to proliferative glomerulonephritis. Immunopathologic studies first called attention to the presence of mesangial IgA deposits in more than 90% of renal biopsy specimens (Counahan and Cameron, 1977). This led to the demonstration of perivascular IgA deposits in 75% to 100% of lesional skin biopsy specimens and even in a high proportion of normal skin specimens from patients with Henoch-Schönlein purpura (Jones and Callen, 1991). These findings, along with the similarity of skin biopsy features to those of the Arthus reaction, have suggested that HSP is caused by deposition of circulating IgA immune complexes.

Treatment

Most cases of Henoch-Schönlein purpura resolve spontaneously. Systemic corticosteroids may improve joint and gastrointestinal symptoms but do not appear to affect the skin or renal disease. No controlled studies of corticosteroid therapy, other immunosuppressive agents, or plasmapheresis are available. Aspirin should be avoided because it may increase gastrointestinal hemorrhage.

ATOPIC DERMATITIS

Atopic dermatitis (eczema) is a chronic inflammatory disease characterized by erythema, papulation, and intense itching, often accompanied by excoriations, lichenification, weeping, and crusting (see Chapter 20). It usually begins in infancy, and 95% of cases begin within the first 5 years of age. The disorder is extremely common, and the incidence has increased from 3% in 1950 to an estimated 10% of infants more recently (Schultz-Larsen et al., 1986). The disease appears to affect all races, although Asians may have the greatest susceptibility. This multifactorial condition may not appear while individuals live in rural or underdeveloped areas, for it is manifested only when the genetically susceptible person moves to an urban locale (Hanifin, 1991). Environmental pollution, psychologic stress, and excess exposure to antigens may exacerbate the disease in susceptible individuals. Atopic dermatitis is also a risk factor for asthma and may be aggravated by exposure to cigarette smoke (Murray and Morrison, 1990). Indeed, persons with atopic dermatitis often have methacholine-reactive airways, which suggests a predisposition to asthma (Barker et al., 1991).

The natural course of atopic dermatitis is one of gradual improvement. Complete clearing occurs in approximately 40% of patients observed over periods from 15 to 25 years (Musgrove and Morgan, 1976), but children with severe atopic dermatitis often have persistent disease.

Pathogenesis

A genetic basis for atopic dermatitis is well established, based on the strong familial association and the high concordance rate in monozygotic twins (Schultz-Larsen et al., 1986). The mode of inheritance is not consistent and may display autosomal dominant, autosomal recessive, and multifactorial inheritance patterns. Studies of gene linkage using immunoglobulin E (IgE) reactivity as a marker have suggested an association with chromosome 11q (Cookson et al., 1989), although these results are disputed (Marsh and Meyers, 1992). Human leukocyte antigen (HLA) associations have shown no consistent patterns. Atopic dermatitis and other atopic conditions, including IgE reactivity to specific antigens, are transferred by bone marrow transplantation; this provides strong evidence for a basic defect in hematopoietic cells rather than in the skin (Agosti et al., 1988). Conversely, transplantation of normal marrow corrects the atopic dermatitis of the Wiskott-Aldrich syndrome (Saurat, 1985).

Two other generalizations can be made about atopic dermatitis: (1) patients have abnormal immune responses and (2) they have a number of pharmacophysiologic abnormalities (Hanifin, 1986).

Immunologic abnormalities include IgE overproduction and altered cell-mediated immune responses. Serum IgE levels are elevated in 80% of patients with atopic dermatitis, but it is important to recognize the crucial 20% exception; the latter patients have normal serum IgE levels and a negative radioallergosorbent test (RAST) and skin test and no asthma or rhinoconjunctivitis (Hanifin and Lobitz, 1977). Thus, IgE reactivity may simply be an epiphenomenon without true pathogenic importance.

Similar caution is needed to avoid overinterpreting the high interleukin-4 (IL-4) production in atopic dermatitis (Chan et al., 1993b). This cytokine, produced by type 2 T helper cells (T_H2 cells) is an important regulator of IgE synthesis and may well contribute to the excessive IgE production in atopic conditions. T_H2 cells also produce interleukin-5 (IL-5), which regulates eosinophils, an important component of the inflammatory infiltrate in atopic dermatitis (Leiferman et al., 1985). In addition to T_H2 cells and eosinophils, abnormal control of cytokine production and perhaps IgE synthesis may originate with atopic monocytes. These cells have abnormal cyclic nucleotide metabolism because of elevated phosphodiesterase (PDE) hydrolysis of cyclic adenosine monophosphate (cyclic AMP), providing a functional state that encourages cellular hyperresponsiveness (Holden et al., 1986). Likewise, studies have shown increased antigen-presenting capabilities of epidermal Langerhans cells (Mudde et al., 1990), which, along with atopic monocytes, express high-affinity FcεI receptors. Thus, the elevated IgE may enhance cellular immune responses to environmental antigens, such as dust mites, animal proteins, and pollens. Allergen interactions with IgE on antigen-presenting cells (APCs) of the skin surface may cause responses analogous to those in allergic contact hypersensitivity. Defective monocyte and dendritic cell cyclic nucleotide metabolism may underlie the wide range of immune abnormalities found in atopic dermatitis. The abnormal PDE activity in these cells and in other inflammatory cells such as basophils, mast cells, and eosinophils may account for some of the aberrant immunologic and pharmacologic reactions characteristic of atopic disease (Chan et al., 1993a).

Clinical Manifestations

Pruritus is the cardinal symptom of atopic dermatitis. Many have paraphrased Jacqet's dictum that "atopic dermatitis is the itch that rashes rather than the rash that itches" (Rajka, 1989), although, in reality, erythema precedes or accompanies the itching. Erythema, edema, papulation, and induration are the primary clinical features of acute atopic dermatitis. It is also characterized by repeated episodes of flaring, sometimes several times a day, sometimes once or twice a month. The secondary clinical features include dryness, scaling, excoriation, weeping, and lichenification. All are caused by the inflammation and itching, which cause intractable, involuntary scratching, rubbing, and slapping of the skin throughout the day and night. Individuals with pigmented skin such as blacks and Asians also present with perifollicular accentuation, giving the skin a pebbled appearance; they also tend to have more severely lichenified skin in areas of rubbing. On some occasions, urticarial-type lesions accompany the flares, but patients with atopy and atopic dermatitis have no increased tendency toward acute or chronic urticaria.

Many pigmentary effects of inflammation occur in patients with atopic dermatitis. These include postinflammatory hypopigmentation (i.e., pityriasis alba) or hyperpigmentation, sometimes reticulated, sometimes patchy and persistent. Occasionally, vitiliginous depigmentation also develops, although this usually occurs in adults. Patients often refer to these pigmentary defects as "scars," but parents should be reassured that atopic dermatitis essentially never leads to scars in the sense of thickened fibrotic lesions.

Dry skin is a nearly universal finding in patients with atopic dermatitis; the only exceptions occur in tropical or other very humid locales (Hanifin and Rajka, 1980; Uehara and Miyauchi, 1984; Rajka, 1989). In pure atopic dermatitis, without associated ichthyosis vulgaris, the dryness and scaling are simply manifestations of preceding inflammation. Ichthyosis is seen frequently in patients with atopic dermatitis and is best appreciated by finding the polygonal "fish scale" skin markings along with dryness and roughness over the anterior tibial areas (Rajka, 1989). The fine, papular, keratotic lesions over the posterior arms, called *keratosis pilaris*, along with palmar hyperlinearity, are typical manifestations of ichthyosis vulgaris, although they are too often considered hallmarks of atopic dermatitis (Hanifin and Rajka, 1980). The relationship between ichthyosis vulgaris and atopic dermatitis is probably functional rather than genetic. The genetic susceptibility to atopy, combined with the defective stratum cor-

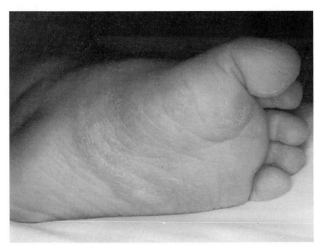

Figure 21–4. Juvenile plantar dermatosis, one of many manifestations of atopic dermatitis that may affect the foot.

neum barrier of ichthyosis, primes the inflammation of atopic dermatitis.

Dryness and scaling over the scalp are typical of atopic dermatitis, but the more greasy scale of seborrheic dermatitis (i.e., cradle cap) can also be a presenting feature, along with periauricular fissures and chapped lips (cheilitis). Less specific parameters include nonspecific hand eczema and foot dermatitis, often called atopic foot or atopic winter foot or juvenile plantar dermatosis (Fig. 21–4). By recognizing this entity one can avoid unnecessary treatment and diagnostic procedures based on misdiagnoses such as contact allergy or athlete's foot. Atopic dermatitis can affect any body region, but it is important to recognize that the diaper area is usually spared (Fig. 21–5) because the moisture maintains a soft, pliable stratum corneum barrier. Atopic infants are not impervious to diaper dermatitis, however. A large study comparing atopic and normal infants found a slightly increased incidence of diaper dermatitis in the former (Seymour et al., 1987).

Cutaneous infection is a frequent concomitant of atopic dermatitis. Staphylococcal infections are the most common, but patients may develop herpes simplex, warts, and molluscum contagiosum (Hanifin and Lobitz, 1977). The increased susceptibility to infection

is due to a mild immune deficit in the skin, heavy colonization with *Staphylococcus aureus*, and chronic excoriation. The colonization is lower in infants than in older patients (Seymour et al., 1987); the prevalence increases with age. A practical management approach is to assume that infants and children with flaring or crusted or weeping lesions are infected and are best treated with systemic antibiotics. Such children usually have enlarged regional lymph nodes. Staphylococcal lesions in atopic dermatitis tend to be superficial and usually arise on the extremities or around the head and neck. These are important distinctions from the findings in hyper-IgE syndrome or other immunodeficiency syndromes, in which patients typically have furuncles and other deep infections. Patients with atopic dermatitis have good resistance to sepsis and other invasive bacterial infections.

Treatment

Therapy of atopic dermatitis first necessitates recognition and reduction of exacerbating factors. These "trigger" factors include dry skin, infection, emotional stress, sweating or overheating, and allergens. Allergen avoidance is overemphasized and of questionable import for most eczematous children. The search for an allergen should not distract from basic management measures such as good moisturizing, antibiotics, and topical corticosteroids.

Children and parents should be educated early about the need for immediate application of emollients after bathing. With that simple requisite, daily baths do no harm and in fact reduce infection and enhance corticosteroid effects. Topical steroids, usually triamcinolone, 0.1% cream or ointment, should be applied twice daily to inflamed or flaring areas at the same time as emollients are used on noninflamed skin areas. When inflammation is controlled, topical steroids should be tapered to twice weekly to prevent steroid skin atrophy, although 1% hydrocortisone can be used more frequently. Oral antibiotics, either erythromycin or a cephalosporin, should be used for 5 days and repeated immediately whenever flaring or infection recurs.

When the child does not respond to this regimen or continues to have flares, allergen avoidance measures should be considered. Unfortunately, allergen identification is imprecise. Careful history and a 1-week restriction of the most suspect foods, including the high-probability foods (eggs, dairy products, peanuts, soy, wheat, and fish) (Sampson and McCaskill, 1985), while optimizing therapy may provide stability; then one food can be added back each day (if there has been no history of anaphylaxis). If this approach does not induce remission, allergy tests are indicated, but the parents should be cautioned that a positive RAST or skin test will show false-positive results up to 80% of the time (Sampson and Albergo, 1984) and do not prove that the allergens causing the positive skin test cause the disease. Foods that trigger eczema are often recognized by parents and then avoided, obviating the need for medical help. Double-blind challenge tests in highly selected patients indicate that temporary itching and

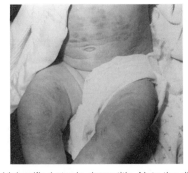

Figure 21–5. Lichenified atopic dermatitis. Note the distribution over the extensor surfaces and sparing of the well-hydrated diaper area.

rash can develop (Sampson and McCaskill, 1985), but such challenges are not practical, possible, or relevant in the practice setting. Food-induced eczema is extremely rare and represents less than 1% of the cases. The physician should be alert for the occasional undetected food allergy but never at the expense of proper general skin therapy.

ALLERGIC CONTACT DERMATITIS

Clinical Manifestations

Allergic contact dermatitis is relatively uncommon in childhood, although not because of lack of sensitizing capability. Infants can be sensitized to the *Rhus* pentadecacatechol antigen even in the newborn period (Epstein, 1961). This highly antigenic moiety of poison ivy and poison oak (*Toxicodendron* species) plants is probably the most common cause of allergic contact dermatitis in both children and adults (see Chapter 20). The acute form of allergic contact dermatitis presents as erythematous papulation or vesiculation with oozing. Those with *T. rhus* dermatitis often have linear streaks of vesiculation. The dermatitis is usually in areas of contact with plants; however, because it can be spread by pets, shoelaces, and clothing, the eruption may affect any body surface.

The chronic form of allergic contact dermatitis is indolent with mild erythema, scaling, and induration, usually well marginated but occasionally diffuse. This subacute or chronic dermatitis occurs as a result of repeated exposure to weaker chemical allergens and may be indistinguishable from atopic dermatitis. Typically, the cause of the dermatitis is evident and avoidance clears up the problem. However, when contact allergy is suspected but the allergen is unknown, patch testing with common contact allergens is necessary to make a diagnosis.

Pathogenesis

The immunologic basis for allergic contact dermatitis has been well delineated through experimental studies in animals. Allergic contact dermatitis involves a sensitization and an elicitation phase. The antigens are low-molecular-weight haptens that conjugate with proteins. These haptens have the ability to penetrate the epidermis and form strong covalent bonds with proteins. Lipid solubility of haptens also enhances sensitization capacity because it leads to better skin penetration. The hapten–protein carrier complex is processed by Langerhans cells or other antigen-presenting cells in the skin. The antigen-bearing Langerhans cells migrate into the dermis and initiate T-lymphocyte sensitization, either locally or in draining lymph nodes (Tron and Sauder, 1991). The sensitization process generally takes 9 to 21 days, but with very strong antigens reactions can occur within 5 days. The elicitation phase occurs in 24 to 48 hours, hence the usual 48-hour duration for patch testing. Histologic features of allergic contact dermatitis are the same as those of any other form of eczema.

Diagnosis

The types of allergen exposure are infinite. A typical list of compounds tested, based on the most probable allergens encountered in North America, has been developed by the North American Contact Dermatitis Group and is shown in Table 21–1. In children, topically applied medications and skin care preparations may be the most common cause of contact allergy. These include benzocaine and other "caine" derivatives, neomycin, preservatives (e.g., parabens, ethylenediamine, thimerosal), fragrances, and balsam of Peru. Rubbers and glues, especially in footwear, are other common sensitizers. Nickel is a common sensitizing antigen because of its presence in earrings and other body-piercing jewelry in our society.

Patch testing involves the application of the suspected antigen to the skin of the back in a nonirritating form for 48 hours. Any adhesive plaster can be used, but most dermatologists now apply antigens under small aluminum disks called Finn chambers held in place with paper tape. Two readings are recommended, the first at 48 hours and the second 4 to 7 days after the application. Clearly positive reactions are easy to discern, but reactions are often ambiguous because of irritation or flaring of surrounding inflamed skin ("angry back" syndrome). If positive reactions are found, patients should be advised about the many cross-reacting substances present in the environment.

Treatment

Treatment consists of anti-inflammatory agents, usually medium potency corticosteroid creams such as 0.1% triamcinolone, although this and 1% hydrocortisone cream are generally inadequate for controlling severe acute allergic contact dermatitis. In such cases, high-potency corticosteroids such as betamethasone propionate may be necessary. For severe widespread contact dermatitis, such as that in patients exposed to

Table 21–1. North American Contact Dermatitis Group Standard Allergens

1. Benzocaine 5% petrolatum	12. Ethylenediamine dihydrochloride 1% petrolatum
2. Mercaptobenzothiazole 1% petrolatum	13. Epoxy resin 1% petrolatum
3. Colophony 20% petrolatum	14. Quaternium-15 2% petrolatum
4. *p*-Phenylenediamine 1% petrolatum	15. *p-tert*-Butylphenol formaldehyde resin 1% petrolatum
5. Imidazolidinyl urea 2% aqueous	16. Mercapto mix 1% petrolatum
6. Cinnamic aldehyde 1% petrolatum	17. Black rubber mix 0.6% petrolatum
7. Lanolin alcohol 30% petrolatum	18. Potassium dichromate 0.25% petrolatum
8. Carba mix 3% petrolatum	19. Balsam of Peru 25% petrolatum
9. Neomycin sulfate 20% petrolatum	20. Nickel sulfate 2.5% petrolatum
10. Thiuram mix 1% petrolatum	
11. Formaldehyde 1% aqueous	

Data from Hermal, Inc., Delmar, New York.

poison ivy or oak, systemic corticosteroids are required. Because reactions can last up to 3 weeks, a course of systemic corticosteroids tapering over a 2-week period may be necessary. Prednisone at 1 mg/kg/day in a single or twice-daily dose, may be used for younger children. In adolescents and adults, a prednisone dose of 1 to 2 mg/kg (e.g., 60 to 80 mg/day) is required to interrupt the severe inflammatory reaction. Preprepared steroid dose packs usually have an inadequate supply to cover the necessary duration of treatment. A simplified plan for a teenager might be prednisone at 60 mg/day for 7 days, followed by 30 mg/day for 7 days. For patients with severe dermatitis, wet dressings or cool baths may provide considerable relief.

Patients and parents must be educated about the need to wash all clothing and about other possible sources of exposure, including family pets, immediately when poison oak dermatitis is recognized. For prevention in patients repeatedly exposed to poison ivy or oak, Stokogard cream, which inactivates the antigen (Orchard et al., 1986) can be used; it is available at industrial supply retailers. If the skin is rinsed with water immediately after contact with the offending plants, the reaction can usually be averted. Encouraging avoidance through education, using pictures of the offending plants, is often helpful.

PSORIASIS

Psoriasis is a papulosquamous inflammatory disease, rare in childhood but common in adults at any age. Girls are affected more frequently than boys (Esterly and Kever, 1978), and a family history is noted in about 50% of cases. The pathogenesis of psoriasis is unknown; for years, faulty control of proliferating epidermal cells was suspected. More recently, immunologic aberration as the cause of psoriasis has been suggested (Krueger, 1989; Cooper, 1990). Langerhans cells and other antigen-presenting cells (APCs) in the epidermis present stimulatory antigens (e.g., microbial products) in association with HLA-DR to specific T-cell receptors on the lymphocytes. Lymphokine production then leads to recruitment of increased numbers of APCs and increased T-cell activation. The lymphokines also stimulate epidermal proliferation and inflammation. Cyclosporine, methotrexate, and ultraviolet light may act on T cells, APCs, or keratinocytes to inhibit the inflammatory process.

Clinical Manifestations

There are two general forms of psoriasis in children. The classic form appears over typical locations of elbows, knees, scalp, and presacrum. Slowly evolving erythematous papules coalesce into well-demarcated plaques overlain by white or silvery scale. Nail pitting and onycholysis are common. The second form is eruptive, guttate psoriasis, which can appear explosively with profuse, small, round or oval lesions over the face, trunk, and proximal extremities. This may follow a streptococcal or other infection but can also be triggered by sunburn or systemic corticosteroid withdrawal. Guttate psoriasis may be of short duration, receding with resolution of infection. Alternatively, patients may progress to erythroderma or pustular psoriasis, necessitating hospitalization. Infantile psoriasis may occur with the subtle onset of lesions in skin folds and periauricular and diaper areas and may be indistinguishable from seborrheic dermatitis. Psoriasis of the diaper region may also be confused with candidiasis or eczematous diaper dermatitis.

Treatment

Therapy for psoriasis varies, depending on the clinical form, location, extent, and intensity of inflammation. Topical corticosteroids are generally the first line of therapy, but for classic, plaque-type lesions the thickened epidermis may prevent adequate drug penetration, necessitating medium to high potency agents or the use of occlusive dressings. A reasonable first-line therapeutic agent is triamcinolone, 0.1% ointment, applied after the bath once or twice daily for 2 weeks. Prolonged use leads to atrophy, so careful monitoring is necessary. Cessation of corticosteroid therapy usually leads to prompt rebound of psoriatic inflammation. Thus, topical corticosteroid therapy should be combined with stabilizers such as tar preparations (e.g., 1% to 5% crude coal tar ointment, 5% to 15% liquor carbonis detergens [LCD]) or ultraviolet light therapy. With seborrheiform psoriasis or inverse psoriasis (affecting mainly folds and genitals), hydrocortisone, 1% cream or ointment, is safe and usually effective. Use of tar preparations in these areas can lead to worsening of inflammation. For the scalp, tar shampoos are quite helpful and, if necessary, twice daily application of a low to medium potency corticosteroid solution is indicated.

Treatment of guttate psoriasis is a challenge. Streptococcal infection should be identified by throat culture and treated with penicillin. Baths and topical corticosteroids are used initially. If the eruption becomes chronic or progresses, systemic therapy or methotrexate may be indicated.

CUTANEOUS MANIFESTATIONS OF PRIMARY IMMUNODEFICIENCIES

A variety of skin abnormalities have been described in children with various immunodeficiency syndromes. Other than the thrombocytopenic purpura of Wiskott-Aldrich syndrome and mucocutaneous candidiasis, these are nonspecific (see Chapter 9). They include pyodermas, oral candidiasis, viral exanthems, and atopic dermatitis (Buckley et al., 1972; Hanifin and Lobitz, 1977). Typical atopic dermatitis occurs in Wiskott-Aldrich syndrome (Saurat, 1985) and in X-linked agammaglobulinemia (Peterson et al., 1962), and atypical eczematous lesions occur in other conditions (Hanifin and Rajka, 1980; Hanifin, 1991). Patients with hyperimmunoglobulinemia E syndrome have coarse facial lesions, furuncles, and intertriginous lesions but seldom atopic dermatitis (Peterson et al., 1962) (see Chapter 13).

References

Agosti JM, Sprenger JD, Lum LG, Witherspoon RP, Fisher LD, Storb R, Henderson WR Jr. Transfer of allergen-specific IgE-mediated hypersensitivity with allogeneic bone marrow transplantation. N Engl J Med 319:1623–1628, 1988.

Allen DM, Diamond LK, Howell DA. Anaphylactoid purpura in children (Schönlein-Henoch syndrome). Am J Dis Child 99:833–853, 1960.

Barker AF, Hirshman CA, D'Silva R, Hanifin JM. Airway responsiveness in atopic dermatitis. J Allergy Clin Immunol 87:780–783, 1991.

Buckley RH, Ray BB, Belmaker EZ. Extreme hyperimmunoglobulinemia-E and undue susceptibility to infection. Pediatrics 49:59–70, 1972.

Champion RH. Disorders of blood vessels. In Champion RH, Burton JL, Ebling FJG, eds. Rook/Wilkinson/Ebling Textbook of Dermatology, 5th ed. Oxford, Blackwell Scientific Publications, 1992, pp. 1839–1840.

Chan SC, Kim J-W, Henderson WR Jr, Hanifin JM. Altered prostaglandin E_2 regulation of cytokine production in atopic dermatitis. J Immunol 151:3345–3352, 1993a.

Chan SC, Li S-H, Hanifin JM. Increased interleukin 4 production by atopic mononuclear leukocytes correlates with increased cyclic AMP–phosphodiesterase activity and is reversible by phosphodiesterase inhibition. J Invest Dermatol 100:681–684, 1993b.

Cookson WOCM, Faux JA, Sharp PA, Hopkin JM. Linkage between immunoglobulin-E responses underlying asthma and rhinitis and chromosome 11q. Lancet 1:1292–1295, 1989.

Cooper KD. Psoriasis: leukocytes and cytokines. Dermatol Clin 8:737–745, 1990.

Cormane RH, Gianetti A. IgA in various dermatoses: immunofluorescence studies. Br J Dermatol 84:523–533, 1971.

Counahan R, Cameron JS. Henoch-Schönlein nephritis. Contrib Nephrol 76:143–165, 1977.

Crumb CK. Renal involvement in Schönlein-Henoch syndrome. In Suki WN, ed. The Kidney in Systemic Disease. New York, John Wiley & Sons, 1976, pp. 43–55.

Eichenfield L, Honig P. Blistering disorders in childhood. Pediatr Clin North Am 38:959–976, 1991.

Epstein WL. Contact-type delayed hypersensitivity in infants and children: induction of *Rhus* sensitivity. Pediatrics 27:51–53, 1961.

Esterly NB, Kever E. Maculopapular eruptions. In Weinberg S, Hoekelman RA, eds. Pediatric Dermatology for the Primary Care Practitioner. New York, McGraw-Hill, 1978, pp. 30–38.

Fried R, Schonberg IL, and Litt JZ. Erythema annulare centrifugum (Darier) in a newborn infant. J Pediatr 50:66–67, 1957.

Fritsch P, Elias P. Erythema multiforme and toxic epidermal necrolysis. In Wolff K, Freedberg I, Austen K, eds. Dermatology in General Medicine, 4th ed. New York, McGraw-Hill, 1993, pp. 585–600.

George P, Tunnessen W. Childhood discoid lupus erythematosus. Arch Dermatol 129:613–617, 1993.

Hall RP III. Henoch-Schönlein purpura. In Jordon RE, ed. Immunologic Diseases of the Skin. East Norwalk, Conn. Appleton & Lange, 1991, p. 451.

Hanifin JM. Pharmacophysiology of atopic dermatitis. Clin Rev Allergy 4:43–65, 1986.

Hanifin JM. Atopic dermatitis in infants and children: pediatric dermatology. Pediatr Clin North Am 38:763–789, 1991.

Hanifin JM, Lobitz WC. Newer concepts of atopic dermatitis. Arch Dermatol 113:663–670, 1977.

Hanifin JM, Rajka G. Diagnostic features of atopic dermatitis. Acta Derm Venereol (Stockh) 92(Suppl.):44–47, 1980.

Holden CA, Chan SC, Hanifin JM. Monocyte localization of elevated cAMP phosphodiesterase activity in atopic dermatitis. J Invest Dermatol 87:372–376, 1986.

Huff CV. Erythema multiforme. In Provost TT, Weston WL, eds. Bullous Diseases. St. Louis, Mosby–Year Book, 1993, pp. 213–256.

Huff JC. Erythema multiforme. In Jordon RE, ed. Immunologic Diseases of the Skin. East Norwalk, Conn., Appleton & Lange, 1991, pp. 463–470.

Hurwitz S. The skin and systemic disease. In Clinical Pediatric Dermatology, 1st ed. Philadelphia, WB Saunders, 1981, pp. 411–413.

Jones EM, Callen JP. Collagen vascular diseases of childhood. Pediatr Clin North Am 38:1033–1038, 1991.

Krueger GG. A perspective on psoriasis as an aberration in skin modified to expression by the inflammatory/repair system. In Norris DA, ed. Immune Mechanisms in Cutaneous Disease. New York, Marcel Dekker, 1989, pp. 425–445.

Lee L. Neonatal lupus erythematosus. J Invest Dermatol 100:9S–13S, 1993.

Leiferman KM, Ackerman SJ, Sampson HA, Haugen H, Venenci PY, Gleich GJ. Dermal deposition of eosinophil-granule major basic protein in atopic dermatitis. N Engl J Med 313:282–285, 1985.

Marks J, Shuster S, Watson AJ. Small bowel changes in dermatitis herpetiformis. Lancet 2:1280–1282, 1966.

Marsden RA. Linear IgA disease of childhood. In Wojnarowska F, Briggaman R, eds. Management of Blistering Diseases. London, Chapman & Hall Medical, 1990, pp. 119–126.

Marsh DG, Meyers DA. A major gene for allergy—fact or fancy? Nat Genet 2:252–254, 1992.

McCord M, Hall R. IgA-mediated autoimmune blistering diseases. In Fine J-D, ed. Topics in Clinical Dermatology: Bullous Diseases. New York, Igaku-Shoin, 1993, pp. 97–120.

McCuistion CH, Schoch EP. Possible discoid lupus erythematosus in a newborn infant; report of a case with subsequent development of acute systemic lupus erythematosus in the mother. Arch Dermatol 70:782–785, 1954.

Mudde GC, Van Reijsen FC, Boland GJ, De Gast GC, Bruinzeel PLB, Bruinzeel-Koomen CAFM. Allergen presentation by epidermal Langerhans cells from patients with atopic dermatitis is mediated by IgE. Immunology 69:335–341, 1990.

Murray AB, Morrison BJ. It is children with atopic dermatitis who develop asthma more frequently if the mother smokes. J Allergy Clin Immunol 86:732–739, 1990.

Musgrove K, Morgan JK. Infantile eczema. Br J Dermatol 95:365–372, 1976.

Orchard S, Fellman JH, Storrs FJ. Poison ivy/oak dermatitis. Arch Dermatol 122:783–789, 1986.

Peterson RDA, Page AR, Good RA. Wheal and erythema allergy in patients with agammaglobulinemia. J Allergy Clin Immunol 33:406–411, 1962.

Prendiville J, Hebert A, Greenwald M, Esterly N. Management of Stevens-Johnson syndrome and toxic epidermolysis in children. J Pediatr 115:881–887, 1989.

Rabinowitz LG, Esterly NB. Inflammatory bullous diseases in children. Dermatol Clin 11:565–581, 1993.

Rajka G. Essential Aspects of Atopic Dermatitis. Berlin, Springer-Verlag, 1989, pp. 1–261.

Rothfield N. Lupus erythematosus. In Fitzpatrick TB, Eisen AZ, Wolff K, Freedberg I, Austen F, eds. Dermatology in General Medicine, 4th ed. New York, McGraw-Hill, 1993, pp. 2137–2148.

Sampson HA, Albergo R. Comparison of results of skin tests, RAST, and double-blind placebo-controlled food challenges in atopic dermatitis. J Allergy Clin Immunol 74:26–33, 1984.

Sampson HA, McCaskill CM. Food hypersensitivity and atopic dermatitis: evaluation of 113 patients. J Pediatr 107:669–675, 1985.

Saurat JH. Eczema in primary immune deficiencies. Clues to the pathogenesis of atopic dermatitis with special reference to the Wiskott-Aldrich syndrome. Acta Derm Venereol (Stockh) 114(Suppl.):125–128, 1985.

Schachner LA, Hansen RC, eds. Erythema chronicum migrans. In Pediatric Dermatology. New York, Churchill Livingstone, 1988, pp. 984–985.

Schultz-Larsen F, Holm NV, Henningsen K. Atopic dermatitis: a genetic-epidemiologic study in a population-based twin sample. J Am Acad Dermatol 15:487–494, 1986.

Seymour JL, Keswick BH, Hanifin JM, Jordan WP, Milligan MC. Clinical effects of diaper types on the skin of normal infants and infants with atopic dermatitis. J Am Acad Dermatol 17:988–997, 1987.

Shapiro ED, Gerber MA, Holabird NB, Berg AT, Feder HM Jr, Bell GL, Rys PN, Persing DH. A controlled trial of antimicrobial prophylaxis for Lyme disease after deer-tick bites. N Engl J Med 327:1769–1773, 1992.

Smith E, Zone JJ. Dermatitis herpetiformis and linear IgA bullous dermatosis. Dermatol Clin 11:373–348, 1993.

Stevens AM, Johnson FC. A new eruptive fever associated with stomatitis and ophthalmia. Am J Dis Child 24:526–533, 1922.

Tron VA, Sauder DN. Allergic contact dermatitis. In Jordon RE, ed. Immunologic Diseases of the Skin. East Norwalk, Conn., Appleton & Lange, 1991, pp. 253–261.

Troy JL, Goetz DM. Erythema nodosum and gyrate erythemas. In Jordon RE, ed. Immunologic Diseases of the Skin. East Norwalk, Conn., Appleton & Lange, 1991, p. 474.

Uehara M, Miyauchi H. The morphologic characteristics of dry skin in atopic dermatitis. Arch Dermatol 120:1186–1190, 1984.

Watson R, Provost T. Neonatal lupus erythematosus. In Beutner E, Chorzelski T, Kumen V, eds. Immunopathology of the Skin, 3rd ed. New York, Churchill Livingstone, 1987, pp. 583–600.

Weston WL, Harmon C, Peebles C, Manchester D, Franco HL, Huff JC, Norris DA. A serologic marker for neonatal lupus erythematosus. Br J Dermatol 107:377–382, 1982.

Zone JJ. Dermatitis herpetiformis. Curr Probl Dermatol 3(1), 1991 (entire issue).

Zone JJ. Dermatitis herpetiformis, linear IgA disease, chronic bullous disease of childhood. In Provost TT, Weston WL, eds. Bullous Diseases. St. Louis, Mosby–Year Book, 1993, pp. 157–212.

Chapter 22

Pulmonary Disorders

John K. Pfaff and Lynn M. Taussig

Exposure of the lungs to inhalant and blood-borne noxious agents has necessitated the development of a complex and diversified pulmonary defense system to prevent disease. These defenses consist of physiologic mechanisms, such as aerodynamic filtration and mucociliary clearance; reflexes, such as cough and bronchoconstriction; immunoglobulins, protease inhibitors and other secretions; and phagocytic cells (Table 22–1). A detailed description of these individual components of the lung's defense against damage is beyond the scope of this chapter, but they have been reviewed by Bienenstock (1984), Bowden (1984), Stuart (1984), Willoughby and Willoughby (1984), Quie (1986), and Daniele and coworkers (1988).

Which of the various defense mechanisms are utilized to defend against a specific inhaled particle depends on the nature of the particle and its final location in the respiratory tract. Deposition site is determined by:

1. Particle size, shape, and density.
2. Aerodynamic, electrostatic, solubility, and surface properties.
3. Airway anatomy.
4. Patterns of flow.

Large particles (greater than 10 μm) tend to fall out in the nose and upper airways, mainly by inertial deposition caused by turbulence, whereas smaller particles (less than 5 μm) deposit in the more peripheral airways and alveoli. Stimulation of cough and irritant receptors located throughout the upper respiratory tract may produce reflex bronchoconstriction (thereby

Table 22–1. Lung Defense Mechanisms

Cells
Lymphocytes (T and B)
Macrophages

Secretions
Transferrin
Alpha₁-antitrypsin
Alpha₂-macroglobulin
Lysozyme
Immunoglobulins (IgG, IgM, IgA, IgE)
Secretory components (bound and free)
C3, C4
Opsonins
Interferon
Mucus
Surfactant

Lymphoid Tissue
Bronchus-associated lymphoid tissue (BALT)
Lymph nodes
Peripheral aggregates of lymphoid tissue

Physiologic Mechanisms
Mucociliary transport
Cough
Reflex bronchoconstriction
Alveolar fluid movement

preventing more peripheral deposition of the agent) and cough clearance. Mucociliary transport is the predominant clearance mechanism in the conducting airways, from the terminal bronchiole to the larynx. Alveolar-bronchiolar clearance is dependent not on mucociliary transport but rather on alveolar fluid movement and macrophages (Newhouse et al., 1976).

Small particles may penetrate epithelial cells, resulting in cell death and eventual transport of debris to the mucociliary escalator or the interstitial space. Paracellular and transcellular passage through the epithelium may occur with subsequent destruction by the phagocytic system or transport to the lymphatics (Clarke and Pavia, 1991).

Lymphocytes and macrophages are the predominant cells in bronchial lavage fluid from normal individuals. Both T and B lymphocytes are found in the airways, and the ratio of T to B cells and of their subtypes appears to be similar to the ratio in the circulation, although the concentration in the lavage fluid is one half that in the lung parenchyma (Hunninghake and Fauci, 1979; Hunninghake et al., 1981). In the normal state, these lymphocytes are probably derived from peripheral aggregates of lymphoid tissue, from bronchus-associated lymphoid tissue (BALT), or from both. In disease states, lymphocyte migration from capillaries quite likely occurs (Kaltreider, 1991). Pulmonary macrophages are derived from two sources; the majority are transformed from monocytes that originate in the bone marrow and arrive via the circulation, and a lesser number derive from resident interstitial cells and multiplication of free macrophages (Bowden, 1984). These cells, in addition to their major phagocytic role, possess specific surface receptors for IgA (Bienenstock, 1984), all IgG subclasses (Naegel et al., 1984), and complement (Reynolds et al., 1974).

Alveolar macrophages, through their ingestion and degradation of particulates, generally protect the lung from immune stimulation (Kaltreider, 1991). These cells are normally suppressive, but under appropriate conditions and following phagocytosis and intracellular processing, they may present antigen to T lymphocytes. The macrophage secretes interleukin 1 (IL-1), which stimulates lymphokine release and activation of T-helper cells. Gamma interferon, a T-lymphocyte product, amplifies antigen processing and may help sustain the immune response (Daniele et al., 1988).

Additionally, the macrophage, through a variety of mediators, recruits neutrophils, eosinophils, and blood monocytes and activates inflammation, thus making it an important element in host defenses in the lung. Despite the secretion of proteolytic agents, such as elastases and collagenases, the macrophage also secretes chemoattractants that aid in mesenchymal repair. Macrophage-derived oxidants, on the other hand, make the extracellular matrix more susceptible to protease degradation (Bowden, 1984; Willoughby and Willoughby, 1984; Crystal, 1991). Eosinophils are found in the lung in a variety of disease states and are discussed later.

The most common immunoglobulins found in the respiratory tract are IgA (mostly in the larger airways) and IgG (mostly in the smaller airways) (Newhouse et al., 1976; Kaltreider, 1991). IgM and IgE are found in lung lavage fluid at approximately the same levels as in serum (Hunninghake et al., 1979). IgD has not been detected in alveolar fluid. IgA is present in normal alveolar fluid in the dimeric form (91% of total) and the monomeric form (9% of total); free secretory piece can also be found in lavage fluid (Hunninghake and Fauci, 1979). IgG may act as an opsonin in the lung. The role of IgA in preventing lung disease is less well defined; it functions poorly as an opsonin and does not fix complement by the classical pathway. However, IgA blocks antigen uptake in the respiratory tract, may be a blocking antibody in allergic reactions, inhibits viral binding and replication, and by binding to lymphocytes, may play a role in mediating antibody-dependent cell cytotoxicity (Bienenstock, 1984). IgE, in addition to its role in hypersensitivity reactions, assists host resistance to parasitic and viral pathogens and modulates immune responses by regulating vascular permeability (Kaltreider, 1991). Complement components are present in low titers in bronchoalveolar lavage fluid and are probably derived from serum, although they can be synthesized by macrophages (Whaley, 1980).

Proteins such as alpha₁-antitrypsin, alpha₂-macroglobulin, and lysozyme protect the lung by destroying or inhibiting the activity of harmful proteases (collagenase and elastase) (Gadek et al., 1984). Deficiency of such antiproteases results in destructive lung disease (e.g., alpha₁-antitrypsin deficiency).

MECHANISMS IN IMMUNOLOGIC LUNG DISEASE

Various derangements in local and systemic defense systems may predispose one to the development of different types of lung disease. The four basic types of immunologic reactions that can produce lung disease are summarized in Table 22–2. These are based on the original classification of Coombs and Gell (1968).

Type I reactions are IgE mediated, disease being produced by the binding of IgE and antigen to mast cells with release of various mediators. Type I reactions are further characterized by immediate type skin reactions and the lack of cytotoxicity.

Lung diseases caused by type II reactions are characterized by tissue destruction (cytotoxicity), the presence of autoantibodies, complement activation, and linear deposition of antibody and complement along basement membranes, as demonstrated by electron microscopy and immunofluorescence. In humans, the most common example of a type II lung disease is Goodpasture's syndrome, in which antiglomerular and antilung basement membrane antibodies can be demonstrated. It should be noted that antilung antibody can be found in other diseases, such as asthma, emphysema, tuberculosis, cystic fibrosis, and interstitial fibrosis. However, in contrast to Goodpasture's syndrome, antilung antibody is not found in the pulmonary lesions of these other lung disorders (McCombs, 1972).

Type III reactions involve the deposition of circulating immune complexes in small blood vessels, activation of complement, and leukocyte-mediated tissue destruction. If the antigen gains access to the lungs via inhalation, alveolitis and granuloma formation predominate; if the complexes are deposited mainly by the circulation, vasculitis is the major histologic finding (Roberts, 1975). Electron microscopy and immunofluorescent studies demonstrate material (e.g., immunoglobulins and complement) along the alveolar capillary basement membranes, as opposed to the linear deposits characteristic of type II reactions. Intermediate (Arthus) skin reactions are representative of a type III immunologic mechanism and indicate the presence of circulating precipitins.

The final immunologic reaction producing lung disease is the cell-mediated type IV reaction, or delayed type hypersensitivity. Delayed skin reactions are the hallmark of type IV reactions. Sensitized lymphocytes interact with antigens, causing release of tissue-injuring toxins. These reactions are most commonly seen with certain viral, bacterial, and fungal infections but are also involved in graft rejection and contact dermatitis. Type IV immunologic principles underlying certain infectious diseases are discussed in Chapter 30.

This chapter emphasizes pulmonary disease in which type II, III, and IV reactions are involved and other diseases in which immunologic mechanisms are operative but the exact nature of which remains undefined. Type II and III diseases are relatively rare, and they manifest similar clinical findings, lung function abnormalities, and chest radiographic appearances. The principal type I disorder to be considered in this chapter is allergic bronchopulmonary aspergillosis. The immunologic aspects of sarcoidosis are reviewed in Chapter 19.

CYSTIC FIBROSIS

Cystic fibrosis (CF) (fibrocystic disease of the pancreas, mucoviscidosis) is the most common lethal genetic disease of whites, occurring in about one of every 2500 births (Boat et al., 1989). It is an autosomal recessive disease, and the heterozygote (carrier) rate is approximately 1:25.

Historical Aspects

Cystic fibrosis was first described as a distinct entity in the late 1930s, and the diagnostic sweat test was discovered in 1953 by di Sant'Agnese and coworkers. The disease is primarily manifested through the exocrine glands of the body, although many other organs are involved. Several investigators have mapped the CF gene to the long arm of chromosome 7 (Emrie and Fisher, 1986), and the gene responsible for CF was isolated from this region (7q31.3) using positional cloning methods (Riordan et al., 1989; Rommens et al., 1989).

Table 22–2. Immunologic Mechanisms of Lung Injury

Mediator	Involves Complement	Cell Type	Skin Test	Tissue Necrosis	Disease Example	Comments
IgE	No	Mast cells	Immediate (10–20 min)	No	Asthma	Release of allergic mediators causes disease manifestations.
IgG, IgM	Yes	PMN	—	Yes	Goodpasture's syndrome	Antibody directed against host tissue and/or haptens bound to host tissue. Circulating antigen-antibody complexes not involved.
IgG, IgM	Yes	PMN	Arthus (16–18 hr)	Yes	Extrinsic allergic alveolitis; collagen disease	Antibody probably directed against host and nonhost antigens. Circulating complexes involved.
T lymphocytes	No	Lymphocyte	Delayed (48 hr)	Yes	Intracellular infection; graft rejection	Antibodies not involved.

Abbreviation: PMN = Polymorphonuclear leukocyte.
Modified from Gell PGH, Coombs RRA, eds. Clinical Aspects of Immunology. Philadelphia, F. A. Davis Co., 1968, pp. 317–337.

Pathogenesis and Clinical Manifestations

The cystic fibrosis gene product is a 1480–amino acid polypeptide called the *cystic fibrosis transmembrane conductance regulator* (CFTR) and structurally belongs to a superfamily of ATP-dependent transport proteins (McIntosh and Cutting, 1992). A three–base pair deletion leading to the omission of a phenylalanine residue at the 508 codon (ΔF508) of the CFTR is responsible for approximately 70% of the CF mutations (Cystic Fibrosis Genetic Analysis Consortium, 1990). To date, more than 300 different mutations have been identified, of which at least 230 may be associated with disease (Crystal, 1995). Transfection of cells from CF patients with CFTR complementary deoxyribonucleic acid (cDNA) corrects the chloride conduction abnormality seen in these patients. Permeability studies strongly support the idea that CFTR is an ion channel rather than a regulator (Collins, 1992; Tsui, 1995).

Expression of the CFTR gene also shows an epithelial distribution (Trezise and Buchwald, 1991). Other studies (Cheng et al., 1990; Gregory et al., 1991) indicate that an associated cellular defect is the inability of the CFTR to leave the endoplasmic reticulum; thus, migration to the cell surface and incorporation into the cell membrane are impaired. Tissues in which CFTR is concentrated include the pancreas, gastrointestinal tract, uterus, and testes. Expression of the gene has also been identified at low levels in the bronchi and bronchioles. Respiratory epithelial cells of CF patients have shown an increase in Na^+ reabsorption and a blockage of chloride efflux. This situation presumably leads to excessive water reabsorption and, hence, the drying of respiratory secretions (Collins, 1992; Tizzano and Buchwald, 1992; Knowles et al., 1995). The clinical presentation of CF follows directly from the organs involved in CFTR expression and improper function of the CFTR.

The abnormal electrolyte concentrations seen in sweat from cystic fibrosis patients allows a diagnosis through sweat chloride quantitation. Obstruction of organ ducts leads to the myriad manifestations, including pancreatic insufficiency with malabsorption, biliary cirrhosis, abnormal gallbladder, small and large bowel obstruction, vas deferens obliteration with sterility, thickened vaginal secretions with decreased female fertility, and bronchiolar and bronchial obstruction (Table 22–3).

Except for some neonates with meconium ileus, the extent of pulmonary involvement usually determines the prognosis. Obstruction of airways by mucus predisposes to pulmonary infections, which produce more secretions, thereby maintaining the vicious (and viscous!) circle. Progressive lung involvement is manifested by chronic productive cough, recurrent pulmonary infections, bronchiectasis, lung abscesses, cysts or bullae, cor pulmonale, digital clubbing, malnutrition, and acute and chronic respiratory failure, which eventually terminate in a premature death. Atelectasis, hemoptysis, and pneumothorax are the typical complications. The lungs in CF patients are usually chronically colonized with *Staphylococcus aureus* and *Pseudomonas*

Table 22–3. Organ Involvement in Cystic Fibrosis

Organ	Clinical Features
Lung	Bronchiolitis, bronchitis, pneumonia, bronchiectasis, atelectasis, abscess, cysts, pneumothorax, hemoptysis, cor pulmonale
Upper airway	Sinusitis, nasal polyps, middle ear obstruction, and conductive hearing loss
Gastrointestinal tract	
Neonate	Meconium ileus, meconium peritonitis, bowel atresia, volvulus
Infant	Hypoalbuminemia, edema, hypoprothrombinemia, rectal prolapse
Child	Meconium ileus equivalent, intussusception
Pancreas	Pancreatic insufficiency, malabsorption, fibrosis resulting in diabetes mellitus
Liver	
Neonate	Prolonged neonatal jaundice
Child	Cirrhosis, portal hypertension
Gallbladder	Cholelithiasis, cystic duct obstruction, small and often filled with secretions
Reproductive tract	Male sterility, decreased female fertility, hydrocele, hernia
Sweat glands	Abnormal sweat electrolytes, heat prostration
Salivary glands	Abnormal electrolytes, enlargement
Heart	Cor pulmonale, fibrosis
Extremities	Hypertrophic osteoarthropathy

aeruginosa. Despite acute pulmonary exacerbations resulting from these organisms, bacteremia and sepsis are rare.

A study by Kronborg and colleagues (1993) demonstrated an increase in cytokine production in the lungs of CF patients, in particular tumor necrosis factor-α (TNF-α) and several interleukins (IL-1α, IL-1β, and IL-6). The associated presence of the IL-1 receptor antagonist peptide (IRAP) in the lungs and serum of CF patients suggests that chronic infection may establish, through immunologic defenses, a balance between stimulatory and inhibitory cytokines. Interestingly, the presence of serum IRAP correlated with failing pulmonary function, but this fall actually preceded the presence of colonization with *P. aeruginosa.*

An emerging concern is colonization of the lungs by *Pseudomonas cepacia*, which has been reported in as many as 30% of patients in some centers (MacLusky and Levison, 1990). Several investigators have associated the presence of this organism with rapid deterioration of pulmonary status, acute necrotizing pneumonia, increased morbidity, and premature death (Thomassen et al., 1985). It is not clear whether colonization is causally related to pulmonary decline or if patients with disease that is more progressed are vulnerable to colonization. Age at colonization is older for *P. cepacia* than for *P. aeruginosa* (13.7 compared with 7.5 years); this finding may reflect increased survival of the patient population (MacLusky and Levison, 1990). Unlike its distant relative *P. aeruginosa*, *P. cepacia* may cause bacterial sepsis (Goldmann and Klinger, 1986).

Host Defenses

Because of the extensive organ involvement in CF and chronic lung infections, host defense mechanisms have been studied extensively (Schiotz, 1981; Moss and Lewiston, 1984; Talamo and Schwartz, 1984; Piedra and Ogra, 1986); however, no unique defect in the host defense system has been found to explain all the manifestations, and many of the immunologic findings have been discrepant (Table 22–4). As the CF transmembrane regulatory protein is expressed by cells of nonepithelial origin, such as fibroblasts, macrophages, and neutrophils (Yoshimura et al., 1991), the possibility of a primary functional defect of certain immune cells must be considered. Immune dysfunction, most of which is attributable to secondary effects, is discussed here. In the future, careful analysis of specific activation and effector pathways may reveal subtle functional abnormalities in immune cell lines (Sorensen et al., 1991).

Immunoglobulins

Serum immunoglobulin levels have generally been found to be elevated, especially IgG and IgA (Schwartz, 1966; Moss and Lewiston, 1980; Pritcher-Wilmot et al., 1982), and to correlate with *P. aeruginosa* pulmonary involvement (Moss and Lewiston, 1980); they may play a protective role against sepsis in these patients. An elevated IgE level is a common finding not clearly correlated with the presence of atopy (Moss and Lewiston, 1980; Tobin et al., 1980). However, a subset of CF patients younger than 10 years of age, with milder lung disease, has been found to have hypogammaglobulinemia-G (Matthews et al., 1980). A 5-year follow-up of this group of patients demonstrated that those with persistently low IgG levels had better lung function, fewer hospitalizations, and less colonization with *P. aeruginosa* (Wheeler et al., 1984).

Hemagglutination-inhibiting antibody responses to influenza vaccine have been reported to be normal (Feery et al., 1979), although its effectiveness in preventing disease in these patients is unproven. The bronchial mucosa in CF patients contains an increased number of IgA-producing cells (Martinez-Tello et al., 1968). Free secretory component of IgA can be found in the serum of one third of CF patients (Wallwork and MacFarlane, 1976), and this finding has led to the proposal that a defect in synthesis of IgA may be the cause of increased allergic symptoms in some patients (Hodson, 1980). The increase in immunoglobulin levels and immunocompetent cells most likely reflects the continuous antigenic stimulation by the bacterial organisms in the tracheobronchial tree.

Salivary IgA levels have been reported to be elevated (Gugler et al., 1968; Wallwork et al., 1974) or normal (South et al., 1967). Elevated IgA levels were found in the meconium of neonates with CF (Rule et al., 1971), and since IgA is not normally produced in large quantities before birth, these authors suggest that this finding may be unique to CF and may have etiologic significance. However, Falchuk and Taussig (1973) demonstrated that IgA production by jejunal mucosa is inversely related to the degree of pancreatic insufficiency. Patients with hereditary pancreatitis and pancreatic insufficiency also had increased jejunal IgA production. Most likely, the increased IgA found in the meconium of CF patients is caused by a local noninfectious antigenic stimulus and probably represents a secondary manifestation.

Pseudomonal Antibodies

Bronchoalveolar lavage fluids from patients with CF and chronic *P. aeruginosa* infection contain higher levels of IgG, IgA, IgE, and C3c than those from normal individuals and chronic bronchitis patients with *P. aeruginosa* infection. Elastolytic activity in the bronchoal-

---

Table 22–4. Host Defense Mechanisms in Cystic Fibrosis

B-Cell Function
Normal to increased number of circulating B cells
Normal to increased serum levels of IgG and IgA
Increased serum levels of precipitins to bacterial species
Increased number of IgA- and IgG-producing cells in bronchial mucosa and bronchial lymph glands
Increased levels of salivary IgA
Increased jejunal production of IgA (pre- and postnatally)
Decreased levels of secretory IgA in sputum
Decreased affinity binding of sputum antibodies
Serum and sputum precipitins to *Pseudomonas aeruginosa* and *Staphylococcus aureus*
CF serum depresses phagocytosis of *P. aeruginosa* (but not of *S. aureus*) by rabbit alveolar macrophages (? defect in IgA opsonic function)
Immune complexes in serum and sputum
Immunoglobulins found in complexes in lungs and pancreas
Increased frequency of antinuclear antibody (ANA)
Increased levels of IgE (? increased incidence of allergy)
High serum precipitin and IgE levels to *Aspergillus fumigatus*

T-Cell Function
Normal to increased number of circulating T cells
Normal skin test reactivity
Normal and abnormal lymphocyte transformation
Abnormal lymphocyte response to *P. aeruginosa* (but not to *S. aureus*)

Complement
Normal to increased C3 levels
Transient depressions of C3, C4, CH_{50} with viral infections
Found in immune complexes in lungs and pancreas
Normal and abnormal alternative pathways
Normal bacterial activation of terminal complement components

Neutrophil Function
Normal to low opsonins
Normal phagocytic and bactericidal activity against *P. aeruginosa*
Increased leukotaxis (related to activity of lung infection)
Increased NBT test (related to activity of lung infection)
Inhibition of leukocyte migration when exposed to certain antigens (lung, pancreas, *A. fumigatus*, *P. aeruginosa*)

Other Host Defense Mechanisms
Depressed tracheal mucociliary transport rates
Sodium reabsorption inhibitory factor
Normal to elevated serum protease inhibitors (e.g., alpha$_1$-antitrypsin)
Decreased lung antiproteases (especially in advanced disease)
Normal levels of secretory piece

Abbreviation: NBT = nitroblue tetrazolium.

veolar lavage (BAL) fluids of these CF patients was reported to be strikingly elevated, whereas alpha$_1$-antitrypsin antigenic levels were normal (Fick et al., 1984).

The chronic colonization of the respiratory tract by *Staphylococcus aureus* and *P. aeruginosa* produces high levels of precipitating antibody to these organisms in the serum. Most of the *Pseudomonas*-specific precipitins are IgG and IgA (Høiby and Hertz, 1979, 1981), although *Pseudomonas*-specific IgE antibodies have been reported (Shen et al., 1981; Pathial et al., 1992). Precipitating antibodies against *Escherichia coli* and *Bacteroides fragilis* are also elevated in patients with CF; however, unlike the case with *Pseudomonas* precipitins, their presence or titers do not correlate with severity of clinical disease (Høiby and Hertz, 1979).

Certain *Pseudomonas* exoprotein-specific antibodies have been shown not only to correlate generally with severity of disease but to rise significantly during active pulmonary infection (exacerbation) and fall with antibiotic treatment (Ganstrom et al., 1984). Antibodies to *Pseudomonas* mucoid exopolysaccharide (Speert et al., 1984) and exoproteins, such as exotoxin A and phospholipase C, can clearly identify the patient with chronic *Pseudomonas* colonization.

Monitoring levels of exoprotein antibody has been proposed as a potentially useful objective guide to treatment of patients with CF (Granstrom et al., 1984). By keeping IgG titers against *P. aeruginosa* in the control range with the use of early and frequent anti-*Pseudomonas* antibiotic therapy, Brett and coworkers (1992) were able to limit sputum conversion to positive for *P. aeruginosa* and improve lung function. The presence of such a large number and variety of antipseudomonal antibodies may explain why immunization with *Pseudomonas* vaccine has not been beneficial in preventing pulmonary exacerbations in CF (Pennington et al., 1975; Wood et al., 1983).

CF sputum has been shown to contain precipitins to *S. aureus, P. aeruginosa,* and *H. influenzae* (Wallwork et al., 1974; Clarke, 1976; Schiller and Millard, 1983; Schiotz and Høiby, 1975, 1979; Schiotz et al., 1979b, 1980). These antibodies are of the IgG and IgA classes and may cross-react with bacteria of the gut and pharyngeal flora, raising the possibility that they are not induced by chronic pulmonary infection alone (Schiotz, 1981). Specific IgA antibody titers may be higher in sputum than in serum, suggesting local production (Schiotz and Høiby, 1979).

The presence of antibodies to specific *Pseudomonas* toxic products has been linked to lung colonization in CF patients (Hollsing et al., 1987; Jagger et al., 1982). The presence of these antibodies may explain the conversion of sputum isolates to mucoid strains that express fewer proteinases than their nonmucoid counterparts (Storey et al., 1992) and would therefore be less vulnerable to opsonization. Attempts to link *P. aeruginosa* toxic products, exotoxin A (*tox* A) and elastase B (*las* B), to isolate types from CF patients using messenger ribonucleic acid (mRNA) transcript and transcript product accumulation have met with limited success (Storey et al., 1992). This method may, however, be used to more clearly elucidate the pattern of lung injury caused by specific *Pseudomonas* toxic products in colonized patients.

The precise function of antibodies found in CF sputum or bronchoalveolar lavage fluid is unknown. IgA is thought to inhibit attachment of bacteria to mucosal cells, and IgG may act as an opsonin (Schiotz, 1981). However, the presence of large amounts of antibody does not necessarily imply normal function. Indeed, the functional ability of IgG antibodies to act as opsonins has been shown to be impaired in CF patients (Fick et al., 1981). Fick and colleagues (1984) found that BAL fluid from CF patients contained as little as 18% intact IgG and that the level of IgG cleavage fragments correlated with impairment of opsonizing ability. This opsonizing defect could be duplicated using proteolytically produced IgG peptide fragments and could be corrected by adding intact IgG to CF BAL fluid specimens.

Moss and coworkers (1986) described a 30-fold increase of *P. aeruginosa* serotype-specific lipopolysaccharide IgG antibodies and elevation of IgG subclass 1–4 antibodies in colonized CF patients compared with uncolonized patients and healthy controls. Elevated levels of IgG antibodies in these CF patients were associated with an isotypic shift in the distribution of IgG subclasses. This shift in IgG subclasses has been substantiated by several investigators, who have shown that IgG subclass IgG2, IgG4, or both against *P. aeruginosa* are increased in the sera of CF patients (Fick et al., 1986; Moss et al., 1986; Shryock et al., 1986). Since alveolar macrophages have surface receptors that bind primarily IgG1 and IgG3 antibodies, excessive production of IgG2 and IgG4 may create a ligand-receptor mismatch for opsonized *P. aeruginosa* (Sorensen et al., 1991).

In colonized patients, serum opsonic capacity for phagocytosis of *P. aeruginosa* was significantly impaired and was correlated with elevated levels of IgG4 subclass antibodies and high concentrations of functional antibody (Moss et al., 1986). Since a major defense mechanism against *Pseudomonas* is provided by IgG *Pseudomonas* antibodies and macrophages with appropriate surface Fc receptors, proteolytic destruction of IgG antibodies or the presence of antibody isotypes that may inhibit efficient macrophage uptake of *Pseudomonas* organisms is potentially very important. Thus, despite the large numbers of anti-*Pseudomonas* precipitins in sera and respiratory tract secretions, their functional capacity is ill defined, and protection of the lungs in CF patients has not been convincingly demonstrated.

Cellular Immunity

Elevated numbers of B and T lymphocytes but a normal B to T cell ratio in patients with CF was reported by Høiby and Mathiesen in 1974. It is, however, generally thought that cell-mediated immunity is normal in CF patients, including lymphocyte numbers and migration, leukocyte migration, and delayed hypersensitivity (Sorensen et al., 1991). One report established a correlation between deteriorating nutritional status, T–helper cell number, and blastogenic responses to mitogens (Smith et al., 1987). If the presence of an abnormal chloride channel in B lymphocytes (Chen et al., 1989) can be confirmed, it may be possible to study the effects of this defect on cellular function. Lymphocytes from CF patients have been found to produce less 3',5'-cyclic monophosphate (cAMP) than normal lymphocytes in response to isoproterenol (Davis et al., 1983), to have increased mitochondrial Ca^{2+} compared with normal cells (Waller et al., 1984), and to produce less IL-10 in response to mitogen concanavalin A [conA] stimulation (Moss et al., 1995). These findings suggest that CF lymphocytes may have abnormalities that could affect their protective capacity in vivo (Sorensen et al., 1991).

Lymphocyte transformation studies (Wallwork et al., 1974) have been normal, but Gibbons and colleagues (1976) demonstrated inhibition of leukocyte migration of CF cells to the lungs, pancreas, and *Aspergillus fumigatus* and *P. aeruginosa* antigens. This inhibition is related to disease severity and is reversed by corticosteroids. Lymphocyte reactivity to *Pseudomonas* has been shown to be impaired in CF patients (Sorensen et al., 1977, 1978, 1979, 1981a, 1981b, 1983) as well as reactivity to *Klebsiella pneumoniae, Serratia marcescens,* and *Proteus mirabilis* (Sorensen et al., 1979). This impaired lymphocyte proliferative response to *Pseudomonas* could not be corrected by incubation of lymphocytes in non-CF serum and could not be induced in non-CF lymphocytes by incubation in CF serum (Sorensen et al., 1981b). Cellular mechanisms to explain this defect in reactivity to *Pseudomonas* have yet to be established (Sorensen et al., 1991). It may be reversible with antibiotic treatment in some patients (Sorensen et al., 1981a).

Alveolar Macrophages

Alveolar macrophages from CF patients are morphologically normal and phagocytize *Pseudomonas* in normal serum (Thomassen et al., 1980). However, serum from patients with CF depresses phagocytosis of *P. aeruginosa* (but not *S. aureus*) by isolated rabbit and human alveolar macrophages (Biggar et al., 1971; Boxerbaum et al., 1973; Thomassen et al., 1980; Fick et al., 1984). In one study, the defect was lessened by concentrated serum (Biggar et al., 1971), whereas in another, the defect was accentuated by increasing the serum concentration (Boxerbaum et al., 1973). In the study by Thomassen and coworkers (1980), phagocytosis by both CF and normal alveolar macrophages was markedly inhibited by CF serum. Suggested explanations include lymphokines, nonopsonizing or blocking antibodies (Høiby and Olling, 1977; Thomassen et al., 1979), and a defect in IgA opsonic function specific for *Pseudomonas* (Biggar et al., 1971). Opsonin-mediated macrophage phagocytosis and intracellular killing of *Pseudomonas* are markedly impaired in the presence of IgG opsonins derived from CF sera (Fick et al., 1981) or respiratory fluids (Fick et al., 1984). In their 1984 study, Fick and colleagues found that this impairment was related to proteolytic fragmentation of IgG opsonins and further showed, as mentioned previously, that abnormal over-representation of IgG2 and IgG4

subclasses to *P. aeruginosa* may prevent normal opsonization of this bacterium by macrophages that primarily bind IgG1 and IgG3 (Fick et al., 1986). None of these studies have correlated the phagocytic defect with the severity of disease.

Increased monocyte oxidase activity with increased superoxide production by macrophages from both CF patients and carriers has lead to speculation that CF gene carriers may have a selective advantage for intracellular microbe killing (Regelmann et al., 1991). On the other hand, as mentioned earlier, the presence of increased macrophage-derived oxidants may make the CF lung extracellular matrix more susceptible to protease degradation (Crystal, 1991; Willoughby and Willoughby, 1984; Bowden, 1984). An in vivo inhibition of macrophage function is suggested by Thomassen and coworkers (1980) on the basis of morphologic studies showing no difference between the appearance of alveolar macrophages from infected CF patients and non-infected normals. In contrast, polymorphonuclear neutrophils (PMNs) from the same CF group were obviously engaged in phagocytic activity, unlike PMNs from non-infected controls. As a potential source of the neutrophil chemoattractant, interleukin-8 (IL-8), the macrophage may provide an important signal for neutrophil recruitment into the lung and may help to explain the elevation of this cytokine in the BAL fluid of patients with CF (Dai et al., 1994).

Neutrophil Function

Neutrophils are the principal effector cells causing damaging inflammation in the cystic fibrosis lung (Bedrossian et al., 1976). Neutrophil function has been shown to be both normal (Biggar et al., 1971; Boxerbaum et al., 1973) and depressed (Holland et al., 1981) in the presence of CF serum. Granulocyte chemiluminescence, a measure of oxidative metabolism, has been used to study granulocyte function in CF. Graft and colleagues (1982) found that the peak response was normal in CF patients but that a more rapid time of onset correlated with the severity of lung disease. They concluded that granulocytes of CF patients seem to be "primed" in their response to a phagocytic stimulus. In the same study, neutrophil concentration and release of β-glucuronidase was found to be similar in controls and CF patients, suggesting normal degranulation.

By contrast, granulocytes from CF patients have been shown to have reduced superoxide degeneration (Waller, 1984), decreased chemiluminescence, and decreased lysosomal β-glucuronidase release in response to N-formyl-methionyl-leucyl-phenylalanine (FMLP) (Kemp et al., 1986). The functional implications of these findings are not yet clear.

Leukotaxis and nitroblue tetrazolium (NBT) dye reduction by CF neutrophils have been reported to be normal (Church et al., 1979, 1980) or above normal (Hill et al., 1974), probably owing to the presence of active pulmonary infection. Random neutrophil migration was normal. The NBT test has been used to search for active bacterial infections in patients with CF (Sullivan et al., 1973), but it has been shown that the test does not always distinguish bacterial from viral infections (Sieber et al., 1976; Berry and Brewster, 1977).

Neutrophil recruitment in the CF lung is thought to occur through cytokine signaling (e.g., via epithelial and possibly macrophage-derived IL-8). In fact, BAL fluid concentrations of IL-8 correlate strongly with disease severity (Dai et al., 1994). Under the influence of the potent activator and chemoattractant macrophage-derived IL-1, neutrophils produce free radicals, leukotriene B$_4$ (LTB$_4$), and proteolytic enzymes. Another indication that neutrophils are highly activated in the lungs of CF patients is the local inactivation of endogenous alpha$_1$-proteinase inhibitor by neutrophil elastase (Goldstein and Döring, 1986). Together with oxidative damage, this mechanism is thought to be one of the primary causes of CF lung damage (Döring et al., 1988).

Complement

McFarlane and coworkers (1975) found deposits of immunoglobulins (IgG, IgA, IgM) and complement (Clq, C3, C4) in various organs in CF patients; such deposits were most prevalent in the lungs and gastrointestinal tract. Serum albumin and staphylococcal hemolysins were two antigens present in the complexes. In addition, 18 of 40 patients had low serum C3 levels. Other studies, however, have demonstrated elevated levels of C3 (Holzhauer et al., 1976; Lieberman, 1975; Polley and Bearn, 1974), but these increased levels may be related to disease severity or sex of the patient. Strunk and coworkers (1977) have shown that C3 and C4 levels are depressed in CF patients (but not in normal children) during documented viral illnesses; these levels return to normal following recovery from the viral illness. The alternative complement pathway was not abnormal in this study or in the one by Lyrene and colleagues (1977) but was abnormal in the study by Polley and Bearn (1974).

Strauss (1979) found the classical and alternative complement pathways to be functionally normal in sera from CF patients, except for the finding that factor B is more readily activated in CF patients than in controls. Complement depression in CF may be secondary to the presence of the antigen-antibody complexes (Döring et al., 1988; McFarlane et al., 1975). Döring and associates (1988) also reported cleavage of complement components, namely, C3 and C5, and of complement receptors, specifically C3b, on human neutrophils by neutrophil elastase. Complement components are appropriately activated by *S. aureus* and *P. aeruginosa* (Buescher and Winkelstein, 1978). Activated complement in the sputum of CF patients has been correlated with colonization by *P. aeruginosa* (Schiotz et al., 1979a).

Autoantibodies

High levels of serum precipitins in CF could participate in a local type III reaction. The antigens could be derived from viruses, altered bacterial components, or lung tissue. Isoantibodies to lung tissue are found in the sputum of CF patients but not in their serum (Stein et al., 1964). There is an increased incidence of antinuclear antibodies (ANAs) in CF serum (Høiby and Wiik, 1975). Smooth muscle autoantibodies were found in a subset of CF patients by Hodson and Turner-Warwick (1981) and were associated with liver involvement. Høiby and Wiik (1975) found no increase in rheumatoid factor (RF) or lupus erythematosus (LE) cells, while Schiotz and colleagues (1979c) have reported a group of CF patients with a high prevalence of IgG-RF cells, which correlated with the number of *P. aeruginosa* precipitins. Adults with chronic bronchitis and repeated infections also have elevated levels of autoantibodies (Hodson and Turner-Warwick, 1976).

Attempts have been made to link the presence of human histocompatibility antigens HLA-DR2 and HLA-DR3 to the rapidly progressive pulmonary disease seen in some CF patients. These HLA types are associated with a variety of autoimmune disorders and show poor Fc-IgG receptor function. So far, no strong association has been demonstrated between HLA type and lung disease in CF (Jones et al., 1989).

Immune Complexes

Numerous investigators have found circulating immune complexes to be present in the serum and/or sputum of 50% to 100% of CF patients (Schiotz et al., 1977; Berdischewsky et al., 1980; Moss et al., 1980, 1981; Church et al., 1981; Manthei et al., 1982; Pritcher-Wilmot et al., 1982; Moss and Hsu, 1982; Disis et al., 1986). Although three investigators found a correlation with exacerbation or deterioration of pulmonary function (Church et al., 1981; Moss et al., 1981; Pritcher-Wilmot et al., 1982), the others found no correlation with severity of illness. Disis and colleagues (1986) found elevated circulating immune complexes in 100% of CF patients studied, which correlated with indices of chronic disease but not with acute exacerbation. Immune complex activity as well as complement activation is usually associated with the presence of chronic *P. aeruginosa* colonization (Schiotz et al., 1977, 1978), and *P. aeruginosa* antigens have been detected in immune complexes (Döring et al., 1988).

In vitro immune complex formation in sera from CF patients infected with *Pseudomonas* but not in sera from noninfected CF patients has been demonstrated (Permin et al., 1982). Moss and Hsu (1982) found circulating immune complexes to *P. aeruginosa*, *S. aureus*, and *Candida albicans* and suggested that circulating immune complex formation specifically corresponds to respiratory tract colonization.

Despite the presence of circulating immune complexes in CF patients, recent immunofluorescence studies of lung tissue at autopsy failed to show strong evidence for immune complex deposition in the lungs of CF patients in the absence of an associated rheumatologic disorder (Tomashefski et al., 1992). Proteolytic cleavage of immune complexes may account for the difficulty in identifying immune complexes and hence problems in correlating immune complexes with patient clinical status (Döring et al., 1988).

In summary, there is suggestive evidence that type II and III reactions may occur in the lungs of CF patients, and it seems clear that a poor prognosis is associated with chronic pseudomonal infection and increased anti-pseudomonal antibodies (Schiotz, 1981); however, the conclusion that type II or type III reactions are of primary importance in the pathogenesis of the progressive lung disease seen in CF is unwarranted at this time.

Relation to Allergy and Asthma

The relationship of allergy and asthma to lung disease in CF remains controversial. It is still unclear if CF patients have an increased incidence of clinically important allergic manifestations. About one third of CF patients have elevated total IgE levels (Wallwork et al., 1974; Tobin et al., 1980; Tacier-Eugster et al., 1980); specific *P. aeruginosa* IgE has been reported (Shen et al., 1981), and about 50% of patients have elevated specific IgE antibodies and/or precipitins to *A. fumigatus* (Schwartz et al., 1970; Warren et al., 1975; Bardana et al., 1975; Galant et al., 1976; Carswell et al., 1979). There appears to be a relationship between levels of *Aspergillus* precipitins and disease severity (Schwartz et al., 1970; Galant et al., 1976). Nelson and colleagues (1979) reported positive *Aspergillus* fungal cultures and sputum eosinophilia in 57% of CF patients who produced sputum, and Tobin and coworkers (1980) found a higher mean eosinophil count in the serum of CF patients compared with controls.

About one third of patients demonstrate type I and III skin reactions to *A. fumigatus*; however, in contrast to patients with allergic bronchopulmonary aspergillosis, CF patients have only a type I response when challenged intranasally with this organism. Pulmonary disease due to *Aspergillus* is uncommon in CF, even though the organism is commonly found in the sputum. Increased skin reactivity and elevated serum precipitins may reflect defective mucosal defenses against these allergens, thereby allowing for increased systemic or local production of antibodies; abnormalities in local IgA protective mechanisms may be involved (McFarlane et al., 1975; Warner et al., 1976; Nelson et al., 1979; Wilmott, 1991).

Although CF patients appear to have increased skin reactivity to numerous allergens and some patients manifest bronchial hyperreactivity, allergic disease and asthma may not occur more frequently (Warren et al., 1975; Wilmott, 1991). Several studies have reported an increased incidence of atopy and/or asthma in CF (Tobin et al., 1980; Tacier-Eugster et al., 1980); however, the criteria for diagnosis of atopy in CF are often based on positive prick skin tests, elevated serum levels of IgE, and bronchial hyperreactivity, all of which may occur in CF patients without allergic disease. No relationship between skin test reactivity and survival has been found in CF (Wilmott, 1991). Survival rates have been negatively associated with skin test reactivity to *P. aeruginosa* but no more so than in patients colonized

with *Pseudomonas* and having a negative skin test. Attempts to use response to exercise in order to distinguish atopic from nonatopic CF patients have not been successful (Zambie et al., 1979; Silverman et al., 1978).

The need for caution in this area was shown by Holzer and coworkers (1981), who evaluated the use of allergy skin tests, exercise challenge, and histamine bronchial challenge in the diagnosis of allergy and asthma in CF patients. They found that although positive results roughly correlated with overall impairment of pulmonary function, 56% of patients had variable responses to exercise, 44% to histamine challenge, and 24% to skin tests. This variability did not correlate with pulmonary disease exacerbation or pulmonary function changes. More recent investigations again show that the association between specific allergic sensitization and deteriorating pulmonary function in CF is weak at best and, when present, may be secondary to increased access of antigen to the diseased airway mucosa (Wilmott, 1991). Again, the only strongly associated finding to explain deterioration of lung function in CF patients was the colonization with, not skin test conversion to, *P. aeruginosa* (Wilmott, 1991).

One must question the validity of using any one of these methods to diagnose allergy or asthma in CF patients. Furthermore, the wheezing noted in CF patients is often due to obstruction by viscid secretions rather than to bronchospasm, although wheezing is said to be more common in "atopic" CF patients (Nelson et al., 1979). In fact, bronchodilators may have an adverse effect on lung function in certain CF patients, possibly by removing any remaining bronchomotor tone in bronchiectatic airways (Landau and Phelan, 1973; Shapiro et al., 1976; Loughlin et al., 1977; Zach et al., 1985). Nasal polyps are relatively common in CF and may be related to mucus obstruction of glands, iodide therapy, or allergies. The suggestion by Rachelefsky and colleagues (1974) that asthma in CF patients tends to protect them from rapid deterioration remains to be confirmed; in fact, some investigators have found that CF patients with positive skin tests to allergens had more severe pulmonary disease (Warner et al., 1976), while others have not (Tobin et al., 1980; Holzer et al., 1981).

The fact that the infections seen in CF are limited to the lung, whereas the ducts and secretions of other organs are also involved, makes an immunologic mechanism an unlikely possibility for the primary defect in CF. CF has been described in patients with agammaglobulinemia, selective IgA deficiency, combined immunodeficiency syndrome, and Wiskott-Aldrich syndrome; these associations are probably coincidental. The identification of an abnormal chloride channel in B lymphocytes should be pursued to determine if functional responses are affected (Chen et al., 1989; Sorensen et al., 1991).

Diagnosis

The diagnosis of cystic fibrosis is based on a history of chronic lung disease, malabsorption, family history of CF, and a positive sweat test (>60 mEq/L of chloride) (Taussig, 1984; Tizzano and Buchwald, 1992). Adequate sweat analysis by the pilocarpine iontophoresis test requires that patients be referred to a laboratory with sufficiently skilled technicians. A relatively new macroductal sweat collection system may allow laboratories to overcome these technical demands and thus make accurate diagnosis more readily available (Hammond et al., 1994). The diagnosis should be considered in any child with recurrent lower respiratory tract illness, chronic diarrhea, and malnutrition. Evaluation of ejaculates (for aspermia) and vaginal secretions (for viscosity) may assist in the diagnosis of older patients.

Several methods are now employed for the prenatal diagnosis of cystic fibrosis. In the case of known mutations, the polymerase chain reaction (PCR) can be used on samples of chorionic villi or cultured amniotic cells. If the most common CF mutation, ΔF508, and other common mutations are not present, the addition of restriction fragment–length polymorphisms (RFLPs) (Spence et al., 1987) in combination with intragenic polymorphisms or repetitive sequences can be utilized. If RFLP analysis is not fully informative, identification of low levels of microvillar intestinal enzymes (alkaline phosphatase intestinal enzyme, leucine aminopeptidase, and gamma-glutamyl transpeptidase) can be helpful (Tizzano and Buchwald, 1992).

Postnatal diagnosis can usually be made for "at risk" infants by obtaining DNA from blood, blood spots, or mouthwashes using commercially available kits. The presence of more than 300 genetic mutations makes general population screening using DNA analysis impractical, but the finding of an increased immunoreactive trypsinogen together with DNA analysis may add specificity to the newborn screening and avoid problems of false-positive results (Gregg et al., 1993).

Treatment

The treatment for the many manifestations of cystic fibrosis is varied and extensive, but proof of efficacy is often lacking (Taussig, 1984; Smith, 1986). The gastrointestinal manifestations are treated with supplemental oral pancreatic enzymes and vitamins. The pulmonary aspects are treated with vigorous pulmonary hygiene (e.g., postural drainage, chest physiotherapy, or breathing exercises), oral and intravenous antibiotics, and aerosolized medications (including mucolytics, bronchodilators, and antibiotics when appropriate) (MacLusky et al., 1986). Conventional chest physiotherapy may be augmented by external high-frequency chest compression (HFCC) devices (Warwick and Hansen, 1991) or endobronchial oscillation ("flutter valve") in efforts to mobilize pulmonary secretions.

Early optimism about the use of chronic steroids to slow progression of chronic lung disease in cystic fibrosis came after the report by Auerbach and colleagues (1985) of decreased morbidity and slowed pulmonary deterioration using alternate-day prednisone at 2 mg/kg. Complications related to glucose abnormalities, cataracts, and growth retardation led to early discontinuation of the high-dose limb of a multicenter

alternate-day steroid trial (Rosenstein and Eigen, 1991). Linear growth retardation was subsequently noted in the low-dose treatment group (1 mg/kg), and the study was stopped (Rosenstein et al., 1993). In conclusion, there is little support for use of chronic steroids in the routine treatment of CF. Other anti-inflammatory drugs, including ibuprofen and inhaled antiproteases, are currently being studied. Ibuprofen, in high dose, when taken consistently for four years slows progression of lung disease, as measured by longitudinal decline of the 1-second forced expiratory volume (FEV$_1$) in patients with mild lung disease (Konstan et al., 1995). Aerosolized leukoprotease inhibitors may decrease lung injury through reductions in neutrophil elastase as well as through modulation of epithelial cell expression of the inflammatory cytokine IL-8 (McElvaney et al., 1992).

Several investigators have observed improved pulmonary function in moderately to severely ill, *Pseudomonas*-colonized patients when they were given intravenous immunoglobulin (IVIG) (Winnie et al., 1989; Bentur et al., 1990). Although they were not sustained, these improvements suggest that phagocytosis of *Pseudomonas* organisms by neutrophils, alveolar macrophages, or both may be stimulated. Identification of specific serum opsonic activity in response to conventional IVIG or *Pseudomonas* hyperimmune globulin (Ps-IVIG) may allow development of adjuncts to conventional therapy, especially in those patients infected with multiply-resistant organisms (Van Wye et al., 1990).

The developing science of transplant immunology has provided an increasing number of CF patients the hope of increased survival and improved quality of life. Several cytokine products of the T$_H$1 subset of CD4$^+$ cells, such as IL-2 and IFN-γ, participate in graft rejection (Nisen, 1993). A more complete understanding of signal transduction pathways leading to transcriptional activation of these cytokines may permit the development of more effective immunsuppressive agents. Biologic response modifiers, such as anti-thymocyte globulin (ATG) and antibodies to specific cell receptor molecules, are especially important in the rescue of acute rejection episodes (Nisen, 1993).

Cystic fibrosis patients present the transplant team with a variety of challenges. Complication rates are increased by chronic malnutrition and colonization of the tracheobronchial tree by multiply resistant organisms (Noyes et al., 1994). Post-transplant infection caused by *P. cepacia* remains a particularly troublesome complication in patients who have previously been colonized. Avoidance of triple-drug immunosuppression, patient-specific tailoring of perioperative antimicrobial therapy, and meticulous intraoperative handling of the bibronchial anastomoses may lessen complication rates (Maurer, 1993; Noyes et al., 1994).

Influenza vaccine may be useful in reducing the potentially serious consequences of that infection on the lung. The potential usefulness of other vaccines in patients with CF is even less well defined. Amantidine may be used to prevent or treat influenza A infections.

Other exciting new prospects exist for the treatment

of cystic fibrosis lung disease (Collins, 1992). Aerosolization of the diuretic amiloride may improve mucus hydration by retarding sodium and water reabsorption. Uridine triphosphate (UTP) by aerosol may recruit alternative Cl^- channels and bypass the need for a functional CFTR; this could produce increased chloride and water secretion, enhancing mucus hydration. The use of human recombinant DNase may help reduce mucus viscosity (Fuchs et al., 1994; Hodson, 1995). The successful development of a transgenic mouse model expressing the abnormal CFTR will provide a valuable tool for testing new therapies (Clarke et al., 1992).

The most exciting prospect for the future in the treatment of CF lung disease is the correction of the ion transport abnormalities by introduction of normal genetic material (e.g., gene therapy) into airway cells of CF patients. A variety of viral, liposomal, and DNA–protein complex vectors are currently being explored as methods for introducing the normal genetic material into host target cells (Collins, 1992). The adenoviral vector systems, with their natural affinity for airway epithelial cells, are the most extensively studied. Human trials using this delivery system have been initiated in patients with CF (Ramsey and Boat, 1994; Korst et al., 1995).

Prognosis

The prognosis for patients with cystic fibrosis has improved considerably over the past 30 years (Davis and di Sant'Agnese, 1984). Approximately half of all patients will live to 29 years of age (McIntosh and Cutting, 1992). For unknown reasons, male patients consistently do better than female patients (Ramsey and Boat, 1994). The prognosis appears to be related to early diagnosis, nutritional status, and genetic variability in the expression of the disease (Gaskin et al., 1982; Kerem et al., 1990; Ramsey and Boat, 1994), and—clearly the most important—the extent of chronic pulmonary involvement.

Kerem and associates (1990) and Johansen and colleagues (1991) defined the extent to which the most common CF mutation, ΔF508, affects severity of disease. Patients who are homozygous (ΔF508/ΔF508) are much more likely to have pancreatic insufficiency than heterozygotes (ΔF508/other) or those without the common mutation (other/other). To date, good correlations noted have not been between genotypes and respiratory function and/or pulmonary symptoms. However, these discoveries have opened an intense new avenue of investigation. Attempts to correlate these and other aspects of disease severity with mutation type may allow better prognostication for patients with certain mutations (Campbell et al., 1991).

PULMONARY INFILTRATES WITH EOSINOPHILIA (PIE Syndrome)

Several respiratory illnesses have been characterized by the term *pulmonary infiltrates with eosinophilia,* or PIE syndrome (Reeder and Goodrich, 1952). PIE syndrome was originally described by Crofton and colleagues (1952) and classified into five categories: simple pulmonary eosinophilia, cryptogenic pulmonary eosinophilia, tropical eosinophilia, vasculitis, and pulmonary eosinophilia with asthma (Liebow and Carrington, 1969). Because of the extensive overlap between the categories and poorly defined nature of many of the illnesses, this classification has been difficult to use (Pepys and Simon, 1973; Citro et al., 1973; Ottesen, 1976). Somewhat later, Schatz and coworkers (1981, 1982) proposed a new classification for PIE syndrome based on clearly definable syndromes (Table 22–5). Although pulmonary eosinophilia is a prominent feature of most of the disorders in Table 22–5, the classification system refers to pulmonary infiltrates with peripheral blood eosinophilia and is thus clinically oriented.

Löffler's syndrome, or simple pulmonary eosinophilia, was formerly defined as transient, migratory pulmonary infiltrates and eosinophila with mild or absent respiratory symptoms. This term is no longer used because most patients probably had undetected parasitic infections, drug reactions, or allergic bronchopulmonary aspergillosis (ABPA), and thus the condition did not constitute a separate entity. Pulmonary eosinophilia with asthma is no longer considered a PIE syndrome disorder (Schatz et al., 1981). Although eosinophilia does occur in patients with asthma, the eosinophil appears to be only one of many pathogenetic agents involved, and most asthmatic patients who were previously thought to have PIE syndrome proba-

Table 22–5. Classification of Pulmonary Infiltrates with Peripheral Eosinophilia

Group	Type of Illness	Specific Examples
Illnesses in which PIE is a major component	Allergic bronchopulmonary aspergillosis	—
	Chronic eosinophilic pneumonia	—
	Drug reaction	Nitrofurantoin and others
	Hypereosinophilic syndrome	—
	Parasitic infestation	Tropical eosinophilia and other parasites
	Polyarteritis nodosa	Churg-Strauss syndrome
Illnesses in which PIE occurs infrequently and is a minor feature	Infection	Bacterial (tuberculosis, brucellosis)
		Fungal (coccidioidomycosis, histoplasmosis)
	Neoplasm	Hodgkin's disease
	Immunologic disorders	Sarcoidosis and rheumatoid lung disease
PIE without features of the other two groups	Unknown	—

Abbreviation: PIE = pulmonary infiltrates with eosinophilia.
Data from Schatz M, Wasserman S, Patterson R. Eosinophils and immunologic lung disease. Med Clin North Am 65:1055–1071, 1981; Schatz M, Wasserman S, Patterson R. The eosinophil and the lung. Arch Intern Med 142:1515–1519, 1982.

bly had allergic bronchopulmonary aspergillosis instead (Leitch, 1979). In addition, reversible obstructive airways disease ("asthma") may be a clinical finding in virtually all PIE syndrome disorders (Leitch, 1979).

Other disorders that may result in a peripheral blood eosinophilia but with less marked lung eosinophilia include neoplasms (e.g., Hodgkin's disease), desquamative interstitial pneumonia, fungal infections (e.g., coccidioidomycosis), sarcoidosis, rheumatoid lung disease, and radiation injury—none of which are discussed in this chapter. Allergic bronchopulmonary aspergillosis is discussed later under that heading.

Chronic Eosinophilic Pneumonia

Chronic eosinophilic pneumonia usually occurs in women between 20 and 30 years of age, but patients younger than 20 years of age represent 6% of cases (Rao et al., 1975; Weller, 1984; Jederlinic et al., 1988). Common manifestations are cough, malaise, dyspnea, fever, night sweats, and weight loss. Wheezing ("asthma"), often of recent onset, and hemoptysis may occur (Schatz et al., 1981). A pattern of restrictive lung disease and a decreased diffusing capacity are common pulmonary function findings, but progression to hypoxemia and respiratory failure can occur (Lopez and Salvaggio, 1991). In some patients, standard spirometry can be used to follow response to therapy, with improved FEV_1 seen in two thirds of patients (Jederlinic et al., 1988).

Chest radiographic changes usually consist of peripheral nonsegmental, nonlobar infiltrates described by Carrington as "the photographic negative of pulmonary edema" (Carrington et al., 1969); however, the chest radiograph may show pleural effusion or cavitation (Lopez and Salvaggio, 1991) or be normal (Dejaegher et al., 1983).

The usual laboratory findings include anemia, a greatly elevated erythrocyte sedimentation rate (ESR), and an increased serum IgE. Peripheral blood eosinophilia occurs but may be absent in one third of the patients, and lung biopsy shows an alveolar and interstitial infiltrate of eosinophils as well as macrophages, lymphocytes, and plasma cells (Weller, 1984; Gonzalez et al., 1986). Clumps of eosinophils that produce "eosinophil abscesses" and granulomas with necrosis may be seen. Many think that the diagnosis can be made on clinical grounds with appropriate support from diagnostic laboratory tests. The use of BAL and computed tomographic (CT) scan may help define the disease and avoid the need for lung biopsy (Jederlinic et al., 1988). The etiology and immunopathogenesis of this disorder are unknown, although the presence of major basic protein (MBP) in lung tissue and pleural fluid suggests that eosinophilic granule constituents may lead to lung damage in this disease (Grantham et al., 1986). A type I mechanism has been suggested but remains unproven (McCarthy and Pepys, 1973; Schatz et al., 1981).

Steroids are of benefit in treating acute episodes (Rogers et al., 1975), but the disease may worsen when steroids are tapered. Recurrence after long periods of remission is not uncommon (Schatz et al., 1981), although prolongation of therapy for 6 months reduces the frequency of relapse (Jederlinic et al., 1988).

Drug Reactions

Many drugs can produce the PIE syndrome; acute nitrofurantoin reaction is characteristic. Beginning within 10 days of the onset of treatment with nitrofurantoin, the patient experiences fever, dyspnea, and cough. Cyanosis and bibasilar crackles are often present, and the chest x-ray usually shows basilar infiltrates and, at times, pleural effusions (Weller, 1984; Schatz et al., 1981). The lung pathology is characterized by a histiocytic and eosinophilic alveolar infiltrate, sometimes with vasculitis, interstitial inflammation, and granuloma formation. Type IV immunologic reactivity is thought to be the mechanism of injury, although antibodies against nitrofurantoin have been found (Schatz et al., 1981). Other drugs reported to cause the PIE syndrome are listed in Table 22–6. Unfortunately, a pattern of interstitial eosinophilia may develop with features of usual interstitial pneumonia (UIP), suggesting progression to fibrosis and chronic disease (Smith, 1990). This occurs more commonly with nitrofurantoin or gold salts, whereas the pattern of acute eosinophilic pneumonia is more typical of reactions to antibiotics. Treatment consists mainly of withdrawal of the offending drug and steroid therapy in severe cases (Schatz et al., 1981).

Hypereosinophilic Syndrome

The hypereosinophilic syndrome is a disease of middle-aged men and is discussed only briefly here. It has been reported to occur in a patient 5 years of age (Chusid et al., 1975). The diagnosis is made when there is marked eosinophilia (>1500 cells/mm³) for more than 6 months, organ infiltration, and no other etiology for the eosinophilia (Chusid et al., 1975; Fauci et al., 1982). Fever, diarrhea, edema, cough, cardiac murmurs, hepatomegaly, splenomegaly, arthralgias, and abdominal pain are common. A restrictive cardiomyopathy occurs and is a major source of morbidity and mortality. There is also nervous system and skin involvement. Histologically, the disease is characterized by infiltrates of mature eosinophils in many organs,

Table 22–6. Drugs Associated with Eosinophilia and Pulmonary Infiltrates

Nitrofurantoin	Captopril
Penicillin	Beclomethasone
Sulfonamides	Tetracycline
Imipramine	Cromolyn
Mephenesin	Para-aminosalicylic acid
Aspirin	Aminosalicylic acid
Methylphenidate	Methotrexate
Carbamazepine	Chlorpropamide
Chloroquine	Chlorpromazine
Gold salts	

Data from Schatz M, Wasserman S, Patterson R. Eosinophils and immunologic lung disease. Med Clin North Am 65:1055–1071, 1981; Smith GJW. The histopathology of pulmonary reactions to drugs. Clin Chest Med 11:95–117, 1990.

but the immunopathogenesis is unknown (Schatz et al., 1981; Fauci et al., 1982). The response to steroid treatment is variable.

Tropical Eosinophilia (Parasitic Infestation)

The life cycles of several helminthic parasites are characterized by transpulmonary migration of larvae. The result may be blood eosinophilia, reversible obstructive airways disease, and transient infiltrates in the lungs. Parasites such as *Ascaris,* hookworm, and *Strongyloides* can cause this clinical picture, and in fact *Ascaris* infestation was probably the etiology in many of Löffler's original patients (Weller, 1984). Other parasites that may cause this syndrome are listed in the review article by Schatz and coworkers (1982).

Tropical eosinophilia is a distinct PIE syndrome caused by infestation with filarial organisms of the genera *Brugia* and *Wuchereria.* It is most commonly found in men during the third and fourth decades of life and is characterized by a dry cough, dyspnea, wheezing (often worse at night), weight loss, and fatigue (Neva and Ottesen, 1978). The chest radiograph may be normal or show linear markings and hilar prominence (98%). Diffuse, finely nodular infiltrates and consolidation are also seen, usually with ill-defined margins and a subsegmental distribution. Restrictive abnormalities are found on pulmonary function testing, although these are superimposed on an obstructive pattern in 30% of cases (Schatz et al., 1981; Lopez and Salvaggio, 1991). Intense eosinophilia (>2000 cells/mm^3), elevated total IgE (>1000 ng/ml), and high titers of antifilarial complement–fixing antibodies in the absence of circulating microfilaria characterize the laboratory findings.

Granulomas may develop and microfilariae can be seen in the lesions. The disease is usually confined to the lungs without peripheral tissue invasion. Type I, III, and IV immune mechanisms are thought to be operative in this form of PIE syndrome (Schatz et al., 1981). Treatment consists of diethylcarbamazine for 2 weeks. The prognosis is usually good.

Churg-Strauss Syndrome (Pulmonary Vasculitis)

Although vasculitis was a category in the original Crofton classification, eosinophilia is characteristic of only one vasculitis syndrome: allergic granulomatous angiitis, or Churg-Strauss syndrome (Weller, 1984). Churg-Strauss syndrome has been considered a variant of polyarteritis nodosa (PAN) (Wolfe and Hunninghake, 1991) but has unique features that may distinguish it from PAN. Asthma, peripheral eosinophilia, involvement of various types and sizes of pulmonary vessels, intravascular and extravascular granuloma formation, and eosinophilic tissue infiltrates characterize Churg-Strauss syndrome. PAN is characterized by occasional asthma and peripheral eosinophilia, neutrophilic cellular infiltrates, involvement of small and medium-sized arteries, and the absence of extravascular granuloma formation (Lopez and Salvaggio, 1991).

The treatment for Churg-Strauss syndrome involves high-dose corticosteroids and cytotoxic agents when necessary. Intravenous immunoglobulin has been reported to be of benefit (Hamilos et al., 1991). Type I, III, and IV reactions may be involved in producing the lung changes seen with vasculitis (Cohen and Ottesen, 1983; Lopez and Salvaggio, 1991), and collagen-vascular disease; such findings are usually minor features of these diseases (Table 22–7).

Allergic Bronchopulmonary Aspergillosis

Aspergillus lung disease occurs in a variety of forms that can be divided into three major groups: (1) invasive, (2) non-invasive (aspergilloma and suppurative aspergillosis), and (3) *Aspergillus* hypersensitivity syndromes, such as extrinsic asthma, extrinsic allergic alveolitis, and allergic bronchopulmonary aspergillosis (Pennington, 1980, 1988).

Invasive aspergillosis is rare in children. A variant form, pseudomembranous necrotizing bronchial aspergillosis, has been reported in a 15-year-old boy with acquired immunodeficiency syndrome (AIDS) (Pervez et al., 1985). Although *Aspergillus* may trigger broncho-

Table 22–7. Immunologic Characteristics of Certain Immunologic Lung Disorders

| Disease Category | Eosino-philia | Precip-itins | Autoanti-bodies | Elevated IgE | Skin Tests | | Lung Immunofluorescence* | | | |
					Immediate	Arthus	IgG	IgM	IgA	Complement
Pulmonary infiltration with eosinophilia (PIE)†	+Δ	±	−	+	−	−	−	−	−	−
Extrinsic allergic alveolitis (EAA)	±	+	−	±	±	+	±	−	−	±
Allergic bronchopulmonary aspergillosis (ABPA)	+	+	−	+	+	+	−	−	−	−
Vasculitides‡	+	−	+	−	−	−	±	±	±	±
Cryptogenic fibrosing alveolitis (CFA)	±	−	+	−	−	−	±	±	−	±

* = Immunofluorescence in capillary and/or bronchial walls.
† = When not associated with one of the vasculitides or ABPA.
+Δ = Usually, but not always, associated with the disease.
± = Occasionally associated, but not a characteristic feature.
− = Rarely or never associated with the disease.
‡ = Includes systemic lupus erythematosus and rheumatoid arthritis.

spasm in the sensitized patient with extrinsic asthma, fever and lung infiltrates are not common. In contrast, ABPA, which usually occurs in atopic and asthmatic patients, comprises a distinct clinical entity with lung infiltrates, fever, and bronchiectasis. Excluding *Aspergillus* as a trigger in extrinsic asthma, the other forms of *Aspergillus* lung disease do not occur more frequently in asthmatics (Pennington, 1980).

ABPA is an allergic bronchopulmonary mycosis characterized by reactive airways disease, *Aspergillus* skin reactivity (immediate), pulmonary infiltrates, increased serum IgE, blood eosinophilia, *Aspergillus* precipitating antibodies, increased IgG/IgE-*Aspergillus* antigen complexes, and proximal bronchiectasis (McCarthy and Pepys, 1971a, 1971b; Greenberger, 1984; Longbottom, 1983; Detjen et al., 1991).

ABPA is much more commonly diagnosed in England than in the United States, and pediatric cases are unusual (Slavin et al., 1970; Wang et al., 1979a). The disease has been reported in several infants younger than two years of age (Katz and Kniker, 1973; Imbeau et al., 1977; Kiefer et al., 1986), and the diagnosis is often delayed, sometimes for years. ABPA may be diagnosed in patients with cystic fibrosis, steroid-dependent asthmatic patients, those with previously diagnosed bronchiectasis, and multiple family members. Some of these patients may have a normal chest radiograph (Greenberger, 1984). The disease may occur at any time in an asthmatic patient, and no specific predisposing events have been elucidated.

Clinical Manifestations

In the asthmatic patient with ABPA, there is a marked increase in wheezing, cough, peripheral eosinophilia, fever, pleuritic chest pain, and sputum production. The sputum contains tenacious, firm, spindle-shaped, yellow-brown mucous plugs. The chest radiograph shows nodular lesions ranging in size from 1.0 cm to entire lobar involvement. Atelectasis and pneumonia-type lesions are migratory, usually resolving within 6 weeks, only to recur later in different lung segments. With numerous recurrences, a characteristic bronchiectasis involving the central airways may develop. The upper lobes are usually more involved (Scadding, 1967). This is in contrast to other causes of bronchiectasis, which usually involve the more distal airways (Pepys and Simon, 1973).

The alveoli are filled with eosinophils and mononuclear cells, and the alveolar septa are engorged with mast cells, fibroblasts, and edematous fluid. Polypoid masses of granulation tissue often protrude into the bronchioles. Some patients with ABPA may develop bronchocentric granulomatosis or bronchial mucoid impaction resulting in distal bronchiolitis obliterans (Bosken et al., 1988). Although fungal hyphae are present in the bronchial mucus and the organism can be easily cultured from this source, bronchial wall invasion is not seen. A lung biopsy will reveal these characteristic changes but is not necessary for diagnosis.

Laboratory Findings

Laboratory results in patients with ABPA have been extensively investigated and are summarized briefly here. *Aspergillus* antigen or mixes should produce an immediate positive reaction upon skin prick or intradermal testing. High levels of specific IgE and IgG precipitins to *Aspergillus* antigens can be found in at least 90% of patients (Patterson and Roberts, 1974; Hart et al., 1976; Pauwels et al., 1976). IgA is also elevated in serum, whereas IgM and complement levels are normal. Serum IgE is almost always elevated in ABPA and rises sharply during exacerbations. Although elevated levels of IgG and IgE antibodies directed against *A. fumigatus* are found in serum of affected patients (IgG-Af, IgE-Af), the markedly elevated IgE level is usually nonspecific and not directed against *Aspergillus* (Detjen et al., 1991). IgE levels decrease with effective therapy and can be used as a diagnostic aid and as a sensitive marker of treatment efficacy (Ricketti et al., 1984). T and B cells are present in normal numbers in stable patients (Greenberger, 1984). Basophils from patients with ABPA have been demonstrated to have markedly increased histamine release in response to *Aspergillus* antigens when compared with mold-sensitive asthmatic patients (Ricketti et al., 1983). Other cellular differences have not been demonstrated. Immunoglobulins are increased in BAL fluid, and concentrations suggest increased local production of IgE, IgA, and possibly IgM (Greenberger, 1984; Kauffman et al., 1984). Peripheral blood eosinophilia is common in untreated patients but may be suppressed or absent with steroid treatment. Sputum cultures may be positive but are not diagnostic. Expectorated mucous plugs reveal mycelium, eosinophils, fibrin, Charcot-Leyden crystals (lysophospholipase), and Curschmann's spirals and are culture-positive for *Aspergillus fumigatus*. Sputum cultures for the organism become negative when the chest roentgenogram clears (Greenberger and Patterson, 1987).

Pathogenesis

Type I, III, and IV immune reactions appear to be involved in the development of various manifestations of ABPA; in fact, evidence suggests that a type I reaction is essential before the type III reaction can occur (Cochrane, 1971; Ottesen, 1976). Dual skin reactions can easily be demonstrated in the patient with ABPA by both skin testing and inhalation challenges. In both types of challenges, an immediate type I reaction is usually followed 4 to 6 hours later by a delayed Arthus (type III) reaction. In nonatopic individuals, only a type III reaction occurs. These patients probably have extrinsic allergic alveolitis rather than ABPA. Granuloma formation and infiltrates of mononuclear cells in the lung suggest that type IV reactions are involved. Furthermore, some patients have lymphocytes that undergo blastogenesis following exposure to *Aspergillus* antigen (Turner et al., 1972; Forman et al., 1978). Immune complex activation of eosinophils to produce leukotriene C_4 (LTC_4) may be involved in the pathogenesis (Cromwell et al., 1988). An interesting case report by Stephens and colleagues (1988) of Churg-Strauss syndrome developing in a woman with a prior history of ABPA also strengthens the potential immunopathogenic link between eosinophilic pneumonia and ABPA. Additional nonimmunologic damage may occur from proteolytic enzymes produced by the *Aspergillus* organisms (Greenberger, 1984).

After a mucous plug is expectorated, the radiographic infiltrates may resolve spontaneously or remain for months if the condition is untreated. Resolution of infiltrates is accelerated by steroid treatment (Greenberger, 1984). The pathogenesis of the bronchiectasis is unknown. It has been noted that the location of the bronchiectatic lesions and the radiographic infiltrates coincide (Scadding, 1967). Although the radiologic abnormalities may be absent in ABPA, the typical finding of proximal bronchiectasis may be defined using CT, in some cases avoiding the need for bronchography (Neeld et al., 1990; Shah et al., 1992).

Diagnosis

The diagnosis of ABPA may be difficult. Many patients, such as those with cystic fibrosis (Schwartz et al., 1970), may be colonized with *Aspergillus fumigatus* without active disease. Furthermore, sputum cultures are positive in only 35% to 65% of all symptomatic patients with ABPA and thus may not be helpful in confirming the diagnosis. Presensitized persons without ABPA may have serum precipitins and positive skin tests (Hart et al., 1976). An asthmatic patient may have an elevated IgE level, positive skin tests, wheezing, peripheral blood eosinophilia, and precipitating antibodies to *Aspergillus* and still not have ABPA. The diagnosis must be based on a constellation of findings, including clinical symptomatology (e.g., wheezing and fever), migratory and transient infiltrates, brown mucous plugs, peripheral eosinophilia, elevated precipitating antibodies, specific IgE and IgG antibodies to *Aspergillus,* positive dual-type skin reactions, and elevated IgE/IgG-*Aspergillus* complexes compared with levels in mold-sensitive asthmatics. This approach, emphasizing *Aspergillus*-specific IgE and IgG indices, has been successfully applied in the diagnosis of ABPA in a 20-month-old child (Kiefer et al., 1986).

Pulmonary function tests may reveal severe restrictive or irreversible obstructive disease, or both. Acute exacerbations are accompanied by a reduction in lung volumes and diffusing capacity. During remission, pulmonary function may return to normal, even in the face of bronchiectatic changes, making such measurements an insensitive indicator of early changes of ABPA (Detjen et al., 1991).

Treatment

Although spontaneous remissions may occur, the treatment of choice is prednisone. Radiographic lesions usually begin resolving by 2 weeks, and a reduction in total serum IgE occurs at 4 to 8 weeks (Greenberger, 1984). In fact, it is recommended that failure to achieve a 35% reduction in total serum IgE after 2 months of corticosteroid therapy should alert the physician to the possibility of noncompliance with medications or incorrect diagnosis (Ricketti et al., 1984). Specific treatment recommendations are published elsewhere (Wang et al., 1979b; Ricketti et al., 1984; Detjen et al., 1991). Other forms of therapy, such as antifungal agents, inhaled steroids, and disodium cromoglycate, have not been as effective as prednisone (Greenberger, 1984). The use of several inhaled antifungal drugs has been attempted with mixed and usually disappointing results (Hostetler et al., 1992). The poor response to specific antifungal therapy reflects the immunologic nature of this disorder. A newer oral antifungal agent, itraconazole, may prove an effective adjunct to steroid therapy by decreasing the antigenic load presented to the airways (Denning et al., 1991; Hostetler et al., 1992). Experience thus far suggests that treatment with steroids is effective in preventing progression to pulmonary fibrosis (Detjen et al., 1991).

Pathogenesis of Eosinophilia

The role of eosinophils in PIE syndrome disorders has not been fully elucidated. However, the many enzymes and cationic polypeptides contained in eosinophilic granules have putative functions that may be of major significance in the development of PIE syndromes (Lopez and Salvaggio, 1991). These include:

1. Major basic protein (MBP) represents 95% of core granule proteins. It mediates eosinophil adhesion and activates mast cells (type I immune reaction).
2. Eosinophil cationic protein (ECP) is found in the granule matrix and alters Hageman factor function, enhances plasmin activity, is helminthicidal, is neurotoxic, and activates mast cells (type I immune reaction).
3. Eosinophil-derived neurotoxin (EDN) and eosinophilic protein–X may be identical polypeptides and are centrally neurotoxic.
4. Eosinophil peroxidase (EPO), a granule matrix enzyme, is microbicidal and activates mast cells (type I immune reaction).
5. Charcot-Leyden crystal protein is a plasma membrane–derived enzyme that inactivates lysophospholipids.
6. Phospholipase D is found in eosinophilic granules and inactivates platelet-activating factor.
7. Histaminase, also found in granules, inactivates histamine.

Activated eosinophils are hypodense and are found in the bronchoalveolar lavage (BAL) fluid of patients with PIE syndromes (Chihara et al., 1985). Hypodense eosinophils exhibit enhanced antibody-mediated cytotoxicity against certain parasites, increased ligand-initiated chemotactic activity, enhanced ionophore-induced generation of LTC_4, increased glucose and O_2 consumption, and enhanced expression of low-affinity IgE receptors and other surface receptors (Lopez and Salvaggio, 1991). Eosinophil chemotactic activity (ECA) is maximal in the lung and is influenced by numerous chemoattractants, such as eosinophil chemotactic factor of anaphylaxis (ECF-A), histamine, platelet-activating factor (PAF), and leukotriene B_4 (LTB_4). Eosinophils are also capable of down-regulating hypersensitivity reactions through prostaglandin E_2(PGE_2)–induced suppression of mast cell–mediator release, ingestion of mast cell granules, inactivation of histamine by histaminase, and heparin-binding by MBP. Despite the obvious beneficial effects on host protection, the presence of these inflammatory cells and their associated mediators may lead to the hypereosinophilic state.

Neutrophil-derived ECF-A–like peptides are implicated in cell-mediated (type IV) reactions (Fantone and Ward, 1983). Eosinophils generate superoxide and hydroxyl radicals, PGE_2 and LTC_4, and several hydroxyeicosatetraneoic acid (HETE) metabolites (Lopez and Salvaggio, 1991). Complement components C3a, C5, C5a, and C567 (a trimolecular complex) are known to assist in the development of eosinophilic states and are important in type II and III reactions (Fantone and Ward, 1983; Ottesen, 1976). Eosinophils alone or in concert with mast cells and macrophages are capable of participating actively in host defenses, promote processes that injure host tissue, and may involve all four immune mechanisms in the development of the hypereosinophilic states.

HYPERSENSITIVITY PNEUMONITIS
(Extrinsic Allergic Alveolitis)

A number of pulmonary disorders produced by an immunologic reaction to inhaled organic dusts have been grouped together under the term hypersensitivity pneumonitis or extrinsic allergic alveolitis (Table 22–8) (Schuyler and Salvaggio, 1984). Although patients may present with recurrent acute respiratory distress, these disorders are easily separable from asthma in that (1) they occur in nonatopic as well as allergic individuals; (2) they are not usually associated with IgE (i.e., they are not type I reactions); (3) they involve the terminal airways and lung parenchyma as well as larger bronchioles and bronchi; and (4) bronchospasm is not a characteristic feature. The importance of exposure to organic dusts in producing lung disease was described by Ramazzini in 1713 (Schlueter, 1974), but it was nearly 200 years later when several groups of investigators demonstrated the relationship of hay and maple bark exposure to the development of pulmonary symptoms. In the 1960s, bird antigens were causally related to pulmonary manifestations (Reed et al., 1965).

Pathogenesis

Although it has been repeatedly demonstrated that inhalation of various organic materials is the cause of acute and chronic lung disorders in susceptible individuals, the immunologic mechanisms underlying the lung damage are still not precisely defined (see Table 22–7). Small dust particles (<5 μm) can penetrate to the distal airways and alveoli, where they may initiate

Table 22–8. Etiologic Agents in Hypersensitivity Pneumonitis*

Disease	Exposure	Antigen
Farmer's lung disease	Moldy hay	*Micropolyspora faeni* *Thermoactinomyces vulgaris* *Aspergillus* sp.
Bagassosis	Moldy pressed sugarcane (bagasse)	Thermophilic actinomycetes *T. sacchari, T. vulgaris*
Suberosis	Moldy cork	*Penicillium* sp.
Maple bark disease	Contaminated maple logs	*Cryptostroma corticale*
Sequoiosis	Contaminated wood dust	*Graphium* sp., *Pullularia* sp.
Humidifier lung disease	Contaminated humidifiers, air conditioners, dehumidifiers	Thermophilic actinomycetes *T. candidus, T. vulgaris* *Penicillium* sp. *Cephalosporium* sp. Amoebae
Familial hypersensitivity pneumonitis	Contaminated wood dust in walls	*Bacillus subtilis*
Thatched roof disease	Dried grasses and leaves	*Saccharomonospora viridis*
Cephalosporium hypersensitivity pneumonitis	Contaminated basement (sewage)	*Cephalosporium* sp.
Sauna taker's disease	Sauna water	*Pullularia* sp.
Pigeon breeder's disease	Pigeon droppings	Altered pigeon serum (probably IgA)
Duck fever	Duck feathers	Duck proteins
Wheat weevil disease (miller's lung)	Wheat flour weevils	*Sitophilus granarius*

*Agents that have been reported to or possibly might produce disease in children. See also Chapter 20.

a complex immunologic reaction. In susceptible individuals, the initial event occurring after acute exposure to antigen inhalation is a transient neutrophil alveolitis, which reverts within 1 week to the well-known pattern of lymphocyte predominance found in patients with chronic hypersensitivity pneumonitis (Fournier et al., 1985). Lung biopsy, usually performed in patients with subacute or chronic disease, reveals interstitial infiltration with lymphocytes, macrophages, and plasma cells. There is often interstitial fibrosis with granulomas containing foam cells (alveolar macrophages with lipid inclusion bodies). Bronchi are inflamed and may be obstructed. Although localized vascular inflammation may be seen, a generalized pulmonary vasculitis does not occur (Schuyler and Salvaggio, 1984). Biopsy specimens may contain antibody, antigen, complement components, and nodular ("lumpy") deposits of proteinaceous material along alveolar capillary basement membranes (Wenzel et al., 1971; McCombs, 1972; Pepys, 1973; Ghose et al., 1974), but evidence for classic immune complex–mediated lung injury is lacking (Fink, 1984; Calvanico et al., 1984; Salvaggio and deShazo, 1986).

The presence of mononuclear cell infiltrates and noncaseating granuloma formation suggest an important role for cell-mediated immunity in the pathogenesis of hypersensitivity pneumonitis. Lymphocytes from the peripheral blood of symptomatic patients respond to tests of in vitro cell-mediated immunity, such as antigen-induced blastogenesis and lymphokine release (Moore et al., 1974; Hansen and Penny, 1974; Purtillo et al., 1975; Schuyler et al., 1978; Fink, 1984, 1992). Bronchial and circulating lymphocytes can produce macrophage inhibitory factor (MIF) (Caldwell et al., 1973), and suppressor cell function may be abnormal (Fink, 1984).

Bronchoalveolar lavage fluid from patients with chronic hypersensitivity pneumonitis contains about 65 percent lymphocytes, most of which are T cells (helper-to-suppressor cell ratios of <1) (Leatherman et al., 1984b; Salvaggio and deShazo, 1986; Semenzato, 1991). This inversion of the CD4:CD8 ratio persists in farm workers with continued exposure to sensitizing antigen but reverts to normal after 6 months in those removed from antigen exposure. The presence of very late activation (VLA-1) antigen on CD8$^+$ T cells from BAL fluid of patients with hypersensitivity pneumonitis suggests the CD8$^+$ cells are an activated homing population in these patients. VLA-1 may be involved in cell-cell interactions and may contribute to cytotoxicity. Strong experimental evidence exists that granuloma formation is associated with the presence of T helper cells and that granulomas resolve under the influence of suppressor/cytotoxic T cells and NK cells (Semenzato, 1991).

Taken together with the finding of activated macrophages in BAL of these patients, it is possible that activation or dampening of suppressor cells by macrophages may be important in the pathogenesis of hypersensitivity pneumonitis (Guzman et al., 1992; Fink, 1992). Thus, current evidence is suggestive of a type IV immunologic mechanism, likely involving genetically determined immunoregulatory abnormalities, but this is not conclusive; some of these findings may occur by nonimmunologic mechanisms in response to inhaled particles.

A type III immune mechanism is suggested by the presence of high levels of precipitating antibodies (IgG, IgM, and IgA classes) (Faux et al., 1971) to the offending antigen (Patterson et al., 1976), the latent period following exposure, and the occasional presence of antibody in bronchial walls. The Arthus reaction to skin testing is also suggestive; however, lung pathology is inconsistent with a type III mechanism, and when susceptible individuals are made symptomatic by inhalation challenge, serum complement levels are not usually lowered. The presence of precipitins and complement-fixing antibodies in asymptomatic individuals suggests an immune response to exposure and not disease. Positive rheumatoid factors and Monospot tests have been reported. Autoantibodies are not present.

The immediate wheal-flare skin testing reaction seen in 80% of patients with pigeon breeder's disease may be mediated by IgG4 subclass short-latent sensitizing antibody (Fink, 1984). Data to support a role for a type I immune mechanism are lacking, since IgE levels are normal and specific IgE antibody has not been found in symptomatic patients. Type II immune reactions are apparently not involved in the pathogenesis of hypersensitivity pneumonitis. Fink (1984) has pointed out that several nonspecific mechanisms of lung injury may be of pathogenetic importance. A wide variety of potentially potent inflammatory agents of microbial, animal, or vegetable origin are present in inhaled organic dusts. These include proteolytic enzymes that may activate kallikrein and complement systems, nonproteolytic complement activators, such as microbial cell wall substances, adjuvants, endotoxins, histamine releasers, and nonspecific precipitins.

Thus, it appears that the immunopathogenesis of hypersensitivity pneumonitis probably involves multiple immunologic and nonimmunologic mechanisms. The factors responsible for the variation in susceptibility to disease are unknown, although several investigators have suggested a genetic basis involving the major histocompatibility complex. Early studies reporting an increased incidence of human leukocyte antigen HLA-B8 in hypersensitivity pneumonitis were not supported by later work; however, HLA-DR3 has been demonstrated to be more common in symptomatic individuals compared with antigen-exposed asymptomatic individuals and has been shown to be closely linked to HLA-B8 (Watters, 1986). Similarly, HLA-Dw6 has been reported to occur more commonly in patients with avian hypersensitivity (Berrill and Rood, 1977). The link, if any, between these findings and the variation in disease susceptibility remains to be defined.

Clinical Manifestations

Most of the reported childhood cases of hypersensitivity pneumonitis have been caused by bird antigens (Stiehm et al., 1967; Shannon et al., 1969; Chandra and Jones, 1972; Cunningham et al., 1976; Chiron et al., 1984), but any of the agents listed in Table 22–8 may potentially produce disease in children. Hypersensitivity pneumonitis may occur as a reaction to *Aspergillus* and has been reported in infancy (Katz and Kniker, 1973; Chiron et al., 1984). The severity of disease is dependent on the duration of exposure to the dust, the type and amount of dust, particle size, and the peculiarities of the individual's immune response.

There are several patterns of illness (Fraser and Paré, 1975; Schuyler and Salvaggio, 1984; Fink, 1984, 1986, 1992). In the acute form, following a period of sensitization, re-exposure produces cough, dyspnea, fever, chills, myalgia, and malaise usually beginning 4 to 6 hours after exposure and lasting 12 to 18 hours, assuming no additional exposure. On physical examination, the patient is acutely ill, toxic, and dyspneic. Crackles (rales) are usually heard in the lung bases at end-expiration; wheezes are not usually heard. The white blood count may be markedly elevated, with a shift to the left; eosinophilia occasionally occurs. IgG, IgM, and IgA levels are elevated, but IgE is normal (in nonatopic patients). Rheumatoid factor in moderate to high titers is present during acute illness, but disappears if re-exposure is avoided.

Chest radiographs may be normal during acute episodes or may demonstrate peripheral bibasilar infiltrates, nodules, or both; the findings are not characteristic of this disease. Pulmonary function tests reveal low lung volumes, reduced dynamic lung compliance, reduced carbon monoxide diffusing capacity, and hypoxemia (Chiron et al., 1984); the findings are typical of a restrictive lung disease. Chest radiographs and pulmonary function abnormalities usually revert to normal within weeks to months after the acute episode. However, Allen and coworkers (1976) demonstrated small airway obstruction in bird breeders who were asymptomatic; in some of these patients, pulmonary function abnormalities progressed despite removal of the antigen.

If the exposure to the dust is chronic and intense, an insidious progressive chronic lung disease may develop, characterized by cyanosis, tachypnea at rest, chronic cough, anorexia, and weight loss. The chest radiograph may demonstrate the typical but nonspecific findings of an interstitial lung disease, usually a reticulonodular pattern with honeycombing throughout all lung fields. In addition to the usual restrictive pattern detected with lung function testing, flow rates may be decreased, especially at low lung volumes, suggesting obstruction of peripheral airways. Lung pathology at this stage consists of interstitial fibrosis with granuloma formation. The alveolar walls are thickened by collagen tissue and infiltrated with lymphocytes, plasma cells, and, rarely, eosinophils. Thickened bronchiolar walls are infiltrated by similar cells; this finding, together with smooth muscle hypertrophy, produces the picture of bronchiolitis obliterans. Alveolar spaces are often filled with plasma cells, engorged alveolar macrophages, and foam cells (which are occasionally found in alveolar walls). The foam cells are generally seen when serum proteins are the antigens. Destructive emphysema and Arthus-type vasculitis are occasional findings but are not characteristic.

Diagnosis

The diagnosis of hypersensitivity pneumonitis is based on the history, presence of serum precipitins, and improvement of symptoms on avoidance of the suspected organic dust. In certain cases, re-exposure may be necessary to confirm the diagnosis. In older patients, bronchial challenge with aerosolized antigen may produce abnormalities in lung function, thereby supporting the diagnosis. Lung biopsy is rarely required and may be supplanted by BAL when suppressor T-cell alveolitis is demonstrated (Fink, 1992). The differential diagnosis of the chronic form includes the vasculitides, sarcoidosis, cryptogenic fibrosing alveolitis, histiocytosis, pulmonary hemosiderosis, prolonged pulmonary eosinophilia, and mycoplasmal and viral infections. Skin tests are generally not useful. Many antigen preparations contain nonspecific irritants, and even when the antigen is pure, a positive skin test does not distinguish between exposure and disease states.

Treatment and Prognosis

Avoidance of the offending antigen is the best therapy. Acute and subacute illness often responds dramatically to oral steroid therapy. There is little demonstrated benefit from inhaled steroids, although cromolyn sodium may be tried in patients with mild inflammation (Fink, 1992). Improvement in lung function, symptoms, and chest radiographs is related to the age of the patient (younger patients do better) (Chiron et al., 1984), ability to avoid continued exposure, and the degree of permanent lung damage that has occurred before onset of treatment (Allen et al., 1976; Fink, 1986, 1992; Grammer et al., 1990).

PULMONARY VASCULITIS (Collagen-Vascular Disease)

Several systemic diseases (Table 22–9) are associated with pulmonary vasculitis, characterized by infiltration of granulocytes and mononuclear cells around the endothelium of small arterioles, venules, and capillaries. Lung involvement may precede other signs and symptoms (e.g., rheumatic pneumonia) or may occur at any time following the onset of other organ involvement. Pulmonary involvement complicating these systemic diseases generally occurs less frequently in children than in adults.

Pathology of the lung in these disorders suggests that both type III and IV immune reactions are involved (Cupps and Fauci, 1981) (see Table 22–7). In most cases, the inciting antigen is unknown (two exceptions are hepatitis B surface antigen and streptococcal protein) (Fulmer and Kaltreider, 1982). Lung damage can be initiated when the antigen reaches the lung via the circulation or is inhaled into the airways. Release of vasoactive amines from clumped platelets can lead to increased vascular permeability; antigen-antibody complexes are trapped in basement membranes; complement is activated; polymorphonuclear cells are attracted; and lysosomal enzymes are released that produce tissue damage (type III reaction). Bronchoalveolar lavage fluid from patients with collagen-vascular disease and lung involvement contains increased levels of IgG, IgM, and IgA immune complexes as well as complement factors (Jansen et al., 1984). In addition, antigen and sensitized lymphocytes combine to attract macrophages, which release lysozymes, damage vessel

Table 22–9. Diseases Associated with Pulmonary Vasculitis

Systemic lupus erythematosus	Wegener's granulomatosis
Rheumatoid arthritis	Churg-Strauss syndrome
Juvenile rheumatoid arthritis	Hypersensitivity pneumonitis
Dermatomyositis	Ulcerative colitis
Polymyositis	Serum sickness
Ankylosing spondylitis	Drug-induced hypersensitivity
Progressive systemic sclerosis	states
Periarteritis nodosa	Mixed connective tissue disease
Sarcoidosis (rare)	(probable)
Henoch-Schönlein purpura	

walls and lung parenchyma, and subsequently produce granulomas (type IV reaction). However, immune complexes can also produce granulomas (Cupps and Fauci, 1981).

The clinical manifestations of many of these diseases are discussed in more detail in Chapters 24 and 25. Pulmonary symptomatology is nonspecific, and in most of the diseases listed in Table 22–9, the patient presents with dyspnea, cough, hemoptysis, and pleuritic pain. Additional clues to the presence of a vasculitic syndrome include fever of unknown cause, glomerulonephritis, palpable purpura, ischemic symptoms, mononeuritis multiplex, and multisystem involvement. Diagnosis is dependent on other organ involvement and specific laboratory tests (e.g., DNA antibodies, rheumatoid factor, immune complexes, and cryoglobulins) (Cupps and Fauci, 1981).

Systemic Lupus Erythematosus

Pulmonary involvement occurs in 50% to 70% of adult and pediatric patients with systemic lupus erythematosus (SLE) and tends to occur more frequently with more severe disease (King et al., 1977; Caciro et al., 1981). Autopsy studies of lung disease in SLE suggest a high frequency of occurrence (Gross et al., 1972; Eisenberg et al., 1973; Matthay et al., 1975; Walravens and Chase, 1976; Doll and Salvaggio, 1984). De Jongste and colleagues (1986) reported a series of eight children with SLE, four of whom initially presented with pulmonary findings. All demonstrated at least one type of pulmonary abnormality during the course of the disease. Lung disease in SLE patients occurs in the absence of renal lesions and may carry a better prognosis (Turner-Warwick, 1984). The usual clinical manifestations include a productive or nonproductive cough, dyspnea, pleuritis, and occasionally hemoptysis. Pleural disease is common, usually painful, and often accompanied by fever.

Nine forms of SLE lung involvement have been described (Hunninghake and Fauci, 1979; Leatherman et al., 1984b; Nadorra and Landing, 1987; Carette, 1988):

1. Pleurisy with or without effusion.
2. Atelectasis.
3. Uremic pulmonary edema.
4. Acute lupus pneumonitis.
5. Diffuse interstitial disease.
6. Diaphragmatic dysfunction with loss of lung volume.
7. Extensive pulmonary hemorrhage.
8. Obstructive bronchiolitis.
9. Pulmonary hypertension.

More than one of these findings may be present in an individual at any one time.

About 50% to 75% of patients with SLE will have pleuritis and/or effusion at some point during their illness. In the report by de Jongste and colleagues (1986), pleural effusion was present in 6 of 8 children at the time of initial presentation. It is, therefore, the most common pleuropulmonary abnormality in SLE and may be an important early manifestation. Pleural disease is usually painful and is associated with systemic disease exacerbation. Pleural effusions may be massive but are usually small and bilateral. The pleural fluid is an exudate with depressed levels of total hemolytic complement, C3 and C4 (Hunder et al., 1972), occasional LE cells, antinuclear antibodies, and elevated levels of DNA-binding antibodies. Glucose levels are normal or slightly depressed, and leukocyte counts are elevated (usually with a lymphocytic predominance) in pleural fluid (Turner-Warwick, 1984; Nadorra and Landing, 1987). Concomitant infection is common, and appropriate diagnostic studies should be obtained before administering corticosteroid treatment (Hunninghake and Fauci, 1979).

Peripheral basilar atelectasis is a commonly seen radiographic finding in SLE, possibly caused by splinting of the chest wall as a result of chronic pleural pain. Others have suggested diaphragmatic dysfunction, direct SLE lung injury, and steroid-induced myopathy as possible causes. Dyspnea and a restrictive pattern of lung disease occur and may seem to be out of proportion to the radiologic findings (Doll and Salvaggio, 1984; Hunninghake and Fauci, 1979).

Pulmonary edema appears on the chest radiograph as fluffy alveolar infiltrates, often more prominent in the lower lobes and perihilar area. The cause of this finding in some SLE patients is unknown. It has been attributed to uremia (Hunninghake and Fauci, 1979), aspiration, congestive heart failure, and infection (Doll and Salvaggio, 1984; Nadorra and Landing, 1987).

Acute lupus pneumonitis is reported in about 10% to 20% of adults with SLE (Matthay et al., 1975); however, the true incidence is difficult to determine since it is a diagnosis of exclusion that may be mimicked by many of the other pleuropulmonary abnormalities (Hunninghake and Fauci, 1979). Chest radiographs are characterized by unilateral or bilateral, poorly defined, acinar infiltrates that are often migratory, and may occasionally be associated with effusions. Acute respiratory difficulties, fever, tachypnea, basilar crackles, and hypoxia characterize the clinical picture. Pathologic findings are not well defined because most studies were conducted post mortem or after steroid therapy. Findings have included vasculitis, interstitial pneumonitis, alveolar hemorrhage, arterial thrombi, and immune complex deposition (Doll and Salvaggio, 1984). Granular deposits of IgG, C3, and DNA have been demonstrated in the interstitium of the alveolar walls and alveolar capillary walls (Inoue et al., 1979). Infection is not the primary cause of pneumonitis in these patients, and antibiotics are usually ineffective. Patients often respond dramatically to corticosteroid treatment, but immunosuppressive agents may be necessary. Even with effective therapy, recurrences are common, and residual restrictive lung disease can result (Hunninghake and Fauci, 1979).

Interstitial lung disease may occur in 1% to 6% of adult patients with SLE, although this rate is disputed and was found in 3 of 8 children reported with SLE (de Jongste et al., 1986). Symptoms include shallow, rapid breathing, dyspnea on exertion, cough, and pleuritic chest pain. Fine inspiratory crackles are heard over the lung bases, and clubbing of the digits is unusual. Chest radiographs show a spectrum of findings from early granular or reticular patterns to an end-stage honeycomb pattern. Pulmonary function testing shows a restrictive defect, a reduced carbon monoxide diffusing capacity, and hypoxemia. The pathology is characterized by alveolar wall thickening and edema and the presence of chronic inflammatory cell infiltrates. Hyperplasia of the alveolar lining cells and intra-alveolar macrophages are also found. In a review of autopsy cases of children by Nadorra and Landing (1987), all 26 patients had some degree of interstitial pneumonitis. Optimal treatment is unknown. Corticosteroids and immunosuppressive agents have been used, but the results are not clear. Long-term oxygen therapy may benefit chronically hypoxemic patients (Eisenberg, 1982).

Diaphragm dysfunction with loss of lung volume occurs in SLE, sometimes associated with a restrictive ventilatory pattern and atelectasis. A diffuse myopathy affecting the diaphragmatic muscles is thought to be the cause. These patients exhibit dyspnea in the supine position, a symptom characteristic of diaphragmatic paralysis. The natural history of this form of SLE pulmonary disease is unknown (Hunninghake and Fauci, 1979).

Pulmonary hemorrhage also occurs in patients with SLE, although rarely as a presenting symptom. It is usually of sudden onset, extensive, associated with active systemic disease, and often fatal (70% mortality rate in one series). Massive intra-alveolar hemorrhage is seen on biopsy or autopsy in addition to the typical pattern of immune complex deposition (Leatherman et al., 1984a), although pulmonary hemorrhage in SLE has been reported to occur in the absence of immune complex deposits in the lungs (Desnoyers et al., 1984). The pathogenesis of extensive alveolar hemorrhage in SLE and its treatment remain undefined (Leatherman et al., 1984a). Alveolar hemorrhage has been linked to lupus anticoagulant in at least one clinical report (Howe et al., 1988).

Pulmonary hypertension is now widely recognized as a complication of SLE. Intimal thickening and fibrosis, medial hypertrophy, and plexiform lesions are similar to those reported for primary pulmonary hypertension. A minority of cases show vasculitis or immune complex deposition. The pathogenesis may include increased vasoreactivity or coagulation abnormalities. The cause may be related to the presence of antiphospholipid antibodies, which theoretically could lead to decreased prostacyclin production or cause recurrent pulmonary thromboembolism. Death usually occurs within 2 years (Carette, 1988).

Bronchiolitis obliterans has been reported in children with SLE (Nadorra and Landing, 1987), as well as the probably distinct entity bronchiolitis obliterans organizing pneumonia (BOOP) (Gammon et al., 1992). Although other causes of these pathologic changes, such as infection or oxygen toxicity, could not be consistently excluded, obstructive bronchiolitis should be considered as a possible cause of chronic lung disease in SLE patients.

Rheumatoid Arthritis

Pleuropulmonary involvement in rheumatoid arthritis (RA) patients is seen in approximately one half of autopsy cases (Hunninghake and Fauci, 1979) and occurs in about 40% of adult patients with RA (Frank et al., 1973). The most common manifestations are pleurisy with or without effusion, necrobiotic nodules (nonpneumoconiotic intrapulmonary rheumatoid nodules), Caplan's syndrome (rheumatoid pneumoconiosis), diffuse interstitial disease, and pulmonary arteritis and hypertension (Hunninghake and Fauci, 1979). The pleural fluid is usually an exudate with many leukocytes, elevated lactate dehydrogenase and rheumatoid factor, depressed glucose levels, and decreased complement activity. Parenchymal involvement begins with a nonspecific interstitial pneumonitis of plasma cells, macrophages, and lymphocytes and can progress to extreme architectural distortion (honeycombed lung) (Hunninghake and Fauci, 1979; MacFarlane et al., 1984). Recruitment of inflammatory cells to the lung may, in part, be under the control of tumor necrosis factor-α (TNF-α) released from activated alveolar macrophages (Gosset et al., 1991). IgM and IgG but not complement have been found along alveolar septa and in capillary walls, but vasculitis is rare (McCombs, 1972; De Horatius et al., 1972). Pulmonary involvement in RA may precede the onset of joint manifestations, and restrictive lung abnormalities can be demonstrated when symptoms are minimal.

Pleuropulmonary involvement also occurs in about 4% to 8% of children with juvenile rheumatoid arthritis (JRA) (see Chapter 24). Although it is most commonly seen with the systemic forms of JRA, it may also occur with the polyarticular and pauciarticular types (Athreya et al., 1980). Pleural disease with effusion is much more common than parenchymal lung disease. The major types of pulmonary disease in children with JRA are pleurisy with effusion, transient patchy infiltrates, lymphoid bronchiolitis, and lymphocytic interstitial pneumonitis. Other reported complications of JRA include idiopathic pulmonary hemosiderosis, amyloidosis, and pulmonary arteritis. Chest radiographic patterns include interstitial reticular and nodular infiltrates, transient pneumonitis, patchy pleural infiltrates, and pleural or pericardial effusions (Athreya et al., 1980). Pulmonary function tests in children may demonstrate decreased air flow, decreased lung volume, decreased diffusing capacity, and ventilation-perfusion mismatching during exercise (Wagener et al., 1981).

Mixed Connective Tissue Disease

Mixed connective tissue disease (MCTD) is a distinct rheumatic syndrome with overlapping clinical features of SLE, polymyositis (PM) and dermatomyositis (DM), antibodies to extractable nuclear antigen (ENA), and high serum titers of speckled-pattern fluorescent antinuclear antibody (Hunninghake and Fauci, 1979). Pulmonary involvement has been reported to occur in 82% of adults (Weiner-Kronish et al., 1981) and about

40% of children with MCTD (Singsen et al., 1977). It usually consists of diffuse interstitial lung disease, pleural effusions, and/or pulmonary hypertension (Prakash, 1988). Shortness of breath, dyspnea on exertion, and cough are common manifestations. Chest radiographic findings include normal lung fields with prominent right hilum, pleural effusions, bibasilar infiltrates, diffuse reticular nodular pattern, and cardiomegaly. Pulmonary function tests show a restrictive pattern, a decreased carbon monoxide diffusing capacity, hypoxemia, and respiratory alkalosis.

Histologically, MCTD lung disease may show widespread proliferative vascular lesions, including intimal thickening in the pulmonary circulation (Singsen et al., 1980), and leukocytic adventitial infiltrates in involved arteries (Wiener-Kronish et al., 1981). Positive granular staining for IgG, C3, and Clq in the blood vessels of the lungs and patchy interstitial fibrosis have been demonstrated, but clear evidence of immune complex deposition (type III reaction) is lacking (Wiener-Kronish et al., 1981). Selective IgA deficiency may be associated with childhood MCTD (Sanders et al., 1973). Children with MCTD and lung involvement usually respond well to corticosteroid therapy (Sanders et al., 1973; Fraga et al., 1978; Singsen et al., 1977).

Scleroderma

Although not clinically apparent, most children with scleroderma have mild pulmonary function abnormalities, such as impaired diffusing capacity, decreasing lung volumes, and decreased alveolocapillary permeability (Falcini et al., 1992). Pleural effusion occurs infrequently (Dabich et al., 1974; Silver and Miller, 1990).

Dermatomyositis and Polymyositis

Diffuse interstitial fibrosis occurs in about 5% of patients with dermatomyositis and polymyositis and is characterized by chronic nonproductive cough and shortness of breath (Hunninghake and Fauci, 1979) (see Chapters 24 and 28). Neuromuscular involvement of the pharyngeal and respiratory muscles often results in a weak and ineffective cough, aspiration pneumonia, and respiratory failure due to muscle weakness. Dermatomyositis may be associated with rapidly progressive, life-threatening interstitial pneumonia (Park and Nyhan, 1975).

Sjögren's Syndrome

Sjögren's syndrome, a chronic inflammatory condition characterized by dry mucous membranes, including the mouth, eyes, and tracheobronchial tree, occurs with a wide variety of rheumatic diseases and has been reported in children (Sanders et al., 1973; Fraga et al., 1978) (see Chapter 24). Pleuropulmonary manifestations are common and include pleurisy and/or effusion, interstitial fibrosis, desiccation of the tracheobronchial tree, and lymphoid interstitial disease. Desiccation of the respiratory tract apparently results in cough,

chronic bronchitis, atelectasis, and pneumonia (Hunninghake and Fauci, 1979). Low CD4:CD8 ratios in BAL fluid in advanced disease are suggestive of alveolitis and thus may correlate with decreased pulmonary function (Dalavanga et al., 1991), but this association has not been strong and deserves further study. The major antigens are thought to be cell nuclei, altered gamma globulin, salivary duct cells, and thyroid antigens. Antinuclear antibodies and rheumatoid factor are found in Sjögren's syndrome, as well as salivary duct and thyroid microsomal antibodies (Turner-Warwick, 1984). Some patients respond to corticosteroid therapy (Hunninghake and Fauci, 1979).

Ankylosing Spondylitis

Ankylosing spondylitis is a chronic inflammatory disease that typically begins between the ages of 15 and 30 and results in a progressive limitation of spinal mobility (see Chapter 24). Upper lobe fibrobullous disease and chest wall restriction are the two major types of respiratory involvement. The chest wall restriction often fixes the thorax at high lung volumes, and functional impairment is usually minimal. Cavities in the fibrobullous type of disease may become secondarily infected with mycobacteria or fungi such as *Aspergillus*, which may result in massive hemoptysis. The cause of the parenchymal lung involvement is unknown (Hunninghake and Fauci, 1979).

Henoch-Schönlein Purpura (Anaphylactoid Purpura)

Henoch-Schönlein purpura (HSP) or syndrome, thought to be IgA immune complex–mediated, is a necrotizing vasculitis syndrome occurring predominantly in children and occasionally involving the lungs with diffuse alveolitis or pneumonia (see Chapters 21, 24, and 25). One patient with fatal HSP pulmonary involvement had extensive deposition of IgA along the alveolar septa with smaller amounts of IgG and fibrinogen (Kathuria and Cheifec, 1982). The mildly decreased lung diffusion capacity occasionally seen in HSP returns to normal as the disease resolves (Chaussain et al., 1992). The rare complication of pulmonary hemorrhage carries a high mortality, but survival is possible with aggressive supportive care (Olson et al., 1992).

Pulmonary Manifestations of Gastrointestinal and Liver Disease

Chronic active hepatitis and primary biliary cirrhosis may be associated with pulmonary manifestations, which are thought to be produced by immunologic mechanisms (see Chapter 23). These patients have alveolitis with or without pleural effusion, alveolar wall thickening, honeycombing, increased pulmonary lymphoid tissue, and complement and immunoglobulin deposits in the lung. Rheumatoid factor and antinuclear, mitochondrial, and smooth muscle autoantibodies are often present (Turner-Warwick, 1974; 1984).

Alveolitis and bronchiectasis are associated with ulcerative colitis and colon mucosal antibodies. A similar mechanism may be involved in the alveolitis and granuloma formation seen in some patients with celiac disease (Turner-Warwick, 1984).

Rheumatic Fever

Numerous reports have established that rheumatic pneumonitis is a distinct clinical manifestation of acute rheumatic fever (ARF), separate from congestive heart failure, acute bacterial pneumonias, or other collagen-vascular diseases (Serlin et al., 1975) (see Chapter 24). Rheumatic pneumonitis occurs in about 10% to 15% of patients and may precede other manifestations of ARF, although it is usually associated with active carditis. Patients with pneumonitis usually have extensive and progressive pulmonary symptoms, with crackles and friction rubs. Chest radiographs show increased lung markings extending from the hila to the midlung areas; often these infiltrates are migratory, and in some survivors, a chronic interstitial pneumonia develops. Pleurisy with pleural effusions has also been associated with rheumatic pneumonitis. At autopsy, the alveoli contain exudate, and there is considerable hemorrhage and necrosis of parenchyma and bronchiolar mucosa. Evidence for arteritis (vasculitis) is usually present. The streptococcal antigen is thought to be responsible for rheumatic pneumonitis, producing a type III immune reaction. These patients are usually unresponsive to steroid therapy, and in some the pulmonary manifestations worsen on steroid therapy. The symptoms improve as other manifestations of ARF improve. However, the prognosis for rheumatic pneumonitis is generally poor, with a high mortality rate.

Wegener's Granulomatosis

Wegener's granulomatosis is characterized by: (1) the development of a necrotizing, granulomatous vasculitis of small vessels, primarily of the upper and lower respiratory tract; (2) a focal glomerulonephritis; and (3) disseminated vasculitis (Fauci, 1976). It is primarily a disease of adults but does occur in childhood (Hansen et al., 1983; Rottem et al., 1993) (see Chapters 24 and 25). Ninety-four percent of adult patients have lung disease; pulmonary infiltrates, sinusitis, fever, otitis, cough, rhinitis, and hemoptysis are the usual respiratory signs and symptoms (Fauci et al., 1983). The complications of subglottic stenosis and nasal deformity are more common in pediatric patients (Rottem et al., 1993). Chest radiographs demonstrate solitary or multiple nodular densities, which are usually bilateral and may be cavitated. CT may aid in identifying cavitary and unidentified opacified lesions in the lung (Cordier et al., 1990). Pleural effusions, atelectasis, and hilar adenopathy are common (Fauci and Wolff, 1973; Landman and Burgener, 1974), as are macroscopic findings at bronchoscopy of inflammation, stenosis, and hemorrhage (Cordier et al., 1990).

Both immune complexes and granulomas have been demonstrated in the glomerular lesions, suggesting that Wegener's granulomatosis may be caused by both type III and type IV immune reactions (Fauci, 1976). Diagnosis has been facilitated by the demonstration of anti-neutrophil cytoplasmic antibodies (ANCAs) in as many as 88% of patients with this disorder (Rottem et al., 1993). However, at least one case of Wegener's granulomatosis was reported in which vascular lymphoid infiltrates consisted predominantly of T cells and monocytes, and IgG, IgM, IgA, and C3 were not found in pulmonary alveoli, septa, or vessels (Gephardt et al., 1983).

In the recent past, the prognosis of Wegener's granulomatosis was extremely grave, with a mean survival of 12.5 months for steroid-treated patients. Long-term remissions can now be induced and maintained with a combination of prednisone and cytotoxic drugs, such as cyclophosphamide or azothiaprine. Serious infections occur in 50% of patients during therapy; therefore, a switch to alternate-day glucocorticoids should take place as soon as possible. Relapse occurs in 38% of children within 5 years of remission (Rottem et al., 1993).

DRUG-INDUCED HYPERSENSITIVITY LUNG DISEASE

Although many drugs are suspected of producing a hypersensitivity reaction in the lung (Table 22–10), there is meager evidence to confirm that the reaction is truly immunologic. In the majority of cases in which an allergic reaction to a drug is suspected, circulating antibodies or sensitized lymphocytes cannot be found. The diagnosis of drug-induced hypersensitivity lung disease is usually made, less than optimally, on the following basis:

1. The reaction observed is not a known pharmacologic effect.
2. The onset of the reaction occurred after a latent period of 7 to 10 days (reactions may occur sooner if the patient has been exposed previously to the same drug or to similar antigenic determinants).
3. The reaction recurred after exposure to the same drug (Rosenow, 1976). Hypersensitivity reactions must be distinguished from other adverse reactions, such as

Table 22–10. Drugs That May Produce Hypersensitivity Lung Diseases

Nitrofurantoin	Methadone
Sulfonamides	Propoxyphene
Penicillin	Pituitary snuff
Busulfan	Methylsergide
Cyclophosphamide	Hexamethonium
Methotrexate	Blood
Bleomycin	Drugs that induce systemic
Procarbazine	lupus erythematosus*
Melphalan	Hydrochlorothiazide
Heroin	Chlordiazapoxide

*See Table 22–11.
Modified from Rosenow EC III. Drug-induced hypersensitivity disease of the lung. In Kirkpatrick CH, Reynolds HY, eds. Immunologic and Infectious Reactions in the Lung. New York, Marcel Dekker, 1976, pp. 261–287.

overdosage, side effects, secondary effects, drug interactions, intolerance, and idiosyncrasy (Rosenow, 1972). The type of drug reaction is usually difficult to determine inasmuch as the clinical manifestations and the pathology are similar to the various types of reactions.

As many as 25% of all drug-induced diseases may be due to hypersensitivity, and many of these illnesses involve the lung. Most drugs have a low molecular mass; thus, to be antigenic, they must bind to proteins. In the lung, these antigens may produce pulmonary edema (increased vascular permeability), bronchospasm, mucus hypersecretion, cellular infiltrates, granulomas, neoplastic changes, and fibrosis (Sostman et al., 1977; Alvarado et al., 1978). All four types of immunologic mechanisms may be involved (not necessarily simultaneously) in producing these pulmonary changes. Conversely, some drugs such as penicillin may, depending on the circumstance, produce all four types of reactions. Type I reactions are thought to be caused by procainamide, hormones, and antitoxins; type II, by quinidine; type III, by penicillin, sulfa drugs, and *p*-aminosalicylic acid; and type IV, by topical drugs such as penicillin (Rosenow, 1976).

Certain drugs, such as nitrofurantoin, may produce acute pulmonary disorders (bronchospasm, eosinophilia, and pleural effusions) as well as chronic ones (interstitial lung disease with fibrosis). The immunologic mechanisms underlying these responses may be different. Nine cases of nitrofurantoin pulmonary toxicity in children have been reported since the drug was introduced in 1953 (Broughton and Wilson, 1986; Coraggio et al., 1989). A large number of drugs (Table 22–11) are implicated in inducing illnesses resembling systemic lupus erythematosus. The disease produced by these drugs differs from SLE in that there is less involvement of the skin and kidneys, more involvement of the lungs, and no depression of serum complement, although antibodies to DNA and other cellular elements are found. Drugs such as pituitary snuff may cause an extrinsic allergic alveolitis with measurable serum antibodies to an extract of the snuff.

Treatment of these drug-induced disorders is discontinuation and future avoidance of the drug and other drugs with similar antigenic structure.

CRYPTOGENIC FIBROSING ALVEOLITIS (Idiopathic Pulmonary Fibrosis)

The term *cryptogenic fibrosing alveolitis* (CFA) is now applied to a group of chronic interstitial lung diseases, which, by definition, are of unknown origin. Hamman and Rich (1944) first described an entity of acute, rapidly progressive interstitial pneumonia in adult patients who usually died within months. Bradley (1956) first described this disorder in children, and numerous cases have been reported since (Hewitt et al., 1977). Several entities, which collectively comprise the CFA disorders and probably constitute a spectrum of disease with varying pathologic features, have been described (Crystal et al., 1976). Familial patterns have also occurred (Hewitt et al., 1977; Farrell et al., 1986); in one family, six affected siblings all carried the immunoglobulin allotype Glm(1), suggesting transmission by a dominantly inherited gene on chromosome 14 (Musk et al., 1986). Although the term *interstitial* appears in the name of these disorders, it should be remembered that alveolitis is an essential feature, and that veins, arteries, and airways may also be involved (Crystal et al., 1981; Cherniack et al., 1991).

Clinical Manifestations

The subclassification of CFA into usual interstitial pneumonitis (UIP), desquamative interstitial pneumonitis (DIP), and lymphoid interstitial pneumonitis (LIP) is given here because these terms were used extensively in earlier literature, especially in studies of treatment and prognosis. However, although this point is still controversial (Reynolds, 1986), it is now thought by many that they are actually different stages of the same disease process. DIP may represent the earlier stages of CFA, whereas UIP represents later stages in which more structural derangement has occurred (Crystal et al., 1976; Patchefsky et al., 1973).

1. *Usual interstitial pneumonia* (UIP) refers to the disorder originally described by Hamman and Rich, also known as idiopathic pulmonary fibrosis, or the *Hamman-Rich syndrome*. Pathologically, it is characterized by alveolar wall necrosis, interstitial edema, hyaline membranes lining the alveoli, interstitial infiltration by monocytes and lymphocytes (occasionally plasma cells and eosinophils), organization with obliteration of air spaces, peribronchial fibrous tissue and inflammatory cells, and finally, honeycombing of the lung. The walls

Table 22–11. Drugs That Can Induce Systemic Lupus Erythematosus

Antiarrhythmic drugs	Antituberculous drugs
practolol	isoniazid
procainamide	para-aminosalicylic acid
quinidine	streptomycin
Antibiotics	Phenothiazines
griseofulvin	chlorpromazine
nitrofurantoin	levomepromazine
penicillin	perazine
sulfonamides	perphenazine
tetracycline	promethazine
	thioridazine
Anticonvulsant drugs	
carbamazepine	Miscellaneous
diphenylhydantoin (phenytoin)	amoproxan
ethosuximide	anthiolimine
mephenytoin	D-penicillamine
phenylethylacetylurea	digitalis
primidone	gold
trimethadione	methysergide
	methylthiouracil
Antihypertensive drugs	oral contraceptives
guanoxan	oxyphenistatin
hydralazine	phenylbutazone
levodopa	propylthiouracil
methyldopa	thiazides
reserpine	

Modified from Ginsburg WW. Drug-induced systemic lupus erythematosus. Semin Respir Med 2:51–58, 1980.

of the muscular pulmonary arteries are thickened, but vasculitis does not occur.

2. *Desquamative interstitial pneumonia* (DIP) was originally described as an entity distinct from UIP in 1965 by Leibow and coworkers. Since then, it has been described in a number of infants and children, the youngest being 7 weeks of age (Schneider et al., 1967; Rosenow et al., 1970; Buchta et al., 1970; Bhagwat et al., 1970; Howatt et al., 1973; Leahy et al., 1985). A familial form, affecting infants as young as 6 months of age, has been described (Farrell et al., 1986). In DIP, there is minimal necrosis of alveolar septa, and honeycombing is much less common. The alveoli are filled with large mononuclear cells, which are both type II pneumocytes and macrophages, and the alveolar walls are lined by proliferating type II cells. Originally, the interstitial infiltrate was described as consisting mainly of plasma cells, eosinophils, monocytes, and lymphocytes; however, neutrophils are difficult to recognize in conventional sections stained with hematoxylin or eosin. Neutrophils are now known to be a prominent feature of the alveolitis (Crystal et al., 1981).

3. *Lymphoid interstitial pneumonia* (LIP) is characterized by interstitial infiltrates of lymphocytes and some plasma cells, high serum IgG and/or IgM levels, and a progressive course usually unresponsive to therapy (Halprin et al., 1972). Familial LIP has been reported (O'Brodovich et al., 1980), and LIP is a characteristic feature of many children with pediatric AIDS; it is discussed further later in this chapter under the heading Pulmonary Manifestations of HIV (Kornstein et al., 1986) and in Chapter 18.

The clinical, radiographic, and physiologic findings are similar in all three conditions. The main symptom is dyspnea, which may be associated with a nonproductive chronic cough, chest pain, anorexia, weight loss, fatigue, and eventually cor pulmonale and heart failure. Late inspiratory crackles ("Velcro crackles") are usually heard, but bronchospasm with wheezing is a less common finding (Hewitt et al., 1977; Olson et al., 1990). Clubbing occurs earlier than in the course of extrinsic allergic alveolitis. Hypoxia and subsequent cyanosis are almost always present.

Chest radiographic abnormalities may lag behind clinical manifestations; in fact, extensive lung histologic changes and dyspnea can be present with a normal chest radiograph (Renzi and Lopez-Mijano, 1976; Epler et al., 1978). Radiographs demonstrate a diffuse reticulonodular pattern, which sometimes obliterates the vascular markings, and hilar adenopathy may be present. In DIP, a characteristic triangular haziness extending from the hila along the heart borders to the lung bases has been described; this appears to occur more frequently in adults than in children (Hewitt et al., 1977).

Pulmonary function tests reveal decreases in lung volumes, increased elastic recoil at high lung volumes, decreased static and dynamic compliance, increased physiologic dead space, and preservation of flow rates determined by large airway function (specific conductance at functional residual capacity [FRC] may be increased) (Zapletal et al., 1985). Decreases in flow rates influenced by small airways have been described in some (Ostrow and Cherniack, 1973) but not all patients (Schofield et al., 1976; Zapletal et al., 1986). Hyperventilation and hypoxia, the latter mainly caused by ventilation-perfusion abnormalities and not diffusion (alveolar-capillary block) problems, are common; increased epithelial permeability may explain the plasma extravasation, which contributes to the hypoxia (Cherniack et al., 1991). Young infants with CFA may have hyperinflation of the chest, suggesting small airway obstruction and air trapping.

Diagnosis

The differential diagnosis of CFA includes connective tissue disorders, sarcoidosis, granulomatous disease, pulmonary hemorrhage syndromes, radiation injury, vasculitis, alveolar proteinosis, histiocytosis, extrinsic allergic alveolitis, and *Mycoplasma pneumoniae* and viral infections. The diagnosis is made by exclusion of other entities with appropriate tests, lack of precipitins for the diagnosis of extrinsic allergic alveolitis (see Table 22–7), lung biopsy, and gallium scan. Supporting evidence is provided by serologic, physiologic, radiographic, and bronchoalveolar lavage findings. High-resolution CT scan may be able to demonstrate fibrotic changes and elucidate the nonhomogeneous distribution of lesions seen in CFA (Cherniack et al., 1991).

BAL fluid analysis can be a useful diagnostic aid in patients with cryptogenic fibrosing alveolitis. In contrast to extrinsic allergic alveolitis (increased lymphocytes, absent neutrophils), BAL fluid from patients with CFA contains an increased proportion of neutrophils and normal proportions of lymphocytes and lymphocyte subpopulations (Crystal et al., 1981). Eosinophil percentages in BAL fluid are higher than in controls, are not usually accompanied by peripheral eosinophilia, and have been associated with a poor prognosis (Haslam et al., 1980; Rudd et al., 1981; Cherniack et al., 1991). Analysis of BAL immune and inflammatory proteins is generally not as useful. IgG is elevated, whereas IgA, IgE, and complement levels are normal in most of the interstitial lung diseases that have been evaluated in extrinsic allergic alveolitis but not in CFA. Patients with CFA, however, may have increased levels of free collagenase (Crystal et al., 1981) and fibronectin (Morgan et al., 1984) in BAL fluid.

Pathogenesis

The cause of CFA is obscure. Toxic agents, collagen-vascular diseases, familial predisposition, and pneumoconioses have all been proposed. A viral etiology was originally proposed by Hamman and Rich (1944). Electron microscopic studies have demonstrated viral-like inclusion bodies in lung tissue (O'Shea and Yardley, 1970; Kawai et al., 1976), and many children with CFA had a previous upper respiratory tract infection, presumably of viral origin.

The general pathogenetic sequence is similar for all of the interstitial lung diseases and can be divided into several stages. First, some type of stimulus, unknown in the CFA disorders, results in an alveolitis characterized by the presence of effector cells (neutrophils, alveolar macrophages, and eosinophils) capable of damaging alveolar structures. Then, "maintenance" of the alveolitis results in chronic, continuous damage, derangement of alveolar structures, and, eventually, irreversible loss of functional alveolar-capillary units (end-stage). These concepts are well supported by the following observations:

1. Serial histologic evaluation has revealed that alveolitis precedes derangement.

2. Alveolitis without structural derangement is present in early interstitial lung disease.

3. Alveolitis is the predecessor of structural alterations in experimental models.

4. Activated effector cells present are clearly capable of causing alveolar derangement (Crystal et al., 1981; Cherniack et al., 1991).

Patients with CFA have the macrophage-neutrophil type of alveolitis, in which macrophages predominate and, most important, neutrophils are chronically present. When properly stained, neutrophils are seen associated with interstitial connective tissue and parenchymal lung cells. B lymphocytes, although present in normal numbers, are secreting immunoglobulin, and macrophages are in an activated state (Hunninghake and Moseley, 1984; Cherniack et al., 1991).

Current understanding of the pathogenesis of CFA alveolitis has been outlined by Hunninghake and Moseley (1984). First, lung mononuclear cells are stimulated by an unknown antigen(s) to produce immunoglobulins, resulting in local immune complex production. Alveolar macrophages respond by producing chemotactic factors that cause influx of neutrophils from the circulation into lung tissues. A study by Carré and associates (1991) correlated expression of alveolar macrophage IL-8 mRNA with the number of neutrophils per milliliter of BAL fluid and with disease severity. Once present, neutrophils are stimulated to release their array of potent mediators of destruction, including reactive oxygen species and collagenase. The result is that lung cells are directly injured, and collagen is constantly being destroyed.

Alveolar macrophages in CFA patients secrete a potent fibroblast growth factor, which induces cell division, and fibronectin, which sets the stage for cell division and is a chemoattractant for lung fibroblasts (it is 1000 times more powerful than serum fibronectin). Thus, collagen is constantly being destroyed and replaced, and the stage is set for structural alveolar derangement (fibrosis). Ultrastructural and immunohistochemical analysis of myofibroblasts suggests active contraction, analogous to wound contraction; this may contribute to the distorted lung architecture (Kuhn and McDonald, 1991).

Although the antigens and immunoglobulin specificities are not known, immunoglobulins may be directed against alveolar components as a result of injury (Hunninghake and Moseley, 1984). Lymphocytes from patients with certain types of CFA show cell-mediated immunity to type I collagen, and some cells produce immunoglobulins specific for type I collagen. There is ample evidence that the resulting immune complexes are produced locally in lung tissue and that circulating immune complexes are not of etiologic significance. Continuous production of antigen or abnormal suppressor T-cell function has been proposed, but the actual mechanisms responsible for maintaining the unremitting immune response are unknown (Morgan et al., 1984). Thus, it appears that the lung damage seen in patients with CFA is produced by a combination of type III and type IV immune mechanisms.

Treatment and Prognosis

Since cryptogenic fibrosing alveolitis is, at least in part, a disease of neutrophil-mediated lung destruction, a hypothesis linking levels of neutrophils in bronchoalveolar lavage fluid with prognosis seems reasonable. Indeed, independent of sex-related differences, a strong correlation exists between prognosis and percentages of neutrophils in BAL fluid (Crystal et al., 1981). This has been more clearly defined by Rudd and colleagues (1981). Patients with increased lymphocytes tended to have a better response to corticosteroids and a good prognosis. Increased neutrophils or eosinophils in BAL fluid were associated with a poor response to treatment, and progressive deterioration was likely in patients with an increased proportion of eosinophils.

CFA has been classified as either high intensity (>10% neutrophils in BAL fluid) or low intensity (<10% neutrophils in BAL fluid) and has been evaluated longitudinally in patients. Those with low-intensity alveolitis had less deterioration of pulmonary function with time, thus providing additional support for the hypothesized link between prognosis and the intensity of the alveolitis (Crystal et al., 1981). Patients classified as having UIP and LIP generally have an unfavorable prognosis and poor response to therapy (55% survive 5 years and 28%, 10 years after onset), compared with those with DIP, who often respond well to steroid treatment and may recover spontaneously (95% survive 5 years, and 70% survive 10 years) (Carrington et al., 1978). The survival pattern for children may be slightly better than for adults (Hewitt et al., 1977).

Ultimately, the morbidity and mortality in patients with CFA are caused by irreversibly deranged, nonfunctional alveolar-capillary units. The main principle of therapy is therefore to arrest or suppress the alveolitis before permanent damage occurs. Since alveolitis is so closely linked to prognosis, the use of gallium scans or bronchoalveolar lavage to stage the activity or intensity of the alveolitis has been recommended (Crystal et al., 1981). However, the use of these techniques in routine clinical practice is still controversial (Morgan et al., 1984; Turner-Warwick and Haslam, 1986; Cherniack et al., 1991).

Treatment with corticosteroids, the standard approach to therapy, will slow the progression of this usually fatal disease and occasionally reverse it (Brown and Turner-Warwick, 1971; Weese et al., 1975; Carrington et al., 1978). Newer treatment regimens use prednisone initially, and long-term treatment is adjusted according to alveolitis intensity as determined by periodic gallium scans and BAL. Patients who do not respond to steroid treatment may benefit from azathioprine, penicillamine, vincristine, chlorambucil, cyclophosphamide (alone or with corticosteroids), or colchicine (Crystal et al., 1981; Turner-Warwick and Haslam, 1986; Peters et al., 1993). One infant apparently responded to treatment with prednisone and chloroquine (Leahy et al., 1985). However, the efficacy for drugs other than corticosteroids has not been proved convincingly, and major adverse reactions have been reported. Indeed, several of these agents may cause interstitial lung disease. Because CFA is a chronic inflammatory lung disease, chest physiotherapy, bronchodilators, and other nonspecific measures are often used. Antibiotics are useful in treating secondary infections, and long-term oxygen therapy may improve the quality of life in hypoxemic patients.

PULMONARY HEMOSIDEROSIS

Pulmonary hemosiderosis results when recurrent pulmonary hemorrhage produces a progressive accumulation of iron (hemosiderin) in the lungs. Certain cardiac and collagen-vascular diseases secondarily produce pulmonary hemosiderosis. However, in a number of disorders pulmonary hemosiderosis is a primary feature of the disease and may have an immunologic basis; they can be classified as follows:

1. Idiopathic pulmonary hemosiderosis.
2. Pulmonary hemosiderosis from sensitivity to cow's milk.
    a. Without upper airway obstruction.
    b. With upper airway obstruction.
3. Pulmonary hemosiderosis with glomerulonephritis (Goodpasture's syndrome).

Idiopathic Pulmonary Hemosiderosis

Idiopathic pulmonary hemosiderosis (IPH), or isolated primary pulmonary hemosiderosis, is the occurrence of diffuse alveolar hemorrhage with accumulation of hemosiderin in lung tissue in the absence of an apparent cause (such as coagulopathy, hemodynamic abnormalities, or infection) or associated systemic disease (Leatherman et al., 1984a; Leatherman, 1991). It is a disease of young children, usually presenting between 1 and 10 years of age, occurring equally in boys and girls, often with a long delay between onset of symptoms and diagnosis (Chryssanthopoulos et al., 1983; Kjellman et al., 1984). Although no specific genetic pattern of disease has been observed and most cases occur sporadically, there are several reports of familial IPH (Beckerman et al., 1979).

Clinical Findings

IPH is characterized by hemoptysis, cough, tachypnea, malaise, weight loss, and iron deficiency anemia.

During an acute hemorrhage, there may be abdominal pain, tachycardia, and leukocytosis, findings compatible with a diagnosis of pneumonia. Following episodes of acute hemorrhage, reticulocytosis and elevated serum bilirubin may be found. IPH is sometimes subclinical because some patients have minimal symptoms and demonstrate only a mild anemia. Hemolysis is not a feature of IPH, and the Coombs' test is usually negative (Leatherman et al., 1984a). Eosinophilia and hepatosplenomegaly are present in about 20% of cases; clubbing is not unusual. Radiographic abnormalities of the chest range from reticular and interstitial patterns to extensive infiltrates with segmental or lobar involvement. Chronic disease produces interstitial fibrosis with a reticulonodular radiographic picture; acute hemorrhage often results in transient infiltrates, which may be unilateral. There may be symptom-radiographic dissociation—that is, radiographic abnormalities of the chest may precede or lag behind clinical symptoms.

Diagnosis

The diagnosis is made by the history of recurrent pulmonary hemorrhages (hemoptysis or transient infiltrates), the presence of iron deficiency anemia, and the finding of hemosiderin-laden macrophages in sputum or early-morning gastric aspirates. Lung biopsy is not always required for diagnosis; moreover, apparently stable patients have rapidly decompensated following lung biopsy (Soergel and Sommers, 1962; Repetto et al., 1967).

Laboratory Findings

There have been only limited studies of lung function in IPH; the findings are consistent with both obstructive and restrictive lung disease (Repetto et al., 1967; Allue et al., 1973; Beckerman et al., 1979). Examination of lung tissue by light microscopy reveals alveolar epithelial hyperplasia with shedding of cells, hemosiderin-laden macrophages in alveoli, erythrocytes in alveoli and the interstitium, and degeneration of elastic fibers (fibrosis). Vasculitis, alveolar septal necrosis, and granuloma formation are usually absent; their presence suggests that the hemosiderosis is secondary to some other disease (e.g., collagen-vascular disease). Electron microscopy has demonstrated intact alveolar-capillary basement membranes (Donlan et al., 1975; Gonzalez-Crussi et al., 1976), breaks in the basement membranes (Hyatt et al., 1972; Donald et al., 1975), thickened basement membranes with reduplication (Gonzalez-Crussi et al., 1976), and the absence of immune complexes and protein deposits in the subendothelial areas (Hyatt et al., 1972; Donlan et al., 1975).

Pathogenesis

Although an immunologic basis for IPH is frequently postulated, no consistent defect has been found. However, an immune basis is suggested by several observations:

1. IgA is elevated in over one half of cases.

2. IPH and celiac sprue have occurred in the same individuals.

3. The alveolar hemorrhage of IPH is similar to that of several immune disorders.

4. Immunosuppressive agents are apparently beneficial in some patients (Leatherman et al., 1984a).

Serum IgA elevation is not accompanied by increased salivary IgA (Valassi-Adam et al., 1975). Other serum immunoglobulins are normal. No immunofluorescence to IgG, IgM, IgA, and C3, and no immune complexes have been found in IPH lung tissue (Irwin et al., 1974; Donald et al., 1975; Donlan et al., 1975). Serum autoantibodies to lung tissue are not detectable (Hyatt et al., 1972).

Treatment

Because of the variability of the clinical course, it has been difficult to assess the various forms of therapy. Splenectomy does not appear to be of benefit (Soergel and Sommers, 1962). Steroids are helpful in the treatment of acute hemorrhage (Soergel and Sommers, 1962); immunosuppressive agents (Byrd and Gracey, 1973) and plasmapheresis (Leatherman et al., 1984a) have apparently been beneficial in a small number of patients. Deferoxamine may be helpful in mobilizing the excessive iron sequestered in the lung. Patients should be given a trial off milk products (in the presence or absence of serum milk precipitins, discussed later); some patients with IPH demonstrate considerable improvement while abstaining from milk and experience recurrence of symptoms when challenged with cow's milk.

Prognosis

The prognosis for patients with IPH is variable; although many patients succumb within the first 2 years after onset of manifestations, others may have a spontaneous remission of variable duration. The rarity of adult patients with IPH suggests that older patients either die or go into a near-permanent remission as they approach adult life. Although males and females are equally represented at the time of presentation, Chryssanthopoulos and coworkers (1983) have reported that females tend to survive longer (M:F = 1:2 among survivors). In addition, they found that younger age at time of onset carries a poor prognosis, severity of disease at the time of onset does not determine outcome, and the current therapeutic modalities do not appear to affect long-term prognosis.

Pulmonary Hemosiderosis from Sensitivity to Cow's Milk (Heiner Syndrome)

Heiner and colleagues (1962) described a disorder similar to IPH in infants who had serum precipitins to cow's milk and positive immediate skin tests to cow's milk proteins. These children (some of whom were as young as 13 to 14 days) also had eosinophilia, growth retardation, recurrent otitis media, chronic rhinitis,

gastrointestinal symptoms (diarrhea and vomiting), and gastrointestinal bleeding; notably, eczema was not a frequent finding. The pulmonary and gastrointestinal manifestations subsided with withdrawal of milk products and recurred when milk was reintroduced. A few patients without milk precipitins also appear to improve when cow's milk is removed, raising the question of what role, if any, these precipitins play in the pathogenesis of the bleeding. The immediate skin tests suggest that IgE (or IgG-mediated) type I reactions may play a role in this syndrome.

Boat and colleagues (1975) described pulmonary hemosiderosis occurring in early infancy associated with eosinophilia; serum precipitins to milk proteins; high IgE levels; normal IgG, IgM, and IgA levels; immediate and delayed skin reactions to milk antigens; chronic nasal discharge; diarrhea with gastrointestinal bleeding; and enlarged adenoids, producing upper airway obstruction and cor pulmonale. This syndrome occurred only in black children of both sexes. (The syndrome described by Heiner and coworkers [1962] also occurred more frequently in black children.) Although a unique immunologic mechanism causing milk-induced pulmonary hemosiderosis was not found in a later study by the same group (Stafford et al., 1977), it was observed that in some infants when milk was stopped, IgE levels and milk precipitin titers dropped markedly, pulmonary and gastrointestinal bleeding subsided, and nasal symptoms improved. The upper and lower respiratory tract disease produced by sensitivity to cow's milk seems to be mediated by both type I (high IgE levels) and type III (milk precipitins) immunologic reactions; the immediate and Arthus-type skin responses tend to confirm this hypothesis. Therapy consists of withdrawal of milk products and adenoidectomy.

Pulmonary Hemosiderosis with Glomerulonephritis (Goodpasture's Syndrome)

Goodpasture's syndrome generally refers to the combination of diffuse alveolar hemorrhage and glomerulonephritis resulting from anti–basement membrane antibody disease (see Chapter 25). It is primarily a disease of adolescents and young adults, although a few cases have been reported in childhood (O'Connell et al., 1964; Rees, 1984). The strong male predominance seen in older series was not found by Rees (1984) (M:F = 29:22).

Clinical Findings

Hemoptysis, anemia, exertional dyspnea, and microscopic hematuria are common findings at the time of presentation (Leatherman et al., 1984a). Azotemia is present in about 55% of patients at diagnosis, and, as with IPH, there is often a considerable delay between the onset of symptoms and correct diagnosis (Leatherman et al., 1984a).

Histology

Historically, Goodpasture's syndrome was thought to typify a type II (cytotoxic) immunologic reaction in the kidneys and lungs. Circulating anti–glomerular basement membrane antibody is present in the sera of most patients. The renal lesions demonstrate linear immunofluorescence along the basement membranes to IgA, IgG, IgM, and C3 (Donald et al., 1975), findings characteristic of a type II reaction. In the lungs, linear deposits of IgG, IgM, and C3 have been found along alveolar septa (Sturgill and Westervelt, 1965; Beirne et al., 1968; Poskitt, 1970); others have not seen such deposits in the lungs (Donald et al., 1975). A case of glomerulonephritis and alveolar hemorrhage with linear deposits of IgA in the lungs and kidneys has been reported (Border et al., 1979). Histologically, the pulmonary findings are diffuse alveolar hemorrhage and hemosiderin-laden macrophages. Recurrent hemorrhage may result in fibrosis. Severe inflammation is unusual, and neither alveolar septal necrosis nor vasculitis is found (Leatherman et al., 1984b).

Pathogenesis

The pathogenesis of the lung involvement is unclear. Anti–basement membrane antibody is specific for only a few basement membranes, including those of the renal tubule, glomerulus, alveolus, and choroid plexus. It is possible that an autoimmune process in one organ may produce antibodies that cross-react with similar basement membranes in other organs (Leatherman, 1991). The antigenic component to which the Goodpasture antibody binds is the α3 (IV) chain of type IV collagen (Gunwar et al., 1991). Anti–basement membrane glomerulonephritis may occur without lung disease in 20% to 40% of patients, but anti–basement membrane antibody lung disease rarely occurs without renal involvement (Rees, 1984). Difficulties with the concept that high levels of circulating anti–basement membrane antibody are solely responsible for the lung disease include the following:

1. New episodes of hemorrhage and their severity do not correlate with serum levels of anti–basement membrane antibody.
2. Anti-basement membrane antibody (in animal experiments) does not appear to bind to alveolar basement membrane in vivo.
3. Most anti–basement membrane glomerulonephritis patients without lung involvement have levels of circulating antibody comparable to those with lung disease.
4. Human anti–basement membrane antibody injected into sheep causes glomerulonephritis but not lung disease (Leatherman et al., 1984a).
5. Alveolar capillaries are usually not permeable to molecules the size of IgG (Rees, 1984).

It is logical, then, to postulate that lung involvement in Goodpasture's syndrome is precipitated by some insult that increases pulmonary capillary permeability, thus allowing circulating antibody to reach the alveolar basement membrane, setting the stage for lung injury (Rees, 1984). Duncan and coworkers (1965) suggested that viruses may be implicated, either by sharing antigens with lung and kidney basement membranes or by altering lung and kidney antigens. Viruses may also be implicated by increasing pulmonary capillary permeability; indeed, about 50% of patients describe an upper respiratory tract infection immediately before presentation (Rees, 1984; Leatherman, 1991). Similarly, smoking may be linked to the lung involvement in Goodpasture's syndrome. Donaghy and Rees (1983) studied 51 patients with anti–basement membrane glomerulonephritis; only 2 of 10 nonsmokers had lung involvement, whereas all of 37 smokers had lung and renal disease. Goodpasture's syndrome is strongly linked to the histocompatibility antigen HLA-DR2, and more severe glomerulonephritis occurs in association with HLA-B7 (Rees, 1984). Thus, the expression of injury in this disorder appears to depend on a complex interrelationship between genetic, immunologic, and environmental influences.

Several adults (Berine et al., 1973; Lewis et al., 1973) and children (Loughlin et al., 1978) show pathologic evidence suggesting that a variant of Goodpasture's syndrome is produced by a type III immunologic process. In these cases, there was no demonstrable circulating anti–basement membrane antibody; the deposits in the kidney along the basement membrane were granular ("lumpy-bumpy"), suggestive of circulating immune complexes that are cleared by the kidney; and immunofluorescent study of the lungs revealed no immunoglobulin or complement (Loughlin et al., 1978).

Diagnosis

Identification of anti–basement membrane antibody (ABMA) in the serum of patients may be done with high specificity and sensitivity by radioimmunoassay, enzyme-linked immunosorbent assay, and indirect immunofluorescence (least sensitive). The hallmark of this disease is the linear staining of IgG along glomerular basement membrane in renal biopsy specimens, and staining should be performed unless strongly contraindicated (Leatherman, 1991).

Treatment and Prognosis

The prognosis is generally poor, with death resulting from massive pulmonary hemorrhage (20%) or renal failure (75%). Plasma exchange and immunosuppressive agents (prednisone, cyclophosphamide, with or without azathioprine) are currently recommended therapy; however, large comparative clinical trials are needed (Rees, 1984; Leatherman, 1991). The results with steroids are less clear. High-dose methylprednisolone has been successfully used to treat alveolar hemorrhage associated with anti–basement membrane disease but not the renal involvement (Briggs et al., 1979). Some clinicians think that alveolar hemorrhage is better controlled with plasma exchange added to steroids. Renal transplant should be postponed until

ABMA has disappeared, since recurrence of glomerular lesions may be noted in up to 30% of renal allografts (Garrick and Neilson, 1988). Nephrectomy, once thought to diminish pulmonary involvement, no longer has a place in the management of Goodpasture's syndrome (Leatherman et al., 1984a).

PULMONARY MANIFESTATIONS OF HUMAN IMMUNODEFICIENCY VIRUS INFECTION

Pulmonary complications occur in two thirds of children infected with the human immunodeficiency virus (HIV) and constitute the most frequent cause of death (Hauger, 1991; Cunningham et al., 1991). The immunopathogenesis of HIV infection is discussed in detail in Chapter 18. Several unique problems related to the respiratory tract deserve mention here.

Lymphocytic Interstitial Pneumonitis

Lymphocytic interstitial pneumonitis (LIP) is the most common respiratory complication of pediatric HIV infection. HIV-associated LIP usually occurs in children older than 20 months of age and is common with perinatally acquired disease (incidence is 30% to 50%). The clinical presentation varies but typically has an indolent onset without fever. A predominance of rales is heard on auscultation, together with low serum lactate dehydrogenase (LDH) levels and mild hypoxia with digital clubbing. Pulmonary function changes are typified by a decrease in lung compliance and expiratory flows. Chest roentgenograms may show a diffuse reticular or reticulonodular pattern with widening of the mediastinum and hilum (Oldam et al., 1989; Cunningham et al., 1991). Patchy alveolar infiltrates and bronchiectasis have been described (Amarosa et al., 1992).

LIP occurs in children with relatively high CD4+ lymphocytes when compared with the child with *Pneumocystis carinii* infection. Lung biopsy specimens demonstrate diffuse interstitial thickening with occasional nodules. When nodules predominate, the pathogenic picture is referred to as pulmonary lymphoid hyperplasia (PLH). Benign, small, noncleaved lymphocytes and plasma cells are found in the alveolar septa, interlobular septa, and subpleural and peribronchial lymph channels. Whereas the pleura, blood vessels, and bronchi are often spared, cellular aggregates may be found around small arteries and distal airways, and pulmonary fibrosis may develop (Oldam et al., 1989; Pitt, 1991).

In adults, immunophenotypic studies have identified both B- and T-lymphocyte infiltrates (Barbera et al., 1992). The Epstein-Barr virus has been implicated as a synergist in the development of LIP and may act by stimulating B-lymphocyte proliferation (Barbera et al., 1992). Since zidovudine causes a positive clinical response in some patients, HIV itself may be a direct causative agent of pulmonary changes (Pitt, 1991). The alveolar macrophage has also been implicated in the pathogenesis of LIP (Semenzato et al., 1991). Bron-

choalveolar lavage may be useful in excluding opportunistic infection and may thereby help confirm the diagnosis of LIP. Treatment consists of supportive care, which may include bronchodilators and supplemental oxygen. Prednisone, human immunoglobulin, and zidovudine have been used in the treatment of LIP but responses have been variable and these agents lack proof of efficacy by clinical trials (Pitt, 1991).

The presence of LIP may represent a period in the natural course of HIV infection when the host's immunoproliferative responses are still somewhat intact; this often precedes the period of vulnerability to opportunistic infection. The median age of survival in HIV-infected children who initially present with LIP is 72 months. Although clinically suspected in the child with chronic interstitial pneumonia, lymphocytosis, hypergammaglobulinemia, and lymphadenopathy or parotid enlargement, a definitive diagnosis of LIP requires a lung biopsy.

Other Interstitial Disorders

Other interstitial diseases have been reported in the HIV-infected child but are less frequent (Joshi and Oleske, 1986; Kornstein et al., 1986). Desquamative interstitial pneumonitis (DIP) differs from LIP in that the normal pulmonary architecture is preserved. Intra-alveolar proliferation of macrophages and cuboidal metaplasia of alveolar type II cells are found on biopsy. Chronic interstitial pneumonitis, a rare complication of HIV infection in children, involves bronchiolar destruction with peribronchiolar interstitial infiltrates of lymphocytes, plasma cells, and macrophages. Treatment of these entities is the same as for LIP.

Malignancies

Immunoblastic sarcoma has been reported in the lung of a child with HIV infection, tumor nodules penetrating the bronchial walls and surrounding pleura (Zimmerman et al., 1987). Kaposi's sarcoma is not found in the lungs of HIV-infected children despite its fairly frequent occurrence in other tissues (Rogers et al., 1987).

Infections

Opportunistic infections are frequent complications in children with HIV infection and are discussed in detail elsewhere (Hauger, 1991; Murray and Mills, 1990) and in Chapters 18 and 31. *Pneumocystis carinii* infection is also discussed (Chapter 18). Pulmonary infection is typically found in the child whose helper (CD4+) lymphocytes are low (<400/mm³), the helper : suppressor (CD4:CD8) ratio is less than 1.0, and total lymphocyte count is less than 1500/mm³ (Inselman, 1990). Bronchoalveolar lavage typically shows increased total lymphocyte numbers, predominantly CD8+ cells, and a low CD4+:CD8+ ratio. Increases in IgA and IgG are found, and the total number of macrophages is low. Although opportunistic infections typically have a more acute onset than the interstitial pneumonitides, differentiation by clinical or radiographic means is rarely possible, and histologic or microbiologic differentiation is often required.

References

Allen DH, Williams GV, Woolcock AJ. Bird breeder's hypersensitivity pneumonitis: progress studies of lung function after cessation of exposure to the provoking antigen. Am Rev Respir Dis 114:555–566, 1976.

Allue X, Wise MB, Beaudry PH. Pulmonary function studies in idiopathic pulmonary hemosiderosis in children. Am Rev Respir Dis 107:410–415, 1973.

Alvarado CS, Boat TF, Newman AJ. Late-onset pulmonary fibrosis and chest deformity in two children treated with cyclophosphamide. J Pediatr 92:443–446, 1978.

Amorosa JK, Miller RW, Laraya-Cuasay L, Gaur S, Marone R, Frenkel L, Nosher JL. Bronchiectasis in children with lymphocytic interstitial pneumonia and acquired immune deficiency syndrome. Pediatr Radiol 22:603–607, 1992.

Athreya BH, Doughty RA, Bookspan M, Schumacher HR, Sewell EM, Chatten J. Pulmonary manifestations of juvenile rheumatoid arthritis: a report of 8 cases and review. Clin Chest Med 1:361–374, 1980.

Auerbach HS, Kirkpatrick JA, Williams M, Colten HR. Alternate-day prednisone reduces morbidity and improves pulmonary function in cystic fibrosis. Lancet 2:686–688, 1985.

Barbera JA, Hayashi S, Hegele RG, Hogg JC. Detection of Epstein-Barr virus in lymphocytic interstitial pneumonia by in situ hybridization. Am Rev Respir Dis 145:940–946, 1992.

Bardana EJ, Sobti KL, Cianciulli FD, Noonan MJ. Aspergillus antibody in patients with cystic fibrosis. Am J Dis Child 129:1164–1167, 1975.

Beckerman RC, Taussig LM, Pinnas LM. Familial idiopathic pulmonary hemosiderosis. Am J Dis Child 133:609–611, 1979.

Bedrossian CWM, Greenberg SD, Singer DB, Hansen JJ, Rosenberg HS. The lung in cystic fibrosis: a qualitative study including the prevalence of pathologic findings among different age groups. Hum Pathol 7:195–204, 1976.

Beirne GJ, Kopp WL, Zimmerman SW. Goodpasture syndrome: dissociation from antibodies to glomerular basement membrane. Arch Intern Med 132:261–263, 1973.

Beirne GJ, Octaviano GN, Kopp WL, Burns RO. Immunohistology of the lung in Goodpasture's syndrome. Ann Intern Med 69:1207–1212, 1968.

Bentur L, McKlusky I, Levison H, Roifman MC. Advanced lung disease in a patient with cystic fibrosis and hypogammaglobulinemia: response to intravenous immune globulin therapy. J Pediatr 117:741–742, 1990.

Berdischewshy M, Pollack M, Young LS, Chia D, Osher AB, Barnett EV. Circulating immune complexes in cystic fibrosis. Pediatr Res 14:830–833, 1980.

Berrill WT, van Rood JJ. HLA-DW6 and avian hypersensitivity. Lancet 2:248–249, 1977.

Berry DH, Brewster MA. Granulocyte NADH oxidase in cystic fibrosis. Ann Allergy 38:316–319, 1977.

Bhagwat AG, Wentworth P, Conen PE. Observations on the relationship of desquamative interstitial pneumonia and pulmonary alveolar proteinosis in childhood: a pathologic and experimental study. Chest 58:326–331, 1970.

Bienenstock J. The lung as an immunologic organ. Annu Rev Med 35:49–62, 1984.

Biggar WD, Holmes B, Good RA. Opsonic defects in patients with cystic fibrosis of the pancreas. Proc Natl Acad Sci 68:1716–1719, 1971.

Boat TF, Polmar SH, Whitman V, Kleinerman JI, Stern RC, Doershuk CF. Hyperreactivity to cow milk in young children with pulmonary hemosiderosis and cor pulmonale secondary to nasopharyngeal obstruction. J Pediatr 87:23–29, 1975.

Boat TF, Welsh MJ, Beaudet AL. Cystic fibrosis. In Beaudet AL, Sly WS, Valle D, eds. Metabolic Basis of Inherited Disease. New York, McGraw-Hill, 1989, pp. 2649–2680.

Border WA, Baehler RW, Bhathena D, Glassock RJ. IgA anti-base-ment membrane nephritis with pulmonary hemorrhage. Ann Intern Med 91:21–25, 1979.

Bosken CH, Myers JL, Greenberger PA, Katzenstein AA. Pathologic features of allergic bronchopulmonary aspergillosis. Am J Surg Pathol 12:216–222, 1988.

Bowden DH. The alveolar macrophage. Environ Health Perspect Monograph on Pulmonary Toxicology, 55:327–347, 1984.

Boxerbaum B, Kagumba M, Matthews LW. Selective inhibition of phagocytic activity of rabbit alveolar macrophages by cystic fibrosis serum. Am Rev Respir Dis 108:777–783, 1973.

Bradley CA. Diffuse interstitial fibrosis of the lungs in children. J Pediatr 48:442–450, 1956.

Brett MM, Simmonds EJ, Ghoneim ATM, Littlewood JM. The value of serum IgG titres against *Pseudomonas aeruginosa* in the management of early pseudomonal infection in cystic fibrosis. Arch Dis Child 67:1086–1088, 1992.

Briggs WA, Johnson JP, Teichman S, Yeagen HC, Wilson CB. Antiglomerular basement membrane antibody-mediated glomerulonephritis and Goodpasture's syndrome. Medicine 58:348, 1979.

Broughton RA, Wilson DH. Nitrofurantoin pulmonary toxicity in a child. Pediatr Infect Dis 5:466–469, 1986.

Brown CH, Turner-Warwick M. Treatment of cryptogenic fibrosing alveolitis with immunosuppressant drugs. Q J Med 40:289–302, 1971.

Buchta RM, Park S, Giammona ST. Desquamative interstitial pneumonia in a 7-week-old infant. Am J Dis Child 120:341–343, 1970.

Buescher ES, Winkelstein JA. The ability of bacteria to activate the terminal complement components in serum of patients with cystic fibrosis. J Pediatr 93:530–531, 1978.

Byrd RB, Gracey DR. Immunosuppressive treatment of idiopathic pulmonary hemosiderosis. JAMA 226:458–459, 1973.

Caciro F, Michielson FMC, Bernstein R, Hughes GRV, Ansell BM. Systemic lupus erythematosus in childhood. Ann Rheum Dis 40:325–331, 1981.

Caldwell JR, Pearce DE, Spencer C, Leder R, Waldman RH. Immunologic mechanisms in hypersensitivity pneumonitis. I. Evidence for cell-mediated immunity and complement fixation in pigeon breeder's disease. J Allergy Clin Immunol 52:225–230, 1973.

Calvanico NJ, Fink JN, Keller RH. Hypersensitivity pneumonitis. In Bienenstock J, ed. Immunology of the Lung and Upper Respiratory Tract. New York: McGraw-Hill, Inc, 1984, pp. 365–385.

Campbell PW, Phillips JA, Krishnamani MRS, Maness KJ, Hazinski TA. Cystic fibrosis: relationship between clinical status and F508 deletion. J Pediatr 118:239–241, 1991.

Carette S. Cardiopulmonary manifestations of systemic lupus erythematosus. Rheum Dis Clin North Am 14:135–147, 1988.

Carré PC, Mortenson RL, King TE, Noble PW, Sable CL, Riches WH. Increased expression of interleukin gene by alveolar macrophages in idiopathic pulmonary fibrosis. J Clin Invest 88:1802–1810, 1991.

Carrington CB, Addington WW, Goff AM, Madoff IM, Marks A, Schwaber JR, Gaensler EA. Chronic eosinophilic pneumonia. N Engl J Med 280:787–798, 1969.

Carrington CB, Gaensler EA, Coutu RE, FitzGerald MX, Gupta RG. Natural history and treated course of usual and desquamative interstitial pneumonia. N Engl J Med 298:801–809, 1978.

Carswell F, Oliver J, Silverman M. Allergy in cystic fibrosis. Clin Exp Immunol 35:141–146, 1979.

Chandra S, Jones HE. Pigeon fancier's lung in children. Arch Dis Child 47:716–718, 1972.

Chaussain M, de Boissieu D, Kalifa G, Epelbaum S, Niaudet P, Badoual J, Gendrel D. Impairment of lung diffusion capacity in Schönlein-Henoch purpura. J Pediatr 121:12–16, 1992.

Chen JK, Schulman H, Gardner P. A cAMP-regulated chloride channel in lymphocytes that is affected in cystic fibrosis. Science 243:657–660, 1989.

Cheng SH, Gregory RJ, Marshall J, Paul S, Souza DW, White GA, O'Riordan CR, Smith AE. Defective intracellular transport and processing of CFTR is the molecular basis of most cystic fibrosis. Cell 63:827–834, 1990.

Cherniack RM, Crystal RG, Kalica AR. Current concepts in idiopathic pulmonary fibrosis: a road map for the future. Am Rev Resp Dis 143:680–683, 1991.

Chihara J, Kino T, Fukuda F. Increases of hypodense eosinophils in bronchoalveolar lavage fluid in patients with PIE syndrome. Jpn J Allergy 34:676, 1985.

Chiron C, Gauthier C, Boule M, Grimfeld A, Girard F. Lung function in children with hypersensitivity pneumonitis. Eur J Respir Dis 65:79–91, 1984.

Chryssanthopoulos C, Cassimos C, Panagiotodou C. Prognostic criteria in idiopathic pulmonary hemosiderosis in children. Eur J Pediatr 140:123–125, 1983.

Church JA, Jordan JC, Keens TG, Wang CI. Circulating immune complexes in cystic fibrosis. Chest 80:405–411, 1981.

Church JA, Keens TG, Wang CI. Neutrophil and monocyte chemotaxis in acutely infected patients with cystic fibrosis. Ann Allergy 45:217–219, 1980.

Church JA, Keens TG, Wang CI, O'Neal M, Richards W. Normal neutrophil and monocyte chemotaxis in patients with cystic fibrosis. J Pediatr 95:272–274, 1979.

Chusid MJ, Dale DC, West BC, Wolff SM. The hypereosinophilic syndrome. Medicine 54:1–27, 1975.

Citro LA, Gordon ME, Miller WT. Eosinophilic lung disease. Am J Roentgenol 117:787–797, 1973.

Clarke CW. Aspects of serum and sputum antibody in chronic airways obstruction. Thorax 31:702–707, 1976.

Clarke LL, Grubb BR, Gabriel SE, Smithies O, Koller BH, Boucher RC. Defective epithelial chloride transport in a gene-targeted mouse model of cystic fibrosis. Science 257:1125–1128, 1992.

Clarke SW, Pavia D. Mucociliary clearance. In Crystal RG, West JB, et al., eds. The Lung: Scientific Foundations. New York, Raven Press, 1991, pp. 1845–1859.

Cochrane CG. Mechanisms involved in the deposition of immune complexes in tissues. J Exp Med 134:755–895, 1971.

Cohen SG, Ottesen EA. The eosinophil, eosinophilia, and eosinophil-related disorders. In Middleton E, Reed CE, Ellis EF, eds. Allergy—Principles and Practice, 2nd ed. St. Louis, C. V. Mosby, 1983, pp. 701–769.

Collins FS. Cystic fibrosis: molecular biology and therapeutic implications. Science 256:774–779, 1992.

Coraggio MJ, Gross TP, Roscelli JD. Nitrofurantoin toxicity in children. Pediatr Infect Dis J 8:163–166, 1989.

Cordier J-F, Valeyre D, Guillevin L, Loire R, Brechot J-M. Pulmonary Wegener's granulomatosis: a clinical and imaging study of 77 cases. Chest 97:906–912, 1990.

Coombs RRA, Gell PGH. The classification of allergic reactions underlying disease. In Gell PGH, Coombs RRA, eds. Clinical Aspects of Immunology. Philadelphia, F. A. Davis, 1968, pp. 317–337.

Crofton JW, Livingstone JL, Oswald NC, Roberts ATM. Pulmonary eosinophilia. Thorax 7:1–35, 1952.

Cromwell O, Moqbel R, Fitzharris P, Kurlak L, Harvey C, Walsh GM, Shaw RJ, Kay AB. Leukotriene C4 generation from human eosinophils stimulated with IgG–*Aspergillus fumigatus* antigen immune complexes. J Allergy Clin Immunol 82:535–544, 1988.

Crystal RG. Alveolar macrophages. In Crystal RG, West JB, et al., eds. The Lung: Scientific Foundations. New York, Raven Press, 1991, pp. 527–538.

Crystal RG. Cystic fibrosis—from the gene to the cure. Am J Respir Crit Care Med 151:S45–S46, 1995.

Crystal RG, Fulmer JD, Roberts WC, Moss ML, Line BR, Reynolds HY. Idiopathic pulmonary hemosiderosis. Ann Intern Med 85:769–788, 1976.

Crystal RG, Gadek JE, Ferrans VJ, Fulmer JD, Line BR, Hunninghake GW. Interstitial lung disease: current concepts of pathogenesis, staging, and therapy. Am J Med 70:542–568, 1981.

Cunningham AS, Fink JN, Schlueter DP. Childhood hypersensitivity pneumonitis due to dove antigens. Pediatrics 58:436–442, 1976.

Cunningham SJ, Crain EF, Bernstein LJ. Evaluating the HIV-infected child with pulmonary signs and symptoms. Pediatr Emerg Care 7:32–37, 1991.

Cupps TR, Fauci AS. The vasculitides. Major problems. Clin Med 21:1–211, 1981.

Cystic Fibrosis Genetic Analysis Consortium. World survey of the delta F508 mutation. Report from the Cystic Fibrosis Genetic Analysis Consortium (CFGAC). Am J Hum Genet 47:354–359, 1990.

Dabich L, Sullivan DB, Cassidy JT. Scleroderma in the child. J Pediatr 85:770–775, 1974.

Dai Y, Dean TP, Church MK, Warner JO, Shute JK. Desensitisation of neutrophil responses by systemic interleukin-8 in cystic fibrosis. Thorax 49:867–871, 1994.

Dalavanga YA, Constantopoulos SH, Galanopoulou V, Zerva L, Moutsopoulos HM. Alveolitis correlates with clinical pulmonary involvement in primary Sjögren's syndrome. Chest 99:1394–1397, 1991.

Daniele RP, Whiteside TL, Rowlands DT. Cells and secretory products of the immune system. In Daniele RP, ed. Immunology and Immunologic Diseases of the Lung. Boston, Blackwell Scientific Publications, 1988, pp. 3–19.

Davis PB, Dieckman L, Boat TF, Stern RC, Doershuk CF. Beta adrenergic receptors in lymphocytes and granulocytes from patients with cystic fibrosis. J Clin Invest 71:1785–1787, 1983.

Davis PB, di Sant'Agnese PA. Diagnosis and treatment of cystic fibrosis: an update. Chest 85:802–809, 1984.

De Horatius RJ, Abruzzo JL, Williams RC Jr. Immunofluorescent and immunologic studies of rheumatoid lung. Arch Intern Med 129:441–446, 1972.

Dejaegher P, Derveaux L, Dubois P, Demedts M. Eosinophilic pneumonia without radiographic infiltrates. Chest 84:637–638, 1983.

De Jongste JC, Neijens HJ, Duiverman EJ, Bogaard JM, Kerrebijn KF. Respiratory tract disease in systemic lupus erythematosus. Arch Dis Child 61:478–483, 1986.

Denning DW, Van Wye JE, Lewiston NJ, Stevens DA. Adjunctive therapy of allergic bronchopulmonary aspergillosis with itraconazole. Chest 100:813–819, 1991.

Desnoyers MR, Bernstein S, Cooper AG, Kopelman RI. Pulmonary hemorrhage in lupus erythematosus without evidence of an immunologic cause. Arch Intern Med 144:1398–1400, 1984.

Detjen PF, Greenberger PA, Patterson R. Allergic bronchopulmonary aspergillosis. In Lynch JP, DeRemee RA, eds. Immunologically Mediated Pulmonary Diseases. Philadelphia, J. B. Lippincott, 1991, pp. 378–398.

di Sant'Agnese PA, Darling RC, Perea GA, Shea E. Abnormal electrolyte composition of sweat in cystic fibrosis of the pancreas. Pediatrics 12:549–563, 1963.

Disis ML, McDonald TL, Colombo JL, Kobayashi R, Angle CR, Murray S. Circulating immune complexes in cystic fibrosis and their correlation to clinical parameters. Pediatr Res 20:385–390, 1986.

Doll NJ, Salvaggio JE. Pulmonary manifestations of the collagen-vascular disease. Semin Respir Med 5:273–281, 1984.

Donaghy M, Rees AJ. Cigarette smoking and lung hemorrhage in glomerulonephritis caused by auto-antibodies to glomerular basement membrane. Lancet 2:1390–1393, 1983.

Donald KJ, Edwards RL, McEvoy JDS. Alveolar capillary basement membrane lesions in Goodpasture's syndrome and idiopathic pulmonary hemosiderosis. Am J Med 59:642–649, 1975.

Donlan CJ Jr, Srodes CH, Duffy FD. Idiopathic pulmonary hemosiderosis: electron microscopic, immunofluorescent, and iron kinetic studies. Chest 68:577–580, 1975.

Döring G, Albus A, Høiby N. Immunologic aspects of cystic fibrosis. Chest 94:109s–114s, 1988.

Duncan DA, Drummond DN, Michael AF, Vernier RL. Pulmonary hemorrhage and glomerulonephritis. Ann Intern Med 62:920–938, 1965.

Eisenberg H. The interstitial lung diseases associated with the collagen vascular disorders. Clin Chest Med 3:565–578, 1982.

Eisenberg H, Dubois EL, Sherwin RP, Balchum OJ. Diffuse interstitial lung disease in systemic lupus erythematosus. Ann Intern Med 79:37–45, 1973.

Emrie P, Fisher JH. Genetic basis of cystic fibrosis. Semin Respir Med 7:359–361, 1986.

Epler GP, McLoud TC, Gaensler EA, Mikus JP, Carrington CB. Normal chest roentgenograms in chronic diffuse infiltrative lung disease. N Engl J Med 298:934–939, 1978.

Falchuk ZM, Taussig LM. IgA synthesis by jejunal biopsies from patients with cystic fibrosis and hereditary pancreatitis. Pediatrics 51:49–54, 1973.

Falcini F, Pigone A, Matucci-Cerinic M, Camiciottoli G, Taccetti G, Trapani S, Zammarchi E, Lombardi A, Bartolozzi G, Cagnoni M. Clinical utility of noninvasive methods in the evaluation of scleroderma lung in pediatric age. Scand J Rheumatol 21:82–84, 1992.

Fantone JC, Ward PA. Chemotactic mechanisms in the lung. In Newball HH, ed. Immunopharmacology of the Lung. New York, Marcel Dekker 1983, pp. 243–272.

Farrell PM, Gilbert EF, Zimmerman JJ, Warner TF, Saari TN. Familial lung disease associated with proliferation and desquamation of type II pneumocytes. Am J Dis Child 140:262–266, 1986.

Fauci A. Pulmonary vasculitis. In Kirkpatrick CH, Reynolds HY, eds. Immunologic and Infectious Reactions in the Lung. New York, Marcel Dekker, 1976, pp. 243–257.

Fauci AS, Wolff SM. Wegener's granulomatosis: studies in eighteen patients and a review of the literature. Medicine 52:535–561, 1973.

Fauci AS, Harley JB, Roberts WC, Ferran VJ, Gralnick HR, Bjornson BH. The idiopathic hypereosinophilic syndrome: clinical, pathophysiologic and therapeutic considerations. Ann Intern Med 97:78–92, 1982.

Fauci AS, Haynes BF, Katz P, Wolff SM. Wegener's granulomatosis: prospective clinical and therapeutic experience with 85 patients for 21 years. Ann Intern Med 98:76–85, 1983.

Faux JA, Wide L, Hargreave FE, Longbottom JL, Pepys J. Immunological aspects of respiratory allergy in budgerigar (*Melopsittacus undulatus*) fanciers. Clin Allergy 1:149–158, 1971.

Feery BJ, Phelan PD, Gallichio HA, Hampson AW. Antibody response to influenza virus vaccine in patients with cystic fibrosis. Aust Paediatr J 15:181–182, 1979.

Fick RB, Naegel GP, Matthay RA, Reynolds HY. Cystic fibrosis pseudomonas opsonins: inhibitory nature in an *in vitro* phagocytic assay. J Clin Invest 68:899–914, 1981.

Fick RB, Naegel GP, Squire SU, Wood RE, Gee JBL, Reynolds HY. Proteins of the cystic fibrosis respiratory tract. J Clin Invest 74:236–248, 1984.

Fick RB, Olchowski J, Squire SU, Merril WW, Reynolds HY. Immunoglobulin-G subclasses in cystic fibrosis. Am Rev Respir Dis 133:418–422, 1986.

Fink JN. Hypersensitivity pneumonitis. J Allergy Clin Immunol 74:1–9, 1984.

Fink JN. Clinical features of hypersensitivity pneumonitis. Chest 89(Suppl.):196s–198s, 1986.

Fink JN. Hypersensitivity pneumonitis. Clin Chest Med 13:303–309, 1992.

Forman SR, Fink JN, Moore VL, Wang J, Patterson R. Humoral and cellular immune responses in *Aspergillus fumigatus* pulmonary disease. J Allergy Clin Immunol 62:131–136, 1978.

Fournier E, Tonnel AB, Gosset PH, Wallaert B, Ameisen JC, Voisin C. Early neutrophil alveolitis after antigen inhalation in hypersensitivity pneumonitis. Chest 88:563–566, 1985.

Fraga A, Gudino J, Ramos-Niembro F, Alarcon-Segovia D. Mixed connective tissue disease in childhood. Am J Dis Child 132:263–265, 1978.

Frank ST, Weg JG, Harkleroad LE, Fitch RF. Pulmonary dysfunction in rheumatoid disease. Chest 63:27–34, 1973.

Fraser RG, Paré JAP. Extrinsic allergy alveolitis. Semin Roentgenol 10:31–42, 1975.

Fuchs HJ, Borowitz DS, Christiansen DH, Morris EM, Nash ML, Ramsey BW, Rosenstein BJ, Smit AL, Wohl ME. Effect of aerosolized recombinant human DNase on exacerbations of respiratory symptoms and on pulmonary function in patients with cystic fibrosis. N Engl J Med 331:637–642, 1994.

Fulmer JD, Kaltreider HB. The pulmonary vasculitides. Chest 82:615–624, 1982.

Gadek JE, Fells GA, Zimmerman RL, Crystal RG. Role of connective tissue proteases in the pathogenesis of chronic infection lung disease. Environ Health Perspect Monograph on Pulmonary Toxicology 55:297–306, 1984.

Galant SP, Rucker RW, Groncy CE, Wells ID, Novey SH. Incidence of serum antibodies to several aspergillus species and to *Candida albicans* in cystic fibrosis. Am Rev Respir Dis 114:325–331, 1976.

Gammon RB, Bridges TA, Al-Nezir H, Alexander CB, Kennedy JI. Bronchiolitis obliterans organizing pneumonia associated with systemic lupus erythematosus. Chest 102:1171–1174, 1992.

Garrick RE, Neilson EG. Anti–basement membrane disease with special reference to Goodpasture's syndrome. In Daniele RP, ed. Immunology and Immunologic Diseases of the Lung. Boston, Blackwell Scientific Publications, 1988, pp. 429–450.

Gaskin K, Gurwitz D, Durie P, Corey M, Levinson H, Forstner G. Improved respiratory prognosis in patients with cystic fibrosis with normal fat malabsorption. J Pediatr 100:857–862, 1982.

Gephardt GN, Ahmad M, Tubbs RR. Pulmonary vasculitis (Wegener's granulomatosis): immunohistochemical study of T and B cell markers. Am J Med 74:700–704,, 1983.

Ghose T, Landrigan P, Killeen R, Dill J. Immunopathological studies in patients with farmer's lung. Clin Allergy 4:119–129, 1974.

Gibbons A, Allan JD, Holzel A, McFarlane H. Cell-mediated immunity in patients with cystic fibrosis. Br Med J 1:120–122, 1976.

Ginsburg WW. Drug-induced systemic lupus erythematosus. Semin Respir Med 2:51–58, 1980.

Goldman DA, Klinger JD. *Pseudomonas cepacia:* Biology, mechanisms of virulence, epidemiology. J Pediatr 108:806–812, 1986.

Goldstein W, Döring G. Lysosomal enzymes from polymorphonuclear leukocytes and proteinase inhibitors in patients with cystic fibrosis. Am Rev Respir Dis 134:49–56, 1986.

Gonzalez-Crussi F, Hull MT, Grosfeld JL. Idiopathic pulmonary hemosiderosis: evidence of capillary basement membrane abnormality. Am Rev Respir Dis 144:689–698, 1976.

Gonzalez EB, Swedo JL, Rajaraman S. Ultrastructural and immunohistochemical evidence for release of eosinophilic granules in vivo: cytotoxic potential in chronic eosinophilic pneumonia. J Allergy Clin Immunol 79:755–762, 1986.

Gosset P, Perez T, Lassalle P, Duquesnoy B, Farre JM, Tonnel AB, Capron A. Increased TNF-alpha secretion by alveolar macrophages from patients with rheumatoid arthritis. Am Rev Respir Dis 143:593–597, 1991.

Graft DF, Mischler E, Farrell PM, Busse WW. Granulocyte chemiluminescence in adolescent patients with cystic fibrosis. Am Rev Respir Dis 125:540–543, 1982.

Grammer LC, Roberts M, Lerner C, Patterson R. Clinical and serologic follow-up of four children and five adults with bird-fancier's lung. J Allergy Clin Immunol 85:655–660, 1990.

Granstrom M, Ericsson A, Strandvik B, Wretlind B, Pavlovskis OR, Berka R, Vasil ML. Relation between antibody response to *Pseudomonas aeruginosa* exoproteins and colonization/infection in patients with cystic fibrosis. Acta Paediatr Scand 73:772–777, 1984.

Grantham JG, Meadows JA, Gleich GJ. Chronic eosinophilic pneumonia—evidence for eosinophil degranulation and release of major basic protein. Am J Med 80:89–94, 1986.

Greenberger PA. Allergic bronchopulmonary aspergillosis. J Allergy Clin Immunol 74:645–653, 1984.

Greenberger PA, Patterson R. Allergic bronchopulmonary aspergillosis: model of bronchopulmonary disease with defined serologic, radiologic, pathologic and clinical findings from asthma to fatal destructive lung disease. Chest 91:165S–171S, 1987.

Gregg RG, Wilfond BS, Farrell PM, Laxova A, Hassemer D, Mischler EH. Application of DNA analysis in a population-screening program for neonatal diagnosis of cystic fibrosis (CF): comparison of screening protocols. Am J Hum Genet 52:616–626, 1993.

Gregory RJ, Rich DP, Cheng SH, Souza DW, Paul S, Manavalan P, Anderson MP, Welsh MJ, Smith AE. Maturation and function of cystic fibrosis transmembrane conductance regulator variants bearing mutations in putative nucleotide-binding domains 1 and 2. Mol Cell Biol 11:3886–3893, 1991.

Gross M, Esterly JR, Earle RH. Pulmonary alterations in systemic lupus erythematosus. Am Rev Respir Dis 105:572–577, 1972.

Gugler E, Pallavicini JC, Swerdlow H, Zipkin I, di Sant'Agnese PA. Immunological studies of submaxillary saliva from patients with cystic fibrosis and from normal children. J Pediatr 73:548–559, 1968.

Gunwar S, Bejarano PA, Kalluri R, Langveld JPM, Wisdom BJ, Noelken ME, Hudson BG. Alveolar basement membrane: molecular properties of the noncollagenous domain (hexamer) of collagen IV and its reactivity with Goodpasture autoantigen. Am J Respir Cell Mol Biol 5:107–112, 1991.

Guzman J, Wang Y-M, Kalaycioglu O, Schoenfeld B, Hamm H, Bartsch W, Costabel U. Increased surfactant protein A content in human alveolar macrophages in hypersensitivity pneumonitis. Acta Cytologica 36:668–673, 1992.

Halprin GM, Ramirez RJ, Pratt PC. Lymphoid interstitial pneumonia. Chest 62:418–423, 1972.

Hamman L, Rich AR. Acute diffuse interstitial fibrosis of the lungs. Bull Johns Hopkins Hosp 74:117–212, 1944

Hansen LP, Jacobsen J, Skytte H. Wegener's granulomatosis in a child. Eur J Respir Dis 64:620–624, 1983.

Hansen PJ, Penny R. Pigeon-breeder's disease. Int Arch Allergy 47:498–507, 1974.

Hart RJ, Patterson R, Sommers H. Hyperimmunoglobulinemia E in a child with allergic bronchopulmonary aspergillosis and bronchiectasis. J Pediatr 89:38–41, 1976.

Haslam PL, Turton CWG, Lukoszek A, Collins JV, Salsbury AJ, Turner-Warwick ME. Bronchoalveolar lavage fluid cell counts in cryptogenic fibrosing alveolitis and their relation to therapy. Thorax 35:328–339, 1980.

Hamilos DL, Christensen J. Treatment of Churg-Strauss syndrome with high-dose intravenous immunoglobulin. J Allergy Clin Immunol 88:823–824, 1991.

Hammond KB, Turcios NL, Gibson LE. Clinical evaluation of the macroduct sweat collection system and conductivity analyzer in the diagnosis of cystic fibrosis. J Pediatr 124:255–260, 1994.

Hauger SB. Approach to the pediatric patient with HIV infection and pulmonary symptoms. J Pediatr 119:S25–S33, 1991.

Heiner DC, Sears JW, Kniker WT. Multiple precipitins to cow's milk in chronic respiratory disease. Am J Dis Child 103:634–654, 1962.

Hewitt CJ, Hull D, Keeling JW. Fibrosing alveolitis in infancy and childhood. Arch Dis Child 52:22–37, 1977.

Hill HR, Warwick WJ, Dettloff J, Quie PG. Neutrophil granulocyte function in patients with pulmonary infection. J Pediatr 84:55–58, 1974.

Hodson ME. Immunologic abnormalities in cystic fibrosis: chicken or egg? Thorax 35:801–806, 1980.

Hodson ME. Aerosolized dornase alfa (rhDNase) for therapy of cystic fibrosis. Am J Respir Crit Care Med 151:S70–S74, 1995.

Hodson ME, Turner-Warwick M. Autoantibodies in patients with chronic bronchitis. Br J Dis Chest 70:83–88, 1976.

Hodson ME, Turner-Warwick M. Autoantibodies in cystic fibrosis. Clin Allergy 11:565–570, 1981.

Hoestetler S, Denning DW, Stevens DA. US experience with itraconazole in *Aspergillus, Cryptococcus* and *Histoplasma* in the immunocompromised host. Chemotherapy 38(Suppl. 1):12–22, 1992.

Høiby N, Hertz JB. Precipitating antibodies against *Escherichia coli, Bacteroides fragilis,* ss. thetaiotaomicron, and *Pseudomonas aeruginosa* in serum from normal persons and cystic fibrosis patients, determined by means of crossed immunoelectrophoresis. Acta Paediatr Scand 68:495–500, 1979.

Høiby N, Hertz JB. Quantitative studies on immunologically specific and non-specific absorption of *Pseudomonas aeruginosa* antibodies in serum from cystic fibrosis patients. Acta Pathol Microbiol Scand 89:185–192, 1981.

Høiby N, Mathiesen L. *Pseudomonas aeruginosa* infection in cystic fibrosis. Acta Pathol Microbiol Scand 82:559–566, 1974.

Høiby N, Olling S. *Pseudomonas aeruginosa* infection in cystic fibrosis. Acta Pathol Microbiol Scand 85:107–114, 1977.

Høiby N, Wiik A. Antibacterial precipitins and autoantibodies in serum of patients with cystic fibrosis. Scand J Respir Dis 56:38–46, 1975.

Holland EJ, Loren AB, Scott PJ, Niwa Y, Yokoyama M. Demonstration of neutrophil dysfunction in the serum of patients with cystic fibrosis. J Clin Lab Immunol 6:137–139, 1981.

Hollsing AE, Granstrom M, Vasil ML, Wretlind B, Strandvik B. Prospective study of serum antibodies to *Pseudomonas aeruginosa* exoproteins in cystic fibrosis. J Clin Microbiol 25:1868–1874, 1987.

Holzer FJ, Olinsky A, Phelan PD. Variability of airways hyper-reactivity and allergy in cystic fibrosis. Arch Dis Child 56:455–459, 1981.

Holzhauer RJ, Van Ess JD, Schwartz RH. Third component of complement in cystic fibrosis. Cystic Fibrosis Club Abstracts 17:22, 1976.

Howard WA. Pulmonary infiltrates with eosinophilia (Löffler syndrome). In Chernick V, Kendig EL, eds. Disorders of the Respiratory Tract in Children, 5th ed. Philadelphia, WB Saunders, 1990, pp. 876–878.

Howatt WF, Heidelberger KP, LeGlovan DP, Schnitzer B. Desquamative interstitial pneumonia: case report of an infant unresponsive to treatment. Am J Dis Child 126:346–348, 1973.

Howe HS, Boey ML, Fong KY, Feng PH. Pulmonary hemorrhage, pulmonary infarction, and the lupus anticoagulant. Ann Rheum Dis 47:869–872, 1988.

Hunder GG, McDuffie FC, Hepper NGG. Pleural fluid complement in systemic lupus erythematosus and rheumatoid arthritis. Arch Intern Med 76:357–363, 1972.

Hunninghake GW, Fauci AS. Pulmonary involvement in the collagen-vascular diseases. Am Rev Respir Dis 119:471–503, 1979.

Hunninghake GW, Gadek JE, Kawanami O, Ferrans VJ, Crystal RG. Infectious and immune processes in the human lung in health and disease: evaluation by bronchoalveolar lavage. Am J Pathol 97:149–206, 1979.

Hunninghake GW, Kawanami O, Ferrans VJ, Young RC, Roberts WC, Crystal RG. Characterization of the inflammatory and immune effector cell in the lung parenchyma of patients with interstitial lung disease. Am Rev Resp Dis 123:407–412, 1981.

Hunninghake GW, Moseley PL. Immunological abnormalities of chronic non-infectious pulmonary diseases. In Bienenstock J, ed. Immunology of the Lung and Upper Respiratory Tract. New York, McGraw-Hill, 1984, pp. 345–364.

Hyatt RW, Adelstein ER, Halazun JF, Lukens JN. Ultrastructure of the lung in idiopathic pulmonary hemosiderosis. Am J Med 52:822–829, 1972.

Imbeau SA, Cohen M, Reed CE. Allergic bronchopulmonary aspergillosis in infants. Am J Dis Child 131:1127–1130, 1977.

Imbeau SA, Nichols D, Flaherty D, Dickie H, Reed C. Relationships between prednisone therapy, disease activity, and the total IgE level in allergic bronchopulmonary aspergillosis. J Allergy Clin Immunol 62:91–95, 1978.

Inoue T, Kanayama Y, Ohe A, Kato N, Horiguchi T, Ishii M, Shiota K. Immunopathologic studies of pneumonitis in systemic lupus erythematosus. Ann Intern Med 91:30–34, 1979.

Inselman LS. Pulmonary disorders in pediatric acquired immunodeficiency syndrome. In Chernick V, Kendig EL, eds. Disorders of the Respiratory Tract in Children, 5th ed. Philadelphia, WB Saunders, 1990, pp. 991–1003.

Irwin RS, Cottrell TS, Hsu KC, Griswold WR, Thomas MH. Idiopathic pulmonary hemosiderosis: an electron microscopic and immunofluorescent study. Chest 65:41–45, 1974.

Jagger KS, Robinson DL, Frantz MN, Warren RL. Detection by enzyme-linked immunosorbent assays of antibody specific for *Pseudomonas* proteinases and exotoxin A in sera from cystic fibrosis patients. J Clin Microbiol 17:55–59, 1982.

Jansen HM, Schutte AJH, Geissen MVB, The TH. Immunoglobulin subclasses in local immune complexes recovered by bronchoalveolar lavage in collagen-vascular disease. Lung 162:287–296, 1984.

Jederlinic PJ, Sicilian L, Gaensler EA. Chronic eosinophilic pneumonia. Medicine 67:154–162, 1988.

Johansen HK, Nir M, Høiby N, Koch C, Schwartz M. Severity of cystic fibrosis in patients homozygous and hetrozygous for ΔF508 mutation. Lancet 337:631–634, 1991.

Jones MM, Seilheimer DK, Pollack MS, Curry M, Crane MM, Rossen RD. Relationship of hypergammaglobulinemia, circulating immune complexes, and histocompatibility antigen profiles in patients with cystic fibrosis. Am Rev Respir Dis 140:1636–1639, 1989.

Joshi VV, Oleske JM. Pulmonary lesions in children with the acquired immunodeficiency syndrome: a reappraisal based on data in additional cases and follow-up study of previously reported cases. Hum Pathol 17:641–642, 1986.

Kathuria S, Cheifec B. Fatal pulmonary Henoch-Schönlein syndrome. Chest 82:654–656, 1982.

Kaltreider HB. Normal immune responses. In Crystal RG, West JB, et al., eds. The Lung: Scientific Foundations. New York, Raven Press, 1991, pp. 499–510.

Katz RM, Kniker WT. Infantile hypersensitivity pneumonitis as a reaction to organic antigens. N Engl J Med 288:233–237, 1973.

Kauffman HF, Beaumont F, de Monchy JGR, Sluiter HJ, de Vries K. Immunologic studies in bronchoalveolar fluid in a patient with bronchopulmonary aspergillosis. J Allergy Clin Immunol 74:835–840, 1984.

Kawai T, Fujiwara T, Aoyama Y, Aizawa Y, Yamada K, Aoyagi T, Mikata A, Kageyama K. Diffuse interstitial fibrosing pneumonitis and adenovirus infection. Chest 69:692–694, 1976.

Kemp T, Schram-Dumont A, van Geffel R, Kram R, Szpirer C. Alteration of the N-formyl-methionyl-leucyl-phenylalanine–induced response in cystic fibrosis neutrophils. Pediatr Res 20:520–526, 1986.

Kerem E, Carey M, Kerem B, Rommens J, Markiewicz D, Levison H, Tsui L, Durie P. The relationship between genotype and phenotype in cystic fibrosis—analysis of the most common mutation (Δ F508). N Engl J Med 323:1517–1522, 1990.

Kiefer TA, Kesarwala HH, Greenberger PA, Sweeney JR Jr, Fischer

TJ. Allergic bronchopulmonary aspergillosis in a young child: diagnostic confirmation by serum IgE and IgG indices. Ann Allergy 56:233–236, 1986.

King KK, Kornreich HK, Bernstein BH, Singsen BH, Hanson V. The clinical spectrum of systemic lupus erythematosus in childhood. Arthritis Rheum 20:287–294, 1977.

Kjellman B, Elinder G, Garwicz S, Svan H. Idiopathic pulmonary haemosiderosis in Swedish children. Acta Paediatr Scand 73:584–588, 1984.

Knowles MR, Olivier K, Noone P, Boucher RC. Pharmacologic modulation of salt and water in the airway epithelium in cystic fibrosis. Am J Respir Crit Care Med 151:S65–S69, 1995.

Konstan MW, Byard PJ, Hoppel CL, Davis PB. Effets of high-dose ibuprofen in patients with cystic fibrosis. N Engl J Med 332:848–854, 1995.

Kornstein MJ, Pietra GG, Hoxie JA, Conley ME. The pathology and treatment of interstitial pneumonitis in two infants with AIDS. Am Rev Respir Dis 133:1196–1198, 1986.

Korst RJ, McElvaney NG, Chu C-S, Rosenfeld MA, Mastrangeli A, Hay J, Brody SL, Eissa NT, Danel C, Jaffe HA, Crystal RB. Gene therapy for the respiratory manifestations of cystic fibrosis. Am J Respir Crit Care Med 151:S75–S87, 1995.

Kronborg G, Hansen MB, Svenson M, Fomsgaard A, Høiby N, Bendtzen K. Cytokines in sputum and serum from patients with cystic fibrosis and chronic *Pseudomonas aeruginosa* infection as markers of destructive inflammation in the lung. Pediatr Pulmonol 15:292–297, 1993.

Kuhn C, McDonald JA. The role of the myofibroblast in idiopathic pulmonary fibrosis: ultrastructural and immunohistochemical features of sites of active extracellular matrix synthesis. Am J Pathol 138:1257–1265, 1991.

Landau LI, Phelan PD. The variable effect of a bronchodilating agent on pulmonary function in cystic fibrosis. J Pediatr 82:863–868, 1973.

Landman S, Burgener F. Pulmonary manifestations in Wegener's granulomatosis. Radiology 122:750–757, 1974.

Leahy F, Pasterkamp H, Tal A. Desquamative interstitial pneumonia responsive to chloraquine. Clin Pediatr 24:230–232, 1985.

Leatherman JW. Diffuse alveolar hemorrhage in immune and idiopathic disorders. In Lynch JP, DeRemee RA, eds. Immunologically Mediated Pulmonary Diseases. Philadelphia, JB Lippincott, 1991, pp. 473–498.

Leatherman JW, Davies SF, Hoidal JR. Alveolar hemorrhage syndromes: diffuse microvascular lung hemorrhage in immune and idiopathic disorders. Medicine 63:343–361, 1984a.

Leatherman JW, Michael AF, Schwartz BA, Hoidal JR. Lung T cells in hypersensitivity pneumonitis. Ann Intern Med 100:390–392, 1984b.

Leitch AG. Pulmonary eosinophilia. Basics Respir Dis 7:1–6, 1979.

Lewis EJ, Schur PH, Busch GJ, Galvanek E, Merrill JP. Immunopathologic features of a patient with glomerulonephritis and pulmonary hemorrhage. Am J Med 54:507–513, 1973.

Lieberman J. Carboxypeptidase B–like activity and C3 in cystic fibrosis. Am Rev Respir Dis 111:100–102, 1975.

Liebow AA, Carrington CB. The eosinophilic pneumonias. Medicine 48:251–285, 1969.

Liebow AA, Steer A, Billingsley JG. Desquamative interstitial pneumonia. Am J Med 39:396–404, 1965.

Longbottom JL. Allergic bronchopulmonary aspergillosis: reactivity of IgE and IgG antibodies with antigenic components of *Aspergillus fumigatus* (IgE/IgG-antigen complexes). J Allergy Clin Immunol 72:668–669, 1983.

Lopez M, Salvaggio JE. Eosinophilic pneumonias. In Lynch JP, DeRemee RA, eds. Immunologically Mediated Pulmonary Diseases. Philadelphia, JB Lippincott, 1991, pp. 413–431.

Loughlin G, Cota K, Taussig LM. The relationship between flow transients and bronchial lability in cystic fibrosis. Am Rev Respir Dis 115:284, 1977.

Loughlin GM, Taussig LM, Murphy SA, Strunk RC, Kohnen PW. Immune-complex–mediated glomerulonephritis and pulmonary hemorrhage simulating Goodpasture syndrome. J Pediatr 93:181–184, 1978.

Lyrene RK, Polhill RB Jr, Guthrie RB, Tiller RE. Alternative complement pathway activity in cystic fibrosis. J Pediatr 91:681–682, 1977.

MacFarlane JD, Franken CK, Van Leeuwen AWFM. Progressive cavitating pulmonary changes in rheumatoid arthritis: a case report. Ann Rheum Dis 43:98–101, 1984.

MacLusky I, Levison H. Cystic fibrosis. In Chernick V, Kendig EL, eds. Disorders of the Respiratory Tract in Children. Philadelphia, WB Saunders, 1990, pp. 692–730.

MacLusky I, Levison H, Gold R, McLaughlin FJ. Inhaled antibiotics in cystic fibrosis: Is there a therapeutic effect? J Pediatr 108:861–865, 1986.

Manthei U, Taussig LM, Beckerman RC, Strunk RC. Circulating immune complexes in cystic fibrosis. Am Rev Respir Dis 126:253–257, 1982.

Martinez-Tello FJ, Braun DG, Blanc WA. Immunoglobulin production in bronchial mucosa and bronchial lymph nodes, particularly in cystic fibrosis of the pancreas. J Immunol 101:989–1003, 1968.

Matthay RA, Schwartz MI, Petty TL, Stanford RE, Gupta RC, Sahn SA, Steigerwald JC. Pulmonary manifestations of systemic lupus erythematosus: a review of 12 cases of acute lupus pneumonitis. Medicine 54:397–409, 1975.

Matthew TH, Hobbs JB, Kalowski S, Sutherland PW, Kincaid-Smith P. Goodpasture's syndrome: normal renal diagnostic findings. Ann Intern Med 82:215–218, 1975.

Matthews WJ, Williams M, Oliphant BO, Geha R, Colten HR. Hypogammaglobulinemia in patients with cystic fibrosis. N Engl J Med 302:245–249, 1980.

Maurer JR. Outcome issues in cystic fibrosis lung transplant recipients. Pediatr Pulmonol S9:199–200, 1993.

McCarthy DS, Pepys J. Allergic bronchopulmonary aspergillosis. Clinical immunology. 1. Clinical features. Clin Allergy 1:261–286, 1971a.

McCarthy DS, Pepys J. Allergic bronchopulmonary aspergillosis. Clinical immunology. 2. Skin, nasal and bronchial tests. Clin Allergy 1:415–432, 1971b.

McCarthy DS, Pepys J. Cryptogenic pulmonary eosinophilias. Clin Allergy 3:339–351, 1973.

McCombs RP. Diseases due to immunologic reactions in the lungs. N Engl J Med 286:1186–1194, 1972.

McElvaney NG, Nakamura H, Birrer P, Hébert CA, Wong WL, Alphonso M, Baker JB, Catalano MA, Crystal RG. Modulation of airway inflammation in cystic fibrosis: In vivo suppression of interleukin-8 on the respiratory epithelial surface by aerosolization of recombinant secretory leukoprotease inhibitor. J Clin Invest 90:1296–1301, 1992.

McFarlane H, Holzel A, Brenchley P, Allan JD, Wallwork JC, Singer BE, Worsley B. Immunologic complexes in cystic fibrosis. Br Med J 1:423–428, 1975.

McIntosh I, Cutting GR. Cystic fibrosis transmembrane conductance regulator and the etiology and pathogenesis of cystic fibrosis. FASEB J 6:2775–2782, 1992.

Moore VL, Fink JN, Barboriok JJ, Ruff LL, Schleuter DP. Immunologic events in pigeon breeder's disease. J Allergy Clin Immunol 53:319–328, 1974.

Morgan JE, Barkman HW, Waring NP. Idiopathic pulmonary fibrosis. Semin Respir Med 5:255–262, 1984.

Moss RB, Bocian RC, Hsu YP, Wei T, Yssel H. Reduced interleukin-10 production by cystic fibrosis (CF) T cell clones. Am J Resp Crit Care Med 151:A248, 1995.

Moss RB, Hsu YP. Isolation and characterization of circulating immune complexes in cystic fibrosis. Clin Exp Immunol 47:301–308, 1982.

Moss RB, Hsu YP, Lewiston NJ. ^{125}I-Clq–binding and specific antibodies as indicators of pulmonary disease activity in cystic fibrosis. J Pediatr 99:215–222, 1981.

Moss RB, Hsu YP, Sullivan MM, Lewiston NJ. Altered antibody isotype in cystic fibrosis: Possible role in opsonic deficiency. Pediatr Res 20:453–459, 1986.

Moss RB, Lewiston NJ. Immune complexes and humoral response to *Pseudomonas aeruginosa* in cystic fibrosis. Am Rev Respir Dis 121:23–29, 1980.

Moss RB, Lewiston NJ. Immunopathology of cystic fibrosis. In Shapira E, Wilson BG, eds. Immunological Aspects of Cystic Fibrosis Boca Raton, FL: CRC Press, 1984, pp. 5–27.

Murray JF, Mills J. Pulmonary infectious complications of human immunodeficiency virus infection. Am Rev Resp Dis 141:1582–1598, 1990.

Musk AW, Zilko PJ, Manners P, Kay PH, Kamboh MI. Genetic studies in familial fibrosing alveolitis. Chest 89:206–210, 1986.

Nadorra RL, Landing BH. Pulmonary lesions in childhood onset systemic lupus erythematosus: analysis of 26 cases, and summary of literature. Pediatr Pathology 7:1–18, 1987.

Naegel GP, Young KR, Reynolds HY. Receptors for human IgG subclasses on human alveolar macrophages. Am Rev Resp Dis 129:413–418, 1984.

Neeld DA, Goodman LR, Gurney JW, Greenberger PA, Fink JN. Computerized tomography in the evaluation of allergic bronchopulmonary aspergillosis. Am Rev Respir Dis 142:1200–1205, 1990.

Nelson LA, Callerame ML, Schwartz RC. Aspergillosis and atopy in cystic fibrosis. Am Rev Respir Dis 120:863–873, 1979.

Neva FA, Ottesen EA. Tropical (filarial) eosinophilia. N Engl J Med 298:1129–1132, 1978.

Newhouse M, Sanchis J, Bienenstock J. Lung defense mechanisms. N Engl J Med 295:1045–1052, 1976.

Nisen PD. Transplant immunology. Pediatr Pulmonol S9:197–198, 1993.

Noyes BE, Kurland G, Orenstein DM, Fricker FJ, Armitage JM. Experience with pediatric lung transplantation. J Pediatr 124:261–268, 1994.

O'Brodovich HM, Moser MM, Lu L. Familial lymphoid interstitial pneumonia: a long-term follow-up. Pediatrics 65:523–528, 1980.

O'Connell EJ, Dower JC, Burke EC, Brown AL Jr, McCaughey WTE. Pulmonary hemorrhage–glomerulonephritis syndrome. Am J Dis Child 108:302–308, 1964.

Oldam SAA, Castillo M, Jacobson FL, Mones JM, Saldana MJ. HIV-associated lymphocytic interstitial pneumonia: radiologic manifestations and pathologic correlation. Radiology 170:83–87, 1989.

Olson JC, Kelly KJ, Pan CG, Wortmann DW. Pulmonary disease with hemorrhage in Henoch-Schönlein purpura. Pediatrics 89:1177–1181, 1992.

Olson J, Colby TV, Elliot CG. Hamman-Rich syndrome revisited. Mayo Clin Proc 65:1538–1548, 1990.

O'Shea PA, Yardley JH. The Hamman-Rich syndrome in infancy: report of a case with virus-like particles by electron microscopy. Johns Hopkins Med J 126:320–336, 1970.

Ostrow D, Cherniak RM. Resistance to airflow in patients with diffuse interstitial lung disease. Am Rev Respir Dis 108:205–210, 1973.

Ottesen EA. Eosinophilia and the lung. In Kirkpatrick CH, Reynolds HY, eds. Immunologic and Infectious Reactions in the Lung. New York, Marcel Dekker, 1976, pp. 289–332.

Park S, Nyhan WL. Fatal pulmonary involvement in dermatomyositis. Am J Dis Child 129:723–726, 1975.

Patchefsky AS, Isreal HL, Hoch WS, Gordon G. Desquamative interstitial pneumonia: relationship to interstitial fibrosis. Thorax 28:680–693, 1973.

Pathial K, Saff R, Murali P, Splaingard M, Biller J, McCarthy K, Fink J, Greenberger P, Kurup V. Immune responses to *Pseudomonas aeruginosa* in cystic fibrosis. J Allergy Clin Immunol 89:167, 1992.

Patterson R, Roberts M. IgE and IgG antibodies against *Aspergillus fumigatus* in sera of patients with bronchopulmonary allergic aspergillosis. Int Arch Allergy Appl Immunol 46:150–160, 1974.

Patterson R, Schatz M, Fink JN, DeSwarte RS, Roberts M, Cugell D. Pigeon breeder's disease. 1. Serum immunoglobulin concentrations; IgG, IgM, IgA, and IgE antibodies against pigeon serum. Am J Med 60:144–151, 1976.

Pauwels R, Stevens EM, van der Straeten M. IgE antibodies in bronchopulmonary aspergillosis. Ann Allergy 37:195–200, 1976.

Pennington JE. *Aspergillus* lung disease. Med Clin North Am 64:475–490, 1980.

Pennington JE. Opportunistic fungal pneumonias: *Aspergillus, Mucor, Candida, Torulopsis*. In Pennington JE, ed. Respiratory Infections: Diagnosis and Management, 2nd ed. New York, Raven Press, 1988, pp. 443–456.

Pennington JE, Reynolds J, Wood RE, Robinson RA, Levine AS. Use of a *Pseudomonas aeruginosa* vaccine in patients with acute leukemia and cystic fibrosis. Am J Med 58:629–636, 1975.

Pepys J. Immunopathology of allergic lung disease. Clin Allergy 3:1–22, 1973.

Pepys J, Simon G. Asthma, pulmonary eosinophilia and allergic alveolitis. Med Clin North Am 57:573–591, 1973.

Permin H, Skov PS, Norn SA, Høiby N, Schiotz PO. Platelet 3H-serotonin releasing immune complexes induced by *Pseudomonas aeruginosa* in cystic fibrosis. Allergy 37:93–100, 1982.

Pervez NK, Kleinerman J, Kattan M, Freed JA, Harris MB, Rosen MJ, Schwartz IS. Pseudomembranous necrotizing bronchial aspergillosis. Am Rev Respir Dis 131:961–963, 1985.

Peters SG, McDougall JC, Douglas WW, Coles DT, DeRemee RA. Colchicine in the treatment of pulmonary fibrosis. Chest 103:101–104, 1993.

Piedra P, Ogra PL. Immunologic aspects of surface infections in the lung. J Pediatr 108:817–823, 1986.

Pitt J. Lymphocytic interstitial pneumonia. Pediatr Clin North Am 38:89–95, 1991.

Polley MJ, Bearn AG. Annotation: cystic fibrosis: current concepts. J Med Genet 11:249–252, 1974.

Poskitt TR. Immunologic and electron microscopic studies in Goodpasture's syndrome. Am J Med 49:250–257, 1970.

Prakash UBS. Pulmonary manifestations in mixed connective tissue disease. Semin Respir Med 9:318–324, 1988.

Pritcher-Wilmot RW, Levinsky RJ, Matthew DJ. Circulating soluble immune complexes containing pseudomonas antigens in cystic fibrosis. Arch Dis Child 57:577–581, 1982.

Purtilo DT, Brem J, Ceccaci L, Fitzpatrick AJ. A family study of pigeon breeder's disease. J Pediatr 86:569–571, 1975.

Quie PG. Lung defense against infection. J Pediatr 108:813–816, 1986.

Rachelefsky GS, Osher A, Dooley RE, Ank B, Stiehm ER. Coexistent respiratory allergy and cystic fibrosis. Am J Dis Child 128:355–359, 1974.

Ramsey BW, Boat TF. Outcome measures for clinical trials in cystic fibrosis: summary of a Cystic Fibrosis Foundation consensus conference. J Pediatr 124:177–192, 1994.

Rao M, Steiner P, Rose JS, Kassner EG, Kottmeier P, Steiner M. Chronic eosinophilic pneumonia in a one-year-old child. Chest 68:118–120, 1975.

Reed CE, Sosman A, Barbee RA. Pigeon-breeder's lung. JAMA 193:261–265, 1965.

Reeder WH, Goodrich BE. Pulmonary infiltration with eosinophilia. Ann Intern Med 36:1217–1240, 1952.

Rees AJ. Pulmonary injury caused by anti–basement membrane antibodies. Semin Respir Med 5:264–272, 1984.

Regelmann WE, Skubitz KM, Herron JM. Increased monocyte oxidase activity in cystic fibrosis heterozygotes and homozygotes. Am J Cell Mol Biol 5:27–33, 1991.

Renzi GD, Lopez-Majano V. Early diagnosis of interstitial fibrosis. Respiration 33:294–302, 1976.

Repetto G, Lisboa C, Emparanza E, Ferretti R, Neira M, Etchart M, Meneghello J. Idiopathic pulmonary hemosiderosis. Pediatrics 40:24–32, 1967.

Reynolds HY. Idiopathic interstitial pulmonary fibrosis. Chest 89(Suppl.):139–144, 1986.

Reynolds HY, Atkinson JP, Newball HH, Frank MM. Receptors for immunoglobulin and complement on human alveolar macrophages. J Immunol 114:1813–1819, 1975.

Ricketti AJ, Greenberger PA, Pruzanshy JJ, Patterson R. Hyperreactivity of mediator-releasing cells from patients with allergic bronchopulmonary aspergillosis as evidenced by basophil histamine release. J Allergy Clin Immunol 72:386–392, 1983.

Ricketti AJ, Greenberger PA, Patterson R. Serum IgE as an important aid in management of allergic bronchopulmonary aspergillosis. J Allergy Clin Immunol 74:68–71, 1984.

Riordan JR, Rommens JM, Kerem B, Alon N, Chou JL, Drumm ML, Iannuzzi MC, Collins FS, Tsui L-C. Identification of the cystic fibrosis gene: cloning and characterization of complementary DNA. Science 245:1066–1073, 1989.

Roberts SR Jr. Immunology and the lung: an overview. Semin Roentgenol 10:7–19, 1975.

Rogers MF, Thomas PA, Starcher ET, Noa MC, Bush TJ, Jaffe HW. Acquired immunodeficiency syndrome in children: report of the Centers for Disease Control national surveillance, 1982 to 1985. Pediatrics 79:1008–1014, 1987.

Rogers RM, Christiansen JR, Coalson JJ, Patterson CD. Eosinophilic pneumonia. Chest 68:665–671, 1975.

Rommens JM, Iannuzzi MC, Kerem B, Drumm ML, Melmer G, Dean M, Rozmahel R, Cole JL, Kennedy D, Hidaka N, Zsiga M, Buchwald

M, Riordan JR, Tsui L-C, Collins FS. Identification of the cystic fibrosis gene: chromosome walking and jumping. Science 245:1059–1065, 1989.

Rosenow EC III. The spectrum of drug-induced pulmonary disease. Ann Intern Med 77:977–991, 1972.

Rosenow EC III. Drug-induced hypersensitivity disease of the lung. In Kirkpatrick CH, Reynolds HY, eds. Immunologic and Infectious Reactions in the Lung. New York, Marcel Dekker, 1976, pp. 261–287.

Rosenow EC III, O'Connell EJ, Harrison EG Jr. Desquamative interstitial pneumonia in children. Am J Dis Child 120:344–348, 1970.

Rosenstein BJ, Eigen H. Risk of alternate-day prednisone in patients with cystic fibrosis. Pediatrics 87:245–246, 1991.

Rosenstein BJ, Eigen H, Schidlow DV. Alternate-day prednisone in patients with cystic fibrosis. Pediatr Res 33:385A, 1993.

Rottem M, Fauci AS, Hallahan CW, Kerr GS, Lebovics R, Leavitt RY, Hoffman GS. Wegener granulomatosis in children and adolescents: clinical presentation and outcome. J Pediatr 122:26–31, 1993.

Rudd RM, Haslam PL, Turner-Warwick M. Cryptogenic fibrosing alveolitis: relationships of pulmonary physiology and bronchoalveolar lavage to response to treatment. Am Rev Respir Dis 124:1–8, 1981.

Rule H, Lawrence D, Hager HJ, Hyslop N Jr, Schwachman H. IgA: presence in meconium obtained from patients with cystic fibrosis. Pediatrics 48:601–604, 1971.

Salvaggio JE, deShazo RD. Pathogenesis of hypersensitivity pneumonitis. Chest 89(Suppl.):190–193, 1986.

Sanders DY, Huntley CC, Sharp GC. Mixed connective tissue disease in a child. J Pediatr 83:642–644, 1973.

Scadding JG. The bronchi in allergic aspergillosis. Scand J Respir Dis 48:372–377, 1967.

Schatz M, Wasserman S, Patterson R. Eosinophils and immunologic lung disease. Med Clin North Am 65:1055–1071, 1981.

Schatz M, Wasserman S, Patterson R. The eosinophil and the lung. Arch Intern Med 142:1515–1519, 1982.

Schiller NL, Millard RL. *Pseudomonas*-infected cystic fibrosis patient sputum inhibits the bactericidal activity of normal human serum. Pediatr Res 17:747–752, 1983.

Shiotz PO. Local humoral immunity and immune reaction in the lungs of patients with cystic fibrosis. Acta Pathol Microbiol Scand 276:1–25, 1981.

Schiotz PO, Clemmensen I, Høiby N. Immunoglobulins and albumin in sputum from patients with cystic fibrosis. Acta Pathol Microbiol Scand 88:275–280, 1980.

Schiotz PO, Egeskjold EM, Høiby N, Permin H. Autoantibodies in serum and sputum from patients with cystic fibrosis. Acta Pathol Microbiol Scand 87:319–324, 1979a.

Schiotz PO, Høiby N. Precipitating antibodies against *Pseudomonas aeruginosa* in sputum from patients with cystic fibrosis: specificities and titres determined by means of crossed immunoelectrophoresis with intermediate gel. Acta Pathol Microbiol Scand 83:469–475, 1975.

Schiotz PO, Høiby N. Precipitating antibodies against *Haemophilus influenzae* and *Staphylococcus aureus* in sputum and serum from patients with cystic fibrosis. Acta Pathol Microbiol Scand 87:345–351, 1979.

Schiotz PO, Høiby N, Juhl F, Permin H, Nielson H, Svehag SE. Immune complexes in cystic fibrosis. Acta Pathol Microbiol Scand 85:57–64, 1977.

Schiotz PO, Høiby N, Permin H, Wiik A. IgA and IgG antibodies against surface antigens of *Pseudomonas aeruginosa* in sputum and serum from patients with cystic fibrosis. Acta Pathol Microbiol Scand 87:229–233, 1979b.

Schiotz PO, Nielsen H, Høiby N, Glikmann G, Svehag HE. Immune complexes in the spectrum of patients with cystic fibrosis suffering from chronic *Pseudomonas aeruginosa* lung infection. Acta Pathol Microbiol Scand 86:37–40, 1978.

Schiotz PO, Sorensen H, Høiby N. Activated complement in the sputum from patients with cystic fibrosis. Acta Pathol Microbiol Scand 87:1–5, 1979c.

Schleuter DP. Response of the lung to inhaled antigens. Am J Med 57:476–492, 1974.

Schneider RM, Neivus DB, Brown HZ. Desquamative interstitial pneumonia in a four-year-old child. N Engl J Med 277:1056–1058, 1967.

Schofield NM, Cameron RJ, Davies IR, Green M. Small airways in fibrosing alveolitis. Am Rev Respir Dis 113:729–735, 1976.

Schuyler M, Salvaggio JE. Hypersensitivity pneumonitis. Semin Respir Med 5:246–254, 1984.

Schuyler MR, Thigpen TP, Salvaggio JE. Local immunity in pigeon breeder's disease. Ann Intern Med 88:355–358, 1978.

Schwartz RH. Serum immunoglobulin levels in cystic fibrosis. Am J Dis Child 111:408–411, 1966.

Schwartz RH, Johnstone DE, Holsclaw DS, Dooley RR. Serum precipitins to *Aspergillus fumigatus* in cystic fibrosis. Am J Dis Child 120:432–433, 1970.

Semenzato G. Immunology of interstitial lung diseases: cellular events taking place in the lung of sarcoidosis, hypersensitivity pneumonitis and HIV infection. Eur Respir J 4:94–102, 1991.

Serlin SP, Rimsza ME, Gay JH. Rheumatic pneumonia: the need for a new approach. Pediatrics 56:1075–1078, 1975.

Shah A, Pant CS, Bhagat R, Panchal N. CT in childhood allergic bronchopulmonary aspergillosis. Pediatr Radiol 22:227–228, 1992.

Shannon DC, Andrews JL, Recavarren S, Kazemi H. Pigeon breeder's lung disease and interstitial pulmonary fibrosis. Am J Dis Child 117:504–510, 1969.

Shapiro GG, Bamman J, Kanarek P, Bierman CW. The paradoxical effect of adrenergic and methylxanthine drugs in cystic fibrosis. Pediatrics 58:740–743, 1976.

Shen J, Brackett R, Fischer T, Holder A, Kellog F, Michael JG. Specific pseudomonas immunoglobulin E antibodies in sera of patients with cystic fibrosis. Infect Immun 32:967–968, 1981.

Shryock TR, Molle JS, Klinger JD, Thomassen MJ. Association with phagocytic inhibition of anti-*Pseudomonas aeruginosa* immunoglobulin G antibody subclass levels in serum from patients with cystic fibrosis. J Clin Microbiol 23:513–516, 1986.

Sieber OF, Wilska ML, Riggin R. Elevated nitroblue tetrazolium dye reduction tests: response in acute viral respiratory disease. Pediatrics 58:122–124, 1976.

Silver RM, Miller S. Lung involvement in systemic sclerosis. Rheum Dis Clin North Am 16:199–216, 1990.

Silverman M, Hobbs FDR, Gordon IRS, Carswell F. Cystic fibrosis, atopy, and airways lability. Arch Dis Child 53:873–877, 1978.

Singsen BH, Bernstein BB, Kornreich HK, King KK, Hanson V, Tan EM. Mixed connective tissue disease in childhood: a clinical and serologic survey. J Pediatr 90:893–900, 1977.

Singsen BH, Swanson VL, Bernstein BH, Heuser ET, Hanson V, Landing BH. A histologic evaluation of mixed connective tissue disease in childhood. Am J Med 68:710–717, 1980.

Slavin RG, Laird TS, Cherry JD. Allergic bronchopulmonary aspergillosis in a child. J Pediatr 76:415–421, 1970.

Smith AL. Antibiotic therapy in cystic fibrosis: evaluation of clinical trials. J Pediatr 108:866–870, 1986.

Smith GJW. The histopathology of pulmonary reactions to drugs. Clin Chest Med 11:95–117, 1990.

Smith MJ, Morris L, Stead RJ, Hodson ME, Batten JC. Lymphocyte subpopulations and function in cystic fibrosis. Eur J Respir Dis 70:300–308, 1987.

Soergel KH, Sommers SC. Idiopathic pulmonary hemosiderosis and related syndromes. Am J Med 32:499–511, 1962.

Sorensen RU, Chase PA, Stern RC, Polmar SH. Influence of cystic fibrosis plasma on lymphocyte responses to *Pseudomonas aeruginosa in vivo*. Pediatr Res 15:14–18, 1981a.

Sorensen RU, Ruuskanen O, Miller K, Stern RC. B-lymphocyte function in cystic fibrosis. Eur J Respir Dis 64:524–533, 1983.

Sorensen RU, Stern RC, Chase PA, Polmar SH. Changes in lymphocyte reactivity to *Pseudomonas aeruginosa* in hospitalized patients with cystic fibrosis. Am Rev Respir Dis 123:37–41, 1981b.

Sorensen RU, Stern RC, Chase P, Polmar SH. Defective cellular immunity to gram-negative bacteria in cystic fibrosis patients. Infect Immunol 23:398–402, 1979.

Sorensen RU, Stern RC, Polmar SH. Cellular immunity to bacteria: impairment of *in vitro* lymphocyte responses to *Pseudomonas aeruginosa* in cystic fibrosis patients. Infect Immunol 18:735–740, 1977.

Sorensen RU, Stern RC, Polmar SH. Lymphocyte responsiveness to *Pseudomonas aeruginosa* in cystic fibrosis: relationship to status of pulmonary disease in sibling pairs. J Pediatr 93:201–205, 1978.

Sorensen RU, Waller RL, Klinger JD. Infection and immunity to *Pseudomonas*. Clin Rev Allergy 9:47–74, 1991.

Sostman HD, Matthay RA, Putman CE. Cytotoxic drug-induced lung disease. Am J Med 62:608–615, 1977.

South MA, Warwick WJ, Wollheim FA, Good RA. The IgA system. III. IgA levels in the serum and saliva of pediatric patients—evidence for a local immunological system. J Pediatr 71:645–653, 1967.

Speert DP, Lawton D, Mutharia LM. Antibody to *Pseudomonas aeruginosa* mucoid exopolysaccharide and to sodium alginate in cystic fibrosis serum. Pediatr Res 18:431–433, 1984.

Spence JE, Buffone GJ, Rosenbloom CI, Fernbach SD, Curry MR, Carpenter RJ, Ledbetter DH, O'Brien WE, Beaudet AL. Prenatal diagnosis of cystic fibrosis using linked DNA markers and microvillar intestinal enzyme analysis. Hum Genet 76:5–10, 1987.

Stafford HA, Polmar SH, Boat TF. Immunologic studies in cow's milk–induced pulmonary hemosiderosis. Pediatr Res 11:898–903, 1977.

Stein AA, Mamlapas FC, Soike KF, Patterson PR. Specific isoantibodies in cystic fibrosis. J Pediatr 65:495–500, 1964.

Stephens M, Reynolds S, Gibbs AR, Davies B. Allergic bronchopulmonary aspergillosis progressing to allergic granulomatosis and angiitis (Churg-Strauss syndrome). Am Rev Respir Dis 137:1226–1228, 1988.

Stiehm ER, Reed CE, Tooley WH. Pigeon breeder's lung in children. Pediatrics 39:904–915, 1967.

Storey DG, Ujack EE, Rabin HR. Population transcript accumulation of *Pseudomonas aeruginosa* exotoxin A and elastase in sputa from patients with cystic fibrosis. Infect Immunol 60:4687–4694, 1992.

Strauss RG. Complement in cystic fibrosis. Helv Paediatr Acta 34:429–435, 1979.

Strunk RC, Sieber O, Taussig LM, Gall E. Serum complement depressions with viral pulmonary illnesses. Arch Dis Child 52:687–690, 1977.

Stuart BO. Deposition and clearance of inhaled particles. Envir Health Perspect Monograph on Pulmonary Toxicology 55:369–392, 1984.

Sturgill BC, Westervelt FB. Immunofluorescence studies in a case of Goodpasture's syndrome. JAMA 194:172–174, 1965.

Sullivan JF, Dolan TF Jr, Meyers A, Treat K. Use of nitroblue tetrazolium dye test. Am J Dis Child 125:702–704, 1973.

Tacier-Eugster H, Wuthrich HM, Meyer H. Atopic allergy, serum IgE and RAST-specific IgE antibodies in patients with cystic fibrosis. Helv Paediatr Acta 35:31–37, 1980.

Talamo RC, Schwartz RH. Immunologic and allergic manifestations. In Taussig LM, ed. Cystic Fibrosis. New York, Thieme-Stratton, 1984, pp. 175–194.

Taussig LM, ed. Cystic Fibrosis. New York, Theime-Stratton, 1984.

Taussig LM, Landau LI. Cystic fibrosis. In Kelley V, ed. Practice of Pediatrics. New York, Harper & Row, 1980, pp. 1–35.

Thomassen MJ, Boxerbaum B, Demko CA, Kuchenbrod PJ, Dearborn DG, Wood RE. Inhibitory effect of cystic fibrosis serum on *Pseudomonas* phagocytosis by rabbit and human alveolar macrophages. Pediatr Res 13:1085–1088, 1979.

Thomassen MJ, Demko CA, Wood RE, Tandler B, Dearborn DG, Boxerbaum B, Kuchenbrod PJ. Ultrastructure and function of alveolar macrophages from cystic fibrosis patients. Pediatr Res 14:715–721, 1980.

Thomassen MJ, Demko CA, Klinger JD, Stern RC. *Pseudomonas cepacia* colonization among patients with cystic fibrosis. Am Rev Respir Dis 131:791–796, 1985.

Tizzano EF, Buchwald M. Cystic fibrosis: beyond the gene to therapy. J Pediatr 120:337–349, 1992.

Tobin MJ, Maguire O, Reen D, Tempany E, Fitzgerald MX. Atopy and bronchial reactivity in older patients with cystic fibrosis. Thorax 35:807–813, 1980.

Tomashefski JF, Abramowsky CR, Chung-Park M, Wisniewska J, Bruce MC. Immunofluorescence studies of lung tissue in cystic fibrosis. Pediatr Pathol 12:313–324, 1992.

Trezise AEO, Buchwald M. In vivo cell-specific expression of the cystic fibrosis transmembrane conductance regulator. Nature 353:434–437, 1991.

Tsui L-C. The cystic fibrosis transmembrane conductance regulator gene. Am J Respir Crit Care Med 151:S47–S53, 1995.

Turner KJ, O'Mahony J, Wetherall JD, Elder J. Hypersensitivity studies in asthmatic patients with bronchopulmonary aspergillosis. Clin Allergy 2:361–372, 1972.

Turner-Warwick M. Immunological aspects of systemic diseases of the lungs. Proc R Soc Med 67:541–547, 1974.

Turner-Warwick M. The lung in systemic diseases. In Bienenstock J, ed. Immunology of the Lung and Upper Respiratory Tract. New York, McGraw-Hill, 1984, pp. 386–396.

Turner-Warwick ME, Haslam PL. Clinical applications of bronchoalveolar lavage: an interim view. Br J Dis Chest 80:105–121, 1986.

Valassi-Adam H, Rouska A, Karpouzas J, Matsaniotis N. Raised IgA in idiopathic pulmonary hemosiderosis. Arch Dis Child 50:320–322, 1975.

Van Wye JE, Collins MS, Baylor M, Pennington JE, Hsu Y, Sampanvejsopa V, Moss RB. *Pseudomonas* hyperimmune globulin passive immunotherapy for pulmonary exacerbations in cystic fibrosis. Pediatr Pulmonol 9:7–18, 1990.

Wagener JS, Taussig LM, DeBenedetti C, Lemen RJ, Loughlin GM. Pulmonary function in juvenile rheumatoid arthritis. J Pediatr 99:108–110, 1981.

Waller RL, Brattin WJ, Dearborn DG. Cytosolic free calcium concentration and intracellular calcium distribution in lymphocytes from cystic fibrosis patients. Life Sci 35:775–781, 1984.

Wallwork JC, Brenchley P, McCarthy J, Allan JD, Moss D, Ward AM, Hozel A, Williams RF, McFarlane H. Some aspects of immunity in patients with cystic fibrosis. Clin Exp Immunol 18:303–320, 1974.

Wallwork JC, MacFarlane H. The SIgA system and hypersensitivity in patients with cystic fibrosis. Clin Allergy 6:349–358, 1976.

Walravens PA, Chase HP. The prognosis of childhood systemic lupus erythematosus. Am J Dis Child 130:929–933, 1976.

Wang JLF, Patterson R, Mintzer R, Roberts M, Rosenberg M. Allergic bronchopulmonary aspergillosis in pediatric practice. J Pediatr 94:376–381, 1979a.

Wang JLF, Patterson R, Roberts M, Ghory AC. The management of allergic bronchopulmonary aspergillosis. Am Rev Respir Dis 120:87–92, 1979b.

Warner JO, Taylor BW, Norman AP, Soothill JF. Association of cystic fibrosis with allergy. Arch Dis Child 51:507–511, 1976.

Warren CPW, Tai E, Batten JC, Hutchcroft BJ, Pepys J. Cystic fibrosis—immunological reactions to *A. fumigatus* and common allergens. Clin Allergy 5:1–12, 1975.

Warwick WJ, Hansen LG. The long-term effect of high-frequency chest compression therapy on pulmonary complications of cystic fibrosis. Pediatr Pulmonol 11:265–271, 1991.

Watters LC. Genetic aspects of idiopathic pulmonary fibrosis and hypersensitivity pneumonitis. Semin Respir Med 7:317–325, 1986.

Weese WC, Levine BW, Kazemi H. Interstitial lung disease resistant to corticosteroid therapy. Report of three cases treated with azathioprine and cyclophosphamide. Chest 67:57–60, 1975.

Weiner-Kronish JP, Solinger AM, Warnock ML, Churg A, Ordonez N, Golden JA. Severe pulmonary involvement in mixed connective tissue disease. Am Rev Respir Dis 124:499–503, 1981.

Weller PF. Eosinophilia. J Allergy Clin Immunol 73:1–10, 1984.

Wenzel FJ, Emanuel DA, Gray RL. Immunofluorescent studies in patients with farmer's lung. J Allergy Clin Immunol 48:224–229, 1971.

Whaley K. Biosynthesis of complement components and the regulatory protein of the alternative complement pathway by human peripheral blood monocytes. J Exp Med 151:501–516, 1980.

Wheeler B, Williams M, Matthews W, Colten H. Progression of cystic fibrosis lung disease as a function of serum immunoglobulin G levels: a 5-yr longitudinal study. J Pediatr 104:695–699, 1984.

Willoughby WF, Willoughby JB. Immunologic mechanisms of lung injury. Environ Health Perspect Monograph on Pulmonary Toxicology 55:239–258, 1984.

Wilmot RW. The relationship between atopy and cystic fibrosis. In Moss RB, ed. Clinical Reviews in Allergy, Vol. 9, Cystic Fibrosis. Clifton, NJ, Humana Press, 1991, pp. 29–46.

Winnie GB, Cowan RG, Wade NA. Intravenous immune globulin treatment of pulmonary exacerbations in cystic fibrosis. J Pediatr 114:309–314, 1989.

Wolfe CA, Hunninghake GW. Vasculitides of the polyarteritis nodosa group. In Lynch JP, DeRemee RA, eds. Immunologically Mediated Pulmonary Diseases. Philadelphia, JB Lippincott, 1991, pp. 234–249.

Wood RE, Pennington JE, Reynolds HY. Intranasal administration of a pseudomonas lipopolysaccharide vaccine in cystic fibrosis patients. Pediatr Infect Dis 2:367–369, 1983.

Wood RE, Wanner A, Hirsch J, Farrell PM. Tracheal mucociliary transport in patients with cystic fibrosis and its stimulation by terbutaline. Am Rev Respir Dis 111:733–738, 1975.

Yoshimura K, Nakamura H, Trapnell BC, Dalemans W, Pavirani A, Lecocq J-P, Crystal RG. The cystic fibrosis gene has a "housekeeping"-type promoter and is expressed at low levels in cells of epithelial origin. J Biol Chem 266:9140–9144, 1991.

Zach MS, Oberwaldner B, Forch G, Polgar G. Bronchodilators increase airway instability in cystic fibrosis. Am Rev Respir Dis 131:537–543, 1985.

Zambie MF, Gupta S, Lemen RJ, Hilman B, Waring WW, Sly RM. Relationship between response to exercise and allergy in patients with cystic fibrosis. Ann Allergy 42:290–294, 1979.

Zapetal A, Houštěk J, Sămánek M, Čopová M, Paul T. Lung function in children and adolescents with idiopathic interstitial pulmonary fibrosis. Pediatr Pulmonol 1:154–166, 1985.

Zimmerman BL, Haller JO, Price AP, Thelmo WL, Fikrig S. Children with AIDS—Is pathologic diagnosis possible based on chest radiographs? Pediatr Radiol 17:303–307, 1987.

Chapter 23

Gastroenterologic and Liver Disorders

Athos Bousvaros and W. Allan Walker

In the past decade, the study of immune responses at epithelial surfaces (mucosal immunology) has emerged as a separate subdiscipline within the broad field of immunology. In the years since the previous edition of this book, scientists have developed increased understanding of the homing of lymphocytes to the gut, the development of oral tolerance, the mechanisms of immunoglobulin A production and secretion, the role of the epithelial cell in immunoregulation, and the ontogeny of the human mucosal immune system. In addition, two previously unrecognized pediatric diseases (autoimmune enteropathy and type II autoimmune chronic active hepatitis) have been identified.

This chapter first briefly discusses the physiology and development of the mucosal immune system, with emphasis on macromolecular transport, immunoglobulin

A synthesis, and the role of nutrition in immunity. For a more detailed review of mucosal immunity, see Chapter 8. The second part reviews gastrointestinal diseases in which immunologic factors play a significant etiologic role (Fig. 23–1).

IMMUNOPHYSIOLOGY OF THE MUCOSAL IMMUNE SYSTEM

Structure of Gut-Associated Lymphoid Tissue

The intestine is challenged with antigenic proteins every day in the form of foods and orally ingested viruses and bacteria. Despite this, clinically significant intestinal inflammation rarely occurs. The intestinal mucosal immune system is able to mount an *immune response* to potentially harmful pathogens and also induce mucosal and systemic *tolerance* to normal bacterial

Dr. Bousvaros' research was supported in part by National Institutes of Health Cap award 2M01 RR 02172.

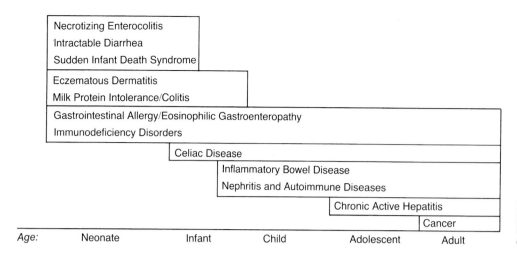

Figure 23–1. Clinical disorders possibly associated with pathologic macromolecular uptake according to age of clinical onset.

flora and food antigens. The gut epithelium and mucosal lymphoid cells constitute a first line of defense against infection and penetration of potentially harmful macromolecules into the systemic circulation (Sanderson and Walker, 1993). The population of lymphoid and other immune cells in the intestine is frequently termed gut-associated lymphoid tissue (GALT); increasingly, the term mucosa-associated lymphoid tissue (MALT) is used to emphasize the interplay between lymphocytes of the gut and other mucosal sites (including respiratory, urinary, and reproductive epithelia) (Kraehenbuhl and Neutra, 1992).

The gut immune system can be arbitrarily divided into two portions (Fig. 23–2). The organized mucosa-associated lymphoid tissue (O-MALT, also called the afferent limb of the mucosal immune system) consists of the dome (follicle-associated) epithelium, Peyer's patches, and mesenteric lymph nodes. Solitary lymphoid aggregates may be seen in the duodenum and jejunum in the human, but Peyer's patches (large groups of lymphoid nodules) are seen almost exclusively in the ileum. Peyer's patches are normally from 0.6 to 3 mm in diameter and are scattered throughout

the intestinal lamina propria. The dome epithelium overlying the Peyer's patches is characterized by a paucity of goblet cells, less intestinal mucin, and the presence of modified epithelial cells (microfold or M cells) that are specialized for antigen uptake (Pabst, 1987).

The putative purpose of the dome epithelium is to provide a portal of entry for antigens to be sampled by antigen-presenting cells in the O-MALT, ultimately resulting in activation of B and T cells in the lymphoid follicles and conversion of naive lymphocytes into memory and effector cells (Waksman and Ozer, 1976; Pabst, 1987; Kraehenbuhl and Neutra, 1992). Regulatory "switch" T cells in the O-MALT may promote B-cell synthesis of immunoglobulin (Kawanishi et al., 1983; Strober and Harriman, 1991).

The diffuse mucosa-associated lymphoid tissue (D-MALT, also called the efferent limb of the mucosal immune system) consists of lymphocytes widely distributed throughout the intestinal lamina propria and other mucosal sites (see Fig. 23–2). Components of the D-MALT include plasma cells; helper, suppressor, and cytotoxic T cells; and intestinal intraepithelial lymphocytes. The majority of T lymphocytes in the intestinal lamina propria are of the phenotype $CD4^+CD45RO^+$ or $CD4^+Leu-8^-$ and provide help for immunoglobulin synthesis by B cells (Morimoto et al., 1985; Kanof et al., 1988b). It has been proposed that secretion of interleukin-5 by T lymphocytes in the lamina propria may promote terminal B-cell differentiation into immunoglobulin A (IgA)–producing plasma cells (Matsumoto et al., 1989). Other immune cells in the lamina propria, including eosinophils, macrophages, and neutrophils, are not traditionally included in the cells constituting the D-MALT but are important as effectors and regulators of the mucosal inflammatory response.

Components of Intestinal Host Defense

There is now abundant evidence that antigenic macromolecules penetrate the intestinal surface in quantities of immunologic significance (Walker and Isselbacher, 1974; Weiner, 1988). This section focuses on mechanisms by which such antigens and pathogens are degraded, processed, inactivated, and eliminated from

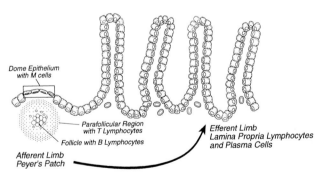

Figure 23–2. Components of intestinal host defense. The afferent limb of the mucosal immune system (left side of figure) samples antigen through modified epithelial cells (M cells). Antigen-presenting cells, "naive" T cells, and B cells within the Peyer's patch sample are activated by antigens taken up by the M cell. In contrast, the efferent limb of the mucosal immune system located in the intestinal lamina propria consists of differentiated "memory" T cells and plasma cells. (From Bousvaros A, Walker WA. Intestinal host defense. In Kirsner J, ed. Inflammatory Bowel Disease, 4th ed. Baltimore, Williams & Wilkins, 1995, pp. 140–161.)

the gut before they enter the systemic circulation. Because immunoglobulin A is the principal mucosal antibody (with over 3 g/d secreted by the human adult intestine), its function is discussed in detail. In addition, because the human responds to most ingested antigens with systemic tolerance, mechanisms of oral tolerance are discussed. Currently recognized components of intestinal host defense are summarized in Figure 23–1 and Table 23–1.

Nonimmunologic Defenses

These defenses prevent antigen penetration into the systemic circulation by either enzymatic degradation of proteins, intestinal transport out of the lumen, or physical blockage of antigen. *Gastric acid* results in a stomach pH cytotoxic to many bacteria and facilitates digestion of proteins by pepsin. Individuals with decreased gastric acid (as a result of medical or surgical reduction of gastric acid output) are more susceptible to gut colonization by pathogenic bacteria (Garvey et al., 1989; Sarker and Gyr, 1992). *Pancreatic secretions,* including proteases, amylase, lipase, and bicarbonate, break down macromolecules and may also have antimicrobial properties (Saffran et al., 1979; Mett et al., 1984). *Intestinal peristalsis* (particularly the spontaneous peristalsis termed the migrating motor complex) is important in transporting bacteria out of the bowel, and bacterial overgrowth is common in patients with aperistaltic intestinal ''blind loops'' or bowel obstruction (Kirsch, 1990; Sarker and Gyr, 1992). The *normal bacterial flora* prevents gut colonization by pathogenic bacteria (e.g., *Clostridium difficile*) and fungi (e.g., *Candida*) through two mechanisms: consumption of intraluminal nutrients and production of volatile fatty acids that inhibit growth of pathogenic bacteria (Hentges, 1986; Tazume et al., 1993).

Physical blockage of antigen passage into the body is prevented by the intestinal mucin layer and the epithelial cell surface barrier. *Intestinal mucins* are highly

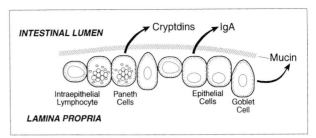

Figure 23–3. The gut epithelium in intestinal host defense. A physical barrier is formed by the enterocytes and their tight junctions that prevents antigen passage into the systemic circulation. In addition, products secreted by the cells of the gut epithelium (including secretory immunoglobulin A transported by the enterocyte, cryptdins synthesized by the Paneth cell, and mucin synthesized by the goblet cell) can prevent invasion by antigens or microbes. (From Bousvaros A, Walker WA. Intestinal host defense. In Kirsner J, ed. Inflammatory Bowel Disease, 4th ed. Baltimore, Williams & Wilkins, 1995, pp. 140–161.)

glycosylated molecules of high molecular weight and consist of a core protein (apomucin) joined to oligosaccharides (including fucose, N-acetylglucosamine, and N-acetylgalactosamine). Cloning of apomucin genes demonstrates homology between bronchial and intestinal mucins, emphasizing again the presence of a common mucosal immune system (Jany et al., 1991; Kim et al., 1991). Intestinal mucin protects the intestine by multiple mechanisms. First, mucin forms a viscoelastic layer over the intestinal epithelium, serving as a physical barrier to proteins and pathogens. Second, glycoproteins on the mucous coat may preferentially bind pathogenic bacteria, thus competitively inhibiting binding of such bacteria to epithelial cells. Lastly, mucin may increase antibody concentration over the epithelial cell layer by acting as a matrix to which secretory immunoglobulins can bind (Snyder and Walker, 1987).

The *intestinal epithelial barrier* is composed principally of five types of cells: enterocytes, goblet cells, intraepithelial lymphocytes, Paneth cells, and neuroendocrine cells (Fig. 23–3) (Pabst, 1987). The enterocytes, joined together by a network of tight junctions, limit antigen passage across the intestine but under certain conditions may take up proteins and present antigenic peptides to T lymphocytes (Bland and Kambarage, 1991). Studies of animals also suggest that during intestinal inflammation, enterocytes can produce cytokines that modulate mucosal immune function (Radema et al., 1991). Other components of the epithelial cell barrier are also important in preventing infection: goblet cells secrete mucins, and Paneth cells secrete the antimicrobial proteins cryptdins and lysozyme (Selsted et al., 1992). Intraepithelial lymphocytes (IELs) are predominantly CD8 cells, and investigators have shown that they may kill virally infected epithelial cells or suppress immune responses in vitro (Ebert, 1990; Cerf-Bensussan and Guy-Grand, 1991; Hoang et al., 1991; Sachdev et al., 1993).

Macromolecular Transport Mechanisms

Four mechanisms have been proposed to account for macromolecular transport across the intact epithelial

Table 23–1. Factors Preventing Antigen Transport from the Gut

Nonimmunologic Factors	
Luminal	*Mucosal*
Gastric acid secretion	Intestinal mucin
Intestinal proteolysis	Epithelial cell maturity
Bile acids	
Early enteral nutrition	
Intestinal flora	
Intestinal motility	

Immunologic Factors		
Mucosal	*Passive Defense*	*Hepatic*
Secretory IgA	Transplacental IgG	Reticuloendothelial cells
Other immunoglobulins (IgG, IgM, and IgE)	Breast milk factors (immune/hormonal)	Immune-complex (IgA) clearance
Cell-mediated immunity		Immune modulation

Table 23–2. Macromolecular Transport Mechanisms

1. Receptor-mediated endocytosis
2. Nonselective endocytosis
3. Direct penetration of cell membrane
4. Passage across tight junctions

cell barrier (Table 23–2) (Gonnella and Walker, 1987; Weiner, 1988; Sanderson and Walker, 1993).

Receptor-Mediated Endocytosis

This refers to the process initiated by the interaction between an intraluminal macromolecule (ligand) and a specific receptor to which it binds on the enterocyte plasma membrane (Fig. 23–4A). The binding stimulates the clustering of additional receptors in a clathrin-coated pit area of the cell, with invagination and internalization of the coated pit, forming a vesicle. Depending on intracellular trafficking, the vesicle and its contents may be either expelled intact from the basolateral membrane of the enterocyte or intracellularly degraded by a lysosome (Walker and Isselbacher, 1974).

Receptor-mediated endocytosis is particularly important in the developing animal for uptake of growth factors and antibodies from breast milk. Suckling rodents absorb immunoglobulin G (IgG) in maternal breast milk through Fc receptors located on enterocytes (Rodewald, 1970); a similar receptor has been isolated from fetal human intestine (Israel et al., 1993). Nerve growth factor and epidermal growth factor (EGF) can also cross the developing epithelium, and specific receptors for EGF have been identified on enterocytes (Siminoski et al., 1986; Thompson, 1988; Sanderson and Walker, 1993). Therefore, intestinal uptake of trophic factors and antibodies by the suckling rodent and possibly the human fetus may promote intestinal growth and differentiation.

Nonselective Endocytosis

In a second mechanism of macromolecular transport, extracellular macromolecules are nonselectively trapped and internalized through invaginations of noncoated regions of cells (Fig. 23–4B). Such a mechanism has been postulated for preferential uptake of macromolecules by microfold cells (M cells). These cells preferentially take up proteins, viruses, and bacteria in the dome epithelium above Peyer's patches (Table 23–3); although pathogens preferentially adhere to M cells, specific receptors for pathogens on the M cell have not yet been identified (Wolf and Bye, 1984). An interaction between a lectin or other adhesion molecule on the surface of the M cell and a corresponding ligand on the viral or bacterial surface may in fact account for this "nonselective endocytosis" (Amerongen et al., 1992). In addition, intraluminal immunoglobulins seem to preferentially adhere to M cells, even though M cells lack Fc receptors (Weltzin et al., 1989).

Direct Penetration

A third means of entry is direct penetration through the epithelial cell membrane. This mechanism may be important for certain bacterial and plant toxins, but its physiologic significance is poorly understood (Goldstein et al., 1979).

Passage Across Tight Junctions (Paracellular Pathway)

In the healthy human, only low-molecular-weight molecules can pass across the tight junction between enterocytes. However, passage of larger macromolecules across the gut has been observed in those with

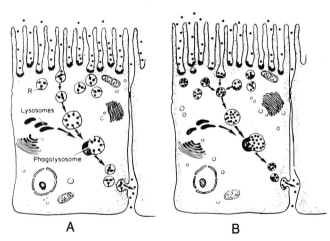

Figure 23–4. Mechanisms of macromolecular absorption in the neonatal mammalian intestine.

A, Selective transport of antigens occurs in the small intestine of the newborn via a specific receptor site (R) present on the microvillus membrane. Antigens thus transported may be protected from intracellular lysosomal digestion because of attachment to the receptor site and would thus be transported in increased quantities out of the cell.

B, A nonselective uptake and transport of other macromolecules occurs throughout the small intestine of most neonatal animals. Immature intestinal absorptive cells engulf large quantities of macromolecules. After intracellular digestion in phagolysosomes, very small quantities are deposited in the intercellular space.

(From Walker WA, Isselbacher KJ. Uptake and transport of macromolecules by the intestine: possible role in clinical disorders. Gastroenterology 67:531–550, 1974.)

Table 23–3. Microorganisms and Nonliving Particles Adherent to M-Cell Apical Membranes

Bacteria	Protozoa
Vibrio cholerae	*Cryptosporidium*
Salmonella typhi	
Yersinia enterocolitica	Nonliving particles
BCG	Carbon particles
Campylobacter jejuni	Latex beads
Shigella flexneri	Copolymer microspheres
RDEC-1 strain of *Escherichia coli*	Hydroxyapatite
Viruses	
Reovirus	
Poliovirus	
HIV-1	

Abbreviations: BCG = bacille Calmette-Guérin; HIV-1 = human immunodeficiency virus type 1.

From Amerongen MH, Weltzin RW, Mack JA, Winner LS, Michetti P, Apter FM, Kraehenbuhl JP, Neutra MR. M cell–mediated antigen transport and monoclonal IgA antibodies for mucosal immune protection. Ann NY Acad Sci 664:18–26, 1992.

intestinal inflammation (including patients with celiac disease, inflammatory bowel disease, and infectious enteritis), suggesting that inflammation may "loosen" the tight junctions (Turck et al., 1987; Hollander, 1992). Investigators have proposed that relatives of patients with inflammatory bowel disease (IBD) may be predisposed to the development of intestinal inflammation because they have increased intestinal permeability to antigens via the paracellular pathway (May et al., 1993).

Antigen Processing and Immunoglobulin Synthesis

Antigens that have penetrated the intestinal epithelium may provoke an immune response (usually characterized by secretory IgA production) or a state of systemic unresponsiveness (tolerance) to antigen. The immunoregulatory mechanisms and cellular interactions within the Peyer's patch have not yet been elucidated. For an antibody response to antigen to occur, naive B cells within the Peyer's patch must differentiate, proliferate, and migrate into the lamina propria, where they become immunoglobulin-producing plasma cells (Fig. 23–5). Signals promoting B-cell activation and differentiation include antigen binding to surface immunoglobulins on the B-cell membrane and soluble cytokines (particularly interleukin-4 and interleukin-5) secreted by helper T cells (Fig. 23–6) (Abbas, 1988).

Helper (CD4) T cells do not recognize antigen directly but do recognize peptide fragments on the surface of antigen-presenting cells (APCs). CD4 cells recognize antigenic peptide in association with major histocompatibility complex (MHC) class II molecules via the T-cell receptor (see Fig. 23–6) (Grey et al., 1989). Macrophages, dendritic cells, and B cells all express surface MHC class II molecules and represent the "professional" antigen-presenting cells within the Peyer's patch. Enterocytes also express MHC class II molecules on their cell surface, particularly during intestinal inflammation, and can present antigen to T lymphocytes in vitro. Some investigators propose that this pathway of antigen presentation is important in the pathogenesis of mucosal inflammation, but its true significance has not been clarified (Bland and Kambarage, 1991). Allan and colleagues (1993) demonstrated that MHC class II molecules are present on M cells in the rat and suggested that M cells can also function as antigen-presenting cells.

The principal immunoglobulin produced by the mucosal immune system is secretory IgA; the plasma cell ratio of IgA-, IgM-, and IgG-producing cells is 20:3:1, almost the reverse of that in the systemic immune system (Brandtzaeg and Baklien, 1977). B cells stimulated in the Peyer's patches undergo isotype switching to IgA, resulting in the preponderance of mucosal IgA-producing plasma cells. The factors controlling isotype switching probably include cell-cell contact (particularly between CD40 on the B-cell surface and gp39, the CD40 ligand on the T-cell surface), antigenic stimulation itself, and secretion of regulatory "switch factor

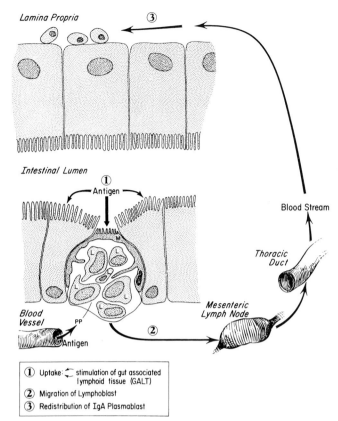

Figure 23–5. Schematic representation of antigen response of lymphoid tissue located in gut-associated lymphoid tissue (GALT) and of homing of stimulated lymphoid cells to intestinal mucosa.

1, Antigen is taken up by M cells and, to a lesser degree, by intestinal epithelial cells. This leads to stimulation of cells within the lymphoepithelial complex and within diffuse lymphoid tissue.

2, After antigen stimulation, cells migrate to mesenteric lymph nodes, where they are "processed" and become lymphoblasts. These lymphoblasts migrate through thoracic duct to systemic circulation, where they "mature."

3, Lymphocytes then "home" to diffuse lymphoid tissue of the gut, lung, breast, and female reproductive tract.

(From Walker WA, Isselbacher KJ. Intestinal antibodies. N Engl J Med 297:767–773, 1977.)

cytokines" (Strober and Harriman, 1991; Fuleihan et al., 1993).

Mucosally secreted immunoglobulin A differs from systemic IgA in several aspects. First, whereas systemic IgA is almost exclusively monomeric IgA of the IgA1 subtype, secretory IgA is a dimer (Conley and Delacroix, 1987). Second, secretory IgA (sIgA) is synthesized from both IgA1 and IgA2; the IgA2 present in sIgA may be more resistant to degradation by bacterial proteases (Meyer et al., 1987). The IgA dimer is synthesized within the plasma cell by coupling the constant regions of two IgA molecules to a linking peptide termed J chain. The J chain–IgA dimer is secreted by lamina propria plasma cells and binds to the polymeric immunoglobulin receptor (also called secretory component or SC) on the basolateral surface of the enterocyte. The IgA dimer–J chain–SC complex is internalized by the enterocyte and secreted into the intestinal lumen (Ahnen et al., 1985). The cytokines interleukin-4 and interferon-γ regulate SC expression by the entero-

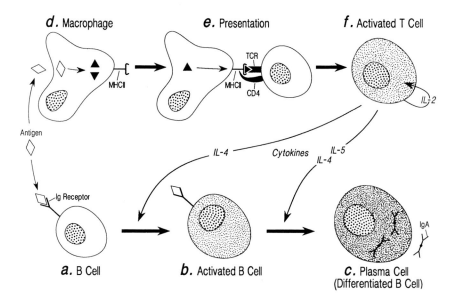

Figure 23–6. Antigen processing in Peyer's patch. Antigen may bind directly to immunoglobulin on the surface of the B cell or may be endocytosed by an antigen-presenting cell (for example, a macrophage) and presented to a helper T cell. The antigen presented to the macrophage is located within a cleft in the MHC class II molecule of the macrophage and is bound by the T-cell receptor of the CD4 T cell. The helper T cell then secretes cytokines that promote B-cell differentiation. (From Bousvaros A, Walker WA. Basic gastrointestinal immunity. In Bouchier IA, et al., eds. Gastroenterology: Clinical Science and Practice, 2nd ed. Philadelphia, WB Saunders, 1993, pp. 577–582.)

cyte and hence may regulate luminal IgA secretion (Philips et al., 1990). Studies of animal models have shown that antigen-specific secretory IgA has potent antimicrobial activity against enteric bacteria and viruses, including *Vibrio cholerae, Salmonella typhimurium,* reovirus, and retroviruses (Kraehenbuhl and Neutra, 1992).

In addition to producing secretory IgA in the same region as the initial antigenic challenge (i.e., the gut), antigen-stimulated B lymphocytes travel through the mesenteric lymph nodes, thoracic duct, and systemic circulation to other mucosal sites (including bronchi, salivary glands, uterus, biliary tree, and mammary gland), as well as returning to the gut (see Fig. 23–5) (Husband and Gowans, 1977). These migratory B cells may therefore serve to transfer immunologic memory from one mucosal site to another, and antigen-specific IgA produced by these B cells can be complexed to secretory component at other epithelial sites and transported into other secretions. Kleinman and Walker (1979) postulated an "enteromammary immune system" in which B cells form IgA to pathogens in the mother's gut and migrate to the mammary gland, where antigen-specific IgA is secreted in breast milk and transferred to the infant (Fig. 23–7).

The Liver: A Second Line of Defense

If an antigen penetrates the gut epithelium and enters the portal circulation, it must pass through the hepatic sinusoids before entering the systemic circulation. The liver Kupffer cells, members of the tissue macrophage family, can phagocytose bacteria, antigens, immune complexes, and tumor cells that have bypassed the intestinal host defenses and entered the portal circulation. Although Kupffer cells do not usually possess specific receptors for bacterial glycoproteins, Kupffer cells can bind fibronectin, the C3b component of complement, and the Fc components of IgG and IgA. These molecules in turn can opsonize bacteria (including Enterobacteriaceae and streptococci) or bind to food antigens in the intestinal lumen, mucosa, or portal circulation. Therefore, antigen-antibody complexes and opsonin-coated bacteria generated in the intestine may be bound through specific Kupffer cell receptors and digested by Kupffer cell lysosomes (Toth and Thomas, 1992). Rodent bile contains high concentrations of secretory immunoglobulin A, but biliary IgA is of little functional importance in the human (Kleinman, 1987).

Oral Tolerance

Whereas orally ingested food antigens can generate a mucosal immune response (e.g., secretory IgA production), a more common systemic response to oral antigen is one of immunologic hyporesponsiveness, or tolerance (see Chapter 8). Tolerance is defined as an antigen-specific inactivation of lymphocytes resulting in the absence of an immune response. An animal exposed to a tolerance-inducing antigen (tolerogen) will not respond to a more immunogenic form of the antigen given systemically.

Two major mechanisms by which tolerance develops have been proposed: (1) clonal deletion or anergy and (2) suppressor cell activation. With clonal deletion and anergy, interaction of the tolerogen with a B or helper T lymphocyte results in death or unresponsiveness of the regulatory cells that promote the proinflammatory response. Clonal anergy usually occurs in helper T cells but may also occur in B cells. The end result is an absence of immunoglobulin-producing cells directed against that specific antigen (Mowat, 1987b; Melamed and Friedman, 1993).

In contrast, suppressor cell activation occurs when antigen processing in the Peyer's patch generates T lymphocytes, which inhibit B cell antibody production; CD8 suppressor T lymphocytes are probably the most important cellular mediators of oral tolerance (Ishii et al., 1993). The generation of suppressor T cells mediating oral tolerance can be abrogated by the administra-

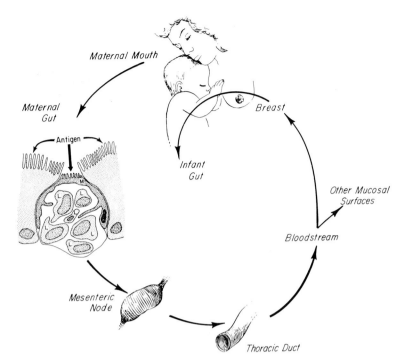

Figure 23–7. Dietary antigen entering the maternal gut reaches lymphoid follicles through specialized transport cells (M cells). This antigen commits the lymphoblasts to production of specific IgAs, and these then migrate via the mesenteric nodes and thoracic duct into the systemic circulation. During the periods of proper hormonal stimulation, such cells populate the breast and secrete sIgA, which then is ingested by and functions in the infant. T cells, B cells, and macrophages are also extruded into the breast milk and are immunologically active. sIgA = secretory immunoglobulin A. (From Kleinman RE, Walker WA. The enteromammary immune system: an important new concept in breast milk host defense. Dig Dis Sci 24:876–882, 1979.)

tion of immunosuppressive agents such as cyclophosphamide (Hoyne et al., 1993).

Studies of oral tolerance are largely confined to animal models, but the induction of systemic tolerance by oral feeding of antigen offers promise in the therapy of human autoimmune disease. In mice, orally administered ovalbumin can generate tolerance to intravenous ovalbumin given as early as 1 hour after the oral immunization; this tolerance is in part dependent on the MHC haplotype of the mouse and can be transferred among syngeneic mice by injecting serum from the orally immunized mouse into an unimmunized mouse (Mowat et al., 1987).

A hypothesis based on these data is that intestinal antigen-processing cells (e.g., macrophages) modify an immunogenic protein (e.g., ovalbumin) into a "tolerogenic" protein that preferentially activates T-suppressor cells in the systemic immune system (Peng et al., 1990). Work by Weiner's group suggests that orally fed myelin basic protein can prevent the development of experimental allergic encephalomyelitis in rats and that tolerance is mediated through the production of immunosuppressive cytokines, including transforming growth factor–beta (Khoury et al., 1992). Similar work suggests that adjuvant arthritis in chickens can be prevented by oral feeding of collagen molecules (Zhang et al., 1990). Treatments utilizing oral tolerance may therefore be of future therapeutic benefit in human diseases such as multiple sclerosis.

Nutrition and Immunity

Enteral nutrition is important in the development of the neonatal mucosal immune system and is essential in the maintenance of systemic and mucosal immunity in the adult. Malnourished children and adults have impaired cell-mediated immunity and increased sus-

ceptibility to infections (Keusch, 1986; Wan et al., 1989) (see Chapter 19). Properties of enteral nutrition that influence immunity are summarized in Table 23–4. These include stimulation of the mucosal immune system through antigen, provision of trophic factors important in mucosal integrity, transfer of passive immunity through breast milk, and provision of micronutrients important in lymphocyte function (Ferguson, 1994; Sanderson and Walker, 1991).

In rodents and humans, feeding may stimulate the maturation of the secretory IgA system. Although T and B lymphocytes are present in the human fetal intestinal mucosa as early as 16 to 18 weeks of gestation, the intestinal mucosa of the term neonate con-

Table 23–4. Nutritional Factors Influencing Immunity

1. Protein antigenic stimulation of mucosal B cells
2. Trophic factors
    Nucleotides
    Glutamine
    Epidermal growth factor
    Nerve growth factor
3. Passive immunity from breast milk
    Lactoferrin
    Lysozyme
    Secretory immunoglobulins (principally secretory
      immunoglobulin A)
    Lipases
    Glycoproteins
    Leukocytes
4. Micronutrients
    Zinc
    Copper
    Iron
    Selenium
    Vitamins

From Sanderson IR, Walker WA. Nutrition and immunity. Curr Opin Gastroenterol 7:463–470, 1991; Slade HB, Schwartz SA. Mucosal immunity: the immunology of breast milk. J Allergy Clin Immunol 80:346–356, 1987.

tains no IgA-producing plasma cells before 10 days of age (Perkkio and Savilahti, 1980). Both cow's milk protein and protein hydrolysate feeding stimulate IgA plasma cell growth in neonatal mice, but the intact protein stimulates plasma cell development to a greater extent (Sagie et al., 1974). Knox (1986) noted that 2-week-old human infants given enteral feedings had IgA and IgM plasma cells in the intestinal lamina propria, whereas infants not yet fed had a paucity of these cells. Thus, dietary antigenic stimulation may be important in promoting mucosal immune maturation.

Trophic factors present in breast milk include epidermal growth factor and nerve growth factor; as stated previously, the neonatal rodent intestine contains specific receptors to transport these substances to the systemic circulation. Other critical trophic substances include dietary nucleotides and the amino acid glutamine (Grimble, 1994). Nunez and colleagues (1990) demonstrated the partial efficacy of nucleotides in promoting epithelial repair in the damaged gut of rodents. Glutamine and nucleotides given to animals receiving total parenteral nutrition increase intestinal villous height, although they do not decrease gut permeability to bacteria (Ogoshi et al., 1985; Deitch, 1994).

Breast milk contains nutrients, growth factors, proteins with antimicrobial properties (including lactoferrin and lysozyme), immunoglobulins (predominantly IgA in the human and IgG in the rodent), and intact leukocytes (including neutrophils, macrophages, and lymphocytes) (Slade and Schwartz, 1987) (see Chapter 8). Trophic factors present in breast milk stimulate the maturation of intestinal epithelial function (Widdowson et al., 1976; Heird and Hansen, 1977) and may decrease intestinal permeability to macromolecules (Weaver et al., 1987).

Studies of women immunized with poliovirus support the hypothesis of an enteromammary immune system by demonstrating that virus-specific IgA can be transferred into breast milk (Svennerholm et al., 1981). Prentice and coworkers (1989) measured fecal IgA and lactoferrin in breast-fed and bottle-fed Gambian children and found 10-fold higher levels in the stools of breast-fed children; they estimated that one third of ingested immunoglobulin escapes digestion. Therefore, ingested IgA from breast milk potentially confers intraluminal antimicrobial activity to the entire small bowel and colon.

Specific micronutrients present in enteral nutrition may also promote mucosal immunity. Various studies suggest beneficial effects on immune function from the addition of vitamin A, vitamin E, copper, selenium, iron, and zinc to the diet (Meydani, 1990; Sanderson and Walker, 1991). Infants with primary acrodermatitis enteropathica (AE), an autosomal recessive defect in intestinal zinc absorption, have an increased susceptibility to infection that is correctable with zinc supplementation.

Summary

The control of macromolecular uptake is dependent on a number of factors within the gut lumen, the mucosal surface, and the intestinal lamina propria. The neonate's intestine may allow increased macromolecular uptake because of decreased gastric acid production, pancreatic function, or epithelial barrier integrity. Nutrition, particularly with mammalian breast milk, confers both antigenic stimulation of the intestine and passive immunity. Immunologic tolerance is essential in the prevention of systemic or mucosal immune responses to dietary antigens, but the cellular and molecular mechanisms resulting in tolerance are just beginning to be unraveled. Disturbances in the permeability of the immature, malnourished, or damaged gut may cause intestinal or systemic disease states as described in the following text.

ALLERGIC AND INFLAMMATORY CONDITIONS OF THE BOWEL

Necrotizing Enterocolitis

Necrotizing enterocolitis (NEC) is an acute fulminating disease of neonates associated with focal or diffuse ulceration of the distal small intestine and colon, often leading to bowel necrosis or perforation (Santulli et al., 1975). The most common acquired gastrointestinal emergency in the newborn, NEC appears to be a common pathologic response of the immature intestine to many injurious factors. It is primarily a disease of premature infants, occurring in approximately 10% of neonates weighing under 1500 g. However, 5% to 10% of cases occur in term infants or infants who have not been fed (MacKendrick and Caplan, 1993).

Pathogenesis

The pathophysiology of necrotizing enterocolitis remains a mystery. A number of factors (including hypoxia/ischemia, hyperosmolar feedings, and intraluminal bacteria) may damage the comparatively immature intestinal barrier of the premature infant. These multiple insults result in epithelial disruption and permeability to potentially pathogenic bacteria, resulting in a vicious circle leading to gut necrosis (Fig. 23–8). Prematurity and enteral feedings are the two risk factors most strongly associated with NEC; delay of enteral feedings in the premature may delay the onset of NEC, but also delays the time of presentation of the disease. Prenatal maternal cocaine use has been identified as a risk factor in term infants, which suggests that the vasoconstrictive properties of cocaine predispose the infant to bowel ischemia (Downing et al., 1991).

Studies of fetal gut blood flow and intestinal maturation in animals provide useful insights into the pathogenesis and potential prevention of necrotizing enterocolitis. To determine whether episodic mesenteric ischemia of the developing neonatal intestine makes the bowel more permeable to potentially toxic macromolecules, Crissinger and Granger (1989) studied the effects of ischemia and reperfusion of the bowel in developing piglets. Piglets 1 to 30 days of age had similar gut permeability to chromium-51–labeled edetic acid (EDTA) (a small molecule) after their bowels had

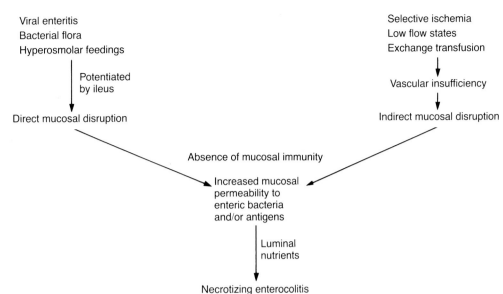

Viral enteritis
Bacterial flora
Hyperosmolar feedings

Selective ischemia
Low flow states
Exchange transfusion

Potentiated
by ileus

Vascular insufficiency

Direct mucosal disruption

Indirect mucosal disruption

Absence of mucosal immunity

Increased mucosal
permeability to
enteric bacteria
and/or antigens

Luminal
nutrients

Necrotizing enterocolitis

Figure 23–8. Proposed pathway for the interaction of multiple factors predisposing to the development of necrotizing enterocolitis. (From Lake AM, Walker WA. Neonatal necrotizing enterocolitis: a disease of altered host defense. Clin Gastroenterol 6:463, 1977.)

been subjected to 1 hour of iatrogenic ischemia. However, feeding of cow's milk–based formula to piglets whose intestines were subjected to ischemia and reperfusion for 1 hour caused significantly greater injury in 1-day-old animals than in older animals. These investigators later demonstrated that the lipid fraction of enteral feed in 1-day-old piglets was responsible for the increased permeability of intestinal mucosa after ischemia and reperfusion (Crissinger and Tso, 1992). Thus, ischemia combined with feeding potentiates intestinal damage by macromolecules in infant pigs, and triglycerides may potentiate the ischemic damage to the neonatal gut.

Microbial agents are responsible for some of the intestinal damage in necrotizing enterocolitis. Epidemics of the disease are frequently reported. The intestinal pneumatosis of NEC is probably due to bacterial fermentation of carbohydrates. Bacterial or viral agents may be isolated from blood or stool of affected infants (Kliegman et al., 1993). Agents commonly reported or isolated from stool or blood include *Klebsiella, Escherichia coli,* rotavirus, *Staphylococcus epidermidis,* and *Clostridium* species (Kliegman and Fanaroff, 1984; Palmer et al., 1989). However, in most cases no specific infectious pathogen is isolated. Furthermore, it is not clear whether the isolated organisms are the primary cause of bowel damage (perhaps through endotoxin production) or are secondary invaders of a damaged gut.

The role of immature host defenses in the pathogenesis of necrotizing enterocolitis requires further study. Several pathogens or toxins require contact with a receptor on the mucosal surface to cause damage; for example, rotavirus may bind to intestinal mucins, and cholera toxin binds to a GM_1 ganglioside on the enterocyte membrane. Diminished degradation or neutralization of these proteins may result in increased binding and intestinal inflammation (Chu and Walker, 1993; Kliegman et al., 1993). The human premature infant has less gastric acid output, less pancreatic enzyme activity, a more permeable gut, and less secretory IgA

than the older infant. Such factors may predispose the neonatal gut to colonization and systemic invasion by viruses or bacteria, with resultant inflammation and sepsis.

Pretreatment of rodent fetuses with either thyroxine or corticosteroids promotes maturation of the gut epithelium, decreases gut permeability, and lessens the occurrence of NEC (Pang et al., 1985; Israel et al., 1987, 1990). Therapeutic attempts to speed gut maturation or to supply exogenous antibody to infants with NEC have met with some success (see later), suggesting that the barrier function of the gut can be augmented pharmacologically.

Inflammatory cytokines may mediate intestinal mucosal damage in necrotizing enterocolitis. Hsueh and coworkers demonstrated that intravenous administration of platelet activating factor (PAF) in a rat model may cause pathologic changes similar to those seen in NEC. The intestinal damage caused by endotoxin may be blocked by platelet activating factor antagonists (Hsueh et al., 1986, 1987). In addition, humans with the disease have significantly higher serum levels of PAF and tumor necrosis factor–alpha (TNF-α) (Kliegman et al., 1993). Although other cytokines are likely to be important in the pathogenesis of NEC, the role of PAF and TNF-α in promoting the disease warrants further investigation.

In summary, although the exact pathogenesis of necrotizing enterocolitis is not known, a combination of bowel immaturity, mesenteric vascular insufficiency, microbial colonization, and early feeding contribute to its development.

Clinical Manifestations

Signs and symptoms of necrotizing enterocolitis are summarized in Table 23–5. The infant with a mild case has mild abdominal distention, vomiting, or hematochezia; the sick infant with NEC has signs consistent with an acute abdomen, bowel perforation, or sepsis. The clinical staging system of Bell and cowork-

Table 23–5. Signs and Symptoms of Necrotizing
Enterocolitis

Mild to Moderate	Severe
Abdominal distention	Peritonitis
Elevated pregavage residuals	Ileus
	Acidosis and hyperkalemia
Vomiting	Hematochezia
Occult blood in stool	Neutropenia and
Temperature instability	thrombocytopenia
Coagulopathy	Portal venous gas
Apnea/bradycardia	Pneumoperitoneum
Abdominal tenderness	
Dilated bowel on radiography	
Pneumatosis intestinalis	

ers(1978), which is still widely used today, utilizes a combination of intestinal and systemic signs plus plain abdominal radiography to grade severity. Necrotizing enterocolitis must be suspected whenever a premature infant exhibits signs of feeding intolerance, regurgitation, apnea, irritability, temperature instability, or hematochezia.

Diagnosis

The diagnosis is then confirmed by a combination of laboratory and radiographic features. A low hematocrit,

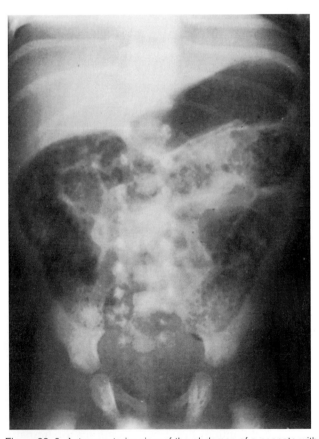

Figure 23–9. Anteroposterior view of the abdomen of a neonate with abdominal distention and vomiting. The radiograph demonstrates areas of intraluminal air (pneumatosis intestinalis) confirming necrotizing enterocolitis. (Courtesy of C. C. Roy, M.D., Montreal, Canada.)

elevated white blood cell count, low platelet count, or elevated prothrombin or partial thromboplastin time may be present. The abdominal radiograph may demonstrate pneumatosis intestinalis, gas in the portal venous system, or frank pneumoperitoneum (Fig. 23–9). The pathologic correlate of these radiographic findings is bowel ischemia with intraluminal gas production by microbes or bowel necrosis with perforation. Necrotizing enterocolitis typically involves the distal ileum and ascending colon, although the entire bowel may be involved (Caplan and MacKendrick, 1993; Kliegman, 1993).

Treatment

The primary treatment for necrotizing enterocolitis is medical and nutritional support, with surgical resection of the bowel reserved for critically ill infants (Table 23–6). Bowel rest up to 3 weeks is recommended for infants with demonstrated (by radiography) NEC and generally necessitates central venous hyperalimentation. Intravenous antibiotics do not cure the bowel disease but may prevent or treat bacteremia and sepsis. Loss of fluid into the bowel may cause oliguria hyponatremia and hypoalbuminemia, and bowel necrosis may cause acidosis and hyperkalemia. To correct these complications, intravenous fluids, albumin, blood, and clotting factors may be required. Infants with clinical or radiographic evidence suggestive of necrotic bowel require laparotomy and bowel resection (Kliegman, 1993).

Prevention

Despite these therapeutic measures, necrotizing enterocolitis is associated with high morbidity and mortality. Thus, efforts to prevent NEC by augmenting intestinal host defenses have been undertaken. Eibl and colleagues (1988) gave premature infants (between 800 and 2000 g) either infant formula alone or formula plus 600 mg of an oral human IgG-IgA preparation. Six cases of NEC occurred in the 91 control infants during refeeding; no cases occurred in the infants receiving oral immunoglobulin. Serum immunoglobulin levels did not differ significantly between the groups, suggesting that the effect of the oral preparation was intraluminal. A similar study showed that oral monomeric IgG can decrease the incidence of the disease in premature infants (Rubaltelli et al., 1991). Enterally administered immunoglobulin could potentially prevent NEC by binding to antigens or microbes intraluminally; such an effect may not occur with donor breast milk because pasteurization may denature antibody.

Another approach to prevention is to accelerate maturation of the infant mucosal barrier by prenatal or postnatal administration of exogenous hormones. Israel and coworkers (1987, 1990) have demonstrated that when either thyroxine or cortisone is injected into pregnant rats, the offspring are less susceptible to ischemic bowel injury and have structurally more mature intestinal mucosal barriers. Oral corticosteroids fed to newborn rats may have a similar effect (Teichberg

Table 23–6. Management of Necrotizing Enterocolitis

Supportive measures
  Nothing by mouth
  Parenteral nutrition
  Antibiotics
  Ventilatory support
  Bicarbonate
  Fresh frozen plasma
  Surgery (if necessary)

Preventive measures
  Oral immunoglobulins A and G
  Prenatal/postnatal corticosteroids
  Thyroxine (in animal models)
  Platelet activating factor antagonist (in animal models)

Data from Caplan MS, MacKendrick WM. Necrotizing enterocolitis: a review of pathogenetic mechanisms and implications for prevention. Pediatr Pathol 13:357–369, 1993; Kliegman RM. Neonatal necrotizing enterocolitis. In Wyllie R, Hyams JS, eds. Gastrointestinal Disease: Pathophysiology, Diagnosis, Management. Philadelphia, WB Saunders, 1993, pp. 788–798.

et al., 1992). A randomized trial of cortisone administration versus placebo administration to 466 premature infants showed that the premature infants receiving cortisone either prenatally or postnatally were less likely to develop necrotizing enterocolitis (Halac et al., 1990).

Food Allergy

Food allergy is an adverse reaction to a food caused by an immunologic reaction to some component of the food (see Chapter 20). Improved diagnostic techniques enable the clinician to distinguish between true food allergy and reaction to food additives, food intolerance, or an erroneous history. The double-blind placebo-controlled food challenge is now the "gold standard" by which the sensitivity and specificity of other diagnostic tests (including skin prick or radioallergosorbent testing) can be measured.

Pathophysiology

At least two types of food allergy are recognized. The first, immediate hypersensitivity, is characterized by clinical symptoms of asthma, urticaria, or anaphylaxis. This is a Gell and Coombs type I hypersensitivity reaction mediated by IgE released when mast cells are degranulated. Although the exact mediators causing food anaphylaxis are not known, Sampson and coworkers (1989) have identified a histamine-releasing factor that interacts with IgE on the mast cell surface to cause degranulation and release of histamine and prostaglandins.

A second type of food allergy is suggestive of a delayed-type hypersensitivity reaction (Gell and Coombs type IV), inasmuch as children develop symptoms 12 to 72 hours after ingestion of offending food. The symptoms differ from those in type I reactions and include vomiting, colitis, abdominal pain, and atopic dermatitis. This form of food allergy may involve antigen presentation to helper T lymphocytes in the intestinal mucosa, with failure of normal immunoregulatory mechanisms to produce systemic tolerance.

Van Sickle and coworkers (1985) demonstrated increased proliferation in response to milk and soy proteins by peripheral blood T lymphocytes from infants with allergic colitis compared with control infants, suggesting in vivo sensitization to these antigens. In other studies, Kondo and colleagues found that lymphocytes of children with atopic dermatitis and egg hypersensitivity cultured with ovalbumin or egg antigens released interferon-γ and interleukin-2 in culture supernatants (Agata et al., 1992; Kondo et al., 1993). Thus, atopic patients have lymphocytes primed to respond to certain food antigens.

Impaired barrier function of the gut may predispose to food hypersensitivity. Children are at highest risk for developing food allergies in the first year of life, when the mucosal barrier may be more permeable to food antigens. Delaying introduction of highly allergenic and prolonged breast feeding may reduce the incidence of food allergy in children with a strong family history of atopy. Viral or bacterial infections may damage gut epithelium and increase intestinal macromolecular absorption and can result in postinfectious allergic enteropathy to cow's milk or soy proteins (Harrison et al., 1976; Schrieber and Walker, 1988).

Clinical Manifestations

The incidence of true food allergy in the pediatric population has been estimated to be 2% to 4%. In contrast, histories of childhood "allergies" are reported by the parents of as many as 28% of children. For this reason, the American Academy of Allergy and Immunology and the National Institutes of Health suggest the following nomenclature (Sampson, 1994). *Adverse food reaction* includes any untoward event that follows ingestion of a food and includes *food intolerance* and *food allergy*. Food intolerance can include food poisoning (secondary to bacterial toxins), pharmacologic effects (such as reflux or arrhythmias secondary to caffeine), enzymatic deficiencies (including galactosemia or hypolactasia), or unknown reactions. Food allergies, in contrast, are thought to be true systemic or mucosal immune responses to ingested food antigens and include type I or type IV hypersensitivity reactions. Foods best known to cause these reactions include milk, soy, peanut, egg, and fish (Sampson, 1994). Celiac disease (gluten-sensitive enteropathy) may also be a type IV hypersensitivity reaction (to wheat proteins); it is considered in a separate section.

Clinical manifestations of food hypersensitivity (Table 23–7) include cutaneous (eczema, urticaria), respiratory (rhinitis, asthma), and gastrointestinal reactions

Table 23–7. Clinical Manifestations of Food Allergy

Asthma	Rhinorrhea
Vomiting	Conjunctivitis
Diarrhea/malabsorption	Urticaria/angioedema
Lactose intolerance	Atopic dermatitis
Abdominal pain	Colic/irritability
Infant colic (questionable)	Migraine headaches
Hematochezia/allergic colitis	Laryngeal edema/anaphylaxis

(allergic colitis, vomiting, and possibly abdominal pain). Hill and coworkers (1986) have identified three types of milk hypersensitivity: patients in group 1 develop cutaneous reactions within 45 minutes of challenge; those in group 2 develop gastrointestinal symptoms between 45 minutes and 20 hours after challenge; and those in group 3 develop both gastrointestinal and respiratory symptoms more than 24 hours after challenge. This chapter focuses on gastrointestinal manifestations of food allergy; food allergy is also discussed in Chapter 20.

Milk- and Soy-Sensitive Enteropathy

Up to 50% of children with milk allergy develop gastrointestinal symptoms, particularly vomiting or diarrhea. Two common subtypes of this enteropathy, allergic colitis and postinfectious protein intolerance, are described in the following. Some infants with milk or soy intolerance develop a severe enteropathy in the neonatal period that can be confused with that of infants having either necrotizing enterocolitis or pyloric stenosis (Schwarzenberg and Whitington, 1983; Snyder et al., 1987). Barium radiography may demonstrate antral narrowing or mucosal thickening of the duodenum and jejunum, and biopsy of an affected area shows a small-bowel eosinophilic infiltrate (Fig. 23–10).

Other infants present in the first months of life with vomiting or chronic diarrhea but without other atopic features; in these patients, celiac disease, giardiasis, cystic fibrosis, or other malabsorptive disorders must be excluded. Biopsies of small intestine in this group may demonstrate partial villous atrophy in a focal or patchy distribution, with or without an eosinophilic infiltrate. In more severe cases, a flat intestinal mucosa resembling that in celiac disease can be seen (Stern, 1991). Similar lesions have been identified with hypersensitivity to soy protein; indeed, 10% to 30% of infants with milk hypersensitivity also react to soy (Ament and Rubin, 1972; Halpin et al., 1977).

Allergic Proctocolitis of Infancy

Infants under 1 year of age may present with bloody diarrhea as the only manifestation of protein allergy. This condition occurs most frequently in infants fed cow's milk formula, although colitis can also occur in infants fed soy formula or breast milk (Powell, 1978; Perisic et al., 1988). Allergic colitis occurs frequently in infants under 3 months of age; presentation before 3 days or after 6 months of age is unusual. The patient is typically a term infant who appears healthy, is afebrile, and appears normal on physical examination; there is often a family history of allergy. The condition must be differentiated from more serious causes of rectal bleeding in the infant, including necrotizing enterocolitis, infectious colitis, or Hirschsprung's enterocolitis. Flexible sigmoidoscopy in the symptomatic infant can establish the diagnosis. Endoscopy identifies an erythematous and friable mucosa, and histologic examination of the affected tissue demonstrates a mucosal eosinophilic infiltrate (more than six eosinophils per high-power field) (Winter et al., 1990; Odze et al., 1993). Despite the mucosal eosinophilic infiltrate, eosinophils and neutrophils are rarely seen in the stool. The infant typically responds promptly to a switch to casein hydrolysate feedings; breast-fed infants may respond to a maternal diet in which milk products are strictly avoided (Lake et al., 1982).

Postinfectious Cow's Milk Protein and Soy Protein Intolerance

After a viral or bacterial enteric illness, an infant or toddler is at increased risk of developing an enteropathy because of immune hypersensitivity to proteins in milk or soy. In 1976, Harrison and coworkers described 25 children with chronic protracted diarrhea after acute gastroenteritis; all but four were under 1 year of age. Small-bowel biopsy demonstrated partial villous atrophy and an inflammatory cell infiltrate. Lactose intolerance was also present but resolved promptly after the illness. These patients improved when fed a protein hydrolysate but redeveloped diarrhea, colitis, urticaria, or wheezing when rechallenged with cow's milk formula (Harrison et al., 1976). Similar illness may occur in infants fed soy formula after enteritis (Iyngkaran et al., 1988). Excess antigen absorption of ovalbumin has been observed in infants with acute gastroenteritis; Walker-Smith (1986) hypothesized that excess antigen overwhelms the tolerance mechanisms of the gut, leading to systemic and mucosal sensitization and food-sensitive enteropathy. This phenomenon may be less common than previously believed; Hager and colleagues (1987) found enteropathy in only 2 of 24 chil-

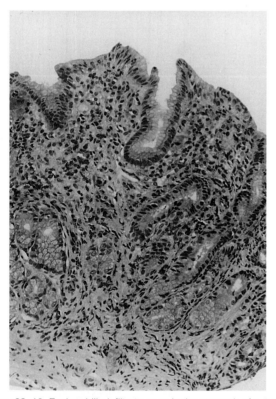

Figure 23–10. Eosinophilic infiltrate seen in the stomach of a 1-year-old with eosinophilic gastroenteritis. (Courtesy of Dr. Asma Nusrat, Department of Pathology, Children's Hospital, Boston.)

dren under 3 months of age who were fed cow's milk formula following a viral infection.

Eosinophilic Gastroenteropathy

Eosinophilic gastroenteropathy is characterized by an eosinophilic infiltrate in one or more parts of the gut, most commonly the gastric antrum, duodenum, or small bowel. Three forms have been described: *mucosal or submucosal involvement* is characterized by abdominal pain, diarrhea, and protein-losing enteropathy; *muscular involvement* is characterized by bowel thickening or obstruction; and *serosal involvement* is characterized by hypoalbuminemia and abdominal ascitic fluid containing eosinophils. Clinical features overlap those of milk-sensitive enteropathy, and the two are frequently confused. Katz and coworkers (1984) have suggested the following characteristics for differentiating between the two entities. Patients with eosinophilic gastroenteropathy are usually older, with a mean age of 4 years. Furthermore, they often have signs of systemic allergy, including rhinitis or urticaria, but a history of food-specific allergy is rarely present. Peripheral blood eosinophilia is seen in 20% to 70% of cases. These patients rarely respond to an elimination diet but respond well to oral corticosteroids, which can then be gradually tapered over time. Case reports suggest that oral disodium cromoglycate may be used to treat this condition (DiGioacchino et al., 1990).

Diagnosis

A combination of history, physical examination, response to elimination diet, and laboratory tests is required to diagnose and treat food allergy. In some cases in which the symptoms are highly suggestive of allergy and the offending agent is easily identified (for example, in an infant receiving cow's milk formula who has allergic colitis), an empirical dietary elimination or formula change is reasonable. In most cases, however, the diagnosis is not simple and the precipitating agent not obvious. Many diagnostic tests are available to identify the food antigens that are causative (Table 23–8) (Van Arsdel and Larson, 1992; Burks and Sampson, 1992). Goldman's regimen of elimination of a food and rechallenge with the same food three times is rarely used today, because of its difficulty and the risk of exposing an atopic child repeatedly to the same antigen (Goldman et al., 1963).

Skin prick tests and radioallergosorbent testing (RAST) are commonly utilized in the outpatient set-

Table 23–8. Diagnostic Tests for Food Allergy

Complete blood count (for peripheral eosinophilia)
Skin testing
Radioallergosorbent (RAST) testing
D-Xylose absorption
Immunoglobulin levels (including immunoglobulin E)
Antigliadin/antiendomysial antibodies (for celiac disease)
Repeated food challenge (Goldman criteria)
Double-blind placebo-controlled food challenge
Intestinal/colonic biopsy

ting. Skin tests have an excellent negative predictive value for IgE-mediated food hypersensitivity; that is, if the skin test result is negative, it is highly unlikely (>95%) that the subject will react to that food antigen (Bock et al., 1978; Sampson and Albergo, 1984; Burks and Sampson, 1992). However, positive prick test results correlate poorly with the presence of clinical food allergy. Radioallergosorbent tests may be performed by nonallergists in the outpatient setting; however, they are somewhat less sensitive and specific than skin tests (Wraith et al., 1979; Sampson and Albergo, 1984; Ortolani et al., 1989). In a study of children with soy hypersensitivity, RAST had a sensitivity of 69%, a specificity of 77%, and a positive predictive value (i.e., likelihood that the patient was truly allergic to soy if the RAST was positive) of only 6% (Giampietro et al., 1992).

Double-blind placebo-controlled food challenges in the hospital or office are the most definitive and safest way to evaluate patients with food hypersensitivity and to control for confounding factors (such as idiopathic urticaria, reactions to food additives, or psychogenic influences). In patients with a history of anaphylaxis, personnel trained in resuscitation and use of emergency drugs (including epinephrine and diphenhydramine) must be present. The challenge involves giving increasing amounts of encapsulated lyophilized food protein or placebo in doses ranging from 125 mg to 10 g (Burks and Sampson, 1992). Reactions should be observed by an objective third person unaware of whether the patient receives placebo or antigen. Although the challenges are used primarily in tertiary care centers, protocols for double-blind food challenges in the hospital or office setting are available (Bock et al., 1988; Metcalfe and Sampson, 1990).

Treatment

When food allergy is diagnosed, the cornerstone of therapy is elimination of the offending food. The elimination diet must be strict and often requires the supervision of a registered dietician, because the offending foods may be present in fillers or additives in processed foods (Leihnas et al., 1987). Most patients have reactions caused by only one or two offending foods, the most common being milk, soy, egg, peanuts, wheat, or fish. However, severe reactions to a great many foods, including rice, are reported (Borchers et al., 1993). Because a milk-allergic infant or child may also react to soy protein, we generally recommend casein hydrolysate formulas for infants with cow's milk intolerance. For older infants and children, we do not recommend an empirical elimination diet, because of the adverse effects on the child's nutrition and growth. Instead, elimination diets should be based on the results of food challenges. Children receiving special diets may require nutritional assessment followed by calcium or vitamin supplementation.

Prevention

Early avoidance of allergenic foods may help to prevent the subsequent development of atopic disease in infants at high risk. Zeiger and coworkers (1989) randomly assigned infants of atopic parents to either a regular diet or a restricted diet. The restricted diet consisted of avoidance of maternal ingestion of cow's milk, soy, and peanuts during the third trimester of pregnancy and during lactation and avoidance of infant ingestion of cow's milk, soy, citrus, wheat, peanuts, corn, egg, and fish for the first year of life. The prevalence of atopic disease was 27% in the control group and 16% in the food-restricted group. A similar study was conducted by Sigurs and coworkers (1992), who found a decrease in the percentage of patients with atopic dermatitis but not other disorders. Thus, avoidance of antigenic foods in the first year of life may prevent the subsequent development of food allergies.

Prognosis

Most children outgrow their food allergies (except for nut allergies). In our experience, less than 10% of infants with allergic colitis develop adverse reactions when challenged with cow's milk protein at 1 year of age. However, one of our patients with allergic colitis developed anaphylaxis after challenge. We thus recommend that a challenge be performed under close observation in a physician's office or procedure unit. Bishop and colleagues (1990) reported a long-term study of 100 children with atopic illness (urticaria, eczema, bronchitis, and diarrhea) associated with cow's milk allergy. Seventy-two percent of children still reacted to milk at 2 years of age, but only 22% of children reacted to milk at age 6 (Bishop et al., 1990). Thus, it may take several years to achieve clinical tolerance. By contrast, children with peanut allergies persist with skin test reactivity and clinical allergy into adolescence (Bock and Atkins, 1989).

Gastroesophageal Reflux

The reflux of small amounts of gastric contents into the lower esophagus is a normal occurrence, particularly after meals. Gastroesophageal reflux (GER) is characterized by an increased number or duration of these episodes, the presence of symptoms, and possibly complications.

Clinical Manifestations

Effortless regurgitation is the usual manifestation in infants, whereas the older child typically complains of retrosternal burning, epigastric discomfort, and heartburn. In a few patients, symptoms are severe enough to impair weight gain and lead to failure to thrive. In a subset of these infants, peptic esophagitis develops, resulting in hematemesis or occult blood loss and iron deficiency anemia. Esophageal strictures may eventually develop if the child remains untreated.

Less common presentations include recurrent aspiration pneumonia, chronic cough, wheezing (often nocturnal), and asthma (Malroot et al., 1987). Apneic spells in the newborn and sudden infant death syndrome have been ascribed to gastroesophageal reflux.

Pseudoneurologic symptoms, including abnormal posturing (Sandifer's syndrome) and rumination, are rare presentations (Bray et al., 1977; Boyle, 1989). Pathologic reflux is common in children with neurologic disabilities as well as in those with congenital malformations of the esophagus.

Diagnosis

The clinician is confronted with a large number of infants who spit up but are otherwise well. Infants who have normal growth and who do not present with any complications of reflux (poor weight gain, occult gastrointestinal bleeding, immunodeficiency, anemia, repeated lower respiratory infections, chronic cough, or wheezing) do not require investigation.

In addition to infants with these complications, infants with significant neurologic disorders or esophageal anomalies (tracheosophageal fistula) or those symptomatic beyond age 2 years require evaluation.

Extended monitoring of the pH of the distal esophagus remains the gold standard in the diagnosis of pathologic reflux. The normal infant has a higher percentage of acid reflux into the esophagus than the adult; thus, caution must be exercised when interpreting pediatric pH studies as normal or abnormal (Vandenplas et al., 1991). The barium swallow is utilized to rule out anatomic abnormalities (e.g., hiatus hernia, pyloric stenosis, or malrotation) or gastric outlet obstruction, but it is a poor test for gastroesophageal reflux. Scintigraphic scanning after the patient ingests tracer-labeled milk is a noninvasive technique involving little radiation. It is more sensitive than radiology in the detection of reflux, but its main utility is in the detection of delayed gastric emptying. Esophageal manometry is useful for demonstrating abnormalities of motility or swallowing. Lower esophageal sphincter pressure does not correlate well with gastroesophageal reflux.

Endoscopy and biopsy demonstrate complications of reflux (esophagitis, strictures, metaplasia, or Barrett's esophagus) and rule out other causes of vomiting (peptic ulcer disease, *Helicobacter pylori* infection, or eosinophilic gastroenteritis). The esophageal histologic findings in a patient with reflux esophagitis include lengthening of the esophageal papillae, hyperplasia of the basal epithelial cell layer, and intraepithelial eosinophils (Vandenplas, 1994). Kelly and coworkers (1994) have proposed that isolated intraepithelial eosinophilia may be caused by food allergy as well as reflux; therefore, the clinician should take a careful history of allergy for any child with eosinophilic esophagitis, and the presence or absence of eosinophils in the gastric antrum should be established by endoscopic biopsy.

Treatment

Medical management of patients with gastroesophageal reflux commences initially by recommending that the parents thicken the formula by adding cereal directly to the bottle and offer smaller and more frequent feedings. Positioning of the child (prone, head tilted up) after feedings and during sleep may also be beneficial (Orenstein et al., 1983). Pharmacotherapy is reserved for either older children or infants with complicated reflux (i.e., children with weight loss, esophagitis, reactive airway disease, apnea, or aspiration). Therapy for gastroesophageal reflux involves treatment with a prokinetic agent, an antacid, or both. Prokinetic agents currently available include bethanechol, metoclopramide, and cisapride (Reynolds and Putnam, 1992). Antacid therapies include coating agents (e.g., Mylanta), histamine-H$_2$ receptor antagonists (cimetidine, ranitidine, famotidine, and nizatidine), and proton-pump antagonists (omeprazole).

Surgery (fundoplication) is reserved for those with severe complications refractory to medical treatment and controls reflux in approximately 90% of patients. Fundoplication has unwanted effects (including delayed gastric emptying or dumping syndrome) in 15% to 20% of patients, so it should be performed in cases of life-threatening reflux or medical treatment failures (Fung et al., 1990).

Gluten-Sensitive Enteropathy (Celiac Sprue, Celiac Disease)

Gluten-sensitive enteropathy (GSE) is a nonallergic abnormal immunologic response to the gliadin fraction of gluten, a protein found in wheat, rye, barley, and oats, and is characterized clinically by malabsorption and histologically by small-intestinal villous atrophy. A gluten-free diet results in normalization of small-bowel histology and clinical improvement, and rechallenge with gluten causes recurrence of the histologic abnormalities and clinical symptoms. The relationship of gluten ingestion to celiac disease was astutely deduced in the early 1950s by Willem-Karel Dicke, a Dutch pediatrician, who observed that GSE diminished during the bread shortage of World War II (Dicke et al., 1953; van Berge-Henegouwen and Mulder, 1993). Diagnosis and follow-up of patients with GSE have changed dramatically in the past 5 years with the widespread utilization of noninvasive serologic testing with antigliadin and antiendomysial antibodies.

Pathogenesis

Several hypotheses have been proposed to explain the gliadin-mediated intestinal mucosal injury of gluten-sensitive enteropathy (Trier, 1991; Kagnoff, 1992). One suggests that an enzyme deficiency may impair digestion of gliadins, with damage to the gut by undegraded noxious proteins; however, no brush border enzyme deficiency has been identified. A second hypothesis suggests that genetic factors are the principal determining features. In support of this hypothesis, there is a strong concordance among identical twins and a strong human leukocyte antigen (HLA) association with celiac disease. A third hypothesis suggests an abnormal immune response to gliadin peptides, resulting in antibody- and cell-mediated immunologic damage to the gut epithelium. Most investigators currently believe that the etiology of GSE includes both a genetic predisposition and excessive immune activation.

There is a 10% incidence of gluten-sensitive enteropathy in first-degree relatives of patients with GSE, a 30% concordance in HLA-identical siblings, and a 70% concordance among identical twins (Mylotte et al., 1974; Mearin and Pena, 1987; Marsh, 1992). Early epidemiologic studies suggested an association of GSE with the class I MHC antigen HLA-B8 (Falchuk et al., 1972; Auricchio et al., 1988). Subsequently, much stronger associations with certain MHC class II molecules have been observed. More than 90% of GSE patients either have HLA-DR3 or are heterozygous for HLA-DR5/DR7 (Ek et al., 1978; De Marchi et al., 1979; Alper et al., 1987; Sollid and Thorsby, 1993). Utilizing oligonucleotide probes that precisely map the MHC class II complex, a strong association between two alleles (DQA1*0501, DQB1*0201) and celiac disease has been noted. These findings have led Sollid and Thorsby (1993) to propose that a specific MHC class II protein, an HLA-DQαβ heterodimer, HLA-DQ(α1*0501,β1*0201), is present on antigen-presenting cells of almost all patients with celiac disease and that this protein complex either preferentially binds or presents gluten peptides to lymphocytes, resulting in immune activation. Although this hypothesis satisfactorily explains the available genetic data, enhanced gluten binding to antigen-presenting cells with this MHC protein complex has not been demonstrated. Furthermore, the incidence of GSF in all subjects with this MHC heterodimer needs to be established.

Considering that concordance for gluten-sensitive enteropathy is not 100% in HLA-identical siblings and twins, environmental factors must also play a role in its activation (Kagnoff, 1992). Because GSE can present at any time between early infancy and old age, it has been postulated that other antigens may trigger gluten sensitivity in genetically predisposed individuals. Kagnoff and colleagues (1984) discovered a 12-amino-acid sequence homology between A-gliadin and the E1b protein of human adenovirus type 12. These investigators subsequently showed that 16 of 18 patients with celiac disease, compared with 6 of 35 control subjects, had been exposed to this virus (Kagnoff et al., 1987). However, another group has not confirmed this association (Howdle et al., 1989).

Humoral and cellular immunologic abnormalities are present in the intestinal mucosa of patients with gluten-sensitive enteropathy. Increased lamina propria plasma cells and increased mucosal IgA and IgM production are observed. The IgA antibody secreted in GSE is primarily dimeric, whereas monomeric IgA is produced in inflammatory bowel disease (Baklien et al., 1977; Colombel et al., 1990). Serum antibodies to gliadin peptides (antigliadin IgG and IgA) and to the membrane of primate smooth muscle (antiendomysial antibodies) are present in patients with GSE (Levenson et al., 1985; Ferreira et al., 1992), but it is not known whether these antibodies play a pathogenic role in GSE (i.e., through antibody-mediated cellular cytotoxicity) or are simply epiphenomena. They are useful in diagnosis and monitoring of GSE (see later).

Intraepithelial lymphocytes (IELs) are in close proximity to gut epithelial cells and may be involved in epithelial damage in patients with gluten-sensitive enteropathy. Russell and coworkers (1993) have demonstrated the presence of the cytotoxic protein nucleolysin TIA-1 within the IELs of patients with active GSE; therefore, IELs possess cytotoxic molecules that could potentially damage enterocytes. Spencer and colleagues (1991) have demonstrated that patients with GSE have an increased percentage (up to 30%) of $CD3^+CD4^-CD8^-$ intraepithelial lymphocytes expressing the gamma/delta T-cell receptor. However, the increase in gamma/delta IEL cells is not specific for GSE, as it is also found in other enteropathies (Spencer et al., 1989, 1991; Halstensen et al., 1989, 1990). Most intraepithelial lymphocytes of patients with GSE bear alpha/beta T-cell receptors, and these decrease significantly in response to a gluten-free diet, whereas the gamma/delta TCR cells remain stable (Kutlu et al., 1993). Thus, both alpha/beta and gamma/delta IELs are present in the mucosa in GSE, but whether either phenotype mediates intestinal damage is not known.

In summary, gluten-sensitive enteropathy occurs when there is an altered mucosal immune response in genetically susceptible individuals. Whether GSE is caused only by an immunologic response to gluten or is initiated by other antigens such as adenovirus type 12 is not known.

Clinical Manifestations

The prevalence of celiac disease ranges from 1 in 300 in western Ireland to 1 in 2000 in other regions. The disease is common in northern Europe and rare in China and Africa (Trier, 1991). Gluten-sensitive enteropathy is rarely diagnosed in developing countries. However, we identified GSE in a child from a well-to-do family from urban Ethiopia who presented with a 2-year history of marasmus, hypocalcemia, and multiple nutritional deficiencies.

Several diseases are associated with gluten-sensitive enteropathy, including diabetes mellitus, Down syndrome, and atopic dermatitis (Auricchio et al., 1988; Murphy and Walker, 1991). Selective IgA deficiency is a frequent association, occurring in 1 of 200 patients with GSE, compared with 1 in 700 in the general population (Cunningham-Rundles, 1988) (see Chapter 14). A study of 75 selective IgA-deficient children found an incidence of GSE near 10% (Savilahti and Pelkonen, 1979).

Patients with gluten-sensitive enteropathy may also develop other immunologic disorders, including arthritis, chronic hepatitis, thyroiditis, aphthous ulcers, and pulmonary hemosiderosis (Auricchio et al., 1988). Dermatitis herpetiformis, an immunologically mediated papulovesicular skin disease, is strongly associated with gluten sensitivity and remission occurs when patients are given a gluten-free diet (Reunala et al., 1977; Gawkrodger et al., 1988). This condition is rare in children (see Chapter 21).

Clinical features of celiac disease are given in Table

Table 23–9. Clinical Features of Celiac Disease

Primary Features	Associated Disorders
Diarrhea	Arthritis
Growth failure	Hepatitis
Anorexia	Pulmonary hemosiderosis
Irritability/lethargy	Diabetes mellitus
Abdominal pain	Thyroid function abnormalities
Constipation	Down syndrome
Pubertal delay	Iritis
Weight loss	Dermatitis herpetiformis
Abdominal distention	Selective IgA deficiency
Buttock wasting	Sarcoidosis
Digital clubbing	IgA nephropathy
Pallor	
Edema	

23–9. Most cases are diagnosed in children 1 to 3 years of age; others are diagnosed throughout childhood, adolescence, and adulthood. The typical infant presents with diarrhea, foul-smelling stools, and poor weight gain, and the disorder is easily recognized. In our experience, however, this classical presentation is uncommon. Infants may also present with refusal to feed, constipation, irritability, lethargy, and iron deficiency anemia. Older children may present with short stature, pubertal delay, malaise, or crampy abdominal pain. In adults, amenorrhea, folate deficiency, and peripheral neuropathy have been described.

Diagnosis

The diagnosis of celiac disease necessitates a small-bowel biopsy and demonstration of villous atrophy, increased intraepithial lymphocytes, epithelial destruction, increased crypt mitotic activity, and infiltration of the lamina propria by plasma cells and lymphocytes (Fig. 23–11). The biopsy may be performed either endoscopically or by use of a swallowed small-bowel biopsy capsule passed into the jejunum. Results of endoscopic biopsies of the duodenum correlate well with jejunal histology. Endoscopy can also visualize the gross morphology of the duodenal folds, which may be flattened or scalloped in patients with active gluten-sensitive enteropathy.

Differential Diagnosis

The histologic appearance is not specific to GSE and can be seen in other diseases, such as milk and soy protein intolerance, malnutrition, immunodeficiency, giardiasis, and viral infections. For this reason, before 1990, the European Society of Pediatric Gastroenterology and Nutrition (ESPGN) recommended that three small-bowel biopsies be performed to establish the diagnosis: one biopsy at initial presentation, a second after 6 months of a gluten-free diet, and a third after gluten rechallenge (to show that the gluten was truly the offending agent and exclude transient gluten intolerance) (Walker-Smith et al., 1990). The cost and invasiveness of these repeated procedures led to the widespread use of empirical "wheat-free" diets. Until recently, noninvasive tests for diagnosis of GSE (Table

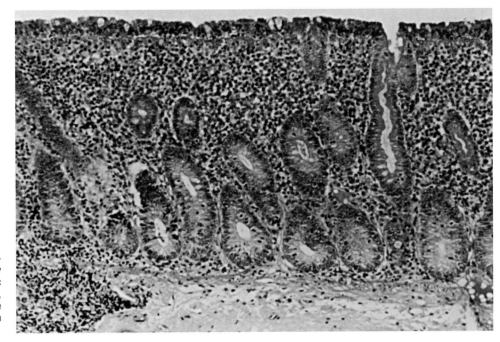

Figure 23–11. Low-power photomicrograph of a small-bowel biopsy specimen in a patient with celiac disease. Complete villous atrophy, increased mitotic activity in the crypts, and increased cellularity in the lamina propria are seen.

23–10) assessed only intestinal mucosal function and lacked sensitivity and specificity for detecting celiac disease.

Antigliadin and Antiendomysial Antibodies

Assays for serum antigliadin and antiendomysial antibodies have greatly facilitated the diagnosis of gluten-sensitive enteropathy, and these tests should be performed on all children when the diagnosis is suspected. In a study of 340 children with untreated celiac disease, Burgin-Wolff and colleagues (1991) found that the combination of antigliadin IgG and IgA antibodies and antiendomysial IgA antibodies detected gluten-sensitive enteropathy in 338 of 340 (99.4%) children with the disease. Therefore, if assays for all three antibodies were negative, GSE was essentially excluded. In this study, the antiendomysial antibody was the most specific, with only 2 of 211 false-positive results; in contrast, the IgG antigliadin antibody had a very high (35%) false-positive rate. A smaller study found the sensitivity and specificity of the antiendomysial antibody alone to approach 100% (Ferreira et al., 1992).

We routinely screen all patients with both antigliadin and antiendomysial antibodies and perform biopsies for all patients with positive antiendomysial antibodies. If a patient has a positive antigliadin IgG and negative antigliadin IgA and antiendomysial IgA antibody, we review the clinical data to see if biopsy is warranted. Selective IgA-deficient patients may not have positive IgA antiendomysial antibodies even if they have celiac disease; thus, immunoglobulin levels are a useful adjunct in the evaluation of the patient in whom GSE is suspected.

Because both false-negative and false-positive antibody results can occur and the diagnosis involves lifelong dietary restriction, an initial biopsy for every patient with suspected celiac disease remains standard. Antibody titers usually decrease upon institution of a gluten-free diet and increase with gluten rechallenge and may be used to follow disease activity (Burgin-Wolff et al., 1991). For this reason, the ESPGN has amended its prior recommendation, stating that three biopsies are no longer necessary in every case of GSE (Walker-Smith et al., 1990). There is currently no consensus regarding which patients warrant repeated biopsies; further studies of the reliability of antibodies in monitoring disease activity are needed before recommendations are made.

Table 23–10. Diagnostic Tests in Celiac Disease

Test	Common Finding
Blood count	Microcytic anemia
Blood chemistries	Hypoalbuminemia
	Hypocalcemia
D-Xylose	Poor absorption (1-hour level < 20 mg/dl)
Lactose breath hydrogen test	Lactose intolerance
Fecal fat	Fat malabsorption
Upper gastrointestinal series with small-bowel follow-through	Loss of small-bowel pattern Flocculation of barium Bowel dilatation
Antigliadin, antireticulin, antiendomysial antibodies*	Elevated titers
Small-bowel biopsy	Villous atrophy

*Most specific antibody for celiac disease.

Treatment

Therapy for gluten-sensitive enteropathy involves the institution of a strict gluten-free diet and the correction of any nutritional deficiencies caused by malabsorption. Even small amounts of dietary gluten (such as in processed foods) can result in villous inflammation and damage. Consultation with a dietician and referral to a celiac support group are recommended. Most patients demonstrate some catch-up growth within a year after diagnosis and treatment, although their ultimate height may be less than that of siblings. If symptoms persist or growth remains poor, the patient's dietary compliance should be evaluated, antibody tests or biopsy repeated, and other causes of malabsorption sought. Adults with celiac disease have a high incidence of intestinal T-cell lymphoma (Nielsen et al., 1985; Logan et al., 1989). A gluten-free diet may decrease the risk of this malignancy by minimizing intestinal inflammation, but this has not been proved.

Inflammatory Bowel Disease

The inflammatory bowel diseases (IBDs) are characterized by persistent chronic intestinal inflammation without an identifiable infectious or dietary cause. In this country, the term inflammatory bowel disease refers to ulcerative colitis (UC) and Crohn's disease (CD). We also discuss Behçet's disease, malacoplakia, and intractable ulcerating enterocolitis of infancy, because these illnesses may have a similar pathophysiology and are often confused clinically with UC and CD. In the United States, 500,000 to 1 million patients are afflicted with either UC or CD.

Etiology and Pathophysiology

Many factors have been linked with inflammatory bowel disease (Table 23–11), but no cause of the disease has been found. Heredity plays a strong role; a patient with ulcerative colitis or Crohn's disease has a 10% chance of having a first-degree relative with IBD, and concordance among monozygotic twins is approximately 65% for CD and 20% for UC (Yang et al., 1992). No strong HLA association has been identified in either CD or UC, but some weak associations have been identified. Specifically, whites with ulcerative colitis have an increased prevalence of HLA-B27, HLA-BW35, and HLA-DR2, and whites with Crohn's disease have an increased incidence of HLA-B2 and HLA-B44 (Schreiber et al., 1992). Of note, patients with certain genetic syndromes, including Turner's syndrome and Hermansky-Pudlak syndrome, appear to be at increased risk for development of IBD (Mendeloff and Calkins, 1988). Several patients with both glycogen storage disease type Ib and IBD have also been described (see Gastrointestinal Manifestations of Primary and Secondary Immunodeficiencies later).

Numerous organisms, including normal bacterial flora, *E. coli*, atypical mycobacteria, *C. difficile*, and measles virus, have been proposed as causes of inflammatory bowel disease. However, no single infectious agent has withstood the test of time as the etiologic agent. The same is true for ingested agents; milk and other foods have been proposed as potential proinflammatory antigens, but little evidence linking dietary substances to exacerbation of IBD exists (Glassman et al., 1990). However, some patients with Crohn's disease may undergo remission when given an elemental diet, suggesting that elimination of food antigens diminishes intestinal inflammation in CD (Logan et al., 1981; Seidman et al., 1987; Kleinman et al., 1989).

Mucosal immunity may be altered in inflammatory bowel disease. Schreiber and coworkers (1992) have proposed that the mucosal immune system in patients with ulcerative colitis and Crohn's disease is in a heightened state of activation. These and other investigators postulate that enhanced intestinal permeability or antigen presentation by intestinal epithelial cells leads to macrophage activation and interleukin-1 secretion within mucosal lymphoid aggregates. This in turn results in helper T-lymphocyte secretion of interleukin-2 (IL-2), IL-4, and IL-5; B-cell activation; immunoglobulin production; and recruitment of effector cells (including eosinophils, mast cells, and neutrophils). The inflammatory response results in intestinal epithelial damage, enhanced antigen absorption, and perpetuation of the inflammatory cascade (Fig. 23–12) (Schreiber et al., 1992).

Much evidence supports abnormal immune activation in inflammatory bowel disease. First, immunosuppressive agents including corticosteroids, 6-mercaptopurine, and cyclosporine are effective therapeutic agents in Crohn's disease and ulcerative colitis. Second, both diseases are associated with other immune disorders, including peripheral arthritis, chronic active hepatitis, uveitis, and primary sclerosing cholangitis. Hollander and colleagues (1986) have demonstrated that some healthy relatives of patients with IBD have increased permeability to macromolecular markers such as lactulose or polyethylene glycol; this may predispose them to IBD. Indeed, some patients with IBD in remission have increased permeability to lactulose, and this may be predictive of disease relapse (Wyatt et al., 1993). Bland and Mayer have demonstrated that epithelial cells express MHC class II molecules and present antigen in vitro to T lymphocytes; such antigen-presenting activity may be augmented in patients with ulcerative colitis and Crohn's disease (Bland and Warren, 1986; Mayer and Eisenhardt, 1990; Mayer et al., 1991). Therefore, evidence exists for abnormal gut permeability and increased antigen presentation in IBD.

There is other evidence of immune activation in the intestinal mucosa of patients with inflammatory bowel disease. Immunohistochemical and flow cytometric studies show increased numbers of activated T cells expressing IL-2 receptors (CD25) in the bowel wall of patients with Crohn's disease and increased numbers

Table 23–11. Associations With and Risk Factors for Inflammatory Bowel Disease

Genetic	Infections
Jewish ancestry	Atypical mycobacteria
Family history	Enteric bacterial flora
Turner's syndrome	Measles virus
Hermansky-Pudlak syndrome	*Clostridium difficile*
Exogenous intake	Immune
Milk consumption	Altered intestinal permeability
Sugar consumption	Associated autoimmune
Smoking	disorders (e.g., sclerosing
Oral contraceptive pill	cholangitis)

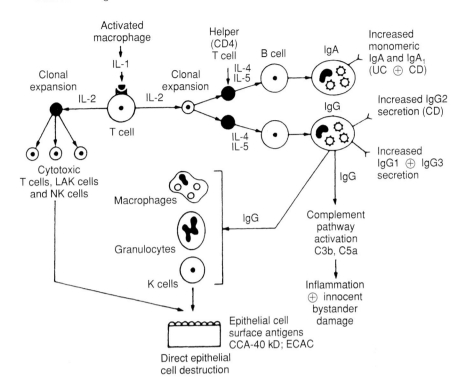

Figure 23–12. Inflammatory cascade postulated in inflammatory bowel disease. The activated T cell secretes cytokines, causing expansion of T-cell populations (e.g., IL-2) and expansion of B-cell populations (e.g., IL-4, IL-5). Cytokines produced by activated T cells can also stimulate cytotoxic T cells, natural killer (NK) cells, and lymphokine-activated killer (LAK) cells, which can damage gut epithelium. The stimulated B cells mature into plasma cells, produce antibodies, and activate complement, which may further recruit other inflammatory cells (neutrophils, mast cells). Alterations of IgA and IgG subclass antibodies may be seen in inflammatory bowel disease. IL-2 = interleukin-2; IgA = immunoglobulin A. (From Baldassano RN, MacDermott RP. Immunologic aspects of inflammatory bowel disease. Semin Pediatr Gastroenterol Nutr 1:5, 1990.)

of activated macrophages in the intestinal mucosa of patients with ulcerative colitis (Choy et al., 1990). Proinflammatory cytokines, including IL-1, IL-2, interferon-γ, IL-6, and IL-8, are elevated in the intestine of patients with IBD (Mahida et al., 1989; Fais et al., 1991; Stevens et al., 1992). Interleukin-8 in particular may be a potent chemotactic factor resulting in neutrophil recruitment. The mucosal plasma cells of patients with IBD have increased local production of IgG and IgA1 (Kett and Brandtzaeg, 1987; Kett et al., 1987). Lastly, messenger ribonucleic acid (mRNA) for granzyme B, a molecular mediator of damage by cytotoxic T cells, is increased in the mucosa of patients with ulcerative colitis (Stevens et al., 1994). These findings suggest that abnormalities of immune regulation are essential steps in the development of the inflammatory state in CD and UC.

To investigate which cytokine abnormalities cause colitis, researchers have developed several transgenic animals that contract colitis. Sadlack and colleagues (1993) have developed an IL-2–deficient mouse that develops colitis at week 10 of life and whose mucosa contains activated T cells. Similarly, colitis develops in transgenic mice lacking the alpha/beta T-cell receptor (Mombaerts et al., 1993). An IL-10–deficient mouse develops both colitis and small-bowel lesions (Kuhn et al., 1993). Lastly, Hammer and colleagues (1990) have reported on a transgenic rat containing multiple copies of the HLA-B27 gene; these rats develop colitis in conjunction with a systemic autoimmune erosive arthropathy. These studies suggest that colitis may be an end result of multiple immune system aberrations rather than a single specific abnormality (Strober and Ehrhardt, 1993).

Circulating autoantibodies to gut epithelium have

been implicated in the pathogenesis of inflammatory bowel disease. Anticolon antibodies are present in the serum of patients with the disease; however, they are nonspecific and are present in those with other inflammatory colitides (Thayer et al., 1969; Shorter et al., 1972). Das and coworkers (1993) have identified a serum antibody directed against tropomyosin that may be specific for ulcerative colitis. Serum antineutrophil cytoplasmic antibodies (ANCA) are also found in 60% to 80% of patients with UC; unlike the cytoplasmic ANCA of Wegener's granulomatosis, ANCA of UC are perinuclear (p-ANCA) (Duerr et al., 1991) (see Chapters 22, 24, and 25). Proujansky and colleagues (1993) have shown that, at least in pediatric IBD, serum ANCA are also present in 20% of patients with Crohn's disease and so do not reliably differentiate between ulcerative colitis and Crohn's disease.

In summary, host defense abnormalities, including increased gut permeability, increased antigen presentation by enterocytes, T-lymphocyte activation, and alterations in immunoglobulin synthesis, are present in both Crohn's disease and ulcerative colitis. The genetic factors predisposing to the antigens initiating the intestinal inflammation are largely undefined.

Clinical Manifestations

In spite of some similarities, ulcerative colitis and Crohn's disease must be considered separate entities. Crohn's disease may involve any part of the gastrointestinal tract from mouth to anus, whereas ulcerative colitis is limited to the large bowel and rectum. Inflammation in CD is transmural and characterized by granulomas, whereas the inflammation in UC is limited to the mucosa and submucosa (Kelts and Grand, 1980).

Clinical and pathologic differences between CD and UC are summarized in Table 23–12.

Diagnosis

Diagnosis of Crohn's disease or ulcerative colitis is established in five separate steps:

1. Clinical suspicion of inflammatory bowel disease must be based on identification of suggestive clinical features, particularly growth failure, anemia, abdominal pain, diarrhea, or arthritis.
2. Other infectious (usually bacterial or parasitic) or immune (Behçet's disease, malacoplakia, or chronic granulomatous disease) causes of intestinal inflammation that can mimic the inflammation in ulcerative colitis or Crohn's disease must be excluded.
3. The disease should be classified as either Crohn's disease or ulcerative colitis on the basis of laboratory, radiographic, and endoscopic studies; in approximately 10% of cases, this is not possible, and the disease is termed indeterminate colitis.
4. The location of the disease should be pinpointed. For ulcerative colitis, this means identifying the segments of the large bowel that are involved; for Crohn's disease, it requires localizing disease to the mouth, esophagus, stomach, small bowel, colon, or anus.
5. Extraintestinal disease should be sought, including peripheral arthritis (present in 10% to 15% of patients with inflammatory bowel disease), liver disease (including chronic active hepatitis and sclerosing cholangitis), eye disease (including episcleritis and uveitis), and skin disease (including pyoderma gangrenosum and erythema nodosum).

A clinical and laboratory evaluation for the patient with suspected ulcerative colitis or Crohn's disease is given in Table 23–13.

Ulcerative Colitis

Among patients under 20 years of age with ulcerative colitis, 50% are over age 16 and fewer than 1% are under age 5. The most common presentation is a subacute illness with diarrhea, rectal bleeding, weak-

Table 23–13. Evaluation of the Patient with Suspected Inflammatory Bowel Disease

1. Weight, height, anthropometrics, and bone age
2. Tanner staging
3. Clinical evidence of
   Clubbing
   Iritis
   Mouth ulcers
   Arthritis
   Back pain/sacroiliitis
   Abdominal mass
   Perianal disease—hemorrhoids, fissures, fistulas
4. Laboratory studies
   Stool guaiac (occult blood)
   Complete blood count with differential, reticulocyte count
   Sedimentation rate
   Albumin, total protein
   Transaminases, alkaline phosphatase, bilirubin
   Gamma-glutamyl transpeptidase
   Serum iron, total iron-binding capacity
   Antigliadin, antiendomysial antibodies (to exclude celiac disease)
5. Purified protein derivative, *Candida* skin tests
6. Stool cultures
   Bacteria (including *Escherichia coli* O157:H7 and *Clostridium difficile*)
   Ova and parasites
   Radiography
   Upper gastrointestinal series (with small-bowel follow-through and antegrade cologram)
   Barium enema (may be useful if colonoscopy unavailable)
7. Flexible sigmoidoscopy or colonoscopy/ileoscopy

ness, anemia, weight loss, and fever. Stool frequency ranges from 2 to 10 bowel movements per day. A minority of patients present with more severe symptoms, including severe abdominal pain, bloody and mucus-filled diarrhea, tenesmus, leukocytosis, hypoalbuminemia, and bowel wall thickening seen on abdominal radiographs; these symptoms must be differentiated from those of acute infectious colitides such as shigellosis or *Campylobacter* diarrhea (Werlin and Grand, 1977).

Extraintestinal manifestations may also be observed at the time of presentation (Table 23–14). Two forms of arthritis are associated with ulcerative colitis (see

Table 23–12. Clinical Characteristics of Inflammatory Bowel Disease

Characteristic	Ulcerative Colitis	Crohn's Disease
Symptoms		
Rectal bleeding	Common	Less frequent
Diarrhea	Often severe	Moderate to absent
Pain	Infrequent	Common
Anorexia	Mild	Often severe
Weight loss	Variable	Common
Extraintestinal symptoms	Not infrequent	Not infrequent
Distribution of the lesions	Colon only; continuous	Throughout the gastrointestinal tract, segmental
Pathologic changes	Mucosal only	Transmural
Clinical course		
Remissions	Relatively common	Difficult to define
Relapse rate after surgery	None following protocolectomy	70%
Cancer risk	20% per decade of disease after the first decade	20% greater than the population at large

Table 23–14. Presenting Features of Crohn's Disease and Ulcerative Colitis in Childhood

Crohn's Disease

Intestinal	Extraintestinal
Growth failure	Arthritis/arthralgia
Weight loss	Erythema nodosum
Diarrhea	Fever
Abdominal pain	Anorexia
Abdominal mass	Oral ulcers
Rectal bleeding	Anemia
Perianal fissures/	Pubertal delay
fistulas	Clubbing
	Liver disease
	Renal stones
	(oxalate)
	Uveitis/episcleritis

Ulcerative Colitis

Intestinal	Extraintestinal
Diarrhea	Anemia
Rectal bleeding	Fever
Abdominal pain	Arthralgias/arthritis
Cramping/tenesmus	Spondyloarthropathy
Fulminant colitis	Erythema nodosum
Growth failure	Pyoderma
	gangrenosum
	Liver disease
	Uveitis/episcleritis

Chapter 24). Peripheral arthritis involving knees, ankles, elbows, and wrists occurs in 10% to 20% of patients, and arthritis tends to wax and wane with disease activity. In contrast, an axial arthritis resembling ankylosing spondylitis occurs in 5% to 10% of patients with UC, progresses despite disease activity, and is associated with HLA-B27 (Gravallese and Kantrowitz, 1988). Primary sclerosing cholangitis, a progressive inflammation and fibrosis of the bile ducts, occurs in 1% to 2% of patients and may progress to cirrhosis and liver transplantation; unfortunately, colectomy does not prevent disease progression (Schrumpf et al., 1988). Erythema nodosum is the most common dermatosis associated with UC and CD

in children. Pyoderma gangrenosum is seen rarely in pediatric UC, although it is not uncommon in adults with long-standing UC.

Diagnosis. After infectious agents have been excluded (see Table 23–13), flexible sigmoidoscopy or colonoscopy with biopsy is the most useful diagnostic procedure to establish the diagnosis of ulcerative colitis. Visual inspection of the colon reveals diffuse erythema, mucosal friability with bleeding, loss of the vascular pattern, purulent exudate, and small superficial ulcerations. In contrast to findings in CD, there is continuous involvement of the colon, without skip areas. One of three patterns of disease localization is usually seen: proctitis limited to the rectosigmoid, left-sided colitis from the rectum to the splenic flexure, or pancolitis involving the entire colon. On microscopic examination, a mucosal infiltrate of polymorphonuclear leukocytes with epithelial cell destruction and crypt abscesses is seen; granulomas are absent (Fig. 23–13). Signs of chronic colitis, including mucin depletion and branching of colonic crypts, help to differentiate ulcerative colitis from an acute enteritis (Kelts and Grand, 1980; Michener and Wyllie, 1990).

Therapy. Therapy for ulcerative colitis is primarily medical and directed at rapidly controlling acute attacks and subsequently maintaining remission. Available therapies are summarized in Table 23–15. Remission is achieved with a potent immunosuppressive agent such as prednisone and maintained with a 5-aminosalicylate derivative (e.g., sulfasalazine or olsalazine sodium [Dipentum]) (Michener and Wyllie, 1990). Corticosteroids must be given cautiously to children and adolescents because of their adverse effects on growth and bone development. Nutritional support may help sustain a patient during an acute flare but will not bring about disease remission. Cyclosporine has been utilized for patients with severe colitis in an attempt to postpone colectomy (Treem et al., 1991).

Surgery is utilized for patients who do not respond or have adverse effects with medical therapy or who

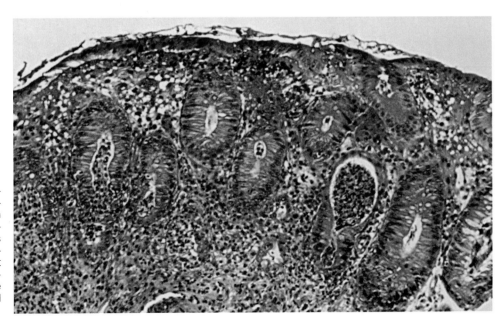

Figure 23–13. Low-power photomicrograph from a child with ulcerative colitis. The colonic epithelium overlying the crypts is partially denuded, with evidence of mucus depletion in the goblet cells. Several crypt abscesses are present with associated necrosis. The lamina propria shows a dense infiltrate of neutrophils, lymphocytes, and plasma cells.

Table 23–15. Therapies for Crohn's Disease and
Ulcerative Colitis

1. Corticosteroids
   Prednisone
   Topical steroid enemas
2. 5-Aminosalicylate derivatives
   Sulfasalazine
   Mesalamine
   Olsalazine
   5-Aminosalicylate enemas
3. Antibiotics
   Metronidazole
   Ciprofloxacin
4. Immunosuppressives
   6-Mercaptopurine
   Azathioprine
   Cyclosporine
5. Enteral nutrition
6. Surgery

develop colonic epithelial dysplasia and thus are at risk of cancer. Colectomy is curative for patients with ulcerative colitis and may be preferable to protracted medical therapy with corticosteroids or other immunosuppressives.

Crohn's Disease

In contrast to patients with ulcerative colitis, those with Crohn's disease (CD) are more likely to present with protean or subtle symptoms, including growth failure, abdominal pain, anemia, or fever of unknown origin. The prominence of growth failure as a presenting feature of CD cannot be overemphasized. Studies suggest that 50% or more of the patients have short stature and growth retardation (Kirschner et al., 1978). Kanof and colleagues (1988a) retrospectively reviewed growth curves of pediatricians' patients with CD; one third had an appreciable falloff in height velocity 1 to 2 years before the onset of any gastrointestinal symptoms. The cause of growth failure is unknown but it is probably decreased caloric intake, although increased caloric requirements and intestinal malabsorption may

be contributing causes. Lenaerts and coworkers (1989) found that one third of pediatric patients with CD had inflammation of the esophagus, stomach, or duodenum; thus, upper gastrointestinal tract inflammation may result in the anorexia of Crohn's disease.

Other atypical presentations of Crohn's disease include isolated perianal disease, with recurrent skin tags and fistulas in the absence of any bowel disease. Biopsy of a perianal skin tag demonstrates a granuloma in up to 30% of cases. In addition, isolated orofacial granulomatosis may be associated with CD in the absence of any bowel involvement. Buccal swelling, mouth ulcers, cheilitis, and cervical adenopathy may be present and mistaken for symptoms of Melkersson-Rosenthal syndrome or hereditary angioedema (Williams et al., 1991). Granulomatous inflammation of the penis occasionally occurs (Ninan et al., 1992). Extraintestinal manifestations including arthritis and dermatoses may also occur; primary sclerosing cholangitis is seen less frequently in Crohn's disease than in ulcerative colitis.

Diagnosis. The diagnosis is more difficult to establish in Crohn's disease than in ulcerative colitis. All patients with suspected CD should have an upper gastrointestinal series with small-bowel follow-through to identify small-bowel nodularity, strictures, or ulceration. In addition, colonoscopy is recommended to look for focal colitis. Lastly, consideration must be given to upper endoscopy or directed biopsy of oral or perianal lesions suspected to be lesions of CD. On occasion, the disease presents with acute right lower quadrant pain indistinguishable from that of appendicitis, and the diagnosis is made by laparotomy; creeping mesenteric fat, adherent intestinal serosa, and thickened ileum are observed at surgery. Histologically, Crohn's disease can be distinguished from ulcerative colitis by the presence of transmural inflammation with fissuring and by the presence of granulomas (Fig. 23–14). Granulomas are present in 50% of surgical resections and 25% of endoscopic biopsy specimens (Jackson and Grand, 1990).

Treatment. As with ulcerative colitis, therapy for Crohn's disease is directed at controlling flares of dis-

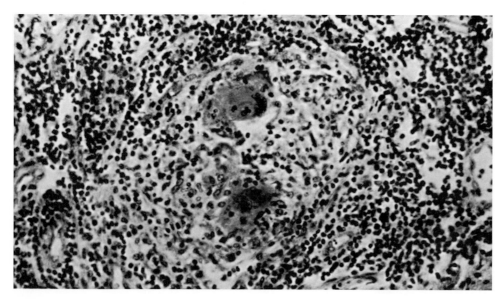

Figure 23–14. Typical noncaseating granuloma found in Crohn's disease. Note the nodular shape of the lesion made up of epithelioid cells surrounding multinucleated giant cells.

ease activity. No medication has any proven efficacy in maintaining remission in CD (see Table 23–15). Prednisone has been utilized for treatment of acute flares, but many patients are resistant to prednisone or have relapses when therapy is stopped. Accordingly, other immunosuppressive drugs have been utilized (Ruderman, 1990). In a randomized placebo-controlled crossover study, Present and colleagues (1980) demonstrated that 6-mercaptopurine induced remission and facilitated tapering of corticosteroid use in 70% of patients with active CD. In a similar study, Brynskov and coworkers (1989) utilized cyclosporine to treat steroid-refractory patients and found a 60% response rate. Cyclosporine works rapidly, with an onset of action within 1 month of initiation of therapy, compared with 3 months for 6-mercaptopurine. Although published experience with immunosuppressives in pediatric CD is limited, the results to date suggest an efficacy similar to that of adult studies (Markowitz et al., 1990; Verhave et al., 1990).

Enteral nutrition is also important in the treatment of patients with Crohn's disease, improving growth and promoting disease remission. In the recent past, parenteral nutrition was utilized to improve nutrition before surgery. It is now recognized that enteral nutrition with liquid formulas is equally efficacious for this purpose. Several studies have demonstrated the efficacy of an elemental diet delivered continuously by nasogastric tube to accelerate weight gain and growth velocity (Belli et al., 1988; Greenberg et al., 1988; Kleinman et al., 1989). Elemental diets may also bring about disease remission and have been suggested as primary therapy for patients with disease flares (Morin et al., 1982; O'Morain et al., 1984; Sanderson et al., 1987). However, relapses occur quickly when the elemental diet is discontinued. In addition, the unpalatability of the elemental diet and the difficulty of nasogastric tube feeding of children have limited its widespread use. Patients with CD may also develop specific micronutrient deficiencies, including folate, zinc, and vitamin B_{12} deficiencies; therefore, blood levels of these nutrients should be monitored (Michener and Wyllie, 1990).

Sulfasalazine and other 5-aminosalicylate (5-ASA) derivatives are utilized frequently for treatment in Crohn's colitis. Newer enteric-coated salicylate preparations such as mesalamine (Pentasa) are designed for release into the small bowel, but their efficacy in small-bowel CD has not been established. Antibiotics have also been utilized. Metronidazole is a useful drug for mild Crohn's ileitis and is the drug of choice for perianal Crohn's disease. However, its utility is limited because peripheral neuropathy may occur with long-term use (Peppercorn, 1990). Other antibiotics including ampicillin, tetracycline, and ciprofloxacin are reported to be efficacious but have not been subjected to controlled studies.

Surgery in CD, unlike UC, is not curative and is accompanied by a high rate of clinical relapse (50% within 5 years). Surgery is therefore a treatment of last resort, reserved for complications such as stricture, fistula, abdominal abscess, or fulminant colitis. The length of small bowel resected should be as small as possible to minimize the risk of development of short-bowel syndrome. Data suggest that if surgery is well timed in prepubertal growth-retarded children, catch-up growth and improved nutritional status will occur (Davies et al., 1990; McLain et al., 1990). However, surgery should be reserved for children who have not responded to optimal medical and nutritional therapy.

Summary

Therapy for pediatric inflammatory bowel disease emphasizes reduced use of corticosteroids and increased use of therapeutic alternatives, including elemental diet, immunosuppressives, antibiotics, and surgery. Medical, nutritional, and surgical management of pediatric ulcerative colitis and Crohn's disease is focused on preventing growth failure and maintaining a good quality of life. For patients with UC, this involves maintenance of remission and timely colectomy in medical failures. For those with CD, aggressive use of immunosuppressive agents and elemental diets is required to prevent complications and the need for surgery.

OTHER INFLAMMATORY DISEASES OF THE GUT

Autoimmune Enteropathy

In 1982 a new disorder, autoimmune enteropathy (AE), characterized by chronic protracted diarrhea of infants and young children associated with gut autoantibodies, was identified (Unsworth et al., 1982; Mirakian et al., 1986; Catassi et al., 1988). Autoimmune enteropathy is characterized by intractable chronic diarrhea, poor response to exclusion diets, absence of infection or immunodeficiency, and the presence of circulating antienterocyte antibodies (Sanderson et al., 1991a). Colletti and coworkers (1991) demonstrated the presence in one patient of autoantibodies that reacted with a 55-kd membrane protein present on the epithelium of both gut and kidney. Other histopathologic abnormalities include villous atrophy, increased expression of MHC class II antigens on bowel epithelium, and the presence of a dense mononuclear inflammatory infiltrate in the lamina propria of the small bowel and colon (Hill et al., 1991).

Patients with autoimmune enteropathy typically present between 2 weeks and 1 year of age with intractable diarrhea unresponsive to nutritional intervention. The stools may contain blood and mucus related to large-bowel inflammation (Hill et al., 1991). At other times, a secretory diarrhea with loss of sodium, potassium, and chloride is seen (Santer and Lebenthal, 1990). Patients may also develop membranous glomerulonephritis, possibly associated with cross-reactive antibodies to renal epithelium (Ellis et al., 1982; Martini et al., 1983; Coletti et al., 1991). Less common autoimmune features include diabetes, hypothyroidism, chronic hepatitis, and hemolytic anemia.

Initial therapy is primarily supportive, including correction of electrolyte abnormalities and placement of a central venous line for parenteral hyperalimentation. Subsequently a trial of immunosuppressives is instituted, with either corticosteroids or, in refractory cases, cyclosporine (Sanderson et al., 1991a). Clinical response is measured by serial intestinal absorptive studies (including stool electrolytes and fat absorption) and improved bowel histology. The short-term outlook for these children has improved with better nutritional support, but their long-term prognosis is guarded.

Malacoplakia

Malacoplakia (malakoplakia) is a multisystem chronic granulomatous inflammatory disorder that primarily involves the urinary tract but may also involve the bowel, skin, and brain. In children, intestinal malacoplakia may be misdiagnosed as Crohn's disease or ulcerative colitis. Clinical findings in intestinal malacoplakia include bloody diarrhea, fever, abdominal pain, and small-bowel fistulas (Harfi et al., 1985). On endoscopy, small or large raised submucosal nodules (plaques) are seen. Biopsy of the nodules demonstrates a diffuse histiocytic infiltrate that may be granulomatous. The mononuclear cells contain concentric spherical intracytoplasmic densities termed Michaelis-Gutmann bodies (Moran et al., 1989).

The etiology of malacoplakia is unknown. Many cases are reported in Arab patients, and the disease often occurs in children below 13 years of age (McClure, 1981). It is also reported in families, in malnourished patients, in immunosuppressed patients, or in association with tuberculosis (Biggar et al., 1985; Satti and Abu-Melha, 1985; el-Mouzan et al., 1988). Biggar and coworkers (1985) reported reversal of malacoplakia in a group of four transplant recipients when immunosuppression was withdrawn, suggesting that immunodeficiency may be important in its pathogenesis. Colonic malacoplakia is associated with adenocarcinoma of the colon in adults (Moran et al., 1989). There is no specific therapy for malacoplakia, although beneficial effects of antibiotics and steroids have been reported anecdotally.

Behçet's Syndrome

Behçet's syndrome is a chronic relapsing vasculitis characterized by recurrent oral aphthous ulcers, recurrent genital ulcers, uveitis or retinitis, and a follicular skin rash (International Study Group for Behçet's Disease, 1990). Associated features include an ulcerative ileocolitis primarily involving the terminal ileum and cecum, thrombophlebitis, meningoencephalitis, seronegative oligoarthritis, axial arthritis, venous and arterial thrombosis (including Budd-Chiari syndrome), and glomerulonephritis. The disease is most common in Japan, Turkey, and other Mediterranean countries, with a prevalence approaching 1 in 10,000 (Ninkovic, 1993). It is rare in North America. The cause of Behçet's disease is unknown.

Gastrointestinal complications occur in 10% of patients with Behçet's disease. The presence of ileal and colonic ulcers, arthritis, recurrent oral ulceration, and elevated serum levels of acute-phase reactants leads to confusion between Behçet's and Crohn's disease. However, perianal disease and granulomas are far more common in Crohn's disease than in Behçet's disease (Lee, 1986). Intestinal involvement without oral ulceration or uveitis is rare in Behçet's disease. Human leukocyte antigen (HLA) typing may be helpful; up to 80% of Turkish patients with Behçet's disease have the MHC antigen HLA-B5 (Chajek, 1987).

Therapy for Behçet's disease is more complicated than that for Crohn's disease, because of its multisystem nature, and usually includes a combination of corticosteroids, cytotoxic drugs, anticoagulation for thrombotic episodes, and topical therapy for skin lesions (Ninkovic, 1993). Although the colitis and oral ulcers can generally be controlled, considerable morbidity is associated with ocular Behçet's disease (which can cause blindness) and central nervous system involvement. Central nervous system involvement warrants immunosuppressive therapy (O'Duffy and Goldstein, 1976). Pulmonary hemorrhage associated with aneurysms of the pulmonary arteries has been described (Raz et al., 1989).

Intractable Ulcerating Enterocolitis of Infancy

Sanderson and coworkers (1991b) described a distinct form of chronic inflammatory bowel disease occurring in five children under 6 months of age. These children were of Middle Eastern or Portuguese descent and presented with growth failure, oral and perirectal (but not genital) ulceration, and inflammatory diarrhea. Concentrations of serum immunoglobulins, particularly IgA, were elevated. Small-bowel biopsies demonstrated partial villous atrophy, and colonoscopy demonstrated deep flask-shaped ulcers. Vasculitis or granulomas were not present. The disease progressed despite treatment with corticosteroids, azathioprine, or cyclosporine. In every case, progression of disease necessitated colectomy (Sanderson et al., 1991b).

GASTROINTESTINAL MANIFESTATIONS OF PRIMARY AND SECONDARY IMMUNODEFICIENCIES

Human Immunodeficiency Virus Infection

The gastrointestinal tract is important in patients with human immunodeficiency virus (HIV) infection for several reasons:

1. The intestinal mucosa may be the portal of entry for HIV in some patients, for example, individuals practicing rectal intercourse.
2. Thirty to fifty percent of patients with acquired immunodeficiency syndrome (AIDS) have chronic diarrhea or enteric infections.
3. The resultant diarrhea and malabsorption may result in chronic malnutrition and further impairment

in cell-mediated immunity (Smith and Mai, 1992; Winter and Miller, 1994).

Inflammation of the hepatobiliary system and pancreas may also occur in HIV infection (see Chapter 18).

Pathogenesis

Human immunodeficiency virus can infect CD4 lymphocytes within Peyer's patches and the lamina propria underlying the intestine. The intestinal epithelium contains primarily CD8 lymphocytes, which are much less susceptible to HIV infection. Delivery of intact HIV virus to CD4 cells in the mucosa may occur via the M cell, which in a murine model transports HIV to underlying lymphoid tissue (Amerongen et al., 1991, 1992). Alternatively, infection of mucosal CD4 cells may occur through systemic spread of HIV-containing lymphocytes in patients infected via blood-borne or perinatal transmission.

Whether epithelial cells are infected with HIV is controversial. Villous atrophy and AIDS enteropathy may occur in the absence of any opportunistic pathogens. In addition, some studies of epithelial cell lines suggest that HIV may infect epithelial cells (Adachi et al., 1987). Heise and coworkers (1991), utilizing in situ hybridization, found HIV RNA in enterocytes of five of nine HIV-infected patients. In contrast, Fox and colleagues (1989), who used a similar technique, concluded that intestinal epithelial cells were infrequently (if ever) infected with HIV. Some cases of idiopathic enteropathy presumed related to HIV are probably due to undiagnosed opportunistic infections, now more readily diagnosed by molecular pathology techniques (Grohmann et al., 1993).

Human immunodeficiency virus infection may result in decreased gastric acid secretion and slow intestinal motility, predisposing the patients to bacterial overgrowth (Lake-Bakaar et al., 1988). Smith and coworkers (1988) found that bacterial colony counts in the proximal small intestine of HIV-infected patients were 10- to 100-fold higher than those of healthy control subjects. The mucosal immune system is also affected by HIV infection. There is a marked deficiency of CD4 cells in the intestinal lamina propria. In addition, few activated T cells are seen in the duodenal mucosa (Ullrich et al., 1990). The CD4 cell depletion presumably results in impaired local antibody production, with decreased numbers of IgA-producing mucosal plasma cells (Kotler et al., 1987). These local host defense deficiencies predispose the patient with HIV infection to multiple opportunistic gastrointestinal pathogens.

Clinical Manifestations

The pediatric patient with HIV infection usually presents to the gastroenterologist with weight loss associated with feeding refusal, increased caloric need, diarrhea, or malabsorption. Because malnutrition aggravates HIV morbidity, an aggressive evaluation is warranted (Table 23–16). The history should include a caloric count by a dietician and inquiries about dyspha-

Table 23–16. Suggested Evaluation for the Child With Immunodeficiency and Chronic Diarrhea

Stool Studies
Culture for enteric pathogens including *Salmonella, Shigella, Yersinia, Campylobacter, Escherichia coli* O157:H7, *Clostridium difficile,* and *Aeromonas*
Ova and parasites (including *Isospora belli* and *Enterocytozoon bieneusi*)
Clostridium difficile toxin
Rotavirus and adenovirus ELISA
Acid-fast stain (for *Cryptosporidium*)
Viral culture (for cytomegalovirus)
Electron microscopy (for other viruses)

Tests of Mucosal Function
D-Xylose
Lactose breath hydrogen test
72-hour fecal fat

Endoscopic Evaluation
Upper endoscopy
 Biopsy for histology, including electron microscopy
 Disaccharidase assay
 Duodenal fluid for *Giardia*
 Bacterial colony count
 Bacterial/viral/fungal cultures
Flexible sigmoidoscopy
 Biopsy for histology, including electron microscopy
 Viral culture

Abbreviation: ELISA = enzyme-linked immunosorbent assay.

gia, odynophagia, or diarrhea. About 50% of symptomatic children with HIV infection have evidence of malnutrition, and diarrhea was present in 44% of 544 children in one study (Italian Multicenter Study, 1988).

Physical examination should include an assessment of mental status and feeding behavior. Children with HIV encephalopathy may be unable to swallow, and children with esophagitis push food away. The oropharynx should be carefully examined for thrush or hairy leukoplakia. Patients with pancreatitis, gastritis, or esophagitis may have pain upon palpation of the midepigastrium. The liver and spleen may be massively enlarged and cause anorexia by gastric compression. The presence of leukocytes or blood in the stool suggests infectious colitis.

The conventional and opportunistic pathogens that cause esophagitis, enteropathy, or colitis in patients with AIDS are summarized in Table 23–17. Many of these pathogens are not detected in routine stool cultures. Thus, for the ill patient for whom the cultures and stool analysis fail to yield an infectious organism, esophagogastroduodenoscopy and colonoscopy may be required (Smith et al., 1988). In the esophagus, white exudate (suggestive of candidiasis) or ulcers (suggestive of herpes or cytomegalovirus esophagitis) may be seen; cultures of the esophagus for fungus and virus should be performed. The stomach and duodenum frequently appear normal; however, light or electron microscopy may identify parasites (including *Cryptosporidium, Isospora belli,* microsporidia, and *Mycobacterium avium-intracellulare*). During duodenoscopy, aspiration of fluid (to test for bacterial overgrowth and *Giardia)* and tissue sampling for viruses, mycobacteria, and fungi should be performed. In a patient with colitis, colonoscopy

Table 23–17. Gastrointestinal Microbes and Associated Illness in Patients with Human Immunodeficiency Virus Infection

Pathogen	Illness
Bacteria	
Salmonella	Diarrhea, enteritis, colitis
Shigella	Diarrhea, enteritis, colitis
Yersinia	Diarrhea, enteritis, colitis
Campylobacter	Diarrhea, enteritis, colitis
Dysgonic fermenter-3	Diarrhea, enteritis, colitis
Escherichia coli	Diarrhea, enteritis, colitis
Clostridium difficile	Diarrhea, enteritis, colitis
Aeromonas	Diarrhea, enteritis, colitis
Neisseria	Proctitis
Chlamydia	Proctitis
Fungi	
Candida albicans	Esophagitis
Torulopsis glabrata	Esophagitis
Histoplasma capsulatum	Ileitis
Parasites	
Cryptosporidium	Diarrhea, enteritis
Isospora belli	Diarrhea, enteritis
Microsporidia (Enterocytozoon bieneusi)	Diarrhea, enteritis
Strongyloides stercoralis	Diarrhea, enteritis
Giardia lamblia	Diarrhea, enteritis
Entamoeba histolytica	Colitis
Pneumocystis	Colitis
Mycobacteria	
Mycobacterium avium-intracellulare	Enteritis
Mycobacterium genavense	Enteritis
Viruses	
Cytomegalovirus	Esophagitis, diarrhea, proctocolitis
Herpes simplex virus	Esophagitis, diarrhea, proctocolitis
Rotaviruses	Diarrhea, enteritis
Norwalk viruses	Diarrhea, enteritis
Adenoviruses	Diarrhea, enteritis
Caliciviruses	Diarrhea, enteritis
Picornaviruses	Diarrhea, enteritis
Astroviruses	Diarrhea, enteritis
Adenovirus	Diarrhea, enteritis
Human immunodeficiency virus	Role in enteropathy unclear

may reveal ulcerations suggestive of bacterial, viral, or fungal disease. Utilizing electron microscopy, cultures, and immunoassays, investigators have identified viral infections in 35% of HIV-infected patients with diarrhea (Grohmann et al., 1993).

Diagnosis

A small-bowel biopsy may reveal villous atrophy, chronic inflammation, or focal vacuolization of duodenal enterocytes (Ullrich et al., 1989; Patterson et al., 1993). The presence of large numbers of periodic acid–Schiff (PAS)–positive macrophages suggests atypical mycobacterial infection. Intestinal function can also be assessed by D-xylose absorption, lactose breath hydrogen testing, and a 72-hour stool fat analysis. Miller and coworkers (1991) performed D-xylose and lactose breath tests for 28 HIV-infected children and demonstrated that, whereas abnormal D-xylose absorption

was found in patients with enteric infections, lactose intolerance was frequently present whether or not children had evidence of infection. Occult lactose intolerance may contribute to the abdominal pain or diarrhea in these children.

Complications

Hepatobiliary and pancreatic complications of HIV infection are listed in Table 23–18 (Cappell, 1991). Primary HIV hepatitis is not known to occur, but other viral hepatitides, opportunistic infections of the liver, or drug-induced hepatitis may occur (Reddy and Jeffers, 1993). Infiltration of the hepatic parenchyma with *M. avium-intracellulare, Mycobacterium tuberculosis, Candida, Cryptococcus, Histoplasma,* herpes simplex virus, *Pneumocystis carinii,* hepatitis viruses, or malignancy results in hepatomegaly and transaminitis. Biliary cryptosporidiosis, microsporidiosis, or cytomegalovirus infection leads to obstructive cholangiopathy, hyperbilirubinemia, and clinical jaundice. In this syndrome, abdominal ultrasonography may show dilated bile ducts, and the patient should undergo endoscopic retrograde cholangiopancreatography for analysis and culture of biliary fluid (Benhamou et al., 1993; Pol et al., 1993). In patients with cholangitis or biliary duct stricture, papillary sphincterotomy may provide symptomatic relief (Benhamou et al., 1993). Pancreatitis occurs in 17% of pediatric patients with HIV infection and is characterized by high serum lipase levels and only mild elevations in amylase (Miller et al., 1992). The presence of pancreatitis is associated with a low CD4 count,

Table 23–18. Causes of Liver Disease in HIV Infection and AIDS

Viral hepatitis
   Hepatitis A, B, C, delta viruses
   Cytomegalovirus
   Epstein-Barr virus
   Herpes simplex virus
   Varicella virus
   Human immunodeficiency virus

Other hepatic infections
   Mycobacterium tuberculosis
   Atypical mycobacteria
   Fungi, including *Candida, Histoplasma,* and *Cryptococcus*
   Parasites, including *Entamoeba histolytica*
   Pyogenic liver abscesses

Cholangiopathy
   Infectious, most commonly due to *Cryptosporidium,* cytomegalovirus, or Microsporidia
   Primary sclerosing cholangitis

Drug-associated
   Amphotericin B
   Clindamycin
   Trimethoprim-sulfamethoxazole
   Rifampin
   Zidovudine

Neoplasm

Abbreviations: HIV = human immunodeficiency virus; AIDS = acquired immunodeficiency syndrome.

Table 23–19. Antimicrobial Therapies for Opportunistic Gastrointestinal Human Immunodeficiency Virus Infections

Pathogen	Therapy
Candida albicans	Nystatin or ketoconazole or fluconazole or amphotericin
Cytomegalovirus (colitis, esophagitis)	Ganciclovir or foscarnet
Mycobacterium avium–intracellulare	Rifampin and ethambutol and clofazimine and ciprofloxacin with or without amikacin Clarithromycin and azithromycin may also be effective
Isospora belli	Trimethoprim-sulfamethoxazole
Giardia lamblia	Metronidazole or furazolidone or quinacrine
Cryptosporidium	No proven therapy Octreotide provides symptomatic relief

Adapted from Med Lett 33:95–102, 1991.

the use of zidovudine and dideoxyinosine, and a poor prognosis (Miller et al., 1992).

Treatment

Treatment of the HIV-infected child with gastrointestinal illness involves identification of and antimicrobial therapy for enteric pathogens, symptomatic relief of diarrhea, and aggressive enteral or parenteral nutritional support. A summary of antimicrobial therapies directed at gastrointestinal pathogens in HIV infection is given in Table 23–19. Many of the common opportunistic pathogens, including cytomegalovirus, atypical mycobacteria, and cryptosporidia, are cleared poorly with current therapy, and diarrhea persists. Plettenberg and colleagues (1993), in an open-label trial, utilized oral bovine colostrum in the treatment of 18 HIV-infected patients with refractory cryptosporidiosis and observed improvement or resolution of diarrhea in 64% of them. Patients with refractory diarrhea may benefit from subcutaneous injections of octreotide, an analog of somatostatin with a long half-life. Octreotide slows bowel motility and decreases electrolyte secretion by the enterocyte; a multicenter clinical trial has demonstrated its efficacy in reducing stool frequency and volume in diarrhea associated with AIDS (Cello et al., 1991).

In addition to symptomatic therapy for intestinal illness, nutritional support of the HIV-infected child is often necessary. Most HIV-infected infants have normal birth weights but postnatally show a falloff in weight and weight for height (Miller et al., 1993). Anorexia and vomiting associated with extraintestinal infections, esophagitis, gastritis, or medications are common. Gastrostomy tube placement may facilitate enteral feedings. For children with pancreatitis, intractable diarrhea, or severe reflux, parenteral nutrition should be considered (Winter and Miller, 1994).

Intestinal Lymphangiectasia

Intestinal lymphangiectasia refers to a primary or secondary impairment of lymphatic drainage variably associated with fat malabsorption and loss of serum proteins and lymphocytes (see Chapters 12 and 19). Primary intestinal lymphangiectasia results from lymphatic dysplasia and may occur as an isolated phenomenon or in association with thoracic lymphatic malformations (chylous ascites) or peripheral lymphedema (lymphedema praecox, Milroy's disease) (Hilliard et al., 1990). In contrast, secondary intestinal lymphangiectasia results from obstruction of lymph flow from the lymphatics and into the heart and may be caused by intestinal inflammatory disorders, increased right-sided heart pressure (e.g., after a Fontan operation for congenital heart disease), obstruction of mesentric lymphatic outflow (e.g., by intermittent bowel volvulus), or obstruction of the thoracic duct (e.g., by an intrathoracic tumor).

Pathogenesis

The resultant lymphatic obstruction leads to loss of serum proteins and lymphocytes from the bowel, villous blunting (Fig. 23–15), fat and fat-soluble vitamin malabsorption, hypoalbuminemia, hypocalcemia, abdominal pain, and growth failure (Vardy et al., 1975; Fonkalsrud, 1977). Immunologic abnormalities are

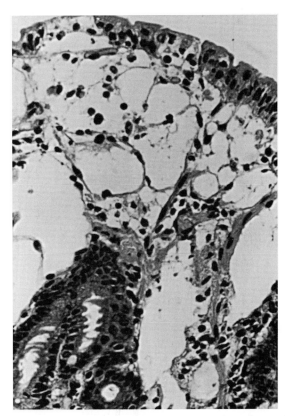

Figure 23–15. Peroral small-intestinal biopsy specimen from a 2½-year-old patient with intestinal lymphangiectasia, manifested by chronic diarrhea, failure to thrive, hypoproteinemia, and lymphedema of one extremity. Villous architecture is distorted; distended lymphatic channels appear to be bursting through the epithelial cells.

present in severe cases of intestinal lymphangiectasia and are due to the loss of immunoglobulins and lymphocytes into the bowel. Although antibody synthesis remains normal, antibody titers are low because of increased losses (Strober et al., 1967). Defects in cell-mediated immunity include lymphopenia, decreased T-cell numbers, impaired in vitro responses to mitogens and specific antigens, cutaneous anergy, and diminished skin graft rejection (Weiden et al., 1972). Yamamoto and coworkers (1989) identified a patient in whom the peripheral blood was depleted of CD4 T cells, although normal numbers B cells were present; they postulated that this patient may have had a selective impairment of T-cell help.

Clinical Manifestations

The clinical severity of intestinal lymphangiectasia ranges from mild edema with hypoalbuminemia to severe malabsorption requiring parenteral nutrition. In severe cases, growth failure, steatorrhea, chylous ascites, and pleural or pericardial effusions develop. Less common intestinal complications include gastrointestinal bleeding and intestinal ileus (Perisic and Kokai, 1991; Lenzhofer et al., 1993). Despite lymphopenia and hypogammaglobulinemia, severe infections in these patients are rare. However, in one of our patients bacterial sepsis and peritonitis developed, and in another patient fatal fulminant sepsis developed.

Diagnosis

Laboratory studies show hypocalcemia, hypogammaglobulinemia, lymphopenia, and increased 72-hour fecal fat excretion. Radiographic contrast studies show thickened intestinal folds consistent with malabsorption in 50% of the patients. A fecal $alpha_1$-antitrypsin level is used to confirm the diagnosis of protein-losing enteropathy (Gleason, 1993). Small-bowel biopsy demonstrates dilated lacteals and distortion of the villous architecture (see Fig. 23–15); several biopsy specimens should be analyzed because of the patchy nature of the lesion.

Treatment

Treatment includes restricting dietary fat, monitoring and correcting deficiencies of fat-soluble vitamins, providing nutritional support, and managing peripheral edema. For infants, Portagen is the formula of choice because it contains no long-chain fat. However, a small amoung of long-chain fat should be given enterally (as safflower oil or Lipomul) to prevent essential fatty acid deficiency (Holt, 1964). For older children, a fat-free diet with added medium-chain triglycerides reduces intestinal protein loss, edema, and ascites and corrects albumin and calcium deficiencies (Vardy et al., 1975). In patients with secondary lymphangiectasia, treatment of the underlying cause may reverse the intestinal abnormalities. Some patients with lymphangiectasia after a Fontan operation have improved with corticosteroid therapy (Rothman and Snyder, 1991). Patients with

recurrent infections and hypogammaglobulinemia may benefit from intravenous immunoglobulin (IVIG) therapy; however, the half-life of IVIG in these patients is shortened because of intestinal loss.

Acrodermatitis Enteropathica

Acrodermatitis enteropathica is an autosomal recessive disorder of zinc absorption, manifested in infancy by severe dermatitis, alopecia, diarrhea, and zinc deficiency (Van Wouwe, 1989). In addition to the congenital form, the term acrodermatitis enteropathica may be applied to secondary zinc deficiency states with similar clinical manifestations. Zinc deficiency in acrodermatitis was first described by Barnes and Moynahan in 1973. Others soon confirmed this observation and described a rapid therapeutic response to oral zinc (Michaelson, 1974; Thyresson, 1974; Nelder and Hambidge, 1975).

Pathogenesis

Patients with congenital acrodermatitis enteropathica have a negative zinc balance and reduced quantities of zinc in the small intestinal mucosa. Although the inherited molecular defect in acrodermatitis is unknown, patients have diminished zinc absorption with a normal diet. Zinc absorption improves when the intraluminal zinc concentration is increased by dietary supplementation.

Acquired zinc deficiency can result from inadequate intake, defective absorption, or excessive loss. Conditions associated with zinc deficiency include Crohn's disease, intractable diarrhea of infancy, long-term parenteral nutrition with inadequate zinc, high output ileostomy, celiac disease, and cystic fibrosis (Silverman and Roy, 1983). Infants with inborn errors of metabolism maintained with a non–animal milk formula or other special formulas may become zinc-deficient.

Zinc deficiency has profound effects on the immune system. In murine models, dietary zinc restriction causes thymic atrophy and depresses humoral responses through loss of helper T-cell function. Patients with acrodermatitis enteropathica demonstrate increased susceptibility to infection because of depressed humoral and cellular immunity (Good et al., 1979). Findings of autopsies in children demonstrate decreased lymphoid tissue (including Peyer's patches) and thymic abnormalities (Rodin and Goldman, 1969; Julius et al., 1973). Golden and colleagues (1977, 1978) have shown that the T-cell immunodeficiency of protein-calorie malnutrition (PCM) is associated with zinc deficiency. One patient with acrodermatitis presented with selective IgG deficiency that resolved with zinc supplementation (Wilson et al., 1982). Zinc treatment for PCM enhances delayed cutaneous hypersensitivity and reverses thymic atrophy. However, the sera of patients with acrodermatitis may also contain autoantibodies (including antinuclear antibodies and rheumatoid factor), and these persist despite zinc supplementation (Anttila et al., 1986).

Clinical Manifestations

Acrodermatitis enteropathica presents in infancy, usually between 4 and 10 weeks of age. The onset is delayed in breast-fed infants but occurs several weeks after weaning. Principal findings include intensive acral and orofacial eczematous vesiculopustular dermatitis, progressive alopecia, and diarrhea. Stomatitis, glossitis, photophobia, corneal opacities, blepharitis, conjunctivitis, angular cheilitis with drooling, hoarseness, paronychia, nail dystrophy, and irritability may also occur. Secondary infection often complicates the illness. Secondary zinc deficiency resulting from chronic diarrhea may also cause immune abnormalities; in one case, there was a return of cell-mediated immunity after correction of the zinc deficiency (Oleske et al., 1979).

Diagnosis

The diagnosis of acrodermatitis enteropathica is based on the clinical features and the presence of abnormally low plasma levels of zinc (less than 50 μg/dl). Care must be taken to avoid contamination of the specimen, which can lead to falsely elevated zinc levels (Garretts and Molokhia, 1977). All tubing and glassware should be acid-washed and ordinary rubber stoppers avoided, because commercially available tubes and stoppers (such as Vacutainers) contain zinc. Zinc levels in hair are not reliable because they are dependent on normal growth; in acrodermatitis, hair growth is slow and hair zinc levels may be only slightly depressed. Urinary zinc levels are also abnormally low and return to normal within 2 to 3 weeks after therapy (Nelder and Hambidge, 1975). They correlate well with plasma levels and can be used to monitor therapy. Serum levels are falsely decreased in the presence of hypoalbuminemia. Serum alkaline phosphatase, a zinc-dependent enzyme, is abnormally low in patients with untreated acrodermatitis and returns to normal with zinc therapy.

Treatment

Oral zinc therapy results in both clinical remission and normalization of immune function. The daily dose of zinc sulfide recommended is 30 to 45 mg (Lungarotti et al., 1976; Silverman and Roy, 1983). No side effects of therapy have been reported.

Prognosis

Oral zinc supplementation must be continued indefinitely in the inborn disorder. Skin improvement begins within several days, with complete healing in weeks. Diarrhea resolves rapidly (1 week), and hair growth recommences within 2 to 3 weeks (Nelder et al., 1978). Prognosis is favorable with therapy, whereas if the patient remains untreated, malnutrition and death may occur, usually by 3 years of age.

Selective IgA Deficiency

Selective IgA deficiency is the most common primary immunodeficiency, with a prevalence as high as 1 in 500 humans (see Chapter 14). The most common gastrointestinal infection associated with secretory IgA deficiency is giardiasis, which may lead to partial villous atrophy and secondary malabsorption (Zinneman and Kaplan, 1972; Cunningham-Rundles, 1988; Morgan and Levinsky, 1988) (Table 23–20). Diagnosis of giardiasis may be difficult; even three stool examinations may miss up to 10% of cases. An enzyme-linked immunosorbent assay (ELISA) for *Giardia* antigen that has become available may increase the sensitivity of detection to 98% (Addiss et al., 1991). For the patient in whom giardiasis is suspected but not found, a string test (sampling duodenal fluid by oral ingestion of a string-coated capsule, followed by withdrawal of the string), endoscopy for duodenal aspirate, or an empirical trial of antibiotic therapy should be considered. Metronidazole, tinidazole, furazolidone, and quinacrine are effective antibiotics for giardiasis, with cure rates in nonimmunocompromised hosts of 60% to 95% (Shepherd and Boreham, 1989). Patients with IgA deficiency frequently have recurrences, necessitating repeated treatment or treatment of family members and pets.

Bacterial overgrowth has also been reported in association with selective IgA deficiency (Pignata et al., 1990).

Patients with selective IgA deficiency have a 10-fold relative risk of developing celiac disease; conversely, 1 in 200 patients with celiac disease has selective IgA deficiency (Cunningham-Rundles, 1988; Collin et al., 1992). Because the antiendomysial antibody used in the diagnosis of celiac disease is an IgA molecule, this test may miss patients with selective IgA deficiency and celiac disease; in contrast, the IgG class antireticulin antibodies are positive in 94% of patients (Collin et al., 1992). It is not known whether the increased incidence of celiac disease in patients with selective IgA deficiency represents genetic linkage of two diseases or whether the defect in IgA secretion predisposes to celiac disease. Rarely, idiopathic villous atrophy without celiac disease is seen in patients with selective IgA deficiency.

Food and systemic allergy may also be present in patients with selective IgA deficiency (Ammann and Hong, 1971). Patients have high titers of serum antibodies to milk, as well as increased circulating immune complexes after milk ingestion (Buckley and Dees, 1969; Cunningham-Rundles et al., 1978). However,

Table 23–20. Gastrointestinal Manifestations of Immunoglobulin A Deficiency

1. None (majority of patients)
2. *Giardia lamblia* infestation (often recurrent)
3. Nodular lymphoid hyperplasia
4. Nonspecific enteropathy ± bacteria overgrowth ± disaccharidase deficiency
5. Increased incidence of circulating antibodies to food antigens
6. Gluten-sensitive enteropathy
7. Pernicious anemia/atrophic gastritis/increased risk of gastric cancer
8. Idiopathic inflammatory bowel disease (Crohn's disease, ulcerative colitis)

there is no correlation between these abnormalities and clinical allergy (Cunningham-Rundles, 1988). Lymphoid nodular hyperplasia and sarcoidosis have also been associated with IgA deficiency (Disdier et al., 1991). Finally, there is an increased risk for the development of certain cancers, particularly lymphoma and gastric adenocarcinoma (Cunningham-Rundles et al., 1980).

X-Linked Agammaglobulinemia

X-linked agammaglobulinemia presents with recurrent infections in male infants after 9 months of age as a result of failure of synthesis of all classes of immunoglobulins (see Chapter 11). In a review of 96 patients, Lederman and Winkelstein (1985) found otitis media, sinusitis, pneumonitis, infectious diarrheas, meningitis, and oligoarticular arthritis to be common complications. Furthermore, 10% of patients developed chronic diarrhea, with rotavirus, *Giardia lamblia, Salmonella,* and enteropathogenic *E. coli* the identified pathogens. Other causes of chronic enteritis in patients with X-linked agammaglobulinemia include bacterial overgrowth, *Campylobacter, Cryptosporidium,* coxsackievirus, and poliovirus (Lederman and Winkelstein, 1985; Arbo and Santos, 1987).

An association with sclerosing cholangitis and sprue-like illness has also been noted, but it is unclear whether autoimmune disease is actually increased in these patients (Stiehm et al., 1986; Sisto et al., 1987). In older patients, amyloidosis, atrophic gastritis, pernicious anemia, and gastric adenocarcinomas are seen (Lavilla et al., 1993; Meysman et al., 1993).

Transient Hypogammaglobulinemia of Infancy

Transient hypogammaglobulinemia of infancy is prolonged and exaggerated symptomatic physiologic hypogammaglobulinemia (see Chapters 10 and 11). Affecting children between 1 and 3 years of age, this disorder is characterized by low levels of serum IgG or IgG subclasses; IgA or IgM levels may also be decreased. McGeady (1986) has postulated that some of these children develop persistent hypogammaglobulinemia or selective IgA deficiency.

Perlmutter and colleagues (1985) reported 55 patients with transient hypogammaglobulinemia and diarrhea; lactose intolerance, *G. lamblia* infestation, and *C. difficile* infection were frequently identified. Recurrent *C. difficile* infection is particularly difficult to manage in these children and causes either pseudomembranous enterocolitis or chronic diarrhea with failure to thrive (Sutphen et al., 1983). In a survey of 43 infants and children with *C. difficile* infection, 35% had hypogammaglobulinemia (Gryboski et al., 1991). Patients with hypogammaglobulinemia may lack the ability to make antibodies to *C. difficile* toxin A, the putative mediator of the enteropathy in *C. difficile* colitis (Triadafilopoulos et al., 1987; Leung et al., 1991).

Fifty percent of patients with transient hypogammaglobulinemia have histologic small-bowel enteritis, ranging from mild inflammation to complete villous atrophy. Antibiotic therapy or a lactose-free diet benefits those with identifiable microbial pathogens or lactose intolerance. For patients with *C. difficile* infection, vancomycin or metronidazole is used. Recurrence of *C. difficile* infection occurs in 20% to 30% of patients and can be treated with a prolonged, tapering course of vancomycin (Peterson and Gerding, 1990). In addition, intravenous immunoglobulin (IVIG) may help prevent recurrences in the immunodeficient patient (Leung et al., 1991). Otherwise, chronic diarrhea may persist for 18 months, and other therapies are rarely necessary (Perlmutter et al., 1985). Some patients have recurrent systemic infections and may benefit from regular IVIG infusions (Benderly et al., 1986; Kosnik et al., 1986).

Common Variable Immunodeficiency

Common variable immunodeficiency (CVID) has an onset in late childhood or adulthood and is characterized by low levels of IgG and the other immunoglobulin classes (see Chapter 11). Recurrent otitis media, bronchitis, pneumonia and sinusitis are the most common presenting features, but gastrointestinal disease occurs in up to 70% of patients and accounts for much morbidity (Table 23–21) (Hausser et al., 1983). The enteropathy can be either infectious or autoimmune (Sperber and Mayer, 1988).

Giardia is the most common gastrointestinal infectious agent, but *Salmonella, Campylobacter, Cryptosporidium,* or rotavirus may also be implicated (Webster, 1980; Sperber and Mayer, 1988). Nodular lymphoid hyperplasia, defined as multiple discrete lymphoid aggregates in the stomach and small bowel, is detected radiographically or endoscopically in up to 20% of patients and may predispose to either malabsorption or gastrointestinal bleeding (Bennett et al., 1987; Bastlein et al., 1988). Massive nodular lymphoid hyperplasia may develop and be difficult to distinguish from lymphoma. Sander and coworkers (1992), utilizing techniques of in situ hybridization for Epstein-Barr virus and immunohistochemical staining for clonality, concluded that the majority of lymphoid lesions in patients with CVID were benign and not associated with Epstein-Barr virus infection. However, 2 of their 17 patients developed malignant lymphoma. One patient with nodular lymphoid hyperplasia had a clonal B-cell population but has been observed for over 4 years without developing lymphoma, suggesting that clonality does not necessarily result in malignancy (Laszewski et al., 1990).

An association between CVID and celiac disease exists, but the risk is less than for patients with selective

Table 23–21. Gastrointestinal Manifestations of Common Variable Immunodeficiency

1. Infectious diarrhea (*Giardia*, bacterial, viral)
2. Bacterial overgrowth syndrome
3. Pernicious anemia/atrophic gastritis/gastric carcinoma
4. Nodular lymphoid hyperplasia
5. Gluten-sensitive enteropathy
6. Nonspecific enteropathy/colitis

IgA deficiency (Webster et al., 1981). Idiopathic sprue with subtotal villous atrophy is also reported in patients with no infections and is generally unresponsive to a gluten-free diet (Conley et al., 1986; Catassi et al., 1988). This "hypogammaglobulinemic sprue" is characterized by decreased brush border enzyme activity and lactose intolerance (Dawson et al., 1986). A granulomatous enteropathy with granulomas scattered throughout the intestine has been reported in adults with CVID (Mike et al., 1991). Patients have a high incidence of gastritis and pernicious anemia–like syndrome, without antibodies to intrinsic factor, gastric parietal cells, or thyroglobulin (Twomey et al., 1970). Other gastrointestinal abnormalities include bacterial overgrowth, aphthous stomatitis, cholelithiasis, malacoplakia, and inflammatory bowel disease (Sperber and Mayer, 1988). Severe malabsorption associated with enteropathy in patients with CVID may result in hyperoxaluria, vitamin B_{12} deficiency, and caloric deprivation and may require parenteral nutrition (Bennett et al., 1987).

Hyper-IgM Syndrome

Immunodeficiency with hyper-IgM is characterized by high serum IgM levels, low IgG and IgA levels, recurrent infections, intermittent leukopenia, lymphoid hyperplasia, and autoimmune disorders. Patients with the hyper-IgM syndrome have recurrent oral ulcers and gingivitis (particularly when they are leukopenic) and less commonly have chronic diarrhea and lymphoid nodular hyperplasia. The lymphoid nodular hyperplasia may be massive enough to cause a functional colon obstruction and require steroid therapy. Esophageal histoplasmosis and small-bowel cryptosporidiosis have also been reported (Stiehm et al., 1986; Tu et al., 1991).

Severe Combined Immunodeficiency

Patients with severe combined immunodeficiency (SCID) have profound antibody and T-cell immune defects and present in the first months of life with chronic diarrhea, failure to thrive, and persistent viral or fungal infections (see Chapter 12). Gastrointestinal illness occurs in 90% of these patients, and intractable diarrhea and oral thrush are common presenting features. Organisms frequently associated with illness include rotavirus, *Candida,* cytomegalovirus, and *E. coli.* Chronic viral infection is the most frequent cause of enteritis (Stephan et al., 1992). Jarvis and coworkers (1983) isolated viral pathogens from the stool in 9 of 12 patients with SCID and chronic diarrhea; the viruses identified included rotavirus, picornavirus, adenovirus type 5, and coxsackievirus A. The viral enteritis was partially or directly responsible for death in 80% of cases. Other less common causes of enteropathy noted include *Salmonella, Shigella,* and *Cryptosporidium* infections. Although candidiasis rarely involves the intestine, candidal esophagitis should be suspected in infants with SCID who have decreased oral intake (Stiehm et al., 1986; Arbo and Santos, 1987).

In some patients with SCID, enteropathy or colitis occurs in the absence of identifiable infection. Some investigators have postulated that this is an immune-mediated enteritis (S. Strobel, personal communication); however, antienterocyte antibodies or antinuclear cytoplasmic antibodies have not been described in patients with SCID. Gilger and colleagues (1992) utilized immunostaining to look for extraintestinal rotavirus infection in infants with SCID. Rotaviral particles were found in the kidney and liver of four patients, leading the investigators to postulate that rotavirus may also cause systemic illness.

Bare Lymphocyte Syndrome

Another cause of profound cellular immunodeficiency phenotypically similar to SCID is the bare lymphocyte syndrome, the absence of MHC class II molecules on the surface of immune cells (see Chapter 12). In a review of 30 patients with the syndrome (Klein et al., 1993), almost all had some form of gastrointestinal illness. Gastrointestinal candidiasis was present in 25 patients, and giardiasis, cryptosporidiosis, and other bacterial enteritides were present. In addition, a high incidence of hepatobiliary abnormalities was noted. Ten patients had evidence of biliary tract disease, including sclerosing cholangitis in four patients (associated with biliary cryptosporidiosis in three of the four). Bacterial cholangitis involving *Pseudomonas, Enterococcus,* and *Streptococcus* was also seen.

Combined Immunodeficiency With Predominant T-Cell Defect

Commonly referred to as *Nezelof syndrome,* this disorder is characterized by absent T-cell function and a variable B-cell defect with some serum immunoglobulin production (Nezelof, 1968) (see Chapter 12). Some of these patients present in late infancy and childhood; others present in early infancy. The literature has limited information regarding their gastrointestinal complications. One older child with a mild variant of Nezelof syndrome presented with recurrent chest infections and chronic malabsorption; a mucosal biopsy demonstrated villous atrophy and a mucosal plasma cell infiltrate (Novis et al., 1985).

Chronic Mucocutaneous Candidiasis

Chronic mucocutaneous candidiasis (CMC) is characterized by a diminished T-cell response to candidal antigens and severe local candidiasis. Infants may present with persistent thrush or candidal dermatitis, failure to thrive, and dystrophic nails (see Chapter 12). The principal gastrointestinal complication is candidal esophagitis, which may result in food refusal (Kirkpatrick, 1989). In a series of 43 patients, chronic active hepatitis and giardiasis developed in 5% of the patients (Herrod, 1990). A polyglandular endocrinopathy syndrome characterized by hypoparathyroidism, hypothyroidism, adrenal insufficiency, and pernicious anemia develops in up to 70% of older children. Malabsorption associated with pancreatic insufficiency contributes to the poor weight gain in 10% of patients and requires pancreatic enzyme supplementation (Herrod, 1990).

Chronic Granulomatous Disease

Chronic granulomatous disease (CGD) is caused by an inability of the patient's phagocytes to generate superoxide, leading to infections with catalase-positive organisms, including *Staphylococcus aureus, Serratia, Aspergillus,* and *Nocardia* (Lehrer et al., 1988) (see Chapter 15). The clinical syndrome includes recurrent infections, multifocal abscesses affecting the skin and liver, lymphadenopathy, hepatosplenomegaly, chronic lung disease, and diarrhea. Small-bowel involvement with inflammatory cells may mimic that in Crohn's disease, with diarrhea, protein-losing enteropathy, pancolitis, small-bowel obstruction, and fistulizing disease. Multifocal abscesses, giant cells, and noncaseating granulomatous colitis are present on endoscopic biopsy specimens of patients who have colonic inflammation (Werlin et al., 1982; Isaacs et al., 1985). The presence of lipid-containing histiocytes in the mucosa and submucosa of colon biopsy specimens suggests CGD rather than Crohn's disease (Werlin et al., 1982; Lindahl et al., 1984). The colitis of patients with CGD may respond to therapy with sulfasalazine or interferon-γ, but surgical resection may be necessary for intractable colitis or acute obstruction (Ezekowitz et al., 1991). High doses of steroids have also been used to treat patients with intestinal or urinary tract obstruction (Chin et al., 1987).

Leukocyte Adhesion Defect

Patients with leukocyte adhesion defect (LAD) have impaired phagocytic function related to deficiencies of adhesion molecules (CD18/Mac-1) necessary for cell migration and interactions (see Chapters 15, 16, and 17). Necrotic infections of the skin (including pyoderma gangrenosum) and mucous membranes, otitis media, and episodes of microbial sepsis are the principal features. (Anderson and Springer, 1987; Voss and Rhodes, 1992). Gastrointestinal complications include intraoral infections and periodontitis, candidal esophagitis, gastritis, appendicitis, necrotizing enterocolitis, and perirectal abcess (Anderson and Springer, 1987; Todd and Freyer, 1988; Roberts and Atkinson, 1990). Fatal necrotizing enterocolitis developed in one child at 18 months of age (Hawkins et al., 1992). Therapy includes antibiotic therapy for infections and bone marrow transplantation in severe cases.

Glycogen Storage Disease Type 1b

Patients who have glycogen storage disease (GSD) type 1b present with severe hypoglycemia, failure to thrive, and hepatomegaly (see Chapters 15, 16, and 19). In contrast to those with von Gierke's disease (GSD type 1a), these patients have severe neutropenia and phagocytic dysfunction (Gitzelmann and Bosshard, 1993). Glycogen storage disease type 1a is characterized

biochemically by absence of glucose-6-phosphatase activity, and GSD type 1b is characterized by absence of the hepatic glucose-6-phosphate transport protein (Nordlie et al., 1993).

The primary intestinal complication of patients with GSD type 1b is an idiopathic colitis clinically indistinguishable from that in Crohn's disease (Roe et al., 1986; Couper et al., 1991). The intestinal manifestations develop in late childhood or adolescence and include oral ulceration, perianal infections, anemia, and transmural colonic inflammation with stricturing. This colitis, as well as that in chronic granulomatous disease and congenital neutropenia, has led Couper and colleagues (1991) to speculate that neutrophil deficiency or dysfunction predisposes to granulomatous colitis. Indeed, Roe and coworkers (1992) utilized granulocyte-macrophage colony-stimulating factor (GM-CSF) in the treatment of two patients with GSD type 1b and noted increased neutrophil counts, decreased sedimentation rates, and decreased bowel inflammation, which suggests that raising the neutrophil count may have a beneficial effect on the bowel lesion.

IMMUNE DISORDERS OF THE LIVER AND BILE DUCTS

Hepatic inflammation arises as an immune response against infectious agents (e.g., in viral hepatitis) or against self-antigens (e.g., in autoimmune chronic active hepatitis). A discussion of viral or other infectious hepatitides can be found elsewhere (Balistreri, 1988; Alter and Sampliner, 1989; Hoofnagle, 1990; Krugman, 1992; Koff, 1993). A partial list of diseases causing chronic hepatitis is given in Table 23–22. We focus on two immune-mediated disorders seen in pediatric patients: autoimmune chronic active hepatitis and primary sclerosing cholangitis.

Chronic Active Hepatitis

Chronic active hepatitis (CAH) is a progressive, destructive inflammatory disease characterized by portal tract infiltration with mononuclear cells and destruc-

Table 23–22. Causes of Chronic Active Hepatitis

Autoimmune	*Drug-related*
Type I and type II	Alcoholic liver disease
	Alpha-methyldopa
Virus-associated	Isoniazid
Hepatitis B	Phenothiazines
Hepatitis C	Oxyphenacetin
Delta hepatitis	Nitrofurantoin
Human immunodeficiency	Halothane
virus	Sulfonamides
	Propylthiouracil
Metabolic	
Wilson's disease	*Miscellaneous*
Alpha₁-antitrypsin deficiency	Non-alcoholic
Hemochromatosis	steatohepatitis
Primary hepatobiliary disorders	
Primary biliary cirrhosis	
Sclerosing cholangitis	

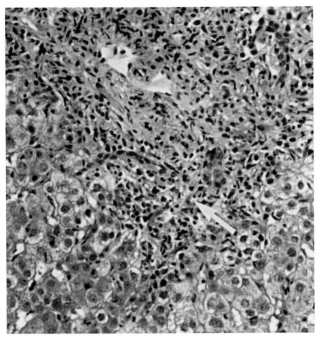

Figure 23–16. Liver biopsy specimen from a 14-year-old girl with chronic active hepatitis unassociated with hepatitis B. The portal tract area is enlarged and demonstrates fibrosis (*upper center*). Infiltration of the portal tract by lymphocytes and plasma cells extends beyond the limiting plate, causing piecemeal necrosis (*arrow*). Hepatocytes surrounding the portal zone demonstrate moderate swelling. (× 250.) (Courtesy of P. Brochu, M.D., Montreal, Canada.)

tion of the limiting plate of hepatocytes surrounding the portal tract. In advanced cases, strands of fibrous tissue connecting portal triads (bridging fibrosis), ultimately progressing to macro- or micronodular cirrhosis, are present (Fig. 23–16). Chronic active hepatitis may occur as a result of viral infection, toxin or drug exposure, metabolic disease, or autoimmune hepatitis (see Table 23–22). Autoimmune CAH is characterized by an extensive periportal hepatic infiltrate, the presence of antibodies against different hepatocyte antigens, association with certain HLA antigens, autoimmune diseases, and a good response to immunosuppressive therapy.

Classification

Autoimmune chronic active hepatitis has now been classified into two major types based on clinical fea-

tures and the types of antibody present (Table 23–23). Type I autoimmune CAH (formerly designated classical CAH or lupoid CAH) occurs predominantly in young women (often in the second or third decade of life) and is characterized by hypergammaglobulinemia and by antibodies to the cytoskeletal protein F-actin (i.e., anti–smooth muscle antibodies).

In contrast, type II autoimmune CAH occurs predominantly in young children and adolescents. It is characterized by the presence of antibodies to the cytochrome P_{450} component IID6 (anti–liver-kidney microsomal antibodies, anti–LKM-1) (Johnson et al., 1991; Boyer and Reuben, 1993). Both disorders are associated with other autoimmune illness (including thyroiditis, diabetes, and vitiligo), and both respond to immunosuppressive therapy. However, initial reports suggest that type II autoimmune CAH may have a worse prognosis, with 80% progression to cirrhosis after 3 years (Homberg et al., 1987). Other variants of autoimmune CAH probably exist, as antibodies to several different liver antigens have been discovered (see later). In addition, a form of CAH has been described that is histologically similar to autoimmune CAH and is corticosteroid responsive but in which antibodies to liver antigens are not present (Czaja et al., 1993a).

Pathogenesis

Like other autoimmune disorders, autoimmune CAH tends to occur in genetically susceptible individuals with an aberrant response to target tissue (in this case, the hepatocytes and biliary epithelium). A genetic predisposition to autoimmune CAH can be identified in one third of European and American patients; type I autoimmune CAH has been associated with two HLA types: HLA-A1/B8/DR3, and HLA-DR4 (Donaldson et al., 1991; Czaja et al., 1993b). Autoimmune CAH associated with HLA-DR4 tends to occur in older patients and is more responsive to corticosteroid therapy, but it is unclear whether there is a better long-term prognosis. Japanese patients with autoimmune CAH are more likely to have the HLA-DR4 allele (Seki et al., 1990; Maddrey, 1993).

Many believe that hepatitis C is an important trigger for type II autoimmune CAH. Lenzi and coworkers (1990, 1991) found that 88% of patients with autoimmune CAH type II (with positive anti–LKM-1 antibody) had evidence of prior hepatitis C infection.

Table 23–23. Antibodies Present in Autoimmune Chronic Active Hepatitis (CAH)

Antibody	Antigen	Disease	Comments
Anti–smooth muscle	P-Actin	CAH type I	Also seen in primary biliary cirrhosis
Anti–liver-kidney microsome 1 (anti–LKM-1)	Cytochrome P_{450} IID6	CAH type II	Predominantly in European children, possible association with hepatitis C
Anti-LKM-2	Cytochrome P_{450}-8	Ticrynafen-induced hepatitis	
Anti-LKM-3	Unknown	Delta virus hepatitis (hepatitis D)	
Antinuclear antibodies (ANA)	Nuclear histones	CAH type I	Nonspecific finding
Anti–soluble liver antigen (anti-SLA)	Hepatocyte cytoplasmic protein	CAH type I Other CAH	Seen in CAH I, may also define a third type of CAH

Data from Maddrey WC. How many types of autoimmune hepatitis are there? Gastroenterology 105:1571–1575, 1993; Johnson PJ, McFarlane IG, Eddleston AL. The natural course and heterogeneity of chronic active hepatitis. Semin Liver Dis 11:187–196, 1991.

Manns (1991) demonstrated a 50% incidence of hepatitis C infection in type II autoimmune CAH, compared with a 0% incidence in type I autoimmune CAH. However, Vergani and Mieli-Vergani (1993) found no association with hepatitis C infection in British patients with autoimmune CAH, leading them to speculate that there is geographic and genetic heterogeneity in autoimmune CAH.

There is even less information on what agents trigger inflammation in type I autoimmune CAH. Vento and coworkers (1991) prospectively monitored 58 healthy relatives of 13 patients with autoimmune CAH type I. Two of the 58 subjects who contracted mild hepatitis A developed type I autoimmune CAH within 5 months of infection. Therefore, hepatitis A may be a risk factor for type I autoimmune CAH in genetically predisposed individuals (Vento et al., 1991).

Several authors have postulated that antibodies to actin, cytochromes, and other liver components are important in the immune-mediated liver damage, either directly or through antibody-dependent cytotoxicity (MacFarlane, 1991; Manns, 1991). The nature and significance of the T-cell infiltrate in autoimmune CAH have not yet been determined. Schlaak and colleagues (1993) isolated and cloned the T cells from liver tissues of patients with autoimmune CAH and found the predominant clones isolated to be IL-4–producing CD4 T cells. In contrast, Li and coworkers (1991), analyzing hepatic T cells from liver tissue in a wide variety of liver diseases, found the proportion of CD8 cells to be increased in autoimmune CAH compared with viral hepatitis.

Clinical Manifestations

Both type I and type II autoimmune chronic active hepatitis are associated with a pronounced female (ranging from 4:1 to 10:1) predominance. Presenting symptoms include fatigue, weakness, jaundice, pruritus, abdominal pain or hepatic tenderness, amenorrhea, arthritis, or rash (Czaja, 1991). Type II autoimmune CAH tends to occur in younger children, whereas type I autoimmune CAH occurs in adolescents and adults; however, there is extensive overlap in the ages of presentation.

Both disorders are associated with other autoimmune disorders, including thyroiditis, diabetes, immune thrombocytopenia purpura, rheumatoid arthritis, inflammatory bowel diseases, and hemolytic anemia. Associated autoimmune disease is probably more common in type II autoimmune CAH, occurring in up to 35% of these patients (Homberg et al., 1987).

On physical examination, jaundice, hepatosplenomegaly, acne, palmar erythema, and spider angiomas may be seen; patients with more advanced cases may have ascites or encephalopathy. The serum bilirubin level is usually elevated. Transaminase activities are frequently 10-fold above normal and often exceed 1000 IU/L; alanine aminotransferase activity is usually higher than aspartate aminotransferase activity. In contrast to enzyme levels in primary sclerosing cholangitis, the alkaline phosphatase activity is less elevated than the transaminase activities (Fitzgerald, 1982). Hypergammaglobulinemia is usually pronounced, and in type I autoimmune CAH the serum IgG level may exceed 4000 mg/dl (Odievre et al., 1983).

Diagnosis

Diagnosis is made by excluding other causes of chronic hepatitis, particularly viral and metabolic liver disease (including Wilson's disease); by determining the presence of specific autoantibodies; by demonstrating a pattern consistent with autoimmune CAH by liver biopsy; and by finding a good response to immunosuppressive therapy. Serologic testing for hepatitis A, B, and C, cytomegalovirus, and Epstein-Barr virus should be done for all patients. To exclude Wilson's disease, ophthalmologic examination for Kayser-Fleischer rings and tests for serum ceruloplasmin and 24-hour urinary copper should be performed, taking into account the fact that copper excretion may be increased in some forms of chronic liver disease. Deficiency of alpha$_1$-antitrypsin should be excluded by obtaining a serum alpha$_1$-antitrypsin level and protease inhibitor phenotype. Antinuclear antibody, anti–smooth muscle antibody, and anti–liver-kidney microsomal antibody testing should be performed; the presence of antimitochondrial antibodies may suggest primary biliary cirrhosis. Finally, a liver biopsy should be obtained before starting therapy; this demonstrates a periportal infiltrate of lymphocytes and plasma cells, necrosis of hepatocytes, and, in advanced disease, fibrosis or cirrhosis.

Treatment

Therapy should be instituted as soon as the diagnosis is established to slow progression of liver disease. Traditionally, hepatitis must be present for longer than 6 months to be termed "chronic" hepatitis. However, if the clinical picture, serologic testing, and biopsy findings are consistent with autoimmune chronic active hepatitis, it is unwise to delay therapy. Patients receive corticosteroids alone or corticosteroids plus azathioprine (Arasu et al., 1979; Maggiore et al., 1984; Czaja, 1991). A clinical and biochemical response usually occurs within a month, with resolution of fatigue and jaundice, falling transaminase levels, declining levels of IgG, and declining autoimmune antibody levels. Relapse may occur in up to 85% of pediatric patients when steroids are tapered (Maggiore et al., 1984). In adults, a randomized trial showed that azathioprine alone was efficacious in preventing relapse after steroids were tapered (Stellon et al., 1988).

Prognosis

Despite the good initial response to therapy, the long-term prognosis for patients with both type I and type II autoimmune chronic active hepatitis remains guarded. In one series of patients with type I autoimmune CAH, 30% of the patients had cirrhosis upon initial presentation and the 5-year mortality was 13%

despite therapy (Keating et al., 1987). Of patients with type II autoimmune CAH, 80% developed cirrhosis within 3 years and mortality was 20% (Homberg et al., 1987). Liver transplantation is of value for patients with autoimmune CAH with advanced liver disease, and recurrence in the transplanted liver is rare.

Primary Sclerosing Cholangitis

Primary sclerosing cholangitis (PSC) is an idiopathic inflammatory disease of the extrahepatic and intrahepatic bile ducts that ultimately results in biliary scarring and stricturing, cholestasis, and hepatic cirrhosis. Primary sclerosing cholangitis must be differentiated from chronic cholangitis associated with infectious agents (such as cytomegalovirus or *Cryptosporidium*), particularly in patients with HIV infection. Although the pathogenesis of PSC is poorly understood, the association of PSC with inflammatory bowel disease and immunodeficiency syndromes in pediatrics suggests an immunologic cause.

Pathophysiology

Suggested causes of primary sclerosing cholangitis include low-grade biliary bacterial infection, abnormal bile acid metabolism, accumulation of a toxin (e.g., copper), viral infection, or ischemia. Another hypothesis suggests that immune-mediated damage to the bile duct occurs in patients with a genetic predisposition. The latter hypothesis is the most likely because toxic, bacterial, or viral causes of biliary injury have largely been excluded (Lindor et al., 1990). The occurrence of PSC in multiple family members suggests a genetic predisposition (Quigley et al., 1983; Jorge et al., 1987). In patients with ulcerative colitis who have the HLA-B8 and HLA-DR3 phenotype, the risk for development of PSC is increased 10-fold (Shepherd et al., 1983). Primary sclerosing cholangitis is also associated with HLA-DRW52a and HLA-DR2 (Eddleston and Williams, 1978; Prochazka et al., 1990).

Several humoral and cellular immune abnormalities have been discovered in patients with PSC (Table 23–24). Because the majority of patients with PSC have an associated disease (such as ulcerative colitis or histiocytosis), it is difficult to determine whether the reported abnormalities are associated with PSC or with the underlying disease (Chapman, 1991). The best-characterized serum abnormality in patients with PSC is the presence of perinuclear antineutrophil cytoplasmic antibodies (p-ANCA). About 75% to 90% of patients with PSC have p-ANCA in their serum (Duerr et al., 1991; Seibold et al., 1992; Mulder et al., 1993). This finding is not specific to PSC, because ANCA can also be seen in those with ulcerative colitis or autoimmune chronic active hepatitis (Mulder et al., 1993). The percentage of those expressing ANCA decreases to 40% in patients with PSC without inflammatory bowel disease (Seibold et al., 1992).

The liver of patients with PSC demonstrates enhanced expression of MHC class II antigens on biliary tract epithelium, suggesting exchanged antigen presen-

Table 23–24. Abnormalities in Primary Sclerosing Cholangitis

Abnormality	References
Peripheral Blood	
Perinuclear antineutrophil cytoplasmic antibodies (p-ANCA)	Seibold et al., 1992
	Mulder et al., 1993
	Duerr et al., 1991
Hypergammaglobulinemia	Chapman et al., 1980
	Mowat, 1987a
Antinuclear antibodies	Zauli et al., 1987
Immune complexes	Bodenheimer et al., 1983
Decreased suppressor/cytotoxic (CD8+) cells	Lindor et al., 1987a
	Snook et al., 1989
Enhanced T-lymphocyte autoreactivity	Lindor et al., 1987b
Tissue	
Increased biliary HLA-DR expression	Chapman et al., 1988
	Broome et al., 1990
Inappropriate biliary expression of blood group antigens A and B	Bloom et al., 1993
Increased T lymphocytes	Whiteside et al., 1985
Increased suppressor/cytotoxic (CD8+) lymphocytes	Senaldi et al., 1992
Increased macrophages	

Abbreviation: HLA = human leukocyte antigen.

tation or interferon-γ production (Chapman et al., 1988). Increased numbers of CD8 cells are present in the hepatic and portal infiltrate of patients with PSC (Senaldi et al., 1992); if these cells are cytotoxic T cells, they could cause the observed damage to the biliary tract epithelium.

Clinical Manifestations

Primary sclerosing cholangitis can occur at any age; one pediatric series at a large tertiary referral center included 56 cases in 29 years (Debray et al., 1994). Patients may be completely asymptomatic, and the disease may be suspected only because of biochemical abnormalities in high risk patients (Porayko et al., 1990). Alternatively, patients may present with intermittent jaundice, right upper quadrant abdominal pain, fever, fatigue, weight loss, xanthomas, or ascites. Certain disorders place the pediatric patient at high risk for the development of PSC (Table 23–25). The principal risk factor for the older adolescent is inflammatory bowel disease; 1% to 2% of patients with ulcerative colitis develop PSC, and 50% of adults with PSC have inflammatory bowel disease. Other associated conditions include histiocytosis X, immunodeficiencies (both cellular and humoral), sickle cell anemia, and psoriasis (Mowat, 1987a; Sisto et al., 1987; Debray et al., 1994).

Diagnosis

Laboratory tests for patients with primary sclerosing cholangitis suggest chronic cholestasis and hepatitis; classically, elevations of alkaline phosphatase and gamma-glutamyl transpeptidase exceed elevations of transaminases. Other signs of cholestasis, including a prolonged prothrombin time, may be seen. Anti–smooth muscle antibodies and antimitochondrial antibodies may be present in a few patients but occur in

Table 23–25. Diseases Associated With Primary Sclerosing Cholangitis in Children and Adults

Inflammatory bowel disease
Histiocytosis X
Cystic fibrosis
Autoimmune hemolytic anemia
Sickle cell disease
Lupus erythematosus
Vasculitis
Thyroiditis
Celiac disease
Bronchiectasis
Psoriasis
Pancreatitis
Rheumatoid arthritis
Reticular cell sarcoma
Immunodeficiency
X-linked agammaglobulinemia
Hyper–immunoglobulin M immunodeficiency
Pure cellular immunodeficiency
Combined humoral and cellular immunodeficiency

Data from Sisto A, Feldman P, Garel L, Seidman E, Brochu P, Morin C, Weber AM, Roy CC. Primary sclerosing cholangitis in children: study of five cases and review of the literature. Pediatrics 80:918–923, 1987; Debray D, Pariente D, Urvoas E, Hadchouel M, Bernard O. Sclerosing cholangitis in children. J Pediatr 124:49–56, 1994; Wiesner RH. Primary sclerosing cholangitis. In Schiff L, Schiff ER, eds. Diseases of the Liver, 7th ed. Philadelphia, JB Lippincott, 1993, pp. 411–426.

low titers (Wiesner and LaRusso, 1980). Liver biopsy may demonstrate periportal inflammation, cholangitis, chronic active hepatitis, or periductular fibrosis; in advanced cases, "onion skin" fibrosis and cirrhosis are seen. A diagnosis of PSC can also be made by using endoscopic retrograde cholangiopancreatography (ERCP), which demonstrates segmental stricturing and dilatation of the intra- and extrahepatic bile ducts (Wiesner et al., 1985).

Treatment

When the diagnosis of primary sclerosing cholangitis is established, therapy is directed primarily at symptomatic relief and monitoring for progression to cirrhosis or cholangiocarcinoma. No treatment has been shown to stop the inexorable progression of the biliary inflammation. Ursodeoxycholic acid promotes bile flow, improves the biochemical parameters of cholestasis, and improves clinical symptoms of jaundice and pruritus in patients with PSC (Chazouilleres et al., 1990). An open-label trial of methotrexate in patients with PSC suggested some efficacy, but a randomized trial did not confirm the initial result (Knox and Kaplan, 1994). In patients with isolated strictures of the bile duct and obstruction, endoscopic stenting of the bile duct or balloon dilation of the stricture may provide long-term symptomatic relief (Martin et al., 1990). Colectomy in patients with ulcerative colitis does not prevent progression, arguing against a role for colonic bacterial translocation in the pathogenesis of PSC (Cangemi et al., 1989). The treatment of choice for advanced cases of PSC with cirrhosis and liver failure is liver transplantation, and the 3-year survival of patients with PSC who undergo liver transplantation is

greater than 80% (McEntee et al., 1991; Rand and Whitington, 1992).

References

Abbas AK. A reassessment of the mechanisms of T cell–dependent B cell activation. Immunol Today 9:89–94, 1988.

Adachi A, Koenig S, Gendelmann HE, Daugherty D, Gatton-Celii S, Fauci AS, Martin MA. Productive, persistent infection of colorectal cell lines with human immunodeficiency virus. J Virol 61:201–213, 1987.

Addiss DG, Mathews HM, Stewart JM, Wahlquist SP, Williams RM, Finton RJ, Spencer HC, Juranek DD. Evaluation of a commercially available ELISA for *Giardia lamblia* antigen in stool. J Clin Microbiol 29:1137–1142, 1991.

Agata H, Kondo N Fukutomi O, Shinoda S, Orii T. Interleukin-2 production of lymphocytes in food sensitive atopic dermatitis. Arch Dis Child 67:280–284, 1992.

Ahnen DJ, Brown WR, Kloppel TM. Secretory component: the polymeric immunoglobulin receptor. Gastroenterology 89:667–682, 1985.

Aiges H, Markowitz J, Rosa J, Daum F. Home nocturnal supplemental nasogastric tube feedings in growth-retarded adolescents with Crohn's disease. Gastroenterology 97:905–910, 1989.

Allan CH, Mendrick DL, Trier JS. Rat intestinal M cells contain acidic endosomal-lysosomal compartments and express class II major histocompatibility complex determinants. Gastroenterology 104:698–708, 1993.

Alper CA, Fleishnick E, Awdeh Z, Katz AJ, Yunis EJ. Extended major histocompatibility complex haplotypes in patients with gluten-sensitive enteropathy. J Clin Invest 79:251–256, 1987.

Alter MJ, Sampliner RE. Hepatitis C: and miles to go before we sleep. N Engl J Med 321:1538–1540, 1989.

Ament ME, Rubin CE. Soy protein—another cause of the flat intestinal lesion. Gastroenterology 62:227–234, 1972.

Amerongen HM, Weltzin R, Farnet CM, Michetti P, Haseltine WA, Neutra MR. Transepithelial transport of HIV-1 by intestinal M cells. J AIDS 4:760–765, 1991.

Amerongen MH, Weltzin RW, Mack JA, Winner LS, Michetti P, Apter FM, Kraehenbuhl JP, Neutra MR. M cell–mediated antigen transport and monoclonal IgA antibodies for mucosal immune protection. Ann NY Acad Sci 664:18–26, 1992.

Ammann AJ, Hong R. Selective IgA deficiency: presentation of 30 cases and a review of the literature. Medicine (Baltimore) 50:223–236, 1971.

Anderson DC, Springer TA. Leukocyte-adhesion deficiency: an inherited defect in the Mac-1, LFA-1, and p150,95 glycoproteins. Annu Rev Med 38:175–194, 1987.

Anttila PH, von Willebrand E, Simell O. Abnormal immune responses during hypozincemia in acrodermatitis enteropathica. Acta Paediatr Scand 75:988–992, 1986.

Arasu TS, Wyllie R, Hatch TF, Fitzgerald JF. Management of chronic aggressive hepatitis in children and adolescents. J Pediatr 95:514–522, 1979.

Arbo A, Santos JI. Diarrheal diseases in the immunocompromised host. Pediatr Infect Dis 6:894–906, 1987.

Auricchio S, Greco L, Troncone R. Gluten-sensitive enteropathy in childhood. Pediatr Clin North Am 35:157–187, 1988.

Baklien K, Brandtzaeg P, Fausa O. Immunoglobulins in jejunal mucosa and serum from patients with adult coeliac disease. Scand J Gastroenterol 12:149–159, 1977.

Balistreri WF. Viral hepatitis. Pediatr Clin North Am 35:375–407, 1988.

Barnes PM, Moynahan EJ. Zinc deficiency in acrodermatitis enteropathica: multiple dietary intolerance treated with synthetic diet. Proc R Soc Med 66:325–333, 1973.

Bastlein C, Burlefinger R, Holzberg E, Voeth C, Garbrecht M, Ottenjann R. Common variable immunodeficiency syndrome and nodular lymphoid hyperplasia in the small intestine. Endoscopy 20:272–275, 1988.

Bell MJ, Ternberg JL, Feigin RD, Keating JP, Marshall R, Barton L, Brotherton T. Neonatal necrotizing enterocolitis: therapeutic decisions based on clinical staging. Ann Surg 187:1–7, 1978.

Belli DC, Seidman E, Bouthillier L, Weber AM, Roy CC, Pletincx

M, Beaulieu M, Morin CL. Chronic intermittent elemental diet improves growth failure in children with Crohn's disease. Gastroenterology 94:603–610, 1988.

Benderly A, Pollack S, Etzioni A. Transient hypogammaglobulinemia of infancy with severe bacterial infections and persistent IgA deficiency. Isr J Med Sci 22:393–396, 1986.

Benhamou Y, Caumes E, Gerosa Y, Cadranel JF, Dohin E, Katlama C, Amouyal P, Canard JM, Azar N, Hoang C, Le Charpentier Y, Gentilini M, Opolon P, Valla D. AIDS related cholangiopathy: critical analysis of a prospective series of 26 patients. Dig Dis Sci 38:1113–1118, 1993.

Bennett WG, Watson RA, Heard JK, Vesely DL. Home hyperalimentation for common variable hypogammaglobulinemia with malabsorption secondary to intestinal nodular lymphoid hyperplasia. Am J Gastroenterol 82:1091–1095, 1987.

Biggar WD, Crawford L, Cardella C, Bear RA, Gladman D, Reynolds WJ. Malakoplakia and immunosuppressive therapy. Reversal of clinical and leukocyte abnormalities after withdrawal of prednisone and azathioprine. Am J Pathol 119:5–11, 1985.

Bishop JM, Hill DJ, Hosking CS. Natural history of cow milk allergy: clinical outcome. J Pediatr 116:862–867, 1990.

Bland PW, Kambarage DM. Antigen handling by the epithelium and lamina propria macrophages. Gastroenterol Clin North Am 20:577–596, 1991.

Bland PW, Warren LG. Antigen presentation by epithelial cells of the rat small intestine. II. Selective induction of suppressor T cells. Immunology 58:9–14, 1986.

Bloom S, Heryet A, Fleming K, Chapman RW. Inappropriate expression of blood group antigens on biliary and colonic epithelia in primary sclerosing cholangitis. Gut 34:977–983, 1993.

Bock SA, Atkins FM. The natural history of peanut allergy. J Allergy Clin Immunol 83:900–904, 1989.

Bock SA, Buckley J, Holst A, May CD. Proper use of skin tests with food extracts in diagnosis of food hypersensitivity. Clin Allergy 8:559–564, 1978.

Bock SA, Sampson HA, Atkins FM, Zeiger RS, Lehrer S, Sachs M, Bush RK, Metcalfe DD. Double-blind placebo controlled food challenges as an office procedure: a manual. J Allergy Clin Immunol 82:986–997, 1988.

Bodenheimer HC, La Russo NF, Thayer WP Jr, Charland C, Staples PJ, Ludwig J. Elevated circulating immune complexes in primary sclerosing cholangitis. Hepatology 3:150–154, 1983.

Borchers SD, Friedman RA, McClung HJ. Rice-induced anaphylactoid reaction. J Pediatr Gastroenterol Nutr 15:321–24, 1993.

Boyer JL, Reuben A. Chronic hepatitis. In Schiff L, Schiff ER, eds. Diseases of the Liver. Philadelphia, JB Lippincott, 1993, pp. 612–619.

Boyle JT. Gastroesophageal reflux in the pediatric patient. Gastroenterol Clin North Am 18:315–337, 1989.

Brandtzaeg P, Baklien K. Intestinal secretion of IgA and IgM: a hypothetical model. Ciba Found Symp 46:77–113, 1977.

Bray PF, Herbert JJ, Johnson DG. Childhood gastroesophageal reflux: neurologic and psychiatric symptoms mimicked. JAMA 237:1342–1345, 1977.

Broome U, Galamann H, Hulterantz R, Forsum U. Distribution of HLA-DR, HLA-DP, HLA-DQ antigens in liver tissue from patients with primary sclerosing cholangitis. Scand J Gastroenterol 25:54–58, 1990.

Brynskov J, Freund L, Rasmussen SN, Lauritsen K, Schaffalitzky de Muckadell O, Williams N, MacDonald A, Taunton R, Molina F, Campanini MC, Bianchi P, Ranzi T, Quarto di Palo F, Malchow-Moller A, Thomsen O, Tage-Jensen U, Binder V, Riis P. A placebo-controlled, double-blind, randomized trial of cyclosporine therapy in active chronic Crohn's disease. N Engl J Med 321:845–850, 1989.

Buckley RH, Dees SC. The correlation of milk precipitins with IgA deficiency. N Engl J Med 281:465–469, 1969.

Burgin-Wolff A, Gaze H, Hadziselimovic F, Huber H, Lentze MJ, Nussle D, Raymond-Berthet C. Antigliadin and antiendomysium antibody determination for coeliac disease. Arch Dis Child 66:941–947, 1991.

Burks AW, Sampson HA. Diagnostic approach to the patient with suspected food allergies. J Pediatr 121:S64–S71, 1992.

Cangemi JR, Wiesner RH, Beaver SJ, Ludwig J, MacCarty RL, Dozois RR, Zinsmeister AR, LaRusso NF. Effect of proctocolectomy for chronic ulcerative colitis on the natural history of primary sclerosing cholangitis. Gastroenterology 96:790–794, 1989.

Caplan MS, MacKendrick WM. Necrotizing enterocolitis: a review of pathogenetic mechanisms and implications for prevention. Pediatr Pathol 13:357–369, 1993.

Cappell MS. Hepatobiliary manifestations of the acquired immune deficiency syndrome. Am J Gastroenterol 86:1–15, 1991.

Catassi C, Mirakian R, Natalini G, Sbarbati A, Cinti S, Coppa GV, Giorgi PL. Unresponsive enteropathy associated with circulating enterocyte antibodies in a boy with common variable hypogammaglobulinemia and type 1 diabetes. J Pediatr Gastroenterol Nutr 7:608–613, 1988.

Cello JP, Grendell JH, Basuk P, Simon D, Weiss L, Wittner M, Rood RP, Wilcox CM, Forsmark CE, Read AE, Satow JA, Weikel CS, Beaumont C. Effect of octreotide on refractory AIDS-associated diarrhea. A prospective, multicenter clinical trial. Ann Intern Med 115:705–710, 1991.

Cerf-Bensussan N, Guy-Grand D. Intestinal intraepithelial lymphocytes. Gastroenterol Clin North Am 20:549–576, 1991.

Chajek T. HLA-B51 may serve as an immunogenetic marker for a subgroup of patients with Behçet's syndrome. Am J Med 83:666–672, 1987.

Chapman RW. Role of immune factors in the pathogenesis of primary sclerosing cholangitis. Semin Liver Dis 11:1–4, 1991.

Chapman RW, Marborgh BA, Rhodes JM, Summerfield JA, Dick R, Scheuer PJ, Sherlock S. Primary sclerosing cholangitis—a review of its clinical features, cholangiography, and hepatic histology. Gut 21:870–877, 1980.

Chapman RW, Kelly P, Heryet A, Jewell DP, Fleming KA. Expression of HLA-DR antigens on bile duct epithelium in primary sclerosing cholangitis. Gut 29:422–427, 1988.

Chazouilleres O, Poupon R, Capron JP, Metman EH, Dhumeauz D, Amouretti M, Couzigou P, Labayle D, Trinchet JC. Ursodeoxycholic acid for primary sclerosing cholangitis. J Hepatol 11:120–123, 1990.

Chin TW, Stiehm ER, Falloon J, Gallin JI. Corticosteroids in treatment of obstructive lesions of chronic granulomatous disease. J Pediatr 111:349–352, 1987.

Choy MY, Walker-Smith JA, Williams CB, Macdonald TT. Differential expression of CD25 (interleukin-2 receptor) on lamina propria T cells and macrophages in the intestinal lesions in Crohn's disease and ulcerative colitis. Gut 31:1365–1390, 1990.

Chu SW, Walker, WA. Bacterial toxin interaction with the developing intestine. Gastroenterology 104:916–925, 1993.

Colletti RB, Guillot AP, Rosen S, Bhan AK, Hobson D, Collins AB, Russell GJ, Winter HS. Autoimmune enteropathy and nephropathy with circulating antiepithelial cell antibodies. J Pediatr 118:858–864, 1991.

Collin P, Maki M, Keyrilainen O, Hallstrom O, Reunala T, Pasternack A. Selective IgA deficiency and celiac disease. Scand J Gastroenterol 27:367–371, 1992.

Colombel JF, Mascart-Lemone F, Nemeth J, Vaerman JP, Dive C, Rambaud JC. Jejunal immunoglobulin and antigliadin antibody secretion in active celiac disease. Gut 31:1345–1349, 1990.

Conley ME, Delacroix DL. Intravascular and mucosal immunoglobulin A: two separate systems of immune defense? Ann Intern Med 106:892–899, 1987.

Conley ME, Park CL, Douglas SD. Childhood common variable immunodeficiency with autoimmune disease. J Pediatr 108:915–922, 1986.

Couper R, Kapelushnik J, Griffiths AM. Neutrophil dysfunction in glycogen storage disease Ib: association with Crohn's like colitis. Gastroenterology 100:549–554, 1991.

Crissinger KD, Granger DN. Mucosal injury induced by ischemia and reperfusion in the piglet intestine: influences of age and feeding. Gastroenterology 97:920–926, 1989.

Crissinger KD, Tso P. The role of lipids in ischemia/reperfusion-induced changes in mucosal permeability in developing piglets. Gastroenterology 102:1693–1699, 1992.

Cunningham-Rundles C. Selective IgA deficiency and the gastrointestinal tract. Immunol Allergy Clin North Am 8:435–449, 1988.

Cunningham-Rundles C, Brandeis WE, Good RA, Day NK. Milk precipitins, circulating immune complexes and IgA deficiency. Proc Natl Acad Sci USA 75:3386–3389, 1978.

Cunningham-Rundles C, Pudifin DJ, Armstrong D, Good RA. Selective IgA deficiency and neoplasia. Vox Sang 38:61–67, 1980.

Czaja AJ. Diagnosis, prognosis and treatment of classical autoimmune chronic active hepatitis. In Krawitt EL, Wiesner RH, eds. Autoimmune Liver Diseases. New York, Raven Press, 1991, pp. 143–166.

Czaja AJ, Carpenter HA, Santrach PJ, Moore B, Homburger HA. The nature and prognosis of severe cryptogenic chronic active hepatitis. Gastroenterology 104:1755–1761, 1993a.

Czaja AJ, Carpenter HA, Santrach PJ, Moore SB. Significance of HLA DR4 in type I autoimmune hepatitis. Gastroenterology 105:1502–1507, 1993b.

Das KM Dasgupta A, Mandal A, Geng X. Autoimmunity to cytoskeletal protein tropomyosin. A clue to the pathogenetic mechanism for ulcerative colitis. J Immunol 150:2487–2493, 1993.

Davies G, Evans CM, Shand WA, Walker-Smith JA. Surgery for Crohn's disease in childhood: influence of site of disease and operative procedure on outcome. Br J Surg 77:891–894, 1990.

Dawson J, Bryant MG, Bloom SR, Peters TJ. Jejunal mucosal enzyme activities, regulatory peptides, and organelle pathology of the enteropathy of common variable immunodeficiency. Gut 27:273–277, 1986.

Debray D, Pariente D, Urvoas E, Hadchouel M, Bernard O. Sclerosing cholangitis in children. J Pediatr 124:49–56, 1994.

Deitch EA. Bacterial translocation: the influence of dietary variables. Gut 35(Suppl.):S23–S27, 1994.

DeMarchi M, Borelli I, Olivetti E, Richiardi P, Wright P, Ansaldi N, Barbera C, Santini B. Two HLA-D and DR alleles are associated with celiac disease. Tissue Antigens 14:309–316, 1979.

Dicke WK, Weijers HA, van de Kamer JH. Coeliac disease. II. The presence in wheat of a factor having a deleterious effect in cases of coeliac disease. Acta Paediatr Scand 42:34–42, 1953.

DiGioacchino M, Pizzicannella G, Fini N, Falusca F, Antinucci R, Masci S, Mezzetti A, Marzio L, Cuccurullo F. Sodium cromoglycate in the treatment of eosinophilic gastroenteritis. Allergy 45:161–166, 1990.

Disdier P, Harle JR, Monges D, Chrestian MA, Horschowski N, Weiller PJ. Duodenal sarcoidosis with selective IgA deficiency and lymphoid nodular hyperplasia. Gastroenterol Clin Biol 15:849–851, 1991.

Donaldson PT, Doherty DG, Hayllar KM, McFarlane IG, Johnson PJ, Williams R. Susceptibility to autoimmune chronic active hepatitis: human leukocyte antigens DR4 and A1-B8-DR3 are independent risk factors. Hepatology 13:701–706, 1991.

Downing GJ, Horner SR, Kilbride HW. Characteristics of perinatal cocaine-exposed infants with necrotizing enterocolitis. Am J Dis Child 145:26–27, 1991.

Duerr RH, Targan SR, Landers CJ, La Russo NF, Lindsay KL, Wiesner RH, Shanahan F. Neutrophil cytoplasmic antibodies: a link between primary sclerosing cholangitis and ulcerative colitis. Gastroenterology 100:1385–1391, 1991.

Ebert EC. Intra-epithelial lymphocytes: interferon-gamma production and suppressor/cytotoxic activities. Clin Exp Immunol 82:81–85, 1990.

Eddleston AL, Williams R. HLA and liver disease. Br Med Bull 34:295–300, 1978.

Eibl MM, Wolf HM, Furnkranz H, Rosenkranz A. Prevention of necrotizing enterocolitis in low birth weight infants by IgG-IgA feeding. N Engl J Med 319:1–7, 1988.

Ek J, Albrechtsen D, Solheim BG, Thorsby E. Strong association between the HLA-Dw3–related B cell alloantigen-DRw3 and celiac disease. Scand J Gastroenterol 13:229–233, 1978.

Ellis D, Fisher SE, Smith WI, Jaffe R. Familial occurrence of renal and intestinal disease associated with tissue autoantibodies. Am J Dis Child 136:323–326, 1982.

el-Mouzan MI, Satti MB, al Quorain AA, el-Ageb A. Colonic malacoplakia—occurrence in a family. Report of cases. Dis Colon Rectum 31:390–393, 1988.

Ezekowitz RAB and the International Chronic Granulomatous Disease Cooperative Study Group. A controlled trial of interferon gamma to prevent infection in chronic granulomatous disease. N Engl J Med 324:509–516, 1991.

Fais S, Capobianchi MR, Pallone F, DiMarco P, Boirivant M, Oianzani F, Torsoli A. Spontaneous release of interferon gamma by intestinal lamina propria lymphocytes in Crohn's disease. Kinetics of in vitro response to interferon gamma inducers. Gut 32:403–407, 1991.

Falchuk ZM, Rogentine GN, Strober W. Predominance of histocompatibility antigen HLA-B8 in patients with gluten-sensitive enteropathy. J Clin Invest 51:1602–1605, 1972.

Ferguson A. Immunological functions of the gut in relation to nutritional state and mode of delivery of nutrients. Gut 35(Suppl.):S10–S12, 1994.

Ferreira M, Lloyd Davies S, Butler M, Scott D, Clark M, Kumar P. Endomysial antibody: is it the best screening test for coeliac disease? Gut 33:1633–1637, 1992.

Fitzgerald JF. Chronic hepatitis. Semin Liver Dis 2:282–290, 1982.

Fonkalsrud EW. A syndrome of congenital lymphedema of the upper extremity and associated systemic lymphatic malformations. Surg Gynecol Obstet 145:228–234, 1977.

Fox CH, Kotler D, Tierney A, Wilson CS, Fauci AS. Detection of HIV-1 RNA in the lamina propria of patients with AIDS and gastrointestinal disease. J Infect Dis 159:467–471, 1989.

Fuleihan R, Ramesh N, Loh R, Jahara H, Rosen RS, Chatila T, Fu SM, Stamenkovic I, Geha RS. Defective expression of the CD40 ligand in X chromosome–linked immunoglobulin deficiency with normal or elevated IgM. Proc Natl Acad Sci USA 90:2170–2173, 1993.

Fung KP, Seagram G, Pasieka J, Trevenen C, Machida H, Scott B. Investigation and outcome of 121 infants and children requiring Nissen fundoplication for the management of gastroesophageal reflux. Clin Invest Med 13:237–246, 1990.

Garretts M, Molokhia M. Acrodermatitis enteropathica without hypozincemia. J Pediatr 91:492–494, 1977.

Garvey BM, McCambley JA, Tuxen DV. Effect of gastric alkalinization on bacterial colonization in critically ill patients. Crit Care Med 17:211–216, 1989.

Gawkrodger DJ, Ferguson A, Barnetson R. Nutritional status in patients with dermatitis herpetiformis. Am J Clin Nutr 48:355–360, 1988.

Giampietro PG, Ragno V, Daniele S, Cantani A, Ferrara M, Businco L. Soy hypersensitivity in children with food allergy. Ann Allergy 69:143–146, 1992.

Gilger MA, Matson DO, Conner ME, Rosenblatt HM, Finegold MJ, Estes MK. Extraintestinal rotavirus infections in children with immunodeficiency. J Pediatr 120:912–917, 1992.

Gitzelmann R, Bosshard NU. Defective neutrophil and monocyte functions in glycogen storage disease type Ib: a literature review. Eur J Pediatr 152(Suppl. 1):S33–S38, 1993.

Glassman MS, Newman LJ, Berezin S, Gryboski JD. Cow's milk protein sensitivity during infancy in patients with inflammatory bowel disease. Am J Gastroenterol 85:838–840, 1990.

Gleason WA. Protein-losing enteropathy. In Hyams JS, Wyllie R, eds. Pediatric Gastrointestinal Disease. Philadelphia, WB Saunders, 1993, pp. 536–543.

Golden MH, Jackson AA, Golden BE. Effect of zinc on the thymus of recently malnourished children. Lancet 2:1057–1059, 1977.

Golden MH, Harland PS, Golden BE, Jackson AA. Zinc and immunocompetence in protein-energy malnutrition. Lancet 1:1226–1227, 1978.

Goldman AS, Anderson DW, Sellers WA, Sapperstein S, Kniker WT, Halpern SR. Milk Allergy I. Oral challenge with milk and isolated proteins in allergic children. Pediatrics 32:425–443, 1963.

Goldstein JL, Anderson RGW, Brown MS. Coated pits, coated vesicles and receptor-mediated endocytosis. Nature 279:679–685, 1979.

Gonnella PA, Walker WA. Macromolecular absorption in the gastrointestinal tract. Adv Drug Delivery Rev 1:235–248, 1987.

Good RA, Fernandes G, West A. Nutrition, immunity and cancer: a review. Part I: Influence of protein or protein caloric malnutrition and zinc deficiency on immunity. Clin Bull 9:3–12, 1979.

Gravallese EM, Kantrowitz FG. Arthritic manifestations of inflammatory bowel disease. Am J Gastroenterol 83:703–709, 1988.

Greenberg GR, Fleming CR, Jeejeebhoy KN, Rosenberg IH, Sales D. Controlled trial of bowel rest and nutritional support in the management of Crohn's disease. Gut 29:1309–1315, 1988.

Grey HM, Sette A, Buus S. How T cells see antigen. Sci Am 261(5):56–64, 1989.

Grimble GK. Dietary nucleotides and gut mucosal defense. Gut 35(Suppl.):S46–S51, 1994.

Grohmann GS, Glass RI, Pereira HG, Monroe SS, Hightower AW, Weber R, Bryan RT. Enteric viruses and diarrhea in HIV-infected patients. N Engl J Med 329:14–20, 1993.

Gryboski JD, Pellerano R, Young N, Edberg S. Positive role of *Clostrid-*

ium difficile infection in diarrhea in infants and children. Am J Gastroenterol 86:685–689, 1991.

Hager C, Faber J, Kaczuni A, Goldstein R, Levy E, Freier S. Prevalence of postenteritis cow's milk protein intolerance. Isr J Med Sci 23:1128–1131, 1987.

Halac E, Halac J, Begue E, Casanas JM, Indiverdi DR, Petit JF, Figueroa MJ, Olmas JM, Rodriguez LA, Obregon RJ, Martinez NV, Grinblat DA, Vilarrodena HO. Prenatal and postnatal corticosteroid therapy to prevent necrotizing enterocolitis: a controlled trial. J Pediatr 117:132–138, 1990.

Halpin TC, Byrne WJ, Ament ME. Colitis, persistent diarrhea, and soy protein intolerance. J Pediatr 91:404–407, 1977.

Halstensen TS, Scott H, Brandtzaeg P. Intraepithelial T cells of the TCR gamma/delta CD8 negative and Vδ1/Jδ1 phenotypes are increased in celiac disease. Scand J Immunol 30:665–672, 1989.

Halstensen TS, Scott H, Brandtzaeg P. Human CD8+ intraepithelial T lymphocytes are mainly CD45A-RB+ and show increased co-expression of CD45RO in celiac disease. Eur J Immunol 20:1825–1830, 1990.

Hammer RE, Maika SD, Richardson JA, Tang JP, Taurog JD. Spontaneous inflammatory disease in transgenic rats expressing HLA-B27 and human β2m: an animal model of HLA-B27 associated human disorders. Cell 63:1099–1112, 1990.

Harfi HA, Akhtar M, Subayti YA, Ali MA, Ferentzi C, Larkworthy W. Gastrointestinal malakoplakia in children. Clin Pediatr (Phila) 24:423–428, 1985.

Harrison M, Kilby A, Walker-Smith J, France N, Wood CB. Cow's milk protein intolerance: a possible association with gastroenteritis, lactose intolerance, and IgA deficiency. Br Med J 1:1501–1508, 1976.

Hausser C, Virelizier JL, Buriot D, Griscelli C. Common variable hypogammaglobulinemia in children. Am J Dis Child 137:833–837, 1983.

Hawkins HK, Heffelfinger SC, Anderson DC. Leukocyte adhesion deficiency: clinical and postmortem observations. Pediatr Pathol 12:119–130, 1992.

Heird WC, Hansen IH. Effect of colostrum on growth of intestinal mucosa. Pediatr Res 11:406A, 1977.

Heise C, Dandekar S, Kumar P, Duplantier R, Donovan RM, Halsted CH. Human immunodeficiency virus infection of enterocytes and mononuclear cells in human jejunal mucosa. Gastroenterology 100:1521–1527, 1991.

Hentges DJ. The protective function of the indigenous intestinal flora. Pediatr Infect Dis 5:S17–S20, 1986.

Herrod HG. Chronic mucocutaneous candidiasis in childhood and complications of non-*Candida* infection. J Pediatr 116:377–382, 1990.

Hill DJ, Firer MA, Shelton MJ, Hosking CS. Manifestations of milk allergy in infancy: clinical and immunologic findings. J Pediatr 109:270–276, 1986.

Hill SM, Milla PJ, Bottazzo GF, Mirakian R. Autoimmune enteropathy and colitis: is there a generalised autoimmune gut disorder? Gut 32:36–42, 1991.

Hilliard RI, McKendry JB, Phillips MJ. Congenital abnormalities of the lymphatic system: a new clinical classification. Pediatrics 86:988–994, 1990.

Hoang P, Dalton HR, Jewell DP. Human colonic intraepithelial lymphocytes are suppressor cells. Clin Exp Immunol 85:498–503, 1991.

Hoefer RA, Ziegler MM, Koop CE, Schnaufer L. Surgical manifestations of eosinophilic gastroenteritis in the pediatric patient. J Pediatr Surg 12:955–962, 1977.

Hollander D, Vadheim CM, Brettholz E, Petersen GM, Delahunty T, Rotter JI. Increased intestinal permeability in patients with Crohn's disease and their relatives: a possible etiologic factor. Ann Intern Med 105:883–885, 1986.

Hollander D. The intestinal permeability barrier. Scand J Gastroenterol 27:721–726, 1992.

Holt PR. Dietary treatment of protein loss in intestinal lymphangiectasia. Pediatrics 34:629–635, 1964.

Homberg JC, Abauf N, Bernard O, Islam S, Alvarez F, Khalil S, Poupon R, Darnis F, Levy VG, Grippon P, Opolon P, Bernuau J, Benhamou JP, Alagille D. Chronic active hepatitis associated with anti liver/kidney microsomal antibody type I: a second type of autoimmune hepatitis. Hepatology 7:1333–1339, 1987.

Hoofnagle JH. Chronic hepatitis B. N Engl J Med 323:337–339, 1990.

Howdle PD, Blair Zajdel ME, Smart CJ, Tresdosiewicz LK, Blair GE, Losowsky MS. Lack of serological response to an E1b protein of adenovirus type 12 in celiac disease. Scand J Gastroenterol 24:282–286, 1989.

Hoyne GF, Callow MG, Kuhlman J, Thomas WR. T-cell lymphokine response to orally administered proteins during priming and unresponsiveness. Immunology 78:534–540, 1993.

Hsueh W, Gonzalez-Crussi F, Arroyave JL, Anderson RC, Lee ML, Houlihan WJ. Platelet activating factor induced ischemic bowel necrosis: the effect of PAF antagonists. Eur J Pharmacol 123:79–83, 1986.

Hsueh W, Gonzalez-Crussi F, Hsueh W. Platelet activating factor is an endogenous mediator for bowel necrosis in endotoxemia. FASEB J 1:403–405, 1987.

Husband AJ, Gowans JL. The origin and antigen-dependent distribution of IgA containing cells in the intestine. J Exp Med 148:1146–1160, 1977.

International Study Group for Behçet's Disease. Criteria for diagnosis of Behçet's disease. Lancet 335:1078–1080, 1990.

Isaacs D, Wright VM, Shaw DG, Raafat F, Walker-Smith JA. Chronic granulomatous disease mimicking Crohn's disease. J Pediatr Gastroenterol Nutr 4:498–501, 1985.

Ishii N, Moriguchi N, Sugita Y, Nakajima H, Tanaka S, Aoki I. Analysis of responsive cells in tolerance by the oral administration of ovalbumin. Immunol Invest 22:451–462, 1993.

Israel EJ, Pang KY, Harmatz PA, Walker WA. Structural and functional maturation of gut mucosal barrier with thyroxine. Am J Physiol 252:G762–G767, 1987.

Israel EJ, Schiffrin E, Carter E, Freiberg E, Walker WA. Prevention of necrotizing enterocolitis in the rat with prenatal cortisone. Gastroenterology 99:1333–1338, 1990.

Israel EJ, Simister N, Freiberg E, Caplan A, Walker WA. Immunoglobulin G binding sites on the human fetal intestine: a possible mechanism for the passive transfer of immunity from mother to infant. Immunology 79:77–81, 1993.

Italian Multicenter Study. Epidemiology and clinical features of pediatric HIV infection: results from an Italian multicenter study on 544 children. Lancet 2:1046–1048, 1988.

Iyngkaran N, Yadav M, Looi L, Boey CG, Kam KL, Balabaaskaran S, Puthucheary S. Effect of soy protein on the small bowel mucosa of young infants recovering from acute gastroenteritis. J Pediatr Gastroenterol Nutr 7:68–79, 1988.

Jackson WD, Grand RJ. Crohn's disease. In Walker WA, Durie PR, Walker-Smith JA, Hamilton JR, Watkins JB, eds. Pediatric Gastrointestinal Disease. Philadelphia, BC Decker, 1990, pp. 592–608.

Jany BH, Gallup MW, Yan PS, Gum JR, Kim YS, Basbaum CB. Human bronchus and intestine express the same mucin gene. J Clin Invest 87:77–82, 1991.

Jarvis WR, Middleton PJ, Gelfand EW. Significance of viral infections in severe combined immunodeficiency disease. Pediatr Infect Dis 2:187–192, 1983.

Johnson PJ, McFarlane IG, Eddleston AL. The natural course and heterogeneity of chronic active hepatitis. Semin Liver Dis 11:187–196, 1991.

Jorge AD, Esley C, Ahumada J. Family incidence of primary sclerosing cholangitis associated with immunologic diseases. Endoscopy 19:114–117, 1987.

Julius R, Schulkind M, Sprinkle T, Rennert O. Acrodermatitis enteropathica with immune deficiency. J Pediatr 83:1007–1011, 1973.

Kagnoff MF. Celiac disease. A gastrointestinal disease with environmental, genetic, and immunologic components. Gastroenterol Clin North Am 21:405–425, 1992.

Kagnoff MF, Austin RK, Hubert JJ, Bernardin JE, Kusarda DD. Possible role for a human adenovirus in the pathogenesis of celiac disease. J Exp Med 160:1544–1547, 1984.

Kagnoff MF, Paterson YJ, Kumar YJ, Kusarda DD, Carbone FR, Unsworth DJ, Austin RK. Evidence for the role of a human intestinal adenovirus in the pathogenesis of celiac disease. Gut 28:995–1001, 1987.

Kanof M, Lake A, Bayless T. Decreased height velocity in children and adolescents before the diagnosis of Crohn's disease. Gastroenterology 95:1523–1527, 1988a.

Kanof ME, Strober W, Fiocchi C, Zeitz M, James SP. CD4 positive Leu-8 negative helper-inducer T cells predominate in the human intestinal lamina propria. J Immunol 141:3029–3036, 1988b.

Katz AJ, Twarog FJ, Zieger RS, Falchuk ZM. Milk-sensitive and eosinophilic gastroenteropathy: similar clinical features with contrasting mechanisms and clinical course. J Allergy Clin Immunol 74:72–78, 1984.

Kawanishi H, Saltzman L, Strober W. Mechanisms regulating IgA class-specific immunoglobulin production in gut-associated lymphoid tissues. I. T cells derived from Peyer's patches that switch sIgM B cells to sIgA B cells in vitro. J Exp Med 157:433–450, 1983.

Keating JJ, O'Brien CJ, Stellon AJ, Portmann BC, Johnson RD, Johnson PJ, Williams R. Influence of aetiology, clinical, and histological features on survival in chronic active hepatitis: an analysis of 204 patients. Q J Med 62:59–66, 1987.

Kelly K, Lazenby A, Yardley J, Perman J, Sampson H. Elemental diet therapy in pediatric patients with chronic reflux symptoms: improvement of esophageal histopathology. Gastroenterology 106:A104, 1994.

Kelts DG, Grand RJ. Inflammatory bowel disease in children and adolescents. Curr Prob Pediatr 10:5–40, 1980.

Kett K, Brandtzaeg P. Local IgA subclass alterations in ulcerative colitis and Crohn's disease of the colon. Gut 28:1013–1021, 1987.

Kett K, Rognum TO, Brandtzaeg P. Mucosal subclass distribution of immunoglobulin G–producing cells is different in ulcerative colitis and Crohn's disease of the colon. Gastroenterology 93:919–924, 1987.

Keusch GT. Nutrition and infection. Annu Rev Nutr 6:131–154, 1986.

Khoury SJ, Hancock WW, Weiner HL. Oral tolerance to myelin basic protein and natural recovery from experimental autoimmune encephalomyelitis are associated with downregulation of inflammatory cytokines and differential upregulation of transforming growth factor-beta, interleukin-4, and prostaglandin E expression in the brain. J Exp Med 176:1355–1364, 1992.

Kim YS, Gum JR, Byrd JC, Toribara NW. The structure of human intestinal apomucins. Am Rev Respir Dis 144:S10–S14, 1991.

Kirkpatrick CH. Chronic mucocutaneous candidiasis. Eur J Clin Microbiol Infect Dis 8:448–456, 1989.

Kirsch M. Bacterial overgrowth. Am J Gastroenterol 85:231–237, 1990.

Kirschner BS, Voinchet O, Rosenberg IH. Growth retardation in inflammatory bowel disease. Gastroenterology 75:504–511, 1978.

Klein C, Lisowska-Grospierre L, LeDiest F, Fischer A, Griscelli C. Major histocompatibility class II deficiency: clinical manifestations, immunologic features and outcome. J Pediatr 123:921–928, 1993.

Kleinman RE. The liver and intestinal immunoglobulin A: up from the "minors"? Gastroenterology 93:650–651, 1987.

Kleinman RE, Walker WA. The enteromammary immune system: an important new concept in breast milk host defense. Dig Dis Sci 24:876–882, 1979.

Kleinman RE, Balisteri WF, Heyman MB, Kirschner BS, Lake AL, Motil KJ, Seidman E, Udall JN. Nutritional support for pediatric patients with inflammatory bowel disease. J Pediatr Gastroenterol Nutr 8:8–12, 1989.

Kliegman RM. Neonatal necrotizing enterocolitis. In Wyllie R, Hyams JS, eds. Pediatric Gastrointestinal Disease: Pathophysiology, Diagnosis, Management. Philadelphia, WB Saunders, 1993, pp. 788–798.

Kliegman RM, Fanaroff AA. Necrotizing enterocolitis. N Engl J Med 310:1093–1103, 1984.

Kliegman RM, Walker WA, Yolken RH. Necrotizing enterocolitis: research agenda for a disease of unknown etiology and pathogenesis. Pediatr Res 34:701–708, 1993.

Knox WF. Restricted feeding and human intestinal plasma cell development. Arch Dis Child 61:744–749, 1986.

Knox TA, Kaplan MM. A double-blind controlled trial of oral pulse methotrexate therapy in the treatment of primary sclerosing cholangitis. Gastroenterology 106:494–499, 1994.

Koff RS. Viral hepatitis. In Schiff L, Shiff ER, eds. Diseases of the Liver, 7th ed. Philadelphia, JB Lippincott, 1993, pp. 492–577.

Kondo N, Fukitomi O, Agata H, Motoyoshi F, Shinoda S, Kobayashi Y, Kuwabara N, Kameyama T, Orii T. The role of T lymphocytes in patients with food sensitive atopic dermatitis. J Allergy Clin Immunol 91:658–668, 1993.

Kosnik EF, Johnson JP, Rennels MB, Caniano DA. Streptococcal sepsis presenting as acute abdomen in a child with transient hypogammaglobulinemia of infancy. J Pediatr Surg 21:975–976, 1986.

Kotler DP, Scholes JV, Tierney AR. Intestinal plasma cell alterations in acquired immunodeficiency syndrome. Dig Dis Sci 32:129–138, 1987.

Kraehenbuhl JP, Neutra MR. Molecular and cellular basis of immune protection of mucosal surfaces. Physiol Rev 72:853–879, 1992.

Krugman S. Viral hepatitis: A,B,C,D,E infection. Pediatr Rev 13:203–212, 1992.

Kuhn R, Lohler J, Rennick D, Rajewsky K, Muller W. Interleukin-10 deficient mice develop chronic enterocolitis. Cell 75:263–274, 1993.

Kutlu T, Brousse N, Rambaud C, LeDiest F, Schmitz J, Cerf-Bensussan N. Numbers of T cell receptor alpha/beta but not of TCR gamma/delta intraepithelial lymphocytes correlate with the grade of villous atrophy on a long term gluten free diet. Gut 34:208–214, 1993.

Lake AM, Whittington PF, Hamilton SR. Dietary protein–induced colitis in breast-fed infants. J Pediatr 101:906–910, 1982.

Lake-Bakaar G, Quadros E, Beidas S, Elsakr M, Tom W, Wilson DE, Dinscoy HP, Cohen P, Straus EW. Gastric secretory failure in patients with the acquired immunodeficiency syndrome. Ann Intern Med 109:502–504, 1988.

Laszewski MJ, Kemp JD, Goeken JA, Mitros FA, Platz CE, Dick FR. Clonal immunoglobulin gene rearrangement in nodular lymphoid hyperplasia of the gastrointestinal tract associated with common variable immunodeficiency. Am J Clin Pathol 94:338–343, 1990.

Lavilla P, Gil A, Rodriguez MC, Dupla ML, Pintado V, Fontan G. X-linked agammaglobulinemia and gastric adenocarcinoma. Cancer 72:1528–1531, 1993.

Lederman HM, Winkelstein JA. X-linked agammaglobulinemia: an analysis of 96 patients. Medicine (Baltimore) 64:145–156, 1985.

Lee RG. The colitis of Behçet's syndrome. Am J Surg Pathol 10:888–893, 1986.

Lehrer RI, Ganz T, Selsted ME, Babior BM, Curnutte JT. Neutrophils and host defense. Ann Intern Med 109:127–142, 1988.

Leihnas JL, McCaskill C, Sampson HA. Food allergy challenges: guidelines and implications. J Am Diet Assoc 87:604–608, 1987.

Lenaerts C, Roy CC, Vaillancourt M, Weber AM, Morin CL, Seidman E. High incidence of upper gastrointestinal tract involvement in children with Crohn disease. Pediatrics 83:777–781, 1989.

Lenzhofer R, Lindner M, Moser A, Berger J, Schuschnigg C, Thurner J. Acute jejunal ileus in intestinal lymphangiectasia. Clin Invest 71:568–571, 1993.

Lenzi M, Ballardini G, Fusconi M, Cassani F, Selleri L, Volat U, Zauli D, Bianchi FB. Type 2 autoimmune hepatitis and hepatitis C virus infection. Lancet 335:258–259, 1990.

Lenzi M, Johnson PJ, McFarlane IG, Ballardini G, Smith HM, McFarlane BM, Bridger C, Vergani D, Bianchi FB, Williams R. Antibodies to hepatitis C virus in autoimmune liver disease: evidence for geographical heterogeneity. Lancet 338:277–280, 1991.

Leung DY, Kelly CP, Boguniewicz M, Pothoulakis C, LaMont JT, Flores A. Treatment with intravenously administered gamma globulin of chronic relapsing colitis induced by Clostridium difficile toxin. J Pediatr 118:633–637, 1991.

Levenson SD, Austin RK, Dietler MD, Kasarda DD, Kagnoff MF. Specificity of antigliadin antibody in celiac disease. Gastroenterology 89:1–5, 1985.

Li XM, Jeffers LJ, Reddy KR, de Medina M, Silva M, Villanueve S, Klimas NG, Esquenazi V, Schiff ER. Immunophenotyping of lymphocytes in liver tissue of patients with chronic liver diseases by flow cytometry. Hepatology 14:121–127, 1991.

Lindahl JA, Williams FH, Newman SL. Small bowel obstruction in chronic granulomatous disease. J Pediatr Gastroenterol Nutr 3:637–640, 1984.

Lindor KD, Wiesner RH, Katzman JA, LaRusso NF, Beaver SJ. Lymphocyte subsets in primary sclerosing cholangitis. Dig Dis Sci 32:720–725, 1987a.

Lindor KD, Wiesner RH, LaRusso NF, Homburger HA. Enhanced autoreactivity of T lymphocytes in primary sclerosing cholangitis. Hepatology 7:884–888, 1987b.

Lindor KD, Wiesner RH, MacCarty RL, Ludwig J, La Russo NF. Advances in primary sclerosing cholangitis. Am J Med 89:73–80, 1990.

Logan RF, Gillon J, Ferrington C, Ferguson A. Reduction of gastrointestinal protein loss by elemental diet in the small bowel. Gut 22:383–387, 1981.

Logan RF, Rifkind EA, Turner ID, Ferguson A. Mortality in celiac disease. Gastroenterology 97:265–271, 1989.

Lungarotti MS, Ruffini S, Calbo A, Mariotti G, Ghebreggzabher M, Monaldi B. Treatment of acrodermatitis enteropathica with zinc sulfate. Helv Paediatr Acta 31:117–121, 1976.

MacFarlane IG. Autoimmunity and hepatotropic viruses. Semin Liver Dis 11:223–233, 1991.

MacKendrick W, Caplan M. Necrotizing enterocolitis. Pediatr Clin North Am 40:1047–1059, 1993.

Maddrey WC. How many types of autoimmune hepatitis are there? Gastroenterology 105:1571–1575, 1993.

Maggiore G, Bernard O, Hadchouel M, Hadchouel P, Odievre M, Alagile D. Treatment of autoimmune chronic active hepatitis in childhood. J Pediatr 104:839–844, 1984.

Mahida YR, Wu K, Jewell DP. Enhanced production of interleukin-1 beta by mononuclear cell isolated from mucosa with active ulcerative colitis of Crohn's disease. Gut 30:835–838, 1989.

Malroot A, Vandenplas Y, Verlinden M, Piepsz A, Dab I. Gastroesophageal reflux and unexplained chronic respiratory disease in children. Pediatr Pulmonol 3:208–213, 1987.

Manns MP. Cytoplasmic autoantigens in autoimmune hepatitis: molecular analysis and clinical relevance. Semin Liver Dis 11:205–214, 1991.

Manuel PD, Walker-Smith JA, France NE. Patchy enteropathy in childhood. Gut 20:211–215, 1979.

Markowitz J, Rosa J, Grancher K, Aiges H, Daum F. Long-term 6-mercaptopurine (6-MP) in adolescents with Crohn's disease. Am J Gastroenterol 94:1347–1351, 1990.

Marsh MN. Gluten, major histocompatibility complex, and the small intestine. Gastroenterology 102:330–354, 1992.

Martin FM, Rossi RL, Nugent FW, Scholz FJ, Jenkins RL, Lewis WD, Gagner M, Foley E, Braasch JW. Surgical aspects of sclerosing cholangitis: results in 178 patients. Ann Surg 212:551–556, 1990.

Martini A, Scotta MS, Notarangelo LD, Maggiore G, Guarnaccia S, DeGiacomo C. Membranous glomerulopathy and chronic small-intestinal enteropathy associated with autoantibodies directed against renal tubular basement membrane and the cytoplasm of intestinal epithelial cells. Acta Paediatr Scand 72:931–934, 1983.

Matsumoto R, Matsumoto M, Mita S, Hitoshi Y, Adno M, Araki S, Yamaguchi N, Tominaga A, Takatsu K. Interleukin-5 induces maturation but not class switching of IgA positive B cells into IgA secreting plasma cells. Immunology 66:32–41, 1989.

May GR, Sutherland LR, Mengs JB. Is small intestinal permeability really increased in relatives of patients with Crohn's disease? Gastroenterology 104:1627–1632, 1993.

Mayer L, Eisenhardt D. Lack of induction of suppressor T cells by intestinal epithelial cells from patients with inflammatory bowel disease. J Clin Invest 86:1255–1260, 1990.

Mayer L, Eisenhardt D, Salomon P, Bauer W, Plous R, Piccinini L. Expression of class II molecules on intestinal epithelial cells in humans. Differences between normal and inflammatory bowel disease. Gastroenterology 100:3–12, 1991.

McClure J. Malakoplakia of the gastrointestinal tract. Postgrad Med J 57:95–103, 1981.

McEntee G, Wiesner RH, Rosen C, Cooper J, Wahlstorm HE. A comparative study of patients undergoing liver transplantation for primary sclerosing cholangitis and primary biliary cirrhosis. Transplant Proc 23:1563–1564, 1991.

McGeady SJ. Transient hypogammaglobulinemia of infancy: need to reconsider name and definition. J Pediatr 110:47–50, 1987.

McLain BI, Davidson PM, Stokes KB, Beasley SW. Growth after gut resection for Crohn's disease. Arch Dis Child 65:760–762, 1990.

Mearin ML, Pena AS. Clinical indications of HLA typing and measurement of antigliadin antibodies in coeliac disease. Neth J Med 31:279–285, 1987.

Melamed D, Friedman A. Direct evidence for anergy in T lymphocytes tolerized by oral administration of ovalbumin. Eur J Immunol 23:935–942, 1993.

Mendeloff AI, Calkins BM. The epidemiology of idiopathic inflammatory bowel disease. In Kirsner J, Shorter RG, eds. Inflammatory Bowel Disease, 3rd ed. Philadelphia, Lea & Febiger, 1988, pp. 3–34.

Metcalfe DD, Sampson HA. Workshop on experimental methodology for clinical studies of adverse reactions to foods and food additives. J Clin Immunol 86:421–442, 1990.

Mett H, Gyr K, Zak O, Vosbeck K. Duodenopancreatic secretions enhance bactericidal activity of antimicrobial drugs. Antimicrob Agents Chemother 26:35–38, 1984.

Meydani SN. Dietary modulation of cytokine production and biologic functions. Nutr Rev 10:361–369, 1990.

Meyer T, Halter R, Pohlner J. Mechanism of extracellular secretion of an IgA protease by gram-negative host cells. Adv Exp Med Biol 216B:1271–1281, 1987.

Meysman M, Debeuckelaer S, Reynaert H, Schoors DF, Dehou MF, Van Camp B. Systemic amyloidosis-induced diarrhea in sex-linked agammaglobulinemia. Am J Gastroenterol 88:1275–1277, 1993.

Michaelson G. Zinc deficiency in acrodermatitis enteropathica. Acta Derm Venereol (Stockh) 54:377–381, 1974.

Michener WM, Wyllie R. Management of children and adolescents with inflammatory bowel disease. Med Clin North Am 74:103–117, 1990.

Mike N, Hansel TT, Newman J, Asquith P. Granulomatous enteropathy in common variable immunodeficiency: a cause of chronic diarrhea. Postgrad Med J 67:446–449, 1991.

Miller TL, Orav EJ, Martin SR, Cooper ER, McIntosh K, Winter HS. Malnutrition and carbohydrate malabsorption in children with vertically transmitted human immunodeficiency virus infection. Gastroenterology 100:1296–1302, 1991.

Miller TL, Winter HS, Luginbuhl LM, Orav EJ, McIntosh K. Pancreatitis in pediatric human immunodeficiency virus infection. J Pediatr 120:223–227, 1992.

Miller TL, Evans SJ, Orav J, Morris V, McIntosh K, Winter HS. Growth and body composition in children infected with the human immunodeficiency virus-1. Am J Clin Nutr 57:588–592, 1993.

Mirakian R, Richardson A, Milla PJ, Walker-Smith JA, Unsworth J, Savage MO, Bottazzo GF. Protracted diarrhea of infancy: evidence in support of an autoimmune variant. Br Med J 293:1132–1136, 1986.

Mombaerts P, Mizoguchi E, Grusby MJ, Glimcher LH, Bhan AH, Tonegawa S. Spontaneous development of inflammatory bowel disease in T cell receptor mutant mice. Cell 75:275–282, 1993.

Moran CA, West B, Schwartz IS. Malacoplakia of the colon in association with colonic adenocarcinoma. Am J Gastroenterol 84:1580–1582, 1989.

Morgan G, Levinsky RJ. Clinical significance of IgA deficiency. Arch Dis Child 63:579–581, 1988.

Morimoto C, Letvin NL, Distaso JA, Aldrich WR, Schlossman S. The isolation and characterization of the human suppressor-inducer T cell subset. J Immunol 134:1508–1515, 1985.

Morin CL, Roulet M, Roy CC, Weber A, LaPointe N. Continuous elemental enteral alimentation in the treatment of children and adolescents with Crohn's disease. J Parenteral Enteral Nutr 6:194–199, 1982.

Mowat AP. Primary sclerosing cholangitis in childhood. Gastroenterology 92:1226–1235, 1987a.

Mowat AM. The regulation of immune responses to dietary protein antigens. Immunol Today 8:93–98, 1987b.

Mowat AM, Lamont AG, Bruce MG. A genetically determined lack of oral tolerance to ovalbumin is due to the failure of the immune system to respond to intestinally derived tolerogen. Eur J Immunol 17:1673–1676, 1987.

Moynahan EJ. Acrodermatitis enteropathica: a lethal inherited human zinc deficiency disorder. Lancet 2:399–400, 1974.

Mulder AH, Horst G, Haagsma EB, Limburg PC, Kleibeuker JH, Kallenberg CG. Prevalence and characterization of neutrophil cytoplasmic antibodies in autoimmune liver disease. Hepatology 17:411–417, 1993.

Murphy MS, Walker WA. Celiac disease. Pediatr Rev 12:325–330, 1991.

Mylotte M, Egan-Mitchell B, Fottrell PF, McNicholl B, McCarthy CF. Family studies in celiac disease. J Med 43:359–369, 1974.

Nelder KH, Hambidge KM. Zinc therapy in acrodermatitis enteropathica. N Engl J Med 292:879–882, 1975.

Nelder KH, Hambidge KM, Walravens BA. Acrodermatitis enteropathica. Int J Dermatol 17:380–387, 1978.

Nezelof C. Thymic dysplasia with normal immunoglobulins and immunologic deficiency: pure alymphocytosis. Birth Defects 4:104–112, 1968.

Nielsen OH, Jacobsen O, Pedersen ER Rasmussen SN, Petri M, Lauland S, Jarnum S. Non-tropical sprue: malignant diseases and mortality rate. Scand J Gastroenterol 20:13–18, 1985.

Ninan T, Aggatt PJ, Smith F, Youngson G, Miller ID. Atypical genital involvement in a child with Crohn's disease. J Pediatr Gastroenterol Nutr 15:330–333, 1992.

Ninkovic M. Behçet's syndrome. In Bouchier IA, Allan RN, Hodgson HJ, Keightey MR, eds. Gastroenterology—Clinical Science and Practice. London, WB Saunders, 1993, pp. 1247–1254.

Nordlie RC, Sukalskie KA, Johnson WT. Human microsomal glucose-6-phosphatase system. Eur J Pediatr 152(Suppl.):S2–S6, 1993.

Novis BH, Gilinsky NH, Wright JP, Price S, Marks IN. Plasma cell infiltration of the small intestine, recurrent pulmonary infections, and cellular immunodeficiency (Nezelof's syndrome). Am J Gastroenterol 80:891–895, 1985.

Nunez MC, Ayudarte MV, Morales D, Suarez MD, Gil A. Effect of dietary nucleotides on intestinal repair in rats with experimental chronic diarrhea. J Parenteral Enteral Nutr 14:598–604, 1990.

Odievre M, Maggiore G, Homberg JC, Saadoun F, Courouce AM, Yvart J, Hadchouel M, Alagille D. Seroimmunologic classification of chronic hepatitis in 57 children. Hepatology 3:407–409, 1983.

O'Duffy JD, Goldstein NP. Neurological involvement in seven patients with Behçet's disease. Am J Med 61:170–178, 1976.

Odze RD, Bines J, Leichtner AM, Goldman H, Antonioli DA. Allergic proctocolitis in infants: a prospective clinicopathologic biopsy study. Hum Pathol 24:668–674, 1993.

Ogoshi S, Iwasa M, Tamiya T. Effect of nucleotide and nucleoside mixture on rats given total parenteral nutrition after 70% hepatectomy. J Parenteral Enteral Nutr 9:339–342, 1985.

Oleske JM, Westphal ML, Shore S, Gorden D, Bogden JD, Nahmias A. Zinc therapy of depressed cellular immunity in acrodermatitis enteropathica. Its correction. Am J Dis Child 133:915–918, 1979.

O'Morain C, Segal AW, Levi AJ. Elemental diet as primary treatment of acute Crohn's disease: a controlled trial. Br Med J 288:1859–1862, 1984.

Orenstein SR, Whittington PF, Orenstein DF. The infant seat as treatment for gastroesophageal reflux. N Engl J Med 309:760–763, 1983.

Ortolani C, Ispano M, Pastorello EA, Ansaloni R, Magri GC. Comparison of results of skin prick tests and RAST in 100 patients with oral allergy syndrome. J Allergy Clin Immunol 83:683–690, 1989.

Pabst R. The anatomic basis for the immune function of the gut. Anat Embryol 176:135–144, 1987.

Palmer SR, Biffin A, Gamsu HR. Outcome of necrotizing enterocolitis. Arch Dis Child 64:388–394, 1989.

Pang KY, Newman AP, Udall JN, Walker WA. Development of gastrointestinal mucosal barrier. VII. In vitro maturation of microvillus surface by cortisone. Am J Physiol 249:G85–G91, 1985.

Patterson BK, Ehrenpreis ED, Yokoo H. Focal enterocyte vacuolization. A new microscopic finding in the acquired immune deficiency syndrome. Am J Clin Pathol 99:24–27, 1993.

Peng HJ, Turner MW, Strobel S. The generation of a tolerogen after the ingestion of ovalbumin. Clin Exp Immunol 81:510–515, 1990.

Peppercorn MA. Advances in drug therapy for inflammatory bowel disease. Ann Intern Med 112:50–60, 1990.

Perisic VN, Kokai G. Bleeding from duodenal lymphangiectasia. Arch Dis Child 66:153–154, 1991.

Perisic VN, Filipovic D, Kokai G. Allergic colitis with rectal bleeding in an exclusively breast-fed neonate. Acta Paediatr Scand 77:163–164, 1988.

Perkkio M, Savilahti E. Time of appearance of immunoglobulin containing cells in the mucosa of the neonatal intestine. Pediatr Res 14:953–955, 1980.

Perlmutter DH, Leichtner AM, Goldmen H, Winter HS. Chronic diarrhea associated with hypogammaglobulinemia and enteropathy in infants and children. Dig Dis Sci 30:1149–1155, 1985.

Peterson LR, Gerding DN. Antimicrobial agents in C. difficile associated intestinal diseases. In Rambaud JC, Ducluzeau R, eds. Clostridium difficile–Associated Intestinal Diseases. New York, Springer-Verlag, 1990, pp. 115–127.

Philips JO, Everson MP, Moldoveanu Z, Lue C, Mestecky J. Synergistic effect of IL-4 and IFN-gamma on the expression of polymeric Ig receptor (secretory component) and IgA binding by human epithelial cells. J Immunol 145:1740–1744, 1990.

Pignata C, Budillon G, Monaco G, Nani E, Cuomo R, Parrilli G, Ciccimara F. Jejunal bacterial overgrowth and intestinal permeability in children with immunodeficiency syndromes. Gut 31:879–882, 1990.

Plettenberg A, Stoehr A, Stellbrink HJ, Albrecht H, Meigel W. A preparation from bovine colostrum in the treatment of HIV positive patients with chronic diarrhea. Clin Invest 71:42–45, 1993.

Pol S, Romana CA, Richard S, Amouyal P, Desportes-Livage D, Carnot F, Pays JF, Berthelot P. Microsporidia infection in patients with the human immunodeficiency virus and unexplained cholangitis. N Engl J Med 328:95–99, 1993.

Porayko MK, Wiesner RH, La Russo NF, Ludwig J, MacCarty RL, Steiner BL, Twomey CK, Zinsmeister AR. Patients with asymptomatic primary sclerosing cholangitis frequently have progressive disease. Gastroenterology 98:1594–1602, 1990.

Powell GK. Milk and soy induced enterocolitis of infancy. Clinical features and standardization of challenge. J Pediatr 93:553–560, 1978.

Prentice A, MacCarthy A, Stirling DM, Vasquez-Velasquez L, Ceesay SM. Breast milk IgA and lactoferrin survival in the gastrointestinal tract: a study in rural Gambian children. Acta Paediatr Scand 78:505–512, 1989.

Present DH, Korelitz BI, Wisch N, Glass JL, Sachar DB, Pasternack BS. Treatment of Crohn's disease with 6-mercaptopurine. N Engl J Med 302:981–987, 1980.

Prochazka EJ, Terasaki PI, Park MS, Goldstein LI, Busutil RW. Association of primary sclerosing cholangitis with HLA-DRW 52a. N Engl J Med 322:1842–1844, 1990.

Proujansky R, Fawcett P, Gibney KM, Treem WR, Hyams JS. Examination of anti-neutrophil cytoplasmic antibodies in childhood inflammatory bowel disease. J Pediatr Gastroenterol Nutr 17:193–197, 1993.

Quigley EMM, La Russo NF, Ludwig J, MacSween RNM, Birnie GG, Watkinson G. Familial occurrence of primary sclerosing cholangitis and ulcerative colitis. Gastroenterology 85:1160–1165, 1983.

Radema SA, Vandeventer SJ, Cerami A. Interleukin-1 beta is expressed predominantly by enterocytes in experimental colitis. Gastroenterology 100:1180–1186, 1991.

Rand EB, Whitington PF. Successful orthotopic liver transplantation in two patients with liver failure due to sclerosing cholangitis with Langerhans cell histiocytosis. J Pediatr Gastroenterol Nutr 15:202–207, 1992.

Raz I, Okon E, Chajek-Shaul T. Pulmonary manifestations in Behçet's syndrome. Chest 95:585–589, 1989.

Reddy KR, Jeffers LJ. Acquired immunodeficiency syndrome and the liver. In Schiff L, Schiff ER, eds. Diseases of the Liver, 7th ed. Philadelphia, JB Lippincott, 1993, pp. 1362–1372.

Reunala T, Blomquist K, Tarpila S, Halme H, Kangas K. Gluten-free diet in dermatitis herpetiformis. Clinical response of skin lesions in 81 patients. Br J Dermatol 97:473–480, 1977.

Reynolds J, Putnam P. Prokinetic agents. Gastroenterol Clin North Am 21:567–596, 1992.

Roberts MW, Atkinson JC. Oral manifestations associated with leukocyte adhesion deficiency: a five year case study. Pediatr Dent 12:107–111, 1990.

Rodewald R. Selective antibody transport in the proximal small intestine of the neonatal rat. J Cell Biol 45:635–640, 1970.

Rodin AE, Goldman AS. Autopsy findings in acrodermatitis enteropathica. Am J Clin Pathol 51:315–320, 1969.

Roe TF, Thomas DW, Gilsanz V, Isaacs H, Atkinson JB. Inflammatory bowel disease in glycogen storage disease type Ib. J Pediatr 109:55–59, 1986.

Roe TF, Coates TD, Thomas DW, Miller JH, Gilsanz V. Brief report: treatment of chronic inflammatory bowel disease in glycogen storage disease type Ib with colony-stimulating factors. N Engl J Med 326:1666–1669, 1992.

Rothman A, Snyder J. Protein-losing enteropathy following the Fontan operation: resolution following prednisone therapy. Am Heart J 121:618–619, 1991.

Rubaltelli FF, Benini F, Sala M. Prevention of necrotizing enterocolitis in neonates at risk by oral administration of monomeric IgG. Dev Pharmacol Ther 17:138–146, 1991.

Ruderman WB. Newer pharmacologic agents for the therapy of inflammatory bowel disease. Med Clin North Am 74:133–153, 1990.

Russell, GJ, Nagler-Anderson C, Anderson C, Anderson P, Bhan AK. Cytotoxic potential of intraepithelial lymphocytes. Presence of TIA-1, the cytolytic granule-associated protein, in human intraepithelial lymphocytes in normal and diseased intestine. Am J Pathol 143:350–354, 1993.

Sachdev GK, Dalton HR, Hoang P, DiPaolo MC, Crotty B, Jewell DP. Human colonic intraepithelial lymphocytes suppress in vitro immunoglobulin synthesis by autologous peripheral blood lymphocytes and lamina propria lymphocytes. Gut 34:257–263, 1993.

Sadlack B, Merz H, Schorle H, Schimpl A, Feller AC, Horak I. Ulcerative colitis like disease in mice with a disrupted interleukin-2 gene. Cell 75:253–261, 1993.

Saffran M, Franco-Saenz R, Kong A, Papahadjopoulos D, Szoka F. A model for the study of oral administration of peptide hormones. Can J Biochem 577:548–553, 1979.

Sagie E, Tarabulus J, Maier DM, Freier S. Diet and development of intestinal IgA in the mouse. Isr J Med Sci 10:532–534, 1974.

Sampson HA. Food allergy. In Shils ME, Olson JA, Shike M, eds. Modern Nutrition in Health and Disease. Baltimore, Lea & Febiger, 1994, pp. 1391–1398.

Sampson HA, Albergo R. Comparison of results of skin tests, RAST, and double-blind placebo controlled food challenges in children with atopic dermatitis. J Allergy Clin Immunol 74:26–33, 1984.

Sampson HA, Broadbent KR, Bernhisel-Broadbent J. Spontaneous release of histamine from basophils and histamine-releasing factor from patients with atopic dermatitis and food hypersensitivity. N Engl J Med 321:228–232, 1989.

Sander CA, Medeiros LJ, Weiss LM, Yano T, Sneller MC, Jaffe ES. Lymphoproliferative lesions in patients with common variable immunodeficiency syndrome. Am J Surg Pathol 16:1170–1182, 1992.

Sanderson IR, Walker WA. Nutrition and immunity. Curr Opin Gastroenterol 7:463–470, 1991.

Sanderson IR, Walker WA. Uptake and transport of macromolecules by the intestine: possible role in clinical disorders. Gastroenterology 104:622–639, 1993.

Sanderson IR, Boulton P, Menzies I, Walker-Smith JA. Improvement of abnormal lactulose/rhamnose permeability in active Crohn's disease of the small bowel by an elemental diet. Gut 28:1073–1076, 1987.

Sanderson IR, Phillips AD, Spencer J, Walker-Smith JA. Response of autoimmune enteropathy to cyclosporin therapy. Gut 32:1421–1425, 1991a.

Sanderson IR, Risdon RA, Walker-Smith JA. Intractable ulcerating enterocolitis of infancy. Arch Dis Child 66:295–299, 1991b.

Santer R, Lebenthal E. Secretory diarrhea in infancy and childhood. In Lebenthal E, Duffy M, eds. Textbook of Secretory Diarrhea. New York, Raven Press, 1990, pp. 337–353.

Santulli TV, Schullinger JN, Heird WC. Acute necrotizing enterocolitis in infancy: a review of 64 cases. Pediatrics 55:376–387, 1975.

Sarker SA, Gyr K. Non-immunological defense mechanisms of the gut. Gut 33:987–993, 1992.

Satti MB, Abu-Melha A. Colonic malakoplakia and abdominal tuberculosis in a child. Dis Colon Rectum 28:353–357, 1985.

Savilahti E, Pelkonen P. Clinical findings and intestinal immunoglobulins in children with partial IgA deficiency. Acta Paediatr Scand 68:513–519, 1979.

Schlaak JF, Lohr H, Gallati H, Meyer zum Buschenfelde KH, Fleischer B. Analysis of the in vitro cytokine production by liver-infiltrating T cells of patients with autoimmune hepatitis. Clin Exp Immunol 94:168–173, 1993.

Schrieber RA, Walker WA. The gastrointestinal barrier: antigen uptake and perinatal immunity. Ann Allergy 61:3–12, 1988.

Schreiber S, Raedler A, Stenson WE, MacDermott RP. The role of the mucosal immune system in inflammatory bowel disease. Gastroenterol Clin North Am 21:451–502, 1992.

Schrumpf E, Fausa O, Elgjo K, Kolmannskog F. Hepatobiliary complications of inflammatory bowel disease. Semin Liver Dis 8:201–209, 1988.

Schwarzenberg SJ, Whitington PF. Colonic stricture complicating formula protein intolerance enterocolitis. J Pediatr Gastroenterol Nutr 2:190–192, 1983.

Seibold F, Weber P, Klein R, Berg PA, Wiedmann KH. Clinical significance of antibodies against neutrophils in patients with inflammatory bowel disease and primary sclerosing cholangitis. Gut 33:657–662, 1992.

Seidman EG, Roy CC, Weber AM, Morin CL. Nutritional therapy of Crohn's disease in childhood. Dig Dis Sci 32(Suppl.):82S–88S, 1987.

Seki T, Kiyosawa K, Inoko H, Ota M. Association of autoimmune hepatitis with HLA-Bw54 and DR4 in Japanese patients. Hepatology 12:1300–1304, 1990.

Selsted ME, Miller SI, Henschen AH, Ouellette AJ. Enteric defensins: antibiotic peptide components of intestinal host defense. J Cell Biol 118:929–936, 1992.

Senaldi G, Portman B, Mowat AP, Mieli-Vergani G, Vergani D. Immunohistochemical features of the portal tract mononuclear cell infiltrate in chronic aggressive hepatitis. Arch Dis Child 67:1447–1453, 1992.

Shepherd HA, Selby WS, Chapman RW, Nolan D, Barbatis C, McGee JO, Jewell DP. Ulcerative colitis and persistent liver dysfunction. Q J Med 52:503–513, 1983.

Shepherd RW, Boreham PFL. Recent advances in the diagnosis and management of giardiasis. Scand J Gastroenterol [Suppl] 169:60–64, 1989.

Shorter RG, Huizenga KA, Spencer RJ. A working hypothesis for the etiology and pathogenesis of inflammatory bowel disease. Am J Dig Dis 17:1024–1032, 1972.

Sigurs N, Hattevig G, Kjellman B. Maternal avoidance of eggs, cow's milk, and fish during lactation: effect on allergic manifestations, skin-prick tests, and specific IgE antibodies in children at age four years. Pediatrics 89:735–739, 1992.

Silverman A, Roy CC. Pediatric Clinical Gastroenterology, 3rd ed. St. Louis, CV Mosby, 1983, pp. 226–228.

Siminoski K, Gonella P, Bernankke J, Owen L, Neutra M, Murphy R. Uptake and transepithelial transport of nerve growth factor in suckling rat ileum. J Cell Biol 103:1979–1990, 1986.

Sisto A, Feldman P, Garel L, Seidman E, Brochu P, Morin C, Weber AM, Roy CC. Primary sclerosing cholangitis in children: study of five cases and review of the literature. Pediatrics 80:918–923, 1987.

Slade HB, Schwartz SA. Mucosal immunity: the immunology of breast milk. J Allergy Clin Immunol 80:346–356, 1987.

Smith PD, Mai UE. Immunopathophysiology of gastrointestinal disease in HIV infection. Gastroenterol Clin North Am 21:331–345, 1992.

Smith PD, Lane HC, Gill VJ, Manischewitz JF, Quinnan GV, Fauci AS, Masur H. Intestinal infections in patients with the acquired immunodeficiency syndrome: etiology and response to therapy. Ann Intern Med 108:328–333, 1988.

Snook JA, Chapman RW, Sachdev GK, Heryet A, Kelly PM, Fleming KA, Jewell DP. Peripheral blood and portal tract lymphocyte populations in primary sclerosing cholangitis. J Hepatol 9:36–41, 1989.

Snyder JD, Walker WA. Structure and function of intestinal mucin: developmental aspects. Int Arch Allergy Appl Immunol 82:351–356, 1987.

Snyder JD, Rosenblum N, Wershil B, Goldman H, Winter HS. Pyloric stenosis and eosinophilic gastroenteritis in infants. J Pediatr Gastroenterol Nutr 6:543–547, 1987.

Sollid LM, Thorsby E. HLA susceptibility genes in celiac disease: genetic mapping and role in pathogenesis. Gastroenterology 105:910–922, 1993.

Spencer J, Isaacson PG, Diss TC, McDonald TT. Expression of disulfide linked and non disulfide linked forms of the T cell receptor heterodimer gamma/delta in human intraepithelial lymphocytes. Eur J Immunol 19:1335–1338, 1989.

Spencer J, Isaacson PG, McDonald TT, Thomas AJ, Walker SJ. Gamma/delta T cells and the diagnosis of celiac disease. Clin Exper Immunol 85:109–113, 1991.

Sperber KE, Mayer L. Gastrointestinal manifestations of common variable immunodeficiency. Immunol Allergy Clin North Am 8:423–434, 1988.

Stellon AJ, Keating JJ, Johnson PJ, McFarlane IG, Williams R. Maintenance of remission in autoimmune chronic active hepatitis with azathioprine after corticosteroid withdrawal. Hepatology 8:781–784, 1988.

Stephan JL, Vlekova V, Lediest F, Blanche S, Donadieu J, Saint-Basile G, Durandy A, Griscelli C, Fischer A. Severe combined immunodeficiency: a single-center study of clinical presentation and outcome in 117 patients. J Pediatr 123:564–572, 1992.

Stern M. Gastrointestinal allergy. In Walker WA, Durie PR, Hamilton JR, Walker-Smith JA, Watkins JB, eds. Pediatric Gastrointestinal Disease. Philadelphia, BC Decker, 1991, pp. 557–573.

Stevens AC, Walz G, Singaram C, Lipman ML, Zanker B, Muggia A, Antonioli D, Peppercorn MA, Strom TB. Tumor necrosis factor alpha, interleukin-1 beta, and interleukin-6 expression in inflammatory bowel disease. Dig Dis Sci 37:818–826, 1992.

Stevens AC, Lipman M, Spivak J, Peppercorn MA, Strom TB. Heightened perforin and granzyme B but not interleukin 2 mRNA transcripts in active ulcerative colitis colonic specimens. Gastroenterology 106:A778, 1994.

Stiehm ER, Chin TW, Haas A, Peerless AG. Infectious complications of the primary immunodeficiencies. Clin Immunol Immunopathol 40:69–86, 1986.

Strober W, Ehrhardt RO. Chronic intestinal inflammation: an unexpected outcome in cytokine or T cell receptor mutant mice. Cell 75:203–205, 1993.

Strober W, Harriman GR. The regulation of IgA B-cell differentiation. Gastroenterol Clin North Am 20:473–494, 1991.

Strober W, Wochner RD, Carbone PP, Waldmann TA. Intestinal lymphangiectasia: a protein losing enteropathy with hypogammaglobulinemia and impaired homograft rejection. J Clin Invest 46:1643–1656, 1967.

Sutphen JL, Grand RJ, Flores A, Chang TW, Bartlett JG. Chronic diarrhea associated with *Clostridium difficile* in children. Am J Dis Child 137:275–278, 1983.

Svennerholm AM, Hanson LA, Holmgren J, Jalil F, Lindblad BS, Khan SR, Nilsson A, Svennerholm B. Antibody responses to live and killed poliovirus vaccines in the milk of Swedish women. J Infect Dis 143:707–711, 1981.

Tazume S, Ozawa A, Yamamoto T, Takahashi Y, Takeshi K, Saidi SM, Ichoroh CG, Waiyaki PG. Ecological study on the intestinal bacterial flora of patients with diarrhea. Clin Infect Dis 16:S77–S82, 1993.

Teichberg S, Isolauri E, Wapnir RA, Moyse J, Lifshitz F. Development of the neonatal rat small intestinal barrier to nonspecific macromolecular absorption. II. Role of dietary corticosterone. Pediatr Res 32:50–57, 1992.

Thayer WR Jr, Brown M, Sangree MH, Katz J, Hersh T. *Escherichia coli* O:14 and and colon hemagglutinating antibodies in inflammatory bowel disease. Gastroenterology 57:311–318, 1969.

Thompson JF. Specific receptors for epidermal growth factor in rat intestinal microvillus membranes. Am J Physiol 254:G429–G435, 1988.

Thyresson N. Acrodermatitis enteropathica. Acta Derm Venereol (Stockh) 54:383–386, 1974.

Todd RF, Freyer DR. The CD11/CD18 leukocyte glycoprotein deficiency. Hematol Oncol Clin North Am 2:13–31, 1988.

Toth CA, Thomas P. Liver endocytosis and Kupffer cells. Hepatology 16:255–266, 1992.

Touraine JL, Marseglia GL, Betuel H, Souillet G, Gebuhrer L. The bare lymphocyte syndrome. Bone Marrow Transplant 9(Suppl. 1):54–56, 1992.

Treem WR, Davis PM, Hyams JS. Cyclosporine treatment of severe ulcerative colitis in children. J Pediatr 119:994–997, 1991.

Triadafilopoulos G, Pothoulakis C, O'Brien MJ, LaMont JT. Differential effects of *Clostridium difficile* toxins A and B on rabbit ileum. Gastroenterology 93:273–279, 1987.

Trier JS. Celiac sprue. N Engl J Med 325:1709–1719, 1991.

Tu RK, Peters ME, Gourley GR, Hong R. Esophageal histoplasmosis in a child with immunodeficiency with hyper-IgM. Am J Roentgenol 157:381–382, 1991.

Turck D, Ythier H, Maquet E, Deveaux M, Marchandise X, Farriaux JP, Fontaine G. Intestinal permeability to [¹⁵Cr]EDTA in children with Crohn's disease and celiac disease. J Pediatr Gastroenterol Nutr 6:535–537, 1987.

Twomey JJ, Jordan PH, Laughter AH, Meuwissen HJ, Good RA. The gastric disorder of immunodeficient patients. Ann Intern Med 72:499–504, 1970.

Ullrich R, Zeitz M, Heise W, L'age M, Hoffken G, Riecken EO. Small intestinal structure and function in patients affected with human immunodeficiency virus. Ann Intern Med 111:15–21, 1989.

Ullrich R, Zeitz M, Heise W, L'age M, Ziegler K, Bergs C, Riecken EO. Mucosal atrophy is associated with loss of activated T cells in the duodenal mucosa of human immunodeficiency virus infected patients. Digestion 46(Suppl. 2):302–307, 1990.

Unsworth DJ, Hutchins P, Mitchell J, Phillips A, Hindocha P, Holborow J, Walker-Smith JA. Flat small intestinal mucosa and autoimmune antibodies against gut epithelium. J Pediatr Gastroenterol Nutr 1:503–513, 1982.

Van Arsdel PP, Larson EB. Diagnostic tests for patients with suspected allergic disease. Ann Intern Med 110:304–312, 1989.

van Berge-Henegouwen GP, Mulder CJ. Pioneer in the gluten free diet: Willem-Karel Dicke 1905–1962. Gut 34:1473–1475, 1993.

Vandenplas Y. Reflux esophagitis in infants and children: a report from the working group on gastro-oesophageal reflux disease of the European Society of Paediatric Gastroenterology and Nutrition. J Pediatr Gastroenterol Nutr 18:413–422, 1994.

Vandenplas Y, Goyvaerts H, Helven R, Sacre L. Gastroesophageal reflux, as measured by 24-hour pH monitoring, in 509 healthy infants screened for risk of sudden infant death syndrome. Pediatrics 88:834–840, 1991.

Van Sickle GJ, Powell GK, McDonald PJ, Goldblum RM. Milk and soy protein–induced enterocolitis: evidence for lymphocyte sensitization to specific food proteins. Gastroenterology 88:1915–1921, 1985.

Van Wouwe JP. Clinical and laboratory diagnosis of acrodermatitis enteropathica. Eur J Pediatr 149:2–8, 1989.

Vardy PA, Lebenthal E, Shwachman H. Intestinal lymphangiectasia: a reappraisal. Pediatrics 55:842–851, 1975.

Vento S, Garofano T, DePerri G, Dolci L, Concia E, Bassetti D. Identification of hepatitis A virus as a trigger for autoimmune chronic hepatitis type I in susceptible individuals. Lancet 337:1183–1187, 1991.

Vergani D, Mieli-Vergani G. Type II autoimmune hepatitis: what is the role of the hepatitis C virus? Gastroenterology 104:1870–1873, 1993.

Verhave M, Winter HS, Grand RJ. Azathioprine in the treatment of children with inflammatory bowel disease. J Pediatr 117:809–814, 1990.

Voss LM, Rhodes KH. Leukocyte adhesion deficiency presenting with recurrent otitis media and persistent leukocytosis. Clin Pediatr 31:442–445, 1992.

Waksman BH, Ozer H. Specialized amplification elements in the immune system. The role of nodular lymphoid organs in the mucous membranes. Prog Allergy 21:1–18, 1976.

Walker WA, Isselbacher KJ. Uptake and transport of macromolecules by the intestine: possible role in clinical disorders. Gastroenterology 67:531–550, 1974.

Walker WA, Isselbacher KJ. Intestinal antibodies. N Engl J Med 297:767–773, 1977.

Walker-Smith JA. Food sensitive enteropathies. Clin Gastroenterol 15:55–69, 1986.

Walker-Smith JA, Guandalini S, Schmitz J, Shmerling D, Visakorpl JK. Revised criteria for the diagnosis of celiac disease. Arch Dis Child 65:909–911, 1990.

Wan JM, Haw MP, Blackburn GL. Nutrition, immune function, and inflammation—an overview. Proc Nutr Soc 48:315–335, 1989.

Weaver LT, Laker MF, Nelson R, Lucas A. Milk feeding and changes in intestinal permeability and morphology in the newborn. J Pediatr Gastroenterol Nutr 6:351–358, 1987.

Webster ADB. Giardiasis and immunodeficiency diseases. Trans R Soc Trop Med Hyg 74:440–443, 1980.

Webster AD, Slavin G, Shiner M, Platts-Mills TA, Asherson GL. Celiac disease with severe hypogammaglobulinemia. Gut 22:153–157, 1981.

Weiden PL, Blaese RM, Strober W, Block JB, Waldmann TA. Impaired lymphocyte transformation in intestinal lymphangiectasia: evidence for at least two functionally distinct populations in man. J Clin Invest 51:1319–1325, 1972.

Weiner ML. Intestinal transport of macromolecules in food. Food Chem Toxicol 26:867–880, 1988.

Weltzin RA, Lucia Jandris P, Michetti P, Fields BN, Kraehenbuhl JP, Neutra MR. Binding and transepithelial transport of immunoglobulins by intestinal M cells. J Cell Biol 108:1673–1685, 1989.

Werlin SL, Grand RJ. Severe colitis in children and adolescents: diagnosis, course, and treatment. Gastroenterology 73:828–832, 1977.

Werlin SL, Chusid MJ, Caya J, Oechler HW. Colitis in Chronic granulomatous disease. Gastroenterology 82:328–331, 1982.

Weston WL, Huff JC, Humbert JR, Hambidge KM, Neldner KH, Walravens PA. Zinc correction of defective chemotaxis in acrodermatitis enteropathica. Arch Dermatol 113:422–425, 1977.

Whiteside TL, Lasky S, Si L, VanThiel DH. Immunohistologic analysis of mononuclear cells in liver tissues and blood of patients with primary sclerosing cholangitis. Hepatology 5:468–474, 1985.

Widdowson EM, Colombo VE, Artavans CA. Changes in the organs of pigs in response to feeding for the first 24 hours after birth. II. The digestive tract. Biol Neonate 28:272–281, 1976.

Wiesner RH. Primary sclerosing cholangitis. In Schiff L, Schiff ER, eds. Diseases of the Liver, 7th ed. Philadelphia, JB Lippincott, 1993, pp. 411–426.

Wiesner RH, LaRusso NF. Clinicopathologic features of the syndrome of primary sclerosing cholangitis. Gastroenterology 79:200–206, 1980.

Wiesner RH, Ludwig J, LaRusso NF, MacCarty RL. Diagnosis and treatment of primary sclerosing cholangitis. Semin Liver Dis 5:241–253, 1985.

Williams AJ, Wray D, Ferguson A. The clinical entity of orofacial Crohn's disease. Q J Med 79:451–458, 1991.

Wilson MC, Fischer TJ, Riordan MM. Isolated IgG hypogammaglobulinemia in acrodermatitis enteropathica: correction with zinc therapy. Ann Allergy 48:288–291, 1982.

Winter HS, Miller TL. Gastrointestinal and nutritional problems in pediatric HIV disease. In Pizzo PA, Wilfert CM, eds. Pediatric AIDS, 2nd ed. Baltimore, Williams & Wilkins, 1994, pp. 513–533.

Winter HS, Antonioli DA, Fukagawa N, Marcial M, Goldman H. Allergy-related proctocolitis in infants: diagnostic usefulness of rectal biopsy. Mod Pathol 3:5–10, 1990.

Wolf JL, Bye WA. The membranous (M) cell and the mucosal immune system. Annu Rev Med 35:95–112, 1984.

Wraith DG, Merret J, Roth A, Yman L, Merrett TG. Recognition of food allergic patients and their allergens by RAST technique and clinical investigation. Clin Allergy 9:25–36, 1979.

Wyatt J, Vogelsang H, Hubl W, Waldjoer T, Lochs H. Intestinal permeability and the prediction of relapse in Crohn's disease. Lancet 341:1437–1439, 1993.

Yamamoto I, Tsutsui T, Mayumi M, Kasakura S. Immunodeficiency associated with selective loss of helper/inducer T cells and hypogammaglobulinemia in a child with intestinal lymphangiectasia. Clin Exp Immunol 75:196–200, 1989.

Yang H, Shohat T, Rotter JI. The genetics of inflammatory bowel disease. In MacDermott R, Stenson W, eds. Inflammatory Bowel Disease. New York, Elsevier, 1992, pp. 17–53.

Zauli D, Schrumpf E, Crespi C, Cussani F, Fausa O, Aadland E. An autoantibody profile in primary sclerosing cholangitis. J Hepatol 5:14–17, 1987.

Zeiger RS, Heller S, Mellon MH, Forsythe AB, O'Connor RD, Hamburger RN, Schatz M. Effect of combined maternal and infant food allergen avoidance on development of atopy in early infancy: a randomized study. J Allergy Clin Immunol 84:72–89, 1989.

Zhang ZY, Lee CS, Lider O, Weiner HL. Suppression of adjuvant arthritis in Lewis rats by oral administration of type II collagen. J Immunol 145:2489–2493, 1990.

Zinneman HH, Kaplan AP. The association of giardiasis with reduced secretory immunoglobulin A. Am J Dig Dis 17:793–797, 1972.

Chapter 24

Rheumatic Disorders

Lori B. Tucker, Laurie C. Miller,
and Jane G. Schaller

The rheumatic diseases are illnesses that share the basic characteristic of chronic inflammation of connective tissue components in the body. The broad variety of clinical syndromes that are grouped together as "rheumatic diseases" result from the involvement of different organ systems and tissues (Table 24–1). The cause of these disorders is generally unknown, but the contributions to disease pathogenesis of genetic susceptibility, infectious agents, and host abnormalities of immune response are the subject of intense investigation. The diagnosis of rheumatic disorders relies heavily on clinical characteristics of the individual disorders; there are few specific laboratory tests. Although rheumatic diseases are frequently associated with the presence of autoantibodies, elevations of serum immunoglobulin and acute-phase reactant levels, and other laboratory signs of activation of the immune system, such as complement consumption, these findings are nonspecific.

In the first section of this chapter, laboratory tests related to the diagnosis of rheumatic diseases are discussed, including acute-phase reactants, antinuclear antibodies, other autoantibodies, rheumatoid factors, serum complement, immunoglobulins, immune complexes, and histocompatibility antigens. Each of the major rheumatic disorders of childhood is discussed in the second section, including juvenile rheumatoid arthritis and the spondyloarthropathies, systemic lupus erythematosus and its variants, dermatomyositis, acute rheumatic fever, vasculitic syndromes, Kawasaki disease, scleroderma, eosinophilic fasciitis, and Lyme disease.

THE ACUTE-PHASE RESPONSE

The acute-phase response is the term given to the coordinated series of events that occur nonspecifically in response to infection, inflammation, or trauma. Clinical signs of the acute-phase response include fever, anorexia, and increased slow wave sleep, and laboratory findings include neutrophilia, hypoalbuminemia, hypozincemia, hypoferremia, and elevations in a number of plasma proteins, termed "acute-phase proteins" (Dinarello, 1984). The acute-phase proteins include C-reactive protein, serum amyloid A protein, fibrinogen, gamma globulins, α_1-globulins, haptoglobin, ceruloplasmin, and the third component of complement (C3). It is now known that these events are controlled through the activity of cytokines, especially interleukin-1 (IL-1) (Dinarello, 1984; Kushner, 1991).

Table 24–1. Rheumatic Disorders of Childhood

Juvenile rheumatoid arthritis
Juvenile spondyloarthropathy syndromes
　Ankylosing spondylitis
　Seronegative enthesopathy
　Arthritis with inflammatory bowel disease
　Reactive arthritis
　Psoriatic arthritis
　Reiter's disease
Rheumatic fever
Lyme disease
Systemic lupus erythematosus
　Mixed connective tissue disease
　Neonatal lupus syndrome
Dermatomyositis
Vasculitis
　Polyarteritis
　Henoch-Schönlein purpura
　Kawasaki disease
　Takayasu's arteritis
　Wegener's granulomatosis and other granulomatous vasculitis
Scleroderma
Eosinophilic fasciitis

The cytokines, acting in a complex cascade, regulate the gene expression of the acute-phase proteins and directly induce the clinical phenomena associated with the acute-phase response (Schultz and Arnold, 1990). IL-6 and IL-11 act synergistically with IL-1 to regulate hepatic acute-phase protein synthesis (Baumann and Schendel, 1991; Oldenburg et al., 1993). The production of cytokines is stringently controlled at the levels of gene transcription and translation. In addition, the biologic activity of some cytokines is further regulated through the expression of receptors on target cells and by cytokine inhibitors, antagonists, and soluble receptors (Dinarello, 1991). For example, IL-1 activity is opposed by IL-1 receptor antagonist, a specific inhibitor that is differentially regulated and lacks agonist activity.

Cytokine biology is the subject of ongoing intense investigation, both in clinical medicine and basic sciences (see Appendix 2). In rheumatic diseases, aberrant regulation of cytokine responses may result in many of the deleterious effects observed in chronic inflammation. For example, induction of IL-1 within the joint space may occur after infection or injury. If IL-1 activity is not appropriately down-regulated, then unopposed IL-1 activity occurs, resulting in the proliferation of synovial cells and fibroblasts, excessive formation of PGE_2, increased collagen synthesis, increased collagenase production, and eventually activation of osteoclasts and subsequent boney erosions (Dinarello, 1991; Miller and Dinarello, 1987). Excess of IL-1 as well as of other cytokines, has been demonstrated in synovial fluid from inflammatory arthritides. Although many cytokine abnormalities have been reported in the rheumatic diseases, direct evidence linking cytokines to the pathogenesis of other rheumatic diseases is lacking. Many of the rheumatic diseases, however, have clinical and laboratory features that reflect activation of the acute-phase response.

Teleologically, the acute-phase response may be seen as the host's means of creating an inhospitable environment for an invading microbe (Dinarello, 1984).

The acute-phase proteins help contain pathogens and their toxins and inactivate microbial proteases and highly reactive O_2 metabolites. They may also contribute to non–antibody-mediated elimination of some pathogens (such as C-reactive protein for pneumococcus), whereas fever itself inhibits the growth of some microbes. Many bacterial pathogens depend on iron and zinc for optimal growth; the acute-phase response "sequesters" the host's stores of these factors from the invading organisms. Enhanced release of neutrophils from the bone marrow increases the availability of these cells to fight infection. Increased sleep may conserve the host's energy at a time of increased metabolic demands.

LABORATORY FINDINGS

Erythrocyte Sedimentation Rate

It has been noted since the time of the ancient Greeks that red blood cells from some ill patients sediment rapidly. It is now recognized that the erythrocyte sedimentation rate (ESR) reflects erythrocyte aggregation (Ballas, 1975; Fahraeus, 1921). Various biomechanical forces influence the degree of aggregation; most important among these is the amount of plasma proteins present, particularly fibrinogen. Elevations of acute-phase proteins, as is seen nonspecifically in inflammatory states, thus increases the ESR.

Several other circumstances may also result in elevations of the ESR. These include anemia, some drugs (including heparin and some oral contraceptives), pregnancy, and the presence of increased quantities of immunoglobulins, such as in multiple myeloma or Waldenström's macroglobulinemia (Bain, 1983; Burton, 1967; Ozanne et al., 1983; Penchas et al., 1978). In contrast, the ESR is "falsely" decreased in patients with polycythemia, in sickle cell disease and other conditions with abnormal red blood cell morphology, and in some patients with congestive heart failure and hemodynamic compromise (Haber et al., 1991; Reinhart, 1989). Sex, age, race, and obesity may also affect the ESR (Dalhoj and Wiggers, 1990; Gillum, 1993; Haber et al., 1991).

The ESR is a simple, inexpensive, and widely available test and may be useful to follow disease activity in some patients with rheumatic diseases. Because patients with rheumatic diseases have an active inflammatory process, elevated sedimentation rates are often present during periods of active disease. The ESR is not invariably elevated with active inflammation in all patients; therefore, a normal ESR does not exclude the possibility of an active rheumatic process. Furthermore, elevated acute-phase proteins are of little diagnostic value: they are present in any condition associated with inflammation (e.g., infection, malignancy, tissue trauma, and tissue necrosis) and do not distinguish the causes of inflammation.

Rheumatoid Factors

Rheumatoid factors are autoantibodies directed against the constant region (Fc) of IgG immunoglobulin molecules (Milgrom, 1988; Moore and Dorner, 1993; Williams, 1992). Although rheumatoid factors were first discovered fortuitously in the sera of patients with classic rheumatoid arthritis in the 1930s, a complete understanding of their pathophysiologic role in disease remains unknown.

Waller (1969) and Rose et al. (1948) first described the antiglobulin activity of sera from patients with rheumatoid arthritis through experiments showing that these sera augmented agglutination reactions of streptococci by rabbit antibody (Ragan, 1961). Subsequent work showed that antiglobulin antibodies (rheumatoid factors) were responsible for these red blood cell agglutination reactions and that their presence in patients with rheumatoid arthritis was useful as a disease marker.

The precise stimuli for the production of rheumatoid factors in rheumatoid arthritis, and the role they may play in the initiation or perpetuation of disease, is largely unknown. Rheumatoid factors from patients with rheumatoid arthritis differ in their genetic derivation from rheumatoid factors that can be found in low titer in normal individuals or in those produced in paraproteinemias (Carson et al., 1991; Vaughan, 1993). Rheumatoid factors found in healthy individuals, called natural autoantibodies, are generally low affinity, low titer, IgM antibodies and appear to derive from germline immunoglobulin genes, with little mutation evident (Chen et al., 1986; Newkirk et al., 1987). Rheumatoid factors from patients with rheumatoid arthritis, however, are high titer, high affinity, and often of the IgM isotype. Genetic analysis of these rheumatoid factors by several groups (Olee et al., 1992; Pascual et al., 1992) has revealed evidence of antigen selection because of a high number of mutations.

One hypothesis for the production of rheumatoid factors in rheumatoid arthritis is that immune complexes of bacterial or viral antigens and autologous immunoglobulin may act as a trigger, perhaps through altering the autologous antibody to render it immunogenic (Milgrom, 1988; Williams, 1992). Others have suggested that rheumatoid factors are anti-idiotype antibodies to autologous anti-bacterial, parasite, or viral antibody (He et al., 1992; Vaughan, 1993).

The preferred binding site on IgG for rheumatoid factors has been localized to an interface between the CH_2 and CH_3 regions (Mannik, 1992; Sasso et al., 1988). Rheumatoid factors from patients with rheumatoid arthritis and juvenile rheumatoid arthritis have the highest specificity for IgG1 and IgG3 subclasses (Moore and Dorner, 1993; Robbins et al., 1986). Formation of immune complexes composed of IgG and rheumatoid factors occurs in rheumatoid arthritis, and these complexes can be detected in affected synovial tissues, blood vessels, cutaneous ulcers, synovial fluid, and phagocytic cells (Cooke et al., 1975; Johnson and Faulk, 1976; Mannik and Nardella, 1985).

Detection of Rheumatoid Factors

A variety of methods exist for the detection of rheumatoid factors, with no one method more specific for a particular disease (Dorner et al., 1987; Waller, 1969). The most common tests for rheumatoid factors use an agglutination reaction. Particles (e.g., latex or red blood cells) are coated with gamma globulin, and in the presence of sera with rheumatoid factor, agglutinate visibly (Fig. 24–1). The quantity of rheumatoid factor is expressed as the highest dilution of serum that still gives detectable results. The use of laser nephelometry, a particle-counting technique, allows exact quantification of results (Moore and Dorner, 1993).

Enzyme-linked immunosorbent assay (ELISA) methods have been developed to improve the sensitivity of testing for IgM rheumatoid factors. Radioimmunoassays are also available but are less frequently used (Koopman and Schrohenloher, 1980). ELISA testing also allows detection of rheumatoid factors of IgG and IgA isotypes (van Leeuwen et al., 1988). These rheumatoid factors are generally not effective agglutinators of IgG-coated particles and therefore may be missed in standard rheumatoid factor testing. In addition, IgG rheumatoid factors may self-associate, and special techniques such as digestion of IgM rheumatoid factors and immune complexes may be necessary to detect these factors. The clinical associations and usefulness of IgG and IgA rheumatoid factors is still debated, however, and IgM rheumatoid factors continue to be the most commonly reported and used.

Hidden rheumatoid factors are 19S IgM rheumatoid factors that do not react in usual agglutination testing because they exist in serum bound to IgG. After subjecting the serum to acid-gel filtration, investigators have reported detecting rheumatoid factors in 65% to 75% of children with traditionally seronegative juvenile rheumatoid arthritis (Magsaam et al., 1987; Moore et al., 1988). Moore and colleagues have suggested a correlation of hidden rheumatoid factor with disease activity in children with juvenile rheumatoid arthritis (Moore et al., 1980, 1982, 1988), although the role of these factors in pathophysiology is not known.

Clinical Significance

Rheumatoid factors, particularly IgM rheumatoid factors, are typically associated with rheumatoid arthritis, especially in adult patients in whom they are often present in high titer and persist over time; but, rheumatoid factors are neither specific for nor diagnostic of rheumatoid arthritis. They are also found in association with a wide variety of other conditions, including acute and chronic infections, malignancy, and a variety of chronic inflammatory conditions (Aho et al., 1967; Carson et al., 1978; Sherry, 1968). Low titer rheumatoid factor can be detected in normal individuals, and this finding increases with age. The most common reason for a positive rheumatoid factor is the presence of infection.

Classically, rheumatoid factors are thought to be associated with rheumatoid arthritis, but one must also consider the possibility of other rheumatic conditions such as systemic lupus, mixed connective tissue disease, or Sjögren's disease. In addition, only 5% to 10% of children with juvenile rheumatoid arthritis are

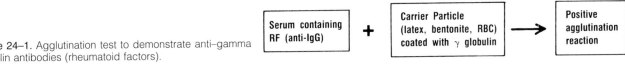

Figure 24–1. Agglutination test to demonstrate anti–gamma globulin antibodies (rheumatoid factors).

seropositive (Petty et al., 1977); thus, rheumatoid factor testing has less importance in the diagnostic evaluation of children with arthritis (Eichenfield et al., 1986a). The presence of rheumatoid factor is associated with more severe and protracted arthritis and vasculitis, both in classic adult rheumatoid arthritis and in seropositive JRA (Panush et al., 1971; Torrigiani et al., 1969).

Lupus Erythematosus Cell

The lupus erythematosus (LE) cell was discovered fortuitously in the early 1940s by Hargraves, who noted the presence of characteristic inclusion-containing cells in the bone marrow of several patients with systemic lupus erythematosus (SLE) (Hargraves et al., 1948; Hargraves, 1969). Soon after Hargraves' description of the LE cell, a factor was found to be present in the serum of these SLE patients that induced LE cell formation (Haserick et al., 1950). This factor was determined to be immunoglobulin that reacted with isolated cell nuclei, leading to phagocytosis. The LE factor is now known to be an antinuclear antibody directed against deoxyribonucleoprotein (DNP) (Holman and Kunkel, 1957). LE cells can be demonstrated in the laboratory by incubating serum containing anti-DNP antibody with cell nuclei, phagocytes, and complement.

Traditionally, the LE cell test was used for the diagnosis of SLE as a crude measure of autoantibody presence in the serum. With the advent of more sensitive and specific fluorescent antinuclear antibody testing, however, the LE test has become less clinically useful. LE cells have been described in patients with conditions other than SLE, including chronic active hepatitis, scleroderma, and Stevens-Johnson syndrome (Rallison et al., 1961; Tuffanelli and Winkelmann, 1961).

Antinuclear Antibodies

The antinuclear antibodies (ANAs) are antibodies that react with various constituents of cell nuclei. The antigenic targets of ANAs include deoxyribonucleic acid (DNA), extractable small nuclear proteins (snRNP), ribonucleic acid (RNA), histones, enzymes, and nucleoli (Beck, 1969; Friou, 1967; Kunkel and Tan, 1964; Nakamura and Tan, 1978; Notman et al., 1975; Seligmann et al., 1965; Sharp et al., 1976; Tan, 1982; Tan et al., 1982b). There has been intense research both to determine the specific molecular components of the antigenic targets of ANAs and to determine the molecular structure of ANAs (Nakamura and Tan, 1992; Tan, 1989). Despite much new information, the stimuli for production of these autoantibodies and understanding of the possible role in pathogenesis of disease remains an enigma. ANAs of all 3 major immuno-

globulin classes (IgG, A, and M) have been identified. An individual serum often contains ANAs reactive with more than one nuclear antigen, either because of antibody cross-reactivity or the presence of a variety of ANAs in the same individual.

Laboratory Detection

Antinuclear antibodies are detected by immunofluorescent staining techniques using a source of cell nuclei, such as a cell line or tissue sections. Although substrates such as mouse or rat liver have been commonly used for ANA testing, current techniques using a human carcinoma cell line (hep 2) have greater sensitivity. In addition, this cell line has higher concentrations of certain nuclear and cytoplasmic antigens, such as Ro and La, which improve the sensitivity and utility of the test (Nakamura and Tan, 1992; Osborn et al., 1984).

The technique of detecting ANAs is outlined in Figure 24–2. Fixed substrate cells on a slide are overlaid with the test serum; antinuclear antibodies in the serum adhere to the cell nuclei. The preparation is washed and layered with a fluorescent-labeled antibody to gammaglobulin, which binds to any areas where ANAs have adhered. Positive preparations appear as fluorescent-stained nuclei. Serum containing ANA is generally titered out, and the result is reported as the highest dilution at which a positive staining is still detected. The ANA titer in patients with rheumatic disease generally does not correlate well with clinical findings, however, and is usually not helpful in following the course of disease. This test detects all types of ANAs and those of all immunoglobulin classes (Gonzalez and Rothfield, 1966). The method is subject to differences in interpretation, depending on laboratory experience, substrate, and kit components. Therefore, test results may vary among laboratories.

Other methods for detecting specific types of ANAs are available. ELISA methods are becoming the most commonly used means of testing for specific autoantibodies (Maddison et al., 1985; Saitta and Keene, 1992). In addition, methods such as counterimmunoelectrophoresis (CIE), precipitation in agar gel (Ouchterlony), and passive hemagglutination are sometimes used.

Antinuclear Antibody (ANA) Patterns

A variety of patterns of ANA staining can be described, including peripheral, homogeneous, speckled, centromere, and nucleolar. The pattern of staining may indicate the type of ANA present or may correlate with a particular disease. A peripheral or homogeneous pattern may be indicative of anti-DNA, RNA, or histone antibodies, and speckled patterns may be indicative of anti-Sm or RNP specificities (Friou, 1967; Sharp et al.,

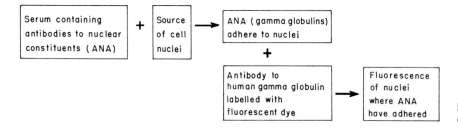

Figure 24–2. Immunofluorescent method for detecting antinuclear antibodies.

1976). Nucleolar and centromere staining are frequently associated with scleroderma (Fritzler et al., 1980; Livingston et al., 1987; Powell et al., 1984).

ANA Specificities

Determination of the antigen specificities of a patient's ANA may be helpful in the diagnosis of autoimmune diseases. Molecular analysis techniques are used to delineate the specificities of autoantibody reactivity with nuclear antigens. Table 24–2 lists clinically important autoantibody reactivities and their recognized disease associations. Many of the antigen targets of rheumatic autoantibodies are molecules with critical cellular functions. It is unknown whether these molecules are the eliciting immunogens for autoantibody formation or whether these autoantibodies are directly pathogenic based on interaction with these intranuclear antigens (Tan, 1989).

The detection in serum of antibodies that react with nuclei may encompass a large range of specific antigen reactivity. The ANA test can be used as a screening test, and if a positive result is obtained, further analysis for autoantibody specificity can be undertaken, depending on the clinical suspicions.

Anti-DNA antibodies are most commonly associated with SLE (see later). Other important ANA specificities include antibodies reactive with RNA and RNA-binding proteins, called Ro, La, Sm, and RNP (see Table 24–2). The Sm and RNP antigens are subcellular particles made up of small nuclear RNA complexed with a set of nuclear nonhistone proteins. These protein and RNA particles have been extensively studied and their struc-

tures have been elucidated through genetic cloning (Craft, 1992; Lerner and Steitz, 1979). Antibodies to Sm and RNP are frequently found together in the same patient and are strongly associated with SLE and mixed connective tissue disease (Borg et al., 1990; Munieus and Schur, 1983; Sharp et al., 1972; Winn et al., 1979). Titers of these autoantibodies may fluctuate during the course of disease, but are rarely useful in the prediction of disease activity.

Antibodies reactive with the Ro antigen were first described in the sera of patients with Sjögren's syndrome (Ben-Chetrit, 1993). The Ro antigen is a complex of protein in association with small cytoplasmic RNA particles. At least five different forms of Ro antigen have been now described, with differing molecular weight forms found in different cell types such as lymphocytes, red blood cells, platelets, and epithelial cells. Autoantibodies have been described that react with only the two major forms of Ro, the 60- and 52-kD forms (Harley et al., 1992). Anti-La is frequently found in association with anti-Ro, and the antigen reactivity is with a 50-kD protein that associates with RNA polymerase proteins which include some of the RNA particles of the Ro antigen (St. Clair, 1992). Both anti-Ro and anti-La are found in some individuals with SLE, Sjögren's syndrome, subacute cutaneous lupus, and C2 complement deficiency and are strongly associated with the neonatal lupus syndrome.

Clinical Significance

The detection of antinuclear antibodies as an isolated laboratory finding is neither diagnostic nor specific for

Table 24–2. Autoantibody Specificities and Disease Associations

Autoantibody	Disease Association	Specificity
DNA	SLE	dsDNA
RNP	SLE, MCTD	Ribosomal nucleoproteins (70, 30, 22 kD) complexed with U1 snRNA
Sm	SLE	Nucleoproteins (9, 11, 13, 16, 28, 29 kD) complexed with U1, U2, U4–6 snRNAs
Histone	SLE, drug-induced SLE, JRA	H1, H2A, B, H3, H4
Ro (SSA)	SLE, Sjögren's syndrome, neonatal SLE	52- or 60-kD protein complexed with RNA particles
La (SSB)	SLE, Sjögren's syndrome, neonatal SLE	48-kD protein complexed with RNA polymerase proteins
Nucleolar	Scleroderma	RNA Pol 1, fibrillarin
Centromere	Scleroderma, CREST	Centromere proteins (17, 80, 140 kD)
SCL-70	Scleroderma	DNA topoisomerase 1
Jo1	Polymyositis	Histidyl tRNA synthetase
PM-Scl	Overlap polymyositis/scleroderma	Complex of 11 polypeptides

Abbreviations: SLE = systemic lupus erythematosus; JRA = juvenile rheumatoid arthritis; CREST = calcinosis, Raynaud's phenomenon, esophageal motility disorders, sclerodactyly, and telangiectasia; SnRNA = small nuclear RNA; tRNA = transfer RNA; MCTD = mixed connective tissue disease; dsDNA = double-stranded DNA.

any one disease. Antinuclear antibodies can be detected in 2% to 9% of healthy children (Allen et al., 1991; Martini et al., 1989). One study (Cabral et al., 1992) found no progression to autoimmune disease among a group of healthy children with positive ANA tests who were carefully followed over an average of 5 years. These data suggest that a child with a positive ANA but no other autoantibodies or clinical findings suggestive of rheumatic illness has little likelihood of developing any rheumatic disease. ANAs are also found in higher frequency among first-degree or second-degree relatives of patients with rheumatic disease (Miles and Isenberg, 1993).

Antinuclear antibodies are not diagnostic of the presence of a rheumatic disease, but do provide valuable information. ANAs are detected in virtually all patients with SLE; the use of human cells for substrate has almost eliminated the occurrence of "ANA-negative" SLE. ANAs are also routinely found in 25% of patients with dermatomyositis and in 50% of patients with scleroderma. In addition, ANAs are often found in children with juvenile rheumatoid arthritis (JRA). Over 50% of young children with pauciarticular onset disease have ANA, often in low titer (Egeskjold et al., 1982; Garcia-De LaTorre and Miranda-Mendez, 1982; Glass et al., 1980). In these children, the ANA is highly associated with an increased risk for chronic iridocyclitis (Glass et al., 1980; Schaller et al., 1974). ANAs are also detected in children with polyarticular onset JRA.

Antinuclear antibodies are found in a variety of other medical conditions. Patients with bacterial, viral, fungal, or parasitic infections may have a positive ANA that persists for a short period of time after recovery. ANAs may also be detected in patients with malignancies (Zuber, 1992). It is therefore important to place the significance of a positive ANA in the context of a patient's clinical presentation to avoid overinterpretation.

Anti-DNA Antibodies

Autoantibodies reactive with DNA are detected most frequently in patients with systemic lupus erythematosus. These antibodies can be detected by a number of different assay systems. The Farr radioimmunoassay detects anti-DNA antibodies using ammonium sulfate precipitation with radiolabeled DNA. Because it is a fluid-phase assay, it detects high avidity anti-DNA antibodies. The ELISA technique is frequently used and is more sensitive than the Farr assay. It detects lower avidity antibodies, however, because the reactivity takes place on a solid support (Tipping et al., 1991). The presence of double-stranded DNA within the kinetoplast of the *Crithidia luciliae* parasite has enabled clinical laboratories to detect anti–double-stranded DNA (dsDNA) antibodies using immunofluorescent methods (Chubick et al., 1978; Crowe and Kushner, 1977).

Anti-dsDNA antibodies are relatively specific for SLE, but occur in only about 60% of SLE patients (Schur and Sandson, 1968; Tan et al., 1966; Weinstein et al., 1983). In contrast, antibodies reactive with the single-stranded form of DNA are detected in 90% of SLE patients, but also are found in a variety of other rheumatic diseases and in conditions such as chronic active hepatitis. In addition to specificity for SLE, the levels of anti-dsDNA antibody detected in many patients correlate well with disease activity and can be used to indicate response to therapy or impending disease flare (Rothfield and Stollar, 1967; Ward et al., 1989). Immune complexes containing anti-dsDNA antibodies have been found in areas of tissue inflammation in lupus glomerulonephritis, implying an important pathogenic role of these antibodies.

Anti-histone Antibodies

Autoantibodies directed against histones, a group of structural proteins associated with DNA, are found in patients with a number of rheumatic conditions, most commonly SLE and drug-induced SLE. Histones are a group of nuclear proteins that function to form DNA into chromatin structures. There are five types of histones that can be separated into two groups: (1) the core particle histones H2A, H2B, H3, and H4; and (2) H1 and variants. In the nucleosome, DNA winds in two superhelical turns around two molecules each of H2A, H2B, H3, and H4; H1 is found associated with the nucleosome in proximity to DNA entering and exiting the nucleosome (Fritzler, 1993; Miller et al., 1992).

The presence of anti-histone antibodies correlates with a positive antinuclear antibody in a homogeneous or diffuse pattern, because histones are a component of the nuclei of any ANA substrate. Early assays to detect anti-histone antibodies used either complement fixation or indirect immunofluorescence of nuclei after acid extraction and resorption of histones (Monestier and Kotzin, 1992). These assays were unreliable, leading to difficulties in interpreting early data. Current techniques include ELISA, radioimmunoassay, or Western blotting using purified histones or chromatin components as antigens. These assays are an improvement, but technical problems still remain. Obtaining purified histone preparations, free of DNA, is difficult. The use of histones from species other than human may lead to reactivity with antigenic epitopes not relevant in the human system. Poorly controlled detecting antisera may allow unacceptable background.

Anti-histone antibodies are found in a majority of patients with SLE, with reactivity most frequent to H1 and H2B (Gioud et al., 1982; Hardin and Thomas, 1983). There is poor correlation of clinical symptoms or course with the presence of anti-histone antibodies. In addition, anti-histone antibodies are found in most individuals who develop a lupus-like syndrome associated with certain medications, most commonly procainamide and hydralazine (Rubin et al., 1985; Totoritis et al., 1988) (see later, Drug-Induced SLE). Anti-histone antibodies have also been found in patients with rheumatoid arthritis, juvenile rheumatoid arthritis (see later), and primary biliary cirrhosis.

Antineutrophil Cytoplasmic Antibodies

Autoantibodies reactive with neutrophil granules were first described by van der Woude and colleagues in 1985. These antibodies, called antineutrophil cytoplasmic antibodies (ANCA), were found in the sera of patients with Wegener's granulomatosis. Since this initial description, there has been intense investigation into the antigenic specificity and clinical applicability of these autoantibodies.

Indirect immunofluorescence using human peripheral blood neutrophils as the substrate is the technique used to detect ANCA in serum. Two patterns of staining can be seen, indicative of reactivity with different antigens and related to different clinical correlations. Cytoplasmic ANCAs (c-ANCA) have a diffuse granular reactivity, whereas the perinuclear ANCAs (p-ANCA) have staining around the nucleus. The autoantigens to which ANCAs are directed are enzymes in the primary and lysosomal granules of neutrophils; c-ANCAs are directed against proteinase 3, a serine protease, and p-ANCAs are primarily reactive with myeloperoxidase but also react with elastase and lactoferrin (Bini et al., 1992; Falk and Jennette, 1988; Goldschmeding et al., 1989). ELISAs specific for these autoantigens are now performed in some laboratories and are a more objective method of detecting ANCA and following the serum titers with accuracy. Immunofluorescence is still the preferred method of screening for ANCA, however, so the pattern of staining can be established (Wiik, 1989).

Antineutrophil cytoplasmic antibody testing is clinically useful in some diagnostic situations. The presence of a c-ANCA is strongly suggestive of Wegener's granulomatosis (Nolle et al., 1989), although it can also be detected in patients with microscopic polyarteritis nodosa and has rarely been reported in Kawasaki disease (Cohen-Tervaert et al., 1991; Falk and Jennette, 1988; Harrison et al., 1989; Savage et al., 1989). ANCA is found in 50% to 96% of patients with Wegener's granulomatosis and can be a useful diagnostic tool (Bleil et al., 1991; Nolle et al., 1989), but definite diagnosis still rests on histologic confirmation. ANCA titers may be useful in following disease activity or predicting flares of disease in patients with Wegener's granulomatosis, thereby guiding therapy (Cohen-Tervaert et al., 1990b; Egner and Chapel, 1990; Halma et al., 1990).

Perinuclear ANCAs are less specific in clinical situations than the c-ANCA. Perinuclear ANCA is found in patients with necrotizing and crescentic glomerulonephritis and granulomatous vasculitic disorders, such as Churg-Strauss syndrome, which are clinically similar to Wegener's granulomatosis (Cohen-Tervaert et al., 1990b, 1991; Halma et al., 1990). p-ANCA has also been reported in patients with ulcerative colitis, primary sclerosing cholangitis, and autoimmune hepatitis (Hardarson et al., 1993). p-ANCA of the IgA isotype has been reported in patients with Henoch-Schönlein nephropathy (van den Wall Bake, 1989). Both p-ANCA and c-ANCA patterns have been recognized in patients with HIV infection (Klaasen et al., 1992).

Anticellular Antibodies

Hematopoietic cells such as red cells, platelets, and lymphocytes may be targets for autoantibodies in patients with rheumatic diseases (Karpatkin et al., 1972; Rustagi et al., 1985; Winfield et al., 1993). Red cell antibodies can be detected by the antiglobulin test (Coombs' test) (Mongan et al., 1967). In the direct Coombs' test, the presence of antibodies on the surface of red cells is routinely detected with the use of antisera to human immunoglobulin, which leads to an agglutination reaction. An indirect Coombs' test can detect free anti–red cell antibody or immune complexes by reacting patient serum with autologous red cells and then observing for agglutination. Red cell antibodies are most commonly associated with idiopathic autoimmune hemolytic anemia. These autoantibodies are also commonly detected in patients with SLE and may result in autoimmune hemolytic anemia. Not all patients with detectable Coombs' antibodies, however, have hemolytic anemia. Autoantibodies reactive with leukocytes and platelets are also found in patients with SLE.

Antiphospholipid Antibodies

Antiphospholipid antibodies (APLAs) represent a class of autoantibody distinct from antinuclear antibodies associated with a spectrum of clinical manifestations. As more has been learned about APLAs, a proliferation of confusing terminology and testing procedures has developed in this area. In 1952, Conley and Hartman first described a unique in vitro anticoagulant phenomenon present in the serum of some patients with SLE. Feinstein and Rapaport designated this factor the lupus anticoagulant, confusing terminology because many patients with this serum factor do not actually have SLE, and the factor is associated with thrombosis, not anticoagulation (Feinstein and Rapaport, 1972). In 1963, Bowie and associates correlated the presence of this anticoagulant property with the occurrence of thrombosis in patients with SLE. It was also recognized that many patients with this serum inhibitor had a false-positive VDRL test. This false-positive serologic test for syphilis occurs because the substrate in the VDRL is phospholipid, primarily cardiolipin. Using an ELISA test, Harris and colleagues (1983) demonstrated that patients with the lupus anticoagulant had autoantibodies reactive with anionic phospholipids such as cardiolipin and suggested a correlation among lupus anticoagulant, antiphospholipid antibodies, and clinical findings of thrombosis, recurrent spontaneous abortion, and thrombocytopenia.

From an immunochemical standpoint, it is important to view APLAs as a class of autoantibodies with a variety of specificities for phospholipids (Sammaritano et al., 1990; Triplett, 1990). Several different laboratory tests can be performed to detect APLAs—the partial prothrombin time (PTT), lupus anticoagulant test, Russell viper venom time, and specific ELISAs for binding to phospholipid. In the PTT, lupus anticoagulant test, and Russell viper venom time, the APLA interferes with the phospholipid-dependent steps of these coagulation assays. In the presence of APLAs, prolongation of coagulation as detected in the laboratory test is not corrected by the addition of normal plasma, in contrast to abnormal coagulation secondary to factor deficiency. Results of ELISA testing for APLAs, although more specific, can vary depending on the phospholipid substrate of the kit used, the expertise of the laboratory, and the scoring of positive results. These factors make it difficult to compare results among laboratories, even when testing is done on the same patient. In addition, because of the heterogeneity of APLAs, patients may have a positive result with one test but negative results with others.

APLAs are detected in patients with autoimmune disease, as well as in other medical conditions. They are rarely detected in normal healthy individuals but are found frequently in patients with infections and malignancy (Kalunian et al., 1988; Love and Santoro, 1990; Sammaritano et al., 1990; Taillan et al., 1989; Vaarala et al., 1986). APLAs are found in 30% to 40% of patients with SLE and when present, especially high titer IgG isotype, may indicate an increased risk of thrombosis, thrombocytopenia, hemolytic anemia, stroke, chorea, transverse myelitis, and cardiac valvular disease (Alarcon-Segovia et al., 1989; Asherson and Hughes, 1988; Asherson et al., 1989a, Cronin et al., 1988; Ford et al., 1988; Harris et al., 1985; Lavalle et al., 1990). Some individuals with clinical manifestations attributable to APLAs do not have SLE; these patients have been classified as having the primary antiphospholipid syndrome (Asherson et al., 1989b; Mackworth-Young et al., 1989). Patients with the primary antiphospholipid syndrome may have one or several of the major clinical manifestations of recurrent thrombosis, recurrent fetal loss, or thrombocytopenia.

There are reports of possible association of APLAs and myocardial infarction or stroke in patients who present with these clinical events at a young age (Fields et al., 1990; Sletnes et al., 1992). Rare cases of isolated deep vein thrombosis in children have been described in association with APLAs (Ravelli et al., 1990).

There has been extensive investigation of the immunochemical nature of APLAs, their derivation, and potential pathogenic mechanisms. APLAs appear to require a cofactor for binding to phospholipids, which has been identified as the plasma protein B2-glycoprotein I (also known as apolipoprotein H) (Roubey et al., 1992). This plasma protein exhibits some anticoagulant properties in vitro, but the exact mechanism of induction of thrombosis by APLAs remains unknown. The immunization of healthy mice or rabbits with the apolipoprotein H cofactor alone results in the induction of APLAs as well as antiapolipoprotein antibodies (Gharavi et al., 1992). Evidence that APLAs have direct pathogenic effects has come from experiments demonstrating a decrease in fecundity and increase in fetal loss in mice injected with monoclonal APLAs (Blank et al., 1990).

Complement

The complement system is comprised of more than 25 plasma proteins, which act in a cascade to perform critical biologic functions of immune cell activation, opsonization of foreign material, and cell injury and lysis (Frank, 1992; Nusinow et al., 1985; Schur and Austen, 1972). There are two components of the complement system, the classical and alternative pathways, each containing unique proteins. In addition to these proteins, inhibitory proteins are present that modulate the system. A complete discussion of the complement system can be found in Chapter 7.

Measurements of complement activity and complement components are useful indicators of activity of certain rheumatic diseases, notably systemic lupus erythematosus, and are also of diagnostic help. In diseases characterized by immune complex formation, depression of serum complement indicates active disease. This is particularly true in immune-mediated nephritis, such as SLE, serum sickness, poststreptococcal glomerulonephritis, and cryoglobulinemia. Some rheumatic diseases associated with nephritis, however, such as Henoch-Schönlein purpura, polyarteritis, and Wegener's granulomatosis, are not associated with depression of serum complement; therefore, determination of serum complement can have diagnostic utility.

Measurement of the total serum hemolytic complement (CH_{50}) is the most useful laboratory test, because it reflects the functional integrity of the entire complement cascade. This test measures the ability of a test serum to hemolyze sensitized (antibody-coated) red blood cells. Measurement of individual complement components, generally C3 and C4, can also be determined by immunodiffusion. One potential difficulty in the interpretation of complement component levels is that they are increased as acute-phase reactants in the presence of active inflammation. Therefore, the actual level may be normal, even with active complement consumption, if accelerated production is occurring (Frank, 1992; Oppermann et al., 1992). In these situations, assessment of complement breakdown products, such as C3d, may be a more accurate measure of complement activation (Buyon et al., 1992; Rother et al., 1993).

Complement Deficiencies and Rheumatic Diseases

Selective deficiency of complement components has been associated with an increase of rheumatic diseases in affected individuals (Table 24–3). In general, deficiency of the early pathway components (C1–C4) is associated with SLE-like conditions (Agnello et al., 1972; Gewurz et al., 1978; Glass et al., 1976; Jasin, 1976; Komine et al., 1992; Moncada et al., 1972; Osterland et al., 1975; Rosenfeld et al., 1976; Schaller et al., 1977; Segurado et al., 1992) (see Chapter 17). These patients frequently present with SLE at a young age, with a history of other affected family members. The association between homozygous complement deficiency and autoimmune disease is strong, particularly in patients with C2 deficiency, in which one third of patients develop systemic or discoid lupus erythematosus. Other rheumatic conditions associated with complement deficiencies include vasculitis and dermatomy-

Table 24–3. Disease Association With Homozygous Complement Deficiencies in Children

Complement Component	Disease Associations
C1q	Systemic lupus erythematosus (SLE), glomerulonephritis
C1r	SLE, glomerulonephritis
C1s	SLE
C2	SLE, glomerulonephritis, Henoch-Schönlein purpura, juvenile rheumatoid arthritis, dermatomyositis
C3	SLE, glomerulonephritis, vasculitis, arthritis
C4	SLE, glomerulonephritis, Henoch-Schönlein purpura
C6–9	Disseminated gonococcal or meningococcal infections; SLE rarely

ositis (Friend et al., 1975; Gelfand et al., 1975; Kolble and Reid, 1993; Leddy et al., 1975). Deficiency of later pathway components (C5–C9) are more frequently associated with infections, particularly with *Neisseria meningitidis* (Wurzner et al., 1992).

The pathogenesis of autoimmune disease in patients with selective complement deficiencies is not clear. It has been suggested that these individuals may have impaired host defense to infections that can act as triggers for autoimmune reactivity. Alternatively, complement deficiency could lead to defective clearance of immune complexes, allowing the development of a chronic inflammatory state. The linkage of genes determining several complement components to the major histocompatibility complex genes may explain associations between complement deficiency and disease susceptibility.

Circulating Immune Complexes

Circulating complexes of antigen and antibody are present in many rheumatic diseases, notably SLE and some forms of vasculitis. Although they participate in disease pathogenesis through tissue deposition and activation of complement, levels of circulating immune complexes are not generally useful in diagnosis or following the course of disease. A variety of laboratory assays are available for detection of immune complexes; results can be difficult to interpret because of poor standardization of assays and interlaboratory variability. Methods of immune complex detection include the following: (1) complement fixation tests, which measure the ability of a serum to consume a standard amount of complement as a result of the presence of aggregates of antigen and antibody; (2) binding of the immune complexes to purified C1q; and (3) the Raji cell assay, a sensitive test, in which circulating complexes bind to a lymphoblastoid cell with a high concentration of complement receptors.

Immunoglobulins

Elevated levels of immunoglobulins are frequently found in the rheumatic diseases in childhood. Patients with SLE often have marked elevations of one or more immunoglobulin classes. Increased levels of immunoglobulins may also occur in JRA, scleroderma, dermatomyositis, and vasculitis, and are related to a generalized inflammatory state, with little diagnostic significance.

IMMUNODEFICIENCY AND RHEUMATIC DISEASES

Selective IgA deficiency has been described in association both with arthritis in children (Ammann and Hong, 1971; Barkley et al., 1979; Cassidy and Burt, 1967; Cassidy et al., 1973; Huntley et al., 1967; Panush et al., 1971; Petty et al., 1977), and with SLE (Cassidy et al., 1969; Takigawa et al., 1976). This association is relatively uncommon. No increased susceptibility to infection has been noted in these patients. One patient with selective IgA deficiency with deletion of the short arm of chromosome 18 had recurrent knee synovitis (Ruvalcaba and Thuline, 1969). An increased prevalence of several chronic inflammatory and autoimmune diseases has been described in patients with IgA deficiency (Ammann and Hong, 1971). The relationship between the IgA deficiency and these diseases is not well understood.

Some patients with hypogammaglobulinemia have been described with arthritis, at times chronic and resembling rheumatoid arthritis (Barnett et al., 1970; Grayzel et al., 1977; Janeway et al., 1956; McLaughlin et al., 1972; Petty et al., 1977; Schaller, 1977b) (see Chapter 11). With immunoglobulin treatment of these patients, however, development of arthritis is now rarely seen. Reasons for this association are not known, but the observation adds weight to the hypothesis that chronic arthritis may result from chronic infection and occur more often in patients predisposed to chronic infections; an alternative explanation suggests faulty regulation of the immune system, resulting in chronic inflammation. Tissue histology resembles that of rheumatoid arthritis, except for a dearth of plasma cells. As expected, such patients usually have negative tests for rheumatoid factors and other autoantibodies; in one child, small amounts of immunoglobulin and a weakly positive latex fixation test were found in the synovial fluid (Barnett et al., 1970).

Other associations between immunodeficiency and rheumatic diseases occur. A dermatomyositis-like syndrome has been reported in patients with hypogammaglobulinemia (Rosen, 1974). ECHO-virus has been isolated from affected muscle, suggesting that this condition represents a viral myositis in immunodeficient hosts (Bardelas et al., 1977; Mease et al., 1981). A lupus-like illness has been described in carrier mothers of boys with chronic granulomatous disease (Schaller, 1972) (see Chapter 15). A chronic arthritis has been described in a family with a granulocyte defect resembling chronic granulomatous disease. Such observations suggest that faulty immune mechanisms and chronic infection may result in diseases that mimic rheumatic diseases and that these mechanisms may be related to the cause of rheumatic disorders.

THE MAJOR HISTOCOMPATIBILITY COMPLEX

The major histocompatibility complex (MHC) is located on the short arm of chromosome 6 and contains genes that encode proteins involved in the control and regulation of the immune response. The study of allograft rejection first brought attention to the role of MHC genes in the regulation of the immune response. MHC-coded molecules, called human leukocyte antigens (HLAs), exist on the surface of most body cells and permit recognition of "self" from "non-self" (Bach and van Rood, 1976; Schaller and Omenn, 1976). Each individual inherits one maternal and one paternal set of MHC genes; a multiplicity of alleles exist for each locus, resulting in widely different capabilities of the immune response for each individual. The prevalence of MHC genes varies among ethnic groups.

The products of the MHC genes can be divided into two distinct classes: HLA-A, HLA-B, and HLA-C molecules are designated class I, and DR, DQ, DP (or Ia) molecules are designated class II. Class III genes, located within the MHC complex but not part of the HLA system, encode some of the complement proteins, the enzyme 21-hydroxylase, and the cytokines tumor necrosis factor alpha and beta (TNF-α and TNF-β). Class I molecules are found essentially on all cells except mature red blood cells, trophoblast, and early embryonic tissue. Expression of class II molecules is normally limited to B cells, monocytes, dendritic cells, and stimulated T cells. Both class I and II molecules are glycoproteins comprised of α and β chains. Structurally, they are distinct. Class I molecules are comprised of an α chain with three domains and a β chain, β_2-microglobulin. Class II molecules are composed of an α and β chain, each of which has two domains. The tertiary structure of class I and II molecules forms an antigen-binding "cleft." Class I molecules preferentially bind cell membranes and react with T-cell receptors on CD8$^+$ cells; class II molecules recognize soluble proteins and react with T-cell receptors on CD4$^+$ cells (Winchester, 1985) (see Chapter 4).

HLA typing requires antisera of known specificity for class I and class II loci. Because of the multiplicity of alleles, over 100 sera are required to type any one individual specifically. Because HLAs are genetically determined traits that can be measured, their identification can be used to provide information concerning disease associations (the occurrence of particular diseases in association with particular HLAs. In addition, HLA haplotype disease linkages can be determined, implying the proximity of genes responsible for such traits to those of the HLA system.

The HLA system is also discussed in Chapters 3 and 4.

HLA and Disease Susceptibility

The contribution of MHC genes to disease susceptibility has been gradually elucidated. It is not yet known whether the relation of a specific HLA locus to a particular disease results from an abnormal gene product, aberrant antigen presentation, closely linked gene or genes, or unrelated genes. Susceptibility to autoimmune disease may also involve genes encoding T-cell receptors, immunoglobulin, complement, peptide transporter proteins, and sex hormones (Carson, 1992). Even when genetic factors play a role, it is clear that other elements, such as gender, age, and environmental exposures, also contribute to disease expression. One hypothesis is that a particular histocompatibility molecule could predispose to autoimmune disease by tightly binding to a self-peptide, thereby increasing its antigenicity. Another possibility is that particular histocompatibility genes preferentially select for the expansion of autoreactive T cells or, alternatively, delete T cells that control infection, allowing chronic immune stimulation and eventual autoreactivity.

HLA Associations with Rheumatic Diseases

HLA-B27 and Rheumatic Disease. The most striking association of HLA and rheumatic disease is that of HLA-B27 with ankylosing spondylitis, first recognized in 1973 (Brewerton et al., 1973a; Schlosstein et al., 1973). Almost 90% of patients with ankylosing spondylitis have HLA-B27, as compared with only about 9% of the white North American population. An individual carrying the HLA-B27 has 70 times the relative risk of developing ankylosing spondylitis as does an HLA-B27 negative individual. It has been estimated that only 3% to 20% of individuals with HLA-B27, however, actually develop ankylosing spondylitis or related diseases (Brewerton, 1976; Calin and Fries, 1975). Other spondyloarthropathies (diseases associated with spondylitis) are also associated with HLA-B27; these include Reiter's syndrome (Arnett et al., 1980; Brewerton et al., 1973b; Morris et al., 1974a), the spondylitis of inflammatory bowel disease (Brewerton et al., 1974b; Lindsley and Schaller, 1974; Morris et al., 1974b), psoriatic spondylitis (Brewerton et al., 1974b; Eastmond and Woodrow, 1977), acute iridocyclitis (Brewerton et al., 1974a), isolated sacroiliitis, pauciarticular arthritis of teenage and adult patients (Schaller and Wedgwood, 1976), and the "reactive" arthritis that follows infections with such organisms as *Salmonella, Shigella, Yersinia enterocolitica, Chlamydia,* and *Campylobacter* (Goldenberg, 1983).

Both reactive arthritis and Reiter's syndrome occur after identifiable environmental events, such as infections; this suggests that genetically predisposed hosts (i.e., those with HLA-B27) exposed to certain environmental insults (e.g., *Shigella* or *Yersinia*) can develop rheumatic diseases (Khan and Kellner, 1992; Petty, 1990). Experiments with transgenic HLA-B27 rats suggest that the HLA locus itself in some way confers disease susceptibility, because these animals spontaneously develop an inflammatory disease with a marked resemblance to spondyloarthropathy (Hammer et al., 1990). Diarrhea is the earliest sign of disease, a reflection of massive infiltration of the intestinal lamina propria with B27-positive T cells. Animals then develop axial and peripheral joint arthritis, as well as nail and skin changes. The affected rats have a high density of B27 on mononuclear cells, possibly allowing presentation of a B27 peptide to a reactive T-cell population that then triggers an arthritogenic response. Interestingly, arthropathy is not evident among rats raised in a germ-free environment (Taurog et al., 1993).

Associations of the spondyloarthropathies with HLA-B27 appear to hold true for various racial groups (Sonozaki et al., 1975), although the association may be weaker for American blacks (Khan et al., 1976). Some B27 subtypes, not always identified on screening tests, are more strongly associated with spondyloarthropathies in different racial groups.

HLA Associations with JRA. The immunogenetic associations of juvenile rheumatoid arthritis continue to be an area of interest, although the haplotype associations are not as clear as in the B27-related diseases. Children with pauciarticular JRA have been shown to exhibit an increase of HLA-A2, DRw8, and DPw2 haplotypes (Glass et al., 1980; Nepom and Glass, 1992; Stasny and Fink, 1979). Using molecular probes to identify disease-specific alleles, within the HLA-DRw8 and DPw2 groups, DRB1*0801 and DPB1*0201 alleles have been found associated with pauciarticular JRA (Malagon et al., 1992). In studies attempting to delineate HLA associations with chronic iridocyclitis in pauciarticular JRA, the presence of HLA-DRB1*1104 was associated with a higher risk for eye disease in one population of children with JRA (Melina-Aldana et al., 1992). Other investigators have suggested that HLA-DRB1*0801 and DRB1*1301 are correlated with progression from a pauciarticular to polyarticular course of disease (Nepom and Glass, 1992).

There is less information concerning HLA associations with subtypes of JRA other than pauciarticular. An association of systemic onset JRA and HLA-DR4, the HLA haplotype found in adults with rheumatoid arthritis has been reported (Bedford et al., 1992). HLA-DR4 has also been reported to be increased in children with rheumatoid factor–positive polyarticular JRA (Vehe et al., 1990). Although these data need further confirmation, they suggest that in time HLA typing may be helpful in predicting disease manifestations and course.

Clinical Value of HLA Typing

HLA typing is not diagnostic of any disease and has little practical use in clinical medicine other than transplantation. HLA-B27 testing has come into vogue in the evaluation of individuals with arthritis but, as noted previously, HLA-B27 is not diagnostic of any of the spondyloarthropathies. Histocompatibility studies remain of great interest in clinical research to classify diseases, to seek possible genetic factors that predispose to disease, and to predict adverse responses to medication.

The most important applications are yet to come. Identification of individuals who are at greatest risk for the development of genetically determined diseases

may allow measures to prevent these diseases. Furthermore, disease associations with the HLA system may permit understanding of basic disease mechanisms. As techniques in molecular genetics improve, investigation of regions of the genome outside of the MHC complex are also being conducted for disease associations.

JUVENILE RHEUMATOID ARTHRITIS

Juvenile rheumatoid arthritis is a disease characterized by chronic arthritis in children. It is termed Still's disease, juvenile chronic polyarthritis, juvenile arthritis, and juvenile chronic arthritis in other countries. The arthritis results from inflammation of synovium, the lining tissue of the joints (Fig. 24–3). The synovitis of rheumatoid arthritis is characteristically chronic, lasting weeks, months, or even years. If chronic synovitis persists long enough, damage to articular cartilage and subchondral bone may result, causing permanent joint damage, because articular cartilage regenerates poorly, if at all. Damage to joint surfaces and to ligaments and tendons surrounding joints may lead to permanent deformities, such as subluxation, fusion, or joint destruction. Deformities may also result from shortening of muscles and other tissues around arthritic joints (contractures), even in the absence of significant damage to the joints themselves. Fortunately, most children with chronic arthritis escape without permanent joint damage or deformity.

Historical Aspects

The occurrence of chronic arthritis in children was first described by an English pediatrician, George Frederick Still, in 1897. He focused attention on the fact that some children with arthritis have manifestations affecting other body systems besides the joints. He was the first to advance the idea that arthritis in children

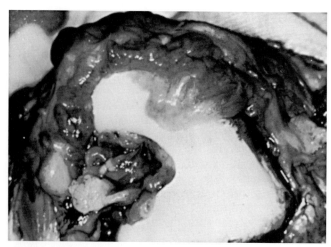

Figure 24–3. Rheumatoid synovitis, visible in a knee joint undergoing surgery. The synovium is greatly hypertrophied, with formation of grape-like projections (villi) and early extensions over the surface of the articular cartilage (pannus formation).

Table 24–4. Subgroups of Juvenile Rheumatoid Arthritis (JRA)

Subgroup	Percent of JRA Patients	Ratio Girls/Boys	Age at Onset	Joints Affected	Laboratory Tests	Extra-articular Manifestations	Prognosis
Systemic onset	20%	8/10	Any age	Many joints, large and small	ANA neg RF neg	High fever, rash, organomegaly, polyserositis, leukocytosis	25% severe arthritis
Rheumatoid factor negative polyarticular	25–30%	8/1	Any age	Many joints, large and small	ANA 25% RF neg	Low-grade fever, mild anemia, malaise	10–15% severe arthritis
Rheumatoid factor positive polyarticular	10%	6/1	Late childhood	Many joints, large and small	ANA 75% RF 100%	Low-grade fever, anemia, malaise; rheumatoid nodules	>50% severe arthritis
Pauciarticular with chronic iridocyclitis (type I)	25%	7/1	Early childhood	Few large joints (hips and sacroiliac joints spared)	ANA 50% RF neg	Few constitutional complaints; chronic iridocyclitis in 50%	Severe arthritis rare; 10–20% ocular damage from iridocyclitis
Pauciarticular with sacroiliitis (type II)	15–20%	1/10	Late childhood	Few large joints (hip and sacroiliac involvement common)	ANA neg RF neg HLA-B27 75%	Few constitutional complaints; acute iridocyclitis in 5–10% during childhood	Some will have spondyloarthropathies as adults

Abbreviations: ANA = antinuclear antibody; RF = rheumatoid factor; HLA-B27 = human leukocyte antigen-B27.

was a different disease than rheumatoid arthritis in adults. Since Still's first description, many series of children with chronic arthritis have been reported, adding to the clinical spectrum of JRA.

Classification

On careful analysis of large series of children with JRA, several fairly distinct clinical subgroups of disease have emerged, with characteristics generally apparent within 6 months of disease onset (Table 24–4). At least five subgroups can be easily identified (Schaller, 1977d, 1977f, 1980): systemic onset disease, polyarticular seronegative disease, polyarticular seropositive disease (rheumatoid factor positive or negative), pauciarticular disease associated with chronic iridocyclitis (type I), and pauciarticular disease associated with sacroiliitis (type II).

The seropositive polyarticular type of disease resembles classic adult-onset rheumatoid arthritis. Seronegative polyarthritis and pauciarticular arthritis associated with sacroiliitis are also well recognized in adults. Systemic onset JRA is rare in adults, however, and pauciarticular disease type I has not been described in adults. It seems that what is called juvenile rheumatoid arthritis is actually more than one disease, but it is also possible that patients with the same basic disease may show several distinct clinical patterns. At any rate, recognition of the five disease subgroups of JRA is useful in the diagnosis and care of affected children.

Epidemiology

Chronic childhood arthritis rarely begins in the first year of life, but may begin at any time thereafter up to adulthood. There are age differences in onset among the different subgroups: seropositive polyarthritis and pauciarticular disease type II are associated with an older age at onset; seronegative polyarthritis and systemic onset diseases may begin at any time during childhood (often in young children); and pauciarticular disease type I generally begins before the age of 6 years. Sex ratios also vary among subgroups; there are strong female preponderances in seronegative polyarthritis, seropositive polyarthritis, and pauciarticular disease type I. There is a male preponderance in pauciarticular disease type II, and systemic onset JRA affects girls and boys equally.

The exact incidence of JRA in the United States is unknown, but it is not rare. It has been estimated that 5% of all rheumatoid arthritis begins in children less than 16 years old and that there are about 250,000 affected children in the United States (Gare and Fasth, 1992; Gare et al., 1987; Gewanter et al., 1983; Towner et al., 1983).

Clinical Manifestations

Systemic Onset Juvenile Rheumatoid Arthritis

About 20% of children with JRA have disease characterized at the onset by prominent extra-articular (systemic) manifestations as well as arthritis. These systemic manifestations include high intermittent fever, rash, hepatosplenomegaly, lymphadenopathy, pericarditis, pleuritis, abdominal pain, leukocytosis, anemia, and occasional disseminated intravascular coagulopathy.

Fever is a prominent characteristic, with one or two daily high elevations (102°F to 107°F) and subsequent rapid return to normal or subnormal levels (Fig. 24–4). Febrile patients may appear very ill, only to improve dramatically as the fever subsides.

The rash (Fig. 24–5) is characteristic of systemic JRA and may be more prominent at times of high fever. Individual lesions are small, evanescent, pale red mac-

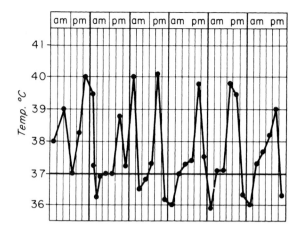

Figure 24–4. Characteristic fever of "systemic" juvenile rheumatoid arthritis. High temperature elevations, occurring once or twice daily are followed by a rapid return to normal or subnormal levels. (From Schaller JG, Beckwith B, Wedgwood RJ. Hepatic involvement in juvenile rheumatoid arthritis. J Pediatr 77:203–210, 1970.)

ules, often with central clearing; they may appear on any part of the body, including the palms and soles. Lesions are occasionally pruritic and often occur in areas of skin trauma, such as scratch marks (isomorphic response). The rash appears more prominent with fever or external application of heat; it generally appears in the evening when the fever is at its maximum and usually disappears by morning (Isdale and Bywaters, 1956; Schaller and Wedgwood, 1970).

Pleuritis and pericarditis are generally mild and often asymptomatic, although some patients may complain of chest pain. (Bernstein et al., 1974; Leitman and

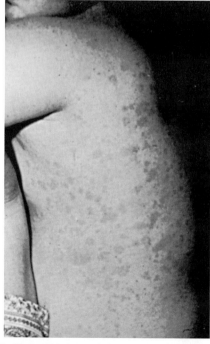

Figure 24–5. Characteristic rash of juvenile rheumatoid arthritis. This rash is also characterized by evanescence and recurrence.

Bywaters, 1963; Wagener et al., 1981). Occasionally, patients may present with large pericardial effusions requiring decompression. Lymphadenopathy and hepatosplenomegaly may be marked, simulating malignancy. There may be mild alternations in liver function tests, which may be associated with active systemic disease; chronic liver disease does not occur (Schaller et al., 1970). When abnormal liver function tests are found, the hepatotoxicity of drug therapy, such as nonsteroidal anti-inflammatory drugs (NSAIDs) or methotrexate, must be differentiated. A few children receiving high dose salicylates during the systemic phase of the illness develop symptoms of hepatotoxicity with concomitant elevation of liver enzymes to dramatic levels, hepatic tenderness, and abnormal coagulation profiles (Koff, 1977). A syndrome of disseminated intravascular coagulation has been described in children with systemic JRA and is a potentially fatal complication if not treated promptly with corticosteroids. This syndrome has been reported in a few cases in association with intramuscular gold treatment in children with active systemic disease (Jacobs et al., 1984; Scott et al., 1985; Silverman et al., 1983).

Severe abdominal pain occurs at times with active systemic JRA, possibly because of mesenteric adenopathy or peritonitis. Peripheral leukocyte counts may be greatly elevated, sometimes exceeding 50,000/mm³. Anemia may be severe and require treatment with corticosteroids. Central nervous system disease with seizures, behavioral disturbances, and abnormal electroencephalograms has been occasionally described (Jan et al., 1972); it is not certain whether such events are actually part of the disease, however. Growth retardation may accompany long-standing active disease (Bernstein et al., 1977). This complication results from the catabolic effects of active inflammation, poor nutritional intake, and the effects of corticosteroids used in some children for treatment.

Initial joint manifestations at the onset of systemic JRA may include overt arthritis or only myalgia and arthralgia. Children are irritable, seem to hurt all over, and may refuse to stand or move about. Joint pain is prominent when the fever is high and may improve when the fever recedes. Systemic manifestations may be so overwhelming that joint problems are initially overlooked. Within a few weeks of onset, however, it usually becomes apparent that the patient has arthritis. Occasionally, overt arthritis does not begin for weeks, months, or even years after systemic manifestations. Multiple joints are generally affected in a polyarticular pattern; a few patients have only a few joints involved.

Systemic manifestations, particularly fever, usually remit after a period of weeks or months; in some patients, however, arthritis becomes chronic, even though systemic manifestations are gone. Systemic manifestations may recur at unpredictable intervals, but rarely after late adolescence. Systemic disease is rarely fatal. The major morbidity of systemic onset JRA lies in the degree and severity of arthritis. Arthritis ultimately involves multiple joints in many patients with systemic onset disease, and 25% of these patients eventually develop severe progressive arthritis with ultimate disability.

Seronegative Polyarticular Juvenile Rheumatoid Arthritis

About 20% to 30% of children with JRA have arthritis involving multiple joints within a few months of onset, without prominent systemic manifestations, and with negative tests for rheumatoid factors. Any joint may be affected, except perhaps those of the lumbothoracic spine. Arthritis may begin in either large joints (knees, ankles, wrists, and elbows) or small joints of the hands (Fig. 24–6) and feet. The cervical spine, temporomandibular joints, and hips are also affected in many patients. Joint involvement is usually symmetric. Affected joints are swollen, warm, and tender, and have decreased motion or pain on motion. Joint effusions and synovitis are often present. Stiffness of joints after inactivity, particularly in the morning, is characteristic in children as in adults.

Although extra-articular manifestations are not as dramatic as in systemic onset JRA, many patients with seronegative polyarthritis have malaise, a low-grade fever, anorexia, growth retardation, irritability, and mild anemia during periods of active disease. Rheumatoid nodules are rarely found.

Prognosis is related to the severity and duration of arthritis and the degree of permanent joint damage. Periods of active arthritis may last for months or years and may recur long after seemingly complete remission (Jeremy et al., 1968). Fortunately, 80% to 90% of children eventually enter remissions or have relatively mild chronic disease and do not develop permanent joint damage or serious disability. A few have severe progressive disease, with joint destruction and permanent disability. Micrognathia with dental deformities and facial asymmetry may result from temporomandibular arthritis in early childhood; occasionally, surgical correction is necessary.

Seropositive Polyarticular Juvenile Rheumatoid Arthritis

About 5% to 10% of children with JRA have polyarticular arthritis associated with positive tests for rheumatoid factors (seropositivity) by standard agglutination techniques (IgM rheumatoid factors) (Schaller, 1980; Schaller and Hansen, 1982a). Rheumatoid factors are present at disease onset and remain usually in high titers. In most seropositive patients, the onset of disease is after 8 years of age. The pattern of joint involvement is similar to that of seronegative polyarthritis and is identical to that in adult onset rheumatoid arthritis. The course of arthritis, however, is severe, with at least 50% of patients (Williams and Ansell, 1985) not responding well to any known methods of treatment. Seropositive patients frequently have subcutaneous rheumatoid nodules similar to those observed in adults and a few develop rheumatoid vasculitis. These patients are also more likely to carry the same HLA association found in adults with rheumatoid arthritis, HLA-DR4 (Barron et al., 1992; Nepom et al., 1982). Sjögren and Felty syndromes have also been described in patients of this subgroup. Patients may have low-grade fever, malaise, and weight loss or growth retardation.

Pauciarticular Juvenile Rheumatoid Arthritis

About 50% of children with JRA have arthritis limited to one or only a few joints during the first 6 months and often during the entire course of their disease. Arthritis generally affects large joints and is spotty rather than symmetric in distribution. It is difficult to define this disease solely by numbers of joints affected; official numbers that are accepted are usually either four or five total joints. This type of disease is referred to as pauciarticular (few joint) arthritis (Bywaters and Ansell, 1965; Cassidy et al., 1967; Schaller, 1977d, 1977f, 1980; Schaller and Hansen, 1982b; Schaller and Wedgwood, 1976). The clinical appear-

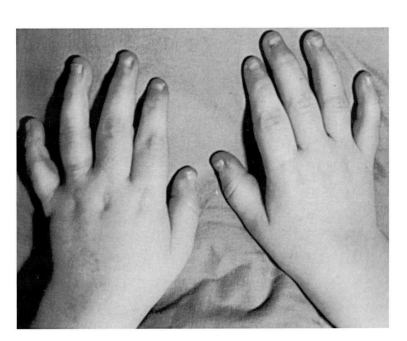

Figure 24–6. Characteristic appearance of the hands of a child with polyarticular rheumatoid arthritis. The proximal interphalangeal joints are swollen ("spindling"), as are the metacarpophalangeal and wrist joints.

ance of affected joints is similar to that of polyarticular disease, as is the synovial histology. At least two subgroups exist within pauciarticular disease (Schaller and Wedgwood, 1976).

Pauciarticular Arthritis Type I. This subgroup predominantly affects young girls and accounts for about 40% to 50% of all JRA cases. Large joint involvement predominates, particularly affecting knees, ankles, and elbows. Small joints of the hands are spared or affected only in a spotty fashion; hip involvement is unusual and sacroiliitis does not occur. The arthritis may be of long duration but is generally mild. Eighty percent or more of patients remain with only pauciarticular joint involvement, and prognosis concerning joint function is good. As many as 20% develop polyarthritis over the years and may incur joint destruction. Local bony overgrowth around affected joints may cause growth disturbances, such as inequality of leg lengths; these generally correct with growth, although a lift to the contralateral shoe may be temporarily required to permit normal function. Disabling flexion contractures can occur around affected joints, particularly the knee and elbow, if proper attention is not given to physical therapy.

The main complication in these patients is chronic iridocyclitis (Merriam et al., 1983; Schaller, 1977c; Smiley et al., 1957). Iridocyclitis occurs occasionally in patients with systemic onset disease or seropositive polyarthritis. Iridocyclitis usually begins insidiously and can be detected early only by slit-lamp examination. One or both eyes may be affected. Unless ocular inflammation is promptly controlled, anterior chamber scarring, secondary glaucoma, cataract formation, and band keratopathy may ensue, with severe or total loss of vision. Reasons for the association of iridocyclitis with pauciarticular arthritis remain unknown. Other extra-articular manifestations are uncommon in this group of patients, although malaise, anorexia, low-grade fever, and mild anemia may occur during periods of active disease.

The outcome for most children with pauciarticular JRA is excellent, but a small percentage of these children progress to a polyarticular course that may be associated with disability and severe disease. It is suggested that up to 15% of children with pauciarticular JRA eventually develop polyarticular disease. There are currently no clinical or genetic parameters to distinguish the children who will progress to a more severe course of disease (Hertzberger-Ten Cate et al., 1992).

Pauciarticular Arthritis Type II. Pauciarticular disease type II affects children, usually boys, who tend to be more than 8 years old at onset; about 15% of all JRA patients fall into this subgroup. Differentiation of children with this form of JRA and spondyloarthropathy is confusing, because there is likely overlap between the two groups (Burgos-Vargas, 1993).

In pauciarticular type II disease, large joints, particularly the hips, knees, and ankles, are predominantly affected; metatarsal joints are sometimes involved, and occasional spotty involvement of the upper extremities may occur as well. Hip girdle symptoms are common; indeed, patients may be rendered nonambulatory by

severe hip pain and stiffness. Some patients have radiographic sacroiliitis at the time of onset; this increases with the duration of disease. Sacroiliitis may be silent, unassociated with clinical symptoms, or may manifest by hip girdle pain or sacroiliac tenderness. Enthesopathy (inflammation at the site of tendon insertions into bones) is common and may differentiate these patients from those with other forms of JRA (Rosenberg and Petty, 1982).

The course of pauciarticular disease type II is variable, and the ultimate outcome for patients in this group is not yet defined. Peripheral arthritis may wax and wane over a period of years or remain chronic with little joint destruction. With time, some of these patients develop one of the spondyloarthropathies, such as ankylosing spondylitis, the spondylitis of inflammatory bowel disease, psoriatic arthritis, or Reiter's syndrome (Arnett et al., 1976; Burgos-Vargas, 1993; Lindsley and Schaller, 1974; Schaller, 1977a; Schaller et al., 1969b; Singsen et al., 1977a). There is often a positive family history of spondyloarthropathy. Some patients have acute self-limited attacks of iridocyclitis that are rarely associated with permanent ocular damage (Kanski, 1977; Schaller, 1977c; Schaller et al., 1974). Other extra-articular complaints are not usual, unless features of the spondyloarthropathies appear, such as Reiter's disease or inflammatory bowel disease.

Pathogenesis

The cause of JRA is not known. The histopathology of affected tissues, notably synovial tissues, shows chronic inflammation, with lymphocytes and plasma cells as the chief inflammatory cells. No histologic differences have been reported among synovial tissues from the various JRA subgroups or adult disease (Wynne-Roberts et al., 1978). Affected synovial tissues, studied chiefly in adult rheumatoid arthritis, may contain organized lymphoid follicles and germinal centers, and plasma cells may be shown by fluorescent antibody or elution techniques to be producing immunoglobulins, including rheumatoid factors.

There are emerging data to suggest a role for genetic susceptibility factors and cellular immune reactivity in the pathogenesis of JRA. Children with JRA often have a variety of autoantibodies present in their serum, although their role in disease onset and pathogenesis is not known. The role of infectious exposure as a trigger for JRA continues to be an appealing hypothesis, but with little direct scientific proof.

Immunogenetics

As increased knowledge has become available concerning the contribution of the MHC locus in immune reactivity, interest has focused on whether specific MHC alleles predispose to autoimmune diseases, including JRA. Reports of JRA occurring in monozygotic twins and siblings (Baum and Fink, 1968; Kapusta et al., 1969) provide a clue that genetic factors may play a role in susceptibility to JRA.

The majority of studies investigating HLA associations in JRA have focused on children with the pauciarticular subtype, because this is the most common form of JRA. There is an increase in HLA-A2, HLA-DR8, HLA-DR5, and HLA-DPw2 in these patients (Glass, et al., 1980; Malagon et al., 1992; Nepom and Glass, 1992; Schaller and Hansen, 1982b; Stasny and Fink, 1979). A particular allele split of HLA-DR5, HLA-DRB1*1104, has been seen in increased frequency in children with pauciarticular JRA who develop iridocyclitis. Correlations of HLA subtype and clinical course of disease to date have been weak and unrevealing.

There is less information available concerning HLA associations with subtypes of JRA other than pauciarticular onset. HLA-DR4 occurs in children with seropositive polyarticular disease (Nepom, et al., 1982), with evidence that children with systemic JRA also have an increased incidence of DR4 (Barron et al., 1992; Bedford, et al., 1992).

Infection as a Pathogenic Factor

Many investigators have been searching for specific infectious triggers in the pathogenesis of JRA. A number of viral and bacterial infections are known to be commonly associated with episodes of transient arthritis. For example, parvovirus B19, the causative agent of childhood Fifth disease, can be associated with transient arthritis that may appear similar to JRA (Nocton et al., 1993). Serologic evidence of antibody titers to rubella virus found in the serum of children with JRA (Linnemann et al., 1975) was followed by reports of active rubella virus being cultured from synovial fluid of children with JRA (Chantler et al., 1985). Episodes of reactive arthritis have a clear association with infectious triggers in many cases, generally with organisms such as *Chlamydia trachomatis, Yersinia enterocolitica, Salmonella, Shigella,* and *Campylobacter.* Studies have shown reactivity of blood and synovial fluid T cells to some of these bacterial pathogens in children with reactive arthritis, but also in some children with pauciarticular type II JRA (Sieper et al., 1992). These data suggest that exposure to common infectious agents may, in susceptible hosts, result in a chronic arthritis such as JRA.

Diagnosis and Laboratory Findings

Diagnosis of JRA rests solely on clinical recognition of the disease (Brewer et al., 1977; Cassidy et al., 1986). It is critical that other disorders associated with arthritis and joint pain be excluded, including septic arthritis, osteomyelitis, Lyme arthritis, other rheumatic diseases, inflammatory bowel disease, malignancies, congenital defects of the musculoskeletal system, and numerous noninflammatory conditions of bones and joints in children (e.g., avascular necrosis of bone, discitis, and slipped capital femoral epiphysis). Other than radiographic changes of joint destruction occurring late in severe disease, there are no diagnostic laboratory tests, but laboratory studies may be useful in the exclusion of other diseases.

Rheumatoid Factors. Rheumatoid factors are demonstrable in virtually 100% of adults with rheumatoid arthritis by standard agglutination techniques, but are found in JRA patients much less frequently (Cassidy and Valkenberg, 1967; Hanson et al., 1969; Jeremy et al., 1968; Laaksonen, 1966; Schaller, 1980; Schaller and Hansen, 1982a). Rheumatoid factor positivity occurs almost exclusively in children who are older than 8 years at disease onset and who have a form of JRA similar to adult-onset rheumatoid arthritis. Patients who are seronegative at disease onset do not become seropositive as they get older, even though active disease continues. The presence of rheumatoid factors detectable by standard agglutination tests correlates with severe joint disease in most patients and with the presence of rheumatoid nodules in both children and adults and with rheumatoid vasculitis in adults (Nepom, et al., 1982; Schaller, 1977d, 1977f, 1980; Schaller and Hansen, 1982a).

The reasons for negative agglutination tests for rheumatoid factors in most cases of childhood onset arthritis are unknown. Rheumatoid factors are not seen in systemic JRA or either of the pauciarticular subgroups. Some investigators have reported the presence of "hidden rheumatoid factors" in children with JRA who are seronegative in usual agglutination testing (see earlier, Rheumatoid Factors) (Moore et al., 1980, 1988). The role of these serum factors is unknown.

Antinuclear Antibodies. Antinuclear antibodies are demonstrable in 20% to 30% of both adults and children with rheumatoid arthritis (Lawrence et al., 1993; Leak, 1988; Rosenberg, 1988; Schaller et al., 1974). The incidence of antinuclear antibodies varies among JRA subgroups, but positive tests are found in 25% of children with seronegative polyarthritis, 50% or more of children with pauciarticular disease type I, and 75% of patients with seropositive polyarthritis (Schaller, 1977d, 1977f; Schaller and Hansen, 1982a). Antinuclear antibodies are rarely, if ever, found in systemic JRA or pauciarticular disease type II.

Antinuclear antibodies occur more frequently in girls, especially in those with early childhood onset of disease; this is consistent with the subgroup distribution. There is no apparent correlation with severity or duration of disease. Antinuclear antibodies in children with the pauciarticular subtype of JRA, however, are associated with the development of chronic iridocyclitis (Egeskjold et al., 1982; Schaller et al., 1974). Positive tests for antinuclear antibodies are thus useful in identifying patients who are at risk for this complication. A high prevalence of reactivity against histones among children with JRA, especially those with iridocyclitis, has been described by a number of investigators (Leak and Woo, 1991; Monestier et al., 1990; Ostenson et al., 1989).

Joint Fluid Analysis. Joint fluid analysis is not diagnostic of juvenile rheumatoid arthritis, but its examination is crucial in the exclusion of septic arthritis or other crystal-induced arthritides such as gout, although rare in children. In JRA, joint fluid is characteristically somewhat turbid and yellow-green in color and contains an increased number of white cells, predominantly polymorphonuclear leukocytes (5,000 to 80,000/mm³). Synovial histology is not specific but resembles that of other rheumatic diseases; a synovial biopsy is sometimes helpful in excluding chronic septic arthritis, tuberculous arthritis, or rare conditions such as sarcoidosis or synovial tumors.

Acute-Phase Reactants. Acute-phase reactants, such as the erythrocyte sedimentation rate, are increased in many children with active JRA. The ESR is frequently normal in children with pauciarticular JRA. Tests of acute-phase reactants are not diagnostic and have only limited value in monitoring the course of disease. Mild anemia is common in children with active disease (Koerper et al., 1978); occasionally, children with severe systemic disease may have severe anemia (Schaller, 1977d, 1977f; Schaller and Hansen, 1982a). The nature of the anemia is poorly understood; hypoproliferation of red blood cells, iron deficiency, gastrointestinal blood loss related to medications, and perhaps increased red cell destruction may all play a role. Reports of success in using recombinant erythropoietin in treating the severe anemia of systemic JRA are promising but need further study (Fantini et al., 1992).

Radiography. Radiographs and other imaging techniques may provide useful information in documenting the extent of joint damage in the individual patient. Radiographs taken within the first year or so of disease show only soft tissue swelling, periarticular osteoporosis, and sometimes juxta-articular periostitis; those taken later in severe disease may show evidence of articular damage, including loss of cartilage space and erosions into subchondral bone. With severe joint destruction, deformities and fusion of adjacent bones may occur. Such radiographic changes are characteristic of seropositive rheumatoid arthritis, particularly in the hands and wrists (Fig. 24–7) (Williams and Ansell, 1985). Chest radiographs may show mild pleuritis and enlargement of the cardiac shadow consistent with pericarditis in children with systemic onset JRA.

Radiographic techniques such as skeletal scintigraphy, ultrasonography, and magnetic resonance imaging (MRI) can also aid in the diagnosis of joint disease in children (Poznanski, 1992). Bone scans are helpful in distinguishing infections of bones or joints and in detecting a malignant process with multiple lesions. Ultrasonography is useful to detect joint effusions or synovial thickening and may detect popliteal cysts in children with knee arthritis (Szer et al., 1992). MRI is a sensitive technique for detecting cartilage loss or bony erosions that are too small to be seen easily in regular radiographs (Poznanski et al., 1988), and synovitis can be detected after injection with gadolinium dye (Herve-Somma et al., 1992). MRI is an expensive procedure, however, and requires sedation in younger children.

Therapy

Therapy must be designed with the realization that the prognosis for most children with JRA is good, although for any given patient the outcome and duration of disease are uncertain. With adequate care during periods of active disease, at least 75% of JRA children avoid significant disability. The physician must avoid harmful drugs, as far as possible, and use a good measure of optimism and reassurance to help children and

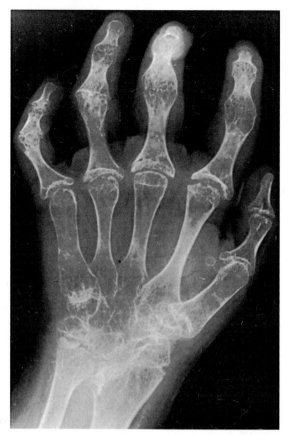

Figure 24–7. Late radiographic appearance of severe juvenile rheumatoid arthritis. There is widespread destruction apparent in the wrist and finger joints, with loss of joint space (articular cartilage), numerous erosions into subchondral bone, and actual fusion of some adjacent bones. Such a radiograph is diagnostic of rheumatoid arthritis, but these changes appear only late in the course of juvenile rheumatoid arthritis. Fortunately, many children with rheumatoid arthritis never incur joint damage severe enough to be visible radiographically.

families cope with this sometimes discouraging, but by no means hopeless, disease. Because the cause and pathogenesis of chronic arthritis are poorly understood, therapy is symptomatic, not curative (Schaller, 1993). Drugs that modify the inflammatory response are employed and ancillary measures, such as physical and occupational therapy, are essential. Care must be taken to avoid psychogenic invalidism and to allow normal growth and development.

Salicylates and Other NSAIDs. Salicylates have been used in the treatment of JRA over many years, with efficacy and safety. Liver function tests should be monitored during salicylate therapy because of the risk of hepatotoxicity (Schaller, 1978). Concern over the development of Reye's syndrome in children receiving salicylates has resulted in recommending discontinuation of the drug on varicella exposure and during flu-like illnesses. If an adequate course of salicylates is not effective, other drugs should be tried.

There are currently a proliferation of NSAIDs used in adults with arthritis, but only tolmetin and naproxen are currently labeled for use in children in the United States. Although none of the NSAIDs have been clearly shown to be more effective than salicylates, they may have the benefit of more convenient dosing schedules. Indomethacin and some of the other nonsteroidal agents are considered useful in the therapy of ankylosing spondylitis and may be helpful in the treatment of pauciarticular disease type II and the other spondyloarthropathies. Hepatotoxicity may occur with NSAIDs as well as with salicylates, and liver function tests should be monitored regularly. Salicylates and other nonsteroidal agents are known to cause gastrointestinal side effects in adults, such as gastritis, microscopic blood loss, or frank ulcers. Children frequently develop gastrointestinal side effects as well (Mulberg et al., 1993), and complaints of stomach upset or unexplained anemia should prompt evaluation.

Sulfasalazine. Encouraging results in using sulfasalazine in adults with rheumatoid arthritis and spondyloarthropathies led to trials of this medication in children with JRA. Sulfasalazine is a combination of 5-aminosalicylic acid and sulfapyridine; the salicylate portion is not absorbed in the gut. Although no placebo-controlled trials have been done, sulfasalazine was effective in open studies, in a significant number of children, particularly those with pauciarticular type II disease or spondyloarthropathy (Joos et al., 1991). Toxicity may include mild gastrointestinal intolerance, leukopenia, or rash. Severe reactions have been reported, however, particularly in children with systemic onset disease (Hertzberger-Ten Cate and Cats, 1991).

Methotrexate. In children whose arthritis is refractory to adequate NSAID therapy, methotrexate is a frequent therapeutic choice. Methotrexate, given in average doses of 10 mg/M^2/week, has been shown to be relatively efficacious in many children with persistent disease activity and erosive changes (Giannini et al., 1992; Rose et al., 1990; Wallace et al., 1993). The side effects of methotrexate are generally mild and reversible, including gastrointestinal upset, oral ulcers, and bone marrow suppression. Liver toxicity is frequently seen by elevations of serum transaminases, but severe permanent liver damage has rarely been reported in children, although cases of cirrhosis have been seen in adults (Keim et al., 1990). Severe pulmonary toxicity with fibrosis is an additional rare complication. With careful laboratory and clinical monitoring, most children tolerate methotrexate well. Few adverse effects have been reported in studies following children who have taken methotrexate as long as 5 years, with no significant liver or pulmonary toxicity seen (Graham et al., 1992). Some investigators are advocating higher doses of methotrexate in children who do not have an adequate clinical response to standard doses (Wallace and Sherry, 1992).

Gold. For patients whose arthritis does not respond to NSAIDs, injections of gold salts may be effective in controlling arthritis. Gold therapy is reasonably safe if given under careful supervision, but a complete blood count, platelet count, and urinalysis must be done before each gold injection, as well as a physical examination for evidence of skin or mucosal lesions. The usual dose of gold (as Myochrysine) is 1 mg/kg, given weekly. Up to a third of children must discontinue gold

salts because of unacceptable side effects (Brewer et al., 1980). Oral gold (auranofin) has not been shown to be more effective than placebo in controlled trials, although side effects occur much less frequently than with the injectable preparation (Giannini et al., 1990).

Antimalarials. Antimalarials may be useful in some rheumatoid patients but must be given with extreme care to children because of possible irreversible retinal toxicity; antimalarials are also poisons, with no antidote in overdosage. The most frequently reported side effect is corneal deposition of the drug; macular degeneration from retinal deposition is the most severe sequela. Regular monitoring of visual fields is required. The usual dose of hydroxychloroquine (Plaquenil) is 5 to 7 mg/kg. Discontinuation of the drug may reverse corneal deposition, but macular degeneration is not reversible and may progress despite drug withdrawal.

Penicillamine. Penicillamine, another slow-acting, disease-modifying agent used in the treatment of adults with rheumatoid arthritis, has been studied in children and is thought to have some efficacy in a few patients (Manners and Ansell, 1986). One blinded study, however, showed no increased efficacy of either penicillamine or hydroxychloroquine as compared to placebo in children with JRA (Brewer et al., 1986).

Corticosteroids. Corticosteroids can be dramatic in relieving symptoms and suppressing signs of arthritis, but their long-term use is fraught with toxic hazard (Schaller, 1977g). Corticosteroids do not cure rheumatoid arthritis; joint destruction may proceed, even during administration. Once started, these drugs may be difficult to discontinue because of severe recurrences of symptoms. Because JRA is usually chronic, corticosteroids may be needed for years and the side effects may be severe. Corticosteroids used alone should be avoided unless all other measures have failed. They are sometimes indicated for severe systemic disease or iridocyclitis. The lowest possible doses sufficient to relieve symptoms should be employed, and long-term usage should be avoided. The use of low-dose alternate-day dosing regimens or intermittent intravenous pulse treatments may be effective in treatment and may prevent some of the major side effects.

Immunosuppressives. Although studies in adult rheumatoid arthritis have shown the effectiveness of drugs such as cyclophosphamide (Ansell, 1993; Pistoia et al., 1993), the use in children with JRA remains experimental and is rarely warranted in a nonfatal disease with a generally good outlook.

Physical Therapy. Physical therapy is extremely important in preserving range of motion and muscle strength. All children with JRA should be started early on a regular program of exercises designed to retain normal joint function and muscle strength (Emery and Bowyer, 1991; Rhodes, 1991). Simple measures such as hot baths in the morning may be helpful in relieving joint stiffness. Exercises and judicious splinting may prevent future and correct existing deformities.

Surgery. Orthopedic surgical procedures are occasionally needed. Early prophylactic removal of inflamed synovium (synovectomy) is of only limited usefulness in children (Granberry, 1977a), although occasional patients may benefit. Total replacement of damaged joints, particularly hips and knees, offers hope of rehabilitation for children with severe joint destruction and disability, but only after they have achieved full growth (Boublik et al., 1993; Ruddlesdin et al., 1986; Scott, 1990; Singsen et al., 1978). Soft tissue releases may be useful in alleviating joint contractures that do not respond to physical therapy (Granberry, 1977b).

Treatment of Iridocyclitis. Therapy of iridocyclitis should be managed in conjunction with an ophthalmologist. Early recognition of this complication is crucial; for this reason, children with JRA, particularly those with pauciarticular JRA type I, should have quarterly slit-lamp examinations. Topical corticosteroids and atropine may be adequate to control ocular inflammation. If not, systemic or locally injected corticosteroids should be tried.

Treatment of Amyloidosis. Chlorambucil has been advocated in the therapy of amyloidosis, a potentially fatal complication that affects as many as 6% of JRA patients in Europe and other parts of the world (David et al., 1993; Schnitzer and Ansell, 1977; Smith et al., 1968). It is rare in the United States.

Complications and Prognosis

The morbidity of JRA is determined by the joint damage and disability that occurs as well as visual loss from iridocyclitis. Prognosis varies from subgroup to subgroup. Between 80% and 90% of children with seronegative polyarthritis do well without serious disability in adulthood, although their disease may be active for a long time. More than 50% of children with seropositive polyarthritis have persistent destructive arthritis with joint disability. The acute manifestations of systemic JRA are in themselves rarely a cause of significant long-term morbidity, but 25% of children with systemic JRA develop severe seronegative arthritis with joint disability. Patients with pauciarticular disease type I have a generally good outlook for joint function, although 10% to 20% ultimately develop multiple joint involvement, which may be severe, and about 30% have chronic iridocyclitis, which may cause ocular damage.

The ultimate prognosis for patients with pauciarticular disease type II is uncertain; a significant number probably have chronic spondyloarthropathy in childhood, although the spondyloarthropathies are usually not associated with severe loss of function.

Overall, more than 75% of children with JRA eventually enter remission without significant residual disability. In any given patient, however, the disease is unpredictable, and recurrences occasionally occur in adulthood after years of remission (Jeremy et al., 1968). Two other causes of long-term morbidity in JRA are iatrogenic damage from drugs, notably corticosteroids, and the psychologic and social disability resulting from chronic disease.

ANKYLOSING SPONDYLITIS AND SPONDYLOARTHROPATHY SYNDROMES

Ankylosing spondylitis (AS) is the prototypic spondyloarthropathy. This seronegative inflammatory arthritis primarily involves the axial skeleton and affects young adult or middle-aged men; however, the onset of this condition can be insidious in childhood (Jacobs, 1963b; Ladd et al., 1971; Schaller et al., 1969). In addition to the *forme fruste* of AS, there are a number of related arthritis syndromes, generally grouped under the heading of "spondyloarthropathies." These syndromes are characterized by occurrence in older children, male predominance, and association with the genetic marker HLA-B27.

In juvenile ankylosing spondylitis (JAS), chronic arthritis of the peripheral joints and axial skeleton occurs, often accompanied by enthesitis. Large joints and joints of the feet are commonly affected, usually in an asymmetric pattern, and often with an indolent or transient and recurrent course. Inflammation of the sacroiliac joints must occur by definition, but this finding may be delayed for years making the diagnosis difficult at onset. Patients with JAS and ankylosing spondylitis are generally seronegative for rheumatoid factors.

Historical and Epidemiologic Aspects

Ankylosing spondylitis was described in the early 1900s, and the names of three early observers (Von Bechterow, Strumpell, and Marie) are still associated with the disease (Bywaters, 1976; Schaller et al., 1969). Criteria for the diagnosis of AS were not established until 1973 (Moll and Wright, 1973). Ankylosing spondylitis differs from rheumatoid arthritis in several important aspects, including the classic sacroiliac and lumbosacral involvement, male predominance, familial nature, and lack of rheumatoid factors. Estimates of the incidence of ankylosing spondylitis in the adult population range from 1% to 6.7% of whites (Khan, 1992). JAS is less common than JRA, but specific estimates of incidence and prevalence are not available.

Juvenile ankylosing spondylitis belongs to a group of related disorders that share genetic features and frequently occur together in certain families. These disorders—AS, Reiter's syndrome, inflammatory bowel disease, reactive arthritis, psoriatic arthritis, and the seronegative enthesopathy syndrome—are all related by the frequent finding of the HLA-B27 genetic marker in affected individuals (Brewerton et al., 1973a, 1973b, 1974b; Morris et al., 1974a, 1974b; Schlosstein et al., 1973). Pauciarticular type II JRA is also logically grouped together with these disorders. HLA-B27 is found in 90% to 94% of patients with JAS, as compared with 6% to 8% of the general white population (Khan and van der Linden, 1990).

Despite this association, the relationship of this genetic marker to disease pathogenesis remains unknown. One might postulate that in HLA-B27 positive individuals there exists a genetically programmed host response to an environmental factor, leading to disease expression. Infectious agents are suspected as a key environmental factor in the development of AS, because there is a close relationship of AS to diseases such as reactive arthritis and Reiter's syndrome, in which they play a triggering role in disease pathogenesis (Keat, 1982, 1983). Some studies implicate molecular mimicry between HLA-B27 and bacterial agents related to spondyloarthropathies, such as *Klebsiella* and *Shigella* (Schwimmbeck et al., 1987).

Clinical Manifestations

Initial joint symptoms in JAS include recurring episodes of pain in the lower back, buttocks, groin, or heels. These early symptoms may be overlooked or misdiagnosed for a long period until more specific symptoms develop.

Peripheral joint complaints may be prominent at the onset of disease, making JAS clinically indistinguishable from JRA initially in some children (Garcia-Morteo et al., 1983; Ginsburg and Cohen, 1983; Marks et al., 1982; Schaller, 1977a). The constellation of clinical clues of male gender, older age of onset, and family history of related disorders, however, may suggest JAS as the correct diagnosis. Pain and stiffness in the hips is common and often a major source of disability. Axial arthritis involving the sacroiliac joints and lumbar spine develops gradually in children with JAS and may not be apparent at disease onset. There may be loss of the normal lumbar lordosis with flattening of the lumbosacral spine and limited forward flexion of the lower spine. Decreased chest expansion related to involvement of the costovertebral joints may be found in early JAS (Schaller et al., 1969).

Episodic attacks of acute iritis occur in 5% to 10% of children with JAS (Garcia-Morteo et al., 1983; Marks et al., 1982). Aortitis has been reported in adult patients with long-standing AS; however, cases of aortic valve insufficiency have been reported rarely in JAS as well (Bulkley and Roberts, 1973; Gore et al., 1981; Kean et al., 1980).

Laboratory and Radiographic Findings

There are no specific laboratory findings in JAS. During active disease, mild anemia and an increased sedimentation rate may be present. Neither rheumatoid factor nor antinuclear antibodies are associated with JAS.

Radiologic findings are considered necessary for the diagnosis of JAS, but these may not be evident for the first several years of disease. Characteristic radiographic changes of the sacroiliac joints include sclerosis, erosions of the joint margins, and widening of the joint space; these may progress to narrowing and ankylosis. Computed tomography (CT) and MRI scanning are more sensitive than plain radiographs in detecting early sacroiliitis (Ahlstrom et al., 1990; Kozin et al., 1981). Late in the disease, radiographic changes of the spine include syndesmophyte formation, apophyseal joint fusions, and eventual calcification, with "bamboo" spine.

Therapy and Prognosis

The treatment of JAS is similar to that of JRA, with the use of NSAIDs to alleviate pain and stiffness and physical therapy to maintain good posture, muscle strength, and joint function. Some patients with JAS respond particularly well to indomethacin. Sulfasalazine may be useful, although there are no controlled studies of its efficacy. Patients with severe articular disease may require advanced treatment with agents such as methotrexate. Corticosteroids are rarely warranted or effective in JAS.

JAS can enter permanent remission at any stage. Progressive loss of vertebral mobility occurs in some patients, but prognosis for overall function is good if good posture can be maintained. Although the peripheral arthritis of JAS is often benign, some patients develop severe hip disease, with reports of up to 15% of patients requiring total hip replacement (Calin et al., 1988).

Reiter's Syndrome

Reiter's syndrome (RS) is defined by the classic triad of arthritis, urethritis, and ocular inflammation. Other common findings include gastroenteritis, mucocutaneous lesions (mouth or penile ulcers), and skin rashes (keratoderma blennorrhagicum). The designation "partial Reiter's syndrome" has been proposed for patients who do not fulfull the entire triad but are thought to belong in this disease category (Wilkens et al., 1982). Although Reiter's syndrome generally occurs in young men, it has been described in childhood (Keat, 1983; Leirisalo et al., 1982; Lockie and Hunder, 1971; Rosenberg and Petty, 1979).

Pathogenesis

The cause of Reiter's syndrome is unknown, but there is much evidence suggesting that this syndrome is postinfectious, or reactive, in nature. In many cases, there is a temporal relationship between the development of RS and enteric infection with *Shigella flexneri*, *Y. enterocolitica*, *Salmonella enteritidis*, *C. trachomatis*, and *Salmonella typhimurium* (Davies et al., 1969; Friis, 1980; Keat, 1983; Russell, 1977; Smith, 1989).

Clinical Manifestations

The arthritis of RS affects predominantly large joints, particularly of the lower extremities. Sacroiliac joint involvement may occur, with subsequent progression to spondylitis similar to that of classic AS (Oates and Young, 1959; Russell et al., 1977). Prominent systemic complaints of fever, malaise, and weight loss can be present with disease flares. Dysuria is a common complaint suggestive of urethritis, and bilateral acute conjunctivitis is present in two thirds of children at onset (Rosenberg and Petty, 1979). Rarely, aortic insufficiency similar to that seen in AS has been reported in childhood onset RS (Hubscher and Susini, 1984).

Arthritis of Inflammatory Bowel Disease

Arthritis and arthralgia are among the most frequent extragastrointestinal complications of inflammatory bowel disease and may be the presenting complaints in some patients (Lindsley and Schaller, 1974) (see Chapter 23). Two distinct forms of arthritis are described: peripheral arthritis, often pauciarticular in distribution, and chronic spondylitis, resembling AS. Only the spondylitis of inflammatory bowel disease is associated with HLA-B27 (Brewerton et al., 1974b; Morris et al., 1974b). Occult inflammatory bowel disease should be suspected as an underlying cause of arthritis in children with seronegative arthritis, unexplained anemia, gastrointestinal symptoms, erythema nodosum, growth failure or weight loss, or mucosal ulcerations.

Psoriatic Arthritis

Psoriasis, a common dermatologic condition, is associated with arthritis in a small percentage of affected children (see Chapter 21). Psoriatic arthritis is well recognized in adulthood but is less frequently described in children (Lambert et al., 1976; Shore and Ansell, 1982). Two forms of psoriatic arthritis have been described—a peripheral form, either pauciarticular or polyarticular, and a spondylitic form, similar to AS. As with inflammatory bowel disease, the spondylitic form may be associated with HLA-B27, whereas peripheral arthritis in children has been associated with HLA-A2 and B17 (Espinoza et al., 1990; Hamilton et al., 1990; Suarez-Almazor and Russell, 1990). The rash of psoriasis may precede arthritis or there may be a long interval between the onset of arthritis and psoriasis (Scarpa et al., 1984). One important clinical finding characteristic of patients with psoriatic arthritis is dactylitis of a single digit, either a finger or toe, caused by inflammation and swelling of the tendon sheath. This is referred to as a "sausage digit" and may help differentiate psoriatic arthritis from JRA. Nail pitting or onycholysis may also be a helpful clinical clue.

RHEUMATIC FEVER

Acute rheumatic fever is a poststreptococcal immunologic disease characterized by nonsuppurative inflammation of various tissues, most characteristically the heart (DiSciascio and Taranta, 1980; Feinstein and Spagnuolo, 1962; Kaplan, 1978; Markowitz, 1977; Markowitz and Gordis, 1972; Special Writing Group, 1992).

Historical Aspects

Rheumatic fever has been recognized since the time of the ancient Greeks, and its occurrence after pharyngitis was first noted in the 1800s. The relationship of rheumatic fever to streptococcal infection was established in the 1930s. In the 1940s, it was demonstrated that rheumatic fever attacks could be prevented by prompt treatment of streptococcal pharyngitis with penicillin (Bland, 1987; Wannamaker et al., 1951).

Rheumatic fever is still the most common cause of acquired heart disease in children and young adults in the world and is the most common cardiovascular cause of death in the first four decades of life (Annegers et al., 1982; Markowitz, 1985; McLaren et al., 1975;

Stollerman, 1982). The incidence of rheumatic fever decreased dramatically in most industrialized countries from the 1950s to the mid-1980s, even before the widespread availability of penicillin (Hicks, 1977; Massell et al., 1988; Quinn, 1989). The use of penicillin, screening and educational programs, improved living standards, and access to medical care undoubtedly contributed to the virtual disappearance of rheumatic fever in the United States.

It was surprising, therefore, that a number of outbreaks of rheumatic fever occurred in the United States in the mid-1980s to late 1980s, predominantly among middle-class individuals with easy access to medical care (Bissenden, 1988; Congeni et al., 1987; Griffiths and Gersony, 1990; Hosier et al., 1987; Kavey and Kaplan, 1989; Markowitz and Kaplan, 1989; Veasy et al., 1987; Wald et al., 1987). Numerous theories, such as changes in "streptococcal rheumatogenicity" (the ability of the organism to induce rheumatic fever) and decreased vigilance in identification and treatment of streptococcal pharyngitis, have been proposed to account for these outbreaks. Rheumatic fever continues to be common, however, and is a major source of morbidity among children in developing third-world countries.

Clinical Manifestations

Rheumatic fever is a disease of children and young adults; it rarely occurs before the third year of life, suggesting that repeated exposure may be necessary to develop the disease. Both sexes are equally affected, but curiously, even in epidemics, only about 3% of individuals develop rheumatic fever after streptococcal pharyngitis (Rammelkamp et al., 1952).

The clinical signs of rheumatic fever vary considerably, depending on the sites of involvement and the severity of disease. In contrast to acute glomerulonephritis, which can follow group A streptococcal pyoderma or pharyngitis, rheumatic fever almost always occurs only after infection in the upper respiratory tract (Wannamaker, 1973). Periods of active disease (attacks) rarely last longer than 6 months if untreated, but may recur periodically if preventive measures are not taken. Attacks of rheumatic fever are always preceded by group A streptococcal pharyngitis, which may be subclinical (Wannamaker, 1973). The streptococcal infection is followed by a latent period of one to several weeks before signs and symptoms of rheumatic fever appear.

The major clinical manifestations of rheumatic fever are carditis, arthritis, chorea, subcutaneous nodules, and erythema marginatum. Fever and arthritis are the most frequent presenting complaints. Evidence of a prior streptococcal infection is a required criterion for diagnosis. A positive throat culture or an elevated titer of antistreptococcal antibodies is acceptable proof of infection (Kaplan, 1978; WHO Study Group, 1987; Special Writing Group, 1992).

Carditis. The carditis of acute rheumatic fever is the most characteristic manifestation of the disease and is the only one leading to permanent organ damage. The incidence of carditis following an initial attack of rheumatic fever is 40% to 50%; it usually appears within the first week or two of the rheumatic attack if it is going to occur (Massell et al., 1958).

The carditis may present as valvulitis (especially mitral or aortic), cardiomegaly, pericarditis, or congestive heart failure. Prolongation of the PR interval on ECG, gallop rhythms, and tachycardia with fever are nonspecific and by themselves are not evidence of rheumatic carditis. A heart murmur may be present in children with carditis of rheumatic fever, but echocardiogram is a more sensitive technique for detecting subtle valvulitis, even without auscultative signs.

Arthritis. Arthritis occurs in about 75% of patients during the initial attack and is usually the chief complaint. Arthritis is manifested by swelling, heat, redness, and tenderness or by pain and limitation of motion of two or more joints. Large joints, especially knees, ankles, elbows, or wrists, are most frequently involved. It may involve several joints simultaneously, or may migrate from joint to joint. The arthritis may be exquisitely painful, but invariably resolves without permanent joint damage. Some patients have only arthralgia without objective arthritis.

Sydenham's Chorea. Purposeless, involuntary, rapid movements often with muscle weakness, and emotional lability characterize chorea. Chorea must be differentiated from athetosis, hyperkinesis, benign tics, Huntington's chorea, systemic lupus erythematosus, or Wilson's disease. Rheumatic chorea is often delayed from several weeks to months after the other manifestations and, if the attack was mild, chorea may be the initial presentation. Other signs of rheumatic fever may have resolved during the long latent period. The relationship of "pure chorea" to acute rheumatic fever, however, is well-established (Berrios et al., 1985; Taranta, 1959).

Erythema Marginatum. A rare manifestation of rheumatic fever, this distinctive pink rash occurs on the trunk and proximal limbs but never on the face. Lesions vary greatly in size and often have pale centers and round or serpiginous margins. The rash is transient, migratory, and may be induced by the application of heat.

Subcutaneous Nodules. Subcutaneous nodules are also rare and are most often associated with severe carditis. These firm, painless nodules occur over pressure points, particularly the elbows, knees, wrists, occiput, and thoracic and lumbar vertebral spinous processes. Clinically, they may resemble rheumatoid nodules, but histologically they are less well organized (Bywaters et al., 1958).

Other Clinical Features. Other less specific manifestations of acute rheumatic fever include fever, malaise, epistaxis, and abdominal pain. Laboratory findings such as leukocytosis, elevated erythrocyte sedimentation rate and C-reactive protein are usually seen (Kaplan, 1978).

Pathogenesis

The occurrence of rheumatic fever as a sequela of group A streptococcal pharyngitis is well established;

no other groups of streptococci or other organisms have been linked to this disease. The exact mechanisms by which streptococcal infections lead to rheumatic fever are unknown. Many serotypes of group A streptococci have been isolated in association with rheumatic fever. The existence of "rheumatogenic" strains of group A streptococcus has been postulated but never proven. Serotyping of streptococci isolated during epidemics of rheumatic fever has shown predominance of a limited number of M types, many of which appear mucoid in appearance on blood agar plates (Marcon et al., 1988). No single serotype has been responsible for all cases in a particular locale, however, emphasizing that rheumatogenicity is not simply related to serotype (Kaplan et al., 1989).

Mechanisms invoked to explain the association of rheumatic fever with the group A streptococcus include the following: (1) persistence of streptococci or their variants; (2) toxic components or products of streptococci; (3) molecular mimicry between the streptococcus and cardiac tissue; and (4) genetic susceptibility or altered immune responsiveness of the host.

No evidence has been found to support the hypothesis that persistent streptococcal infections cause rheumatic fever (Wannamaker et al., 1951). Although streptococci must be eradicated within 10 days to prevent rheumatic fever, established rheumatic heart disease cannot be ameliorated with massive doses of penicillin (Vaisman et al., 1965). Group A streptococci contain enzymes and other extracellular products that conceivably are cardiotoxic, yet none have been directly implicated in the pathogenesis of rheumatic fever.

Molecular mimicry of antigens of the streptococcus may be a pathogenic mechanism in rheumatic fever (Williams, 1985). More than 30 years ago, antibodies in the sera of rheumatic fever patients were found to react with heart muscle as well as with skeletal muscle, cardiac valve fibroblasts, and basal ganglia neurons (Goldstein et al., 1968; Gulizia et al., 1991; Hess et al., 1964; Husby et al., 1976; Kaplan, 1963; Kaplan et al., 1961; Kaplan and Svee, 1964; Zabriskie et al., 1970). Cross-reactivity of antibody to purified streptococcal M proteins with cardiac myosin has been demonstrated (Bronze et al., 1988; Cunningham et al., 1986; Cunningham et al., 1988; Dale and Beachey, 1984, 1986; Manjula et al., 1985; Sargent et al., 1987). For some M types, the cross-reactive epitope cannot be physically or immunologically separated from the region that elicits protective antibody. This suggests that an effective host response of protective antibody to certain M types may result in antibodies reactive with epitopes of cardiac tissue as well.

A genetic predisposition to rheumatic fever most likely contributes to the increased incidence within certain population groups, such as the Maori of New Zealand (116/100,000), or even within a single family. HLA typing studies have shown variable results in different racial groups. These include the following: in Martinique, increased HLA-B35, decreased B14 and Bw42; in India, increased HLA-DR3, decreased HLA-DR2; in American blacks, increased HLA-DR2; and in

American whites, increased HLA-DR4 (both of these latter also associated with persistent elevation of anti-group A carbohydrate titers) (Alarcon-Riquelme et al., 1990; Ayoub et al., 1986; Hafez et al., 1989, 1990; Khanna et al., 1989; Manjula et al., 1985; Rajapakse et al., 1990; Rich et al., 1988). A specific B-cell alloantigen (an inherited marker on B cells) has been associated with increased susceptibility to rheumatic fever (Khanna et al., 1989; Patarroyo et al., 1979); thus, inherited differences in B-cell populations may contribute to susceptibility to rheumatic fever.

A variety of aberrant cellular immune responses to streptococci or streptococcal products have been found in rheumatic fever patients, including increased leukocyte migration inhibition, decreased blastogenesis and proliferation, and increased natural killer cell cytotoxicity (Gray et al., 1981; Regelmann et al., 1987). Decreased blastogenic and proliferative responses to streptococcal antigens have also been found in unaffected family members of rheumatic fever patients. Furthermore, abnormal immune responses of tonsillar mononuclear cells from rheumatic fever patients have been reported, supporting the idea of a "localized" immune abnormality in the pharynx that predisposes to rheumatic fever (Miller et al., 1989).

Diagnosis

The diagnosis of rheumatic fever is a clinical one and should not be lightly made in view of the therapeutic implications (WHO Study Group, 1987). There is no single diagnostic sign or laboratory test. The revised modified Jones criteria shown in Table 24–5 are valuable diagnostic guides (Special Writing Group, 1992). Two major or one major and two minor criteria indicate a high probability of acute rheumatic fever, if supported by the evidence of prior streptococcal infection. Rising titers of antibodies to streptolysin O or DNAse B are particularly useful, whereas commercial slide agglutination tests using multiple streptococcal antigens, such as Streptozyme, are less well standardized. Only patients with "pure chorea" may properly be diagnosed with rheumatic fever in the absence of evidence of prior streptococcal infection, because the interval from infection to presentation may be pro-

longed. Some children develop poststreptococcal arthritis but do not fulfill Jones criteria, yet later develop evident rheumatic fever. This suggests the importance of close follow-up of these patients (De Cunto et al., 1988; Herold and Shulman, 1988).

Pathologic findings in the heart in rheumatic fever include the Aschoff body, a small granulomatous lesion. Its genesis is poorly understood. Aschoff bodies may persist for years after the last attack of rheumatic fever, often in association with a mononuclear cell infiltrate (Chopra et al., 1988). An association between anticardiolipin antibodies and rheumatic carditis and chorea has been suggested (Figueroa et al., 1992).

Treatment

Therapy of acute rheumatic fever begins with an initial course of antibiotic therapy to eradicate any group A streptococci that might be present (Wood et al., 1964). This is known as "primary" prophylaxis and must be followed by "secondary" prophylaxis, the carefully monitored long-term administration of antibiotics to prevent recolonization or reinfection with group A streptococci.

Both primary and secondary prophylaxis may most effectively be accomplished by the use of intramuscular benzathine penicillin G in nonallergic patients. Recommendations regarding the frequency of administration of secondary prophylaxis vary from every 3 to 4 weeks (Dajani et al., 1988). The duration of secondary prophylaxis is long-term and continues until adulthood (WHO Study Group, 1987). A low recurrence rate of rheumatic fever has been reported in patients without carditis whose penicillin prophylaxis was discontinued at age 18 (Berrios et al., 1993).

Additional treatment may be beneficial during the acute attack of rheumatic fever. Both salicylates and corticosteroids have been advocated for the treatment of acute carditis, although there is little substantive evidence that these reduce the incidence of subsequent rheumatic heart disease (Combined Rheumatic Fever Study Group, 1960, 1965). Mild carditis without congestive heart failure may be treated with salicylates to achieve a serum salicylate level of 15 to 20 mg/dl for 3 to 4 weeks, and then at a reduced dose for an additional 6 to 8 weeks. In patients with congestive heart failure, most clinicians add prednisone, 2 to 3 mg/kg/day, in divided doses, with reduction in the dose by tapering as soon as there is clinical improvement. Some physicians believe that rheumatic fever patients are more sensitive to digitalis preparations; although this has not been proven, smaller doses of these preparations are often given. There appears to be little rationale for prolonged bed rest for children with carditis (Grossman, 1968). Evidence of inflammation may be monitored by erythrocyte sedimentation rate or C-reactive protein.

The arthritis associated with rheumatic fever responds dramatically to salicylates. Some question the diagnosis of rheumatic fever in a patient whose arthritis does not respond within 24 to 36 hours. Therapy for chorea is supportive; diazepam or haloperidol is some-

Table 24–5. Modified (Revised) Jones Criteria for Acute Rheumatic Fever

Major Criteria	Minor Criteria
Carditis	Fever
Polyarthritis	Arthralgia
Chorea	Prolonged PR interval
Erythema marginatum	Increased erythrocyte
Subcutaneous nodules	sedimentation rate or
	C-reactive protein

Plus: Supporting evidence of prior streptococcal infection:
  Positive throat culture for group A streptococci or rapid
    streptococcal antigen test
  Elevated or rising titer of antistreptococcal antibodies (e.g.,
    antistreptolysin O [ASO], anti-DNAse B)

From Special Writing Group, Committee on Rheumatic Fever, 1992.

times recommended. A role for corticosteroids in this situation is uncertain (Kaplan, 1978). The value of intravenous immunoglobulin for treatment of chorea is under study.

Complications and Prognosis

During an initial attack of rheumatic fever, death can result from fulminating carditis; this can now largely be prevented by corticosteroids. The only potentially damaging sequela of acute rheumatic fever is residual cardiac damage. For the 50% to 60% of patients without demonstrable carditis at presentation, long-term prognosis is excellent, with complete recovery the rule. About one third of patients with carditis at onset also are spared residual rheumatic heart disease.

The incidence and severity of residual heart disease are related to the severity of carditis at onset (Combined Rheumatic Fever Study Group, 1960, 1965). Patients without carditis during the initial attack do not usually develop significant heart disease on follow-up, prompting some to call for minimizing secondary prophylaxis duration in these patients (Berrios et al., 1993; Majeed et al., 1990). Patients who have had carditis initially may suffer further heart damage with subsequent attacks (Feinstein et al., 1964). Much of the disability and death in rheumatic fever is related to recurrent attacks. The prognosis in rheumatic fever is therefore dependent on the the success of secondary prophylaxis.

LYME DISEASE

Lyme disease is a tick-borne illness with multisystem manifestations, including rheumatic complaints, caused by the spirochete *Borrelia burgdorferi*. There are three different genomic species of *Borrelia* that occur in Europe; only one has been identified in the United States (Baranton et al., 1992).

Although the skin manifestations of Lyme disease had been described in Europe since the early 1900s, Lyme arthritis was first recognized and described in 1977 in the United States (Burgdorfer et al., 1982; Steere et al., 1977). Since epidemiologic surveillance of Lyme disease in the United States was initiated by the Centers for Disease Control (1991) in 1982, increasing numbers of cases have been recognized, as well as geographic spread of the spirochete. In the United States, Lyme disease is most frequent in coastal New England and the upper Midwest.

Clinical Manifestations

Lyme disease occurs in stages, generally described as early localized disease (stage 1), early disseminated disease (stage 2), and late persistent disease (stage 3). Many individuals have only early localized disease, which is either treated successfully or resolves spontaneously. Some patients only become symptomatic in stage 2 or 3, presenting with arthritis, heart block, or neurologic complaints (Cooper and Schoen, 1992; Steere, 1989).

After inoculation through the tick bite, *Borrelia* spreads through the skin to result in the classic skin lesion of Lyme disease, erythema migrans. Erythema migrans lesions often begin as a small, red papule and enlarge in a ring-like pattern, with central clearing and an erythematous margin. The lesions can occur anywhere on the body, and multiple lesions are often present (Asbrink, 1991). The skin lesions are frequently accompanied by mild, flu-like symptoms of fatigue, fever, arthralgia, or headache. Even in untreated patients, the skin lesions resolve over 3 to 4 weeks spontaneously (Steere, 1989; Steere et al., 1983).

Within days to weeks of the early phase of disease, the spirochete spreads hematogenously and results in clinical manifestations involving the heart, nervous system, or musculoskeletal system. Neurologic manifestations occur in 20% of patients, with the most common findings of aseptic meningitis or Bell's palsy. Less frequently, peripheral neuritis may occur (Finkel and Halpern, 1991; Halpern et al., 1991). Cardiac manifestations of atrioventricular block, or rarely myocarditis or pericarditis, occur in 10% of patients (Steere et al., 1980). The AV block resolves with antibiotic treatment of Lyme disease, and therefore patients generally do not require the placement of permanent pacemakers. Musculoskeletal complaints are common, developing in 60% of patients. An average of 6 months after the onset of the illness, brief recurrent attacks of asymmetric oligoarthritis develop (Eichenfield et al., 1986b; Steere et al., 1979). This presentation can mimic that of juvenile rheumatoid arthritis, and therefore Lyme arthritis needs to be carefully considered in the evaluation of all children with new onset arthritis.

Late persistent disease manifests months to years after the onset of disease. Although uncommon, an unknown percentage of patients with Lyme disease go on to develop subtle late neurologic findings of encephalomyelitis or polyneuritis (Logigian et al., 1990). In Europe, investigators have described patients with late Lyme disease who present with progressive encephalomyelitis including paraparesis, ataxia, cognitive and memory impairment, and dementia (Krupp et al., 1991). The demonstration of specific intrathecal production of anti-*Borrelia* antibody is a helpful diagnostic clue for the presence of central nervous system (CNS) Lyme disease.

Although the vast majority of patients with Lyme arthritis have complete resolution of their disease, the arthritis may persist for years (Steere et al., 1987; Szer, et al., 1991). A small number of patients with Lyme arthritis have persistent joint disease which responds poorly to antibiotic treatment, and in some cases can become erosive. The development of chronic Lyme arthritis is associated with an increased frequency of HLA-DR4 and DR2, the same genetic haplotypes associated with classic rheumatoid arthritis (Steere et al., 1979, 1990).

Diagnosis

The diagnosis of Lyme disease rests on serologic determination, because the routine culturing of *Borrelia* is difficult and impractical. Serodiagnosis is generally performed using ELISA-based systems; however, there is wide variance of reliability and little standardization among kits and laboratories performing Lyme testing, leading to inaccuracy and confusion (Luger and Krauss, 1990). It is important to determine both IgM and IgG titers to *Borrelia* to help distinguish early active disease from late or previous illness.

Antibodies to *Borrelia* are not detectable within the first several weeks of infection. In addition, early treatment of either tick bites or erythema migrans lesions may abrogate the antibody response, resulting in negative results later in disease. Within 2 to 4 weeks of erythema migrans lesions, IgM anti-*Borrelia* antibodies develop, peaking within 6 to 8 weeks of the illness and declining by 4 to 6 months. IgG antibodies develop later, 6 to 8 weeks after onset of illness and peaking within 4 to 6 months. IgG antibodies remain strongly elevated in patients with late persistent disease (Rahn and Malawista, 1991; Sigal, 1992; Steere, 1989).

Difficulties with definitive diagnosis of Lyme disease using ELISA results can be addressed with Western blotting, in which serum reactivity to specific *Borrelia* proteins can be detected. A negative Western blot test in the face of equivocal ELISA results is strong evidence against the diagnosis of Lyme disease (Rose et al., 1991; Zoller et al., 1991).

Treatment

The early disease manifestations of Lyme disease can be effectively treated in most cases with oral antibiotics (Salazar et al., 1993). Oral doxycycline or amoxicillin is recommended for adults, and amoxicillin or erythromycin for children, for a course of 10 to 30 days. Central nervous system disease, cardiac manifestations, or persistent arthritis may require a course of intravenous antibiotics for resolution. Some reports (Plotkin et al., 1991; Rahn and Malawista, 1991; Sigal, 1992) provide specific details of recommended treatment regimens. Complete resolution of signs and symptoms may not occur for several weeks after a course of therapy, so one should not conclude that the treatment has failed if the individual still has persistent symptoms immediately after treatment.

LUPUS ERYTHEMATOSUS

Lupus erythematosus (LE) is the prototype of human autoimmune disease. Systemic lupus erythematosus (SLE) refers to the form of the disease that can involve multiple organ systems. This illness has a widely variable presentation, course, and outcome; it may be mild or severe and potentially fatal. The hallmark of SLE is the production of autoantibodies reactive with body tissue constituents that can lead to organ system damage. In the past, most children with SLE died of their disease, whereas with modern treatment and disease recognition the prognosis is now good for most patients.

Historical Aspects

The name lupus, which derives from the Latin term for wolf, refers to the cutaneous lesions of LE, which can ulcerate and thus resemble the bite of an animal. Skin lesions of LE were recognized as early as the thirteenth century (Virchow, 1865). In the 1800s, lupus was recognized to have systemic as well as cutaneous manifestations by Osler (1895, 1900). The description of the LE cell by Hargraves and colleagues in 1948 (Hargraves, 1969) led to the discovery of the prominent role of autoantibodies in patients with SLE.

Pathogenesis

Although the cause of SLE remains unknown, much has been learned about its pathogenesis and immune abnormalities. Clearly, genetically inherited susceptibility factors contribute to the potential to develop SLE. Hormonal, environmental, or other factors may also trigger or mediate disease, but their relative importance in promoting disease remains a mystery. Intense investigation has led to the hypothesis that disease-inciting triggers interact to promote the production of autoantibodies, abnormalities of lymphocyte function, and the development of immune complexes and their deposition in organs, with resultant complement activation and eventual tissue damage.

Role of Abnormal B and T cells

Numerous abnormalities of lymphocyte function have been described in murine and human SLE. A central feature in the development of SLE is the loss of tolerance to self-antigens, and both B and T cells may play a critical role in initiating and perpetuating escape from tolerance. B cells of patients with SLE are hyperactive, spontaneously secreting large amounts of polyclonal immunoglobulin (Blaese et al., 1980). In addition, B cells that recognize self-antigens, normally suppressed or deleted, are able in lupus patients to escape tolerance, proliferate, and produce pathogenic autoantibodies (Blaese et al., 1980).

The T-cell system plays an important role in allowing autoantibody-producing B cells to develop in patients with SLE, although the specific details of the mechanisms are not understood. Circulating T cells in patients with SLE are activated in higher numbers than in healthy individuals. There is conflicting evidence concerning whether there is an increased CD4[+] helper T-cell population, or merely "abnormal" help (Inghirami et al., 1988; Shivakumar et al., 1989). Decreased numbers of CD8[+] (suppressor) T cells have been noted in SLE. In addition, CD8[+] T cells might be functionally impaired in SLE because they appear unable to downregulate the abnormal immunoglobulin and autoantibody synthesis (Linker-Israeli et al., 1990).

Autoantibody Formation in SLE

A key pathogenic finding characteristic of SLE is the production of autoantibodies. One central question is whether they arise nonspecifically as a result of polyclonal activation or as a clonally specific product of antigen selection (Schwartz and Stollar, 1985). The relationship between lupus autoantibodies and protective antibodies produced in normal immune responses has been studied to address this question (Shoenfeld et al., 1983). It is clear that lupus autoantibodies derive from the same antibody genes used in normal responses. For example, in the mouse, the genes that encode anti-DNA antibodies are found in normal mice as well as in those with autoimmune disease (Naparstek et al., 1986). Evidence that lupus autoantibodies can arise from somatic mutation of genes used to encode antibodies of the normal immune response has led some to suggest that autoantigens might themselves be the immune stimulus in SLE (Davidson et al., 1987).

Role of Immune Complexes

The tissue damage that occurs in SLE is generally a result of formation of immune complexes. These complexes are able to fix complement and deposit in tissues such as the renal glomeruli, causing tissue damage (Davis et al., 1978; Koffler et al., 1967, 1971; Kohler and Bensel, 1969; Schur and Sandson, 1968b). Normally, circulating immune complexes are rapidly cleared by fixation to red blood cell complement receptors and phagocytic destruction (Davies et al., 1990). Patients with SLE have defects in immune complex fixation, with low numbers of CR1 receptors and saturation of available receptors by excess immune complexes (Walport and Lachmann, 1988; Wilson and Fearon, 1984). Clearance of complexes by phagocytes has been shown to be impaired in patients with active SLE (Kimberly et al., 1983). Both of these abnormalities favor the persistence of free immune complexes and subsequent tissue deposition. Immune complexes can also be formed in situ in patients with SLE, either through direct binding of autoantibody to tissue antigens or binding of antigen with sequential binding of autoantibody (Madaio et al., 1987).

The important role of immune complexes in perpetuating the tissue damage in SLE is supported by the presence of complexes and complement in affected tissues such as glomeruli and skin (Davis et al., 1978; Koffler et al., 1967, 1969). The direct role of autoantibodies in pathogenic immune complexes is supported by the finding that anti-DNA antibodies have been eluted from kidney tissue of patients with active SLE nephritis (Kalunian et al., 1989; Madaio et al., 1987; Winfield et al., 1977).

Although circulating immune complex levels are often elevated in patients with active SLE, there is no clear correlation between disease activity and the absolute level of immune complexes.

Epidemiology

The prevalence of SLE is not precisely known; in the United States, it is somewhere between 15 and 50 cases/100,000 persons. The estimated annual incidence of SLE in childhood is 0.6/100,000 (DeNardo et al., 1994; Siegel and Lee, 1973), so SLE is a relatively uncommon disease. Approximately 20% of SLE cases begin in childhood, with the majority presenting at age 8 or older. SLE rarely is seen in children under age 5 (Emery, 1986; Fish et al., 1977; Lehman et al., 1989).

There is a striking preponderance of females affected with SLE; in adults, there are approximately eight women affected to one man. In prepubertal children, the ratio is three girls to one boy affected (Emery, 1986; Kaslow and Masi, 1978; Koster-King et al., 1977; Masi and Kaslow, 1978; Meislin and Rothfield, 1968). These statistics suggest that sex hormones play a role in the susceptibility and development of SLE. Further evidence to support this hypothesis is the finding of a higher than expected prevalence of Klinefelter's syndrome among males with SLE (Stern et al., 1977; Wenkert et al., 1991). In murine SLE, female mice develop earlier and more severe disease. Androgen treatment of female mice ameliorates the onset of nephritis, whereas orchiectomizing male mice leads to earlier, more severe disease (Roubinian et al., 1979, 1983).

Racial differences in the distribution of SLE are seen, with a higher incidence among American black, Hispanic, Native American, and Asian populations (DeNardo et al., 1994; Kaslow and Masi, 1978; Koster-King et al., 1977). The reasons for these patterns are unknown.

Genetic influences clearly contribute to susceptibility to SLE. Monozygotic twins have a concordance rate of 60% but in dizygotic twins the concordance rate is only 5% (Block et al., 1975, 1976; Brunner et al., 1971; Lieberman et al., 1968). There is an increased frequency of SLE among first-degree and second-degree relatives of patients, with rates of 17% to 27% reported for patients with childhood onset disease. In addition, positive antinuclear antibody tests are found in 20% to 30% of unaffected first-degree relatives of lupus patients, compared with less than 5% of controls (Miles and Isenberg, 1993).

Histocompatibility antigen associations in SLE have been described in detail (Stasny, 1978). Overall, HLA-DR2 and -DR3 are most common, with DR2 more prevalent among patients with early onset SLE (Schur et al., 1982; Stasny, 1978). Thus far, there is little evidence to suggest any strong association of HLA haplotypes and specific clinical manifestations of SLE (Hochberg et al., 1985). There is an association noted between certain HLA haplotypes and autoantibody production. The production of anti-Ro and -La antibodies has been associated with HLA-B8/DR3 and -DQw2 as well as with the co-occurrence of HLA-DR2 and -DR3 (Bell and Maddison, 1980).

Clinical Manifestations

Lupus erythematosus in childhood is generally of the systemic form, involving multiple organ systems, and appears to be more acute and of greater severity than in adults. Often, children may present with the sudden appearance of multisystem disease; however, some children may have the insidious onset of vague symptoms for some time before the diagnosis becomes clear (Cassidy et al., 1977a; Cook et al., 1960; Emery, 1986; Glidden et al., 1983; Gribetz and Henley, 1959; Hagge et al., 1967; Jacobs, 1963a; Lehman et al., 1989; Nepom and Schaller, 1984; Norris et al., 1977; Platt et al., 1982; Wallace et al., 1978; Walravens and Chase, 1976; Zetterstrom and Berglund, 1956). Constitutional features include malaise, weight loss, fever, rash, arthritis, and arthralgia.

Cutaneous manifestations affect most patients at some time during the course of disease (see Chapter 21). The characteristic facial "butterfly" rash of SLE is seen on the cheeks and over the bridge of the nose, often sparing the nasolabial folds (Fig. 24–8). The malar rash often has a thickened or scaly quality, and may be photosensitive. Similar macular lesions may involve the extremities and trunk. Distinct purplish erythematous macules may be seen on the palms, soles, or distal digits and are secondary to small vessel vasculitis or thrombosis; infarction of tissue can occur. Raynaud's phenomenon is present in many patients and may precede other symptoms. Erythematous or ulcerative lesions frequently occur on the oral and nasal mucous membranes. Alopecia, either patchy or generalized, may occur during active disease. Other skin lesions include erythema nodosum, purpura, and erythema multiforme.

Musculoskeletal complaints are common, and arthralgia or arthritis may be the presenting complaints. Severe arthritis may mimic JRA, although the joint involvement is typically nondeforming and rarely erosive. Myositis, with muscle weakness, pain, and ele-

vated serum muscle enzyme levels, occurs in some patients.

Polyserositis, with pleuritis, pericarditis, or peritonitis, is frequent and can be the sole presenting symptom of SLE in children. Cardiac manifestations of SLE include myocarditis, pericarditis, verrucous nonbacterial endocarditis (Libman-Sacks endocarditis) and, less commonly, myocardial infarction related to coronary artery vasculitis. Cardiac valvular abnormalities and dysfunction occur in active SLE, and are best identified by echocardiography (Cervera et al., 1992; Crozier et al., 1990; Galve et al., 1988; Tucker et al., 1992). The increased risk of early atherosclerotic heart disease among some young patients with SLE is likely related to coronary vasculitis and abnormal lipid profiles resulting from steroid therapy (Homcy et al., 1982; Hosenpud et al., 1983). Pulmonary manifestations of SLE range from gradual interstitial disease, pneumonitis and pulmonary infiltrates, to pulmonary hemorrhage, a severe complication with high mortality (Delgado et al., 1990; Miller et al., 1986).

Renal involvement occurs in the majority of children with SLE and represents one of the most serious disease manifestations (Koster-King et al., 1977; Wallace et al., 1979). Signs of renal involvement include abnormal urine sediment with proteinuria, hematuria, or cellular casts, hypertension, nephrotic syndrome, or renal insufficiency. Hypertension may be an ominous sign in patients with SLE and may be associated with a poor prognosis. Histologic morphology of renal disease in children with SLE has shown greater than 50% incidence of diffuse proliferative glomerulonephritis, a severe lesion with high potential for progression to renal failure. Progression from mild focal lesions to more severe lesions has been documented in some patients (Garin et al., 1976; Lee et al., 1984; Pollak et al., 1964; Tejani et al., 1983; Woolf et al., 1979). Lupus nephritis is discussed extensively in Chapter 25.

Involvement of the nervous system in SLE is frequent. Children with SLE often have CNS manifestations at onset (Yancey et al., 1981). Seizures and psychosis are the classic CNS manifestations of SLE as accepted in the criteria for SLE diagnosis (Silber et al., 1984), but intracerebral hemorrhage and coma may also occur. Peripheral neuritis, cranial nerve abnormalities, and chorea may be seen, but are less frequent (Herd et al., 1978). Transverse myelitis, a rare complication of SLE, is associated with the presence of antiphospholipid antibodies in many patients (Provenzale and Bouldin, 1992). Ocular findings may consist of cytoid bodies (resembling cotton wool exudates) secondary to retinal abnormalities, uveitis, or episcleritis.

Hepatosplenomegaly and generalized lymphadenopathy are common. An acute abdominal crisis, caused by vasculitis of the bowel, can occur and have significant morbidity.

Hematologic abnormalities are common and include the anemia of chronic illness, autoimmune hemolytic anemia, leukopenia, lymphopenia, and thrombocytopenia. Autoantibodies to red cells, platelets, and lymphocytes may be present. Patients with antiphospholipid antibodies or a lupus anticoagulant often have a

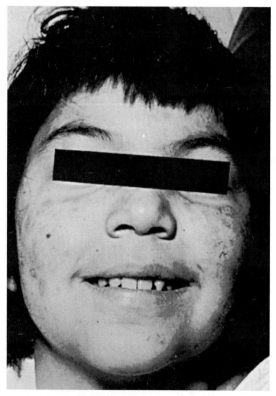

Figure 24–8. Facial rash of systemic lupus erythematosus with characteristic butterfly distribution. This patient also had generalized alopecia and brittle, fragmented hair, which is apparent in the frontal area ("fractured forelocks").

prolonged PTT or false-positive VDRL. Clinical manifestations associated with antiphospholipid antibodies include recurrent venous or arterial thrombosis, thrombocytopenia, recurrent spontaneous abortions, transient ischemic attacks, stroke, myocardial ischemia or infarction, and cardiac valvulitis.

Isolated discoid lupus erythematosus is a chronic skin disease characterized by scarring plaques on the hands and upper body. Discoid lupus rarely affects children and is usually not accompanied by progression to the systemic form of lupus (George and Tunnessen, 1993; Winkelmann, 1968).

Diagnosis and Laboratory Findings

The diagnosis of SLE relies primarily on clinical findings of multisystem disease, with confirmation by laboratory and serologic studies. The diagnosis of SLE can be made with 96% sensitivity and specificity when the diagnostic criteria developed by Tan and colleagues (1982a) are fulfilled (Table 24–6).

Serologic Studies

Serologic findings provide helpful clues in suggesting and confirming the diagnosis of SLE. The antinuclear antibody test is the single most useful test for SLE, because it is almost always positive in the presence of active disease. It must be emphasized, however, that antinuclear antibodies are not specifically diagnostic for SLE. ANA-negative SLE has been described, although the incidence of negative tests has diminished with the use of the more sensitive hep-2 substrate for ANA testing (Ferreiro et al., 1984; Fessel, 1978). Some ANA-negative patients may have circulating anticytoplasmic antibodies (Provost et al., 1977).

The presence of antibodies to native DNA is a fairly specific laboratory finding for SLE, because these autoantibodies are rarely seen in other conditions. Not all patients with SLE have detectable anti-DNA antibodies, however, so the lack of these antibodies does not rule out the diagnosis of SLE. In patients with detectable anti-DNA titers, the serum level generally fluctuates with disease activity and provides a clinical marker for treatment response or impending disease flare (Emlen et al., 1986; Pincus et al., 1969, 1971; Schur and Sandson, 1968a; Ward et al., 1989).

There are many other serologic abnormalities in SLE, including polyclonal elevation of serum immunoglobulins, positive rheumatoid factor tests, positive Coombs' test, false-positive serologic test for syphilis, and circulating anticoagulants. Organ-specific autoantibodies such as antithyroid antibodies may also be detected.

Serum complement levels are low in patients with active immune complex disease (Schur and Sandson, 1968a; Singsen et al., 1976); measurement of serum complement is useful to follow the course of disease, because levels return to normal as disease activity abates (Appel et al., 1978; Laitman et al., 1989). In patients with SLE whose complement levels remain depressed despite other evidence of improving disease, evaluation for a complement deficiency state should be considered.

Renal Pathology

The histologic classification of renal lesions in patients with SLE can aid in the diagnosis, prognosis, and evaluation of treatment protocols. Several different histologic patterns of renal pathology are seen in SLE, including mesangial immune deposits with or without proliferation, focal or diffuse proliferative nephritis, or membranous lesions (Baldwin et al., 1970, 1977; Ginzler et al., 1974; Koffler et al., 1969; Lowenstein et al., 1970; Southwest Pediatric Nephrology Group, 1986). Mesangial or focal proliferative lesions represent milder forms of lupus nephritis, with potential for good response to treatment and outcome. Mild lesions can progress to a more severe form, however, with correspondingly poor outcome (Baldwin et al., 1977; Ginzler et al., 1974). The diffuse proliferative lesion of lupus nephritis may be associated with severe clinical manifestations, such as hypertension, abnormal urinary sediment, and varying degrees of renal insufficiency. Membranous lupus nephritis is often characterized by persistent nephrotic syndrome, with risk of subsequent renal failure.

The histologic characterization alone may be insufficient to predict response to therapy and outcome (Fries et al., 1978). The degree of chronic changes present in the renal biopsy, as assessed by a chronicity index, is useful to predict potential response to immunosuppressive therapy (Carette et al., 1983) and eventual renal outcome.

Other Laboratory Findings

Hematologic studies frequently show anemia, thrombocytopenia, and leukopenia (Budman and Steinberg,

---

Table 24–6. Criteria for the Classification of Systemic Lupus Erythematosus (SLE)*

Malar rash
Discoid lupus rash
Photosensitivity
Oral or nasal mucocutaneous ulcerations
Nonerosive arthritis
Nephritis
   Proteinuria >0.5 g/day
   Cellular casts
Central nervous system manifestations
   Psychosis
   Seizures
Serositis
   Pleuritis
     or
   Pericarditis
Hematologic manifestations
   Coombs'-positive hemolytic anemia
     or
   Lymphopenia <1500 cells/mm³ or leukopenia <4000 cells/mm³
     or
   Thrombocytopenia
Positive antinuclear antibody
Positive autoantibodies
   Antibodies to double-stranded DNA or Sm
     or
   Positive LE cell preparation
     or
   Biologic false-positive test for syphilis

*The presence of 4 of these 11 criteria confers 96% sensitivity and 96% specificity for the diagnosis of SLE.

1977). Acute-phase reactants are present during periods of active disease, although this is not universal. The erythrocyte sedimentation rate may be elevated, but this is not generally helpful in following disease activity. Liver function tests are frequently mildly abnormal during active disease; patients with SLE appear to be especially sensitive to hepatotoxicity of salicylates; thus, transaminase levels must be carefully monitored (Seaman and Ishak, 1974). Myositis may be present, with elevations in serum muscle enzyme levels.

Assessment of organ systems for damage often aids in determining the degree of active disease and guiding therapy. Pulmonary function tests, electrocardiograms, and echocardiography may reveal subtle tissue damage prior to clinical symptoms (Tucker et al., 1992). Diagnosis of central nervous system SLE is difficult, because abnormalities of cerebrospinal fluid, electroencephalograms, CT, or MRI may not correlate well with clinical signs and symptoms (Sibbitt et al., 1989).

Treatment

Therapy in SLE is initially aimed at reducing inflammation. The extent of systemic involvement determines the treatment required in the individual patient. In patients with renal disease, a renal biopsy may be helpful to indicate the severity and activity of disease.

For individuals with mild SLE without nephritis and with normal levels of serum complement, symptomatic therapy with NSAIDs, antimalarials, or possibly low dose corticosteroids may be sufficient. Careful follow-up, including evaluation of organ status, is crucial to detect early disease flares. For individuals with more severe disease with evidence of organ system damage and low levels of serum complement, aggressive therapy is warranted.

High-dose corticosteroids provide the first line of treatment in patients with active SLE. It is critical to control active disease as quickly and completely as possible to prevent tissue damage. The most useful indication of adequate control of disease is normalization of serum complement levels and decrease of DNA antibodies (Laitman et al., 1989; Schur and Sandson, 1968a; Urman and Rothchild, 1977). Whenever possible, once acute disease is controlled, alternate-day steroid therapy should be used in children to minimize growth retardation and cushingoid features.

Immunosuppressive drugs such as azathioprine and cyclophosphamide play an important role in the treatment of SLE. These drugs are helpful in controlling active disease in patients with incomplete response to steroids, in patients who present with fulminant disease, and in patients with unacceptable side effects of long-term, high-dose steroid treatment. Long-term outcome in patients with SLE nephritis is improved by intravenous pulse cyclophosphamide treatment in addition to steroids as compared with steroid treatment alone (Austin et al., 1986; Felson and Anderson, 1984; Lehman et al., 1988). The potential complications and side effects of these medications, however, including severe disseminated infection, possible increased risk of malignancy, and damage to reproductive potential,

make careful consideration essential before undertaking a course of treatment.

Complications and Prognosis

The prognosis of SLE is related to the extent and severity of systemic involvement in each individual patient. SLE is a potentially fatal disease; however, some patients have relatively mild systemic involvement, which is compatible with long-term, morbidity-free survival. Some patients have prolonged remissions of their disease. Causes of mortality in SLE have changed with the advent of aggressive treatment for renal disease—fewer patients are developing renal failure, but mortality from fulminant disease, pulmonary hemorrhage, myocardial infarction, and infection still occurs. Infection in particular is emerging as the major cause of morbidity and mortality in patients with SLE as more aggressive immunosuppressive protocols are used in treatment (Lacks and White, 1990). Early atherosclerotic heart disease is emerging as a potential cause of morbidity and mortality among young patients surviving SLE (Homcy et al., 1982; Hosenpud et al., 1983).

Nonetheless, the prognosis for patients with SLE is greatly improved over the past, with 5-year survival in most centers exceeding 90%. Early aggressive therapy and meticulous attention to follow-up are important factors in ensuring improved outcome for patients with SLE.

Neonatal Lupus Syndrome

The neonatal lupus syndrome (NLS) is an illness that occurs in infants born to mothers with SLE, Sjögren's syndrome, other rheumatic diseases, or asymptomatic mothers who have antibodies to Ro(SSA) and/or La(SSB) in their serum. During gestation, these autoantibodies are transmitted to the infants, resulting in transient clinical manifestations of rash and cytopenias and permanent complete congenital heart block. NLS is an important model of organ injury mediated by lupus autoantibodies (Buyon and Winchester, 1990; Reed et al., 1983; Weston et al., 1982).

Clinical Manifestations

The clinical features of NLS are variable, but most infants have only mild skin findings. In general, infants have either skin or cardiac manifestations; it is rare to find both manifestations in the same infant. The skin rash is an annular, scaly, erythematous eruption that develops in patches on the face, scalp, extremities, or trunk. The rash is often photosensitive and is similar to lesions of subacute cutaneous lupus (Epstein and Litt, 1961; Jackson, 1964; McCuistion and Schoch, 1954; Schaller, 1977e). The lesions nearly always resolve by 6 to 8 months, coincident with decreasing titers of maternal IgG. Transient cytopenias can also occur in NLS, with thrombocytopenia most frequently reported. Mild hemolytic anemia and leukopenia can be seen (Seip, 1960; Watson et al., 1988). Less frequently, hepatic abnormalities, hepatosplenomegaly, or severe cytopenias have been reported (Bremers et al., 1979; Draznin et al., 1979; Laxer et al., 1990).

The most significant manifestation of NLS is complete congenital heart block, because this is a permanent sequela. Neonatal lupus syndrome accounts for the majority of cases of congenital heart block; even if the mother does not have a diagnosed rheumatic condition, she usually has serum anti-Ro or anti-La antibodies. Most infants with congenital heart block require a pacemaker. Overall mortality is as high as 15% to 20% (McCue et al., 1977; McCune et al., 1987). Lesser degrees of heart block have been seen in NLS, with evidence in rare cases of postnatal progression (Geggel et al., 1988). Endomyocardial fibroelastosis, myocarditis, or cardiomyopathy has also been reported in NLS (Hogg, 1957; Hull et al., 1966).

Pathogenesis and Risk Factors

It is generally believed that the clinical manifestations of NLS result from the passage of high titers of anti-Ro and anti-La antibodies from the mother into the developing fetus, with resultant inflammation of tissues such as the heart and skin (Buyon and Winchester, 1990; Harley et al., 1985; Lee and Weston, 1984; Litsey et al., 1985; Reed et al., 1983; Scott et al., 1983). The Ro and La antigens are present in high quantities in fetal heart tissue and skin, which may explain the predilection of involvement of these organs in NLS (Horsfall, 1991).

Many mothers of infants with NLS have SLE, but a large percentage have no known rheumatic illness (Schaller et al., 1979). Careful questioning of these mothers frequently reveals rheumatic symptoms, and some of these "well" mothers develop SLE or Sjögren's syndrome subsequently (McCue et al., 1977). Interestingly, not all pregnancies of women with anti-Ro and anti-La antibodies result in affected infants, and in fact, most offspring of these women are completely normal. A 1988 study by Lockshin and colleagues showed that only 10% of infants born to a group of women with SLE and anti-Ro/La antibodies developed NLS and none had heart block. Although there is an increased risk of a second affected infant, the magnitude of this risk is not precisely known. There have been dizygotic twin pregnancies of women with anti-Ro or anti-La antibodies who were discordant for NLS (Lockshin et al., 1988). Although anti-Ro and anti-La are the most commonly identified antibodies associated with NLS, several cases associated with anti-RNP (ribonucleoprotein) antibodies have been reported (Provost et al., 1987).

The specificities of the autoantibodies involved in NLS have been explored. There is a strong association of maternal anti–48-kD La antibody with the development of NLS. The combination of anti–52-kD Ro and anti–48-kD La antibody has the highest risk of having an affected infant (Buyon et al., 1989). These studies explain why not all infants born to women with anti-Ro/La antibodies develop NLS, and may permit identification of pregnancies at risk in utero.

Genetic factors of both mothers and infants have been investigated in hopes of defining additional risk factors in the development of NLS. The haplotype of HLA-B8, -DR3, -DQw2, -DRw52 was present in 75% of a group of 20 mothers of infants with neonatal lupus syndrome (Alexander et al., 1989). HLA-DR3 in particular is strongly associated with neonatal lupus syndrome in mothers with anti-Ro or anti-La antibodies. No infant haplotype was identified that predisposes to NLS.

Prognosis and Treatment

The skin lesions of NLS require no specific treatment; they resolve spontaneously as the maternal autoantibodies disappear from the infant's circulation. No specific treatment reverses the congenital heart block, once present. Infants with NLS who are seriously ill, however, with evidence of myocardial dysfunction, should be considered for aggressive immunosuppressive therapy (Rider et al., 1993; Silverman, 1993). There is controversy over whether identifying infants at risk for NLS in utero and offering aggressive treatment of their mothers to decrease their autoantibody titer improves the outcome (Buyon et al., 1987; Carreira et al., 1993).

Although most infants with NLS recover without sequelae, a few infants develop SLE later in childhood or early adulthood (Fox et al., 1979; Jackson and Gulliver, 1979; Lanham et al., 1983).

Mixed Connective Tissue Disease

Mixed connective tissue disease (MCTD) is an overlap syndrome closely related to SLE, first described in 1972 in a group of patients with clinical features of a number of rheumatic conditions who had high titers of antibodies to extractable nuclear antigens, particularly nuclear RNP (Sharp et al., 1972). The variability of clinical manifestations and lack of specificity of anti-RNP antibodies for MCTD have led to difficulties in identifying MCTD as a truly distinct disorder. In fact, there remains significant controversy about whether MCTD is a distinctive entity (Black and Isenberg, 1992).

Clinical Manifestations

Clinical features of MCTD combine those of SLE, dermatomyositis, scleroderma, and chronic arthritis. (Hoffman et al., 1993; Oetgen et al., 1981; Sanders et al., 1973; Singsen et al., 1977b; Tiddens et al., 1993). Presentation may mimic any of these disorders; the presence of a high titer, speckled-pattern ANA should suggest investigation for the presence of anti-RNP antibodies and further study for clinical features of MCTD (Hoffman et al., 1993). Polyarthritis may be mild or severe; some patients may develop erosive disease (Halla and Hardin, 1978). Raynaud's phenomenon may be the early presenting feature of MCTD and scleroderma-like changes of the skin, especially involving distal extremities, can be seen. Some patients have a classic dermatomyositis rash and myositis. Esophageal dysmotility is common and frequently asymptomatic. Mild pulmonary abnormalities are often present, but patients with severe pulmonary hypertension have also been reported (Derderian et al., 1985; Prakash et al., 1985; Rosenberg et al., 1979). Other clinical features include rashes suggestive of SLE, overt vasculitis, fever, lymphadenopathy and organomegaly, thrombocytopenia, and serositis. Early studies suggested that renal disease was less frequent in this group of patients, but this has proved untrue on longer follow-up of adult patients (Nimelstein et al., 1980).

Treatment and Prognosis

Treatment of MCTD should be similar to that of SLE in general. Patients with mild disease manifestations may only require NSAIDs, antimalarials, and physical therapy. Patients with severe progressive arthritis can be treated as for JRA with methotrexate, although no formal therapeutic trials have been done. For more severe systemic involvement, corticosteroids or cytotoxic agents may be required.

The prognosis of MCTD was originally considered to be good, with the perception that it was a milder disease than SLE. Many patients evolve over time, however, to a course more consistent with either SLE, scleroderma, or RA, and the mortality is considerably higher than previously believed (Black and Isenberg, 1992; Nimelstein et al., 1980). Certainly, there is potential for long-term morbidity, justifying close follow-up and treatment.

DERMATOMYOSITIS

Dermatomyositis is a rheumatic disorder characterized by inflammation of striated muscle and specific skin lesions, with occlusive small vessel vasculitis as the characteristic pathologic finding (Ansell, 1984; Banker and Victor, 1966; Bitnum et al., 1964; Bohan and Peter, 1975; Hanson and Kornreich, 1967; Schaller, 1971; Sullivan et al., 1972, 1977; Wallace et al., 1985). In polymyositis, which is extremely rare in children, cutaneous lesions are lacking.

Clinical Manifestations

The myositis characteristically involves the proximal limb and trunk muscles. Although the disease may occasionally present acutely, more typically weakness develops over weeks to months, and the first symptoms may be decreased endurance or fatigue. Myositis classically involves proximal muscle groups, including the neck, abdominal muscle, shoulder, and hip girdles, more than distal muscles. Involvement of palatal or respiratory muscles may occur as well, with the onset of a nasal voice or, less commonly, difficulty swallowing or handling oral secretions. Myalgias, arthralgias, and arthritis may also be present.

The characteristic cutaneous lesions include a violaceous erythema of the upper eyelids ("heliotrope"

hue) and extensor surfaces of the joints, especially the small joints of the hands ("Gottron's sign"). Dilated periungual capillary loops can readily be seen and may be an accurate indicator of active disease (Nussbaum et al., 1983; Silver and Maricq, 1989). Facial and truncal rashes may also be present.

Vasculitis of the gastrointestinal tract may result in abdominal pain or bleeding, and perforation can occur at any level. Calcinosis of subcutaneous tissue, fascia, and muscle occurs in 20% to 30% of patients, largely in those with inadequate early treatment of disease. Other systemic complications of dermatomyositis are exceedingly rare. Cardiac arrhythmias, pericarditis, tamponade, and myocarditis have been reported. Pronounced weakness may cause restrictive pulmonary disease; interstitial lung disease or pulmonary hemorrhage is uncommon in children. A small number of children with dermatomyositis have developed an acquired lipodystrophy associated with insulin resistance and other endocrine abnormalities late in the course of severe disease (Tucker et al., 1995).

Diagnosis

Criteria for diagnosis of dermatomyositis include the presence of symmetric proximal muscle weakness, characteristic rash, elevated muscle enzyme levels (aldolase, creatine phosphokinase, alanine aminotransferase, aspartate aminotransferase, lactate dehydrogenase), myopathic findings on electromyogram, and typical muscle biopsy histology. In patients without typical rash, EMG and biopsy are necessary to exclude other forms of myopathy. Pathologically, muscle biopsies show fiber necrosis, variation in fiber size, endothelial swelling, and occlusive vasculitis; perivascular inflammatory infiltrates are minimal as compared to findings in polymyositis. Vasculitis may also be seen in other involved tissues (Crowe et al., 1982). The erythrocyte sedimentation rate is often normal. Antinuclear antibodies are sometimes found (Friedman et al., 1983; Mellins et al., 1982, Pachman and Cooke, 1980, Pachman et al., 1985).

In adults with dermatomyositis, antibodies to several amino-acyl transfer RNA synthetases have identified patients with an increased risk for interstitial pneumonitis (Dalakas and Plotz, 1989; Dalakas, 1991). These include antibodies to Jo-1 (antihistidyl tRNA synthetase), PL-7 (antithreonyl tRNA synthetase), PL-12 (antialanyl tRNA synthetase), and anti-isoleucyl and antiglycyl-tRNA synthetases. Autoantibodies to signal recognition peptide are found in adults with polymyositis (Targoff et al., 1990). Analysis of adults with inflammatory myositis has shown that determination of autoantibody reactivity correlated well with specific clinical manifestations and response to therapy (Love et al., 1991). To date, analysis of the prevalence and clinical associations of these autoantibodies in children with inflammatory myopathies has not been done.

Pathogenesis

The cause of dermatomyositis is not known. Humoral and cellular abnormalities have been described, including cytotoxicity of patient lymphocytes and serum to muscle tissue in vitro, excess proliferative responses of peripheral blood mononuclear cells to muscle cells, and abnormal deposition of complement components, immunoglobulin, and activated leukocytes in muscle tissue (Dawkins and Mastaglia, 1973; Johnson et al., 1972; Kalovidouris et al., 1989; Kissel et al., 1986; Whitaker and Engel, 1972). Various infectious agents, including coxsackievirus, echovirus, picornavirus, retroviruses, and toxoplasmosis have been proposed, but not proven, to have a role in the pathogenesis of dermatomyositis (Leff et al., 1992; Rosenberg et al., 1989). One theory is that some tRNA synthetases may become immunogenic after binding to viral DNA. Genetic factors may also contribute to pathogenesis. An increased incidence of HLA-DR3 and -B8 has been found, most strikingly among white patients (Friedman et al., 1983; Malleson, 1990; Pachman et al., 1985). In one study, children with dermatomyositis were found to have an increased incidence of C4 null genes (Moulds et al., 1990).

Some adult patients with dermatomyositis have associated malignancy, usually carcinomas; the muscle disease may remit with treatment of the tumor (Richardson and Callen, 1989; Sigurgeirsson et al., 1992). This curious relation has not been noted with childhood dermatomyositis.

Treatment

Dermatomyositis and polymyositis generally respond well to therapy with corticosteroids and have a good prognosis if treated early and vigorously (Hanson and Kornreich, 1967; Schaller, 1971; Sullivan et al., 1972, 1977; Ansell, 1984, 1992). High doses of oral or intravenous steroids are the usual first choice for treatment. Adjunctive therapy is necessary for some patients, including those with severe onset disease (extreme muscle weakness, severe systemic involvement), those with a relapsing course, or those with chronic persistent disease (Malleson, 1990). Adjunctive therapy may also provide significant steroid-sparing effect. Azathioprine, methotrexate, hydroxychloroquine, and cyclosporin A have all been reported to have beneficial effects (Ansell, 1992; Fischer et al., 1979; Heckmatt et al., 1989; Jacobs, 1977; Lueck et al., 1991; Miller et al., 1992; Olson and Lindsley, 1989; Wallace et al., 1985).

Other treatments, including high dose intravenous immunoglobulin (IVIG), have been tried in children with recalcitrant disease, with some promising results (Barron et al., 1992; Cherin et al., 1991; Dalakas et al., 1993). The mechanism of action of IVIG may be the prevention of deposition of activated complement components in the capillaries of the muscle tissue (Basta and Dalakas, 1994).

A controlled trial of leukapheresis and plasma exchange in 39 adult patients with dermatomyositis or polymyositis found no difference between these treatments and sham pheresis (Miller et al., 1992).

Physical therapy is an important component of treatment for children with dermatomyositis to maintain range of motion and eventually to improve endurance and muscle strength.

VASCULITIS SYNDROMES

Henoch-Schönlein purpura, Kawasaki disease, polyarteritis nodosa, and their variants are inflammatory diseases of blood vessels. The vasculitis syndromes may result in various insults to blood vessels, including immune complex deposition in endothelial cells from cell-mediated immune injury to blood vessels or, as has been shown in animal models of vasculitis, through direct infection of endothelium (Haynes and Fauci, 1978). In contrast to other rheumatic diseases, the vasculitis syndromes affect males slightly more frequently than females. Henoch-Schönlein purpura and Kawasaki disease are the most common vasculitides in childhood and affect medium-sized vessels. Polyarteritis nodosa, allergic granulomatosis (Churg-Strauss disease), and Wegener's granulomatosis are relatively rare in children. Takayasu's arteritis is the only large-vessel vasculitis occurring in childhood. Other forms of vasculitis, including Behçet's syndrome, Cogan's syndrome, and lymphomatoid granulomatosis are even more uncommon.

Henoch-Schönlein Purpura

Henoch-Schönlein purpura (HSP; also known as anaphylactoid purpura) is a relatively common form of vasculitis of childhood characterized by purpuric rash, gastrointestinal findings, and renal disease (Allen et al., 1960; Ayoub and Hoyer, 1970; Bywaters et al., 1957; Emery et al., 1977; Vernier et al., 1961) (see Chapters 21, 22, and 25).

Clinical Manifestations

The clinical picture of HSP is distinctive. A rash of erythematous macules, which may progress to purpura, is invariably present, most commonly over the extensor surfaces of the legs and buttocks, but sometimes involving the arms, face, and trunk as well (Fig. 24–9). The rash may initially appear urticarial and may be accompanied by localized edema of the dorsum of the hands, the feet, face, and scalp. Joint symptoms precede other signs of HSP in 25% of patients. Large joints, especially knees, ankles, wrists, and elbows, are preferentially involved, often in a migratory fashion. The arthritis always resolves completely. Colicky abdominal pain, often with melena, is the most common gastrointestinal symptom and may precede the rash. In patients who have undergone surgery, purpuric lesions of the small bowel serosa and segmental edema of the bowel walls are found (Martinez-Frontanilla et al., 1984). Generally, the gastrointestinal manifestations of HSP resolve spontaneously; however, intussusception, bowel infarction, and other intestinal complications have all been reported.

Renal involvement in HSP ranges from microscopic or gross hematuria to glomerulonephritis, with or

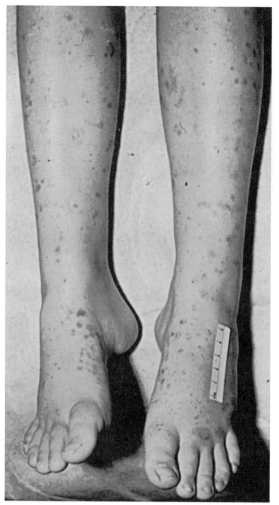

Figure 24–9. Characteristic rash of Schönlein-Henoch vasculitis. Small erythematous maculae, purpuric spots, and petechiae are distributed over the lower extremities. In contrast to the evanescent rash of juvenile rheumatoid arthritis, skin lesions in Schönlein-Henoch vasculitis resolve over a period of days to weeks.

gies, vaccination, anesthesia, or malignancy (Maggiore et al., 1984). Evidence of preceding streptococcal infection was found in more than 50% of patients in one study, suggesting that strep may act as a trigger for some patients with HSP, but follow-up studies found no difference from healthy children (Ayoub and Hoyer, 1970; Bywaters et al., 1957).

Thirty to fifty percent of HSP patients have elevated serum levels of IgA (Trygstad and Stiehm, 1971). Increased numbers of IgA-bearing lymphocytes and IgA-containing immune complexes or cryoglobulins are found in the circulation during active disease (Hall et al., 1980; Kauffman et al., 1980; Kuno-Sakai et al., 1979; Saulsbury, 1992). Lymphocytes from HSP patients spontaneously synthesize excessive amounts of IgA (Beale et al., 1982). IgA immune deposits are found in renal mesangium, skin, and intestinal capillaries (André et al., 1980; Conley et al., 1980). Similar abnormalities are found in patients with IgA nephropathy (Berger's disease), which has been called "monosymptomatic" HSP (Mihatsch et al., 1984; Nakamoto et al., 1978). IgA nephropathy has occurred in renal transplants done after renal failure from HSP (Weiss, 1978). The relationship between the two diseases is further illustrated by a report of identical twin boys with adenovirus infection, followed a few days later by typical HSP in one twin and IgA nephropathy in the second twin (Meadow and Scott, 1985) (see Chapter 25).

Diagnosis and Laboratory Findings

The diagnosis of HSP is clinical and cannot be made in the absence of the characteristic rash. By definition, the purpura is not associated with thrombocytopenia; rather, thrombocytosis is more often observed. Leukocytosis and an elevated sedimentation rate are usually seen. Although not usually measured clinically, activation of the alternate complement pathway is reflected in decreased circulating levels of properdin, properdin convertase, and Factor B (Garcia-Fuentes et al., 1978). Measurements of CH_{50}, C3, and C4 are normal, and antinuclear antibodies are not present.

Treatment and Prognosis

Treatment of HSP is symptomatic. The disease usually resolves in days to weeks. Occasionally, a short course of corticosteroids may be warranted for significant gastrointestinal involvement. Some centers advocate the use of corticosteroids, sometimes supplemented by cytotoxic drugs, for 6 to 12 months to treat proliferative glomerulonephritis when there is evidence of renal decompensation (Michael et al., 1967). No controlled studies have been reported and the number of patients who have received these drugs is small.

The prognosis for patients with HSP is excellent with full recovery without residua occurring in most patients. Many children have recurrences of HSP, with a waxing and waning course over 6 months. The eventual outcome is related to the degree of renal involve-

without concomitant nephrotic syndrome. The incidence of renal disease is not known; various series report 10% to 90% of patients with HSP have renal manifestations. Rapidly progressive glomerulonephritis with renal insufficiency can occur (Ansell, 1970; Austin and Balow, 1983; Counahan et al., 1977; Hurley and Drummond, 1972; Kauffman et al., 1980; Levy et al., 1976; Urizar et al., 1968; Vernier et al., 1961). Although the rash, arthritis, and gastrointestinal symptoms may recur episodically, especially in the first month of the disease, renal manifestations may persist for months to years, even in patients who eventually recover completely.

Pulmonary, cardiac, and central nervous system involvement also have rarely been reported in HSP.

Pathogenesis

The cause of HSP is unknown, although numerous antecedent events have been invoked as "triggers," including bacterial or viral infections, drugs, food aller-

ment, but even many children with severe renal involvement have complete recovery.

Kawasaki Disease

Kawasaki disease (formerly called mucocutaneous lymph node syndrome) is an acute systemic inflammatory disease affecting infants and young children, first described by Kawasaki in Japan in 1967 (Kawasaki, 1967; Kawasaki et al., 1974). More than 80,000 cases of Kawasaki disease have subsequently been recognized in Japan, and thousands reported worldwide, making Kawasaki disease one of the most common vasculitic diseases of childhood (Bell et al., 1983; Dean et al., 1982; Meade and Brandt, 1982; Melish et al., 1976; Rowley et al., 1988a).

Epidemiology

Kawasaki disease is an illness of young children, with most patients younger than 5 years. The disease is less common in teenagers and rare in adulthood. There is a slight male preponderance, with a boy:girl ratio of 1.5:1 (Rowley et al., 1988b). Kawasaki disease does not appear to be spread through contact, because it is rare to have multiple cases in a family or school class.

The epidemiologic characteristics of Kawasaki disease are suggestive of an infectious cause, because there are epidemics in different geographic areas and cases are most frequent in the late winter and spring months (Dean et al., 1982; Meade and Brandt, 1982; Rowley et al., 1988a).

Clinical Manifestations

Kawasaki disease is characterized by prolonged high fever, nonpurulent conjunctivitis, stomatitis, swelling and erythema of hands and feet with subsequent desquamation of the skin (particularly of the distal phalanges, beginning 2 to 3 weeks after onset of the disease), nonsuppurative lymphadenopathy, and polymorphous exanthems. The cardiovascular system is prominently involved in many patients with Kawasaki disease (see later). Other clinical features described in patients with Kawasaki disease include arthralgia or arthritis, sterile pyuria, aseptic meningitis, mild hepatitis, hydrops of the gallbladder, and diarrhea.

No specific diagnostic test exists for Kawasaki disease, and establishment of the diagnosis rests on the fulfillment of clinical criteria developed by the American Heart Association in 1990. The criteria for the diagnosis of Kawasaki disease are listed in Table 24–7. Fever and at least four of these five features should be present to establish the diagnosis of Kawasaki disease with certainty; however, patients with documented coronary artery disease and fewer than four clinical features are considered to have atypical disease. Increasing cases of atypical Kawasaki disease are being reported, in which patients do not fulfill criteria (Levy and Koren, 1990). The majority of patients with atypical disease are younger than 1 year old. Children with a prolonged unexplained febrile illness, particularly with

Table 24–7. Criteria for the Diagnosis of Kawasaki Disease

Fever for 5 days or more, plus four of the following five:
1. Changes of the peripheral extremities—erythema of the palms and soles, diffuse edema of the hands and feet, subsequent desquamation of the fingertips
2. Polymorphous exanthem
3. Bilateral nonpurulent conjunctival congestion
4. Changes of the lips and oral mucosa—red, dry, cracked lips, strawberry tongue, injection of the oral and pharyngeal mucosa
5. Acute, nonpurulent cervical lymphadenopathy >1.5 cm in size

features of desquamating rash, mucosal changes, and thrombocytosis, should be investigated for Kawasaki disease with cardiac echo, in order not to miss unusual cases that warrant treatment.

The clinical criteria for diagnosis of Kawasaki disease are sufficiently nonspecific to possibly include children with other childhood illnesses. Clinicians should take care to exclude infectious diseases, such as measles, streptococcal disease, viral infections, and toxic shock syndrome (Burns et al., 1991).

Cardiovascular manifestations of Kawasaki disease are the most serious, because it is recognized that without treatment, up to 2% of children die from the complications of coronary vasculitis such as myocardial infarction. Coronary aneurysms develop in up to 20% of untreated children with Kawasaki disease (Kato et al., 1975; Koren et al., 1986; Munro-Faure, 1959; Rose, 1990) and are best diagnosed by echocardiography (Yoshikawa et al., 1979). The size of aneurysms is a helpful prognostic factor; patients who develop giant aneurysms (>8 mm) are at the highest risk for myocardial infarction secondary to thrombosis or stenosis of healing vessels (Nakano et al., 1986; Yanagisawa et al., 1974).

Other cardiovascular manifestions seen less commonly in the acute stage of Kawasaki disease include myocarditis, pericarditis, valvulitis, and arrhythmias (Dean et al., 1982; Gidding et al., 1986; Imakita et al., 1984; Nakano et al., 1985). Even less frequently, vasculitis and aneurysms affect other medium-sized arteries throughout the body, such as brachial, hepatic, or iliac arteries (Fukushige et al., 1980).

The natural history of coronary artery aneurysms in Kawasaki disease is eventual regression, with 50% resolved by 1 year after onset of disease, as detected by echocardiogram (Akagi et al., 1992; Dean et al., 1982; Takahashi et al., 1987). However, residual abnormalities may remain in these vessels and predispose to future complications. Pathologic findings of abnormalities in coronary vessels of children who recovered from Kawasaki disease and died of unrelated causes support these concerns (Fijiwara et al., 1988; Naoe et al., 1987). The coronary arteries of some children with Kawasaki disease and resolved aneurysms have poor vasodilatory responses to infusion of isosorbide dinitrate, suggesting residual dysfunction (Anderson et al., 1985; Sugimura et al., 1992). Increasing numbers of early anginal symptoms, ischemic disease, and sudden death are being reported among patients who have had Kawasaki disease in childhood (Gersony, 1992; Ishiwata et al., 1990; Kohr, 1986; Suzuki et al., 1990). Long-term follow-up is necessary to determine the risk of early atherosclerotic heart disease in children after Kawasaki disease.

Laboratory Findings

There are no diagnostic laboratory tests for Kawasaki disease. The erythrocyte sedimentation rate is elevated, and leukocytosis and anemia are common. Tests for antinuclear antibody and rheumatoid factors are negative, but circulating immune complexes have been detected in some patients (Rowley et al., 1988a). Elevated levels of IgE have been reported (Kasakawa and Heiner, 1976). Dramatic elevation of the platelet count is the most helpful laboratory clue, generally occurring in the second week of illness and reaching levels as high as 1 to 2 million/mm³.

Etiology

There is continued interest and speculation about the cause of Kawasaki disease. Patients with Kawasaki disease exhibit numerous immunoregulatory abnormalities, including overall decreased numbers of T cells, with increased CD4⁺ activated T-helper cells and decreased CD8⁺ cytotoxic T cells, polyclonal B-cell activation, and increased production of cytokines (interferon-γ, IL-1, TNF-α, and IL-6) (Leung, 1990; Leung et al., 1982; Ono et al., 1985). A selective expansion of a subset of T cells in children with acute Kawasaki disease has been reported; this subset is usually expanded in reaction to toxins which act as superantigens (Abe et al., 1993). These investigators have been able to culture toxic shock syndrome toxin-secreting *Staphylococcus aureus* from a majority of children with Kawasaki syndrome as compared with control children, suggesting a possible causative mechanism (Leung et al., 1993).

Treatment

Treatment of Kawasaki disease is aimed at preventing or decreasing inflammation of coronary vessels and preventing thrombosis in inflamed vessels. Initially, high-dose salicylate treatment was the only available therapy, used to control fever and to prevent thrombosis (Koren et al., 1985), but salicylate therapy did not prevent the development of coronary aneurysms.

High-dose intravenous immunoglobulin (IVIG) has been shown to decrease the incidence of coronary vessel aneurysms, first by Furusho and colleagues in Japan in 1984 and confirmed by the U.S. Multicenter Kawasaki Syndrome studies (Newburger et al., 1986; Rowley, 1991). Treatment with IVIG resulted in rapid clinical improvement and in a decrease in the prevalence of aneurysms and development of giant aneurysms (Chung, 1989; Kato et al., 1979; Rowley et al., 1988b). Further studies have shown that a single infusion of 2 g/kg of IVIG and administration of aspirin (80–100 mg/

kg/day for 14 days, then 3–5 mg/kg/day) is as effective as multiple-day IVIG infusions (Barron et al., 1990; Engle et al., 1989; Newburger et al., 1991).

The mechanism of action of IVIG in Kawasaki disease is unknown, with hypotheses including Fc receptor blockade, toxin neutralization, direct inflammatory response blockade, anti-idiotypic effects, or provision of specific antibodies against some as yet unknown pathogen or its superantigens.

Polyarteritis Nodosa

Polyarteritis nodosa (PAN) is a diffuse vasculitis of medium-sized muscular arteries; adjacent veins may be involved. Antecedent infections may trigger the disease; PAN has been reported to occur in association with hepatitis B or streptococcal infections (Blau et al., 1977; Fink, 1978; Gocke et al., 1970). In some cases, hepatitis B antigen and immune globulins were found deposited in affected blood vessels, and the disease was thought to be immune complex–mediated (Gocke et al., 1970). However, most cases of PAN are of unknown cause.

Clinically, multiple organ systems are involved, with skin rash and renal involvement (often manifesting as hypertension) most common. Gastrointestinal involvement may progress to visceral infarction. Neurologic involvement is typically mononeuritis multiplex. Skin involvement is usually limited to nodules or livedo reticularis. Vasculitis affecting the testes, epididymis, bladder, or ovaries may occur.

Diagnosis of PAN requires angiography to demonstrate the characteristic aneurysmal dilatation of blood vessels. Biopsies of affected tissues reveal vasculitis. The prognosis of PAN is much worse than HSP. PAN should be treated with corticosteroids, supplemented if necessary by cytotoxic therapy.

Wegener's Granulomatosis

Wegener's granulomatosis is a necrotizing vasculitis associated with granulomas involving the upper and lower respiratory tracts and kidneys (Fauci et al., 1983; Hall et al., 1985; Orlowski et al., 1978; Ozen et al., 1992). A possible genetic predisposition has been reported with an increased incidence of HLA-B8 and -DR2.

In addition to constitutional symptoms, patients may have sinusitis, serous otitis media, and rhinitis. A saddle-nose deformity may develop. Necrotizing glomerulonephritis and pulmonary infiltrates (often asymptomatic) are characteristic. Purpura, episcleritis, and neurologic and cardiac involvement may also occur. Laboratory tests for antineutrophil cytoplasmic antibodies (van der Wonde et al., 1985; Cohen-Tervaert et al., 1991) may aid in the diagnosis of Wegener's (Falk and Jennette, 1988). In the past, Wegener's was nearly always fatal, but treatment with cyclophosphamide may reverse the disorder in most patients (Fauci et al., 1979; Moorthy et al., 1977; Novack and Pearson, 1971).

SCLERODERMA

Scleroderma, a disease characterized by hardening of the skin and subcutaneous tissues, occurs in localized forms (morphea, linear scleroderma) and a generalized cutaneous and systemic form (progressive systemic sclerosis) (Ansell et al., 1976; Cassidy et al., 1977b; Kornreich et al., 1977; Winkelmann et al., 1971).

Clinical Manifestations

The appearance and the histology of cutaneous lesions are similar in the localized and generalized forms. The affected skin becomes shiny, indurated, and eventually bound down to underlying structures; patchy hyperpigmentation or vitiligo may be present. The localized cutaneous forms (morphea and linear scleroderma) rarely progress to generalized disease; the relationship between localized cutaneous scleroderma and progressive systemic sclerosis (PSS) is not defined.

Systemic manifestations of progressive systemic sclerosis include involvement of the esophagus, bowel, lung, kidney, and heart (Suarez-Almazor et al., 1985). Raynaud's phenomenon is nearly always present and may precede typical skin changes by months or even years. Capillaroscopy of nail beds has revealed varying patterns of nail fold capillary changes; an active pattern characterized by destruction and loss of capillaries, with reorganization of the nail fold capillary bed, seems to be associated with a rapidly progressive form of the disease as opposed to enlargement and/or telangiectasis, which may herald a milder disease course (Chen, et al., 1984; Spencer-Green et al., 1983).

Diagnosis is made on clinical grounds with the aid of laboratory techniques seeking specific organ involvement, such as pulmonary function tests, echocardiography, and esophageal motility studies (Follansbee et al., 1984; Peters-Golden et al., 1984).

Pathogenesis

The pathogenesis of scleroderma is not understood, but, a number of immunologic, vascular, and connective tissue abnormalities have been described. Many patients with scleroderma produce antibodies rather specific for these disorders. Antitopoisomerase I (Scl-70) antibodies are seen in patients with systemic sclerosis. Patients with the CREST form of scleroderma (a more limited form with subcutaneous calcinosis, Raynaud's phenomenon, esophageal dysmotility, sclerodactyly, and telangiectasias) frequently have anticentromere antibodies. Studies of MHC association in scleroderma have shown an increase in HLA-DR1, -DR3, -DR5, and -C4 null alleles in particular disease subsets, although results differ among ethnic groups and different countries (Black, 1993; Briggs et al., 1993).

Abnormalities of microvasculature are postulated to play a role in disease pathogenesis. The development of Raynaud's phenomenon, a hyperreactive vascular state, often long before obvious clinical signs of scleroderma, suggests vascular changes may take place early in disease course. There is histologic evidence of endothelial cell necrosis early in scleroderma, with arterial intimal proliferation and inflammatory perivascular infiltration (Fleischmajer and Perlish, 1980).

The classic pathologic finding in scleroderma is the increase in normal extracellular matrix and fibrosis. In scleroderma, certain types of collagen are overproduced, and the gene message for these collagen molecules has been shown to be increased. Cytokines may play a role in abnormal regulation of fibroblasts in scleroderma, but no direct evidence to support this is available (Black, 1993).

Several clinical conditions resembling scleroderma have been described. A scleroderma-like state occurs in some patients after bone marrow transplant (van Vloten et al., 1977), often related to chronic graft-versus-host disease (Jaffe and Claman, 1983). Likewise, symptoms and signs suggestive of scleroderma have been described as part of the Spanish toxic oil syndrome (Kilbourne et al., 1983). There are reports of women with silicone breast implants developing scleroderma (Spiera and Kerr, 1993; Varga et al., 1989); however, the degree of this association and extent of risk of silicone implants for development of rheumatic disease is still not well explained (Sanchez-Guerro et al., 1994).

Treatment

In contrast to the other rheumatic diseases, scleroderma responds poorly, if at all, to even vigorous therapy with potent anti-inflammatory drugs, such as corticosteroids. Many experimental drugs have been used to treat this disease without success. Such drugs as penicillamine, which result in an increase of soluble collagen components, have been tried, but the results have not been dramatic. Some suggest, however, that treatment with penicillamine over long periods of time results in improved survival and slowing of pulmonary involvement (Jimenez and Sigal, 1991). Therapy with chlorambucil has also been proposed, but its efficacy is uncertain. Voluntary control of digital temperatures using biofeedback has proved helpful in controlling Raynaud's phenomenon. Nifedipine and other calcium channel blockers are considered useful agents for treatment, with action on the vascular abnormalities postulated in scleroderma. New treatment trials in scleroderma are being undertaken with agents such as recombinant interferon-γ (Freundlich et al., 1992) and extracorporeal photopheresis. With improved knowledge of scleroderma pathogenesis, there is hope for improved directed therapeutic approaches.

Prognosis

The prognosis of scleroderma is uncertain. The cutaneous forms are often self-limited but may cause extensive crippling. Progressive systemic sclerosis is inexorably severe but may sometimes develop slowly enough so that the prognosis is not entirely gloomy.

EOSINOPHILIC FASCIITIS

Eosinophilic fasciitis is a rare entity characterized by inflammation of fascia with an eosinophilic infiltrate (Bennett et al., 1977; Grisanti et al., 1989; Michet et al., 1981; Shulman, 1977).

Clinical Manifestations

Eosinophilic fasciitis resembles scleroderma in both its diffuse and localized forms but, unlike those disorders, the onset is acute, with widespread inflammation and sclerosis of the deep fascia, and without associated Raynaud's phenomenon (Rodnan et al., 1975). Affected fascial tissues are infiltrated with plasma cells, lymphocytes, and often eosinophils. Because fascia is affected and overlying skin is spared, there is often superficial puckering of the skin, with hardening and tenderness of the underlying tissues. The face is characteristically spared; tissues of the limbs and sometimes the trunk are predominantly affected. Visceral involvement is uncommon, but symmetric polyarthritis has been described (Rosenthal and Benson, 1980). In a number of patients, fasciitis has occurred after vigorous physical activity, suggesting that it may be an aberrant response to the overuse of muscles. It has been described after allogeneic bone marrow transplantation (Markusse et al., 1990), in an HLA-identical sibling pair (Thomson et al., 1989).

Diagnosis and Laboratory Findings

There are no diagnostic laboratory tests. Antinuclear antibodies and rheumatoid factors are not present; however, immunoglobulin levels are usually elevated. The clinical picture is reasonably distinctive, although there may be confusion with scleroderma, scleredema, or dermatomyositis. Eosinophilic fasciitis must be differentiated from the recently described eosinophilia-myalgia syndrome related to tryptophan ingestion (Silver et al., 1990). Diagnosis rests on demonstration of histologic fasciitis by appropriate deep biopsies. Eosinophilia may be present in either tissue sections or peripheral blood. MRI may be helpful diagnostically and in guiding biopsies (De Clerck et al., 1989).

Treatment and Prognosis

Most patients respond well to corticosteroids. Children with more extensive disease and a younger age of onset appear to have increased risk of development of residual cutaneous fibrosis resembling localized scleroderma (Farrington et al., 1993). Progressive flexion contractures (especially of the small joints of the hands), localized morphea, or carpal tunnel syndrome may occur. Penicillamine, cimetidine, colchicine, cyclosporine, methotrexate, and chloroquine have been used as therapeutic agents with variable results. Physical and occupational therapy are important to maintain strength, range of motion, and flexibility.

In some patients, prognosis is excellent with nearly complete resolution over a period of 2 to 5 years (Rodnan et al., 1975). In others, however, systemic involvement similar to that of scleroderma occurs. In a few patients, serious associated disease, such as aplastic anemia or thrombocytopenic purpura, has been described (Shulman et al., 1979).

References

Abe J, Kotzin BL, Meissner C, Melish ME, Takahashi M, Fulton D, Romagne F, Malissen B, Leung DYM. Characterization of T cell repertoire changes in acute Kawasaki disease. J Exp Med 177:791–796, 1993.

Agnello V, DeBracco M, Kunkel H. Hereditary C2 deficiency with some manifestations of systemic lupus erythematosus. J Immunol 108:837–840, 1972.

Ahlstrom H, Feltelius N, Nyman R, Hallgren R. Magnetic resonance imaging of sacroiliac joint inflammation. Arthritis Rheum 33:1763–1769, 1990.

Aho K, Somer T, Salo OP. Rheumatoid factor and immunoconglutinin responses following various vaccinations. Proc Soc Exp Biol Med 124:229–233, 1967.

Akagi T, Rose V, Berson LN, Newman A, Freedom RM. Outcome of coronary artery aneurysms after Kawasaki disease. J Pediatr 121:689–694, 1992.

Alarcon-Riquelme ME, Alarcon-Segovia D, Loredo-Abdala A, Alcocer-Varela J. T lymphocyte subsets, suppressor and contrasuppressor cell functions, and production of interleukin-2 in the peripheral blood of rheumatic fever patients and their apparently healthy siblings. Clin Immunol Immunopathol 55:120–128, 1990.

Alarcon-Segovia D, Deleze M, Oria C, Sanchez-Guerrero J, Gomez-Pacheco L, Cabiedes J, Fernandez L, Ponce de Leon S. Antiphospholipid antibodies and the antiphospholipid syndrome in systemic lupus erythematosus. Medicine 68:353–365, 1989.

Alexander EL, McNichall J, Watson RM, Bias W, Reichlin M, Provost TT. The immunogenetic relationship between anti-Ro(SSA)/La(SSB) antibody-positive Sjögren's/lupus erythematosus overlap. J Invest Dermatol 93:751, 1989.

Allen DM, Diamond LK, Howell DA. Anaphylactoid purpura in children (Schönlein-Henoch syndrome). Am J Dis Child 99:833–854, 1960.

Allen RC, Dewez P, Stuart L, Gatenby PA, Sturgess A. Antinuclear antibodies using HEP-2 cells in normal children and in children with common infections. J Paediatr Child Health 27:39–42, 1991.

Ammann A, Hong R. Selective IgA deficiency: presentation of thirty cases and review of the literature. Medicine 50:223–236, 1971.

Anderson TM, Meyer RA, Kaplan S. Long-term echocardiographic evaluation of cardiac size and function in patients with Kawasaki disease. Am Heart J 110:107–115, 1985.

André C, Berthoux FC, Andre F. Prevalence of IgA2 deposits in IgA nephropathies. N Engl J Med 303:1343–1346, 1980.

Annegers JF, Pillman NL, Weidman WH, Kurland LT. Rheumatic fever in Rochester, Minnesota, 1935–1978. Mayo Clin Proc 57:753–757, 1982.

Ansell BM. Henoch-Schönlein purpura with particular reference to the prognosis of the renal lesion. Br J Dermatol 82:211–215, 1970.

Ansell BM. Management of polymyositis and dermatomyositis. Clin Rheum Dis 10:205–213, 1984.

Ansell BM. Juvenile dermatomyositis. J Rheumatol 19 (Suppl 33):60–62, 1992.

Ansell BM. Cyclosporin A in paediatric rheumatology. Clin Exp Rheumatol 11:113–115, 1993.

Ansell BM, Nasseh GA, Bywaters EGL. Scleroderma in childhood. Ann Rheum Dis 35:189–197, 1976.

Appel AE, Sablay LB, Golden RA, Bartland P, Grayzel AI, Bank N. The effect of normalization of serum complement and anti-DNA antibody on the course of lupus nephritis. Am J Med 64:274–283, 1978.

Arnett FC, McCluskey OE, Schacter BZ, Lordon RE. Incomplete Reiter's syndrome: discriminating features and HL-A w27 in diagnosis. Ann Intern Med 84:8–12, 1976.

Arnett FC, Bias WB, Stevens MB. Juvenile-onset chronic arthritis. Clinical and roentgenographic features of a unique HLA-B27 subset. Am J Med 69:369–376, 1980.

Asbrink E. Cutaneous manifestations of Lyme borreliosis. Scand J Infect Dis 77 (Suppl):44–50, 1991.

Asherson RA, Hughes GRV. Antiphospholipid antibodies and chorea. J Rheumatol 15:377–379, 1988.

Asherson RA, Khamashta MA, Gil A. Cerebrovascular disease and antiphospholipid antibodies in systemic lupus erythematosus, lupus-like disease, and the primary antiphospholipid antibody syndrome. Am J Med 86:391–399, 1989a.

Asherson RA, Khamashta MA, Ordi-Ros J, Derksen RHWM, Machin SJ, Path FRC, Barquinero J, Outt HH, Harris EN, Vilardell-Torres M, Hughes GRV. The "primary" antiphospholipid syndrome: major clinical and serological features. Medicine 68:366–374, 1989b.

Austin HA, Balow JE. Henoch-Schönlein nephritis: prognosis features and the challenge of therapy. Am J Kidney Dis 2:512–520, 1983.

Austin HA, Klippel JH, Balow JE, LeRiche NG, Steinberg AD, Plotz PH, Decker JL. Therapy of lupus nephritis. Controlled trial of prednisone and cytotoxic drugs. N Engl J Med 314:614–619, 1986.

Ayoub EM, Hoyer J. Anaphylactoid purpura: streptococcal antibody titers and beta$_{1c}$ globulin levels. J Pediatr 75:193–201, 1970.

Ayoub EM, Barrett DJ, Maclaren NK, Krischer JP. Association of class II human histocompatibility leukocyte antigens with rheumatic fever. J Clin Invest 77:2019–2026, 1986.

Bach FH, van Rood JJ. The major histocompatibility complex—genetics and biology. N Engl J Med 295:806–936, 1976.

Bain BJ. Some influences on the ESR and the fibrinogen level in healthy subjects. Clinical Lab Haematol 5:45–54, 1983.

Baldwin DS, Lowenstein J, Rothfield NF, Gallo G, McCluskey RT. The clinical course of the proliferative and membranous forms of lupus nephritis. Ann Intern Med 73:929–942, 1970.

Baldwin DS, Gluck MC, Lowenstein J, Gallo GR. Lupus nephritis. Clinical course as related to morphologic forms and their transitions. Am J Med 62:12–30, 1977.

Ballas SK. The erythrocyte sedimentation rate, rouleaux formation and hyperviscosity syndrome. Theory and fact. Am J Clin Pathol 63:45–48, 1975.

Banker BQ, Victor M. Dermatomyositis (systemic angiopathy) of childhood. Medicine 45:261–289, 1966.

Baranton G, Postic D, Saint Girons I, Boerlin P, Piffaretti JC, Assous M, Grimont PAD. Delineation of *Borrelia burgdorferi* sensu stricto, *Borrelia Garinii* sp. nov., and group VS461 associated with Lyme borreliosis. Int J Syst Bacteriol 42:378–383, 1992.

Bardelas J, Winkelstein J, Seto D, Tsai T, Rogol A. Fatal ECHO 24 infection in a patient with hypogammaglobulinemia: relationship to dermatomyositis-like syndrome. J Pediatr 90:396–399, 1977.

Barkley D, Hohermuth H, Howard A, Webster D, Ansell B. IgA deficiency in juvenile chronic polyarthritis. J Rheumatol 6:219–224, 1979.

Barnett E, Winkelstein A, Weinberger H. Agammaglobulinemia with polyarthritis and subcutaneous nodules. Am J Med 48:40–47, 1970.

Barron KS, Murphy DJ, Silverman ED. Treatment of Kawasaki syndrome: a comparison of two dosage regimens of intravenously administered immune globulin. J Pediatr 117:638–644, 1990.

Barron KS, Sher MR, Silverman ED. Intravenous immunoglobulin therapy: magic or black magic? J Rheumatol 19 (Suppl 33):94–97, 1992.

Barron KS, Silverman ED, Gonzales JC, Owerbach D, Reveille JD. DNA analysis of HLA-DR, DQ, and DP alleles in children with polyarticular juvenile rheumatoid arthritis. J Rheumatol 19:1611–1616, 1992.

Basta M, Dalakas MC. High-dose intravenous immunoglobulin exerts its beneficial effect in patients with dermatomyositis by blocking endomysial deposition of activated complement fragments. J Clin Invest 94:1729–1735, 1994.

Baum J, Fink C. Juvenile rheumatoid arthritis in monozygotic twins: a case report and review of the literature. Arthritis Rheum 11:33–36, 1968.

Baumann H, Schendel P. Interleukin-11 regulates the hepatic expression of the same plasma protein genes as interleukin-6. J Biol Chem 266:20424–20427, 1991.

Beale MG, Nash GS, Bertorich MJ. Similar disturbances in B cell activity and regulatory T-cell function in Henoch-Schönlein purpura and systemic lupus erythematosus. J Immunol 128:486–491, 1982.

Beck JS. Antinuclear antibodies: methods of detection and significance. Mayo Clin Proc 44:600–619, 1969.

Bedford PA, Ansell BM, Hall PJ, Woo P. Increased frequency of DR4 in systemic onset juvenile rheumatoid arthritis. Clin Exp Rheumatol 10:189–193, 1992.

Bell DA, Maddison PJ. Serologic subsets in systemic lupus erythematosus: the examination of autoantibodies in relationship to clinical features of disease and HLA antigens. Arthritis Rheum 23:1268–1273, 1980.

Bell DM, Morens DM, Holman RC, Hurwitz ES, Hunter MK. Kawasaki syndrome in the United States. Am J Dis Child 137:211–214, 1983.

Ben-Chetrit E. The molecular basis of the SSA/Ro antigens and the clinical significance of their autoantibodies. Br J Rheumatol 32:396–402, 1993.

Bennett RM, Herron A, Keogh L. Eosinophilic fasciitis. Ann Rheum Dis 36:354–357, 1977.

Bernstein B, Takahashi M, Hanson V. Cardiac involvement in juvenile rheumatoid arthritis. J Pediatr 85:313–317, 1974.

Bernstein BH, Stobie D, Singsen BH, Koster-King K, Kornreich HK, Hanson V. Growth retardation in juvenile rheumatoid arthritis (JRA). Arthritis Rheum 20:212–216, 1977.

Berrios X, Quesney F, Morales A, Blazquez J, Bisno AL. Are all recurrences of "pure" Sydenham chorea true recurrences of acute rheumatic fever? J Pediatr 107:867–872, 1985.

Berrios X, del Campo E, Guzman B, Bisno AL. Discontinuing rheumatic fever prophylaxis in selected adolescents and young adults. Ann Intern Med 118:401–406, 1993.

Bini P, Gabay JE, Melchior M, Zhou JL, Elkon KB. Antineutrophil cytoplasmic autoantibodies in Wegener's granulomatosis recognize conformational epitope(s) on proteinase 3. J Immunol 149:1409–1415, 1992.

Bissenden JG. Transatlantic warning bells sound on rheumatic fever. Br Med J 296:13, 1988.

Bitnum S, Daeschner CW, Travis LB, Dodge HC. Dermatomyositis. J Pediatr 64:101–131, 1964.

Black C, Isenberg DA. Mixed connective tissue disease—goodbye to all that. Br J Rheumatol 31:695–700, 1992.

Black CM. The aetiopathogenesis of systemic sclerosis. J Int Med 234:3–8, 1993.

Blaese RM, Grayson J, Steinberg AD. Elevated immunoglobulin secreting cells in the blood of patients with active systemic lupus erythematosus: correlation of laboratory and clinical assessment of disease activity. Am J Med 69:345–350, 1980.

Bland EF. Rheumatic fever: the way it was. Circulation 76:1190–1195, 1987.

Blank M, Cohen J, Toder V, Shoenfeld Y. Induction of antiphospholipid syndrome in naive mice with mouse lupus monoclonal and human polyclonal anti-cardiolipin antibodies. Proc Natl Acad Sci USA 88:3069–3073, 1990.

Blau EB, Morris RF, Yunis EJ. Polyarteritis nodosa in older children. Pediatrics 60:227–234, 1977.

Bleil L, Manger B, Winkler T, Herrman M, Burmester G, Krapf F, Kalden J. The role of antineutrophil cytoplasm antibodies, anticardiolipin antibodies, von Willebrand factor antigen, and fibronectin for the diagnosis of systemic vasculitis. J Rheumatol 18:1199–1206, 1991.

Block SR, Winfield JB, Lockshin MD, D'Angelo WA, Christian CL. Studies of twins with systemic lupus erythematosus. A review of the literature and presentation of 12 additional sets. Am J Med 59:533–552, 1975.

Block SR, Lockshin MD, Winfield JB, Weksler ME, Imamura M, Winchester RJ, Mellors RC, Christian CL. Immunologic observations on 9 sets of twins either concordant or discordant for SLE. Arthritis Rheum 19:545–554, 1976.

Bohan A, Peter JB. Polymyositis and dermatomyositis. N Engl J Med 292:344–347, 1975.

Borg E, Groen H, Horst G, Limburg P, Wouda A, Kallenberg C. Clinical associations of antiribonucleoprotein antibodies in patients with systemic lupus erythematosus. Semin Arthritis Rheum 20:163–173, 1990.

Boublik M, Tsahakis PJ, Scott RD. Cementless total knee arthroplasty in juvenile onset rheumatoid arthritis. J Clin Orthop Rel Res 286:88–93, 1993.

Bowie EJW, Thompson JH, Pascuzzi CA, Owen CAJ. Thrombosis in systemic lupus erythematosus despite circulating anticoagulant. J Lab Clin Med 62:416–430, 1963.

Bremers HH, Golitz LE, Weston WL, Hays WG. Neonatal lupus erythematosus. Cutis 24:287, 1979.

Brewer EJJ, Bass J, Baum J, Cassidy JT, Fink C, Jacobs J, Hanson V, Levinson JE, Schaller J, Stillman JS. Current proposed revision of juvenile rheumatoid arthritis criteria. Arthritis Rheum 20 (Suppl):195–199, 1977.

Brewer EJJ, Giannini EH, Barkley E. Gold therapy in the management of juvenile rheumatoid arthritis. Arthritis Rheum 23:404–411, 1980.

Brewer EJ, Giannini EH, Kuzmina N, Alekseev L. Penicillamine and hydroxychloroquine in the treatment of severe juvenile rheumatoid arthritis. N Engl J Med 314:1270–1276, 1986.

Brewerton DA. HLA-B27 and the inheritance of susceptibility to rheumatic disease. Arthritis Rheum 19:656–668, 1976.

Brewerton DA, Hart FD, Nicholls A, Caffrey M, James DC, Sturrock RD. Ankylosing spondylitis and HLA-B27. Lancet 1:904–907, 1973a.

Brewerton DA, Nicholls A, Oates JK, Caffrey M, Walters D, James DCO. Reiter's disease and HL-A27. Lancet 2:996–998, 1973b.

Brewerton DA, Caffrey M, Nicholls A, Walters D, James DCO. Acute anterior uveitis and HL-A27. Lancet 1:464, 1974a.

Brewerton DA, Nicholls A, Caffrey M, Walters D, James DCO. HL-A27 and arthropathies associated with ulcerative colitis and psoriasis. Lancet 1:956–958, 1974b.

Briggs D, Stephens C, Vaughan R, Welsh K, Black C. A molecular and serologic analysis of the major histocompatibility complex and complement component C4 in systemic sclerosis. Arthritis Rheum 36:943–954, 1993.

Bronze MS, Beachey EH, Dale JB. Protective and heart-cross reactive epitopes located within the NH$_2$ terminus of type 19 streptococcal M protein. J Exp Med 167:1849–1859, 1988.

Brunner CM, Horwitz DA, Davis JS. Identical twins discordant for SLE: an experiment in nature. Arthritis Rheum 14:373, 1971.

Budman DR, Steinberg AD. Hematologic aspects of systemic lupus erythematosus. Ann Intern Med 86:220–229, 1977.

Bulkley BH, Roberts WC. Ankylosing spondylitis and aortic regurgitation. Circulation 48:1014–1027, 1973.

Burgdorfer W, Barbour A, Hayes S, Benach J, Grunwaldt E, Davis J. Lyme disease: a tick-borne spirochetosis? Science 216:1317–1319, 1982.

Burgos-Vargas R. Spondyloarthropathies and psoriatic arthritis in children. Curr Opin Rheumatol 5:634–643, 1993.

Burns JC, Mason WH, Glode MP, Shulman ST, Melish ME, Meissner C, Bastian J, Beiser AS, Myerson HM, Newburger JW. Clinical and epidemiologic characteristics of patients referred for evaluation of possible Kawasaki's disease. J Pediatr 118:680–686, 1991.

Burton JL. Effect of oral contraceptives on erythrocyte sedimentation rate in healthy young women. Br Med J 3:214–215, 1967.

Buyon JP, Winchester R. Congenital complete heart block. Arthritis Rheum 33:609–614, 1990.

Buyon JP, Swersky SH, Fox HE, Bierman FZ, Winchester RJ. Intrauterine therapy for presumptive fetal myocarditis with acquired heart block due to systemic lupus erythematosus. Arthritis Rheum 30:44–49, 1987.

Buyon JP, Ben-Chetrit E, Karp S, Roubey RAS, Pompeo L, Reeves WH, Tan EM, Winchester R. Acquired congenital heart block: pattern of maternal antibody response to biochemically defined antigens of the SSA/Ro-SSB/La system in neonatal lupus. J Clin Invest 84:627–634, 1989.

Buyon J, Tamerius J, Belmont H, Abramson S. Assessment of disease activity and impending flare in patients with systemic lupus erythematosus. Comparison of the use of complement split products and conventional measurements of complement. Arthritis Rheum 35:1028–1037, 1992.

Bywaters EGL. Ankylosing spondylitis in childhood. Clin Rheum Dis 2:387–396, 1976.

Bywaters EGL, Ansell BM. Monarticular arthritis in children. Ann Rheum Dis 24:116–122, 1965.

Bywaters EGL, Isdale I, Kempton JJ. Schönlein-Henoch purpura evidence for a group A B hemolytic streptococcal etiology. Q J Med 26:161–175, 1957.

Bywaters EGL, Glynn LE, Zeldis A. Subcutaneous nodules of Still's disease. Ann Rheum Dis 17:278–285, 1958.

Cabral D, Petty R, Fung M, Malleson P. Persistent antinuclear antibodies in children without identifiable inflammatory rheumatic or autoimmune disease. Pediatrics 89:441–444, 1992.

Calin A, Fries JF. Striking prevalence of ankylosing spondylitis in "healthy" W27 positive males and females. N Engl J Med 293:835–839, 1975.

Calin A, Elswood J, Rigg S, Skevington SM. Ankylosing spondylitis—an analytical review of 1500 patients: the changing pattern of disease. J Rheumatol 15:1234–1238, 1988.

Carette S, Klippel JH, Decker JL, Austin HA, Plotz PH, Steinberg AD, Balow JE. Controlled studies of oral immunosuppressive drugs in lupus nephritis. A long-term follow-up. Ann Intern Med 99:1–8, 1983.

Carreira PE, Gutierrez-Larraya F, Gomez-Reino JJ. Successful intrauterine therapy with dexamethasone for fetal myocarditis and heart block in a woman with systemic lupus erythematosus. J Rheumatol 20:1204–1207, 1993.

Carson DA. Genetic factors in the etiology and pathogenesis of autoimmunity. FASEB J 6:2800–2805, 1992.

Carson DA, Bayer AS, Eisenberg PA, Lawrence S, Theofilopoulos A. IgG rheumatoid factor in subacute bacterial endocarditis: relationship of IgM rheumatoid factor and circulating immune complexes. Clin Exp Immunol 31:100–103, 1978.

Carson DA, Chen PP, Kipps TJ. New roles for rheumatoid factor. J Clin Invest 87:379–383, 1991.

Cassidy J, Burt A. Isolated IgA deficiency in juvenile rheumatoid arthritis. Arthritis Rheum 10:272, 1967.

Cassidy JT, Valkenberg HA. A five-year prospective study of rheumatoid factor tests in juvenile rheumatoid arthritis. Arthritis Rheum 10:83–90, 1967.

Cassidy JT, Brody GL, Martel W. Monoarticular juvenile rheumatoid arthritis. J Pediatr 70:867–875, 1967.

Cassidy J, Burt A, Petty R, Sullivan D. Selective IgA deficiency in connective tissue diseases. N Engl J Med 280:275, 1969.

Cassidy J, Petty R, Sullivan D. Abnormalities in the distribution of serum immunoglobulin concentrations in juvenile rheumatoid arthritis. J Clin Invest 52:1931–1936, 1973.

Cassidy JT, Sullivan DB, Petty RE, Ragsdale C. Lupus nephritis and encephalopathy. Prognosis in 58 children. Arthritis Rheum 20:315–322, 1977a.

Cassidy JT, Sullivan DB, Dabich L, Petty RE. Scleroderma in children. Arthritis Rheum 20:351–354, 1977b.

Cassidy JT, Levinson JE, Bass JC, Baum J, Brewer EJJ, Fink CW, Hanson V, Jacobs JC, Masi AT, Schaller JG, Fries JF, McShane D, Young E. A study of classification criteria for a diagnosis of juvenile rheumatoid arthritis. Arthritis Rheum 29:274–281, 1986.

Centers for Disease Control. Lyme disease surveillance: United States, 1989–1990. MMWR 40:417–421, 1991.

Cervera R, Font J, Pare C, Azqueta M, Perez-Villa F, Lopez-Soto A, Ingelmo M. Cardiac disease in systemic lupus erythematosus: prospective study in 70 patients. Ann Rheum Dis 51:156–159, 1992.

Chantler JK, Tingle AJ, Petty RE. Persistent rubella virus infection associated with chronic arthritis in children. N Engl J Med 313:1117–1123, 1985.

Chen PP, Albrandt K, Orida NK, Radoux V, Chen EY, Schrantz R, Liu F-T, Carson DA. Genetic basis for the cross-reactive idiotypes on the light chains of human IgM anti-IgG autoantibodies. Proc Natl Acad Sci USA 83:8318–8322, 1986.

Chen ZY, Silver RM, Ainsworth SK, Dobson RL, Rust P, Maricq HR. Association between fluorescent antinuclear antibodies, capillary patterns, and clinical features in scleroderma spectrum disorders. Am J Med 77:812–822, 1984.

Cherin P, Herson S, Wechsler B, Piette J, Bletry O, Coutellier A, Ziza J, Godeau P. Efficacy of intravenous gammaglobulin therapy in chronic refractory polymyositis and dermatomyositis: an open study with 20 adult patients. Am J Med 91:162–168, 1991.

Chopra P, Narula J, Kumar AS, Sachdeva S, Bhatia ML. Immunohistochemical characterisation of Aschoff nodules and endomyocardial inflammatory infiltrates in left atrial appendages from patients with chronic rheumatic heart disease. Int J Cardiol 20:99–105, 1988.

Chubick A, Sontheimer RD, Gilliam JN, Ziff M. An appraisal of tests for native DNA antibodies in connective tissue diseases: clinical usefulness of *Crithidia luciliae* assay. Ann Intern Med 89:186–192, 1978.

Chung KJ, U.S. Multicenter Kawasaki Disease Study. Incidence and prognosis of giant coronary artery aneurysms in Kawasaki disease. Circulation, 80:282, 1989.

Cohen-Tervaert JW, Goldschmeding R, Elema JD. Association of autoantibodies to myeloperoxidase with different forms of vasculitis. Arthritis Rheum 33:1264–1272, 1990a.

Cohen-Tervaert JW, Huitema MG, Hene RJ, Sluiter WJ, The TH, van der Hem GK, Kallenberg CGM. Prevention of relapses in Wegener's granulomatosis by treatment based on antineutrophil cytoplasmic antibody titre. Lancet 336:709–711, 1990b.

Cohen-Tervaert JW, Limburg PC, Elema JD, Huitema MG, Horst G, The H, Kallenberg CGM. Detection of autoantibodies against myeloid lysosomal enzymes: a useful adjunct to classification of patients with biopsy-proven necrotizing arteritis. Am J Med 91:59–66, 1991.

Combined Rheumatic Fever Study Group. A comparison of the effect of prednisone and acetylsalicylic acid on the incidence of residual rheumatic heart disease. N Engl J Med 262:895–902, 1960.

Combined Rheumatic Fever Study Group. A comparison of short-term, intensive prednisone and acetylsalicylic acid therapy in the treatment of acute rheumatic fever. N Engl J Med 272:63–70, 1965.

Congeni B, Rizzo C, Congeni J, Sreenivasan VV. Outbreak of acute rheumatic fever in Northeast Ohio. J Pediatr 111:176–179, 1987.

Conley CL, Hartman RC. A hemorrhagic disorder caused by circulating anticoagulant in patients with disseminated lupus erythematosus. J Clin Invest 31:621–622, 1952.

Conley ME, Cooper MD, Michael AF. Selective deposition of immunoglobulin A, in immunoglobulin A nephropathy, anaphylactoid purpura nephritis, and systemic lupus erythematosus. J Clin Invest 66:1432–1435, 1980.

Cook CD, Wedgwood RJ, Craig JM, Hartmann JR, Janeway CA. Systemic lupus erythematosus. Description of 37 cases in children and a discussion of endocrine therapy in 32 of the cases. Pediatrics 26:570–585, 1960.

Cooke TD, Hurd ER, Jasin HE, Bienenstock J, Ziff M. Identification of immunoglobulins and complement in rheumatoid articular collagenous tissues. Arthritis Rheum 18:541–551, 1975.

Cooper JD, Schoen RT. Epidemiology, clinical features, and diagnosis of Lyme disease. Curr Opin Rheumatol 4:520–528, 1992.

Counahan R, Winterborn MH, White RHR. Prognosis of Henoch-Schönlein nephritis in children. Br Med J 2:11–14, 1977.

Craft J. Antibodies to snRNPs in systemic lupus erythematosus. Rheum Dis Clin North Am 18:311–336, 1992.

Cronin ME, Biswas RM, van der Straeton C. IgG and IgM anticardiolipin antibodies in patients with lupus with anticardiolipin antibody-associated clinical syndromes. J Rheumatol 15:795–798, 1988.

Crowe W, Kushner I. An immunofluorescent method using *Crithidia luciliae* to detect antibodies to double-stranded DNA. Arthritis Rheum 20:811–814, 1977.

Crowe WE, Bove KE, Levinson JE, Hilton PK. Clinical and pathogenetic implications of histopathology in childhood polydermatomyositis. Arthritis Rheum 25:126–139, 1982.

Crozier IG, Li E, Milne MJ, Nicholls MG. Cardiac involvement in systemic lupus erythematosus detected by echocardiography. Am J Cardiol 65:1145–1148, 1990.

Cunningham MW, Hall NK, Krisher KK, Spanier AM. A study of anti–group A streptococcal monoclonal antibodies cross-reactive with myosin. J Immunol 136:293–298, 1986.

Cunningham MW, McCormack JM, Talaber LR, Ayoub EM, Muneer RS, Chun LT, Reddy DV. Human monoclonal antibodies reactive with antigens of the group A streptococcus and human heart. J Immunol 141:2760–2766, 1988.

Dajani AS, Bisno AL, Chung KJ, Durack DT, Gerber MA, Kaplan EL, Millard HD, Randolph MF, Shulman ST, Watanakunakorn C. Prevention of rheumatic fever: A statement for health professionals by the Committee on Rheumatic Fever, Endocarditis, and Kawasaki Disease of the Council on Cardiovascular Disease in the Young, the American Heart Association. Circulation 78:1082–1086, 1988.

Dalakas MC. Polymyositis, dermatomyositis, and inclusion-body myositis. N Engl J Med 325:1487–1498, 1991.

Dalakas M, Plotz PH. Current concepts in the idiopathic inflammatory myopathies: polymyositis, dermatomyositis, and related disorders. Ann Intern Med 111:143–157, 1989.

Dalakas M, Illa I, Dambrosia J, Soueidan S, Stein D, Otero C, Dinsmore S, McCrosky S. A controlled trial of high-dose intravenous immune globulin infusions as treatment for dermatomyositis. N Engl J Med 329:1993–2000, 1993.

Dale JB, Beachey EH. Unique and common protective epitopes among different serotypes of group A streptococcal M proteins defined with hybridoma antibodies. Infect Immun 46:267–269, 1984.

Dale JB, Beachey EH. Sequence of myosin–cross reactive epitopes of streptococcal M protein. J Exp Med 164:1785–1790, 1986.

Dalhoj J, Wiggers P. Blood sedimentation rate in healthy persons. Ugeskr Laeger 152:456–459, 1990.

David J, Vouyiouka O, Ansell BM, Hall A, Woo P. Amyloidosis in juvenile chronic arthritis: a morbidity and mortality study. Clin Exp Rheumatol 11:85–90, 1993.

Davidson A, Shefner R, Livneh A, Diamond B. The role of somatic mutation of immunoglobulin genes in autoimmunity. Ann Rev Immunol 5:85–108, 1987.

Davies KA, Hird V, Stewart S, Sivolapenko GB, Jose P, Epenetos AA. A study of *in vivo* immune complex formation and clearance in man. J Immunol 144:4613–4620, 1990.

Davies NE, Haverty JR, Boatwright M. Reiter's disease associated with shigellosis. South Med J 62:1101–1104, 1969.

Davis JS, Godfrey SM, Winfield JB. Direct evidence for circulating DNA/anti-DNA complexes in systemic lupus erythematosus. Arthritis Rheum 21:17–22, 1978.

Dawkins RL, Mastaglia FL. Cell-mediated cytotoxicity to muscle in polymyositis. N Engl J Med 288:434–438, 1973.

De Clerck LS, Degryse HR, Wonters E, Van Offel JR, De Schepper AM, Martin JJ, Stevens WJ. Magnetic resonance imaging in the evaluation of patient with eosinophilic fasciitis. J Rheumatol 16:1270–1273, 1989.

De Cunto CL, Giannini EH, Fink CW, Brewer KJ, Person DA. Prognosis of children with poststreptococcal reactive arthritis. Pediatr Infect Dis J 7:683–686, 1988.

Dean AG, Melish ME, Hicks R, Palumbo NE. An epidemic of Kawasaki syndrome in Hawaii. J Pediatr 100:552–557, 1982.

Delgado EA, Malleson PN, Pirie GE, Petty RE. The pulmonary manifestations of childhood onset systemic lupus erythematosus. Semin Arthritis Rheum 19:285–293, 1990.

DeNardo BA, Tucker LB, Miller LC, Szer IS, Schaller JG, Affiliated Children's Arthritis Centers of New England. Demography of a regional pediatric rheumatology patient population. J Rheumatol 21:1553–1561, 1994.

Derderian SS, Tellis CJ, Abbrecht PH, Welton RC, Rajagopol HR. Pulmonary involvement in mixed connective disease. Chest 88:45–48, 1985.

Dinarello CA. Interleukin-1. Rev Infect Dis 6:51–95, 1984.

Dinarello CA. Interleukin-1 and interleukin-1 antagonism. Blood 77:1–26, 1991.

DiSciascio G, Taranta A. Rheumatic fever in children. Am Heart J 99:635–658, 1980.

Dorner RW, Alexander RL, Moore TL. Rheumatoid factors. Clin Chim Acta 167:1–21, 1987.

Draznin TH, Esterly NB, Furey NL, DeBofsky H. Neonatal lupus erythematosus. J Am Acad Dermatol 1:437–442, 1979.

Eastmond C, Woodrow J. The HLA system and the anthropathies associated with psoriasis. Ann Rheum Dis 36:112–121, 1977.

Egeskjold EM, Permin AJH, Hoyeraal HM, Sorenson T. The significance of antinuclear antibodies in juvenile rheumatoid arthritis associated with chronic bilateral iridocyclitis. Acta Paediatr Scand 71:615–620, 1982.

Egner W, Chapel HM. Titration of antibodies against neutrophil cytoplasmic antigens is useful in monitoring disease activity in systemic vasculitides. Clin Exp Immunol 82:244–249, 1990.

Eichenfield AH, Athreya BH, Doughty RA, Cebul RD. Utility of rheumatoid factor in the diagnosis of juvenile rheumatoid arthritis. Pediatrics 78:480–484, 1986a.

Eichenfield AH, Goldsmith DP, Benach JL, Ross AH, Loeb FX, Doughty RA, Athreya BH. Childhood Lyme arthritis: experience in an endemic area. J Pediatr 109:753–758, 1986b.

Emery H. Clinical aspects of systemic lupus erythematosus in childhood. Pediatr Clin North Am 33:1177–1190, 1986.

Emery HM, Bowyer SL. Physical modalities of therapy in pediatric rheumatic diseases. Rheum Dis Clin North Am 17:1001–1014, 1991.

Emery H, Larter W, Schaller JG. Henoch-Schönlein vasculitis. Arthritis Rheum 20:385–388, 1977.

Emlen W, Pisetsky DS, Taylor RP. Antibodies to DNA. A perspective. J Pediatr 78:981–984, 1986.

Engle MA, Fatica NS, Bussel JB. Clinical trial of single-dose intravenous gamma globulin in acute Kawasaki disease. Am J Dis Child 143:1300–1304, 1989.

Epstein HC, Litt JZ. Discoid lupus erythematosus in a newborn infant. N Engl J Med 265:1106–1107, 1961.

Espinoza LR, Vasey FB, Oh JH, Wilkinson R, Osterland CK. Association between HLA-BW38 and peripheral psoriatic arthritis. Arthritis Rheum 21:72–75, 1990.

Fahraeus R. The suspension stability of the blood. Acta Med Scand, 55:223–228, 1921.

Falk RJ, Jennette JC. Anti-neutrophil cytoplasmic autoantibodies with specificity for myeloperoxidase in patients with systemic vasculitis and idiopathic necrotizing and crescentic glomerulonephritis. N Engl J Med 318:1651–1657, 1988.

Fantini F, Gattinara M, Gerloni V, Bergoni P, Cirla E. Severe anemia associated with active systemic onset juvenile rheumatoid arthritis successfully treated with recombinant human erythropoietin: a pilot study. Arthritis Rheum 35:724–726, 1992.

Farrington ML, Haas JE, Nazar-Stewart V, Mellins ED. Eosinophilic fasciitis in children frequently progresses to scleroderma-like cutaneous fibrosis. J Rheumatol 20:128–132, 1993.

Fauci AS, Katz P, Hayes BF, Wolfe SM. Cyclophosphamide therapy of severe systemic necrotizing vasculitis. N Engl J Med 301:235–238, 1979.

Fauci AS, Hayes BF, Katz P, Wolff SM. Wegener's granulomatosis: prospective clinical and therapeutic experience with 85 patients for 21 years. Ann Intern Med 98:76–85, 1983.

Feinstein AR, Spagnuolo M. The clinical patterns of acute rheumatic fever: a reappraisal. Medicine 41:279–305, 1962.

Feinstein AR, Wood HF, Spagnuolo M, Taranta A, Jonas S, Kleinberg E, Tursky E. Rheumatic fever in children and adolescents. VII. Cardiac changes and sequelae. Ann Intern Med 60 (Suppl 5):87–123, 1964.

Feinstein DI, Rapaport SI. Acquired inhibitors of blood coagulation. Prog Hemost Thromb 1:75–95, 1972.

Felson DT, Anderson J. Evidence for superiority of immunosuppressive drugs and prednisone over prednisone alone in lupus nephritis: results of a pooled analysis. N Engl J Med 311:1528–1533, 1984.

Ferreiro JE, Reiter WM, Saldana MJ. Systemic lupus erythematosus presenting as a chronic serositis with no demonstrable antinuclear antibodies. Am J Med 76:1100–1105, 1984.

Fessel WJ. ANA-negative systemic lupus erythematosus. Am J Med 64:80–86, 1978.

Fields RA, Sibbitt WL, Toubbeh H, Bankhurst AD. Neuropsychiatric lupus erythematosus, cerebral infarctions, and anticardiolipin antibodies. Ann Rheum Dis 49:114–117, 1990.

Figueroa F, Berrios X, Gutierrez M, Carrion F, Goycolea JP, Riedel I, Jacobelli S. Anticardiolipin antibodies in acute rheumatic fever. J Rheumatol 19:1175–1180, 1992.

Fink CW. Polyarteritis and streptococcal infection. Pediatrics 61:675, 1978.

Finkel M, Halpern J. Nervous system Lyme borreliosis. Arch Neurol 49:102–107, 1991.

Fischer TJ, Rachelefsky GS, Klein RB, Paulus HE, Stiehm ER. Childhood dermatomyositis and polymyositis: treatment with methotrexate and prednisone. Am J Dis Child 133:386–389, 1979.

Fish AJ, Blau EB, Westberg NG, Burke BA, Vernier RL, Michael AF. Systemic lupus erythematosus within the first two decades of life. Am J Med 62:99–117, 1977.

Fleischmajer R, Perlish JS. Capillary alterations in scleroderma. J Am Acad Dermatol 2:161–170, 1980.

Follansbee WP, Curtiss EI, Medsger TA, Steen VD, Uretsky BF, Owens GR, Rodnan GP. Physiologic abnormalities of cardiac function in progressive systemic sclerosis with diffuse scleroderma. N Engl J Med 310:142–148, 1984.

Ford PM, Ford SE, Lillicrap DP. Association of lupus anticoagulant and severe valvular heart disease in systemic lupus erythematosus. J Rheumatol 15:597–600, 1988.

Fox RJJ, McCuiston CH, Schoch EPJ. Systemic lupus erythematosus association with previous neonatal lupus erythematosus. Arch Dermatol 115:340, 1979.

Frank M. Detection of complement in relation to disease. J Allergy Clin Immunol 89:641–648, 1992.

Freundlich B, Jimenez SA, Steen VD, Medsger TAJ, Szkolnicki M, Jaffe HS. Treatment of systemic sclerosis with recombinant interferon-gamma. A phase I/II clinical trial. Arthritis Rheum 35:1134–1142, 1992.

Friedman JM, Pachman LM, Maryjowski ML, Radvany RM, Crowe WE, Hanson V, Levinson JE, Spencer CH. Immunogenetic studies of juvenile dermatomyositis: HLA-DR antigen frequencies. Arthritis Rheum 26:214–216, 1983.

Friend P, Repine J, Kim Y, Clawson C, Michael A. Deficiency of the second component of complement (C2) with chronic vasculitis. Ann Intern Med 82:813–816, 1975.

Fries JF, Porta J, Liang HM. Marginal benefit of renal biopsy in systemic lupus erythematosus. Arch Intern Med 138:1386–1389, 1978.

Friis J. Reiter's disease with childhood onset having special reference to HLA-B27. Scand J Rheumatol 9:250–252, 1980.

Friou GJ. Antinuclear antibodies: diagnostic significance and methods. Arthritis Rheum 10:151–159, 1967.

Fritzler MJ. Histone antibodies. In Wallace DJ, Hahn BH, eds. Dubois' Lupus Erythematosus, 4th ed. Philadelphia, Lea & Febiger, 1993, pp. 202–215.

Fritzler MJ, Kinsella TD, Garbutt E. The CREST syndrome: a distinct serologic entity with anticentromere antibodies. Am J Med 69:520–526, 1980.

Fujiwara T, Fujiwara H, Nakano H. Pathological features of coronary arteries in children with Kawasaki disease in which coronary arterial aneurysm was absent at autopsy. Circulation 78:345–350, 1988.

Fukushige J, Nihill MR, McNamara DG. Spectrum of cardiovascular lesions in mucocutaneous lymph node syndrome: analysis of eight cases. Am J Cardiol 45:98–107, 1980.

Furusho K, Kamiya T, Nakano H, Kiyosawa N, Shinomiya K, Hayashidera T, Tamura T, Hirose O, Manabe Y, Yokoyama T, et al. High-dose intravenous gammaglobulin for Kawasaki disease. Lancet 2:1055–1057, 1984.

Galve E, Candell-Riera J, Pigrau C, Permanyer-Miralda G, Garcia-Del-Castillo H, Soler-Solerl J. Prevalence, morphologic types, and evolution of cardiac valvular disease in systemic lupus erythematosus. N Engl J Med 319:817–823, 1988.

Garcia-De LaTorre I, Miranda-Mendez L. Studies of antinuclear antibodies in juvenile rheumatoid arthritis. J Rheumatol 9:603–606, 1982.

Garcia-Fuentes M, Martin A, Chantler C. Serum complement components in Henoch-Schönlein purpura. Arch Dis Child 53:417–419, 1978.

Garcia-Morteo O, Maldonado-Coco JA, Suarez-Almazor ME. Ankylosing spondylitis of juvenile onset: comparison with adult onset disease. Scand J Rheumatol 12:246–248, 1983.

Gare BA, Fasth A. Epidemiology of juvenile chronic arthritis in southwestern Sweden: a 5-year prospective population study. Pediatrics 90:950–958, 1992.

Gare BA, Fasth A, Andersson J, Berglund G, Eksktrom M, Hammaren L, Holmquist L, Ronge E, Thilen A. Incidence and prevalence of juvenile chronic arthritis: a population survey. Ann Rheum Dis 46:277–281, 1987.

Garin EH, Donnelly WH, Fennell RS, Richard GA. Nephritis in systemic lupus erythematosus in children. J Pediatr 89:366–371, 1976.

Geggel RL, Tucker L, Szer I. Postnatal progression from second- to third-degree heart block in neonatal lupus syndrome. J Pediatr 113:1049–1052, 1988.

Gelfand E, Clarkson J, Minta J. Selective deficiency of the second component of complement in a patient with anaphylactoid purpura. Clin Immunol Immunopathol 4:269–276, 1975.

George PM, Tunnessen WWJ. Childhood discoid lupus erythematosus. Arch Dermatol 129:613–617, 1993.

Gersony WM. Long-term issues in Kawasaki disease. J Pediatr 121:731–733, 1992.

Gewanter HL, Roghmann KJ, Baum J. The prevalence of juvenile arthritis. Arthritis Rheum 26:599–603, 1983.

Gewurz A, Lint T, Roberts J, Zeitz H, Gewurz H. Homozygous C2 deficiency with fulminant lupus erythematosus. Arthritis Rheum 21:28–36, 1978.

Gharavi AE, Sammaritano LR, Wen J, Eikon KB. Induction of anti-phospholipid autoantibodies by immunization with B2 glycoprotein I (apolipoprotein H). J Clin Invest 90:1105–1109, 1992.

Giannini EH, Brewer EJ, Kuzmina N, Shaikov A, Wallin B. Auranofin in the treatment of juvenile rheumatoid arthritis. Results of the USA-USSR double-blind, placebo-controlled trial. Arthritis Rheum 33:466–476, 1990.

Giannini EH, Brewer EJ, Kuzmina N, Shaikov A, Maximov A, Vorontsov I, Fink CW, Newman AJ, Cassidy JT, Zemel LS. Methotrexate in resistant juvenile rheumatoid arthritis. Results of the USA-USSR double-blind, placebo-controlled trial. N Engl J Med 326:1043–1049, 1992.

Gidding SS, Shulman ST, Ilbawi M, Crussi F, Duffy CF. Mucocutaneous lymph node syndrome (Kawasaki disease): delayed aortic and mitral insufficiency secondary to active valvulitis. J Am Coll Cardiol 7:894–897, 1986.

Gillum RF. A racial difference in erythrocyte sedimentation. J Natl Med Assoc 85:47–50, 1993.

Ginsburg WW, Cohen MD. Peripheral arthritis in ankylosing spondylitis. A review of 209 patients followed up for more than 20 years. Mayo Clin Proc 58:593–596, 1983.

Ginzler EM, Nicastri AD, Chen CK, Friedman EA, Diamond HS, Kaplant D. Progression of mesangial and focal to diffuse lupus nephritis. Ann Intern Med 291:693–696, 1974.

Gioud M, Kaci MA, Monier JC. Histone antibodies in systemic lupus erythematosus. Arthritis Rheum 25:407–413, 1982.

Glass D, Raum D, Gibson D, Stillman JS, Schur PH. Inherited deficiency of the second component of complement. J Clin Invest 58:853–861, 1976.

Glass D, Litvin D, Wallace K, Chylack L, Garovoy M, Carpenter CB, Schur PH. Early onset pauciarticular juvenile rheumatoid arthritis associated with human leukocyte antigen DRw5, iritis, and antinuclear antibodies. J Clin Invest 66:426–429, 1980.

Glidden RS, Mantzouranis EC, Borel Y. Systemic lupus erythematosus in childhood: clinical manifestations and improved survival in fifty-five patients. Clin Immunol Immunopathol 29:196–210, 1983.

Gocke DJ, Hsu K, Morgan C, Bombardiere S, Lockshin M, Christian CL. Association between polyarteritis and Australia antigen. Lancet 2:1149–1153, 1970.

Goldenberg DL. "Post-infectious" arthritis—new look at an old concept with particular attention to disseminated gonococcal infection. Am J Med 74:925–928, 1983.

Goldschmeding R, Cohen TJW, van der Schoot CE, van der Veen C, Kallen CGM, con dem Borne AEG. ANCA, antimyeloperoxidase and antielastase: three members of a novel class of autoantibodies against myeloid lysosomal enzymes. Acta Pathol Microbiol Immunol Scand 97 (Suppl 6):48, 1989.

Goldstein I, Rebeyotte P, Parlebas J, Halpern B. Isolation from heart valves of glycopeptides which share immunological properties with streptococcus haemolyticus group A polysaccharides. Nature 219:866–868, 1968.

Gonzalez EN, Rothfield NF. Immunoglobulin class and pattern of nuclear fluorescence in systemic lupus erythematosus. N Engl J Med 274:1333–1338, 1966.

Gore JE, Vizcarrondo FE, Rieffel CN. Juvenile ankylosing spondylitis and aortic regurgitation: a case presentation. Pediatrics 68:423–426, 1981.

Graham L, Myones B, Rivas-Chacon R, Pachman L. Morbidity associated with long-term methotrexate therapy in juvenile rheumatoid arthritis. J Pediatr 120:468–473, 1992.

Granberry W. Synovectomy in juvenile rheumatoid arthritis. Arthritis Rheum 20:561–564, 1977a.

Granberry G. Soft tissue release in children with juvenile rheumatoid arthritis. Arthritis Rheum 20:565–566, 1977b.

Gray ED, Wannamaker LW, Ayoub EM, El Kholy A, Abdin ZH. Cellular immune responses to extracellular streptococcal products in rheumatic heart disease. J Clin Invest 68:665–671, 1981.

Grayzel AI, Marcus R, Stern R, Winchester RJ. Chronic polyarthritis associated with hypogammaglobulinemia. Arthritis Rheum 20:887–894, 1977.

Gribetz D, Henley WL. Systemic lupus erythematosus in childhood. J Mt Sinai Hosp NY 26:289–306, 1959.

Griffiths SP, Gersony WM. Acute rheumatic fever in New York City (1969 to 1988): a comparative study of two decades. J Pediatr 116:882–887, 1990.

Grisanti MW, Moore TL, Osborn TG, Haber PL. Eosinophilic fasciitis in children. Semin Arthritis Rheum 19:151–157, 1989.

Grossman BJ. Early ambulation in the treatment of acute rheumatic fever. Am J Dis Child 115:557–569, 1968.

Gulizia JM, Cunningham MW, McManus BM. Immunoreactivity of anti-streptococcal monoclonal antibodies to human heart valves. Am J Pathol 138:285–301, 1991.

Haber HL, Leavy JA, Kessler PD, Kukin ML, Gottleib SS, Packer M. The erythrocyte sedimentation rate in congestive heart failure. N Engl J Med 324:353–358, 1991.

Hafez M, El-Battoty MF, Hawas S, Al-Tonbary Y, Sheishaa A, El-Sallab SH, El-Morsi Z, El-Ziny M, Hawas SE. Evidence of inherited susceptibility of increased streptococcal adherence to pharyngeal cells of children with rheumatic fever. Br J Rheumatol 28:304–309, 1989.

Hafez M, Abdalla A, El-Shennawy F, Al-Tonbary Y, Sheishaa A, El-Moris Z, Tawfik SH, Settien A, El-Khair M. Immunogenetic study of the response to streptococcal carbohydrate antigen of the cell wall in rheumatic fever. Ann Rheum Dis 49:708–714, 1990.

Hagge WW, Burke EC, Stickler GB. Treatment of systemic lupus erythematosus complicated by nephritis in children. Pediatrics 40:822–827, 1967.

Hall RP, Lawley TJ, Heck JA. IgA-containing circulating immune complexes in dermatitis herpetiformis, Henoch-Schönlein purpura, systemic lupus erythematosus, and other diseases. Clin Exp Immunol 40:431–437, 1980.

Hall SL, Miller LC, Duggan E, Mauer SM, Beatty EC, Hellerstein S. Wegener's granulomatosis in pediatric patients. J Pediatr 106:739–744, 1985.

Halla JF, Hardin JG. Clinical features of the arthritis of mixed connective tissue disease. Arthritis Rheum 21:497–503, 1978.

Halma C, Daha M, Schrama E, Hermans J, van Es LA. Value of anti-neutrophil cytoplasmic autoantibodies and other laboratory parameters in follow-up of vasculitis. Scand J Rheumatol 19:392–397, 1990.

Halpern J, Volkman D, Wu P. Central nervous system abnormalities in Lyme neuroborreliosis. Neurology 41:1571–1582, 1991.

Hamilton ML, Gladman DD, Shore A, Laxer RM, Silverman ED. Juvenile psoriatic arthritis and HLA antigens. Ann Rheum Dis 49:694–697, 1990.

Hammer RE, Maika SD, Richardson JA, Tang JP, Taurog JD. Spontaneous inflammatory disease in transgenic rats expressing HLA-B27 and human beta 2m: an animal model of HLA-B27 associated with human disorders. Cell 63:1099–1112, 1990.

Hanson V, Kornreich H. Systemic rheumatic disorders ("collagen disease") in childhood. Bull Rheum Dis 17:435–446, 1967.

Hanson V, Drexler E, Kornreich H. The relationship of rheumatoid factor to age of onset in juvenile rheumatoid arthritis. Arthritis Rheum 12:82–86, 1969.

Hardarson S, LaBrecque DR, Mitros FA, Neil GA, Goeken JA. Antineutrophil cytoplasmic antibody in inflammatory bowel and hepatobiliary diseases. Clin Microbiol Immunol 99:277–281, 1993.

Hardin JA, Thomas JO. Antibodies to histones in systemic lupus erythematosus: Localization of prominent autoantigens on histones H1 and H2B. Proc Natl Acad Sci USA 80:7410–7416, 1983.

Hargraves MM. Discovery of the LE cell and its morphology. Mayo Clin Proc 44:579–599, 1969.

Hargraves MM, Richmond H, Morton R. Presentation of two bone marrow elements, the "tart" cell and the "LE" cell. Mayo Clin Proc 23:25–28, 1948.

Harley JB, Kaine JL, Fox OF, Reichlin M, Gruber B. Ro(SS-A) antibody and antigen in a patient with congenital complete heart block. Arthritis Rheum 28:1321–1325, 1985.

Harley JB, Scofield RH, Reichlin M. Anti-Ro in Sjögren's syndrome and systemic lupus erythematosus. Rheum Dis Clin North Am 18:337–358, 1992.

Harris EN, Gharavi AE, Boey ML. Anticardiolipin antibodies: detection by radioimmunoassay and association with thrombosis in systemic lupus erythematosus. Lancet 2:1211–1214, 1983.

Harris EN, Asherson RA, Gharavi AE. Thrombocytopenia in SLE and related autoimmune disorders: association with anticardiolipin antibody. Br J Haematol 59:227–230, 1985.

Harrison DJ, Simpson R, Kharbanda R, Abernethy VE, Nimmo G. Antibodies to neutrophil cytoplasmic antigens in Wegener's granulomatosis and other conditions. Thorax 44:373–377, 1989.

Haserick JR, Lewis LA, Bortz DW. Blood factor in acute disseminated lupus erythematosus: determination of gammaglobulin as specific plasma fraction. Am J Med Sci 219:660–663, 1950.

Haynes BF, Fauci AS. The spectrum of vasculitis. Ann Intern Med 89:660–676, 1978.

He X, Goronzy J, Weyand C. Selective induction of rheumatoid factors by superantigens and human helper T cells. J Clin Invest 89:673–680, 1992.

Heckmatt J, Saunders C, Peters AM, Rose M, Hasson N, Thompson N, Cambridge G, Hyde SA, Dubowitz V. Cyclosporin in juvenile dermatomyositis. Lancet 1063–1066, 1989.

Herd JK, Medhi M, Uzendoski DM, Saldivar VA. Chorea associated with systemic lupus erythematosus: report of 2 cases and review of literature. Pediatrics 61:308–315, 1978.

Herold BC, Shulman ST. Poststreptococcal arthritis. Pediatr Infect Dis J 7:681–682, 1988.

Hertzberger-Ten Cate R, Cats A. Toxicity of sulfasalazine in systemic juvenile chronic arthritis. Clin Exp Rheum 9:85–88, 1991.

Hertzberger-Ten Cate R, Dervlugt BCMD, Van Suijlekomsmit LWA, Cats A. Disease patterns in early onset pauciarticular juvenile chronic arthritis. Eur J Pediatr 151:339–341, 1992.

Herve-Somma C, Touzet P, Lallemand D, Prieur AM. Gd-DOTA enhanced MR imaging in juvenile chronic arthritis (JCA) before and after intraarticular therapy (abstract). J Rheumatol 19:A66, 1992.

Hess EV, Fink CS, Taranta A, Ziff M. Heart muscle antibodies in rheumatic fever and other diseases. J Clin Invest 43:886–893, 1964.

Hicks RM. Rheumatic fever in Hawaii. Arthritis Rheum 20:375–376, 1977.

Hochberg MC, Boyd RE, Ahearn JM, Arnett FC, Bias WB, Provost TT, Stevens MD. Systemic lupus erythematosus: a review of clinic-laboratory features and immunogenetic markers in 150 patients with emphasis on demographic subsets. Medicine 64:285–295, 1985.

Hoffman RW, Cassidy JT, Takeda Y, Smith-Jones EI, Wang GS, Sharp GC. U1-70-kd autoantibody-positive mixed connective tissue disease in children. Arthritis Rheum 36:1599–1602, 1993.

Hogg GR. Congenital lupus erythematosus associated with subendocardial fibroelastosis. Am J Clin Pathol 28:648–654, 1957.

Holman HR, Kunkel HG. Affinity between the lupus erythematosus serum factor and cell nuclei and nucleoprotein. Science 126:162–163, 1957.

Homcy CJ, Liberthson RR, Fallon JT, Gross S, Miller LM. Ischemic heart disease in systemic lupus erythematosus in the young patient: report of 6 cases. Am J Cardiol 49:478–484, 1982.

Horsfall, AC, Venables PJW, Taylor PV, Maini RN. Ro and La antigens and maternal anti-La idiotype on the surface of myocardial fibers in congenital heart block. J Autoimmun 4:165–176, 1991.

Hosenpud JD, Montanaro A, Hart MV, Haines JE, Specht HD, Bennett RM, Kloster FE. Myocardial perfusion abnormalities in asymptomatic patients with systemic lupus erythematosus. Am J Med 77:286–292, 1983.

Hosier DM, Craenen JM, Teske DW, Wheller JJ. Resurgence of acute rheumatic fever. Am J Dis Child 141:730–733, 1987.

Hubscher O, Susini JG. Aortic insufficiency in Reiter's syndrome of juvenile onset. J Rheumatol 11:94–95, 1984.

Hull D, Binns BOA, Joyce D. Congenital heart block and widespread fibrosis due to maternal lupus erythematosus. Arch Dis Child 41:688–690, 1966.

Huntley CC, Thorpe DP, Lyerly AD, Kelsey WM. Rheumatoid arthritis with IgA deficiency. Am J Dis Child 113:411–418, 1967.

Hurley RM, Drummond KN. Anaphylactoid purpura nephritis: clinicopathological correlations. J Pediatr 81:904–911, 1972.

Husby G, van de Rijn I, Zabriskie JB, Abdin ZH, Williams RCJ. Antibodies reacting with cytoplasm of subthalamic and caudate nuclei neurons in chorea and acute rheumatic fever. J Exp Med 144:1094–1110, 1976.

Imakita M, Sasaki Y, Misugi K, Miyazawa Y, Hyodo Y. Kawasaki disease complicated with mitral insufficiency. Autopsy findings with special reference to valvular lesion. Acta Pathol Jpn 34:605–616, 1984.

Inghirami G, Simon J, Balow JE, Tsokos GC. Activated T lymphocytes in the peripheral blood of patients with systemic lupus erythematosus induce B cells to produce immunoglobulin. Clin Exp Rheumatol 6:269–276, 1988.

Isdale IC, Bywaters EGL. The rash of rheumatic arthritis and Still's disease. Q J Med 25:377–387, 1956.

Ishiwata S, Nishiyama S, Nakanishi S, Seki A, Watanabe Y, Konishi T, Fuse K. Coronary artery disease and internal mammary artery aneurysms in a young woman: possible sequelae of Kawasaki disease. Am Heart J 120:213–217, 1990.

Jackson R. Discoid lupus in a newborn infant of a mother with lupus erythematosus. Pediatrics 33:425–430, 1964.

Jackson R, Gulliver M. Neonatal lupus erythematosus progressing into systemic lupus erythematosus. Br J Dermatol 101:81–83, 1979.

Jacobs JC. Systemic lupus erythematosus in childhood. Report of 35 cases with discussion of seven apparently induced by anticonvulsant medication and of prognosis and treatment. Pediatrics 32:257–264, 1963a.

Jacobs JC. Treatment of dermatomyositis. Arthritis Rheum 20:338–341, 1977.

Jacobs JC, Gorin LJ, Hanissian AS, Simon JL, Smithwick EM, Sullivan D. Consumption coagulopathy after gold therapy for juvenile rheumatoid arthritis (letter). J Pediatr 105:674–675, 1984.

Jacobs P. Ankylosing spondylitis in children and adolescents. Arch Dis Child 38:492–499, 1963b.

Jaffe BD, Claman HN. Chronic graft-versus-host disease (GVHD) as a model for scleroderma. Cell Immunol 77:1–12, 1983.

Jan JE, Hill RH, Low MD. Cerebral complications in juvenile rheumatoid arthritis. Can Med Assoc J 107:623–625, 1972.

Janeway CA, Gitlin D, Craig M, Grice DS. Collagen disease in patients with congenital agammaglobulinemia. Trans Assoc Am Physicians 69:93–97, 1956.

Jasin HE. Absence of the eighth component of complement (C8) and SLE-like disease. Arthritis Rheum 19:803–804, 1976.

Jeremy R, Schaller J, Arkless R, Wedgwood RJ, Healey LA. Juvenile rheumatoid arthritis persisting into adulthood. Am J Med 45:419–434, 1968.

Jimenez SA, Sigal SH. A 15-year prospective study of treatment of rapidly progressive systemic sclerosis with D-penicillamine. J Rheumatol 18:1496–1503, 1991.

Johnson PM, Faulk WP. Rheumatoid factor: its nature, specificity, and production of rheumatoid arthritis. Clin Immunol Immunopathol 6:414–430, 1976.

Johnson RL, Fink CW, Ziff M. Lymphotoxin formation by lymphocytes and muscle in polymyositis. J Clin Invest 51:2435–2449, 1972.

Joos R, Veys EM, Mielants H, van Werveke S, Goemaere S. Sulfasalazine treatment in juvenile chronic arthritis: an open study. J Rheumatol 18:880–884, 1991.

Kalovidouris AE, Pourmand R, Passo MH, Plotkin Z. Proliferative response of peripheral blood mononuclear cells to autologous and allogeneic muscle in patients with polymyositis/dermatomyositis. Arthritis Rheum 32:446–453, 1989.

Kalunian KC, Peter JB, Middlekauf HR. Clinical significance of a single test for anticardiolipin antibodies. Am J Med 85:602–608, 1988.

Kalunian KC, Panosian-Sahakian N, Ebling FM, Cohen AH, Louie JS, Kaine J, Hahn BH. Idiotypic characteristics of immunoglobulins associated with human systemic lupus erythematosus. Studies of antibodies deposited in glomeruli of humans. Arthritis Rheum 32:513–522, 1989.

Kanski JJ. Anterior uveitis in juvenile rheumatoid arthritis. Arch Ophthalmol 95:1794–1797, 1977.

Kaplan EL. Acute rheumatic fever. Pediatr Clin North Am 25:817–829, 1978.

Kaplan E, Johnson DR, Cleary PP. Group A streptococcal serotypes isolated from patients and sibling contacts during the resurgence of rheumatic fever in the United States in the mid-1980s. J Infect Dis 159:101–103, 1989.

Kaplan MH. Immunologic relation of streptococcal and tissue antigens. I. Properties of an antigen in certain strains of group A streptococci exhibiting an immunologic cross-reaction with human tissue. J Immunol 90:595–606, 1963.

Kaplan MH, Svee KH. Immunologic relation of streptococcal and tissue antigens. III. Presence in human sera of streptococcal antibody cross-reactive with heart tissue. Association with streptococcal infection, rheumatic fever, and glomerulonephritis. J Exp Med 119:651–666, 1964.

Kaplan MH, Meyeserian M, Kushner I. Immunologic studies of heart tissue. IV. Serologic reactions with human heart tissue as revealed by immunofluorescent methods. J Exp Med 113:17–36, 1961.

Kapusta MA, Metrakos JD, Pinsky L. Juvenile rheumatoid arthritis in a mother and her identical twin sons. Arthritis Rheum 12:411–414, 1969.

Karpatkin S, Strick N, Karpatkin M. Cumulative experience in the detection of antiplatelet antibody in 234 patients with idiopathic thrombocytopenic purpura, systemic lupus erythematosus and other clinical disorders. Am J Med 52:776–785, 1972.

Kasakawa S, Heiner DC. Elevated levels of immunoglobulin E in the acute febrile mucocutaneous lymph node syndrome. Pediatr Res 10:108–111, 1976.

Kaslow RA, Masi AT. Age, sex and race effects on mortality from systemic lupus erythematosus in the United States. Arthritis Rheum 21:473–479, 1978.

Kato H, Koike S, Yamamoto M, Ito Y, Yano E. Coronary aneurysms in infants and young children with acute febrile mucocutaneous lymph node syndrome. J Pediatr 86:892–898, 1975.

Kato H, Koike S, Yokoyama T. Kawasaki disease: effect of treatment on coronary artery involvement. Pediatrics 63:175–179, 1979.

Kauffman RH, Herrmann WA, Meyer CJ. Circulating IgA-immune complexes in Henoch-Schönlein purpura. Am J Med 69:859–866, 1980.

Kavey RW, Kaplan EL. Resurgence of acute rheumatic fever. Pediatrics 84:585–586, 1989.

Kawasaki T. Acute febrile mucocutaneous syndrome with lymphoid involvement with specific desquamation of the fingers and toes. Arerugi 16:178–222, 1967.

Kawasaki T, Kosaki F, Okawa S, Shigematsu I, Yanagawa H. A new infantile acute febrile mucocutaneous lymph node syndrome (MLNS) prevailing in Japan. Pediatrics 54:271–276, 1974.

Kean WF, Anastassiades TP, Ford PM. Aortic incompetence in HLA-B27-positive juvenile arthritis. Ann Rheum Dis 39:294–295, 1980.

Keat A. HLA-linked disease susceptibility and reactive arthritis. J Infect Dis 5:227–239, 1982.

Keat A. Reiter's syndrome and reactive arthritis in perspective. N Engl J Med 309:1606–1615, 1983.

Keim D, Ragsdale C, Heidelberger K, Sullivan D. Hepatic fibrosis with the use of methotrexate for juvenile rheumatoid arthritis. J Rheumatol 17:846–848, 1990.

Khan MA. An overview of clinical spectrum and heterogeneity of spondyloarthropathies. Rheum Dis Clin North Am 18:1–10, 1992.

Khan MA, van der Linden SM. Ankylosing spondylitis and other spondyloarthropathies. Rheum Dis Clin North Am 16:551–579, 1990.

Khan MA, Kellner H. Immunogenetics of spondyloarthropathies. Rheum Dis Clin North Am 18:837–864, 1992.

Khan MA, Kushner I, Braun WE. Low incidence of HLA-B27 in American blacks with spondyloarthropathies. Lancet 1:483–485, 1976.

Khanna AK, Buskirk DR, Williams RCJ, Gibofsky A, Crow MK, Menon A, Fotina M, Reid HM, Poon-King T, Rubinstein P, Zabriskie JB. Presence of a non-HLA B cell antigen in rheumatic fever patients and their families as defined by a monoclonal antibody. J Clin Invest 83:1710–1716, 1989.

Kilbourne EM, Rigau-Perez JG, Heath CWJ, Zack MM, Falk H, Martin-Marcos M, de Carlos A. Clinical epidemiology of toxic-oil syndrome: manifestations of a new illness. N Engl J Med 309:1408–1414, 1983.

Kimberly RP, Parris TM, Inman RD, McDougal JS. Dynamics of mononuclear phagocyte system Fc receptor function in systemic lupus erythematosus. Relation to disease activity and circulating immune complexes. Clin Exp Immunol 51:261–268, 1983.

Kissel JT, Mendell JR, Ramohan KW. Microvascular deposition of complement membrane attack complex in dermatomyositis. N Engl J Med 314:329–334, 1986.

Klaasen RJ, Goldschmeding R, Dolman KM, Vlekke AB, Weigel HM, Eeftinck Schattenkerk JK, Mulder JW, Westedt ML, von dem Borne AE. Anti-neutrophil cytoplasmic autoantibodies in patients with symptomatic HIV infection. Clin Exp Immunol 87:24–30, 1992.

Koerper MA, Stempel DA, Dallman PR. Anemia in patients with juvenile rheumatoid arthritis. J Pediatr 92:930–933, 1978.

Koff RS. Case records of the Massachusetts General Hospital. N Engl J Med 296:1337–1346, 1977.

Koffler D, Schur PH, Kunkel HG. Immunological studies concerning the nephritis of systemic lupus erythematosus. J Exp Med 126:607–623, 1967.

Koffler D, Agnello V, Carr RI, Kunkel HG. Variable patterns of immunoglobulin and complement deposition in the kidneys of patients with systemic lupus erythematosus. Am J Pathol 56:305–316, 1969.

Koffler D, Agnello V, Thoburn R, Kunkel HG. Systemic lupus erythematosus: prototype of immune complex nephritis in man. J Exp Med 134:169–179, 1971.

Kohler PF, Bensel R. Serial complement component alterations in acute glomerulonephritis and systemic lupus erythematosus. Clin Exp Immunol 4:191–202, 1969.

Kohr RM. Progressive asymptomatic coronary artery disease as a fatal sequela of Kawasaki disease. J Pediatr 108:256–259, 1986.

Kolble K, Reid KB. Genetic deficiencies of the complement system and association with disease—early components. Int Rev Immunol 10:17–36, 1993.

Komine M, Matsuyama T, Nojima Y, Minoda S, Furue M, Tsuchida T, Sakai S, Ishibashi Y. Systemic lupus erythematosus with hereditary deficiency of the fourth component of complement. Int J Dermatol 31:653–656, 1992.

Koopman WJ, Schrohenloher RE. A sensitive radioimmunoassay for quantitation of IgM rheumatoid factor. Arthritis Rheum 23:302–308, 1980.

Koren G, Rose V, Lavi S. Probable efficacy of high-dose salicylates in reducing coronary involvement in Kawasaki disease. JAMA 254:767–769, 1985.

Koren G, Lavi S, Rose V, Rowe R. Kawasaki disease: review of risk factors for coronary aneurysms. J Pediatr 108:388–392, 1986.

Kornreich HK, King KK, Bernstein BH, Singsen BH, Hanson V. Scleroderma in childhood. Arthritis Rheum 20:343–350, 1977.

Koster-King K, Kornreich HK, Bernstein BH, Singsen BH, Hanson V. The clinical spectrum of systemic lupus erythematosus in childhood. Arthritis Rheum 20:287–294, 1977.

Kozin F, Carrera GF, Ryan LM, Foley D, Lawson TL. Computed tomography in the diagnosis of sacroiliitis. Arthritis Rheum 24:1479–1485, 1981.

Krupp L, Masur D, Schwartz J, Coyle P, Langenbach L, Fernquist S, Jandorf L, Halperin J. Cognitive functioning in late Lyme borreliosis. Arch Neurol 48:1125–1129, 1991.

Kunkel HG, Tan EM. Autoantibodies and disease. Adv Immunol 4:351–395, 1964.

Kuno-Sakai H, Sakai H, Nomoto Y. Increase of IgA-bearing peripheral blood lymphocytes in children with Henoch-Schönlein purpura. Pediatrics 64:918–922, 1979.

Kushner I. The acute phase response: from Hippocrates to cytokine biology. Eur Cytokine Network 2:75–80, 1991.

Laaksonen A. A prognostic study of juvenile rheumatoid arthritis. Acta Paediatr Scand 166 (Suppl):1–16, 1966.

Lacks S, White P. Morbidity associated with childhood systemic lupus erythematosus. J Rheumatol 17:941–945, 1990.

Ladd JR, Cassidy JT, Martel W. Juvenile ankylosing spondylitis. Arthritis Rheum 14:579–590, 1971.

Laitman RS, Glicklich D, Sablay LB, Grayzel AI, Bartland P, Bank N. Effect of long-term normalization of serum complement levels on the course of lupus nephritis. Am J Med 87:132–138, 1989.

Lambert JR, Ansell BM, Stephenson E, Wright V. Psoriatic arthritis in childhood. Clin Rheum Dis 2:339–352, 1976.

Lanham JG, Walport MJ, Hughes GRV. Congenital heart block and familial connective tissue disease. J Rheumatol 10:823–825, 1983.

Lavalle C, Pizzaro S, Drenkard C. A manifestation of systemic lupus erythematosus strongly associated with antiphospholipid antibodies. J Rheumatol 17:34–37, 1990.

Lawrence JM, Moore TL, Osborn TG, Nesher G, Madson KL, Kinsella MB. Autoantibody studies in juvenile rheumatoid arthritis. Semin Arthritis Rheum 22:265–274, 1993.

Laxer RM, Roberts EA, Gross KR, Britton JR, Cutz E, Dimmick J, Petty RE, Silverman ED. Liver disease and neonatal lupus erythematosus. J Pediatr 116:238–242, 1990.

Leak A. Autoantibody profile in juvenile chronic arthritis. Ann Rheum Dis 47:178–182, 1988.

Leak AM, Woo P. Juvenile chronic arthritis, chronic iridocyclitis, and reactivity to histones. Ann Rheum Dis 50:653–657, 1991.

Leddy JP, Griggs RC, Klemperer MR, Frank MM. Hereditary complement (C2) deficiency with dermatomyositis. Am J Med 58:83–91, 1975.

Lee HS, Mujais SK, Kasinath BS, Spargo BH, Katz AI. Course of renal pathology in patients with systemic lupus erythematosus. Am J Med 77:612–620, 1984.

Lee LA, Weston WI. New findings in neonatal lupus syndrome. Am J Dis Child 138:233–236, 1984.

Leff RL, Love LA, Miller FW, Greenberg SJ, Klein EA, Dalakas MC, Plotz PH. Viruses in idiopathic inflammatory myopathies: absence of candidate viral genomes in muscle. Lancet 339:1192–1195, 1992.

Lehman TJA, Sherry DD, Wagner-Weiner L, McCurdy DK, Emery HM, Magilavy DB, Kovalesky A. Intermittent intravenous cyclophosphamide therapy for lupus nephritis. J Pediatr 114:1055–1066, 1988.

Lehman TJA, McCurdy DK, Bernstein BH, King KK, Hanson V. Systemic lupus erythematosus in the first decade of life. Pediatrics 83:235–239, 1989.

Leirisalo M, Skylv G, Kousa M, Voipio-Pulkki LM, Suoranta H, Nissila M, Hvidman L, Nielsen ED, Svejaard A, Tilikainen A, Laitinen O. Follow-up study on patients with Reiter's disease and reactive arthritis with special reference to HLA-B27. Arthritis Rheum 25:249–259, 1982.

Leitman PS, Bywaters EGL. Pericarditis in juvenile rheumatoid arthritis. Pediatrics 32:855–860, 1963.

Lerner MR, Steitz JA. Antibodies to small nuclear RNAs complexed with proteins are produced by patients with systemic lupus erythematosus. Proc Natl Acad Sci U S A 76:5495–5499, 1979.

Leung DY. Immunologic aspects of Kawasaki syndrome. J Rheumatol 17 (Suppl 24):15–18, 1990.

Leung DY, Siegel RL, Grady S, Krensky A, Meade R, Reinherz EL, Geha RS. Immunoregulatory abnormalities in mucocutaneous lymph node syndrome. Clin Immunol Immunopathol 23:100–112, 1982.

Leung DYM, Meissner HC, Fulton DR, Murray DL, Kotzin BL, Schlievert PM. Toxic shock syndrome toxin-secreting *Staphylococcus aureus* in Kawasaki syndrome. Lancet 342:1385–1388, 1993.

Levy M, Koren G. Atypical Kawasaki's disease: analysis of clinical presentation and diagnostic clues. Pediatr Infect Dis J 9:122–126, 1990.

Levy M, Broyer M, Arsan A. Anaphylactoid purpura nephritis in childhood: natural history and immunopathology. Adv Nephrol 6:183–228, 1976.

Lieberman E, Heuser E, Hanson V, Kornreich H, Donnell GN, Landing BH. Identical three-year-old twins with disseminated lupus erythematosus: one with nephrosis and one with nephritis. Arthritis Rheum 11:22–32, 1968.

Lindsley CB, Schaller JG. Arthritis associated with inflammatory bowel disease in children. J Pediatr 84:16–20, 1974.

Linker-Israeli M, Quismorio FPJ, Horwitz DA. CD8+ lymphocytes from patients with systemic lupus erythematosus sustain, rather than suppress, spontaneous polyclonal IgG production and synergize with CD4+ cells to support autoantibody synthesis. Arthritis Rheum 33:1216–1225, 1990.

Linnemann CCJ, Levinson JE, Buncher CR, Schiff GM. Rubella antibody levels in juvenile rheumatoid arthritis. Ann Rheum Dis 34:354–358, 1975.

Litsey SE, Noonan JA, O'Connor WN, Cottrill CM, Mitchell B. Maternal connective tissue disease and congenital heart block. Demonstration of immunoglobulin in cardiac tissue. N Engl J Med 312:98–100, 1985.

Livingston JZ, Scott TE, Wigley FM, Anhelt GJ, Bias WB, McLean RH, Hochberg MC. Systemic sclerosis (scleroderma): clinical, genetic, and serologic subsets. J Rheumatol 14:512–518, 1987.

Lockie GN, Hunder GG. Reiter's syndrome in children: a case report and review. Arthritis Rheum 14:767–772, 1971.

Lockshin MD, Bonfa E, Elkon K, Druzin ML. Neonatal lupus risk to newborns of mothers with systemic lupus erythematosus. Arthritis Rheum 31:697–701, 1988.

Logigian EL, Kaplan RF, Steere AC. Chronic neurologic manifestations of Lyme disease. N Engl J Med 323:1438–1444, 1990.

Love LA, Leff RL, Targoff IN, Dalakas M, Plotz PH, Miller FW. A new approach to the classification of idiopathic inflammatory myopathy: myositis-specific autoantibodies define useful homogeneous patient groups. Medicine 70:360–374, 1991.

Love PE, Santoro SA. Antiphospholipid antibodies: anticardiolipin and the lupus anticoagulant in systemic lupus erythematosus (SLE) and in non-SLE disorders. Ann Intern Med 112:682–698, 1990.

Lowenstein J, Rothfield NF, Gallo C, McCluskey RT. The clinical course of proliferative and membranous forms of lupus nephritis. Ann Intern Med 73:929–942, 1970.

Lueck CJ, Trend P, Swash M. Cyclosporin in the management of polymyositis and dermatomyositis. J Neurol 54:1007–1008, 1991.

Luger S, Krauss E. Serological tests for Lyme disease: interlaboratory variability. Arch Intern Med 150:761–763, 1990.

Mackworth-Young CG, Loizou S, Walport MJ. Primary antiphospholipid syndrome: features of patients with raised anticardiolipin antibodies and no other disorder. Ann Rheum Dis 48:362–367, 1989.

Madaio MP, Carlson J, Cataldo J, Ucci A, Migliorini P, Pankewycs O. Murine monoclonal anti-DNA antibodies bind directly to glomerular antigens and form immune deposits. J Immunol 138:2883–2893, 1987.

Maddison PF, Skinner RP, Vlachoyiannopoulos P. Antibodies to nRNP, Sm, Ro(SSA) and La(SSB) detected by ELISA: their specificity and inter-relations in connective tissue disease sera. Clin Exp Immunol 62:337–345, 1985.

Maggiore G, Martin A, Crifeo S. Hepatitis B virus infection and Schönlein-Henoch purpura. Am J Dis Child 138:681–682, 1984.

Magsaam J, Ferjencik P, Tempels M. A new method for the detection of hidden IgM rheumatoid factor in patients with juvenile rheumatoid arthritis. J Rheumatol 14:757–762, 1987.

Majeed HA, Khuffash FA, Bhatnagar S, Farwana S, Yusuf AR, Yousof AM. Acute rheumatic polyarthritis. Am J Dis Child, 144:831–833, 1990.

Malagon C, Vankerckhove C, Giannini EH, Taylor J, Lovell DJ, Levinson JE, Passo MH, Ginsberg J, Burke MJ, Glass DN. The iridocyclitis of early onset pauciarticular juvenile rheumatoid arthritis: outcome in immunogenetically characterized patients. J Rheumatol 19:160–163, 1992.

Malleson PN. Controversies in juvenile dermatomyositis. J Rheumatol 17 (Suppl 22):1–6, 1990.

Manjula BN, Trus BL, Fischetti VA. Presence of two distinct regions in the coiled-coil structure of the streptococcal Pep M5 protein: relationship to mammalian coiled-coil proteins and implications to its biological properties. Proc Natl Acad Sci USA 82:1064–1068, 1985.

Manners JP, Ansell BM. Slow acting antirheumatic drug use in systemic onset juvenile chronic arthritis. Pediatrics 77:99–103, 1986.

Mannik M. Rheumatoid factors in the pathogenesis of rheumatoid arthritis. J Rheumatol 19 (Suppl 32):46–49, 1992.

Mannik M, Nardella FA. IgG rheumatoid factors and self-association of these antibodies. Clin Rheum Dis 11:551–572, 1985.

Marcon MJ, Hribar MM, Hosier DM, Powell DA, Brady MT, Hamoudi AC, Kaplan EL. Occurrence of mucoid M-18 *Streptococcus pyogenes* in a central Ohio pediatric population. J Clin Microbiol 26:1539–1542, 1988.

Markowitz M. The changing picture of rheumatic fever. Arthritis Rheum 20:369–374, 1977.

Markowitz M. The decline of rheumatic fever: role of medical intervention. J Pediatr 106:545–550, 1985.

Markowitz M, Gordis L. Rheumatic Fever, 2nd ed. Philadelphia, WB Saunders, 1972.

Markowitz M, Kaplan E. Reappearance of rheumatic fever. Adv Pediatr 36:39–66, 1989.

Marks SH, Barnett M, Calin A. A case-control study of juvenile and adult onset ankylosing spondylitis. J Rheumatol 9:739–741, 1982.

Markusse HM, Dijkmans BA, Fibbe W. Eosinophilic fasciitis after allogeneic bone marrow transplantation. J Rheumatol 17:692–694, 1990.

Martinez-Frontanilla LA, Haase GM, Ernster JA. Surgical complications in Henoch-Schönlein purpura. J Pediatr Surg 19:434–436, 1984.

Martini A, Lorini R, Zanaboni D, Ravelli A, Burgio R. Frequency of autoantibodies in normal children. Am J Dis Child 143:493–496, 1989.

Masi AT, Kaslow RA. Sex effects in systemic lupus erythematosus. Arthritis Rheum 21:480–484, 1978.

Massell BF, Fyler DC, Roy SB. The clinical picture of rheumatic fever.

Diagnosis, immediate prognosis, course and therapeutic implications. Am J Cardiol 1:436–449, 1958.

Massell BF, Chute CG, Walker AM, Kurland GS. Penicillin and the marked decrease in morbidity and mortality from rheumatic fever in the United States. N Engl J Med 318:280–286, 1988.

McCue CM, Mantakas ME, Tingelstad JB, Ruddy S. Congenital heart block in newborns of mothers with connective tissue disease. Circulation 56:82–90, 1977.

McCuistion CH, Schoch EP. Possible discoid lupus erythematosus in newborn infant. Report of a case with subsequent development of acute systemic lupus erythematosus in mother. Arch Dermatol 70:782–785, 1954.

McCune AB, Weston WI, Lee LA. Maternal and fetal outcome in neonatal lupus erythematosus. Ann Intern Med 106:518–523, 1987.

McLaren MJ, Hawkins DM, Koornhof HJ, Bloom KR, Bramwell-Jones DM, Cohen E, Gale GE, Kannrek K, Lachman AS, Lakier JB, Pocock WA, Barlow JB. Epidemiology of rheumatic heart disease in black school children of Soweto, Johannesburg. Br Med J 3:474–478, 1975.

McLaughlin JF, Schaller J, Wedgwood RJ. Arthritis and immunodeficiency. J Pediatr 81:801–803, 1972.

Meade RH, Brandt L. Manifestations of Kawasaki disease in New England outbreak of 1980. J Pediatr 100:558–562, 1982.

Meadow SR, Scott DG. Berger disease: Henoch-Schönlein syndrome without the rash. J Pediatr 106:27–52, 1985.

Mease P, Ochs H, Wedgwood R. Successful treatment of echovirus meningoencephalitis and myositis-fasciitis with intravenous immune globulin therapy in a patient with X-linked agammaglobulinemia. N Engl J Med 304:1278–1281, 1981.

Meislin AG, Rothfield N. Systemic lupus erythematosus in childhood. Pediatrics 42:37–49, 1968.

Melina-Aldana H, Giannini EH, Taylor J, Lovell DJ, Levinson JE, Passo MH, Ginsberg J, Burke MJ, Glass DN. Human leukocyte antigen-DRB1*1104 in the chronic iridocyclitis of pauciarticular juvenile rheumatoid arthritis. J Pediatr 121:56–60, 1992.

Melish ME, Hicks RM, Larson EJ. Mucocutaneous lymph node syndrome in the United States. Am J Dis Child 130:599–607, 1976.

Mellins E, Malleson P, Schaller JG, Hansen J. Childhood dermatomyositis: immunogenetic and family studies. VIII Pan-American Congress of Rheumatology. Arthritis Rheum 25:S151, 1982.

Merriam JC, Chylack LT, Albert DM. Early-onset pauciarticular juvenile rheumatoid arthritis: a histopathologic study. Arch Ophthalmol 101:1085–1092, 1983.

Michael AF, Vernier RL, Drummond KN, Levitt JI, Herdman RC, Fish AJ, Good RA. Immunosuppressive therapy of chronic renal disease. N Engl J Med 276:817–828, 1967.

Michet CJJ, Doyle JA, Ginsburg WW. Eosinophilic fasciitis. Mayo Clin Proc 56:27–34, 1981.

Mihatsch MJ, Imbasciati E, Fogazzi G, Giani M, Ghio L, Gaboardi F. Ultrastructural lesions of Henoch-Schönlein syndrome and the IgA nephropathy: similarities and differences. Contrib Nephrol 40:255–263, 1984.

Miles S, Isenberg DA. A review of serological abnormalities in relatives of SLE patients. Lupus 2:145–150, 1993.

Milgrom F. Development of rheumatoid factor research through 50 years. Scand J Rheumatol (Suppl)75:2–12, 1988.

Miller FW, Leitman SF, Cronin ME, Hicks JE, Leff RL, Wesley R, Fraser DD, Dalakas M, Plotz PH. Controlled trial of plasma exchange and leukapheresis in polymyositis and dermatomyositis. N Engl J Med 326:1380–1384, 1992.

Miller LC, Dinarello CA. Biologic activities of interleukin-1 relevant to rheumatic diseases. Pathol Immunopathol 6:22–36, 1987.

Miller LC, Gray ED, Regelmann WE. Cytokines and immunoglobulin in rheumatic heart disease: production by blood and tonsillar mononuclear cells. J Rheumatol 16:1436–1442, 1989.

Miller LC, Sisson BA, Tucker LB, DeNardo BA, Schaller JG. Methotrexate treatment of recalcitrant childhood dermatomyositis. Arthritis Rheum 35:1143–1149, 1992.

Miller RW, Salcedo JR, Fink RJ, Murphy TM, Magilavy DB. Pulmonary hemorrhage in pediatric patients with systemic lupus erythematosus. J Pediatr 108:576–579, 1986.

Moll JMH, Wright V. New York clinical criteria for ankylosing spondylitis. Ann Rheum Dis 32:354–363, 1973.

Moncada B, Day NK, Good RA, Windhorst DB. Lupus-erythemato-sus-like syndrome with a familial defect of complement. N Engl J Med 286:689–693, 1972.

Monestier M, Kotzin BL. Antibodies to histones in systemic lupus erythematosus and drug-induced lupus syndromes. Rheum Dis Clin North Am 18:415–436, 1992.

Monestier M, Losman JA, Fasy TM, Debbas ME, Massa M, Albani S, Bohn L, Martini A. Antihistone antibodies in antinuclear antibody-positive juvenile arthritis. Arthritis Rheum 33:1836–1841, 1990.

Mongan ES, Leddy JP, Atwater EC, Barnett EV. Direct antiglobulin (Coombs) reactions in patients with connective tissue diseases. Arthritis Rheum 10:502–508, 1967.

Moore TL, Dorner RW. Rheumatoid factors. Clin Biochem 26:75–84, 1993.

Moore TL, Dorner RW, Weiss TD. Hidden 19S IgM rheumatoid factor in juvenile rheumatoid arthritis. J Rheumatol 9:599–602, 1980.

Moore TL, Dorner RW, Sheridan PW. Longitudinal study of the presence of hidden 19S IgM rheumatoid factor in juvenile rheumatoid arthritis. J Rheumatol 9:599–602, 1982.

Moore TL, Dorner RW, Osborn TG, Zuckner J. Hidden 19S IgM rheumatoid factors. Semin Arthritis Rheum 18:72–75, 1988.

Moorthy AV, Chesney RW, Segar WE, Groshong T. Wegener granulomatosis in childhood: prolonged survival following cytotoxic therapy. J Pediatr 91:616–618, 1977.

Morris R, Metzger AL, Bluestone R, Terasaki PI. HL-AW27—a clue to the diagnosis and pathogenesis of Reiter's syndrome. N Engl J Med 290:554–556, 1974a.

Morris R, Metzger AL, Bluestone R, Terasaki PI. HL-AW27—a useful discriminator in the arthropathies of inflammatory bowel disease. N Engl J Med 290:1117–1119, 1974b.

Moulds JM, Rolih C, Goldstein R, Whittington KF, Warner NB, Targoff IN, Reichlin M, Arnett FC. C4 null genes in American whites and blacks with myositis. J Rheumatol 17:331–334, 1990.

Mulberg AE, Linz C, Bern E, Tucker LB, Verhave M, Grand RJ. Identification of nonsteroidal antiinflammatory drug–induced gastroduodenal injury in children with juvenile rheumatoid arthritis. J Pediatr 122:647–649, 1993.

Munieus EF, Schur PH. Antibodies to Sm and RNP: prognosticators of disease involvement. Arthritis Rheum 26:848–853, 1983.

Munro-Faure H. Necrotizing arteries of the coronary vessels in infancy. Pediatrics 23:914–926, 1959.

Nakamoto Y, Asano Y, Dohi K, Fujioka M, Iida H, Kida H, Kibe Y, Hattori N, Takeuchi J. Primary IgA glomerulonephritis and Schönlein-Henoch purpura nephritis: clinicopathological and immunohistological characteristics. Q J Med 47:495–516, 1978.

Nakamura RM, Tan EM. Recent progress in the study of autoantibodies to nuclear antigens. Hum Pathol 9:85–91, 1978.

Nakamura RM, Tan EM. Update on autoantibodies to intracellular antigens in systemic rheumatic diseases. Clin Lab Med 12:1–23, 1992.

Nakano H, Nojima K, Saito A, Ueda K. High incidence of aortic regurgitation following Kawasaki disease. J Pediatr 107:59–63, 1985.

Nakano H, Saito A, Ueda K, Nojima K. Clinical characteristics of myocardial infarction following Kawasaki disease: report of 11 cases. J Pediatr 108:198–203, 1986.

Naoe S, Takahashi K, Masuda H, Tanaka N. Coronary findings post Kawasaki disease in children who died of other causes. In Shulman ST, ed. Kawasaki Disease. New York, Alan R Liss, 1987, pp. 341–346.

Naparstek K, Andre-Schwartz J, Manser T, Wysocki L, Breitman L, Stollar BD, Schwartz RS. A single V_H germline gene segment of normal A/J mice encodes autoantibodies characteristic of systemic lupus erythematosus. J Exp Med 164:614–626, 1986.

Nepom BS, Glass D. Juvenile rheumatoid arthritis and HLA—report of the Park City III Workshop. J Rheumatol 19:70–74, 1992.

Nepom BS, Schaller JG. Childhood systemic lupus erythematosus. In Cohen AS, ed. Progress in Clinical Rheumatology. Orlando, Fla., Grune & Stratton, 1984, pp. 33–69.

Nepom BS, Nepom GT, Michelson E, Schaller JG, Antonelli P, Hansen JA. Specific HLA-Dr4 associated histocompatibility molecules characterize patients with juvenile rheumatoid arthritis. J Clin Invest 74:287–291, 1982.

Newburger JW, Takahashi M, Burns JC, Beiser AS, Chung KJ, Duffy CE, Glode MP, Mason WH, Reddy V, Sanders SP, Shulman ST, Wiggins JW, Hicks RV, Fulton DR, Lewis AB, Leung DYM, Colton

T, Rosen FS, Melish ME. The treatment of Kawasaki syndrome with intravenous gamma globulin. N Engl J Med 315:342–347, 1986.

Newburger J, Takahashi M, Beiser A, Burns J, Bastian J, Chung K, Colan S, Duffy E, Fulton D, Glode M, Mason W, Meissner C, Rowley A, Shulman S, Reddy V, Sundel R, Wiggens J, Colton T, Melish M, Rosen F. A single intravenous infusion of gamma globulin as compared with four infusions in the treatment of acute Kawasaki's syndrome. N Engl J Med 324:1633–1639, 1991.

Newkirk MM, Mageed RA, Jefferis R, Chen PP, Capra JD. Complete amino acid sequences of variable regions of two human IgM rheumatoid factors, BOR and KAS of the Wa idiotypic family, reveal restricted use of heavy and light chain variable and joining region gene segments. J Exp Med 166:550–564, 1987.

Nimelstein SH, Brody S, McShane D, Holman HR. Mixed connective tissue disease: a subsequent evaluation of the original 25 patients. Medicine 59:239–248, 1980.

Nocton JJ, Miller LC, Tucker LB, Schaller JG. Human parvovirus B19–associated arthritis in children. J Pediatr 122:186–190, 1993.

Nolle B, Specks U, Ludemann J, Rohrbach MS, DeRemee RA, Gross WL. Anticytoplasmic autoantibodies: their immunodiagnostic value in Wegener's granulomatosis. Ann Intern Med 111:28–40, 1989.

Norris DG, Colon AR, Stickler GB. Systemic lupus erythematosus in children. Clin Pediatr 16:774–778, 1977.

Notman DD, Kurata N, Tan EM. Profiles of antinuclear antibodies in systemic rheumatic disease. Ann Intern Med 83:464–469, 1975.

Novack SN, Pearson CM. Cyclophosphamide therapy in Wegener's granulomatosis. N Engl J Med 284:938–942, 1971.

Nusinow SR, Zuraw BL, Curd JG. The hereditary and acquired deficiencies of complement. Med Clin North Am 69:487–504, 1985.

Nussbaum AI, Silver RM, Maricq HR. Serial changes in nailfold capillary morphology in childhood dermatomyositis. Arthritis Rheum 26:1169–1172, 1983.

Oates JK, Young AC. Sacro-iliitis in Reiter's disease. Br Med J 1:1013–1015, 1959.

Oetgen WJ, Boice JA, Lawless OJ. Mixed connective tissue disease in children and adolescents. Pediatrics 67:333–337, 1981.

Oldenburg HS, Rogy MA, Lazarus DD, Van Zee KJ, Keeler BP, Chizzonite RA, Lowry SF, Moldawer LL. Cachexia and the acute-phase protein response in inflammation are regulated by interleukin-6. Eur J Immunol 23:1889–1894, 1993.

Olee T, Lu EW, Huang D-F, Soto-Gil RW, Deftos M, Kozin F, Carson DA, Chen PP. Genetic analysis of self-associating IgC rheumatoid factors from two rheumatoid synovia implicates an antigen driven response. J Exp Med 175:831–842, 1992.

Olson NY, Lindsley CB. Adjunctive use of hydroxychloroquine in childhood dermatomyositis. J Rheumatol 16:1545–1547, 1989.

Ono S, Onimaru T, Kawakami K, Hokonohara M, Miyata K. Impaired granulocyte chemotaxis and increased circulatory immune complexes in Kawasaki disease. J Pediatr 106:567–570, 1985.

Oppermann M, Hopken U, Gotze O. Assessment of complement activation in vivo. Immunopharmacology 24:119–134, 1992.

Orlowski JP, Clough JD, Dymet PG. Wegener's granulomatosis in the pediatric age group. Pediatrics 61:83–90, 1978.

Osborn TG, Patel NJ, Moore TL, Zuckner J. Use of the Hep-2 cell substrate in the detection of antinuclear antibodies in juvenile rheumatoid arthritis. Arthritis Rheum 27:1286–1289, 1984.

Osler W. On the visceral complications of erythema exudativum multiforme. Am J Med Sci 110:629–646, 1895.

Osler W. The visceral lesions of the erythema group. Br J Dermatol 12:227–245, 1900.

Ostenson M, Fredriksen K, Kass E, Rekvig O. Identification of anti-histone antibodies in subsets of juvenile chronic arthritis. Ann Rheum Dis 48:114–117, 1989.

Osterland CK, Espinoza L, Parker LP, Schur PH. Inherited C2 deficiency and systemic lupus erythematosus: studies on a family. Ann Intern Med 822:323–328, 1975.

Ozanne P, Linderkamp O, Miller FC, Meiselman HJ. Erythrocyte aggregation during normal pregnancy. Am J Obstet Gynecol 147:576–583, 1983.

Ozen S, Besbas N, Saatci U, Bakkaloglu A. Diagnostic criteria for polyarteritis nodosa in childhood. J Pediatr 120:206–209, 1992.

Pachman LM, Cooke N. Juvenile dermatomyositis: a clinical and immunologic study. J Pediatr 96:226–234, 1980.

Pachman LM, Friedman JM, Maryjowski-Sweeney ML, Jonnason O, Radvany RM, Sharp GC, Cobb MA, Battles ND, Crowe WE, Fink CW, Hanson V, Levinson J, Spencer C, Sullivan D. Immunogenetic studies of juvenile dermatomyositis. III. Study of antibody to organ-specific and nuclear antigens. Arthritis Rheum 28:151–157, 1985.

Panush RS, Bianco NE, Schur PH. Serum and synovial fluid IgG, IgA and IgM antigammaglobulins in rheumatoid arthritis. Arthritis Rheum 14:737–747, 1971.

Pascual V, Victor K, Randen I, Thompson K, Natvig JB, Capra JD. IgM rheumatoid factors in patients with rheumatoid arthritis derive from a diverse array of germline immunoglobulin genes and display little evidence of somatic variation. J Rheumatol 19 (Suppl 32):50–53, 1992.

Patarroyo ME, Winchester RJ, Vejerano A, Gibofsky A, Chalem F, Zabriskie JB, Kunkel HG. Association of a B-cell alloantigen with susceptibility to rheumatic fever. Nature 278:173–174, 1979.

Penchas S, Stern Z, Bar-Or D. Heparin and the ESR. Arch Intern Med 138:1864–1865, 1978.

Peters-Golden M, Wise RA, Hochberg MC, Stevens MB, Wigley FM. Carbon monoxide diffusing capacity as predictor of outcome in systemic sclerosis. Am J Med 77:1027–1034, 1984.

Petty RE. HLA-B27 and rheumatic diseases of childhood. J Rheumatol 17 (Suppl 26):7–10, 1990.

Petty RE, Cassidy JT, Tubergen DG. Association of arthritis with hypogammaglobulinemia. Arthritis Rheum 20:441–443, 1977.

Pincus T, Schur PH, Rose JA, Decker JL, Talal N. Measurement of serum DNA binding activity in systemic lupus erythematosus. N Engl J Med 281:701–705, 1969.

Pincus T, Hughes GRV, Pincus D, Tina LU, Bellanti JA. Antibodies to DNA in childhood systemic lupus erythematosus. J Pediatr 78:981–984, 1971.

Pistoia V, Buoncompagni A, Scribanis R, Fasce L, Alpigiani G, Cordone G, Ferrarini M, Barrone C, Cottafava F. Cyclosporin A in the treatment of juvenile chronic arthritis and childhood polymyositis-dermatomyositis. Results of a preliminary study. Clin Exp Rheumatol 11:203–208, 1993.

Platt JL, Burke BA, Fish AJ, Kim Y, Michael AF. Systemic lupus erythematosus in the first two decades of life. Am J Kidney Dis 2 (Suppl 1):212–222, 1982.

Plotkin SA, Peter G, Committee on Infectious Diseases. Treatment for Lyme borreliosis. Pediatrics 88:177–179, 1991.

Pollak VE, Pirani CL, Schwartz FD. The natural history of the renal manifestations of systemic lupus erythematosus. J Lab Clin Med 63:537–550, 1964.

Powell FC, Winkelmann RK, Venencie-LeMarchand F, Spurbeck JL, Schroeter AL. The anticentromere antibody: disease specificity and clinical significance. Mayo Clin Proc 59:700–706, 1984.

Poznanski AK. Radiologic approaches to pediatric joint disease. J Rheumatol 19:78–93, 1992.

Poznanski AK, Glass RBJ, Feinstein KA, Pachman LM, Fisher MR, Hayford JR. Magnetic resonance imaging in juvenile rheumatoid arthritis. Int Pediatr 3:304–311, 1988.

Prakash UBS, Luthra HS, Divertie MB. Intrathoracic manifestations in mixed connective tissue disease. Mayo Clin Proc 60:813–821, 1985.

Provenzale J, Bouldin TW. Lupus-related myelopathy: report of three cases and review of the literature. J Neurol Neurosurg Psychiatry 55:830–835, 1992.

Provost TT, Ahmed AR, Maddison PJ, Reichlin M. Antibodies to cytoplasmic antigens in lupus erythematosus. Serologic marker for systemic disease. Arthritis Rheum 20:1457–1463, 1977.

Provost TT, Watson R, Gammon WR, Radowsky M, Harley JB, Reichlin M. The neonatal lupus syndrome associated with U₁RNP (nRNP) antibodies. N Engl J Med 315:1135–1139, 1987.

Quinn RW. Comprehensive review of morbidity and mortality trends for rheumatic fever, streptococcal disease, and scarlet fever: the decline of rheumatic fever. Rev Infect Dis 11:928–953, 1989.

Ragan C. The history of the rheumatoid factor. Arthritis Rheum 4:571–573, 1961.

Rahn DW, Malawista SE. Lyme disease: recommendations for diagnosis and treatment. Ann Intern Med 114:472–481, 1991.

Rajapakse C, Al Balla S, Al-Dallan A, Kamal H. Streptococcal antibody cross-reactivity with HLA-DR4⁺ B-lymphocytes. Basis of the DR4 associated genetic predisposition to rheumatic fever and rheumatic heart disease? Br J Rheumatol 29:468–470, 1990.

Rallison ML, Carlisle JW, Lee REJ, Vernier RL, Good RA. Lupus erythematosus and Stevens-Johnson syndrome. Occurrence as reactions to anticonvulsant therapy. Am J Dis Child 101:725–738, 1961.

Rammelkamp CH, Wannamaker LW, Kenny FW. The epidemiology and prevention of rheumatic fever. Bull N Y Acad Med 28:321–334, 1952.

Ravelli A, Caporali R, Bianchi E, Violi S, Solmi M, Montecucco C, Martini A. Anticardiolipin syndrome in childhood: a report of two cases. Clin Exp Rheum 8:95–98, 1990.

Reed BR, Lee LA, Harmon C, Wolfe R, Wiggins J, Peebles C, Weston WL. Autoantibodies to SS-A/Ro in infants with congenital heart block. J Pediatr 103:889–891, 1983.

Regelmann WE, Gray ED, Wannamaker LW, Lebien TW, Mansour M, El Kholy A, Abdin Z. Lymphocyte subpopulations. J Rheumatol 14:23–27, 1987.

Reinhart W. Red blood aggregation and sedimentation: the role of the cell shape. Br J Haematol 73:551–556, 1989.

Rhodes V. Physical therapy management of patients with juvenile rheumatoid arthritis. Phys Ther 71:910–919, 1991.

Rich SS, Gray ED, Talbot R, Martin D, Cairns L, Zabriskie JB, Braun D, Regelmann WE. Cell surface markers and cellular immune response associated with rheumatic heart disease: complex segregation analysis. Genetic Epidemiol 5:463–470, 1988.

Richardson JB, Callen JP. Dermatomyositis and malignancy. Med Clin North Am 73:1211–1220, 1989.

Rider LG, Buyon JP, Rutledge J, Sherry DD. Treatment of neonatal lupus: case report and review of the literature. J Rheumatol 20:1208–1211, 1993.

Robbins DL, Skilling J, Benisek WF, Wistar R. Estimation of the relative avidity of 19S IgM rheumatoid factor secreted by rheumatoid synovial cells for human IgG subclasses. Arthritis Rheum 29:722–729, 1986.

Rodnan GP, DiBartolomeo AG, Medsger TA. Eosinophilic fasciitis. Report of 7 cases of a newly recognized scleroderma-like syndrome. Arthritis Rheum 18:422–423, 1975.

Rose CD, Singsen BH, Eichenfield AH, Goldsmith DP, Athreya BH. Safety and efficacy of methotrexate therapy for juvenile rheumatoid arthritis. J Pediatr 117:653–659, 1990.

Rose CD, Fawcett PT, Singsen BH, Dubbs SB, Doughty RA. Use of Western blot and enzyme-linked immunosorbent assays to assist in the diagnosis of Lyme disease. Pediatrics 88:465–470, 1991.

Rose HM, Ragan C, Pearce E, Lipman MO. Differential agglutination of normal and sensitized sheep erythrocytes by sera of patients with rheumatoid arthritis. Proc Soc Exp Biol Med 68:1–6, 1948.

Rose V. Kawasaki syndrome—cardiovascular manifestations. J Rheumatol 17 (Suppl 24):11–14, 1990.

Rosen FS. Primary immunodeficiency. Pediatr Clin North Am 21:533–549, 1974.

Rosenberg AM. The clinical associations of antinuclear antibodies in juvenile rheumatoid arthritis. Clin Immunol Immunopathol 49:19–27, 1988.

Rosenberg AM, Petty RE. Reiter's disease in children. Am J Dis Child 133:394–398, 1979.

Rosenberg AM, Petty RE. A syndrome of seronegative enthesopathy and arthropathy in children. Arthritis Rheum 25:1041–1047, 1982.

Rosenberg AM, Petty RE, Cumming GR, Koehler BE. Pulmonary hypertension in a child with MCTD. J Rheumatol 6:700–704, 1979.

Rosenberg NL, Rotbart HA, Abzug MJ, Ringel SP, Levin MJ. Evidence for a novel picornavirus in human dermatomyositis. Ann Neurol 26:204–209, 1989.

Rosenfeld SI, Kelly ME, Leddy JP. Hereditary deficiency of the fifth component of complement in man. J Clin Invest 57:1626–1634, 1976.

Rosenthal J, Benson MD. Diffuse fasciitis and eosinophilia with symmetric polyarthritis. Ann Intern Med 92:507–509, 1980.

Rother E, Lang B, Coldeway R, Hartung K, Peter HH. Complement split product C3d as an indicator of disease activity in systemic lupus erythematosus. Clin Rheumatol 12:31–35, 1993.

Rothfield NF, Stollar BD. The relation of immunoglobulin class, pattern of anti-nuclear antibody, and complement-fixing antibodies to DNA in sera from patients with systemic lupus erythematosus. J Clin Invest 46:1785–1794, 1967.

Roubey RAS, Pratt CW, Buyon JP, Winfield JB. Lupus anticoagulant activity of autoimmune antiphospholipid antibodies is dependent upon B2-glycoprotein I. J Clin Invest 90:1100–1104, 1992.

Roubinian JR, Talal N, Greenspan JS, Goodman JR, Siiteri PK. Delayed androgen treatment prolongs survival in murine lupus. J Clin Invest 63:902–911, 1979.

Roubinian JR, Talal N, Greenspan JR, Siiteri PK. Effect of castration and sex hormone treatment on survival, anti-nucleic acid antibodies and glomerulonephritis in NZB/NZW F1 mice. J Exp Med 147:1568–1583, 1983.

Rowley AH. Current therapy for acute Kawasaki syndrome. J Pediatr 118:987–991, 1991.

Rowley AH, Duffy CE, Shulman ST. Prevention of giant coronary artery aneurysms in Kawasaki disease by intravenous gammaglobulin therapy. J Pediatr 113:290–294, 1988a.

Rowley AH, Gonzalez-Crussi F, Shulman ST. Kawasaki syndrome. Rev Infect Dis 10:1–15, 1988b.

Rubin RL, McNally EM, Nusinow SR, Robinson CA, Tan EM. IgG antibodies to the histone complex H2A-H2B characterize procainamide-induced lupus. Clin Immunol Immunopathol 36:46–59, 1985.

Ruddlesdin C, Ansell BM, Arden GP, Swann M. Total hip replacement in children with juvenile chronic arthritis. J Bone Joint Surg 68B:218–222, 1986.

Russell AS. Reiter's syndrome in children following infection with *Yersinia enterocolitica* and *Shigella*. Arthritis Rheum 20:471–474, 1977.

Russell AS, Davis P, Percy JS, Lentle B. The sacroiliitis of acute Reiter's syndrome. J Rheumatol 4:293–296, 1977.

Rustagi A, Currie M, Logue G. Complement-activating antineutrophil antibody in systemic lupus erythematosus. Am J Med 78:971–977, 1985.

Ruvalcaba RH, Thuline HC. IgA absence associated with short arm deletion of chromosome No. 18. J Pediatr 74:964–965, 1969.

Saitta MR, Keene JD. Molecular biology of nuclear autoantigens. Rheum Dis Clin North Am 18:283–310, 1992.

Salazar JC, Gerber MA, Goff CW. Long-term outcome of Lyme disease in children given early treatment. J Pediatr 122:591–593, 1993.

Sammaritano LR, Gharavi AE, Lockshin MD. Antiphospholipid antibody syndrome: immunologic and clinical aspects. Semin Arthritis Rheum 20:81–96, 1990.

Sanchez-Guerro J, Schur PH, Sergent JS, Liang MH. Silicone breast implants and rheumatic disease. Arthritis Rheum 37:158–168, 1994.

Sanders DY, Huntley CC, Sharp GC. Mixed connective tissue disease in a child. J Pediatr 83:642–645, 1973.

Sargent SJ, Beachey EH, Corbett CE, Dale JB. Sequence of protective epitopes of streptococcal M proteins shared with cardiac sarcolemmal membranes. J Immunol 139:1285–1290, 1987.

Sasso EH, Barber CV, Nardella FA, Yount WJ, Mannik M. Antigenic specificities of human monoclonal and polyclonal IgM rheumatoid factors: the C2-C3 interface region contains the major determinants. J Immunol 140:3098–3107, 1988.

Saulsbury FT. Heavy and light chain composition of serum IgA and IgA rheumatoid factor in Henoch-Schönlein purpura. Arthritis Rheum 35:1377–1380, 1992.

Savage COS, Tizard J, Lockwood JD, Dillon MJ. Antineutrophil cytoplasm antibodies in Kawasaki disease. Arch Dis Child 64:360–363, 1989.

Scarpa R, Oriente P, Pucino A, Torella M, Vigone L, Riccio A, Biondi-Oriente C. Psoriatic arthritis in psoriatic patients. Br J Rheum 23:246–250, 1984.

Schaller JG. Dermatomyositis. J Pediatr 83:699–702, 1971.

Schaller JG. Illness resembling lupus erythematosus in mothers of boys with chronic granulomatous disease. Ann Intern Med 76:747–750, 1972.

Schaller JG. Ankylosing spondylitis of childhood onset. Arthritis Rheum 20:398–401, 1977a.

Schaller JG. Arthritis and immunodeficiency. Arthritis Rheum 20:443–445, 1977b.

Schaller JG. Iridocyclitis. Arthritis Rheum 20:227–228, 1977c.

Schaller JG. Juvenile rheumatoid arthritis: series I. Arthritis Rheum 20:165–170, 1977d.

Schaller JG. Lupus phenomena in the newborn. Arthritis Rheum 20:312–314, 1977e.

Schaller JG. The diversity of JRA: a 1976 look at the subgroups of chronic childhood arthritis. Arthritis Rheum 20 (Suppl):S52–S61, 1977f.

Schaller JG. Corticosteroids in juvenile rheumatoid arthritis. Arthritis Rheum 20:537–543, 1977g.

Schaller JG. Chronic salicylate administration in juvenile rheumatoid arthritis. Aspirin "hepatitis" and its clinical significance. Pediatrics 62:916–925, 1978.

Schaller JG. Juvenile rheumatoid arthritis. Pediatr Rev 2:163–174, 1980.

Schaller JG. Therapy for childhood rheumatic diseases. Have we been doing enough? Arthritis Rheum 36:65–70, 1993.

Schaller JG, Hansen J. Rheumatoid factor-positive juvenile rheumatoid arthritis: the childhood equivalent of classic adult rheumatoid arthritis. Arthritis Rheum 25:S18, 1982a.

Schaller JG, Hansen J. Early childhood pauciarticular juvenile rheumatoid arthritis: clinical and immunogenetic studies. Arthritis Rheum 25:S63, 1982b.

Schaller JG, Omenn GS. The histocompatibility system and human disease. J Pediatr 88:913–926, 1976.

Schaller JG, Wedgwood RJ. Pruritus associated with the rash of juvenile rheumatoid arthritis. Pediatrics 45:296–298, 1970.

Schaller JG, Wedgwood RJ. Pauciarticular childhood arthritis: identification of two distinct subgroups. Arthritis Rheum 19:820–821, 1976.

Schaller JG, Bitnum S, Wedgwood RJ. Ankylosing spondylitis with childhood onset. J Pediatr 74:505–515, 1969.

Schaller JG, Beckwith B, Wedgwood RJ. Hepatic involvement in juvenile rheumatoid arthritis. J Pediatr 77:203–210, 1970.

Schaller JG, Johnson GD, Holborow EJ, Ansell BM, Smiley WK. The association of antinuclear antibodies with the chronic iridocyclitis of juvenile arthritis (Still's disease). Arthritis Rheum 17:409–416, 1974.

Schaller JG, Gilliland GC, Ochs HD, Leddy JP, Agodoa LCY, Rosenfeld SI. Severe systemic lupus erythematosus with nephritis in a boy with deficiency of the fourth component of complement. Arthritis Rheum 20:1519–1525, 1977.

Schaller JG, Wallace C, Stamm S, Morgan BC, Patterson M. The occurrence of congenital heart block in infants of mothers with clinical or serological evidence of rheumatic disease. Arthritis Rheum 22:656, 1979.

Schlosstein L, Terasaki PI, Bluestone R, Pearson CM. High association of an HL-A antigen, W27, with ankylosing spondylitis. N Engl J Med 288:704–706, 1973.

Schnitzer TJ, Ansell BM. Amyloidosis in juvenile chronic polyarthritis. Arthritis Rheum 20:245–252, 1977.

Schultz DR, Arnold PI. Properties of four acute phase proteins: C-reactive protein, serum amyloid A protein, alpha 1-acid glycoprotein, and fibrinogen. Semin Arthritis Rheum 20:129–147, 1990.

Schur PH, Austen KF. Complement in the rheumatic diseases. Bull Rheum Dis 22:666–673, 1972.

Schur PH, Sandson J. Immunologic factors and clinical activity in systemic lupus erythematosus. N Engl J Med 278:533–538, 1968.

Schur PH, Meyer I, Garovoy M, Carpenter CB. Associations between systemic lupus erythematosus and the MHC: clinical and immunological considerations. Clin Immunol Immunopathol 24:263–275, 1982.

Schwartz RS, Stollar BD. Origins of anti-DNA antibodies. J Clin Invest 75:321–327, 1985.

Schwimmbeck PL, Yu DT, Oldstone MB. Autoantibodies to HLA B27 in the sera of HLA B27 patients with ankylosing spondylitis and Reiter's syndrome. Molecular mimicry with *Klebsiella pneumoniae* as potential mechanism of autoimmune disease. J Exp Med 166:173–181, 1987.

Scott J, Gerber P, Maryjowski MC, Pachman L. Evidence for intravascular coagulation in systemic onset but not polyarticular juvenile rheumatoid arthritis. Arthritis Rheum 28:256–261, 1985.

Scott JS, Maddison PJ, Taylor PV, Esscher E, Scott O, Skinner RP. Connective-tissue disease, antibodies to ribonucleoprotein, and congenital heart block. N Engl J Med 309:209–212, 1983.

Scott RD. Total hip and knee arthroplasty in juvenile rheumatoid arthritis. J Clin Orthop Rel Res 259:83–91, 1990.

Seaman WE, Ishak AD. Aspirin-induced hepatotoxicity in patients with systemic lupus erythematosus. Ann Intern Med 80:1, 1974.

Segurado OG, Arnaiz-Villena AA, Iglesias-Casarrubios P, Martinez-Laso J, Vicario JL, Fontan G, Lopez-Trascasa M. Combined total deficiency of C7 and C4B with systemic lupus erythematosus (SLE). Clin Exp Immunol 87:410–414, 1992.

Seip M. SLE in pregnancy with haemolytic anemia, leucopenia and thrombocytopenia in the mother and her newborn infant. Arch Dis Child 35:364–366, 1960.

Seligmann M, Cannat A, Hamard M. Studies on antinuclear antibodies. Ann N Y Acad Sci 124:816–832, 1965.

Sharp GC, Irvin WS, Tan EM, Gould RG, Holman HR. Mixed connective tissue disease: an apparently distinct rheumatic disease syndrome associated with a specific antibody to an extractable nuclear antigen (ENA). Am J Med 52:148–159, 1972.

Sharp GC, Irvin WS, May CM, Holman HR, McDuffie FC, Hess EV, Schmid FR. Association of antibodies to ribonucleoprotein and Sm antigens with mixed connective tissue disease, systemic lupus erythematosus and other rheumatic diseases. N Engl J Med 295:1149–1154, 1976.

Sherry MG. The incidence of positive RA tests in Hodgkin's disease and leukemia. Am J Clin Pathol 50:398–400, 1968.

Shivakumar S, Tsokos GC, Datta SK. T cell receptor alpha/beta expressing double negative (CD4$^-$/CD8$^-$) and CD4$^+$ T helper cells in humans augment the production of pathogenic anti-DNA autoantibodies associated with lupus nephritis. J Immunol 143:103–112, 1989.

Shoenfeld Y, Rauch J, Masicotte I, Datta SK, Andre-Schwartz J, Stollar BD, Schwartz RS. Polyspecificity of monoclonal lupus autoantibodies produced by human-human hybridomas. N Engl J Med 303:414–420, 1983.

Shore A, Ansell BM. Juvenile psoriatic arthritis—an analysis of 60 cases. J Pediatr 100:529–535, 1982.

Shulman LE. Diffuse fasciitis with hypergammaglobulinemia and eosinophilia: A new syndrome? Arthritis Rheum 20 (Suppl 6):205–215, 1977.

Shulman LE, Hoffman R, Dainiak N, Nesbitt J, Adelman HM, Lawless OJ, Lindsey SM. Antibody-mediated aplastic anemia and thrombocytopenic purpura in diffuse eosinophilic fasciitis. Arthritis Rheum 22:659–661, 1979.

Sibbitt WLJ, Sibbitt RR, Griffey RH, Eckel C, Bankhurst AD. Magnetic resonance and computed tomographic imaging in the evolution of acute neuropsychiatric disease in systemic lupus erythematosus. Ann Rheum Dis 48:1014–1022, 1989.

Siegel M, Lee SL. The epidemiology of SLE. Semin Arthritis Rheum 3:1–54, 1973.

Sieper J, Braun J, Doring E, Wu P, Heesemann J, Trehame J, Kingsley G. Aetiological role of bacteria associated with reactive arthritis in pauciarticular juvenile chronic arthritis. Ann Rheum Dis 51:1208–1214, 1992.

Sigal LH. Current recommendations for the treatment of Lyme disease. Drugs 43:683–699, 1992.

Sigurgeirsson B, Lindelof B, Edhag O, Allander E. Risk of cancer in patients with dermatomyositis or polymyositis. N Engl J Med 326:363–367, 1992.

Silber TJ, Chatoor I, White PH. Psychiatric manifestations of systemic lupus erythematosus in children and adolescents. Clin Pediatr 23:331–335, 1984.

Silver RM, Maricq HR. Childhood dermatomyositis: serial microvascular studies. Pediatrics 83:278–283, 1989.

Silver RM, Heyes MP, Maize JC, Quearry B, Vionnet-Fuasset M, Sternberg EM. Scleroderma, fasciitis, and eosinophilia associated with the ingestion of tryptophan. N Engl J Med 322:869–873, 1990.

Silverman ED. Congenital heart block and neonatal lupus erythematosus: prevention is the goal. J Rheumatol 20:1101–1104, 1993.

Silverman ED, Miller JJ, Bernstein B, Shafai T. Consumption coagulopathy associated with systemic juvenile rheumatoid arthritis. J Pediatr 103:872–876, 1983.

Singsen BH, Bernstein BH, King KK, Hanson V. Systemic lupus erythematosus in childhood: correlations between changes in disease activity and serum complement levels. J Pediatr 89:358–365, 1976.

Singsen BH, Bernstein BH, Koster-King KG, Glovsky MM, Hansen V. Reiter's syndrome in childhood. Arthritis Rheum 20 (Suppl):402–407, 1977a.

Singsen BH, Bernstein BH, Kornreich HK, King KK, Hansen V. Mixed connective tissue disease in childhood. A clinical and serologic survey. J Pediatr 90:893–900, 1977b.

Singsen BH, Isaacson AS, Bernstein BH, Patzakis MJ, Kornreich HK, King KK, Hansen V. Total hip replacement in children with arthritis. Arthritis Rheum 21:401–406, 1978.

Sletnes KE, Smith P, Abdelnoor M, Arnesen H, Wisloff F. Antiphospholipid antibodies after myocardial infarction and their relation to mortality, reinfarction, and non-haemorrhagic stroke. Lancet 339:451–453, 1992.

Smiley WK, May E, Bywaters EGL. Ocular presentations of Still's disease and their treatment. Ann Rheum Dis 16:371–382, 1957.

Smith ME, Ansell BM, Bywaters EGL. Mortality and prognosis related to the amyloidosis of Still's disease. Ann Rheum Dis 27:137–145, 1968.

Smith RJ. Evidence of *Chlamydia trachomata* and *Ureaplasma urealyticum* in a patient with Reiter's disease. J Adol Health Care 10:155–159, 1989.

Sonozaki H, Seki H, Chang S, Okuyama M, Juji T. Human lymphocyte antigen, HL-A27, in Japanese patients with ankylosing spondylitis. Tissue Antigens 5:131–136, 1975.

Southwest Pediatric Nephrology Group. Comparison of idiopathic and systemic lupus erythematosus–associated membranous glomerulonephropathy in children. Am J Kidney Dis 7:115–124, 1986.

Special Writing Group of the Committee on Rheumatic Fever, Endocarditis, and Kawasaki Disease of the Council on Cardiovascular Disease in the Young of the American Heart Association: Guidelines for the diagnosis of rheumatic fever. JAMA 268:2069–2073, 1992.

Spencer-Green G, Schlesinger M, Bove KE, Levinson JE, Schaller JG, Hanson V, Crowe WE. Nailfold capillary abnormalities in childhood rheumatic diseases. J Pediatr 102:341–346, 1983.

Spiera H, Kerr LD. Scleroderma following silicone implantation: a cumulative experience of 11 cases. J Rheumatol 20:958–961, 1993.

St. Clair EW. Anti-La antibodies. Rheum Dis Clin North Am 18:359–376, 1992.

Stasny P. HLA-D and Ia antigens in rheumatoid arthritis and systemic lupus erythematosus. Arthritis Rheum 21:1728, 1978.

Stasny P, Fink CW. Different HLA-D associations in adult and juvenile rheumatoid arthritis. J Clin Invest 63:124–130, 1979.

Steere AC. Lyme disease. N Engl J Med 321:586–596, 1989.

Steere A, Malawista S, Snydman D, Shope R, Andiman W, Ross M, Steele F. Lyme arthritis: an epidemic of oligoarticular arthritis in children and adults in three Connecticut communities. Arthritis Rheum 20:7–17, 1977.

Steere AC, Gibofsky A, Patarroyo ME, Winchester RJ, Hardin JA, Malawista SE. Chronic Lyme arthritis. Ann Intern Med 90:896–901, 1979.

Steere AC, Batsford WP, Weinberg M, Alexander J, Berger HJ, Wolfson S, Malawista SE. Lyme carditis: cardiac abnormalities of Lyme disease. Ann Intern Med 93 (Part 1):8–16, 1980.

Steere AC, Bartenhagen NH, Craft JE, Hutchinson GJ, Newman JH, Rahn DW, Sigal LH, Spieler PN, Stenn KS, Malawista SE. The early clinical manifestations of Lyme Disease. Ann Intern Med 99:76–82, 1983.

Steere A, Schoen R, Taylor E. The clinical evolution of Lyme arthritis. Ann Intern Med 107:725–731, 1987.

Steere A, Dwyer E, Winchester R. Association of chronic Lyme arthritis with HLA-DR4 and HLA-DR2 alleles. N Engl J Med 323:219–223, 1990.

Stern R, Fishman J, Brusman H, Kunkel HG. Systemic lupus erythematosus associated with Klinefelter's syndrome. Arthritis Rheum 20:18–22, 1977.

Still GF. On a form of chronic joint disease in children. Med Chir Trans 80:47–59, 1897.

Stimmler MM, Coletti PM, Quismorio FPJ. Magnetic resonance imaging of the brain in neuropsychiatric systemic lupus erythematosus. Sem Arthritis Rheum 22:335–349, 1993.

Stollerman GH. Global Changes in Group A Streptococcal Diseases and Strategies for Their Prevention. Chicago, Year Book Medical Publishers, 1982, pp. 373–406.

Suarez-Almazor ME, Russell AS. Sacroiliitis in psoriasis: relationship to peripheral arthritis and HLA-B27. J Rheumatol 17:804–808, 1990.

Suarez-Almazor ME, Cataggio LJ, Maldonado-Cocco JA, Cuttica R, Garcia-Morteo O. Juvenile progressive systemic sclerosis: clinical and serologic findings. Arthritis Rheum 28:699–702, 1985.

Sugimura T, Kato H, Inoue O, Takagi J, Fukuda T, Sato N. Vasodilatory response of the coronary arteries after Kawasaki disease: evaluation by intracoronary injection of isosorbide dinitrate. J Pediatr 121:684–688, 1992.

Sullivan DB, Cassidy JT, Petty RE, Burt MT. Prognosis in childhood dermatomyositis. J Pediatr 80:555–563, 1972.

Sullivan DB, Cassidy JT, Petty RE. Dermatomyositis in the pediatric patient. Arthritis Rheum 20:327–331, 1977.

Suzuki A, Kamiya T, Ono Y, Okuno M, Yagihara T. Aorto-coronary bypass surgery for coronary arterial lesions resulting from Kawasaki disease. J Pediatr 116:567–573, 1990.

Szer IS, Taylor E, Steere AC. The long-term course of Lyme arthritis in children. N Engl J Med 325:159–163, 1991.

Szer IS, Klein-Gitelman M, DeNardo BA, McCauley R. Ultrasonography in the study of prevalence and clinical evolution of popliteal cysts in children with knee effusions. J Rheumatol 19:458–462, 1992.

Taillan B, Roul C, Fuzibet JG. Circulating anticoagulant in patients seropositive for human immunodeficiency virus. Am J Med 87:238, 1989.

Takahashi M, Mason W, Lewis A. Regression of coronary aneurysms in patients with Kawasaki syndrome. Circulation 75:387–394, 1987.

Takigawa M, Kanoh T, Imamura S, Takahashi C. IgA deficiency and systemic lupus erythematosus. Arch Dermatol 112:845–849, 1976.

Tan EM. Autoantibodies to nuclear antigens (ANA), their immunobiology and medicine. Adv Immunol 33:167–240, 1982.

Tan EM. Interactions between autoimmunity and molecular and cell biology. J Clin Invest 84:1–6, 1989.

Tan EM, Schur PH, Carr RI, Kunkel HG. Deoxyribonucleic acid (DNA) and antibodies to DNA in the serum of patients with systemic lupus erythematosus. J Clin Invest 45:1732–1740, 1966.

Tan EM, Cohen AS, Fries JF, Masi AT, McShane DJ, Rothfield NF, Schaller JG, Talal N, Winchester RJ. The 1982 revised criteria for the classification of systemic lupus erythematosus. Arthritis Rheum 25:1271–1277, 1982a.

Tan EM, Fritzler MJ, McDougal JS, McDuffie FC, Nakamura RM, Reichlin M, Reimer CB, Sharp GC, Schur PH, Wilson MR, Winchester RJ. Reference sera for antinuclear antibodies. I. Antibodies to native DNA, Sm nuclear RNP, and Ss-B/La. Arthritis Rheum 25:1003–1005, 1982b.

Taranta A. Relation of isolated recurrences of Sydenham's chorea to preceding streptococcal infections. N Engl J Med 260:1204–1210, 1959.

Targoff IN, Johnson AE, Miller FW. Antibody to signal recognition particle in polymyositis. Arthritis Rheum 33:1361–1370, 1990.

Taurog JD, Hammer RE, Montanez S, Hadavand R, Breban M, Croft JT, Balish E. Effect of the germfree state on the inflammatory disease of HLA-B27 transgenic rats: a split result. Arthritis Rheum 36:S46, 1993.

Tejani A, Nicastri AD, Chen CK, Fikrig S, Gurumurthy K. Lupus nephritis in black and hispanic children. Am J Dis Child 137:481–483, 1983.

Thomson GT, MacDougall B, Watson PH, Chalmers IM. Eosinophilic fasciitis in a pair of siblings. Arthritis Rheum 32:96–99, 1989.

Tiddens HA, van der Net JJ, de Graeff-Meeder ER, Fiselier TJ, de Rooij DJ, van Luijk MH, Herzberger R, van Suijlekom LW, van Venrooij WJ, Zegers BJ. Juvenile-onset mixed connective tissue disease: longitudinal follow-up. J Pediatr 152:191–197, 1993.

Tipping PG, Buchanan RC, Riglar AG, Dimech WJ, Littlejohn GO, Holdsworth SR. Measurement of anti-DNA antibodies by ELISA: a comparative study with *Crithidia* and a Farr assay. Pathology 23:21–24, 1991.

Torrigiani G, Ansell BM, Chown EEA, Roitt IM. Raised IgG antiglobulin factors in Still's disease. Ann Rheum Dis 28:424–427, 1969.

Totoritis MC, Tan EM, McNally EM, Rubin RL. Association of antibody to histone complex H2A-H2B with symptomatic procainamide-induced lupus. N Engl J Med 318:1431–1436, 1988.

Towner SR, Michet CJ, O'Fallon WM, Nelson AM. The epidemiology of juvenile arthritis in Rochester, Minnesota, 1960–79. Arthritis Rheum 26:1208–1213, 1983.

Triplett DA. Laboratory diagnosis of lupus anticoagulants. Semin Thromb Hemost 16:182–192, 1990.

Trygstad CW, Stiehm ER. Elevated serum IgA globulin in anaphylactoid purpura. Pediatrics 47:1023–1028, 1971.

Tucker LB, Miller LC, Marx G, Dorkin HL, Schaller JG. Cardiopulmonary followup during the course of childhood systemic lupus erythematosus (SLE) (abstract). Arthritis Rheum 35 (Suppl 9):D81, 1992.

Tucker LB, Sadeghi-Nejad A, Schaller JG. The association of acquired generalized lipodystrophy with juvenile dermatomyositis. Arthritis Rheum in press, 1995.

Tuffanelli DL, Winkelmann RK. Systemic scleroderma. A clinical study of 727 cases. Arch Dermatol 84:359–371, 1961.

Urizar RE, Michael AF, Sisson S. Anaphylactoid purpura. II. Immunofluorescent and electron microscopic studies of the glomerular lesions. Lab Invest 19:437–450, 1968.

Urman JD, Rothchild NF. Corticosteroid treatment in systemic lupus erythematosus. Survival studies. JAMA 238:2272–2276, 1977.

U.S. and U.K. Joint Report. The evolution of rheumatic heart disease in children: five year report of a cooperative clinical trial of ACTH, cortisone and aspirin. Circulation 22:503–515, 1960.

Vaarala O, Palusuo T, Kleemola M. Anticardiolipin response in acute infections. Clin Immunol Immunopathol 41:8–15, 1986.

Vaisman S, Guasch J, Vignan A, Correa E, Schuster A, Mortimer EA, Rammelkamp CH. Failure of penicillin to alter acute rheumatic valvulitis. JAMA 194:1284–1286, 1965.

van den Wall Bake AWL. IgA class anti-neutrophil cytoplasmic antibodies (IgA-ANCA) in primary IgA nephropathy. Acta Pathol Microbiol Immunol Scand 97 (Suppl 6):25–26, 1989.

van der Woude FJ, Rasmussen N, Lobatto S. Autoantibodies against neutrophils and monocytes: tool for diagnosis and marker of disease activity in Wegener's granulomatosis. Lancet 1:425–429, 1985.

van Leeuwen MA, Westra J, Limburg PC, deJong HJ, Marrink J, van Rijswijk MH. Quantification of IgM, IgA, and IgG rheumatoid factors by ELISA in rheumatoid arthritis and other rheumatic disorders. Scand J Rheumatol 75:25–31, 1988.

van Vloten WA, Scheffer E, Dooren LJ. Localized scleroderma-like lesions after bone marrow transplantation in man. A chronic graft-vs-host reaction. Br J Dermatol 96:337–341, 1977.

Varga J, Schumacher HR, Jimenez SA. Systemic sclerosis after augmentation mammoplasty with silicone implants. Ann Intern Med 111:377–383, 1989.

Vaughan JH. Pathogenetic concepts and origins of rheumatoid factor in rheumatoid arthritis. Arthritis Rheum 36:1–6, 1993.

Veasy LG, Weidmeier SE, Orsmond GS, Ruttenberg HD, Boucek MM, Roth SJ, Tait VF, Thompson JA, Daly JA, Kaplan EL, Hill HR. Resurgence of acute rheumatic fever in the intermountain area of the United States. N Engl J Med 316:421–427, 1987.

Vehe RK, Begovich AB, Nepom BS. HLA susceptibility genes in rheumatoid factor positive juvenile rheumatoid arthritis. J Rheumatol 17 (Suppl 26):11–15, 1990.

Vernier RL, Worthen HG, Peterson RD, Colle E, Good RA. Anaphylactoid purpura: pathology of the skin and kidney and frequency of streptococcal infection. Pediatrics 27:181–193, 1961.

Virchow R. Historical note on lupus. Arch Pathol Anat 32:139–143, 1865.

Wagener JS, Taussig LM, DeBenedetti C. Pulmonary function in juvenile rheumatoid arthritis. J Pediatr 99:108–110, 1981.

Wald ER, Dashefsky MD, Feidt C, Chiponis D, Myers C. Acute rheumatic fever in western Pennsylvania and the tristate area. Pediatrics 80:371–374, 1987.

Wallace CA, Sherry DD. Preliminary report of higher dose methotrexate treatment in juvenile rheumatoid arthritis. J Rheumatol 19:1604–1607, 1992.

Wallace C, Schaller JG, Emery H, Wedgwood R. Prospective study of childhood systemic lupus erythematosus (SLE). Arthritis Rheum 21:599–600, 1978.

Wallace C, Striker G, Schaller JG, Wedgwood RJ, Emery HM. Renal histology and subsequent course in childhood systemic lupus erythematosus (SLE). Arthritis Rheum 22:669, 1979.

Wallace CA, Sherry DD, Mellins ED, Aiken RP. Predicting remission in juvenile rheumatoid arthritis with methotrexate treatment. J Rheumatol 20:118–122, 1993.

Wallace DJ, Metzger AL, White K. Combination immunosuppressive treatment of steroid resistant dermatomyositis/polymyositis. Arthritis Rheum 28:590–592, 1985.

Waller M. Methods of measurement of rheumatoid factor. Ann N Y Acad Sci 168:5–17, 1969.

Walport MJ, Lachmann PJ. Erythrocyte complement receptor type 1, immune complexes, and the rheumatic diseases. Arthritis Rheum 31:153–158, 1988.

Walravens PA, Chase HP. The prognosis of childhood systemic lupus erythematosus. Am J Dis Child 130:929–933, 1976.

Wannamaker LW. The chain that links the heart to the throat. Circulation 48:9–18, 1973.

Wannamaker LW, Rammelkamp CH, Deny FW, Brink WR, Houser HB, Hahn EO, Dingle JH. Prophylaxis of acute rheumatic fever by treatment of the preceding streptococcal infection with various amounts of depot penicillin. Am J Med 10:673–695, 1951.

Ward MM, Pisetsky DS, Christenson VD. Antidouble-stranded DNA antibody assays in systemic lupus erythematosus: correlations of longitudinal antibody measurements. J Rheumatol 16:609–613, 1989.

Watson R, Kang JE, Kudak M, Kickler T, Provost TT. Thrombocytopenia in the neonatal lupus syndrome. Arch Dermatol 124:560–563, 1988.

Weinstein A, Bordwell B, Stone B, Tibbetts C, Rothfield NF. Antibodies to native DNA and serum complement (C3) levels. Application to diagnosis and classification of systemic lupus erythematosus. Am J Med 74:206–216, 1983.

Weiss JA. Possible relationship between Henoch-Schönlein syndrome and IgA nephropathy. Nephron 22:589–595, 1978.

Wenkert D, Miller LC, Tucker LB, Szer IS, Schaller JG. Chromosomal abnormalities in boys with systemic lupus erythematosus. Arthritis Rheum 34:A169, 1991.

Weston WL, Harmon C, Peebles C, Manchester D, Franco HL, Huff JC, Norris DA. A serological marker for neonatal lupus erythematosus. Br J Dermatol 107:377–382, 1982.

Whitaker JN, Engel WK. Vascular deposits of immunoglobulins and complement in idiopathic inflammatory myopathy. N Engl J Med 286:333–338, 1972.

WHO Study Group on Rheumatic Fever and Rheumatic Heart Disease. Rheumatic fever and rheumatic heart disease: report of a WHO study group. WHO Technical Report, 1987, pp. 4–58.

Wiik A. Delineation of a standard procedure for indirect immunofluorescence detection of ANCA. Acta Pathol Microbiol Immunol Scand 97 (Suppl 6):12–13, 1989.

Wilkens RF, Arnett FC, Bitter T. Reiter's syndrome: evaluation of preliminary criteria for definite disease. Bull Rheum Dis 32:31–34, 1982.

Williams RA, Ansell BM. Radiological findings in seropositive juvenile chronic arthritis (juvenile rheumatoid arthritis) with particular reference to progression. Ann Rheum Dis 44:685–693, 1985.

Williams RCJ. Molecular mimicry and rheumatic fever. Clin Rheum Dis 11:573–590, 1985.

Williams RCJ. Rheumatoid factors: historical perspective, origins and possible role in disease. J Rheumatol 19 (Suppl 32):42–45, 1992.

Wilson JG, Fearon DT. Altered expression of complement receptors as a pathogenic factor in systemic lupus erythematosus. Arthritis Rheum 27:1321–1328, 1984.

Winchester RJ. The major histocompatibility complex. In Kelley WN, Harris ED, Ruddy S, Sledge CB, eds. Textbook of Rheumatology, 2nd ed. Philadelphia, WB Saunders, 1985, pp. 36–54.

Winfield JB, Faiferman I, Koffler D. Avidity of anti-DNA antibodies in serum and IgG glomerular eluates from patients with systemic lupus erythematosus. Association of high avidity antinative DNA antibody with glomerulonephritis. J Clin Invest 59:90–96, 1977.

Winfield JB, Mimura T, Fernsten PD. Antilymphocyte autoantibodies. In Wallace DJ, Hahn BH, eds. Dubois' Lupus Erythematosus, 4th ed. Philadelphia, Lea & Febiger, 1993, pp. 254–259.

Winkelmann RK. Chronic discoid lupus erythematosus in children. JAMA 205:675–678, 1968.

Winkelmann RK, Kierland RR, Perry HO, Muller SA, Sams WM. Symposium on scleroderma. Mayo Clin Proc 46:77–134, 1971.

Winn DM, Wolfe JF, Lindberg D, Fristoe EA, Kingsland L, Sharp GC. Identification of a clinical subset of systemic lupus erythematosus by antibodies to Sm antigen. Arthritis Rheum 22:1334–1337, 1979.

Wood HW, Feinstein AR, Taranta A, Epstein JA, Simpson R. Comparative effectiveness of 3 prophylaxis regimens in preventing streptococcal infections and rheumatic recurrences. Ann Intern Med 60: (Suppl 5):31–46, 1964.

Woolf A, Croker B, Osofsky SG, Kredich DW. Nephritis in children and young adults with systemic lupus erythematosus and normal urinary sediment. Pediatrics 64:678–685, 1979.

Wurzner R, Orran A, Lalchmann PJ. Inherited deficiencies of the terminal components of human complement. Immunodefic Rev 3:123–147, 1992.

Wynne-Roberts CR, Anderson CH, Turano AM, Baron M. Light

and electron-microscopic findings in juvenile rheumatoid arthritis synovium: comparison with normal juvenile synovium. Semin Arthritis Rheum 7:287–302, 1978.

Yanagisawa M, Kobayashi N, Matsuya S. Myocardial infarction due to coronary thromboarteritis, following acute febrile mucocutaneous lymph node syndrome (MLNS) in an infant. Pediatrics 54:277–281, 1974.

Yancey CL, Doughty RA, Athreya BH. Central nervous system involvement in childhood systemic lupus erythematosus. Arthritis Rheum 24:1389–1395, 1981.

Yoshikawa J, Yanagihara K, Owaki T, Kato H, Takagi Y, Okumachi F, Fukaya T, Tomita Y, Baba K. Cross-sectional echocardiographic diagnosis of coronary artery aneurysms in patients with the mucocutaneous lymph node syndrome. Circulation 59:133–139, 1979.

Zabriskie JB, Hsu KC, Seegal BC. Heart-reactive antibody associated with rheumatic fever: characterization and diagnostic significance. Clin Exp Immunol 7:147–159, 1970.

Zetterstrom R, Berglund G. Systemic lupus erythematosus in childhood. A clinical study. Acta Pediatr 45:189–204, 1956.

Zoller L, Burkard S, Schafer H. Validity of Western immunoblot band patterns in the serodiagnosis of Lyme borreliosis. J Clin Microbiol 29:174–182, 1991.

Zuber M. Positive antinuclear antibodies in malignancies. Ann Rheum Dis 51:573–574, 1992.

Chapter 25

Renal Disorders

Alfred J. Fish and Beth A. Vogt

IMMUNOLOGIC MECHANISMS IN EXPERIMENTAL AND HUMAN RENAL DISEASE

Although the causes of most forms of human renal disease are unknown, there is reason to believe that immunologic mechanisms play a prominent role in the pathogenesis of the various types of glomerulonephritis. Evidence is derived from a number of sources:

- The demonstration that the morphology and immunopathology of the kidney in certain forms of experimentally induced immune renal disease are similar to those in human glomerulonephritis
- The occurrence of serum complement or complement component abnormalities in some renal disorders

- Immunopathologic techniques demonstrating immune reactants (immunoglobulins and complement components) in glomerular capillaries
- The presence of certain autoantibodies with reactivity for basement membranes and other renal structures

Experimentally Induced Immune Glomerulonephritis

Structure and Biochemistry of the Glomerular Capillary Wall

Immune injury to the glomerular capillary wall should be examined in context of its structure and

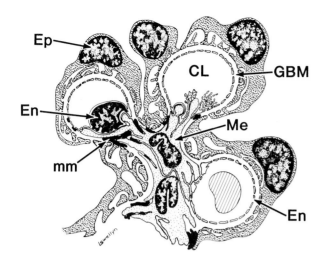

Figure 25–1. Schematic view of the glomerular lobule with three glomerular capillaries supported by mesangial cells (Me) with their network of mesangial matrix (mm). The capillary wall is composed of fenestrated endothelial cells (En), basement membrane (GBM), and the podocytes of epithelial cells (Ep). CL = capillary lumen. (Modified from Vernier RL, Resnick JS, Mauer SM. Recurrent hematuria and focal glomerulonephritis. Kidney Int 7:224–231, 1975.)

composition. The glomerular capillary bed is unique in design and function; while handling a high blood blow, it maintains its major function of glomerular filtration. The glomerular structure is designed to minimize the response to noxious immune assault to preserve function.

The glomerular capillary wall features a specialized basement membrane (GBM), lined by the fenestrated glomerular capillary endothelium and bounded on the outside by the podocytic epithelial cells of the glomerulus (Fig. 25–1). The glomerular capillaries are supported by a network of smooth muscle cells that form the mesangium; this cellular conglomerate has a separate system of intercellular channels composed of mesangial matrix resembling GBM (Michael et al., 1980). The 1.1 antigen present on thymocytes and lymphocytes has also been detected on rat mesangial cells (Bagchus et al., 1986). Ia-positive phagocytic cells of bone marrow origin are also found in the mesangium of rat glomeruli (Schreiner et al., 1981).

The GBM has certain biochemically characterized components (Fish et al., 1979) (Fig. 25–2). The major structural protein of the GBM is type IV collagen, which differs from interstitial and tendon collagen to accommodate the increased flexibility and other functional properties of the GBM (Timpl 1986; Yurchenco and Schittny 1990). Five subunit alpha chains of type IV collagen have been defined: alpha-1, and alpha-2 type IV collagen chains are present in the mesangium and subendothelium (Butkowski et al., 1989); alpha-3 through alpha-5 type IV collagen chains are present predominantly in the lamina densa of the GBM (Kleppel et al., 1986, 1992; Hudson et al., 1989; Morrison et al., 1991; Turner et al., 1992; Zhou et al., 1993; Kashtan and Michael, 1993). The subendothelium of the glomerular capillary wall also contains type V collagen

and fibronectin, which are also present in the mesangium (Scheinman et al., 1980; Michael et al., 1984).

Since the initial characterization of laminin (Beck et al., 1990) and its localization to GBM and other renal basement membranes, it has become known that multiple laminin isoforms exist. The laminin B2 chain is common to all isoforms, and along with laminin S chain are the predominant laminin components of the GBM and mesangium (Desjardins and Bendayan, 1989; Sanes et al., 1990). Entactin (also called nidogen) is present in the GBM and mesangium (Aumailley et al., 1989; Katz et al., 1991) and is bound to laminin.

Negatively charged heparan sulfate proteoglycans (Kanwar, 1984) present within the GBM may contribute to its permeability barrier, which is responsible for sieving during glomerular filtration (Vernier et al., 1983; Mohan and Spiro, 1991; van den Born et al., 1991; Hagen et al., 1993). Heparan sulfate, along with chondroitin sulfate, is present in the mesangium. Anionic plasma proteins like albumin, IgG4, and amyloid P protein appear to be trapped in the GBM (Melvin et al., 1984a; Eddy and Michael, 1992; Fujigaki et al., 1993). A highly negatively charged sialic acid–rich polyanion (also called *podocalyxin*) (Nevins and Michael, 1981; Kerjaschki et al., 1984b) coats glomerular epithelial cells. At the base of glomerular epithelial cell foot processes, where contact with the GBM occurs, there are concavities known as *cathrin-coated pits*; they contain a 330-kD glycoprotein called *gp330*, which is also known as *Fx1A* or *Heymann antigen* (Kerjaschki et al., 1987; Antonovych et al., 1992).

Immune injury involves perturbations of these glomerular components with resultant changes in function and permeability and in proteinuria (Table 25–1).

Anti–Glomerular Basement Membrane Antibody Disorders

Numerous studies by many investigators have defined two general types of immunologic assault on

Table 25–1. Immunologic Mechanisms in Renal Disease

Immune Complex Disease
Deposition of circulating antigen–antibody complexes in glomeruli and vessels
   Includes most forms of glomerulonephritis
   Antigens
     Host (e.g., DNA in lupus)
     Bacterial, viral, fungal, parasitic
Interaction of antibody with a fixed antigen (in situ complex disease)
   Passive Heymann's nephritis
   Planted antigens (concanavalin A, cationized proteins)

Anti–Basement Membrane Antibody Disease
Interaction of antibody with glomerular basement membrane (GBM) (e.g., Goodpasture's syndrome)
Interaction of antibody with tubular basement membrane (e.g., tubulointerstitial nephritis)

Cellular Mechanisms
Participation of polymorphonuclear leukocytes and monocytes in tissue injury induced by immune complexes or anti-GBM antibody
Possible role of antineutrophil cytoplasmic antibodies

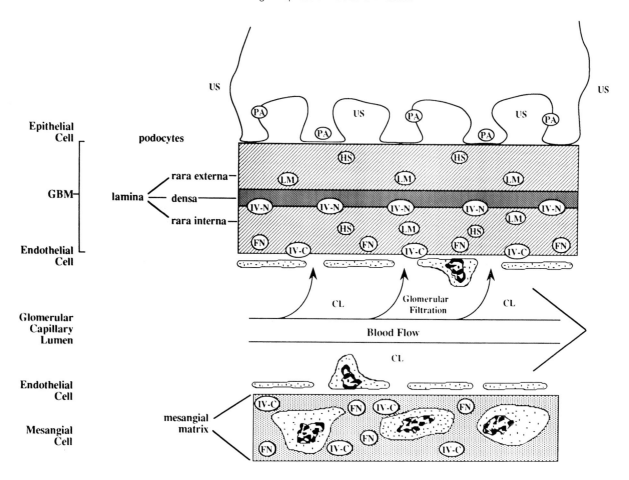

Figure 25–2. Schematic representation of the position of glomerular capillary wall components in relation to the capillary lumen (CL), mesangium (cell and matrix), endothelial cell, glomerular basement membrane (GBM) with lamina rara interna, externa, and lamina densa, epithelium, and urinary space (US). IV = type IV collagen; HS = heparan sulfate proteoglycan; GP = Goodpasture antigen; FN = fibronectin; PA = polyanionic sialoproteins on the epithelial cell; LM = laminin; IV-C = (α1, α2 classic type IV collagen); IV-N = (α3, α4, α5 novel type IV collagen).

the kidney (Eddy and Michael, 1992). In *nephrotoxic nephritis* or *anti-GBM antibody disease*, antikidney antibody experimentally administered to an animal results in glomerulonephritis due to fixation of heterologous IgG and host complement in the GBM. After several days, the host's own IgG becomes fixed to the deposited heterologous IgG with accentuation of the disease. The first (heterologous antibody fixation) and second (autologous antibody fixation) stages of this disease each depend on complement activation for the immunologic injury. The role of circulating inflammatory cells, both polymorphonuclear leukocytes and monocytes, is described later. Other experimental models that depend on anti-GBM antibody formation and fixation include Steblay's nephritis in sheep (Steblay et al., 1962; Lerner et al., 1967) and autoimmune nephritis in rabbits. In the former, sheep are immunized with GBM from another species and produce antibodies that fix to their own GBM (Jeraj et al., 1982).

Heteroantisera made to whole GBM preparations react against multiple GBM antigens (Fish et al., 1979); thus, antigenic specificity of Steblay nephritis antibodies is unknown. Antilaminin (Abrahamson et al., 1982)

and antitype IV collagen antibodies (Wick et al., 1982) have induced experimental glomerular injury.

Immunopathologic studies of anti-GBM antibody disease reveal immunoglobulin and complement components in a linear distribution on the GBM, analogous to that seen in Goodpasture's disease and in certain types of rapidly progressive glomerulonephritis in humans; autoantibodies to the NC1 domain of type IV collagen alpha-3 chain are present as described later.

Brown Norway rats and rabbits injected with mercuric chloride develop anti-GBM antibodies and glomerulonephritis. After several weeks, the glomerular injury changes to a pattern type of membranous glomerulopathy with immune deposits typical of antigen–antibody complexes (Houssin et al., 1983). The nature of the antigens involved and the autoantibodies formed are unknown (Fukatsu et al., 1987; Pelletier et al., 1987).

Antigen–Antibody Complex Nephritis

The classic prototype of the second kind of experimental disease is acute or chronic serum sickness nephritis. In the *acute* form, one dose of a protein antigen (such as bovine serum albumin) is administered to a rabbit (Fish et al., 1966). After 10 to 14 days, the animal begins to produce antibody in an antigen-rich environment, thus favoring the production of soluble antigen–antibody complexes. These complexes have a number of important biologic properties, including the ability to activate the complement system.

The reason for the localization within glomeruli is not known, although it may be related to physiologic factors, uptake by the glomerular mesangium, the influence of certain chemical mediators known to localize complexes to the subendothelial region of vessels, or the size and physiochemical properties of the complexes (Cochrane, 1971). Localized complexes and complement (Yamamoto and Wilson, 1987) result in a number of important effects, including cell injury, monocyte infiltration (Hunsicker et al., 1979), and activation of the coagulation mechanism, resulting in the morphologic picture of glomerulonephritis.

In the *chronic* form of experimental serum sickness, frequent injections of antigen are administered to maintain a state of antigen excess and chronic exposure to immune complexes (Dixon et al., 1961). The disease produced in this circumstance is similar to chronic glomerulonephritis in humans.

Molecular weight, antibody avidity, antigen charge, and plasma concentration of immune complexes are important determinants governing glomerular localization; complexes of low-avidity antibody are small and localize in the peripheral capillary loop, whereas high-avidity antibodies result in high-molecular-weight complexes that are taken up by the mesangium (Ooi et al., 1977a, 1977b; Iskander et al., 1983). In general, sequestration of immune complexes in the mesangium protects the peripheral glomerular capillary loops from injury. Plasma concentration of complexes, an important factor in renal localization, is a balance between reticuloendothelial and monocytic phagocytosis. The latter is a function of binding by Fc and complement receptors (Holdsworth, 1983). Complexes made with reduced and alkylated antibody are poorly phagocytosed by mononuclear cells, attain a higher plasma level, and are more likely to localize in the glomeruli (Haakenstad et al., 1976). Because the GBM is known to have negatively charged heparan sulfate–rich moieties, enhanced localization of positively charged complexes is formed from cationized antigens (Gallo et al., 1981, 1983). Similarly, chronic serum sickness in rabbits induced with cationized bovine serum albumin leads to the development of membranous glomerulopathy with peripheral glomerular loop localization (Border et al., 1982).

Immune complexes enter the mesangium at the endothelial–mesangial cell interface. Numerous physiologic factors, including blood flow, presence of renal artery stenosis, angiotensin II (Raij et al., 1984), hypertension, nephrotic proteinuria, and immune complex injury, affect the afferent limb of mesangial uptake. Egress routes from the mesangium are uncertain; macromolecules leave the mesangium by means of the glomerular stalk area and pass into the renal interstitium or tubule or recycle into the circulation.

Another model of complex disease is *Heymann's autologous immune complex nephritis*. In this case, rats immunized with the proximal tubular antigen Fx1A in Freund's adjuvant develop a chronic, ongoing nephritis (Heymann et al., 1959; Edgington et al., 1968; Miettinen et al., 1980). Passive administration of antibody to Fx1A results in immediate fixation of IgG to the glomerular capillary and appearance of epimembranous deposits. This has been shown to be an example of in situ immune complex disease (Couser et al., 1978; Van Damme et al., 1978; Couser and Salant, 1980; Madaio et al., 1983; Jeraj et al., 1984).

Passive administration of heterologous antibody results in binding to the Fx1A antigen within the glomerular capillary wall, leading to proteinuria and complement activation but without stimulation of circulating inflammatory cells (Salant et al., 1980). The fixed glomerular antigen and the tubular cell epithelial brush border antigens appear to be related if not identical (Kerjaschki and Farquhar, 1982). A glycoprotein (gp330) that is present within coated pits on glomerular epithelial cells has been characterized as the Heymann antigen (Kerjaschki et al., 1984a, 1987).

In analogous experimental circumstances, antigens planted within the glomerulus passively reacted with administered antibody. Foreign proteins in a macromolecular form (e.g., heat-aggregated IgG) given intravenously localize in the mesangium (Mauer et al., 1973). The kidney containing mesangial deposits of aggregated IgG is transplanted to another animal, which is then given an intravenous injection of antibody against the aggregated IgG. Diffuse exudative mesangial inflammation results. Marked mesangial hypercellularity and mesangial deposits of IgG, C3, and fibrin are seen. When concanavalin A (Golbus and Wilson, 1979), cationized ferritin, or IgG (Oite et al., 1982, 1983) is injected into experimental animals followed by antibody to the respective antigens, glomerulonephritis develops, with binding of specific antibody to the previously in situ planted antigens. However, no human renal disease of in situ complex injury has been identified. Acute poststreptococcal glomerulonephritis in humans may be a form of in situ immune complex injury, although the relation with streptococcal infection is not understood.

In both the acute and chronic forms of experimental complex disease, immunopathologic and electron microscopic studies reveal numerous deposits of immunoglobulin, antigen, and complement on both sides of or within the GBM. Serum complement levels may be depressed during the period of antigen removal from the circulation. Polyclonal B-cell stimulation to autologous and exogenous antigens has been postulated as a pathogenetic mechanism of immune complex formation (Pelletier et al., 1987; Bruijn et al., 1990).

Cell-Mediated Glomerular Injury

Although T-cell regulatory mechanisms affect the humoral mechanism described earlier, evidence is accumulating to support the role of T-cell immunity in renal disease (Fillit and Zabriskie, 1984; Eddy and Michael, 1992). A resident population of bone marrow–derived phagocytes bearing Ia antigens has been observed in the rat glomerulus (Schreiner and Cotran, 1982).

Light and electron microscopic studies have demonstrated mononuclear cells in the kidneys of patients and experimental animals (Holdsworth et al., 1981; Atkins et al., 1982). Monocytes play an active role in the glomerular injury of nephrotoxic serum nephritis in rats (Schreiner et al., 1978; Kreisberg et al., 1979; Dubois et al., 1981; Sterzl and Pabst 1982; Parra et al., 1990) and in acute serum sickness nephritis in rabbits (Hunsicker et al., 1979; Holdsworth et al., 1981). Sensitized lymphocytes may augment glomerular injury in experimental nephritis (Mauer et al., 1975; Bhan et al., 1978, 1979). Using leukocyte migration inhibition and lymphocyte blastogenesis, it has been shown that lymphoid cells from patients with glomerulonephritis react against GBM antigens (Fillit et al., 1978; Fillit and Zabriskie, 1982). Although idiopathic nephrotic syndrome of childhood is not mediated by humoral antibody, some evidence links altered cellular immunity to this condition (see later).

Monocytic infiltration in glomeruli of patients with various forms of glomerulonephritis has been observed. Glomerular monocytes have been prominently observed in poststreptococcal glomerulonephritis (Parra et al., 1984) and chronic glomerulonephritis (Monga et al., 1981; Stachura et al., 1984). Monocytes may be attracted to immune complexes in glomeruli via surface receptors for complement components, or the Fc fragment of IgG. These cells may bind extracellular matrix components such as fibronectin and collagen through cell surface integrin receptors. Fibrin in glomerular crescents appears to be a chemoattractant for monocytes.

Renal Injury and Complement Activation

The complement system is a complex interaction of serum proteins that have a multiplicity of effects on host defense mechanisms, including inflammation, coagulation, capillary permeability, chemotaxis, and phagocytosis. Because the complement activation sequence is reviewed in Chapter 7, only the relation of complement activation to renal disorders is discussed here.

Activation of the classical and alternate complement pathways in some renal disorders can be attributed to circulating antibody or antigen–antibody complexes (Couser et al., 1985). In some renal diseases, however, complement deposition is present but antibody or complexes are not evident. Control of spontaneous complement activation is regulated by inhibitors that affect the complement cascade at different points. The final pathway of complement activation (C5 through C9) is the result of C3 activation by C3 convertase. Classical pathway activation is generated through C1 (q, r, and s), C4, and C2 to form the classical pathway convertase. Activators of the classical pathway include antigen–antibody complexes. The Fc portions of IgG1, IgG3, and IgM are responsible for the initial activation of

C1q. By contrast, the alternate complement pathway is activated without antibody (although aggregated IgE and IgA may do so) by such agents as bacteria (Gewurz et al., 1968b), yeasts, and viruses. Properdin, factor D, and factor B participate in the formation of the alternate pathway C3 convertase C3bBb. Both C3 convertases cause hydrolysis of an internal thioester bond of C3 with formation of C3b, the active molecule.

A depression in the level of serum hemolytic complement in acute poststreptococcal glomerulonephritis is regularly observed (Lange et al., 1960; West et al., 1964; Gewurz et al., 1968a; Lewis et al., 1971). Other diseases in which complement levels are depressed include systemic lupus erythematosus (SLE) (Kohler and Ten Bensel, 1969), membranoproliferative glomerulonephritis (MPGN), serum sickness, cryoglobulinemia, and the glomerulonephritis associated with certain infections (Table 25–2) (see also Chapter 17).

The serum complement level in each illness depends on the course of the disease. Levels of individual complement components may show certain distinctive features in these diseases. In type II MPGN, primarily alternative pathway activation is seen with depression of C3 and normal levels of C1 and C4. The serum contains an autoantibody against the C3 convertase (C3bBb). In lupus erythematosus, on the other hand, classical and alternative activation coexists. Evidence suggests that the alternative complement pathway may be operative in various forms of glomerulonephritis. Changes in complement-control proteins, such as factor H (βIH) and C3 INA have been observed in some forms of glomerulonephritis (Wyatt et al., 1979).

The biologic effects of complement activation are partially expressed by the release of small peptides from C3, C4, and C5. C3a peptide is an anaphylatoxin that causes mast cells to release histamine, which in turn increases membrane permeability. C5a peptide both acts on mast cells and stimulates PMN chemotaxis; its release may impair pulmonary function during hemodialysis. C3e peptide may cause PMN release from the bone marrow.

Three other observations link the complement system to renal disorders. There is a high incidence of glomerulonephritis in several genetic complement deficiencies (Praz et al., 1984). Activation of the classical and alternate pathways in the final stages of renal injury has been observed (Velosa et al., 1976). This can

Table 25–2. Diseases Usually Associated with Reduction in Whole Serum Complement (CH$_{50}$) and Serum C3

Poststreptococcal glomerulonephritis
Glomerulonephritis with systemic infection
Membranoproliferative glomerulonephritis
    Type I
    Type II (dense-deposit disease)*
    Type III
Lupus erythematosus
Cryoglobulinemia

---

*In type II membranoproliferative glomerulonephritis serum contains C3NeF (autoantibody to C3bBb) and early complement components (C1 and C4) are often normal; it may be associated with partial lipodystrophy.

occur without the presence of antibody, similar to the situations in type II MPGN and acute glomerulonephritis (Kim and Michael, 1980). Finally, complement component C9, in the form of C9 neoantigen, has been identified on basement membranes in various forms of renal injury (Falk et al., 1983; Michael et al., 1984; Hinglais et al., 1986). C9 neoantigen is the final pathway of C5-9 activation and results in the formation of the membrane attack complex (Cybulsky et al., 1988). This complex induces a reorganization of cell membrane lipid bilayers and the formation of a transmembrane channel; its role in pathogenesis of immune glomerular injury is unknown (Falk et al., 1983; Lai et al., 1989a, 1989b).

Immunopathology

The distribution of immunoglobulins (IgG, IgM, and IgA) and certain complement components (C3, C1q, C2, C4) along the GBM or in the mesangium has been useful in forming concepts about the pathogenesis of certain forms of glomerulonephritis (Fig. 25–3). The thin, linear, nongranular deposition of immunoglobulins on the GBM (anti-GBM antibody) characteristic of Goodpasture's disease is rare in renal tissue from children. The granular or nodular distribution of IgG and C3 along the GBM in such diseases as acute poststreptococcal glomerulonephritis, lupus nephritis, and glomerulonephritis and associated with infection suggesting an immune complex form of renal injury is much more common in children. In other diseases, the location and form of glomerular immunoreactants, although not similar to anti-GBM antibody, also are not identical to those seen in experimental complex disease. Characterization of these diseases as complex mediated, therefore, is speculative.

Circulating Immune Complexes

Assays to detect immune complexes include binding to radiolabeled C1q (Digeon et al., 1977; Ooi et al., 1977a, 1977b; Woodroffe et al., 1977); C1q deviation tests (Sobel et al., 1976); fixation to the C3b receptor of lymphoblastoid lines (Raji cells) (Bayer et al., 1976; Theofilopoulos et al., 1976; Woodroffe et al., 1977); and the bovine conglutinin assay (Eisenberg et al., 1977). Immune complexes have been found in nephrotic syndrome (Allison et al., 1969) and acute glomerulonephritis (Solling, 1983) but rarely in IgA-IgG nephropathy or membranous glomerulonephritis (Tung et al., 1978).

The levels of circulating immune complexes in these disorders vary, depending on the assay used (Lambert et al., 1978; Border, 1983). Presence of immune complexes depends on a balance between production and the rate of uptake by circulating monocytes or fixed macrophages of the mononuclear phagocytic system (MPS). The receptor function of the MPS measured by the clearance of IgG-coated erythrocytes is diminished in SLE (Frank et al., 1979; van Es and Daha, 1984). Circulating immune complexes have been observed occasionally in idiopathic nephrotic syndrome, a disorder

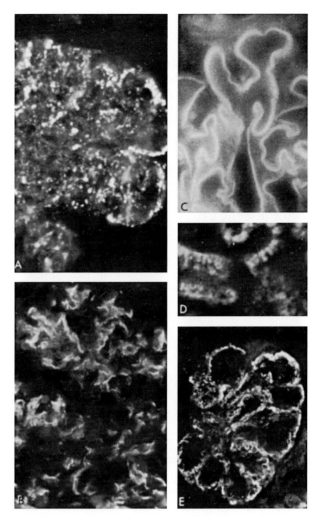

Figure 25–3. Immunofluorescent studies illustrating the various distributions of protein deposits in the glomerulus in different forms of glomerulonephritis.

A, Acute glomerulonephritis (AGN) and hypocomplementemia associated with severe staphylococcal infection. Note the isolated granular and nodular deposits along the capillary loop (C3 ×400).

B, Anaphylactoid glomerulonephritis. Fibrin is present within the mesangium in a distribution similar to that of C3 and IgG. Note the absence of basement membrane–oriented fluorescence (fibrin ×530).

C, Goodpasture's syndrome. There is ultralinear continuous glomerular basement membrane (GBM) fluorescence for IgG, with no isolated deposits (IgG ×1400).

D, Membranous glomerulopathy. Nodular epimembranous deposits are visualized along the epithelial aspect of the basement membrane (IgG ×1300).

E, Membranoproliferative glomerulonephritis (type I). C3 is present in a peripheral lobular distribution. Note the absence of fluorescence in the centers (mesangium) of the lobules (C3 ×220).

(*A–E*, From Michael AF, Westberg NG, Fish AJ, Vernier RL. Studies on chronic membranoproliferative glomerulonephritis with hypocomplementemia. J Exp Med 134(Suppl):208s–227s, 1971.)

not thought to have an immune complex–mediated pathogenesis. The presence of immune complexes is of some diagnostic value but of limited value in the management of glomerulonephritis or SLE.

Immune-Related Glomerulonephritis

On the basis of this evidence, a number of forms of human glomerulonephritis can be tentatively classified as immune-related, as described in Table 25–3. It must be remembered that the exact pathogenesis of these diseases is unknown and that a certain license is taken in presenting this classification. The list is by no means inclusive, since there are unusual forms of chronic glomerulonephritis with a presumed immune pathogenesis that cannot be easily categorized. This discussion includes only the more important and easily recognizable forms of glomerulonephritis (Michael, 1984).

ACUTE POSTSTREPTOCOCCAL GLOMERULONEPHRITIS

Acute poststreptococcal glomerulonephritis (AGN) is a form of acute glomerular injury that is a delayed sequela of infection with certain nephritogenic strains of group A β-hemolytic streptococci. Documentation of streptococcal infection (positive throat culture or elevated titers of antibody to certain extracellular antigens such as streptolysin O, DNase B, NADase, hyaluronidase) is a prerequisite for establishing the diagnosis. The urinalysis usually reveals proteinuria, hematuria, and the presence of red blood cell casts. Frequently, after onset of this disease, serum CH_{50} complement titers and C3 levels are markedly depressed. Hypertension, azotemia, and oliguria are usually mild but are severe in a small percentage of patients. AGN is generally a nonprogressive disease in children, leading to complete recovery. Baldwin and colleagues (1974) presented evidence of progressive glomerular sclerosis, hypertension, and decreasing renal function in some patients years after AGN. However, this has not been completely verified by other investigators. Recurrent attacks of this disease occur, with repeated streptococcal infections (Roy et al., 1969; Fish et al., 1970).

Historical Aspects

As early as 1914, Gunn observed that immunologic mechanisms are active in the pathogenesis of AGN,

Table 25–3. Classification of Human Immune-Mediated Glomerulonephritis

---

Immune Complex Disease (proven or presumed)
    Acute poststreptococcal glomerulonephritis
    Glomerulonephritis associated with infections
    Serum-sickness glomerulonephritis
    Lupus erythematosus
    Membranous glomerulopathy
    Membranoproliferative glomerulonephritis types I, II, and III
    Drugs (e.g., gold and penicillamine)
    Rapidly progressive nephritis (certain types)
    Glomerulonephritis associated with cancer
    Focal glomerulitis and vasculitis (e.g., Henoch-Schönlein)
    Cryoglobulinemia
    IgA nephropathy

Anti–Basement Membrane Antibody Nephritis
    Anti–glomerular basement membrane antibody
    Goodpasture's syndrome
    Rapidly progressive nephritis (certain types)
    Anti–tubular basement membrane antibody
    Acute tubulointerstitial nephritis

---

and he described depression of serum complement in four patients with scarlatinal nephritis; this was confirmed by multiple observers during the next 50 years (Fischel and Gajdusek, 1952; Ellis and Walton, 1958; Lange et al., 1960). Immunoglobulins were detected on glomeruli in acute glomerulonephritis by Freedman and coworkers in 1960; this observation was later confirmed by Lachmann and associates (1962). Glomerular deposition of complement (C3) was first described by Lachmann and associates in 1962.

It was observed by electron microscopy that discrete, dense deposits were present on the epithelial side of the GBM associated with AGN. With refinement and improvement of immunofluorescent microscopic techniques, as well as the application of these methods to percutaneous renal biopsy specimens, Michael and coworkers (1966) saw that discrete immunoprotein deposits were a constant feature in this disease (see Fig. 25–3).

Pathogenesis

By immunopathologic analysis, it appears that glomerular injury in AGN may be mediated by soluble immune complexes. The soluble immune complex injury during serum-sickness nephritis in rabbits results in the presence of discrete GBM deposits, a finding similar to that seen in AGN (Fish et al., 1966). The latent period after streptococcal infection to the onset of acute glomerulonephritis in humans is similar to that after antigen administration and the appearance of experimental serum-sickness nephritis. Soluble immune complexes have been detected in the circulation of some patients with AGN (Ooi et al., 1977a; Mohammed et al., 1977; Tung et al., 1978; Verroust et al., 1979). In addition, the characteristic lesions that are the hallmark of soluble immune complex injury are regularly observed, namely, discrete deposits of IgG and C3 on the epithelial side of the GBM (Michael et al., 1966; Burkholder and Bradford, 1969).

By electron microscopy, these deposits are electron-dense and are observed projecting from the epithelial side of the basement membrane. If soluble antigen–antibody complexes localize in the glomerulus, one would expect to find streptococcal antigens present in the deposits. There have been reports (Seegal et al., 1965; Michael et al., 1966; Seligson et al., 1985) of streptococcal antigens within the glomerulus. These findings have been inconsistent, but, when streptococcal products have been detected, their distribution has not paralleled the distribution of IgG and C3 localization (Lange et al., 1983). In situ immune complex formation is an attractive hypothesis to explain immune glomerular injury in AGN; along with the cationic nature of streptococcal antigens, which may fix to the glomerular capillary wall, antibody binding and immune complex formation is possible (Vogt, 1984).

Cellular immunity to GBM antigens (Fillit et al., 1978, 1982, 1984) altered T-cell function (Williams et al., 1981), and glomerular localization of T-helper and -suppressor lymphocytes (Monga et al., 1981; Parra et al., 1984; Nolasco et al., 1987) have been observed in poststreptococcal glomerulonephritis. Altered C3 synthesis and catabolism also have been described (Endre et al., 1984). The presence of streptococcal neuraminidase, which affects serum sialic acid levels and antiglobulin formation, has been noted (Rodriguez-Iturbe et al., 1981; Asami et al., 1985).

Fish and associates (1970) investigated an epidemic of glomerulonephritis involving 27 children with streptococcal pyoderma. The children with the severest symptoms had classical nodular immunoprotein deposits; patients with milder forms of the disease had only focal, interrupted, linear deposition of C3 along the GBM and within the mesangium, and no immune deposits were observed. It was possible to study the whole spectrum of acute glomerulonephritis, including the milder asymptomatic cases. Long-term follow-up studies of epidemic glomerulonephritis have revealed similar findings (Garcia et al., 1981; Potter et al., 1982).

Symptomatic AGN has been associated predominantly with type 12 (throat) and type 49 (skin) β-hemolytic streptococcal infections (Wannamaker, 1967). These organisms have been administered to experimental animals in different forms using various methods of inoculation (Michael et al., 1972a). Although there are some reports of glomerular injury in these experiments, no consistent model is yet available to experimentally induce in humans the lesions observed by immunofluorescent and electron microscopy.

Diagnosis

The diagnosis of AGN is usually established by detecting evidence of streptococcal infection (positive culture or elevated antistreptococcal antibody titers) and by demonstrating depressed complement levels (Rodriguez-Iturbe, 1984), although the latter may not always be present. Percutaneous renal biopsy, in conjunction with the findings gained by light, immunofluorescent, and electron microscopy, is occasionally necessary in atypical clinical situations to establish definitively the diagnosis of an immune complex disease.

Treatment

Only supportive care is recommended in the treatment of AGN. Careful salt and water restriction in the oliguric phases and adequate antihypertensive therapy are essential. The prognosis is excellent, and mortality is low. Occasionally, with severe oliguria and azotemia, dialysis is necessary.

SYSTEMIC LUPUS ERYTHEMATOSUS

Systemic lupus erythematosus (SLE) is a multisystem disease characterized by arthritis, facial rash, and glomerulonephritis (see Chapter 24). Frequently, there is associated cardiac, central nervous system, and pulmonary involvement resulting from vasculitis. Autoimmune hemolytic anemia, leukopenia, and thrombocytopenia are often observed. Antinuclear antibodies and depression of serum complement titers are present. The renal injury is often progressive, ultimately leading to azotemia and hypertension in untreated patients. Corticosteroids and perhaps immunosuppressive therapy effectively suppress the disease. It is doubtful whether SLE of childhood can be completely cured. Exceptions to this rule include patients with drug-induced lupus erythematosus, in which case the disease can be completely controlled by removal of the offending agent.

Historical Aspects

For many years, it has been appreciated that immune mechanisms are active in lupus erythematosus. Low serum complement titers, hyperglobulinemia, an elevated rheumatoid factor, a positive Wassermann test, and Coombs'-positive hemolytic anemia all point to heightened immunologic activity in these patients. In 1957, Mellors and colleagues demonstrated glomerular immunoglobulin deposition by immunofluorescent microscopy. This was followed in 1962 by the observations of Lachmann and colleagues that C3 is also deposited in the glomerulus. Freedman and Markowitz (1962), using citrate buffer at low pH, eluted immunoglobulins from isolated glomeruli obtained from autopsy kidneys of patients with lupus erythematosus and observed that the eluted immunoglobulins possessed antinuclear antibody activity similar to that present in the sera of patients with this disease. By electron microscopy, the glomerular capillary loops in patients with SLE contain electron-dense deposits in the GBM as well as in subendothelial and subepithelial loci. These lesions are similar to the ultrastructural alterations in experimental chronic antigen–antibody complex nephritis (Dixon et al., 1961).

Pathogenesis

The granular and nodular deposition of IgG and C3 within the GBM, glomerular capillary endothelium, and mesangium is a frequent and almost constant feature of SLE, especially in children. From experimental models of nephritis, these lesions are suggestive of an immune complex pathogenesis.

During the acute stage of active lupus erythematosus (before treatment or during exacerbations), serum anti-DNA titers are elevated. Tan and colleagues (1966) observed that during the acute phase of the disease, anti-DNA titers are absent and small amounts of DNA are detectable within the circulation, presumably in the form of a soluble antigen–antibody complex as DNA–anti-DNA in some patients. IgG eluted from lupus glomeruli has immunologic specificity for DNA and nucleoprotein (Krishnan and Kaplan, 1967).

Koffler and associates (1967) provided further evidence of immune complex injury in lupus nephritis by showing that the deposited IgG could be removed from the glomerulus by treating frozen tissue sections with deoxyribonuclease; enzymatic treatment of this nature releases IgG, which is associated with native DNA and single-stranded DNA as an immune complex deposit. Partial elution of IgG in lupus nephritis immune deposits using 2.0-M NaCl uncovered DNA antigen within glomerular deposits in patients when the sections were stained with fluorescein-labeled antibody to DNA. These findings are similar to the observations in SLE-like nephropathy in New Zealand black/New Zealand white (NZB/NZW) mice.

The evidence points strongly toward immune complex injury. The antigen is DNA, of either host or possibly viral origin. Other antigens may play a similar role. Koffler and colleagues (1971) clearly demonstrated the unique specificity of antibody to native DNA in lupus erythematosus; native DNA–anti-native DNA complexes appear to be operative in most patients with the disease. Other autoantibodies to nuclear antigens are present in lupus erythematosus, including anti-Sm antibody, which is elevated and correlates with disease activity (Tan, 1989).

Hanauer and Christian (1967) showed that C1q, a portion of the first component of complement, is regularly depressed in patients with lupus erythematosus. This is in agreement with the findings of Gewurz and others (1968a) that all complement components are depressed in lupus erythematosus since the complement cascade is activated at C1. Agnello and coworkers (1970) took advantage of the known property of C1q binding to aggregated IgG or soluble complexes by reacting serum samples from patients with lupus erythematosus in gel diffusion against purified preparations of C1q and obtained precipitin bands, thereby detecting the presence of circulating immune complexes. Using more refined techniques, immune complexes are regularly detected (Ooi et al., 1977a, 1977b; Woodroffe et al., 1977; Tung et al., 1978).

Electron microscopic studies by several researchers (Kawano et al., 1969; Norton, 1969; Grausz et al., 1970; Pincus, 1982) have drawn attention to the presence of cytoplasmic microtubular elements in glomerular endothelial cells in patients with lupus nephritis. These structures, which resemble virus particles, have been observed in other renal diseases but are more apparent in SLE (Garancis et al., 1971). The role of viruses and their relation to immune complex formation in SLE must await further investigation (Christian, 1982; Pincus, 1982).

In SLE, the production of autoantibodies reflects a generalized polyclonal B-cell expansion. The formation of immune complexes may be secondary to the release of host tissue antigens, such as nuclear components and extranuclear antigens, which combine with autoantibodies; complex localization to the glomerular capillary bed may be due to defective Fc-mediated clearance (Frank et al., 1983; Abrass et al., 1980b). Other factors include the female gender and sex hormone metabolism, familial clustering, and association with complement and IgA deficiencies (Arnett and Shulman, 1976; Lahita et al., 1982; Rynes, 1982; Schwartz, 1981; Reveille et al., 1983). The excessive autoantibody production in SLE appears to be a consequence of defective immunoregulation by T cells. Increased ratios of helper to suppressor T cells (Smolen et al., 1982; Hardin, 1986) and other manifestations of altered cellular immunity are evident (Steinberg, 1984).

Increasing attention is being focused on the roles of autoimmune-mediated vascular thrombosis in patients with SLE. The lupus anticoagulant detected in the sera of these patients was first defined by its ability to prolong the prothrombin time of normal plasma and is now known to be an antiphospholipid (anticardiolipin) autoantibody (Asherson et al., 1985; Alarcon-Segovia et al., 1989). Vascular thrombotic events and complications have also been correlated with the presence of antiphospholipid autoantibodies in patients without evidence of typical SLE (Hughes et al., 1986).

Diagnosis

The diagnosis of lupus erythematosus is established by finding elevated antinuclear antibody titers, especially anti–native DNA (Notman et al., 1975; Synkowski et al., 1980; Morrow et al., 1982; Eaton et al., 1983), and depression of the serum complement level. The presence of leukopenia, thrombocytopenia, Coombs'-positive hemolytic anemia, rheumatoid factor, a positive Wassermann test, and antithyroid antibodies provides confirmatory data. Renal biopsy specimens reveal a wide variety of glomerular lesions, with varying degrees of endothelial and mesangial cell proliferation and basement membrane thickening. Immunofluorescent studies uniformly reveal immunoprotein deposition (Baldwin et al., 1977; Appel et al., 1978; Cameron et al., 1979; Glassock et al., 1981; Morris et al., 1981; Wallace et al., 1982; Schwartz et al., 1989).

Treatment

Successful management of lupus nephritis with resolution and healing of the glomerular lesions can be accomplished with high doses of steroids, often with the addition of immunosuppressive drugs, such as azathioprine (Michael et al., 1967; Ginzler et al., 1975; Fish et al., 1977) or cyclophosphamide (Steinberg et al., 1974; Balow et al., 1984). Intravenous pulse cyclophosphamide has been advocated in patients with SLE to permit reduction in steroid therapy (Austin et al., 1986; Lehman et al., 1989; Boumpas et al., 1992). Aggressive therapy aimed at reversing the abnormal immunologic features of the disease is highly effective during the first two decades of life (Fish et al., 1977; Platt et al., 1982). The presence or absence of renal disease is the most important predictor of long-term survival (Ginzler et al., 1982; Rosner et al., 1982; Magil et al., 1988; Esdaile et al., 1989). When end-stage renal failure develops, patients often experience remission of the disease and then are at low risk for lupus nephropathy in a transplanted kidney.

Although SLE is an incurable disorder, current therapy has improved survival dramatically, which has permitted most young patients to live into adulthood with normal renal function and to safely negotiate childbearing (Houser et al., 1980; Lockshin et al., 1984). The risk of an infant of a mother with lupus erythematosus for development of congenital heart block is correlated with the presence of maternal anti-Ro (SS-A ribonucleoprotein) autoantibodies (Scott et al., 1983). Long-term survival in adults is limited by the increased risk of atherosclerotic cardiovascular disease. Intravenous pulse cyclophosphamide has been advocated in patients with SLE to permit reduction in steroid therapy (Austin et al., 1986; Lehman et al., 1989; Boumpas et al., 1992).

GLOMERULONEPHRITIS ASSOCIATED WITH INFECTION

Glomerulonephritis may appear as a concomitant of systemic infection, associated with hypocomplementemia. In some infections, an acute form of nephritis develops; in other infections, a picture similar to chronic glomerulonephritis with nephrotic syndrome is seen (Table 25–4) (Kim and Michael, 1978a, 1978b).

Historical Aspects and Etiology

The development of diffuse glomerulonephritis in patients with subacute bacterial endocarditis was recognized for many years, especially in the pre-antibiotic era. The demonstration of hypocomplementemia and immune reactants in the glomeruli of these patients suggested an immune pathogenesis rather than simple bacterial embolization (Williams and Kunkel, 1962; Cordeiro et al., 1965; Tu et al., 1969).

Significant glomerulonephritis has been described associated with *Staphylococcus albus* infections of the subarachnoid–jugular shunt (Black et al., 1965; Stickler et al., 1968; Dobrin et al., 1975a); staphylococcal and pneumococcal bacteremia (Michael et al., 1972a; Boul-

ton-Jones et al., 1986; Bayer and Theofilopoulos, 1990; Rodriguez-Garcia et al., 1990); intra-abdominal bacterial sepsis (Beaufils, 1981; Andrews et al., 1989); osteomyelitis (Boonshaft et al., 1970); malaria (Kibukamusoke et al., 1967); and syphilis (Falls et al., 1965; Braunstein et al., 1970).

Hypocomplementemia has been seen, especially in patients with associated bacterial infections. Rheumatoid factor, cryoglobulinemia, and circulating immune complexes containing bacterial antigens have been observed in bacterial endocarditis (Inman et al., 1982) and in infected ventricular shunts (Schena et al., 1983; Narchi et al., 1988). Immunopathologic studies have demonstrated immunoglobulin, C3, and properdin in glomeruli and, in the case of malaria, malarial antigens. The morphology of the glomeruli may resemble that of either an acute diffuse proliferative glomerulonephritis or a chronic membranoproliferative glomerulonephritis.

It is likely that this syndrome is caused by antigen–antibody complexes, although this has not been proven. Any infection that is of sufficiently low pathogenicity not to kill the host, but that readily presents its organism or antigens to the circulation over a long enough period, may have the potential to cause glomerulonephritis. The various bacterial infections associated with glomerulonephritis are presented in Table 25–4.

The concurrence of joint disease, vasculitis, and alteration in serum C3 in certain instances of HBsAg-positive hepatitis suggests that complexes may be an important mediator of vascular injury in certain viral

Table 25–4. Bacterial Infection and Nephritis

Clinical Condition	Renal Pathology	Infectious Agents
Endocarditis	Proliferative glomerulonephritis	*Streptococcus* viridans *Staphylococcus aureus* Enterococcus Pneumococcus *Haemophilus influenzae* Gonococcus *Bacteroides* *Brucella suis* *Propionibacterium acnes*
Infected ventriculoatrial shunt	Membranoproliferative glomerulonephritis	*Staphylococcus albus* *Corynebacterium bovis* *Staphylococcus aureus* *Listeria monocytogenes*
Syphilis (congenital and acquired)	Proliferative glomerulonephritis	*Treponema pallidum*
Typhoid fever	Mesangioproliferative glomerulonephritis Interstitial nephritis	*Salmonella typhi*
Leprosy	Proliferative glomerulonephritis	*Mycobacterium leprae*
Tuberculosis	Proliferative glomerulonephritis	*Mycobacterium tuberculosis*
Osteomyelitis	Membranoproliferative glomerulonephritis	*Staphylococcus aureus*
Abdominal abscess	Membranoproliferative glomerulonephritis	*Staphylococcus aureus* *Moraxella alcaligens*
	Focal proliferative glomerulonephritis	*Pseudomonas aeruginosa* *Escherichia coli*
	Extracapillary glomerulonephritis	*Proteus mirabilis*
Pneumonia	Membranoproliferative glomerulonephritis	Pneumococcus

From Kim Y, Michael AF. Chronic bacteremia and nephritis. Annu Rev Med 29:319–325, 1978.

diseases (Gocke et al., 1970; Combes et al., 1971; Onion et al., 1971; Prince and Trepo, 1971).

The renal disease occurring in association with infectious mononucleosis is usually interstitial nephritis rather than glomerulonephritis (Woodroffe et al., 1974).

Diagnosis

The important diagnostic feature is the demonstration of infection in a patient with clinical evidence of glomerulonephritis. The syndrome can take two forms. In some patients, the renal disease resembles acute poststreptococcal nephritis, with a sudden onset of hematuria, proteinuria, cylindruria, and hypertension. This is often associated with a bacterial infection.

Histologic studies reveal a diffuse proliferative glomerulonephritis. In other patients, the clinical picture resembles that of chronic glomerulonephritis or nephrotic syndrome. This has been described in chronic subarachnoid–jugular shunt infection, malaria, and congenital and acquired syphilis.

Pathologic studies often demonstrate a membranoproliferative glomerulonephritis or focal mesangial proliferation. Immunoglobulin and C3 can also be demonstrated in the glomeruli in both types of the syndrome along with dense immune deposits by electron microscopy. A thorough search for infection should be made in every patient with glomerulonephritis. Determination of serum complement or C3 levels can also be helpful.

Treatment

Eradication of the infection is often associated with spontaneous improvement. This is especially true if mild glomerulitis is present, whereas more severe glomerular injury may not be reversible.

MEMBRANOPROLIFERATIVE GLOMERULONEPHRITIS

Membranoproliferative glomerulonephritis (MPGN) with hypocomplementemia, also called mesangiocapillary glomerulonephritis, is a syndrome with distinct clinical, pathologic, and immunologic features (Table 25–5) (Herdman et al., 1970; Michael et al., 1971; Habib et al., 1973a; Peters et al., 1973; Cameron et al., 1983; Yoshikawa et al., 1988; McEnery, 1990). Three forms of MPGN are recognized: types I, II, and III (West, 1992).

Historical Aspects

The initial descriptions of MPGN with hypocomplementemia as an entity were made in 1965 (Gotoff et al., 1965; West et al., 1965). The histologic appearance of the kidney was previously described as lobular glomerulonephritis, mixed membranous and proliferative nephritis, mesangiocapillary glomerulonephritis, and latent chronic glomerulonephritis. In some studies,

Table 25–5. Summary of Clinical, Pathologic, and Immunologic Features of Type I and Type II (Dense-Deposit Disease) Membranoproliferative Glomerulonephritis

Clinical Presentation
  Onset usually between 4 and 30 years of age
  Asymptomatic proteinuria and hematuria
  Nephrotic syndrome
  Gross hematuria or acute nephritis syndrome
  Variably progressive; hypertension frequent
  Moderate to poor selectivity of proteinuria
  Association of partial lipodystrophy and type II

Pathology
  Both types I and II show mesangial proliferation, increased matrix, glomerular lobulation, and enlargement
  Type I—interposition of mesangial fibrils and cytoplasm between endothelium and GBM (splitting); endothelial- and GBM-oriented immune deposits
  Type II—electron-dense linear deposits (nonimmune) within the GBM and TBM. In addition, immune deposits are present as in type I.

Immunology
  Type I—capillary loop immune deposits of C3 and properdin and usually IgG and IgM; peripheral lobular distribution
  Type II—basement membrane electron-dense deposits do not contain immunoglobulin or complement components. C3 outlines the dense deposits in GBM (railroad tracks) and mesangium (rings).

Complement and Plasma Factors
  Type I—often decrease in C3 and variable decrease in C1 and C4
  Type II—usual decrease in C3; early components (C1, C2, and C4) often normal; C3NeF (autoantibody to C3bBb) usually present

Abbreviation: GBM = glomerular basement membrane; TBM = tubular basement membrane.

this morphology was depicted as being related to acute poststreptococcal glomerulonephritis and latent chronic glomerulonephritis. However, this syndrome is quite distinct from AGN, although it may mimic it morphologically.

Earlier studies demonstrated relatively normal concentrations of C1, C2, and C4 in the presence of reduced levels of C3 (Gewurz et al., 1968a) and revealed evidence of in vivo breakdown of C3 to C3d (West et al., 1967). The presence of a factor in the patient's serum, the C3 nephritic factor (C3NeF), was also described and partially characterized (Spitzer et al., 1969; Vallota et al., 1970, 1971). A similar factor was also found in the sera of some patients with partial lipodystrophy, some of whom have MPGN (Peters et al., 1973). The reason for the association of C3NeF, MPGN, and partial lipodystrophy is unknown. It has been suggested that the hypocomplementemia may be the primary defect predisposing to chronic low-grade infection with chronic immune complex formation and deposition. C3NeF has been characterized as a 7S globulin (Schreiber et al., 1976) and shown to be an autoantibody to C3bBb, the alternative pathway convertase (Daha et al., 1978).

The uniform demonstration of C3 and properdin in the glomeruli, most frequently in a peripheral lobular distribution, has been described; immunoglobulins and early complement components (C1q and C4) are found less frequently (see Fig. 25-3) (Michael et al., 1969, 1971; Herdman et al., 1970; Westberg et al., 1971).

Clinical Features

Two or three distinct types of MPGN are recognized; the similarities and differences are outlined in Table 25-5. Approximately 75% of patients have type I MPGN, and the remainder have either type II, also called *dense-deposit disease*, or type III MPGN, which is the least common.

Type I MPGN

Type I MPGN is characterized morphologically by GBM thickening, mesangial proliferation, apparent splitting of the basement membrane due to interposition of mesangial cell cytoplasm between the GBM and the endothelium, and immune deposits along the endothelial aspect of the glomerular capillary. Immunofluorescent studies of the kidney reveal granular deposits of C3 and properdin along the endothelial region of the GBM; earlier complement components, IgM, and IgG are found less frequently (Bannister et al., 1983). Serologically, there is often a reduction in whole complement components; C3NeF is usually not present.

Type II MPGN

Type II MPGN was initially recognized by electron microscopic studies of the kidney (Berger and Galle, 1963; Antoine and Faye, 1972; Habib et al., 1973a, 1974). Morphologically, electron-dense alteration of the GBM, tubular basement membrane, and glomerular afferent arteriolar walls is present. Immunofluorescent studies do not reveal any immunoglobulin or complement components within the nonimmune electron-dense deposit, although C3 can be seen adjacent to the dense material in the GBM ("railroad track") and mesangium ("mesangial ring") (Kim et al., 1977). Immune deposits containing C3 and Ig can also be observed but are less intense than in type I. Serologically, these patients usually have reduced complement (CH_{50}) and C3, with relatively normal early complement components. C3NeF, an autoantibody to the alternative pathway convertase, C3bBb, is usually present (Daha et al., 1979). This syndrome is often associated with partial lipodystrophy. Recurrence of dense-deposit disease in the transplanted kidney has been well documented (Zimmerman et al., 1974; Galle and Mahieu, 1975; Mathew et al., 1975; McCoy et al., 1975; McLean et al., 1976). Low levels of C3NeF may be associated with a better prognosis (Klein et al., 1983), although C3NeF did not correlate with the risk of recurrence in the transplanted kidney (Leibowitch et al., 1979). Other nephritic factors that are autoantibodies to alternative and classical pathway complements have also been characterized (Tanuma et al., 1990; West, 1992).

Type III MPGN

An additional variety of MPGN (type III) has been described and has certain unique characteristic morphologic features (Strife et al., 1977). Typically, type III shows the basic features of type I with increased immune complex deposits.

Pathogenesis

Whether type I or II disease is a result of antigen–antibody complexes has not been settled, although immune complexes have been found in the sera of some patients (Ooi, 1977a; Woodroffe et al., 1977; Davis et al., 1981). Histologically, similar features have been seen in certain instances of MPGN associated with bacterial infection (see earlier), and it is possible that an infection due to an undefined agent is responsible for the immunologic features in MPGN and that a unique type of immune complex is involved. MPGN has been found in individuals with various inherited complement component deficiencies (Coleman et al., 1983). A B-cell alloantigen has been described in patients with type I MPGN, suggesting linkage to the major histocompatibility locus—and possibly implicating an association with unique immune responses (Friend et al., 1977). The cause of the GBM dense-deposit alteration in type II MPGN is unknown, but it may be a consequence of an alteration in GBM metabolism. Whether this is caused by a highly specific and unique immune injury that leads to alternative pathway activation is unknown.

Diagnosis

In most circumstances, patients with MPGN present clinically with proteinuria, nephrotic syndrome, or an acute nephritic picture, often with hematuria and hypertension (more frequent in type II). Laboratory studies reveal moderate to marked proteinuria with microscopic hematuria and pyuria; the glomerular filtration rate is normal or reduced. Features of mild nephrotic syndrome (hypoalbuminemia and hypercholesterolemia) may also be present. The serum levels of CH_{50} and C3 are usually reduced, especially in children (Ooi et al., 1976; Cameron et al., 1983; Watson et al., 1984; Varade et al., 1990). Both classical and alternate pathways of complement activation in MPGN are evident, although the latter is predominant. C3NeF activity may be demonstrated, usually in type II disease (Schena et al., 1982), and uniformly results in hypocomplementemia. However, patients with type I MPGN may have normal complement values, especially adults, and hypocomplementemia is not an essential criterion for the diagnosis. Sequential studies have demonstrated a subsequent fall in the complement level in some patients in whom initial values were normal, as well as an increase to normal in other patients in whom initial values were low (Cameron et al., 1970).

Treatment

No proven therapy exists, but various regimens (e.g., prednisone, prednisone and azathioprine, and cyclophosphamide and anticoagulants) have been used. The reader is referred to reviews of this information by Donadio and Offord (1989) and Donadio (1993). Evidence suggests that alternate-day prednisone therapy may help some patients (McEnery et al., 1986; Ford et al., 1992).

Complications and Prognosis

MPGN is usually progressive, with renal insufficiency developing most commonly in patients with type II disease within 4 or 5 years; there may be less activity in type I MPGN over a longer period. Recurrence of both types of MPGN in transplanted kidneys has been described (McCoy et al., 1975; Cameron et al., 1983).

MEMBRANOUS GLOMERULOPATHY

Historical Aspects

Early studies of membranous glomerulopathy defined this condition in patients with nephrotic syndrome. Diffuse thickening of the GBM was seen by light microscopy without significant cellular proliferation. Milder cases of this condition could not be differentiated from nil lesion nephrotic syndrome. With the advent of silver staining and electron microscopy, the characteristic diffuse spike projections of the GBM lamina densa provided a unique finding for the diagnosis of this condition. By immunofluorescence, epimembranous immune deposits were observed between the GBM spike lesions.

Pathogenesis

Membranous glomerulopathy is a relatively rare syndrome in children in which proteinuria and the nephrotic syndrome are associated with a characteristic glomerular histology (Habib et al., 1973b; Olbing et al., 1973; Latham et al., 1982). Numerous epimembranous deposits of immunoglobulin and C3 are present along the epithelial surface of the GBM, which becomes progressively thickened. Little or no glomerular proliferation is present. The micronodular immune deposits are similar to those seen in an experimental form of antigen–antibody complex nephritis called *Heymann's autologous immune complex disease* (see earlier, Antigen–Antibody Complex Nephritis). Studies of membranous glomerulopathy have not detected the gp330 antigen of the Heymann model in human glomerular lesions (Collins et al., 1981). The GBM spike lesions are derived from the lamina densa as defined by the presence of laminin (Fukatsu et al., 1988), entactin (Katz et al., 1991), and novel type IV collagen (Kim et al., 1991) in these structures.

Diagnosis

The diagnosis of membranous glomerulopathy should be suspected in any patient with persistent proteinuria or nephrotic syndrome, especially if either appears in adolescence or late childhood. Rarely, hematuria is observed. The serum complement is normal. The diagnosis is made by light and immunofluorescent microscopy (Donadio et al., 1988). This clinical and pathologic syndrome can also be associated with renal vein thrombosis. Although in the past renal venous occlusion was considered a cause of nephrotic syndrome, it is probable that in most instances the immune complex injury was responsible for the proteinuria and antedated the venous occlusion. Lupus erythematosus may on occasion produce a similar lesion and must be excluded.

The following systemic disorders have been associated with membranous glomerulopathy: hepatitis B antigenemia, syphilis, malaria (Allison et al., 1969), lymphoma, leukemia, and sickle cell anemia (Kleinknecht et al., 1979). Membranous glomerulopathy has also been associated with therapy in patients receiving gold salts, penicillamine, and captopril. The reader is referred to a comprehensive review of the multiple causes of this condition (Coggins, 1993).

Prognosis

The prognosis of the patient with membranous glomerulopathy is variable, with reversal of the nephrotic syndrome in some patients, although the GBM remains thickened. In other patients, progressive glomerular destruction occurs. There is no known effective therapy.

ANTI–BASEMENT MEMBRANE NEPHRITIS (Goodpasture's Syndrome)

Anti–glomerular basement membrane (anti-GBM) nephritis is most common in men; however, occasional cases have been observed in older children. It frequently leads to irreversible renal failure, although recovery with immunosuppressive therapy and plasmapheresis may occur. Goodpasture's syndrome (pulmonary hemorrhage and glomerulonephritis) is mediated by circulating anti-GBM antibodies, which are the cause of progressive glomerular injury and, in some patients, pulmonary hemorrhage. Anti-GBM nephritis can occur in the absence of lung hemorrhage.

Historical Aspects

The immunopathologic lesion characteristic of Goodpasture's syndrome consists of diffuse linear deposition of IgG and C3 along with GBM (Duncan et al., 1965; Michael et al., 1966). The distribution and nature of immunoprotein disposition in the glomerulus are similar to those observed in experimental anti-GBM or nephrotoxic nephritis. Deposition of IgG and C3 along the alveolar capillary basement membranes has been demonstrated in some patients (Beirne et al., 1968; Koffler et al., 1969); the antibody eluted from lung tissue showed specificity for lung and GBM.

Lerner and coworkers (1967) removed the deposited immunoglobulin from glomeruli in autopsy kidneys from patients with Goodpasture's syndrome by treatment with low pH citrate buffer. The immunoglobulin eluted in this manner was shown to have anti-GBM antibody activity by overlaying the eluates on normal kidney sections and demonstrating fixation of antibody to GBM. When examined by immunofluorescent microscopy, the eluted Goodpasture antibody was shown to fix not only to GBM but also to Bowman's capsule and tubular basement membranes. When the eluted antibody was administered intravenously to squirrel monkeys, proteinuria and proliferative nephritis with progressive uremia developed immediately, and the animals died in 2 weeks. Immunofluorescent analysis of the diseased kidneys in these animals showed the same linear distribution along the GBM as seen in patients with Goodpasture's syndrome. These investigations provided strong evidence that anti-GBM glomerulonephritis is an autoimmune disease mediated by antibody interaction with host GBM.

Pathogenesis

In most instances, Goodpasture's syndrome is a one-pulse injury because anti-GBM antibodies disappear from the circulation over time. The diagnosis of Goodpasture's syndrome should be suspected in any patient with rapidly progressive glomerulonephritis or with hemoptysis and radiologic evidence of progressive pulmonary infiltration associated with glomerulonephritis and renal failure. Serum complement levels are always normal. Immunofluorescent analysis of percutaneous renal biopsy material showing diffuse linear deposition of IgG and, less frequently, C3 along the GBM provides strong evidence in support of this diagnosis (see Fig. 25–3). Circulating anti-GBM antibodies are present in the serum and can be detected by indirect immunofluorescent methods on sections of normal human kidney. The latter is an insensitive method in contrast to radioimmunoassays (Mahieu and Winand, 1973; Wilson, 1980) or enzyme-linked immunosorbent assays (ELISAs) (Wheeler and Sussman, 1981; Wieslander et al., 1983; Fish et al., 1985).

Collagenase digestion of isolated GBM preparations releases Goodpasture antigen (Marquardt et al., 1973). Western blotting of collagenase digests reveals that Goodpasture antibodies are reactive with 54- and 28-kd proteins (Fish et al., 1984; Wieslander et al., 1984a). These components are derived from the carboxy-terminal noncollagenous (NC domain) propeptides of the alpha-3 type IV collagen chain (Wieslander et al., 1984a, 1984; Butkowski et al., 1985; Yoshioka et al., 1985; Kleppel et al., 1986). This work led to the specific characterization of the alpha-3 type IV collagen chain as a component of the GBM lamina densa (Butkowski et al., 1989, 1990a; Hudson et al., 1989). The alpha-3 chain, along with the alpha-4 and alpha-5 type IV collagen (novel) chains has been cloned and found to have unique cDNA sequences (Morrison et al, 1991; Turner et al., 1992; Kashtan and Michael, 1993). The novel alpha type IV collagen chains have a specialized organization and network within the GBM lamina densa; these chains differ in composition from classic alpha-1 and alpha-2 type IV collagen in the lamina rara interna (Butkowski et al., 1989; Kleppel et al., 1992).

Patients with Alport's syndrome, or familial nephritis, have reduced detectable Goodpasture antigen or alpha-3 type IV collagen (McCoy et al., 1975), and some of these patients develop anti-GBM antibodies after renal transplantation (Olson et al., 1980; Jeraj et al., 1983). These antibodies are directed against the NC1 domain of the alpha-5 type IV collagen chain (Kleppel et al., 1992). These studies have led to cloning of the COL4A5 alpha-5 type IV collagen gene defects in different families with Alport's syndrome (Reeders, 1992; Kashtan and Michael, 1993; Nomura et al., 1993; Tryggvason et al., 1993; Zhou et al., 1993; Ding et al., 1994).

Treatment

Patients with Goodpasture's syndrome are successfully treated with cyclophosphamide alone or together with azathioprine and plasma exchange (Peters et al., 1982; Simpson et al., 1982; Johnson et al., 1985; Walker et al., 1985; Turner et al., 1993). If it is necessary to remove the kidneys, transplantation should not be done until circulating anti-GBM antibodies have disappeared from the circulation.

HENOCH-SCHÖNLEIN PURPURA NEPHRITIS (Anaphylactoid Purpura)

Henoch-Schönlein purpura (HSP) is a disorder characterized by vasculitis of the small vessels, producing a purpuric rash of the extremities and buttocks, often accompanied by arthritis or arthralgia, gastrointestinal pain and bleeding, and glomerular disease. The syndrome predominates in the 2- to 15-year age group and in males over females by nearly a 2:1 ratio (see Chapters 14, 21, and 24).

When renal involvement occurs, it follows the other symptoms within 4 to 8 weeks of onset of illness. Although microscopic hematuria is reported to be present in all children with HSP (Meadow et al., 1972), 20% to 30% have macroscopic hematuria, and 30% to 70% have proteinuria or hematuria lasting longer than 1 week (Meadow, 1978; Farine et al., 1986; Walker et al., 1986). Acute nephritis, hypertension, and nephrotic syndrome are occasionally present. Chronic renal disease and insufficiency develop in 2% of patients with HSP (Koskimies et al., 1981), but end-stage HSP nephritis accounts for 5% to 10% of patients who enter pediatric dialysis programs.

Although a few children with HSP nephritis have histologically normal glomeruli, the typical lesion by light microscopy consists of focal, segmental, or diffuse mesangial proliferation. Mesangial proliferation may be accompanied by a focal, segmental endocapillary or extracapillary glomerulonephritis with monocyte infiltration (Yoshioka et al., 1989), sclerosis, adhesions, and crescents. The severity of mesangial proliferation and crescent formation correlates with the clinical picture at time of biopsy. Immunofluorescent studies (Urizar et al., 1968; Vernier et al., 1971) have demonstrated that fibrin and IgA are consistently deposited while IgG, IgM, and C3 are more variably observed in the glomerular mesangium. Immunoglobulin and fibrin deposits can also occur in the peripheral capillary in clinically severe disease.

Electron microscopy reveals dense deposits in the mesangium and occasionally in the subendothelium and subepithelium. The latter deposits, as well as "lead shot" microparticles in the mesangial matrix, have been associated with severe clinical disease and outcome (Yoshikawa et al., 1981).

Skin histologic findings usually demonstrate pronounced leukocytic perivascular infiltrates, microthromboses containing leukocytes and platelets (Vernier et al., 1961), and granular IgA and C3 deposits of the dermal capillaries (Baart de la Faille-Kuyper et al., 1976).

Diagnosis

There are no specific laboratory tests to make a conclusive diagnosis of HSP. The history and physical findings of a characteristic purpuric eruption usually establish the diagnosis. However, in older patients with atypical rashes and nephritis, it is important to exclude SLE and acute postinfectious glomerulonephritis with complement levels and appropriate serologic studies. Complement and C3 levels in patients with HSP are normal or high. Renal biopsy provides confirmatory evidence, although the light and immunofluorescent microscopic findings of HSP may be present in other forms of glomerulonephritis.

Pathogenesis

Although the precise immunologic mechanisms involved in HSP are unknown, the presence of elevated serum IgA levels and circulating immune complexes containing IgA during the initial or active phase of disease (Coppo et al., 1982) suggests that deposition of immune complexes is responsible for the skin and renal abnormalities. Activation of the alternate complement pathway by IgA immune complexes (as suggested by the presence of C3 or properdin and the absence of C1q or C4 by immunofluorescence) may be responsible for renal injury; IgG and IgM immune complexes and classic complement activation may occur in later stages of the disease (Kauffmann et al., 1980). Because IgA has both humoral and mucosal origins, there is considerable controversy about the predominant subclass (IgA1 or IgA2) and molecular size of IgA in the immune complexes and mesangial deposits (André et al., 1980; Conley et al., 1980). The seasonal occurrence of HSP during late winter and the occurrence of a preceding upper respiratory infection in 80% of cases have led to the speculation that the IgA immune complexes result from a mucosal defect of antigen exclusion or processing (Cameron, 1979; Habib and Cameron, 1982).

There is considerable interest in the immunologic and histologic features shared by patients with HSP nephritis and IgA nephropathy. These two conditions

have occurred simultaneously after adenovirus infection in HLA-identical twin boys (Meadow and Scott, 1985). Some have proposed that HSP is the systemic form of IgA nephropathy (Nakamoto et al., 1978).

Prognosis

The prognosis for most children with HSP nephritis is excellent, but clinical features that suggest chronic renal disease or insufficiency include recurrent purpuric episodes, nephrotic syndrome, and presentation with acute nephritis, particularly if a combined nephritic-nephrotic state is present. Histologic features that suggest an unfavorable outcome are crescent formation in more than 50% of the glomeruli and the presence of subepithelial dense deposits by electron microscopy. Because some children with severe disease undergo complete remission and some children with mild disease initially progress to severe renal involvement (Bunchman et al., 1988; Peratoner et al., 1990; Goldstein et al., 1992), however, none of these indicators is completely reliable.

Treatment

Supportive care, including salt restriction, diuretic therapy, and antihypertensive therapy, is indicated in rare patients with hypertension and edema. In patients with progressive deterioration or an unfavorable histologic pattern on biopsy (>50% crescentic glomeruli), a trial of therapy is probably warranted. In noncontrolled studies, some observers have reported a beneficial effect from prednisone and azathioprine. Anticoagulation therapy and plasmapheresis have also been used despite the risks of hemorrhage or infectious complications.

Patients with end-stage renal disease have undergone successful renal transplantation. Recurrence of HSP nephritis in the graft has been reported in only 3 of more than 100 patients worldwide. Asymptomatic recurrence of mesangial IgA deposits has been observed in seven of nine patients who underwent biopsy after transplantation (Habib and Cameron, 1982).

VASCULITIS

Uncommon in childhood, vasculitis encompasses a spectrum of conditions characterized by inflammation of blood vessel walls. Kidney involvement is frequently present in affected patients and commonly is described as a pauci-immune necrotizing crescentic glomerulonephritis. Three vasculitic syndromes with significant renal involvement occur in childhood: Wegener's granulomatosis, microscopic polyarteritis nodosa, and idiopathic crescentic glomerulonephritis. Classification of these forms of vasculitis is confusing, since there is considerable overlap in clinical symptoms and histopathologic findings. However, the discovery of antineutrophil cytoplasmic autoantibodies (ANCAs) offers a new approach to understanding the vasculitic syndromes of childhood, an approach in which these vasculitides are viewed as a continuum of disease rather than as distinct disease entities (see Chapter 24).

Clinical Features

Wegener's Granulomatosis

Although involvement of nearly all organ systems has been described, Wegener's granulomatosis has traditionally been defined as a necrotizing, granulomatous inflammatory process of small to medium-sized vessels in the upper respiratory tract, the lungs, and the kidneys. Upper respiratory tract symptoms include epistaxis, sinusitis, and rhinorrhea, whereas lower respiratory tract involvement is characterized by cough, dyspnea, hemoptysis, chest pain, and pulmonary infiltrates (see Chapters 22 and 24). Glomerulonephritis, ranging clinically from minimal renal dysfunction to severe rapidly progressive irreversible renal failure, is reported in 61% of cases of Wegener's granulomatosis in childhood, although only a minority of children (9%) have renal involvement at presentation (Rottem et al., 1993). Typical renal histopathology is a pauci-immune necrotizing crescentic glomerulonephritis, frequently associated with granuloma formation.

Microscopic Polyarteritis Nodosa

Microscopic polyarteritis nodosa is a necrotizing vasculitis of small and medium-sized arteries that is occasionally seen in children but predominantly affects middle-aged adults (see Chapter 24). A retrospective analysis of 31 children with polyarteritis nodosa describes multisystem involvement and defines involvement of the kidney and musculoskeletal system as major criteria of this disease (Ozen et al., 1992). Minor criteria include cutaneous findings, gastrointestinal disturbances, peripheral neuropathy, central nervous system disease, hypertension, cardiac involvement, lung involvement, constitutional symptoms, elevation of acute-phase reactants, and presence of HbsAg in some patients. Renal involvement is reported in 65% of patients and ranges from isolated proteinuria, hematuria and proteinuria, and nephrotic syndrome with hematuria, to rapidly progressive glomerulonephritis. As in Wegener's granulomatosis, renal histopathology reveals a pauci-immune necrotizing crescentic glomerulonephritis.

Idiopathic Crescentic Glomerulonephritis

Idiopathic crescentic glomerulonephritis is a vasculitis of small to medium-sized vessels that is confined to the kidney and that results in the clinical syndrome of rapidly progressive glomerulonephritis in the absence of systemic signs and symptoms. As in Wegener's granulomatosis and microscopic polyarteritis nodosa, renal histopathology reveals a pauci-immune glomerulonephritis.

Pathogenesis

Although each of the previously described vasculitic syndromes has traditionally been recognized as a dis-

tinct disease process, the recent association of ANCA as a serologic marker of vasculitis allows recognition of these illnesses as related processes on a pathologic continuum. ANCAs are autoantibodies directed toward cytoplasmic components of neutrophil primary granules and monocyte lysosomes (Jennette and Falk, 1990). Of patients with pauci-immune crescentic glomerulonephritis, 80% have positive ANCAs; 70% of these patients have systemic involvement (i.e., Wegener's granulomatosis or microscopic polyarteritis nodosa), and 30% have idiopathic crescentic glomerulonephritis (Jennette and Falk, 1990).

Two distinct classes of ANCAs are defined by indirect immunofluorescence staining patterns on alcohol-fixed neutrophils. P-ANCAs are characterized by artifactual perinuclear (P) staining, whereas C-ANCAs demonstrate cytoplasmic (C) staining. Although both P-ANCAs and C-ANCAs can have multiple specificities for neutrophil and monocyte antigens, 90% of P-ANCAs have specificity for myeloperoxidase and most C-ANCAs are specific for proteinase 3 (Jennette and Falk, 1990). The pattern of ANCA staining correlates to a degree with the distribution of vascular injury. Of 23 patients with idiopathic crescentic glomerulonephritis, in which renal disease occurs in the absence of systemic involvement, 83% had P-ANCAs and only 17% had C-ANCAs. On the other hand, C-ANCAs are present in more than 90% of patients with untreated classically defined Wegener's granulomatosis in which pauci-immune crescentic glomerulonephritis is accompanied by lung and sinus disease. P-ANCAs and C-ANCAs are seen in nearly equal frequency in patients with non-Wegener's systemic vasculitis (i.e., microscopic polyarteritis nodosa) (Jennette et al., 1989; Jennette and Falk, 1990).

ANCAs not only are a serologic marker of vasculitis but also are implicated in the pathogenesis of disease. Falk and associates (1990a, 1990b) proposed that ANCAs recognize cytoplasmic antigens that have been presented to the neutrophil cell surface in response to cytokine-mediated "priming." The resulting neutrophil respiratory burst releases toxic reactive oxygen species and lytic cellular enzymes that damage the vascular endothelial cell (Falk et al., 1990b). Indeed, ANCAs have been shown to damage human endothelial cells in vitro after priming with cytokines and endotoxin (Ewert et al., 1992).

In ANCA-positive glomerulonephritis, the most frequent renal histopathology is a pauci-immune necrotizing crescentic glomerulonephritis, identical to that previously described in Wegener's granulomatosis, polyarteritis nodosa, and idiopathic crescentic glomerulonephritis. Immunofluorescent and electron microscopic studies demonstrate absent deposition of immunoproteins; periglomerular granulomatous response to injury is occasionally present, and necrotizing arteritis is demonstrable in a minority (12%) of renal biopsy specimens.

Treatment

The optimal therapy for the three vasculitic syndromes described here and for ANCA-positive pauci-immune necrotizing crescentic glomerulonephritis has not been well established. The use of cyclophosphamide in conjunction with corticosteroids has been effective in inducing remission in Wegener's granulomatosis (Hoffman et al., 1990, 1992), systemic necrotizing vasculitis (Fauci et al., 1979), and idiopathic crescentic glomerulonephritis (Kunis et al., 1992). Although both therapies have been used in the treatment of renal vasculitis, there is evidence for the superior efficacy of pulse intravenous methylprednisolone therapy over oral corticosteroids (Bolton et al., 1989). Oral and intravenous cyclophosphamide are equally efficacious in association with treatment with oral corticosteroids (Falk et al., 1990a). Present treatment regimens advise the concurrent use of corticosteroids, either oral or intravenous, and a cytotoxic agent, most commonly cyclophosphamide. Data using this approach document a greater than 70% 2-year patient and renal survival rate in those with ANCA-positive glomerulonephritis with and without systemic involvement (Jennette and Falk, 1990).

Several other modes of treatment have been used to manage renal vasculitis. Intravenous immunoglobulin administration was successful in inducing remission in patients resistant to standard therapy (Jayne et al., 1991, 1993; Tuso et al., 1992). A controlled multicenter study failed to show additional benefit from the addition of plasmapheresis to conventional immunosuppressant therapy (Glöckner et al., 1988). Renal transplantation is successful in patients with ANCA-associated pauci-immune crescentic necrotizing glomerulonephritis (Montalbert et al., 1980; Morin et al., 1993), although recurrence of the original disease in the allograft is reported (Oberhuber et al., 1988; Jacquot et al., 1990).

IgA NEPHROPATHY (Berger's Disease)

IgA nephropathy, first described by Berger, is a distinct primary glomerular disorder characterized by the presence of mesangial deposits of IgA under immunofluorescent microscopy (Berger, 1969). In addition to renal biopsy, clinical and laboratory exclusion of SLE, anaphylactoid purpura, and cirrhosis are required for diagnosis, since similarly intense glomerular deposition of IgA can be exhibited in these diseases.

Although its peak incidence is in the second and third decades, IgA nephropathy has been identified in younger children undergoing biopsy for asymptomatic hematuria (Michalk et al., 1980). Males are more frequently affected by a nearly 3:1 ratio.

Clinical Features

The most common presenting clinical manifestation of IgA nephropathy in childhood is recurrent macroscopic hematuria often preceded by an upper respiratory infection (Levy et al., 1973; Michalk et al., 1980). Between episodes of gross hematuria, urinalysis may be normal but patients usually show intermittent or persistent microhematuria or proteinuria. Less commonly, patients with IgA nephropathy present with isolated microhematuria and heavy proteinuria, or nephrotic syndrome, renal insufficiency, or hypertension. These latter symptoms are more common in adults (D'Amico et al., 1985; D'Amico, 1987). Loin pain may also accompany macroscopic hematuria in adults (Kincaid-Smith and Nicholls, 1983).

The immunofluorescent hallmark of IgA nephropathy is granular deposition of IgA and, less frequently, C3. There is variable staining for IgG, IgM, fibrin, and properdin, but C1q and C4 are rarely present. IgA deposition may extend to the peripheral capillary in severe disease (Waldherr et al., 1984). Light microscopy reveals a spectrum of histologic change (Sinniah et al., 1981), including the following:

- Normal glomeruli
- Mild and focal increase in mesangial matrix and cellularity
- Focal and segmental mesangial proliferation and glomerulonephritis (with segmental sclerosis and fibrinoid necrosis)
- Diffuse proliferative glomerulonephritis (either mesangial or endocapillary and extracapillary proliferation with crescents)
- Diffuse sclerosing glomerulonephritis

In general, children with intermittent microscopic hematuria and mild proteinuria have normal or minimally affected glomeruli, whereas those with repeated episodes of gross hematuria, heavy proteinuria, or acute nephritis at time of biopsy tend to have diffuse mesangial proliferation, with sclerosis and crescents.

Electron microscopy consistently shows dense deposits in the mesangium and, occasionally, in subendothelial and subepithelial locations. Ultrastructural changes of peripheral glomerular capillary wall thinning, splitting, and lamination correlate closely with the histologic appearance of proliferative glomerulonephritis and heavy proteinuria (Hogg, 1982).

Pathogenesis

Clinical and experimental findings support the presence of IgA-containing circulating immune complexes as the source of mesangial deposition in IgA nephropathy (Woodroffe et al., 1980). In some studies, the levels of immune complexes correlate with clinical activity (Coppo et al., 1982, 1984; Feehally et al., 1986; Chui et al., 1991). Elevated levels of serum IgA (and less commonly IgG and IgM) are observed in many patients but do not parallel disease activity. Serum complement levels are consistently normal, but deposited IgA–immune complexes can cause glomerular injury through activation of the alternate complement pathway. Indeed, C3, properdin, and C9 are frequently seen, and C1q and C4 are rarely noted on immunofluorescence. In situ activation of the alternate pathway, presumably by mesangial IgA deposits, has been demonstrated in renal biopsy specimens from affected patients after incubation with guinea pig serum (Tomino et al., 1981).

Characterization of the IgA in both the immune

complexes and glomerular mesangium to identify its origin (humoral or mucosal) has been attempted. Most studies indicate that IgA1 is the predominant IgA subclass involved (Conley et al., 1980; Tomino et al., 1982; Katz et al., 1984; Valentijn et al., 1984; Rajaraman et al., 1986; van den Wall Bake et al., 1993). However, IgA2 was found to be the main subclass in two studies (André et al., 1980; Bene et al., 1982). There is also disagreement concerning the monomeric versus polymeric nature of IgA and the presence or absence of secretory component (SC) and J chain in glomerular deposits. Although some evidence (Valentijn et al., 1984) demonstrates that the mesangial antibody is dimeric IgA1 capable of binding free SC, other investigators have not found SC and J chain in mesangial deposits (Dobrin et al., 1975b). However, a mucosal origin for the IgA antibody seems likely, since tonsillar tissue from patients with IgA nephropathy has an increased percentage of IgA-secreting plasma cells (patients, 37% IgG, 56% IgA; controls, 65% IgG, 29% IgA) as well as an increased number of dimeric IgA-secreting cells (identified by a J chain) (Bene et al., 1983).

The possible mechanisms responsible for the presence of immune complexes in IgA nephropathy have been reviewed (Clarkson et al., 1984). The temporal relation of respiratory infection to symptom exacerbation in this disease—as well as the occurrence of IgA mesangial deposits in such systemic disorders as celiac sprue, dermatitis herpetiformis, and Crohn's disease—has suggested a mucosal defect in antigen exclusion as the stimulus for antibody production and immune complex formation (Czerkinsky et al., 1986; Schena et al., 1989b). Alternatively, a reduced rate of clearance of formed antibody or complexes may be a contributing factor, as can occur in the mesangial IgA deposition of alcoholic cirrhosis. Circulating IgA–fibronectin complexes have been detected in this disorder (Cederholm et al., 1988; Davin et al., 1991; Jennette et al., 1991). An intrinsic derangement in the autoregulation of IgA production has also been proposed, since there is an increase in IgA-bearing peripheral blood lymphocytes (Nomoto et al., 1979; Hale et al., 1986) and an increase in IgA-specific helper T cells (Sakai et al., 1982), as well as a decrease in IgA-specific suppressor T-cell activity (Sakai et al., 1979, 1989; Rothschild and Chatenoud, 1984; Fortune et al., 1992; Layward et al., 1992). Altered interleukin-2 activity has also been reported in this disease (Lai et al., 1989a; McGhee et al., 1989; Schena et al., 1989a; Parera et al., 1992).

There is a geographic variation in IgA nephropathy, suggesting environmental or genetic influences, with more cases in Japan, France, and Australia than in the United Kingdom or the United States. Genetic factors are also suggested by several familial cases of IgA nephropathy (Levy and Lesavre, 1992). Julian and co-workers (1985) reported three pedigrees (possibly related) in which 14 patients had biopsy-documented IgA nephropathy, 17 had glomerulonephritis, and 6 others had chronic nephritis. There also is an increased frequency of HLA-B35 and HLA-DR4 antigens in patients with IgA nephropathy (Berthoux et al., 1984). HLA-DQ gene polymorphism also has been observed

in nephropathy patients with IgA (Moore et al., 1990). In view of the multiple factors that may play a role in IgA nephropathy, it is prudent to guard against assuming a single pathogenetic mechanism (van Es, 1992; Williams, 1993).

Prognosis

Initially believed to be benign and static without significant sequelae, IgA nephropathy exhibits variable rates of progression. Although a few patients progress rapidly to acute renal failure (Kincaid-Smith and Nicholls, 1983), most have slowly progressive disease (Johnston et al., 1992). In a series of 374 predominantly adult patients, D'Amico and colleagues (1985) found that 25% were on maintenance dialysis 20 years after onset of disease. The fact that the course appears to be more benign in children (renal insufficiency in less than 10%) may reflect glomerular resistance to injury or the short duration of follow-up (Linné et al., 1991). In an ongoing multicenter pediatric study in which 39 children were followed up for 2 years or longer after biopsy, 5% had hypertension and 15% showed reduced glomerular filtration rates (Hogg, 1982). These trends have been reported in other pediatric series (Berg and Widstam-Attorps, 1993; Hogg and Browne, 1993).

Clinical indicators of poor outcome in children are heavy proteinuria, hypertension, and reduced renal function. Histologic indicators of poor outcome are diffuse crescents involving more than 30% of glomeruli, capillary wall splitting and lamination on electron microscopy, and the presence of tubular atrophy and interstitial fibrosis. There is no means to determine which patients with mild or moderate clinical and histologic disease are at risk for further progression.

Treatment

The treatment of IgA nephropathy is limited to supportive measures for patients with hypertension, nephrotic syndrome, or renal insufficiency. Control of hypertension and diet are important measures in reducing the rate of progressive renal impairment. Specific therapies are of unproven success, although Andreoli and Bergstein (1989) reported beneficial results using prednisone and azathioprine, and Donadio and colleagues (1994) reported that fish oil retarded the rate of loss of renal function. Renal transplantation has been performed on patients with end-stage disease, but recurrence of IgA deposits has occurred in some allografts (Berger et al., 1975; Berger, 1988).

NEPHROTIC SYNDROME

Nephrotic syndrome is characterized by marked proteinuria, hypoalbuminemia, edema, and hypercholesterolemia. All of the manifestations of this pathophysiologic state are related to proteinuria. Although numerous causes for the nephrotic syndrome have been described (Table 25–6), it is probable that most of these depend on increased permeability of the glomerular capillary to protein. Some biochemical and structural factors that determine the impermeability of the glomerular capillary are known. It seems clear, however, that a number of different pathogenetic mechanisms could injure this filter, leading to proteinuria (Michael et al., 1972b; Melvin et al., 1984b; Kanwar, 1984).

The immune-related diseases discussed earlier are major causes of proteinuria. The exact mechanism by which immune glomerular injury leads to increased capillary permeability in humans is unknown. Lysosomal proteinase derived from white cells, circulating monocytes (Beale et al., 1983), chemical mediators, and complement-induced membrane injury seem to play a role.

Diagnosis

The most common type of nephrotic syndrome in childhood is that which has been variously termed *lipoid* or *idiopathic nephrosis, nil* or *minimal lesion nephrotic syndrome*. This disorder, which appears most commonly in early childhood, occurs abruptly and is not usually associated with either hypertension or hematuria. If the glomerular filtration rate is depressed, it is almost always associated with a low plasma volume and decreased renal perfusion. The urinalysis reveals proteinuria with the absence of formed elements; the serum complement levels are normal.

Pathogenesis

The etiology of idiopathic nephrosis is unknown. Histologic studies generally reveal normal or minimally abnormal glomeruli by light microscopy and foot process fusion alone, unassociated with immune deposits by electron microscopy; no GBM-oriented deposition of immunoglobulin or complement can be demonstrated (Roy et al., 1973a; Yang et al., 1984). Serum comple-

Table 25–6. Causes of Nephrotic Syndrome in the First Two Decades of Life

Idiopathic Nephrotic Syndrome
  With normal or minimally abnormal histology, usually with corticosteroid responsiveness
  With mesangial proliferation
  With focal and segmental sclerosis, often with corticosteroid resistance

Immunologically Mediated Glomerulonephritis
  Membranoproliferative glomerulonephritis (types I, II, or III)
  Membranous nephropathy
  Poststreptococcal glomerulonephritis
  Glomerulonephritis with systemic infection
  Anaphylactoid (Henoch-Schönlein) purpura
  Rapidly progressive glomerulonephritis
  Drug related (e.g., gold, penicillamine)

Other Causes
  Familial nephritis
  Congenital (genetic)
  Diabetic nephropathy
  Amyloidosis

ment components are generally normal, although slight depression of the C1q globulin has been reported (Lewis et al., 1971), as well as decrease in factor B (McLean et al., 1977). The latter is probably a consequence of urinary loss.

Although immunologic abnormalities as a cause of increased glomerular capillary permeability have not been conclusively demonstrated, some lines of evidence suggest that immune factors play a role. The presence of circulating non–complement-fixing immune complexes have been detected by inhibition of agglutination of IgG-coated latex particles by rabbit IgM anti-IgG (Levinsky et al., 1978; Abrass et al., 1980a; Cairns et al., 1982). Production of lymphokines by nephrotic lymphocytes that increase vessel permeability of skin has been observed (Lagrue et al., 1975). Altered T-cell function, possibly secondary to the elevated lipid levels, has been associated with the nephrotic syndrome (reviewed by Fillit and Zabriski, 1982; Barna et al., 1983; Melvin et al., 1984b). Altered CD4 and CD8 T-cell populations have been reported (Feehally et al., 1984; Nagata et al., 1984), with increased CD8 suppressor and decreased activated CD4 helper cells (Arnold et al., 1990). A lymphokine (soluble immune response suppressor) has been demonstrated in elevated amounts in serum and urine of patients with steroid-responsive nephrotic syndrome, which stimulates $CD8^+$ suppressor cells and depresses immune reactivity (Schnaper and Aune, 1987; Schnaper, 1989, 1990).

The suggestion that an alteration in immune function may be causally related to the nil lesion nephrotic syndrome has also been made on the basis of recurrence associated with infection; induction of remission by measles infection; association of Hodgkin's disease, thymoma, bone marrow transplantation, interferon therapy, and acquired immune deficiency disease (Rao et al., 1984); and responsiveness to cyclophosphamide, chlorambucil, cyclosporine, and nitrogen mustard. It has been observed that the use of immunostimulant drugs, such as levamisole, are effective in sustaining steroid-induced remissions of proteinuria (British Association for Paediatric Nephrology, 1991) in idiopathic nephrotic syndrome. About 95% of these patients are responsive to corticosteroid therapy, with complete cessation of proteinuria and reversal of the nephrotic state. Relapses may be relatively frequent in some patients and are often precipitated by minor viral infections.

Treatment

A subgroup of patients with idiopathic nephrotic syndrome show evidence of focal and segmental *glomerular sclerosis* at the time of the initial biopsy, or show progression from minimal lesion nephrotic syndrome to glomerular sclerosis. These patients are generally unresponsive to corticosteroid therapy, and renal failure develops in a certain percentage. Evidence that immunologic mechanisms are operative in this group of patients is suggested by treatment responses using bolus methylprednisolone (Mendoza et al., 1990), cyclophosphamide (Melvin et al., 1984b; Ingulli and Tejani, 1992), and cyclosporine (Ponticelli et al., 1993; Tanaka et al., 1993). Recurrence of this type of nephrotic syndrome in the transplanted kidney in some patients has occurred (Hoyer et al., 1972; Maizel et al., 1981).

Prognosis

Patients with nil lesion nephrotic syndrome have excellent prognoses; the main risks are infection and complications of steroid therapy. These patients are usually responsive to steroid therapy, and although there may be relapses after cessation of therapy, they ultimately outgrow this disorder. The steroid-dependent state can be ameliorated with a course of cyclophosphamide therapy.

A much less favorable outcome is seen in patients with nephrotic syndrome due to focal glomerulosclerosis. As indicated earlier, the nephrotic state of these patients is resistant to steroid therapy, and progressive renal failure frequently occurs. Evidence indicates that therapy with cyclosporine may ameliorate the proteinuria and slow the rate of progression to renal failure.

TUBULOINTERSTITIAL NEPHRITIS

Tubulointerstitial nephritis (TIN) is evident when the primary injury to the kidney is in the interstitium with relative sparing of glomerular structures. Although this region of the kidney can be injured by a variety of acquired agents, such as drugs, chemicals, and infection, the discussion here relates to immune injury. TIN may be mediated by immune complexes or by autoantibodies to TIN antigen, which is localized to the proximal tubule basement membrane. Tubular immune complexes have been produced experimentally by immunization of rats with Tamm-Horsfall protein (Friedman et al., 1982), and this lesion is also found in humans (McCluskey, 1983) with lupus erythematosus (Lehman et al., 1974) or with conditions such as cryoglobulinemia, Sjögren's syndrome, and IgA nephropathy, as well as in persons with renal allografts (Kelly et al., 1991; Wilson, 1991).

Pathogenesis

Autoantibodies to TIN antigen have been studied experimentally in rats and guinea pigs, in which immunization with tubular basement membrane (TBM) in Freund's adjuvant results in TIN with uniform linear deposition of IgG along the tubular basement membrane (Lehman et al., 1974). Passive transfer of experimental TIN can be achieved using sera from affected animals that have circulating anti-TBM antibodies (Bannister and Wilson 1985).

Diagnosis

The development of anti-TIN antigen nephritis in humans is uncommon but is associated with acute renal failure and the presence of anti-TIN antibodies (Klassen et al., 1973; Lehman et al., 1975; Spital et al., 1987; Neilson, 1989). Pathologic findings reveal acute TIN with linear tubular basement membrane deposition of IgG (Brentjens et al., 1989). Anti-TIN nephritis has been observed in certain patients with associated membranous glomerulopathy (Katz et al., 1992).

The target antigen in the renal proximal tubule to which anti-TIN antibodies have been directed is a glycoprotein of variable molecular weight (Clayman et al., 1986; Fliger et al., 1987; Neilson et al., 1991). TIN antigen has been found in other basement membranes and shown to exist in multiple forms of higher molecular weight (Butkowski et al., 1990b, 1990c; Yoshioka et al., 1992; Crary et al., 1993).

Treatment and Prognosis

Patients with anti-TBM–mediated tubulointerstitial nephritis are treated with plasmapheresis, steroids, and immunosuppression with variable response. The outcome is poor in some patients, including chronic renal failure and end-stage renal disease.

References

Abrahamson DR, Caulfield JP. Proteinuria and structural alterations in rat glomerular basement membranes induced by intravenously injected antilaminin immunoglobulin G. J Exp Med 156:128–145, 1982.

Abrass CK, Hall CL, Border WA, Brown CA, Glassock RJ, Coggins CH. Circulating immune complexes in adults with idiopathic nephrotic syndrome. Kidney Int 17:545–553, 1980a.

Abrass CK, Nies KM, Louis JS, Border WA, Glassock RJ. Correlation and predictive accuracy of circulating immune complexes with disease activity in patients with systemic lupus erythematosus. Arthritis Rheum 23:273–282, 1980b.

Agnello V, Winchester RJ, Kunkel HG. Precipitin reactions of the C1q component of complement with aggregated γ-globulin and immune complexes in gel diffusion. Immunology 19:909–919, 1970.

Alarcon-Segovia D, Deleze M, Oria CV, Sanchez-Guerrero J, Gomez-Pacheco L, Cabiedes J, Fernandez L, Ponce de Leon L. Antiphospholipid antibodies and the antiphospholipid syndrome in systemic lupus erythematosus: a prospective analysis of 500 patients. Medicine 68:353–365, 1989.

Allison AC, Hendrickse RG, Edgington GM, Houba V, de Petris S, Adeniyi A. Immune complexes in the nephrotic syndrome of African children. Lancet 1:1232–1238, 1969.

André C, Berthoux FC, André F, Gillon J, Genin C, Sabatier J-C. Prevalence of IgA2 deposits in IgA nephropathies. N Engl J Med 303:1343–1346, 1980.

Andreoli SP, Bergstein JM. Treatment of severe IgA nephropathy in children. Pediatr Nephrol 3:248–253, 1989.

Andrews PI, Kainer G, Yong LC, Tobias VH, Rosenberg AR. Glomerulonephritis, pulmonary hemorrhage and anemia associated with Campylobacter jejuni infection. Aust NZ J Med 19:721–723, 1989.

Antoine B, Faye C. The clinical course associated with dense deposits in the kidney basement membranes. Kidney Int 1:420–427, 1972.

Antonovych TT, MacKay K, Boumpas DT, Balow JE. Membranous nephropathy. Ann Intern Med 116:672–682, 1992.

Appel GB, Silva FG, Pirani CL, Meltzer JI, Ester D. Renal involvement in systemic lupus erythematosus (SLE). Medicine 57:371–410, 1978.

Arnett FC, Shulman LE. Studies in familial systemic lupus erythematosus. Medicine 55:313–322, 1976.

Arnold WC, Fisher RT, Carlton RK, Steele RW, Childress SH. Two color flow cytometric analysis of T-lymphocyte subsets in pediatric minimal change nephrotic syndrome. J Am Soc Nephrol 1:557, 1990.

Asami T, Tanaka T, Gunji T, Sakai K. Elevated serum and urine sialic acid levels in renal diseases of childhood. Clin Nephrol 23:112–119, 1985.

Asherson RA, Mackworth-Young CG, Harris EN, Gharavi AE, Hughes GRV. Multiple venous and arterial thrombosis associated with the lupus anticoagulant and antibodies to cardiolipin in absence of SLE. Rheumatol Int 5:91–93, 1985.

Atkins RC, Holdsworth SR, Hancock WW, Thomson NW, Glasgow EF. Cellular immune mechanisms in human glomerulonephritis: the role of mononuclear leukocytes. Springer Semin Immunopathol 5:269–296, 1982.

Austin HA, Klippel JH, Balow JE, le Riche NGH, Steinberg AD, Plotz PH, Decker JL. Therapy of lupus nephritis: controlled trial of prednisone and cytotoxic drugs. N Engl J Med 314:614–619, 1986.

Aumailley M, Wiedemann H, Mann K, Timpl R. Binding of nidogen and the laminin–nidogen complex to basement membrane collagen type IV. Eur J Biochem 184:241–248, 1989.

Baart de la Faille-Kuyper EH, Kater L, Kuijten J, Kooiker CJ, Wagenaar, SS, van der Zouwen P, Dorhout Mees EJ. Occurrence of vascular IgA deposits in clinically normal skin of patients with renal disease. Kidney Int 9:424–429, 1976.

Bagchus WM, Hoedemaeker PJ, Rozing J, Bakker WW. Glomerulonephritis induced by monoclonal anti-Thy 1.1 antibodies. Lab Invest 55:680–687, 1986.

Baldwin DS, Gluck MC, Schacht RG, Gallo G. The long-term course of poststreptococcal glomerulonephritis. Ann Intern Med 80:342–358, 1974.

Baldwin DS, Gluck MC, Lowenstein J, Gallo GR. Lupus nephritis: clinical course as related to morphologic forms and their transitions. Am J Med 62:12–30, 1977.

Balow JE, Austin HA, Muenz LF, Joyce KM, Antonovych TT, Klippel JH, Steinberg AD, Plotz PH, Decker JL. Effect of treatment on the evolution of renal abnormalities in lupus nephritis. N Engl J Med 311:491–495, 1984.

Bannister KM, Howarth GS, Clarkson AR, Woodroffe AJ. Glomerular IgG subclass distribution in human glomerulonephritis. Clin Nephrol 19:161–165, 1983.

Bannister KM, Wilson CB. Transfer of tubulointerstitial nephritis in the brown Norway rat with anti–tubular basement membrane antibody: quantitation and kinetics of binding and effect of decomplementation. J Immunol 135:3911–3917, 1985.

Barna BP, Makker S, Kallen R, Valenzuela R, Deodhar SD, Yeip IM, Leto D, Verbic MA, Rajaraman S, Govidaragan S. A lymphocytotoxic factor(s) in plasma of patients with minimal change nephrotic syndrome: partial characterization. Clin Immunol Immunopathol 27:272–282, 1983.

Bayer AS, Theofilopoulos AN. Immunopathogenic aspects of infective endocarditis. Chest 97:204–212, 1990.

Bayer AS, Theofilopoulos AN, Eisenberg R, Dixon FJ, Guze LB. Circulating immune complexes in infective endocarditis. N Engl J Med 295:1500–1505, 1976.

Beale MG, Nash GS, Bertovich MJ, MacDermott RP. Immunoglobulin synthesis by peripheral blood mononuclear cells in minimal change nephrotic syndrome. Kidney Int 23:380–386, 1983.

Beaufils M. Glomerular disease complicating abdominal sepsis. Kidney Int 19:609–618, 1981.

Beck K, Hunter I, Engel J. Structure and function of laminin: anatomy of a multidomain glycoprotein. FASEB J 4:148–160, 1990.

Beirne GJ, Octaviano GN, Koop WL, Burns RO. Immunohistology of the lung in Goodpasture's syndrome. Ann Intern Med 69:1207–1212, 1968.

Bene M-C, Faure G, Levy M, Duheille J. Nephropathies à IgA: identification de la sous-classe IgA1 et/ou IgA2 des dépôts mesangiaux d'IgA. Nouv Presse Med 11:2639–2640, 1982.

Bene M-C, Faure G, Hurault de Ligny B, Kessler M, Duheille J. Immunoglobulin A nephropathy: quantitative immunohistomorphometry of the tonsillar plasma cells evidences an inversion of the immunoglobulin A versus immunoglobulin G secreting cell balance. J Clin Invest 71:1342–1347, 1983.

Berg V, Widstam-Attorps V. Follow-up of renal function and urinary protein excretion in childhood IgA nephropathy. Pediatr Nephrol 7:123–129, 1993.

Berger J. IgA glomerular deposits in renal disease. Transplant Proc 1:939–944, 1969.

Berger J. Recurrence of IgA nephropathy in renal allografts. Am J Kidney Dis 12:371–372, 1988.

Berger J, Galle P. Dèpôts dense au sein des basales du rein. Presse Med 71:2251–2254, 1963.

Berger J, Yaneva H, Nabarra B, Barbanel C. Recurrence of mesangial deposition of IgA after renal transplantation. Kidney Int 7:232–241, 1975.

Berthoux FC, Genin C, LePetit J-C, Laurent B. Immunogenetics of mesangial IgA nephritis. In D'Amico G, Minetti L, Ponticelli C, eds. Contributions to Nephrology. Vol. 40. Basel, Karger, 1984, pp. 118–123.

Bhan AK, Schneeberger EE, Collins AB, McCluskey RT. Evidence for a pathogenic role of a cell mediated immune mechanism in experimental glomerulonephritis. J Exp Med 148:246–260, 1978.

Bhan AK, Collins AB, Schneeberger EE, McCluskey RT. A cell mediated reaction against glomerular bound immune complexes. J Exp Med 150:1410–1420, 1979.

Black JA, Challacombe DN, Ockenden BG. Nephrotic syndrome associated with bacteraemia after shunt operations for hydrocephalus. Lancet 2:921–924, 1965.

Bolton WK, Sturgill BC. Methylprednisolone therapy for acute crescentic rapidly progressive glomerulonephritis. Am J Nephrol 9:368–375, 1989.

Boonshaft B, Maher JF, Schreiner GE. Nephrotic syndrome associated with osteomyelitis without secondary amyloidosis. Arch Intern Med 125:322–327, 1970.

Border WA. Results of immune complex detection in glomerular diseases. In Cummings NB, Michael AF, Wilson CB, eds. Immune Mechanisms in Renal Disease. New York, Plenum, 1983, pp. 225–231.

Border WA, Wilson CB, Götze O. Nephritic factor: description of a new quantitative assay and findings in glomerulonephritis. Kidney Int 10:311–318, 1976.

Border WA, Ward HJ, Kamil ES, Cohen AH. Induction of membranous nephropathy in rabbits by administration of an exogenous cationic antigen. J Clin Invest 69:451–461, 1982.

Boulton-Jones JM, Davison AM. Persistant infection as a cause of renal disease in patients submitted to renal biopsy: a report from the glomerulonephritis registry of the United Kingdom MRC. Q J Med 58:123–132, 1986.

Boumpas DT, Austin HA III, Vaughn EM, Klippel JH, Steinberg AD, Yarboro CH, Balow JE. Controlled trial of pulse methylprednisolone versus two regimens of pulse cyclophosphamide in severe lupus nephritis. Lancet 340:741–745, 1992.

Braunstein GD, Lewis EJ, Galvanek EG, Hamilton A, Bell WR. The nephrotic syndrome associated with secondary syphilis: an immune deposit disease. Am J Med 48:643–648, 1970.

Brentjens JR, Matsuo S, Fukatsu A, Min I, Kohli R, Anthone R, Anthone S, Biesecker G, Andres G. Immunologic studies in two patients with antitubular basement membrane nephritis. Am J Med 86:603–608, 1989.

British Association for Paediatric Nephrology. Levamisole for corticosteroid-dependent nephrotic syndrome in childhood. Lancet 337:1555–1557, 1991.

Bruijn JA, Hoedemaeker PJ, Fleuren GJ. Pathogenesis of anti-basement membrane glomerulopathy and immune-complex glomerulonephritis: dichotomy dissolved. In Rubin E, Damjanov I, eds. Pathology Reviews. Clifton, NJ, Humana Press, 1990, pp 143–151.

Bunchman TE, Mauer SM, Sibley RK, Vernier RL. Anaphylactoid purpura: characteristics of 16 patients who progressed to renal failure. Pediatr Nephrol 2:393–397, 1988.

Burkholder PM, Bradford WD. Proliferative glomerulonephritis in children: a correlation of varied clinical and pathologic patterns utilizing light, immunofluorescent and electron microscopy. Am J Pathol 56:423–467, 1969.

Butkowski RJ, Wieslander J, Wiscom BJ, Barr JF, Noelken ME, Hudson BG. Properties of the globular domain of type IV collagen and its relationship to the Goodpasture antigen. J Biol Chem 260:3739–3747, 1985.

Butkowski RJ, Wieslander J, Kleppel M, Michael AF, Fish AJ. Basement membrane collagen in the kidney: regional localization of novel chains related to collagen IV. Kidney Int 35:1195–1202, 1989.

Butkowski RJ, Shen G-Q, Wieslander J, Michael AF, Fish AJ. Characterization of type IV collagen NC1 monomers and Goodpasture antigen in human renal basement membranes. J Lab Clin Med 115:365–373, 1990a.

Butkowski RJ, Kleppel MM, Katz A, Michael AF, Fish AJ. Distribution in renal and extrarenal tissues of glycoprotein (TIN antigen) associated with anti-tubular basement membrane nephritis: identification of high molecular weight forms. Kidney Int 40:838–846, 1990b.

Butkowski RJ, Langeveldt JPM, Wieslander J, Brentjens JR, Andres GA. Characterization of a tubular basement membrane component reactive with autoantibodies associated with tubulointerstitial nephritis. J Biol Chem 265:21,091–21,098, 1990c.

Cairns SA, London RA, Mallick NP. Circulating immune complexes in idiopathic glomerular disease. Kidney Int 21:507–512, 1982.

Cameron JS. The nephritis of Schönlein-Henoch purpura: current problems. In Kincaid-Smith P, D'Apice AJP, Adkins RC, eds. Progress in Glomerulonephritis. New York, John Wiley & Sons, 1979, pp. 283–309.

Cameron JS, Glascow EF, Ogg CS, White R. Membranoproliferative glomerulonephritis and persistent hypocomplementemia. Br Med J 4:7–14, 1970.

Cameron JS, Turner DR, Ogg CS, Williams DG, Lessof MH, Chantler C, Leibowitz S. Systemic lupus with nephritis: a long term study. Q J Med 48:1–24, 1979.

Cameron JS, Turner DR, Heaton J, Gwyn Williams D, Ogg CS, Chantler C, Haycock GB, Hicks J. Idiopathic mesangiocapillary glomerulonephritis: comparison of types I and II in children and adults and long term prognosis. Am J Med 74:175–192, 1983.

Cederholm B, Wieslander J, Bygren P, Heinegard D. Circulating complexes containing IgA and fibronectin in patients with primary IgA nephropathy. Proc Natl Acad Sci USA 85:4865–4868, 1988.

Christian CL. Role of viruses in etiology of systemic lupus erythematosus. Am J Kidney Dis 2(Suppl.):114–118, 1982.

Chui SH, Lam CWK, Lewis WHP, Lai KN. Light-chain ratio of serum IgA1 in IgA nephropathy. J Clin Immunol 11:219–223, 1991.

Clayman MD, Michaud L, Brentjens J, Andres GA, Kefalides NA, Neilson EG. Isolation of the target antigen of human anti–tubular basement membrane antibody–associated interstitial nephritis. J Clin Invest 77:1143–1147, 1986.

Cochrane CG. Mechanisms involved in the deposition of immune complexes in tissue. J Exp Med 134:75s–89s, 1971.

Coggins CH. Membranous glomerulopathy. In Schrier RW, Gottschalk CW, eds. Diseases of the Kidney. 5th ed. Boston, Little Brown, 1993, pp. 1785–1813.

Coleman TH, Forristal J, Kosaka T, West CD. Inherited complement component deficiencies and membranoproliferative glomerulonephritis. Kidney Int 24:681–690, 1983.

Collins AB, Andres GA, McCluskey RT. Lack of evidence for a role of renal tubular antigen in human membranous glomerulonephritis. Nephron 27:297–301, 1981.

Combes B, Stastny P, Shorey J, Eigenbrodt EH, Barrera A, Hull AR, Carter NW. Glomerulonephritis with deposition of Australia antigen–antibody complexes in basement membrane. Lancet 2:234–237, 1971.

Conley ME, Cooper MD, Michael AF. Selective deposition of immunoglobulin A1 in immunoglobulin A nephropathy, anaphylactoid purpura nephritis, and systemic lupus erythematosus. J Clin Invest 66:1432–1436, 1980.

Coppo R, Basolo B, Martina G, Rollino C, DeMarchi M, Giacchino F, Mazzucco G, Messina M, Piccoli G. Circulating immune complexes containing IgA, IgG, and IgM in patients with primary IgA nephropathy and with Henoch-Schönlein nephritis: correlation with clinical and histologic signs of activity. Clin Nephrol 18:230–239, 1982.

Coppo R, Basolo B, Piccoli G, Mazzucco G, Bulzomi MR, Roccatello D, De Marchi M, Carbonara AO, DiBelgiojoso GB. IgA1 and IgA2 immune complexes in primary IgA nephropathy and Henoch-Schönlein nephritis. Clin Exp Immunol 57:583–590, 1984.

Cordeiro A, Costa H, Laginha F. Immunologic phase of subacute bacterial endocarditis. Am J Cardiol 16:477–481, 1965.

Couser W. Rapidly progressive glomerulonephritis: classification, pathogenic mechanisms, and therapy. Am J Kidney Dis 11:449–464, 1988.

Couser WG, Steinmuller DR, Stilmant M, Salant DJ, Lowenstein LM. Experimental glomerulonephritis in the isolated perfused rat kidney. J Clin Invest 63:1275–1287, 1978.

Couser WG, Salant D. In situ complex formation and glomerular injury. Kidney Int 17:1–13, 1980.

Couser WG, Baker PJ, Adler S. Complement and the direct mediation of immune glomerular injury: a new perspective. Kidney Int 28:879–890, 1985.

Crary GS, Katz A, Fish AJ, Michael AF, Butkowski RJ. Role of a basement membrane glycoprotein in anti–tubular basement membrane nephritis. Kidney Int 43:140–146, 1993.

Cybulsky AV, Quigg RJ, Salant DJ. Role of the complement membrane attack complex in glomerular injury. In Wilson CB, Brenner BM, Stein JH, eds. Immunopathology of Renal Disease. New York, Churchill Livingstone, 1988, pp. 57–86.

Czerkinsky C, Koopman WJ, Jackson S, Collins JE, Crago SS, Schrohenloher RE, Julian BA, Galla JH, Mestecky J. Circulating immune complexes and immunoglobulin A rheumatoid factor in patients with mesangial immunoglobulin A nephropathies. J Clin Invest 77:1931–1938, 1986.

Daha MR, Austen KF, Fearon DT. Heterogeneity, polypeptide chain composition and antigenic reactivity of C3 nephritic factor. J Immunol 120:1389–1394, 1978.

Daha MR, van Es, LA. Further evidence for the antibody nature of C3 nephritic factor (C3Nef). J Immunol 123:755–758, 1979.

D'Amico G. The commonest glomerulonephritis in the world: IgA nephropathy. Q J Med 64:709–727, 1987.

D'Amico G, Imbasciati E, DiBelgiojoso GB, Bertoli S, Fogazzi G, Ferrario F, Fellini G, Ragni A, Colasanti G, Minetti L, Ponticelli C. Idiopathic IgA mesangial nephropathy: clinical and historical study of 374 patients. Medicine 64:49–60, 1985.

Davin J-C, Li-Vecchi M, Nagy J, Foidart JM, Foidart JB, Barbagallo Sangiorgi G, Malaise M, Mahieu P. Evidence that the interaction between circulating IgA and fibronectin is a normal process enhanced in primary IgA nephropathy. J Clin Immunol 11:78–94, 1991.

Davis CA, Marder H, West CD. Circulating immune complexes in membranoproliferative glomerulonephritis. Kidney Int 20:728–732, 1981.

Desjardins M, Bendayan M. Heterogenous distribution of type IV collagen, entactin, heparan sulfate proteoglycan, and laminin among renal basement membranes as demonstrated by quantitative immunocytochemistry. J Histochem Cytochem 37:885–897, 1989.

Digeon M, Laver M, Riza J, Bach JF. Detection of circulating immune complexes in human sera by simplified assays with polyethylene glycol. J Immunol Methods 16:165–183, 1977.

Ding J, Kashtan CE, Fan WW, Sun MJ, Neilson EG, Michael AF. A monoclonal antibody marker for Alport syndrome identifies the alpha 5 chain of type IV collagen. Kidney Int 46:1504–1506, 1994.

Dixon FJ, Feldman FD, Vazquez JJ. Experimental glomerulonephritis: the pathogenesis of a laboratory model resembling the spectrum of human glomerulonephritis. J Exp Med 113:899–920, 1961.

Dobrin RS, Day NK, Quie PG, Moore HL, Vernier RL, Michael AF, Fish AJ. The role of complement, immunoglobulin and bacterial antigen in coagulase-negative staphylococcal shunt nephritis. Am J Med 59:660–673, 1975a.

Dobrin RS, Knudson FE, Michael AF. The secretory immune system and renal disease. Clin Exp Immunol 21:318–328, 1975b.

Donadio JV Jr. Membranoproliferative glomerulonephritis. In Schrier RW, Gottschalk CW, eds. Diseases of the Kidney. Boston, Little, Brown, 1993, pp. 1815–1837.

Donadio JV, Torres VE, Velosa JA, Wagoner RD, Holley KE, Okamura M, Ilstrup DM, Chu C-P. Idiopathic membranous nephropathy: the natural history of untreated patients. Kidney Int 33:708–715, 1988.

Donadio JV, Offord KP. Reassessment of treatment results in membranoproliferative glomerulonephritis with emphasis on life table analysis. Am J Kidney Dis 14:445–451, 1989.

Donadio JV, Bergstralh EJ, Offord KP, Spencer DC, Holley KE, for the Mayo Nephrology Collaborative Group. A controlled trial of fish oil in IgA nephropathy. N Engl J Med 331:1194–1199, 1994.

Dubois CH, Foidart JB, Hautier MB, Dechenne CA, Lemaire MJ, Mahieu PR. Proliferative glomerulonephritis in rats: evidence that mononuclear phagocytes infiltrating the glomeruli stimulate the proliferation of endothelial and mesangial cells. Eur J Clin Invest 11:91–104, 1981.

Duncan DA, Drummond KN, Michael AF, Vernier RL. Pulmonary hemorrhage and glomerulonephritis: report of six cases and study of the renal lesion by fluorescent antibody technique and electron microscopy. Ann Intern Med 62:920–938, 1965.

Eaton RB, Schneider G, Schur PH. Enzyme immunoassay for antibodies to native DNA: specificity and quality of antibodies. Arthritis Rheum 26:52–62, 1983.

Eddy A, Michael AF. Immune mechanisms of renal injury. In Edelmann CM, ed. Pediatric Kidney Disease. 2nd ed. Boston, Little, Brown, 1992, pp. 329–397.

Edgington TS, Glassock RJ, Dixon FJ. Autologous immune complex nephritis induced with renal tubular antigen: I. Identification and isolation of the pathogenetic antigen. J Exp Med 127:555–572, 1968.

Eisenberg R, Theofilopoulos AN, Dixon FJ. Use of bovine conglutinin for the assay of immune complexes. J Immunol 118:1428–1434, 1977.

Ellis HA, Walton KW. Variations in serum complement in the nephrotic syndrome and other forms of renal disease. Immunology 1:234–250, 1958.

Endre ZH, Pussell BA, Charlesworth JA, Coovadia HM, Seedat YK. C3 metabolism in acute glomerulonephritis: implications for sites of complement activation. Kidney Int 25:937–941, 1984.

Esdaile JM, Levinton C, Federgreen W, Hayslett JP, Kashgarian M. The clinical and renal biopsy predictors of long term outcome in lupus nephritis: a study of 57 patients and review of the literature. Q J Med 72:779–833, 1989.

Ewert BH, Jennette JC, Falk RJ. Anti-myeloperoxidase antibodies stimulate neutrophils to damage human endothelial cells. Kidney Int 41:375–383, 1992.

Falk RJ, Dalmasso AP, Kim Y, Tsai CH, Scheinman JI, Gewurz H, Michael AF. Neoantigen of the polymerized ninth component of complement: characterization of a monoclonal antibody and immunohistochemical localization in renal disease. J Clin Invest 72:560–573, 1983.

Falk RJ, Hogan SV, Carey TS, Jennett JC. Clinical course of anti-neutrophil cytoplasmic autoantibody–associated glomerulonephritis and systemic vasculitis. Ann Intern Med 113:656–663, 1990a.

Falk RJ, Terrell RS, Charles LA, Jennette JC. Anti-neutrophil cytoplasmic autoantibodies induce neutrophils to degranulate and produce oxygen radicals in vitro. Proc Natl Acad Sci U S A 87:4115–4119, 1990b.

Falls WF Jr, Ford KL, Ashworth CT, Carter NW. The nephrotic syndrome in secondary syphilis: a report of a case with renal biopsy findings. Ann Intern Med 63:1047–1058, 1965.

Farine M, Poucell S, Geary D, Baumal R. Prognostic significance of urinary findings and renal biopsies in children with Henoch-Schönlein nephritis. Clin Pediatr 25:257–259, 1986.

Fauci AS, Katz P, Haynes BF, Wolff SM. Cyclophosphamide therapy of severe systemic necrotizing vasculitis. N Engl J Med 301:235–238, 1979.

Feehally J, Beattie TJ, Brenchley PEC, Coupes BM, Houston IB, Mallick NP, Postlethwaite RJ. Modulation of cellular immune function by cyclophosphamide in children with minimal-change nephropathy. N Engl J Med 310:415–420, 1984.

Feehally J, Beattie TJ, Brenchley PEC, Coupes BM, Mallick N. Postlethwaite RJ. Sequential study of the IgA system in relapsing IgA nephropathy. Kidney Int 30:924–931, 1986.

Fillit HM, Read SE, Sherman RL, Zabriskie JB, van de Rijn I. Cellular reactivity to altered glomerular basement membrane in glomerulonephritis. N Engl J Med 298:861–868, 1978.

Fillit HM, Zabriskie JB. Cellular immunity in glomerulonephritis. Am J Pathol 109:227–243, 1982.

Fillit HM, Zabriskie JB. New concepts of glomerular injury. Lab Invest 51:117–119, 1984.

Fischel EE, Gajdusek DC. Serum complement in acute glomerulonephritis and other renal diseases. Am J Med 12:190–196, 1952.

Fish AJ, Michael AF, Vernier RL, Good RA. Acute serum sickness nephritis in the rabbit: an immune deposit disease. Am J Pathol 49:997–1022, 1966.

Fish AJ, Herdman RC, Michael AF, Pickering RJ, Good RA. Epidemic acute glomerulonephritis associated with type 49 streptococcal pyoderma. II. Correlative study of light, immunofluorescent and electron microscopic findings. Am J Med 48:28–39, 1970.

Fish AJ, Blau EB, Westberg NG, Burke B, Vernier RL, Michael AF. Systemic lupus erythematosus within the first two decades of life. Am J Med 62:99–117, 1977.

Fish AJ, Carmody KM, Michael AF. Spatial orientation and distribution of antigens within human glomerular basement membrane. J Lab Clin Med 94:447–457, 1979.

Fish AJ, Lockwood MC, Wong M, Price RG. Detection of Goodpasture antigen in fractions prepared from collagenase digests of human glomerular basement membrane. Clin Exp Immunol 55:58–66, 1984.

Fish AJ, Kleppel M, Jeraj K, Michael AF. Enzyme immunoassay of antiglomerular basement membrane antibodies. J Lab Clin Med 105:700–705, 1985.

Fliger FD, Wieslander J, Brentjens JR, Andres GA, Butkowski RJ. Identification of a target antigen in human anti–tubular basement membrane nephritis. Kidney Int 31:800–807, 1987.

Ford DM, Briscoe DM, Shanley PF, Lum GM. Childhood membranoproliferative glomerulonephritis type I: limited steroid therapy. Kidney Int 41:1606–1612, 1992.

Fortune F, Courteau M, Williams DG, Lehner T. T and B cell responses following immunization with tetanus toxoid in IgA nephropathy. Clin Exp Immunol 88:62–67, 1992.

Frank MM, Hamburger MI, Lawley TJ, Kimberly RF, Plotz PH. Defective reticuloendothelial system Fc-receptor function in systemic lupus erythematosus. N Engl J Med 300:518–523, 1979.

Frank MM, Lawley TJ, Hamburger MI, Brown EJ. NIH Conference: immunoglobulin G Fc receptor–mediated clearance in autoimmune diseases. Ann Intern Med 98:206–218, 1983.

Freedman P, Peters JH, Kark RM. Localization of gamma globulin in the diseased kidney. AMA Arch Intern Med 105:524–535, 1960.

Freedman P, Markowitz AS. Isolation of antibody-like gammaglobulin from lupus glomeruli. Br Med J 5286:1175–1178, 1962.

Friedman J, Hoyer JR, Seiler MW. Formation and clearance of tubulointerstitial immune complexes in kidneys of rats immunized with heterologous antisera to Tamm-Horsfall protein. Kidney Int 21:575–582, 1982.

Friend PS, Noreen HJ, Yunis EJ, Michael AF. B-cell alloantigen associated with chronic mesangiocapillary glomerulonephritis. Lancet 1:562–564, 1977.

Fujigaki Y, Nagase M, Kobayasi S, Hidaka S, Shimomura M, Hishida A. Intra-GBM site of the functional filtration barrier for endogenous proteins in rats. Kidney Int 43:567–574, 1993.

Fukatsu A, Brentjens JR, Killen PD, Kleinman HK, Martin GR, Andres GA. Studies on the formation of glomerular immune deposits in brown Norway rats injected with mercuric chloride. Clin Immunol Immunopathol 45:35–47, 1987.

Fukatsu A, Matsuo S, Killen PD, Martin GR, Andres GA, Brentjens JR. The glomerular distribution of type IV collagen and laminin in human membranous glomerulonephritis. Hum Pathol 19:64–68, 1988.

Galle P, Mahieu P. Electron dense alteration of kidney basement membranes: a renal lesion specific of a systemic disease. Am J Med 58:749–764, 1975.

Gallo GR, Caulin-Glaser T, Lamm ME. Charge circulating immune complexes as a factor in glomerular basement membrane localization in mice. J Clin Invest 67:1305–1313, 1981.

Gallo GR, Caulin-Glaser T, Emancipator SN, Lamm ME. Nephritogenicity and differential distribution of glomerular immune complexes related to immunogen charge. Lab Invest 48:353–362, 1983.

Garancis JC, Konorowsku RA, Bernhard GC, Straumfjord JV. Significance of cytoplasmic microtubules in lupus nephritis. Am J Pathol 64:1–12, 1971.

Garcia R, Rubio L, Rodriguez-Iturbe B. Long-term prognosis of epidemic poststreptococcal glomerulonephritis in Maracaibo: follow-up studies 11–12 years after the acute episode. Clin Nephrol 15:291–298, 1981.

Gewurz H, Pickering RJ, Mergenhagen SE, Good RA. The complement profile in acute glomerulonephritis systemic lupus erythematosus and hypocomplementemic chronic glomerulonephritis: contrasts and experimental correlations. Int Arch Allergy 34:556–570, 1968a.

Gewurz H, Shin HS, Mergenhagen SE. Interactions of the complement system with endotoxic lipopolysaccharide: consumption of each of the six terminal complement components. J Exp Med 128:1049–1057, 1968b.

Ginzler E, Sharon E, Diamond H. Long-term maintenance therapy with azathioprine in systemic lupus erythematosus. Arthritis Rheum 18:27–34, 1975.

Ginzler EM, Diamond HS, Weiner M, Schlesinger M, Fries JF, Wasner C, Medsger JA Jr, Zeiger G, Klippel JH, Hadler NM, Albert DA, Hess EV, Spencer-Green G, Grazel A, Worth D, Hahn BH, Barnett EV. A multicenter study of outcome in systemic lupus erythematosus. I. Entry variables as predictors of prognosis. Arthritis Rheum 25:601–611, 1982.

Glassock RJ, Goldstein DA, Finlander P, Koss M, Kitridou R, Border WA. Glomerulonephritis in systemic lupus erythematosus. Am J Nephrol 1:53–67, 1981.

Glöckner WM, Sieberth HG, Wichmann HE, Backes E, Bambauer R, Boesken WH, Bohle A, Daul A, Graben N, Keller F, Klehr HU, Köhler H, Metz U, Schultz W, Thoenes W, Vlaho M. Plasma exchange and immunosuppression in rapidly progressive glomerulonephritis: a controlled, multi-center study. Clin Nephrol 29:1–8, 1988.

Gocke DJ, Hsu K, Morgan C, Bombardieri S, Lockshin M, Christian CL. Association between polyarteritis and Australia antigen. Lancet 2:1149–1153, 1970.

Golbus SM, Wilson CB. Experimental glomerulonephritis induced by in situ formation of immune complexes in glomerular capillary wall. Kidney Int 16:148–157, 1979.

Goldstein AR, White RHR, Akuse R, Chantler C. Long term follow up of childhood Henoch-Schönlein nephritis. Lancet 339:280–282, 1992.

Gotoff SP, Fellers FX, Vawter GF, Janeway CA, Rosen FS. The beta-1C globulin in childhood nephrotic syndrome: laboratory diagnosis of progressive glomerulonephritis. N Engl J Med 273:524–529, 1965.

Grausz H, Earley LE, Stephens BG, Lee JC, Hooper J. Diagnostic import of virus-like particles in the glomerular endothelium of patients with systemic lupus erythematosus. N Engl J Med 283:506–511, 1970.

Gunn WC. Variation in the amount of complement in blood in some acute infectious disease and its relationship to the clinical features. J Pathol Bacteriol 19:155–181, 1914.

Haakenstad AO, Striker GE, Mannik M. The glomerular deposition of soluble immune complexes prepared with reduced and alklyated antibodies and with intact antibodies in mice. Lab Invest 35:293–301, 1976.

Habib R, Kleinknecht C, Gubler MC, Levy M. Idiopathic membrano-proliferative glomerulonephritis in children: report of 105 cases. Clin Nephrol 1:194–214, 1973a.

Habib R, Kleinknecht C, Gubler MC. Extramembranous glomerulo-nephritis in children: report of 50 cases. J Pediatr 82:754–766, 1973b.

Habib R, Loirat C, Gubler M, Levy M. Morphology and serum complement levels in membranoproliferative glomerulonephritis. In Hamburger J, Crosnier J, Maxwell MH, eds. Advances in Nephrology. Vol. 4. Chicago, Year Book Medical Publishers 1974, pp. 109–136.

Habib R, Cameron JS. Schönlein-Henoch purpura. In Bacon PA, Hadler NM, eds.The Kidney and Rheumatic Disease. London Butterworths 1982, pp. 178–201.

Hagen SG, Michael AF, Butkowski RJ. Immunochemical and biochemical evidence for distinct basement membrane heparan sulfate proteoglycans. J Biol Chem 268:7261–7269, 1993.

Hale GM, McIntosh SL, Hiki Y, Clarkson AR, Woodroffe AJ. Evidence for IgA-specific B cell hyperactivity in patients with IgA nephropathy. Kidney Int 29:718–724, 1986.

Hanauer LB, Christian CL. Clinical studies of hemolytic complement and the 11S component. Am J Med 42:882–890, 1967.

Hardin JA. The lupus autoantigen and the pathogenesis of systemic lupus erythematosus. Arthritis Rheum 29:457–460, 1986.

Herdman RC, Pickering RJ, Michael AF, Vernier RL, Fish AJ, Gewurz H, Good RA. Chronic glomerulonephritis associated with low serum complement activity (chronic hypocomplementemic glomerulonephritis). Medicine (Balt) 49:207–226, 1970.

Heymann W, Hackle DB, Harwood S, Wilson SG, Hunter JL. Production of nephrotic syndrome in rats by Freund's adjuvant and rat kidney suspensions. Proc Soc Exp Biol Med 100:660–664, 1959.

Hinglais N, Kazatchkine MD, Bhakdi S, Appay M-D, Mandet C, Grossetete J, Bariety J. Immunohistochemical study of the C5b-9 complex of complement in human kidneys. Kidney Int 30:399–410, 1986.

Hoffman GS, Leavitt RY, Fleisher TA, Minor JR, Fauci AS. Treatment of Wegener's granulomatosis with intermittent high-dose intravenous cyclophosphamide. Am J Med 89:403–410, 1990.

Hoffman GS, Kerr GS, Leavitt RY, Hallahan CW, Lebovics RS, Travis WD, Rottem M, Fauci AS. Wegener granulomatosis: an analysis of 158 patients. Ann Intern Med 116:488–498, 1992.

Hogg RJ. A multicenter study of IgA nephropathy in children: a report of the Southwest Pediatric Nephrology Study Group. Kidney Int 22:643–652, 1982.

Hogg RJ, Browne R. Prognostication in children with renal disease—with an emphasis on IgA nephropathy. Pediatr Nephrol 7:130–131, 1993.

Holdsworth SR. Fc dependence of macrophage accumulation and subsequent injury in experimental glomerulonephritis. J Immunol 130:735–739, 1983.

Holdsworth SR, Neale TJ, Wilson CB. Abrogation of macrophage-dependent injury in experimental glomerulonephritis in the rabbit: use of an antimacrophage serum. J Clin Invest 68:686–698, 1981.

Houser MT, Fish AJ, Tagatz GE, Williams PP, Michael AF. Pregnancy and systemic lupus erythematosus. Am J Obstet Gynecol 138:409–413, 1980.

Houssin D, Druet E, Hinglais N, Verroust P, Grossetete J, Bariety J, Druet P. Glomerular and vascular IgG deposits in HgCl$_2$ nephritis: role of circulating antibodies and of immune complexes. Clin Immunol Immunopathol 29:167–180, 1983.

Hoyer J, Raij L, Vernier RL, Simmons RL, Najarian JS, Michael AF. Recurrence of idiopathic nephrotic syndrome following renal transplantation. Lancet 2:343–348, 1972.

Hudson BG, Wieslander J, Wisdom BJ Jr, Noelken ME. Biology of disease: Goodpasture syndrome—molecular architecture and function of basement membrane antigen. Lab Invest 61:256–269, 1989.

Hughes GRV, Harris NN, Gharavi AE. The anticardiolipin syndrome. J Rheumatol 13:486–489, 1986.

Hunsicker L, Shearer T, Plattner SB, Weisenburger D. The role of monocytes in serum sickness nephritis. J Exp Med 150:413–425, 1979.

Ingulli E, Tejani A. Severe hypercholesterolemia inhibits cyclosporin A efficacy in a dose-dependent manner in children with nephrotic syndrome. J Am Soc Nephrol 3:254–259, 1992.

Inman RD, Redecha PB, Knechtle SJ, Schned ES, van de Rijn I, Christian CL. Identification of bacterial antigens in circulating immune complexes of infective endocarditis. J Clin Invest 70:271–280, 1982.

Iskander SS, Jennette JC. Influence of antibody avidity on glomerular immune complex localization. Am J Pathol 112:155–159, 1983.

Jacquot C, Thoua Y, Dupont E, Vereerstraeten P. Récidive de granulomatose de Wegener sur une greffe de rein de cadavre. Néphrologie 11:97–103, 1990.

Jayne DRW, Davies MJ, Fox CJV, Black CM, Lockwood, CM. Treatment of systemic vasculitis with pooled intravenous immunoglobulin. Lancet 337:1137–1139, 1991.

Jayne DRW, Esnault VLM, Lockwood CM. ANCA anti-idiotype antibodies and the treatment of systemic vasculitis with intravenous immunoglobulin. J Autoimmun 2:207–219, 1993.

Jennette JC, Wilkman AS, Falk RJ. Anti–neutrophil cytoplasmic autoantibody–associated glomerulonephritis and vasculitis. Am J Pathol 135:921–930, 1989.

Jennette JC, Falk RJ. Antineutrophil cytoplasmic autoantibodies and associated diseases: a review. Am J Kidney Dis 15:517–529, 1990.

Jennette JC, Wieslander J, Tuttle R, Falk RJ. Serum IgA-fibronectin aggregates in patients with IgA nephropathy and Henoch-Schönlein purpura: diagnostic value and pathogenic implications: the glomerular disease collaborative network. Am J Kidney Dis 18:466–471, 1991.

Jeraj K, Michael AF, Fish AJ. Immunologic similarities between Goodpasture's and Steblay's antibodies. Clin Immunol Immunopathol 23:408–413, 1982.

Jeraj K, Kim Y, Vernier RL, Fish AJ, Michael AF. Absence of Goodpasture's antigen in male patients with familial nephritis. Am J Dis Kidney 2:626–629, 1983.

Jeraj K, Vernier RL, Sisson SP, Michael AF. A new glomerular antigen in passive Heymann's nephritis. Br J Exp Pathol 65:485–498, 1984.

Johnson JP, Moore J, Austin HA, Balow JE, Antonovych TT, Wilson CB. Therapy of anti-glomerular basement antibody disease: analysis of prognostic significance of clinical pathologic treatment factors. Medicine 64:219–227, 1985.

Johnston PA, Brown JS, Braumholtz DA, Davidson AM. Clinicopathological correlations and long-term follow-up of 253 United Kingdom patients with IgA nephropathy: a report from the MRC glomerulonephritis registry. Q J Med 84:619–627, 1992.

Julian BA, Quiggins PA, Thompson JS, Woodford SY, Gleason K, Wyatt RJ. Familial IgA nephropathy: evidence of an inherited mechanism of disease. N Engl J Med 312:202–208, 1985.

Kanwar YS. Biophysiology of glomerular filtration and proteinuria. Lab Invest 51:7–21, 1984.

Kashtan CE, Michael AF. Alport syndrome: from bedside to genome to bedside. Am J Kidney Dis 22:627–640, 1993.

Katz A, Fish AJ, Kleppel MM, Hagen SG, Michael AF, Butkowski RJ. Renal entactin (nidogen): isolation, characterization and tissue distribution. Kidney Int 40:643–652, 1991.

Katz A, Newkirk MM, Klein MH. Circulating and mesangial IgA in IgA nephropathy. In D'Amico G, Minetti L, Ponticelli C, eds. Contributions to Nephrology. Vol. 40. Basel, Karger, 1984, pp. 74–79.

Katz A. Fish AJ, Santamaria P, Nevins TE, Kim Y, Butkowski RJ. Role of antibodies to tubulointerstitial nephritis antigen in human anti-tubular basement membrane nephritis associated with membranous nephropathy. Am J Med 93:691–698, 1992.

Kaufmann RH, Herrmann WA, Mëyer CJLM, Daha M, Van Es LA. Circulating IgA-immune complexes in Henoch-Schönlein purpura. Am J Med 69:859–866, 1980.

Kawano K, Miller L, Kimmelstiel P. Virus-like structures in lupus erythematosus. N Engl J Med 281:1228–1229, 1969.

Kelly CJ, Roth DA, Meyers CM. Immune recognition and response to the renal interstitium. Kidney Int 31:518–530, 1991.

Kerjaschki D, Farquhar MG. The pathogenetic antigen of Heymann nephritis is a membrane glycoprotein of the renal proximal tubule brush border. Proc Natl Acad Sci USA 79:5557–5581, 1982.

Kerjaschki D, Noronha-Blob L, Sacktor B, Farquhar MG. Micro domains of distinctive glycoprotein composition in the kidney proximal tubule brush border. J Cell Biol 98:1505–1513, 1984a.

Kerjaschki D, Sharkey DJ, Farquhar MG. Identification and characterization of podocalyxin: the major sialoprotein of the renal glomerular epithelial cell. J Cell Biol 98:1591–1596, 1984b.

Kerjaschki D, Miettinen A, Farquhar MG. Initial events in the formation of immune deposits in passive Heymann nephritis: gp330–anti-gp330 immune complexes form in epithelial coated pits and rapidly become attached to the glomerular basement membrane. J Exp Med 166:109–128, 1987.

Kibukamusoke JW, Hutt MSR, Wilks NE. The nephrotic syndrome in Uganda and its association with quartan malaria. Q J Med 36:393–408, 1967.

Kim Y, Michael AF. Idiopathic membranoproliferative glomerulonephritis. Annu Rev Med 31:273–288, 1980.

Kim Y, Michael AF. Infection and nephritis. In Edelmann, C, ed. Pediatric Kidney Disease. Boston, Little, Brown, 1978a, pp. 828–837.

Kim Y, Michael AF. Chronic bacteremia and nephritis. Annu Rev Med 29:319–325, 1978b.

Kim Y, Vernier RL, Michael AF. C3 in mesangial rings (MR) and railroad tracks (RRT): specificity for dense deposit disease (DDD). Lab Invest 12:514, 1977.

Kim Y, Butkowski R, Burke B, Kleppel MM, Crosson J, Katz A, Michael AF. Differential expression of basement membrane collagen in membranous nephropathy. Am J Pathol 139:1381–1388, 1991.

Kincaid-Smith P, Nicholls K. Mesangial IgA nephropathy. Am J Kidney Dis 3:90–102, 1983.

Klassen J, Kano K, Milgrom F, Menno AB, Anthone S, Anthone R, Sepulveda M, Elwood CM, Andres GA. Tubular lesions produced by autoantibodies to tubular basement membrane in human renal allografts. Int Arch Allergy 45:675–689, 1973.

Klein M, Poucell S, Arbus GS, McGraw M, Rance CP, Yoon S-J, Baumal R. Characteristics of a benign subtype of dense deposit disease: comparison with the progressive form of this disease. Clin Nephrol 20:163–171, 1983.

Kleinknecht C, Levy M, Gagnadoux M-F, Habib R. Membranous glomerulonephritis with extra-renal disorders in children. Medicine 58:219–228, 1979.

Kleppel MM, Michael AF, Fish AJ. Antibody specificity of human glomerular basement membrane type IV collagen NC1 subunits. J Biol Chem 261:16547–16552, 1986.

Kleppel MM, Fan WW, Cheong HI, Michael AF. Evidence for separate networks of classical and novel basement membrane collagen: characterization of α3(IV)–Alport antigen heterodimer. J Biol Chem 267:4137–4142, 1992.

Koffler D, Schur PH, Kunkel HG. Immunological studies concerning the nephritis of systemic lupus erythematosus. J Exp Med 126:607–624, 1967.

Koffler D, Sandson J, Carr R, Kunkel HG. Immunologic studies concerning the pulmonary lesion in Goodpasture's syndrome. Am J Pathol 54:293–305, 1969.

Koffler D, Agnello V, Thoburn R, Kunkel H. Systemic lupus erythematosus: prototype of immune complex nephritis in man. J Exp Med 134:169s–179s, 1971.

Kohler PF, Ten Bensel R. Serial complement component alterations in acute glomerulonephritis and systemic lupus erythematosus. Clin Exp Immunol 4:191–202, 1969.

Koskimies O, Mir S, Rapola J, Vilska J. Henoch-Schönlein nephritis: long term prognosis of unselected patients. Arch Dis Child 56:482–484, 1981.

Kreisberg JI, Wayne DB, Karnovsky MJ. Rapid and focal loss of negative charge associated with mononuclear cell infiltration early in nephrotoxic serum nephritis. Kidney Int 16:290–300, 1979.

Krishnan C, Kaplan MH. Immunopathologic studies of systemic lupus erythematosus. II. Antinuclear reaction of γ-globulin eluted from homogenates and isolated glomeruli of kidneys from patients with lupus nephritis. J Clin Invest 46:569–579, 1967.

Kunis CL, Kiss B, Williams G, D'Agati V, Appel GB. Intravenous "pulse" cyclophosphamide therapy of crescentic glomerulonephritis. Clin Nephrol 37:1–7, 1992.

Lachmann PJ, Müller-Eberhard HJ, Kunkel HG, Paronetto F. The localization of the in vivo bound complement in tissue sections. J Exp Med 115:63–82, 1962.

Lagrue G, Xheneumont S, Branellec A, Hirbec G, Weil BA. vascular permeability factor elaborated from lymphocytes. I. Demonstration in patients with nephrotic syndrome. Biomedicine 23:37–40, 1975.

Lahita RG, Bradlow HL, Fishman J, Kunkel HG. Abnormal estrogen and androgen metabolism in the human with systemic lupus erythematosus. Am J Kidney Dis 2(Suppl.):206–211, 1982.

Lai KN, Leung JCK, Lai FM, Tam JS. T-lymphocyte activation in IgA nephropathy: serum soluble interleukin-2 receptor level, interleukin-2 production and interleukin-2 receptor expression by cultured lymphocytes. J Clin Immunol 9:485–492, 1989a.

Lai KN, Lo STH, Lai FM-M. Immunohistochemical study of the membrane attack complex of complement and S-protein in idiopathic and secondary membranous nephropathy. Am J Pathol 135:469–476, 1989b.

Lambert PH, Dixon FJ, Zubler RH, Agnell V, Cambiaso C, Casali P, Clarke J, Courdery JS, McDuffie FC, Hay, FC, Maclennan ICM, Masson P, Müller-Eberhard HJ, Penttinen K, Smith M, Tappeiner G, Theofilopoulos AN, Verroust PA. WHO collaborative study for the evaluation of eighteen methods for detecting immune complexes in serum. J Clin Lab Immunol 1:1–15, 1978.

Lange K, Wasserman E, Slobody LB. The significance of serum complement levels for the diagnosis and prognosis of acute and subacute glomerulonephritis and lupus erythematosus disseminatus. Ann Intern Med 53:636–646, 1960.

Lange K, Seligson G, Cronin W. Evidence for the in situ origin of poststreptococcal glomerulonephritis: glomerular localization of endostreptosin and the clinical significance of the subsequent antibody response. Clin Nephrol 19:3–10, 1983.

Latham P, Poucell S, Koresaar A, Arbus G, Baumal R. Idiopathic membranous glomerulopathy in Canadian children: a clinicopathologic study. J Pediatr 101:682–685, 1982.

Layward L, Allen AC, Harper SJ, Hattersley JM, and Feehally J. Increased and prolonged production of specific polymeric IgA after systemic immunization with tetanus toxoid in IgA nephropathy. Clin Exp Immunol 88:394–398, 1992.

Lehman DH, Wilson CB, Dixon FJ. Interstitial nephritis in rats immunized with heterologous tubular basement membrane. Kidney Int 5:187–195, 1974.

Lehman DH, Wilson CB, Dixon FJ. Extraglomerular immunoglobulin deposits in human nephritis. Am J Med 58:765–786, 1975.

Lehman TJA, Sherry DD, Wagner-Weiner L, McCurdy DK, Emery HM, Magilavy DB,Kovalesky A. Intermittent intravenous cyclophosphamide for lupus nephritis. J Pediatr 114:1055–1060, 1989.

Leibowitch J, Halbwachs L, Wattel S, Gaillard M-H, Droz D. Recurrence of dense deposits in the transplanted kidney: II. Serum complement and nephritic factor profiles. Kidney Int 15:396–403, 1979.

Lerner RA, Glassock RJ, Dixon FJ. The role of antiglomerular basement membrane antibody in the pathogenesis of human glomerulonephritis. J Exp Med 126:989–1004, 1967.

Levinsky R, Malleson PN, Barratt TM, Soothill J. Circulating immune complexes in steroid-responsive nephrotic syndrome. N Engl J Med 298:126–129, 1978.

Levy M, Beaufils H, Gubler MC, Habib R. Idiopathic recurrent macroscopic hematuria and mesangial IgA-IgG deposits in children (Berger's disease). Clin Nephrol 1:63–69, 1973.

Levy M, Lesavre P. Genetic factors in IgA nephropathy (Berger's disease). In Grünfeld J-P, Bach JF, Kivalis H, Maxwell MH, eds. Advances in Nephrology. Chicago, Mosby–Year Book, 1992, pp. 23–51.

Lewis EJ, Carpenter CB, Schur PH. Serum complement component levels in human glomerulonephritis. Ann Intern Med 75:555–560, 1971.

Linné T, Berg V, Bohman S-O, Sigström L. Course and long-term outcome of idiopathic IgA nephropathy in children. Pediatr Nephrol 5:383–386, 1991.

Lloyd W, Schur PH. Immune complexes, complement, and anti-DNA in exacerbations of systemic lupus erythematosus (SLE). Medicine 60:208–217, 1981.

Lockshin MD, Reinitz E, Druzin ML, Murrman M, Estes D. Lupus pregnancy: case control prospective study demonstrating absence of lupus exacerbation during or after pregnancy. Am J Med 77:893–898, 1984.

Madaio MP, Salant DJ, Cohen AJ, Adler S, Couser WG. Comparative study of in situ immune deposit formation in active and passive Heymann's nephritis. Kidney Int 23:498–505, 1983.

Magil AB, Puterman ML, Ballon HS, Chan V, Lirenman DS, Rar A, Sutton RA. Prognostic factors in diffuse lupus glomerulonephritis. Kidney Int 34:511–517, 1988.

Mahieu PM, Winand RJ. Carbohydrate and amino acid composition of human glomerular-basement-membrane fractions purified by affinity chromatography. Eur J Biochem 37:157–163, 1973.

Maizel SE, Sibley RK, Horstman JP, Kjellstrand CM, Simmons RL. Incidence and significance of recurrent focal segmental glomerulosclerosis in renal allograft recipients. Transplantation 32:512–516, 1981.

Marquardt H, Wilson CB, Dixon FJ. Isolation and immunological characterization of human glomerular basement membrane antigens. Kidney Int 3:57–65, 1973.

Mathew TH, Mathews DC, Hobbs JB, Kincaid-Smith P. Glomerular lesions after renal transplantation. Am J Med 59:177–190, 1975.

Mauer SM, Sutherland DER, Howard RJ, Fish AJ, Najarian JS, Michael AF. The glomerular mesangium: III. Acute immune mesangial injury: a new model of glomerulonephritis. J Exp Med 137:553–570, 1973.

Mauer SM, Lee CS, Goren G, Sutherland DER, Howard RJ, Hoyer JR, Michael AF. Inability of the lymphocyte to induce glomerular injury. Transplant Proc 7:315–320, 1975.

McCluskey RT. Immunologically mediated tubulointerstitial nephritis. In Brenner BM, Stein JH, Cotran RS, eds. Contemporary Issues in Nephrology. Vol. 10. New York, Churchill Livingstone, 1983, pp. 121–149.

McCoy RC, Clapp J, Seigel HF. Membranoproliferative glomerulonephritis: progression from the pure form to the crescentic form with recurrence after transplantation. Am J Med 59:288–292, 1975.

McCoy RC, Johnson HK, Stone WJ, Wilson CB. Absence of nephritogenic GBM antigen(s) in some patients with hereditary nephritis. Kidney Int 21:642–652, 1982.

McEnery PT. Membranoproliferative glomerulonephritis: the Cincinnati experience—cumulative renal survival from 1957 to 1989. J Pediatr 116:S109–S114, 1990.

McEnery PT, McAdams AJ, West CD. The effect of prednisone in a high-dose alternate day regimen on the natural history of idiopathic membranoproliferative glomerulonephritis. Medicine (Balt), 401–425, 1986.

McGhee JR, Mestecky J, Elson CO, Kiyono H. Regulation of IgA synthesis and immune response by T cells and interleukins. J Clin Immunol 9:175–199, 1989.

McLean RH, Geiger H, Burke S, Simmons R, Najarian JS, Vernier RL, Michael AF. Recurrence of membranoproliferative glomerulonephritis following kidney transplantation. Am J Med 60:60–72, 1976.

McLean RH, Forsgren A, Björkstén B, Kim Y, Quie PG, Michael AF. Decreased serum factor B concentration associated with decreased opsonization of E. coli in the idiopathic nephrotic syndrome. Pediatr Res 11:910–916, 1977.

Meadow SR. The prognosis of Henoch-Schönlein nephritis. Clin Nephrol 9:87–90, 1978.

Meadow SR, Glasgow EF, White RHR, Moncrieff MW, Cameron JS, Ogg CS. Schönlein-Henoch nephritis. Q J Med 41:241–258, 1972.

Meadow SR, Scott DG. Berger disease: Henoch-Schönlein syndrome without the rash. J Pediatr 106:27–32, 1985.

Mellors RC, Ortega LG, Holman HR. Role of gamma globulins in pathogenesis of renal lesions in systemic lupus erythematosus and chronic membranous glomerulonephritis, with an observation on the lupus erythematosus cell reaction. J Exp Med 106:191–202, 1957.

Melvin T, Kim Y, Michael AF. Selective binding of IgG4 and other negatively charged plasma proteins in normal and diabetic human kidneys. Am J Pathol 115:443–446, 1984a.

Melvin T, Sibley R, Michael AF. Nephrotic syndrome. In Tune BM, Mendoza SA, Brenner BM, Stein JH, eds. Contemporary Issues in Nephrology. Edinburgh, Churchill Livingstone, 1984b, pp. 191–230.

Mendoza SA, Reznik VM, Griswold WR, Krensky AM, Yorgin PD, Tune BM. Treatment of steroid-resistant focal segmental glomerulosclerosis with pulse methylprednisolone and alkylating agents. Pediatr Nephrol 4:303–307, 1990.

Michael AF Jr. In Immunologic Mechanisms in Renal Disease: An Overview. Proceedings of IXth International Congress of Nephrology. New York, Springer-Verlag, 1984, pp. 485–503.

Michael AF Jr, Drummond KN, Good RA, Vernier RL. Acute poststreptococcalglomerulonephritis: immune deposit disease. J Clin Invest 45:237–248, 1966.

Michael AF Jr, Vernier RL, Drummond KN, Levitt JI, Herdman RC, Fish AJ, Good, R. A. Immunosuppressive therapy of chronic renal disease. N Engl J Med 276:817–828, 1967.

Michael AF Jr, Herdman RC, Fish AJ, Pickering RJ, Vernier RL. Chronic membranoproliferative glomerulonephritis with hypocomplementemia. Transplant Proc 1:925–932, 1969.

Michael AF Jr, Westberg NG, Fish AJ, Vernier RL. Studies on chronic membranoproliferative glomerulonephritis with hypocomplementemia. J Exp Med 134(Suppl.):207s–227s, 1971.

Michael AF Jr, Hoyer J, Westberg NG, Fish AJ. Experimental models for the pathogenesis of acute post-streptococcal glomerulonephritis. In Wannamaker LW, Matsen JM, eds. Streptococci and Streptococcal Diseases. New York, Academic Press, 1972a, pp. 481–500.

Michael AF, Blau E, Mauer SM, Hoyer JR. Glomerular capillary permeability and experimental nephrotic syndrome. In Day S, Good RA, eds. Membranes and Viruses in Immunopathology. New York, Academic Press, 1972b, pp. 477–501.

Michael AF, Keane W, Raij L, Vernier RL, Mauer SM. The glomerular mesangium. Kidney Int 17:141–154, 1980.

Michael AF, Falk RJ, Platt JL, Melvin T, Yang J-Y. Antigens of the human glomerulus. In Advances in Nephrology. Vol. 13. Chicago, Year Book Medical Publishers 1984, pp. 203–218.

Michalk D, Waldherr R, Seelig HP, Weber HP, Scharer K. Idiopathic mesangial IgA-glomerulonephritis in childhood: description of 19 pediatric cases and review of the literature. Eur J Pediatr 134:13–22, 1980.

Miettinen A, Törnroth T, Tikkanen I. Virtanen I., Linder, E. Heymann nephritis induced by kidney brush border glycoproteins. Lab Invest 43:547–555, 1980.

Mohammed I, Ansell BM, Holborow EJ, Bryceson ADM. Circulating immune complexes in subacute infective endocarditis and post-streptococcal glomerulonephritis. J Clin Pathol 30:308–311, 1977.

Mohan PS, and Spiro RG. Characterization of heparan sulfate proteoglycan from calf lens capsule and proteoglycans synthesized by cultured lens epithelial cells: comparison with other basement membrane proteoglycans. J Biol Chem 266:8567–8575, 1991.

Monga G, Mazzucco G, Di Belgiojoso GB, Busnach G. Monocyte infiltration and glomerular hypercellularity in human acute and persistent glomerulonephritis: light and electron microscopic, immunofluorescence and histochemical investigation of twenty-eight cases. Lab Invest 44:381–387, 1981.

Montalbert C, Carvallo A, Broumand B, Noble D, Anstine LA, Currier CB Jr. Successful renal transplantation in polyarteritis nodosa. Clin Nephrol 14:206–209, 1980.

Moore RH, Hitman GA, Lucas EY, Richards NT, Venning MC, Papiha S, Goodship TH, Fidler A, Awad J, Festenstein H. HLA DQ region gene polymorphism associated with primary IgA nephropathy. Kidney Int 37:991–995, 1990.

Morin M-P, Thervet E, Legendre C, Page B, Kreis H, Noel L-H. Successful kidney transplantation in a patient with microscopic polyarteritis and positive ANCA (letter). Nephrol Dial Transplant 8:287–288, 1993.

Morris MC, Cameron JS, Chantler C, Turner DR. Systemic lupus erythematosus with nephritis. Arch Dis Child 56:779–783, 1981.

Morrison KE, Germino GG, Reeders ST. Use of the polymerase chain reaction to clone and sequence a cDNA encoding the bovine α3 chain of type IV collagen. J Biol Chem 266:34–39, 1991.

Morrow WJW, Isenberg DA, Todd-Pokropek A, Parry HF, Snaith ML. Useful laboratory measurements in the management of systemic lupus erythematosus. Q J Med 51:125–138, 1982.

Nagata K, Platt JL, Michael AF. Interstitial and glomerular immune cell populations in idiopathic nephrotic syndrome. Kidney Int 25:88–93, 1984.

Nakamoto Y, Asano Y, Dohi K, Fujioka M, Iida H, Kida H, Kibe Y, Hattori N, Takeuchi J. Primary IgA glomerulonephritis and Schönlein-Henoch purpura nephritis: clinicopathological and immunohistological characteristics. Q J Med 47:495–516, 1978.

Narchi H, Taylor R, Azmy AF, Murphy AV, Beattie TJ. Shunt nephritis. J Pediatr Surg 23:839–841, 1988.

Neilson EG. Pathogenesis and therapy of interstitial nephritis. Kidney Int 35:1257–1270, 1989.

Neilson EG, Sun MJ, Kelly CJ, Hines WH, Haverty TP, Clayman MD, Cooke N E. Molecular characterization of a major nephritogenic domain in the autoantigen of anti–tubular basement membrane disease. Proc Natl Acad Sci U S A 88:2006–2010, 1991.

Nevins TE, Michael AF. Isolation of rat glomerular polyanion. Kidney Int 19:553–563, 1981.

Nolasco FEB, Cameron JS, Hartley B, Coelho A, Hildreth G, Reuben R. Intraglomerular T cells and monocytes in nephritis: study with monoclonal antibodies. Kidney Int 31:1160–1166, 1987.

Nomoto Y, Sakai H, Arimori S. Increase of IgA-bearing lymphocytes in peripheral blood from patients with IgA nephropathy. Am J Clin Pathol 71:158–166, 1979.

Nomura S, Osawa G, Sai T, Harano T, Harano K. A splicing mutation in the alpha 5(IV) collagen gene of a family with Alport's syndrome. Kidney Int 43:1116–1124, 1993.

Norton W. Endothelial inclusions in active lesions of systemic lupus erythematosus. J Lab Clin Med 74:369–379, 1969.

Notman DD, Kurata N, Tan EM. Profiles of antinuclear antibodies in systemic rheumatic diseases. Ann Intern Med 83:464–469, 1975.

Oberhuber G, Prior C, Bösmüller C, Dietze O, Margreiter R. Early recurrence of Wegener's granulomatosis in a kidney allograft under cyclosporine treatment. Transplant Int 1:49–50, 1988.

Oite T, Batsford SR, Mihatsch MJ, Takamiya M, Vogt A. Quantitative studies of in situ immune complex glomerulonephritis in the rat induced by planted cationized antigen. J Exp Med 155:460–474, 1982.

Oite T, Schimizu F, Kihara I, Batsford SR, Vogt A. An active model of immune complex glomerulonephritis in the rat employing cationized antigen. Am J Pathol 112:185–194, 1983.

Olbing H, Greifer I, Bennett BP, Bernstein J, Spitzer A. Idiopathic membranous nephropathy in children. Kidney Int 3:381–390, 1973.

Olson DL, Anand SK, Landing BH, Heuser E, Grushkin CM, Lieberman E. Diagnosis of hereditary nephritis by failure of glomeruli to bind anti-glomerular basement membrane antibodies. J Pediatr 96:697–699, 1980.

Onion KD, Crumpacker CS, Gilliland BC. Arthritis of hepatitis associated with Australia antigen. Ann Intern Med 75:29–33, 1971.

Ooi Y M, Vallota EH, West CD. Classical complement pathway activation in membrane proliferative glomerulonephritis. Kidney Int 9:46–53, 1976.

Ooi YM, Vallota EH, West CD. Serum immune complexes in membranoproliferative and other glomerulonephritis. Kidney Int 11:275–283, 1977a.

Ooi YM, Ooi BS, Pollak VE. Relationship of levels of circulating immune complexes to histologic patterns of nephritis: a comparative study of membranous glomerulopathy and diffuse proliferative glomerulonephritis. J Lab Clin Med 90:891–898, 1977b.

Ozen S, Besbas N, Saatci U, Bakkaloglu A. Diagnostic criteria for polyarteritis nodosa in childhood. J Pediatr 120:206–209, 1992.

Parera M, Rivera F, Egido J, Campos A. The role of interleukin 2 (IL-2) and serum-soluble IL-2 receptor cells in idiopathic IgA nephropathy. Clin Immunol Immunopathol 63:196–199, 1992.

Parra G, Platt JL, Falk RJ, Rodriguez-Iturbe B, Michael AF. Cell populations and membrane attack complex in glomeruli of patients with poststreptococcal glomerulonephritis: identification using monoclonal antibodies by indirect immunofluorescence. Clin Immunol Immunopathol 33:324–332, 1984.

Parra G, Mosquera J, Rodriguez-Iturbe B. Migration inhibition factor in acute serum sickness nephritis. Kidney Int 38:1118–1124, 1990.

Pelletier L, Hirsch F, Rossert J, Druet E, Druet P. Experimental mercury-induced glomerulonephritis. Springer Semin Immunopathol 9:359–369, 1987.

Peratoner L, Longo F, Lepore L, Freschi P. Prophylaxis and therapy of glomerulonephritis in the course of anaphylactoid purpura: the results of a polycentric clinical trial. Acta Paediatr Scand 79:976–977, 1990.

Peters DK, Williams DG, Charlesworth JA, Boulton-Jones JM, Sissons JGP, Evans DJ, Kourilsky O, Morel-Maroger L. Mesangiocapillary glomerulonephritis, partial lipodystrophy and hypocomplementemia. Lancet, 2:535–538, 1973.

Peters DK, Rees AJ, Lockwood CM, Pusey CD. Treatment and prognosis in antibasement membrane antibody–mediated nephritis. Transplant Proc 14:513–521, 1982.

Pincus T. Studies regarding a possible function for viruses in the pathogenesis of systemic lupus erythematosus. Arthritis Rheum 25:847–856, 1982.

Platt JL, Burke BA, Fish AJ, Kim Y, Michael AF. Systemic lupus erythematosus in the first two decades of life. Am J Kidney Dis 2(Suppl.):212–222, 1982.

Ponticelli C, Rizzoni G, Edefonti A, Altieri P, Rivolta E, Rinaldi S, Ghio L, Lusvaghi E, Gusmano R, Locatelli F, Pasquali S, Castellani A, Casa-Alberighi OD. A randomized trial of cyclosporine in steroid-resistant idiopathic nephrotic syndrome. Kidney Int 43:1377–1384, 1993.

Potter EV, Lipshultz SA, Abidh S, Poon-King T, Earle DP. Twelve to seventeen year follow-up of patients with poststreptococcal acute glomerulonephritis in Trinidad. N Engl J Med 307:725–729, 1982.

Praz F, Halbwachs L, Lesavre P. Genetic aspects of complement and glomerulonephritis. In Grunfeld JP, Maxwell MH, eds. Advances in Nephrology. Vol 13. Chicago, Year Book Medical Publishers 1984, pp. 271–296.

Prince AM, Trepo C. Role of immune complexes involving SH antigen in pathogenesis of chronic active hepatitis and polyarteritis nodosa. Lancet 1:1309–1312, 1971.

Raij L, Azar S, Keane W. Mesangial immune injury, hypertension, and progressive glomerular damage in Dahl rats. Kidney Int 26:137–143, 1984.

Rajaraman S, Goldblum RM, Cavallo T. IgA associated glomerulonephritis: a study with monoclonal antibodies. Clin Immunol Immunopathol 39:514–522, 1986.

Rao TKS, Filippone EJ, Nicastri AD, Landesman SH, Frank E, Chen CK, Friedman EA. Associated focal and segmental glomerulosclerosis in the acquired immunodeficiency syndrome. N Engl J Med 310:669–673, 1984.

Reeders, S. T. Molecular genetics of hereditary nephritis. Kidney Int 42:783–792, 1992.

Reveille JD, Bias WB, Winkelstein JA, Provost TT, Dorsch CA, Arnett FC. Familial systemic lupus erythematosus: immunogenetic studies in eight families. Medicine 62:21–35, 1983.

Rodriguez-Garcia JL, Fraile G, Mampaso F, Teruel JL. Pulmonary tuberculosis associated with membranous nephropathy (letter). Nephron 55:218–219, 1990.

Rodriguez-Iturbe B. Nephrology forum: epidemic poststreptococcal glomerulonephritis. Kidney Int 25:129–136, 1984.

Rodriguez-Iturbe B, Katiyar VN, Coello J. Neuraminidase activity and free sialic acid levels in the serum of patients with acute poststreptococcal glomerulonephritis. N Engl J Med 304:1506–1510, 1981.

Rosner S, Ginzler EM, Diamond HS, Weiner M, Schlesinger M, Fries JF, Wasner C, Medsger TA Jr, Zeiger G, Klippel JH, Hadler NM, Albert DA, Hess EV, Spencer-Green G, Grayzel A, Worth D, Hahn BH, Barnett EV. A multicenter study of outcome in systemic lupus erythematosus. II. Causes of death. Arthritis Rheum 25:612–617, 1982.

Rothschild E, Chatenoud L. T cell subset modulation of immunoglobulin production in IgA nephropathy and membranous glomerulonephritis. Kidney Int 25:557–564, 1984.

Rottem M, Fauci AS, Hallahan CW, Kerr GS, Lebovics R, Leavitt RY, Hoffman GS. Wegener granulomatosis in children and adolescents: clinical presentation and outcome. J Pediatr 122:26–31, 1993.

Roy LP, Westberg NG, Michael AF. Nephrotic syndrome: no evidence for a role for IgE. Clin Exp Immunol 13:553–559, 1973a.

Roy LP, Fish AJ, Vernier RL, Michael AF. Recurrent macroscopic hematuria, focal nephritis, and mesangial deposition of immunoglobulin and complement. J Pediatr 82:767–772, 1973b.

Roy S, Wall HP, Etteldorf JN. Second attacks of acute glomerulonephritis. J Pediatr 75:758–767, 1969.

Rynes RI. Inherited complement deficiency states and SLE. Clin Rheum Dis 8:29–47, 1982.

Sakai H, Nomoto Y, Arimori S. Decrease of IgA-specific suppressor T cell activity in patients with IgA nephropathy. Clin Exp Immunol 38:243–248, 1979.

Sakai H, Endoh M, Tomino Y, Nomoto Y. Increase of IgA specific helper $T\alpha$ cells in patients with IgA nephropathy. Clin Exp Immunol 50:77–82, 1982.

Sakai H, Miyazaki M, Endoh M, Nomoto Y. Increase of IgA-specific switch T cells in patients with IgA nephropathy. Clin Exp Immunol 78:378–382, 1989.

Salant DJ, Belok S, Madaio MP, Couser WG. A new role for complement in experimental membranous nephropathy in rats. J Clin Invest 66:1339–1350, 1980.

Sanes JR, Engvall E, Butkowski R, Hunter DD. Molecular heterogeneity of basal laminae: isoforms of laminin and collagen IV at the neuromuscular junction and elsewhere. J Cell Biol 111:1685–1699, 1990.

Scheinman JI, Foidart J-M, Gehran-Robey P, Fish AJ, Michael AF. The immunohistology of glomerular antigens. IV. Laminin, a defined non-collagen basement membrane glycoprotein. Clin. Immunol. Immunopathol 15:175–189, 1980.

Schena FP, Pertosa G, Stanziale P, Vox E, Pecoraro C, Andreucci VE. Biological significance of C3 nephritic factor in membranoproliferative glomerulonephritis. Clin Nephrol 18:240–246, 1982.

Schena FP, Pertosa G, Pastore A, de Tommasi A, Montagna MT, Bonomo L. Circulating immune complexes in infected venticuloatrial and ventriculoperitoneal shunts. J Clin Immunol 3:173–177, 1983.

Schena FP, Mastrolitti G, Jirillo, E, Munno, I, Pellegrino N, Fracasso AR, Aventaggiato L. Increased production of interleukin-2 and IL-2 receptor in primary IgA nephropathy. Kidney Int 35:875–879, 1989a.

Schena FP, Pastore A, Ludovico N, Sinico RA, Benuzzi S, Montinaro V. Increased serum levels of IgG1-IgG immune complexes and anti-F (ab')2 antibodies in patients with primary nephropathy. Clin Exp Immunol 77:15–20, 1989b.

Schnaper HW. The immune system in minimal change nephrotic syndrome. Pediatr Nephrol 3:101–110, 1989.

Schnaper HW. A regulatory system for soluble immune response suppressor production in steroid-responsive nephrotic syndrome. Kidney Int 38:151–159, 1990.

Schnaper HW, Aune TM. Steroid-sensitive mechanism of soluble immune response suppressor production in steroid-responsive nephrotic syndrome. J Clin Invest 79:257–264, 1987.

Schreiber RD, Götze O, Müller-Eberhard HS. Alternative pathway of complement: demonstration and characterization of initiation factor and its properdin-independent function. J Exp Med 144:1062–1075, 1976.

Schreiner GF, Cotran RS, Pardo V, Unanue AR. A mononuclear cell component in experimental immunological glomerulonephritis. J Exp Med 147:369–384, 1978.

Schreiner GF, Kiely JM, Cotran RS, Unanue ER. Characterization of resident glomerular cells in the rat expressing Ia determinants and manifesting genetically restricted interactions with lymphocytes. J Clin Invest 68:920–931, 1981.

Schreiner GF, Cotran RS. Localization of an Ia-bearing glomerular cell in the mesangium. J Cell Biol 94:483–488, 1982.

Schur PH. Complement and lupus erythematosus. Arthritis Rheum 25:793–798, 1982.

Schwartz MM, Bernstein J, Hill GS, Holley K Phillips EA. Predictive value of renal pathology in diffuse proliferative lupus glomerulonephritis nephritis: lupus nephritis collaborative study group. Kidney Int 36:891–896, 1989.

Schwartz RS. Immunologic and genetic aspects of systemic lupus erythematosus. Kidney Int 19:474–484, 1981.

Scott JS, Maddison PJ, Taylor PV, Esscher E, Scott O, Skinner RP. Connective tissue disease, antibodies to ribonucleoprotein and congenital heart block. N Engl J Med 309:209–212, 1983.

Seegal BC, Andres GA, Hsu KC, Zabriskie JB. Studies on the pathogenesis of acute and progressive glomerulonephritis in man by immunofluorescein and immunoferritin techniques. Fed Proc 24:100–108, 1965.

Seligson G, Lange K, Majeed HA, Deol H, Cronin W, Bovie R. Significance of endostreptosin antibody titers in poststreptococcal glomerulonephritis. Clin Nephrol 24:69–75, 1985.

Simpson IJ, Doak PB, Williams LC, Blacklock HA, Hill RS, Teague CA, Herdson PB, Wilson CB. Plasma exchange in Goodpasture's syndrome. Am J Nephrol 2:301–311, 1982.

Sinniah R, Javier AR, Ku G. The pathology of mesangial IgA nephritis with clinical correlation. Histopathology 5:469–490, 1981.

Smolen JS, Chused TM, Leiserson WM, Reeves JP, Alling D, Steinberg AD. Heterogeneity of immunoregulatory T-cell subsets in systemic lupus erythematosus. Am J Med 72:783–790, 1982.

Sobel A, Gabay Y, Largue G. Recherche de complexes immuns circulants par le test de déviation de la fraction C1q du complément: premières application à l'étude des glomerulopathies humaines. Nouv Presse Med 5:1465–1469, 1976.

Solling J. Circulating immune complexes in glomerulonephritis: a longitudinal study. Clin Nephrol 20:177–183, 1983.

Spital A, Panner BJ, Sterns RH. Acute idiopathic tubulointerstitial nephritis: report of two cases and review of the literature. Am J Kidney Dis 9:71–78, 1987.

Spitzer RE, Vallota EH, Forristal J, Sudora E, Stitzel A, Davis NC, West CD. Serum C'3 lytic system in patients with glomerulonephritis. Science 164:436–437, 1969.

Stachura I, Si L, Madan E, Whiteside T. Mononuclear cell subsets in human renal disease: enumeration in tissue sections with monoclonal antibodies. Clin Immunol Immunopathol 30:362–373, 1984.

Steblay RW. Glomerulonephritis induced in sheep by injections of heterologous glomerular basement membrane and Freund's complete adjuvant. J Exp Med 116:253–272, 1962.

Steinberg AD. Recent advances on the mechanisms and genetic aspects of lupus erythematosus. Adv Nephrol 14:305–332, 1984.

Steinberg AD, Decker JL. A double-blind controlled trial comparing cyclophosphamide, azathioprine and placebo in the treatment of lupus glomerulonephritis. Arthritis Rheum 17:923–937, 1974.

Sterzl RD, Pabst R. The temporal relationship between glomerular cell proliferation and monocyte infiltration in experimental glomerulonephritis. Virchow Arch Cell Pathol 38:337–350, 1982.

Stickler GB, Shin MH, Burke EC, Holley KE, Miller RH, Segar WE. Diffuse glomerulonephritis associated with infected ventriculoatrial shunt. N Engl J Med 279:1077–1082, 1968.

Strife CF, McEnery PT, McAdams AJ, West CD. Membranoproliferative glomerulonephritis with disruption of the glomerular basement membrane. Clin Nephrol 7:65–72, 1977.

Synkowski DR, Mogavero HS, Provost TT. Lupus erythematosus: laboratory testing and clinical subsets in the evaluation of patients. Med Clin North Am 64:921–940, 1980.

Tan EM. Interactions between autoimmunity and molecular and cell triology: bridges between clinical and basic sciences. J Clin Invest 84:1–6, 1989.

Tan EM, Schur PH, Carr RI, Kunkel HG. Deoxyribonucleic acid (DNA) and antibodies to DNA in the serum of patients with systemic lupus erythematosus. J Clin Invest 45:1732–1740, 1966.

Tanaka R, Yoshikawa N, Kitano Y, Ito H, Nakamura H. Long-term cyclosporine treatment in children with steroid-dependent nephrotic syndrome. Pediatr Nephrol 7:249–252, 1993.

Tanuma T, Ohi H, Hatano M. Two types of C3 nephritic factor: properdin-dependent C3NeF and properdin-independent C3NeF. Clin Immunol Immunopathol 56:226–238, 1990.

Theofilopoulos AN, Wilson CB, Dixon FJ. The Raji cell radioimmune assay for detecting immune complexes in human sera. J Clin Invest 57:169–182, 1976.

Timpl R. Recent advances in the biochemistry of glomerular basement membrane. Kidney Int 30:293–298, 1986.

Tomino Y, Endoh M, Nomoto Y, Sakai H. Activation of complement by renal tissues from patients with IgA nephropathy. J Clin Pathol 34:35–40, 1981.

Tomino Y, Endoh M, Nomoto Y, Sakai H. Immunoglobulin A1 in IgA nephropathy (letter). N Engl J Med 305:1159–1160, 1982.

Tryggvason K, Zhou J, Hostikka SL, Shows TB. Molecular genetics of Alport sydrome. Kidney Int 43:38–44, 1993.

Tu WH, Shearn MA, Lee JC. Acute diffuse glomerulonephritis in acute staphylococcal endocarditis. Ann Intern Med 71:335–341, 1969.

Tung KS, Woodroffe AJ, Ahlin TD, Williams RC Jr, Wilson CB. Application of the solid phase C1q and Raji cell radioimmunoassays for the detection of circulating immune complexes in glomerulonephritis. J Clin Invest 62:61–72, 1978.

Turner N, Lockwood CM, Rees AJ. Antiglomerular basement membrane antibody–mediated nephritis. In Schrier RW, Gottschalk CW, eds. Diseases of the Kidney. Boston, Little, Brown, 1993, pp. 1865–1894.

Turner N, Mason PJ, Brown R, Fox M, Povey S, Rees A, Pusey CD. Molecular cloning of the human Goodpasture antigen demonstrates it to be the α3 chain of type IV collagen. J Clin Invest 89:592–601, 1992.

Tuso P, Moudgil A, Hay J, Goodman D, Kamil E, Koyyana R, Jordan SC. Treatment of antineutrophil cytoplasmic autoantibody–positive systemic vasculitis and glomerulonephritis with pooled intravenous gammaglobulin. Am J Kidney Dis 20:504–508, 1992.

Urizar RE, Michael AF, Sisson S, Vernier RL. Anaphylactoid purpura. II. Immunofluorescent and electron microscopic studies of the glomerular lesions. Lab Invest 19:437–450, 1968.

Urizar RE, Herdman RC. Anaphylactoid purpura. III. Early morphologic glomerular changes. Am J Clin Pathol 53:258–266, 1970.

Valentijn RM, Radl J, Haayman JJ, Vermeer BJ, Weening JJ, Kauffmann RH, Daha MR, van Es LA. Macromolecular IgA1 in the circulation and mesangial deposits in patients with primary IgA nephropathy. In D'Amico G, Minetti L, Ponticelli C, eds. Contributions to Nephrology. Vol. 40. Basel Karger 1984, pp. 87–92.

Vallota EH, Forristal J, Spitzer RE, Davis NC, West CD. Characteristics of a non–complement-dependent C3-reactive complex formed from factors in nephritis and normal serum. J Exp Med 131:1306–1324, 1970.

Vallota EH, Forristal J, Spitzer R, Davis NC, West CD. Continuing C3 breakdown after bilateral nephrectomy in patients with membrano-proliferative glomerulonephritis. J Clin Invest 50:552–558, 1971.

Van Damme BJC, Fleuren GJ, Bakker WW, Vernier RL, Hoedemaeker Ph J. Experimental glomerulonephritis in the rat induced by antibodies directed against tubular antigens. V. Fixed glomerular antigens in the pathogenesis of heterologous immune complex glomerulonephritis. Lab Invest 38:502–510, 1978.

van den Born J, van den Heuvel L, Bakker MAH, Veerkamp JH, Assmann KJM, Weening JJ, Berden JHM. Distribution of GBM heparan sulfate proteoglycan core protein and side chains in human glomerular diseases. Kidney Int 43:454–463, 1991.

van den Wall Bake AWL, Bruijn JA, Accavitti MA, Crowley-Norwick PA, Schrohenloher RE, Julian BA, Jackson S, Kubagawa H, Cooper MD, Daha MR, Mestecky J. Shared idiotypes in mesangial deposits in IgA nephropathy are not disease-specific. Kidney Int 44:65–74, 1993.

van Es LA. Pathogenesis of IgA nephropathy (clinical conference). Kidney Int 41:1720–1729, 1992.

van Es LA, Daha MR. Factors influencing the endocytosis of immune complexes. In Grunfeld JP, Maxwell MH, eds. Advances in Nephrology. Vol. 13. Chicago, Year Book Medical Publishers 1984, pp. 341–367.

Varade WS, Forristal J, West CD. Patterns of complement activation in idiopathic membranoproliferative glomerulonephritis, types I, II and III. Am J Kidney Dis 14:196–206, 1990.

Velosa J, Miller K, Michael AF. Immunopathology of the end-stage kidney: immunoglobulins and complement component deposition in non-immune disease. Am J Pathol 84:149–162, 1976.

Vernier RL, Worthen HG, Peterson RD, Colle E, Good RA. Anaphylactoid purpura: I. Pathology of the skin and kidney and frequency of streptococcal infection. Pediatrics 27:181–193, 1961.

Vernier RL, Mauer SM, Fish AJ, Michael AF. The mesangial cell in glomerulonephritis. In Hamburger J, Crosnier J, Maxwell MH, eds. Advances in Nephrology. Vol 1. Chicago, Year Book Medical Publishers 1971, pp. 31–46.

Vernier RL, Klein DJ, Sisson SP, Mahan JD, Oegema TR, Brown DM. Heparan sulfate–rich anionic sites in the human glomerular basement membrane: decreased concentration in congenital nephrotic syndrome. N Engl J Med 309:1001–1009, 1983.

Verroust P, Ben-Maiz H, Morel-Morager L, Mahford A, Geniteau M, Benayed H, Richet G. A clinical and immunopathological study of 304 cases of glomerulonephritis in Tunisia. Eur J Clin Invest 9:75–79, 1979.

Vogt, A. New aspects of the pathogenesis of immune complex glomerulonephritis: formation of subepithelial deposits. Clin Nephrol 21:15–20, 1984.

Waldherr R, Rambausek M, Rauterberg W, Andrassy K, Ritz E. Immunohistochemical features of mesangial IgA glomerulonephritis. In D'Amico G, Minetti L, Ponticelli C, eds. Contributions to Nephrology. Vol. 40. Basel Karger 1984, pp. 99–106.

Walker RG, Scheinkestel C, Becker GJ, Owen JE, Dowling JP, Kincaid-Smith P: Clinical and morphological aspects of management of crescentic anti-glomerular basement membrane (anti-GBM) nephritis/Goodpasture's syndrome. Q J Med 54:75–89, 1985.

Walker RG, Bailey R, Lynn K, Swainson C. Outcome of patients with Henoch-Schönlein nephritis (abstract). Kidney Int 30:624, 1986.

Wallace DJ, Podell TE, Weiner JM, Cox MB, Klinenberg JR, Foronzesh S, Dubois EL. Lupus nephritis: experience with 230 patients in a private practice from 1950 to 1980. Am J Med 72:209–220, 1982.

Wannamaker LW. Epidemiology of acute glomerulonephritis. In Acute glomerulonephritis. Proceedings of the Seventeenth Annual Conference on the Kidney. Boston, Little, Brown, 1967, pp. 29–67.

Watson AR, Poucell S, Thorner P, Arbus GS, Rance CP, Baumal R. Membranoproliferative glomerulonephritis type I in children: correlation of clinical features with pathologic subtypes. Am J Kidney Dis 4:141–146, 1984.

West CD. Idiopathic membranoproliferative glomerulonephritis in childhood. Pediatr Nephrol 6:96–103, 1992.

West CD, Northway JD, Davis NC. Serum levels of beta-1C globulin, a complement component in the nephrites lipoid nephrosis and other conditions. J Clin Invest 43:1507–1517, 1964.

West CD, McAdams AJ, McConville JM, Davis NC, Holland NH. Hypocomplementemic and normocomplementemic persistent (chronic) glomerulonephritis: clinical and pathologic characteristics. J Pediatr 67:1089–1112, 1965.

West CD, Winter S, Forristal J, McConville JM, Davis NC. Evidence for in vivo breakdown of beta-1C globulin in hypocomplementemic glomerulonephritis. J Clin Invest 46:539–548, 1967.

Westberg NG, Naff GB, Bover JT, Michael AF. Glomerular deposition of properdin in acute and chronic glomerulonephritis with hypocomplementemia. J Clin Invest 50:642–649, 1971.

Wheeler J, Sussman M. Enzyme linked immunosorbent assay for circulating anti–glomerular basement membrane antibodies. Clin Exp Immunol 45:271–278, 1981.

Wick G, Müller PV, Timpl R. In vivo localization and pathological effects of passively transferred antibodies to type IV collagen and laminin in mice. Clin Immunol Immunopathol 23:656–665, 1982.

Wieslander J, Bygren P, Heinegard D. Anti–glomerular basement membrane antibody: antibody specificity in different forms of glomerulonephritis. Kidney Int 23:855–861, 1983.

Wieslander J, Bygren P, Heinegard D, Barr JF, Butkowski R J, Edwards SJ, Hudson BG. Goodpasture's antigen of the glomerular basement membrane: localization to non-collagenous regions of type IV collagen. Proc Natl Acad Sci U S A 81:3838–3842, 1984a.

Wieslander J, Bygren P, Heinegard D. Isolation of the specific glomerular basement membrane antigen involved in Goodpasture syndrome. Proc Natl Acad Sci U S A 81:1544–1548, 1984b.

Williams DG. Pathogenesis of idiopathic IgA nephropathy. Pediatr Nephrol 7:303–311, 1993.

Williams RC Jr, Kunkel HG. Rheumatoid factor, complement, and conglutinin aberrations in patients with subacute bacterial endocarditis. J Clin Invest 41:666–675, 1962.

Williams RC Jr, van de Rijn I, Reid H, Poon-King T, Zabriskie JB. Lymphocyte cell subpopulations during acute post-streptococcal glomerulonephritis: cell surface antigens and binding of streptococcal membrane antigens and C reactive protein. Clin Exp Immunol 46:397–405, 1981.

Wilson CB. Antitubular basement membrane antibodies after renal transplantation. Transplantation 19:447–452, 1974.

Wilson CB. Radioimmunoassay for anti-glomerular basement membrane antibodies. In Rose NR, Friedman H, eds. Manual of Clinical Immunology. Washington DC, American Society for Microbiology, 1980, pp. 376–379.

Wilson CB. Antibody reactions with native or planted glomerular antigens producing nephritogenic immune deposits or selective glomerular cell injury. In Wilson, CB, Brenner BM, Stein JH, eds.Immunopathology of Renal Disease. New York, Churchill Livingstone 1988, pp 1–34.

Wilson CB. Nephritogenic tubulointerstitial antigens. Kidney Int 39:501–517, 1991.

Woodroffe AJ, Row PG, Meadows R, Lawrence JR. Nephritis in infectious mononucleosis. Q J Med 43:451–460, 1974.

Woodroffe AJ, Border WA, Theofilopoulos AN, Götze O, Glassock RJ, Dixon RJ, Wilson CB. Detection of circulating immune complexes in patients with glomerulonephritis. Kidney Int 12:268–278, 1977.

Woodroffe AJ, Gormly AA, McKenzie PE, Wootton AM, Thompson AJ, Seymour AE, Clarkson AR. Immunologic studies in IgA nephropathy. Kidney Int 18:366–374, 1980.

Wyatt RJ, McAdams AJ, Forristal J, Snyder J, West CD. Glomerular deposition of complement-control proteins in acute and chronic glomerulonephritis. Kidney Int 16:505–512, 1979.

Yamamoto T, Wilson CB. Complement dependence of antibody-induced mesangial cell injury in the rat. J Immunol 138:3758–3765, 1987.

Yang J-Y, Melvin T, Sibley R, Michael AF. No evidence for a specific role of IgM in mesangial proliferation. Kidney Int 25:100–106, 1984.

Yoshikawa N, White RHR, Cameron AH. Prognostic significance of the glomerular changes in Henoch-Schönlein nephritis. Clin Nephrol 16:223–229, 1981.

Yoshikawa N, Yoshiara S, Yoshiya K, Matsuo T, Matsuyama S, Okada S. Focal and diffuse membranoproliferative glomerulonephritis in children. Am J Nephrol 8:102–107, 1988.

Yoshioka K, Kleppel M, Michael AF, Fish AJ. Analysis of nephritogenic antigens in human glomerular basement membrane by two dimensional gel electrophoresis. J Immunol 134:3831–3837, 1985.

Yoshioka K, Takemura T, Aya N, Akano N, Miyamoto H, Maki S. Monocyte infiltration and cross-linked fibrin deposition in IgA nephritis and Henoch-Schönlein purpura nephritis. Clin Nephrol 32:107–112, 1989.

Yoshioka K, Hino S, Takemura T, Miyasato H, Honda E, Maki S. Isolation and characterization of the tubular basement membrane antigen associated with human tubulo-interstitial nephritis. Clin Exp Immunol 90:319–325, 1992.

Yurchenco PD, Schittny JC. Molecular architecture of basement membranes. FASEB J 4:1577–1590, 1990.

Zhou J, Mochizuki T, Smeets H, Antignac C, Laurila P, de Paepe A, Tryggvason K, Reeders ST. Deletion of the paired α5(IV) and α6(IV) collagen genes in inherited smooth muscle tumors. Science 261:1167–1169, 1993.

Zimmerman SW, Hyman LR, Uehling DT, Burkholder PM. Recurrent membranoproliferative glomerulonephritis with glomerular properdin deposition in allografts. Ann Intern Med 80:169–175, 1974.

Chapter 26

Autoimmune Endocrinopathies

William Ernest Winter and Noel K. Maclaren

AUTOIMMUNITY: AN OVERVIEW

Immune recognition of self-antigens normally results in immunologic *tolerance,* the process that prevents autoimmunity in health. Physiologic immune recognition is part of the normal immune response, and pathologic immune recognition with failure of tolerance leads to autoimmunity (Table 26–1) (Theofilopoulous and Dixon, 1982).

Tolerance is primarily a function of T cells and their T-cell receptors (Nossal, 1989). The mechanisms of tolerance include thymic clonal deletion and peripheral clonal anergy. During thymic T-cell development, self-peptides lead to clonal deletion of autoreactive T-cell

Table 26–1. Classification of Immune
Self-Recognition

Physiologic
Class I MHC antigen-directed: T killer cell ↔ target cell
interaction (e.g., lysis of virally infected cells or aberrant tumor
cells)

Class II MHC antigen-directed: Macrophage ↔ T-cell interaction
(e.g., antigen presentation)

Adhesion (addressin) molecules

Pathologic
Autoimmune reactions (autoantibodies, self-reactive cell-
mediated immunity)

Autoimmune disease (clinically evident disruption of organ or
tissue function and/or structure)

Abbreviation: MHC = major histocompatibility complex.

clones. However, not all self-antigens are expressed in the thymus. Because autoreactive T cells to self-antigens can leave the thymus, extrathymic pathways controlling autoimmunity have evolved (Ramsdell and Fowlkes, 1990). Clonal anergy (Kappler et al., 1989; Markmann et al., 1988; Blackman et al., 1990) occurs in the periphery when autoreactive T cells encounter self-antigens, yet do not receive all of the normal excitatory signals needed to proliferate and differentiate. Peripheral anergy results when antigens (e.g., self-peptides) are presented *without* the proper costimulatory cytokine exposure (e.g., interleukin-1 [IL-1]) or proper cell contact interaction (e.g., absence of B7 expression on the antigen-presenting cell [APC]).

Autoimmunity can develop when tolerance to a self-antigen has not been established or when tolerance to self has been lost or bypassed. Failure to acquire tolerance may be due to:

1. A failure of clonal deletion of autoreactive cells.
2. A failure of clonal anergy.
3. Release of a sequestered antigen to which tolerance has not been developed.
4. Alteration of a self-antigen, such that it becomes recognized as non-self.
5. Molecular mimicry between an environmental immunogen and self.
6. Aberrant class II MHC (major histocompatibility complex) expression.
7. Superantigen stimulation of otherwise anergic autoreactive clones.

We believe that failure of peripheral tolerance is the most likely explanation for the autoimmunities discussed in this chapter that are most likely a result of molecular mimicry between an environmental antigen and a self-antigen.

In molecular mimicry, damage to the host occurs during the immune response to a microbial invader because the self-antigen is unintentionally targeted. Kaufman and coworkers (1992) have described primary sequence homology between portions of glutamic acid decarboxylase (an autoantigen in insulin-dependent diabetes) and the P_2-C protein expressed by coxsackievirus. Likewise, homology between a retroviral protein p73 found in non-obese diabetic mouse islets and insulin has been demonstrated. Rheumatic fever resulting from group A β-hemolytic streptococcal pharyngitis is an excellent example of molecular mimicry leading to an immunologic disease, in this case, to the heart, joints, and choroidal plexus. Environmental as well as genetic factors influence the development of autoimmune disorders, as seen in studies of identical twins. Autoimmune damage to self may trigger a variety of effector pathways (Table 26–2).

Findings highly suggestive of an autoimmune disease include:

1. Evidence of anti-self humoral (e.g., autoantibodies) or cell-mediated autoimmune responses (e.g., lymphocytic infiltration of the host target).
2. Ability to transfer disease with either serum or lymphocytes (e.g., usually done in experimental animal models of disease or human disease observed in neonates from transplacentally passed maternal autoantibodies).
3. The ability to prevent, ameliorate, or cure disease with immune intervention therapy.
4. Disease recurrence when target tissue, organ, or cells are transplanted into an individual affected by the disease (e.g., pancreatic transplantation in a patient with long-standing insulin-dependent diabetes).

Common findings that support an autoimmune cause of disease include:

1. Disease associations with particular human leukocyte antigen (HLA) alleles.
2. Disease associations with other autoimmune diseases.
3. Increased disease frequency in females.
4. Increased disease frequency with increasing age.
5. Associated immune aberrancies, such as abnor-

Table 26–2. Effector Mechanisms in Autoimmune Disease

Autoantibodies
Complement fixing—cell lysis
Antibody-dependent—cell cytotoxicity
Immune complexes—local and systemic inflammation
Target cell receptor disruption (e.g., myasthenia gravis) or stimulation (e.g., Graves disease)

Cell-mediated autoimmunity
CD8⁺ T killer cells (cytotoxic T cells, or CTLs)—cell lysis

Table 26–3. Autoimmune Endocrinopathies

Pancreas
1. Autoimmune diabetes mellitus
2. Alpha cell autoimmunity
3. Autoimmune hypoglycemia
4. Type B acanthosis nigricans—insulin resistance syndrome
5. Insulinomimetic insulin receptor autoantibodies
6. Autoimmune beta cell stimulation producing hyperinsulinism

Thyroid
1. Hashimoto thyroiditis, goitrous and atrophic
2. Graves disease
3. Thyroid hormone autoantibodies

Adrenal and gonad (Addison disease and autoimmune hypogonadism)

Anterior pituitary and hypothalamus

malities of T-cell subsets, increased levels of activated T cells, hypergammaglobulinemia, or IgA deficiency.

The following topics cover endocrinopathies resulting from suspected autoimmune processes arranged by the organ affected (Table 26–3). An approach to the patient with autoimmune disorders is discussed in the last section of this chapter.

PANCREATIC AUTOIMMUNITY

Autoimmune abnormalities of the pancreas include (1) autoimmune destruction of the beta cells causing diabetes, (2) alpha cell autoimmunity, (3) autoimmune hypoglycemia, (4) autoimmunity to the insulin receptor producing the type B acanthosis nigricans–insulin resistance syndrome, (5) hypoglycemia secondary to insulinomimetic insulin receptor autoantibodies, and, reportedly, (6) autoimmune stimulation of the beta cell, leading to hyperinsulinism and hypoglycemia.

Insulin-dependent diabetes (IDD) results from autoimmune destruction of pancreatic beta cells. Autoantibodies against the glucagon (alpha)-producing and somatostatin (delta)-producing cells of the islet have been described; however, no ill effects from such autoantibodies have yet been identified. Autoantibodies to circulating insulin can develop spontaneously before the first insulin injection in IDD. Insulin autoantibodies can also provide an insulin reservoir that can inappropriately release excessive amounts of insulin and produce "autoimmune" hypoglycemia. Insulin receptor autoantibodies can block endogenous insulin action causing insulin resistance and diabetes. Alternatively, they can stimulate the receptor by mimicking the action of insulin producing hypoglycemia. Wilkin et al. (1988) described autoantibodies that stimulate insulin release. Confirmatory evidence of such autoantibodies is lacking, and the issue demands further study.

Insulin-Dependent Diabetes (Type I)

Insulin-dependent diabetes results from the failure of the pancreas to produce sufficient quantities of insulin because of pancreatic beta cell destruction. In most cases, beta cell destruction is the result of an autoimmune process (Cahill and McDevitt, 1981; Lernmark and Baekkeskov, 1981; Doniach et al., 1983; Marx, 1984; Atkinson and Maclaren, 1990). Insulinopenia and secondary hyperglucagonemia produce hyperglycemia, unrestrained fat breakdown, and hyperlipidemia leading to ketosis (Sperling, 1979). When the blood glucose level exceeds the renal threshold, glycosuria occurs, producing polyuria and resultant polydipsia. Marked catabolism leads to weight loss and inanition. Untreated, IDD produces ketoacidosis accompanied by dehydration, acidosis, coma, and eventual circulatory failure culminating in death. Although IDD most frequently presents in the first two decades of life, it can develop at any age.

Non–Insulin-Dependent Diabetes (Type II)

In contrast to IDD, type II or non–insulin-dependent diabetes (NIDD) is predominantly a disease of individuals over age 40. Of all NIDD subjects, 80% are obese. Minorities, including Native Americans, African Americans, and Hispanics, are affected more often than whites. Relative insulinopenia and insulin resistance contribute to glucose intolerance and diabetes in NIDD. Insulin levels are variable, but mild fasting hyperinsulinism is typical, indicating insulin resistance as a major biochemical defect (Landau, 1984). NIDD can also be seen in association with a large number of rare genetic syndromes (Rotter and Rimoin, 1981). Specific HLA types are not associated with NIDD.

Although there is no evidence for an autoimmune etiology in most cases of NIDD, a subset of NIDD patients do suffer from slowly progressive autoimmune beta cell destruction. From 4% to 17% of these patients have serologic evidence of beta cell autoimmunity (islet cell autoantibodies [ICAs]) (Irvine et al., 1977; Di Mario et al., 1983; Ohgawara and Hirata, 1984; Niskanen et al., 1991). The ICA titer strongly predicts later insulin dependence and a more severe degree of insulinopenia (Gray et al., 1980; Betterle et al., 1982). Autoimmune IDD masquerading as NIDD is probably as common as classic IDD. If the frequency of classic IDD is 1 in 300 and the United States population is 250,000,000, then 750,000 Americans are affected with IDD. If NIDD conservatively affects 2% of the general population (5 million patients) and 15% of these NIDD patients have beta cell autoimmunity, there are 750,000 NIDD patients with autoimmune diabetes, a figure equal to that for classic IDD. Altogether, 1.5 million Americans could have autoimmune diabetes.

IDD is usually distinguished from NIDD on both clinical and immunologic grounds (Table 26–4) (Skyler and Cahill, 1981). In IDD, most patients at clinical onset have ICA (70% to 80% ICA-positive) (Neufeld et al., 1980b) and antibodies to a 64-kD autoantigen. Lesser numbers of patients (~40%) have insulin autoantibodies (IAAs) (Atkinson et al., 1986). In addition, IDD is significantly associated with the HLA antigens DR3 and DR4 (Cudworth and Woodrow, 1976; Cudworth and Wolf, 1982) as well as the haplotype-associated DQB1*0201, DQB1*0302, DQA1*0501, or DQA1*0301 alleles.

Atypical Diabetes (Type 1.5)

Whereas only 5% of whites with IDD lack high-risk HLA DRB1*03 and DRB1*04 alleles, about 30% of African-Americans with youth-onset diabetes lack both DR3 and DR4 (Maclaren et al., 1982; Winter et al., 1984a, 1987). Many of these DR3- and DR4-negative patients appear to have a different form of diabetes in which insulin is required at diagnosis, but a non–insulin-dependent course develops months to years later (Winter, 1991). Of 26 such patients with "atypical" or type 1.5 diabetes, none of the probands were heterozygous for DR3 and DR4 and none had ICA; insulin secretion, as measured by C-peptide production, was significantly greater than that of classical IDD patients (Winter et al., 1987). In addition, insulin secretion, as measured by Sustacal-stimulated C peptide/glucose ratios, was significantly less than in nondiabetic controls. In contrast to autoimmune IDD, diabetes in the families of atypical diabetes probands is inherited in an autosomal dominant pattern. There was no apparent increase in the frequency of thyroid autoimmunity in these patients, as is the case with IDD.

African-Americans with atypical diabetes differ in several respects from maturity-onset diabetes of youth (MODY) patients. Atypical diabetes patients present with severe symptoms, often including ketosis, that requires early insulin therapy consistent with the diagnosis of IDD. Subjects with MODY are usually diagnosed only by oral glucose tolerance testing and do not display ketosis or require insulin treatment. In contrast to patients with MODY, patients with atypical diabetes have insulin secretion that is generally subnormal. Later in life, patients with atypical diabetes often suffer significant diabetes-related complications, in contrast to families with the Mason-type MODY (Tattersall, 1974). However, other patients with MODY may develop diabetic complications not unlike those more often seen in IDD and NIDD patients.

Historic Aspects

The classical insulitis lesions observed in the pancreata of newly diagnosed patients with IDD were observed as early as 1910 (Cecil, 1910), and were specifically described in 1940 by Von Meyenburg and later confirmed by Gepts (1965). Insulitis was not found in longstanding IDD. Disturbed frequencies of HLA were initially observed by Singal and Blajchmann (1973) and were confirmed and expanded by Nerup et al. (1974) and Cudworth and Woodrow (1976). Bottazzo and associates (1974) described ICAs in patients with autoimmune polyglandular syndromes, and Lendrum and colleagues (1975) later reported that ICAs were common in patients with IDD near the time of diagnosis. Maclaren and Huang (1975) described islet cell surface antibodies (ICSA) in IDD patients; in 1980, they reported the presence of anti-insulinoma autoreactive lymphocytes in IDD (Maclaren and Huang, 1980).

Table 26–4. Clinical and Immunologic Comparison of Insulin-Dependent (Type I) and Non–Insulin-Dependent (Type II) Diabetes

Features	Type of Diabetes	
	Insulin-Dependent	*Non–Insulin-Dependent*
Clinical		
Age of onset	<18 yr of age (in 75%)	>40 yr of age
Insulin-requiring	+	−
Associated with obesity	−	+
Ketosis	+	−
Family history	+/−	+
Immunologic		
ICAs	70%–80% (at diagnosis)	10%
Association with HLA antigens		
DR3 and DR4	+	−
DQB1*0201, DQB1*0302	+	−

Abbreviations: ICAs = islet cell autoantibodies; HLA = human leukocyte antigen.

By the early 1980s, the first successes with immunosuppressive therapy in IDD were reported. In the mid and late 1980s, great advances were made in the identification of the autoantigens of IDD and in the associations between DQB1 and DQA1 alleles with IDD susceptibility.

Pathogenesis

Almost all cases of IDD result from autoimmune destruction of the pancreatic beta cells (Nerup and Lernmark, 1983; Bottazzo et al., 1984a; Atkinson and Maclaren, 1990, 1994; Winter et al., 1991a) (Fig. 26–1). A minority of cases result from toxin ingestion (e.g., the rodenticide Vacor), severe chronic pancreatitis,

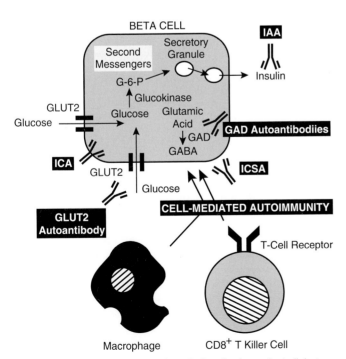

Figure 26–1. Autoimmune reactions in insulin-dependent diabetes. ISCA, islet cell surface antibody; ICA = islet cell cytoplasmic autoantibody; GAD = glutamic acid decarboxylase; GABA = gamma-aminobutyric acid; IAA = insulin autoantibody.

congenital malformation of the pancreas (Winter, 1986), or viral infection of the beta cells (Forrest et al., 1971; Yoon et al., 1979). Most evidence supporting a viral cause of IDD is epidemiologic, and there are few cases in which viral insulitis has been proven. However, there are several good animal models (encephalomyocarditis virus-D variant, reovirus, mengovirus, Kilham's rat virus) to support a role for viruses in IDD. Viruses implicated in human IDD have included coxsackievirus A, coxsackievirus B, cytomegalovirus, echovirus, Epstein-Barr virus, rubella, mumps, and retroviruses.

There is a significant environmental component in the pathogenesis of IDD, since identical twin studies show a concordance rate of only one third. A rising incidence of IDD has been recognized in several countries (Rewers et al., 1987; Diabetes Epidemiology Research International Group, 1990), which suggests some role for diet or novel infectious agents as initiators or inducers of beta cell autoimmunity. Potential toxins include alloxan, streptozotocin, Vacor (Pont et al., 1979; Karam et al., 1980; Kenney et al., 1981), pentamidine (Hauser et al., 1991), and smoked or cured mutton.

Exposure to bovine serum albumin has been implicated as a potentiator of IDD by Karjalainen et al. (1992), but other researchers have not duplicated their findings. There is conflicting data whether breast-feeding is protective against IDD (Fort et al., 1986; Virtanen et al., 1991; Mayer et al., 1988; Bognetti et al., 1992; Kyvik et al., 1992; Metcalfe et al., 1992). At present, however, there is no compelling reason to eliminate cow's milk from children's diets (Maclaren and Atkinson, 1992). The environmental factors that trigger IDD have yet to be identified, but a prior inductive event by an enteroviral infection may be involved (Atkinson and Maclaren, 1994).

There is abundant evidence for autoimmunity in IDD. Humoral and cell-mediated autoimmunity against the islets of Langerhans have been recognized for two decades. Insulitis, the pathognomonic inflammatory cell infiltrate observed in IDD, has been known for almost 90 years.

Islet Cell Cytoplasmic Autoantibodies

As detected by indirect immunofluorescence on unfixed sections of human pancreas, IgG antibodies to islet cell cytoplasm (islet cell cytoplasmic autoantibodies [ICAs]) have been found in 70% to 80% of newly diagnosed white patients with IDD (Lendrum, 1976; Neufeld et al., 1980b). ICAs are islet-specific but are not beta cell–specific. In contrast, ICAs are present at diagnosis in only 40% of African Americans with youth-onset diabetes. This suggests that unknown factors other than autoimmunity (e.g., atypical [type 1.5] diabetes) cause many of the cases of youth-onset diabetes in African Americans (Neufeld et al., 1980a; Winter et al., 1987).

Bottazzo and associates (1980a) have suggested that complement-fixing ICAs (CF-ICA) in nondiabetic individuals are more predictive of acute diabetes onset than are ICAs alone. However, other investigators found that CF-ICAs represent higher-titer ICAs and were not fundamentally different from non–CF-ICAs (Riley et al., 1980a; Bruining et al., 1984). Following diagnosis, the frequency of ICAs falls, so that by 5 years' duration, fewer than 25% of patients remain ICA-positive and after 10 years, fewer than 5% remain ICA-positive.

ICAs have been reported to react with a sialoglycoconjugate target antigen (Nayak et al., 1985) as well as with the enzyme glutamic acid decarboxylase (GAD). When ICAs react with the human pancreas alone, they are often auto-GAD$_{65}$ autoantibodies; when they also react with rodent pancreatic sections, non-GAD ICAs predominate. ICAs are polyclonal (Schatz et al., 1988). Quantitation and reproducibility of ICA assays have been assisted by ICA workshops (Gleichmann and Bottazzo, 1987). Beta cell–specific ICAs have been described using non-human pancreas substrates (Gianani et al., 1992); this requires confirmation by other laboratories. Traditional ICAs in high titer are highly predictive of IDD, especially in first-degree relatives of patients with IDD (Riley et al., 1990). Work in progress suggests that GAD ICAs are usually due to reactivity with a tyrosine phosphatase isolated from insulinoma cells (e.g., IA-2).

Islet Cell Surface Autoantibodies

Surface antibodies to islet cells (ICSAs) were first identified using a human insulinoma line as a target (Maclaren and Huang, 1980). ICSAs can be demonstrated by indirect immunofluorescence (Lernmark et al., 1978) or by ^{51}Cr release (Eisenbarth et al., 1981) from labeled islets. Most investigators employ rat insulinoma cells as targets for ICSAs because of the unavailability of human islet cell lines. ICSAs are carried in the gammaglobulin serum fraction; they suppress glucose-stimulated insulin release from isolated murine islets, probably by killing islet cells (Sai et al., 1981), and from intact murine pancreata after perfusion with ICSA-positive sera (Svenningsen et al., 1983). ICSAs can initiate antibody-dependent cell cytotoxity (Maruyama et al., 1984), and they preferentially bind to beta cells rather than to other pancreatic islet cell types (Van Der Winkel et al., 1982). ICSAs are too difficult

to measure routinely and thus are not useful for IDD risk assessment. They may react to the IA-2 antigen mentioned above.

Glutamic Acid Decarboxylase Autoantibodies

Sera from BB (BioBreeding) rats, non-obese diabetic mice, and diabetic humans can immunoprecipitate unique cell surface proteins (Lernmark and Baekkeskov, 1981; Baekkeskov et al., 1982, 1984) of 64,000 daltons. These 64-kD autoantibodies are at least as common as ICA at disease onset and are highly predictive of IDD (Atkinson et al., 1990). In 1990, Baekkeskov and colleagues identified at least one component of the 64-kD autoantigen to be GAD.

GAD is found in abundance in several areas of the central nervous system (CNS) and catalyzes the conversion of glutamic acid to gamma-aminobutyric acid (GABA), an inhibitory neurotransmitter. GAD enzymatic activity is a result of separate GAD enzymes: GAD$_{65}$ (65,000 kD) and GAD$_{67}$ (67,000 kD) that are coded by genes on two separate chromosomes. One isoform of GAD (GAD$_{64}$, which is equivalent to GAD$_{65}$) may be solely expressed in human islets, and autoimmune activity may be restricted mainly to GAD$_{65}$ (Petersen et al., 1993). However, Kaufman and coworkers (1992) detected autoimmunity to both forms of GAD in subjects with IDD.

The GAD epitope recognized by diabetic sera appears to be a conformational determinant because diabetic sera does not recognize linear GAD peptides. Upon trypsinization of the 64-kD autoantigen, Christie and colleagues (1992) provided data that antibodies to a 37/40 kD beta cell protein derived from the 64 kD autoantigen may be most predictive of IDD. Using purified autoantigens, automated assays, such as enzyme-linked immunosorbent assay (ELISA), for GAD autoantibodies should appear soon. Cellular reactivity to GAD has been demonstrated by Atkinson and others (1992). Harrison and coworkers (1993) suggested that humoral and cellular reactivity to GAD are inversely related to the risk for IDD.

Besides the islet cell sialoglycoconjugate and GAD, several other autoantigens and autoantibodies have been detected in IDD (Table 26–5). Of note, another putative target enzyme in IDD is carboxypeptidase H, which cleaves proinsulin to insulin.

Insulin Autoantibodies

Prior to exogenous insulin therapy, insulin autoantibodies (IAAs) can be found in subjects with IDD (Palmer et al., 1983; Wilkin et al., 1985). Atkinson and colleagues (1986) found that about 40% of newly diagnosed patients have IAAs. IAAs are much more common in children than adults prior to diagnosis of IDD. By themselves, IAAs are minimally predictive of IDD because the frequency of IAAs in the population is higher than that of ICAs (Yassin et al., 1991). However, IAAs in conjunction with ICAs greatly improve the predictive value of ICAs (Atkinson et al., 1986).

Numerous other autoantigens and autoantibodies in IDD are under study. Only ICA, IAA, and anti-64 kd/GAD autoantibodies have been tested in large numbers of diabetic and prediabetic individuals. The role of the

Table 26–5. Autoimmunity and Autoantigens in Insulin-Dependent Diabetes

	Method of Detection	Autoantigen
Autoimmunity to islet cells		
Islet cell cytoplasmic autoantibodies (ICAs)	IFA	Sialoglycoconjugate and GAD
64-kD autoantibodies	IPP	Islet cell protein(s) of 64-kD (includes GAD)
GAD autoantibodies	IPP, ELISA	GAD
37/40-kD autoantibodies	IPP	Tryptic digest of 64-kD islet cell protein(s)
Autoantibodies that block beta cell glucose uptake	Bioassay	GLUT-2
52-kD RIN (rat insulinoma) autoantibodies	WB	Rubella virus–related protein (Karounos et al., 1990)
38-kD autoantibodies	WB	38-kD autoantigen (Pak et al., 1990)
Cellular autoreactivity to GAD	LPA	GAD$_{65}$
Cellular autoreactivity to 38-kD autoantigen	LPA	Insulin secretory granule protein (Roep et al., 1990, 1991)
IA-2 autoantibody	IFA	Transmembrane tyrosine phosphatase
Autoimmunity to beta cell products		
Insulin autoantibodies (IAA)	IPP	Insulin
Anti-proinsulin autoantibodies	IPP	Proinsulin
Anti-carboxypeptidase H autoantibodies	WB	Carboxypeptidase H (Castano et al., 1991)
Autoimmunity to the insulin receptor		
Anti-insulin receptor autoantibodies	RRCA	Insulin receptor

Abbreviations: GAD = glutamic acid decarboxylase (two different forms of the GAD enzyme [GAD$_{65}$ (65,000 kD) and GAD$_{67}$ (67,000 kD)] are coded for by two separate genes; ELISA = enzyme-linked immunosorbent assay; IFA = indirect immunofluorescent assay; IPP = immunoprecipitation assay; LPA = lymphocyte proliferation assay (lymphocytes plus antigen; measure ^{3}H-thymidine incorporation); RRCA = radioreceptor competition assay; WB = Western blot assay.

other autoantibodies in the prediction of IDD is yet to be determined (see Table 26–5).

Other Autoimmune Autoantibodies

Other humoral immune abnormalities include the presence of immune complexes (Virella et al., 1981); antinuclear antibodies; lymphocytotoxic antibodies (Serjeantson et al., 1981), and insulin receptor autoantibodies (Maron et al., 1983). In long-standing IDD, immune complexes composed of insulin antibodies and exogenous insulin may play a role in microvascular disease (Virella et al., 1981). Wilkin and coworkers (1988) have provided data for an autoantibody that stimulates the beta cell to release insulin. However, this observation awaits confirmation.

Specific T-Cell Abnormalities

Evidence for cell-mediated autoimmunity in IDD includes the ability of IDD lymphocytes to kill cultured human insulinoma cells in vitro (Maclaren and Huang, 1980). Likewise, in a rat insulinoma system, IDD lymphocytes suppress insulin secretion (Boitard et al., 1980). IDD lymphocytes produce macrophage inhibition factor when exposed to islet antigens. Several studies suggest a functional deficiency in T-suppressor cells (Lederman et al., 1981; Topliss et al., 1983). Charles and colleagues (1983) have suggested that in vitro islet cell destruction mediated by immune cells may correlate with clinical disease activity. Lang and colleagues (1987) have resurrected some interest in T cell-mediated beta cell destruction as a pathogenic mechanism for IDD.

Insulitis, a mononuclear cell (lymphocyte and macrophage) infiltrate of the pancreatic islets, is found in at least 60% of patients with IDD who come to autopsy within 6 months of diagnosis (Gepts and Lecompte, 1981; Foulis and Stewart, 1984). Foulis and others

(1986) recognized insulitis in 78% of IDD cases, and Foulis and Stewart (1984) described insulitis in 88% of their patients. As determined by histochemical staining, as many as 90% of the pancreatic beta cells have been destroyed by the time of diagnosis.

A pancreas from a patient newly diagnosed with IDD was examined with the use of monoclonal antibody probes (Bottazzo et al., 1985). The infiltrating lymphocytes were activated T lymphocytes expressing DR antigen. The T lymphocytes were predominantly of the CD8$^+$ phenotype, which suggested cell-mediated cytotoxicity as the etiology of the beta cell destruction. It is unknown how long insulitis persists after the clinical diagnosis of IDD. Hanafusa and coworkers (1983) did not find insulitis in seven IDD patients undergoing pancreatic biopsy 2 to 4 months after onset of IDD.

Nonspecific T-Cell Abnormalities

Other cellular immune abnormalities have been described. IDD lymphocytes produce subnormal levels of interleukin-2 (IL-2) (Rodman, 1984; Zier et al., 1984). In comparison with controls, mitogen-stimulated lymphocytes from subjects with IDD provide subnormal cytokine help to B cells (Schatz et al., 1991). Faustman and colleagues (1991) have suggested that class I MHC expression in IDD is deficient in IDD humans and nonobese diabetic mice; however, others have challenged their findings.

Prior to and at the time of diagnosis of IDD, activated T cells have been found (Jackson et al., 1982a, 1984; Alviggi et al., 1984) using anti–class II MHC monoclonal and Tac monoclonal antibodies (MAb) (Hayward and Herberger, 1984). The Tac MAb recognizes IL-2 receptors present on activated T cells. Many groups have described abnormalities in the CD4:CD8 ratio (Horita et al., 1982; Pozzilli et al., 1983; Galluzzo et al., 1984; Ilonen et al., 1984; Hitchcock et al., 1986;

Faustman et al., 1989). Elevated numbers of natural killer (NK) cells may be present at the time of diagnosis (Pozzilli et al., 1979). All of these observations remain controversial.

Bottazzo and coworkers (1983) proposed that endocrine cells aberrantly express class II MHC antigens, permitting the target to "commit suicide" by *autopresentation* of self-antigens (Londei et al., 1984). However, most studies support a primary immunologic abnormality, as opposed to a primary target organ abnormality, as the initiating event in IDD.

Other Autoimmune Diseases Associated with IDD

Insulin-dependent diabetes is associated with other autoimmune diseases (Neufeld et al., 1980b). Thyroid microsomal autoantibodies (TMAs) indicative of *Hashimoto thyroiditis* are found in 20% to 25% of female patients with IDD (Riley et al., 1981). About 10% of male subjects with IDD are TMA-positive. About 50% of the TMA-positive IDD subjects go on to have clinical thyroid disease (20%, Graves disease; 80%, hypothyroidism). About 10% of IDD patients also have gastric parietal cell autoantibodies. These are markers for atrophic gastritis that can lead to achlorhydria and iron deficiency anemia (Riley et al., 1982). Prolonged intrinsic factor deficiency leads to vitamin B_{12} deficiency and pernicious anemia in mid to later life. Thyroid microsomal and parietal cell autoantibodies occur together in about 5% of IDD patients. Autoimmune Addison disease occurs in 1 of 300 patients with IDD, often in association with thyroid and gastric autoimmunity.

Genetic Susceptibility to IDD and HLA Associations

Insulin-dependent diabetes is a polygenic disorder triggered by an environmental insult (Winter et al., 1991b, 1993). HLA antigens have a great influence on susceptibility to IDD.

HLA-DR

Insulin-dependent diabetes is highly associated with the serologically defined HLA-DR class II antigens DRB1*03 and DRB1*04. These are termed *risk,* or *susceptibility, alleles.* More than 95% of white patients with IDD have one or more of these antigens, in contrast to about 50% of a control non-IDD population (Cudworth and Wolf, 1982). Nearly 40% of IDD patients are DRB1*03/04 heterozygotes; the majority of the remainder are DRB1*03-(25%) or DRB1*04- (30%) positive. Only 3% of the control population are heterozygous for DRB1*03/04. As with ICA positivity, 30% of African Americans but only 5% of whites with the IDD clinical phenotype at diagnosis lack both of these alleles (Winter et al., 1987).

DRB1*15 and DRB1*11 both are protective against IDD (Maclaren et al., 1988). These protective alleles are usually dominant over risk alleles (Nepom et al., 1990). DRB1*01 is a risk allele when associated with

03 or 04 (Maclaren et al., 1988). DRB1*07 may also be a risk allele in African Americans. DRB1*09 in the Japanese population replaces 03 as a risk allele (Kida et al., 1989). Using primed lymphocyte typing lines, Sheehy et al. (1985) defined particular subsets of DRB1*04 alleles that are more predictive of IDD than the serologically defined 04 antigen.

The risk for development of IDD over a lifetime is about 1 in 300 for the general population. The presence of a lone DR03 or DR04 allele increases the absolute risk for IDD only slightly. However, this figure is considerably above the 1-in-5000 risk for individuals with neither allele. Individuals with both alleles have a markedly increased risk for IDD (about 1 in 20) (Maclaren et al., 1984).

Some 5% to 15% of patients with IDD have a first-degree relative with IDD. For subjects with a first-degree relative with IDD, the risk for IDD is between 5% and 10%. Fathers with IDD are more likely than mothers with IDD to pass on diabetogenic-HLA alleles and to have children affected with IDD (Warram et al., 1984; Vadheim et al., 1986).

HLA-DQ

In the 1980s, it was shown that alleles at the DQB1 and DQA1 loci were even more strongly associated with susceptibility to IDD than the DR alleles (Owerbach et al., 1983, 1984; Henson et al., 1987; Michelsen and Lernmark, 1987; Horn et al., 1988). DQ and DR alleles are in strong linkage disequilibrium (e.g., very likely to be inherited as a pair). The IDD risk in non-diabetic siblings positive for both DQB1*0201 and DQB1*0302 may be near 1 in 4, which approaches the risk for an identical twin of an IDD patient (1 in 3). Studies of different populations demonstrate that both the DQA1 and DQB1 loci provide susceptibility to IDD. Extended chromosome 6 haplotypes, including the glycerol oxidase (GLO) locus through the MHC complex, have also been implicated in susceptibility to IDD (Raum et al., 1984).

In 1987, Todd and coworkers recognized that certain DQB1 alleles that are protective for IDD (e.g., DQB1 *0602; DQB1*0301) had an aspartic acid at position 57 of the DQβ chain. In contrast, DQB1 alleles associated with IDD susceptibility (e.g., DQB1*0302; DQB1 *0201; DQB1*0501) lack aspartic acid at DQβ position 57. Morel and colleagues (1988) reported that DQB1 non-asp/non-asp homozygotes had a relative risk for IDD of about 100. In France, DQB1*0201/DQB1*0302 heterozygotes have a relative risk for IDD of about 50. However, non-asp/non-asp homozygosity was less predictive of IDD in the French (relative risk, ~13), Finns (relative risk, ~18), Norwegians (relative risk, ~12), and in residents of the United States (relative risk, ~4) (Baisch et al., 1990).

Other investigators (Fletcher et al., 1988; Deschamps et al., 1990) have recognized that arginine in position 52 of the DQα chain was associated with DQA1 alleles that increased susceptibility to IDD (e.g., DQA1*0301; DQA1*0501). Hypothetically, the interaction of aspartic acid and arginine (Owerbach et al., 1988) would form DQA1-DQB1 ionic bond (or "salt bridge") across one end of the antigen-binding cleft in nonsusceptible DQα-DQβ combinations that would be lacking in the susceptible DQα-DQβ combinations. This, in turn, would alter the shape of the class II MHC antigen-binding cleft and the spectrum of antigen-derived peptides that could be presented to T lymphocytes.

Gutierrez-Lopez and coworkers (1992) reported that DQA1 arginine 52 and DQB1 non-asp increase the risk for IDD tenfold. Khalil et al. (1990) found that their IDD patients carried both a DQA1 arginine 52 and a DQB1 non-aspartic acid 57 susceptibility allele. DQA1 and DQB1 alleles may interact to increase susceptibility to IDD either in the "cis" or "trans" position (Khalil et al., 1992). "Cis" refers to alleles located on the same maternal- or paternal-derived chromosome, and "trans" refers to alleles not located on the same maternal or paternal chromosome. The DQA1*0301/DQB1*0302/DQA1*0501/DQB1*0201 genotype provides a relative risk for IDD of 35 as reported by Heimberg et al. (1992). A combination of particular DR4 subtypes (defined by homozygous typing cell reagents) and DQB1*0302 alleles may further increase risk for IDD over DR4 or DQB1*0302 alone (Sheehy et al., 1985, and 1989a). In Asian populations, specifically the Japanese, DQB1 alleles may not influence IDD susceptibility; however, DQA1 alleles appear to control proclivity to IDD (Yamagata et al., 1989, 1991; Ikegami et al., 1990; Jacobs et al., 1992; Tanaka et al., 1992). Interestingly, certain subtypes of DRB1*04 (DRB1*0406/0403) are strongly protective against IDD, even in haplotypes that contain susceptible DQ alleles.

In families with more than one IDD child, haplotype sharing increases the subsequent risk for IDD in unaffected siblings. HLA identity (both haplotypes shared) is found in 60% of affected sibling pairs, as opposed to the randomly expected rate of 25%, whereas the majority of the remaining sibling pairs with IDD share one HLA haplotype (haploidentical) (Cudworth and Wolf, 1982).

HLA antigens may affect genetic susceptibility through several mechanisms (Bottazzo et al., 1984b). First, HLA antigens present antigen-derived peptide fragments to T-cell receptors. Specific HLA alleles might be more adept at presenting autoantigens than other alleles and thus would elicit a stronger autoimmune response. Second, self-antigens, such as the HLA molecules, shape the T-cell receptor repertoire in the thymus as anti–self T-cell receptors are eliminated during T-cell ontogeny. Third, other genes in linkage disequilibrium with the HLA alleles may be the real susceptibility genes.

Other Genetic Polymorphisms

Although the hypervariable region 5′ of the insulin gene is also important (Bell et al., 1984), polymorphisms of the insulin gene in noncoding regions may have a major impact on IDD susceptibility (Julier et al., 1991) independent of the DR type of the individual (Bain et al., 1992). Particular immunoglobulin (Adams et al., 1984) and complement allotypes, complement-extended MHC haplotypes (Raum et al., 1984; Rittner and Bertrams, 1981), and T-cell receptor alpha or beta

polymorphisms have also been implicated as risk factors for IDD.

Other data do not confirm these loci as involved in genetic predisposition to IDD (Sheehy et al., 1989b; Field et al., 1989; Boehm et al., 1990; Concannon et al., 1990; Niven et al., 1990; Aparicio, 1991; Martinez-Naves et al., 1991). More recently, studies of affected sibling pairs by microsatellite mapping techniques have identified at least eight genomic intervals that contain genes relevant to susceptibility to IDD (Todd et al., 1994).

Natural History

Insulin-dependent diabetes resembles other autoimmune endocrinopathies in that beta cell destruction proceeds over a period of months to years before clinical presentation (Fig. 26–2) (Gorsuch et al., 1981). As markers of the autoimmune process, ICAs can appear months to years prior to diagnosis (Riley et al., 1984, 1990). ICA signifies islet cell autoreactivity because about 30% of ICA-positive first-degree relatives of IDD subjects will develop IDD within 5 years. The predictive importance of ICAs and IAAs for IDD are greater in children than in adults. Indeed, children with both autoantibodies almost always develop IDD.

The Prediabetic State

The prediabetic period can be roughly divided into four stages:

Stage 1. Before there is evidence of beta cell autoimmunity or metabolic dysfunction, there is genetic susceptibility (stage 1).

Stage 2. Immune abnormalities (ICA, IAA, or anti-GAD autoantibodies) are present without detectable metabolic disturbances.

Stage 3. Beta cell destruction becomes evident with abnormally low first-phase insulin responses to intravenous glucose (Srikanta et al., 1983a, 1983b, 1983c). In the intravenous glucose tolerance test (IVGTT), beta cell health is assessed by ensuring the insulin concentrations at 1 and 3 minutes (the first-phase insulin release) following intravenous glucose. In ICA-positive

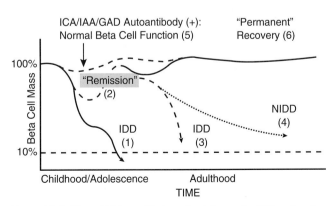

Figure 26–2. Natural history of beta cell autoimmunity. IDD = insulin-dependent diabetes; NIDD = non–insulin-dependent diabetes; ICA = islet cell cytoplasmic autoantibody; GAD = glutamic acid decarboxylase; IAA = insulin autoautobody.

individuals who eventually have IDD, first-phase insulin responses decline at a rate of 20 to 40 µU/ml per year (Srikanta et al., 1984a; 1984b). Insulin response to intravenous glucagon, arginine, and tolbutamide may be preserved despite deficient insulin secretion (Ganda et al., 1984).

Stage 4. Insulitis progresses, and more extensive beta cell destruction occurs. Insulin reserve becomes deficient and oral glucose tolerance deteriorates. Once the oral glucose tolerance test is abnormal, the clinical findings of diabetes (polyuria, polydipsia, and weight loss) generally appear within a year or two.

Patients are said to have been "prediabetic" only retrospectively when IDD develops in people with ICA, IAA, anti-64 kD, or anti-GAD$_{65}$ antibodies. Individuals with humoral beta cell autoimmunity who do not have diabetes may or may not be prediabetic, since not all autoantibody-positive (ICA, IAA, anti-64 kD, or anti-GAD antibodies) subjects develop IDD. When low titers of IDD-related autoantibodies are present, the autoantibodies may disappear spontaneously or may persist at low titers for years or decades without progression to IDD, particularly in adults. ICAs probably do not participate in beta cell damage; however, they serve as useful markers of beta cell damage.

Although ICAs may disappear with time, the body's ability to respond to islet cell antigens can be retained for at least 20 years after diagnosis. This is illustrated in the studies of Sutherland and coworkers (1984a, 1984b) in pancreas transplantation between sets of identical twins discordant for IDD. Immediately following transplantation, all recipient twins showed amelioration of IDD. However, 6 to 8 weeks after transplantation in twins who were not immunosuppressed, insulitis occurred and the patients became frankly diabetic and required insulin treatment. In one of the recipient twins, ICA appeared following the pancreas transplant. This indicates that humoral as well as cell-mediated autoimmunity was aroused following re-exposure of the immune system to the islet cell antigens of the transplanted pancreas. When the recipient twin was immunosuppressed, there was no recurrence of insulitis or IDD.

Diagnosis

The presence of insulin-dependent, ketosis-prone diabetes in association with ICA, IAA (prior to insulin treatment), anti-64 kD or GAD autoantibodies and IDD-associated alleles (e.g., HLA DRB1*03, DRB1*04, DQB1*0201, or DQB1*0302) are virtually diagnostic of autoimmune (type I) diabetes. Additional supportive evidence for an autoimmune pathogenesis includes:

1. Associated autoantibodies (thyroid microsomal, gastric parietal cell, and/or adrenal cell autoantibodies).
2. HLA haplotype sharing with an affected sibling.
3. A positive family history of IDD in a first-degree relative.

If a child shares a DRB1*03/04 haplotype with an affected sibling, the absolute risk for IDD rises to 1 in

4. In the absence of serologic evidence of beta cell autoimmunity (e.g., ICA or IAA), HLA typing has been of limited use in predicting IDD in the general population. In nondiabetic individuals, ICA and GAD$_{65}$ autoantibodies also have powerful predictive values for IDD.

Treatment

Since Banting and Best discovered insulin (1922), the treatment for IDD has been subcutaneously injected insulin. Oral hypoglycemic agents have no role in the treatment of IDD.

Novel therapies involve the following:

1. New approaches to insulin delivery (i.e., insulin pumps, intraportal insulin delivery, closed-loop insulin infusion with a glucose sensor, intranasal insulin).
2. Pancreatic transplantation.
3. Islet transplantation.
4. Immunomodulation (induction of immunologic tolerance) in prediabetes.

Of particular immunologic interest are the last three approaches. Pancreatic transplantation was first attempted in the late 1960s (Sutherland et al., 1984c). Because of early technical failures, interest in transplantation waned until the late 1970s and early 1980s. Now the favored approach is segmental or whole pancreas transplantation with either intestinal or external drainage of the exocrine pancreatic secretions (Sutherland et al., 1984c). Currently, up to 70% of pancreas transplant procedures have been successful.

Human islet cell transplantation has not yet achieved long-term islet cell graft survival. Elimination of carrier lymphocytes within the transplanted pancreas that are capable of stimulating an immune response and encapsulation of islets may improve the future prospects of such therapy (Lafferty et al., 1986).

A wide variety of immunotherapies have been applied to newly diagnosed IDD patients, including:

- Plasmapheresis (Spencer et al., 1982, Ludvigsson et al., 1982)
- Interferon (Rand et al., 1981; Koivisto et al., 1984)
- Levamisole (Cobb et al., 1980)
- Glucocorticoids (Leslie and Pyke, 1980; Najemnik et al., 1980; Elliot et al., 1981; Jackson et al., 1982a; Ludvigsson et al., 1983; Silverstein et al., 1983; Sotos et al., 1984)
- Antithymocyte globulin (Eisenbarth et al., 1983)
- Inosiplex (Gries et al., 1983)
- Azathioprine (Silverstein et al., 1988)
- Cyclosporine A (Stiller et al., 1984; Assan et al., 1985)

Such studies are based on the premise that IDD is an autoimmune disorder and suppression of the immune response may diminish beta cell destruction (Winter and Maclaren, 1985). Such measures are nonspecific (i.e., not aimed exclusively at the autoreactive clones). Most studies have also been uncontrolled and include only a small number of patients.

Specific anti–T-cell monoclonals (i.e., anti-T3, anti-

T12) may target immunosuppression to specific cell types. The use of monoclonal antibodies to class II MHC DR or DQ molecules has been proposed as another way of inhibiting the immune system. DR or DQ antibodies might interfere with antigen presentation and intercellular communication (i.e., macrophage to T cell or B cell). Monoclonal antibodies may be made more effective if they are coupled to immunotoxins such as ricin. However, mouse monoclonal antibodies may themselves be immunogenic, thus negating their benefit.

Cyclosporin (Stiller et al., 1984; Assan et al., 1985; Bougneres et al., 1988) or azathioprine (Harrison et al., 1985; Silverstein et al., 1988) may be effective in producing a non–insulin-requiring state if therapy is begun close to the time of diagnosis. However, cyclosporine can produce serious, irreversible nephrotoxicity (Myers et al., 1984) and therefore is not the agent of choice for long-term immunosuppression. Lymphoma poses a slight risk (~1 in 1000 patients treated) in patients receiving azathioprine. If a remission could be achieved with cyclosporine, less toxic maintenance immunotherapy might be instituted (i.e., azathioprine). At most, only 50% of newly diagnosed patients with IDD respond initially to cyclosporin or azathioprine, and this response diminishes with time. On discontinuing cyclosporin or azathioprine, the subjects again become insulin-dependent.

Because of the toxicity of these agents, they are not suitable for the prevention of IDD. Immunomodulation may be more successful if given prior to clinical diagnosis when a greater beta cell mass is still present. Some researchers now propose prophylactic oral or subcutaneous insulin therapy to prevent IDD. Alternatively, oral immunization of autoantibody-positive individuals with IDD autoantigens has been proposed to induce tolerance to the beta cell. Insulin is expected to be the first autoantigen to be tested in this manner, but GAD may also be used, now that GAD can be produced by recombinant DNA methods. Tolerization should present few risks.

With advances in gene therapy, it may be possible to create new beta cells or to allow cells to provide constitutive levels of insulin that would partially ameliorate the metabolic defect in IDD.

Prognosis

Even with insulin therapy after 15 to 20 years, significant vascular complications develop in most patients with IDD (Rosenbloom, 1983). Since complications do not occur in the absence of overt diabetes, there is a need for prevention or cure. Diabetic microvascular disease is a leading cause of blindness and kidney failure. Macrovascular disease results in accelerated atherosclerosis and early myocardial infarction, stroke, and peripheral vascular disease.

Pancreatic and islet cell transplantation are still in their infancy. These therapeutic modalities may eventually prove successful if (1) tissue rejection can be overcome and (2) an adequate source of pancreata and islets can be found. The use of immunotherapy in prevention necessitates an increased understanding of the natural history of IDD.

Alpha Cell Autoantibody Syndrome

Alpha cell autoantibodies (ACAs) react with the cytoplasm of the glucagon-producing cells of the pancreatic islet. They can be detected only in the absence of ICAs, since ICAs react with all cells of the islet. ACAs are visualized by indirect immunofluorescence on unfixed cryocut human pancreas. A rim-like pattern of islet cell fluorescence is produced because alpha cells are located mainly at the perimeter of the normal islet. Double staining of these cells with rabbit glucagon antisera proves that the reactive rim-pattern cells are alpha cells. A few patients thought to have ACAs in fact have delta cell autoantibodies. Delta cells are most abundant between the central beta cells and peripheral alpha cells of islet and are recognized by staining with somatostatin antisera. Delta cells produce somatostatin whose paracrine effect is to suppress both insulin and glucagon secretion.

History

Bottazzo and Lendrum first described ACAs and delta cell autoantibodies in 1976. The first report of metabolic studies in ACA-positive patients was completed by Del Prete and colleagues in 1978. Winter and coworkers (1984b) have reported a larger series of patients.

Pathogenesis

Little is known about the pathogenesis of alpha cell autoantibodies. The frequency of ACAs in the relatives of patients with IDD is no higher than in the general population. Similarly, there is no apparent increase in associated autoimmunity (i.e., thyroid and gastric autoantibodies, adrenal autoantibodies) in ACA-positive patients. ACAs are as common in the general pediatric population as are ICA (~1 in 250 children tested) (Winter et al., 1984b). Unlike ICAs, ACAs are not associated with particular HLA types. According to clinical studies, ACAs do not reflect alpha cell damage, in contrast to ICAs, which reflect beta cell damage (Riley et al., 1984). ACAs can be present in considerable titer and persist for a long time.

Clinical Course

Normal glucagon secretion following intravenous arginine in ACA-positive patients has been described in two reports (Del Prete et al., 1978; Winter et al., 1984b). In the later study, the patient with the lowest glucagon response to arginine was fasted for 30 hours without the development of hypoglycemia (Winter et al., 1984b). Deficient glucagon response to hypoglycemia occurs in those with long-standing IDD; however, this appears to be a complication of IDD resulting from defective autonomic control of glucagon release (Cryer and Gerich, 1983) rather than autoimmune destruction of the alpha cells. True glucagon deficiency is apparently rare. There has been only one well-documented case of neonatal glucagon deficiency (Vidnes and Oyaseter, 1977). Because glucagon is a key counterregulatory hormone when insulin secretion is present, glucagon deficiency may be incompatible with life.

Diagnosis and Prognosis

ACAs are detected by indirect immunofluorescence using unfixed sections of human pancreas. ACAs are usually identified incidentally during screening for ICAs. The prognosis for patients with ACA appears excellent. Nonpathologic autoantibodies to circulating glucagon have been described in patients never treated with exogenous insulin (which contains minute amounts of glucagon). They may be associated with the use of tolbutamide or methimazole (Baba et al., 1976; Sanke et al., 1983).

Autoimmune Hypoglycemia

To a large extent, steroid and thyroid hormones are present in the circulation bound to carrier proteins. In contrast, all protein hormones exist unbound in the circulation except for the insulin-like growth factors *(somatomedins)*. Insulin antibodies develop in diabetic patients treated with exogenous insulin, especially in those without HLA-DRB1*03 alleles. This occurs regardless of the species source of insulin administered, be it porcine, bovine, or human. These antibodies do not substantially complicate the clinical course of the diabetic patient. However, spontaneously occurring insulin autoantibodies (IAA) arising in individuals not exposed to exogenous insulin can rarely result in spontaneous hypoglycemia or glucose intolerance. This is termed the *autoimmune hypoglycemia syndrome*. Autoimmune hypoglycemia is characterized as a clinical syndrome of hyperinsulinism in the absence of an insulinoma associated with insulin antibodies.

History

In 1972, studies from Japan and Norway reported IAA in individuals affected with hypoglycemia who had not previously been treated with exogenous insulin (Takayama-Hasumi et al., 1990). Autoimmune hypoglycemia has been reported outside of Japan only rarely (Burch et al., 1992; Meschi et al., 1992).

Pathogenesis

A presumed defect in immune surveillance results in the spontaneous production of autoantibodies that bind to circulating insulin and act as carrier proteins (Goldman et al., 1979). Seino and colleagues (1984) have suggested that in some patients there may be molecular abnormalities of insulin. A marked elevation in the total immunoreactive insulin level occurs. The large reservoir of circulating autoantibody-bound insulin can spontaneously release insulin, leading to acute elevations in free insulin levels inappropriate for metabolic needs. This can cause hypoglycemia even after feeding. These insulin autoantibodies can also bind secreted insulin and decrease free insulin in the circulation, thus producing glucose intolerance. Spontaneous insulin autoantibodies are polyclonal antibodies (Dozio et al., 1991) directed against human insulin and not porcine or bovine insulins.

Other autoimmune diseases (e.g., Graves disease) may develop in affected patients. Drugs may also elicit insulin autoantibodies, specifically methimazole (Hirata, 1983; Chen et al., 1990). Japanese investigators have suggested that up to 15% of their patients with spontaneous hypoglycemia have autoimmune hypoglycemia (Takayama and Hirata, 1983; Takayama-Hasumi et al., 1990). The syndrome is associated with HLA-DR4 (Uchigata et al., 1992), especially with the DRB1*0406 subtype that is strongly protective against IDD. Although insulin autoantibodies may also occur in subjects before they have IDD, there appears to be no relationship between the two diseases.

Diagnosis and Treatment

Autoimmune hypoglycemia is diagnosed by the findings of hyperinsulinism and insulin antibodies in the absence of prior therapy with exogenous insulin. Insulinoma should be excluded. Because autoimmune hypoglycemia is antibody-mediated, immunosuppressive therapy may be of theoretical benefit, although it has not yet been attempted. Present treatment consists of frequent high-carbohydrate meals and avoidance of fasting.

Acanthosis Nigricans with Insulin Resistance (Type B)

Acanthosis nigricans is a skin disease in which waxy raised pigmented plaques occur especially about the neck and upper trunk. Insulin resistance in association with acanthosis nigricans has been reported in three forms. One (type B) is an autoimmune disorder (Flier et al., 1979). In type A disease, there is a primary decrease in insulin receptor number. Most patients are female and display the clinical findings of polycystic ovary disease (i.e., hirsutism and amenorrhea) and accelerated growth. Type C disease is not immunologically mediated, and insulin binding to its receptor is normal, suggesting a non-immunologic post-receptor defect.

Acanthosis nigricans–insulin resistance (type B) results from spontaneous autoantibodies directed against the insulin receptor that interfere with insulin action (Fig. 26–3) (Kahn et al., 1976). Type B patients may have other findings that suggest abnormal immunoregulation (i.e., antinuclear antibodies, anti-DNA antibodies, periodic hypocomplementemia, hypergammaglobulinemia, and leukopenia). Several patients with type B have suffered from ataxia-telangiectasia, systemic lupus erythematosus, scleroderma, and Sjögren's syndrome (Bloise et al., 1989).

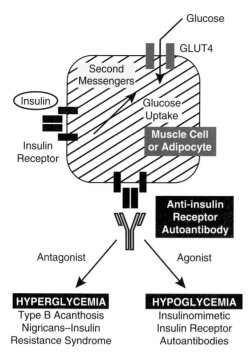

Figure 26–3. Anti-insulin receptor autoimmunity.

Pathogenesis

The peripheral blood monocytes of type B patients display decreased affinity of insulin for its receptor, whereas insulin receptor number is normal (Flier et al., 1979). In type B disease, the receptor appears to be blocked by the antagonistic autoantibody but not destroyed by the autoantibody, as is the case in myasthenia gravis. In myasthenia gravis, motor end-plate autoantibodies lead to increased receptor turnover, with a net loss in numbers of motor end-plate acetylcholine receptors. If normal monocytes are incubated with type B sera, insulin binding is blocked, confirming the presence of insulin receptor autoantibodies. Insulin receptor autoantibodies from different individuals may react with different antigenic determinants. In vitro, insulin receptor autoantibody binding may transiently mimic the action of insulin; on chronic exposure, however, the insulin receptor autoantibody antagonizes the metabolic effects of insulin. De Pirro and colleagues (1984) have reported several different insulin receptor autoantibodies in the same patient.

There is no explanation for the association between acanthosis nigricans and insulin receptor antibodies. Vitiligo also affects some patients; however, melanocyte autoantibodies have not been reported.

Clinical Course

Insulin receptor autoantibodies that block insulin action lead to glucose intolerance and hyperglycemia. Exogenous insulin, in doses exceeding 20,000 units per day, may be ineffective in controlling hyperglycemia. Ketosis is unusual. Insulin resistance produces endogenous hyperinsulinism with insulin levels up to 40,000 IU/ml or higher. Patients may experience symptoms suggestive of hypoglycemia early in the clinical course of the disease consistent with the acute in vitro insulinomimetic properties of these antibodies. Because insulin resistance may resolve spontaneously, reports of amelioration of insulin resistance with immunosuppressive therapy are difficult to interpret (Duncan et al., 1983). Up-regulation of insulin receptor number may occur as a compensatory phenomenon.

Diagnosis

Patients with insulin-resistant diabetes, immune abnormalities, and acanthosis nigricans must be suspected of having type B disease. Insulin receptor autoantibodies can be identified with radioreceptor binding studies. Other findings can include hypergammaglobulinemia, elevated erythrocyte sedimentation rate, hypocomplementemia, and ANA and anti-DNA antibodies. Insulin autoantibodies are generally not found; if they are present, their titers are usually low.

Treatment and Prognosis

Phenomenal doses of exogenous insulin may be required to control hyperglycemia. Duncan and coworkers (1983) successfully used prednisone in treating a teenaged male with type B disease with severe insulin resistance. Patients with type B insulin resistance have the same potential for long-term complications as patients with IDD or NIDD. Further studies concerning the value of immunosuppressive therapy are indicated.

Insulinomimetic Insulin Receptor Autoantibodies

Early in their clinical course, patients with acanthosis nigricans–insulin resistance type B may have symptoms of hypoglycemia (see Fig. 26–3). In 1982, Taylor et al. reported a 60-year-old black female with spontaneous hypoglycemia due to insulinomimetic insulin receptor autoantibodies. Based on these findings, insulin receptor autoantibodies must be considered as a possible cause of hypoglycemia particularly in individuals with autoimmune disease, low insulin levels, and hypoglycemia. Insulinomimetic insulin receptor autoantibodies have been described in a child (Elias et al., 1987) and in adults with lupus erythematosus (Moller et al., 1988; Varga et al., 1990) and Hodgkin's disease (Braund et al., 1987).

AUTOIMMUNE THYROID DISORDERS

Autoimmunity to the thyroid gland results in a wide clinical spectrum of disease spanning Hashimoto thyroiditis (chronic lymphocytic thyroiditis [CLT]) to Graves disease (Editorial, 1981; Strakosch et al., 1982; Fisher et al., 1987) (Fig. 26–4). In CLT, thyroid follicular cells are destroyed by autoimmune mechanisms. In Graves disease, autoantibodies, known as thyroid-stimulating immunoglobulins (TSIs), bind to and stimulate the thyroid-stimulating hormone (TSH) receptor

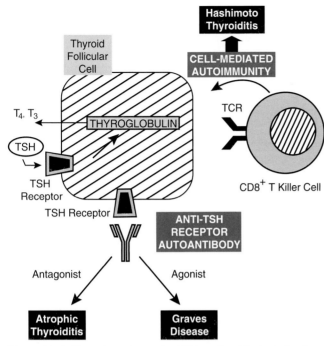

Figure 26–4. Thyroid autoimmunity. TSH = thyroid-stimulating hormone; TCR = T-cell receptor; T_4 = thyroxine; T_3 = triiodothyronine.

to release thyroid hormone and produce clinical hyperthyroidism.

Autoantibodies to thyroid hormone are often present in autoimmune thyroid disease. Occasionally autoantibodies against thyroid hormone elevate thyroid hormone levels. Such autoantibodies do not cause hyperthyroidism, as the unbound or free fraction of thyroid hormone remains normal.

Chronic Lymphocytic (Hashimoto) Thyroiditis

In the broadest sense, any person with thyroid autoantibodies in the absence of hyperthyroidism can be considered to have chronic lymphocytic (Hashimoto) thyroiditis, since biopsy studies show strong correlation between thyroid autoantibodies and histologic CLT. Transient hyperthyroidism can be seen in CLT as a result of thyroid follicular cell destruction with release of thyroid hormone. However, most individuals with CLT are initially euthyroid but up to 50% will develop hypothyroidism with increasing age and continued thyroid follicular cell destruction (Tunbridge et al., 1981). CLT is differentiated from colloid goiter by the presence of lymphoid aggregates on a biopsy specimen and by the presence of associated thyroid autoantibodies in CLT.

Two forms of thyroiditis are recognized: *goitrous* and *atrophic*. When TSH receptor autoantibodies block TSH binding without stimulating the thyroid, the gland atrophies, producing the same potential for hypothyroidism as seen in goitrous CLT (Okamura et al., 1990). A goiter develops in goitrous CLT because of lymphocytic infiltration and follicular cell hyperplasia. The latter may be due to growth-promoting thyroid autoantibodies as well as pituitary TSH stimulation in the face of diminished glandular function.

History

Hashimoto (1912) identified four elderly patients with lymphocytic thyroiditis in 1901. In 1956, Roitt and associates found high titers of serum thyroglobulin autoantibodies in patients with Hashimoto thyroiditis. In that same year, Adams and Purves (1956) described a substance in the sera of patients with Graves disease that was later termed *long-acting thyroid stimulator* (LATS). LATS was the first thyroid-stimulating immunoglobulin to be identified.

Pathogenesis

An autoimmune etiology for chronic lymphocytic thyroiditis (Strakosch et al., 1982) is suggested by (1) lymphocytic infiltration of the thyroid gland, (2) autoantibodies to the thyroid follicular cells, (3) disordered cell mediated immunity directed against the thyroid, (4) associated autoantibodies to pancreatic islets, gastric parietal cells, and adrenal gland, and (5) particular HLA associations (Weetman et al., 1990).

Infiltrating lymphocytes are found throughout the thyroid gland in the interfollicular spaces (Hahn et al., 1965). At times, lymphocyte follicles may be formed. Pujol-Borrell and coworkers (1983) reported that lectins can induce HLA-DR expression on thyroid follicular cells, raising the possibility of self-autoantigen presentation by thyroid cells in affected patients. Indeed, thyrocytes express MHC class II antigens in autoimmune thyroid diseases (Hanafusa et al., 1983).

Thyroid Autoantibodies

Autoantibodies to thyroglobulin (TGAs), the follicular cell microsomes (thyroid microsomal autoantibodies [TMAs]), and a thyroid colloidal antigen have been described (Doniach, 1975). TMAs are cytoplasmic reactive autoantibodies that identify thyroperoxidase (TPO) (Ruf et al., 1987; Mariotti et al. 1990, Banga et al., 1991). TPO catalyzes the conversion of inorganic iodide (I^-) to organic iodine (I^o) that is then covalently bound to the phenolic tyrosine rings of thyroglobulin. TPO is clustered near the apical pole of the thyrocyte (Pinchera et al., 1987). TGA and TMA can be detected by a variety of methods, including indirect immunofluorescence, hemagglutination, radioimmunoassay, complement fixation, and enzyme-linked immunosorbent assay (ELISA) techniques. Vakeva and coworkers (1992) have stressed the need to improve TPO autoantibody assays because of frequent false-negative and false-positive results. Surface autoantibodies to follicular cells have been observed using suspensions of follicular cells as targets. In CLT but not Graves disease, antibody-dependent cell-mediated cytotoxicity to these cells has been demonstrated (Bogner et al., 1984).

It was initially believed that TGA developed because thyroglobulin was released into the circulation following thyroid follicular cell damage, thus exposing the immune system to a previously sequestered antigen.

However, sensitive radioimmunoassays have shown that thyroglobulin is present in normal sera, and thus thyroglobulin is not a sequestered antigen. More than 95% of patients with histologic CLT have TMA and/or TGA/TPO autoantibodies, making them excellent markers for CLT (Doniach, 1975). TMA is more common at the time of diagnosis, whereas TGAs usually appear later in the disease.

In atrophic CLT, autoantibodies may be found that block thyroid cell receptor binding by TSH. Such autoantibodies can cross the placenta and may result in congenital hypothyroidism (Matsuura et al., 1980; Iseki et al., 1983; Van Der Gaag et al., 1985a). However, the maternal thyroid autoantibodies (e.g., TMA and TGA) account for only an occasional case of congenital hypothyroidism (Dussault et al., 1980). Transient congenital hypothyroidism may be due to transplacental TSH receptor autoantibodies (Francis and Riley, 1987).

Using an assay measuring stimulation of thyroid cell growth in vitro, thyroid growth-promoting antibodies (TGPAs) have been recognized (Valente et al., 1984; Van Der Gaag et al., 1985b). TGPA are sometimes present in both Graves disease and CLT. These antibodies stimulate tritiated thymidine uptake, a measure of cellular proliferation, without increasing cyclic adenosine monophosphate (cAMP) generation, a measure of TSH-like stimulation. The TSH receptor-stimulating autoantibodies (TSIs) stimulate cAMP production as well as thyroid hormone production and release.

Many believe that the formation of thyroid autoantibodies results from deficient T-lymphocyte suppressor numbers and function (Okita et al., 1981a, 1981b). Current theory holds that autoreactive B-cell clones arise frequently but are usually held in check by suppressor T cells (Tao et al., 1985). Alternatively, autoreactive clones may be unable to respond to autoantigen because of a lack of helper T cells that supply B-cell growth factors and other lymphokines for B-cell proliferation. This hypothesis is controversial, however, since not all investigators have identified decreased suppressor T-cell function or numbers (MacLean et al., 1981).

Cellular Autoimmunity

In both Graves disease and CLT, local infiltrating lymphocytes may be the major source of thyroid autoantibodies (Canonica et al., 1983). Variable numbers of intrathyroidal T and B lymphocytes are seen in both Hashimoto thyroiditis and Graves disease (Utiger, 1991). Disordered cell-mediated autoimmunity is seen in CTL, with increased secretion of lymphocyte macrophage inhibition factor (Okita et al., 1981c). Mixing experiments support the thesis of decreased T-suppressor cell activity in CLT and Graves disease.

Several studies have shown decreased numbers of circulating (Iwatani et al., 1983; Sridama et al., 1982) and intrathyroidal suppressor (CD8$^+$) or suppressor-inducer (CD4$^+$ CD45RA$^+$) cells (Jansson et al., 1983b; Kawakami et al., 1991). However, Canonica and co-workers (1981) found no T subset abnormalities. Paschke et al. (1991) recorded increased numbers of

intraepithelial CD45RO$^+$ (memory) T lymphocytes and immunoglobulin-producing lymphocytes.

CLT is associated with other autoimmune diseases, including IDD, atrophic gastritis/pernicious anemia (Irvine, 1975), vitiligo, and adrenalitis/Addison disease (Riley et al., 1981). Thyroid autoimmunity, if present, is usually coincident with IDD onset (Riley et al., 1983). As discussed elsewhere in this chapter, CLT is a component of the type II autoimmune polyglandular syndrome.

HLA Associations in Chronic Lymphocytic Thyroiditis

Although the HLA associations are not as impressive as those present in IDD, goitrous CLT appears to be associated with an increased frequency of HLA-DRB1*11 (Doniach et al., 1979) and atrophic CLT is associated with HLA-DRB1*03 (Weissel et al., 1980; Farid et al., 1981). The DRB1*03 association with atrophic CLT is of interest because Graves disease is strongly associated with this HLA allele. This suggests that HLA-DRB1*03 is associated with TSH receptor autoantibody formation that can either stimulate or block the TSH receptor. In spite of these HLA associations, in multigenerational families with autoimmune thyroid disease, apparent autosomal dominant inheritance does not segregate with HLA haplotype (Gorsuch et al., 1980; Phillips et al., 1990; Roman et al., 1992). HLA type may influence the clinical expression of autosomal dominant thyroid autoimmunity (Wick, 1987) to develop into Hashimoto thyroiditis or else to develop into Graves disease when HLA-DRB1*03 is present. DQ alleles may also influence susceptibility to thyroid autoimmunity (Badenhoop et al., 1990).

Combined Thyroid and Gastric Autoimmunities

Because of the frequent association of CLT with gastric parietal cell autoimmunity, the term *thyrogastric autoimmunity* has been coined. We hypothesize that a single gene outside the HLA complex predisposes one to both autoimmune disorders. The expression of this gene is gender-influenced, since more women than men manifest CLT, Graves disease, and thyroid or gastric autoantibodies. The frequency of TMA and gastric parietal cell autoantibodies steadily increases with advancing age (Maclaren and Riley, 1985; Mariotti et al., 1992). If the thyrogastric autoimmunity gene frequencies equal the associated autoantibody frequencies fully expressed in the elderly, it may approach 30% of the population. Because of the frequency of thyrogastric autoantibodies at the time of IDD diagnosis, we hypothesize that IDD subjects are prematurely expressing their genetic predisposition to thyrogastric autoimmunity. The corollary suggests that thyroid and gastric autoimmunities predispose to IDD.

Clinical Manifestations

The most common presenting complaint in thyroid autoimmune disease is goiter (Reiter et al., 1981). Patients may have difficulty swallowing or a sense of fullness in the neck. Neck pain is more characteristic of acute (bacterial) or subacute (viral) thyroiditis. With extensive destruction of the thyroid follicular cells, a fall in thyroid hormone production elicits the secretion of TSH from the pituitary. This trophic stimulation may further increase the size of the gland. Follicular cell destruction may transiently release excessive amounts of thyroid hormone, producing a temporary hyperthyroidism. Dubbed "Hashitoxicosis," (or "Toximoto" disease), this state is differentiated from Graves disease by its transient nature and by its relatively low radioactive iodine uptake. Typically, the thyroid scan reveals patchy uptake of iodide in CLT. In CLT, the gland has a "pebbly" feel, as opposed to the "boggy" gland of Graves disease.

With continued destruction of the follicular cells, thyroid hormone production may become deficient in spite of marked elevations in TSH. Clinical hypothyroidism then develops, often insidiously. Patients with hypothyroidism may manifest brittle hair; dry skin; a puffy, dull appearance; a hoarse voice; bradycardia; constipation; intolerance to cold; and "hung-up" reflexes. In children, cessation or slowing of growth may be the only manifestation of hypothyroidism.

In some patients, CLT results only in goiter; in others, it may progress to hypothyroidism. The clinical course may be punctuated by remissions and exacerbations. Permanent remission with disappearance of the goiter is occasionally seen. In adults with CLT, hypothyroidism develops in about 5% per year (Tunbridge et al., 1981).

Diagnosis

CLT is diagnosed by the presence of goiter and thyroid microsomal autoantibodies (TMAs), TPO autoantibodies and/or thyroglobulin autoantibodies (TGAs) (Doniach et al., 1979). Occasional patients without these autoantibodies may have autoantibodies to the colloid antigen CA-2 or gastric parietal cell autoantibodies. Although their measurement is not widely available, thyroid growth-promoting autoantibodies are supportive of the diagnosis of CLT. Because the treatment for hypothyroidism is simple and straightforward (thyroxine), a thyroid biopsy is rarely indicated. Goiter in CLT may gradually resolve after thyroid hormone replacement.

Treatment

For goiter unaccompanied by TSH elevation, no therapy is required. Once the TSH becomes elevated, with or without clinical hypothyroidism, thyroid hormone replacement is indicated (thyroxine, 100 μg/M^2/day). Because of its high efficacy and safety, immunomodulatory therapy is not indicated.

Prognosis

For appropriately treated patients, the prognosis for CLT is excellent. However, sometimes the goiter may be recalcitrant to hormonal replacement, contrary to the impression portrayed in many textbooks. In adults, untreated hypothyroidism can progress to myxedema with cardiac decompensation and/or coma. In children, the most serious consequence of hypothyroidism is growth retardation. An increased risk of thyroid lymphoma in CLT has been suggested; however, the overall frequency of cancer in patients with CLT is not increased (Holm et al., 1985).

Graves Disease

Hyperthyroidism is the clinical state resulting from inappropriate and excessive release of thyroid hormone. Graves disease is present when hyperthyroidism results from stimulatory autoantibodies produced against the TSH receptor (Strakosch et al., 1982). Thyroid autoimmunity (TMA and TGA), thyroid-stimulating immunoglobulins (TSIs), and lymphocyte infiltration of the thyroid are the hallmarks of Graves disease (McKenzie et al., 1975). Exophthalmos and/or proptosis of the eyes is frequently associated with Graves disease but may occur independently without thyroid enlargement or disease.

Pathogenesis

An autoimmune etiology for Graves disease is firmly based. Most patients with Graves disease have thyroid autoantibodies, including TSIs (e.g., a long-acting thyroid stimulator, LATS), thyroid microsomal autoantibodies (TMA), and/or thyroglobulin autoantibodies (TGA). Biopsy specimens reveal lymphocytic infiltration of the gland along with diffuse follicular cell hyperplasia and colloid absorption. Aberrant expression of HLA-DR antigens on the surface of the follicular cells in Graves disease has been described (Hanafusa et al., 1983).

Autoantibodies

In most patients with Graves disease, TSIs can be detected (Strakosch et al., 1982). Several assays have been used. The first were in vivo bioassays that detected the LATS TSI, using guinea pigs and mice (McKenzie, 1968; Kendall-Taylor, 1975). The animals were iodine-depleted, then prescribed thyroid hormone to suppress TSH and given radioactive iodine. Sera from Graves patients injected into these animals caused the release of increased amounts of ^{131}I from the thyroid. However, the peak response was 10 to 12 hours after injection, significantly different from the peak response at 3 hours produced by TSH injection. This delay accounts for the term "long-acting thyroid stimulator." This phenomenon was described prior to its recognition as an autoantibody.

An in vitro variant of this assay measures radioactive iodine release from thyroid tissue slices (Ekins and Ellis, 1975). Cyclic AMP response to TSIs has also been measured in human thyroid cell monolayers (Rapoport et al., 1982). Using cultured human thyroid cells, Rapoport et al. (1984) report a 93% frequency of TSIs in patients with Graves disease. The failure to find TSIs in all Graves patients might be the result of bioassay insensitivity (Davies et al., 1983) or the presence of specific human TSIs. Human-specific autoantibodies were initially termed "LATS protector," an IgG that blocks LATS neutralization by human thyroid protein (Adams and Kennedy, 1971). TSH receptor autoantibodies can react to different epitopes on the TSH receptor (Shishiba et al., 1982; Dayan et al., 1991); however, most are directed to the extracellular domains of the molecule.

In other assays, radioreceptor techniques are used to measure TSH binding inhibition by sera from Graves patients (TSH binding inhibitory immunoglobulin, TBII; Brown et al., 1986). Other assays for TSIs measure colloid droplet formation in follicular cells, glucose oxidation, incorporation of ^{32}P into phospholipids, cAMP accumulation, and adenyl cyclase activity. The lymphocytes infiltrating the thyroid gland may be the chief source of TSIs (Kendall-Taylor et al., 1984). Carbamizole, a drug that blocks thyroid hormone biosynthesis, may also inhibit thyroid autoantibody production by a suppressive effect on thyroid lymphocytes (McGregor et al., 1980a). However, Jansson et al. (1983a) found intrathyroidal concentrations of methimazole, the breakdown product of carbamizole, to be less immunosuppressive than previously reported (Weiss and Davies, 1981).

Cellular Autoimmunity

Cell-mediated autoimmunity in Graves disease is suggested by elevated levels of lymphocyte migration inhibition factor (Okita et al., 1981c; Topliss et al., 1983). Abnormal suppressor T-cell numbers or functions have been suggested involving H_2 histamine receptor bearing (Okita et al., 1981a) and/or IgG-Fc receptor bearing T lymphocytes (Mori et al., 1982).

Other immune abnormalities in Graves disease include decreased T-suppressor numbers (Okita et al., 1981b; Sridama et al., 1982) and Ia-positive T cells (Jackson et al., 1984). However, the cause-and-effect relationship of immune abnormalities to hyperthyroidism has not been firmly established (Grubeck-Loebenstein et al., 1985).

Graves disease is often associated with other autoimmune diseases, particularly lymphocytic atrophic gastritis and IDD. Interestingly, in patients with Graves and IDD, the hyperthyroidism usually precedes the diabetes (Riley et al., 1981). Graves disease is highly associated with HLA-DRB1*03, as some two of every three patients with Graves disease carry this allele.

Exophthalmos

The relationship of Graves disease to exophthalmos is unclear (Solomon et al., 1977; Gorman, 1983; Schifferdecker et al., 1989; Weetman, 1991, 1992). The two conditions may exist together or independently. Some authors suggest that most patients with ophthalmopathy have some form of thyroid autoimmunity (Salvi et al., 1990).

Exophthalmos may result from autoimmunity to retrobulbar structures that is independent of Graves disease however. Hyperthyroidism increases the body's sensitivity to endogenous catecholamines. Lid retraction, which can result from the sympathetic effects of hyperthyroidism, should not be confused with exophthalmos resulting from retrobulbar inflammation and lymphocytic infiltration. An autoimmune etiology for the exophthalmos with or without coexistent Graves disease is postulated (Doniach and Florin-Christensen, 1975). Because the thyroid lymphatic drainage traverses the retro-orbital space, thyroglobulin-antithyroglobulin complexes may be carried to the retro-orbital muscles. Here, they attach to the sarcolemma and, with the participation of complement, induce extraocular muscle damage and inflammation. Thus the retro-orbital extraocular muscles are "innocent bystanders" to an immune complex disorder generated by the thyroid disease. Sensitized T cells, autoantibody-producing B cells, and other thyroid proteins could also be carried to the retrobulbar space as above.

Thyroglobulin-containing immune complexes are not the explanation for all cases of exophthalmos (Ohtaki et al., 1981); indeed, some patients with Graves disease have no thyroglobulin autoantibodies. Further, exophthalmos is rare in uncomplicated CLT despite the high frequencies of thyroglobulin autoantibodies found in that disease. Autoantibodies to a soluble eye muscle antigen have been detected in almost 75% of patients with Graves exophthalmos (Kodama et al., 1982). TSH does not interfere with the binding of autoantibodies to the orbital antigens (Waring et al., 1983). Since adipocytes have TSH receptors, TSI stimulation may contribute to exophthalmos by inducing retro-orbital adipose cell hyperplasia. However, the absence of TSIs in some patients with exophthalmos weighs against this thesis. Most investigators have not found a firm relationship between TSIs-LATS and exophthalmos.

Other causes of exophthalmos include "ophthalmopathic immunoglobulin," as reported by Atkinson and colleagues (1984). Molecular mimicry between thyroid and orbital targets has also been proposed (Weightman and Kendall-Taylor, 1989; Wall et al., 1991). Nevertheless, there is no evidence that TGA, TMA (anti-TPO), or TSH receptor autoantibodies react with orbital targets (Schifferdecker et al., 1989; Weetman, 1991). Dobyns and Wilson (1954) described an exophthalmos-producing substance (EPS) (Der Kinderen, 1967). The sera from Graves disease patients injected into fish caused exophthalmos. Several other groups confirmed these findings, but the exophthalmos was only transitory and associated with retrobulbar lymph sac distention. EPS is reportedly of pituitary origin. Multiple autoantigens have been discovered with immunoblotting techniques (e.g., 110 kD, 95 kD, 64 kD, 55 kD, 23 kD) (Kadlubowski et al., 1987; Bahn et al., 1989; Bernard et al., 1991; Kendler et al., 1991).

The coexistence of Graves disease and exophthalmos may be much closer than previously recognized. Gamblin et al. (1983) sought subclinical ophthalmopathy in Graves patients and found elevated (>3 mm Hg) intraocular pressure on upward gaze in 76% of their patients. Since only 26% had overt exophthalmos, about 50 percent had undetected ophthalmopathy.

Euthyroid patients with exophthalmos often have thyroid autoantibodies, suggesting a spectrum of coexistent disorders (Ahmann and Burman, 1987).

Other Clinical Manifestations

Other than exophthalmos and pretibial myxedema, thyrotoxicosis in Graves disease does not differ clinically from other forms of hyperthyroidism. Symptoms include fine hair, smooth skin, tachycardia, sweating, diarrhea, weight loss, hyperreflexia, insomnia, and neuropsychologic disorders.

As in Hashimoto thyroiditis, there may be autosomal dominant inheritance of Graves disease. Hashimoto thyroiditis and Graves disease often coexist in families, and both are highly associated with gastric parietal cell autoimmunity. In family studies, co-inheritance of heavy-chain immunoglobulin allotypes and Graves disease has been reported (Tamai et al., 1985).

Diagnosis

Graves disease is diagnosed by the presence of persistent hyperthyroidism with evidence of thyroid autoimmunity. Exophthalmos supports the diagnosis, and a diffusely enlarged thyroid gland is typically found. Because TSIs induce excessive thyroid gland activity, pituitary TSH response to TRH is blunted as a result of negative feedback inhibition. Total and unbound thyroxine (T_4) and triiodothyronine (T_3) are markedly elevated. In cases of iodine deficiency, isolated T_3 toxicosis may result with high T_3 but normal T_4 levels (Hollander et al., 1972). Alternatively, if significant nonthyroidal illness coexists, T_4 may be elevated without elevations of T_3. This may occur because of a relatively deficient T_4 to T_3 conversion, especially in elderly patients. There is a marked predominance of females affected with Graves disease; indeed, female predominance is usual for most autoimmune disorders except for IDD.

The differential diagnosis includes thyrotoxicosis factitia (Mariotti et al., 1982), toxic nodular goiter (Plummer disease), and thyroid neoplasia. Rare cases of TSH-secreting pituitary tumors have been reported (Kourides et al., 1977). In several conditions, high thyroid hormone levels are found in the absence of clinical hyperthyroidism. These disorders fall into two categories: (1) resistance to thyroid hormone (Linde et al., 1982) and (2) elevated levels of circulating thyroid-binding proteins or aberrant carrier proteins. With thyroid hormone resistance, both total and free thyroid hormone levels are elevated but the patient is clinically euthyroid with normal thyroid-binding globulin (TBG) levels. Defects of the thyroid cell nuclear T_3 receptor as well as post-receptor defects have been described.

When there is pituitary thyroid hormone resistance but normal peripheral sensitivity, clinical hyperthyroidism is evident (Norvogroder et al., 1977). Total T_4 and T_3 levels can be elevated because of increased thyroid hormone carrier proteins. Here the unbound hormone levels remain normal and the patient is euthyroid. Most commonly, this is the result of a congenital excess of TBG. TBG elevation can also be induced by pregnancy, estrogen administration, and acute liver disease. Congenital TBG excess can be inherited as an autosomal dominant trait.

Rarer syndromes similar to TBG excess include familial dysalbuminemic hyperthyroxinemia (Ruiz et al., 1982) and euthyroid hyperthyroxinemia with abnormal prealbumin (Moses et al., 1982). Here, TBG levels are normal; however, an abnormal albumin or prealbumin carries supranormal amounts of thyroid hormone, producing an elevation in total thyroid hormone levels, particularly T_4.

Treatment

Oral antithyroid medications, such as the thioureas propylthiouracil and methimazole, which inhibit thyroid hormone biosynthesis, are used to induce and maintain a clinical remission. Because of their short duration of action (6 to 8 hours), good compliance is crucial. After 1 to 2 years, therapy should be tapered and stopped because 50% of patients with Graves disease enter a permanent remission.

Controversy exists as to whether the presence of HLA-DR3 and/or TBII decreases the likelihood of remission (McGregor et al., 1980b). In a prospective study (Allannic et al., 1984), HLA typing did not predict relapse. For those who do experience relapse, radioactive iodine is more efficacious and safer than thyroidectomy (Becker, 1984; Hamburger, 1985). Hypothyroidism is, however, common following radioiodine therapy. In centers skilled in thyroid surgery, thyroidectomy may be preferred.

Exophthalmos may worsen with treatment for hyperthyroidism, especially following ^{131}I ablative therapy. It is unclear whether this is the result of thyroid antigen release or a result of an immunologic alteration with treatment. The treatment of exophthalmos depends on its severity. No treatment is indicated for mild exophthalmos. For advanced or progressing eye disease, oral corticosteroids, orbital irradiation, eye muscle surgery, and orbital decompression are used. Early thyroid hormone replacement following thyroid ablation therapy may minimize the induced exophthalmos.

Prognosis

Untreated, Graves disease can produce life-threatening, high-output cardiac failure. Similarly, *thyroid storm* can produce heart failure. Short of the above, hyperthyroidism can produce severe inanition, fatigue, sleeplessness, diarrhea, and personality changes. Appropriately treated, Graves disease can be controlled or even cured. However, long-term personality changes may persist. Likewise, proptosis may not disappear completely because of fibrosis in the retro-orbital space.

Thyroid Hormone Autoantibodies

Spontaneous anti-T_4 and -T_3 autoantibodies can be recognized in Hashimoto thyroiditis and Graves disease (Volpe, 1991) but usually have no clinical consequences (Nakamura et al., 1989). Occasionally, such autoantibodies can elevate total thyroid hormone levels without producing clinical disease or can depress free hormone levels, leading to hypothyroidism (Trimarchi et al., 1982). Anti-T$_4$ autoantibodies may lead to spuriously high unbound T$_4$ determinations (Fukasawa et al., 1991). Most are polyclonal, but oligoclonal and monoclonal autoantibodies have been reported (Moroz et al., 1983). Autoantibodies to bovine TSH (Eto et al., 1984) and human TSH have also been described (Raines et al., 1985).

AUTOIMMUNE DISORDERS OF THE ADRENALS AND GONADS

Because autoimmunity to the adrenal gland and gonads often occurs concomitantly, these autoimmune disorders are discussed together.

Addison Disease

Addison disease results from the destruction of the adrenal cortex to a degree that clinical problems from loss of glucocorticoid and mineralocorticoid hormones result (Fig. 26–5). Clinical features include weight loss, weakness, fatigue, dehydration, hypoglycemia, and, at a late stage, vascular collapse. A diffuse, ''muddy'' hyperpigmentation results from pituitary hypersecretion of adrenocorticotropic hormone (ACTH) and melanocyte-stimulating hormone (MSH), which are stimulatory to melanocytes.

Autoimmune Addison disease is defined by the absence of known causes of adrenocortical destruction (e.g., tuberculosis, histoplasmosis, hemorrhage, carci-

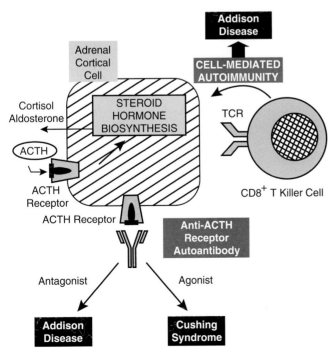

Figure 26–5. Adrenal autoimmunity. ACTH = adrenocorticotropic hormone; TCR = T-cell receptor.

nomatosis), the presence of adrenocortical autoantibodies, and lymphocytic infiltration of the adrenal cortices (Betterle et al., 1989). It is more likely to occur in patients with other autoimmune illnesses (e.g., autoimmune thyroid disease, IDD), especially in those with an HLA phenotype that includes the DRB1*03/ DQB1*0201 haplotype. In other states of adrenocortical insufficiency, such as ACTH deficiency (hypopituitarism), ACTH unresponsiveness, or enzymatic defects of cortisol biosynthesis (congenital adrenal hyperplasia), the term Addison disease is not applicable. In a study conducted during the 1960s in northeast London, nontuberculous Addison disease was found at a rate of 27 cases per million (Doniach and Bottazzo, 1981).

Autoimmune hypogonadism is the loss of hormone-producing cells from the ovary or testes. Autoimmune cellular ablation is suggested by loss of follicles from the ovary, lymphocytic infiltrates of either ovary or testis, and the presence of steroidal cell autoantibodies. Affected individuals may have coexistent Addison disease or other organ-specific autoimmune antibodies. Characteristically, acquired hypergonadotropic hypogonadism (with raised plasma follicle-stimulating hormone [FSH] and luteinizing hormone [LH] levels) and infertility result.

Historic Aspects

In 1849, Thomas Addison, a physician at Guy's Hospital in London, described three patients with severe anemia and loss of the suprarenal capsules. Addison's classic work, published in 1855, reported 11 additional autopsy cases. Four patients had tuberculosis, four had probable malignancy, and three had unexplained adrenal cortical atrophy. One of the latter three patients had extensive vitiligo, and perhaps all three had autoimmune disease.

In 1862, Wilks proposed that the suprarenal syndrome that involved vascular collapse should be termed Addison disease. Nontuberculous Addison disease was relatively rare. Schmidt (1926) described the concurrence of lymphocytic infiltrates of the thyroid gland and adrenal cortices in autopsies of two patients dying of addisonian crisis *(Schmidt syndrome)*. In 1928, Brenner identified that Addison disease results from loss of the adrenal cortex and not the medulla.

Following a report by Beaven and associates (1959), Carpenter and coworkers (1964) described the association between IDD and Schmidt syndrome. Doniach and Roitt (1957) provided evidence that these diseases had an autoimmune basis by identifying precipitating autoantibodies to thyroglobulin in patients with Hashimoto disease.

Anderson and colleagues (1957) and Blizzard and Kyle (1963) described adrenal autoantibodies in patients with idiopathic Addison disease. Anderson and others (1968) recognized that some adrenocortical autoantibodies also reacted with steroid hormone–producing gonadal cells, and Irvine and colleagues (1968) reported hypogonadism associated with these antibodies.

Autoimmune Polyglandular Syndromes

In 1981, Neufeld and coworkers proposed that Addison disease was a part of two (type 1 and type 2) autoimmune polyglandular syndromes (APSs) (Table 26–6):

Type I APS refers to the association of mucocutaneous candidiasis, hypoparathyroidism, and Addison disease. Two of three disorders must be present for diagnosis. They usually present in the order stated; if one condition is absent, it only rarely appears at a later date.

Type II APS is the association of Addison disease with Hashimoto thyroiditis and/or insulin-dependent diabetes (IDD) (Carpenter et al., 1964). About 50% of patients with Addison disease have type II APS (Papadopoulos and Hallengren, 1990).

Other autoimmune diseases may occur in association with either type I or type II APS. Cushing syndrome with anti-ACTH receptor autoantibodies has been described (Carstensen et al., 1989; Teding van Berkhout et al., 1989; Jones, 1990; Wilkin, 1990).

Pathogenesis

Early in the course of Addison disease, *adrenalitis*, a characteristic lymphocytic infiltration of the adrenal cortex, is noted in association with necrosis of adrenocortical cells. As inflammation subsides, fibrosis surrounding regenerating nodules results. Later, complete cortical atrophy with dense fibrosis occurs while the medulla remains relatively intact (Petra and Nerup, 1971). These pathologic changes suggest autoimmune destruction of adrenocortical cells, probably directed against a unique cortical antigen. Also supporting an autoimmune cause is the fact that patients with Addison disease often have associated disorders such as Hashimoto thyroiditis. Finally, Addison patients have autoantibodies (Blizzard and Kyle, 1963) and cell-mediated reactions to adrenal tissue.

Adrenal Autoantibodies

Adrenal IgG autoantibodies can be readily detected by indirect immunofluorescence that react with a cytoplasmic antigen present in sections of unfixed human adrenal glands (Heinonen and Krohn, 1977). They are reactive with all layers of the adrenal cortex but not with the adrenal medulla. These autoantibodies may not be pathogenic because they react with a cytoplasmic antigen not present on the surface of adrenal cells. Nonetheless, they are useful markers for the autoimmune process (Leisti et al., 1983). As IgG autoantibodies, they bind complement (Betterle et al., 1983).

Autoantibodies to an adrenal cell surface antigen also occur in Addison disease and were detected in 33 of 38 individuals with adrenocortical cytoplasmic autoantibodies (Khoury et al., 1981). Surface autoantibodies may be pathogenic by complement-dependent lysis or by antibody-dependent cellular cytotoxicity. There is one reported case of neonatal Addison disease associated with maternal transplacental adrenocortical autoantibodies (Irvine and Barnes, 1975).

The cytoplasmic adrenocortical autoantigen is organ-specific but not species-specific. However, human tissue is best for demonstrating cytoplasmic autoantibody (Elder et al., 1981). The antigen was thought to be a lipoprotein found primarily in adrenocortical cell microsomes (Anderson et al., 1968). Immunoblotting techniques have demonstrated adrenal autoantigens of 45, 55, and 70 kD (Freeman and Weetman, 1992). Some of these proteins may elicit T lymphocyte proliferation. The adrenal enzyme, 17α-hydroxylase (55 kD), was shown to be a target autoantigen in addisonian patients with type I APS (Krohn et al., 1992). Baumann-Antczak et al. (1992) reported that the 21α-hydroxylase enzyme was also an autoantigen in Addison disease, and recently confirmed by Song et al. (1995). The side chain cleavage enzyme (20,22-desmolase) also appears to be an autoantigen in type I APS.

Table 26–6. Autoimmune Polyglandular Syndromes

Features	Type I	Type II
Addison disease	+ + +	+ + +
Hypoparathyroidism	+ + +	–
Chronic mucocutaneous candidiasis	+ + +	–
Hypogonadism	+ +	±
Chronic active hepatitis	+ +	±
Alopecia	+ +	±
Vitiligo	+	±
Malabsorption syndromes	+	–
Pernicious anemia	+ + (juvenile onset)	± (late onset)
Atrophic thyroiditis	–	+ +
Goitrous thyroiditis	–	+ + +
Graves disease	–	+ + +
Insulin-dependent diabetes	±	+ + +
Sjögren's syndrome	+ +	
Immunogenetics	No known association; pedigree segregation independent of HLA haplotypes	Strong association with DR3 and/or DR4; segregation with HLA haplotypes
Early age of onset	+ + +	+ +
Onset in midlife	±	+ + +

Abbreviation: HLA = human leukocyte antigen.
Key: – = absent; + = rarely present; ± = occasionally present; + + = frequently present; + + + = very common.

Frequency of Autoantibodies

Adrenal autoantibodies are rare in the general population (~0.5%). However, they are common among patients with IDD (~2%) and autoimmune thyroid disease (~4%) (Riley et al., 1980b). Since the frequency of autoimmune Addison disease is estimated at only 1 in 30,000 persons, clinical Addison disease will not often develop in individuals with the autoantibody. In nontuberculous Addison disease, adrenal autoantibodies (cytoplasmic type) are present in 38% to 74% of patients (Irvine and Barnes, 1975). The latter figure represents the autoantibody frequency at diagnosis and is less frequent thereafter.

Betterle and colleagues (1983) found that Addison disease developed in four of nine of their asymptomatic patients with adrenocortical autoantibodies after 1 to 31 months of observation. Clinical disease was more likely to develop in individuals with complement-fixing autoantibodies (Betterle et al., 1983). Scherbaum and coworkers (1982) reported that 10% of women (3 of 30) with adrenocortical autoantibodies and thyroid autoimmunity developed Addison disease over 3 years of observation. Our own experience has been similar (Riley et al., 1980a). Thus, in a small percentage of patients with cytoplasmic adrenocortical autoantibodies, symptomatic Addison disease develops each year. We also have found that many asymptomatic patients with autoantibody often show biochemical evidence for adrenocortical insufficiency. Such patients had elevated basal plasma ACTH levels. Further, their renin levels were elevated when recumbent and when salt intake was unrestricted (Ketchum et al., 1984). An increase in ACTH may compensate for the ongoing autoimmune destruction of adrenocortical cells.

Gonadal Autoimmune Disorders

Steroidal cell autoantibodies closely resemble the cytoplasmic type of adrenocortical autoantibodies described above. However, they also react with other steroid hormone–producing cells, including the placental syncytiotrophoblast, the Leydig cells of the testes, the theca interna/granulosa cell layers of the graafian follicles, and the corpora lutea of the ovaries (Sotsiou et al., 1980; Elder et al., 1983). Steroidal cell autoantibodies are most commonly reported (up to 60%) in addisonian patients with secondary amenorrhea (Blizzard et al., 1967; Nerup, 1974; Irvine and Barnes, 1975). Since the steroidal cell antigens are cytoplasmic and not present on the cell membrane, these antibodies are probably not pathogenic; however, they are markers for an underlying autoimmune process causing gonadal destruction. The target antigens appear to be P450 enzymes involved in sex hormonogenesis. McNatty and colleagues (1975) have described a cytotoxic effect on cultured human granulosa cells by nine of 23 sera from patients with Addison disease and ovarian failure.

Cellular Autoimmunity

The early pathologic lesion of Addison disease is a lymphocytic adrenalitis with inflammation surrounding regenerating nodules. Nerup and colleagues (1969) demonstrated specific antiadrenal cellular hypersensitivity in human Addison disease using a leukocyte migration inhibition assay. Rabinowe and colleagues (1984) reported activated Ia$^+$ (DR$^+$) T cells in newly diagnosed Addison disease. In animals, adrenalitis can be induced by immunization with adrenal extracts in Freund's adjuvant. Once induced, adrenalitis can be passively transferred to other animals by immune lymphocytes (Witebsky and Milgram, 1962; Levine and Wank, 1968; Fujii et al., 1992). Despite these clinical and animal observations, proof of a major contribution of T-cell participation in human autoimmune Addison disease is lacking.

HLA Associations

Thompson and colleagues (1975) reported that 70% of patients with Addison disease were HLA-B8 positive in contrast to 24% of controls. Most patients were also Dw3-positive as determined by mixed leukocyte reaction (MLR) typing.

In our patients, we found a strong association between Addison disease and HLA-DRB1*03 and HLA-DRB1*04 antigens reminiscent of the associations seen with IDD (Maclaren and Riley, 1986). Ten of our patients had type I APS, and the frequencies of HLA-DR antigens were normal in this subgroup. Most of the other patients had at least one DR3 or DR4 allele. Furthermore, as with IDD, a negative association was seen with DR2, DR5, and DR7 alleles. We therefore believe that Addison disease is HLA-associated, except when a component of type I APS. Our recent studies, however, showed that the HLA-DRB1*04/DQB1*0302 association was entirely a consequence of concurrent pancreatic beta cell autoimmunity. This suggests diverse pathogeneses for these variants.

Clinical Manifestations

The clinical picture of Addison disease is a result of deficiencies in cortisol, aldosterone, and adrenal sex hormones. Aldosterone deficiency results in urinary sodium loss and potassium retention. Salt craving may develop, and increased salt intake may keep the patient in electrolyte balance until anorexia or vomiting occurs. Salt depletion leads to hypovolemia, weight loss, hypotension, muscular weakness, fatigue, postural syncopy, prerenal azotemia, and—as a preterminal event—vascular collapse. Cortisol deficiency, which may follow aldosterone deficiency, results in adipose wasting, apathy, weakness, deficient energy metabolism with fasting hypoglycemia, ketosis, hypoalaninemia, and deficient glucagon response, inability to excrete a water load, and impaired response to stress. Gastrointestinal symptoms are common and include anorexia, nausea, vomiting, abdominal pain, and weight loss. With a lack of negative feedback by cortisol, there is unrestrained secretion of pituitary ACTH and MSH, resulting in the classical ''muddy'' hyperpigmentation of the skin and buccal mucosa. Vitiligo is also common and generally believed to be an autoimmune etiology (Betterle et al.,

1984, 1985). We have shown that vitiligo in some patients is associated with autoantibodies to tyrosinase, an enzyme important in melanin formation (Song et al., 1994).

Diagnosis

The onset of autoimmune Addison disease is usually insidious, and the diagnosis made only during a crisis situation. In an addisonian crisis, severe dehydration and vascular collapse develop. Laboratory values reflect the sodium loss and potassium retention and prerenal azotemia—elevated serum potassium, blood urea nitrogen (BUN), and creatinine; low serum bicarbonate/pCO_2/pH; normal to low serum sodium; greatly elevated plasma renin and ACTH; hypoglycemia; and inappropriately normal to low plasma cortisol and aldosterone levels. Relative lymphocytosis and modest eosinophilia are also often found.

At an earlier stage, sodium wasting may be reflected by hyperkalemia and mild acidosis and by a subnormal rise of plasma cortisol following ACTH infusion. Persons with adrenocortical autoantibodies without clinical Addison disease may show elevated basal levels of plasma renin and/or ACTH as the only biochemical evidence of adrenocortical compromise.

At diagnosis, adrenocortical autoantibodies are found in about two thirds of patients with idiopathic Addison disease, and these diminish with time.

The diagnosis of autoimmune hypogonadism is based on the findings of elevated gonadotropin levels (especially FSH) and a characteristic gonadal biopsy or the presence of steroidal cell autoantibodies. The gonadal biopsy specimen typically shows lymphocytic infiltration and follicular loss.

Prognosis

The prognosis for appropriately treated patients is good. Replacement therapy with 9α-fluorohydrocortisone (0.05 to 0.15 mg/day) and oral hydrocortisone (12 to 15 mg/M^2/day in divided doses) is indicated. Extraoral cortisol or parenteral hydrocortisone is given during periods of stress, nausea, and vomiting. In general, the prognosis depends on the associated disorder. The most significant associated problem in type I APS is chronic active hepatitis, which often progresses to cirrhosis. Hypocalcemia of concurrent hypoparathyroidism may be masked until initiation of cortisol replacement therapy for Addison disease. Associated disorders should be sought yearly. In patients with Addison disease that is not associated with type I APS, thyroid, pancreatic islet, and gastric parietal cell autoantibodies should be sought.

Autoimmune Disorders of the Anterior Pituitary and Hypothalamus

Anterior Pituitary Autoimmunity

Autoantibodies reacting with the prolactin and/or growth hormone–producing cells of the anterior pituitary have been detected by indirect immunofluorescence in some patients with autoimmune disease (Bottazzo et al., 1975). Such autoantibodies, in concert with reports of lymphocytic hypophysitis (Mayfield et al., 1980), suggest that autoimmunity to certain cells of the anterior pituitary can lead to clinical problems; mass lesions may result from lymphocytic infiltration (Supler and Mickle, 1992).

Pituitary autoimmunity has also been implicated in some cases of growth hormone deficiency (Bottazzo et al., 1980b) and Sheehan syndrome (Engelberth and Jezkova, 1965). Because their height may be increased at diagnosis, Mirakian et al. (1982) studied newly diagnosed IDD patients for pituitary autoantibodies. More than 15% of such patients tested positive, but no control subject showed positive results. In long-standing IDD, only 2% of patients exhibited positive results, suggesting that pituitary autoimmunity may be transient. These findings have yet to be confirmed.

Hypothalamic Autoimmunity

Diabetes insipidus (DI) results when the hypothalamic cells that produce antidiuretic hormone (ADH) are destroyed. In addition, sufficient damage to the posterior pituitary or to the axons leading from the hypothalamus to the posterior pituitary can also produce DI. Scherbaum and Bottazzo (1983) sought autoantibodies to the ADH-producing cells of the hypothalamus in 30 patients with idiopathic DI. About one third of patients with idiopathic DI and no controls were autoantibody-positive. Associated autoimmune endocrine disorders were present in 60% of their patients. These autoantibodies were not directed against antidiuretic hormone, oxytocin, or the neurophysins. The investigators proposed that the autoimmune polyglandular syndromes (APSs) should also include hypothalamic autoimmunity. Autoimmune DI may occur in children (Scherbaum et al., 1985).

AN APPROACH TO THE PATIENT WITH AUTOIMMUNE ENDOCRINOPATHY

Knowledge of common disease associations and mode of disease inheritance is most important for proper management of autoimmune endocrinopathies (Winter and Maclaren, 1987). The following is a practical guide to aid the physician in planning appropriate patient and family evaluation.

Insulin-Dependent Diabetes

At the time of diagnosis of IDD, thyroid microsomal (TMA/TPO), thyroglobulin (TGA), and gastric parietal cell (PCA) autoantibodies should be sought (Neufeld et al., 1980). Patients with TMA/TPO and/or TGA should have yearly studies of TSH and free T_4 levels in search of primary hypothyroidism, especially during early to middle adulthood (Riley et al., 1981); those with PCAs should have annual determinations of vitamin B_{12} and ferritin levels (Riley et al., 1982). In atrophic gastritis, parietal cell damage can result in deficient intrinsic factor production, leading to vitamin B_{12} malabsorption, deficient acid secretion, and poor iron absorption. Family members, especially females, should also be screened for thyroid and gastric autoantibodies.

If TMA/TPOs or PCAs are detected, the patient should be further tested for adrenal autoantibodies as predictors of Addison disease. In patients with adrenal autoantibodies, yearly determinations of fasting ACTH levels and supine renin levels are indicated (Ketchum et al., 1984). Those with elevations of both should be considered as having incipient Addison disease. Such biochemical abnormalities provide early evidence of failing adrenocortical function and warrant early treatment.

When regimens to prevent IDD are available, all first-degree relatives of IDD patients should be screened for ICAs, IAAs, and/or anti-GAD autoantibodies as indicators of a potential prediabetic state. Once recognized, appropriate metabolic measurements of pancreatic beta cell function (oral or intravenous glucose tolerance tests) may be done on a serial basis. If progressive loss of beta cell function is identified, insulin injection prior to the development of frank IDD may prevent or forestall the disease. At present, such preventive therapy is strictly investigational. Periodic screening of children for anti-GAD autoantibodies may become practical with the advent of automated methods.

Thyroid and Gastric Autoimmunity

When either thyroid or gastric autoimmune disease is identified, the other disorder should be sought. Appropriate metabolic evaluations should be carried out as described earlier. Thyrogastric autoimmunity appears to be inherited as an autosomal dominant trait, and therefore all first-degree relatives should be screened for TMAs/TPOs and PCAs.

Addison Disease and the Autoimmune Polyglandular Syndromes

In individuals with mucocutaneous candidiasis, hypoparathyroidism and autoimmune Addison disease, other conditions associated with APS type I should be sought. Specifically, steroidal cell autoantibodies are predictive of autoimmune hypergonadotropic hypogonadism, whereas mitochondrial and/or smooth muscle autoantibodies indicate the possibility of non-B chronic active hepatitis. Hypergonadotropic hypogonadism is normally seen at adolescence; however, elevated FSH and LH levels may not occur if malnutrition is also present. Liver enzymes (AST, ALT, GGTP), bilirubin, albumin, and immunoglobulin levels may be assayed to assess liver function. Hypergammaglobulinemia is common. Elevated levels of plasma unconjugated bile acids are sensitive indicators of liver dysfunction but are usually available only as send-out tests.

Addison disease without hypoparathyroidism or mucocutaneous candidiasis may exist as part of APS type II, necessitating screening for thyroid (TMA/TPO) and

Table 26–7. Target Enzymes in Autoimmune Disorders Other Than Insulin-Dependent Diabetes

Disorder	Enzyme Autoantigen
Hashimoto thyroiditis	Thyroperoxidase (TPO)
Chronic atrophic gastritis	H^+/K^+-ATPase (proton) pump (Karlsson et al., 1988)
Adrenalitis	17-hydroxylase, side chain cleavage enzyme (type I APS)
	21-hydroxylase (type II APS, isolated Addison disease)
Gonaditis	17-hydroxylase, side chain cleavage enzyme
Chronic active hepatitis	Cytochrome P_{450} (Manns et al., 1989, 1991)

pancreatic beta cell (ICA) autoantibodies in patients and their families.

In the future, induction of immunologic tolerance to prevent autoimmune disorders will be attempted. Many autoantigens have been identified as enzymes (Table 26–7). In summary, when one autoimmune endocrinopathy is discovered, associated endocrine and nonendocrine autoimmune diseases should be sought. In this way, preclinical disease may be detected and subsequent symptoms prevented. This may prove especially important in the future management of latent insulin-dependent diabetes.

References

Adams DD, Kennedy TH. Evidence to suggest that LATS protector stimulates the human thyroid gland. J Clin Endocrinol 33:47–51, 1971.

Adams DD, Purves HD. Abnormal responses in the assay for thyrotropin. Proc Univ Otaga Med School 34:11–12, 1956.

Adams DD, Adams YJ, Knight JG, McCall J, White P, Horrocks R, Van Loghem E. A solution to the genetic and environmental puzzles of insulin-dependent diabetes mellitus. Lancet 1:420–424, 1984.

Addison T. Anemia—disease of the supra-renal capsules. London Med Gazette 43:517–518, 1849.

Addison T. On the Constitution and Local Effects of the Disease of the Supra-renal Capsules. London, Samuel Highley, 1855; 43.

Ahmann A, Burman KD. The role of T lymphocytes in autoimmune thyroid disease. Endocrinol Metab Clin North Am 16:287–326, 1987.

Allannic H, Fauchet R, Lorcy Y, Gueguen M, LeGuerrier A-M, Genetet B. A prospective study of the relationship between relapse of hyperthyroid Graves disease after antithyroid drugs and HLA haplotype. J Clin Endocrinol Metab 57:719–722, 1984.

Alviggi L, Johnston C, Hoskins PJ, Tee DEH, Pyke DA, Leslie RDG, Vengani D. Pathogenesis of insulin-dependent diabetes: a role for activated T lymphocytes. Lancet 2:4–6, 1984.

Anderson J, Goudie R, Gray K, Stuart-Smith D. Immunological features of idiopathic Addison disease: an autoantibody to cells producing steroid hormones. Clin Exp Immunol 3:107–112, 1968.

Anderson J, Goudie R, Gray K, Timbury G. Autoantibodies in Addison disease. Lancet 1:1123–1124, 1957.

Aparicio JM. HLA and non-HLA genetic factors in Japanese IDDM. Hokkaido Igaku Zasshi 66:780–793, 1991.

Assan R, Feutren G, Debray-Sachs M, Quiniou-Debrie MD, Laborie C, Thomas G, Chatenoud L, Bach JF. Metabolic and immunological effects of cyclosporin in recently diagnosed type I diabetes mellitus. Lancet 1:67–71, 1985.

Atkinson MA, Maclaren NK. What causes diabetes? Sci Am 262:62–71, 1990.

Atkinson MA, Maclaren N. The pathogenesis of insulin-dependent diabetes mellitus. N Engl J Med 331:1428–1436, 1994.

Atkinson MA, Maclaren NK, Riley WJ, Winter WE, Fisk DD, Spillar RP. Are insulin autoantibodies markers for insulin-dependent diabetes mellitus? Diabetes 35:894–898, 1986.

Atkinson MA, Maclaren NK, Scharp DW, Lacy PE, Riley WJ. 64,000 M$_r$ autoantibodies as predictors of insulin-dependent diabetes. Lancet 335:1357–1360, 1990.

Atkinson MA, Kaufman DL, Campbell L, Gibbs KA, Shah SC, Bu DF, Erlander MG, Tobin AJ, Maclaren NK. Response of peripheral blood mononuclear cells to glutamate decarboxylase in insulin-dependent diabetes. Lancet 339:458–459, 1992.

Atkinson S, Holcombe M, Kendall-Taylor P. Ophthalmopathic immunoglobulin in patients with Graves ophthalmopathy. Lancet 2:374–376, 1984.

Baba S, Morita S, Mizuno N, Okada K. Autoimmunity to glucagon in a diabetic not on insulin. Lancet 2:585, 1976.

Badenhoop K, Schwarz G, Walfish PG, Drummond V, Usadel KH, Bottazzo GF. Susceptibility to thyroid autoimmune disease: molecular analysis of HLA-D region genes identifies new markers for goitrous Hashimoto thyroiditis. J Clin Endocrinol Metab 71(5):1131–1137, 1990.

Baekkeskov S, Aanstoot HJ, Christgau S, Reetz A, Solimena M, Cascalho M, Folli F, Richter-Olesen H, DeCamilli P, Camilli PD. Identification of the 64K autoantigen in insulin-dependent diabetes as the GABA-synthesizing enzyme glutamic acid decarboxylase. Nature 347:151–156, 1990.

Baekkeskov S, Dryberg T, Lernmark A. Autoantibodies to a 64-kilodalton islet cell protein precede the onset of spontaneous diabetes in the BB rat. Science 224:1348–1350, 1984.

Baekkeskov S, Nielson JH, Marner B, Bilde T, Ludvigsson J, Lernmark A. Autoantibodies in newly diagnosed diabetic children immunoprecipitate human pancreatic islet cell proteins. Nature 298:167–169, 1982.

Bahn RS, Gorman CA, Johnson CM, Smith TJ. Presence of antibodies in the sera of patients with Graves disease recognizing a 23 kilodalton fibroblast protein. J Clin Endocrinol Metab 69:622–628, 1989.

Bain SC, Prins JB, Hearne CM, Rodrigues NR, Rowe BR, Pritchard LE, Ritchie RJ, Hall JRS, Undlien DE, Ronningen KS, Dunger DB, Barnett AH, Todd JA. Insulin gene region-encoded susceptibility to type 1 diabetes is not restricted to HLA-DR4-positive individuals. Nat Genet 2:212–215, 1992.

Baisch JM, Weeks T, Giles R, Hoover M, Stastny P, Capra JD. Analysis of HLA-DQ genotypes and susceptibility in insulin-dependent diabetes mellitus. N Engl J Med 322:1836–1841, 1990.

Banga JP, Barnett PS, McGregor AM. Immunological and molecular characteristics of the thyroid peroxidase autoantigen. Autoimmunity 8:335–343, 1991.

Banting FG, Best CH. The internal secretion of the pancreas. J Lab Clin Med 7:465–480, 1922.

Baumann-Antczak A, Wedlock N, Bednarek J, Kiso Y, Krishnan H, Fowler S, Smith BR, Furmaniak J. Autoimmune Addison disease and 21-hydroxylase. Lancet 340:429–430, 1992.

Beaven D, Nelson D, Renold A, Thorn G. Diabetes mellitus and Addison disease: a report on eight patients and a review of 55 cases in the literature. N Engl J Med 261:443–454, 1959.

Becker DV. Choice of therapy for Graves hyperthyroidism. N Engl J Med 311:464–466, 1984.

Bell GI, Horita S, Karam JH. A polymorphic locus near the human insulin gene is associated with insulin-dependent diabetes. Diabetes 33:176–183, 1984.

Bernard NF, Ertug F, Teboul N, Zhang ZG, Salvi M, Wall JR. Isotype and immunoglobulin subclass distribution of eye muscle membrane reactive antibodies in the serum of patients with thyroid-associated ophthalmopathy as detected in Western blotting. Autoimmunity 10:57–63, 1991.

Betterle C, Zanette F, Tiengo A, Trevisan A. Five-year follow-up on non-diabetes with islet-cell antibodies. Lancet 1:284–285, 1982.

Betterle C, Zanette F, Zanchetta R, Pedine B, Trevisan A, Manten F, Rigon F. Complement fixing adrenal autoantibodies: a marker for predicting the onset of idiopathic Addison disease. Lancet 1:1238–1240, 1983.

Betterle C, Mirakian R, Doniach D, Bottazzo GF, Riley W, Maclaren NK. Antibodies to melanocytes in vitiligo. Lancet 1:159, 1984.

Betterle C, Caretto A, De Zio A, Pedini B, Veller Fornasa C, Cecchetto A, Accordi F, Peserico A. Incidence and significance of organ-specific autoimmune disorders (clinical, latent or only autoantibodies) in patients with vitiligo. Dermatologica 171:419–423, 1985.

Betterle C, Scalici C, Pedini B, Mantero F. Addison disease: principal clinical associations and description of natural history of the disease. Ann Ital Med Int 4:195–206, 1989.

Blackman M, Kappler J, Marrack P. The role of the T cell receptor in positive and negative selection of developing T cells. Science 248:1335–1341, 1990.

Blizzard R, Chee D, Davis W. The incidence of adrenal and other antibodies in the sera of patients with idiopathic adrenal insufficiency (Addison disease). Clin Exp Immunol 2:19–24, 1967.

Blizzard R, Kyle M. Studies of the adrenal antigens and antibodies in Addison disease. J Clin Invest 42:1653–1657, 1963.

Bloise W, Wajchenberg BL, Moncada VY, Marcus Samuels B, Taylor SI. Atypical antiinsulin receptor antibodies in a patient with type B insulin resistance and scleroderma. J Clin Endocrinol Metab 68:227–231, 1989.

Boehm BO, Manfras BJ, Rosak C, Kuehnl P, Schoffling K, Trucco M. TcR-alpha and TcR-beta diallelic RFLPs in insulin-dependent (type I) Caucasian diabetic patients. Diabetes Res 15:63–67, 1990.

Bogner U, Schleusener H, Wall JR. Antibody-dependent cell mediated cytotoxicity against human thyroid cells in Hashimoto thyroiditis but not Graves disease. J Clin Endocrinol Metab 59:734–738, 1984.

Bognetti E, Meschi F, Malavasi C, Pastore MR, Sergi A, Illeni MT, Maffeis C, Pinelli L, Chiumello G. HLA-antigens in Italian type 1 diabetic patients: role of DR3/DR4 antigens and breast feeding in the onset of the disease. Acta Diabetol 28:229–232, 1992.

Boitard C, Debray-Sachs M, Pouplard A, Assan R. Inhibition of insulin release by lymphocytes from diabetic patients in vitro. Diabetologia 19:259, 1980.

Bottazzo GF, Lendrum R. Separate autoantibodies to human pancreatic glucagon and somatostatin cells. Lancet 2:873–876, 1976.

Bottazzo GF, Florin-Christensen A, Doniach D. Islet-cell autoantibodies in diabetes mellitus with autoimmune polyendocrine deficiencies. Lancet 2:1279–1283, 1974.

Bottazzo GF, Pouplard A, Florin-Christensen A, Doniach D. Autoantibodies to prolactin-secreting cells of human pituitary. Lancet 2:97–101, 1975.

Bottazzo GF, Dean BM, Gorsuch AN, Cudworth AG, Doniach D. Complement-fixing islet-cell antibodies in type-I diabetes: possible monitors of active beta-cell damage. Lancet 1:668–672, 1980a.

Bottazzo GF, McIntosh C, Stanford W, Preece M. Growth hormone cell antibodies and partial growth hormone deficiency in a girl with Turner's syndrome. Clin Endocrinol 12:1–9, 1980b.

Bottazzo GF, Pujol-Borrell R, Hanafusa T, Feldmann M. Role of aberrant HLA-DR expression and antigen presentation in induction of endocrine autoimmunity. Lancet 2(8359):1115–1119, 1983.

Bottazzo GF, Pozzilli P, Mirakian R, Dean BM, Doniach D. Early immunological events in diabetes. In Andreani D, Mario U, Federlin KF, Heding LG, eds. Immunology in Diabetes. London, Klimpton Medical Publications, 1984a, pp. 95–104.

Bottazzo GF, Todd I, Pujol-Borrell R. Hypotheses on genetic contributions to the aetiology of diabetes mellitus. Immunol Today 5:230–231, 1984b.

Bottazzo GF, Dean BM, McNally JM, MacKay EH, Swift PGF, Gamble DR. In situ characterization of autoimmune phenomena and expression of HLA molecules in the pancreas in diabetic insulitis. N Engl J Med 313:353–360, 1985.

Bougneres PF, Carel JC, Castano L, Boitard C, Gardin JP, Landais P, Hors J, Mihatsch MJ, Paillard M, Chaussain JL, Bach JF. Factors associated with early remission of type I diabetes in children treated with cyclosporine. N Engl J Med 318:663–670, 1980.

Braund WJ, Naylor BA, Williamson DH, Buley ID, Clark A, Chapel HM, Turner RC. Autoimmunity to insulin receptor and hypoglycaemia in patient with Hodgkin's disease. Lancet 1:237–240, 1987.

Brenner O. Addison disease with atrophy of the cortex of the suprarenals. Q J Med 22:121–125, 1928.

Brown RS, Kertiles LP, Rosenfield C, Kleinmann RE, Crigler JF. Thyrotropin-receptor autoantibodies in children and young adults with Graves disease. Am J Dis Child 140:238–241, 1986.

Bruining GJ, Molenaar J, Tuk CW, Lindeman J, Braining HA, Marner B. Clinical time-course and characteristics of islet cell cytoplasmic antibodies in childhood diabetes. Diabetologia 26:24–29, 1984.

Burch HB, Clement S, Sokol MS, Landry F. Reactive hypoglycemic coma due to insulin autoimmune syndrome: case report and literature review. Am J Med 92:681–685, 1992.

Cahill GF, McDevitt HO. Insulin-dependent diabetes mellitus: the initial lesion. N Engl J Med 304:1454–1465, 1981.

Canonica GW, Bagnasco M, Moretta L, Cocco R, Ferrini O, Giordano G. Human T-lymphocyte subpopulations in Hashimoto disease. J Clin Endocrinol Metab 52:553–556, 1981.

Canonica GW, Bagnasco M, Cosulich ME, Torre G, McLachlan SM, Smith BR. Why thyroid is major site of thyroid autoantibody synthesis in autoimmune thyroid disease. Lancet 1:1163, 1983.

Carpenter C, Solomon N, Silverberg S, Bledsoe T, Northcutt R, Klinenberg J, Bennett I, Harvey A. Schmidt's syndrome (thyroid and adrenal insufficiency): a review of the literature and a report of fifteen new cases including ten instances of coexistent diabetes mellitus. Medicine 43:153–180, 1964.

Carstensen H, Krabbe S, Wulffraat NM, Nielsen MD, Ralfkiaer E, Drexhage HA. Autoimmune involvement in Cushing syndrome due to primary adrenocortical nodular dysplasia. Eur J Pediatr 149:84–87, 1989.

Castano L, Russo E, Zhou L, Lipes MA, Eisenbarth GS. Identification and cloning of a granule autoantigen (carboxypeptidase-H) associated with type I diabetes. J Clin Endocrinol Metab 73:1197–1201, 1991.

Cecil RL. A study of the pathological anatomy of the pancreas in ninety cases of diabetes mellitus. J Exp Med 11:266–290, 1910.

Charles MA, Suzuki M, Waldeck N, Dodson LE, Slater L, Ong K, Kershnar A, Buckingham B, Golden M. Immune islet killing mechanisms associated with insulin-dependent diabetes: In vitro expression of cellular and antibody-mediated islet cell cytotoxicity in humans. J Immunol 130:1189–1194, 1983.

Chen CH, Huang MJ, Huang BY, Liu RT, Juang JH, Lin JD, Huang HS. Insulin autoimmune syndrome as a cause of hypoglycemia—report of four cases. Chang Keng I Hsueh 13:134–142, 1990.

Christie MR, Tun RY, Lo SS, Cassidy D, Brown TJ, Hollands J, Shattock M, Bottazzo GF, Leslie RD. Antibodies to GAD and tryptic fragments of islet 64K antigen as distinct markers for development of IDDM: studies with identical twins. Diabetes 41:782–787, 1992.

Cobb WE, Molitch M, Reichlin S. Levamisole in insulin-dependent diabetes mellitus. N Engl J Med 303:1065–1066, 1980.

Concannon P, Wright JA, Wright LG, Sylvester DR, Spielman RS. T-cell receptor genes and insulin-dependent diabetes mellitus (IDDM): no evidence for linkage from affected sib pairs. Am J Hum Genet 47:45–52, 1990.

Cryer PE, Gerich JE. Relevance of glucose counterregulatory systems to patients with diabetes: critical roles of glucagon and epinephrine. Diabetes Care 6:95–99, 1983.

Cudworth AG, Wolf E. The genetic susceptibility to type I (insulin-dependent) diabetes mellitus. Clin Endocrinol Metab 11:389–407, 1982.

Cudworth AG, Woodrow JC. Genetic susceptibility in diabetes mellitus: analysis of the HLA association. Br Med J 2:846–848, 1976.

Davies TF, Platzer M, Schwartz A, Friedman E. Functionality of thyroid-stimulating antibodies assessed by cryopreserved human thyroid cell bioassay. J Clin Endocrinol Metab 57:1021–1027, 1983.

Dayan CM, Londei M, Corcoran AE, Grubeck-Loebenstein B, James RF, Rapoport B, Feldmann M. Autoantigen recognition by thyroid-infiltrating T cells in Graves disease. Proc Natl Acad Sci U S A 88:7415–7419, 1991.

Del Prete GF, Tiengo A, Nosadini R, Bottazzo GF, Betterle C, Bersani G. Glucagon secretion in two patients with autoantibodies to glucagon-producing cells. Horm Metab Res 10:260–261, 1978.

DePirro R, Roth RA, Rossetti L, Goldfine ID. Characterization of the serum from a patient with insulin resistance and hypoglycemia. Diabetes 33:301–304, 1984.

Der Kinderen PJ. EPS, LATS and exophthalmos. In Irvine WJ, ed. *Thyrotoxicosis.* Baltimore, Williams & Wilkins, 1967, pp. 221–234.

Deschamps I, Kahalil I, Lepage V, Gardais E, Hors J. The diagnostic value of DQA-DQB oligonucleotide typing for the prediction of risk of type I diabetes. Diabetes in the Young 24:14, 1990.

Diabetes Epidemiology Research International Group. Secular trends in incidence of childhood IDDM in 10 countries. Diabetes 39:858–864, 1990.

Di Mario U, Irvine WJ, Borsey DQ, Kyner JL, Weston J, Galfo C. Immune abnormalities in diabetic patients not requiring insulin at diagnosis. Diabetologia 25:392–395, 1983.

Doniach D. Humoral and genetic aspects of thyroid autoimmunity. Clin Endocrinol Metab 4:267–285, 1975.

Doniach D, Roitt I. Autoimmunity in Hashimoto's disease and its complications. J Clin Endocrinol Metab 17:1293–1304, 1957.

Doniach D, Bottazzo G. Polyendocrine autoimmunity. In Franklin EC, ed. Clinical Immunology Update. New York, Elsevier, 1981, pp. 95–102.

Doniach D, Florin-Christensen A. Autoimmunity in the pathogenesis of endocrine exophthalmos. Med Clin North Am 4:341–350, 1975.

Doniach D, Bottazzo GF, Russell RCG. Goitrous autoimmune thyroiditis (Hashimoto's disease). Clin Endocrinol Metab 8:63–80, 1979.

Doniach D, Bottazzo GF, Cudworth AG. Etiology of type I diabetes mellitus: heterogeneity and immunological events leading to clinical onset. Ann Rev Med 34:13–20, 1983.

Dozio N, Sodoyez Goffaux, F, Koch M, Ziegler B, Sodoyez JC. Polymorphism of insulin antibodies in six patients with insulin-immune hypoglycaemic syndrome. Clin Exp Immunol 85:282–287, 1991.

Duncan JA, Shah SC, Shulman DI, Siegel RL, Kappy MS, Malone JI. Type b insulin resistance in a 15-year-old white youth. J Pediatr 103:421–424, 1983.

Dussault JH, Letarte J, Guyda H, Laberge C. Lack of influence of thyroid antibodies on thyroid function in the newborn infant and on a mass screening program for congenital hypothyroidism. J Pediatr 96:385–389, 1980.

Editorial: Thyroid autoimmune disease: a broad spectrum. Lancet 1:874–875, 1981.

Ekins RP, Ellis SM. The radioimmunoassay of free thyroid hormones in serum. In Robbins J, Braverman LE, eds. Thyroid Research. Amsterdam, Excerpta Medica, 1975, p. 597.

Eisenbarth GS, Morris MA, Scearrace RM. Cytotoxic antibodies to cloned islet cells in serum of patients with diabetes mellitus. J Clin Invest 67:403–408, 1981.

Eisenbarth GS, Srikanta S, Jackson R, Dolinar R, Morris M. Immunotherapy of recent onset type I diabetes mellitus. Clin Res 31:500A, 1983.

Elder M, Maclaren N, Riley W. Gonadal autoantibodies in patients with hypogonadism and/or Addison's disease. J Clin Endocrinol Metab 52:1137–1142, 1981.

Elias D, Cohen IR, Schechter Y, Spirer Z, Golander A. Antibodies to insulin receptor followed by anti-idiotype: antibodies to insulin in child with hypoglycemia. Diabetes 36:348–354, 1987.

Elliot RB, Crossly JR, Berryman CC, James AG. Partial preservation of pancreatic B-cell function in children with diabetes. Lancet 2:1–4, 1981.

Engelberth O, Jezkova Z. Autoantibodies in Scheehan's syndrome. Lancet 1:1075, 1965.

Eto S, Fujihira T, Ohnami S, Suzuki H. Autoantibody to bovine TSH in Hashimoto's thyroiditis. Lancet 1:520, 1984.

Farid NR, Sampson L, Moens H, Barnard JM. The association of goitrous autoimmune thyroiditis with HLA-DR5. Tissue Antigens 17:265–268, 1981.

Faustman D, Eisenbarth G, Daley J, Breitmeyer J. Abnormal T-lymphocyte subsets in type I diabetes. Diabetes 38:1462–1468, 1989.

Faustman D, Li X, Lin H, Fu Y, Eisenbarth G, Avruch J, Guo J. Linkage of faulty major histocompatibility class I to autoimmune disease. Science 254:1756–1761, 1991.

Field LL, Dugoujon J-M. Immunoglobulin allotyping (Gm, Km) of GAW5 families. Genet Epidemiol 6:31–33, 1989.

Fisher DA, Pandian MR, Carlton E. Autoimmune thyroid disease: an expanding spectrum. Pediatr Clin North Am 34:907–918, 1987.

Fletcher J, Mijovic C, Odugbesan O, Jenkins D, Bradwell AR, Barnett AH. Transracial studies implicate HLA-DQ as a component of genetic susceptibility to type 1 (insulin-dependent) diabetes. Diabetologia 31:864–870, 1988.

Flier JS, Kahn DR, Roth J. Receptors, antireceptor antibodies and mechanisms of insulin resistance. N Engl J Med 330:413–419, 1979.

Forrest JM, Menser MA, Burgess JA. High frequency of diabetes mellitus in young adults with congenital rubella. Lancet 2:332–334, 1971.

Fort P, Lanes R, Dahlem S, Recker B, Weyman Daum M, Pugliese M, Lifshitz F. Breast feeding and insulin-dependent diabetes mellitus in children. J Am Coll Nutr 5:439–441, 1986.

Foulis AK, Stewart JA. The pancreas in recent-onset type 1 (insulin-dependent) diabetes mellitus: insulin content of islets, insulitis and associated changes in the exocrine acinar tissue. Diabetologia 26:456–461, 1984.

Foulis AK, Liddle CN, Farquharson MA, Richmond JA, Weir RS. The histopathology of the the the pancreas in Type 1 (insulin-dependent) diabetes mellitus: a 25-year review of deaths in patients under 20 years of age in the United Kingdom. Diabetologia 29:267–274, 1986.

Francis G, Riley W. Congenital familial transient hypothyroidism secondary to transplacental thyrotropin-blocking autoantibodies. Am J Dis Child 141:1081–1083, 1987.

Freeman M, Weetman AP. T and B cell reactivity to adrenal antigens in autoimmune Addison's disease. Clin Exp Immunol 88:275–279, 1992.

Fujii Y, Kato N, Kito J, Asai J, Yokochi T. Experimental autoimmune adrenalitis: a murine model for Addison's disease. Autoimmunity 12:47–52, 1992.

Fukasawa N, Iitaka M, Hara Y, Yanagisawa M, Hase K, Miura S, Sakatume Y, Ishii J. Studies on thyroid hormone autoantibody (THAA) in 2 cases of Graves' disease with spuriously high free thyroxine values. Nippon Naibunpi Gakkai Zasshi 67:75–83, 1991.

Galluzzo A, Giordino C, Rubino G, Bompiani GD. Immunoregulatory T-lymphocyte subset deficiency in newly diagnosed type-1 (insulin-dependent) diabetes mellitus. Diabetologia 26:426–430, 1984.

Gamblin GT, Harper DG, Galentine P, Buck DR, Chernow B, Eil C. Prevalence of increased intraocular pressure in Graves' disease-evidence of frequent subclinical ophthalmopathy. N Engl J Med 308:420–424, 1983.

Ganda OP, Srikanta S, Brink SJ, Morris MA, Gleason RE, Soeldner JS, Eisenbarth GS. Differential sensitivity to beta-cell secretagogues in early, type 1 diabetes mellitus. Diabetes 33:516–521, 1984.

Gepts W. Pathologic anatomy of the pancreas in juvenile diabetes mellitus. Diabetes 14:619–633, 1965.

Gepts W, Lecompte PM. The pancreatic islets in diabetes. Am J Med 70:105–115, 1981.

Gianani R, Pugliese A, Bonner-Weir S, Shiffrin AJ, Soeldner JS, Erlich H, Awdeh Z, Alper CA, Jackson RA, Eisenbarth GS. Prognostically significant heterogeneity of cytoplasmic islet cell antibodies in relatives of patients with type I diabetes. Diabetes 41:347–353, 1992.

Gleichmann H, Bottazzo GF. Progress toward standardization of cytoplasmic islet cell-antibody assay. Diabetes 36:578–584, 1987.

Goldman J, Baldwin D, Rubenstein AH, Klink DD, Blackard WG, Fisher LK, Roe TF, Schnure JJ. Characterization of circulating insulin and proinsulin-binding antibodies in autoimmune hypoglycemia. J Clin Invest 63:1050–1059, 1979.

Gorman C. Ophthalmopathy of Graves' disease. N Engl J Med 308:453–454, 1983.

Gorsuch AN, Dean BM, Bottazzo GF, Lister J, Cudworth AG. Evidence that type I diabetes and thyrogastric autoimmunity have different genetic determinants. Br Med J 280:145–147, 1980.

Gorsuch AN, Spencer KM, Lister J, McNally JM, Dean BM, Bottazzo GF, Cudworth AG. Evidence for a long prediabetic period in type I (insulin-dependent) diabetes mellitus. Lancet 2:1363–1365, 1981.

Gray RS, Irvine WJ, Cameron EH, Duncan LJ. Glucose and insulin responses to oral glucose in overt non-insulin-dependent diabetics with and without the islet cell antibody. Diabetes 29:312–316, 1980.

Gries FA, Standl E, Lander T, Greulich B, Gerbitz K-D, Bertrams J, Kolb H. Immunointervention studies in newly diagnosed type 1 diabetics. Diabetes 32:151A, 1983.

Grubeck-Loebenstein B, Derfler K, Kassal H, Knapp W, Krisch K, Liszka K, Smyth PPA, Waldhausl W. Immunological features of nonimmunological hyperthyroidism. J Clin Endocrinol Metab 60:150–155, 1985.

Gutierrez-Lopez MD, Bertera S, Chantres MT, Vavassori C, Dorman JS, Trucco M, Serrano-Rios M. Susceptibility to type I (insulin-dependent) diabetes mellitus in Spanish patients correlates quantitatively with expression of HLA-DQ alpha Arg 52 and HLA-DQ beta non-Asp 57 alleles. Diabetologia 35:583–588, 1992.

Hahn HB, Hayles AB, Woolmer LB. Lymphocytic thyroiditis in children. J Pediatr 66:73–78, 1965.

Hamburger JI. Management of hyperthyroidism in children and adolescents. J Clin Endocrinol Metab 60:1019–1024, 1985.

Hanafusa T, Pujol-Borrell R, Chiavoto L, Russell RCG, Doniach D, Bottazzo GF. Aberrant expression of HLA DR antigen on thyrocytes in Graves' disease: relevance to autoimmunity. Lancet 2:1111–1115, 1983.

Harrison LC, Colman PG, Dean B, Baxter R, Martin FI. Increase in remission rate in newly diagnosed type I diabetic subjects treated with azathioprine. Diabetes 34:1306–1308, 1985.

Harrison LC, Honyman MC, DeAizpurua HJ, Schmidli RS, Colman PG, Tait BD, Cram DS. Inverse relation between humoral and cellular immunity to glutamic acid decarboxylase in subjects at risk of insulin-dependent diabetes. Lancet 431:1365–1369, 1993.

Hashimoto H. Zur kenntnis der lymphomatosa veranderung der schilddruse (Struma lymphomatosa). Acta Klin Chir 97:219–248, 1912.

Hauser L, Sheehan P, Simpkins H. Pancreatic pathology in pentamidine-induced diabetes in acquired immunodeficiency syndrome patients. Hum Pathol 229:926–929, 1991.

Hayward AR, Herberger M. Culture and phenotype of activated T-cells from patients with type-1 diabetes mellitus. Diabetes 33:319–323, 1984.

Heimberg H, Nagy ZP, Somers G, De-Leeuw I, Schuit FC. Complementation of HLA-DQA and -DQB genes confers susceptibility and protection to insulin-dependent diabetes mellitus. Hum Immunol 33:10–17, 1992.

Heinonen E, Krohn K. Studies on an adrenal antigen common to man and different animals. Med Biol 55:48–53, 1977.

Henson V, Maclaren N, Riley W, Wakeland EK. Polymorphisms of DQβ genes in HLA-DR4 haplotypes from healthy and diabetic individuals. Immunogenetics 25:152–160, 1987.

Hirata Y. Methamizole and insulin autoimmune syndrome with hypoglycemia. Lancet 2:1037–1038, 1983.

Hitchcock CL, Riley WJ, Alamo A, Pyka R, Maclaren NK. Lymphocyte subsets and activation in prediabetes. Diabetes 35:1416–1422, 1986.

Hollander CS, Stevenson C, Mitsuma T, Pineda G, Shenkman L, Silva E. T₃ toxicosis in an iodine-deficient area. Lancet 2:1276–1278, 1972.

Holm L-E, Blomgren H, Lowhagen T. Cancer risks in patients with chronic lymphocytic thyroiditis. N Engl J Med 312:601–604, 1985.

Horita M, Suzuki H, Onodera T, Ginsberg-Fellner F, Fauci AS, Notkins AL. Abnormalities of immunoregulatory T cell subsets in patients with insulin-dependent diabetes mellitus. J Immunol 129:1426–1429, 1982.

Horn GT, Bugawan TL, Long CM, Erlich HA. Allelic sequence variation of the HLA-DQ loci: relationship to serology and insulin-dependent diabetes susceptibility. Proc Natl Acad Sci U S A 85:6012–6016, 1988.

Ikegami H, Tahara Y, Topyon C, Yamato E, Ogihara T, Noma Y, Shima K. Aspartic acid at position 57 of the HLA-DQβ chain is not protective against insulin-dependent diabetes mellitus in Japanese people. J Autoimmun 3:167–174, 1990.

Ilonen J, Surcel H-M, Mustonen A, Kaar M-L, Akerblom HK. Lymphocyte subpopulations at the onset of type I (insulin-dependent) diabetes. Diabetologia 27:106–108, 1984.

Irvine WJ. The association of atrophic gastritis with autoimmune thyroid disease. Clin Endocrinol Metab 4:351–377, 1975.

Irvine WJ, Barnes EW. Addison's disease, ovarian failure and hypoparathyroidism. Clin Endocrinol Metab 4:379–434, 1975.

Irvine W, Chann MMW, Scarth L, Kolb F, Hartog M, Bayliss R, Drury M. Immunologic aspects of premature ovarian failure associated with idiopathic Addison's disease. Lancet 2:883–887, 1968.

Irvine WJ, Gray RS, McCallum CJ. Pancreatic islet-cell antibody as a marker for asymptomatic and latent diabetes and prediabetes. Lancet 2:1097–1102, 1976.

Irvine WJ, McCallum CJ, Gray RS, Duncan LJP. Clinical and pathogenic significance of pancreatic islet-cell antibodies in diabetics treated with oral hypoglycemic agents. Lancet 1:1025–1027, 1977.

Iseki M, Shimizu M, Oikawa T, Hojo H, Arikawa K, Ichikawa Y, Momotani N, Ito K. Sequential serum measurements of thyrotropin binding inhibitor immunoglobulin G in transient familial neonatal hypothyroidism. J Clin Endocrinol Metab 57:384–387, 1983.

Iwatani Y, Amino N, Mori H, Asari S, Izumiguchi Y, Kumahara Y, Miyai K. T lymphocyte subsets in autoimmune thyroid diseases and subacute thyroiditis detected with monoclonal antibodies. J Clin Endocrinol Metab 56:251–254, 1983.

Jackson RA, Morris MA, Haynes BF, Eisenbarth GS. Increased circulating Ia-antigen bearing T-cells in type I diabetes mellitus. N Engl J Med 306:785–788, 1982a.

Jackson RA, Dolinar R, Srikanta S, Morris M, Eisenbarth GS. Prednisone therapy in early type I diabetes: immunological effects. Diabetes 31:48A, 1982b.

Jackson RA, Haynes BF, Burch WM, Shimizu K, Bowring MA, Eisenbarth GS. Ia$^+$T cells in new onset Graves' disease. J Clin Endocrinol Metab 59:187–190, 1984.

Jacobs KH, Jenkins D, Mijovic C, Penny M, Uchigata Y, Cavan D, Hirata Y, Otani T, Fletcher J, Barnett AH. An investigation of Japanese subjects maps susceptibility to type 1 (insulin-dependent) diabetes mellitus close to the DQA1 gene. Hum Immunol 33:24–28, 1992.

Jansson R, Dahlberg PA, Johansson H, Lindstrom B. Intrathyroidal concentrations of methimazote in patients with Graves' disease. J Clin Endocrinol Metab 57:129–132, 1983a.

Jansson R, Totterman TH, Sallstrom J, Dahlberg PA. Thyroid-infiltrating T lymphocyte subsets in Hashimoto's thyroiditis. J Clin Endocrinol Metab 56:1164–1168, 1983b.

Jones KL. The Cushing syndromes. Pediatr Clin North Am 37:1313–1332, 1990.

Julier C, Hyer RN, Davies J, Merlin F, Soularue P, Briant L, Cathelineau G, Deschamps I, Rotter JI, Froguel P, Boitard C, Bell JI, and Lathrop GM. Insulin-IGF2 region on chromosome 11p encodes a gene implicated in HLA-DR4-dependent diabetes susceptibility. Nature 354:155–159, 1991.

Kadlubowski M, Irvine WJ, Rowland AC. Anti-muscle antibodies in Graves' ophthalmopathy. J Clin Lab Immunol 24:105–111, 1987.

Kahn CR, Flier JS, Bar RS, Archer JA, Gorden P, Martin MM, Roth J. The syndromes of insulin resistance and acanthosis nigricans. N Engl J Med 294:739–745, 1976.

Kappler JW, Staerz U, White J, Marrack P. Self-tolerance eliminates T cells specific for MIs-modified products of the major histocompatibility complex. Nature 332:35–45, 1989.

Karam JH, Lewitt PA, Young CW, Nowlain RE, Frankel BJ, Fujiya H, Freedman ZR, Grodsky GM. Insulinopenic diabetes after rodenticide (Vacor) ingestion: a unique model of acquired diabetes in man. Diabetes 29:971–978, 1980.

Karjalainen J, Martin J, Knip M, Ilonen J, Robinson BH, Savilahti E, Akerblom HK, Dosch HM. A bovine albumin peptide as a possible trigger of insulin-dependent diabetes mellitus. N Engl J Med 327:302–307, 1992.

Karlsson FA, Burman P, Loof L, Mardh S. Major parietal cell antigen in autoimmune gastritis with pernicious anemia is the acid-producing H+, K+-adenosine triphosphatase of the stomach. J Clin Invest 81:475–479, 1988.

Karounos DG, Thomas JW. Recognition of common islet antigen by autoantibodies from NOD mice and humans with IDDM. Diabetes 39:1085–1090, 1990.

Kaufman DL, Erlander MG, Clare-Salzler M, Atkinson MA, Maclaren NK, Tobin AJ. Autoimmunity to two forms of glutamate decarboxylase in insulin-dependent diabetes mellitus. J Clin Invest 89:283–292, 1992.

Kawakami A, Eguchi K, Matsunaga M, Tezuka H, Ueki Y, Shimomura C, Otsubo T, Nakao H, Migita K, Ishikawa N, Itok I, Nagataki S. CD4$^+$ CD45RA$^+$ cells (suppressor-inducer T cells) in thyroid tissue from patients with Graves' disease. Acta Endocrinol Copenh 125:687–693, 1991.

Kendall-Taylor P. LATS and human-specific thyroid stimulator: their relation to Graves' disease. Clin Endocrinol Metab 4:319–339, 1975.

Kendall-Taylor P, Knox AJ, Steel NR, Atkinson S. Evidence that thyroid-stimulating antibody is produced in the thyroid gland. Lancet 1:654–656, 1984.

Kendler DL, Rootman J, Huber GK, Davies TF. A 64 kDa membrane antigen is a recurrent epitope for natural autoantibodies in patients with Graves' thyroid and ophthalmic diseases. Clin Endocrinol Oxf 35:539–547, 1991.

Kenney RM, Michaels IA, Flomenbaum NE, Yu GS. Poisoning with N-3-pyridylmethyl-N'-p-nitrophenylurea (Vacor): immunoperoxidase demonstration of beta-cell destruction. Arch Pathol Lab Med 105:367–370, 1981.

Ketchum C, Riley W, Maclaren N. Adrenal dysfunction in asymptomatic patients with adrenocortical autoantibodies. J Clin Endocrinol Metab 58:1–5, 1984.

Khalil I, Deschamps I, Lepage V, al-Daccak R, Degos L, Hors J. Dose effect of cis-and trans-encoded HLA-DQ alpha beta heterodimers in IDDM susceptibility. Diabetes 41:378–384, 1992.

Khoury E, Hammond L, Bottazzo, G Doniach D. Surface reactive antibodies to human adrenal cells in Addison's disease. Clin Exp Immunol 45:48–55, 1981.

Kida K, Mimura G, Kobayashi T, Nakamura K, Sonoda S, Inouye H, Tsuji K. Immunogenetic heterogeneity in type I (insulin-dependent) diabetes among Japanese-HLA antigens and organ-specific autoantibodies. Diabetologia 32:34–39, 1989.

Kodama K, Sikorska H, Bandy-Dafoe P, Bayly R, Wall JR. Demonstration of a circulating autoantibody against a soluble eye-muscle antigen in Graves' ophthalmopathy. Lancet 2:1353–1356, 1982.

Koivisto VA, Aro A, Cantell K, Haataja M, Huttunen J, Karonen S-L, Mustajoki P, Velkonen R, Seppala P. Remissions in newly diagnosed type I (insulin-dependent) diabetes: influence of interferon as an adjunct to insulin therapy. Bulletin of the International Study Group for Diabetes in the Young 10:16, 1984.

Kourides IA, Ridgeway EC, Weintraub BD, Bigos ST, Gershengorn MC, Maloof F. Thyrotropin-induced hyperthyroidism: Use of alpha and beta subunit levels to identify patients with pituitary tumors. J Clin Endocrinol Metab 45:534–543, 1977.

Krohn K, Uibo R, Aavik E, Peterson P, Savilahti K. Identification by molecular cloning of an autoantigen associated with Addison's disease as steroid 17 alpha-hydroxylase. Lancet 339:770–773, 1992.

Kyvik KO, Green A, Svendsen A, Mortensen K. Breast feeding and the development of type 1 diabetes mellitus. Diabet Med 9:233–235, 1992.

Lafferty KJ, Babcock SK, Gill RG. Prevention of rejection by treatment of the graft: an overview. Prog Clin Biol Res 224:87–117, 1986.

Landau RL. Endocrinology and metabolism. JAMA 252:2172–2176, 1984.

Lang, F, Maugendre D, Houssaint E, Charbonnel B, Sai P. Cytoadherence of lymphocytes from type I diabetic subjects to insulin-secreting cells, a marker of anti-β-cell cellular immunity. Diabetes 36:1356–1364, 1987.

Lederman MM, Ellner JJ, Rodman HM. Defective suppressor cell generation in juvenile onset diabetes. J Immunol 127:2051–2059, 1981.

Leisti S, Ahonen P, Perheentupa J. The diagnosis and staging of hypocortisolism in progressing autoimmune adrenalitis. Pediatr Res 17:861–867, 1983.

Lendrum R, Walker G, Gamble DR. Islet-cell antibodies in juvenile diabetes mellitus of recent onset. Lancet i:880–883, 1975.

Lendrum R, Walker G, Cudworth AG, Theophanides C, Pyke DA, Bloom A, Gamble DR. Islet-cell antibodies in diabetes mellitus. Lancet 2:1273–1276, 1976.

Lernmark A, Baekkeskov S. Islet cell antibodies: theoretical and practical implications. Diabetologia 21:431–435, 1981.

Lernmark A, Freedman ZR, Hofmann C, Rubenstein AH, Steiner DF, Jackson RL, Winter RJ, Traisman, HS. Islet-cell-surface antibodies in juvenile diabetes mellitus. N Engl J Med 299:375–380, 1978.

Leslie RDG, Pyke DA. Immunosuppression of acute insulin-dependent diabetes. In Irvine WJ ed. The Immunology of Diabetes. Edinburgh, Tevoit Scientific Publications, 1980, pp. 345–347.

Levine S, Wenk E. The production and passive transfer of allergic adrenalitis. Am J Pathol 52:41–44, 1968.

Linde R, Alexander N, Island DP, Rabin D. Familial insensitivity of the pituitary and periphery to thyroid hormone: a case report in two generations and a review of the literature. Metabolism 31:510–513, 1982.

Londei M, Lamb JR, Bottazzo GF, Feldman M. Epithelial cells expressing aberrant MHC class II determinants can present antigen to cloned human T cells. Nature 312:639–641, 1984.

Ludgate M, Dong Q, Dreyfus PA, Zakut H, Taylor P, Vassart G, Soreq H. Definition, at the molecular level, of a thyroglobulin-acetylcholinesterase shared epitope: study of its pathophysiological significance in patients with Graves' ophthalmopathy. Autoimmunity 3:167–176, 1989.

Ludvigsson J, Heding L, Lernmark A, Lieden G. An attempt to break the autoimmune process at the onset of IDDM by the use of plasmapheresis and high doses of prednisolone. Bulletin of the International Study Group for Diabetes in the Young 6:11–12, 1982.

Ludvigsson J, Heding L, Gudrun L, Marner B, Lernmark A. Plasmapheresis in the initial treatment of insulin-dependent diabetes mellitus in children. Br Med J 286:176–178, 1983.

Maclaren NK, Atkinson MA. Is insulin-dependent diabetes mellitus environmentally induced? N Engl J Med 327:347–349, 1992.

Maclaren NK, Huang S-W. Antibody to cultured human insulinoma cells in insulin-dependent diabetes. Lancet 1:997–999, 1975.

Maclaren NK, Huang S-W. Cell-mediated immunity in insulin dependent diabetes. In Irvine WJ, ed. The Immunology of Diabetes. Edinburgh, Tevoit Scientific Publications, 1980, pp. 185–193.

Maclaren NK, Riley WJ. Thyroid, gastric, and adrenal autimmunities associated with insulin-dependent diabetes mellitus. Diabetes Care 8(Suppl 1):34–38, 1985.

Maclaren NK, Riley WJ. Inherited susceptibility to autoimmune Addison's disease is linked to human leukocyte antigens-DR3 and/or DR4. J Clin Endocrinol Metab 62:455–459, 1986.

Maclaren N, Riley W, Rosenbloom A, Elder M, Spillar R, Cuddeback J. The heterogeneity of Black insulin dependent diabetes. Diabetes 31:65A, 1982.

Maclaren N, Riley W, Skordis N, Atkinson M, Spillar R, Silverstein J, Klein R, Vadheim C, Rotter J. Inherited susceptibility to insulin-dependent diabetes is associated with HLA-DR1, while DR5 is protective. Autoimmunity 1:197–205, 1988.

MacLean DB, Miller KB, Brown R, Reichlin S. Normal immunoregulation of in vitro antibody secretion in autoimmune thyroid disease. J Clin Endocrinol Metab 53:801–805, 1981.

Manns M. Autoantibodies and antigens in liver diseases—updated. J Hepatol 9:272–280, 1989.

Manns MP, Johnson EF. Identification of human cytochrome P450s as autoantigens. Methods Enzymol 206:210–220, 1991.

Mariotti S, Martino E, Cupini C, Lasie R, Giani C, Baschieri L, Pinchera A. Low serum thyroglobulin as a clue to the diagnosis of thyrotoxicosis factitia. N Engl J Med 307:410–412, 1982.

Mariotti S, Caturegli P, Piccolo P, Barbesino G, Pinchera A. Antithyroid peroxidase autoantibodies in thyroid diseases. J Clin Endocrinol Metab 71:661–669, 1990.

Mariotti S, Sansoni P, Barbesino G, Caturegli P, Monti D, Cossarizza A, Giacomelli T, Passeri G, Fagiolo U, Pinchera A, Franceschi C. Thyroid and other organ-specific autoantibodies in healthy centenarians. Lancet 339:1506–1508, 1992.

Markmann J, Lo D, Naji A, Palmiter RD, Brinster RL, Heber-Katz E. Antigen presenting function of class II MHC expressing pancreatic beta cells. Nature 2:476–479, 1988.

Maron R, Elias D, DeJongh BM, Bruining GF, VanRood JJ, Shechter Y, Cohen IR. Autoantibodies to the insulin receptor in juvenile onset insulin-dependent diabetes. Nature 303:817–818, 1983.

Martinez-Naves E, Coto E, Gutierrez V, Urra JM, Setien F, Dominguez O, Hood L, Lopez-Larrea C. Germline repertoire of T-cell receptor beta-chain genes in patients with insulin-dependent diabetes mellitus. Hum Immunol 31:77–80, 1991.

Maruyama T, Takei I, Matsuba I, Tsuruoka A, Taniyama M, Ikeda Y, Kataoka K, Abe M, Matsuki S. Cell-mediated cytotoxic islet cell surface antibodies to human pancreatic beta cells. Diabetologia 26:30–33, 1884.

Marx JZ. Diabetes: a possible autoimmune disease. Science 225:1381–1383, 1984.

Matsuura N, Yamada Y, Nohara Y, Konishi J, Kasagi K, Endo K, Kojima H, Wataya K. Familial neonatal transient hypothyroidism due to maternal TSH-binding inhibitor immunoglobulins. N Engl J Med 303:738–741, 1980.

Mayer EJ, Hamman RF, Gay EC, Lezotte DC, Savitz DA, Klingensmith GJ. Reduced risk of IDDM among breast-fed children: the Colorado IDDM Registry. Diabetes 37:1625–1632, 1988.

Mayfield RK, Levine JH, Gordon L, Powers J, Galbraith RM, Rawe SE. Lymphoid adenohypophysitis presenting as a pituitary tumor. Am J Med 69:619–623, 1980.

McGregor AM, Petersen MM, McLachlan SM, Rooke P, Smith BR, Hall R. Carbamizole and the autoimmune response in Graves' disease. N Engl J Med 303:302–307, 1980a.

McGregor AM, Smith BR, Hall R, Petersen MM, Miller M, Dewar PJ. Prediction of relapse in hyperthyroid Graves' disease. Lancet 1:1101–1103, 1980b.

McKenzie JM. Humoral factors in the pathogenesis of Graves' disease. Physiol Rev 48:252–310, 1968.

McKenzie JM, Zakarija M, Bonnyns M. Graves' disease. Med Clin North Am 59:1177–1192, 1975.

McNatty K, Short R, Barnes E, Irvine W. The cytotoxic effect of serum from patients with Addison's disease and autoimmune ovarian failure on human granulosa cells in culture. Clin Exp Immunol 22:378–383, 1975.

Meschi F, Dozio N, Bognetti E, Carra M, Cofano D, Chiumello G. An unusual case of recurrent hypoglycaemia: 10-year follow up of a child with insulin autoimmunity. Eur J Pediatr 151:32–34, 1992.

Metcalfe MA, Baum JD. Family characteristics and insulin dependent diabetes. Arch Dis Child 67:731–736, 1992.

Michelsen B, Lernmark A. Molecular cloning of a polymorphic DNA endonuclease fragment associates insulin-dependent diabetes mellitus with HLA-DQ. J Clin Invest 79:1144, 1987.

Mirakian R, Cudworth AG, Bottazzo GF, Richardson CA, Doniach D. Autoimmunity to anterior pituitary cells and the pathogenesis of insulin-dependent diabetes mellitus. Lancet 1:755–759, 1982.

Moller DE, Ratner RE, Borenstein DG, Taylor SI. Autoantibodies to the insulin receptor as a cause of autoimmune hypoglycemia in systemic lupus erythematosus. Am J Med 84:334–338, 1988.

Morel PA, Dorman JS, Todd JA, McDevitt HO, Trucco M. Aspartic acid at position 57 of the HLA-DQβ chain protects against type I diabetes: a family study. Proc Natl Acad Sci U S A 85:8111–8115, 1988.

Mori H, Amino N, Iwatani Y, Asari S, Izumiguchi Y, Kumahara Y, Miyai K. Decrease of immunoglobulin G-Fc receptor-bearing T lymphocytes in Graves' disease. J Clin Endocrinol Metab 55:399–402, 1982.

Moroz LA, Meltzer SJ, Bastomsky CH. Thyroid disease with monoclonal (immunoglobulin lambda) antibody to triiodothyronine and thyroxine. J Clin Endocrinol Metab 56:1009–1015, 1983.

Moses AC, Lawlor J, Haddow J, Jackson IMD. Familial euthyroid hyperthyroxinemia resulting from increased thyroxine binding to thyroxine-binding prealbumin. N Engl J Med 306:966–969, 1982.

Myers BD, Ross J, Newton L, Luetscher J, Perlroth M. Cyclosporin associated chronic nephropathy. N Engl J Med 311:699–705, 1984.

Najemnik C, Kritz H, Kaspar L, Irsigler K. Remission phase: prospective study to induce or prolong remission (REM) with closed and open-loop treatment (effect of additional cortisone treatment). Diabetologia 29:301, 1980.

Nakamura S, Sakata S, Komaki T, Kamikubo K, Miura K. Thyroid hormone autoantibodies (THAA) in three sisters: a four-year follow up. J Endocrinol Invest 12:421–427, 1989.

Nayak RC, Omar MAK, Rabizadeh A, Srikanta S, Eisenbarth GS. Cytoplasmic islet cell antibodies. Diabetes 34:617–619, 1985.

Nepom GT. A unified hypothesis for the complex genetics of HLA associations with IDDM. Diabetes 39:1153–1157, 1990.

Nerup J. Addison's disease: serological studies. Acta Endocrinol 76:142–160, 1974.

Nerup J, Anderson V, Bendixen G. Antiadrenal cellular hypersensitivity in Addison's disease. Clin Exp Immunol 4:355–358, 1969.

Nerup J, Lernmark A. Autoimmunity in insulin-dependent diabetes mellitus. Am J Med 70:135–141, 1983.

Nerup J, Platz P, Andersen OO. HL-A antigens and diabetes mellitus. Lancet 2:864–866, 1974.

Neufeld MR, Maclaren NK, Riley WJ. HLA in American blacks with juvenile diabetes. N Engl J Med 303:111–112, 1980a.

Neufeld M, Maclaren NK, Riley WJ, Lezotte D, McLaughlin JV, Silverstein J, Rosenbloom AL. Islet cell and other organ-specific autoantibodies in U.S. Caucasians and Blacks with insulin-dependent diabetes mellitus. Diabetes 29:589–592, 1980b.

Neufeld M, Maclaren N, Blizzard R. Two types of autoimmune Addison's disease associated with polyglandular syndromes. Medicine 60:355–362, 1981.

Niskanen L, Karjalainen J, Sarlund H, Siitonen O, Uusitupa M. Five year follow-up of islet-cell antibodies in type 2 (non-insulin dependent) diabetes mellitus. Diabetologia 34:402–408, 1991.

Niven MJ, Caffrey C, Moore RH, Sachs JA, Mohan V, Festenstein H, Hoover ML, Hitman GA. T-cell receptor beta-subunit gene polymorphism and autoimmune disease. Hum Immunol 27:360–367, 1990.

Nossal GJV. Immunologic tolerance: collaboration between antigen and lymphokines. Science 245:147–153, 1989.

Novogroder M, Utiger R, Boyar R, and Levine LS. Juvenile hyperthyroidism with elevated thyrotropin (TSH) and normal 24 hour FSH, LH, GH, and prolactin secretory patterns. J Clin Endocrinol Metab 45:1053–1059, 1977.

Ohgawara H, Hirata Y. Islet cell surface antibodies in diabetes and their possible influence on glucose tolerance. Tohoku J Exp Med 142:211–216, 1984.

Ohtaki S, Endo Y, Horinouchi K, Yoshitake S, Ishikawa E. Circulating thyroglobulin-antithyroglobulin immune complex in thyroid diseases using enzyme-linked immunoassays. J Clin Endocrinol Metab 52:239–246, 1981.

Okamura K, Sato K, Yoshinari M, Ikenoue H, Kuroda T, Nakagawa M, Tsuji H, Washio M, Fujishima M. Recovery of the thyroid function in patients with atrophic hypothyroidism and blocking type TSH binding inhibitor immunoglobulin. Acta Endocrinol Copenh 122:107–114, 1990.

Okita N, How J, Topliss D, Lewis M, Row VV, Volpe R. Suppressor T lymphocyte dysfunction in Graves' disease: role of the H-2 histamine receptor-bearing suppressor T lymphocytes. J Clin Endocrinol Metab 53:1002–1007, 1981a.

Okita N, Row VV, Volpe R. Suppressor T-lymphocyte deficiency in Graves' disease and Hashimoto's thyroiditis. J Clin Endocrinol Metab 52:528–533, 1981b.

Okita N, Topliss D, Lewis M, Row VV, Volpe R. T-lymphocyte sensitization in Graves' and Hashimoto's diseases confirmed by an indirect migration inhibition factor test. J Clin Endocrinol Metab 52:523–527, 1981c.

Owerbach D, Lernmark A, Platz P, Ryder LP, Rask L, Peterson PA, Ludvigsson J. HLA-D region beta-chain DNA endonuclease fragments differ between HLA-DR identical healthy and insulin-dependent diabetic individuals. Nature 303:815–817, 1983.

Owerbach D, Gunn S, Ty G, Wible L, Gabby KH. Oligonucleotide probes for HLA-DQA and DQB genes define susceptibility to type 1 (insulin-dependent) diabetes mellitus. Diabetologia 31:751–757, 1988.

Owerbach D, Hagglof B, Lernmark A, Holmgren G. Susceptibility to insulin-dependent diabetes defined by restriction enzyme polymorphism of HLA-D region genomic DNA. Diabetes 33:958–965, 1984.

Pak CY, Cha CY, Rajotte RV, McArthur RG, Yoon JW. Human pancreatic islet cell specific 38 kilodalton autoantigen identified by cytomegalovirus-induced monoclonal islet cell autoantibody. Diabetologia 33:569–572, 1990.

Palmer JP, Asplin CM, Raghu PK, Clemons P, Lyen K, Tatpati O, McKnight B, Paquette T. Anti-insulin antibodies in insulin dependent diabetes before insulin treatment: a new marker for autoimmune B cell damage. Diabetes 32:76A, 1983.

Papadopoulos KI, Hallengren B. Polyglandular autoimmune syndrome type II in patients with idiopathic Addison's disease. Acta Endocrinol Copenh 122:472–478, 1990.

Paschke R, Bruckner N, Schmeidl R, Pfiester P, Usadel KH. Predominant intraepithelial localization of primed T cells and immunoglobulin-producing lymphocytes in Graves' disease. Acta Endocrinol Copenh 124:630–636, 1991.

Petersen JS, Russel S, Marshall MO, Kofod H, Buschard K, Cambon N, Karlsen AE, Boel E, Hagopian WA, Hejnaes KR, Moody A, Dryberg T, Lernmark A, Madsen OD, Michelsen BK. Differential expression of glutamic acid decarboxylase in rat and human islets. Diabetes 42:484–495, 1993.

Petra W, Nerup J. Addison's adrenalitis. Acta Pathol Microbiol Scand 79:381–388, 1971.

Phillips D, McLachlan S, Stephenson A, Roberts D, Moffitt S, McDonald D, Ad'Hiah A, Stratton A, Young E, Clark F, Beever K, Bradbury J, Rees-Smith B. Autosomal dominant transmission of autoantibodies to thyroglobulin and thyroid peroxidase. J Clin Endocrinol Metab 70:742–746, 1990.

Pinchera A, Mariotti S, Chiovato L, Vitti P, Lopez G, Lombardi A, Anelli S, Bechi R, Carayon P. Cellular localization of the microsomal antigen and the thyroid peroxidase antigen. Acta Endocrinol Suppl Copenh 281:57–62, 1987.

Pont A, Rubino JM, Bishop D, Peal R. Diabetes mellitus and neuropathy following Vacor ingestion in man. Arch Intern Med 139:185–187, 1979.

Pozzilli P, Sensi M, Gorsuch A, Bottazzo GF, Cudworth AG. Evidence of raised K-cell levels in type-1 diabetes. Lancet 2:173–175, 1979.

Pozzilli P, Zuccarini O, Iavicoli M, Andreani D, Sensi M, Spencer KM, Bottazzo GF, Beverly PCL, Kyner JL, Cudworth AG. Monoclonal antibodies defined abnormalities of T-lymphocytes in type 1 (insulin-dependent) diabetes. Diabetes 32:91–94, 1983.

Pujol-Borrell R, Hanafusa T, Chiovata L, Bottazzo GF. Lectin-induced expression of DR antigen on human cultured follicular thyroid cells. Nature 304:71–73, 1983.

Rabinowe SL, Jackson RA, Sluhy RG, Williams GH. Ia + T lymphocytes and recently diagnosed idiopathic Addison's disease. Am J Med 77:597–601, 1984.

Raines KB, Baker JR, Lukes YG, Wartofsky L, Burman KD. Antithyrotropin antibodies in the sera of Graves' disease patients. J Clin Endocrinol Metab 61:217–222, 1985.

Ramsdell F, Fowlkes BJ. Clonal deletion versus clonal anergy. the role of the thymus in inducing self tolerance. Science 248:1342–1348, 1990.

Rand KH, Rosenbloom AL, Maclaren NK, Silverstein JH, Riley WJ, Butterworth BE, Yoon JW, Rubenstein AH, Merigan TC. Human leukocyte interferon treatment of two children with insulin-dependent diabetes. Diabetologia 21:116–119, 1981.

Rapoport B, Filetti S, Takai H, Seto P, Halverson G. Studies on the cyclic AMP response to thyroid stimulating immunoglobulin (TSI) and thyrotropin (TSH) in human thyroid cell monolayers. Metabolism 11:1159–1167, 1982.

Rapoport B, Greenspan FS, Filetti S, Pepitone M. Clinical experience with a human thyroid cell bioassay for thyroid-stimulating immunoglobulin. J Clin Endocrinol Metab 58:332–338, 1984.

Raum D, Awdeh Z, Yunis EJ, Alper CA, Gabbay KH. Extended major histocompatibility complex haplotypes in type 1 diabetes mellitus. J Clin Invest 74:449–454, 1984.

Reiter EO, Root AW, Rettig K, Vargas A. Childhood thyromegaly: recent developments. J Pediatr 99:501–518, 1981.

Rewers M, LaPorte RE, Walczak M, Dmochowski K, Bogaczynska E. Apparent epidemic of insulin-dependent diabetes mellitus in Midwestern Poland. Diabetes 36:106–113, 1987.

Riley WJ, Neufeld M, Maclaren NK. Complement-fixing islet-cell antibodies: a separate species? Lancet 1:1133, 1980a.

Riley W, Maclaren N, Neufeld M. Adrenal autoantibodies and Addison's disease in insulin dependent diabetes mellitus. J Pediatr 97:191–195, 1980b.

Riley WJ, Maclaren NK, Lezotte D, Spillar RP, Rosenbloom AL. Thyroid autoimmunity in insulin-dependent diabetes mellitus: the case for routine screening. J Pediatr 98:350–354, 1981.

Riley WJ, Toskes PP, Maclaren NK, Silverstein JS. Predictive value of gastric parietal cell autoantibodies as a marker for gastric and hematological abnormalities associated with insulin-dependent diabetes. Diabetes 32:1051–1055, 1982.

Riley WJ, Winer A, Goldstein D. Coincident presence of thyrogastric autoimmunity at onset of type 1 (insulin-dependent) diabetes. Diabetologia 24:418–421, 1983.

Riley WJ, Spillar RP, Waltz J, Brody B. Predictive value of islet cell antibodies (ICA): 6 years experience. Diabetes 33:44A, 1984.

Riley WJ, Maclaren NK, Krischer J, Spillar RP, Silverstein JH, Schatz DA, Schwartz S, Malone J, Shah S, Vadheim C, Rotter JI. A prospective study of the development of diabetes in relatives of patients with insulin-dependent diabetes. N Engl J Med 323:1167–1172, 1990.

Rittner C, Bertrams J. On the significance of C2, C4, and factor B polymorphisms in disease. Hum Genet 56:235–247, 1981.

Rodman HM. Deficient interleukin-2 synthesis in type 1 diabetes. Diabetes 33:11A, 1984.

Roep BO, Kallan AA, Hazenbos WL, Bruining GJ, Bailyes EM, Arden SD, Hutton JC, de-Vries RR. T-cell reactivity to 38 kD insulin-secretory-granule protein in patients with recent-onset type 1 diabetes. Lancet 337:1439–1441, 1991.

Roitt IM, Doniach D, Campbell PN, Hudson RV. Autoantibodies in Hashimoto's disease (lymphadenoid goitre). Lancet 2:820–821, 1956.

Roman SH, Greenberg D, Rubinstein P, Wallenstein S, Davies TF. Genetics of autoimmune thyroid disease: lack of evidence for linkage to HLA within families. J Clin Endocrinol Metab 74:496–503, 1992.

Rosenbloom AL. Long term complications of type 1 (insulin-dependent) diabetes mellitus. Pediatr Ann 12:655–683, 1983.

Rotter JI, Rimoin DL. The genetics of the glucose intolerance disorders. Am J Med 70:116–126, 1981.

Ruf J, Czarnocka B, De Micco C, Dutoit C, Ferrand M, Carayon P. Thyroid peroxidase is the organ-specific ''microsomal'' autoantigen involved in thyroid autoimmunity. Acta Endocrinol Suppl Copenh 281:49–56, 1987.

Ruiz M, Rajatanavin R, Young RA, Taylor C, Brown R, Braverman LE, Ingbar SH. Familial dysalbuminemic hyperthyroxinemia. N Engl J Med 306:635–639, 1982.

Sai P, Boitard C, Debray-Sachs M, Pouplard A, Assan R, Hamburger J. Complement-fixing islet cell antibodies from some diabetic patients alter insulin release in vitro. Diabetes 30:1051–1057, 1981.

Salvi M, Zhang ZG, Haegert D, Woo M, Liberman A, Cadarso L, Wall JR. Patients with endocrine ophthalmopathy not associated with overt thyroid disease have multiple thyroid immunological abnormalities. J Clin Endocrinol Metab 70:89–94, 1990.

Sanke T, Kondo M, Moriyama Y, Nanjo K, Iwo K, Miyamura K. Glucagon binding autoantibodies in a patient with hyperthyroidism treated with methimazole. J Clin Endocrinol Metab 57:1140–1144, 1983.

Schatz DA, Barrett DJ, Maclaren NK, Riley WJ. Polyclonal nature of islet cell antibodies in insulin-dependent diabetes. Autoimmunity 1:45–50, 1988.

Schatz DA, Riley WJ, Maclaren NK, Barrett DJ. Defective inducer T-cell function before the onset of insulin-dependent diabetes mellitus. J Autoimmun 4:125–136, 1991.

Scherbaum W, Berge P. Development of adrenocortical failure in non-Addisonian patients with antibodies to adrenal cortex. Clin Endocrinol 16:345–352, 1982.

Scherbaum WA, Bottazzo GF. Autoantibodies to vasopressin cells in idiopathic diabetes insipidus: evidence for an autoimmune variant. Lancet 1:897–901, 1983.

Scherbaum WA, Czernichow P, Bottazzo GF, Doniach D. Diabetes insipidus in children: IV. A possible autoimmune type with vasopressin cell antibodies. J Pediatr 107:922–925, 1985.

Schifferdecker E, Ketzler-Sasse U, Boehm BO, Ronsheimer HB, Scherbaum WA, Schoffling K. Re-evaluation of eye muscle autoantibody determination in Graves' ophthalmopathy: failure to detect a specific antigen by use of enzyme-linked immunosorbent assay, indirect immunofluorescence, and immunoblotting techniques. Acta Endocrinol Copenh 121:643–650, 1989.

Schmidt M. Eine Biglandulane Erkrangkung (Nebennieren und Schilddruse) bei Morbus Addisonii. Verh Etsch Pathol Ges 21:212–221, 1926.

Seino S, Fu ZZ, Vinik AI. Insulin autoimmune syndrome and molecular abnormalities in insulin. Diabetes 33:61A, 1984.

Serjeantson S, Theophilus J, Zimmet P, Court J, Corssley JR, Elliott RB. Lymphocytotoxic antibodies and histocompatibility antigens in juvenile-onset diabetes mellitus. Diabetes 30:26–29, 1981.

Sheehy MJ, Rowe JR, MacDonald MJ. A particular subset of HLA-DR4 accounts for all or most of the DR4 association in type I diabetes. Diabetes 34:942–944, 1985.

Sheehy MJ, Meske LM, Emler CA, Rowe JR, Neme-de-Gimenez MH, Ingle CA, Chan A, Trucco M, Mak TW. Allelic T-cell receptor alpha complexes have little or no influence on susceptibility to type 1 diabetes. Hum Immunol 26:261–271, 1989a.

Sheehy MJ, Scharf SJ, Rowe JR, Neme-de-Gimenez MH, Meske LM, Erlich HA, Nepom BS. Diabetes-susceptible HLA haplotype is best defined to a combination of HLA-DR and DQ alleles. J Clin Invest 83:830–835, 1989b.

Shishiba Y, Ozawa Y, Ohtsuki N, Shimizu T. Discrepancy between thyroid-stimulating and thyrotropin-binding inhibitory activities of Graves' immunoglobulin G assessed in the mouse. J Clin Endocrinol Metab 54:858–862, 1982.

Silverstein J, Riley W, Barrett D, Maclaren N, Rosenbloom A. Immunosuppressive therapy (IT) for newly diagnosed insulin dependent diabetes mellitus (IDD) with antithymocyte globulin (ATG) and prednisone (pred.). Pediatr Res 71:295A, 1983.

Silverstein J, Maclaren N, Riley W, Spillar R, Radjenovic D, Johnson S. Immunosuppression with azathioprine and prednisone in recent-onset insulin-dependent diabetes mellitus. N Engl J Med 319:599–604, 1988.

Singal DP, Blajchmann MA. Histocompatibility (HL-A) antigens, lymphocytotoxic antibodies and tissue antibodies in patients with diabetes mellitus. Diabetes 22:429–432, 1973.

Skyler JS, Cahill GF. Diabetes mellitus: progress and directions. Am J Med 70:101–104, 1981.

Solomon DH, Chopra IJ, Chopra U, Smith FJ. Identification of subgroups of euthyroid Graves' ophthalmopathy. N Engl J Med 296:181–186, 1977.

Song Y-H, Connor E, Yangxin L, Zorovich B, Balducci P, Maclaren N. The role of tyrosinase in autoimmune vitiligo. Lancet 344:1049–1052, 1994.

Song Y-H, Connor E, Muir A, She JX, Zorovich B, Brooke D, Maclaren N. Antibody epitope mapping of the 21-hydroxylase antigen in autoimmune Addison disease. J Clin Endocrinol Metab 78:1108–1112, 1995.

Sotos JF, Romshe CA, Zipf WB. Immunosuppressive pulse treatment in IDDM of recent onset. Bulletin of the International Study Group for Diabetes in the Young 10:19, 1984.

Sotsiou F, Bottazzo G, Doniach D. Immunofluorescence studies in autoantibodies to steroid producing cells and to germline cells in endocrine disease and infertility. Clin Exp Immunol 39:97–111, 1980.

Spencer KM, Dian BM, Bottazzo GF, Medbak S, Cudworth AG. Preliminary evidence for a possible therapeutic intervention in early type I (insulin-dependent) diabetes. Diabetologia 20:474, 1982.

Sperling MA. Diabetes mellitus. Pediatr Clin North Am 26:149–170, 1979.

Sridama V, Pacini F, DeGrout L. Decreased suppressor T-lymphocytes in autoimmune thyroid diseases detected by monoclonal antibodies. J Clin Endocrinol Metab 54:316–319, 1982.

Srikanta S, Ganda OP. Chronic progressive beta cell dysfunction in relatives of patients with type 1 diabetes. Diabetes 32:51A, 1983a.

Srikanta S, Ganda OP, Eisenbarth GS, Soeldner JS. Islet-cell antibodies and beta-cell function in monozygotic triplets and twins initially discordant for type I diabetes mellitus. N Engl J Med 308:322–325, 1983b.

Srikanta S, Ganda OP, Jackson RA, Gleason RE, Kaldany A, Garovoy MR, Milford EL, Carpenter CB, Soeldner JS, Eisenbarth GS. Type 1 diabetes mellitus in monozygotic twins: chronic progressive beta cell dysfunction. Ann Intern Med 99:320–326, 1983c.

Srikanta S, Ganda OP, Gleason RE, Jackson RA, Soeldner JS, Eisenbarth GS. Pre-type 1 diabetes, linear loss of beta cell response to intravenous glucose. Diabetes 33:717–720, 1984a.

Srikanta S, Ganda OP, Jackson RA, Brink SJ, Fleischnick E, Yunis E, Alpen C, Soeldner JS, Eisenbarth GS. Pre-type 1 (insulin-dependent) diabetes: common endocrinological course despite immunological and immunogenetic heterogeneity. Diabetologia 27:146–148, 1984b.

Stiller CR, Dupre J, Gent M, Jenner MR, Keown PA, Laupacis A, Martell R, Rodger NW, Graffenreid B, Wolfe BMJ. Effects of cyclosporin immunosuppression in insulin-dependent diabetes mellitus of recent onset. Science 223:1362–1367, 1984.

Strakosch CR, Wenzel BE, Row VV, Volpe R. Immunology of autoimmune thyroid diseases. N Engl J Med 301:1499–1507, 1982.

Supler M, Mickle JP. Lymphocytic hypophysitis: report of a case in a man with cavernous sinus involvement. Surg Neurol 37:472–476, 1992.

Sutherland DE, Goetz FC, Najarian JS. Pancreas transplants from related donors. Transplantation 38:625–633, 1984a.

Sutherland DE, Sibley R, Xu XZ, Michael A, Srikanta AM, Taub F, Najarian J, Goetz FC. Twin-to-twin pancreas transplantation: reversal and reenactment of the pathogenesis of type I diabetes. Trans Assoc Am Physicians 97:80–87, 1984b.

Sutherland DER, Goetz FC, Najarian JS. Recent experience with 89 pancreas transplants at a single institution. Diabetologia 27:149–153, 1984c.

Sutherland DE, Gores PF, Farney AC, Wahoff DC, Matas AJ, Dunn DL, Gruessner RW, Najarian JS. Evolution of kidney, pancreas, and islet transplantation for patients with diabetes at the University of Minnesota. Am J Surg 166:456–491, 1993.

Svenningsen A, Dyrberg T, Gerling I, Lernmark A, Mackay P, Rabinovitch A. Inhibition of insulin release after passive transfer of immunoglobulin from insulin-dependent diabetic children to mice. J Clin Endocrinol Metab 57:1301–1304, 1983.

Takayama S, Hirata Y. Incidence of insulin autoimmune hypoglycemia in Japan during the three-year period from 1979 to 1981. Diabetes 32:150A, 1983.

Takayama S, Eguchi Y, Sato A, Morita C, Hirata Y. Insulin autoimmune syndrome is the third leading cause of spontaneous hypoglycemic attacks in Japan. Diabetes Res Clin Pract 10:211–214, 1990.

Tamai H, Uno H, Hirota Y, Matsubayashi S, Kuma K, Matsumoto H, Kumagai LF, Sasazuki T, Nagataki S. Immunogenetics of Hashimoto's and Graves' diseases. J Clin Endocrinol Metab 60:62–66, 1985.

Tanaka M, Abe J, Kohsaka T, Tanae A. Analysis of HLA-DQA1 in Japanese patients with type 1 diabetes mellitus, using DNA-PCR-RFLP typing. Acta Paediatr Jpn 34:46–51, 1992.

Tao TW, Leu SL, Kriss JP. Peripheral blood lymphocytes from normal individuals can be induced to secrete immunoglobulin G antibodies against self-antigen thyroglobulin in vitro. J Clin Endocrinol Metab 60:279–282, 1985.

Tattersall RB. Mild familial diabetes with dominant inheritance. Q J Med 43:339–357, 1974.

Taylor SI, Grunberger G, Marcus-Samuels B, Underhill LH, Dons RF, Ryan J, Roddam RF, Rupe CE, Gorden P. Hypoglycemia associated with antibodies to the insulin receptor. N Engl J Med 307:1422–1425, 1982.

Teding van Berkhout F, Croughs RJ, Wulffraat NM, Drexhage HA. Familial Cushing's syndrome due to nodular adrenocortical dysplasia is an inherited disease of immunological origin. Clin Endocrinol Oxf 31:185–191, 1989.

Theofilopoulos AN, Dixon FJ. Autoimmune diseases, immunopathology and etiopathogenesis. Am J Pathol 108:321–356, 1982.

Thompson M, Platz P, Anderson O, Christy M, Lyngsoe J, Nerup J, Rasmusson K, Ryder L, Nielson L, Svejgaard A. MLC typing in juvenile diabetes mellitus and idiopathic Addison's disease. Transplant Rev 22:125–147, 1975.

Todd JA, Aitman TJ, Cornall RJ, Ghosh S, Hall J, Hearne CM, Knight A, Love J, McAleer MA, Prins JB, et al. Genetic analysis of a complex, multifactorial disease, autoimmune type 1 (insulin-dependent) diabetes. Res Immunol 142:483, 1991.

Todd JA, Bell JI, McDevitt HO. HLA-DQβ gene contributes to susceptibility and resistance to insulin-dependent diabetes mellitus. Nature 329:599–604, 1987.

Topliss D, How J, Lewis M, Row V, Volpe R. Evidence for cell-mediated immunity and specific suppressor T lymphocyte dysfunction in Graves' disease and diabetes mellitus. J Clin Endocrinol Metab 57:700–705, 1983.

Trimarchi F, Benvenga S, Fenzi G, Mariotti S, Consolo F. Immunoglobulin binding of thyroid hormones in a case of Waldenström's macroglobulinemia. J Clin Endocrinol Metab 54:1045–1050, 1982.

Tunbridge WMG, Brewis M, French JM, Appleton D, Bird T, Clark F, Evered DC, Evans JG, Hall R, Smith P, Stephenson J, Young E. Natural history of autoimmune thyroiditis. Br Med J 282:258–262, 1981.

Uchigata Y, Kuwata S, Tokunaga K, Eguchi Y, Takayama Hasumi S, Miyamoto M, Omori Y, Juji T, Hirata Y. Strong association of insulin autoimmune syndrome with HLA-DR4. Lancet 339:393–394, 1992.

Utiger RD. The pathogenesis of autoimmune thyroid disease. N Engl J Med 325:278–279, 1991.

Vadheim CM, Rotter JI, Maclaren NK, Riley WJ, Anderson CE. Preferential transmission of diabetic alleles within the HLA gene complex. N Engl J Med 315:1314–1318, 1986.

Vakeva A, Kontiainen S, Miettinen A, Schlenzka A, Maenpaa J. Thyroid peroxidase antibodies in children with autoimmune thyroiditis. J Clin Pathol 45:106–109, 1992.

Valente WA, Vitti P, Rotella CM, Vaughan MM, Aloj SM, Grollman EE, Ambesi-Impiombato FS, Kohn LD. Antibodies that promote thyroid growth. N Engl J Med 309:1028–1034, 1983.

Van Der Gaag RD, Drexhage HA, Dussault, JH. Role of maternal immunoglobulins blocking TSH-induced thyroid growth in sporadic forms of congenital hypothyroidism. Lancet 1:246–250, 1985a.

Van Der Gaag RD, Drexhage HA, Wiersinga WM, Brown RS, Docter R, Bottazzo GF, Doniach D. Further studies on thyroid growth-stimulating immunoglobulins in euthyroid nonepidemic goiter. J Clin Endocrinol Metab 60:972–979, 1985b.

Van Der Winkel M, Smets G, Gepts W. Islet cell surface antibodies from insulin-dependent diabetics bind specifically to pancreatic cells. J Clin Invest 70:41–49, 1982.

Varga J, Lopatin M, Boden G. Hypoglycemia due to antiinsulin receptor antibodies in systemic lupus erythematosus. J Rheumatol 17:1226–1229, 1990.

Vidnes J, Oyaseter S. Glucagon deficiency causing severe neonatal hypoglycemia in a patient with normal insulin secretion. Pediatr Res 11:943–949, 1977.

Virella G, Wohltmann H, Sagel J, Lopes-Virella MFL, Kilpatrick M, Phillips C, Colwell J. Soluble immune complexes in patients with diabetes mellitus: detection and pathological significance. Diabetologia 21:184–191, 1981.

Virtanen SM, Rasanen L, Aro A, Lindstrom J, Sippola H, Lounamaa R, Toivanen L, Tuomilehto J, Akerblom HK. Infant feeding in Finnish children less than 7 yr of age with newly diagnosed IDDM: Childhood Diabetes in Finland Study Group. Diabetes Care 14:415–417, 1991.

Volpe R. Autoimmunity causing thyroid dysfunction. Endocrinol Metab Clin North Am 20:565–587, 1991.

Von Meyenburg H. Ueber "insulitis" bei diabetes. Schwiz Med Wochenschr 24:554–557, 1940.

Wall JR, Salvi M, Bernard NF, Boucher A, Haegert, D. Thyroid-associated ophthalmopathy: a model for the association of organ-specific autoimmune disorders. Immunol Today 12:150–153, 1991.

Waring S, Kodama K, Sikorska H, Wall JR. TSH and orbital antibodies. Lancet 2:224–225, 1983.

Warram JH, Krolewski AS, Gottlieb MS, Kahn CR. Differences in risk of insulin-dependent diabetes in offspring of diabetic mothers and diabetic fathers. N Engl J Med 311:149–152, 1984.

Weetman AP. Thyroid-associated eye disease: pathophysiology. Lancet 338:25–32, 1991.

Weetman AP. Update. Thyroid-associated ophthalmopathy. Autoimmunity 12:215–222, 1992.

Weetman AP, Zhang L, Webb S, Shine B. Analysis of HLA-DQB and HLA-DPB alleles in Graves' disease by oligonucleotide probing of enzymatically amplified DNA. Clin Endocrinol Oxf 33:65–71, 1990.

Weightman D, Kendall-Taylor P. Cross-reaction of eye muscle antibodies with thyroid tissue in thyroid-associated ophthalmopathy. J Endocrinol 122:201–206, 1989.

Weiss I, Davies TF. Inhibition of immunoglobulin-secreting cells by antithyroid drugs. J Clin Endocrinol Metab 53:1223–1228, 1981.

Weissel M, Hoffer R, Zasmeta H, Mayr, W. HLA-DR and Hashimoto's thyroiditis. Tissue Antigens 16:256–257, 1980.

Wick G. Concept of a multigenic basis for the pathogenesis of spontaneous autoimmune thyroiditis. Acta Endocrinol Suppl Copenh 281:63–69, 1987.

Wilkin TJ. Receptor autoimmunity in endocrine disorders. N Engl J Med 323:1318–1324, 1990.

Wilkin T, Hoskins PJ, Armitage M, Rodier M, Casey C, Diaz J-L, Pyke DA, Leslie RDG. Value of insulin autoantibodies as serum markers for insulin-dependent diabetes mellitus. Lancet 1:480–482, 1985.

Wilkin TJ, Hammonds P, Mirza I, Bone AJ, Webster K. Graves' disease of the beta cell: glucose dysregulation due to islet-cell stimulating antibodies. Lancet 2:1155–1158, 1988.

Wilks S. On disease of the suprarenal capsules or morbus Addisonnii. Guy's Hosp Report 8:1, 1962.

Winter WE. Atypical diabetes in Blacks. Clin Diabetes 9:49–56, 1991.

Winter WE, Maclaren NK. Type I insulin dependent diabetes: an autoimmune disease that can be arrested or prevented with immunotherapy? In Barness L, ed. Advances in Pediatrics. Chicago, Year Book Medical Publishers, 1985, pp. 159–175.

Winter WE, Maclaren NK. To what extent is "polyendocrine" serology related to the clinical expression of disease. In Doniach D, Bottazzo GF, eds. Baillière Clinical Immunology and Allergy, Vol. 1. London, Baillière Tindall, 1987, pp. 109–123.

Winter WE, Maclaren NK, Riley WJ, Kappy MS, Jensen J, Spillar R. A novel diabetes syndrome in American Blacks (type 1.5 diabetes): insulin secretory and binding studies. Pediatr Res 18:303A, 1984a.

Winter WE, Maclaren NK, Riley WJ, Unger RH, Neufeld M, Ozand PT. Pancreatic alpha cell autoantibodies and glucagon response to arginine. Diabetes 33:435–437, 1984b.

Winter WE, Maclaren NK, Riley WJ, Andres J, Toskes RP, Rosenbloom AL. Congenital pancreatic hypoplasia: a novel diabetes syndrome of exocrine and endocrine pancreatic insufficiency. Pediatrics 109:465–469, 1986.

Winter WE, Maclaren NK, Riley WJ, Clarke DW, Kappy MS, Spillar RP. Maturity-onset diabetes of youth in Black Americans. N Engl J Med 316:285–291, 1987.

Winter WE, Obata M, Maclaren NK. Clinical and molecular aspects of autoimmune diseases. Vol. 8. In Cruse JM, Lewis RE, eds. Clinical and Molecular Aspects of Autoimmune Endocrine Disease. Basel, S. Karger, 1991a, pp. 189–221.

Winter WE, Obata M, Muir A, Maclaren NK. Heritable origins of type I insulin dependent diabetes mellitus. Growth Genet Horm 7:1–6, 1991b.

Winter WE, Chihara T, Schatz DA. The genetics of autoimmune diabetes. Am J Dis Child 147:1282–1290, 1993.

Witebsky E, Milgram F. Immunological studies on adrenal glands, II. Immunization with adrenals of the same species. Immunology 5:67–72, 1962.

Wolf BM, Bottazzo GF, Cudworth AG. Evidence of a long prediabetic period in type I (insulin-dependent) diabetes mellitus. Lancet 2:1363–1365, 1981.

Yamagata K, Hanafusa T, Nakajima H, Sada M, Amemiya H, Tomita K, Miyagawa J, Noguchi T, Tanaka T, Kono N, Tarui S. HLA-DP and susceptibility to insulin-dependent diabetes mellitus in Japanese. Tissue Antigens 38:107–110, 1991.

Yamagata K, Nakajimi H, Hanafusa T, Noguchi T, Miyazaki A, Miyagawa J, Sada M, Amemiya H, Tanaka T, Kono N, Tarui S. Aspartic acid at position 57 of DQβ chain does not protect against type I (insulin-dependent) diabetes mellitus in Japanese subjects. Diabetologia 32:762–763, 1989.

Yassin N, Seissler J, Gluck M, Boehm BO, Heinze E, Pfeiffer EF, Scherbaum WA. Insulin autoantibodies as determined by competitive radiobinding assay are positively correlated with impaired beta-cell function—the Ulm-Frankfurt Population Study. Klin Wochenschr 69:736–741, 1991.

Yoon J-W, Austin M, Onodera T, Notkins AL. Virus-induced diabetes mellitus. N Engl J Med 300:1173–1179, 1979.

Zier KS, Keo MM, Speilman RS, Baker L. Decreased synthesis of interleukin-2 (IL-2) in insulin-dependent diabetes mellitus. Diabetes 33:552–555, 1984.

Chapter 27

Immune-Mediated Hematologic and Oncologic Disorders, Including Epstein-Barr Virus Infection

Alexandra H. Filipovich, Thomas Gross,
Harumi Jyonouchi, and Ralph S. Shapiro

In this chapter, immune-mediated hematologic and oncologic disorders affecting children are discussed. Particular attention is paid to autoimmune hematologic and malignant diseases affecting children with primary and secondary immunodeficiencies, including the mechanisms that may predispose these patients to autoimmunity.

Also reviewed in depth are infections with Epstein-Barr virus (EBV) and the immunologic abnormalities that accompany infectious mononucleosis, X-linked lymphoproliferative syndrome, and malignant disorders. Finally, the hemophagocytic syndromes and malignant disorders occurring in immunodeficiency are detailed.

Autoimmune hematologic disorders occur in apparently immunocompetent children but are encountered with a higher than normal incidence in primary or secondary immunodeficiency. Although the course of autoimmune hematologic disorders in the general pediatric population is often self-limited or readily responsive to simple therapies, some immunodeficient patients may experience more than one of these autoimmune manifestations simultaneously or sequentially; and the risk of development of autoimmune complications appears to increase with age in certain categories of immunodeficiency.

AUTOIMMUNE HEMOLYTIC ANEMIA

Immune hemolysis is defined as destruction of red blood cells (RBCs) by immunologic mechanisms that involve antibody and complement components acting in concert or alone. In general, there are two types of immune hemolysis: autoimmune and isoimmune.

Autoimmune hemolysis occurs when a person forms antibodies that bind to his or her own red blood cells. For this discussion, drug-induced immune hemolysis is considered to be a form of autoimmune hemolysis. *Isoimmune hemolysis* occurs when a person forms antibody to erythrocyte antigens not present on his or her own cells. Hemolysis results when the antibody is transferred to a second person whose RBCs possess the antigen in question, such as in erythroblastosis fetalis, or when a sensitized individual receives appropriately antigenic RBCs, such as in a transfusion reaction.

To diagnose immune hemolysis, one must demonstrate (1) accelerated destruction of RBCs and (2) immunoglobulins, complement components, or both on RBC membranes.

Pathogenesis

The possibility that acquired hemolytic anemia might be caused by autoantibodies was described in the early 1900s, but it was not until 1945—when Coombs and associates described "a new test for the detection of weak and incomplete Rh agglutinins"—that the routine detection of autoantibodies became possible (Coombs et al., 1945). The *Coombs' test*, or the direct antiglobulin reaction, detects globulins on the surface of erythrocytes by agglutinating immunoglobulin or complement-coated cells with an anti-human globulin serum prepared by immunizing rabbits with human serum proteins. A positive *direct* Coombs' test occurs in almost all cases of immune hemolysis. If serum antibodies binding to normal O$^+$ RBCs are demonstrated by this technique, the *indirect* Coombs' test is said to be positive.

Since 1945, modified antiglobulin sera (Coombs' reagents) that are specific for immunoglobulin classes as well as for some of the components of complement have been prepared. Several studies have disclosed that IgG, IgM, IgA, and C3 may be found together or alone on erythrocytes from patients with autoimmune hemolytic anemia (Dacie, 1967; Dacie and Worlledge, 1969;

Vaughan et al., 1966; Engelfriet et al., 1974; Petz and Garratty, 1980).

An enlarged concept of immune hemolysis emerged with documentation of the first case of drug-induced immune hemolysis in a patient taking the antihelminthic drug stibophen (Harris, 1956). Since that time a number of drugs have been implicated in immune hemolysis (Table 27-1). The use of the electron and scanning electron microscope to study immune reactions involving erythrocytes has elucidated membrane abnormalities that occur in agglutination (Salsbury et al., 1968), complement-mediated lysis (Dourmashkin and Rosse, 1966) and the binding of IgG-coated erythrocytes to mononuclear phagocytes (LoBuglio et al., 1967; Abramson et al., 1970).

Patients with autoimmune hemolytic anemia (AHA) are clinically and immunologically heterogeneous. The erythrocyte antibodies in AHA are heterogeneous with respect to immunoglobulin class, serologic properties, biologic activity, and associated clinical disease, but they are divided into two groups according to the type of antibody generated:

- Warm-reacting autoantibodies, seen in 80% to 90% of AHA cases, which react with erythrocytes at 37°C
- Cold-reacting autoantibodies, also known as *cold agglutinins,* which have enhanced reaction at temperatures below 37°C

Warm Antibody Disease

In a patient with warm antibody AHA, erythrocytes are coated with IgG antibody (Ab) with or without complement (C). The antibody (Ab) is usually directed to the Rh erythrocyte antigens, but its precise specificity is often difficult to define. Red blood cells coated with large amounts of IgG Ab or complement are easily phagocytosed in the spleen and liver by macrophages and other phagocytic cells. Cells of the monocyte-macrophage lineage express receptors for the Fc portion of IgG (FcγRI and FcγRIII) and complement receptors (CR1, CR3, and CR4), which facilitate trapping and

Table 27–1. Drugs Reported To Induce Immune Hemolytic Anemia

Drug	Year Described
Quinidine	1956
Para-aminosalicylic acid (PAS)	1956
Quinine	1958
Phenacetin	1958
Penicillin	1959
Insecticides	1959
Sulfonamides	1960
Isonicotinic acid hydrazide (INH)	1960
Chlorpromazine	1961
Cephalosporins	1967
Rifampin	1971
Tetracycline	1974
Acetaminophen	1976

Data from Dacie, 1967; Worlledge, 1973; Gralnick et al., 1971; and Petz and Garratty, 1980.

phagocytosis of antibody-coated red blood cells (Frank, 1989; Van De Winkel and Capel, 1993). This results in a complete or partial phagocytosis. Partially phagocytosed RBCs (those that have lost a certain portion of their cell membrane) become more rigid and are more readily destroyed in the microvasculature.

Cold Agglutinin Disease

Cold agglutinin disease is defined as hemolytic disease caused by autoantibodies agglutinating RBCs at temperatures below 37°C to 5°C. This occurs less frequently than warm antibody AHA and often is associated with infection (*Mycoplasma pneumoniae* and Epstein-Barr virus) in young adults and with lymphoproliferative diseases in older patients. The cold Ab (cold agglutinin) is typically IgM Ab directed against the RBC antigens of the I/i system. IgM Abs bound to the RBC membrane activate the classical complement pathway, leading to the deposition of C3b on the erythrocyte membrane. Complement-coated RBCs are then phagocytosed by macrophage lineage cells in the liver. Thus, hemolysis caused by cold agglutinins is generally less severe and often self-limited. Differences in agglutination are related to the density of the antigens on the RBC surface. It is known that erythrocyte Rh antigens are widely dispersed and are fewer in number than A determinants, for example.

Antibody Specificity

The specificity of the IgG eluted from sensitized RBCs in idiopathic AHA has been studied. In many instances, no specificity is found (Vaughan et al., 1966), and the patient is said to have a "panagglutinin." When specificity can be demonstrated, the antibodies are usually directed against an Rh antigen and, in particular, the c, e, and ce antigens (Habibi et al, 1974). Cold agglutinins almost always show anti-I specificity. Antibody specificity in AHA in children has not been studied extensively. Such studies can provide insight into the cause of the patient's disease and can aid in the selection of blood donors.

Consequences of Antibody Bound to Erythrocytes

When antibodies bind to erythrocytes, the net negative charge present on the cell membrane decreases. Agglutination occurs when the distance between cells, maintained by electrostatic repulsive charges, is bridged by bivalent antibodies (Rosse and Lauf, 1970). The structural changes that occur when RBCs agglutinate have been studied using the scanning electron microscope (Salsbury et al., 1968). It was observed that when RBCs are agglutinated, the surfaces of the erythrocytes first roughen, then develop protrusions, and then are linked by fine finger-like processes (Fig. 27–1). When cold agglutinins are studied, these events reverse as the agglutinates are warmed to 37°C. Incomplete (nonagglutinating) antibody produces similar changes, al-

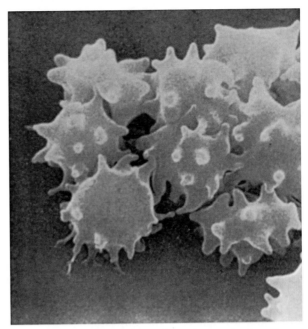

Figure 27–1. Scanning electron photomicrograph of erythrocytes undergoing agglutination with anti-A. Note the membrane protrusions and finger-like processes that link the cells together. (From Salsbury A, Clarke JA. Rev Franc Etud Clin Biol 12:981–986, 1967.)

though more slowly, and progression of the membrane protrusions to finger-like processes does not occur.

The blood of patients with many types of immune hemolysis contains microspherocytes (Fig. 27–2) and exhibits increased osmotic and mechanical fragility in vitro.

The presence of complement components on the RBCs in the absence of antibody suggests that the alternative pathway of complement activation may be involved in some instances of autoimmune hemolysis (Pickering et al., 1969; Gotze and Müller-Eberhard, 1970; Thompson and Lachmann, 1970). Such activated complement components may then attach to the sur-

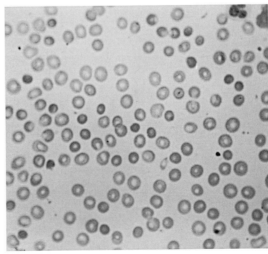

Figure 27–2. Peripheral blood smear from a patient with autoimmune hemolytic anemia. Note microspherocytes (×430).

face of the RBC and bind the remaining components and cause lysis. Alternatively, if complement binding has not proceeded through a complete lytic sequence, one would find intact cells with complement components but no antibody on their surfaces.

In vivo, RBCs coated with antibody, complement, or both are rapidly sequestered in the reticuloendothelial system (RES) and removed from the circulation. The organs involved and the speed at which this occurs vary with the quality and the quantity of the bound antibodies. The rate of hemolysis is proportional to the concentration of cell-bound antibody (Jandl and Kaplan, 1960; Rosse, 1971; Mollison, 1970c). RBCs coated with isoantibodies (such as anti-Rh) would neither lyse nor agglutinate but are sequestered almost completely in the spleen. In patients with enlarged spleens, hemolysis is accelerated. In splenectomized individuals, clearance of sensitized cells is greatly prolonged (Mollison, 1970a). If, in addition, complement components through C3 are fixed to the RBCs, the rate of clearance is increased still further (Mollison, 1970b). If the RBCs are coated with still larger or near-lytic amounts of antibody, intravascular hemolysis results, with the deposition of hemoglobin throughout the RES and kidneys. In subjects with a specific hemolysin, the destruction of RBCs is virtually instantaneous.

Clinical Manifestations

Autoimmune hemolytic anemia occurs in children of all ages and has been reported in premature infants. The clinical features that characterize the onset of disease are determined largely by the rate and location of hemolysis.

Rapid intravascular hemolysis is associated with the abrupt onset of shaking chills, fever, and frequently pain in the back and abdomen. Pallor and weakness may progress to the point of prostration. The urine may vary in color from pink to red to dark brown. If the syndrome is caused by a cold-reacting antibody (paroxysmal cold hemoglobinuria or cold agglutinin disease), a recent exposure to cold may have occurred. Physical examination usually does not disclose the presence of enlarged liver, spleen, or lymph nodes; jaundice is not prominent (Pirofsky, 1976).

Usually, hemolysis occurs more slowly when erythrocytes are destroyed extravascularly in the RES. Patients so afflicted become symptomatic gradually, and their pallor, weakness, and jaundice are determined by the depth of their anemia. Low-grade fever is common. Physical examination usually reveals an enlarged spleen. The liver may be moderately enlarged, but the lymph nodes are not. The presence of additional signs, such as purpura, rash, lymphadenopathy, or massive splenomegaly, usually indicates that hemolysis is secondary to another underlying disease.

In adults, autoimmune diseases and malignancies are often associated with AHA in addition to infectious causes. In children, viral and respiratory infections are most commonly associated with AHA (Table 27–2). It is also noted that AHA in pediatric patients is often associated with immunoregulatory disorders and pri-

Table 27–2. Underlying Conditions Associated with Autoimmune Hemolytic Anemia

Infections
Hepatitis B
Herpes simplex
Mononucleosis
Infections
Cytomegalovirus
Syphilis
Tuberculosis
Mycoplasma
Bacterial infections

Other Autoimmune Disorders
Systemic lupus erythematosus
Rheumatoid arthritis
Periarteritis nodosa
Dermatomyositis
Immune thrombocytopenic purpura (Evans' syndrome)
Inflammatory bowel disease
Scleroderma

Tumors
Leukemia
Lymphoma
Hodgkin's disease
Carcinoma
Kaposi's sarcoma

Primary Immunodeficiencies
Common variable immunodeficiency
Selective IgA deficiency
IgG subclass deficiency
Hyper-IgM immunodeficiency
X-linked agammaglobulinemia
Wiskott-Aldrich syndrome
DiGeorge anomalad
Familial erythrophagocytic lymphohistiocytosis/
   hemophagocytic lymphohistiocytosis

Data from Githers and Hathaway, 1962; Dacie and Worlledge, 1969; Zuelzer et al., 1970; and Petz and Garratty, 1980.

mary immunodeficiencies, as discussed later (Schreiber and Frank, 1988).

Treatment

Treatment of AHA has improved considerably in the past two decades. Initially, an effort should be made to diagnose an underlying disease or to determine whether hemolysis is related to drug exposure. Appropriate therapy of the underlying disease or discontinuing the offending drug may promptly reverse hemolysis.

Most children have warm antibody AHA without an obvious underlying cause. Treatment is directed toward supporting the patient and stopping hemolysis.

Blood Transfusions

Initially, blood transfusions may be required. These should be employed sparingly, since it often is difficult to find compatible blood, and normal erythrocytes usually survive poorly in these patients. If the anemia is life-threatening, the least incompatible blood should be transfused in small amounts as packed RBCs. In emergencies, exchange transfusion may be utilized. In patients with cold agglutinin–mediated disease, plasmapheresis has been reported to be useful.

Corticosteroids

Adrenocortical steroids are the drugs of choice. These inhibit the sequestration of sensitized cells by the RES (Rosse, 1971; Kaplan and Jandl, 1961; Schreiber et al., 1975), promote the dissociation of antibody from sensitized erythrocytes, and decrease both specific antibody titers and serum immunoglobulin levels (Murphy and LoBuglio, 1976). Prednisone is used at a dose of 2 mg/kg/day in divided doses. If the patient is too ill for oral medication, equivalent or greater doses of hydrocortisone, prednisolone, or dexamethasone may be given intravenously in four to six daily divided doses. Because many children recover rapidly following a single episode of hemolysis and since the side effects of steroids occur so regularly, prednisone therapy should be tapered and then discontinued as soon as remission has occurred. Prednisone may be given every other day to the patient who experiences relapse on low doses.

Intravenous Immunoglobulin

During the past decade, high-dose intravenous immunoglobulin (IVIG) has been used in patients with AHA with encouraging results (Flores et al., 1993; Bussel and Baumgartner, 1984). Because of the safety of IVIG, an early trial (400 mg/kg/day for 5 days) is probably indicated. If corticosteroids or IVIG do not control hemolysis, or if steroid side effects (e.g., fluid retention, hypertension, diabetes, growth failure) are severe, alternative therapy may be required. At this juncture, many physicians advise splenectomy.

Immunosuppression

A trial of azathioprine may be used before proceeding to splenectomy, since it produces fewer effects than does 6-mercaptopurine or thioguanine. It is given orally in doses of 2 to 4 mg/kg/day. Frequent white blood cell (WBC) and platelet counts must be performed and observations made for side effects (mouth ulcers, oral moniliasis, skin infections). Because the amount of drug tolerated by a given child is variable, treatment must be individualized. In adults, a success rate of about 50% has been reported (Parker and Vavra, 1969). Similar results have been reported in children (Johnson and Abildgaard, 1976), but the number of reported cases is small and controlled studies have not been carried out.

Splenectomy

The rationale for splenectomy in patients with AHA has been reviewed (Bowdler, 1976). Selecting patients for splenectomy and deciding when this is to be undertaken are difficult decisions. In vitro studies have disclosed that if the patient's antibody is IgG, the spleen is probably responsible for most or all of the RBC destruction. Thus, splenectomy should benefit or cure such patients. If the patient has an IgM antibody, most RBC destruction will be occurring outside the spleen and the chances for improvement following splenectomy are likely to be poor.

Second, the results of scanning the liver and spleen following a ^{51}Cr RBC survival study can be helpful. It has been reported that if, at the half-survival time, the ratio of radioactive counts in the spleen to counts in the liver is greater than 2.3:1, significant splenic sequestration is occurring (Goldberg et al., 1966; Allgood and Chaplin, 1967). Splenectomy, therefore, is expected to be beneficial.

Following splenectomy, children are predisposed to overwhelming sepsis and should be given prophylactic doses of penicillin or trimethoprim-sulfamethoxazole until they are 7 or 8 years old (see Chapter 19). This must be emphasized, particularly if there is an underlying immunodeficiency. These children should also benefit from immunization with the meningococcal, pneumococcal, and *Haemophilus influenzae B* vaccines (at least 1 month) prior to splenectomy and perhaps subsequently.

Other Therapy

Other therapy that has occasionally been beneficial includes danazol, heparin, penicillamine, and thymectomy, with resulting anecdotal improvement.

Prognosis

The prognosis in childhood AHA depends largely on whether the hemolysis is acute (lasting less than 3 months) or chronic and whether it is an isolated phenomenon or associated with other abnormalities. An acute, self-limited form of AHA exists that apparently responds well to steroid therapy, although no prospective controlled trials have been performed. For this group, the survival-recovery rate was 94% (August et al., 1989).

A chronic form of AHA is frequently associated with neutropenia, thrombocytopenia, immunodeficiency, wider autoimmune diseases, or neoplasms. Death occurs more frequently (27%) in these patients but is likely to result from an infectious complication of the underlying disorder or its therapy rather than from hemolysis itself.

In most pediatric series, cold antibody disease and secondary AHA are rare. Cold antibody hemolytic anemia in children is usually associated with a viral infection and is self-limited and mild. In secondary AHA, the prognosis is usually that of the associated illness.

ERYTHROBLASTOSIS FETALIS

Erythroblastosis fetalis (EBF), or hemolytic disease of the newborn, is a disease in which the life span of the newborn's erythrocytes is shortened by the action of specific antibodies formed in the mother and transferred to the infant through the placenta. The mother is stimulated to produce antibodies when exposed to a red blood cell antigen that her erythrocytes do not possess. This process, called *alloimmunization,* is initiated by small leaks of fetal RBCs across the placenta.

The blood group isoantibodies that may cause EBF are of the IgG class and freely cross the placenta. The most important antibody clinically is anti-D (anti-Rh), which accounts for about 95% of antibodies found in women who give birth to an infant with a positive direct Coombs' result. Anti-C and anti-E account for about 6% (Mollison, 1972). Therefore, the best diagnostic test for EBF is a positive direct Coombs' test in the infant. With careful technique and slight modification of the antiglobulin reaction, the direct Coombs' test will be positive in essentially all cases of ABO disease as well.

Emphasis must be placed on prevention of Rh isoimmunization. Administration of anti-D antibody (rhesus immune globulin, RhIG) to the Rh-negative mother of an Rh-positive infant at any time when leaks of fetal cells into the maternal circulation are possible prevents the primary sensitization of the mother.

The indications for use of RhIG in Rh-negative women include the following:

- After delivery of a Rh(D) or Du-positive infant
- After antepartum hemorrhage
- After abortion
- After ectopic pregnancy
- After amniocentesis
- After fetal death
- After molar evacuation
- Before external version
- After Rh-positive blood or platelet transfusions
- After post-partum sterilization

If RhIG is not administered, alloimmunization occurs in about 15% of Rh-negative women.

PERNICIOUS ANEMIA

Pernicious anemia (PA) is a megaloblastic anemia caused by a deficiency of vitamin B_{12}; it is caused by defective absorption of the vitamin as a result of diminished or absent gastric secretion of intrinsic factor. PA is a rare disorder in childhood and is most often associated with an underlying immunodeficiency. The presence of parietal cell antibodies, the high incidence of PA in thyroid disease (in which autoimmune phenomena are common), and the lymphocytic infiltration of the stomach wall of patients with PA also suggest the importance of immune factors. Pernicious anemia with gastric achlorhydria has been described in children.

A group of young children with megaloblastic anemia and normal acid secretions have also been identified. In the latter group, there is a congenital absence of intrinsic factor (IF), and both parietal cell and IF antibodies are lacking as a result of an autosomal recessive disorder. They have juvenile PA, differentiated from adult PA, which is characterized by achlorhydria and the presence of parietal cell and IF antibodies. Some pediatric patients may have the adult type. In a

third form of PA, termed *Imerslund's syndrome,* IF is present but the vitamin B_{12}–IF complex is not absorbed from the intestinal lumen (Imerslund and Bjornstad, 1963).

Pathogenesis

Intrinsic factor is a glycoprotein secreted by the parietal cells of the gastric mucosa; it avidly binds the small amounts of vitamin B_{12} found in most foods of animal origin that is released during peptic digestion. The vitamin B_{12}–IF complex is absorbed within the microvilli of the intestinal cell before the vitamin is released intracellularly and reaches the blood stream.

Antibodies to parietal cells and IF are detected in the serum and gastric juice of most patients with adult PA. Although parietal cell antibodies are present in approximately 80% of patients, they are nonspecific and are also detected in many other patients. These IgG antibodies are directed against a lipoprotein antigen located on the microvilli of parietal cell secretory canaliculi. Their relationship to gastric inflammation and the development of PA is unclear.

Both IF and parietal cell antibodies can be demonstrated using gastric biopsies (Baur et al., 1968). Gastric IF antibodies are of two subtypes—blocking and binding antibodies, both of which are IgG antibodies. Blocking antibodies combine with IF at or near the vitamin B_{12}–binding site and inhibit the formation of the vitamin B_{12}–IF complex. These antibodies are present in approximately 60% of patients with PA. Binding antibodies combine with IF at a location remote from the vitamin B_{12}–binding site and are present in approximately 30% of patients with PA.

Juvenile Pernicious Anemia

Children with juvenile PA have a congenital IF deficiency. This is an autosomal recessive disorder; the heterozygotes manifest no clinical or laboratory abnormalities. In these patients, gastric acid and pepsin secretion is normal. Patients manifest no evidence of gastritis, and they lack antiparietal cell or anti-IF antibodies (McIntyre et al., 1965; Miller et al., 1966). Because this disorder shares none of the pathogenetic features of adult PA, it must be considered a separate disorder. These children may develop mild gastritis and reduced gastric acid production if they are not maintained on parenteral vitamin B_{12} injections (Lillibridge et al., 1967).

Adult Pernicious Anemia

As a result of the loss of IF-secreting cells from an atrophic gastric mucosa, adult PA is rare in children. Those factors that lead to gastric atrophy are not known; a genetic predisposition is suggested by a higher incidence of PA in the relatives of affected individuals than in the general population. Relatives have an increased incidence of achlorhydria, chronic gastritis, and vitamin B_{12} malabsorption, manifested by a decreased uptake of oral radioactive vitamin B_{12}

(Callender and Denborough, 1957). Adult PA may be due to a genetically determined defect in immunologic tolerance for antigens of the stomach. As a result, committed immunocytes may destroy the gastric mucosa by cell-mediated or antibody-mediated reactions, thus abolishing the parietal cells that synthesize IF. These immune reactions may be initiated spontaneously or as a result of injury to gastric cells by a subclinical infection that renders them antigenic.

It is of note that PA occurs more frequently in patients with common variable hypogammaglobulinemia (Twomey et al., 1969). Rheumatoid arthritis and other autoimmune diseases occur frequently in PA (Good et al., 1957). PA often occurs in familial juvenile polyendocrinopathy. These children have a genetically determined tendency to develop organ-specific autoantibodies; many, however, lack parietal cell antibodies, even in the presence of IF antibodies.

Diagnosis

The clinical and laboratory findings in juvenile PA secondary to congenital IF deficiency have been reviewed by Chanarin (1969). Megaloblastic anemia presents between the fourth and 28th month, except for one case in a 13-year-old (Lampkin and Schubert, 1968). After a normal infancy, nonspecific symptoms of pallor, weakness, anorexia, and failure to thrive may develop. Stomatitis develops, and the tongue becomes depapillated. Splenomegaly may develop. Ataxia, defective speech, loss of vibratory sense, brisk knee jerks, and extensor plantar reflexes may become manifested.

The stomach is histologically normal; acid and pepsin secretion is normal (Lillibridge et al., 1967). Intrinsic factor is low to absent, and antibodies to parietal cells and IF are absent. Vitamin B_{12} absorption is impaired and is corrected by the oral administration of intrinsic factor. Serum vitamin B_{12} levels are markedly reduced.

In children, acquired or adult PA usually occurs in late childhood or adolescence. There is achlorhydria, absence of IF, and histologic evidence of atrophic gastritis. Antibodies to parietal cells and IF are present. These children should be investigated for the possibility of a coexistent disorder such as familial juvenile polyendocrinopathy or immunodeficiency.

In any child with a vitamin B_{12}–responsive megaloblastic anemia, the possibility of generalized intestinal malabsorption (celiac disease), chronic ileal disease (Crohn's disease), congenital or acquired strictures, stagnant loop syndrome, distal ileal resection, or fistulous bypass should be considered. Congenital malabsorption of vitamin B_{12} in infants (Imerslund and Bjornstad, 1963) and transcobalamin II deficiency (Hakami et al., 1971) are rare disorders that must be excluded.

Treatment

After the diagnosis of pernicious anemia has been established, parenteral vitamin B_{12} injections are given. Initial therapeutic doses range from 30 to 1000 μg daily for 7 days. Thereafter, monthly injections of 50 to 1000 μg of vitamin B_{12} should be continued indefinitely. These will maintain a normal hemogram and neurologic function.

Prognosis

Long-term follow-up on these patients is not available.

IDIOPATHIC (IMMUNE) THROMBOCYTOPENIC PURPURA

Idiopathic (immune) thrombocytopenic purpura (ITP) is a generalized hemorrhagic disorder characterized by decreased numbers of platelets in the presence of a normal-appearing bone marrow, which usually contains increased numbers of megakaryocytes. Systemic diseases capable of producing thrombocytopenia are not present, and evidence for an immunologic pathogenesis (platelet antibodies and shortened platelet life span) can often be demonstrated.

Classification

ITP is classified as either the childhood disease or "post-viral" ITP (definite preceding viral illness) or the "true" adult-type ITP (no preceding viral illness known). Approximately 50% of cases fall into each category. The "true" adult-type disease (chronic, no preceding infection) tends to occur more frequently in older children and adolescents.

Childhood ITP is frequently related to a preceding (1 to 4 weeks) viral infection. Up to 80% of pediatric cases in one study were preceded by rubella, rubeola, varicella, or viral-like upper respiratory or gastrointestinal illnesses and infectious mononucleosis (Lusher and Zuelzer, 1966). Experimental and clinical evidence supports the concept of immune-mediated platelet destruction in post-viral childhood ITP (Feusner et al., 1979).

Clinical Manifestations

Children with ITP usually present with an acute onset of easy bruising and petechiae following a viral illness. The bleeding tendency may be generalized and severe and may include epistaxis, hematuria, and melena. Life-threatening, intracranial bleeding is seen in about 1% of cases. The parents should be specifically questioned regarding drug ingestion (e.g., quinine, phenytoin [Dilantin], quinidine, choroquine, trimethoprim-sulfamethoxazole, digitoxin). Heparin administration is occasionally associated with thrombocytopenia, and occasionally live virus vaccinations may be associated with thrombocytopenia. Except for evidence of the hemorrhagic tendency, the physical examination is usually unrevealing. In particular, the presence of lymphadenopathy or splenomegaly should alert one to other diagnostic possibilities.

Diagnosis

The blood count shows thrombocytopenia, a normal or slightly elevated WBC with a normal differential count, and no anemia unless the bleeding has been severe. The blood smear shows decreased numbers of platelets (often large in size) and occasionally increased numbers of atypical lymphocytes related to the preceding viral infection. Coagulation tests are normal except for a prolonged bleeding time and impaired clot retraction. Tourniquet tests should not be performed if the patient shows obvious petechiae. The most helpful test is the bone marrow examination, which shows increased numbers of megakaryocytes in an otherwise normal marrow. Bone marrow examination should be performed to confirm the diagnosis in all cases.

On suspicion, other causes of thrombocytopenia associated with a normal marrow should be evaluated by appropriate studies. This differential diagnosis includes infectious mononucleosis, chronic infections, familial thrombocytopenia, human immunodeficiency virus (HIV) infection, chronic thrombotic thrombocytopenic purpura (Moake et al., 1982), hyperthyroidism, systemic lupus erythematosus (SLE), other collagen-vascular disorders, malignancies, and Wiskott-Aldrich syndrome.

Platelet Antibodies

A knowledge of the presence and type of platelet antigens and antibodies is helpful in the differential diagnosis and therapeutic consideration of thrombocytopenic syndromes. Two kinds of platelet antibodies are of importance: *autoimmune* and *alloimmune (isoimmune)*.

Autoimmune Platelet Antibodies

The relationship of platelet-associated immunoglobulins (PA IgG, PA IgM) to ITP, SLE, and other diseases with increased platelet destruction has been extensively reviewed (Karpatkin, 1980; McMillan, 1981; Kelton and Gibbons, 1982). In most patients with ITP, increased amounts of IgG are present on the platelet surface; this is thought to be responsible for the rapid platelet destruction by the RES leading to thrombocytopenia, although the amount of PA IgG may not necessarily correlate with the severity of ITP. Larger amounts of PA IgG as well as IgM and complement (Myers et al., 1982) have been seen in acute ITP compared with chronic ITP in children; however, increased PA IgG is also found in many other disorders, such as chronic active hepatitis, cancer, and infections (Mueller-Eckhardt et al., 1980; Kernoff and Malan, 1983).

Alloimmune (Isoimmune) Platelet Antibodies

Isoimmune platelet antibodies are found in patients who have had previous exposure to human leukocyte antigens (HLA) or specific platelet antigens (PLA system) that are not their own. These antibodies, measured as platelet-associated immunoglobulins, are implicated in the following clinical situations.

Neonatal Thrombocytopenic Purpura. The platelet antibody results from active immunization of the mother from the father's antigens on the platelets of the fetus and is transferred to the baby transplacentally. Although thrombocytopenia in the infant may be severe, the maternal platelet count is normal. Usually, the maternal antibody is directed against the platelet antigen PLA-1. Only 2% of the population is PLA-1–negative; therefore, the disorder is uncommon, affecting only 1 to 2 per 10,000 live births. Other antibodies (anti-Duzo, anti–PLE-2, anti-BakA), including anti-HLA, may occasionally be implicated.

Blood Transfusions. Routine blood and platelet transfusions induce alloimmunization in recipients with bone marrow failure (aplasia, leukemia) in 50% to 90% of patients (Brand et al., 1984). Several maneuvers, including HLA-matched donors, single-donor platelet pheresis, or use of leukocyte-poor blood products (frozen RBCs and freshly prepared platelet packs), can be used to decrease this incidence of platelet sensitization and, therefore, to increase the effectiveness of platelet transfusions.

Post-transfusion Purpura. This rare syndrome is characterized by acute onset of severe thrombocytopenia associated with an anamnestic response to blood transfusion in a previously alloimmunized patient; alloimmune antibody with anti–PLA-1 specificity has been demonstrated in most cases. Plasmapheresis may be of benefit in therapy of the acute episode (Lau et al., 1980).

Treatment

Because childhood ITP is usually self-limited and only rarely recurrent, a conservative attitude should be taken. If the bleeding is not severe, no specific therapy is given regardless of the level of the platelet count. The parents and patient are advised that the patient should avoid trauma, contact sports, acetylsalicylic acid ingestion, or any other drug known to decrease platelet function. An attitude of watchful waiting is assumed.

Corticosteroids

If the patient shows significant and repeated episodes of skin bleeding or epistaxis or evidence of internal bleeding, therapy with corticosteroids should be considered. A randomized cooperative study published in 1994 supports the use of a short course of steroids, because platelet counts may rise more quickly with this approach (Sartorius, 1984).

A typical dose of prednisone is 2 mg/kg/day in three divided doses for 2 weeks. Even if the platelet count does not rise significantly, bleeding usually ceases after institution of this treatment. Then, regardless of the platelet count, the drug can be tapered and discontinued after 2 weeks.

Intravenous Immunoglobulin

The therapeutic benefit of IVIG in immune thrombocytopenia was first reported by Imbach and associates in 1985 in several children with agammaglobulinemia and Wiskott-Aldrich syndrome whose thrombocytopenia improved following IVIG therapy. When this therapy was extended to other pediatric patients with thrombocytopenia, higher platelet counts were noted and bleeding diminished following the administration of IVIG to patients with ITP. Since then, high-dose IVIG (at least 400 mg/kg/day for 3 to 5 days) has been used extensively in both acute and chronic ITP in children and adults (Bussel et al., 1983a; Fehr et al., 1982). Several different commercial IVIG preparations have been used successfully (Uchino et al., 1984); they are probably therapeutically equivalent.

Acute ITP

In children with acute ITP, the risk of life-threatening hemorrhage early in the disease is the major concern. Therefore, attention has focused on how rapidly a sustained rise in platelets has been achieved in patients treated with IVIG. Bussel and coworkers (1985) treated 29 patients with IVIG (1 g/kg/day for 3 days); all experienced a marked increase in the platelet count within 24 hours. Imbach and colleagues (1985) compared 47 children with acute ITP who were treated with IVIG (400 mg/kg/day for 5 days) to 47 children treated with corticosteroids. In most patients (62%), the response to either therapy was equally rapid, but in the remainder (38%) patients treated with IVIG achieved remission sooner. The incidence of progression to chronic thrombocytopenic purpura was the same in both groups (about 20%).

Because the risk of severe hemorrhage is greatest with extremely low platelet counts, IVIG has been recommended in acute thrombocytopenic purpura when the platelet count falls below 10,000/μl (Bussel, 1986). One strategy has been to treat these children with corticosteroids first because of the ease of administration. If steroids do not cause a prompt increase in the platelet count, IVIG can be added to bring about a more rapid remission.

Chronic ITP

IVIG has also been used in chronic ITP when conventional therapy has been relatively ineffective; children with this disease may respond better than adults. Bussel and colleagues (1983b) gave IVIG to 12 children with chronic ITP who were also receiving corticosteroid therapy and were being considered for splenectomy. IVIG was given at doses of 400 mg/kg/day for 5 days followed by single infusions of 400 mg/kg/day, first weekly and then monthly as needed to maintain the platelet count over 40,000/μl. All patients responded with an immediate rise from an average pre-treatment platelet count of 24,000/μl to an average peak post-treatment count of 266,000/μl. At follow-up at least 4 months after maintenance therapy was stopped, one of 12 patients had achieved complete remission and four of 12 had maintained platelet counts more than 40,000/μl. Thus, IVIG may permit the postponement or avoidance of splenectomy in some children. It may also permit the discontinuation of immunosuppressive medication that is causing undesirable side effects.

Mori and coworkers (1983) studied 25 children with chronic ITP given IVIG (400 mg/kg/day for 5 days without subsequent infusions); the results, however, were less dramatic. Twenty responded with significantly increased platelet counts, but in only three did platelet counts remain over 100,000/μl for at least 4 months. In the remaining 17, the platelet count returned to pre-treatment values within 1 to 4 weeks. There were no untreated controls in either study, so it is difficult to determine whether IVIG truly deferred the need for splenectomy.

Mechanisms of Action

Several mechanisms of action for the beneficial effects of IVIG in thrombocytopenia have been proposed. IVIG delays the clearance of antibody-coated autologous erythrocytes; this parallels an increase in the platelet count, suggesting a competitive blockade of reticuloendothelial Fc receptors (Nydegger and Spycher, 1986).

Platelet-associated immune globulin also decreases after successful IVIG therapy (Bussel and Baumgartner, 1984; Bussel, 1986; Ball et al., 1985), suggesting that antiplatelet antibody production is decreased by IVIG. IVIG also inhibits pokeweed mitogen (PWM)–induced B-cell differentiation, presumably by an antigen-nonspecific effect on antibody production (Stohl, 1986). Alternatively, the presence of anti-idiotypic antibodies in IVIG may successfully downregulate antibody production (Nydegger and Spycher, 1986). IVIG may also interfere with the interaction of platelets with immune complexes, antiplatelet antibodies, or both (Bussel and Baumgartner, 1984).

Other Thrombocytopenias

The success of IVIG in ITP has prompted its use in several other immunologically mediated thrombocytopenias. IVIG given to patients who are sensitized and refractory to random donor platelets prolongs the survival of exogenous platelets during episodes of active bleeding (Becton et al., 1984; Junghans and Ahn, 1984). Neonatal thrombocytopenic purpura secondary to maternal ITP and transplacental maternal antibody has been successfully reversed with IVIG (Chirico et al., 1983). IVIG given prenatally to mothers with thrombocytopenic purpura has prevented neonatal thrombocytopenic purpura in some, but not all, reports, despite attainment of normal maternal platelet counts (Davies et al., 1986).

Post-transfusion purpura has responded to IVIG (Mueller-Eckhardt et al., 1983; Berney et al., 1985), as have thrombotic thrombocytopenic purpura (Viero et al., 1986), gold-induced purpura (Goldstein et al., 1986), and isoimmune neonatal thrombocytopenia (Massey et al., 1987). Finally, IVIG has been used successfully in post-infectious thrombocytopenia—that associated with either varicella-zoster infection (DiTuro et al., 1986) or HIV infection (Ordi et al., 1986).

Rh (Anti-D) Immune Globulin

Rh (anti-D) immune globulin has also been used in the treatment of acute and chronic ITP in Rh-positive patients. Presumably, the antibody attaches to some erythrocytes (not enough to cause significant hemolysis) and the coated erythrocytes block Fc receptors—similar to the effect of IVIG (Salama and Mueller-Eckhardt, 1992). One regimen utilizes 25 μg/kg on days 1, 2, and 7; 35 μg/kg on day 14; and 55 μg/kg on day 21 and is then repeated as necessary (Andrew et al., 1992). A single dose of RhIg for intramuscular use contains 300 μg. An intravenous preparation of the antibody has been used (Andrew et al., 1992); others use the commercially available intramuscular product (Gringeri et al., 1992, Borgna-Pignatti et al., 1994). Although the intramuscular form is safe, easy, and inexpensive compared with IVIG, its use is reserved for steroid-resistant, IVIG-resistant patients with ITP and not as a first-choice agent (Blanchette et al., 1994).

Splenectomy

Splenectomy must be considered in children with ITP who have suspected intracranial hemorrhage and in those with chronic ITP. Splenectomy reverses the thrombocytopenia in over half the cases of chronic ITP (those children who are still thrombocytopenic 6 to 12 months after onset). Whenever possible, splenectomy is delayed for at least a year. In the child under age 5 years, particular effort should be made to delay splenectomy because of the risk of overwhelming infection. One should be sure that the child does not have a hereditary thrombocytopenia or a Wiskott-Aldrich variant (Weiden and Blaese, 1972). The platelet count rises promptly after splenectomy, and this is why these patients do not bleed excessively at the time of surgery. The platelet count may increase to $2 \times 10^6/\mu l$ following splenectomy. This is usually temporary and rarely leads to thrombotic complications. Patients who have previously received prednisone should be given supportive steroid therapy during and immediately after surgery.

Platelet Transfusions

Platelet transfusions are seldom indicated in acute ITP. In the child with severe bleeding, platelet concentrates provide temporary hemostasis while steroid therapy is being instituted. The usual dosage is one platelet concentrate or pack (prepared from 1 unit of fresh blood) per 5 to 6 kg of body weight. Because of the shortened life span of transfused platelets in ITP, it may be necessary to repeat this dose every 12 to 24 hours to achieve hemostasis. Patients with chronic ITP who require emergency surgical procedures may occasionally need intermittent platelet transfusions in the operative and postoperative period.

Immunosuppressive Therapy

Immunosuppressive therapy with azathioprine, cyclophosphamide, or vincristine may be considered as a last resort in the refractory patient; a successful outcome is not assured (Ahn et al., 1974; Joseph and Evans, 1982).

Neonatal Thrombocytopenic Purpura

As noted earlier, neonatal thrombocytopenia may occur as a result of the transplacental passage of specific platelet alloantibodies or maternal autoantibodies (ITP, SLE). Because the management of the thrombocytopenic infants is different for each type, a careful approach to the differential diagnosis is indicated.

Neonatal Autoimmune Thrombocytopenia. This disorder occurs in infants whose mothers have ITP or SLE. The mothers are variably thrombocytopenic, may have had a previous splenectomy, and usually show increased amounts of platelet-associated IgG (platelets and serum). The severity of the infant's thrombocytopenia is difficult to predict from maternal platelet count or platelet antibody titers; however, maternal platelet-associated IgG is predictive of affected infants (Kelton et al., 1982). Fetal scalp blood platelet counts (obtained during labor) are helpful in prediction of the infant's platelet count (Scott et al., 1980).

Neonatal Isoimmune (Alloimmune) Thrombocytopenia. This is a much less common disorder and is usually due to maternal antibodies directed against the platelet-specific antigen PLA-1. The mother's platelet count and platelet-associated IgG are normal. Her serum contains increased platelet-bindable IgG; this observation (platelet IgG normal and serum platelet-associated IgG increased) can be used to differentiate between ITP and alloimmunization (Kelton et al., 1980). Isoimmune neonatal thrombocytopenia can occur with the first pregnancy and may recur with subsequent pregnancies. If the diagnosis is suspected (severe thrombocytopenia in an otherwise healthy infant), antibody studies should be performed so that future pregnancies may be managed optimally.

Treatment. Management of both disorders includes delivery by the most atraumatic mode possible. Prenatal steroids 10 to 14 days prior to delivery in ITP mothers may be helpful in producing a higher platelet count in the newborn (Karpatkin et al., 1981). IVIG has also been given prior to delivery (Tchernia et al., 1984; Wenske et al., 1983). Close observation of the infant, including ultrasound examinations for occult hemorrhage, should be done until the platelet count reaches a safe level. Prednisone (2 to 4 mg/kg divided twice daily) administered to the infant may be helpful in raising the platelet count and decreasing the bleeding tendency (Karpatkin, 1984).

Alternatively, IVIG can be given (400 mg/kg/day for 5 days) (Chirico et al., 1983). Massey and associates (1987) treated three newborns with isoimmune thrombocytopenia with IVIG and obtained a prompt therapeutic response in all three patients.

Serious bleeding or extremely low platelet counts ($<10,000/\mu l$) are treated by (1) washed maternal platelet concentrates (or platelets from donors without the specific antigen) in alloimmune disease or (2) exchange transfusion followed by random platelets as in autoimmune thrombocytopenia.

COAGULATION FACTOR INHIBITORS

Coagulation factor inhibitors are antibodies directed against specific coagulation factors or coagulants that may produce a clinical bleeding disorder and/or an abnormality in coagulation tests. Most circulating anticoagulants that occur in children are against factor VIII or are of the "lupus" type. Rarely, inhibitors to factor IX (Berman et al., 1981) or heparin-like anticoagulants have been reported (Bussel et al., 1984).

Historical Aspects

The first non-hemophiliac with an acquired anticoagulant was described in 1940 (Lozner et al.), and a hemophiliac with an inhibitor was noted in 1941 (Lawrence and Johnson). In 1961, Margolius and coworkers presented the first comprehensive review of 40 patients with circulating anticoagulants. Since that time, acquired inhibitors to coagulation factors I, II, V, VII, VIII, IX, X, XI, and XII have been described (Margolius et al., 1961; Bidwell, 1969; Feinstein and Rapaport, 1972; Shapiro and Hultin, 1975).

Pathogenesis

Nearly all the factor VIII antibodies in children are found in classic hemophiliacs. Their incidence varies with the series and the sensitivity of the assay. In Shapiro and Hultin's (1975) review of 11 published series, the incidence of inhibitors in hemophilia A was 3.6% to 21.4%. The usual frequency was 8% to 14%. The American Cooperative Study found a prevalence rate of 14.2% in 1522 patients (Shapiro, 1984). In patients of any age with classic hemophilia, an inhibitor may develop; patients who do not have an inhibitor after 90 to 100 days of exposure to factor VIII infusions would probably not acquire the inhibitor on subsequent infusions. Antibodies to factor VIII may develop in both mild and severe hemophiliacs (Shapiro and Hultin, 1975).

As discussed by Shapiro (1984), several lines of reasoning support the concept that there is a genetic component to factor VIII inhibitor formation in hemophilia A. As already noted, patients appear destined to develop an inhibitor after a finite amount of exposure to transfused factor VIII. As discussed later, inhibitor patients tend to fall into two groups: low responders and high responders, based on their anamnestic response. Also, an increased distribution of inhibitors in sibships with hemophilia cannot be explained on chance alone. Evidence suggests possible segregation of the immune response genes with inhibitor development in hemophilia (Shapiro, 1984; Frommel et al., 1977; Mayr et al., 1984).

Diagnosis

Patients with obscure hemorrhagic diatheses and hemophiliacs who do not respond to conventional therapy should be evaluated for the presence of a coagulation inhibitor. In addition, factor VIII inhibitor determinations should be done on all severe hemophiliacs at yearly intervals. A standardized assay for factor VIII inhibitors in hemophilia has been described (Kasper et al., 1975). With this assay a unit of inhibitor is defined as that amount reducing the factor VIII content of the incubation mixture to 50% of the control in 2 hours at 37°C (Bethesda unit, BU). The assay or similar ones should be used in all hemophiliac patients.

Treatment

Patients with factor VIII inhibitors can be divided into two groups: high responders and low responders (Allain and Frommel, 1976). The high responders show a rapid and often extreme anamnestic rise in antibody titer after infusion with factor VIII material; by contast, the low responders may be infused repeatedly without marked changes in antibody affinity or titer. Because of the stimulatory effect of the factor VIII antigen on antibody production, high responder patients should not be infused with factor VIII material unless absolutely necessary. By contrast, low responders may be treated with factor VIII–containing material (cryoprecipitates or concentrates) as indicated for bleeding episodes.

An additional therapeutic measure for patients with factor VIII inhibitors is the use of prothrombin complex concentrates (PC) (Konyne, Proplex); these may halt acute bleeding episodes even though antibody titers and factor VIII levels remain unchanged (Lusher et al., 1980). These products are heat inactivated to kill HIV and other viruses. Activated prothrombin complex concentrates are also available for specific therapy of inhibitor patients (Abildgaard et al., 1980; Hilgartner et al., 1983). Rarely, the antibody titer may rise after transfusion with prothrombin-complex concentrates owing to their trace contamination with factor VIII (Kasper, 1979). Since this material may be thrombogenic, repeated or extremely high doses should be used with caution (Sullivan et al., 1984a).

For all patients with factor VIII inhibitor, conservative management, including immobilization of the bleeding joint, ice packs, and avoidance of acetylsalicylic acid and other agents that may decrease platelet function, should be instituted at the first sign of hemorrhage. Further recommendations for serious or life-threatening hemorrhage are dependent on their clinical classification.

Low Responders

For patients with persistently low inhibitor titers after infusion of factor VIII–containing material, appropriate amounts of factor VIII material should be infused in order to obtain hemostasis. Higher doses of factor VIII than usual may be necessary to neutralize the antibodies and obtain a hemostatic level of factor VIII. These patients may be candidates for *immunotherapy*.

High Responders

For patients with a strong anamnestic response to factor VIII infusions, leading to the development of high levels of inhibitors, therapy must be individualized, depending on the baseline titer of antibody.

Patients with a baseline *low titer of antibody* may be given APC (Feiba, Autoplex) or PC (Konyne, Proplex) during acute bleeding episodes without causing an anamnestic response, depending on the patient's response and the severity of the hemorrhage. The dosage for these products is 50 to 75 units/kg, given not more frequently than every 12 to 24 hours. Low antibody titers (less than 10 BU) may be overcome by large doses of factor VIII concentrate, usually given continuously (Blatt et al., 1977). In 5 days, when the anamnestic response occurs, further therapy may involve activated prothrombin complex concentrates.

Patients with a *high antibody titer* should be given APC or PC concentrates as described above. In addition, the antibody titer should be reduced to less than 5 to 10 BU by repeated plasmapheresis. Then the patient is treated with continuous factor VIII infusions, followed by APC or PC as needed (Slocombe et al., 1981; Leggett et al., 1984).

Immunosuppression and Immunotherapy

Many factor VIII inhibitor patients have been treated with corticosteroids, 6-mercaptopurine, azathioprine, or cyclophosphamide. In general, the effect of such therapy in decreasing factor VIII antibody levels and ameliorating bleeding episodes has been disappointing. Specific immunotherapy, including induction of tolerance (Stenbjerg et al., 1984) and high-dose intravenous gamma globulin (Sultan et al., 1984), has been used with initial success in a few patients. This therapy may be more effective in low responders (Hultin et al., 1976).

Acquired Inhibitors in Other Hereditary Disorders

Rarely, an antibody to the von Willebrand portion of the factor VIII molecule develops in an individual; the patient presents with a bleeding diathesis associated with decreased factor VIII activity and a prolonged bleeding time (Stableforth et al., 1976). Factor VIII–related antigen and ristocetin-induced platelet aggregation may also be reduced in these patients. Handin and coworkers (1976) described a patient with an acquired inhibitor against the von Willebrand portion of the factor VIII molecule. Factor VIII procoagulant activity and antigen were reduced but not absent, even in the presence of antibody. Multimeric analysis of von Willebrand factor revealed a selective loss of the larger forms in a patient with acquired von Willebrand disease (Meyer et al., 1979). Antibodies to von Willebrand factor that affect therapy can develop in patients with severe type 3 von Willebrand's disease following multiple transfusions (Mannucci et al., 1981).

Inhibitors may also develop in hemophiliacs with factor IX deficiency, but the incidence is much less than that seen in classic hemophilia (Shapiro and Hultin, 1975).

Lupus Anticoagulants

Lupus anticoagulants (Thiagarajan and Shapiro, 1983) are antibodies that inhibit prothrombin activation in phospholipid-dependent coagulation tests such as the partial thromboplastin times (PTT) and, rarely, the prothrombin time (PT). These inhibitors are found in patients with SLE and other conditions such as infections and after antibiotic therapy in children (Brodeur et al., 1980; Orris et al., 1980; Muntean and Petek, 1980). The lupus anticoagulant is suspected when the prolonged PTT does not correct on 1:1 mixing with normal plasma and must be differentiated from specific factor inhibitors (factors VIII, IX, XI, prothrombin) by appropriate assays. Interestingly, the lupus inhibitor does not produce a hemorrhagic diathesis but has been noted in association with deep vein thrombosis (St. Clair et al., 1981; MacKay et al., 1982). Occasionally, a child with a lupus anticoagulant also has a prolonged bleeding time as a result of associated platelet antibodies and, therefore, is prone to bleeding.

IMMUNE NEUTROPENIA

Immune neutropenic syndromes may result from alloimmunization secondary to blood transfusions or maternal-fetal incompatibility or from autoimmunity secondary to the spontaneous occurrence of leukoagglutinins not specific for known leukocyte antigens. Leukocyte antigens are of two types: (1) those shared with other tissues, i.e., HLA antigens; and (2) those present only on the neutrophil (NA1, NA2, NB1) (Lalezari and Radel, 1974). Leukoagglutinin tests, neutrophil opsonic assays, radiolabeled antiglobulin tests and fluorescein-labeled staphylococcal protein A assays have been used to detect neutrophil antibodies.

Isoimmune Neonatal Neutropenia

The clinical findings in 19 cases of isoimmune neonatal neutropenia (INN) were reviewed by Lalezari and Radel (1974). The 19 infants were seen in ten families. Most of the patients were studied after infection had resulted. Signs included skin abscesses, omphalitis, pneumonias, and sepsis. The neutropenia was severe, ranging from 1 to 1900 polymorphonuclear neutrophils (PMNs)/μl. In 12 of the infants, there was complete absence of PMNs for part of their course. Relative monocytosis was common. The bone marrow usually showed hypercellularity with an arrest at the metamyelocyte or band stage. Two infants died; the neutrophil count recovered in the remainder after 2 to 17 weeks (mean 7 weeks). The neutrophil antigen was NA1 in four families, NA2 in one family, NB1 in four families, and Vaz in one family. Corticosteroids were used in four infants, and in only one of these did they seem helpful. HLA isoimmunization as a cause for INN is doubtful because the placenta has the same HLA antigens as the fetus and absorbs the antibodies.

Blood transfusions can be associated with febrile reactions due to leukocyte agglutinins of both the HLA system and specific leukocyte antigens (Mollison, 1972). This is a familiar complication in the frequently transfused patient unless the neutrophils are removed prior to administration of the blood product.

Autoimmune Neutropenia

Several patients with autoimmune chronic neutropenia have been reported who have neutrophil antibodies apparently unrelated to alloimmunization (Boxer et al., 1975; Lalezari et al., 1975). One child had a leukocyte agglutinin with an NA2 specificity. The other five patients, ranging in age from 8 months to 72 years, had serum factors that opsonized normal neutrophils and caused them to be ingested by rabbit macrophages. In four of the patients, corticosteroids raised the neutrophil count. Using a radiolabeled antiglobulin test, Cines and colleagues (1982) demonstrated neutrophil-associated IgG in neutropenic patients with an underlying immunologic disorder (SLE, ITP, AHA, rheumatoid arthritis). In children, autoimmune neutropenia usually occurs after viral infection and is often self-limited.

Treatment

In INN, supportive care and careful attention to infections are indicated while one is waiting for the antibody to disappear. In extreme cases, transfusion of granulocytes lacking the involved antigen may be lifesaving. In autoimmune neutropenia, a cautious trial of corticosteroids should be undertaken; vincristine has been used successfully in some patients with autoimmune neutropenia (Webster et al., 1981). Intravenous immune globulin has been used successfully in a few newborns and older patients with autoimmune neutropenia (Bussel et al., 1983c; Pollack et al., 1982). The mechanism is the same as in ITP.

AUTOIMMUNE PANCYTOPENIA WITH APLASTIC ANEMIA

Autoantibodies against hematopoietic precursors occasionally cause pancytopenia, resembling aplastic anemia. The presence of such an autoantibody can be demonstrated by the growth suppression of normal hematopoietic cells following the addition of sera from the affected patients (Warkentin et al., 1980). Generation of cytotoxic T cells has also been proposed as a cause of aplastic anemia. In such cases, T cells from patients' marrow suppress the growth of normal and patients' hematopoietic cells (Shadduck et al., 1979; Nissen et al., 1980).

Pathogenesis

The possibility that acquired aplastic anemia might occur on an immune basis was suggested years ago by observations, both in experimental animal models (Simonsen, 1962) and in humans (Hathaway et al., 1965), that graft-versus-host reactions were associated with the development of bone marrow failure. Evidence of a different sort began to emerge from experience in human bone marrow transplantation. In 1974, Jeannet and coworkers reported two patients with aplastic anemia who recovered after treatment with antilymphocyte globulin (ALG) and transplantation with semi-incompatible bone marrow. Subsequent studies of red cell antigens, as well as sex chromosomes, failed to show any evidence for the engraftment of donor marrow. In 1976, two instances of recovery of autologous marrow following transplantation of allogeneic marrow and subsequent graft rejection were reported (Thomas et al., 1976; Speck et al., 1976). Other cases have been reported (Warkentin et al., 1980). Subsequently, it began to be suspected that the critical element in the recovery of these patients was immunosuppression.

Stimulated by these case reports, Ascensao and colleagues (1976) initiated studies of the effect of antithymocyte globulin (ATG) and complement on the growth in vitro of bone marrow cells of patients with aplastic anemia. Later, these investigators and others reported the results of coculture experiments wherein bone marrow cells or peripheral blood lymphocytes of patients with aplastic anemia suppressed the growth of myeloid colonies obtained from normal marrow. These studies have been comprehensively summarized (Warkentin et al., 1980).

Treatment

Although histocompatible bone marrow transplantation is the treatment of choice for severe aplastic anemia, several patients with aplastic anemia without an HLA-identical marrow donor have been successfully treated with ATG. About 50% of both children (Cairo and Baehner, 1982) and adults (Champlin et al., 1983) respond to ATG. A 50% response rate was also seen in patients treated with high-dose (20 mg/kg/day) bolus methylprednisolone (Bacigalupo et al., 1981); the response was correlated with in vitro myeloid colony formation and the presence of suppressor T cells. Thus, children with severe idiopathic aplastic anemia without a suitable sibling donor should be given a trial of immunosuppression with ATG, probably preceded by a trial of high-dose prednisone.

PRIMARY IMMUNODEFICIENCY AND AUTOIMMUNE HEMATOLOGIC DISORDERS

The association of autoimmune disease with various primary immunodeficiency diseases is now clearly recognized. Both antibody- and T cell–deficient patients may have autoimmune illness. Two groups are described: (1) antibody deficiencies and (2) T-cell and combined immunodeficiencies.

Antibody Deficiencies

Primary hypogammaglobulinemia includes IgA deficiency, common variable immunodeficiency (CVID), and X-linked agammaglobulinemia and several other syndromes (see Chapter 11).

In a study of 103 CVID patients, autoimmune diseases developed in 22% of the patients, more commonly females. ITP and AHA were the most common autoimmune diseases noted. In 11% of the patients, other family members were IgA deficient or hypogammaglobulinemic (Cunningham-Rundles, 1989). Other rheumatic diseases, including rheumatoid arthritis (RA), juvenile rheumatoid arthritis (JRA), primary biliary cirrhosis, chronic active hepatitis, sicca complex, SLE, pernicious anemia, and thyroid disease, have also been reported in patients with CVID.

In selective IgA deficiency, autoimmune diseases, such as SLE, JRA, and RA, are common (see Chapter 14). The risk for development of these autoimmune diseases for IgA-deficient patients is 10 to 20 times higher than in the general population (Klemola, 1987; Ryser et al., 1988). Autoimmune hemolytic anemia and immune thrombocytopenic purpura have been reported in patients with selective IgA deficiency, but the incidence of immunohematologic disorders does not appear to be markedly elevated.

In patients with IgG subclass deficiency, the association with autoimmune disorders is not clearly established, although anecdotal case reports have been published (Villiger et al, 1992).

Several mechanisms may explain the association of antibody deficiencies with autoimmune disorders, as described next.

Lack of Antigenic Exclusion

A lack of antibody, especially IgA, in the mucosa of the airway and gastrointestinal tract permits microbial antigens and dietary proteins to enter the circulation, thus activating the immune system. Antibodies against certain food and viral antigens are common in IgA-deficient individuals. The frequent infections in hypogammaglobulinemic patients also increase their antigen load.

Increased exposure to foreign antigen induces expression of major histocompatibility complex (MHC) class I and class II antigens on tissues secondary to the increased cytokine production, produced in response to external antigen exposure. In turn, MHC class I and II expression may provoke autoimmune responses. Local inflammatory reactions may also activate autoreactive T- and B-cell clones nonspecifically.

Entry of foreign antigens can lead to circulating immune complexes, which provoke tissue damage and initiate secondary autoimmunity (Cunningham-Rundles et al., 1979).

Stimulation of the immune system by microbial or food antigens may cause autoimmunity by molecular mimicry. If there is cross-reactivity between exogenous and autoantigens or perturbation of the idiotypic network, the antibody to the exogenous antigen may mimic or share the idiotype of an autoantibody.

Chronic polyclonal T- and B-cell activation by microbial antigens may result in the development of autoreactive lymphocytes, which results in autoimmune responses. Polyclonal T-cell activation can be induced by superantigens, which have been implicated in the pathogenesis of rheumatic diseases. Polyclonal B-cell activation often follows exposure to endotoxins (lipopolysaccharide) or Epstein-Barr virus, which may result in systemic autoimmune diseases, including AHA and ITP. As in normal individuals, autoimmune hematologic diseases in hypogammaglobulinemic patients are often preceded by viral infections.

Shared Genetic Factors

The association of autoimmune disease with certain HLA alleles is well established. The HLA-A1, -B8, -DR3 haplotype is common in IgA deficiency but is also associated with SLE, insulin-dependent diabetes mellitus (IDD), and other autoimmune diseases. A high frequency of C4A null alleles (C4A: gene coding for complement C4) and C4A and 21-hydroxylase gene deletions have been reported in both selective IgA deficiency and CVID (Schaffer et al., 1989). Systemic autoimmune diseases, such as SLE, have also been associated with C4A and C4B null alleles (Batchelor et al., 1987; Kumar et al., 1991). It is possible that genes regulating serum Ig levels, especially IgA, are located within the MHC, close to the C4 genes, and that defective expression of these genes leads to an imbalance of Ig production and autoimmunity (French and Dawkins, 1990).

Abnormality in T-Cell Regulation

A regulatory T-cell abnormality may result in both immunodeficiency and autoimmunity. For example, certain drugs, such as dilantin, that dysregulate T-cell immunity cause selective IgA deficiency and various autoimmune symptoms (Anderson and Mosekild, 1977). The CD40 ligand (gp39), expressed on the T-cell surface, is crucial for T- and B-cell interaction and regulates B-cell differentiation and isotype switching in the presence of certain cytokines (Noelle et al., 1992; Armitage et al., 1993; Roy et al., 1993). In patients with hyper-IgM syndrome, abnormalities of the gp39 (CD40 ligand) gene have been confirmed and this illness is associated with several autoimmune syndromes, particularly AHA (see Chapter 11).

T-Cell and Combined Immunodeficiencies

Patients with Wiskott-Aldrich syndrome (WAS) are at risk for autoimmune disorders. The molecular basis of WAS is not completely defined, but T cells in these patients are morphologically abnormal, and there are membrane and signal transduction abnormalities (Molina et al., 1993) (see Chapter 12).

In patients with DiGeorge anomalad, autoimmune disorders also develop, especially as the patient enters the second and third decades of life following successful heart surgery (see Chapter 12). AHA and ITP are most frequently reported in patients with WAS and DiGeorge anomalad. Autoimmunity in these patients is probably secondary to regulatory T-cell abnormalities.

SECONDARY IMMUNODEFICIENCY AND AUTOIMMUNE HEMATOLOGIC DISORDERS

An association between secondary immunodeficiency and autoimmune diseases is well exemplified by HIV infection. Thrombocytopenia is common in HIV patients, as is AHA and neutropenia. HIV-related thrombocytopenia may be related to the production of antiplatelet antibody, immune complex formation, direct viral suppression of thrombopoiesis, antiviral medication, or autoimmunity against megakaryocytes. HIV infection results in a profound imbalance of the lymphokine network, specifically T_H1 and T_H2 helper cell responses (Clerici and Shearer, 1993), causing immune dysregulation. Altered functions of antigen-presenting cells (APCs) (which also become infected by HIV through their CD4 receptors) and secondary infections with *Mycoplasma*, EBV, and cytomegalovirus (CMV) may also play a role in promoting autoimmune thrombocytopenia.

Chronic graft-versus-host disease following bone marrow transplantation is associated with autoimmune hematologic disorders, including AHA and ITP (Atkinson, 1992).

Treatment of autoimmune hematologic disorders in patients with immunodeficiencies usually consists of steroids and/or IVIG. Treatment resistance occurs more often in these patients; further, they are less capable of tolerating immunosuppressive therapy and splenectomy than normal children. The development of life-threatening autoimmune hematologic disorders should be considered as an indication for corrective marrow transplantation in suitable pediatric candidates with primary immunodeficiencies.

HEMOPHAGOCYTIC SYNDROMES

Hemophagocytic lymphohistiocytosis (HLH), a term adopted by the Histiocyte Society (Henter et al., 1991), describes a life-threatening hemodestructive syndrome occurring as a congenital disease termed familial hemophagocytic lymphohistiocytosis (FHL) (Farquhar and Claireaux, 1952) and an acquired disease termed viral- or infection-associated hemophagocytic syndrome (VAHS or IAHS) (Risdall et al., 1979).

Clinical Manifestations

Clinical manifestations include prolonged fever, failure to thrive, and hepatosplenomegaly. Laboratory features include pancytopenia, hypertriglyceridemia, and hypofibrinogenemia. The characteristic histopathologic feature is diffuse infiltration with activated non-Langerhans histocytes that are phagocytizing erythrocytes in the liver, spleen, bone marrow, lymph nodes, and brain (Fig. 27–3).

Viral and infectious syndromes (VAHS/IAHS) can occur at any age, are triggered by viral illness or other infection, and are often associated with immunosuppression, drug-induced secondary immunodeficiency, or malignancy (Zuazu et al., 1979; Risdall et al., 1984).

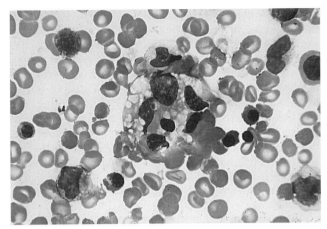

Figure 27–3. Erythrophagocytic histiocyte in hemophagocytic lymphohistiocytosis (HLH). This is the characteristic histopathologic feature of the HLH syndrome.

The familial form (FHL) generally presents in previously well infants who have a family history of hemophagocytic disease. The inheritance pattern suggests an autosomal recessive disorder (Gencik et al., 1984). Distinguishing the familial syndrome from the secondary form in a young child without a predisposing factor or family history is difficult. Infants born with HLH symptoms have been reported (Parker et al., 1989).

Diagnosis

Because there is no specific diagnostic test for HLH, guidelines have been proposed by the FHL working group of the Histiocyte Society, based on clinical features with histologic and laboratory supporting data (Table 27–3). The sine qua non is the demonstration of a benign, non-Langerhans histiocytosis associated

---

Table 27–3. Diagnostic Guidelines for Hemophagocytic Lymphohistiocytosis (HLH) and Familial Hemophagocytic Lymphohistiocytosis (FHL)

Clinical and Laboratory Criteria

Fever (≥7 days' duration 38.5°C)
Splenomegaly (≥3 cm below costal margin)
Cytopenia (≥2 of 3 lineages in peripheral blood and not caused by a hypocellular or dysplastic bone marrow):
    Hemoglobin (<9.0 g/dl)
    Platelets (<100,000/μl)
    Neutrophils (<1000/μl)
Hypertriglyceridemia and/or hypofibrinogenemia
    Fasting triglycerides ≥3 SD above the normal average for age
    Fibrinogen ≤3 SD below normal

Histologic Criteria

Hemophagocytosis* in
    Bone marrow
    Spleen
    Lymph node
No evidence of malignancy

Diagnose HLH if above criteria are present. The diagnosis is FHL/HLH if there *also* is a family history of HLH. Parental consanguinity strongly suggests a diagnosis of FHL/HLH.

*If hemophagocytic activity is not found at presentation, a continued search for hemophagocytosis is indicated (spleen, lymph nodes, serial bone marrows).

As proposed by Henter JI, et al. Diagnostic guidelines for hemophagocytic lymphohistiocytosis. Semin Oncol 18:29–33, 1991.

with hemophagocytosis. The bone marrow is the easiest site for a biopsy specimen, but initial marrow examination may show little histiocytic infiltrate or active hemophagocytosis. In most cases, repeated biopsy findings show increasing numbers of histiocytes and hemophagocytosis. This is also true of liver and lymph node biopsies. Lack of a positive biopsy result does not rule out the diagnosis.

Radiographic evaluation of the central nervous system (CNS) is helpful in monitoring patients with HLH. In a retrospective evaluation of magnetic resonance imaging (MRI) and computed tomography (CT) studies of 12 consecutive patients with HLH, nonfocal parenchymal volume loss was the most common finding in addition to intracerebral and intraventricular hemorrhages, areas of infarction, and diffuse increase in white matter signal on T2-weighted images. Although these changes are nonspecific, their presence is consistent with the diagnosis of HLH. Because of better definition of white matter changes, an MRI scan may be preferred for the evaluation and monitoring of CNS involvement in HLH (Fig. 27–4).

Pathogenesis

It is currently believed that HLH represents an exaggerated immune response that fails normal regulatory control mechanisms (Stark et al., 1987). Hemophagocytosis progressively destroys the bone marrow, while the lymphohistiocytic infiltrates compromise other vital organs and often lead to death. The immune dysregulation may be primary, as in the inherited FHL, or secondary, as in VAHS/IAHS. In malignancy-associated HLH, tumor-derived factors have been identified that suppress normal immune responses or stimulate hemophagocytosis (Jaffe et al., 1983).

Persistent T-cell activation with overproduction of cytokines may contribute to the pathophysiology of HLH. Patients with active disease have evidence of T-cell activation, including MHC class II expression by T cells, elevated serum soluble interleukin-2 (IL-2) receptors (Komp et al., 1989), elevated soluble CD8 (Henter et al., 1991), and elevated neopterin levels (Howells et al., 1990; Henter and Elinder, 1992). Inflammatory cytokines such as serum interferon-γ, IL-6, and tumor necrosis factor are also elevated and often correlate with disease activity (Holtman et al., 1982).

The most consistent immunologic abnormality described in HLH is impaired natural killer (NK) function (Perez et al., 1984; Arico et al., 1988; Eife et al., 1989; Kataoka et al., 1990). NK cell numbers and phenotype are usually normal (McClain et al., 1988). In patients with Chédiak-Higashi syndrome, a congenital immunodeficiency that includes impaired NK function, a fatal hemophagocytic process frequently develops in response to EBV infection, which is clinically indistinguishable from HLH (Ladisch et al., 1976). Some patients with HLH may recover NK function when in remission (Arico et al., 1988), which suggests that this is a secondary and not a primary immunologic abnormality. Cytotoxic T-cell function, lymphokine-activated killer (LAK) cell function, and antibody-mediated cellular cytotoxicity are also decreased (McClain et al., 1988; Ladisch et al., 1976).

Treatment

HLH is difficult to treat and is usually fatal. VAHS/IAHS has a better prognosis, and there are occasional

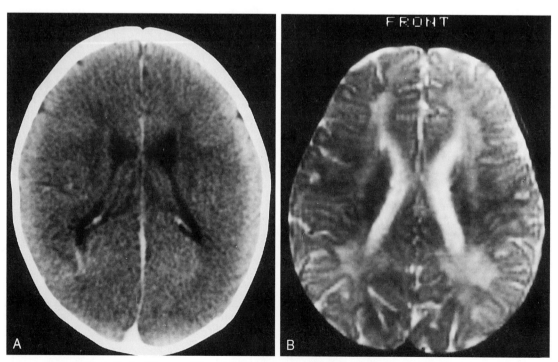

Figure 27–4. Brain CT scan *(A)* and MRI scan *(B)* of patient with HLH. MRI is preferable for radiographic CNS evaluation because it provides better definition of white matter changes.

survivors, especially when the immunodeficient state can be reversed. Of 121 cases of HLH reviewed in 1983, only four long-term survivors were identified (Janka, 1983). Clinical and laboratory remissions were first reported in 1980 using etoposide (VP16–324) (Ambruso et al., 1980). Other podophyllotoxin derivatives, such as teniposide (VM26), also are effective (Henter et al., 1986), although responses to other therapies have been described (Ladisch et al., 1982; Fischer et al., 1985; Alvarado et al., 1986; Becton et al., 1987; Henter and Elinder, 1991); however, podophyllotoxins remain the most effective drugs to induce remission (Blanche et al., 1991). Treatment of CNS disease utilizes intrathecal methotrexate; there are responses to thiotepa, cytosine arabinoside, steroids, and irradiation as well (Alvarado et al., 1986; Blanche et al., 1991).

Maintenance is achieved by repeated dosing with VP-16. Concern has been raised regarding the risk of secondary acute myelocytic leukemia (AML) following extended administration of podophyllotoxins for treatment of childhood malignancies (Fischer et al., 1985; Pui et al., 1989, 1990). Immunosuppressive therapy consisting of prednisone, cyclosporine, and intermittent intrathecal methotrexate has been successful in maintaining clinical and laboratory remission (Loechelt et al., 1994). Bone marrow transplantation is curative (Blanche et al., 1991; Stephan et al., 1993). A report of success with antithymocyte globulin, steroids, and cyclosporine offers support for the use of immunosuppressive rather than myeloablative therapy (Stephan et al., 1993).

A successful outcome with bone marrow transplantation is more likely if the patient is in remission and if the donor is an HLA-matched sibling. Because most children with FHL lack HLA-matched sibling donors, use of closely matched unrelated donors as an alternative marrow source is being explored with early success (Filipovich et al., 1994). Bone marrow transplantation for patients with active disease or from haploidentical or mismatched donors has been disappointing.

EPSTEIN-BARR VIRUS–ASSOCIATED DISORDERS

Epstein-Barr virus is one of eight known DNA viruses belonging to the human herpesvirus family. The only natural host for the virus is a human, although a few species of New World primates are infectable (Miller et al., 1977). In developing countries, more than 90% of the population is infected before age 2 years (Levy and Henle, 1968). In industrialized countries, such as the United States, only 25% to 40% of children are infected by age 2, but up to 75% to 90% of individuals are infected by age 25 (Evans et al., 1968).

Generally, a person is exposed by salivary contact with a virus-shedding host (Morgan et al., 1979), although infections from blood transfusions (Straus and Fleisher, 1989), organ transplants (Cen et al., 1991), or bone marrow (Gratama et al., 1992) have occurred. Perinatal infection is not thought to occur, despite a

few anecdotal reports (Goldberg et al., 1981). In children, primary EBV infection is usually asymptomatic, but if it occurs during adolescence or later in life, infectious mononucleosis (IM) is the most frequent manifestation.

EBV has been associated with several malignancies: Burkitt's lymphoma (BL), other lymphomas (including Hodgkin's disease), and nasopharyngeal carcinoma.

EBV infection in the immunocompromised host may pose additional problems. In HIV-infected children, EBV infection has been associated with lymphoid interstitial pneumonitis (Katz et al., 1992), CNS disease, and B-cell lymphoma (Cohen, 1991; Del Mistro et al., 1990). Individuals affected with certain primary immunodeficiencies are at increased risk for an EBV-associated lymphoproliferative disorder or "lymphoma" (see later). A rare X-linked defect results in an ineffective response to EBV infection, resulting in a rapidly fatal course of IM (Purtilo, 1991) (see Chapter 12).

Infectious Mononucleosis

Henle and colleagues (1968) made the critical observation that a technician in their laboratory seroconverted for EBV, while suffering from infectious mononucleosis (IM). IM is usually a self-limited syndrome characterized by the clinical triad of fever, pharyngitis, and generalized adenopathy, with an atypical lymphocytosis (>20%) and presence of heterophile antibodies (HA) (Henle and Henle, 1979b). EBV causes about 90% of such cases, with cytomegalovirus, toxoplasmosis, human herpesvirus type 6, and acute HIV infections the leading causes of the remainder of cases (Straus, 1992). Usually, IM occurs only once in a lifetime, but recurrences have been reported (Bender, 1962; Change and Maddow, 1980), and exacerbations of unresolved infection or transition to a chronic course may occur (Straus, 1992).

Pathogenesis

Following salivary exposure to an individual shedding virus, the virus appears to infect cells through the complement C3d receptor (CR2, CD21) (Fingeroth et al., 1984), which is expressed on B lymphocytes, and epithelium of the oral and nasopharynx (Sixby et al., 1987). Viral replication occurs in the oropharyngeal epithelial cells, and, presumably, released virions infect B lymphocytes in the lymphoid tissue of Waldeyer's ring. The incubation period is generally thought to be 4 to 6 weeks; during that time, increased numbers of B lymphocytes are infected, disseminate throughout the body, and proliferate in the germinal centers of lymph nodes as well as the spleen and sinusoidal and periportal areas of the liver (Downey and Stasney, 1936; Henle and Henle, 1979a).

In response to this proliferation and dissemination of infected B lymphocytes, there is a well-orchestrated immune response consisting of humoral responses (Henle and Henle, 1979a), antibody-dependent cellular cytotoxicity (Pearson and Orr, 1984), NK activity (Blazar et al., 1980), and cytokine production (IFN-α and IFN-γ) (Kure et al., 1986; Magrath et al., 1991); however, T lymphocytes predominate, mainly suppressor cytotoxic CD8$^+$ cells. These CD8$^+$ lymphocytes account for the majority of the cells in the lymphocytosis of IM (Horwitz et al., 1981; Tomkinson et al., 1987). These cells are highly activated, evidenced by elevated serum levels of soluble IL-2 receptors and soluble CD8 (Tomkinson et al., 1987). The large, pleomorphic, atypical lymphocytes *(Downey cells)* characteristic of IM (Kumar et al., 1991) are cytotoxic to EBV-positive lymphoblastoid lines in vitro (Hutt et al., 1975; Royston et al., 1975; Svedmyr and Jondal, 1975). However, immunologic and cytochemical studies suggest that most are activated suppressor cells that inhibit B-lymphocyte proliferation (Tosato et al., 1979; Hirt et al., 1981; Way et al., 1986).

This oligoclonal T-cell response may be stimulated through a superantigen effect (Smith et al., 1993). In this response, all T cells expressing a specific variable region of the beta chain of the T-cell receptor complex are stimulated without presensitization. How EBV triggers such a response in not known. Thus, the symptoms of IM can be largely attributed to T-cell activation with release of inflammatory cytokines rather than an effect of proliferating EBV-infected B lymphocytes.

As with other herpesviruses, an infected individual carries the virus for life. Viral replication and shedding into salivary secretions are present in at least 15% of seropositive people at any given time (Gerber et al., 1972). An estimated 10^5 to 10^6 latently infected B lymphocytes can be found in the peripheral blood, lymph nodes, and bone marrow of a seropositive individual (Tosato et al., 1984). EBV latently infected B cells can undergo spontaneous transformation in vitro and be established into immortal lymphoblastoid cell lines (Nilsson et al., 1971). How the body maintains latency without uncontrolled B-cell proliferation is uncertain. Though anti-EBV antibodies persist for life, it is believed that cytotoxic memory T cells are critical in controlling latent infection (Klein et al., 1981; Moss et al., 1981).

Infectious mononucleosis is a disease of adolescents and young adults and is present almost exclusively in higher socioeconomic classes in developed countries. The conditions of crowding and poverty in underdeveloped countries predispose to early infection (Henle and Henle, 1970). Why younger children do not experience the symptoms of IM following primary EBV infection is not known, but it does suggest that the massive response seen during IM is not essential for controlling primary infection and viral latency.

Clinical Manifestations

In infants or young children, primary EBV infection is either subclinical or associated with upper respiratory tract symptoms and rashes (Henle and Henle, 1970). Classically, IM first presents with a prodrome of malaise, fever, and headache and is often associated with an exudate. Generalized adenopathy and hepatosplenomegaly are characteristic. The duration and se-

verity of symptoms are variable, but they usually resolve in 2 to 8 weeks. Laboratory findings include a relative lymphocytosis (total leukocyte count can be decreased, increased, or normal), abnormal liver function tests, and positive tests for heterophil antibody and EBV-specific antibody (Henle and Henle, 1979a, 1979b; Sumaya and Ench, 1986).

Complications

Complications occur frequently but are rarely serious. Skin rashes are common, especially following administration of ampicillin and, less frequently, other penicillins. Hematopoietic complications may include anemia, autoimmunity, viral marrow suppression (Worlledge and Dacie, 1969), and the virus-associated hemophagocytic syndrome (VAHS) (Risdall et al., 1979; Wilson et al., 1981). Neutropenia and thrombocytopenia has been reported, especially in young children (Henle and Henle, 1970), or with the VAHS syndrome. Hepatitis with elevated liver enzymes is almost universal, but clinical jaundice occurs in only 25% of patients. Splenomegaly with splenic rupture is potentially life-threatening; however, it is extremely rare (1:1000 to 2000) (Bartley et al., 1989).

A variety of neurologic disorders have been associated with IM, including meningoencephalitis, Guillain-Barré syndrome, Bell's palsy, and cerebellar ataxia (Grose et al., 1975). Ophthalmologic complications (e.g., oculoglandular syndrome, conjunctivitis, keratitis, and uveitis) can occur in up to 40% of IM cases (Tanner, 1952; Matoba, 1990). Carditis, arthritis, nephritis, and pneumonitis have all been documented in IM (Bartley et al., 1989); all are probably associated with transient immune dysfunction.

Laboratory Findings

Heterophil Antibodies

Heterophil antibodies (HAs) are IgM antibodies formed in response to infection with one species, but they combine with antigens from a second unrelated species (Carter and Penman, 1969). During the course of infectious mononucleosis, many heterophil antibodies unrelated to EBV appear; among them the Paul-Bunnell-Davidsohn heterophil antibody is highly specific for IM (Paul and Bonnell, 1932). This antibody agglutinates sheep erythrocytes (SRBCs) or horse erythrocytes; its ability to agglutinate SRBC is absorbed by bovine erythrocytes but is not absorbed by Forssman antigen, a substance found in RBCs and tissue cells of many species (Davidsohn and Walker, 1935). Low levels of antibodies to SRBC occur in many normal individuals. Higher levels (i.e., ≥1:56) appear in a variety of acute illnesses (Schultz, 1948), but these do not show the absorption pattern characteristic of IM; the SRBC agglutinins are not absorbed by Forssman antigen (Davidsohn and Lee, 1969).

Paul-Bunnell HA arises in most cases of EBV-induced IM but not in other viral illnesses characterized by atypical lymphocytosis, such as cytomegalovirus infection, adenovirus infection, or hepatitis. Furthermore, heterophil is often absent in infants and toddlers (Horwitz et al., 1981). Although HA is specific for primary EBV infection, it has not been possible to demonstrate any antigens on the surface of EBV-containing lymphoblastoid cells that cross-react with SRBC or heterophil antigens, nor is there any interaction between heterophil antibody and EBV lymphoblastoid cells lines in vitro (Henle et al., 1974b). The antigenic stimulus for HA production is unknown.

Epstein-Barr Virus–Specific Antibodies

Many EBV-specific antibodies have been described during the acute and convalescent phases of IM (Henle et al., 1974a). After primary EBV infection in the immunologically normal host, the levels of antibodies rise and fall or rise but remain within a fairly narrow range of titers. The antibodies are directed against antigens on the surface of the virus particle itself, against EBV-related antigens that appear on the cell surfaces or within the nuclei of lymphoblastoid cell lines, or against virally coded cellular proteins. The majority of antibodies are measured by direct or indirect immunofluorescence (Henle et al., 1974a, 1974b). Those antibodies used routinely to diagnose acute IM are represented in Figure 27–5 and are described next.

The EBV-specific antibodies used clinically are:

- IgG and IgM to the viral capsid antigen (VCA)
- IgG to the early antigen (EA)
- IgG to the Epstein-Barr virus nuclear antigen (EBNA)

Anti-VCA IgM is the first detectable EBV-specific antibody produced following EBV infection and is present during acute IM or occasionally during viral reactivation. Anti-VCA IgG is also detectable early in the course of IM, and both IgG and IgM to VCA are often present by the time a person seeks medical attention. Anti-VCA IgG usually peaks 1 to 2 months into the clinical illness and then gradually falls off, but it persists for life.

Anti-EA shows two distinct staining patterns: diffuse (D), appearing during acute IM and viral reactivation; and restricted (R), which occurs more often in young children and immunocompromised individuals.

Anti-EBNA IgG rises slowly over 1 to 2 years; most normal individuals have detectable IgG to EBNA by 6 months following EBV infection, and anti-EBNA antibodies persist for life. In the immunocompromised patient, a different pattern is present: anti-VCA IgG titers are greatly elevated, EA titers may persist, and anti-EBNA titers are low or often absent (Morgan, 1991), suggesting a lack of normal true convalescence.

Other Antibodies

Wasserman antibody, rheumatoid factor, antinuclear antibody, leukoagglutinins, anti-thyroid antibodies, and antibodies to mitochondria, lymphocyte surface antigens, and liver nuclei also appear in some cases of IM (Carter and Penman, 1969). The antigenic stimulus for these antibodies in IM is not known. These antibodies may all be heterophils, for which the cross-reacting antigenic stimulus has yet to be discovered. Alternatively, as with anti-SRBC and anti-i antibodies, some of these antibodies may be present at undetectable levels prior to IM. Then, since EBV is a polyclonal B-cell mitogen, the proliferation of antibody-producing B cells proportionately increases the amount of antibodies to measurable levels. All classes of immunoglobulins, in fact, do increase during early IM (MacKinney, 1968): rises of IgM to 300%, IgA to 130%, and IgG to 170% of normal are found in the first 3 weeks of illness (Wollheim, 1969).

Atypical Lymphocytes

Atypical lymphocytes are large fragile pleomorphic mononuclear cells. Although atypical lymphocytes are one of the classic hallmarks of IM, they are also seen in cytomegalovirus infection, rubella, hepatitis, and toxoplasmosis. They are seen in young children with IM even in the absence of symptoms or heterophil antibody (Horwitz et al., 1981). Early in the course of IM, both B- and T-lymphocytes are found among the atypical lymphocytes (Denman and Pelton, 1974; Enberg et al., 1974; Magni et al., 1974). Later in the illness, the majority of atypical lymphocytes form rosettes with sheep erythrocytes (Sheldon et al., 1973),

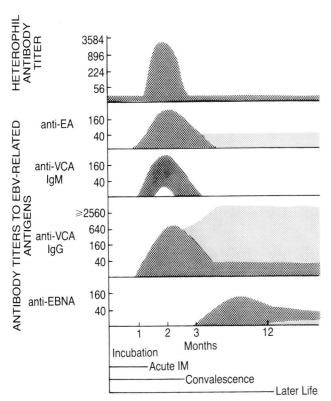

Figure 27–5. Laboratory findings during and after infectious mononucleosis (IM). The densely hatched areas include the ranges of antibody found in the normal host; the finely hatched areas define the ranges of antibody seen in compromised hosts. EBV = Epstein-Barr virus; EA = early antigen; VCA = viral capsid antigen; EBNA = Epstein-Barr nuclear antigen. (Adapted in part from Henle W, et al. Epstein-Barr virus–specific diagnostic tests in infectious mononucleosis. Hum Pathol 5:551–565, 1974.)

have human T-specific surface antigens (Pattengale et al., 1974), and thus appear to be T cells.

In vitro, the atypical lymphocytes are cytotoxic to lymphoblastoid cells that contain the EBV genome but not to cell lines that are EBV-negative (Hutt et al., 1975; Royston et al., 1975; Svedmyr and Jondal, 1975). Thus, in vitro, atypical lymphocytes are engaged in the destruction of cells that are either infected with or are transformed by EBV. Immunologic, cytochemical, and cytokinetic studies of patients' cells show that most atypical lymphocytes are activated suppressor cells; a minority are proliferating helper cells (Hirt et al., 1981). The suppressor cells inhibit B-lymphocyte proliferation (Tosato et al., 1979).

Cell-Mediated Immunity

Defects in cell-mediated immunity (CMI) have been recognized in IM. Cutaneous anergy to tuberculin (Haider et al., 1973), *Candida,* and streptokinase-streptodornase (Magni et al., 1974) appear during acute IM and resolve during convalescence. Peripheral blood lymphocytes respond poorly to stimulation with plant mitogens (Sheldon et al., 1973) and in mixed leukocyte cultures (Twomey, 1974) but return to normal levels within 3 to 5 weeks (Pattengale et al., 1974; Twomey, 1974). The unstimulated lymphocytes show substantial increases in spontaneous DNA synthesis, which subsides at the time mitogen-induced increases in DNA synthesis returns (Pattengale et al., 1974). Migration inhibition of leukocytes in the presence of EBV antigen is defective during IM, but adults who have had past IM demonstrate normal migration inhibition (Lai et al., 1974). On the other hand, T-cell-mediated killing of EBV-containing lymphoblasts is enhanced during IM (Svedmyr and Jondal, 1975; Hutt et al., 1975). The defects in cell-mediated immunity that occur in IM are thought to be an indirect consequence of excessive suppressor T-cell activity. The suppressor T cells limit primary EBV infection and prevent overgrowth of EBV-transformed B lymphocytes (Tosato et al., 1979; Haynes et al., 1979; Hirt et al., 1981).

In patients with chronic EBV infection, there is persistence of alterations in T-cell function that occurs transiently in patients with acute IM. Among persistent defects are depressed IL-2 and interferon production after mitogen stimulation and reduced natural killing of fractionated mononuclear leukocytes (Kibler et al., 1985).

Treatment

Infectious mononucleosis is usually self-limited, and no specific treatment is required. Corticosteroids have been used for life-threatening complications, such as airway obstruction, carditis, or cerebral edema. Their efficacy is largely anecdotal and presumably a result of their anti-inflammatory and lympholytic properties. Double-blind controlled studies of steroid treatment suggest a decreased duration of fever and pharyngitis using corticosteroids (Bender, 1967). However, there is a reluctance to use steroids during a viral infection for fear of predisposing to additional complications.

EBV is exquisitely sensitive to acyclovir in vitro (Colby et al., 1980). Trials of acyclovir in the treatment of IM have demonstrated a complete but transient inhibition of oropharyngeal viral replication and shedding (Sullivan et al., 1984b; Andersson et al., 1986). A study using the combination of acyclovir plus corticosteroids in patients with severe symptoms of IM reported dramatic improvement of fever and oropharyngeal symptoms but no effect on the hepatitis (Sullivan et al., 1984b).

A viral protein vaccine has been developed that protects marmosets from the development of lymphoproliferative disease (Morgan, 1991), and human clinical trials may begin soon. However, the utility for the vaccine in prevention of IM is controversial, although it may be beneficial in endemic areas of Burkitt's lymphoma or nasopharyngeal carcinoma.

Chronic Fatigue Syndrome

Chronic EBV infections (CEBVs) are rare and should be differentiated from chronic mononucleosis or the *chronic fatigue syndrome* (CFS). CFS is characterized by recurrent fever, persistent hepatosplenomegaly, hematologic abnormalities, myalgias, headaches, and often debilitating fatigue (Holmes et al., 1988). Because of the similar symptoms and early reports of elevated anti-VCA and EA titers, EBV was thought to be the etiologic agent in CFS (Jones et al., 1985). In controlled studies, no specific pattern of EBV serologies differentiates patients with CFS from controls (Holmes et al., 1987). CFS has been associated with other infections (viral and bacterial), and therefore should not be considered a disease caused by EBV. Suggested early criteria for the diagnosis of CFS are outlined in Table 27–4.

A new working definition of CFS has been developed recently to aid in both diagnosis and further studies (Fukuda et al., 1994). This definition includes:

1. Self-reported, and fully evaluated, persistent,

Table 27–4. Original Chronic Fatigue Syndrome: Diagnostic Criteria (1988)*

Major Criteria
1. Persistent or relapsing fatigue
   a. >6 months in duration
   b. Impairs daily activity to <50%
2. Exclusion of other clinical conditions that may produce similar symptoms

Minor Criteria
1. Mild fever
2. Pharyngitis
3. Painful cervical or axillary adenopathy
4. Generalized weakness
5. Myalgias
6. Prolonged fatigue (>24 hours)
7. Generalized headaches
8. Migratory arthralgias
9. Neuropsychologic complaints (photophobia, forgetfulness, irritability, confusion, inability to concentrate, depression)
10. Sleep disturbance

Note: The patient must fulfill major criteria and six of the minor criteria.
*A simplified definition has recently been proposed; see text.
Modified from Holmes GP, Kaplan JE, Glantz NM. Chronic fatigue syndrome: a working case definition. Ann Intern Med 108:387–389, 1988. Reproduced with permission.

or relapsing fatigue lasting 6 or more consecutive months and causing significant impairment of normal activities, not resolving with bed rest.

2. Concurrent occurrence of four or more of the following symptoms, all of which must have persisted or recurred during six or more consecutive months of illness and must not have predated the fatigue:

a. Self-reported impairment in short term memory or concentration contributing to inability to perform daily tasks.

b. Sore throat.

c. Tender cervical or axillary lymph nodes.

d. Muscle pain or polyarthralgia.

e. Headaches of a new type, pattern, or severity.

f. Unrefreshing sleep.

g. Postexertional malaise lasting more than 24 hours.

Treatment

Therapy for chronic fatigue syndrome is controversial. In a placebo-controlled trial of acyclovir, clinical improvement was seen as frequently with the placebo (Straus et al., 1988).

Chronic Epstein-Barr Virus Infection

There are only rare instances in which patients do not experience resolution of their IM symptoms. Patients with true chronic or progressive EBV infections have been reported to have immunologic abnormalities, such as deficient NK cell activity (Joncas et al., 1989), decreased or absent EBNA antibodies, and elevated titers of anti-VCA and anti-EA (Okano et al., 1988). However, specific immunologic abnormalities have not been identified. These infections are more likely to occur in children and young adults (Okano et al., 1991). These patients can experience life-threatening complications, including B- and T-cell lymphoproliferative diseases (Alfiere and Loncas, 1987; Jones et al., 1988; Kikuta et al., 1988; Okano et al., 1991). The diagnosis of progressive or chronic EBV is difficult; suggested criteria are shown in Table 27–5.

Mechanisms responsible for chronic EBV infections are unclear. The magnitude of the EBV antibody response to antigens of the replicative cycle of the virus (e.g., VCA and EA) suggests uncontrolled EBV replication. A defective nontransforming strain of EBV has been detected in some of these patients (Straus, 1992). Chronic infection with adenovirus type 2 has also been reported (Okano et al., 1990b); the adenovirus may stimulate EBV in latently infected cells to undergo viral replication. Since EBV replication results in cell lysis, this does not explain the associated lymphoproliferation of chronic EBV. Chronic infection with EBV may occur when there is a deficiency in the immune response, which allows a dysregulated state of viral latency with increased viral replication and/or uncontrolled cellular proliferation.

Treatment

In chronic EBV as in other EBV-related disease, antiviral therapy (i.e., acyclovir) has not provided signifi-

Table 27–5. Progressive or Chronic Epstein-Barr Virus (EBV) Infections: Suggested Diagnostic Criteria

---

Evidence of Severe, Progressive EBV Illness

1. Began as a primary EBV infection, or fourfold or greater increase in EBV specific antibody titers

2. IgG anti-VCA ≥1:5120, anti-EA ≥1:640, and/or anti-EBNA <1:2, greater than 6 months following primary EBV infection

and/or

Histologic Evidence of Major Organ Involvement by EBV

1. Organ involvement
   a. Persistent lymphadenopathy
   b. Persistent hepatitis
   c. Splenomegaly
   d. Interstitial pneumonitis
   e. Hypoplasia of one or more cell lineage of the bone marrow

2. Detection of EBV in affected tissues
   a. Immunofluorescence staining for EBNA
   b. Immunoperoxidase staining with monoclonal antibodies for EBV specific proteins, i.e., LMP* or EBNA-2†
   c. In situ hybridization for EBERs‡

---

*Latent membrane protein.
†EBV nuclear antigen.
‡EBV early RNAs.
Data from the New England Journal of Medicine. Straus SE, et al. Acyclovir treatment of the chronic fatigue syndrome: lack of efficacy in a placebo-controlled trial. 319:1692–1698, 1988.

cant benefit (Okano et al., 1990a, 1991). The newer antiviral agents ganciclovir and foscarnet may be more efficacious. However, the most encouraging results utilize immunomodulating therapies. Transient improvement using IL-2 has been reported (Kawa-Ha et al., 1987); one patient achieved a clinical remission with restoration of normal NK activity. Further understanding of the factors (e.g., immunologic deficits) that predispose to such infections may lead to better therapeutic strategies.

X-Linked Lymphoproliferative Syndrome

Some males carry an X-linked recessive gene that renders them exquisitely vulnerable to life-threatening complications of EBV infections (Bar et al., 1974; Provisor et al., 1975) (see Chapters 12 and 16). In 1975, Purtilo described a family with three brothers and three additional maternally related males who died of complications of EBV infection (Purtilo et al., 1975). The syndrome originally carried the name of the kindred, "Duncan disease." X-linked lymphoproliferative syndrome (XLP) is now recognized by the World Health Organization (WHO) as a primary deficiency.

Diagnosis

Purtilo suggested that the diagnosis of XLP requires two or more maternally related males demonstrating one or more of the classic phenotypes (fatal IM, malignant lymphoma, agammaglobulinemia or hypogammaglobulinemia, aplastic anemia) following EBV infection (Purtilo et al., 1977; Purtilo and Grierson, 1991). The defective gene has been localized to the long arm of the X chromosome, Xq25–26 (Skare et al., 1987). XLP is rare and is probably underdiagnosed because of the inability to make a definitive diagnosis in families with only a single male exhibiting the phenotype. The estimated incidence worldwide is approximately 1 per million males (Purtilo, 1981).

The diagnosis of additional XLP males and female carriers in a known affected kindred is now possible by restriction fragment–linked polymorphism (RFLP) linkage analysis. Until the gene is cloned, definitive diagnosis of XLP must rely on clinical criteria, but a presumptive diagnosis may be made with certain history and laboratory findings (Table 27–6).

Until an affected person encounters EBV, there are no consistent clinical or laboratory abnormalities that define XLP (Sullivan et al., 1983). In some, subtle abnormalities of the immune system have been noted. Unusual infections (e.g., vaccinia following smallpox vaccination and pneumonitis following measles vaccination) have been reported in affected males prior to EBV infection. A failure to switch from IgM to IgG upon secondary challenge with bacteriophage ϕX174 has been reported (Ochs et al., 1983; Sullivan et al., 1984b). A study comparing 13 RFLP-positive, EBV-negative XLP males with 14 RFLP-positive, EBV-positive males demonstrated that all XLP genotypic males had elevated IgA or IgM and/or deficient IgG (IgG1 and/or IgG3) (Grierson et al., 1991). Although suggestive, these findings are not diagnostic for XLP.

Unlike the normal immune response that leads to resolution of symptoms and lifetime control of latently infected B cells, patients with XLP generate a vigorous immune response to EBV that may result in fatal IM. A "triphasic" process develops in the marrow of these patients (Purtilo, 1991). Initially, the leukocyte count is elevated with atypical lymphocytes and a hyperplastic marrow. Pancytopenia develops as the marrow shows extensive infiltration by lymphoid cells and erythrophagocytosis by histiocytes. Terminally, the marrow shows massive necrosis, cellular depletion, and marked histiocytic hemophagocytosis (Mroczek et al., 1987). Similar reactions probably occur in other organs—e.g., liver, spleen, lungs, brain, and lymph nodes. The lymphocytic infiltration is composed of polyclonal EBV-positive B cells and activated T cells, both CD8+ and CD4+. The T lymphocytes, activated by proliferating B cells, secrete cytokines that activate macrophages. This process is similar to IM, but the response is uncontrolled, leading to a total clinical course indistinguishable from HLH.

Clinical Manifestations and Prognosis

The prognosis for patients with XLP has been extremely poor; 70% have died (60% before the age of 10 years), and no one has lived past 40 years of age (Purtilo et al., 1991). The mean age of fatal IM is 2.5 years, with death occurring within months of onset. One third of patients survive but ultimately die of immunodeficiency, bone marrow failure, or lymphoma.

About a third of patients with XLP present with hypogammaglobulinemia prior to infection with EBV (Sullivan et al., 1983). In addition, hyper-IgM, hyper-IgA, lymphoid vasculitis, or granulomatosis may develop (Mroczek et al., 1987; Purtilo et al., 1991; Loeffel et al., 1985). Occasionally, XLP presents as malignant lymphoma, but usually this is seen in long-term survivors (Harrington et al., 1987). These lymphomas are generally high-grade B-cell lymphomas that present in extranodal sites. True Burkitt's lymphoma has been reported, but it is rare. Agammaglobulinemia or aplastic anemia can also be the presenting manifestation, although these occur more commonly in long-term survivors (Purtilo et al., 1977).

Long-term survivors of XLP invariably demonstrate cellular and humoral immune deficits after EBV infections. One third of patients become hypogammaglobulinemic, and one third become agammaglobulinemic (Grierson et al., 1991). Patients have deficient antibody responses to VCA and EA and make no antibody response to EBNA (Sakamoto et al., 1981). Caution is needed when one is using these diagnostic criteria because anti-EBNA is produced slowly in the normal individual. Most normal subjects have anti-EBNA by 6 months after infection, but a delay of up to 3 years in normal children has been reported (Sumaya, 1986). Patients with XLP also display decreased NK activity and cytotoxic T-cell function following EBV infection (Harada et al., 1982).

Treatment

Prevention of EBV infection seems a reasonable and rational approach to treating XLP. IVIG prophylaxis to prevent or lessen the effect of EBV infection has been used in individuals with XLP who had been diagnosed prior to EBV infection. Patients have died of IM while receiving prophylactic IVIG; thus, its benefit is uncertain (Okano et al., 1990a). Patients with XLP may be excellent candidates for an EBV vaccine, if they are capable of producing neutralizing antibodies. However, the stimulus for T-cell activation is unknown, and the

---

Table 27–6. Diagnostic Criteria for X-Linked Lymphoproliferative (XLP) Disease

Definitive Diagnosis
1. Two or more maternally related males manifesting XLP phenotype(s) associated with EBV infection
   or
2. A maternally related male in an XLP family who has strong genetic (RFLP) linkage to the XLP locus

XLP Phenotypes
Fatal infectious mononucleosis
Hypo- or agammaglobulinemia
Malignant lymphoma (usually B-cell, non-Hodgkin's lymphoma)
Aplastic anemia

Presumptive Diagnosis
XLP phenotype in a male following EBV infection with:
1. Absent or low titer anti-EBNA response
   and
2. IgG subclass deficiency (IgG1 and/or IgG3) and/or hyper-IgA and/or hyper-IgM

Males at Risk
Any male maternally related to a male manifesting the XLP phenotype

Modified from Seemayer TA, Grierson H, Pirrueauello SJ, et al. X-linked lymphoproliferative disease. Am J Dis Child 147:1242–1247, 1993. Copyright 1993, American Medical Association.

immunogen may trigger a potentially fatal activation of T cells in such subjects. Better understanding of the immune response to EBV is needed before immunization is recommended for XLP.

The longest survivors who have XLP have the hypo-gammaglobulinemia or agammaglobulinemia phenotype. Replacement immunoglobulin therapy is necessary in these patients, but ultimately aplastic anemia, lymphoma, or fulminant IM develops. Treating patients who have malignant lymphoma with conventional therapies (surgery, irradiation, and/or chemotherapy) has had limited success (Harrington et al., 1987). Severe bone marrow suppression tends to develop following conventional doses of cytoreductive drugs, and relapse is common.

As in other EBV infections, antiviral agents (acy-clovir, ganciclovir), high-dose IVIG therapy, and corticosteroids have not been of benefit. Treatment with interferons (both α and γ) has been tried without success (Okano et al., 1989, 1990a). To date, at least eight patients have received bone marrow transplants for XLP: four died early of non–EBV-related complications of bone marrow transplantation; the remaining four have survived between 18 and 40 months (Williams et al., 1993; Pracher et al., 1994). The response to bone marrow transplantation has been encouraging. One child received a cord blood stem cell transplantation from an HLA-identical sibling (Vowels et al., 1993). Identification of the XLP gene and bone marrow transplantation may provide effective therapy for management of this currently fatal condition.

Burkitt's Lymphoma

Burkitt's lymphoma is a malignant neoplasm in which malignant pre–B lymphocytes form tumors in the jaws, lymphoid tissues of tonsils, bowels, ovaries, or other organs of children or young adults (Burkitt, 1958). Burkitt's lymphoma is a rare tumor except in tropical Africa (Burkitt and O'Conor, 1961; O'Conor, 1970). African patients manifest extraordinarily high titers of EBV viral capsid antigen (VCA) and early antigen (EA) antibodies and somewhat less high titers to EBV nuclear antigen and membrane antigen. The antibody to EA is restricted (R) to a rim of fluorescence around the periphery of the cytoplasm, almost like capping (Henle et al., 1969, 1971).

The extraordinarily high titers to EBV in Burkitt's lymphoma, along with the known ability of EBV to transform cells into lymphoblasts, led to the almost too obvious conclusion that EBV was the cause of Burkitt's lymphoma. This conclusion was supported by the demonstration of EBV genomes in biopsy specimens of nearly all African Burkitt's tumors (Zur Hausen et al., 1970; Lindahl et al., 1974). However, tumors morphologically identical to African Burkitt's do occur elsewhere in the world; in American Burkitt's tumors, the EBV genome is present in only 10% to 15% of the cases and EBV antibodies are usually not exceptionally high (Pagano et al., 1973). Furthermore, chromosomal translocations and oncogene activation, which are also associated with Burkitt's lymphoma, are unrelated to EBV.

It is not yet possible to answer the question of whether EBV is the cause of African Burkitt's lymphoma. Interest has focused on malaria as a possible cofactor in the induction of Burkitt's lymphoma in Africa (O'Conor, 1970). The endemic area of Burkitt's lymphoma is the same as that of malaria. Malaria, like IM, produces lymphoid hyperplasia and elevated immunoglobulins. The combination of EBV and malaria-induced lymphoproliferation could lead to an EBV-containing tumor mass which the host can no longer contain and which, therefore, behaves as a malignant tumor. It is also possible, however, that both malarial and EBV infection augment a third oncogenic factor endemic in Africa and that EBV is only incidentally part of a B-cell tumor because it happens to be integrated into B-cell DNA as a result of IM in the distant past.

Nasopharyngeal Carcinoma

Nasopharyngeal carcinoma (NPC) in China, as Burkitt's lymphoma in Africa, is a malignant neoplasm that is associated with disproportionately high EBV antibody titers and with the presence of EBV DNA in the tumor itself (Zur Hausen et al., 1970). The problem of causality is even more perplexing for NPC because the malignant cell is an epithelial cell, not a lymphoid cell, but more recent studies suggest EBV can enter epithelial cells also (Sixby et al., 1984). Elevated anti-EBV VCA IgA antibody titers occur in NPC and are of prognostic and diagnostic value (Schryver et al., 1969; Henle et al., 1977).

Epstein-Barr Virus Infection in Other Compromised Hosts

A number of patients with severe combined immunodeficiency have developed B-cell lymphomas following thymic or marrow engraftment; at least one case was positive for EBV nuclear antigen (Reece et al., 1980). Likewise, patients with ataxia-telangiectasia develop non-Hodgkin's lymphomas, and again EBNA has been detected in tumor tissue (Saemundson et al., 1981). Primary brain lymphomas have been found in renal and bone marrow transplant recipients and patients with ataxia-telangiectasia and Wiskott-Aldrich syndrome (Rosen et al, 1977; Hanto et al., 1982; Schubach et al., 1982; Ziegler et al., 1982). More recently, similar tumors occurring in normal hosts were proven to have EBV genomes and patients had antibody titers consistent with recently acquired primary infections or less often ongoing infections (Hochberg et al., 1983). It appears that EBV may be the etiologic agent in these tumors.

The accelerated phase of Chédiak-Higashi syndrome may be a result of acute IM in an EBV-mediated hemophagocytic lymphohistiocytosis (Rubin et al., 1985).

MALIGNANT COMPLICATIONS OF IMMUNODEFICIENCIES

Tumors, particularly lymphoproliferative disorders, are the second most common cause of death in persons with primary immunodeficiencies, exceeded only by infections (Mueller and Pizzo, 1995). The incidence of tumors for three major primary immunodeficiencies—Wiskott-Aldrich syndrome (WAS), ataxia-telangiectasia (AT), and common variable immunodeficiency (CVID)—is between 15% and 25%. The risk for lymphoma is particularly high in these three disorders and may be 100-fold that of control subjects (Perry et al., 1980; Cunningham-Rundles et al., 1987). In certain immunodeficiencies, the risk of cancer appears to increase with age (Perry et al., 1980).

Table 27–7 outlines genetically determined immunodeficiencies associated with an increased risk of cancer (WHO Scientific Group on Immunodeficiency, 1989).

An international registry of tumors in patients with primary immunodeficiencies was conceived in the early 1970s (Gatti and Good, 1971). With support from the National Cancer Institute, the Immunodeficiency Cancer Registry (ICR) was maintained for a number of years at the University of Minnesota. The ICR cases have been identified through literature review and voluntary case reports (Filipovich et al., 1980). Table 27–8 shows the distribution of cancers in the ICR according to immunodeficiency diagnoses.

Although lymphoproliferative disorders, including non-Hodgkin's lymphomas, Hodgkin's disease, and lymphoid leukemias, predominate in congenital immunodeficiencies, other cancers occur with increased frequency in different immunodeficiencies. In particular, gastrointestinal carcinomas are found in IgA deficiency and CVID and Kaposi sarcoma is seen in HIV infection (Mueller and Pizzo, 1995).

Non-Hodgkin's Lymphoma/B-Cell Lymphoproliferative Disorders

Clinicopathologic Characteristics

Non-Hodgkin's lymphoma/B-cell lymphoproliferative disorders (NHL/BLPD) are the predominant tumors in patients with both primary and secondary immunodeficiencies (e.g., following allografting or during HIV infection). However, non-Hodgkin's lymphoma in previously normal individuals, unlike that in immunodeficiency, often shows histologic evidence of high-grade malignancy (Filipovich et al., 1990). The development of NHL/BLPD in immunodeficient patients is frequently preceded by polyclonal reactive B-cell hyperplasia in lymphoid tissues. The lesions may show oligoclonal features. Clinical deterioration or death may

Table 27–7. Genetically Determined Immunodeficiencies* Associated with an Increased Risk of Malignancy

Disorder	Inheritance	B-Cell Function	T-Cell Function	Other Defects	Predominant Tumors
I. *Combined immunodeficiencies*					
Severe combined immunodeficiency	X,AR	↓↓	↓↓	Dwarfism, skeletal	Lymphoma △
Purine nucleoside phosphorylase deficiency	AR	Normal	↓↓	—	Lymphoma
II. *Predominantly antibody deficiencies*					
X-linked agammaglobulinemia	X	↓↓	Normal	—	Lymphoma
Selective IgA deficiency	AR,AD,S	↓	Normal	Autoimmune disease	Lymphoma, gastrointestinal carcinoma
Common variable immunodeficiency disease	AR,S	↓↓	↓↓-normal	Autoimmune disease	Lymphoma △, gastrointestinal carcinoma
Hyper-IgM syndrome	X,AR	↓↓	↓-normal		Lymphoma
↓ IgG subclass deficiency	AR,S	↓	↓-normal	Autoimmune disease	Lymphoma
III. *Well-defined immunodeficiencies*					
Wiskott-Aldrich syndrome	X	↓	↓	Thrombocytopenia, autoimmune	Lymphoma △
Ataxia-telangiectasia	AR	↓	↓	Endocrine, neurologic	Lymphoma, gastrointestinal carcinoma
DiGeorge anomalad	AD,S	↓-normal	↓↓-↓	Endocrine, cardiac, skeletal	Lymphoma
IV. *Other immunodeficiencies*					
Hyper-IgE syndrome	S	↓	↓	Secondary neutrophil dysfunction	Lymphoma
X-linked lymphoproliferative disease	X	↓	↓	Cardiac and neurologic defects in kindred	Lymphoma △
V. *Phagocytic defects*					
Chédiak-Higashi syndrome	AR	Normal	↓	Albinism, phagocyte dysfunction	Lymphoma △

*Listed according to WHO categories.
X = X-linked; AR = autosomal recessive; AD = autosomal dominant; S = sporadic; △ = known to be frequently associated with Epstein-Barr virus (EBV).

Table 27–8. Immunodeficiency Cancer Registry Cases: Distribution of Tumors and Immunodeficiencies

Immunodeficiency	Adenocarcinoma	Lymphoma	Hodgkin's Disease	Leukemia	Other Tumors	Total Tumors
Severe combined immunodeficiency	1 (2.4%)	31 (73.8%)	4 (9.5%)	5 (11.9%)	1 (2.4%)	42 (8.4%)
Hypogammaglobulinemia	3 (14.3%)	7 (33.3%)	3 (14.3%)	7 (33.3%)	1 (4.8%)	21 (4.2%)
Common variable immunodeficiency	20 (16.7%)	55 (45.8%)	8 (6.7%)	8 (6.7%)	29 (24.2%)	120 (24.0%)
IgA deficiency	8 (21.1%)	6 (15.8%)	3 (7.9%)	0 (0%)	21 (55.3%)	38 (7.6%)
Hyper-IgM syndrome	0 (0%)	9 (56.3%)	4 (25.0%)	0 (0%)	3 (18.8%)	16 (3.2%)
Wiskott-Aldrich syndrome	0 (0%)	59 (75.6%)	3 (3.8%)	7 (9.0%)	9 (11.5%)	78 (15.6%)
Ataxia-telangiectasia	13 (8.7%)	69 (46.0%)	16 (10.7%)	32 (21.3%)	20 (13.3%)	150 (30.0%)
Other immunodeficiencies	1 (4.0%)	12 (48.0%)	1 (4.0%)	4 (16.0%)	7 (28.0%)	25 (5.0%)
Total immunodeficiency categories	46 (9.2%)	252 (50.4%)	43 (8.6%)	63 (12.6%)	96 (19.2%)	500 (100%)

occur irrespective of clonality of tumors (Shapiro et al., 1988).

In contrast to non-Hodgkin's lymphoma in the general population, in immunodeficient hosts this tumor is often first detected at extranodal sites, including the CNS and gastrointestinal tract and is widespread at the time of diagnosis. Table 27–9 summarizes the primary sites of lymphoproliferative disorders, age at diagnosis and sex distribution for the 240 cases of NHL/BLPD collected by the Immunodeficiency Cancer Registry. The median age at diagnosis was only 7.1 years. The overall male predominance reflects the contribution of patients with several X-linked disorders, including severe combined immunodeficiency and Wiskott-Aldrich syndrome. There is an unexplained male predominance in ataxia-telangiectasia, an autosomal recessive disorder.

Etiology

Several biologic factors, occurring alone or in conjunction with others, contribute to the high incidence of B-cell lymphoproliferative disorders in immunodeficient hosts. These include (1) the ubiquity of EBV, (2) host defects in immunoregulation, and (3) imprecise or ineffective rearrangement of immunoglobulin and T-cell receptor genes during lymphopoiesis.

EBV infection is a major cofactor in many, but not all, B-cell lymphoproliferative tumors. Immunodeficient hosts can acquire EBV through primary infection, transplantation, or transfusion.

EBV is often reactivated during immunosuppressive therapy. During primary infection, EBV immortalizes B lymphocytes in vivo, resulting in polyclonal B-cell activation and proliferation. BCRF1, one of the EBV genes, is similar to human IL-10 (Moore et al., 1990). It inhibits the production of TNF and interferon-γ by host T lymphocytes–lymphokines, which normally synergize to kill virus-infected cells and, in this way, may protect the EBV-infected cells from destruction. Unlike a normal person, in whom EBV-specific immunologic control maintains EBV in latency following primary infection, the immunodeficient host has defective suppressor and cytotoxic function. Under these circumstances, the production of regulatory cytokines that maintain viral latency are unbalanced and EBV-infected B cells continue to proliferate.

It is hypothesized that B cells that are already EBV-transformed may have a growth advantage during polyclonal lymphocyte proliferation. The high mitotic index of EBV-transformed cells increases the probability of genetic mutations, giving rise to populations of B cells that may carry specific cytogenetic rearrangements and are not susceptible to regulatory stimuli.

EBV is present in virtually all tumors of post-transplant BLPD both solid organ (Shapiro et al., 1988) and bone marrow (Ambinder et al., 1992). In a retrospec-

Table 27–9. Characteristics of Non-Hodgkin's Lymphomas in the Immunodeficiency Cancer Registry (ICR)*

Immunodeficiency	N	Sex M:F‡	Median Age at Diagnosis (yr)	Brain CNS	Gastrointestinal Tract	Lymph Node	Multiple
Severe combined immunodeficiency	31	23:7	1.6	6.5	3.2	9.7	48.4
Hypogammaglobulinemia	7	7:0	1.2	0	14.3	14.3	14.3
Common variable immunodeficiency	55	30:23	23.0	1.8	12.7	12.7	25.5
IgA deficiency	6	4:1	9.4	16.7	0	0	0
Hyper-IgM syndrome	9	7:2	7.8	11.1	22.2	22.2	0
Wiskott-Aldrich syndrome	59	59:0	6.2	23.7	6.8	8.5	20.3
Ataxia-telangiectasia	69	40:24	8.5	0	8.7	10.1	14.5
Other immunodeficiencies	4	4:0	4.0	0	0	0	0
Total immunodeficiency categories	240	174:57	7.1 yr	7.9%	8.8%	10.4%	21.7%

*Primary Tumor Sites (%)†

*This table excludes cases of non-Hodgkin's lymphoma in immunodeficiency categories with fewer than two cases reported.
†For 51.3% of ICR cases, primary tumor site is other or unknown.
‡Sex reported where known.

tive analysis of archival material from the Immunodeficiency Cancer Registry, NHL/BLPD tumors from patients with severe combined immunodeficiency and Wiskott-Aldrich syndrome were also all EBV-positive (by in situ EBER probes), whereas some tumors in patients with ataxia-telangiectasia and CVID were not (Filipovich et al., 1990).

A second factor favoring the development of B-cell lymphoproliferative disorders in immunodeficiencies is defective immunoregulation following B-cell and T-cell activation. Although their number, subset distribution, and functional repertoire may not be normal, virtually all immunodeficient patients (except with certain forms of SCID) possess B and/or T cells capable of activation. Indeed, because of circumstances peculiar to the immunodeficient settings, stimulation of lymphocytes may be unusually intense or prolonged. Most patients with primary immunodeficiencies have deficient antibody functions, persistent respiratory and gastrointestinal pathogens, and chronic antigenic stimulation.

Chronically activated T cells produce lymphokines that favor lymphocyte multiplication, formation of cytotoxic T cells, and B-cell proliferation. Unbalanced cytokine production may lead to EBV-associated BLPD.

Another mechanism predisposing to tumorigenesis is exemplified in ataxia-telangiectasia (Hecht and McCaw, 1977). AT is an autosomal recessive disorder associated with excess chromosomal breakage and susceptibility to lymphoid malignancies (Hecht and McCaw, 1977). Following exposure to DNA-damaging agents, such as X-irradiation, AT cells fail to pause and repair damage but rush on to DNA replication. In AT, a decreased number of lymphocytes carry productive rearrangements of immunoglobulin and T-cell receptor chains. This finding may explain the variable development of the immune repertoire and the continuous predisposition to acquired cytogenetic changes that can lead to malignant transformation of lymphocytes (Hecht and Hecht, 1987) in this disorder.

Prevention and Treatment

Several distinct approaches can be used to prevent lymphoproliferative disorders associated with immunodeficiency. One approach is to produce full immunoreconstitution in patients with primary immunodeficiency. Failing that, enhancing immune competence may be effective. Finally, avoiding exposure or increasing resistance to the viral cofactors implicated in the lymphoproliferation may be possible.

Bone marrow transplantation from a histocompatible donor is the treatment of choice for immunoreconstitution of patients with otherwise lethal primary immunodeficiencies. Patients receiving transplants for SCID have now been observed for longer than 20 years after bone marrow transplantation, and no cases of lymphoid cancer have developed (Neudorf et al., 1984). In contrast, partial or transient immunoreconstitution in SCID with the use of thymic epithelial transplants or haploidentical T-depleted marrow grafts (Shapiro et al., 1988) does not necessarily confer resis-

tance to subsequent lymphoproliferative complications. Patients who have received matched unrelated transplants have not been followed long enough to determine whether lymphoproliferative disorders will develop.

IVIG and acyclovir have been used in an attempt to prevent primary EBV infection and/or reduce reactivation of latent virus with minimal success.

Treatment of lymphoproliferative disorders with conventional combination chemotherapy, radiation therapy, or both has been disappointing in patients with immunodeficiency. Poor outcome has been attributed to poor tumor responses, excessive toxicity, and the high risk of fatal infections (Shearer et al., 1984).

In a pilot study, five patients with partial immunodeficiency received IFN-α for therapy of EBV-associated lymphoproliferative disease (Shapiro and Filipovich, 1991). Two had developed a B-cell lymphoproliferative disorder following marrow transplant, and three had antibody deficiency. Four of the five patients demonstrated complete clinical resolution of their lymphoproliferative disorders with IFN-α (at a dose of 2 to 3 million U/M^2/day) as the primary therapy, given in conjunction with weekly IVIG. Interferon-α may act by several mechanisms, including (1) a direct antiviral effect, (2) an antiproliferative effect on EBV-infected B cells, or (3) modulation of the host effector (cytotoxic) cells.

Anti–B-cell monoclonal antibody therapy has shown promise in nonclonal B-cell lymphoproliferative disease in secondary immunodeficiencies (Blanche et al., 1988).

Future treatment for BLPD will be determined by improved understanding of the pathophysiology of BLPD and availability of newer therapeutic agents. Perhaps combination therapy with antiviral drugs, cytokines, antibodies, and cellular therapies will be effective. There is great potential for anti-sense oligonucleotides, which may inhibit essential viral or cellular genes involved in transformation and proliferation of B cells latently infected with EBV.

Hodgkin's Disease

Forty-three cases of Hodgkin's disease have been recorded by the Immunodeficiency Cancer Registry, making up 8.6% of the cases. Hodgkin's disease accounts for approximately 10% of tumors in several primary immunodeficiencies, including hypogammaglobulinemia, SCID, ataxia-telangiectasia, and hyper-IgM syndrome. Preliminary studies using in situ probes suggest an association between EBV and Hodgkin's disease in immunodeficient hosts (Moore et al., 1990).

The median age at tumor diagnosis was 10.9 years, reflecting the contribution of four cases identified in very young children with SCID whose median age at tumor diagnosis was 4 months. In contrast to the male predominance observed for B-cell lymphoproliferative disorders, there is no gender dominance.

In 1986, the Immunodeficiency Cancer Registry performed a case-control study (Robison et al., 1987) comparing Hodgkin's disease in immunodeficient and previously well children. The objective of this study was to determine whether differences existed. Patients were compared with previously well "controls" who developed Hodgkin's disease ascertained by the Late Effects Study Group (LESG). Patients with immunodeficiency were significantly younger at diagnosis (mean age 7.8 years) compared with LESG controls (mean age 11.5 years). Immunodeficiencies were significantly less likely to achieve an initial remission, and survival was significantly poorer, with 5-year survival rate of 18% for Immunodeficiency Cancer Registry compared with 84% for LESG controls. The immunodeficient patients who achieved a complete remission had a 5-year survival rate of 53% compared with 86% in the control group.

Tissue specimens from 12 of the Immunodeficiency Cancer Registry patients were reviewed and demonstrated an unusual distribution of histologic subtypes. Compared with previously reported series, Immunodeficiency Cancer Registry patients showed a larger proportion of cases with mixed cellularity (42%) or lymphocyte depletion (33%). Interestingly, these histologic patterns are closely associated with Hodgkin's disease with EBV in the nonimmunodeficient pediatric population.

The response to treatment of Hodgkin's disease has been disappointing in children with primary immunodeficiencies. Survival data in 25 patients of Hodgkin's disease in the Immunodeficiency Cancer Registry are available. Five patients are currently alive, three of them in remission. Overall, eight patients achieved complete remission and seven achieved partial remission. The median duration of survival after diagnosis was 13.6 months. Infection was identified as the predominant cause of death, followed by progressive or recurrent tumor.

Carcinomas

Gastric carcinomas are the most common epithelial tumors reported in patients with primary immunodeficiencies. There are 25 cases of gastric carcinoma in the Immunodeficiency Cancer Registry; 72% (18/25) of these malignancies arose in patients with CVID at a median age of 54 years (range, 15 to 67 years). In addition to the IgA deficiency that was present in all cases, a significant number of these patients had a prior history of pernicious anemia, nodular lymphoid hyperplasia, or atrophic gastritis (Filipovich and Shapiro, 1991).

Gastric carcinoma has also been reported in children with ataxia-telangiectasia IgA deficiency, and selective IgA deficiency. Theoretically, IgA deficiency can result in excess stimulation and hyperplasia of intestinal epithelial and lymphoid structures because of the chronic persistence of pathogens such as *Giardia lamblia* and enteroviruses. More recently, *Helicobacter pylori* has emerged as the most common predisposing factor in nonimmunodeficient individuals with gastric carcinomas (Eurogast Study Group, 1993). *H. pylori* infection is nearly always associated with chronic gastritis, with atrophy and metaplasia of the gastric epithelium. Re-

sultant hypochlorhydria permits gastric colonization with bacteria producing potentially mutagenic N-nitrous compounds. Inflammation from *H. pylori* also generates cytokines that promote proliferation of epithelial cells and lymphoid tissues. Since production of specific IgA antibodies against *H. pylori* is critical to its immunologic control, it is not surprising that patients with inadequate IgA synthesis are particularly vulnerable to this tumor pathogen.

In immunodeficient patients, complete excision of gastric carcinomas has resulted in prolonged tumor-free survival (Filipovich and Shapiro, 1991). Knowledge of the role of *H. pylori* in the pathogenesis of this genetic carcinoma suggests that antibiotic therapy may prevent this disease.

References

Abildgaard CF, Penner JA, Watson-Williams EJ. Anti-inhibitor coagulant complex (autoplex) for treatment of factor VIII inhibitors in hemophilia. Blood 56:978–984, 1980.

Abramson N, LoBuglio AF, Jandl JH, Cotran RS. The interaction between human monocytes and red cells. Binding characteristics. J Exp Med 132:1191–1206, 1970.

Ahn YS, Harrington WJ, Seelman RL, Eytel CS. Vincristine therapy of idiopathic and secondary thrombocytopenias. N Engl J Med 291:376–380, 1974.

Alfiere C, Loncas JH. Biomolecular analysis of a defective nontransforming Epstein-Barr virus (EBV) from a patient with chronic active EBV infection. J Virol 61:3306–3309, 1987.

Allain JP, Frommel D. Antibodies to factor VIII. Patterns of immune response to factor VIII in hemophilia A. Blood 47:973–982, 1976.

Allgood JW, Chaplin H. Idiopathic acquired autoimmune hemolytic anemia. Am J Med 43:254–273, 1967.

Alvarado CS, Buchanan GR, Kim TH, Zaatara G, Sartain P, Ragab AH. Use of VP-a6-213 in the treatment of familial erythrophagocytic lymphohistiocytosis. Cancer 57:1097–1100, 1986.

Ambinder RF, Mann RB, Barletta JM, Murray P, Shapiro RS, Ling Y, Filipovich AH. Association of Epstein-Barr virus (EBV) with Hodgkin's disease (HD) in patients with primary immunodeficiency and frequent detection of EBV in lymphoid tissue without neoplastic involvement in Wiskott-Aldrich syndrome (WAS): a survey of EBV in archival tissues from the Immunodeficiency Cancer Registry (ICR). Blood 80(10 Suppl. 1):118a, 1992.

Ambruso DR, Hays T, Zwartjes WJ, Tubergen D, Favara B. Successful treatment of lymphohistiocytic reticulosis with phagocytosis with epipodophyllotoxin VP-16-213. Cancer 45:2516–2520, 1980.

Anderson P, Mosekild L. Immunoglobulin levels and autoantibodies in epileptics on long-term anticonvulsant therapy. Acta Med Scand 201:69–74, 1977.

Andersson J, Britton S, Ernberg I. Effect of acyclovir on infectious mononucleosis: a double-blind placebo-controlled study. J Infect Dis 153:283–290, 1986.

Andrew M, Blanchette VS, Adams M, Ali K, Barnard D, Chan KW, deVeber LB, Esseltine D, Israels S, Korbrinsky N, Luke B, Milner RA, Woloski BMR, Vegh P. A multicenter study of the treatment of childhood chronic idiopathic thrombocytopenic purpura with anti-D. J Pediatr 120:522–527, 1992.

Arico M, Nespoli L, Maccario R, Montagna D, Bonetti F, Caseli D, Burgio GR. Natural cytotoxicity impairment in familial haemophagocytic lymphohistiocytosis. Arch Dis Child 63:292–296, 1988.

Armitage RJ, Macduff BM, Spriggs MK, Fanslow WC. Human B cell proliferation and Ig secretion induced by recombinant CD40 ligand are modulated by soluble cytokines. J Immunol 150:3671–3680, 1993.

Ascensao J, Kagan W, Moore M, Rajendra P, Hansen J, Good R: Aplastic anemia: evidence for an immunologic mechanism. Lancet 1:669–671, 1976.

Atkinson K. Chronic graft-versus-host disease following marrow transplantation. Marrow Transplant Rev 1–7, 1992.

August CS, Hathaway WE, Lange B. Hematologic disorders. In

Stiehm ER, ed. Immunologic Disorders in Infants and Children, 3rd ed. Philadelphia, WB Saunders, 1989, pp. 634–665.

Bacigalupo A, Podesta M, van Lint MT, Vimereati R, Cerri R, Rossi E, Risso M, Carella A, Santini G, Damasio E, Giordano D, Marmont AM. Severe aplastic anaemia: correlation of in vitro tests with clinical response to immunosuppression in 20 patients. Br J Haematol 47:423–433, 1981.

Ball S, Zuiable A, Roster BLT, Hedge, UM. Changes in platelet immunoprotein levels during therapy in adult immune thrombocytopenia. Br J Haematol 60:631–633, 1985.

Bar RS, DeLor CJ, Clausen KP, Hurtubise P, Henle W, Hewetson JF. Fatal infectious mononucleosis in a family. N Engl J Med 290:363–367, 1974.

Bartley DC, Del Rio C, Shulman JA. "Clinical complications." In Schlossberg D, ed. Infectious Mononucleosis, 2nd ed. Berlin, Springer-Verlag, 1989, pp. 35–48.

Batchelor JR, Fielder AH, Walport MJ, David J, Lord DK, Davery N, Dodi IA, Malasit P, Wanachiwanawin W, Bernstein R, Mackworth-Young C, Isenberg D. Family study of the major histocompatibility complex in HLA-DR3 negative patients with systemic lupus erythematosus. Clin Exp Immunol 70:364–371, 1987.

Baur S, Fisher JM, Strickland RC, Taylor KB. Autoantibody-containing cells in the gastric mucosa in pernicious anemia. Lancet 2:887–890, 1968.

Becton, DL, Kinney TR, Chaffee S, Kurtzberg J, Friedman HS, Falletta JM. High-dose intravenous immunoglobulin for severe platelet alloimmunization. Pediatrics 73:1120–1122, 1984.

Becton DL, Kurtzberg J, Kinney TR, Friedman HS, Chaffee S, Falletta JM. Treatment of lymphohistiocytic erythrophagocytosis with VP-16 and aziridinylbenzoquinone. Med Pediatr Oncol 15:58–61, 1987.

Bender CE. Recurrent mononucleosis. JAMA 182:954–956, 1962.

Bender CE. The value of corticosteroids in the treatment of infectious mononucleosis. JAMA 199:529–531, 1967.

Berman BW, McIntosh S, Clyne LP, Goldberg B, Lobel J, Komp DM. Spontaneously acquired factor IX inhibitors in childhood. Am J Pediatr Hematol Oncol 3:377–381, 1981.

Berney SL, Metcalfe P, Wathen NC, Waters AH. Post-transfusion purpura responding to high dose intravenous IgG. Further observations on pathogenesis. Br J Haematol 61:627–632, 1985.

Bidwell E. Acquired inhibitors of coagulants. Annu Rev Med 20:63–74, 1969.

Blanche S, Le Deist F, Veber F, Lenoir G, Fischer AM, Brochier J, Boucheix C, Delaage M, Griscelli C, Fischer A. Treatment of severe Epstein-Barr virus–induced polyclonal B-lymphocyte proliferation by anti-B-cell monoclonal antibodies: two cases after HLA-mismatched bone marrow transplantation. Ann Intern Med 108:199–203, 1988.

Blanche S, Caniglia M, Girault D, Landman J, Griscelli C, Fischer A. Treatment of hemophagocytic lymphohistiocytosis with chemotherapy and bone marrow transplantation: a single center study of 22 cases. Blood 78:51–54, 1991.

Blanchette V, Imbach P, Andrew M, Adams M, McMillan J, Wang E, Milner R, Ali K, Barnard D, Bernstein M, Chan KW, Esseltine D, deVeber B, Israels S, Kobrinsky N, Luke B. Randomised trial of intravenous immunoglobulin G, intravenous anti-D and oral prednisone in childhood acute immune thrombocytopenic purpura. Lancet 344:703–707, 1994.

Blatt PM, White GC, McMillan CW, Roberts HR. Treatment of antifactor VIII antibodies. Thromb Haemost 38:514–523, 1977.

Blazar BA, Patarvoyo M, Klein E, Klein G. Increased sensitivity of human lymphoid lines to natural killer cells after induction of the Epstein-Barr viral cycle by superinfection or sodium butyrate. J Exp Med 151:614, 1980.

Borgna-Pignatti C, Battisti L, Zecca M, Locatelli F. Treatment of chronic childhood immune thrombocytopenic purpura with intramuscular anti-D immunoglobulins. Br J Haematol 88:618–620, 1994.

Boxer LA, Greenberg MS, Boxer GJ, Stossel TP. Autoimmune neutropenia. N Engl J Med 293:748–753, 1975.

Bowdler AJ. The role of the spleen and splenectomy in autoimmune hemolytic disease. Semin Hematol 13:335–348, 1976.

Brand A, Claas FHJ, Falkenburg JHF, van Rood JJ, Eernisse JG. Blood component therapy in bone marrow transplantation. Semin Hematol 21:141–155, 1984.

Brodeur GM, O'Neill PJ, Williams JA. Acquired inhibitors of coagulation in nonhemophiliac children. J Pediatr 96:439–441, 1980.

Burkitt D. A sarcoma involving the jaws in African children. Br J Surg 46:218–223, 1958.

Burkitt D, O'Conor GT. A malignant lymphoma in African children. I. A clinical syndrome. Cancer 14:258–269, 1961.

Bussel JB. Treatment of acute idiopathic thrombocytopenic purpura. J Pediatr 108:326–327, 1986.

Bussel JB, Baumgartner MW. The use and mechanism of action of intravenous immunoglobulin in the treatment of immune hematologic disease. Br J Haematol 56:1–7, 1984.

Bussel JB, Kimberly BP, Inman RD, Schulman I, Cunningham-Rundles C, Cheung N, Smithwick EM, O'Malley J, Barandun S, Hilgartner MW. Intravenous gammaglobulin treatment of chronic idiopathic thrombocytopenic purpura. Blood 62:480–486, 1983a.

Bussel JB, Schulman I, Hilgartner MW, Barandun S. Intravenous use of gammaglobulin in the treatment of chronic immune thrombocytopenic purpura as a means to defer splenectomy. J Pediatr 103:651–653, 1983b.

Bussel JB, Lalezari P, Hilgartner M, Partin J, Fikrig S, O'Malley J, Barandun S. Reversal of neutropenia with intravenous gammaglobulin in autoimmune neutropenia of infancy. Blood 62:398–400, 1983c.

Bussel JB, Steinherz PG, Miller DR, Hilgartner MW. A heparinlike anticoagulant in an 8-month-old boy with acute monoblastic leukemia. Am J Hematol 16:83–90, 1984.

Bussel JB, Goldman A, Imbach P, Schulman I, Hilgartner MW. Treatment of acute idiopathic thrombocytopenia of childhood with intravenous infusions of gammaglobulin. J Pediatr 106:886–890, 1985.

Cairo MS, Baehner RL. The use of antithymocyte globulin in the treatment of severe aplastic anemia in children. J Pediatr 100:307–311, 1982.

Callender ST, Denborough MA. Family study of pernicious anemia. Br J Haematol 3:88–106, 1957.

Carter RL, Penman GH. Histopathology of infectious mononucleosis. In Carter RL, Penman HG, eds. Infectious Mononucleosis. Oxford, Blackwell Scientific Publications, 1969, pp. 146–161.

Cen H, Breinig MC, Atchiyom RW, Ho M, McCorplet JLC. Epstein-Barr virus transmission via donor organs in solid organ transplantation polymerase chain reaction and restriction fragment length polymorphism analysis of IR2, IR3 and IR4. J Virol 65:976–980, 1991.

Champlin R, Ho W, Gale RP. Antithymocyte globulin treatment in patients with aplastic anemia: a prospective randomized trial. N Engl J Med 308:113–118, 1983.

Change RS, Maddow R. Recurrence of infectious mononucleosis. Lancet 1:704, 1980.

Chanarin I. The Megaloblastic Anemias. Oxford, Blackwell Scientific Publications, 1969.

Chirico G, Duse M, Ugazio AG, Rondini G. Clinical and laboratory observations: high-dose intravenous gammaglobulin therapy for passive immune thrombocytopenia in the neonate. J Pediatr 103:654–655, 1983.

Clerici M, Shearer GM. A Th1–Th2 switch is a critical step in the etiology of HIV infection. Immunol Today 14:107–110, 1993.

Cines DB, Passero F, Guerry D IV, Bina M, Dusak B, Schreiber AD. Granulocyte-associated IgG in neutropenic disorders. Blood 59:124–132, 1982.

Cohen JI. Epstein-Barr virus lymphoproliferative disease associated with acquired immunodeficiency. Medicine 70:137–160, 1991.

Colby BM, Shaw JE, Elion GB, Pagano JS. Effect of acyclovir (9-[2-hydroxyethoxymethyl] guanidine) on Epstein-Barr virus DNA replication. J Virol 34:560–568, 1980.

Coombs RRA, Mourant AE, Race RR. A new test for the detection of weak and "incomplete" Rh agglutinins. Br J Exp Pathol 26:255–268, 1945.

Cunningham-Rundles C. Clinical and immunologic analyses of 103 patients with common variable immunodeficiency. J Clin Immunol 9:22–33, 1989.

Cunninghum-Rundles C, Brandeis WE, Good RA, Day NK. Bovine antigens and the formation of circulating immune complexes in selective IgA deficiency. J Clin Invest 64:272–279, 1979.

Cunningham-Rundles C, Siegal FP, Cunningham-Rundles S, Lieberman P. Incidence of cancer in 98 patients with common variable immunodeficiency. J Clin Immunol 7:294–301, 1987.

Dacie JV. The haemolytic anemias: Congenital and acquired. Part

III. Drug Induced Haemolytic Anaemias, 2nd ed. London, J & A Churchill, 1967, pp. 710–991.

Dacie JV, Worlledge SM. Autoimmune hemolytic anemias. Prog Hematol 6:82–120, 1969.

Davidsohn I, Walker PH. The nature of heterophile antibodies in infectious mononucleosis. Am J Clin Pathol 5:455–465, 1935.

Davidsohn I, Lee CL. The clinical serology of infectious mononucleosis. In Carter RL, Penman HG, eds. Infectious Mononucleosis. Oxford, Blackwell Scientific, 1969, pp. 177–200.

Del Mistro A, Laverda A, Calabrese F, DeMartino M, Calabri G, Cogo P, Coech P, D'Andre E, DeRossi A, Giaquinto C, Giurdano R, Nizri RM, Salvi G, Pennelli N, Chicco-Giandu L. Primary lymphoma of the central nervous system in two children with acquired immune deficiency syndrome. Am J Clin Pathol 94:722–728, 1990.

Denman AM, Pelton BK. Control mechanisms in infectious mononucleosis. Clin Exp Immunol 18:13–25, 1974.

DiTuro WJ, Goldsmith PM, Frenkel LD, Jadeja NG, Dennis TR. Intravenous gammaglobulin treatment of profound herpes varicella zoster associated thrombocytopenia. Ann Allergy 56:206, 241–243, 1986.

Dourmashkin RR, Rosse WF. Morphologic changes in the membranes of red blood cells undergoing hemolysis. Am J Med 41:699–710, 1966.

Downey H, Stasney J. The pathology of lymph nodes in infectious mononucleosis. Fol Haematol 54:417–438, 1936.

Eife R, Janka GE, Belohradsky BN, Holtmann H. Natural killer cell function and interferon production in familial hemophagocytic lymphohistiocytosis. Pediatr Hematol Oncol 6:265–272, 1989.

Enberg RN, Eberle BJ, Williams RC. T- and B-cells in peripheral blood during infectious mononucleosis. J Infect Dis 130:104–111, 1974.

Engelfriet CP, van der Borne AE, Beckers D, van Loghem JJ. Autoimmune haemolytic anemia: serologic and immunochemical characteristics of the auto-antibodies, mechanisms of cell destruction. Ser Haematol 7:328–347, 1974.

Eurogast Study Group. An international association between *Helicobacter pylori* infection and gastric cancer. Lancet 341:1359, 1993.

Evans AS, Neiderman JC, McCollum RW. Seroepidemiologic studies of infectious mononucleosis with EB virus. N Engl J Med 279:1121–1127, 1968.

Farquhar JW, Claireaux AF. Familial hemophagocytic reticulosis. Arch Dis Child 27:519–525, 1952.

Fehr J, Hofmann V, Kappeler U. Transient reversal of thrombocytopenia in idiopathic thrombocytopenic purpura by high-dose intravenous gammaglobulin. N Engl J Med 306:1254–1258, 1982.

Feinstein DI, Rapaport SI. Acquired inhibitors of blood coagulation. Prog Hemost Thromb 1:75–95, 1972.

Feusner JH, Slichter SJ, Harker LA. Mechanisms of thrombocytopenia in varicella. Am J Hematol 7:255–264, 1979.

Filipovich AH, Porta F, Kollmann C. Unrelated donor (URD) bone marrow transplantation (BMT) for primary immunodeficiencies: an international review. Blood 84 (10 Suppl. 1):394a, 1994.

Filipovich AH, Shapiro RS. Tumors in patients with common variable immunodeficiency. J Immunol Immunopharmacol 11:43–46, 1991.

Filipovich AH, Shapiro RS, Robinson L, Mertens A, Frizzera G. Lymphoproliferative disorders associated with immunodeficiency. In Magrath IT, ed. The Non-Hodgkin's Lymphomas. London, Edward Arnold, 1990, pp. 135–154.

Filipovich AH, Spector BSD, Frizzera G, Kersey JH. Malignancy in immunocompromised humans. In Giraldo G, Beth E, eds. The Role of Viruses in Human Cancer. New York, Elsevier North Holland, 1980, pp. 237–253.

Fingeroth JD, Weis JJ, Tedder TF, Strominger JL, Biro PA, Fearon DT. Epstein-Barr virus receptor of human B lymphocytes is the C3d receptor CR2. Proc Natl Acad Sci U S A 81:4510–4516, 1984.

Fischer A, Virelizier JL, Arenzana-Seisdedos R, Perez N, Nezelof C, Griscelli C. Treatment of four patients with erythrophagocytic lymphohistiocytosis by a combination of epidophyllotoxin, steroids, intrathecal methotrexate, and cranial irradiation. Pediatrics 76:263–268, 1985.

Flores G, Cunningham-Rundles C, Newland AC, Bussel JB. Efficacy of intravenous immunoglobulin in the treatment of autoimmune hemoytic anemia: results in 73 patients. Am J Hematol 44:237–242, 1993.

Frank MM. Complement: a brief review. J Allergy Clin Immunol 84:411–420, 1989.

French MAH, Dawkins RL. Central MHC genes, IgA deficiency and autoimmune disease. Immunol Today 11:271–274, 1990.

Frommel D, Muller JY, Prou-Wartelle O, Allain JP. Possible linkage between the major histocompatibility complex and the immune response to factor VIII in classic haemophilia. Vox Sang 33:270–272, 1977.

Fukuda K, Straus SE, Hickie I, Sharpe MC, Dobbins JG, Komaroff A, and the International Chronic Fatigue Syndrome Study Group. The chronic fatigue syndrome: a comprehensive approach to its definition and study. Ann Intern Med 121:953–959, 1994.

Gatti RA, Good RA. Occurrence of malignancy in immunodeficiencies. Cancer 28:89–98, 1971.

Gencik A, Signer E, Muller H. Genetic analysis of familial erythrophagocytic lymphohistiocytosis. Eur J Pediatr 142:248–252, 1984.

Gerber P, Nonyama M, Lucas D, Perlin E, Golstein LI. Oral execretion of Epstein-Barr viruses by healthy subjects and patients with infectious mononucleosis. Lancet 2:988, 1972.

Goldberg A, Hutchinson HE, MacDonald E. Radiochromium in the selection of patients with haemolytic anemia for splenectomy. Lancet 1:109–113, 1966.

Goldberg GN, Fulginiti VA, Ray CG, Ferry P, Jones JF, Cross H, Minnich L. In utero Epstein-Barr virus (infectious mononucleosis) infection. JAMA 246:1579–1581, 1981.

Goldstein R, Blanchette VS, Huebsch LB, McKendry RJR. Treatment of gold-induced thrombocytopenia by high-dose intravenous gamma globulin. Arthritis Rheum 29:426–430, 1986.

Good RA, Rotstein J, Mazzitello WF. The simultaneous occurrence of rheumatoid arthritis and agammaglobulinemia. J Lab Clin Med 49:343–357, 1957.

Gotze O, Müller-Eberhard HJ. Lysis of erythrocytes by complement in the absence of antibody. J Exp Med 132:898–913, 1970.

Gralnick HR, McGinnis M, Elton W, McCurdy P. Hemolytic anemia associated with cephalothin. JAMA 217:1193–1197, 1971.

Gratama JW, Lennette ET, Lonnquist B, Oosterveer MAP, Klein G, Ringden D, Ernberg I. Detection of multiple Epstein-Barr viral strains in allogeneic bone marrow transplant recipients. J Med Virol 37:39–47, 1992.

Grierson HL, Skare J, Hawk JI, Pauza M, Purtilo DT. Immunoglobulin class and subclass deficiencies prior to Epstein-Barr virus (EBV) infection in males with X-linked lymphoproliferative disease. Am J Med Genet 40:294–297, 1991.

Gringeri A, Cattaneo M, Santagostino E, Mannucci PM. Intramuscular anti-D immunoglobulins for home treatment of chronic immune thrombocytopenic purpura. Br J Haematol 80:337–340, 1992.

Grose C, Henle W, Henle G, Feorino P. Primary Epstein-Barr virus infections in acute neurologic diseases. N Engl J Med 292:392–395, 1975.

Habibi B, Homberg JC, Schaison G, Salmon C. Autoimmune hemolytic anemia in children: a review of 80 cases. Am J Med 56:61–69, 1974.

Haider S, del Contino M, Edmond RTD, Sutton RNP. Tubercular anergy and infectious mononucleosis. Lancet 2:74, 1973.

Hakami N, Neiman PE, Canellos GP, Lazerson J. Neonatal megaloblastic anemia due to inherited transcobalamin II deficiency in two siblings. N Engl J Med 285:1163–1170, 1971.

Handin RI, Martin V, Moloney WC. Antibody-induced von Willebrand's disease: a newly defined inhibitor syndrome. Blood 48:393–405, 1976.

Hanto DW, Frizzera G, Gayl-Pecksalska J, Sakamoto K, Purtilo DT, Balfour HH, Simmons RJ, Najarian JS. Epstein-Barr virus B-cell lymphoma after renal transplantation: acyclovir therapy and transition from polyclonal to monoclonal B-cell proliferation. N Engl J Med 306:913–918, 1982.

Harada S, Bechtold T, Seeley TK, Purtilo DT. Cell-mediated immunity to Epstein-Barr virus (EBV) and natural killer (NK)–cell activity in X-linked lymphoproliferative syndrome. Int J Cancer 216:739–744, 1982.

Harrington DS, Weisenburger DD, Purtilo DT. Malignant lymphomas in the X-linked lymphoproliferative syndrome. Cancer 59:1419–1429, 1987.

Harris JW. Studies on the mechanism of a drug-induced hemolytic anemia. J Lab Clin Med 47:760–775, 1956.

Hathaway WE, Blackburn WH, Fulginiti V, Kempe CH. Aplastic anemia, histiocytosis, and erythroderma in immunologically deficient children: probable human runt disease. N Engl J Med 273:953–958, 1965.

Haynes BF, Schooley RT, Payling-Wright CR, Grouse JE, Dolin R, Fauci AS. Emergence of suppressor cells of immunoglobulin synthesis during acute Epstein-Barr virus–induced infectious mononucleosis. J Immunol 123:2095–2101, 1979.

Hecht F, Hecht BKM. Chromosome changes connect immunodeficiency and cancer in ataxia-telangiectasia. Am J Pediatr Hematol Oncol 9:185–188, 1987.

Hecht F, McCaw BK. Chromosome instability syndromes. In Mulvihill JJ, Miller RW, Fraumeni JF, eds. Genetics of Human Cancer. New York, Raven Press, 1977, pp. 105–124.

Henle G, Henle W. Observations on childhood infections with Epstein-Barr virus. J Infect Dis 121:303–310, 1970.

Henle G, Henle W. The virus as the etiologic agent of infectious mononucleosis. In Epstein MA, Achong BG, eds. The Epstein-Barr Virus. Berlin, Springer-Verlag, 1979a, pp. 297–320.

Henle W, Henle G. Seroepidemiology of the virus. In Epstein MA, Achong BG, eds. The Epstein-Barr Virus. Berlin, Springer-Verlag, 1979b, pp. 61–78.

Henle G, Henle W, Diehl V. Relation of Burkitt's tumor–associated herpes-type virus to infectious mononucleosis. Proc Natl Acad Sci U S A 59:94–101, 1968.

Henle G, Henle W, Klein G, Gunven P, Clifford P, Morrow RH, Zeigler JL. Antibodies to early Epstein-Barr virus-induced antigens in Burkitt's lymphoma. J Natl Canc Inst 46:861–871, 1971.

Henle G, Henle W, Clifford P, Diehl V, Kafuko GW, Kirya BG, Klein G, Morrow RH, Munube GMR, Pike P, Tukei PM, Zeigler JL. Antibodies to Epstein-Barr virus in Burkitt's lymphoma and control groups. J Natl Canc Inst 42:1147–1157, 1969.

Henle W, Henle G, Horwitz CA. Epstein-Barr virus–specific diagnostic tests in infectious mononucleosis. Hum Pathol 5:551–565, 1974a.

Henle W, Henle G, Hewetson J, Rocchi G, Leikola J. Failure to detect heterophil antigens in Epstein-Barr virus infected cells and to demonstrate interaction of heterophil antibodies with Epstein-Barr virus. Clin Exp Immunol 19:281–286, 1974b.

Henle W, Ho JCH, Henle G, Chau JCW, Kwan HC. Nasopharyngeal carcinoma: significance of changes in Epstein-Barr virus related antibody patterns following therapy. Int J Cancer 20:663–672, 1977.

Henter JI, Elinder G. Familial hemophagocytic lymphohistiocytosis—clinical review based on the findings in seven children. Acta Paediatr Scand 80:269–277, 1991.

Henter JI, Elinder G. Cerebromeningeal haemophagocytic lymphohistiocytosis. Lancet 1339:104–107, 1992.

Henter JI, Elinder G, Ost A, and the FHL Study group of the Histiocyte Society. Diagnostic guidelines for hemophagocytic lymphohistiocytosis. Semin Oncol 18:29–33, 1991.

Henter JI, Elinder G, Soder O, Hansson M, Andersson B, Andersson U. Hypercytokinemia in familial hemophagocytic lymphohistiocytosis. Blood 78:2918–2922, 1991.

Henter JI, Elinder G, Soder O, Ost A. Successful induction with chemotherapy including teniposide in familial erythrophagocytic lymphohistiocytosis. Lancet 2:1402, 1986.

Hilgartner MW, Knatterud GL, and the FEIBA Study Group. The use of factor eight inhibitor by-passing activity (FEIBA immuno) product for treatment of bleeding episodes in hemophiliacs with inhibitors. Blood 61:36–40, 1983.

Hirt A, Imbach P, Morell A, Wagner HP. Infectious mononucleosis: sequential immunologic, cytochemical and cytokenetic studies on single lymphoid cells in peripheral blood. Blood 58:602–606, 1981.

Hochberg FH, Miller G, Schooley RT, Hirsch MS, Feorino P, Henle W. Central nervous system lymphoma related to Epstein-Barr virus. N Engl J Med 309:745–748, 1983.

Holmes GP, Daplan JE, Stewart JA, Nunt G, Pinsky PF, Schonberge LB. A cluster of patients with a chronic mononucleosis-like syndrome: is Epstein-Barr virus the cause? JAMA 257:2297–2302, 1987.

Holmes GP, Kaplan JE, Glantz NM, Komaroff AL, Schonberger LB, Straus SE, Jones JF, Dubois RE, Cunningham-Rundles C, Pahwa S, Tosato G, Zegans LS, Purtilo DT, Brown N, Schooley RT, Burs I. Chronic fatigue syndrome: a working case definition. Ann Intern Med 108:387–389, 1988.

Holtman H, Janka GE, Weidner E, Eife R. Impaired natural killer cell function in familial hemophagocytic lymphohistiocytosis. Immunology 162:364–371, 1982.

Horwitz CA, Henle W, Henle G, Goldfarb M, Kubic P, Gehr RC, Balfour H, Pleisher GR, Krivit W. Clinical and laboratory evaluation of infants and children with Epstein-Barr virus induced infectious mononucleosis: report of 32 patients (aged 10–48 months). Blood 57:933–938, 1981.

Howells DW, Strobel S, Smith I, Levinsky RJ, Hyland K. Central nervous system involvement in the erythrophagocytic disorders of infancy: the role of cerebrospinal fluid neopterins in their differential diagnosis and clinical management. Pediatr Res 28:116–119, 1990.

Hultin MB, Shapiro SS, Bowman HS, Gill FM, Andrews AT, Martinez J, Eyster ME, Sherwood WC. Immunosuppressive therapy of factor VIII inhibitors. Blood 48:95–108, 1976.

Hutt LM, Huang YT, Dascomb HE, Pagano J. Enhanced destruction of lymphoid cell lines by peripheral blood leukocytes taken from patients with acute infectious mononucleosis. J Immunol 115:243–248, 1975.

Imbach P, Berchtold W, Hirt A, Mueller-Eckbardt C, Rossi E, Wagner HP, Gaedicke G, Joller P, Muller B, Barandun S. Intravenous immunoglobulin versus oral corticosteroids in acute immune thrombocytopenic purpura in childhood. Lancet 2:464–468, 1985.

Imerslund O, Bjornstad P. Familial vitamin B$_{12}$ malabsorption. Acta Haematol (Basel) 30:1–7, 1963.

Jaffe ES, Costa J, Fauci AS, Cossman J, Tsokos M. Malignant lymphoma and erythrophagocytosis simulating malignant histiocytosis. Am J Med 75:741–749, 1983.

Jandl JH, Kaplan ME. The destruction of red cells by antibodies in man. III. Quantitative factors influencing the patterns of hemolysis in vivo. J Clin Invest 39:1145–1156, 1960.

Janka GE. Familial hemophagocytic lymphohistiocytosis. Eur J Pediatr 140:221–230, 1983.

Jeannet M, Rubenstein AA, Pelet B, Kummer H. Prolonged remission of severe aplastic anemia after ALG pretreatment and HLA semi-incompatible bone-marrow cell transfusion. Transplant Proc 6:359–363, 1974.

Johnson CA, Abildgaard CF. Treatment of idiopathic autoimmune hemolytic anemia in children. Acta Paediatr Scand 65:375–379, 1976.

Joncas J, Monczak Y, Ghibu F, Alfieri C, Bonin A, Ahronheim G, Rivard G. Brief report: killer cell defect and persistent immunological abnormalities in two patients with chronic active Epstein-Barr virus infection. J Med Virol 28:110–117, 1989.

Jones JF, Ray CG, Minnich LL, Hicks MJ, Kibler RA, Lucas DO. Evidence for active Epstein-Barr virus infection in patients with persistent unexplained illnesses: elevated anti-early antigen antibodies. Ann Intern Med 102:1–7, 1985.

Jones JF, Shurin S, Abramowsky C, Tubbs RR, Sciotto CG, Wahl R, Sands J, Gottman D, Katz BZ, Sklar J. T-cell lymphomas containing Epstein Barr viral DNA inputs with chronic Epstein Barr virus infections. N Engl J Med 318:733–741, 1988.

Joseph A, Evans DIK. Immunosuppressive treatment of idiopathic thrombocytopenic purpura in children. Acta Paediatr Scand 71:467–469, 1982.

Junghans RP, Ahn YS. High-dose intravenous gammaglobulin to suppress alloimmune destruction of donor platelets. Am J Med 76:204–208, 1984.

Kaplan ME, Jandl JH. Inhibition of red cell sequestration by cortisone. J Exp Med 114:921–937, 1961.

Karpatkin M. Corticosteroid therapy in thrombocytopenic infants of women with autoimmune thrombocytopenia. J Pediatr 105:623–625, 1984.

Karpatkin M, Porges RF, Karpatkin S. Platelet counts in infants of women with autoimmune thrombocytopenia. N Engl J Med 305:936–939, 1981.

Karpatkin S. Autoimmune thrombocytopenic purpura. Blood 56:329–343, 1980.

Kasper CK, Aledort LM, Counts RR, Edson JR, Fratantoni J, Green D, Hampton JW, Shapiro SS, Shulman NR, van Eys J. A more uniform measurement of factor VIII inhibitors. Thrombos Diathes Haemorrh 34:869–872, 1975.

Kasper CK, and the Hemophilia Study Group. Effect of prothrombin complex concentrates on factor VIII inhibitor levels. Blood 54:1358–1368, 1979.

Kataoka Y, Todo S, Marioka Y, Sugie K, Natamura Y, Yodoi J, Imashuku S. Impaired natural killer activity and expression of interleukin-2 receptor antigen in familial erythrophagocytic lymphohistiocytosis. Cancer 65:1976–2041, 1990.

Katz BZ, Berlman AB, Shapiro ED. Serologic evidence of active Epstein-Barr virus infection in EBV-associated lymphoproliferative disorders of children with acquired immunodeficiency syndrome. J Pediatr 120:228–232, 1992.

Kawa-Ha K, Franco E, Doi S, Yumara K, Ishihar S, Tawa A, Yabuuchi H. Successful treatment of chronic active Epstein-Barr virus infection with recombinant interleukin-2. Lancet 1:154, 1987.

Kelton JG, Gibbons S. Autoimmune platelet destruction: idiopathic thrombocytopenic purpura. Semin Thromb Hemost 8:83–104, 1982.

Kelton JG, Blanchette VS, Wilson WE, Powers P, Mohan Pai KR, Effer SB, Barr RD. Neonatal thrombocytopenia due to passive immunization. Prenatal diagnosis and distinction between maternal platelet alloantibodies and autoantibodies. N Engl J Med 302:1401–1403, 1980.

Kelton JG, Inwood MJ, Barr RM, Effer SB, Hunter D, Wilson WE, Ginsburg DA, Powers PJ. The prenatal prediction of thrombocytopenia in infants of mothers with clinically diagnosed immune thrombocytopenia. Am J Obstet Gynecol 144:449–454, 1982.

Kernoff LM, Malan E. Platelet antibody levels do not correlate with response to therapy in idiopathic thrombocytopenic purpura. Br J Haematol 53:559–562, 1983.

Kibler R, Lucas DO, Hicks MJ, Poulos BT, Jones JF. Immune function in chronic active Epstein-Barr virus infection. J Clin Immunol 5:46–54, 1985.

Kikuta H, Taguchi Y, Tomiqawa K, Kojima K, Kawamura N, Ishizaba A, Sakiyama Y, Matsumoto S, Imai S, Kinoshita T, Koizumi S, Osato T, Kobayashi I, Hamada I, Hirai K. Epstein-Barr virus genome-positive T lymphocytes in a boy with chronic active EBV infection associated with Kawasaki-like disease. Nature 333:455–457, 1988.

Klein E, Ernberg I, Masucci MG, Szigeti R, Wu YT, Masucci G, Suedmyr E. T-cell response to B-cells and Epstein-Barr virus antigens in infectious mononucleosis. Cancer Res 41:4210–4215, 1981.

Klemola T. Deficiency of immunoglobulin A. Ann Clin Res 19:248–257, 1987.

Komp DM, McNamara J, Buckley P. Elevated soluble interleukin-2 receptor in childhood hemophagocytic histiocytic syndromes. Blood 73:2128–2132, 1989.

Kumar A, Kumar P, Schur PH. DR3 and non-DR3 associated complement component C4A deficiency in systemic lupus erythematosus. Clin Immunol Immunopathol 60:55–64, 1991.

Kure S, Tada K, Wada J, Yoshie O. Inhibition of Epstein-Barr virus infection in vitro by recombinant human interferons α and γ. Virus Res 5:377–390, 1986.

Ladisch S, Ho W, Matheson D, Pikington R, Hartman G. Immunologic and clinical effects of repeated blood exchange in familial erythrophagocytic lymphohistiocytosis. Blood 60:814–882, 1982.

Ladisch S, Poplack DG, Holiman B, Blaese RM. Immunodeficiency in familial erythrophagocytic lymphohistiocytosis. Lancet 1:581–583, 1976.

Lai PK, Mackay-Scollay EM, Fimmel PJ, Alpers MP, Keast D. Cell-mediated immunity to Epstein-Barr virus and a blocking factor in patients with infectious mononucleosis. Nature 252:608–610, 1974.

Lalezari P, Jiang AF, Yegen L, Santorineou M. Chronic autoimmune neutropenia due to anti-NA2 antibody. N Engl J Med 293:744–747, 1975.

Lalezari P, Radel E. Neutrophil-specific antigens: immunology and clinical significance. Semin Hematol 11:381–290, 1974.

Lampkin BC, Schubert WK. Pernicious anemia in the second decade of life. J Pediatr 72:387–390, 1968.

Lau P, Sholtis CM, Aster RH. Post-transfusion purpura: an enigma of alloimmunization. Am J Hematol 9:331–336, 1980.

Lawrence JS, Johnson JB. The presence of a circulating anticoagulant in a male member of a hemophiliac family. Trans Am Clin Climat Assoc 57:223–231, 1941.

Leggett PL, Doyle D, Smith WB, Culpepper W, Cooper S, Ochsner JL. Elective cardiac operation in a patient with severe hemophilia and acquired factor VIII antibodies. J Thoracic Cardiovasc Surg 87:556–560, 1984.

Levy JA, Henle G. Indirect immunofluorescence tests with sera from African children and cultured Burkitt lymphoma cells. J Bacteriol 92:2275–2276, 1968.

Lillibridge CB, Brandborg LL, Rubin CE. Childhood pernicious anemia. Gastroenterology 52:792–809, 1967.

Lindahl T, Klein G, Reedman BM, Johansson B, Singh S. Relationship between Epstein-Barr virus (EBV) DNA and EBV-determined nuclear antigen (EBNA) in Burkitt lymphoma biopsies and other lymphoproliferative malignancies. Int J Cancer 13:764–772, 1974.

LoBuglio AF, Cotran RS, Jandl JH. Red cells coated with immunoglobulin G: binding and sphering by mononuclear cells in man. Science 158:1582–1585, 1967.

Loechelt BJ, Egeler RM, Filipovich AH, Jyonouchi H, Shapiro RS. Immunosuppression: an alternative maintenance therapy for familial hemophagocytic lymphohistiocytosis (FHL)—preliminary results. Med Pediatr Oncol 22:325–328, 1994.

Loeffel S, Chang CH, Heyn R, Harada S, Lipscomb H, Purtilo DT. Necrotizing lymphoid vasculitis in the X-linked lymphoproliferative syndrome. Arch Pathol Lab Med 109:546, 1985.

Lozner EL, Jolliffe LS, Taylor FHL. Hemorrhagic diathesis with prolonged coagulation time associated with a circulating anticoagulant. Am J Med Sci 199:318–327, 1940.

Lusher JM, Zuelzer WW. Idiopathic thrombocytopenic purpura in childhood. J Pediatr 68:971–979, 1966.

Lusher JM, Shapiro SS, Palascak JE, Rao AV, Levine PH, Blatt PM, the Hemophilia Study Group. Efficacy of prothrombin-complex concentrates in hemophiliacs with antibodies to factor VIII: a multicenter therapeutic trial. N Engl J Med 303:421–425, 1980.

MacKay RJ, Menahem S, Ekert H. Deep vein thrombosis in association with a circulating endogenous anticoagulant. J Pediatr 101:75–77, 1982.

Magrath IT, Rowe M, Filipovich AH, Shapiro R, Su IJ, Sculley T. Advances in the understanding of EBV-associated lymphoproliferative disorders. In Ablasi DV, Huang AT, Pagano JS, Pearson GR, Yang CS, eds. Epstein-Barr Virus and Human Disease 1990. Clifton, NJ, Humana Press, 1991, pp. 405–438.

Magni RJ, Neiderman JC, Kelleher JE, Dwyer JM, Evans AS, Kantor FS. Depression of cell-mediated immunity during acute infectious mononucleosis. N Engl J Med 291:1149–1153, 1974.

Mannucci PM, Ruggeri ZM, Ciavarella N, Kazatchkine MD, Mobray JF. Precipitating antibodies to factor VIII/von Willebrand factor in von Willebrand's disease: effects on replacement therapy. Blood 57:25–31, 1981.

Margolius A Jr, Jackson DP, Ratnoff OD. Circulating anticoagulants. A study of 40 cases and a review of the literature. Medicine 40:145–212, 1961.

Massey GV, McWilliams NB, Mueller DG, Napolitano A, Maurer HM. Intravenous immunoglobulin in neonatal isoimmune thrombocytopenia. J Pediatr 111:133–135, 1987.

Matoba AY. Ocular disease associated with Epstein-Barr virus infection. Surv Ophthalmol 35:145–150, 1990.

Mayr WR, Lechner K, Niessner H, Pabinger-Fasching I. HLA-DR and factor VIII antibodies in hemophilia A (letter). Thromb Haemost 51:293, 1984.

McClain K, Gehrz R, Grierson H, Purtilo D, Filipovich AH. Virus-associated histicytic proliferations in children: frequent association with Epstein-Barr virus and congenital or acquired immunodeficiencies. Am J Pediatr Hemat Oncol 10:196–205, 1988.

McIntyre OR, Sullivan LW, Jeffries GH, Silver RH. Pernicious anemia in childhood. N Engl J Med 272:981–986, 1965.

McMillan R. Chronic idiopathic thrombocytopenic purpura. N Engl J Med 304:1135–1147, 1981.

Meyer D, Frommel D, Larrieu MJ, Zimmerman TS. Selective absence of large forms of factor VIII/von Willebrand factor in acquired von Willebrand's syndrome. Response to transfusion. Blood 54:600–606, 1979.

Miller G, Shope T, Coope D, Waters L, Pagano J, Bornkamm G, Henle W. Lymphoma in cotton-top marmosets after inoculation with Epstein-Barr virus: tumor incidence, histologic spectrum, antibody responses, demonstration of viral DNA, and characterization of viruses. J Exp Med 145:948–967, 1977.

Miller DR, Bloom GE, Streiff RR, LoBuglio AF, Diamond LK. Juvenile congenital pernicious anemia. Clinical and immunologic studies. N Engl J Med 275:978–983, 1966.

Moake JL, Rudy CK, Troll JH, Weinstein MJ, Colannino NM, Azocar

J, Seder RH, Hong SL, Deykin D. Unusually large plasma factor VIII; von Willebrand factor multimers in chronic relapsing thrombotic thrombocytopenic purpura. N Engl J Med 307:1432–1435, 1982.

Molina IJ, Kenney DM, Rosen RS, Remold-O'Donnell E. T cell lines characterize events in the pathogenesis of the Wiskott-Aldrich syndrome. J Exp Med 176:867–874, 1993.

Mollison PL. The effects of isoantibodies on red cell survival. Ann NY Acad Sci 169:199–216, 1970a.

Mollison PL. The role of complement in antibody-mediated red cell destruction. Br J Haematol 18:249–255, 1970b.

Mollison PL. Blood Transfusion in Clinical Medicine 5th ed. Oxford, Blackwell Scientific Publications, 1972c, pp. 1–830.

Moore KW, Lieiza P, Fiorention DF, Trounstine ML, Khan TA, Mosmann TR. Homology of cytokine synthesis inhibitory factor (IL-10) to the Epstein-Barr virus gene BCRF1. Science 248:1230–1234, 1990.

Morgan AJ. Control of viral disease: the development of Epstein-Barr virus vaccines. Springer Semin Immunopathol 13:249–262, 1991.

Morgan DG, Niederman JC, Miller G, Smith HW, Dowaliby JM. Site of Epstein-Barr virus replication in the oropharynx. Lancet 1:1154–1157, 1979.

Morrell D, Cromartie E, Swift M. Mortality and cancer in 263 patients with ataxia telangiectasia. J Natl Cancer Inst 77:89–92, 1986.

Moss DJ, Wallace LE, Rickinson AB, Epstein MA. Cytotoxic T cell recognition of Epstein-Barr virus–infected B cells. I. Specificity and HLA restriction of effector cells reactivated in vitro. Eur J Immunol 11:686–693, 1981.

Mroczek E, Weisenburger DD, Grierson HL, Markin R, Purtilo DT. Fatal infectious mononucleosis and virus-associated hemophagocytic syndrome. Arch Pathol Lab Med 111:530, 1987.

Mueller BU, Pizzo PA. Medical progress: cancer in children with primary or secondary immunodeficiencies. J Pediatr 126:1–10, 1995.

Mueller-Eckhardt C, Kayser W, Mersch-Baumert K, Mueller-Eckhardt G, Breidenbach M, Kugel HG, Graubner M. The clinical significance of platelet-associated IgG: a study on 298 patients with various disorders. Br J Haematol 46:123–131, 1980.

Mueller-Eckhardt C, Kuenzlen E, Thilo-Korner D, Pralie H. High-dose intravenous immunoglobulin for post-transfusion purpura. N Engl J Med 308:287, 1983.

Muntean W, Petek W. Lupus anticoagulant after measles. Eur J Pediatr 134:135–138, 1980.

Murphy S, LoBuglio AF. Drug therapy of autoimmune hemolytic anemia. Semin Hematol 13:323–334, 1976.

Myers TJ, Kim BK, Steiner M, Baldini MG. Platelet-associated complement C3 in immune thrombocytopenic purpura. Blood 59:1023–1028, 1982.

Neudorf SML, Filipovich AH, Kersey JH. Successful immunoreconstitution following bone marrow transplantation decreases the risk of developing lymphoreticular tumors in Wiskott-Aldrich syndrome and severe combined immune deficiency: a retrospective analysis. In Purtilo DT, ed. Immune Deficiency and Cancer: Epstein-Barr Virus and Lymphoproliferative Malignancies. New York, Plenum Press, 1984, pp. 471–480.

Nilsson K, Klein G, Henle W, Henle G. The establishment of lymphoblastoid lines from adult and fetal lymphoid tissue and its dependence on EBV. Int J Cancer 8:443–450, 1971.

Nissen C, Cornu P, Gratwhol A, Speck B. Peripheral blood cells from patients with aplastic anemia in partial remission suppress growth of their own bone marrow precursors in culture. Br J Haematol 45:233, 1980.

Noelle RJ, Roy M, Shepherd DM, Stamenkovic I, Ledbetter JA, Aruffo A. A 39-kDa protein on activated helper T cells binds CD40 and transduces the signal for cognate activation of B cells. Proc Natl Acad Sci U S A 89:6550–6554, 1992.

Nydegger UE, Spycher MO. Polyclonal polyspecific antibody mixtures from random donors as therapeutic tools in autoimmune disease. In Morell A, Nydegger UE, eds. Clinical Use of Intravenous Immunoglobulins. London, Academic Press, 1986, pp. 431–441.

Ochs HD, Sullivan JL, Wedgwood RJ, Seeley JK, Sakamoto K, Purtilo DT. X-linked lymphoproliferative syndrome: abnormal antibody responses to bacteriophage ϕX174. Birth Defects 19:321–323, 1983.

O'Conor GT. Persistent immunologic stimulation as a factor in oncogenesis with special reference to Burkitt's tumor. Am J Med 48:279–285, 1970.

Okano M, Thiele GM, Davis JR, Grierson HL, Purtilo DT. Epstein-Barr virus and human diseases: recent advances in diagnosis. Clin Microbiol Rev 1:300–312, 1988.

Okano M, Thiele GM, Kobayashi RH, Davis JR, Synovec MS, Grierson HL, Jaffe E, Purtilo DT. Interferon-gamma in a family with acute Epstein-Barr virus infection. J Clin Immunol 9:48–54, 1989.

Okano M, Pirruccello SJ, Grierson HL, Johnson DR, Thiele GM, Purtilo DT. Immunovirological studies of fatal infectious mononucleosis in a patient with X-linked lymphoproliferative syndrome treated with intravenous immunoglobulin and interferon-α. Clin Immunol Immunopathol 54:410, 1990a.

Okano M, Thiele G, Purtilo DT. Severe chronic active Epstein-Barr virus infection syndrome and adenovirus type-2 infection. Am J Pediatr Hematol Oncol 12:168–173, 1990b.

Okano M, Matsumoto S, Osata T, Sakiyama Y, Thiele GM, Purtilo DT. Severe chronic active Epstein-Barr virus infection syndrome. Clin Microbiol Rev 4:129–135, 1991.

Ordi J, Vilardell M, Alijotas J, Barquinero J, Vila M. Serum thrombocytopenia and high-dose immunoglobulin treatment. Ann Intern Med 104:282–283, 1986.

Orris DJ, Lewis JH, Spero JA, Hasiba U. Blocking coagulation inhibitors in children taking penicillin. J Pediatr 97:426–429, 1980.

Pagano JS, Huang CH, Levine P. Absence of Epstein-Barr virus DNA in American Burkitt's lymphoma. N Engl J Med 289:1395–1399, 1973.

Parker CW, Vavra JD. Immunosuppression. Prog Hematol 6:1–82, 1969.

Parker P, Escalon EE, Reeves-Garcia J, Gonzalez R. A newborn with fever, hepatosplenomegaly, and thrombocytopenia. Int Pediatr 4:380–383, 1989.

Pattengale PK, Smith RW, Perlin E. Atypical lymphocytes in acute infectious mononucleosis. N Engl J Med 291:1145–1148, 1974.

Paul JR, Bunnell WW. The presence of heterophil antibodies in infectious mononucleosis. Am J Med Sci 183:90–104, 1932.

Pearson GR, Orr TW. Antibody-dependent lymphocyte cytotoxicity against cells experiencing Epstein-Barr virus antigens. J Natl Cancer Inst 56:485–488, 1984.

Perez N, Virelizier JL, Arenazana-Seisdedos F, Fischer A, Griscelli C. Impaired natural killer activity in lymphohistiocytosis syndrome. J Pediatr 104:469–573, 1984.

Perry GS III, Spector BD, Schuman LM, Mandel JS, Anderson VE, McHugh RB, Hanson MR, Fahlstrom SM, Krivit W, Kersey JH. The Wiskott-Aldrich syndrome in the United States and Canada (1892–1979). J Pediatr 97:72–78, 1980.

Petz LD, Garratty G. Acquired Immune Hemolytic Anemias. New York, Churchill Livingstone, 1980.

Pickering RJ, Wolfson MR, Good RA, Gewurz H. Passive hemolysis by serum and cobra venom factor: a new mechanism inducing membrane damage by complement. Proc Natl Acad Sci U S A 62:521–527, 1969.

Pirofsky B. Clinical aspects of autoimmune hemolytic anemia. Semin Hematol 13:251–265, 1976.

Pollack S, Cunningham-Rundles C, Smithwick EM, Barandun S, Good RA. High-dose intravenous gammaglobulin for autoimmune neutropenia. N Engl J Med 307:253, 1982.

Pracher E, Panzer-Grümayer ER, Zoubek A, Peters C, Gadner H. Successful bone marrow transplantation in a boy with X-linked lymphoproliferative syndrome and acute severe infectious mononucleosis. Bone Marrow Transplantation 13:655–658, 1994.

Provisor AJ, Iacuone JJ, Chilocote RR, Neiburger RG, Curssi FG, Baehner RL. Acquired agammaglobulinemia after life-threatening illness with clinical and laboratory features of infectious mononucleosis in three related male children. N Engl J Med 293:62–65, 1975.

Pui CH, Hancock ML, Raimondi SC, Head DR, Thompson E, Wilimas J, Kun LE, Bowman LC, Crist WM, Pratt CB. Myeloid neoplasia in children treated for solid tumors. Lancet 336:417–421, 1990.

Pui CH, Behm FG, Raimondi SC, Dodge RK, George SL, Rivera GK, Mirro J, Kalwinsky DK, Dahl GV, Murphy SB, Crist WM, Williams DL. Secondary acute myeloid leukemia in children treated for acute lymphoid leukemia. N Engl J Med 321:136–142, 1989.

Purtilo DT. X-linked lymphoproliferative syndrome: an immunodeficiency disorder with acquired agammaglobulinemia, fatal infectious mononucleosis or malignant lymphoma. Arch Pathol Med 105:119–121, 1981.

Purtilo DT. X-linked lymphoproliferative disease (XLP) as a model of Epstein-Barr virus-induced immunopathology. Springer Semin Immunopath 13:181–197, 1991.

Purtilo DT, Cassel CK, Yang JPS, Harper R, Stephenson SR, Landing BH, Vawter GF. X-linked recessive progressive variable immunodeficiency (Duncan's disease). Lancet 1:935–941, 1975.

Purtilo DT, DeFlorio D, Hutt LU, Yang JPS, Otto R, Edwards W. Variable phenotypic expression of an X-linked recessive lymphoproliferative syndrome. N Engl J Med 297:1077–1081, 1977.

Purtilo DT, Grierson HL, Davis JR, Okano M. The X-linked lymphoproliferative disease: from autopsy toward cloning the genes 1975–1990. Pediatr Pathol 11:685–710, 1991.

Reece ER, Gartner JG, Seemayer JA, Joncas JH. Lymphoma after thymus transplantation. N Engl J Med 302:302, 1980.

Risdall RJ, Brunning RD, Hernandez JI, Gordon DH. Bacteria-associated hemophagocytic syndrome. Cancer 54:2968–2973, 1984.

Risdall RJ, McKenna RW, Nesbit ME, Krivit W, Balfour HH, Simmons RL, Brunning RD. Virus-associated hemophagocytic syndrome: a benign histiocytic proliferation distinct from malignant histiocytosis. Cancer 44:993–1002, 1979.

Robison L, Stoker V, Frizzera G, Heinitz KJ, Meadows AT, Filipovich AH. Hodgkin's disease in pediatric patients with naturally occurring immunodeficiency. Am J Ped Hem Onc 92:189–192, 1987.

Rosen A, Gergely P, Jondal M, Klein G, Britton S. Polyclonal IgG production after Epstein-Barr virus infection in human lymphocytes in vitro. Nature, 267:52–54, 1977.

Rosse WF. Quantitative immunology of immune hemolytic anemia. II. The relationship of cell-bound antibody to hemolysis and the effect of treatment. J Clin Invest 50:734–743, 1971.

Rosse WF, Lauf PK. Effects of immune reactions on the red cell membrane. Semin Hematol 7:323–340, 1970.

Roy M, Waldschmidt T, Aruffo A, Ledbetter JA, Noelle RJ. The regulation of the expression of gp39, the CD40 ligand, on normal and cloned CD4+ T cells. J Immunol 151:2497–2510, 1993.

Royston I, Sullivan JL, Periman PO, Perlin E. Cell-mediated immunity to Epstein-Barr virus transformed lymphoblastoid cells in acute infectious mononucleosis. N Engl J Med 293:1159–1163, 1975.

Rubin CM, Burke BA, McKenna RW, McClain KL, White JG, Nesbit ME, Filipovitch A. The accelerated phase of Chédiak-Higashi syndrome: an expression of virus associated hemophagocytic syndrome. Cancer 56:524–530, 1985.

Rubinson AB. The biology of Epstein-Barr virus persistence: a reappraisal. Adv Exp Med Biol 278:137–146, 1990.

Ryser O, Morell A, Hitzig W. Primary immunodeficiencies in Switzerland: first report of the national registry in adults and children. J Clin Immunol 8:479–485, 1988.

Saemundson AK, Berkel AI, Henle W. Epstein-Barr virus carrying lymphoma in a patient with ataxia-telangiectasia. Br Med J 282:425–427, 1981.

Sakamoto K, Sexton J, Purtilo DT. Long-term studies of Epstein-Barr virus (EBV) antibody responses in X-linked lymphoproliferative syndrome (XLP). Fed Proc 40:1122, 1981.

Salama A, Mueller-Eckhardt C. Use of Rh antibodies in the treatment of autoimmune thrombocytopenia. Transfusion Med Rev 6:17–25, 1992.

Salsbury AJ, Clarke JA, Shand WS. Red cell surface changes in cold agglutination. Clin Exp Immunol 3:313–322, 1968.

Sartorius JA. Steroid treatment of idiopathic thrombocytopenic purpura in children: preliminary results of a randomized cooperative study. Am J Pediatr Hematol Oncol 6:165–169, 1984.

Schaffer FM, Palermos J, Zhu ZB, Barger BO, Cooper MD, Volanakis JE. Individuals with IgA deficiency and common variable immunodeficiency share polymorphisms of major histocompatibility complex class III genes. Proc Natl Acad Sci U S A 86:8015–8019, 1989.

Schreiber AD, Parsons J, McDermott P, Cooper RA. Effect of corticosteroids on the human monocyte IgG and complement receptors. J Clin Invest 56:1189, 1975.

Schreiber AD, Frank MM. Autoimmune hemolytic anemia. In Samter M, Talmage DW, Frank MM, Austen KF, Claman HM, eds. Immunological Diseases, 4th ed. Boston, Little, Brown, 1988, pp. 1609–1629.

Schryver A, Friberg S, Klein G, Henle W, Henle G, DeThe G, Clifford P, Ho HC. Epstein-Barr virus–associated antibody patterns in carcinoma of the post-nasal space. Clin Exp Immunol 5:443–449, 1969.

Schubach WH, Hackman R, Neiman PE, Miller G, Thomas ED. A monoclonal immunoblastic sarcoma in donor cells bearing Epstein-Barr virus genomes following allogeneic marrow grafting for acute lymphoblastic leukemia. Blood 60:180–187, 1982.

Schultz LE. Heterophile antibody titer in diseases other than infectious mononucleosis. Arch Intern Med 81:328–333, 1948.

Scott JR, Cruikshank DP, Kochenour NK, Pitkin RM, Warenski JC. Fetal platelet counts in the obstetric management of immunologic thrombocytopenic purpura. Am J Obstet Gynecol 136:495–499, 1980.

Seemayer TA, Grierson H, Pirrueaello SJ, Gross TB, Weisenberger DO, Davis J, Spiegel K, Briehauk B, Semugi J. X-linked lymphoproliferative disease. Am J Dis Child 147:1242–1247, 1993.

Shadduck RK, Winkelstein A, Zeigler Z, Lichter J, Goldstein M, Michaels M, Rabin B. Aplastic anemia following infectious mononucleosis: possible immune etiology. Exp Hematol 7:264–271, 1979.

Shapiro RS, Filipovich AH. Successful therapy for EBV associated B cell lymphoproliferative disorders in immunodeficiency using alpha interferon and intravenous immunoglobulin. In Ablasi DV, Faggioni A, Kruger GRF, et al., eds. Epstein-Barr Virus and Human Disease II. Clifton, NJ, Humana Press, 1991, pp. 355–360.

Shapiro RS, McClain K, Frizzera G, Gajl-Peczalska KJ, Kersey JH, Blazar BR, Arthur DC, Patton DF, Greenberg JS, Burke B, Ramsay NKC, McGlave P, Filipovich AH. Epstein-Barr virus associated B cell lymphoproliferative disorders following bone marrow transplantation. Blood 71:1234–1243, 1988.

Shapiro SS, Hultin M. Acquired inhibitors to the blood coagulation factors. Semin Thromb Hemost 1:336–385, 1975.

Shapiro SS. Markers for the factor VIII antibody response in hemophilia A. Scand J Haematol (Suppl. 40)33:181–185, 1984.

Shearer WT, Ritz J, Finegold MJ, Guerra IC, Rosenblatt HM, Lewis DE, Pollack MS, Taber LH, Sumaya CV, Grumet FC, Cleary ML, Warnke R, Sklar J. Epstein-Barr virus associated B cell proliferations of diverse clonal origins after bone marrow transplantation in a 12-year-old patient with severe combined immunodeficiency. N Engl J Med 312:4–49, 1984.

Sheldon PJ, Hemsted EH, Papamichail M, Halboron EJ. Thymic origin of atypical lymphoid cells in infectious mononucleosis. Lancet 1:1153–1155, 1973.

Simonsen M. Graft versus host reactions. Their natural history, and applicability as tools of research. Progr Allergy 6:349–467, 1962.

Sixby JW, Davis DS, Young LS, Hutt-Fletcher L, Tedder TF, Rickinson AB. Human epithelial cell expression of an Epstein-Barr virus receptor. J Gen Virol 678:805–811, 1987.

Sixby JW, Nedrud JG, Raab-Traub N, Hanes RA, Pagano JS. Epstein-Barr virus replication in oropharyngeal epithelial cells. N Engl J Med 310:1225–1230, 1984.

Skare JC, Milunsky A, Byron KS, Sullivan JL. Mapping the X-linked lymphoproliferative syndrome. Proc Natl Acad Sci U S A 84:2015–2018, 1987.

Slocombe GW, Newland AC, Colvin MP, Colvin BT. The role of intensive plasma exchange in the prevention and management of haemorrhage in patients with inhibitors to factor VIII. Br J Haematol 47:577–585, 1981.

Smith TJ, Terada N, Robinson CC, Gelfand EW. Acute infectious mononucleosis stimulates the selective expression/expansion of Vβ6.1–3 and Vβ7 T cells. Blood 81:1521–1526, 1993.

Speck B, Cornu P, Jeannet M, Nissen C, Burri HP, Groff P, Nagel GA, Buckner CD. Autologous marrow recovery following allogeneic marrow transplantation in a patient with severe aplastic anemia. Exp Hematol 4:131–137, 1976.

St. Clair W, Jones B, Rogers JS, Crouch M, Hrabovsky E. Deep venous thrombosis and a circulating anticoagulant in systemic lupus erythematosus. Am J Dis Child 135:230–232, 1981.

Stableforth P, Tamagnini GL, Dormandt KM. Acquired von Willebrand's syndrome with inhibitors both to factor VIII clotting activity and ristocetin-induced platelet aggregation. Br J Haematol 33:565–573, 1976.

Stark B, Cohen IJ, Pecht M, Umiel T, Apte RN, Friedman E, Levin S, Vogel R, Schlesinger M, Zaizov R. Immunologic dysregulation in a patient with familial hemophagocytic lymphohistiocytosis. Cancer 60:2629–2636, 1987.

Stenbjerg S, Ingerslev J, Zachariae E. Factor VIII inhibitor treatment with high doses of F VIII. Thromb Res 34:533–539, 1984.

Stephan JL, Donadieu J, Ledeist F, Blanche S, Griscelli C, Fischer A. Treatment of familial hemophagocytic lymphohistiocytosis with antithymocyte globulins, steroids, and cyclosporin A. Blood 82:2319–2323, 1993.

Stohl W. Cellular mechanisms in the in vitro inhibition of pokeweed mitogen-induced B cell differentiation by immunoglobulin for intravenous use. J Immunol 136:4407–4413, 1986.

Straus SE. Acute progressive Epstein-Barr virus infection. Annu Rev Med 43:437–449, 1992.

Straus SE, Dale JK, Tobi M, Lawley T, Preble O, Blaese RM, Hallahan C, Henle W. Acyclovir treatment of the chronic fatigue syndrome: lack of efficacy in a placebo-controlled trial. N Engl J Med 319:1692–1698, 1988.

Straus SE, Fleisher GR. Infectious mononucleosis, epidemiology and pathogenesis. In Schlossberg D, ed. Infectious mononucleosis, 2nd ed. Berlin, Springer Verlag, 1989, pp. 8–28.

Sullivan JL, Byron KS, Brewster FE, Baker SM, Ochs HD. X-linked lymphoproliferative syndrome: natural history of the immunodeficiency. J Clin Invest 71:1765–1778, 1983.

Sullivan DW, Purdy LJ, Billingham M, Glader BE. Fatal myocardial infarction following therapy with prothrombin complex concentrates in a young man with hemophilia A. Pediatrics 74:279–281, 1984a.

Sullivan JL, Medveesky P, Forman SJ, Baker SM, Monroe JE, Mulder C. Epstein-Barr virus induced lymphoproliferation: implications for antiviral chemotherapy. N Engl J Med 311:1163–1167, 1984b.

Sultan Y, Maisonneuve P, Kazatchkine MD, Nydegger UE. Anti-idiotypic suppression of autoantibodies to factor VIII (anti-haemophilic factor) by high-dose intravenous gammaglobulin. Lancet 2:765–768, 1984.

Sumaya CV. Epstein-Barr virus serologic testing: diagnostic indications and interpretations. Pediatr Infect Dis 5:337–342, 1986.

Svedmyr E, Jondal M. Cytotoxic effector cells specific for B cell lines transformed by Epstein-Barr virus are present in patients with infectious mononucleosis. Proc Natl Acad Sci U S A 72:1622–1626, 1975.

Tanner DR. Ocular manifestations of infectious mononucleosis. Arch Ophthalmol 51:229, 1952.

Tchernia G, Dreyfus M, Laurian Y, Dercyke M, Mirica C, Kerbrat G. Management of immune thrombocytopenia in pregnancy: response to infusions of immunoglobulins. Am J Obstet Gynecol 148:225–226, 1984.

Thiagarajan P, Shapiro SS. Lupus anticoagulants. In Colman RW, ed. Disorders of Thrombin Formation. New York, Churchill Livingstone, 1983, pp. 101–108.

Thomas ED, Storb R, Giblett ER, Longpre B, Weiden PL, Fefer A, Witherspoon R, Clift RA, Buckner CD. Recovery from aplastic anemia following attempted marrow transplantation. Exp Hematol 4:97–102, 1976.

Thompson RD, Lachmann PJ. Reactive lysis: the complement-mediated lysis of unsensitized cells. I. The characterization of the indicator factor and its identification as C7. J Exp Med 131:629–641, 1970.

Tomkinson BE, Wagner DK, Nelson DL, Sullivan JL. Activated lymphocytes during acute Epstein-Barr virus infection. J Immunol 139:3802–3807, 1987.

Tosato G, Magrath I, Koski I, Dooley N, Blaese M. Activation of suppressor T-cells during Epstein-Barr virus–induced infectious mononucleosis. N Engl J Med 30:1133–1137, 1979.

Tosato G, Steinberg AD, Yarchoan R, Heilman CH, Pike SE, DeSeur V, Blaese RM. Abnormally elevated frequency of Epstein-Barr virus–infected B cells in the blood of patients with rheumatoid arthritis. J Clin Invest 73:1789–1795, 1984.

Twomey JJ, Jordan PH, Jarrold T, Trubowitz S, Ritz ND, Conn HO. The syndrome of immunoglobulin deficiency and pernicious anemia. Am J Med 47:340–350, 1969.

Twomey JJ. Abnormalities in the mixed leukocyte reaction during infectious mononucleosis. J Immunol 112:2278–2281, 1974.

Uchino H, Yasunaga K, Akatsuka JI. A cooperative clinical trial of high-dose immunoglobulin therapy in 177 cases of idiopathic thrombocytopenic purpura. Thomb Haemost 51:182–185, 1984.

Van De Winkel JHJ, Capel PJA: Human IgG Fc receptor heterogeneity: molecular aspects and clinical implication. Immunol Today 14:215–221, 1993.

Vaughan JH, Barnett EV, Leddy JP. Autosensitivity diseases: immunologic and pathogenetic concepts in lupus erythematosus, rheumatoid arthritis and hemolytic anemia. N Engl J Med 275:1486–1494, 1966.

Viero P, Cortelazzo S, Buelli M, Comotti B, Minetti B, Bassan R, Barbui T. Thrombotic thrombocytopenic purpura and high-dose immunoglobulin treatment. Ann Intern Med 104:282, 1986.

Villiger PM, Feg MF, Lotz M, Tobler A. IgG4 subclass deficiency and Evan's syndrome in an adult patient. J Allergy Clin Immunol 90:693–694, 1992.

Vowels MR, Lam-Po-Tang R, Berdoukas V, Ford D, Thierry D, Purtilo D, Gluckman E. Brief report: correction of X-linked lymphoproliferative disease by transplantation of cord-blood stem cells. N Engl J Med 329:1623–1625, 1993.

Warkentin PI, Ramsay NKC, Krivit W, Coccia PF, Nesbit ME, Condie R, Kersey JR. Immunosuppressive therapy for severe aplastic anemia. Am J Pediatr Hematol Oncol 2:327–339, 1980.

Way F, Blaese RM, Zoom KC, Tosato G. Suppressor T-cell clones from patients with acute Epstein-Barr virus–induced infectious mononucleosis. J Clin Invest 77:7–14, 1986.

Webster ADB, Platts-Mills TAE, Jannossy G, Morgan M, Asherson GL. Autoimmune blood dyscrasias in five patients with hypogammaglobulinemia: response of neutropenia to vincristine. J Clin Immunol 1:113–118, 1981.

Weiden PI, Blaese RM. Hereditary thrombocytopenia: relation to Wiskott-Aldrich syndrome with special reference to splenectomy. J Pediatr 80:226–234, 1972.

Wenske C, Gaedicke G, Kuenzlen E, Heyes H, Mueller-Eckhardt C, Kleinhauer E, Lauritzine C. Treatment of idiopathic thrombocytopenic purpura in pregnancy by high-dose intravenous immunoglobulin. Blut 46:347–353, 1983.

WHO Scientific Group on Immunodeficiency. Primary immunodeficiency diseases. Immunodefic Rev 1:173–205, 1989.

Williams LL, Rooney CM, Conley ME, Brenner MK, Krance RA, Heslop HE. Correction of Duncan's syndrome by allogeneic bone marrow transplantation. Lancet 342:587–588, 1993.

Wilson ER, Malluh A, Stagno S, Crist WM. Fatal Epstein-Barr virus–associated hemophagocytic syndrome. J Pediatr 98:260–262, 1981.

Wollheim FA. Immunoglobulin changes in the course of infectious mononucleosis. Scand J Haematol 5:97–107, 1969.

Worlledge SM. Immune drug-induced haemolytic anemias. Semin Hematol 10:327–344, 1973.

Worlledge SM, Dacie JV. Hemolytic and other anemias in infectious mononucleosis. In Carter RL, Penman HG, eds. Infectious Mononucleosis. Oxford, Blackwell Scientific Publications, 1969, pp. 82–98.

Ziegler JL, Drew WL, Miner RC. Outbreak of Burkitt's-like lymphoma in homosexual men. Lancet 2:631–633, 1982.

Zuazu JP, Duran JW, Julia AF. Hemophagocytosis in acute brucellosis. N Engl J Med 301:1185–1186, 1979.

Zur Hausen H, Schulte-Holthausen H, Klein G, Henle W, Henle G, Clifford P, Santesson L. EB virus DNA in biopsies of Burkitt's tumors and anaplastic carcinoma of the nasopharynx. Nature 228:1056–1058, 1970.

Chapter 28

Immunologic Diseases of the Nervous System

Robert S. Rust and John O. Fleming

Immunologic abnormalities are prominent in several pediatric neurologic diseases. In these disorders, the immune and nervous systems interact in complex, reciprocal patterns. Although overlap exists, it is clinically useful to consider these diseases as predominantly affecting either the peripheral or the central nervous system (Table 28–1).

INFLAMMATORY MYOPATHIES (Polymyositis and Dermatomyositis)

Historic Aspects

Polymyositis (PM) was first described by Wagner in 1863, and in 1887 Unverricht appreciated the distinc-

Table 28–1. Neuroimmunologic Disorders

Conditions Primarily Affecting the Peripheral Nervous System

Muscle
  Inflammatory myopathies
    Polymyositis
    Dermatomyositis
    Inclusion body myositis

Neuromuscular Junction
  Myasthenia gravis
  Lambert-Eaton myasthenic syndrome

Peripheral Nerve
  Guillain-Barré syndrome
  Chronic inflammatory demyelinating polyradiculoneuropathy
  Bell's palsy
  Other immune-mediated peripheral neuropathies

Conditions Primarily Affecting the Central Nervous System

White Matter
  Acute disseminated encephalomyelitis
  Optic neuritis
  Acute transverse myelitis
  Devic's syndrome
  Acute cerebellar ataxia
  Multiple sclerosis
  Ataxia telangiectasia

Gray Matter
  Sydenham's chorea
  Thrombotic thrombocytopenic purpura/hemolytic-uremic
    syndrome
  Rasmussen's encephalitis
  Paraneoplastic syndromes

tive features of dermatomyositis (DM). Both disorders are associated with weakness, but whereas the inflammatory changes of PM are limited to muscle, DM involves other tissues, particularly the skin. More recently, a related entity, inclusion body myositis (IBM), has been delineated (Lotz et al., 1989; Mikol and Engel, 1994). The common features of these three conditions

have led Dalakas (1991) and others to group them as "inflammatory myopathies." DM is relatively common, PM is rare, and IBM rarely, if ever, occurs in children and adolescents. These disorders must be distinguished from an additional rare inflammatory entity, congenital, or infantile, myositis (CM/IM).

Pathogenesis

Although the pathogenesis of inflammatory myopathies is unknown, it is thought that they may result when toxins, medications, or viruses trigger an autoimmune response. The nature of the immune response and the particular targets attacked produce distinctive patterns of immunopathology and associated clinical findings (Table 28–2).

DM is the result of a small-vessel angiopathy mediated by humoral immunity (Silver and Mericq, 1989; Dalakas, 1991; Engel et al., 1994). Inflammatory elements, including B cells and complement components, such as the C5b-9 membrane attack complex, are restricted to the perivascular region, with little or no lymphocytic invasion within muscle fascicles themselves. Muscle fiber necrosis occurs at the margins of fascicles, in proximity to the perivascular exudate. The microvasculature is the primary target of an autoimmune response in which the myofibrillar injury is secondary to angiitic ischemia. Similar changes may occur in small nerves, skin, connective tissues, the gastrointestinal tract, and lungs.

By contrast, PM is largely mediated by cellular autoimmunity directed against muscle fibers (Dalakas, 1991; Engel et al., 1994). Inflammation and necrosis are not limited to the perivascular region as in PM but involve direct invasion of muscle fascicles by inflammatory cells, particularly CD8$^+$ T lymphocytes and

Table 28–2. Features of Inflammatory Myopathies

	Dermatomyositis (DM)	Polymyositis (PM)	Inclusion Body Myositis (IBM)
Diagnosis	Characteristic rash	By exclusion*	Poor response to conventional therapy; inclusions seen on muscle biopsy
Pathogenesis	Antibody and complement damage to microvasculature with secondary muscle fiber ischemia	Cytotoxic damage to muscle fibers	Cytotoxic damage to muscle fibers?
Associations			
Autoimmunity	Infrequent	Frequent	Infrequent
Malignancies	In adults, not in children	No	No
Muscle biopsy	Prominent inflammation *around* microvasculature and periphery of muscle fascicles; microinfarcts and perivascular atrophy	Lymphocytic infiltrates *within* muscle fascicles; scattered muscle fiber loss	Resembles PM; characteristic inclusions
Response to			
Prednisone	Often good	Often good	Poor
Immunosuppressive drugs	Sometimes effective	Sometimes effective	Poor
Intravenous immunoglobulin	Excellent	Promising	Uncertain

*The diagnosis of PM cannot be made in the presence of any of the following: rash, involvement of eye and facial muscles, family history of neuromuscular disease, history of exposure to myotoxic drugs or toxins, endocrinopathy, neurogenic disease or dystrophy, biochemical muscle disease, or muscle biopsy features of IBM (Dalakas, 1991).

macrophages. Predisposition to cytotoxic T-cell attack may be the result of abnormally high expression of class I major histocompatibility antigens in muscle. In fact, T cells derived from muscle biopsies of PM patients show strong cytotoxic responses to autologous myotubules in vitro (Hohlfield and Engel, 1991). In most cases of PM, T cells predominately bear the $\alpha\beta$ T-cell receptor (TCR), although an instructive case of PM has been reported, in which the T cells bore the $\gamma\delta$ TCR, as well as high expression of heat shock proteins (Hohlfield and Engel, 1991). Studies of PM-derived T cells suggest that they may be oligoclonal (Engel et al., 1994).

The pathogenesis of inclusion body myositis (IBM) may also involve cellular autoimmunity; however, the immunopathologic factors that make IBM resistant to immunosuppressive therapy are not understood. In IBM, muscle fascicles include a mixture of necrotic and regenerating myofibers, mononuclear infiltration, and the pathognomonic sarcoplasmic vacuoles containing eosinophilic inclusions (Lotz et al., 1989). Askanas and colleagues (1993, 1994) have demonstrated that the IBM inclusions contain β-amyloid protein, ubiquitin, hyperphosphorylated tau protein, and prion protein, raising the possibility that IBM may share common pathogenic mechanisms with Alzheimer's disease and the infectious spongiform encephalopathies.

Congenital/infantile myositis (CM/IM) affects infants between birth and 1 year of age and is characterized by generalized weakness with diffuse muscular inflammation, myofibrillar necrosis, and connective tissue proliferation on biopsy. The etiology and relationship to the other inflammatory myopathies remain obscure (Shevell et al., 1990).

Clinical Features

The inflammatory myopathies are characterized by acquired muscular weakness, usually subacute in onset, with variable accompanying features that clinically differentiate the subtypes.

Dermatomyositis

Dermatomyositis (DM) can occur at any age, although most cases manifest in children 5 to 10 years of age. The onset of weakness is usually insidious and is often associated with prominent muscle aching, stiffness, and systemic features such as malaise or fever. The discomfort and irritability are usually prominent enough to justify the aphorism that in children misery plus weakness equals dermatomyositis. Weakness is usually proximal and greater in the legs than the arms, but younger children may show generalized weakness. Muscles may be tender and slightly indurated, and contractures are often present early (Hanissian et al., 1983; Bruguier et al., 1984). Ocular and facial muscles are rarely affected.

The gastrointestinal tract is involved in 20% of DM patients, who have ulceration throughout the bowel; this is a frequent cause of death (Bowyer et al., 1982). Occasionally, the myocardium may be involved, or pul-

monary interstitial fibrosis may develop. The skin manifestations of DM are variable and often occur late in the disease. The classic heliotrope rash may require weeks to months to develop and consists of violaceous discoloration of the upper lids and malar region of the face, often with associated scaling and periorbital edema. A similar rash with even more prominent scaling may occur over pressure areas such as the knees, elbows, and malleoli of the ankles, and a characteristic papular scaling may involve the dorsal surfaces of the fingers over the interphalangeal joints (Gottram's papules). Perhaps the most constant dermatologic finding is the presence of a subtle reticular rash on the extensor surfaces of the arms, occasionally punctuated by fine telangiectasia. Subcutaneous calcification occurs in fully half of children with DM.

Polymyositis

Childhood polymyositis (PM) exhibits similar clinical features, particularly the insidious onset of proximal weakness and misery; malaise and mild fever are variable. Systemic complaints may be minimal, and slowly evolving PM can readily be mistaken for limb-girdle dystrophy (Mastaglia and Ojeda, 1985). Periods of spontaneous arrest and remission are observed.

Inclusion Body Myopathy

Inclusion body myopathy (IBM) rarely, if ever, occurs in childhood and is manifested by indolent proximal weakness. Thus, it may also be mistaken for limb-girdle dystrophy.

Congenital/Infantile Myositis

Congenital/infantile myositis is a striking disorder of infants who present with generalized areflexia, weakness, and hypotonia, often so marked as to require resuscitation and ventilatory support. The clinical appearance is that of severe congenital myopathy or spinal muscular atrophy; muscle biopsy is essential to diagnose this treatable disorder (Thompson, 1982; Roddy et al., 1986).

Associated Disorders

Inflammatory myopathies may be associated with other immunologic conditions. In particular, DM has been associated with scleroderma and mixed connective tissue disease (Mastaglia and Ojeda, 1985; Tymms and Webb, 1985). PM is frequently associated with autoimmune diseases, such as systemic lupus erythematosus, rheumatoid arthritis, and Sjögren's syndrome (Tymms and Webb, 1985; Mimori, 1987). Many authorities insist on a firm nosologic distinction between pure, or classic, PM and inflammatory myopathies occurring as part of a known systemic vasculitis that produces clinical features resembling PM. Although adults with DM have an increased risk of neoplasm, tumors occurring in 15% (Callen 1988; Richardson and Callen, 1989; Dalakas 1991; Engel et al., 1994), no such association has yet been documented for children. Childhood DM is occasionally associated with X-linked agammaglobulinemia.

Diagnosis

The differential diagnosis of inflammatory myopathies includes inherited and metabolic diseases of muscle, disorders of the neuromuscular junction, diseases of the motor neurons or peripheral nerves, and weakness associated with endocrinopathies. Genetic disorders of muscle, including muscular dystrophies and myopathies, are rarely associated with fever and muscle pain and may show relentless progression as compared with the fluctuating course frequently observed in inflammatory myopathies. As noted, limb-girdle dystrophy is particularly difficult to distinguish from cases of PM and IBM when toxic symptoms are minimal. CM/IM must be distinguished from spinal muscular atrophy and congenital myopathies.

Disorders of the neuromuscular junction, such as myasthenia gravis, are marked by fatigable weakness and prominent involvement of the ocular and facial muscles. Lower motor neuron diseases are distinguished by the absence or reduction of deep tendon reflexes; upper motor neuron diseases, by long-tract signs; and peripheral neuropathy, by sensory changes. Endocrinopathies, such as thyrotoxicosis, usually cause widespread systemic disturbances in addition to weakness. *Toxoplasma gondii* infestation may occasionally produce a condition resembling DM or PM (Topi et al., 1979). Viral myositis, especially that caused by coxsackievirus B, may closely resemble DM.

The diagnosis of inflammatory myopathy is established after consideration of clinical features, muscle enzyme determinations, electrodiagnostic studies, and muscle biopsy (Dalakas, 1991). For DM, diagnostic features include the following:

1. Proximal symmetric weakness.
2. Typical rash.
3. Increased creatine phosphokinase (CPK).
4. Typical EMG findings.
5. Typical results of biopsy.

Diagnosis is established when four or more of these features are present. CPK is released from injured muscle cells, but the CPK elevation corresponds only roughly with the clinical course. Thus, CPK is usually a sensitive and reliable screen for muscle injury, but levels may be normal in active inflammatory myopathy, particularly late in the clinical course (Kagen and Aram, 1987).

The electromyogram (EMG) usually shows typical myopathic features, including insertional activity, fibrillation and positive waves at rest, with short-duration, low-amplitude polyphasic potentials during voluntary contraction. However, the EMG may also be normal in exceptional cases. Muscle biopsy should be undertaken in all patients in whom there is a suspicion of inflammatory myopathy, and analysis of the biopsy specimen will usually permit a definitive diagnosis. Rarely, results of the biopsy may fail to show cellular infiltrates in active inflammatory myopathy; in this case, biopsy performed at another site should be considered.

Treatment

Prednisone is the mainstay of treatment for DM and is used, albeit less successfully, in other inflammatory myopathies. This treatment has reduced DM mortality from 30% to less than 10% (Fischer et al., 1979; Bowyer et al., 1982). Moreover, early prednisone therapy reduces contracture formation and calcinosis. Most authorities start with high-dose prednisone each morning, ranging from 1 to 2.5 mg/kg/day. After approximately 1 month, the dose is tapered to alternate-day therapy, diminishing the dose to 5 to 10 mg/month, depending on the clinical response (Miller et al., 1983; Aicardi, 1992). Therapy must be continued for long periods, usually 1 or more years. Response is best judged by muscle strength rather than CPK levels. A common treatment mistake is to "chase" muscle enzyme levels rather than to follow muscle power. At times the positive effects of prednisone on pain, mood, and cooperativeness may falsely enhance the clinical perception of muscle strength.

Prednisone may paradoxically cause increased weakness as a result of "steroid myopathy" (Dalakas, 1991). In some patients, the distinction between increased disease activity and prednisone toxicity may be difficult; in this case, the pattern of response to past treatment should be carefully reviewed. On occasion, the dose of prednisone must be raised or lowered arbitrarily; in such circumstances, the response over several weeks will usually indicate the correct therapeutic course to follow. The response of PM to prednisone is less clear, and remissions may occur even without therapy.

Although congenital/infantile myositis is clearly steroid-responsive, prednisone should be tapered aggressively in order to avoid side effects, such as infection. IBM is not responsive to prednisone.

Up to 20% of children with DM fail to improve significantly on prednisone. Immunosuppressive agents should be considered for these children, as well as for patients (1) who have poorly responsive PM, (2) who have IBM, or (3) who experience unacceptable prednisone toxicity (Engel et al., 1994). Methotrexate (10 to 20 mg/M², oral or intravenous, two times/week) is effective in 75% of resistant DM or PM cases (Hanissian et al., 1983; Miller et al., 1983). Treatment should be started immediately in very ill patients, since many weeks may elapse before improvement is seen. Azathioprine may also be effective. Cyclophosphamide has been advocated for patients with pulmonary involvement, a group with particularly poor outcome (al-Janadi et al., 1989). Pulse methylprednisolone (Laxer et al., 1987) and plasmapheresis (Dau and Bennington, 1981) have also been advocated, but efficacy remains unproven.

A small, controlled double-blind study has shown that high-dose intravenous immunoglobulin (IVIG) is a safe and effective treatment for DM, and open trials have suggested that immunoglobulin treatment may be effective in PM as well (Dalakas et al., 1993). These encouraging results, if confirmed, may suggest a new therapeutic approach to the inflammatory myopathies. A small, uncontrolled study of IVIG in IBM did not show objective improvement (Amato et al., 1994).

Prognosis

Inflammatory myopathies are serious conditions in which aggressive treatment is warranted. Although most DM and PM patients improve on prednisone therapy, IBM is usually resistant to all current therapy. Patients with pulmonary involvement or extensive gastrointestinal ulceration have particularly poor prognoses. IVIG has been used successfully on some refractory patients, thus improving their long-term prognosis and may have an increased role in most cases of inflammatory myopathy in the future.

MYASTHENIA GRAVIS

Myasthenia gravis (MG) is a disorder characterized by weakness associated with fatigue of voluntary muscles (i.e., worsening with repetitive activity) and by the striking tendency to recover motor power following rest or administration of anticholinesterase medications. There is now general agreement that MG is an autoimmune disease in which antibodies are produced against nicotinic acetylcholine receptors (AChRs) in skeletal muscle. Several major types of MG may be distinguished (Table 28–3). Engel (1992, 1994a) and Drachman (1994) have provided comprehensive reviews.

Historic Aspects

Sir Thomas Willis in 1672 first described "asthenia of voluntary muscle" with recovery on resting. Jolly (1895) named the syndrome *myasthenia gravis pseudo-paralytica*. Although tumors of the thymus were described in patients with MG by Laquer and Diegert in 1901, a possible link between this immunologically central organ and the pathogenesis of MG was not considered until relatively recently. Simpson (1960) suggested an autoimmune pathogenesis based on the clinical and pathologic study of 440 patients who had MG. Nastuk and coworkers (1960) described fluctuation of serum complement with exacerbations and remissions of MG, which suggested an antigen-antibody interaction. Strauss and colleagues (1960) used immunofluorescent and complement-fixation techniques to show that gamma globulin from myasthenic patients binds to muscle. These seminal findings have influenced much of MG research in subsequent decades.

Pathogenesis

Normal voluntary motor activity depends on the release of acetylcholine by presynaptic nerve terminals at the neuromuscular junction. These terminals abut nicotinic receptors for acetylcholine (AChR), which are grouped on postsynaptic folds on the muscle surface. When sufficient acetylcholine is bound to the AChR, intracellular events leading to muscle contraction occur. Normally, this reaction is rapidly terminated by extracellular acetylcholinesterase, which degrades residual synaptic acetylcholine. This action "clears" the neuromuscular junction, which again becomes receptive to new signals and effective modulation of motor activity.

The AChR itself consists of a doughnut-shaped aggregate of five types of polypeptide subunits. Each AChR contains two α-subunits, one β-subunit, one δ-subunit, and one γ- or ε-subunit (Drachman, 1994). The α-subunits contain the sites that actually bind molecules of acetylcholine; these sites are the antigenic targets most frequently recognized by anti-AChR antibodies. Genomic and complementary deoxyribonucleic acid (cDNA) clones encoding the human muscle AChRs have been isolated and sequenced (Beesen et al., 1993). Ultrastructural studies show that each AChR has a central pit, probably the channel through which cations flow after acetylcholine-mediated activation. The basic defect in all forms of MG (except congenital MG or the familial myasthenic syndromes, see later) is a reduction in number of the postsynaptic receptors of the neuromuscular junction (Engel, 1992), presumably the result of the action of autoantibodies.

Immunology

Anti-AChR Antibodies

The central role of antibodies to AChR has been shown in clinical studies of MG patients and in experimental animal models of MG (see later). Antibody to AChR can be detected in approximately 84% of patients with MG (Engel, 1992). Immunoglobulin from MG patients causes weakness and AChR depletion on passive transfer to mice (Engel, 1992; Kuncl et al., 1993). Moreover, the adoptive transfer of peripheral

Table 28–3. Classification of Myasthenia Gravis

Type	Onset	Etiology
Neonatal	Birth	Adoptive transfer of anti-AChR antibodies from mother; MG is transient
Congenital*	Birth	Genetic defects in neuromuscular junction; weakness is usually permanent, and anti-AChR antibodies are present
Juvenile	Early childhood or puberty	Autoimmune; anti-AChR antibodies are pathogenic
Adult	After puberty	Autoimmune; anti-AChR antibodies are pathogenic

*Although congenital myasthenic syndromes have traditionally been classified as variants of MG, these syndromes have a genetic, rather than immune, pathogenesis (Engel, 1992). For this reason, congenital myasthenic syndromes should be distinguished from MG nosologically, even though the distinction may clinically be difficult to make. Most genetic myasthenic syndromes are apparent at birth, but some cases may have an onset in childhood or adult life.

blood lymphocytes from patients with MG (even patients who are seronegative for anti-AChR antibodies) induces MG and anti-AChR antibodies in recipient immunodeficient mice (Martino et al., 1993). Taken together, this evidence indicates that autoimmune effector mechanisms in MG are primarily humoral.

Despite these observations, the relationship between clinical MG and anti-AChR antibodies is not simple. As noted, approximately 16% of patients with clear-cut MG are seronegative when tested by commercially available assays. In certain subsets of patients who have MG, such as those with exclusively ocular manifestations, the proportion of patients who are seronegative may be as high as 50%. Also, among different patients, the anti-AChR titers correlate poorly with clinical severity. Nonetheless, in an individual patient, a substantial reduction in antibody titer over time usually is associated with clinical improvement (Engel, 1992). These discrepancies may reflect technical factors in the assay for anti-AChR antibody, the effects of anti-AChR antibodies of different fine specificities, sequestration of antibody at the neuromuscular junction, or the existence of different subtypes of MG, including some in which the disorder is either not autoimmune or in which the antibody is directed against antigenic determinants other than the AChR.

Anti-AChR antibodies may exert their effect in MG by at least three mechanisms (Seybold, 1983; Engel, 1992; Drachman, 1994). First, binding of the antibody to AChR may directly affect its function as a mediator between nerve impulse and muscle contraction; second, antibody cross-linking of AChR may increase receptor degradation and depletion; third, the antibody-AChR interaction may bind complement, with subsequent damage to the AChR-containing postsynaptic membrane folds.

The relative contribution of these mechanisms and the mode of antibody-mediated damage is not known (Richman et al., 1993). Studies of the fine specificities of anti-AChR antibodies show that different MG patients have different humoral responses to AChR—that is, immunoglobulins are not directed against only a few immunodominant epitopes on AChR. This heterogeneity of anti-AChR antibodies may complicate attempts to design specific, targeted immunotherapy (Drachman, 1994).

The Thymus and Cell-Mediated Immunity

Although humoral immunity clearly predominates as the autoimmune effector mechanism in MG, a significant role for cell-mediated immunity and the thymus, particularly during the inductive phase of the illness, has been proposed (Wekerle, 1993; Drachman, 1994). Thus, lymphocytes are common in MG muscle biopsies, and the thymus is histologically abnormal in 70% to 90% of patients with MG (Castleman, 1966). Since myoid, or muscle-like, cells are present in the thymus, it is possible that the presence of these AChR-bearing cells and lymphocytes in the thymus during maturation of the immune system may initiate autoimmunity in MG.

In view of the production of anti-AChR antibodies in MG, one might expect thymic cells to show an excess of T-helper cells. This has been sought and has only inconsistently been found (Seybold and Lindstrom, 1982). The favorable clinical response to thymectomy usually supports the role of the thymus in MG pathogenesis. Kuroda and colleagues (1984) reported a patient with MG in whom thymectomy led to clinical worsening and an increase in anti-AChR antibodies. T cells in the removed thymoma had primarily T-suppressor phenotypes.

HLA and Disease Associations

The genetics of MG has been extensively reviewed (Lisak and Barchi, 1982; Kerzin-Storrar et al., 1988). MG shows a modest association with HLA antigens B8 and DRw3 and a strong but unconfirmed association with DQw2 (Drachman, 1994). Family studies have shown a prevalence of MG in the relatives of as many as 2% of congenital and juvenile MG patients, prompting the observation that those "who are most genetically prone to develop myasthenia do so early in life" (Bundey et al., 1972). Adult patients with MG have an increased incidence of thyroid disease, rheumatoid arthritis, systemic lupus erythematosus, and pernicious anemia, all autoimmune in nature. Studies of monozygotic and dizygotic twins have concordance rates of approximately 40% and 0%, respectively. It is concluded that both genetic and environmental factors are involved in MG.

Experimental Myasthenia Gravis

Patrick and Lindstrom (1973), while attempting to raise antibodies to AChR, noted that injected rabbits developed an illness characterized by weakness of skeletal muscle. This disease, termed *experimental autoimmune myasthenia gravis* (EAMG), has been induced in other species and shows marked similarity to the clinical, electrophysiologic, immunologic, and pathologic features of MG. EAMG has contributed much to the understanding of MG (Lindstrom et al., 1988), particularly with regard to the antigenic specificity and action of anti-AChR antibodies (Krolick et al., 1993).

Etiology

Although the central role of anti-AChR antibodies in MG is generally accepted, the putative factors that may initiate or trigger MG, such as viral infections and thymic myoid cells, are poorly understood. Molecular mimicry between the AChR and microbial (especially viral) antigenic determinants may exist and could trigger an autoimmune reaction (Drachman, 1994); however, surgically removed MG thymus glands reveal no evidence of viral infection (Aoki et al., 1985). Proximity of thymic myoid cells to thymic centers for T-lymphocyte production may result in sensitization to muscle cell antigens, as noted earlier.

A third consideration is based on the observation that low levels of anti-AChR antibodies and AChR-specific T-helper cells can be detected in apparently healthy individuals (Melms et al., 1993). These findings prompted the suggestion that a "few cells secreting antibodies (Ab) at subpathologic levels could be a normal occurrence and that activation and expansion of these clones may be involved in initiation of the MG disease process" (Mittag et al., 1984). MG developing after bone marrow transplantation may be a result of such clonal expansion of normal cells under unusual circumstances (Smith et al., 1983).

Clinical Manifestations

The hallmark of MG is excessive fatigability. Variable weakness manifests differently in each subtype of MG (see Table 28–3).

Neonatal Myasthenia Gravis

In *neonatal MG*, weakness develops transiently in 10% to 25% of children born to mothers who are myasthenic as a result of the passive transfer of maternal antibodies to the fetal circulation (Fenichel, 1978; Barlow, 1981; Morel et al., 1988). The factors that make one fetus more vulnerable than another are unknown. Thus, the chances of delivering an affected child may vary from pregnancy to pregnancy for any given mother. Therefore, every newborn of a woman with MG should be considered at risk and observed meticulously. Although neonatal MG most frequently develops the day after birth, it may occur as late as 1 week of age. The signs of neonatal MG include weak sucking, crying, and swallowing; facial diplegia; respiratory difficulty; extremity weakness; hypotonia; and depressed reflexes. Unlike the manifestations in adults, ptosis and ophthalmoplegia are rare in neonatal MG. Neonatal MG may also occur in mothers with latent or undiagnosed MG.

Congenital Myasthenia Gravis

Several different *congenital* myasthenic syndromes resembling neonatal MG have been recognized, which (1) do not appear to share the immune-mediation of other forms of MG (i.e., AChR antibodies are not found, and infants are not responsive to immunotherapy); (2) may develop after the neonatal period; and (3) are heritable rather than autoimmune. Several features help to distinguish congenital myasthenic syndromes from neonatal MG, including the following:

1. A nonmyasthenic mother.
2. The lack of antibodies to AChR.
3. A relatively benign course involving mostly ocular muscles.
4. A high incidence of affected family members (Fenichel, 1978; Engel, 1992, 1994b).

This distinction is an important one, since the treatment of the two conditions is different.

Juvenile Myasthenia Gravis

Juvenile MG is so similar to adult MG in its manifestations that most authorities consider the conditions to be one disease with different ages of onset (Lisak and Barchi, 1982).

Diagnosis

The diagnosis of MG is usually apparent from the clinical features previously noted, especially when symptoms are maximal at the end of the day or after exercise. Confirmation of the diagnosis should be sought by assessing serum anti-AChR antibodies and neuromuscular function, the latter by the edrophonium chloride (Tensilon) test and repetitive nerve stimulation (Jolly test) (Linton and Philcox, 1990; Engel, 1992). The Tensilon test may be negative in some cases of MG, especially in the ocular form (Seybold, 1986). There is a slight risk of serious side effects. Although anti-AChR antibodies are demonstrable in most MG patients, seronegative cases occur and respond to immunotherapy.

EMG testing with repetitive stimulation at low frequency (2 to 3 Hz) should be performed and is one of the most reliable ways to diagnose MG. This should also be done at high frequency (20 Hz) if some other neuromuscular blockade syndrome (e.g., botulism) is suspected. A decremental response (>20% amplitude reduction of the muscle-evoked potential) is observed at either frequency in MG. This can be seen even in children whose clinical manifestations of MG are confined to the extraocular muscles, especially if the extensor digitorum brevis muscles are studied. Resolution of the abnormality with edrophonium administration is diagnostic. In obscure cases, single-fiber electromyography, in vitro microelectrode studies of neuromuscular transmission, and immunocytochemical analyses may be necessary (Engel, 1992). A search for the presence of a thymoma in juvenile and adult MG should be made by chest radiographs and computed tomography, or magnetic resonance imaging, of the superior mediastinum (Linton and Philcox, 1990).

The differential diagnosis of MG includes all conditions causing acute or subacute weakness (see Guillain-Barré syndrome later). The important diseases to exclude are neurasthenia, botulism, brain stem lesions, acquired myopathies, and the *Lambert-Eaton myasthenic syndrome* (LEMS) (see later). Neurasthenia is usually indicated by the lack of objective clinical and laboratory findings, as well as the presence of variable, "give way" weakness at the bedside. Botulism typically has an abrupt onset, accompanying gastrointestinal symptoms, and prominent visual findings, including abnormal or absent pupillary responses to light. Brain stem lesions usually produce widespread lower cranial nerve dysfunction associated with definite signs of central nervous system involvement, such as involvement of long-motor and sensory tracts. Thyroiditis or hyperthyroidism may mimic or coexist with MG; recognition of these is important because thyroid abnormalities may exacerbate MG (Drachman, 1994).

Exogenous substances may produce illnesses resembling MG, such as a prolonged myasthenic state that may occur after neuromuscular blockade (Benzing et al., 1990). Other exogenous substances to consider include arthropod, snake, and insect venoms; trimethadione and phenytoin; aminoglycosides and polymyxins; magnesium; and quinine and carnitine (Masters et al., 1977; Swift, 1981; Bazzato et al., 1981).

Treatment

Treatment depends on the type and severity of MG. This subject has been reviewed extensively (Lisak and Barchi, 1982; Lindstrom et al., 1988; Linton and Philcox, 1990; Engel, 1992, 1994a; Shah and Lisak, 1993). Neonatal MG is treated with supportive care and anticholinesterase drugs; neostigmine, 0.05 mg IM prior to feedings, is often sufficient. Since neonatal MG is transient and disappears when the passively transferred maternal anti-AChR antibodies are metabolized, the amount of medication should be gradually diminished to avoid cholinergic overdose. Exchange transfusions may be useful in severe cases (Pasternak et al., 1981).

Juvenile and adult forms of MG are the result of ongoing humoral immunopathology. Current treatments have not been studied in controlled clinical trials, and all remain controversial (Engel, 1992). There are, however, several accepted approaches (Table 28–4).

First, many mild cases and cases with exclusively ocular manifestations will respond adequately to anticholinesterase agents, such as neostigmine or pyridostigmine. This treatment increases the half-life of acetylcholine within the synaptic cleft, thereby increasing the likelihood of binding to the sparse postsynaptic receptors. Common side effects include nausea, vomiting, intestinal cramping, bradycardia, and diaphoresis. Long-term use of anticholinesterase therapy carries the theoretical risk of additional injury to the motor endplate (Hudson et al., 1978).

If an adequate trial of anticholinesterase treatment is not effective (an adequate trial may require up to a year), thymectomy should be considered in most adults, many children, and a few elderly patients (the latter reservation is due to increased complications and limited benefit). Although available studies show that early thymectomy apparently has no adverse effects on the maturation of the immune system (Seybold et al., 1971) and results in clinical remission in as many as two thirds of children with MG (Aicardi, 1992), some clinicians suggest that thymectomy should be avoided until after puberty if possible (Drachman, 1994). On the other hand, long-term drug therapy is not without risks, risks that may be avoided in many patients after thymectomy. Drachman (1994) has recently reviewed practical strategies for preoperative and postoperative management of MG patients undergoing thymectomy.

In patients who cannot undergo thymectomy or who are poorly responsive to thymectomy, other therapies can be considered, including plasmapheresis, alternate-day corticosteroid, intravenous immunoglobulin (IVIG), and immunosuppressive medications (azathioprine, cyclosporine) (Drachman, 1994). IVIG, in particular, shows promise because of its ease, safety, and efficacy; it is, however, extremely expensive (Drachman, 1994). Immunosuppressives can stabilize patients prior to thymectomy (Snead et al., 1987). Before such therapy is initiated, patients should have a tuberculin test, a chest radiograph, and a fasting blood glucose determination.

Patients with MG may experience periods of sudden, severe worsening with respiratory and bulbar compromise, called *crisis*. Crisis may be due to excessive *(cholinergic crisis)* or insufficient *(myasthenic crisis)* anticholinesterase medication, the initiation of corticosteroid therapy, physical or emotional stress, concurrent infection, or administration of drugs, such as aminoglycosides, quinidine, procainamide, phenytoin, chlorpromazine, D-penicillamine, neuromuscular blocking agents, and others. Because deterioration may develop rapidly into a life-threatening state, patients with significant worsening, particularly of bulbar or respiratory function, are at risk of crisis and should immediately be admitted to an intensive care unit.

Although the edrophonium test was formerly used to distinguish crisis caused by undermedication from that resulting from overmedication, all authorities currently recommend admitting the patient to an intensive care unit, stopping anticholinesterase treatment for 48 to 72 hours, providing respiratory support if needed, and searching for a reversible precipitant of the crisis. After stabilization, treatment may include reinstitution of anticholinesterase medication, plasmapheresis, IVIG, and corticosteroids (Lisak and Barchi, 1982; Fink, 1993).

In children with MG who respond poorly to immunotherapy, have a family history of neuromuscular disorder, lack antibodies to AChR, or have dysmorphic appearance, a congenital myasthenic syndrome should be considered. Congenital myasthenic conditions may be caused by diverse defects in the neuromuscular apparatus (Engel, 1992). Furthermore, the response to therapy varies widely in these conditions, and in some instances, conventional treatment may result in clinical worsening. When a congenital myasthenic syndrome is suspected, referral to a specialized center is advisable.

Prognosis

Jolly (1895) introduced the term *gravis* to emphasize the poor outlook in untreated MG. With modern therapy, the prognosis is relatively good, although mortality rates still range from 3% to 30% (Aicardi, 1992; Engel, 1994a). On the other hand, 30% of children

---

Table 28–4. Therapeutic Principles in Juvenile and Adult Myasthenia Gravis (MG)

1. Anticholinesterase medications are useful in most forms of MG.*
2. Anticholinesterase medications are the mainstay of treatment for MG limited to ocular weakness.
3. Plasmapheresis should be reserved for short-term use in severely ill patients or those with intractable MG.
4. Thymectomy is absolutely indicated if a thymoma is demonstrated.

*Except for congenital MG or myasthenic syndromes.
Modified from Engel AG. Myasthenia gravis and syndromes. In Rowland LP, DiMauro S, eds. Handbook of Clinical Neurology. New York, Elsevier, 1992, pp. 391–455.

experience spontaneous remission, particularly those with MG confined to the extraocular muscles.

LAMBERT-EATON MYASTHENIC SYNDROME

Lambert-Eaton myasthenic syndrome (LEMS) is usually associated with a malignancy, often small-cell carcinoma of the lung (O'Neill et al., 1988; Engel, 1994b). LEMS usually occurs in adults; however, two apparently similar but rare illnesses have been described in children: (1) a congenital myasthenic syndrome (Bady et al., 1987) and (2) a juvenile form with features of limb-girdle–distributed myopathy and LEMS (Husain et al., 1989). Neither has been associated with malignancy.

Unlike MG, patients with LEMS usually do not have prominent ocular symptoms, and they often develop increased strength with repetitive effort (Eaton and Lambert, 1957). Electrophysiologic studies show incremental evoked muscle responses at high rates of repetitive stimulation (>50 Hz) in contrast to the decremental responses characteristic of MG.

LEMS in adults is associated with antibodies directed against voltage-gated calcium channels on the presynaptic nerve terminals of the neuromuscular junctions (Lang et al., 1993; Wray and Porter, 1993). Also, diagnostic tests for LEMS measure antibody binding to isolated components of the presynaptic calcium channels (Posner, 1991). The treatment of LEMS has been reviewed by Posner (1991) and Engel (1992, 1994b). In general, antitumor therapy and alternate-day prednisone are recommended for neoplastic LEMS, and azathioprine and alternate-day prednisone are recommended for non-neoplastic LEMS. Plasmapheresis may also be of benefit. Treatment with 3,4-diaminopyridine may also lead to increased release of acetylcholine and symptomatic improvement. IVIG is frequently used and may result in dramatic improvement.

GUILLAIN-BARRÉ SYNDROME

Historic Aspects

Guillain-Barré syndrome (GBS), also denoted idiopathic, parainfectious, or inflammatory polyneuritis and acute inflammatory demyelinating polyradiculopathy, was first described by Landry in 1859. He noted that the symmetric weakness and extent of recovery set this condition apart from another, almost contemporaneously described acute areflexic paralysis, poliomyelitis. Guillain and coworkers (1916) further refined this distinction, noting that although both illnesses result in elevations in cerebrospinal fluid (CSF) protein, poliomyelitis produced CSF pleocytosis, whereas the CSF of patients who had GBS contained few or no cells, a finding they called *albuminocytologic dissociation*. GBS was originally presumed to be infectious (Bradford et al., 1919) but has subsequently been shown to result from inflammatory demyelination of peripheral nerves

and nerve roots. Excellent reviews of GBS are available (Arnason, 1984; Koski, 1984; Parry, 1993; Arnason and Soliven, 1993).

Pathology

Pathologic changes are primarily confined to the peripheral nervous system, involving motor, sensory, and autonomic nerves and nerve roots (including the portions of cranial nerves that are coated with peripheral-type myelin). Changes may be found anywhere from the dorsal and ventral spinal roots to the most distal twigs of peripheral nerves, but proximal nerve trunks are generally more involved than spinal roots or distal nerves (Prineas, 1981; Thomas et al., 1992; Arnason and Soliven, 1993). The pathologic hallmark of GBS is segmental demyelination. An inflammatory infiltration surrounding the vasae nervosa (blood vessels supplying the nerves) is also present and includes polymorphonuclear leukocytes, lymphocytes (CD4[+] and CD8[+] T cells and B cells), macrophages, and plasma cells.

Pathogenesis

In most patients with GBS, a clear antecedent can be identified; this might include infection, vaccination, surgery, and systemic illnesses such as malignancy, systemic lupus erythematosus (SLE), transplantation, thyroiditis, and Addison's disease (reviewed by Parry, 1993). Among viral infections, an association between GBS and cytomegalovirus and Epstein-Barr virus, and between GBS and human immunodeficiency virus (HIV), varicella-zoster, and vaccinia-smallpox, is thought probable. Among bacterial infections, *Campylobacter jejuni* and *Mycoplasma pneumoniae* are regarded as definite causes of GBS, and typhoid, *Borrelia burgdorferi* (Lyme disease), *Listeria*, *Chlamydia*, *Brucella*, and others are considered probable causes.

Although these infections may directly affect peripheral nerves, it is more likely that they provoke an autoimmune reaction with secondary demyelination of peripheral nerves. Moreover, the fact that GBS follows vaccinations in approximately 5% of cases also suggests that GBS is the result of a dysregulated response to foreign antigens introduced at the time of inoculation. GBS has been linked to rabies vaccine prepared from neural tissue (not the current tissue culture–derived rabies vaccine) and the 1976 and 1977 swine A/influenza vaccine; a possible link to other vaccines, such as poliovirus, *Haemophilus influenzae*, typhoid, and tetanus, has also been reported (reviewed in Parry, 1993). GBS may also develop after bee or wasp stings (Van Antwerpen et al., 1988).

Numerous investigators have implicated immunopathologic mechanisms in GBS (Arnason and Soliven, 1993). GBS is thought to result when an inciting agent, such as a virus, induces an aberrant immune response that is directed against peripheral nerve myelin. Ample evidence indicates both B- and T-cell immune responses in GBS, although their relative contributions have not been established.

As noted, the pathology of GBS shows prominent involvement of cell-mediated immunity, especially the presence of activated T cells and macrophages. Morphologically, GBS lesions resemble a typical delayed type hypersensitive (DTH) response. In this regard, increases in serum IL-2, as well as IL-2 receptor and transferrin receptor expression on T cells are seen, indicating T-cell activation in GBS (Hartung et al., 1990, 1991; Arnason and Soliven, 1993). In turn, T cells release interferon gamma and other factors that activate macrophages; finally, activated macrophages release proteases, reactive oxygen intermediates, and other molecules that result in demyelination.

Arnason and Soliven (1993) believe the following mechanisms are central to GBS immunopathology:

1. Bystander damage, in which an immune response directed against a microbe or other agent incorporated into host cell membranes damages nearby myelin.

2. Molecular mimicry, in which the inciting agent and peripheral myelin share cross-reacting antigenic determinants.

3. Anamnestic stimulation, in which the inciting agent boosts a pre-existing, subclinical sensitivity to peripheral myelin to cause significant disease.

A defect in humoral immunity in GBS is suggested by the favorable response to plasmapheresis. There is some evidence for the presence of anti–microbial and anti–myelin antibodies (Linington and Brostoff, 1993) in GBS (reviewed in Parry, 1993; Arnason and Soliven, 1993). Also, patients' sera have been shown to cause demyelination when injected into the peripheral nerves of experimental animals (Feasby et al., 1982); however, this observation has been difficult to reproduce. The most significant humoral abnormality is the presence of antibodies directed to peripheral nerve carbohydrate residues that are similar to those of the Forssman antigen, a determinant found in microbes and mammalian tissues but not in humans (Koski et al., 1989; Koski, 1990); these antibodies have been found in a high proportion of GBS patients, and their titer parallels disease activity. However, this finding is not supported by studies such as that of Ilyas and colleagues (1988). Finally, it should be pointed out that plasmapheresis also removes nonantibody serum components, such as cytokines. Arnason and Soliven (1993) conclude that a definite role for an antibody in GBS pathogenesis is unproven.

The immunopathogenesis of GBS continues to be investigated in several animal models, including experimental allergic neuritis, produced by inoculation of peripheral nerve or by antigens; Marek's disease, caused by a herpes-type virus in fowl; and coonhound paralysis, occurring in dogs following raccoon bites.

Macrophages are the first cells to penetrate the basement membrane of nerve fibers; thus, they may be critical effector cells in myelin damage. Although Schwann cells and axons are spared relative to myelin, both may be lost in regions of intense inflammation. Within weeks of onset of illness, the nerve fibers show evidence of repair, including proliferation of Schwann cells and remyelination (Arnason, 1984).

In some cases of GBS, clinical features or neuroimaging have suggested that the central nervous system (CNS) may be involved; however, a review of autopsy cases of typical GBS found no evidence of CNS pathology (Ropper, 1983).

Clinical Manifestations

Most childhood cases present with the symmetric ascending paralysis described by Landry (1859). The first symptom in most cases is exercise-dependent muscle ache or cramping, involving the thighs, buttocks, or back. Meningeal signs are present in more than half of these children (Roca-Gonzalez et al., 1993). Young children are often irritable and resistant to manipulation. Because this irritability may interfere with a thorough examination and the pain is similar to that in tenosynovitis, myositis, or osteomyelitis, early GBS may be misdiagnosed, particularly if the cerebrospinal fluid (CSF) protein is normal (Manners and Murray, 1992). Fever is usually absent.

Paralysis usually ascends over days to weeks and may wax and wane. Fewer than half of affected children show progression beyond 2 weeks (Koski, 1984), and less than 10% progress after 4 weeks (Rostami, 1993). A clinical plateau follows, lasting approximately as long as the period of deterioration in untreated patients. Deep tendon reflexes (DTRs) are absent in more than 80% of cases, including areas in which there is little detectable weakness.

Cranial nerve involvement is seen in half of children with GBS, most commonly facial nerve paresis (Cebreros-Garcia et al., 1990; Aicardi, 1992; Roca-Gonzalez, 1993). Bulbar nerves become involved in 15% to 25% of children, although less than 15% require respiratory support. Ophthalmoparesis occurs in about 3% of patients with GBS (Dehaene et al., 1986). Other than dysesthesia and pain, sensory changes are usually less apparent during the acute illness than weakness or autonomic dysfunction, but may persist after recovery, particularly in the toes. Autonomic dysfunction occurs in half of children with GBS; it is more common and severe than in adults (Winer et al., 1988). Manifestations include labile hypertension, ECG abnormalities, abnormal sweating, cardiac arrhythmias, and gastrointestinal disturbances, such as colicky abdominal pain.

In addition to classic GBS, there are several variants, which account for about 3% of all cases of acute or chronic inflammatory polyneuropathy. These variants include the Miller-Fisher syndrome (Fisher, 1956), in which paralysis is descending and ophthalmoplegia is prominent.

Diagnosis

The diagnosis of GBS is made by (1) the characteristic history and physical examination, (2) cerebrospinal fluid (CSF) analysis and/or physiologic testing of peripheral nerve function, (3) exclusion of alternative conditions. The typical CSF of GBS includes elevation of protein out of proportion to the degree of pleocytosis; indeed, CSF is usually acellular. Early in the course of the GBS, the lumbar puncture may not show protein elevation.

Almost all children with GBS show abnormalities of

peripheral nerve electrophysiologic studies, including reduction and dispersion of the distal compound muscle action potential, but these may not occur until after several weeks of illness. Moreover, as GBS pathology is patchy, electrophysiologic sampling should be widespread.

The differential diagnosis of GBS includes poliomyelitis, diphtheritic polyneuritis, acquired immunodeficiency syndrome (AIDS), Lyme disease, tick bite paralysis, botulism, intoxications, acute intermittent porphyria, and the autosomal dominant form of hypokalemic periodic paralysis. Poliomyelitis and diphtheritic polyneuritis are rare in well-immunized populations, but remain common in developing nations. Of 246 children with flaccid paralysis presenting to a referral center in Mexico City, 63% had GBS and 17% had poliomyelitis (Alcala, 1993). Poliomyelitis does occur in North America in the following instances:

- Immunocompromised infants who receive live-attenuated (Sabin) vaccine or are exposed to a recent vaccinee
- Unimmunized recent immigrants
- As nonepidemic poliomyelitis resulting from viruses such as coxsackie B virus or echovirus

Meningismus, extremely high fever, and gastrointestinal findings are common at onset of paralysis. The tendency of poliomyelitis to asymmetrically affect the limbs and show CSF pleocytosis (often polymorphonuclear) help distinguish it from GBS. Diphtheritic polyneuritis can be distinguished from GBS by the characteristic pharyngitis; severe cranial nerve involvement, especially involving the palate; and visual blurring.

Polyneuropathy associated with AIDS and Lyme disease may have identical pathophysiology to GBS, that is, peripheral nerve and nerve root demyelination. In developing countries with a high prevalence of AIDS, as many as one third of patients presenting with clinical findings compatible with GBS are human immunodeficiency virus (HIV)-positive (Chinyanga and Danha, 1992). AIDS should be considered in Western urban centers where seroprevalence is high. Tick bite paralysis closely resembles GBS but is the result of a toxin secreted by the gravid female tick. Diagnosis rests on the discovery of a feeding tick, usually in the scalp or groin; clinical abnormalities resolve within hours to days after its removal (Henderson, 1961). Botulism can be distinguished from GBS by its epidemic tendency and by early ophthalmoparesis, a rare finding in GBS (except in the Miller-Fisher syndrome) (Brown, 1984). Infantile botulism (caused by honeyed formula) often manifests with subacute onset of progressive weakness and is difficult to distinguish from infantile GBS without the aid of electrodiagnostic studies (Carroll et al., 1977). Lyme disease, tick bite paralysis, and botulism all have well-defined regional limits within the United States. Heavy metal (especially lead) and industrial solvent intoxications (organophosphates, n-hexane, and methyl n-butyl ketone) may also mimic GBS (Schaumburg and Berger, 1993).

Treatment

The mainstay of GBS therapy is meticulous supportive care. The major challenges include (1) inadequate breathing, (2) clinically significant autonomic dysfunction, and (3) neurogenic bladder. Impending bulbar and respiratory muscle dysfunction is suggested by ascending motor or sensory dysfunction, changes in timbre and intensity of the voice, choking, or drooling. Tracheostomy should be performed in severe cases in which prolonged mechanical ventilation is anticipated.

Since the prognosis is favorable for children treated with supportive care, the use of anti-inflammatory agents is not recommended. Parry (1993) reviewed the use of corticosteroids and cytotoxic agents in GBS and could find no convincing value to treatment, although significant adverse effects occurred.

Two large, controlled prospective studies have shown the beneficial effects of plasmapheresis in GBS with a shortening of the duration of mechanical ventilation and hospital stay (Guillain-Barré Syndrome Study Group, 1985; French Cooperative Group, 1987). Only a few children were included in these studies, but subsequent nonrandomized trials in children with GBS have indicated that plasmapheresis is safe and effective in children as young as 11 months (Epstein and Sladky, 1990; LaMont et al., 1991). Although plasmapheresis is relatively safe, it is only effective if begun early.

An attractive alternative to plasmapheresis is the use of high-dose IVIG. Early reports on IVIG in GBS, including childhood GBS, are encouraging (Kleyweg et al., 1988; Shahar et al., 1990; Notarangelo et al., 1993, Arakawa et al., 1993; Leititis, 1993). A prospective randomized trial in adults indicate that IVIG is more effective and better tolerated than plasmapheresis (van der Meche et al., 1992). The mechanism of action of IVIG in GBS is unknown, but neutralization of anti-idiotypic antibodies that block autoimmune demyelination is possible (Shahar and Brand, 1991). Rarely, IVIG is associated with aseptic meningitis, cerebral thrombosis, relapse of GBS (Irani et al., 1993), and renal failure. Parry (1993) reviews these complications but endorses IVIG because of its efficacy, acceptance by patients, and safety.

Prognosis

Up to 75% to 80% of children with GBS attain significant recovery of function, and more than 40% recover completely, especially those that begin to improve within 2 to 4 weeks. Little improvement is seen after 2 years from onset of disease (Ropper, 1983). Factors associated with a good prognosis include the following:

- Young age
- No need for respiratory assistance
- Slow progression of illness
- Normal electrophysiologic studies
- Treatment with plasmapheresis (McKhann, 1990) or IVIG (van der Meche et al., 1992)

One study demonstrated a relationship between CSF

antibodies to neuron-specific enolase and the S-100b protein and severity and duration of illness (Mokuno et al., 1994).

Relapses occur in about 5% of patients who have GBS usually as a single acute episode; however, they typically respond to retreatment with plasmapheresis or IVIG (Kleyweg and van der Meche, 1991). The mortality rate of all patients is approximately 5% and is 2% in children (Arnason, 1984). Deaths in children usually result from autonomic instability or sudden cardiac arrest.

CHRONIC INFLAMMATORY DEMYELINATING POLYRADICULONEUROPATHY

Clinical Findings

Chronic inflammatory demyelinating polyradiculo-neuropathy (CIDP) exhibits a close clinical, immuno-logic, and pathologic resemblance to GBS. Unlike GBS, CIDP usually has an indolent onset and a progressive or relapsing course. GBS typically is associated with spontaneous recovery and lack of responsiveness to corticosteroids; almost paradoxically, CIDP is respon-sive to corticosteroids but has a relatively poor long-term prognosis (Parry, 1993; Dyck et al., 1993).

Pathogenesis

The pathology of CIDP resembles GBS or acute in-flammatory demyelinating polyradiculopathy (AIDP) in segmental demyelination, but differs in the amount of remyelinative "onion-bulb" formation surrounding axons and in the relative paucity of inflammatory cells, consistent with the chronicity of the process (Prineas and McLeod, 1976; Barohn et al., 1989; Dyck et al., 1993). Unlike GBS, in which no human leukocyte antigen (HLA) associations have been identified, CIDP is associated with HLA-B8, -DR3, and -Dw3 (Tiwari and Terasaki, 1985). Antibodies directed at GM1, GD1b, and asialo-GM1 glycolipids have been identified in some cases, suggesting that the galactosyl (beta 1–3) N-acetylgalactosaminyl moiety of myelin may be a tar-get antigen (Yoshino et al., 1992).

Circulating autoantibodies have been detected in some patients with CIDP by their reaction with neuro-blastoma cell lines. These antineural autoantibodies may themselves be neutralized by the F(ab')$_2$ fraction of polyvalent immunoglobulin and by the serum of at least one patient recovering from GBS. This suggests that circulating neutralizing immunoglobulin may de-termine whether the demyelinative illness is self-lim-ited or chronic (Van Doorn et al., 1990). Nevertheless, the exact mechanism of CIDP demyelinization is not known (Lisak and Brown, 1987; Rostami, 1993). As many as 20% to 30% of patients with CIDP studied with MRI, EEG, and evoked responses show CNS involvement (Ohtake et al., 1990), but pathologic con-firmation is lacking. Occasionally, patients have fea-tures of CIDP and multiple sclerosis (Thomas et al., 1987; Dyck et al., 1993).

Diagnosis

During the symptomatic phase of CIDP, the spinal fluid is acellular with an elevated protein, often ex-ceeding 100 mg/dl (Dalakas and Engel, 1981). Motor nerve conduction velocities are slow, and sensory po-tentials typically are absent (Dyck et al., 1975; Barohn et al., 1989). The differential diagnosis includes (1) hereditary sensory-motor neuropathies, (2) toxic neu-ropathies, (3) monoradicular or polyradicular gammop-athies, and (4) polyneuropathy associated with sys-temic autoimmune or inflammatory conditions. The electrophysiologic findings of conduction block, tempo-ral dispersion, and focal slowing distinguish CIDP from most heritable neuropathies (Uncini et al., 1991); in difficult cases, it may be necessary to establish the correct diagnosis by performing a nerve biopsy (Parry, 1993).

Treatment

Corticosteroid therapy for CIDP is of benefit in both children and adults (Uncini et al., 1991). Prednisone at doses of 1.5 to 2.0 mg/kg/day is the usual initial ther-apy although some authorities recommend initial plas-mapheresis (Dyck et al., 1993). Prednisone is tapered to alternate-day therapy over several weeks and then tapered off over several additional weeks. Almost all children respond to steroids, although some may re-lapse during the taper, necessitating retreatment and slower tapering. Functional recovery is expected in 50% to 80% of patients.

The adverse effects of chronic steroid administration have prompted the use of plasmapheresis and IVIG as alternatives. Beydoun and associates (1990) report that plasmapheresis for children with CIDP is safe and effec-tive. A small, double-blind, placebo-controlled cross-over study has also shown the benefit of IVIG in CIDP (Van Doorn et al., 1990). Case reports have described the benefits of azathioprine, cyclophosphamide, and cyclosporine; these are reserved for refractory cases (Parry, 1993).

BELL'S PALSY

Clinical Aspects

Acute idiopathic dysfunction of the facial nerve (usu-ally postinfectious), is called Bell's palsy (BP) after Sir Charles Bell, who described the condition in 1821 (Ni-parko, 1994). Facial nerve abnormalities include (1) decreased facial motor movement (e.g., facial expres-sion, lid closure), (2) denervation of the tensor tympani (resulting in failure to damp the eardrum to loud noises), (3) decreased taste sensation of the anterior two thirds of the tongue, and (4) abnormal lacrimal and salivary function. Little is known about the acute pathology of BP, but it is assumed to be inflammatory, with nerve swelling and compression.

As with GBS and acute disseminated encephalomy-elitis (see later), BP often follows an upper respiratory illness. Most cases are unilateral, but asymmetric bilateral BP is occasionally encountered, often as an early manifestation of GBS. Facial weakness is often heralded by ear pain.

Peripheral white blood cell count and the sedimentation rate are normal, but CSF pleocytosis and elevation of CSF protein and IgG may be present; these are consistent with transient inflammation and blood-brain barrier disturbance. To assess the possibility of other illnesses, such as GBS, a search for polyneuropathy and involvement of other cranial or peripheral nerves is indicated.

Treatment and Prognosis

Symptomatic therapy with artificial tears and eye patches should be used for incomplete eye closure. The use of corticosteroids in BP is controversial; if given early, they may lessen pain with minimal side effects. Nonetheless, prospective controlled studies have not demonstrated objective benefit from corticosteroid treatment (Prescott, 1988; Karnes, 1993). Complications of BP include persistent facial weakness and aberrant facial nerve fiber regeneration, resulting in peculiarities of facial mimesis.

OTHER IMMUNOLOGICALLY MEDIATED PERIPHERAL NEUROPATHIES

Other rare, chronic, immune-mediated polyneuropathies of childhood (Linington and Brostoff, 1993) include neuropathies associated with neoplasms, lymphoma, leukemia, and polycythemia vera (McLeod, 1993a, 1993b); monoclonal gammopathies (Kyle and Dyck, 1993); systemic vasculitides (Chalk et al., 1993); and idiopathic inflammatory conditions (Smith et al., 1993). In some of these disorders, autoantibodies can be identified in the serum or CSF or by immunohistochemical study of peripheral nerve biopsies.

ACUTE DISSEMINATED ENCEPHALOMYELITIS

Historic Aspects

Illnesses resembling acute disseminated encephalomyelitis (ADEM) were first recognized in the nineteenth century by Osler and others, who were struck by the circumstance of an occasional child who developed a severe, acute, multifocal encephalitis followed by a remarkable recovery. Many cases occurred during the influenza epidemic after World War I. The characteristic pathology in these cases was also seen in children following common exanthems or vaccinations (Greenfield, 1930).

Pathology

The prominent pathologic features of ADEM are perivenular inflammatory infiltration and periaxial demyelination, that is, destruction of myelin with relative preservation of nerve fiber axons (Allen and Kirk, 1992). These findings resemble those in multiple sclerosis (MS) and distinguish them from viral encephalitis. Several pathologic stages are recognized, including:

- Venular hyperemia
- Perivascular and subendothelial inflammatory cell infiltration and edema
- Vascular necrosis
- Demyelination with or without hemorrhage
- Astrocytic response with remyelination and gliosis

The initial infiltrate consists of polymorphonuclear leukocytes, but over time lymphocytes predominate. As demyelination occurs, microglial cells become admixed with lymphocytes, as do phagocytes containing lipid byproducts of myelin degradation. Meningeal inflammation may also be found. Brain involvement is symmetric. Reactive changes in the spleen have also been demonstrated (Turnbull and McIntosh, 1926). In severe cases there are disseminated hemorrhages, a syndrome called *acute hemorrhagic encephalopathy* (AHE).

Pathogenesis

The possibility that a CNS viral infection causes ADEM is suggested by its occurrence following viral infection and by the induction of experimental encephalomyelitis by viruses. Prior to widespread immunization, measles was the most common prodromal illness; ADEM occurred in 1 of 800 cases of measles. ADEM can also occur following herpes simplex encephalitis (Koenig et al., 1979), and many other DNA and RNA viruses have also been associated with ADEM.

The occurrence of ADEM after administration of vaccine, including rabies, pertussis, measles, tetanus, and influenza vaccines, spirochetal illnesses (e.g., Lyme disease), and noninvasive bacteria (e.g., *Bordetella pertussis*) suggests that ADEM is not associated with productive infection (Fenichel, 1982; Corsellis et al., 1983). More likely, these exposures mimic critical CNS antigens and induce subsequent immune injury. Similar immune injury and demyelination occur during subacute and chronic CNS infections caused by herpes simplex virus (Sarchielli et al., 1993), human T-cell leukemia/lymphoma virus (HTLV)-1 (tropical spastic paraparesis) (Tachi et al., 1992), and HIV (AIDS) (Rhodes, 1993).

Vascular Changes

Vascular changes may precede an inflammatory perivenular exudate and demyelination, mimicking the vasculitis of serum sickness and immune complex disease. Injury to capillary vascular endothelial cells at the capillary level may result in impairment of the blood-brain barrier.

A role for adhesion molecules in the vascular phase of ADEM has been proposed. They may attract inflammatory cells and may have either positive or negative consequences, depending on whether the cells clear infection or aggravate inflammatory demyelination (Simmons and Cattle, 1992). Enhanced expression of adhesion molecules occurs during experimental relapsing experimental autoimmune encephalomyelitis (Cannella et al., 1990).

Humoral Immunology

Circulating immune complexes are present in some children with ADEM, resulting in immune complex injury to some organs, resulting in myalgia, rash, and proteinuria (Stricker et al., 1992).

Cellular Immunology

The pathologic changes in ADEM resemble those of experimental allergic encephalomyelitis (EAE) (Rivers et al., 1993). In this model, CNS demyelination is induced by repeated inoculation of "encephalitogenic" antigens (e.g., whole spinal cord homogenate, myelin basic protein, or proteolipid protein) into a susceptible animal. The resulting illness, EAE, shares many pathologic features with human demyelinating diseases, including ADEM and MS (Waksman and Adams, 1955).

Wekerle and coworkers (1994) believe the major lessons gained from the study of EAE are that the CNS is not a privileged or isolated immunologic site; that activated T cells penetrate the blood-brain barrier; and that autoaggressive, anti-CNS T cells exist. However, the triggers that activate autoaggressive T cells during naturally occurring demyelination in animals and humans have not been identified. There is growing evidence that autoaggressive T cells may have a restricted T-cell receptor gene usage and epitope specificity. Finally, Wekerle and coworkers (1994) point out that EAE can be initiated by injections of several different CNS antigens, not only of myelin basic protein.

Clinical Aspects

ADEM usually occurs 2 to 20 days after a febrile illness (Miller et al., 1957; de Vries, 1960; Scott, 1967; Croft, 1969). ADEM is more common in winter, when childhood respiratory and gastrointestinal viral illnesses are common. ADEM typically begins in children recovering from a viral illness who abruptly develop irritability and lethargy. Most children have fever during the viral prodrome; at onset of ADEM itself, fever is variable. About 15% of affected children have no prodrome. In a few children, there may be a prolonged fever of unknown origin. Diffuse neurologic signs develop rapidly along with mental status changes and long-tract signs. Seizures occur in 25%. All portions of the CNS may be involved, but the optic nerves and spinal cord are most commonly affected.

Diagnosis

Evaluation of children with ADEM is initially aimed at excluding other causes of diffuse CNS dysfunction, such as intoxication, infection (encephalitis, parasitic conditions), and systemic vasculitis. Prior to magnetic resonance imaging (MRI), encephalitis was difficult to distinguish from ADEM. On MRI, the diagnostic test of choice, patients who have ADEM typically show multiple areas of increased signal intensity on T2 weighting, characteristically at the gray-white junction. When these signs are present, the differential diagnosis is narrowed to ADEM, MS, and systemic lupus erythematosus (Valk and van der Knapp, 1989; Kesselring et al., 1990). The clinical course and ancillary tests distinguish between these conditions.

Other laboratory tests of value include the electroencephalogram (EEG) and cerebrospinal fluid (CSF) analysis. The EEG usually shows slowing while awake; the absence of slowing suggests an ultimate diagnosis of MS. The CSF in ADEM suggests an inflammatory reaction, with elevated IgG, oligoclonal bands, and a moderate lymphocytosis (Valk and van der Knapp, 1989).

Treatment

Although large, controlled trials have not been performed, most clinicians favor treatment of ADEM with corticosteroids. Clinical response may occur within hours of initiation of therapy, particularly when high-dose (15 to 20 mg/kg/day) intravenous methylprednisolone is used. Relapse may occur when steroids are tapered; some relapsing children respond well to a slower taper, but a few may require prolonged steroid therapy (months or years). In patients resistant to high-dose corticosteroids, plasmapheresis, IVIG, or cyclosporine may be employed. ADEM patients in coma have been successfully treated with plasmapheresis (Stricker et al., 1995).

Prognosis

The outlook for complete recovery is excellent. Although some older series report a 10% mortality, only 2% of our 60 cases died because of ADEM-related complications (Rust, unpublished observations, 1995). Recovery is unrelated to severity of initial signs, and complete recovery may occur even in patients who are blind, comatose, and quadriparetic during the nadir of ADEM. Prognosis is poorest in children under age 2 years, many of whom have persistent motor and mental defects. These patients may display generalized abnormalities on MRI and are sometimes labeled acute toxic encephalopathy. For older children, fixed deficits are uncommon. After ten years, approximately 25% of ADEM patients develop MS. ADEM patients are more likely to develop MS if they are (1) afebrile, (2) have no mental status change, (3) have no prodromal "viral" illness or immunization, (4) have no generalized EEG slowing, and (5) have abnormal CSF (Rust, unpublished observations, 1995).

OPTIC NEURITIS

Childhood optic neuritis may be an isolated finding or may be associated with other inflammatory and demyelinative illnesses. Many children with ADEM and a few children with GBS have clinical and laboratory findings consistent with optic neuritis (ON); also, ON commonly is the presenting symptom of MS. In addition, ON may be associated with transverse myelitis, a combination that is called *Devic's syndrome*. The frequency and age at diagnosis of isolated ON (rare in the first years of life, more common at ages 6 to 14) are similar to ADEM. In approximately 70% of children, visual loss occurs days to weeks after a viral illness (especially measles, mumps, and varicella) or immunization (Purvin et al., 1988; Riikonen, 1989).

Diagnosis

The diagnosis of optic neuritis is made on the basis of acute, unilateral diminution in visual acuity not attributed to nutritional deficiency, ischemia, vasculitis, or a compressive lesion. ON can usually be diagnosed by characteristic clinical findings, so that an extensive evaluation is rarely indicated (Beck et al., 1992). When a progressive course, associated neurologic signs, or other orbital findings suggest optic nerve compression, MRI should be performed. Routine neuroimaging of all patients with optic neuritis is not warranted, and may lead to a diagnosis of subclinical multiple sclerosis, which has no therapeutic implications but does have a major psychosocial and insurability impact.

Treatment and Prognosis

Because of pathologic similarities to other demyelinating conditions, ON probably results from similar mechanisms present in GBS, ADEM, and MS. In most childhood ON cases, spontaneous recovery may be expected, although the rate may be slow (Good et al., 1992). The value of corticosteroids in ON is uncertain. A large, multicenter study of corticosteroid use in adult ON (Beck et al., 1992, 1993) indicates the following:

1. IV methylprednisolone speeds recovery from acute exacerbations.
2. Oral prednisone is ineffective in acute exacerbations and probably increases the risk of subsequent relapse.
3. IV methylprednisolone may increase the time interval to development of disseminated MS in patients presenting with isolated optic neuritis.

Some of these conclusions, in particular the third, remain controversial (Silberberg, 1993) and will be subject to further studies. There are no similar trials in childhood ON.

ON may recur, and some children with ON will develop MS. The precise likelihood of MS developing in infants and children with ON is not known but is lower than in adolescents or adults with ON. The risk for MS is higher in unilateral ON and is rare in bilateral ON (Parkin et al., 1984). In one series, 50% of children with ON with poor or incomplete visual recovery were ultimately diagnosed as having MS (Good et al., 1992). Other studies have shown a 0% to 60% risk of MS after childhood ON followed for 8 to 18 years (Parkin

et al., 1984; Kriss et al., 1988; Riikonen et al., 1988). When ON is associated with ADEM, GBS, or Devic's syndrome, visual recovery is likely, and the neurologic prognosis is that of the underlying syndrome.

ACUTE TRANSVERSE MYELITIS

Clinical Manifestations

Acute transverse myelitis (ATM) is an acute disorder manifesting with CNS dysfunction at a discrete level of the spinal cord. ATM often occurs days to weeks (1) after infection with one of the viruses associated with GBS and ADEM, (2) as a complication of vaccination, or (3) as a manifestation of Lyme disease (Tyler et al., 1986; Rousseau et al., 1986; Byrne and Waxman, 1990). ATM may occur in isolation or in association with features suggesting GBS, ADEM, or MS. The pathology of ATM shows prevenular inflammatory changes with demyelination similar to that of ADEM; in severe cases, spinal cord necrosis may occur (Aicardi, 1992). Although the pathogenesis of ATM is unknown, it is probably identical to other postinfectious inflammatory conditions, i.e., immune dysregulation or bystander inflammation.

Diagnosis

The diagnosis of ATM is made by exclusion of tumor, compressive injury, vascular malformation, hemorrhage, stroke, or radiation injury. Spinal cord imaging by MRI with gadolinium enhancement is indicated. With contrast enhancement, neuroimaging may show changes at the appropriate spinal level and cord swelling (Miller et al., 1987). MRI scanning of the head may disclose clinically silent lesions; the significance of these findings in children is uncertain and does not necessarily imply a diagnosis of MS. In some cases, myelography may be useful.

Lyme disease, syphilis, parasitic infection (cysticercosis), and AIDS must be considered; serologic studies and CSF sampling are helpful. CSF pleocytosis is present in 25%, and increased CSF protein is present in 50% of patients (Aicardi, 1992). The vacuolar myelopathy of AIDS that resembles acute transverse myelitis (ATM) has thus far been limited to adults (Rosenblum et al., 1989). Tropical spastic paraparesis, a progressive myelopathy caused by human T-cell lymphotrophic virus (HTLV)-1 infection, occurs in children and may produce MRI changes indistinguishable from ATM, although HTLV-1 lesions often are disseminated throughout the cord (Newton et al., 1987; Link et al., 1989); also, the clinical course of HTLV-1 myelopathy is slower than that of ATM.

Therapy

No therapy, including corticosteroids, is of proven efficacy in the treatment of ATM. Nonetheless, in severe cases, intravenous corticosteroids are often used, sometimes with a dramatic response. Otherwise, management is supportive. Some degree of recovery occurs in 80% to 90% of children but may require weeks to months. Approximately 50% of children with ATM show excellent recovery; however, 10% to 20% develop cord necrosis and remain severely paralyzed. The remainder have variable residua (Ropper and Poskanzer, 1978; Berman et al., 1981). The most important prognostic factor is acuteness of onset; recovery is poor with a hyperacute onset. Ultimately, a diagnosis of MS is made in about 10% of adults who experience ATM; the occurrence of MS after isolated childhood ATM is exceptional (Aicardi, 1992).

DEVIC'S SYNDROME

The combination of optic neuritis (ON) and acute transverse myelitis (ATM), first described by Devic in 1894, is called *neuromyelitis optica*, or Devic's syndrome (DS). The signs of ON and ATM may develop simultaneously or in rapid succession, often after a viral illness or immunization. ON is often bilateral, and fundoscopic changes of papillitis are usually present. Clinical features are otherwise similar to the conditions in isolation. The clinical syndrome is distinct, and the differential diagnosis includes only other inflammatory CNS demyelinating disorders, (i.e., ADEM and MS) (Haslam, 1987).

As in ON and ATM, corticosteroid therapy is often used, particularly when optic nerve or spinal cord swelling is marked and when the cervical cord dysfunction is severe or respiratory symptoms occur. The prognosis may be more guarded for each component of Devic's syndrome than for ON and ATM occurring in isolation (Whitham and Brey, 1985).

ACUTE CEREBELLAR ATAXIA

Historic and Clinical Aspects

Acute cerebellar ataxia (ACA), first described by Batten in 1907, usually develops days to weeks after a viral illness, particularly chickenpox. In the largest series (Connolly et al., 1994), 26% of patients had chickenpox, 3% had Epstein-Barr virus infection, 49% had other viral illnesses, 19% had no prodrome, and 3% developed ACA after immunizations. Other preceding infections include measles, mumps, herpes simplex virus, cocksackievirus, echovirus, poliovirus, *M. pneumoniae*, and *Legionella pneumophila* (Kuban et al., 1983; Aicardi, 1992).

ACA usually occurs in children between 2 and 5 years of age and is rare in adolescents and adults. Epstein-Barr virus infection and immunizations are the most common causes in these older patients (Connolly et al., 1994). Some ataxia is seen in all children who have ACA, and 20% to 50% of patients are unable to walk. Finger dysmetria is seen in two thirds of these children but is strikingly mild compared with the gait ataxia (Connolly et al., 1994). Nystagmus was present in less than 20% of Connolly's (1994) patients,

whereas 45% of Weiss and Carter's patients had nystagmus (1959). Transient behavioral alterations and school difficulties are seen in at least one third of children with ACA.

Given the variety of antecedents, it is likely that ACA is mediated by a common immunoinflammatory process. In this respect, a recent report has identified antineuronal antibodies in ACA following Epstein-Barr virus infection (Ito et al., 1994). CSF pleocytosis occurs in 25% to 50% of children, almost always with a lymphocytic predominance (Weiss and Carter, 1959; Connolly et al., 1994). The CSF IgG index is elevated in 50% of these children, and oligoclonal bands are present in 10% to 17%.

Prognosis

In rare cases without complete recovery, atrophy of the cerebellar hemispheres or other conditions, such as cerebellar tumor or intoxication, should be expected. As with ADEM, children with ACA may develop transient emotional lability and decreased attention span.

MULTIPLE SCLEROSIS

Multiple sclerosis (MS), also known as disseminated sclerosis or *sclerose en plaques*, is the principal immune-mediated demyelinating disease of humans (Matthews, 1991). Although primarily a disorder of young adults, MS has been pathologically verified in infancy (Shaw and Alvord, 1987; Hanefeld et al., 1993). In childhood, MS is less common than ADEM. MS and ADEM may be difficult to distinguish, particularly at the onset of symptoms.

Historic Aspects

The pathologic lesions of MS were reported by Cruveilhier and Carswell in the early nineteenth century. In 1849, Frerichs first made a clinical diagnosis of MS. Charcot (1868) distilled these observations into a coherent and recognizable clinical entity. A detailed account of the history of MS is available (De Jong, 1970).

Pathogenesis

MS primarily affects young adults (Sadovnick and Ebers, 1993). The peak age of onset is 25 to 30 years. In one study, only 125 of 4632 cases (3%) had an onset before age 16 years; the mean age of onset in these cases was 13 years, and only eight had signs or symptoms before age 11 (Duquette et al., 1987). The female:male ratio is 3:2, and whites are at greater risk than blacks. The risk of MS is related to the latitude in which individuals spend their childhood; the risk increases in proportion to the distance from the equator.

A viral pathogenesis of MS is suggested by several lines of evidence (Johnson, 1994). First, the epidemiology suggests exposure to an environmental agent that parallels the prevalence of common viral infections.

Second, CSF immunoglobulin from MS patients may have antibodies to several viruses, notably measles virus; also, viruses have occasionally been isolated from MS tissue. Third, certain animal viruses, such as visna, JHM, Theiler, and canine distemper viruses, cause similar demyelinating diseases (reviewed by Dal Canto, 1990).

Several MS clusters and epidemics provide support for an infectious pathogenesis and genetic susceptibility (Sadovnick and Ebers, 1993). The introduction of MS to the Faroe Islands during World War II suggests that an infectious agent was introduced to a genetically susceptible population.

Racial variation in MS susceptibility also suggests that there is a genetic aspect to MS. There is also a small but definite increase in MS risk among close relatives of index cases. In about 10% to 15% of MS cases, another family member also has MS. Overall, the risk of MS in relatives of an index case is approximately 0.5% for offspring, 0.6% for parents, 1.2% in siblings, 2% to 4% in dizygotic twins, and 25% to 27% in monozygotic twins (Compston, 1991; Mumford, 1994; Ebers, 1994a). These studies indicate the importance of genetics in MS susceptibility; however, since concordance in monozygotic twins is considerably less than 100%, environmental factors remain important.

HLA studies showed that HLA-A3, -B7, -DR2, and -Dw2 are increased, whereas HLA-A2, -B12,-DR7, and -Dw7 were decreased in northern whites with MS (Visscher et al., 1979; Oger and Arnason, 1984; Tiwari and Terasaki, 1985). Other HLA antigens are increased in MS in other racial groups. Hillert (1994) has reviewed these HLA associations but concludes that HLA genes play a minor role in MS risk. Phillips (1993), using a mathematical model, concludes that genetic susceptibility is due to 10 to 15 interacting genes.

Pathology

The characteristic MS pathologic lesions are small areas of perivenular demyelination and large plaques of confluent demyelination with relative axon sparing (Prineas, 1990; Allen, 1991a; Allen and Kirk, 1992; Raine, 1994b). The perivenular demyelination resembles that present in ADEM. The demyelination coalesces to form the typical macroscopic MS plaques. These well-demarcated plaques may be located in any area of the CNS but have a predilection for white matter in the periventricular zones, centrum semiovale, optic nerves, and the spinal cord.

Microscopically, acute plaques have intense cellular infiltrates with lymphocytes, plasma cells, reactive astrocytes, microglia, and macrophages present. Older plaques appear quiescent, with severe loss of myelin and myelin-producing oligodendroglia cells. Established plaques are sclerotic with reactive astrocytosis. Plaques of varying activity generally occur in any given case. Remyelination occurs, but these areas may be particularly susceptible to recurrent demyelination. Electron microscopy shows that demyelination occurs at the margins of active MS plaques; destruction and engulfment of the myelin sheaths occurs outward to inward.

Immunology

There is no systemic immune dysfunction, such as autoimmunity, immunodeficiency, or susceptibility to malignancy in MS (Reder and Arnason, 1985; Allen, 1991b). The increase in glial cell malignancies in MS is too slight to suggest a defect of immune surveillance. Antibody responses and delayed hypersensitivity are normal. Nevertheless, localized immune disturbances in the demyelinating plaque involving both humoral and cellular immunity may be present (Olsson, 1992; Raine, 1994b).

Immunoglobulin abnormalities in CSF have been a consistent finding in MS (Mehta, 1991; Olsson, 1994), including (1) elevated immunoglobulin levels, (2) increased immunoglobulin synthesis, (3) presence of oligoclonal bands on electrophoresis, and (4) increased levels of immunoglobulin components, such as kappa chains (Rudick et al., 1989). Although IgG1 subclass elevation is most common, other subclasses and classes are also elevated. The antigenic specificity of these immunoglobulins is usually not identified, although reactivity with viruses or other microbes has inconsistently been identified.

The MS experimental model EAE suggests that activated lymphocytes mediate demyelination, since both the monophasic and chronic relapsing forms of EAE can be transferred by lymphocytes but not by serum. T-cell subset abnormalities, particularly decreased numbers of CD8 cells, have been reported in children and adults with MS (Reder and Arnason, 1985; Allen, 1991b). Also, in coronavirus-induced demyelination, adoptive transfer of splenic Thy 1+ cells causes paralysis and myelin loss (Fleming et al., 1993). Together with the lymphocytic infiltration present in MS lesions, these findings suggest a local T-cell abnormality in MS. The roles of T-cell activation and the T-cell receptor (TCR) specificity in MS have been reviewed (Olsson, 1992; ffrench-Constant, 1994; Utz and McFarland, 1994; Raine, 1994b).

There is enhanced expression of major histocompatibility (MHC) antigens in MS lesions, particularly class II MHC antigens, on the surface of microglia and macrophages (Ransohoff and Estes, 1991; Raine, 1994a). MHC expression in astrocytes but not oligodendrocytes has also been noted (Raine, 1994b).

The target antigen(s) of MS is not known but may include myelin, viruses, and heat-shock proteins (ffrench-Constant, 1994). Whereas demyelination in EAE is associated with reactivity to myelin constituents such as myelin basic protein, cellular immunity to myelin in MS has not been conclusively demonstrated (Raine, 1994b).

T-cell receptor (TCR) germline polymorphisms in MS have been investigated to determine if certain genes contribute to MS susceptibility; to date, these studies are inconclusive (Olsson, 1992; Utz and McFarland, 1994; Vandevyver et al., 1994). Others have sought restricted TCR elements in MS lesions, but these studies are also inconclusive (reviewed in Utz and McFarland, 1994; Raine, 1994a).

The cellular infiltrates of MS lesions have a predominance of CD4[+] T cells at the leading edge of active lesions, whereas CD8[+] cells are more frequent in less active areas. Most T cells in MS lesions bear TCRαβ-chains, although some T cells bear TCRγδ-chains, particularly in chronic lesions (Raine, 1994b). Chronic lesions also contain reactive oligodendroglia, expressing the 65-kD heat shock protein, hsp 65, a known stimulus for TCRγδ T cells. This may explain the depletion of oligodendrocytes present in chronic MS lesions (Selmaj et al., 1991). Raine (1994b) suggests that TCRαβ cells may initiate inflammation, whereas TCRγδ cells down-regulate the TCRαβ response and perpetuate chronic active lesions.

Immunohistochemical studies of MS lesions demonstrate enhanced expression of adhesion molecules and cytokines (Olsson, 1992; ffrench-Constant, 1994; Raine, 1994a, 1994b). The former include intercellular adhesion molecule-1 (ICAM-1) on the endothelium and leukocyte function–associated antigen-1 (LFA-1) on lymphocytes, both of which facilitate inflammatory cell trafficking into the MS lesions. MS lesions contain proinflammatory cytokines, such as interleukin-2 (IL-2), tumor necrosis factor-α (TNF-α), and interferon-γ (IFN-γ) that are associated with a T_H1 response. Circulating lymphocytes from MS patients show increased production of these proinflammatory cytokines and a diminution of anti-inflammatory cytokines, such as transforming growth factor-β (TGF-β) (Mokhtarian et al., 1994; Link et al., 1994).

Clinical Manifestations

Childhood and adolescent patients who have MS present with a variety of symptoms and signs and have a relapsing-remitting course (Hanefeld et al., 1993). Initially, MS is difficult to distinguish from ADEM. Ultimately, about 25% of children with ADEM develop MS (Rust, unpublished observations, 1995).

The most common initial manifestation of MS is a sensory disturbance (26%). Other features include optic neuritis (17%), other visual disturbances (diplopia or blurred vision) (17%), pure motor disturbance (11%), abnormal gait (8%), cerebellar ataxia or combined sensorimotor disturbances (5%), myelitis (3%), vestibular abnormalities (2%), and sphincter disturbances (1%) (Duquette et al., 1987).

Diagnosis

Diagnostic criteria for MS have been proposed (Matthews, 1991). They require temporal and spatial dissemination of lesions, exclusion of other illness, and a clinical course typical of MS (i.e., chronic relapsing, chronic progressive, or acute fulminant). The role of laboratory tests, such as brain imaging and CSF analysis, in diagnosis has been discussed by Kurtzke (1988).

Rudick and colleagues (1986) studied patients misdiagnosed as MS and suggested some findings that cast doubt on an MS diagnosis: (1) absence of eye findings (optic nerve or oculomotor), (2) absence of clinical remissions, (3) localized disease, (4) absence of sensory or bladder abnormalities, and (5) absence of CSF abnormalities.

The differential diagnosis of MS includes focal conditions, multifocal diseases, and systemic degenerative diseases. Focal conditions to be excluded are tumors of the optic nerve, hypothalamus, or sella turcica; Arnold-Chiari malformation, brain stem glioma, spinal cord tumors, vascular malformations, syrinx, and arachnoiditis. Multifocal diseases to be excluded include SLE, sarcoidosis, Behçet's syndrome, Lyme disease, moyamoya, granulomatous angiitis, and central-type neurofibromatosis. Degenerative diseases to be excluded include metabolic ataxias, spinocerebellar degeneration, late-onset leukodystrophies, mitochondrial cytopathies, and beriberi. Vitamin B_{12} deficiency, an important condition to exclude in adult MS, is rare in children.

Ancillary tests in MS include (1) neuroimaging, particularly MRI, (2) CSF testing, and (3) evoked potential studies. The CSF in children with MS usually has a lymphocyte count of 50 to 100 cells/mm³, higher than that present in adults (Rust et al., 1988; Whitaker et al., 1990; Hanefeld et al., 1993). CSF myelin basic protein levels are elevated in 70% to 90% of acute MS exacerbations, but this is a nonspecific abnormality (Cohen et al., 1980). CSF immunoglobulin abnormalities (IgG index, IgG synthetic rate, light chain levels, oligoclonal bands) are present in 85% to 90% of children with clinically definite MS (Boutin et al., 1988; Hanefeld et al., 1993) and in 25% to 30% of patients with possible or suspected MS (Francis et al., 1991).

Treatment

Therapy for MS is unsatisfactory (Matthews, 1991; Ebers, 1994b; Goodkin, 1994). Corticosteroids are used extensively (Milligan et al., 1987; Compston, 1988; Capildeo, 1989). Controlled studies in acute ON (Beck et al., 1992, 1993) suggest that oral corticosteroids alone may be contraindicated in acute MS, whereas short courses of intravenous corticosteroids may be beneficial. Multicenter trials of corticosteroids in MS are in progress.

Supportive measures include antispasticity medications, urologic management, control of pain, and psychologic support (Matthews, 1991; Mertin, 1994). A recent cooperative study of IFN-β in relapsing-remitting MS showed a reduced frequency of clinical attacks (IFN-β Multiple Sclerosis Study Group, 1993) and a tendency to MRI stabilization (Paty and Li, 1993). The FDA has approved this drug for ambulatory patients. Similar beneficial effects have been noted in a recent study of copolymer (Johnson, personal communication, 1995) in relapsing-remitting MS. A preliminary study (Sipe et al., 1994) has shown that cladrabine may be of benefit in chronic progressive multiple sclerosis. In severe cases, in which rapid deterioration is occurring, cyclophosphamide, cyclosporine, methotrexate, azathioprine, and IVIG may be employed, although benefit is uncertain (Ebers, 1994b).

Prognosis

The "5-year rule" (Kurtzke et al., 1985) states that the degree of disability after 5 years correlates well with disability at 10 and 15 years. Since most pediatric cases have few fixed defects after 5 years, the prognosis is often relatively good.

ATAXIA-TELANGIECTASIA

Ataxia-telangiectasia (see Chapter 12) is associated with prominent neurologic features (Chung et al., 1994), including cerebellar ataxia, choreoathetosis, and dystonia. Neuroimaging shows atrophy of the cerebellar hemispheres and vermis, although white matter abnormalities mimicking a leukodystrophy or primary demyelinating disease have been described. Prognosis is poor, and progression is relentless.

SYDENHAM'S CHOREA

Sydenham's chorea (SC) (St. Vitus' dance) was first described by Thomas Sydenham in the seventeenth century; its association with rheumatic carditis was first noted in the nineteenth century. SC is the major neurologic manifestation of rheumatic fever (RF) (Swedo et al., 1993). Most cases are preceded by clear evidence for a group A β-hemolytic streptococcal infection. The incidence of SC declined dramatically as antibiotic treatment for streptococcal infection became widespread. There has been a resurgence of both RF and SC (Ayoub, 1992).

Sydenham's chorea presumably results from an immune response to streptococcal antigens. Antineuronal antibodies have been identified in patients with SC (Bronze and Dale, 1993) and may be associated with other childhood movement disorders, such as Tourette's syndrome and motor or vocal tics (Kiessling et al., 1993). Limited autopsy studies disclose mild neuronal injury and perivascular inflammatory infiltrates. Aschoff bodies are not present in the brain.

The onset of SC is insidious, marked by fidgeting, clumsiness, and facial grimacing. The chorea may be unilateral or bilateral. Movements are sudden and jerky or slow and writhing. Exotic, dance-like movements of the trunk and hips, making use of the extremities impossible, may be seen. The speech is often dysarthric and explosive, and swallowing is difficult. Emotional lability may be prominent. Physical examination discloses hypotonia and spooning of the hands.

The clinical course worsens for several weeks, and then gradually improves over several months. Relentless deterioration should suggest an alternative diagnosis (e.g., SLE, Wilson's disease, Tourette's syndrome). Daoud and colleagues (1990) found that valproate is of value in treating the choreiform movements in SC; in resistant cases, haloperidol may be effective, although its use is associated with significant adverse effects, such as tardive dyskinesia (al-Eissa, 1993). Streptococcal prophylaxis is indicated.

THROMBOTIC THROMBOCYTOPENIC PURPURA/HEMOLYTIC-UREMIC SYNDROME

Historic Aspects

Thrombotic thrombocytopenic purpura (TTP), first described by Moschcowitz in 1925, is characterized by fever, hemolytic anemia, renal failure, and neurologic dysfunction. The pathology consists of small-vessel hyaline thromboses. Diagnosis requires at least two major criteria (thrombocytopenia, microangiopathic anemia, neurologic dysfunction) and two minor criteria (fever, renal dysfunction, circulating thrombi) (Ridolfi and Bell, 1981; Bukowski, 1982). Hemolytic-uremic syndrome (HUS) may have any or all of these same findings. In fact, there are no objective criteria except for age to distinguish these two illnesses; they appear to represent a continuum (Fong et al., 1982). Usually, if the patient is older and neurologic findings predominate, TTP is diagnosed; if the patient is younger and renal involvement is prominent, HUS is diagnosed.

Pathogenesis

Both TTP and HUS are associated with vascular endothelial injury. Bacterial toxins have been implicated as a cause of HUS (Karmali et al., 1983). Antiendothelial antibodies have been identified in some cases of TTP (Wall and Harker, 1980). Blood vessel injury may lead to platelet adhesion, complement activation, and coagulation initiation. Platelet-derived plasma P-selectin may be a useful clinical marker of this process (Chong et al., 1994).

TTP/HUS may occur spontaneously or may be secondary to inflammatory diseases (rheumatoid arthritis, polyarteritis nodosa, lupus, Sjögren's), lymphoma, endocarditis, and drugs and poisons (sulfa, iodine, birth control pills) (Remuzzi and Bertani, 1988). TTP/HUS is more common in females than in males (ratio 3:2), and the peak incidence is in the third decade. Cases in neonates and young children have been described (Kennedy et al., 1980).

Clinical Manifestations and Treatment

Symptoms of TTP/HUS develop over 7 to 10 days. Purpura is the initial finding in more than 90% of patients; fever is usually present early. Hemorrhages (retinal, choroidal, nasal, gingival, gastrointestinal, and genitourinary), pallor, abdominal pain, arthralgia, and pancreatitis may develop. Neurologic findings include fatigue, confusion, headache, and visual and language dysfunction. Since TTP/HUS primarily affects the microvasculature, major stroke-like events are uncommon. Laboratory findings include microangiopathic hemolytic anemia, thrombocytopenia, proteinuria, and microscopic hematuria. Pathologic findings include capillary and arteriolar thrombi. Prognosis for patients with TTP/HUS is guarded. Survival has increased from 5% to 50% over the past few decades.

Treatment includes aspirin, corticosteroids, splenectomy, and plasma exchange (Hayward et al., 1994).

Table 28–5. Remote Effects of Cancer on the Nervous System

Syndrome	Most Frequently Associated Neoplasm	Neuropathology	Autoantibody
Cerebellar degeneration	Lung, ovarian, Hodgkin's	Purkinje cell loss in cerebellum	Anti-Yo
Opsoclonus-myoclonus	Neuroblastoma	Variable, sometimes none apparent	Anti-Ri*
Retinal degeneration	Small cell lung cancer	Photoreceptor cell loss	Uncertain
Sensory neuropathy/ encephalomyelitis	Hodgkin's, others	Inflammatory infiltrates	Anti-Hu†
Subacute motor neuropathy	Hodgkin's, other lymphomas	Neuronal loss in spinal cord	Unknown
Sensorineural peripheral neuropathy	Lung cancer	Axonal degeneration	IgM paraprotein or anti-MAG

*The association of anti-Ri antibodies and opsoclonus-myoclonus is based on a small number of reports and is currently under investigation.
†The syndromes associated with anti-Hu are diverse, including sensory neuropathy, motor neuron dysfunction, cerebellar symptoms, brain stem symptoms, autonomic dysfunction, and limbic encephalopathy (characterized by dementia, agitation, and seizures). There is multifocal involvement of the nervous system clinically and pathologically, with the syndromes listed named for the area of *predominant* dysfunction.
Abbreviation: MAG = myelin-associated glycoprotein.

Successful outcome is associated with early diagnosis and prompt use of plasma exchange (Scully, 1994).

RASMUSSEN'S ENCEPHALITIS

Rasmussen's encephalitis (RE) is a rare progressive gray matter disease of children (Vining et al., 1993) that manifests in the first decade of life and is characterized by intractable focal epilepsy (epilepsia partialis continua), progressive hemiparesis, cerebral atrophy, and dementia.

Molecular probes have identified cytomegalovirus (CMV) genomes in resected RE tissue (Power et al., 1990; McLachlan et al., 1993). Treatment of one RE patient with the antiviral agent zidovudine resulted in a dramatic improvement of seizure frequency (De-Toledo and Smith, 1994).

Rogers and associates (1994) attempted to raise antibodies to recombinant glutamate receptors (GluR) in rabbits and observed that some rabbits developed anorexia and seizures. Pathologic findings in the rabbits resembled those of RE in humans. Subsequent studies showed that only rabbits immunized with one of the five GluR subtypes (GluR3) were affected. These investigators then found anti-GluR3 antibodies in two of four patients with RE. Plasma exchange performed in one child with RE resulted in a decrease in GluR3 antibody titer, decreased seizure frequency, and improved neurologic function.

Conventional therapy consists of anticonvulsant medication and resection of the involved tissue (Vining et al., 1993); in the future, antiviral, IVIG, or corticosteroid therapies may be helpful (Hart et al., 1994).

PARANEOPLASTIC SYNDROMES

Children and adults with malignancies may develop severe neurologic dysfunction not attributable to either the neoplasm itself (e.g., metastases or local invasion) or treatment complications. These conditions, called paraneoplastic or remote effects of cancer, are clinically heterogeneous and include neurologic findings such as truncal ataxia, myoclonus, and opsoclonus. The neurologic features may precede diagnosis of the tumor (Table 28–5). The clinical features of paraneoplastic syndromes have been reviewed by Posner (1991) and Dalmau and coworkers (1992). The Lambert-Eaton myasthenic syndrome, dermatomyositis, and Guillain-Barré syndrome are sometimes associated with central nervous system tumors (Posner, 1991). There may be a dramatic response to antitumor treatment, corticosteroids, or plasmapheresis (Posner, 1991).

References

Acheson ED. The epidemiology of multiple sclerosis. In Matthews WB, ed. McAlpine's Multiple Sclerosis. Oxford, Churchill Livingstone, 1985, pp. 3–46.

Aicardi J. Diseases of the Nervous System in Childhood. London, MacKeith Press, 1992.

Alcala H. The differential diagnosis of poliomyelitis and other acute flaccid paralyses. Boletin Medico del Hospital Infantil de Mexico 50:136–144, 1993.

al-Eissa A. Sydenham's chorea: a new look at an old disease. Br J Clin Pract 41:14–16, 1993.

al-Janadi M, Smith CD, Karhs J. Cyclophosphamide treatment of interstitial pulmonary fibrosis in polymyositis/dermatomyositis. J Rheumatol 16:1592–1596, 1989.

Allen IV. Pathology of multiple sclerosis. In Matthews WB, ed. McAlpine's Multiple Sclerosis. Oxford, Churchill Livingston, 1991a, pp. 341–378.

Allen IV. Aetiological hypotheses for multiple sclerosis: evidence from human and experimental diseases. In Matthews WB, ed. McAlpine's Multiple Sclerosis. Oxford, Churchill Livingstone, 1991b, pp. 379–390.

Allen IV, Kirk J. Demyelinating diseases. In Adams JH, Duchen LW, eds. Greenfield's Neuropathology New York, Oxford University Press, 1992, pp. 447–620.

Amato AA, Barohn RJ, Jackson CE, Pappert EJ, Sahenk Z, Kissel JT. Inclusion body myositis: treatment with intravenous immunoglobulin. Neurology 44:1516–1518, 1994.

Aoki T, Drachman DB, Asher DM, Gibbs CJ Jr, Habhmanyar S, Wolinsky JS. Attempts to implicate viruses in myasthenia gravis. Neurology 35:185–192, 1985.

al-Qudah AA, Shahar E, Logan WJ, Murphy EG. Neonatal Guillain-Barré syndrome. Pediatr Neurol 4:255–256, 1988.

Arakawa Y, Yoshimura M, Kobayashi S, Ichihashi K, Miyao M,

Momoi MY. The use of intravenous immunoglobulin in Miller-Fisher syndrome. Brain Dev 15:231–233, 1993.

Arnason BGW. Acute inflammatory demyelinating polyradiculoneuropathies. In Dyck PJ, Thomas PK, Lambert EH, Bunge R, eds. Peripheral Neuropathy. Philadelphia, WB Saunders, 1984, pp. 2050–2100.

Arnason BGW, Soliven B. Acute inflammatory demyelinating polyradiculoneuropathy. In Dyck PJ, Thomas PK, eds. Peripheral Neuropathy. Philadelphia, WB Saunders, 1993, pp. 1437–1497.

Askanas V, Engel WK. New advances in inclusion body myositis. Curr Opin Rheumatol 5:732–741, 1993.

Askanas V, Engel WK, Bilak M, Alvarez RB, Selkoe DJ. Twisted tubulofilaments of inclusion body myositis muscle resemble paired helical filaments of Alzheimer brain and contain hyperphosphorylated tau. Am J Pathol 144:177–187, 1994.

Ayoub EM. Resurgence of rheumatic fever in the United States: the changing picture of a preventable illness. Postgrad Med 92:133–136, 1992.

Bady B, Chauplannaz G, Carrier H. Congenital Lambert-Eaton myasthenic syndrome. J Neurol Neurosurg Psychiatry 50:476–478, 1987.

Barlow CF. Neonatal myasthenia gravis. Am J Dis Child 135:209, 1981.

Barohn RJ, Kissel JT, Warmolts JR, Mendell JR. Chronic inflammatory demyelinating polyradiculoneuropathy. Arch Neurol 46:878–884, 1989.

Batten FE. A case of acute ataxia. Trans Clin Soc London 40:276–277, 1907.

Bazzato C, Coli U, Landini S, Mezzina C, Ciman M. Myasthenia-like syndrome after D,L- but not L-carnitine. Lancet 1:1209, 1981.

Beck RW, Cleary PA, Anderson MM, Keltner JL, Shults WT, Kaufman DL, Buckley EG, Corbett JJ, Kuppersmith MJ, Miller NR, Savino PJ, Guy JA, Trobe JD, McCrary JA, Smith CH, Chrousos GA, Thompson S, Katz BJ, Brodsky MC, Goodwin JA, Atwell CW, and the Optic Neuritis Study Group. A randomized, controlled trial of corticosteroids in the treatment of acute optic neuritis. N Engl J Med 326:581–588, 1992.

Beck RW, Cleary PA, Trobe JD, Kaufman DI, Kuppersmith MJ, Paty DW, Brown CH, and the Optic Neuritis Study Group. The effect of corticosteroids for acute optic neuritis on the subsequent development of multiple sclerosis. N Engl J Med 329:1764–1769, 1993.

Beeson D, Vincent A, Morris A, Brydson M, Jacobson L, Baggi F, Jeremiah S, Povey S, Newsom-Davis J. cDNA and genomic clones encoding the human muscle acetylcholine receptor. Ann NY Acad Sci 681:165–167, 1993.

Benzing G, Iannacone ST, Bove KE, Keebler PJ, Shockley LL. Prolonged myasthenic syndrome after one week of muscle relaxants. Pediatr Neurol 6:190–196, 1990.

Berman M, Feldman S, Alter M, Ziber N, Kahana E. Acute transverse myelitis: incidence and etiologic considerations. Neurology 31:966–971, 1981.

Beydoun SR, Engel WK, Karossky P, Swartz MU. Long-term plasmapheresis therapy is effective and safe in children with chronic relapsing dysimmune polyneuropathy. Rev Neurol 146:123–127, 1990.

Boutin B, Esquivel E, Mayer M, Chaumet S, Ponsot G, Arthuis M. Multiple sclerosis in children: report of clinical and paraclinical features of 19 cases. Neuropediatrics 19:118–123, 1988.

Bowyer SL, Blane CE, Sullivan DB, Cassidy JT. Childhood dermatomyositis: factors predicting functional outcome and development of dystrophic calcification. J Pediatr 103:882–888, l982.

Bradford JR, Bashford EF, Wilson JA. Acute infective polyneuritis. Q J Med 12:88–103, 1919.

Bradshaw DY, Jones HR Jr. Guillain-Barré syndrome in children: clinical course, electrodiagnosis and prognosis. Muscle Nerve 15:500–506, 1992.

Bronze MS, Dale JB. Epitopes of streptococcal M proteins that evoke antibodies that cross-react with human brain. J Immunol 151:2820–2828, 1993.

Brown LW. Infant botulism. Pediatr Ann 13:135–148, 1984.

Bruguier AI, Texier P, Clement MC, Dulac O, Ponsot G, Arthuis M. Dermatomyosite infantile. Àpropos de 28 observations. Arch Franc Pédiatr 41:9–14, 1984.

Bukowski RM. Thrombotic thrombocytopenic purpura: a review. Prog Hemost Thromb 287–337, 1982.

Bundey S, Doniach D, Soothill JF. Immunological studies in patients with juvenile-onset myasthenia gravis and in their relatives. Clin Exp Immunol 11:321–332, 1972.

Byrne TN, Waxman SG. Spinal Cord Compression. Philadelphia, FA Davis, 1990, pp. 229–231.

Calleja MA. Autonomic dysfunction and Guillain-Barré syndrome. The use of esmolol in its management. Anaesthesia 45:736–737, 1990.

Callen JP. Malignancy in polymyositis/dermatomyositis. Clin Dermatol 2:55–63, 1988.

Cannella B, Cross AH, Raine CS. Upregulation and coexpression of adhesion molecules correlate with relapsing autoimmune demyelination in the central nervous system. J Exp Med 172:1521–1524, 1990.

Capildeo R, ed. Steroids in Disease of the Central Nervous System. Chichester, England, John Wiley & Sons, 1989.

Carroll BA, Lane B, Norman D, Enzmann D. Diagnosis of progressive multifocal leukoencephalopathy by computed tomography. Radiology 122:137–141, 1977.

Castleman B. The pathology of the thymus gland in myasthenia gravis. Ann NY Acad Sci 135:496–503, 1966.

Cebreros GM, Torres MJ, Simon de las Heras R, Mateos B, Sanchez F, Diaz J. Guillain-Barré syndrome: fifteen pediatric cases. An Esp Pediatr 33:120–123, 1990.

Chalk CH, Dyck PJ, Conn DL. Vasculitic neuropathy. In Dyck PJ, Thomas PK, eds. Peripheral Neuropathy. Philadelphia, WB Saunders, 1993, pp. 1424–1435.

Charcot JM. Histologie de la sclérose en plaques. Gaz Hop (Paris) 41:554–566, 1868.

Chinyanga HM, Danha RF. Human immunodeficiency virus and Guillain-Barré syndrome in intensive care unit patients. Cent Afr J Med 38:86–88, 1992.

Chong BH, Murray B, Berndt MC, Dunlop LC, Brighton T, Chesterman CN. Plasma P-selectin is increased in thrombotic consumptive platelet disorders. Blood 83:1535–1541, 1994.

Chung EO, Bodensteiner JB, Noorani PA, Schochet SS. Cerebral white matter changes suggesting leukodystrophy in ataxia telangiectasia. J Child Neurol 9:31–35, 1994.

Claudio L, Brosnan CF. Effects of prazosin on the blood-brain barrier during experimental autoimmune encephalomyelitis. Brain Res 594:233–243, 1992.

Cohen SR, Brooks BR, Herndon RM, McKhann G. A diagnostic index of active demyelination: myelin basic protein in cerebrospinal fluid. Ann Neurol 8:25–31, 1980.

Compston A. The modern management of multiple sclerosis. Br J Hosp Med 36:200–201, 1986.

Compston A. Methylprednisolone and multiple sclerosis. Arch Neurol 45:669–670, 1988.

Compston DAS. Genetic susceptibility to multiple sclerosis. In Matthews WB, ed. McAlpine's Multiple Sclerosis. Edinburgh, Churchill Livingstone, 1991, pp. 301–319.

Connolly AM, Dodson EW, Prensky AL, Rust RS. Course and outcome of acute cerebellar ataxia. Ann Neurol 35:673–679, 1994.

Corsellis JAN, Janota I, Marshall AK. Immunization against whooping cough: a neuropathological review. Neuropathol Appl Neurobiol 9:261–270, 1983.

Croft PB. Para-infectious and post-vaccinial encephalomyelitis. Postgrad Med J 43:392–400, 1969.

Dalakas MC. Polymyositis, dermatomyositis, and inclusion-body myositis. N Engl J Med 325:1487–1498, 1991.

Dalakas MC, Engel WK. Chronic relapsing (dysimmune) polyneuropathy: pathogenesis and treatment. Ann Neurol 9(Suppl):134–145, 1981.

Dalakas MC, Icca I, Dambrosia JM, Soveidan SA, Stein DP, Otero C, Dinsmore ST, McCrosky S. A controlled trial of high-dose intravenous immune globulin infusions as treatment for dermatomyositis. N Engl J Med 329:1993–2000, 1993.

Dal Canto MC. Experimental models of virus-induced demyelination. In Cook SD, ed. Handbook of Multiple Sclerosis. New York, Marcel Dekker, 1990, pp. 63–100.

Dalmau J, Graus F, Rosenblum MK, Posner JB. Anti-Hu-associated paraneoplastic encephalomyelitis/sensory neuronopathy. A clinical study of 71 patients. Medicine 71:59–72, 1992.

Daoud AS, Zaki M, Shakir R, Al-Saleh Q. Effectiveness of sodium valproate in the treatment of Sydenham's chorea. Neurology 40:1140–1, 1990.

Dau PC, Bennington JL. Plasmapheresis in childhood dermatomyositis. J Pediatr 93:237–240, 1981.

Dehaene I, Martin JJ, Greens K, Cras P. Guillain-Barré syndrome with ophthalmoplegia: clinicopathologic study of the central and peripheral nervous systems, including the oculomotor nerves. Neurology 36:851–854, 1986.

De Jong RN. Multiple sclerosis. History, definition and general considerations. In Vinken PJ, Bruyn GW, eds. Handbook of Clinical Neurology, Vol. 9. Amsterdam, North Holland Publishing Co., 1970, pp. 45–62.

De la Monte SM, Gabuzda DH, Ho DD. Peripheral neuropathy in the acquired immunodeficiency syndrome. Ann Neurol 23:485–492, 1988.

DeToledo JC, Smith DB. Partially successful treatment of Rasmussen's encephalitis with zidovudine: symptomatic improvement followed by involvement of the contralateral hemisphere. Epilepsia 35:352–355, 1994.

Dévic ME. Myélite subaiguë compliquée de névrite optique. Bull Médical (Paris) 8:1033, 1894.

de Vries E. Postvaccinial perivenous encephalitis. Amsterdam, Elsevier, 1960.

Dowling PC, Bosch VV, Cooks SD, Chmel H. Serum immunoglobulins in Guillain-Barré syndrome. J Neurol Sci 57:435–440, 1982.

Drachman DB. Myasthenia gravis. N Engl J Med 330:1797–1810, 1994.

Duquette P, Murray TJ, Pleines J, Ebers GC, Sadovnik D, Weldon P, Warren S, Paty DW, Upton A, Hader W, Nelson R, Auty A, Neufeld B, Meltzer C. Multiple sclerosis in childhood: clinical profile in 125 patients. J Pediatr 111:359–363, 1987.

Dyck PJ, Lais AC, Ohta M, Bastron JA, Okazaki H, Groover RL. Chronic inflammatory polyradiculoneuropathy. Mayo Clin Proc 50:621–627, 1975.

Dyck PJ, Prineas J, Pollard J. Chronic inflammatory demyelinating polyradiculoneuropathy. In Dyck PJ, Thomas PK, eds. Peripheral Neuropathy. Philadelphia, WB Saunders 1993, pp. 1498–1517.

Eaton LM, Lambert EH. Electromyography and electrical stimulation of nerves in diseases of the motor unit: observations on a myasthenic syndrome associated with malignant tumors. JAMA 163:1117–1124, 1957.

Ebers GC. Genetics and multiple sclerosis: an overview. Ann Neurol 36:512–514, 1994a.

Ebers GC. Treatment of multiple sclerosis. Lancet 343:275–279, 1994b.

Engel AG. Myasthenia gravis and syndromes. In Rowland LP, DiMauro S, eds. Handbook of Clinical Neurology. New York, Elsevier, 1992, pp. 391–455.

Engel AG. Acquired autoimmune myasthenia gravis. In Engel AG, Franzin-Armstrong C, eds. Myology. New York, McGraw-Hill, 1994a, pp. 1769–1797.

Engel AG. Myasthenic syndromes. In Engel AG, Franzini-Armstrong C, eds. Myology. New York, McGraw-Hill, 1994b, pp. 1798–1835.

Engel AG, Hohlfield R, Banker BQ. Inflammatory myopathies. In Engel AG, Franzini-Armstrong C, eds. Myology. New York, McGraw Hill, 1994, pp. 1335–1383.

Epstein MA, Sladky JT. The role of plasmapheresis in childhood Guillain-Barré syndrome. Ann Neurol 28:65–69, 1990.

Feasby TE, Hahn AF, Gilbert JJ. Passive transfer studies in Guillain-Barré polyneuropathy. Neurology 32:1159–1167, 1982.

Fenichel GM. Clinical syndromes of myasthenia in infancy and childhood. Arch Neurol 35:97–103, 1978.

Fenichel GM. Neurological complications of immunization. Ann Neurol 12:119–128, 1982.

ffrench-Constant C. Pathogenesis of multiple sclerosis. Lancet 343:271–275, 1994.

Fink ME. Treatment of the critically ill patient with myasthenia gravis. In Ropper AH. Neurological and Neurosurgical Intensive Care. New York, Raven Press, 1993, pp. 351–362.

Fischer TJ, Rachelefsky GS, Klein RB, Paulus HE, Stiehm ER. Childhood dermatomyositis and polymyositis. Treatment with methotrexate and prednisone. Am J Dis Child 133:386–389, 1979.

Fisher M. An unusual variant of acute idiopathic polyneuritis (syndrome of ophthalmoplegia, ataxia, and areflexia). N Engl J Med 255:57–65, 1956.

Fleming JO, Wang FI, Trousdale MD, Hinton DR, Stohlman SA. Interaction of immune and central nervous systems: contribution of anti-viral Thy-1$^+$ cells to demyelination induced by coronavirus JHM. Reg Immunol 51:37–43, 1993.

Flory E, Pfleiderer M, Stuhler A, Wege H. Induction of protective immunity against coronavirus-induced encephalomyelitis: evidence for an important role of CD8$^+$ T cells in vivo. Eur J Immunol 23:1757–1761, 1993.

Fong JS, de Chadarevian JP, Kaplan BS. Hemolytic-uremic syndrome. Current concepts and management. Pediatr Clin North Am 29:835–856, 1982.

Francis GS, Antel JP, Duquette P. Inflammatory demyelinating diseases of the central nervous system. In Bradley WG, Daroff RB, Fenichel GM, Marsden DC, eds. Neurology in Clinical Practice. Boston, Butterworth-Heinemann, 1991, pp. 1133–1166.

French Cooperative Group on Plasma Exchange in Guillain-Barré Syndrome. Efficiency of plasma exchange in Guillain-Barré syndrome: role of replacement fluids. Ann Neurol 22:753–761, 1987.

Frerichs FT. Ueber Hirnsklerose. Arch Ges Med 10:334–347, 1849.

Geczy C, Raper R, Roberts LM, Meyer P, Bernard CCA. Macrophage procoagulant activity as a measure of cell-mediated immunity to P2 protein of peripheral nerves in the Guillain-Barré syndrome. J Neuroimmunol 9:179–191, 1985.

Gendelman HE, Wolinsky JS, Johnson RT, Pressman NJ, Pezeshkpour GH, Boisset GF. Measles encephalitis: lack of evidence of viral invasion of the central nervous system and quantitative study of the nature of demyelination. Ann Neurol 15:353–360, 1984.

Gibbels E, Giebisch U. Natural course of acute and chronic monophasic inflammatory demyelinating polyneuropathies (IDP). A retrospective analysis of 266 cases. Acta Scand 85:282–291, 1992.

Golden GS, Woody RC. The role of nuclear magnetic resonance imaging in the diagnosis of MS in childhood. Neurology 37:689–693, 1987.

Good WV, Muci-Mendoza R, Berg BO, Frederick DR, Hoyt CS. Optic neuritis in children with poor recovery of vision. Aust N Z J Ophthalmol 20:319–323, 1992.

Goodkin DE. Role of steroids and immunosuppression and effects of interferon beta-1b in multiple sclerosis. West J Med 161:292–298, 1994.

Greenfield JG. Acute disseminated encephalomyelitis and sequel to influenza. J Pathol Bacteriol 33:453–462, 1930.

Grob D, Brunner NB, Namba T. The natural history of myasthenia gravis and effect of therapeutic measures. Ann N Y Acad Sci 377:652–669, 1981.

Guillain G, Barré JA, Strohl A. Sur un syndrome de radiculonéurite avec hyperalbuminose du liquide céphalo-rachidien sans réaction cellulaire: Remarques sur les caractégres cliniques et graphiques des réflexes tendineux. Bull Soc Med Hop (Paris) 40:1462–1470, 1916.

Guillain-Barré Syndrome Study Group. Plasmapheresis and acute Guillain-Barré syndrome. Neurology 35:1096–1104, 1985.

Haas G, Schroth G, Krägeloh-Mann I, Buchwald-Saal M. Magnetic resonance imaging of the brain of children with multiple sclerosis. Dev Med Child Neurol 29:586–591, 1987.

Hanefeld FA, Christen HJ, Kruse B, Bauer HJ. Childhood and juvenile multiple sclerosis. In Bauer HJ, Hanefled FA, eds. Multiple Sclerosis: Its Impact from Childhood to Old Age. Philadelphia, WB Saunders, 1993, pp. 14–52.

Hanissian AS, Masi AT, Pitner G, Cape CC, Medsger TA. Polymyositis and dermatomyositis in children: an epidemiologic and clinical analysis. J Rheumatol 9:390–394, 1983.

Hantson P, DeConinck B, Horn JL, Ketelslegers JM, Mahieu P. Polyuria during Guillain-Barré syndrome. Acta Neurol Belg 92:77–82, 1992.

Hart YM, Cortez M, Andermann F, Hwang P, Fish DR, Dulac O, Silver K, Fejerman N, Cross H, Sherwin A, Caraballo R. Medical treatment of Rasmussen's syndrome (chronic encephalitis and epilepsy): effect of high-dose steroids or immunoglobulins in 19 patients. Neurology 44:1030–1036, 1994.

Hartung HP, Hughes RAC, Taylor WA, Heininger K, Reiners K, Toyka KV. T cell activation in Guillain-Barré syndrome and in MS: elevated serum levels of soluble IL-2 receptors. Neurology 40:215–218, 1990.

Hartung HP, Reiners K, Schmidt B, Stoll G, Toyka KV. Serum interleukin-2 concentrations in Guillain-Barré syndrome and chronic idiopathic demyelinating polyradiculoneuropathy: comparison with other neurological diseases of presumed immunopathogenesis. Ann Neurol 30:48–53, 1991.

Hartung HP, Schwenke C, Bitter-Suermann D. Guillain-Barré syndrome: activated complement components C3a and C5a in CSF. Neurology 37:1106–1109, 1987.

Haslam RHA. Multiple sclerosis: experience at the Hospital for Sick Children. Int Pediatr 2:163–167, 1987.

Hayward CPM, Sutton DMC, Carter WH, Campbell ED, Scott JG, Francombe WH, Shumak KH, Baker MA. Treatment outcomes in patients with adult thrombotic thrombocytopenic purpura–hemolytic uremic syndrome. Arch Intern Med 154:982–987, 1994.

Henderson FW. Tick paralysis. JAMA 175:615–617, 1961.

Hillert J. Human leukocyte antigen studies multiple sclerosis. Ann Neurol 36:515–517, 1994.

Hohlfield R, Engel AG. Coculture with autologous myotubes of cytotoxic T cells isolated from muscle in inflammatory myopathies. Ann Neurol 29:498–507, 1991.

Houba V, Allison AC, Adeniyi A, Houba J-E. Immunoglobulin classes and complement in biopsies of Nigerian children with nephrotic syndrome. Clin Exp Immunol 8:761–764, 1971.

Hudson CC, Rash JE, Tiedt TN, Albuquerque EX. Neostigmine-induced alterations at the mammalian neuromuscular junction. II. Ultrastructure. J Pharmacol Exp Ther 205:340–355, 1978.

Hughes RAC, Newsom-Davis JM, Perkin GD, Pierce JM. Controlled trial of prednisolone in acute polyneuropathy. Lancet 2:750–753, 1978.

Hurwitz ES, Holman RC, Nelson DB, Schoenberger LB. National surveillance for Guillain-Barré syndrome—January 1978–March 1979. Neurology 33:156–157, 1983.

Husain F, Ryan NJ, Hogan GR. Concurrence of limb-girdle muscular dystrophy and myasthenia gravis. Arch Neurol 46:101–102, 1989.

IFN-β Multiple Sclerosis Study Group. Interferon beta-1b is effective in relapsing-remitting multiple sclerosis. I. Clinical results of a multicenter, randomized, double-blind, placebo-controlled trial. Neurology 43:665–661, 1993.

Ilyas AA, Mithen FA, Chen ZW, Cook SD. Search for antibodies to neutral glycolipids in sera of patients with Guillain-Barré syndrome. J Neurol Sci 102:67–75, 1991.

Ilyas AA, Willison HJ, Quarles RH, Jungalwala FB, Cornblath DR, Trapp BD, Griffin DE, Griffin JW, McKhann GM. Serum antibodies to gangliosides in Guillain-Barré syndrome. Ann Neurol 23:440–447, 1988.

Iqbal A, Oger J-F, Arnson BGW. Cell-mediated immunity in idiopathic polyneuritis. Ann Neurol 9(Suppl.):65–69, 1981.

Irani DN, Cornblath DR, Chaudhry V, Borel C, Hanley DF. Relapse in Guillain-Barré syndrome after treatment with human immune globulin. Neurology 43:872–875, 1993.

Ishihara O, Yamaguchi Y, Matsuishi T, Yano E, Nakamura Y, Tateishi J, Yamashita F. Multiple ring enhancement in a case of acute reversible demyelinating disease in childhood suggestive of acute multiple sclerosis. Brain Dev 6:401–406, 1984.

Ito H, Sayama S, Irie S, Kanazawa N, Saito T, Kowa H, Haga S, Ikeda K. Antineuronal antibodies in acute cerebellar ataxia following Epstein-Barr virus infection. Neurology 44:1506–1507, 1994.

Jacobson S, Gupta A, Mattson D, Mingioli E, McFarlin DE. Immunological studies in tropical spastic paraparesis. Ann Neurol 27:149–156, 1990.

Johnson AB, Bornstein MB. Myelin-binding antibodies in vitro. Immunoperoxidase studies with experimental allergic encephalomyelitis, anti-galactocerebrosidase, and multiple sclerosis sera. Brain Res 159:173–82, 1978.

Johnson RT. The virology of demyelinating diseases. Ann Neurol 36:S54–S60, 1994.

Johnson RT, Griffin DE, Hirsch RL, Wolinsky JS, Roedenbeck S, Lindo de Soriano I, Vaisberg A. Measles encephalomyelitis—clinical and immunologic studies. N Engl J Med 310:137–141, 1984.

Jolly F. Über myasthenia gravis pseudoparalytica. Berl Klin Wochenschr 32:1–7, 1895.

Kagen LJ, Aram S. Creatine kinase activity inhibitor in sera from patients with muscle disease. Arthritis Rheum 30:213–217, 1987.

Karmali MA, Steele BT, Petric M, Lion C. Sporadic cases of haemolyticuraemic syndrome associated with faecal cytotoxin and cytotoxin-producing Escherichia coli in stools. Lancet 1:619–620, 1983.

Karnes WE. Diseases of the seventh cranial nerve. In Dyk JP, Thomas PK, eds. Pheripheral Neuropathy. Philadelphia, WB Saunders, 1993, pp. 818–836.

Kennedy CR, Webster ADB. Measles encephalitis. N Engl J Med 311:330–331, 1984.

Kennedy SS, Zacharski LR, Beck JR. Thrombotic thrombocytopenic purpura: analysis of 48 unselected cases. Semin Thromb Hemost 6:341–349, 1980.

Kerzin-Storrar L, Metcalfe RA, Dyer PA, Kowalska G, Ferguson I, Harris R. Genetic factors in myasthenia gravis: a family study. Neurology 38:38–42, 1988.

Kesselring J, Miller DH, Robb SA, Kendall BE, Moseley IF, Kingsley D, du Boulay EPGH, McDonald I. Acute disseminated encephalomyelitis MRI: findings and the distinction from multiple sclerosis. Brain 113:291–302, 1990.

Kiessling LS, Marcotte AC, Culpepper L. Antineuronal antibodies in movement disorders. Pediatrics 92:29–43, 1993.

Kleyweg RP, van der Meche FG. Treatment-related fluctuations in Guillain-Barré syndrome after high-dose immunoglobulins or plasma exchange. J Neurol Neurosurg Psychiatry 54:957–960, 1991.

Kleyweg RP, van der Meche FGA, Meulstee J. Treatment of Guillain-Barré syndrome with high-dose gammaglobulin. Neurology 38:1639–1641, 1988.

Klingman WO, Hodges RS. Acute ataxia of unknown origin in children. J Pediatr 24:536–543, 1944.

Koenig H, Rabinowitz SG, Day E, Miller V. Post-infectious encephalomyelitis after successful treatment of herpes simplex encephalitis with adenine arabinoside. N Engl J Med 300:1089–1093, 1979.

Kornips HM, Verhagen WI, Prick MJ. Acute disseminated encephalomyelitis probably related to a Mycoplasma pneumoniae infection. Clin Neurol Neurosurg 95:59–63, 1993.

Koski CL. Guillain-Barré syndrome. Neurol Clin 2:355–366, 1984.

Koski CL. Characterization of complement-fixing antibodies to peripheral nerve myelin in Guillain-Barré syndrome. Ann Neurol 27 (Suppl):544–547, 1990.

Koski CL, Chou DKH, Jungalwala FB. Anti–peripheral nerve myelin antibodies in Guillain-Barré syndrome bind a neutral glycolipid of peripheral myelin and cross-react with Forssman antigen. J Clin Invest 84:280–287, 1989.

Kriss A, Francis DA, Cuendet F, Halliday AM, Taylor DS, Wilson J, Keast-Butler J, Batchelor JR, McDonald IW. Recovery after optic neuritis in childhood. J Neurol Neurosurg Psychiatry 51:1253–1258, 1988.

Krolick KA, Thompson PA, Zoda TE, Yeh T-M: Influence of immunological fine-specificity on the induction of experimental myasthenia gravis. Ann N Y Acad Sci 681:179–197, 1993.

Kuban KC, Ephros MA, Freeman RL, Laffell LB, Bresnan MJ. Syndrome of opsoclonus-myoclonus caused by Coxsackie B3 infection. Ann Neurol 13:69–71, 1983.

Kuncl RW, Wittstein I, Adams RN, Wiggins WW, Avila O, Pestronk A, McIntosh K, Lucas D, DeSilva S, Lehar M, Drachman DB. A novel therapy for myasthenia gravis by reducing the endocytosis of acetylcholine receptors. Ann N Y Acad Sci 681:298–302, 1993.

Kuroda Y, Oda D, Neshiege R, Shibasaki H. Exacerbation of myasthenia gravis after removal of a thymoma having a membrane phenotype of suppressor T cells. Ann Neurol 15:400–402, 1984.

Kurtzke JF. Epidemiology of multiple sclerosis. In Vinken PJ, Bruyn GW, Klawans HL, Koetsier JC, eds. Handbook of Clinical Neurology, Vol. 47. Amsterdam, Elsevier Science 1985, pp. 259–287.

Kurtzke JF. Multiple sclerosis: what's in a name? Neurology 38:309–316, 1988.

Kyle RA, Dyck PJ. Neuropathy associated with the monoclonal gammopathies. In Dyck PJ, Thomas PK, eds. Peripheral Neuropathy. Philadelphia, WB Saunders, 1993, pp. 1275–1287.

Lamont PJ, Johnston HM, Berdoukas VA. Plasmapheresis in children with Guillain-Barré syndrome. Neurology 41:1928–1931, 1991.

Landry O. Note sur la paralysic ascendante aigue. Gaz Hebd Med Chir 6:472–474, 1859.

Lang B, Johnston I, Leys K, Elrington G, Marqueze G, Leveque C, Martin-Moutot N, Seagar M, Hoshino T, Takahashi M, Sugimori M, Cherksey BD, Llinas R, Newson-Davis J. Antibody specificities in Lambert-Eaton myasthenic syndrome. Ann N Y Acad Sci 681:382–393, 1993.

Laxer RM, Stein LD, Petty RE. Intravenous pulse methyl-prednisolone treatment of juvenile dermatomyositis. Arthritis Rheum 30:328–334, 1987.

Leititis JU. Preventive and therapeutic use of intravenous administration of immunoglobulins in intensive care patients in pediatrics. Infusionstherapie Transfusionsmed 20 (Suppl.) 1:29–34, 1993.

Lindstrom SJ, Shelton D, Fujii Y. Myasthenia gravis. Adv Immunol 42:233–284, 1988.

Linington C, Brostoff SW. Peripheral nerve antigens. In Dyck PJ, Thomas PK, eds. Peripheral Neuropathy. Philadelphia, WB Saunders, 1993, pp. 404–417.

Linington C, Izumo S, Suzuki M, Uyemura K, Meyermann R, Wekerle H. A permanent rat T–cell line that mediates experimental allergic neuritis in the Lewis rat in vivo. J Immunol 133:1946–1950, 1984.

Link H, Cruz M, Gessain A, Gout O, De Thé G, Kam-Hansen S. Chronic progressive myelopathy associated with HTLV-1: oligoclonal IgG and anti–HTLV-1 IgG antibodies in cerebrospinal fluid and serum. Neurology 39:1566–1572, 1989.

Link J, Soderstrom M, Olsson T, Hojeberg B, Ljungdahl A, Line H. Increased transforming growth factor-β, interleukin-4, and interferon-γ in multiple sclerosis. Ann Neurol 36:379–386, 1994.

Linton DM, Philcox D. Myasthenia gravis. Dis Mon 36:595–637, 1990.

Lisak RP, Barchi RL, eds. Myasthenia Gravis. Philadelphia, WB Saunders, 1982.

Lisak RP, Brown MJ. Acquired demyelinating polyneuropathies. Semin Neurol 7:40–48, 1987.

Lisak RP, Kuchmy D, Armati-Gulson PJ, Brown MJ, Sumner AJ. Serum-medicated Schwann cell cytotoxicity in the Guillain-Barré syndrome. Neurology 34:1240–1243, 1984.

Lotz BP, Engel AG, Nishisno H, Stevens JC, Litcy WJ. Inclusion body myositis. Brain 112:727–742, 1989.

Maeda Y, Kitamoto I, Kurokawa T, Ueda K, Hasuo K. Infantile multiple sclerosis with extensive white matter lesions. Pediatr Neurol 5:317–319, 1989.

Manners PJ, Murray KJ. Guillian-Barré syndrome presenting with severe musculoskeletal pain. Acta Paediatr 81:1049–1051, 1992.

Martino G, Grimaldi Luigi ME, Wollmann RL, Bongioanni P, Quintans J, Arnason BGW, Barry GW. The hu-SCID myasthenic mouse: a new tool for the investigation of seronegative myasthenia gravis. Ann N Y Acad Sci 681:303–305, 1993.

Martyn C. Epidemiology. In Matthews WB, ed. McAlpine's Multiple Sclerosis. Edinbugh, Churchill Livingstone, 1991, pp. 3–40.

Mastaglia FL, Ojeda VJ. Inflammatory myopathies. Ann Neurol 17:215–227; 317–323, 1985.

Masters CL, Dawkins RL, Zilko PJ, Simpson JA, Leedman RJ, Lindstrom J. Penicillamine-associated myasthenia gravis, antiacetylcholine receptor and antistriatal antibodies. Am J Med 63:689–694, 1977.

Matsumoto Y, Hanawa H, Tsuchida M, Abo T. In situ inactivation of infiltrating T cells in the central nervous system with autoimmune encephalomyelitis. The role of astrocytes. Immunology 79:381–390, 1993.

Matthews WB, ed. McAlpine's Multiple Sclerosis. Edinburgh, Churchill Livingstone, 1991.

McKhann GM. Guillain-Barré syndrome: clinical and therapeutic observations. Ann Neurol 27(Suppl.):13–16, 1990.

McLachlan RS, Girvin JP, Blume WT, Reichman H. Rasmussen's chronic encephalitis in adults. Arch Neurol 50:269–274, 1993.

McLeod JG. Paraneoplastic neuropathies. In Dyck PJ, Thomas PK, eds. Peripheral Neuropathy. Philadelphia, WB Saunders, 1993a, pp. 1583–1590.

McLeod JG. Peripheral neuropathy associated with lymphomas, leukemias, and polycythemia vera. In Dyck PJ, Thomas PK, eds. Peripheral Neuropathy. Philadelphia, WB Saunders 1993b, pp. 1591–1598.

Mehta PD. Diagnostic usefulness of cerebrospinal fluid in multiple sclerosis. Crit Rev Clin Lab Sci 28:233–251, 1991.

Melms A, Malcherek G, Schoepfer R, Sommer N, Kalbacher H, Lindstrom J. Acetylcholine receptor–specific T cells as present in the normal immune repertoire: a study with recombinant polypeptides of the human acetylocholine receptor-subunit. Ann N Y Acad Sci 681:310–312, 1993.

Mertin J. Rehabilitation in multiple sclerosis. Ann Neurol 36:5130–5133, 1994.

Mikol J, Engel AG. Inclusion body myositis. In Engel AG, Franzini-Armstrong C. eds. Myology, 2nd ed. New York, McGraw-Hill, 1994, pp. 1384–1398.

Miller A, Hafler DA, Weiner HL. Tolerance and suppressor mechanisms in experimental autoimmune encephalomyelitis: implica-tions for immunotherapy of human autoimmune diseases. FASEB J 5:2560–2566, 1991.

Miller DH, McDonald WI, Blomhardt LD, Duboulay GH, Halliday AM, Johnson G, Kendall BE, Kingsley DPE, MacManus DG, Moseley IF, Rudge P, Sandercock PAG. Magnetic resonance imaging in isolated noncompressive spinal cord syndrome. Ann Neurol 22:714–723, 1987.

Miller G, Heckmatt JZ, Dubowitz V. Drug treatment of juvenile dermatomyositis. Arch Dis Child 58:445–450, 1983.

Miller HG, Stanton JB, Gibbons JL. Acute disseminated encephalomyelitis and related syndromes. Br Med J 1:668–671, 1957.

Miller RG, Peterson GW, Daube JR. Prognostic value of electrodiagnosis in Guillain-Barré syndrome. Muscle Nerve 11:769–774, 1988.

Milligan NM, Newcombe R, Compston DAS. A double-blind controlled trial of high dose methylprednisolone in patients with multiple sclerosis. 1. Clinical effects. J Neurol Neurosurg Psychiatry 50:511–516, 1987.

Millner MM, Ebner F, Justich E, Urban C. Multiple sclerosis in childhood: contribution of serial MRI to earlier diagnosis. Dev Med Child Neurol 32:769–777, 1990.

Mimori T. Scleroderma-polymyositis overlap syndrome: clinical and serologic aspects. Int J Dermatol 26:419–425, 1987.

Mittag TW, Xu X, Moshoyiannis H, Kornfeld P, Genkins G. Analysis of false negative results in the immunoassay for anti-acetylcholine receptor antibodies in myasthenia gravis. Clin Immunol Immunopathol 31:191–201, 1984.

Mokhtarian F, Shi Y, Shirazian D, Morgante L, Miller A, Grob D. Defective production of anti-inflammatory cytokine, TGF-β by T cell lines of patients with active multiple sclerosis. J Immunol 152:6003, 6010, 1994.

Mokuno K, Kiyosawa K, Sugimura K, Yasuda T, Riku S, Murayama T. Prognostic value of cerebrospinal fluid neuron–specific enolase and S-100b. Acta Neurol Scand 89:27–30, 1994.

Morel E, Eymard B, Vernet D, Garabedian B, Pannier C, Dulac O, Bach JF. Neonatal myasthenia gravis: a new clinical and immunologic appraisal on 30 cases. Neurology 38:138–142, 1988.

Morimoto T, Nagao H, Sano N, Habara S, Takahashi M, Matsuda H, Beppu K, Shoda T. A case of multiple sclerosis with multi–ring-like and butterfly-like enhancement on computerized tomography. Brain Dev 7:43–45, 1985.

Moschcowitz E. An acute febrile pleiochromic anemia with hyaline thrombosis of the terminal arterioles and capillaries. Arch Intern Med 36:89–95, 1925.

Mumford C. Possible significance of familial aggregations of multiple sclerosis. Br J Hosp Med 46:55–57, 1991.

Mumford CS, Wood NW, Kellar-Wood H, Thorpe JW, Miller DH, Compston DAS. The British Isles survey of multiple sclerosis in twins. Neurology 44:11–15, 1994.

Munn R, Farrell K, Cimolai N. Acute encephalomyelitis: extending the neurological manifestations of acute rheumatic fever? Neuropediatrics 23:196–198, 1992.

Najim al-Din AS, Anderson M, Eeg-Ologsson O, Trontelj JV. Neuro-ophthalmic manifestations of the syndrome of ophthalmoplegia, ataxia and areflexia. Observations of 20 patients. Acta Neurol Scand 89:87–94, 1994.

Nasralla CA, Pay N, Goodpasture HC, Lin JJ, Svoboda WB. Postinfectious encephalopathy in a child following *Campylobacter jejuni* enteritis. AJNR 14:444–448, 1993.

Nastuk WL, Plescia OJ, Osserman KE. Changes in serum complement activity in patients with myasthenia gravis. Proc Soc Exp Biol Med 105:177–184, 1960.

Nesbit GM, Forbes GS, Scheithauer BW, Okazaki H, Rodriguez M. Multiple sclerosis: histopathologic and MR and/or CT correlation in 37 cases at biopsy and three cases at autopsy. Radiology 180:467–474, 1991.

Newton M, Cruickshank EK, Miller D, Dalgleish A, Rudge P, Clayden S, Moseley I. Antibody to human T-lymphotrophic virus type 1 in West Indian–born UK residents with spastic paraparesis. Lancet 1:415–416, 1987.

Niparko JK. The acute facial palsies. In Jackler RK, Brackmann DE, eds. Neurotology. St. Louis, CV Mosby, 1994, pp. 1291–1319.

Notarangelo LD, Duse M, Tiberti S, Guarneri B, Brunori A, Negrini A, Ugazio AG. Intravenous immunoglobulin in two children with Guillain-Barré syndrome. Eur J Pediatr 152:372–374, 1993.

Offenbacher H, Fazekas F, Schmidt R, Freidl W, Flooh E, Payer F, Lechner H. Assessment of MRI criteria for a diagnosis of MS. Neurology 43:905–909, 1993.

Oger JF, Arnason BGW. Immunogenetics of multiple sclerosis. In Panayi GS, David CS, eds. Immunogenetics. London, Butterworth, 1984, pp. 177–206.

Ohtake T, Komori T, Hirose K, Tanabe H. CNS involvement in Japanese patients with chronic inflammatory demyelinating polyradiculoneuropathy. Acta Neurol Scand 81:108–112, 1990.

Olsson T. Immunology of multiple sclerosis. Curr Opin Neurol Neurosurg 5:195–202, 1992.

Olsson T. Cerebrospinal fluid. Ann Neurol 36:S100–S102, 1994.

O'Neill JH, Murray NMF, Newsom-Davis J. The Lambert-Eaton myasthenic syndrome: a review of 50 cases. Brain 111:577–596, 1988.

Oosterhuis HJGH. The natural course of myasthenia gravis: a longterm follow-up study. J Neurol Neurosurg Psychiatry 52:1121–1127, 1989.

Ormerod IEC, Miller DH, McDonald WI, Du Boulay EPGH, Rudge P, Kendall BE, Moseley IF, Johnson Tofts PS, Halliday AM, Bronstein AM, Scaravilli F, Harding F, Barnes D, Zilkha KJ. The role of NMR imaging in the assessment of multiple sclerosis and isolated neurological lesions. A quantitative study. Brain 110:1579–1616, 1987.

Ormerod IEC, Roberts RC, Du Boulay EPGH, McDonald WI, Callanan MM, Halliday AM, Johnson G, Kendall BE, Logsdail SS, McManus DG, Moseley IF, Ron MA, Rudge P, and Zilkha KJ. NMR in multiple sclerosis and cerebral vascular disease. Lancet 2:1334–1335, 1984.

Parkin PJ, Hierons R, McDonald WI. Bilateral optic neuritis: a longterm follow-up. Brain 107:951, 1984.

Parry GJ. Guillain-Barré Syndrome. New York, Thieme Verlag, 1993.

Pasternak JF, Hageman J, Adams A, Philip AGS, Gardner TH. Exchange transfusion in neonatal myasthenia. J Pediatr 99:644–646, 1981.

Patrick J, Lindstrom J. Autoimmune response to acetylcholine receptor. Science 180:871–872, 1973.

Paty DW, Li DK. Interferon beta-1b is effective in relapsing-remitting multiple sclerosis. II. MRI analysis results of a multicenter, randomized, double-blind, placebo-controlled trial. Neurology 43:662–667, 1993.

Paty DW, Oger JJF, Kastrukoff LF, Hashimoto SA, Hodge JP, Eisen AA, Eisen KA, Purves SJ, Low MD, Brandejs V, Robertson WD, Li DKB. MRI in the diagnosis of MS: a prospective study with comparison of clinical evaluation, evoked potentials, oligoclonal banding, and CT. Neurology 38:180–185, 1988.

Phillips JT. Genetic susceptibility models in multiple sclerosis. In Rosenberg RN, ed. The Molecular and Genetic Basis of Neurological Disease 2. Boston, Butterworth-Heinemann, 1993, pp. 41–46.

Phillips MS, Stewart S, Anderson JR. Neuropathological findings in Miller-Fisher syndrome. J Neurol Neurosurg Psychiatry 47:492–495, 1984.

Posner JB. Paraneoplastic syndromes. Neurol Clin 9:919–953, 1991.

Power C, Poland SD, Blume WT, Girvin JP, Rice GP. Cytomegalovirus and Rasmussen's encephalitis. Lancet 336:1282–1284, 1990.

Prescott CAJ. Idiopathic facial nerve palsy (the effect of treatment with steroids). J Laryngol Otol 102:403–407, 1988.

Prineas JW. Pathology of the Guillain-Barré syndrome. Ann Neurol 9(Suppl.):6–19, 1981.

Prineas JW. Pathology of multiple sclerosis. In Cook SD, ed. Handbook of Multiple Sclerosis. New York, Marcel Dekker, 1990, pp. 187–218.

Prineas JW, McLeod JG. Chronic relapsing polyneuritis. J Neurol Sci 27:427–458, 1976.

Purvin V, Hrisolamos N, Dunn D. Varicella optic neuritis. Neurology 38:501–503, 1988.

Raine CS. Multiple sclerosis: immune system molecule expression in the central nervous system. J Neuropathol Exp Neurol 53:328–337, 1994a.

Raine CS. The immunology of the multiple sclerosis lesion. Ann Neurol 36:S61–S72, 1994b.

Ransohoff RM, Estes ML. Astrocyte expression of major histocompatibility complex gene products in multiple sclerosis brain tissue obtained by stereotactic biopsy. Arch Neurol 48:1244–1246, 1991.

Rantala H, Uhari M, Niemela M. Occurrence, clinical manifestations, and prognosis of Guillain-Barré syndrome. Arch Dis Child 66:706–709, 1991.

Rebaudengo N, Bianco C, Ferrero P, Troni W, Bergamasco B. Associated polyneuropathy and demyelinating disease. Case report. Ital J Neurol Sci 13:793–796, 1992.

Reder AT, Arnason BGW. Immunology of multiple sclerosis. In Koetsier JC, ed. Handbook of Clinical Neurology, Vol. 47, Demyelinating Diseases. Amsterdam, Elsevier, 1985, pp. 337–395.

Remuzzi G, Bertani T. Thrombotic thrombocytopenic purpura, hemolytic uremic syndrome, and acute cortical necrosis. In Schrier RD, ed. Diseases of the Kidney, 4th ed. Boston, Little, Brown, 1988, pp. 2301–2348.

Rhodes RH. Histopathologic features in the central nervous system of 400 acquired immunodeficiency syndrome cases: implications of rates of occurrence. Hum Pathol 24:1189–1198, 1993.

Richardson JB, Callen JP. Dermatomyositis and malignancy. Med Clin North Am 73:2111–2120, 1989.

Richman DP, Wollmann RL, Maselli RA, Gomez CM, Corey AL, Agius MA, Fairclough RH. Effector mechanisms of myasthenic antibodies. Ann N Y Acad Sci 681:264–273, 1993.

Ridolfi RL, Bell MD. Thrombotic thrombocytopenic purpura: report of 25 cases and review of literature. Medicine 60:413, 1981.

Riikonen R. The role of infection and vaccination in the genesis of optic neuritis and multiple sclerosis in children. Acta Neurol Scand 80:425–431, 1989.

Riikonen R, Donner M, Erkkila H. Optic neuritis in children and its relationship to multiple sclerosis: a clinical study of 21 children. Dev Med Child Neurol 30:349–359, 1988.

Rivers TM, Sprunt DH, Berry G. Observations on attempts to produce disseminated encephalomyelitis in monkeys. J Exp Med 58:39–53, 1933.

Roca-Gonzalez A, Palomeque Rico A, Pastor Duran X, Molinero EC. Guillain-Barré syndrome: a study of 13 children. An Esp Pediatr 39:513–516, 1993.

Roddy SM, Ashwal S, Peckham N. Infantile myositis: a case diagnosis in neonatal period. Pediatr Neurol 2:241–243, 1986.

Rogers SW, Andrews P, Gahring CC, Whisenand T, Cauley K, Crain B, Hughes TE, Heinemann SF, MacNamara JO. Antibodies to glutamate receptor GluR3 in Rasmussen's encephalitis. Science 265:648–651, 1994.

Ropper AH. The CNS in Guillain-Barré syndrome. Arch Neurol 40:397–398, 1983.

Ropper AH, Poskanzer DC. The prognosis of acute and subacute transverse myelopathy based on early signs and symptoms. Ann Neurol 4:51–59, 1978.

Rosen JL, Brown MJ, Hickey WF, Rostami AM. Early myelin lesions in experimental allergic neuritis. Muscle Nerve 13:629–636, 1990.

Rosenblum M, Scheck AC, Cronin K, Brew BJ, Khan A, Paul M, Price RW. Dissociation of AIDS-related vacuolar myelopathy and productive HIV-1 infection of the spinal cord. Neurology 39:892–896, 1989.

Rostami AM. Pathogenesis of immune-mediated neuropathies. Pediatr Res 33(Suppl.):90–94, 1993.

Rostami AM, Gregorian SK, Brown MJ, Pleasure DE. Induction of severe experimental autoimmune neuritis with a synthetic peptide corresponding to the 53-78 amino acid sequence of the myelin P_2 protein. J Neuroimmunol 30:145–151, 1990.

Rousseau JJ, Lust C, Zangerle PF. Acute transverse myelitis as presenting neurological feature of Lyme disease. Lancet 2:1222–1223, 1986.

Rudick RA. Helping patients live with multiple sclerosis—what primary care physicians can do. Postgrad Med 88:197–207, 1990.

Rudick RA, French CA, Breton D, Williams GW. Relative diagnostic value of cerebrospinal fluid kappa chains in MS: comparison with other immunoglobulin tests. Neurology 39:964–968, 1989.

Rudick RA, Schiffer RB, Schwetz KM. Multiple sclerosis: the problem of incorrect diagnosis. Arch Neurol 43:578–583, 1986.

Rudnicki S, Vriesendorp F, Koski CL, Mayer RF. Electrophysiologic studies in the Guillain-Barré syndrome: effects of plasma exchange and antibody rebound. Muscle Nerve 15:57–62, 1992.

Rust RS, Dodson WE, Trotter JS. Cerebrospinal fluid IgG in childhood: establishment of reference values. Ann Neurol 23:406–410, 1988.

Sadovnick AD, Ebers GC. Epidemiology of multiple sclerosis: a critical review. Can J Neurol Sci 20:17–29, 1993.

Sarchielli P, Trequattrini A, Usai F, Murasecco D, Gallai V. Role of viruses in the etiopathogenesis of multiple sclerosis. Acta Neurol (Napoli) 15:363–81, 1993.

Schapiro RT. Symptom Management in Multiple Sclerosis. New York, Oemos, 1987.

Schaumburg H, Berger AR. Human toxic neuropathy due to industrial agents. In Dyck PF, Thomas PK, eds. Peripheral Neuropathy. Philadelphia, WB Saunders 1993, pp. 1533–1548.

Schmidt B, Stoll G, Hartung HP, Heininger K, Schafer B, Toyka KV. Macrophages but not Schwann cells express Ia antigen in experimental autoimmune neuritis. Ann Neurol 28:70–77, 1990.

Schonberger LB, Hurwitz ES, Katona P, Holman RC, Bregman DJ, Gullain-Barré syndrome: its epidemiology and associations with influenza vaccination. Ann Neurol 9(Suppl.):31–38, 1981.

Scott TF McN. Postinfectious and vaccinial encephalitis. Med Clin North Am 51:701–717, 1967.

Scully RE. Case records of the Massachusetts General Hospital. Case 33—1994. N Engl J Med 331:661–667, 1994.

Searles RP, Davis LE, Hermanson S, Froelich CJ. Lymphocytotoxic antibodies in Guillain-Barré syndrome. Lancet 1:273, 1981.

Selmaj K, Brosnan CF, Raine CS. Colocalization of TCRγδ lymphocytes and hsp-65+ oligodendrocytes in multiple sclerosis. Proc Natl Acad Sci U S A 88:6452–6456, 1991.

Seybold ME. Myasthenia gravis: a clinical and basic science review. JAMA 250:2516–2521, 1983.

Seybold ME. The office Tensilon test for ocular myasthenia gravis. Arch Neurol 43:842–844, 1986.

Seybold ME, Howard FM Jr, Duane DD, Payne WS, Harrison EG Jr. Thymectomy in juvenile myasthenia gravis. Arch Neurol 25:385–392, 1971.

Seybold ME, Lindstrom JM. Immunopathology of acetylcholine receptors in myasthenia gravis. Semin Immunopathol 5:389–412, 1982.

Shah A, Lisak RP. Immunopharmacologic therapy in myasthenia gravis. Clin Neuropharmacology 16:97–103, 1993.

Shahani BT, Day TJ, Cros D, Khalil N, Kneebone CS. RR interval variation and the sympathetic skin response in the assessment of autonomic function in peripheral neuropathy. Arch Neurol 47:659–664, 1990.

Shahar E, Brand N. High-dose immunoglobulins in children with Guillain-Barré syndrome. Harefuah 121:225–228, 1991.

Shahar E, Murphy EG, Roifman CM. Benefit of intravenously administered immune serum globulin in patients with Guillain-Barré syndrome. J Pediatr 116:141–144, 1990.

Shaw CM, Alvord EC. Multiple sclerosis beginning in infancy. J Child Neurol 2:252–256, 1987.

Shevell M, Rosenblatt B, Silver K, Carpenter S, Karpati G. Congenital inflammatory myopathy. Neurology 40:1111–1114, 1990.

Silberberg DH. Corticosteroids and optic neuritis. N Engl J Med 329:1808–1810, 1993.

Silver RM, Maricq HR. Childhood dermatomyositis: serial microvascular studies. Pediatrics 83:278–283, 1989.

Simmons RD, Cattle BA. Sialyl ligands facilitate lymphocyte accumulation during inflammation of the central nervous system. J Neuroimmunol 41:123–130, 1992.

Simpson JA. Myasthenia gravis: a new hypothesis. Scott Med J 5:419–436, 1960.

Sipe JC, Romine JS, Koziol JA, McMillan R, Zyroff J, Beutler E. Cladribine in treatment of chronic progressive multiple sclerosis. Lancet 344:9–13, 1994.

Sladky JT. Neuropathy in childhood. Semin Neurol 7:65–75, 1987.

Smith BE, Windebank AJ, Dyck PJ. Nonmalignant inflammatory sensory polyganglionopathy. In Dyck PJ, Thomas PK, eds. Peripheral Neuropathy. Philadelphia, WB Saunders, 1993, pp. 1525–1531.

Smith CIE, Aarli JA, Biberfeld P, Bolme P, Christensson B, Gahrton G, Hammarstrom L, Lefvert AK, Longqvist B, Matell G, Pirskanen R, Ringden OI, Svanborg E. Myasthenia gravis after bone-marrow transplantation: evidence for a donor origin. N Engl J Med 309:1565–1569, 1983.

Snead OC, Kohaut EC, Oh SJ, Bradley RJ. Plasmapheresis for myasthenia gravis in a young child. J Pediatr 110:740–742, 1987.

Sriram S, Steinman L. Postinfectious and postvaccinial encephalomyelitis. Neurol Clin 2:341–353, 1984.

Strauss AJ, Seegal BC, Hsu KC, Burkholder PM, Nastuk WL, Osserman KE. Immunofluorescence demonstration of a muscle-binding complement-fixing serum globulin fraction in myasthenia gravis. Proc Soc Exp Biol Med 105:184–191, 1960.

Stricker RB, Miller RG, Kiprov DD. Role of plasmapheresis in acute disseminated (postinfectious) encephalomyelitis. J Clin Apheresis 7:173–179, 1992.

Sugita K, Suzuki N, Shimizu N, Takanashi J, Ishii M, Niimi N. Involvement of cytokines in N-methyl-n'-nitro-N-nitrosoguanidine–induced plasminogen activator activity in acute disseminated encephalomyelitis and multiple sclerosis lymphocytes. Eur Neurol 33:358–362, 1993.

Swedo SE, Leonard HL, Schapiro MB, Casey BJ, Mannheim GB, Lenane MC, Rettew DC. Sydenham's chorea: physical and psychological symptoms of St. Vitus dance. Pediatrics 91:706–713, 1993.

Swift TR. Disorders of neuromuscular transmission other than myasthenia gravis. Muscle Nerve 4:334–353, 1981.

Tachi N, Watanabe T, Wakai S, Sato T, Chiba S. Acute disseminated encephalomyelitis following HTLV-I associated myelopathy (letter). J Neurol Sci 110:234–235, 1992.

Thomas PK, Landon DN, King RHM. Guillain-Barré syndrome. In Adams HJ, Duchen LW, eds. Greenfield's Neuropathology. New York, Oxford University Press, 1992, pp. 1200–1202.

Thomas PK, LaScelles RG, Hallpike JF. Recurrent and chronic relapsing Guillain-Barré polyneuritis. Brain 92:589–606, 1969.

Thomas PK, Walker RWH, Rudge P, Morgan-Hughes JA, King RH, Jacobs JM, Mills KR, Ormerod IE, Murray NM, McDonald WI. Chronic demyelinating peripheral neuropathy associated with multifocal central nervous system demyelination. Brain 110:53–76, 1987.

Thompson CE. Infantile myositis. Dev Med Child Neurol 24:307–313, 1982.

Tippett DS, Fishman PS, Panitch HS. Relapsing transverse myelitis. Neurology 41:703–706, 1991.

Tiwari JL, Terasaki PI. HLA and Disease Associations. New York, Springer-Verlag, 1985, pp. 152–184.

Topi GC, D'Alessandro L, Catricala C, Zardi O. Dermatomyositis-like syndrome due to *Toxoplasma*. Br J Derm 101:589–591, 1979.

Turnbull HM, McIntosh J. Encephalomyelitis following vaccination. Br J Exp Pathol 7:181–222, 1926.

Tyler KL, Gross RA, Cascino GD. Unusual viral causes of transverse myelitis: hepatitis A virus and cytomegalovirus. Neurology 36:855–858, 1986.

Tymms KE, Webb J. Dermatopolymyositis and other connective tissue diseases: a review of 105 cases. J Rheumatol 12:1140–1148, 1985.

Uncini A, Parano E, Lange DJ, De Vivo DC, Lovelace RE. Chronic progressive polyneuropathy in childhood: clinical and electrophysiological features. Childs Nerv Sys 7:191–196, 1991.

Unverricht H. Polymyositis acuta progressiva. Z Klin Med 12:533–541, 1887.

Utz U, McFarland HF. The role of T cells in multiple sclerosis: implications for therapies targeting the T cell receptor. J Neuropathol Exp Neurol 53:351–358, 1994.

Valk J, van der Knapp MS. Magnetic resonance of myelin, myelination, and myelin disorders. Heidelberg, Springer-Verlag, 1989, pp. 206–214.

Van Antwerpen CL, Gospe SM, Wade N. Myeloradiculopathy associated with wasp sting. Pediatr Neurol 4:379–380, 1988.

van der Mech FGA, Schmitz PIM, the Dutch Guillain-Barré Study Group. A randomized trial comparing intravenous immune globulin and plasma exchange in Guillain-Barré syndrome. N Engl J Med 326:1123–1129, 1992.

Vandevyver C, Buyse I, Philippaerts L, Ghabanbasni Z, Medaer R, Carton H, Cassiman JJ, Raus J. HLA and T-cell receptor polymorphisms in Belgian multiple sclerosis patients: no evidence for disease association with the T-cell receptor. J Neuroimmunol 52:25–32, 1994.

Van Doorn PA, Brand A, Vermeulen M. Clinical significance of antibodies against peripheral nerve tissue in inflammatory polyneuropathy. Neurology 37:1798–1802, 1987.

Van Doorn PA, Rossi F, Brand A, Van Lint M, Vermeulen M, Kazatchkine MD. In the mechanism of high-dose intravenous immunoglobulin treatment of patients with chronic inflammatory demyelinating polyneuropathy. J Neuroimmunol 29:57–64, 1990.

Vining EP, Freeman JM, Brandt J, Carson BS, Vematsu S. Progressive unilateral encephalopathy of childhood (Rasmussen's syndrome): a reappraisal. Epilepsia 34:639–650, 1993.

Visscher BR, Myers LW, Ellison GW, Malmgren RM, Detels R, Lucia

MV, Madden DL, Sever JL, Park MS, Coulson AH. HLA types and immunity in multiple sclerosis. Neurology 29:1561–1565, 1979.

Vriesendorp FJ, Mayer RF, Koski CL. Kinetics of anti-peripheral nerve myelin antibody in patients with Guillain-Barré syndrome treated and not treated with plasmapheresis. Arch Neurol 48:858–861, 1991.

Wagner E. Fall einer seltnen Muskelkrankheit. Arch Heilk 4:282–283, 1863.

Waksman BH, Adams RD. Allergic neuritis: an experimental disease of rabbits induced by the injection of peripheral nervous tissue and adjuvants. J Exp Med 102:213–235, 1955.

Wall RT, Harker LA. The endothelium and thrombosis. Ann Rev Med 31:361, 1980.

Wege H, Winter J, Korner H, Flory E, Zimprich F, Lassmann H. Coronavirus-induced demyelinating encephalomyelitis in rats: immunopathological aspects of viral persistency. Adv Exp Med Biol 276:637–645, 1990.

Weiss S, Carter S. Course and prognosis of acute cerebellar ataxia in childhood. Neurology 9:711–712, 1959.

Wekerle H. The thymus in myasthenia gravis. Ann N Y Acad Sci 681:47–55, 1993.

Weklerle H, Kojima K, Lannes-Vieira J, Lassmann H, Linington C. Animal models. Ann Neurol 36(Suppl):547–553, 1994.

Wekerle H, Schwab M, Linington C, Meyermann R. Antigen presentation in the peripheral nervous system: Schwann cells present endogenous myelin autoantigens to lymphocytes. Eur J Immunol 16:1551–1557, 1986.

Whitaker JN, Benveniste EN, Zhou S. Cerebrospinal fluid. In Cook SD, ed. Handbook of Multiple Sclerosis. New York, Marcel Dekker, 1990, pp. 251–270.

Whitham RH, Brey RL. Neuromyelitis optica: two new cases and review of the literature. J Clin Neurol Ophthalmol 5:263–269, 1985.

Winer JB, Hughes RAC, Osmond C. A prospective study of acute idiopathic neuropathy. I. Clinical features and their prognostic value. J Neurol Neurosurg Psychiatry 51:605–612, 1988.

Wray D, Porter V. Calcium channel types at the neuromuscular junction. Ann N Y Acad Sci 681:356–367, 1993.

Yoshino H, Inuzuka T, Miyatake T. IgG antibody against GM1, GD1b and asialo-GM1 in chronic polyneuropathy following *Mycoplasma pneumoniae* infection. Eur Neurol 32:28–31, 1992.

Zweiman B, Rostami AM, Lisak RP. Immune responses to P2 protein in the human inflammatory demyelinative neuropathies. Neurology 33:234–237, 1983.

Chapter 29

Active and Passive Immunization in the Prevention of Infectious Diseases

Mark W. Kline and William T. Shearer

Prevention of disease by immunization predates knowledge of infection or immunology by many centuries. Inoculation of smallpox material intranasally in an effort to prevent smallpox was first noted in 590 B.C. in the Sung Dynasty (Dixon, 1962). From such empiric beginnings are derived current immunization practices, built on a long history of painstaking observation, intuition, and scientific experiment. This chapter summarizes present practices, underlying theories, and future directions of immunization.

Current immunization practice is based on immunologic aspects of the host response, the state of microbiologic technology, the restraints of practicality and economics, and ethical and medicolegal considerations. Immunizations can change the world. The elimination of smallpox is the most recent chapter of a 2500-year history of vaccination, which has included all of the above factors (Fenner, 1982).

Immunization programs in the United States have been highly successful for two reasons: (1) the nationwide Childhood Immunization Initiative, begun in 1977, effectively mobilized the public and private sectors; and (2) subsequent state laws required routine immunizations for admission to school (Centers for Disease Control [CDC], 1982b). All states and the District of Columbia now have such laws, and more than 95% of children entering school have routinely received the recommended immunizations. Unfortunately, immunization levels among preschool-aged children are considerably lower (CDC, 1992a). The recent resurgence of measles in the United States is attributable largely to failure to vaccinate children at the recommended age of 12 to 15 months (National Vaccine Advisory Committee, 1991).

The decrease in the natural occurrence of vaccine-preventable diseases has increased the visibility of the rare adverse reactions to vaccination. For the benefit of society, state laws require childhood immunization. Those who suffer serious sequelae from immunization may seek compensation through a judicial system that does not allow optimal recourse for the injured or for the private manufacturers and suppliers of immunizing agents. The result has been ever-increasing costs of vaccination and a reluctance on the part of manufacturers to continue producing vaccines.

A National Childhood Vaccine Injury Compensation Act was passed by the United States Congress in 1986. It sought to improve record-keeping about vaccine administration and complications, to provide parents or guardians with standardized statements on the benefits and risks of vaccines, and to establish a federal Vaccine Injury Compensation Program (Peter, 1992). An additional goal was to stabilize vaccine supply and cost (Smith, 1988). Since passage of the act, the number of vaccine injury cases in the civil courts has declined and vaccine prices have stabilized.

Other standard pediatric immunization practices have recently been summarized (CDC, 1993a).

ACTIVE IMMUNIZATION

Active immunization is based on the premise that immunologic mechanisms appropriate to the body's defense against certain microorganisms can be evoked without significant infectious risk to the host. The degree to which this is achieved depends in part on knowledge of natural immunity for the particular disease involved. For example, it is known that circulating antibody directed against pneumococcus prevents serious pneumococcal disease by virtue of its capacity to render the organisms susceptible to phagocytosis (Wood, 1941). This natural phenomenon is possible because the pneumococcal polysaccharide contained within the cell wall can be extracted and used to evoke protective antibody without exposure to the actual infection (Austrian et al., 1976). Ideally, such precise immunologic information should be available for each immunization. However, for many infections, there is limited or no knowledge of specific immune mechanisms, and the procedures employed are based entirely on empiric observations.

Exposure to an infectious agent initiates a variety of cellular and molecular responses. Collectively, these responses are termed the *active immune response*, which is usually characterized by (1) specificity, (2) variety, (3) a molecular sequence, and (4) memory. In some cases, such as the mechanisms of pertussis immunity, these elements are not well understood. In other cases, such as the IgG toxin-neutralizing antibody response in tetanus, the mechanism has been well characterized.

The specificity of an active immune response is related to unique antigenic structures of the infectious agent or one of its chemical products. After immunization, a variety of antibodies are synthesized and directed against a limited number of antigens present on the immunizing substance. On exposure to an antigen, B lymphocytes multiply and produce immunoglobulin molecules, which can react with the antigen or a portion of the antigen; this is the *primary response*. T lymphocytes are also stimulated and influence the capacity of B lymphocytes to respond to the antigen. These cells do not elaborate antibody but do contain an antigen recognition mechanism. Sensitized T cells are capable of effective immunologic action directly by means of the cell-mediated immune response. They may also influence other cells (macrophages or granulocytes) and release lymphokines, such as interleukin-2 and interferon. The role of the cell-mediated immune response to some immunizing agents has been increasingly recognized.

After initial antigen challenge, both B and T cells are capable of memory, as manifested by the continued presence of active immunity beyond the original exposure and the development of a secondary (anamnestic) response. The latter is characterized by rapid response to re-exposure of greater magnitude than that observed in the primary response, often to a lesser quantity of antigen.

To be useful, a vaccine must stimulate B or T cells or both to a degree sufficient to produce effective resistance against a virulent agent. Attenuated measles virus fulfills this criterion and offers protection against natural measles. By contrast, the parainfluenza virus vaccines fail to evoke active immunity despite demonstration of some immunologic responses (Fulginiti et al., 1969).

In addition, memory T and B cells must be stimulated to ensure long-lasting, even lifetime, immunity. Lifelong immunity can occur after certain immunizations, such as with attenuated measles virus vaccine, whereas other immunizations, such as pertussis, have relatively short-lived immunity, probably as a result of inadequate memory stimulation. Thus, the goal in most immunizations is to mimic natural immunity by evoking an active immune response similar to that following natural infection.

PASSIVE IMMUNIZATION

Passive immunity is achieved by antibody administration. Passive immunity occurs in infancy by transplacental transfer of maternal IgG antibody, which affords temporary protection against some infectious diseases. Once the maternal IgG disappears, the infant is susceptible unless he or she has already developed active immunity.

Medical practice has long sought to mimic this model of passive immunity. Initially, animal antisera were raised against specific infectious agents and infused into susceptible individuals on exposure to the infectious agent or after disease was established. Only limited success was achieved with this method, especially if done late in incubation or after the appearance of the disease. A further limitation was the hypersensitivity to animal antigens evoked in many humans.

Human Gamma Globulin

During World War II, human immune serum globulin (ISG) from pooled adult plasma became available and was used in the prevention of poliomyelitis, measles, and hepatitis. Later, gamma globulin derived from plasma lots selected for their high titer of a specific antibody or from subjects deliberately immunized or convalescing from disease was prepared. These special ISGs are useful in the prevention of tetanus, hepatitis B, varicella-zoster virus infection (chickenpox), and several other disorders.

Human gamma globulin preparations intended for intramuscular administration are concentrated solutions of electrophoretically similar globulins, usually prepared by cold alcohol fractionation (Cohn method). They contain high concentrations of IgG molecules with minimal amounts of IgA and IgM. A spectrum of antibodies generally is represented based on the immunologic experience of the adults from whom the pool of plasma was obtained. These preparations contain aggregates of IgG that can cause anaphylactoid reactions if given intravenously.

Eight intravenous immunoglobulin (IVIG) products are licensed for use in the United States (see Table 9–23 in Chapter 9). Three general strategies—enzymatic degradation, chemical modification, and physical purification—have been used to eliminate aggregated IgG from these preparations. Each IVIG lot is derived from thousands of adult donors. In addition, special hyperimmune IVIGs are available or are in development, most notably for immunocompromised patients at risk for cytomegalovirus, varicella-zoster, respiratory syncytial virus, or *Pseudomonas* infection. The properties and risks of IVIG recently have been reviewed (Pacheco, 1992; Sandberg, 1992).

Whenever gamma globulin is administered simultaneously with an immunizing antigen, active immunity may be suppressed. The specific antibody in the gamma globulin combines with the antigen to reduce the net amount of antigen given. In addition, central inhibition of antibody synthesis by the passive antibody may occur, necessitating additional doses of antigen.

Animal Sera

Another way to transfer passive immunity is by administering sera prepared from animal sources, usually horses. These preparations differ not only in their antibody content but also in their specific antigenic composition.

The chief disadvantage of antiserum is the risk of serum reactions, both immediate and delayed. This possibility must be considered each time horse serum is used. Appropriate medications to treat anaphylactic shock should be readily available, including epinephrine drawn up in a syringe for instant administration. The possibility of serum sickness that may develop later should also be kept in mind.

Before administration of animal serum, the following steps are completed (Table 29–1):

1. A careful history of previous use of horse serum products and of subsequent reactions is sought.

2. A history of other allergies or allergic symptoms from contact with horses or horse dander is sought. Although this history is rarely elicited, it can serve as a warning to proceed with extreme caution.

3. Skin or conjunctival tests are performed.

Because a severe reaction occasionally ensues from the testing procedure, one should be prepared to intervene. Most experts believe that conjunctival testing cannot be used because the irritant effect of the material placed in the conjunctival sac often produces a false-positive reaction. For this reason, skin tests are preferred, using 0.1 ml of a 1:100 saline dilution of the serum injected intradermally. In allergic individuals, the dose is reduced to 0.05 ml of a 1:1000 dilution. The appearance of a wheal in 10 to 30 minutes indicates hypersensitivity.

If there is no history of allergy and no reaction to the serum, the appropriate intramuscular dose of the horse serum can be given. For intravenous administration, 0.5 ml of serum in 10 ml of fluid is given initially; if no reaction occurs within 30 minutes, the remainder of the dose is given in a 1:20 dilution. If the patient has a history of allergy or a positive reaction to the skin test but the use of serum is imperative, desensitiza-

Table 29–1. Steps Necessary Before Horse Serum Administration

History—specific inquiries
1. Allergy in general
2. Receipt of horse serum in past
3. Allergic reaction to horse serum or to other horse antigen (e.g., dander)

Perform skin tests*
1. Scratch test first; intradermal test if scratch test is negative
2. Administer
   a. 0.1 ml of 1:100 saline dilution of serum to be used. Reduce dose to 0.05 ml of 1:1000 in allergic individuals.
   b. Appearance of wheal in 10 to 30 minutes indicates hypersensitivity.

Procedure
1. History and skin tests negative
   a. Give appropriate intramuscular dose *or*
   b. Give 0.5 ml serum intravenously in 10 ml saline; with no reaction in 30 minutes, give remainder of dose as 1:20 dilution.
2. History or skin test positive
   a. Give 1.0 ml of 1:10 dilution subcutaneously; with no reaction proceed as in 3a.
3. History and skin test positive:†
   a. Use only if imperative.
   b. Give 0.05 ml of 1:20 dilution subcutaneously.
   c. With no reaction, increase dose every 15 minutes as follows:
      (1) 0.1 ml of 1:10 dilution
      (2) 0.3 ml of 1:10 dilution
      (3) 0.1 ml of undiluted
      (4) 0.2 ml of undiluted
      (5) 0.5 ml of undiluted
      (6) Remainder of dose

*Conjunctival tests are unreliable because of irritant effect.
†If a positive reaction occurs at any stage, reduce dose by half.

tion must be accomplished. Initially, 0.05 ml of a 1:20 dilution is given subcutaneously. If there is no reaction, the dose is increased every 15 minutes as follows: 0.1 ml of a 1:10 dilution, 0.3 ml of a 1:10 dilution, 0.1 ml undiluted, 0.2 ml undiluted, 0.5 ml undiluted; finally, the remainder of the dose is administered. If an adverse reaction develops at any step, the dose should be reduced by one half. If this fails to stop reactivity, the preparation cannot be used.

VACCINE DEVELOPMENT AND USE

The Ideal Vaccine

The ideal immunizing agent has the following characteristics:

1. The antigen is pure and defined.
2. The specific response protects the individual against the disease.
3. The antigen is given in a simple, painless, one-step procedure.
4. The protection afforded is lifelong without the need for boosters.
5. There are no adverse immediate or long-range side effects.
6. The vaccine is acceptable to recipients and parents or guardians.
7. The vaccine is inexpensive.

The degree to which a vaccine fulfills these characteristics is the major issue confronting the practitioner in selection or use of a vaccine. As increasing numbers of vaccines, antisera, and gamma globulin preparations become available, the physician must assess the value of each preparation before using it for the individual patient.

The product brochure carries a complete description of the product and its use. The recommendations of the Committee on Infectious Diseases of the American Academy of Pediatrics *(The Red Book)* and the Advisory Committee on Immunization Practices of the CDC *(Morbidity and Mortality Weekly Report)* should be consulted. Whenever a new vaccine is introduced, these sources offer an authoritative description of the product, the positive and negative attributes, and recommendations for its use in children and adults.

Vaccine Composition

There is no typical vaccine, but the following categories of components are listed:

1. *The principal antigen.* This may be whole bacteria, bacterial products (e.g., toxins or hemolysins), whole viruses, or substructures of viruses.
2. *Host-derived antigens.* These are proteins or other constituents of host tissue that are carried along with or intimately associated with viral particles.
3. *Altered antigens.* These are denatured proteins and other substances that result from the viral infection of the cells on which the virus is grown.
4. *Preservatives and stabilizers.* These are chemical compounds added to prevent bacterial growth or to stabilize the antigen (e.g., thimerosal [Merthiolate] and glycerine).
5. *Antibiotics.* Trace amounts may be present in viral vaccines from the media used in their growth. The same vaccine from different manufacturers may contain different antibiotics.
6. *Menstruum.* The fluid phase of the vaccine suspension or solution may consist of saline or a complex tissue culture medium.
7. *Unwanted or unknown constituents.* Despite elaborate precautions in preparing vaccines, viruses or other unwanted antigens may be present.
8. *Adjuvant.* This is a substance, such as alum, aluminum phosphate, or aluminum hydroxide, that enhances the antigenicity of the principal antigen. Adjuvants often retain the antigen at the depot site and release it slowly.

This list points out the complexities of some vaccines and the difficulty in attributing an unusual reaction to a specific component.

Specific Antigens

Antigens vary in their ability to stimulate the desired immunologic response. For a given antigen, the response is variable, with some individuals responding poorly and a few not at all. Some children who receive a vaccine under optimal circumstances simply do not respond and contract the disease on exposure. This failing should not condemn the vaccine for other children, because it can protect most.

In general, adjuvant (depot type) vaccines are preferred over fluid vaccines because they provide more prolonged immunity, greater antigenic stimulation, and fewer systemic effects. For example, DTP vaccine stimulates prolonged antitoxin production against diphtheria and tetanus and enhances the antibody response to pertussis, particularly in early infancy (Kendrick, 1943). Fluid or aqueous preparations may achieve earlier immunity and are less likely to produce local reactions at the injection site but generally offer no clinically significant advantages.

Dose of Vaccine

Most vaccine schedules are determined by trial and error until an appropriate dose is selected. What is sought is a dose large enough to produce the desired immune response in most or all recipients yet small enough to be harmless, economical, and easy to administer. Although it is tempting to reduce the usual dose for reasons of economy, convenience, or comfort, this practice may result in inadequate immunization. Increasing the dose may be accompanied by toxic effects or unwanted complications.

Route of Immunization

The route of vaccine administration is a critical determinant of both effectiveness and safety and may determine the type and duration of immunologic response. For example, an intramuscular injection of inactivated poliomyelitis virus vaccine induces serum antibody production and systemic immunity. However, it fails to evoke local antibody in the form of secretory IgA and thus does not prevent subsequent gastrointestinal infection.

Live attenuated oral polio vaccine induces both local gastrointestinal and systemic antibody production; therefore, immunization by the oral route may be preferred. Oral or intramuscular administration of a vaccine meant to be given subcutaneously may result in ineffective immunization. Occasionally, the side effects of a subcutaneous vaccine may be diminished by intracutaneous inoculation, but this should be done only if the efficacy of this route has been established. In general, strict adherence to the recommended dose and route is advisable.

Timing of Immunization

In a disease prevalent in infants (e.g., pertussis), immunization must be undertaken early enough to be effective and preventive, yet late enough so that an adequate immune response occurs. Thus, epidemiologic factors of the disease help to determine the timing of vaccine administration.

Some circumstances warrant administration of vaccine coincident with or shortly after exposure. Rabies immunization at the time of a bite is the prime example, but live measles virus vaccination in a just-exposed susceptible person also can be done (Fulginiti, 1964). The incubation period of rabies is long (weeks to months), providing ample time to actively immunize an exposed individual. The incubation period of natural measles is about 11 days and that of the attenuated virus infection is 7 days (Katz et al., 1960), so the vaccine must be given within a few days of exposure.

With some vaccines, booster doses are required if long-term immunity is to be maintained. The precise timing of these additional doses is determined by both theory and experience. Some vaccines require multiple, frequent doses over the life span of an individual (e.g., cholera). Others can be given infrequently at long intervals (e.g., yellow fever). In general, inactivated vaccines require repetitive administration, whereas live vaccines do not. In general, intervals between multiple doses of an antigen (e.g., oral polio vaccine) that are longer than those recommended do not lead to a reduction in overall immunity achieved at the completion of the immunization series. Usually, it is not necessary to restart an interrupted series or to add doses in addition to those recommended. In contrast, the provision of multiple vaccine doses of an antigen at less than the recommended interval may lessen the immune response; doses given at less than the recommended interval should not be counted as part of the primary series. Accurate record keeping on the part of physicians is imperative, and an up-to-date immunization record should be kept by parents (American Academy of Pediatrics, 1994).

Combination of Antigens

Vaccines are often combined to facilitate immunization. Early studies suggested the following:

1. There were limits to the responsiveness of an individual to multiple antigens.
2. Specific vaccine combinations, particularly viral vaccines, were mutually inhibitory, thus diminishing their efficacy.
3. Additive adverse effects were likely to occur.

However, experience with certain vaccine combinations has failed to substantiate these theoretical risks. Thus, DTP and oral poliovirus vaccines, a combination of six antigens, are given together with no decrease in immune response or increase in adverse consequences. Measles, mumps, and rubella virus vaccines can be administered together, without adverse consequences or diminished effect. It is essential that only proven combinations be employed; there is no guarantee of efficacy or safety if the physician mixes other combinations from components designed for individual use.

Rapid sequential administration of certain vaccines has the potential for viral interference. For example, live measles vaccine given 1 week before smallpox vaccine inhibited the latter to some extent (Merigan et al., 1965). Thus, care must be taken to observe acceptable intervals between vaccines. For viral vaccines, interferon stimulation and subsequent viral inhibition is a potential problem. In general, 4 or more weeks should separate administrations of live virus vaccine.

Safety of Vaccines

Most available vaccines are generally safe and effective. Undesirable side effects can be anticipated in a small number of subjects with any of the available vaccines; a small but definite risk is associated with the administration of every immunizing agent. The benefits to the child as well as to society and the risks of vaccine administration should be explained to parents, patients, or both before vaccine administration, and informed consent should be obtained. The risk of adverse reactions associated with vaccine administration always must be compared with the risk of natural acquisition of the disease and its complications. For example, primary immunization with oral polio vaccine in individuals more than 18 years old is associated with a definite risk of vaccine-associated poliomyelitis. Because this risk may be greater than the risk of naturally acquiring the disease, such immunization is not recommended routinely. Similarly, since pertussis acquired by individuals older than 6 years of age carries with it a relatively small risk of morbid complications, immunization is not recommended for older children and adults.

To improve overall knowledge about adverse reactions, all temporally associated events severe enough to require the patient to seek medical attention should be evaluated and reported in detail to local and state health officials as well as the vaccine manufacturer. Frequently, cause-and-effect relationships are impossible to establish when untoward events occur after immunization. Scientific trials designed to document the incidence and nature of adverse reactions to already available or newly introduced vaccines are of critical importance to ensure a scientific rationale for vaccine usage recommendations as well as to ensure optimal public and professional vaccine acceptance.

Vaccine Administration

Injectable vaccines should be administered at a body site relatively free from risk of nerve or vascular injury. The best sites for intramuscular or subcutaneous injections are the anterolateral thigh (in infants) and the deltoid area of the upper arm (in older children and adults). Intragluteal injections carry the risk of sciatic nerve damage.

Vaccines containing adjuvants must be injected deep into a large muscle mass; subcutaneous or intracutaneous injection or leakage should be avoided because of the risk of local irritation, inflammation, and necrosis. Vaccines requiring intramuscular injection include DTP, DT, Td, hepatitis B, and rabies (human diploid cell). Immune globulin preparations also require intramuscular injection.

Contraindications for Vaccines

Contraindications to live virus vaccine administration include conditions associated with high risk for replication of viruses. Immunodeficient patients are at risk, especially those with profound B-cell or T-cell defects. Both congenital and acquired immunodeficiencies (e.g., AIDS, lymphomas, immunosuppressive therapy) are associated with such risks.

Severe reactions, such as extreme somnolence, seizures, or high fever, may represent a contraindication to subsequent immunization with the same antigen. Because scientific data do not support their safety or efficacy, fractional doses of the immunizing agent that elicited the reaction are not recommended to complete an immunization schedule. Minor illness is not an indication for deferral of childhood immunizations, regardless of the degree of accompanying fever (American Academy of Pediatrics, 1994).

Allergic diseases may pose special problems in immunization. Certain vaccine antigens produced in biologic systems containing allergenic substances (e.g., antigens derived from embryonated chick eggs) may cause hypersensitivity reactions, including anaphylaxis, when the final vaccine contains a substantial amount of the allergen (e.g., yellow fever vaccine) (CDC, 1983g). Influenza vaccine antigens, although prepared from viruses grown in embryonated eggs, are highly purified during preparation and only rarely have been associated with hypersensitivity reactions. Similarly, hypersensitivity reactions to measles vaccine rarely have been reported in persons with anaphylactic hypersensitivity to eggs. A history of ability to eat eggs without anaphylaxis excludes most individuals at risk for hypersensitivity reactions to measles, mumps, or influenza vaccines. Furthermore, some vaccines contain preservatives (e.g., thimerosal, a mercurial) or trace amounts of antibiotics (e.g., neomycin) to which individuals may be hypersensitive. Patients with known anaphylactic hypersensitivity to preservatives or antibiotics indicated in the package inserts should not receive these vaccines.

Because of theoretical risks to the developing fetus, live viral vaccines are usually not recommended for pregnant women or those likely to become pregnant within 3 months after receiving the immunizing agent. With respect to some of these vaccines (e.g., rubella, measles, and mumps), pregnancy is an absolute contraindication. Other agents, such as yellow fever and oral polio vaccines, can be given safely to pregnant women who are at substantial risk of exposure to natural infection. When vaccine must be given during pregnancy, a reasonable precaution is to wait until the second or third trimester to minimize concerns about teratogenicity (CDC, 1983g). Further specific information about immunization of pregnant women is provided with each immunizing agent discussed in this chapter.

RECOMMENDATIONS FOR VACCINES IN COMMON USE

Diphtheria Immunization

Rationale for Active Immunization

Historically, diphtheria has always represented a potentially serious pediatric disease. In the prevaccine era, 5% to 10% of reported respiratory cases were fatal, and the highest case-fatality ratios were in the very young and the elderly. The introduction of diphtheria toxoid more than half a century ago has led to a dramatic reduction in the incidence of diphtheria in the United States. More recently, no more than five cases have been reported annually (CDC, 1990). However, diphtheria may continue to represent a potentially significant public health issue because (1) serologic surveys in the United States suggest that many adults are not currently immunized adequately (Crossley et al., 1979); and (2) adequate immunization does not completely eliminate the potential for transmission of *Corynebacterium diphtheriae* (Miller et al., 1972).

Diphtheria is caused by infection with *C. diphtheriae*. Multiplication of the organism is less important than the local elaboration and systemic distribution of a powerful exotoxin. Toxin production is associated with strains of the organism infected with a specific bacteriophage.

Immunity to diphtheria is dependent on the presence of adequate levels of circulating antitoxin. Neutralization of diphtheria toxin prevents the severe manifestations of disease and helps reduce infection. Because the toxin plays a major role in permitting the bacterium to establish itself in the host, neutralization by antitoxin reduces infectious risk and also prevents the severe manifestations of disease. Immunization stimulates the formation of circulating antitoxin and sensitizes the immune system so that additional antitoxin can be synthesized rapidly.

Immunizing Antigen

The immunizing antigen is a toxoid prepared by chemical alteration of toxin to remove its toxicity but maintain antigenicity (Edsall et al., 1951). Diphtheria toxoid is available at two levels of potency, regular (D) and adult (d) and in combination with tetanus (T) as DT (diphtheria and tetanus, pediatric) or Td (diphtheria and tetanus, adult), and with tetanus and pertussis (DTP). Primary immunization of children under 7 years old is accomplished with preparations containing 7 to 25 Lf units of toxoid, the regular toxoid dose (DT or DTP). Because this antigen concentration is too toxic for older children and adults, a preparation containing no more than 2 Lf of toxoid is given (Td) after age 6. These antigens are absorbed to an alum-type adjuvant to provide maximal stimulation. A fluid toxoid is also available but rarely indicated or used. Toxoid should be given deep into a large muscle mass (CDC, 1981a).

Immunity

Immunization of children with diphtheria toxoid does not provide 100% protection but instead brings about a fivefold to tenfold reduction in incidence of subsequent disease. Further, few severe (or fatal) cases of diphtheria occur among fully immunized individuals.

Immunity is correlated with the presence of circulating antitoxin, which can be precisely measured only in specialized laboratories but is not practical for routine testing. In past years, the Schick test has been used to estimate the amount of circulating antitoxin. Diphtheria toxin, 0.1 ml, and a toxoid control are injected intradermally at different sites. A positive test, consisting of erythema at the site of toxin injection in 48 to 96 hours and little or no reaction at the control site, indicates 0.01 to 0.05 units of circulating antitoxin per milliliter of blood and solid immunity. A hypersensitivity reaction, indicated by equivalent reactions to toxoid and control, is occasionally noted.

Diphtheria immunity is of longer duration than previously thought. Booster doses used to be recommended every 4 to 6 years; it is now believed that 10-year intervals are adequate.

Vaccine Usage

The CDC (1981a, 1983g, 1985a) have made the following recommendations for use of DTP.

Primary Immunization in Infancy. Three 0.5-ml doses of DTP are given intramuscularly at 2-month intervals, beginning as early as 2 months of age. Additional DTP doses are given at the age of 15 to 18 months and 4 to 6 years (Table 29–2).

Primary Immunization After 6 Years of Age. This is accomplished with two 0.5-ml doses of tetanus toxoid combined with the lower adult dose of diphtheria toxoid (Td) given at least 4 weeks apart, and followed by a booster 1 year later.

Recall Immunization. Tetanus toxoid should be given with diphtheria toxoid as Td every 10 years. If a dose is given sooner as part of wound management

Table 29–2. Immunization Schedule Suggested for Healthy Infants and Children*

Age	Immunization
At birth	HBV
1–2 mo	HBV
2 mo	DTP, HbCV, OPV
4 mo	DTP, HbCV, OPV
6 mo	DTP, HbCV†
6–18 mo	HBV, OPV
12–15 mo	MMR, HbCV†, VVV
15–18 mo	DTaP or DTP
4–6 yr	DTaP or DTP, OPV
11–12 yr	MMR‡
14–16 yr	Td

*See text for more detail.

†The first two vaccine doses are given at 2 and 4 months of age. If either HbOC or PRP-T is used, a third dose is given at age 6 months. A booster vaccination is given at 12 to 15 months of age.

‡The second dose of MMR can be given at school entry rather than at age 11 to 12 years.

DTaP = diphtheria, tetanus, and acellular pertussis; DTP = diphtheria, tetanus, and pertussis; HbCV = *H. influenzae* type b conjugate vaccine; HBV = hepatitis B vaccine; MMR = measles, mumps, and rubella vaccine; OPV = oral polio vaccine; Td = diphtheria and tetanus vaccine for adults; VVV = varicella virus vaccine.

Adapted from American Academy of Pediatrics. In Peter G, ed. 1994 Red Book: Report of the Committee on Infectious Diseases, 23rd ed. Elk Grove Village, Ill., American Academy of Pediatrics, 1994.

(Td is preferred over tetanus toxoid alone), the next booster is not needed for 10 years thereafter.

Lapsed Immunization. If doses are missed in the primary series, regardless of the interval, additional doses are given until a primary series of doses is completed. Interruption of the recommended schedule or delay in administering subsequent doses during primary immunization does not reduce ultimate immunity; there is no need to restart a series regardless of the time elasped between doses (Table 29–3).

Special Circumstances. Household contacts of patients with suspected respiratory diphtheria should re-

Table 29–3. Primary Immunization Schedule Suggested for Children Not Immunized in the First Year of Life*

Younger than 7 years of age	
Initial visit	DTP, OPV, MMR, HbCV†, HBV
Interval after initial visit	
1 mo	DTP, HBV
2 mo	DTP, OPV, HbCV†
4 mo	DTP
>8 mo	DTP, or DTaP‡, HBV, OPV
4–6 yr (at or before school entry)	DTP, or DTaP, OPV
11–12 yr	MMR
10 yr later	Td
7 years of age and older	
Initial visit	Td, OPV, MMR, HBV
Interval after initial visit	
2 mo	Td, OPV, HBV
8–14 mo	Td, OPV, HBV
11–12 yr	MMR
10 yr later	Td

*See text for more detail.

†HbCV is indicated in children under 60 months of age. A second dose is indicated only in children who received the first dose before 15 months.

‡DTaP at 15+ mo.

DTP = diphtheria, tetanus, and pertussis; HbCV = *Haemophilus influenzae* type b conjugate vaccine; MMR = measles, mumps, and rubella vaccine; OPV = oral polio vaccine; Td = diphtheria and tetanus vaccine for adults.

Adapted from American Academy of Pediatrics. In Peter G, ed. 1994 Red Book: Report of the Committee on Infectious Diseases, 23rd ed. Elk Grove Village, Ill., American Academy of Pediatrics, 1994.

ceive an injection of a diphtheria toxoid–containing preparation appropriate for age and should be evaluated closely. Those who have previously received at least three doses of diphtheria toxoid, including at least one dose during the previous 5 years, need not be vaccinated. Additionally, asymptomatic unimmunized or inadequately immunized household contacts should receive prompt chemoprophylaxis with either an intramuscular injection of benzathine penicillin (600,000 units for persons under 6 years old and 1,200,000 units for those 6 years or older) or a 7-day course of erythromycin. Primary immunization should be completed in all persons who have received fewer than the recommended number of vaccine doses. For patients convalescing from diphtheria infection, complete active immunization should be performed, because infection does not necessarily confer immunity. The only specific contraindication to diphtheria toxoid administration is a history of neurologic or severe hypersensitivity reaction following a previous dose. Vaccination should be deferred during acute illness with high-grade fever.

The use of equine diphtheria antitoxin in unimmunized diphtheria contacts generally is not recommended because of the potential for immediate hypersensitivity reactions. However, for treatment of infected individuals (except those with cutaneous diphtheria), administration of antitoxin should be considered (CDC, 1981a, 1985a; American Academy of Pediatrics, 1994). The dose of antitoxin is empiric and should be administered as soon as diphtheria is diagnosed, even before positive cultures are obtained. Suggested doses are:

- Pharyngeal or laryngeal diphtheria (less than 48 hours—20,000 to 40,000 units
- Nasopharyngeal—40,000 to 60,000 units
- Extensive disease present for over 72 hours—80,000 to 100,000 units
- Brawny neck edema—80,000 to 100,000 units

These doses are empiric and may be modified depending on the site and size of the membrane, the severity of symptoms, and the duration of illness. Cervical adenitis frequently reflects toxin absorption; soft and diffuse adenopathy indicates moderate to severe toxicity.

Before administering antitoxin, sensitivity tests must be done. A 1:10 dilution of antitoxin in the eye or a 1:100 dilution in the skin is used. Desensitization is accomplished as previously described. Antimicrobial therapy must not be substituted for antitoxin; instead, the antitoxin and antibiotics should be used together.

Tetanus Immunization

Rationale for Active Immunization

Tetanus is caused by the neurotoxicity of a potent exotoxin elaborated by *Clostridium tetani,* a ubiquitous organism found throughout nature and particularly in animal excreta. *C. tetani* remains in the spore form until entry into a wound. The spores germinate if an anaerobic environment is established. Common circumstances that lead to tetanus infection include:

- Contamination of the umbilicus of the neonate, especially in areas of the world where poultices of animal dung are applied to the stump
- Wounds that result in pockets of anaerobiosis (the wound may be trivial or obvious)
- Insect bites
- Contaminated surgical wounds, particularly those exposed to gastrointestinal contents

Routine immunization of civilian populations in this country with tetanus toxoid has resulted in a dramatic decrease in the incidence of tetanus. Of further importance has been the near elimination of neonatal tetanus in the United States, although it continues to represent a significant cause of morbidity and mortality in many parts of the world. Most tetanus cases in the United States now occur in individuals over 50 years old, and, in virtually all cases, the disease has been reported only in unimmunized or inadequately immunized individuals (CDC, 1981a). Because it provides long-lasting protection and is relatively safe in human populations, tetanus toxoid has proved to be a nearly ideal immunizing agent.

Immunization is aimed at stimulating the development of antitoxin similar to that in diphtheria immunization. Tetanus is also prevented by prompt and appropriate treatment of injuries and wounds, rather than relying on immunization. Immunization against tetanus provides personal protection but does not provide community protection.

Immunizing Antigen

Tetanospasmin, the toxin of *C. tetani,* is modified by chemical treatment to provide a stable nontoxic agent for immunization. A potent antigen with minimal toxicity, tetanus toxoid is used alone or in combination with diphtheria (DT, Td) and pertussis vaccine (DTP). It is one of the most effective vaccine antigens, and a complete primary series provides long-lasting immunity.

Because toxoid evokes a potent antibody response, too-frequent immunizations can result in severe local necrotic Arthus reactions. The high levels of serum antibody result in antigen–antibody complexes at the injection site with resultant inflammation and vasculitis.

Immunity

The presence of antitoxin appears to be the sole factor in protection from the disease. As little as 0.01 IU/ml of antitoxin is protective (Goldsmith et al., 1962). Primary immunization is so effective that values above this protective level have been observed as long as 35 years after primary immunization (Peebles et al., 1969). Further, a booster dose results in a brisk anamnestic response. Although it may not always be necessary, 10-year boosters are recommended to maintain protective levels of antitoxin.

Vaccine Usage

The CDC (1981a, 1983g) and American Academy of Pediatrics (1994) have made the following recommendations for tetanus toxoid.

Primary Immunization in Infancy. Three doses of tetanus toxoid, usually as DTP, are administered intramuscularly at 2-month intervals, beginning as early as 2 months of age, with booster doses given at 15 to 18 months and 4 to 6 years of age (see Table 29–2).

Primary Immunization at 7 Years of Age or Older. Two doses of either tetanus toxoid alone (0.5 ml) or as Td are administered 2 months apart, with a booster dose 6 months to 1 year later (see Table 29–3).

Lapsed Immunization. If doses are missed, the next dose in the series is administered regardless of interval. It is not necessary to begin the series anew (see Table 29–3).

Recall Immunization. Tetanus toxoid (Td) should be given every 10 years to maintain immunity. Usually, a booster dose is given on school entry and every 10 years thereafter. If a dose is administered sooner as part of wound management, the next routine booster is not needed until 10 years later. In the United States, when the risk of neonatal tetanus is significant, antenatal immunization is recommended for previously unimmunized pregnant women using two properly spaced doses of Td. Booster injections of Td may be used in previously immunized pregnant women. In other regions of the world, adsorbed preparations containing higher concentrations of tetanus toxoid may be available for use in the antenatal immunization of previously unimmunized mothers (CDC, 1981a, 1985a; Chen et al., 1983).

Immunization Associated With Wound Management or Tetanus Infection. Active immunization may not be necessary as part of wound management for trauma or injury (Table 29–4). Adequate primary immunization provides sufficient protective titers of antitoxin for at least 10 years and ensures prompt, anamnestic responses to booster injections for several years longer (Peebles et al., 1969). The prolonged immunity afforded in addition to the known increased incidence of hypersensitivity reactions associated with frequent booster injections supports a conservative approach to the use of tetanus toxoid in wound management. Specific recommendations depend on the individual's immunization status, the nature of the wound, and the duration of time before evaluation and treatment of the injury. In individuals who are immunized adequately, it is not necessary to provide tetanus toxoid more than every 5 years. Tetanus immune globulin (TIG) is indicated only for individuals who have received fewer than two previous doses of tetanus toxoid or those in whom a tetanus-prone wound has been unattended for more than 24 hours. Generally, DT (Td in patients 7 years of age and older) is recommended for wound prophylaxis instead of tetanus toxoid alone to ensure additional immunity to diphtheria (American Academy of Pediatrics, 1994). Subsequent to prophylaxis, primary immunization should be completed in those incompletely immunized.

The exact dose of tetanus immune globulin for therapeutic use is not known. At least 140 units/kg given intramuscularly is recommended, with higher doses used in more severe cases. Patients convalescing from tetanus infection should receive active immunization because infection often does not confer immunity (CDC, 1981a).

Adverse Effects of Immunization

Tetanus toxoid is an extremely safe biological rarely associated with local or systemic reactions. A local Arthus reaction may occur if too many doses are given (Edsall et al., 1967). A history of neurologic or severe hypersensitivity reactions to tetanus toxoid–containing preparations contraindicates subsequent tetanus toxoid use; skin testing may be helpful in the rare patient demonstrating a severe allergic reaction (Jacobs et al., 1982).

Pertussis Immunization

Rationale for Active Immunization

Pertussis (whooping cough) continues to account for significant morbidity and mortality among pediatric patients worldwide, including the United States. Serious complications (e.g., seizures, encephalopathy, and, not uncommonly, death) still occur, especially in children younger than 1 year old. Thus, primary prevention programs in the United States emphasize early active immunization of all infants. Since the introduction of pertussis vaccine in the United States in the 1940s, a dramatic decline in the incidence of clinical pertussis has been documented (Mortimer et al., 1979). While more than 265,000 pertussis cases, including 7518 deaths, were reported in the United States in 1934, only 4570 cases were reported during 1990 (CDC, 1990).

Recent epidemiologic studies have clearly demon-

Table 29–4. Recommended Use of Tetanus Toxoid and Tetanus Immune Globulin in Wound Management

History of Tetanus Immunization (Doses)	Clean, Minor Wounds		Tetanus-Prone* Wounds	
	Td†	TIG‡	Td	TIG
Uncertain, less than three	Yes	No	Yes	Yes
Three or more	No§	No	No‖	No

*"Tetanus-prone" generally refers to wounds that yield anaerobic conditions or are incurred under conditions in which exposure to tetanus species is probable (puncture wound, severe necrotizing soft tissue wound, or wound contaminated with animal excreta).

†Tetanus and diphtheria toxoids (DT recommended for children under 7 years old).

‡Human tetanus immunoglobulin (250 to 500 units intramuscularly).

§Unless more than 10 years since the last dose.

‖Unless more than 5 years since the last dose.

Td = diphtheria and tetanus vaccine for adults; TIG = tetanus immune globulin vaccine.

Modified from American Academy of Pediatrics. In Peter G, ed. 1994 Red Book: Report of the Committee on Infectious Diseases, 23rd ed. Elk Grove Village, Ill., American Academy of Pediatrics, 1994.

strated the protective efficacy of pertussis vaccine in this country. In one study (Broome and Fraser, 1981), attack rates among household contacts younger than 10 years of age declined from 67% for unvaccinated individuals to 4% for those who had received three or more vaccinations (calculated vaccine efficacy of 94% for children younger than 5 years of age). Since children in the United States do not receive three doses of vaccine until 6 months of age under the current vaccination schedule, not all cases of pertussis are preventable. However, the morbidity of clinical disease among incompletely immunized infants and children is related inversely to the number of vaccine doses they have received (CDC, 1982g). Furthermore, the risk of infection in infants under 6 months old may be reduced indirectly by achieving high levels of immunity.

Concerns about pertussis vaccine toxicity and controversies about the relative risks and benefits of routine immunization have diminished vaccine acceptance rates in other countries. For example, in the United Kingdom, accounts of neurologic sequelae associated with vaccine use accounted for a drop in vaccine acceptance rates from 77% in 1974 to 30% in 1978. Not unexpectedly, an outbreak of 102,500 cases of pertussis with 36 fatalities occurred in that country during 1977 to 1979 (Miller et al., 1982). Vaccine acceptance in Japan dropped from 77% in 1974 to 13% in 1976 after two fatalities associated with vaccine use. Only 393 pertussis cases and no deaths had been reported in that country in 1974, but 13,000 cases and 41 deaths were reported in 1979 (Kanal, 1980). Such experience clearly indicates that, although immunization with the whole-cell pertussis vaccine is associated with a measurable risk (Cody et al., 1981), this risk is far outweighed by the benefit of disease prevention (Hinman and Koplan, 1984). An acellular vaccine developed in Japan appears to have equal efficacy but fewer side effects compared with conventional whole-cell vaccines (Sato et al., 1984).

Immunizing Antigen

The pertussis vaccine in use for many years consisted of killed whole *Bordetella pertussis* and fragments of organisms. The precise antigen responsible for protection is not known. New pertussis vaccines, composed of purified components of *B. pertussis*, rather than whole-cell vaccines prepared from inactivated organisms, have been licensed for use in the United States (Peter, 1992). These new vaccines are termed *acellular* pertussis vaccines (aP).

Potency of pertussis vaccine is a critical issue. The standard test is a mouse-protective model developed in the 1940s that correlates well with human protection. Vaccines used in England and elsewhere before 1968 were of low potency as measured by this procedure (Stewart, 1977). The poor results of immunization in England that led to the suggestion that pertussis vaccine should be abandoned were probably a result of ineffective vaccine. Potent vaccine, as judged by mouse-protective units, is capable of providing active immunity and 85% to 90% protection when 12 protec-

tive units are administered in three equal doses given at 4- to 8-week intervals (Broome and Fraser, 1981).

Whole-cell pertussis vaccine can be administered alone or in combination with diphtheria and tetanus toxoids (DTP). It is available as a "plain" preparation or absorbed to alum. The adjuvant vaccine contains four protective units per 0.5-ml dose, whereas the plain vaccine contains somewhat more antigen. There is no indication for the use of plain pertussis vaccine; it offers no immunologic advantage nor improved safety. Acellular pertussis vaccine is combined with diphtheria and tetanus toxoids in a preparation called DTaP.

Immunity

Although several antigens have been isolated from *Bordetella pertussis* and several antibodies occur after immunization, the precise mechanism of immunity is unknown. Almost total protection has been associated with high antibody titers (>1:320) in humans and monkeys (Sako, 1947). However, some protection (approximately 60%) occurs at serum antibody levels below this and may even occur in the absence of antibody. Thus, a role for cell-mediated immunity may exist.

Solid immunity usually follows natural disease, although second cases of proven disease have occurred. Protection following vaccine is relatively short-lived, so adults likely to be at risk (e.g., health personnel) need booster doses of vaccine to maintain immunity.

Complicating assessment of vaccine efficacy is the occurrence of pertussis caused by agents other than *B. pertussis* (Lewis et al., 1973). Parapertussis may account for up to 2% of cases attributed to pertussis. There is no cross-immunity between these organisms. Adenoviruses and other viral agents may also cause pertussis-like syndromes. Thus, evaluation of the efficacy of pertussis vaccine necessitates precise laboratory diagnosis.

Vaccine Usage

American Academy of Pediatrics (1994) and the CDC (1981a, 1983g, 1985a) have made the following recommendations for pertussis vaccination.

Primary Immunization in Infancy. Pertussis vaccine is usually combined with diphtheria and tetanus toxoids as DTP. Each dose of DTP contains 4 units of pertussis vaccine. Three doses of DTP (a total of 12 units) are given intramuscularly at 2-month intervals, beginning at 2 months of age; a booster is given at 15 to 18 months of age (see Table 29–2). Routine recall booster doses are suggested when the child enters school. The two currently licensed acellular pertussis vaccines are approved for the fourth and fifth doses of the pertussis immunization schedule and are recommended only for children 15 months to 7 years of age (CDC, 1992b; American Academy of Pediatrics, 1992a).

Primary Immunization After 6 Years of Age. A somewhat similar schedule of primary immunization can be used for children not immunized in early infancy and those under 7 years old (see Table 29–3). Because of the risks of pertussis immunization and the overall decreased morbidity from pertussis in older individuals, pertussis vaccine is generally recommended only for those under 7 years old. The adult diphtheria and tetanus toxoids (Td) preparation may be used for older patients.

Special Circumstances. In areas of high endemicity or during epidemics, immunization can begin earlier; the vaccine (DTP or pertussis, adsorbed) is begun at 4 to 6 weeks of age, and three doses are given 1 month apart. Rarely, in severe epidemics affecting very young infants, pertussis immunization can be initiated in the first few days or weeks of life.

During pertussis outbreaks, certain exposed individuals require special consideration. Close contacts under 7 years old (e.g., siblings and classmates) who were previously immunized but who have not received a pertussis immunization within the last 6 months should be re-immunized. In this setting, chemoprophylaxis with oral erythromycin also can be considered, especially in those under 1 year of age and unimmunized patients.

Although pertussis vaccine is not recommended routinely for persons over 7 years old, a booster dose (0.25 ml of pertussis vaccine, adsorbed) can be given to older patients with chronic pulmonary disease who are exposed to pertussis, or to health care personnel exposed during outbreaks. Prophylactic chemotherapy can also be considered in such persons. Chemotherapy of the index case may decrease the period of infectivity, but it will not alleviate the clinical course. Individuals who recover from bacteriologically confirmed pertussis require no further pertussis immunization (CDC, 1981a, 1985a; American Academy of Pediatrics, 1994).

After intimate exposure to pertussis or during epidemics, children under 7 years old should receive a 0.5-ml dose. Older patients should receive a half dose (0.25 ml) of either DTP or pertussis adsorbed vaccine.

Adverse Effects of Immunization

Both local and systemic adverse effects may occur following administration of preparations containing pertussis vaccine. Reported reactions following the use of DTP cannot be related certainly to the pertussis component. However, since the incidence of adverse reactions after administration of pediatric diphtheria and tetanus toxoids is markedly less, most serious adverse reactions to DTP are more likely to be from the pertussis vaccine rather than the toxoid components (Cody et al., 1981).

Local reactions to DTP, including erythema, swelling, and pain, are seen in about two thirds of recipients and occur more commonly with repeated immunization.

Occasionally, a sterile abscess may develop at the injection site. Systemic reactions, such as a fever as high as 40.4°C, occur in as many as 50% of DTP recipients. Systemic reactions can be accompanied by mild lethargy, irritability, or vomiting. Such symptoms usually appear within hours and last 1 to 2 days after immunization (Cody et al., 1981).

More serious but very rare systemic reactions include persistent crying, pronounced fever (≥40.5°C), and collapse or shock-like states during which the infant is pale, hypotonic, and unresponsive. Such symptoms characteristically occur within hours after vaccination and last several minutes to hours. Importantly, affected infants generally recover completely. The latter complication occurred in 9 of 15,752 DTP doses administered by Cody and colleagues (1981). Convulsions, primarily brief major motor seizures, also occurred at a rate of 1 per 1750 DTP doses administered. Encephalopathy, with or without convulsions, characterized by a change in level of consciousness, focal neurologic signs, or a bulging fontanelle, has been reported to occur at a rate of 1.3 to 30 per million DTP doses (CDC, 1981a).

The significance of vaccine reactions in terms of permanent neurologic sequelae is not well defined. The National Childhood Encephalopathy Study performed in the United Kingdom estimated that the risk of an acute neurologic disorder occurring in a previously healthy child within 7 days of DTP immunization was 1 per 110,000 doses administered, with sequelae persisting at least 1 year in 1 per 310,000 doses administered (Miller et al., 1981).

Precise estimates of the risk of serious reactions to pertussis vaccine are difficult to determine because the incidence of temporally related reactions is so low that it is difficult to differentiate them from the background incidence of similar syndromes seen in unvaccinated children. Adsorbed vaccines are associated with fewer reactions than those without adjuvant, and reaction rates vary among preparations from different manufacturers of pertussis vaccine (Mortimer and Jones, 1979). DTaP is associated with lower rates of local reactions, fever, and common systemic reactions than is DTP. For children who have had a febrile or afebrile seizure not temporally associated with DTP administration, and for those with seizure disorders in the immediate family, DTaP is preferred over DTP whenever possible (CDC, 1992b).

Precautions and Contraindications

Most reactions following DTP administration do not represent contraindications to further pertussis vaccination. When reactions not contraindicating further pertussis immunization occur, some health care providers divide the remaining inoculations into multiple small doses. No definitive clinical or serologic studies to evaluate the efficacy of such schedules or the effects on the subsequent frequency and severity of adverse reactions have been performed. Thus, the use of fractional doses cannot be recommended at this time (Barkin et al., 1984). Reporting of adverse reactions temporally related to vaccine administration by parents and physicians should be encouraged.

Each of the following reactions to pertussis vaccine represents an absolute contraindication to subsequent pertussis immunization:

- Fever ≥40.5°C within 48 hours
- Persistent screaming or crying of 3 or more hours or an unusual, high-pitched cry
- Collapse or shock-like state

- Generalized or focal neurologic signs or severe alterations of consciousness
- Convulsions with or without fever occurring within 72 hours after immunization
- Systemic allergic reactions

Children under 7 years old in whom further pertussis vaccine is contraindicated may complete the necessary immunization schedule with the DT preparation (CDC, 1984; American Academy of Pediatrics, 1994).

Seizures following pertussis immunization occur more commonly in those with a history of a previous seizure disorder, but they appear to be similar to febrile seizures and are associated with a benign outcome (Cody et al., 1981; Hirtz et al., 1983). In patients with a seizure disorder, pertussis immunization should be deferred until it can be determined whether there is an evolving neurologic disease. Patients with stable neurologic disorders, including well-controlled seizures, may receive pertussis vaccine. Furthermore, a family history of seizures or other neurologic disease is not a contraindication to pertussis immunization (CDC, 1984).

Poliomyelitis Immunization

Rationale for Immunization

The efficacy of primary prevention through active immunization is perhaps most convincingly demonstrated by the near extinction of poliomyelitis in the United States since the introduction of polio vaccines. In contrast to the prevaccine era, when more than 18,000 cases of paralytic disease occurred in this country each year, only 7 cases of paralytic disease were reported in 1990. Although small outbreaks of wild poliovirus-associated paralytic disease continue to occur, they are seen almost exclusively in those who refuse vaccine or as a result of importation. The most recent epidemic of wild virus paralytic polio occurred in 1979 and accounted for 13 cases among unvaccinated Amish (Schonberger et al., 1984).

From 1980 to 1982, 18 cases of paralytic polio were associated with the use of the live attenuated oral poliovirus vaccine (OPV) (Schonberger et al., 1984), continuing the previous decade's average incidence of approximately 1 case per 3.2 million doses of OPV (CDC, 1982i). Approximately two thirds of these cases occurred among vaccinees' contacts (mostly adults) (Moore et al., 1982).

Active immunity can be achieved with either inactivated or attenuated poliovirus vaccines. For maximal effectiveness, polio immunization must involve a large segment of the population, which reduces the spread of wild poliovirus in the community and provides protection to unimmunized individuals. This so-called herd immunity may be more theoretical than practical because unimmunized individuals remain susceptible and wild poliovirus may not be totally eliminated.

The relative safety and efficacy of the inactivated versus the live attenuated poliovirus vaccine has become a topic of controversy among scientists, laypeople, and politicians (Nightingale, 1977). Proponents of use of inactivated polio vaccine (IPV) have suggested that IPV, which does not cause vaccine-associated disease, should replace OPV as the vaccine of choice in the United States (Salk, 1980b). Before the introduction of OPV from 1961 to 1963, IPV, which had been available since 1955, had reduced the incidence of paralytic polio by more than 90% (Salk, 1980a). Further, other countries, such as Sweden (Bottiger, 1984), Finland (Lapinieimu, 1984), and The Netherlands (Bijkerk, 1984), achieved eradication of indigenous polio with the use of IPV exclusively. OPV continues to be the vaccine of choice for primary immunization of children in the United States, as recommended by the American Academy of Pediatrics (1994) and the CDC (1982i) for the following reasons:

1. It induces local (intestinal) immunity.
2. It is simple to administer and therefore well accepted by patients.
3. It contributes to herd immunity by secondarily immunizing some contacts.
4. It has essentially eliminated clinically recognized polio in this country (Fox, 1980).

Underdeveloped countries with tropical and subtropical climates continue to record disease rates higher than those during the prevaccine era in the United States. About 40% of such cases are recognized in the first year of life (Sabin, 1984). While annual mass vaccination programs with OPV have been successful in a limited number of underdeveloped countries, the recent development of an IPV that can be produced more economically on an industrial scale (Van Wezel et al., 1984) and that can provide long-lasting immunity after two or even a single injection (Grenier et al., 1984) may promote more effective polio prevention programs worldwide.

Immunizing Antigens

Inactivated Poliovirus Vaccines. A polyvalent vaccine containing formalin-inactivated poliovirus types 1, 2, and 3 grown in monkey kidney tissue culture was introduced into the United States in 1955 (Salk, 1953; Salk and Salk, 1977). This conventional IPV was widely used until the OPV became available during the period from 1961 to 1964. A method of producing a more potent IPV with greater antigenic content was developed in 1978 and led to the newly licensed IPV, which is produced in human diploid cells (Von Seefried et al., 1984; Bernier et al., 1986). This enhanced-potency IPV, which is manufactured and distributed by Connaught Laboratories Ltd, is currently recommended when IPV immunization is indicated (CDC, 1987). Stringent manufacturing and testing precautions have made it highly unlikely that the infamous "Cutter incident," in which recipients developed poliomyelitis because of a failure to inactivate live poliovirus in certain batches, can recur.

Attenuated Oral Poliovirus Vaccine. Trivalent OPV (TOPV) is a mixture of polioviruses types 1, 2, and 3, grown either in monkey kidney tissue culture or human-fetal-diploid tissue culture (CDC, 1982i; Sabin,

1984). Usually, the dose of type 2 poliovirus is reduced to equalize the antigenicity with types 1 and 3. Monovalent OPV containing a single poliovirus type is usually reserved for epidemics and stockpiled for this purpose.

Immunity

There are two phases of poliovirus immunity, a mucosal phase and a systemic phase (Nathanson and Bodian, 1962; Ogra et al., 1968). Secretory IgA poliovirus antibody, the chief component of topical mucosal immunity in the pharynx and possibly in the intestinal mucosa, serves to neutralize poliovirus and either prevents or limits infection. Serum antibody also provides protection, and titers are correlated with immunity to systemic disease.

Systemic immunity follows both IPV and OPV immunization and natural disease, and local immunity occurs following OPV immunization. Thus, wild poliovirus may replicate asymptomatically in the gastrointestinal tract of IPV recipients despite the presence of serum antibody.

Poliovirus immunity is type-specific and, following natural disease, is lifelong. OPV is also associated with prolonged immunity and perhaps is lifelong. There is disagreement as to the duration of immunity after IPV, but Salk maintains that immunity is long-lived, particularly with the newer, more potent IPV (Salk and Salk, 1977). Others suggest that booster doses of IPV may be necessary every 2 to 5 years.

Vaccine Usage

For primary immunization of infants with TOPV, doses of vaccine are recommended at 2 months and 4 months of age followed by an additional dose at 15 to 18 months. In areas of high endemicity, the administration of an additional dose of TOPV at about 6 months of age may be advisable. Children who have received a full primary series should receive an additional (recall) booster dose of TOPV on entering school, between 4 and 6 years of age (see Table 29–2).

In cases in which the time interval between the doses of the primary series has been longer than recommended, no additional doses are required and primary immunization may be resumed after any time lapse. Children and adolescents who were not immunized in infancy should receive an initial dose of TOPV and subsequent doses at 2-month and 8- to 14-month intervals (see Table 29–3).

Routine immunization of adults (18 years of age or older) in the United States is not necessary, because most adults are immune and little or no transmission of wild poliovirus occurs in this country. Persons traveling to countries where poliomyelitis may be epidemic or endemic and health care workers in close contact with patients who may excrete poliovirus should be vaccinated. In these instances, a single booster dose of TOPV may be given to those who previously have completed a primary series. Incompletely immunized adults should complete the primary series with either

TOPV or enhanced-potency IPV, depending on which was previously received. Enhanced-potency IPV should be given only to those undergoing primary immunization, except when there is insufficient time to give a series of IPV before anticipated exposure or when poliomyelitis is endemic or epidemic in the community. Four (0.5-ml) subcutaneous doses of enhanced-potency IPV are recommended. The first three are given at intervals of 1 to 2 months followed by a fourth dose 6 to 12 months after the third. Those who receive primary immunization with IPV may require a booster dose every 5 years (CDC, 1982i, 1987).

Adults not adequately immunized with either vaccine who reside in a household with a child who receives TOPV are at very small risk of developing vaccine-associated paralytic poliomyelitis, estimated to be one case per 5.5 million doses of OPV distributed. Because of the general importance of achieving prompt and complete immunization of children, the CDC recommends that children receive TOPV regardless of the immunization status of their household members; susceptible adults should be informed of the small risks involved. If there is definite assurance that full immunization will occur in a reasonable time, the adult can be immunized according to the schedule above before the administration of TOPV to the child (CDC, 1982i, 1987).

Precautions and Contraindications

TOPV usage is contraindicated in individuals with altered immune states, including suspected or proven primary immunodeficiency (both humoral and cellular immunodeficiency disease), human immunodeficiency virus (HIV) infection, malignancy, or immunosuppressive therapy (corticosteroids, cytotoxic agents, or radiation therapy). Enhanced-potency IPV should be given if immunization is necessary. TOPV should not be given to household contacts of immunodeficient patients. Administration of TOPV to even healthy hospitalized children is not advisable because of inherent risks to immunocompromised patients in that setting. TOPV should not be given to pregnant women because of a theoretical (but unproven) risk to the fetus, but it is recommended for pregnant women if immediate protection against poliomyelitis is required. Because conventional and enhanced-potency IPV contains streptomycin and neomycin, neither preparation should be administered to individuals demonstrating anaphylactic hypersensitivity to these antibiotics (CDC, 1982i, 1987; American Academy of Pediatrics, 1994).

Measles (Rubeola) Immunization

Rationale for Active Immunization

Measles virus produces a severe systemic infection involving multiple organs that lasts for 7 days or more. Complications are frequent; 5% to 15% develop bacterial infections and 1 in 1000 patients develops encephalitis (Kempe and Fulginiti, 1964). In developing countries, morbidity and mortality from measles remain high. Worldwide, approximately one million children die each year as a result of measles. The highest occurrence and death rates affect those under 1 year old. The licensure and distribution of killed (1963), live (Edmonston B) (1963), and further attenuated measles vaccines (1965) has had a staggering impact on the prevalence of measles and its associated morbidity and mortality in the United States. The Department of Health, Education and Welfare (now Health and Human Services; HHS) predicted the elimination of indigenous measles in this country by October 1, 1982 (CDC, 1978c). Although this goal was not realized, the incidence of measles in the United States was reduced by 99.7% from the prevaccine era in which some 500,000 cases were reported each year (Hinman et al., 1983; CDC, 1984g). A major factor for the successful measles immunization effort in this country was new state legislation to enforce immunization requirements for school entrance. By the 1982–1983 school year, 97% of children entering school had documented measles immunity. Most of the 1163 measles cases recognized in 1983 occurred in a limited number of outbreaks, largely among susceptible preschool or college-aged individuals who were not affected directly by existing state laws (CDC, 1984d, 1984g). Since 1983, the incidence of measles in the United States has increased annually, with nearly 28,000 cases reported in 1990 (CDC, 1990). The recent resurgence of measles is attributable to low measles vaccination rates among preschool-aged children (National Vaccine Advisory Committee, 1991).

Immunizing Antigens

Killed Measles Virus Vaccine (KMV). Although no longer available in the United States, KMV has been administered to more than 600,000 children, and its adverse effects are still being observed. KMV was prepared by inactivating live virus grown in tissue culture and adding adjuvant (Fulginiti et al., 1963). The usual series consisted of two or three doses of KMV followed by boosters of KMV or a dose of live measles virus vaccine.

KMV produced only short-lived antibody production (Fulginiti et al., 1963). After 6 months, KMV recipients exposed to attenuated measles vaccine developed local reactions (heat, induration, pain, and rash at the inoculation site) or systemic reactions (fever, regional adenopathy, headache, and malaise) (Fulginiti et al., 1968). Exposure to wild virus resulted in bizarre atypical eruptions (peripheral accentuation and onset of the rash, vesicles, petechiae, and purpura); severe systemic manifestations (fever, headache, and lethargy); and organ involvement (pneumonia, serositis, pleuritis, peritonitis, and central nervous system symptoms) (Rauh and Schmidt, 1965; Fulginiti et al., 1967). Extremely high antibody titers were also noted. This "atypical measles syndrome" can occur up to 17 or more years after administration of KMV.

Live Measles Virus Vaccine (LMV). Two types of LMV have been developed. The original LMV was developed by Enders and colleagues (1960) from the Edmonston strain of measles virus isolated by Enders. An attenuated Edmonston B virus, obtained after many passages in chick embryo tissue culture, produced mild symptoms and reliable immunity. However, the 15% incidence of rash and 80% incidence of fever were judged too severe. Thus, injection of human measles immune globulin (MIG) at a different site was given to reduce the incidence of rash and fever without significantly reducing immunogenicity.

Schwarz (1964) developed a second attenuated virus by further passages in chick embryo tissue culture. This further attenuated measles virus (FAMV) produces fewer febrile and exanthematous reactions, but antibody levels are lower and decrease more rapidly than with the Edmonston B vaccine. Despite these lower antibody responses, the vaccine appears to be equally protective against measles. FAMV vaccine does not require the simultaneous administration of MIG.

Although millions of children received these vaccines, the vaccine available today in the United States is the Moraten strain developed by Merck, Sharp and Dohme (Hilleman et al., 1968a). It resembles the Schwarz strain and is considered an FAMV.

LMV is supplied in lyophilized form for reconstitution just before immunization. The manufacturer's directions should be followed explicitly in its storage, reconstitution, and administration. The virus is fragile and can be inactivated if any of these steps is omitted or changed. Heating the vaccine, adding improper diluent, using glass syringes, and mixing with immune globulin all may inactivate the virus and result in vaccine failure. Before reconstitution, LMV must be stored between 2° and 8°C or colder and protected from light, which inactivates the virus. LMV is most often used in combination with mumps and rubella vaccines.

Immunity

Recovery from measles is independent of antibody formation, inasmuch as agammaglobulinemic patients with intact cell-mediated immunity usually have a normal course of measles (Good et al., 1962). Immunity to measles on subsequent exposure is, however, well correlated with the presence of antibody. Other factors, notably cell-mediated immunity, may be important, but antibody alone seems sufficient, since passive administration of antibody can prevent measles in a susceptible subject.

Immunity following natural measles is lifelong, as evidenced by measles in isolated communities in which individuals have been exposed at intervals as long as 65 years apart (Christensen et al., 1953). Immunity following LMV immunization is probably equivalent to that resulting from natural disease. Although vaccine-induced antibody titers are lower than those following natural disease, persistence of protective titers at least 16 years after vaccine administration has been demonstrated (Krugman, 1983). Further, more than 20 years have elapsed since FAMV has been in use, and immunity and protection have been sustained during this period.

When measles occurs in vaccine recipients, one of the following factors is usually the cause:

- *Administration of LMV before 15 months of age.* LMV was originally recommended for infants 12 months of age and younger; it is now known that LMV may be ineffective because of persistent maternal antibody, even though it is undetected in the infant's serum. If LMV is given with immune globulin or before 1 year of age, the likelihood of vaccine failure is increased. As many as 35% of infants given LMV at 9 months of age may not be immunized. The data conflict on the efficacy of immunization at 12 months of age. Some studies show failure rates of 15% to 22% at 12 months of age and others show a failure rate as low as 3% to 5% (Krugman, 1977; Yeager et al., 1977; Wilkins and Wehrle, 1978).
- *Use of impotent vaccine.* Several factors, as previously mentioned, may result in LMV inactivation before administration.
- *The natural failure rate.* LMV does not immunize all recipients; 3% to 5% may not develop antibody despite potent vaccine and optimal technique.
- *"True" vaccine failure.* Studies by Cherry and colleagues (1972, 1973) suggest that true vaccine failures occur, that is, vaccine-induced immunity wanes with time. This seems to be rare and accounts for only occasional failure.

Vaccine Usage

For primary immunization, a single dose of FAMV Moraten or Attenuvax is given subcutaneously at 15 months of age or older (see Table 29–2). A second vaccine dose is recommended either at school entry or at entry to junior high school or middle school (i.e., at 11 or 12 years of age) (CDC, 1989; American Academy of Pediatrics, 1994). FAMV can be given most conveniently by a measles, mumps, and rubella (MMR) combination vaccine, although monovalent and measles and rubella (MR) preparations are also available. The antibody responses to MMR vaccine may be inhibited for up to several months after administration of immunoglobulin (Siber et al., 1993).

Adults born before 1957 can be considered immune. Those who have not had clinical measles documented by a physician or who have not received a previous LMV vaccine preparation also should receive a single dose of FAMV. Any child immunized before 12 months of age, at a time when persistence of maternal antibody may have interfered with successful immunization, should be re-immunized with FAMV. During outbreaks, when the likelihood of exposure is high, infants as young as 6 months of age should be immunized. These children then should be revaccinated at 15 months and 11 or 12 years of age. Wilkins and Wehrle (1978) noted, however, that patients initially vaccinated before 1 year of age may respond poorly to subsequent revaccination.

Individuals previously immunized with KMV or those who received a vaccine of unknown type before 1968 should be re-immunized with FAMV, even if a dose of LMV was given within 3 months after a killed or unknown vaccine type. These children may experience untoward reactions to LMV and are susceptible to atypical measles on exposure to wild virus. Thus, discussion with parents and consent for further measles vaccination should be obtained. These children should then be given a single cutaneous dose of FAMV. In 10% to 50% of children, local heat, induration, and tenderness occur. In 3% to 10%, systemic symptoms of fever, malaise, and regional adenopathy occur (Fulginiti and Arthur, 1969). No evidence of an enhanced risk of vaccine-associated reactions exists for those receiving LMV after previous LMV immunization or natural measles infection (CDC, 1982e).

If an unimmunized child is exposed to measles, prompt LMV administration may prevent measles. This protection occurs because LMV has a shorter incubation period than natural measles (7 as opposed to 11 days). LMV given within 72 hours of exposure can provide protection. If exposure does not result in infection, immunization protects against future infection. Human immune serum globulin (ISG), which can prevent or modify disease if given within 6 days of exposure, is indicated for susceptible household contacts under 1 year old who are at highest risk for complications. Then, FAMV should be given at least 3 months later when passive measles antibody titers have waned and the child is at least 15 months old. HISG can be given to exposed immunocompromised hosts (CDC, 1982e).

Children who received their original LMV before 12 months of age should be given a second dose of LMV after 15 months of age because protection from the first dose is uncertain. Considerable confusion exists about the necessity for re-immunizing children who previously received their LMV at 12 months of age. Because the data are conflicting and the risk appears small, routine re-immunization is not recommended. If risk for natural disease is high, re-immunization may be warranted.

In measles epidemics or endemic areas of the world, newborn infants are at high risk. Under these circumstances, infants should be given LMV as early as 6 months of age. Since some of these infants are not successfully immunized because of the immunosuppressive effect of transplacental antibody, they should be re-immunized at or after 15 months of age. For individuals who cannot be given LMV because of an underlying disease, a preventive dose of HISG can be given when necessary.

Precautions and Contraindications

Certain precautions must be observed with LMV. Because disseminated disease and death can result from LMV given to subjects with depressed cellular immunity, live attenuated measles vaccine should not be administered to individuals with suspected or proven primary immunodeficiency disease, as well as disorders or therapeutic regimens associated with secondary immunodeficiency states, with the exception of HIV infection (or AIDS). Severe and even fatal measles has occurred among HIV-infected children, and serious vaccine-associated complications have not been observed (American Academy of Pediatrics, 1994). Lymphoreticular or other generalized malignancies and use of corticosteroids and cytotoxic or radiation therapy represent specific contraindications to LMV administration.

The LMV used for immunization is not communicable. Therefore, contacts of immunocompromised patients should be vaccinated to prevent the spread of natural measles to such patients. Although no direct evidence exists demonstrating that live measles vaccine is harmful to the pregnant female or her fetus, it should not be administered to pregnant women because of the theoretical risk of fetal infection associated with a live virus vaccine.

Because measles vaccination may diminish cutaneous manifestations of cell-mediated immunity temporarily, a tuberculin test performed several days to 6 weeks after immunization may yield a false-negative result. Although natural measles infection may exacerbate tuberculosis, no evidence exists that measles vaccination is associated with such an effect. Thus, tuberculin skin testing is not a prerequisite for LMV immunization because the risk of natural measles far outweighs the theoretical hazard of exacerbating undiagnosed tuberculosis (CDC, 1982e).

Acute illness with high-grade fever justifies postponement of LMV administration, but commonly observed minor respiratory illness associated with low-grade fever does not preclude immunization. LMV immunization also should be postponed for 3 months in persons who have received whole blood, plasma, or HISG because these products may contain sufficient measles antibody to neutralize the vaccine virus.

Measles vaccine contains chick embryo tissue culture protein. Patients with known anaphylactic reactions to egg whites may be at increased risk for a similar reaction from LMV. Skin testing may help evaluate the possibility of immunizing these patients (Herman et al., 1983). Those with a history of minor reactions to egg whites are not at increased risk (CDC, 1982e). Because measles vaccine preparations contain neomycin, patients with a history of anaphylactic reaction to neomycin should not receive measles vaccine.

Passive Immunization

Human immune serum globulin contains a variable amount of measles antibody. Measles immune globulin contained 4000 measles virus–neutralizing units per milliliter, but it is no longer available.

ISG can be used to prevent or modify measles in exposed, susceptible individuals. Regardless of vaccination status, symptomatic HIV-infected persons who are exposed to measles also should receive ISG prophylaxis. Prevention with a dose of 0.25 ml/kg or 0.5 ml/kg (immunocompromised hosts; maximum dose of 15 ml) is recommended, followed by LMV immunization (if not already done) in 5 or 6 months.

ISG is given intramuscularly deep in a large muscle mass; no more than 5 ml is given at one site (CDC, 1982e; American Academy of Pediatrics, 1994).

Rubella (German Measles) Immunization
Rationale for Active Immunization

Largely as a consequence of a major epidemic in the United States in 1964 (more than 20,000 cases of congenital rubella), active immunization programs with attenuated rubella vaccines were initiated in 1969 in hopes of preventing an epidemic expected in the early 1970s. A decision at the time to immunize all children 1 to 12 years old represented an attempt to reduce the reservoir and transmission of wild rubella virus and, secondarily, to diminish the risk of rubella in susceptible pregnant women. This national policy contrasted with the immunization strategy in the United Kingdom, where only susceptible adolescent girls were immunized (Preblud et al., 1980). Proponents of the British policy in this country have argued that (1) natural rubella infection confers lifelong immunity and is therefore more effective than vaccine-induced protection of uncertain duration; and (2) despite rubella vaccine programs, continued outbreaks of rubella in the United States (largely in older children and young adults) attest to the difficulty in achieving herd immunity for this disease. Although 60% to 80% of English girls approaching puberty have received rubella vaccine, there has been no demonstrable decrease to date in either postnatal or congenital rubella in that country.

In contrast, the incidence of congenital rubella in the United States has diminished markedly since rubella vaccines were introduced in 1969; fewer than 15 cases of congenital rubella have been reported each year in infants born since 1980, and only 1125 cases were reported in 1990 (CDC, 1990). Because 95% of all children entering school in the United States continue to be immunized (CDC, 1982j), rubella is likely to be eradicated from this country in the next 10 to 30 years (Orenstein et al., 1984). However, as was true in the prevaccine era, 15% of women of childbearing age remain susceptible. Therefore, efforts to immunize this group must be intensified to prevent congenital rubella associated with continued outbreaks of rubella before its eventual disappearance.

Immunizing Antigens

Live attenuated rubella vaccines licensed for use in the United States in 1969 included HPV-77:DE-5, grown in duck embryo tissue culture; HPV-77:DK-12, grown in dog kidney tissue culture (neither was available after 1979); and Cendehill, grown primarily in rabbit kidney cells and not available after 1976. RA 27/3 (rubella abortus, 27th specimen, third extract) prepared in human diploid tissue culture is the only vaccine now available in the United States. This live attenuated vaccine induces higher antibody titers that more closely parallel the immune response following natural infection than previous vaccines (Lerman et al., 1981; Orenstein, 1984). Monovalent and combination preparations—including measles and rubella (MR), rubella and mumps, and measles, mumps, and rubella (MMR) vaccines—are available. The MMR combination vaccine is used for routine infant immunization programs. Rubella vaccine must be kept at 2°C to 8°C or colder during storage and should be protected from light to avoid virus inactivation. Once reconstituted, it should be used within 8 hours.

Immunity

At least 95% of susceptible vaccinees 12 months of age or older develop antibody titers that are protective although not as high as those resulting from natural infection. The exact duration of protection is uncertain, but antibody levels have waned only slightly after 10 years in the initial group of children receiving the RA 27/3 vaccine (Herrman et al., 1982). Lifelong protection against clinical re-infection or subclinical viremia or both probably results from a single dose of vaccine early in childhood. Therefore, routine rubella re-immunization is not recommended.

In some cases, vaccinees exposed to natural rubella develop a rise of antibody titer unassociated with clinical symptoms. "Re-infection" (≥ fourfold rise of rubella HAI antibody titer) is associated only rarely with viremia. Significant pharyngeal shedding also is observed infrequently. Similarly, re-infection can be observed in individuals with previous natural rubella. Cell-mediated immunity is probably responsible for recovery from and immunity to rubella; this is emphasized by the fact that infection has occurred in individuals with circulating antibody.

Infants with congenital rubella may have persistent viremia despite high levels of transplacentally acquired serum antibodies. Persistent rubella infection may result from direct viral infection of lymphocytes, rendering them unresponsive to rubella antibody. When lymphocyte infection ends, cell-mediated immunity is restored and the virus is eradicated. The fetus initially offers no defense to the virus, but with persistence of the virus, specific IgM antibody develops. Thus, the neonate with congenital rubella has both virus and antibody present. A syndrome analogous to subacute sclerosing panencephalitis has been observed following congenital rubella (Townsend et al., 1975). This suggests that rubella virus becomes latent in brain cells, despite a persistent and brisk antibody response.

Vaccine Usage

For primary immunization, any child, from 15 months old to prepuberty, is a candidate for rubella immunization. The American Academy of Pediatrics (1994) recommends immunization at 15 months of age along with measles vaccination (see Table 29–2). In conjunction with the recently recommended two-dose measles immunization schedule, two doses of rubella vaccine now are recommended (American Academy of Pediatrics, 1994). There is a need to identify unimmunized children on entry into school and at intervals thereafter. All states have adopted mandatory rubella immunization as part of their health code. Concerns about potential transmission of disease from immunized children to susceptible contacts (including preg-

nant women) have not been supported by studies of susceptible household contacts. Therefore, susceptible children whose household contacts are pregnant can be vaccinated (CDC, 1984p). Rubella vaccine is given as a single subcutaneous injection of the antigen (0.5-ml dose given subcutaneously) or as part of a combined vaccine (such as MMR).

Rubella vaccine also should be administered to adolescent and adult women of childbearing age who have not been previously immunized. Premarital screening, routine gynecologic examinations, and the immediate postpartum period are excellent settings for immunization. Rubella vaccine should not be given 2 weeks before to 3 months after administration of HISG. It can be given after anti-Rho(D) immune globulin administration, but if it is given after the administration of blood products, seroconversion should be documented 6 to 8 weeks after vaccination. When practical, potential vaccinees can be screened for susceptibility. However, vaccination of women of childbearing age is justifiable and may be preferable without prior serologic testing in women not known to be pregnant. There is no increased risk of complications in individuals who are vaccinated but already immune (CDC, 1984p).

Women of childbearing age should be vaccinated only when they deny being pregnant and after they are counseled not to become pregnant for 3 months after vaccination. The theoretical risks to the fetus should be explained to them (discussed later).

Students or employees of childbearing age in educational or training institutions, such as colleges and military installations, should be considered for immunization on the basis of prior documented vaccination or serologic testing. Individuals working in hospitals or other health care facilities or any setting where women of childbearing age congregate should be immunized to avoid transmission to susceptible women. Men need not receive routine serologic screening before immunization. During rubella outbreaks, all susceptible individuals should be vaccinated promptly, except those for whom live viral vaccine is contraindicated. Although immunization after exposure probably does not prevent illness, it is not harmful and, if natural infection does not occur, vaccination ensures future immunity. International travelers should have documented rubella immunity.

Adverse Effects of Vaccine

Rubella vaccines generally are well tolerated. Rash, fever, or lymphadenopathy may occur in susceptible children. Arthralgia and arthritis occur in 1% to 5% of all children immunized (CDC, 1984p). The arthritis can occur several weeks after immunization, so its association with the vaccine is often overlooked. Because symptoms resemble rheumatoid arthritis or other related disorders, costly diagnostic evaluations often are undertaken. Arthralgia and arthritis are more frequent in older girls and women; 10% to 30% of these recipients experience these complications.

Unusual pain syndromes occur infrequently in recipients of rubella vaccine. Nonlocalized pain about the joints of the upper and lower extremities is believed to be caused by neuropathy induced by the vaccine. Two forms have been described: one involves the arms, with severe recurrent pain, usually at night, and the other involves the legs, with pain relieved by crouching (catcher's crouch syndrome). The time of onset is variable but can be as late as 70 days after vaccination. Episodes recur at varying intervals; one patient in Arizona had recurrent symptoms in the lower extremities for almost 2 years.

In a report of 214 susceptible women who inadvertently received a live attenuated rubella vaccine within 3 months before or after conception and carried their pregnancy to term, none of their infants had defects compatible with congenital rubella syndrome, although a small number showed serologic evidence of intrauterine infection (CDC, 1984q). Because rubella virus has been isolated from the products of conception of women vaccinated during pregnancy, continued caution with respect to vaccination during pregnancy is advised. However, based on the available evidence, the CDC (1984p) suggests that inadvertent rubella vaccination during pregnancy does not ordinarily represent a reason to consider interruption of pregnancy.

Precautions and Contraindications

Specific contraindications of live rubella vaccine administration include:

- Pregnancy
- Immunodeficiency states (malignancy, primary immunodeficiency disease, immunosuppressive or corticosteroid therapy, and radiation therapy)
- Severe febrile illness
- Known history of anaphylactic reaction to neomycin, a component of the vaccine

Mumps Immunization

Rationale for Active Immunization

Mumps is a viral disease of glandular tissue mostly affecting preteenagers. It usually is mild but can be severe, and complications occur often enough to warrant immunization. Mumps is a risk for postpubertal males, since 20% develop orchitis, a painful, incapacitating disease, although sterility is extremely rare (Candel, 1951).

Mumps is a leading cause of clinical meningoencephalitis and, in even greater numbers, a cause of subclinical meningoencephalitis (Wilfert, 1969). Mumps has also been suspected as a cause of juvenile diabetes mellitus, based on its predilection for infecting the pancreas and the concordance between waves of mumps infection followed by juvenile diabetes mellitus 2 to 4 years later (Sultz, et al., 1975).

Originally, there was some reluctance to recommend mumps vaccine routinely for all infants; authorities preferred instead to restrict its use to prepubertal boys and susceptible men. Since 1967, these restraints have been modified, accounting for a marked reduction in epidemic parotitis. Five thousand two hundred ninety-two cases were reported in 1990, which represents a 97% reduction from the 185,691 cases reported in 1967 (CDC, 1984h). The routine inclusion of mumps vaccine as part of the MMR immunization has conferred mumps immunity to 95% of those entering school in the school year 1982–1983 (CDC, 1983b). In most states, immunity to mumps is required for school entry; states without this requirement have a twofold higher incidence of reported mumps than those that have this legislation. The occurrence of recent outbreaks among children 10 to 14 years old reflects in part an emphasis on selective immunization laws aimed only at children entering school (CDC, 1982f, 1984n).

Immunizing Antigen

A mumps virus isolated from Dr. Maurice Hilleman's daughter, Jeryl Lynn (hence the term *Jeryl Lynn strain*), was attenuated by passage in chick embryo tissue culture (Hilleman et al., 1968b) and used for the vaccine. After testing in 6000 children, it was licensed in 1967. It produces no significant symptoms, and over 96% of recipients develop antibody titers (lower than that following natural infection), which persist for more than 15 years (CDC, 1982f, 1983b, 1984h). Reported clinical vaccine efficacies have ranged from 75% to 90% (CDC, 1982f, 1983b, 1984h). A lack of immunity after mumps immunization can be caused by improperly stored vaccine. Before reconstitution, mumps vaccine must be stored at 2°C to 8°C or colder and protected from light. After reconstitution, the vaccine should be used within 8 hours or discarded.

Immunity

Mumps is one of the few viruses for which cell-mediated immunity can be evaluated, since mumps virus antigens injected intradermally provoke a delayed hypersensitivity response. Although the exact role of cell-mediated immunity is unknown, there is evidence that it plays a role in the disease as well as in recovery. Immunity is associated with the presence of serum antibody that occurs following natural disease or vaccination. Two or more episodes of mumps are best explained by other viral agents that produce parotitis.

Vaccine Usage

For primary immunization in infants, mumps virus vaccine is routinely included in pediatric immunization schedules (CDC, 1982f; American Academy of Pediatrics, 1994). A single dose of mumps vaccine, either alone or as MMR, is injected subcutaneously at 15 months of age. A second dose of MMR now is recommended at 11 or 12 years of age (American Academy of Pediatrics, 1994).

Mumps virus vaccine can be administered to boys and men. A history of mumps can be misleading, since other viruses can produce parotitis. Further, failure to recall mumps is no guarantee that one has not been infected; 30% of childhood mumps cases are asymptomatic.

Susceptible individuals exposed to mumps, particularly male adolescents or men, can be immunized with mumps vaccine, but there is no guarantee that mumps will be averted. However, if mumps does not occur, the individual is protected against subsequent exposures.

Precautions and Contraindications

The use of mumps vaccine is associated with few side effects. The frequency of reported central nervous system dysfunction after vaccination may be even lower than the observed background rate in the unimmunized. Anyone with a history of anaphylactic reaction to egg ingestion should be vaccinated only with extreme caution. Individuals with histories of nonanaphylactic reactions to egg ingestion or allergies to chicken or feathers are not at increased risk of vaccine-associated reactions. A person with a history of anaphylactic reaction to neomycin, which is present in the vaccine, should not be vaccinated. However, those with cutaneous hypersensitivity (contact dermatitis) to neomycin may be vaccinated.

Because of the theoretical risk of fetal damage, mumps vaccine should not be administered to pregnant women. Lymphoreticular or other generalized malignancy and primary or secondary immunodeficiency states represent other specific contraindications for this live viral vaccine. Since infection after vaccination is noncommunicable, mumps vaccine may be given to susceptible close contacts of immunosuppressed patients to help reduce the likelihood of exposure to natural measles. Mumps vaccination generally should be avoided during acute illness with high-grade fever. In addition, it should not be given until 3 months after the administration of immune serum globulin because passively acquired antibody may interfere with the active immune response (CDC, 1982f).

Haemophilus influenzae Type b Immunization

Rationale for Active Immunization

Haemophilus influenzae type b (Hib) is the leading cause of bacterial meningitis in this country, accounting for one half of all cases. More than 90% of meningitis cases from Hib occur in children under 5 years old (11,000 cases annually). Among these cases, 80% occur in children under 2 years old, and most of these are in children younger than 18 months old. The peak attack rate occurs in children 6 to 8 months old. Hib meningitis is fatal in 3% to 10% of cases, and neurologic sequelae occur in 20% to 35% of survivors. Hib also is the primary cause of epiglottitis and a common cause of sepsis, pneumonia, septic arthritis, and cellulitis in children, accounting for about 7300 cases of nonmeningeal invasive disease annually (Cochi et al., 1985).

Groups at high risk for Hib disease include Native Americans, Alaskan natives, blacks, persons of low socioeconomic status, patients with anatomic or functional asplenia, including sickle cell disease, and those with immunodeficiency states, including Hodgkin's disease and primary antibody deficiency syndromes. Day care center attendees (Redmond and Pichichero, 1984; Fleming et al., 1985) and those under 4 years old who are household contacts of patients with invasive Hib disease (Ward et al., 1979) also may be at high risk. Recommendations for the prevention of secondary cases in such settings through the use of rifampin are available (American Academy of Pediatrics, 1994).

Immunizing Antigens

Haemophilus **Type b Polysaccharide Vaccine.** The first Hib vaccine, licensed for use in the United States in April 1985, contained the purified Hib capsular polysaccharide polyribosyl-ribitol phosphate (PRP) (b-CAPSE I vaccine, Praxis Biologics). Development of this vaccine was based on observations that serum antibodies directed against PRP provide protection against Hib disease. Whereas the protective level of Hib capsular antibody in the unimmunized may be greater than 0.15 µg/ml, data suggest that a serum level of at least 1.0 µg/ml 3 weeks after immunization correlates with subsequent protection (Kaythy et al., 1983). As with other polysaccharide vaccines, immunogenicity of the Hib vaccine in children is age dependent. Vaccine responsiveness increases markedly at about 16 to 20 months of age. Protective antibody levels are observed after vaccination in 45% of children 12 to 17 months old, 75% of vaccinees 18 to 23 months old, and 90% of those 24 to 35 months old. Furthermore, the duration of protective antibody levels is related to the age of vaccinees. In those vaccinated before 18 months of age, serum antibody levels are less than protective within 6 months. Protective antibody levels remain for at least 1½ but not 3½ years after immunization in those 18 to 35 months of age, whereas protective levels remain at least 3½ years in those vaccinated at 3 to 5 years of age (Kaythy et al., 1984).

The clinical efficacy of the first-generation Hib PRP vaccine was prospectively evaluated in Finland in a double-blind study (Peltola et al., 1977a) on children 3 to 71 months of age. In this study, approximately 50,000 children received an Hib vaccine similar to that later licensed in the United States and 50,000 received group A meningococcal vaccine. In this trial, protection was correlated with the production of an anticapsular antibody concentration that exceeded 1.0 µg/ml in serum obtained 3 weeks after immunization. In children immunized at 18 to 71 months of age, the protective efficacy was 90%; among those immunized at 18 to 23 months of age, the small number of cases in the vaccine and the control group precluded a definitive conclusion. In 8453 children immunized at 2 years of age (24 to 35 months), the efficacy was 80% (Daum and Granoff, 1985). No efficacy was observed in children 3 to 17 months. These data led the Committee on Infectious Diseases to recommend immunization with PRP for all children at 24 months of age. The results of post-marketing case-control studies after licensure in

1985 indicated that PRP is effective, although its efficacy in 2-year-old American children may be lower than that found in Finland. Lack of efficacy was reported in Minnesota (Osterholm et al., 1987), and several investigators have suggested that an excess of infections occurred during the week after immunization with PRP (Black et al., 1987; CDC, 1988).

***Haemophilus* Type b Conjugate Vaccine (Diphtheria Toxoid Conjugate).** With the ultimate goal of providing an effective vaccine for infants and younger children, Schneerson and coworkers (1985) covalently linked the capsular polysaccharide of *H. influenzae* to a protein carrier. Several manufacturers have prepared "conjugate" vaccines suitable for use in children. The first of these, the diphtheria toxoid conjugate vaccine (PRP-D), is approved for use in children 15 months of age or older. The immunogenicity of PRP-D is significantly greater than that observed with PRP in children 18 months of age or older (Pincus et al., 1982; CDC, 1982, 1988; Berkowitz et al., 1987).

During 1990, the U.S. Food and Drug Administration (FDA) approved two *H. influenzae* type b conjugate vaccines for use in infants 2 months of age and older. The carrier protein for one (HbOC) is a nontoxic mutant diphtheria toxin, whereas the carrier for the other vaccine (PRP-OMP) consists of an outer membrane protein complex of *Neisseria meningitidis*. Approval was based in part on a review of two large studies in the United States that demonstrated the protective efficacy of these vaccines (Black et al., 1991; Santosham et al., 1991). In one of these studies, more than 20,000 infants were given HbOC vaccine at 2, 4, and 6 months of age. Three cases of invasive *H. influenzae* type b disease occurred among infants who had received only one dose of vaccine; invasive disease was not reported in any infant who had received at least two doses.

Another *H. influenzae* type b conjugate vaccine, which uses tetanus toxoid as the carrier protein (PRP-T), has been approved for use in infants as young as 2 months of age. In addition, the oligosaccharide conjugate vaccine (HbOC) has been combined with DTP for ease of administration to young infants.

Vaccine Usage

The routine schedule for *H. influenzae* type b immunization during infancy is shown in Table 29–2. The same conjugate vaccine should be used for all doses administered to infants under 12 months of age. Only HbOC, PRP-OMP, or PRP-T should be given to children younger than age 12 months. The first two vaccine doses are given at 2 and 4 months of age. If either HbOC or PRP-T is used, a third dose is given at age 6 months. A booster vaccination is given at 12 to 15 months of age.

Unimmunized children between the ages of 15 and 60 months should receive one dose of any licensed conjugate vaccine. Immunization against *H. influenzae* type b generally is not indicated in children older than age 5; however, a single dose of any licensed conjugate vaccine is recommended for children over age 5 who have chronic illnesses associated with an increased risk of *H. influenzae* type b disease. Unimmunized children younger than 24 months of age who experience invasive *H. influenzae* type b disease should be immunized beginning 1 to 2 months after recovery from the acute illness. Children who have such disease at 24 months of age or older generally do not require immunization because of natural disease-induced immunity.

All of the conjugate vaccines appear to be safe and well tolerated. No increased incidence of invasive *H. influenzae* type b disease in the weeks after immunization has been reported.

Hepatitis B Immunization

Rationale for Active Immunization

Hepatitis B is reported in about 16,000 persons annually in the United States (CDC, 1994). About 1% of reported cases are associated with fulminant disease and death. There are about 1 million chronic carriers of hepatitis B in this country, many of whom ultimately develop cirrhosis or hepatic carcinoma.

Children become infected with hepatitis B in a variety of ways. The risk of perinatal hepatitis B infection among infants born to mothers with hepatitis B ranges from 10% to 85%, depending on maternal factors. Infants with perinatal hepatitis B infection have a 90% risk of chronic infection, and up to 25% die of chronic liver disease.

Because selective screening of pregnant women fails to identify a high percentage of those infected with hepatitis B, universal screening of all pregnant women for hepatitis B is recommended (CDC, 1991b). The continuing occurrence of hepatitis B infections despite the availability, since 1982, of an effective vaccine has led to a recommendation for universal childhood immunization against hepatitis B (CDC, 1991b; American Academy of Pediatrics, 1992b).

Immunizing Antigen

The first licensed hepatitis B vaccine was a suspension of inactivated and purified plasma–derived hepatitis B surface antigen. It is no longer produced in the United States, and its use is limited to hemodialysis patients, immunocompromised hosts, and persons with known allergy to yeast. The plasma-derived vaccine is immunogenic, effective, and safe.

The available recombinant hepatitis B vaccines are produced using hepatitis B surface antigen synthesized by *Saccharomyces cerevisiae* (baker's yeast) into which a plasmid containing the hepatitis B surface antigen gene has been inserted. The purified product is obtained by lysis of the yeast and chemical and physical separation. Hepatitis B vaccines contain 10 to 40 µg of hepatitis B surface antigen protein per milliliter after adsorption to aluminum hydroxide (0.5 mg/ml). Thimerosal (1:20,000 concentration) is included as a preservative. The yeast protein content is 5% or less of the final product.

A three-dose schedule of recombinant hepatitis B vaccine produces adequate antibody responses in 90%

to 95% of healthy recipients. Field trials of the vaccines licensed in the United States have shown 80% to 95% protective efficacy. The most common side effect is soreness at the injection site; hypersensitivity to yeast or thimerosal has been reported.

Vaccine Usage

Primary immunization against hepatitis B should be administered using a three-dose schedule beginning in early infancy (CDC, 1991). The first vaccine dose can be administered at birth before hospital discharge, with subsequent doses administered at 1 to 2 and 6 to 18 months of age. Alternatively, the three vaccine doses can be administered at 1 to 2, 4, and 6 to 18 months of age. Because hepatitis B vaccine can be administered simultaneously with other vaccines, the latter schedule has the advantage of minimizing the required number of health care visits.

In addition to its routine use during infancy, hepatitis B immunization is indicated in certain other groups at high risk of hepatitis B infection:

1. Adolescents who have multiple sex partners or who are injecting drugs, and those who reside in communities where such activity is prevalent.
2. Persons with occupational risk for infection (health care or public safety workers).
3. Clients and staff of institutions for the developmentally disabled.
4. Hemodialysis patients.
5. Recipients of certain blood products (e.g., clotting factor concentrates).
6. Household contacts and sex partners of chronic hepatitis B carriers.
7. Adoptees from countries where hepatitis B infection is endemic.
8. International travelers.
9. Users of injection drugs.
10. Sexually active homosexual and bisexual men.
11. Sexually active heterosexual men and women.
12. Inmates of long-term correctional facilities.

A three-dose vaccine schedule similar to that employed during infancy is recommended.

The doses of recombinant hepatitis B vaccines used in children and adults vary by patient age and the vaccine preparation used; package inserts should be consulted.

The immunogenicity and efficacy of hepatitis B vaccines in hemodialysis patients are lower than in healthy individuals; larger doses of the standard recombinant or plasma-derived vaccines should be used. A more concentrated formulation of recombinant vaccine (Recombivax HB) is also available for use in dialysis patients. Vaccine is administered intramuscularly. In older children and adults, the deltoid area of the upper arm is the recommended site for vaccination because of reduced immunogenicity when vaccine is administered in the buttocks. The anterolateral thigh is preferred for infants.

The schedules outlined above are appropriate only for hepatitis B pre-exposure prophylaxis. Postexposure prophylaxis entails administration not only of hepatitis B vaccine but also of hepatitis B immunoglobulin (HBIG). In the case of infants born to mothers with hepatitis B infection, HBIG (0.5 ml, intramuscularly) should be administered as soon as possible after birth (preferably within 12 hours). In addition to HBIG, hepatitis B vaccination should be initiated within 7 days (preferably within 12 hours) of birth. The first dose of hepatitis B vaccine can be given simultaneously with HBIG, provided it is given with a separate syringe and at a different body site.

Influenza Immunization

Influenza outbreaks occur each year in the United States and the potential for epidemic (pandemic) spread of this disease in susceptible human populations is well recognized. Periodic minor antigenic shifts of influenza A or B virus account for most influenzal disease yearly; these outbreaks generally are limited in magnitude, although the extent of morbidity and mortality remains unacceptably high. Major antigenic changes of influenza A virus, as occurred in 1957 and 1958 (Asian strain) and again in 1968 and 1969 (Hong Kong variant), account for pandemic spread of disease associated with greater overall morbidity and mortality in highly susceptible populations.

With respect to most prevailing influenza A and B viruses in civilian populations, primary prevention with available vaccines has been directed only at individuals and patient groups at high risk as a result of underlying systemic disease. Prophylaxis may be achieved in the most cost-effective manner by vaccinating individuals in whom there is a higher than average potential for infection and in whom infection can have severe consequences (Paisley et al., 1978; Glezen, 1980; Glezen et al., 1983; CDC, 1993b). Difficulties in identifying new antigenic variants (multiple minor variants may be prevalent simultaneously) and the subsequent preparation, testing, and provision of new vaccines have precluded routine mass immunization for most influenza strains.

In the United States, only inactivated vaccines are licensed for prevention of influenza. Since their introduction more than 40 years ago, refinements in their production have largely eliminated the toxic manifestations commonly observed after vaccination in the past. After receiving the vaccine by parenteral administration, nearly all young adults develop hemagglutination-inhibition antibody titers that are likely to be protective. If provided under optimal conditions (i.e., at an appropriate time and against the prevailing influenzal strain), these vaccines can reduce the incidence of disease by 75% to 80% (Glezen, 1980). Unfortunately, protection afforded by inactivated vaccine is transient; yearly injections are necessary even when no significant antigenic changes of a prevailing influenzal strain have occurred. As a result of rapid and repeated changes in policy, health care personnel should refer to current statements by the CDC (1993b) published periodically in *Morbidity and Mortality Weekly Report*.

Vaccine Usage

Available inactivated vaccines include whole, intact virus particles and split-product preparations derived by disrupting whole virus with organic solvents. In newer preparations, immunogenicity and reactogenicity of split and whole virus vaccines have been shown to be similar in adults (CDC, 1993b), but field studies of the efficacy of split-product vaccines in children are lacking (Glezen, 1980). Because protective influenza vaccines must contain strains antigenically similar to those strains expected to be prevalent during a given respiratory season, the formulation of vaccines is changed periodically. Recommended formulations generally include multivalent products containing recent antigenic variants of influenza A and influenza B strains.

Influenza vaccine is recommended for patients 6 months of age or older who are at high risk for disease, for their medical care personnel, and for anyone who wishes to decrease the risk of illness from influenza. Annual vaccination against influenza is recommended for individuals at high risk of lower respiratory tract complications or death following influenza infection. These high-risk groups have been classified further on the basis of priority into defined target groups for which vaccination is most necessary and include the following (CDC, 1993b):

1. Persons 65 years or older.
2. Residents of nursing homes and other chronic care facilities.
3. Adults and children with chronic disorders of the pulmonary or cardiovascular systems, including children with asthma.
4. Adults and children who have required regular medical follow-up or hospitalization during the preceding year because of chronic metabolic disease, renal dysfunction, hematoglobinopathies, or immunosuppression.
5. Children and teenagers who are receiving long-term aspirin therapy and therefore may be at risk for Reye syndrome.

Medical personnel can transmit influenza infections to their high-risk patients while they are themselves incubating an infection, undergoing subclinical infection, or working despite the existence of symptoms (Glezen, 1980). The potential for introducing influenza to high-risk groups with compromised cardiopulmonary or immune systems or infants in neonatal intensive care units should be reduced by vaccination programs targeted at medical personnel. Annual influenza vaccination of physicians, nurses, and other personnel who have extensive contact with high-risk patient groups is recommended (CDC, 1993b).

Persons who provide essential community services (e.g., fire and police department personnel and health care workers), although not at increased risk of serious influenzal disease, may be offered vaccine to minimize disruption of services during outbreaks. Furthermore, any person wishing to reduce the risk of acquiring influenza infections should be vaccinated (CDC, 1993b).

Current influenza vaccines generally are well tolerated; fewer than one third of vaccines have been reported to develop local redness or induration for 1 to 2 days at the injection site. Systemic reactions, including fever, chills, headache, and malaise, although infrequent, most often affect children who have had no previous exposure to the influenza virus antigens contained in the vaccine. These reactions, attributable to influenza antigens, generally begin 6 to 12 hours after vaccination and persist for only 1 to 2 days. As a result of its diminished potential for causing febrile reactions, only split (subviron) vaccine is recommended for use in children under 13 years old. However, a single dose of split-product vaccine may be significantly less immunogenic than a single dose of whole virus preparation. Therefore, the administration of two doses of the available split-product vaccine separated by at least 4 weeks is recommended for children who have not received vaccines previously (CDC, 1993b). Variable immunogenicity of influenza vaccine has been reported among immunocompromised individuals, including those with malignancy; successful immunologic responses in these populations are most likely to occur when these individuals have been immunized with antigenically similar influenzal strains (Gross et al., 1978; Lange et al., 1979).

Recommended dosage of split-product influenza vaccine is 0.25 ml for patients 6 to 35 months of age and 0.5 ml for older patients. Whole virus vaccine preparations should be administered at a dosage of 0.5 ml. The vaccines should be administered into the deltoid muscle whenever possible. Infants and young children can be vaccinated in the anterolateral thigh muscle (CDC, 1993b).

Chemoprophylaxis or chemotherapy also should be considered, but it should not replace active immunization against influenza. Both amantadine and rimantidine are approved for prophylaxis of influenza A virus infections in children and adults. Rimantidine is as effective as amantadine and has fewer side effects (e.g., agitation, insomnia, or seizures). Although not effective against influenza B, amantadine or rimantidine prophylaxis can be considered for use during influenza A outbreaks:

• When the vaccine may be relatively ineffective or unavailable
• As an adjunct to late immunization of high-risk individuals until the immune response to the vaccine has developed (a period of 6 weeks for primary immunization of young children [two doses of vaccine, 4 weeks apart] and 2 weeks for booster immunization)
• To supplement protection afforded by vaccination of high-risk patients in whom a poor immunologic response may be expected
• To protect those few high-risk individuals for whom influenza vaccine is contraindicated because of anaphylactic hypersensitivity or a previous severe reaction to influenza vaccine
• To protect high-risk patients in the hospital from developing nosocomial influenza A infection

• As chemoprophylaxis of medical personnel who have extensive contact with high-risk patients but have not been vaccinated (CDC, 1993b)

Amantadine or rimantidine also should be considered for therapeutic use in high-risk patients (regardless of vaccine status) who develop an illness compatible with influenza during a period of influenza A activity in the community. In such patients, the drug should be given within 24 to 48 hours of onset of illness and continued until 48 hours after resolution of symptoms. Amantadine should be used with caution in patients with impaired renal function or active seizure disorders (CDC, 1985e). Use of amantadine or rimantidine in infants less than 1 year of age has not been evaluated adequately.

Precautions and Contraindications

Because influenza vaccine is prepared in embryonated chick eggs, persons with known anaphylactic hypersensitivity to egg protein should not be vaccinated. Even though current influenza vaccines contain only a small quantity of egg protein, severe hypersensitivity reactions occur rarely and probably are attributable to sensitivity to residual egg protein (CDC, 1993b). Despite concerns about a theoretical risk of vaccine-associated Guillain-Barré syndrome, there is essentially no risk of developing the syndrome after vaccination.

Hepatitis A Immunization

Rationale for Active Immunization

Hepatitis A is the most prevalent form of infectious hepatitis in the United States. In 1992, 23,112 cases of hepatitis A were reported to the CDC (CDC, 1994); the death rate from fulminant hepatitis A was estimated to be about 0.7%. The cost associated with hepatitis A infection is about $200 million dollars annually.

Hepatitis A infection is acquired via fecal-oral transmission. Poor sanitation, contamination of drinking water, and improper sewage disposal contribute to spread of the virus. As a consequence, the incidence and age at acquisition of hepatitis A vary greatly in different geographic locales. In the developing world, acquisition of hepatitis A in childhood is the rule, whereas only about 40% of United States residents are infected with the virus by age 20 years (CDC, 1994). About one in five reported cases in the United States occurs in children younger than 10 years of age. Because asymptomatic disease is common in children, case report data undoubtedly underestimate the true prevalence of infection in the pediatric age group.

Children often are implicated in transmission of hepatitis A to older siblings and adults. Icterus is observed in 70% to 80% of young adults with hepatitis A infection. In contrast, 10% or fewer of children younger than 5 years of age become icteric.

Immunizing Antigen

Hepatitis A vaccine is prepared by propagation of human-derived virus strain HM175 in human diploid cells, followed by purification and inactivation with formalin. Each 1-ml adult dose of vaccine contains not less than 1440 ELISA units (EL.U.) of viral antigen, adsorbed on aluminum hydroxide. Each 0.5-ml pediatric dose of vaccine contains not less than 360 EL.U. of viral antigen, also adsorbed on aluminum hydroxide. The vaccine contains 2-phenoxyethanol as a preservative.

Two inactivated hepatitis A vaccines, including the currently licensed product, have been demonstrated to be highly efficacious in placebo-controlled trials in children older than age 2 (Werzberger et al., 1992; Innis et al., 1994). The vaccines are usually associated with only mild local reactions; systemic reactions are very rare. Vaccination appears to be protective for at least 3 years, and extrapolation models suggest protection for a minimum of 10 years (CDC, 1994; Berger and Just, 1992).

Vaccine Usage

Hepatitis A vaccine is administered by the intramuscular route. The deltoid region of the upper arm is the preferred site of injection; gluteal injection may result in a suboptimal antibody response. Primary vaccination of adults consists of a single adult vaccine dose (1440 EL.U.). Primary vaccination of children aged 2 to 18 years consists of two pediatric vaccine doses (360 EL.U.) given at least 1 month apart. A booster dose, given 6 to 12 months after initiation of primary vaccination, is recommended for both adults and children in order to ensure high anti–hepatitis A antibody titers.

Immunocompromised individuals may not develop adequate antibody titers in response to routine vaccination. Such individuals may require additional vaccine doses.

Hepatitis A immunization is indicated for adults and children at least 2 years of age who desire protection against hepatitis A. Individuals who are at high risk for hepatitis A and therefore might be particularly good candidates for vaccination include the following:

1. Travelers to areas endemic for hepatitis A.
2. Military personnel.
3. Individuals residing in areas of high endemicity.
4. Certain ethnic and geographic populations that experience cyclic hepatitis A epidemics, including Native Americans and Alaskan natives.
5. Other high-risk individuals, including homosexual males, users of illicit injectable drugs, and residents of a community experiencing a hepatitis A outbreak.
6. Individuals exposed to hepatitis A (immune serum globulin should be given concomitantly).

Varicella Virus Immunization

Rationale for Active Immunization

About 3.9 million cases of varicella (chickenpox) occur annually in the United States (American Academy of Pediatrics, 1995). Varicella typically occurs in children younger than 10 years of age, but 5% to 10% of adults are susceptible.

Most cases of varicella in otherwise healthy children are self-limited and free of complications. Possible complications include bacterial superinfection, Reye syndrome, pneumonitis, and encephalitis. The CDC receives reports of about 90 fatal cases of varicella annually in the United States, mostly in otherwise healthy children. Severe varicella infections are observed with increased frequency in certain groups of individuals, including adults, and children immunocompromised by cancer chemotherapy, corticosteroid therapy, or congenital or acquired immunodeficiency states. A congenital varicella syndrome occurs in about 2% of infants born to mothers who have varicella in the first or second trimester of pregnancy.

The economic costs associated with varicella are substantial. In a study published in 1985, it was estimated that the annual health care costs for varicella were $399 million (Preblud et al. 1985). A cost-benefit analysis published in 1994 concluded that routine varicella vaccination at 1 year of age could result in savings of $384 million annually in the United States (Lieu et al., 1994).

Immunizing Antigen

The vaccine is a cell-free, live, attenuated preparation of the Oka strain of varicella-zoster virus. The virus was obtained initially from a child with natural varicella and was propagated sequentially in human embryonic lung cell cultures, embryonic guinea pig cell cultures, and human diploid cell cultures. Each 0.5-ml vaccine dose contains a minimum of 1350 plaque-forming units of varicella-zoster virus.

Varicella vaccine is supplied as a lyophilized product containing sucrose, phosphate, glutamate, and processed gelatin as stabilizers as well as trace amounts of neomycin. It must be stored frozen at a temperature of $-15°C$ ($+5°F$) or colder. The storage life is up to 18 months. To ensure viral potency, vaccine must be administered within 30 minutes of reconstitution.

The vaccine is efficacious in adults and children 1 year of age or older. All studies demonstrate high rates of protection against severe disease ($>95\%$ protection after household exposure) (American Academy of Pediatrics, 1995). Vaccinees, as compared with unvaccinated children, experience much milder cases of varicella, with fewer skin lesions, less fever, and more rapid recovery. During 8 years of study, the annual rate of varicella among vaccinees has averaged from less than 1% to 3% after exposure to wild virus compared with an annual rate of 7% to 8% in unvaccinated children (Asano et al., 1985; Watson et al., 1993). Waning immunity has not been demonstrated.

Adverse events occur uncommonly after varicella immunization, consisting predominantly of mild maculopapular or varicelliform rash (fewer than 10% of vaccine recipients) and mild local reactions at the injection site (about 20% of children and 25% to 35% of adolescents and adults). Zoster occurs with lower frequency after immunization than after natural disease and reported cases have been mild. Transmission of vaccine strain varicella-zoster virus by vaccinees is a theoretical possibility. Clinical cases of varicella from contact with healthy vaccinees have not been reported. Spread of vaccine virus by vaccinees with leukemia and vaccine-associated rash has been reported; contact cases had subclinical or mild illness (Tsolia et al., 1990).

Vaccine Usage

Varicella vaccine is administered subcutaneously. The outer aspect of the upper arm (deltoid) is the preferred site of injection. Primary immunization of children aged 12 months to 12 years consists of a single 0.5-ml vaccine dose. Individuals 13 years of age or older should receive two 0.5-ml vaccine doses separated by at least 4 to 8 weeks. Varicella vaccine may be given simultaneously with MMR vaccine, but separate syringes and injection sites should be used. If not done simultaneously, administration of varicella vaccine and MMR should be separated by an interval of at least one month. There is no evidence to suggest that varicella vaccine and any other routine vaccines interact in any way that would adversely affect immune responses to vaccination.

Varicella vaccination is contraindicated in the following individuals (American Academy of Pediatrics, 1995):

1. Immunocompromised children, including those with congenital immunodeficiency, blood dyscrasias, leukemia, lymphoma, HIV infection, and malignancy for which they are receiving immunosuppressive therapy.
2. Individuals who have been receiving high-dose systemic corticosteroids for greater than one month.
3. Pregnant women.
4. Individuals with a history of anaphylactoid reactions to neomycin.

The vaccine should not be administered within 5 months of receipt of intravenous immune globulin or other blood products. Because of the theoretical risk of vaccine-associated Reye syndrome, the manufacturer recommends avoidance of salicylates for 6 weeks following immunization.

VACCINES INFREQUENTLY INDICATED FOR SELECTED INDIVIDUALS

Anthrax Vaccine

Anthrax is of public health importance only to select, high-risk, occupationally related segments of the United States population, including veterinarians, those working with *Bacillus anthracis* in the laboratory, and persons who process potentially contaminated animal products, such as textile and felt mill workers. The use of anthrax vaccine among these high-risk groups has significantly reduced anthrax-related morbidity. Of primary importance in the prevention of this disease is a continued awareness of the potential for transmission of anthrax to those at risk and surveillance of anthrax disease among animal populations. Frequent cleaning of working facilities, decontamination of potentially contaminated raw materials, and optimal personal hygiene are other effective preventive measures.

Anthrax vaccine is available from the Michigan Department of Public Health, Lansing, or through the CDC (1984a). It consists of an aluminum hydroxide–adsorbed concentrate of "protective antigen" prepared from a nonencapsulated strain of *B. anthracis* (Puziss and Wright, 1963). Field trials using similar vaccines in human populations have demonstrated their effectiveness (92%) with minimal local reactions (Brachman et al., 1962). Anthrax vaccine should be considered for individuals in high-risk occupations. A basic series consists of six 0.5-ml injections given subcutaneously, the first three at 2-week intervals and the next three at 6-month intervals. When continued occupation-associated exposure is anticipated, booster injections (0.5 ml) are recommended yearly (CDC, 1984a).

BCG Vaccine

The incidence of tuberculosis is increasing in the United States. Nevertheless, the overall prevalence of tuberculosis in this country is not sufficient to justify routine primary prevention through active immunization programs. Almost 26,300 cases of tuberculosis were reported to the CDC in 1991 (Jereb et al., 1993). Furthermore, the number of cases recognized in pediatric age groups continues to represent only a small proportion of total cases (1662 cases in children under 15 years old in 1991). Efforts to recognize and control tuberculosis in the United States are directed primarily at the early identification and treatment of active cases followed by surveillance of closely related individuals and the institution of appropriate preventive measures for those at high risk. In only selected instances, the risk of exposure to recognized cases is significant enough to consider primary immunization with bacille Calmette-Guérin (BCG) vaccine. Of importance to the pediatrician is the risk to infants born to tuberculous mothers or to those living in a household with an identified tuberculous individual (Avery and Wotsdorf, 1968).

BCG is a live, attenuated strain derived from *Mycobacterium bovis*. All available BCG vaccines are derived from the original strain but vary in their immunogenic and reactogenic properties. Efficacy trials before 1955 of previously available liquid BCG vaccines demonstrated variable efficacy from 0% to 80% (Luelmo, 1982; Clemens et al., 1983), but freeze-dried preparations available in the United States represent further attenuated strains; their efficacy has not been demonstrated in controlled clinical trials. BCG preparations have been associated with localized reactions (ulceration, lymphadenitis, or both in 1% to 10%) and osteomyelitis (1 per million vaccinees and possibly higher in newborns). Fatal or disseminated BCG infection (1 to 10 per 10 million vaccinees) occurs almost exclusively in immunocompromised children (CDC, 1979b).

BCG administration represents only an ancillary measure in the public health armamentarium designed to identify, treat, and prevent tuberculosis in this country. Individuals with negative tuberculin skin tests who have had or are likely to have repeated exposure to untreated or ineffectively treated, sputum-positive pulmonary tuberculosis are candidates for BCG. Immunization should be considered for those at risk in well-defined communities or groups in which high infectivity rates have been demonstrated and in which therapeutic or preventive measures are difficult to implement (e.g., medically indigent or migrant populations). Some health workers may be at increased risk of repeated exposure, especially those working in settings where the prevalence of tuberculosis is relatively high (CDC, 1979b; Thompson et al., 1979).

Vaccination with BCG should be considered only for uninfected children who are at unavoidable risk for continued exposure to tuberculosis and for whom other prevention strategies are not feasible. Recommended vaccine recipients include infants and children who have negative tuberculin skin tests, who live in households with repeated or persistent exposure to infectious cases of tuberculosis, and who live in groups with a rate of new tuberculous infections exceeding 1% per year if other control strategies have failed (American Academy of Pediatrics, 1994).

BCG should be given only to individuals who are skin-test negative to 5 tuberculin units (TU) of tuberculin purified protein derivative (PPD). Preparations available in the United States can be administered either percutaneously or intradermally. Recommended dosages are 0.05 ml for infants under 1 month of age and 0.1 ml for older infants, children, and adolescents. Recipients of BCG should have follow-up tuberculin skin tests 2 to 3 months later to establish that tuberculin sensitivity has been acquired; failure to react dictates the need for another BCG injection. In general, the tuberculin reaction to BCG vaccine measures 7 to 15 mm of induration and diminishes gradually over 5 years.

BCG should not be administered to individuals with primary or secondary immunodeficiency states, including chronic granulomatous disease. Leukemia, lymphoma, or other generalized malignancies; HIV infection; immunosuppressive therapy (cytotoxic agents, corticosteroids, or irradiation); disseminated skin infections; and burns all constitute specific contraindications to BCG administration. Although no harmful effects of BCG have been documented in the fetus, it is reasonable to avoid vaccination during pregnancy unless an immediate excessive risk of exposure is unavoidable.

Subsequent to immunization with BCG, it may be difficult to distinguish between a tuberculin reaction representing acquired tuberculous suprainfection and persisting postvaccination sensitivity. Because the degree and duration of protection against tuberculous disease afforded by BCG is uncertain, a positive tuberculin reaction must always be suspected to be disease-related, especially if a recent exposure to active tuberculosis is identified (CDC, 1979b; Fox and Lepow, 1983; American Academy of Pediatrics, 1994).

Cholera Vaccine

Cholera vaccines are of limited value. Only rare cases of cholera have been recognized in the United States in the past decade, although cholera remains a significant public health concern in African and Asian countries. Even in these countries, however, the risk to American travelers is low, and persons following tourist itineraries who use standard accommodations are at virtually no risk. A traveler's best protection against contracting cholera is to avoid food and water that may be contaminated. Cholera vaccination is indicated only for travelers to countries that require evidence of cholera vaccination for entry, although the World Health Organization no longer recommends cholera vaccination for any travelers. The available vaccines are phenol-inactivated suspensions of several strains of *Vibrio cholerae*. In field trials conducted in cholera-endemic regions, these vaccines have been shown to be only about 50% effective in reducing the incidence of clinical illness for 3 to 6 months after vaccination (CDC, 1978a, 1984b, 1984c).

Travelers to countries with entry requirements should obtain a validated international certificate of vaccination documenting receipt of vaccine 6 days to 6 months before entry. Most city, county, and state health departments can validate certificates. Only a single dose is needed to satisfy international health regulations for most countries. A full primary series, recommended only for special high-risk groups working and living in endemic areas, includes two subcutaneous or intramuscular doses administered 1 week to 1 month or more apart. The dosage depends on age (6 months to 4 years, 0.2 ml; 5 to 10 years, 0.3 ml; >10 years, 0.5 ml). The vaccine also can be administered intradermally (0.2 ml) to individuals 5 years of age or older. These dosages are appropriate for all primary and booster immunizations. Booster doses are recommended at 6 months after primary immunization and at 6-month intervals thereafter when necessary. Vaccine is not recommended for infants under 6 months of age. Cholera and yellow fever vaccinations should be separated by at least 3 weeks. If time constraints preclude this, they can be given simultaneously (Felsenfeld et al., 1973; CDC, 1978a, 1984b).

Side effects of cholera vaccine include fever, malaise, headache, and tenderness, erythema, and induration at the injection site for 1 or 2 days. Serious reactions after cholera vaccine are rare but contraindicate revaccination.

Meningococcal Vaccine

Significant morbidity and mortality secondary to *Neisseria meningitidis* (purulent meningitis or septicemia) occur disproportionately in children; those under 5 years old account for half of all cases (CDC, 1993c), with the peak age incidence and mortality occurring during the first year of life. Serogroups B and C account for about 90% of the cases (CDC, 1993c). In children under 5 years old, serogroup B can account for over 70% of meningococcal disease (Band et al., 1983).

Routine immunization of civilians against meningococcal disease is not recommended for several reasons:

1. The overall risk of acquiring meningococcal disease in civilian populations is low.

2. No vaccine is currently available for serogroup B.
3. The current vaccines may be of little benefit in those at highest risk (infants).

Routine vaccination is recommended only for those who may be at high risk for meningococcal disease because of an underlying abnormality, such as deficiency of the terminal components of serum complement (Ellison et al., 1983), or anatomic or functional asplenia (CDC, 1985c).

However, preventive measures must be considered for selected contacts of identified meningococcal cases. Significant secondary attack rates occur in susceptible household contacts (3 per 1000); during epidemic conditions, household secondary attack rates can reach 10% (Munford et al., 1974; Meningococcal Disease Surveillance Group, 1976). Other selected groups, including contacts of cases in day care centers (Jacobson et al., 1977) or schools (Feigin et al., 1982), and hospital personnel who have intimate contact with patients before antimicrobials are administered, also may be at high risk (American Academy of Pediatrics, 1994).

Active immunization should be considered to control epidemic outbreaks of meningococcal disease. Although chemoprophylaxis is the primary means of limiting the spread of sporadic disease, active immunization of close contacts also can be considered in such cases, especially when additional cases are likely to occur during an extended period (American Academy of Pediatrics, 1994). About half of secondary household cases occur 5 or more days after the primary case (Greenwood et al., 1978), thereby allowing time for benefit from vaccination. Furthermore, unless chemoprophylaxis completely eliminates the transmission of *N. meningitidis* within an "epidemiologic unit" (clearly, often not possible), additional secondary cases among susceptible individuals will occur unless active immunization is provided.

Immunizing Antigens

Four preparations derived from the capsular polysaccharides of *N. meningitidis* are licensed for use in the United States: group A, group C, bivalent A/C, and quadrivalent A/C/Y/W135. The meningococcal vaccines consist of 50 μg of each respective capsular polysaccharide and induce group-specific antibody or antibodies within 1 week after parenteral administration; the duration of protection is unknown. Untoward reactions have been reported infrequently and consist primarily of localized erythema and tenderness (Peltola et al., 1977; CDC, 1978; Hankins et al., 1982; American Academy of Pediatrics, 1994).

Serogroup A vaccine has been shown under epidemic conditions to be effective in infants and children 3 months to 5 years old in Finland, and to be highly effective and safe in Egyptian school children 6 to 15 years old (Wahdan et al., 1973). Serogroup C vaccine, used during a Brazilian epidemic, was protective in children 24 to 35 months old, but not in those under

24 months old (Taunay et al., 1974). These observations are in agreement with other investigations demonstrating a strong age-dependent association with serum antibody response (Gold et al., 1979; Wilkins and Wehrle, 1979; Kaythy et al., 1980). The capsular polysaccharides of serogroups Y and W135 are safe and immunogenic in children over 2 years old, although clinical efficacy has not been demonstrated for these antigens. Controlled trials using meningococcal vaccines in household or day care contacts of sporadic cases have not been performed, so their ultimate protective value in this setting is unknown.

Vaccine Usage

The quadrivalent meningococcal vaccine should be administered subcutaneously in a single 0.5-ml dose. Routine immunization is not recommended for civilian populations because of insufficient evidence of its value when the overall risk of infections is low. Routine immunization using the quadrivalent vaccine is recommended only for certain high-risk groups, including those with deficiencies of the terminal components of serum complement and those with anatomic or functional asplenia (CDC, 1985c).

When an outbreak of meningococcal disease occurs, the etiologic serogroup should be determined, and, if represented in the vaccine, the population at risk should be immunized. Definition of the presence and scope of epidemics when they occur should be carried out in conjunction with local health authorities or officials at the CDC before extensive vaccination. When sporadic cases of meningococcal disease are identified, vaccination in addition to chemoprophylaxis should be considered for household or day care contacts, especially when cases occur over an extended period.

Vaccination of individuals before travel to countries in which epidemic meningococcal disease is present also should be considered. The quadrivalent vaccine is given to all United States military recruits. Although the meningococcal polysaccharide vaccines may be safe to give pregnant women, they should not be administered because of theoretical considerations unless there is a substantial risk of disease. Children first immunized when under 4 years of age should be considered for revaccination after they are 2 or 3 years old if they remain at high risk. The necessity of revaccinating older patients currently is not known (CDC, 1985c; American Academy of Pediatrics, 1994).

Plague Vaccine

Plague is an enzootic infection of many wild rodent species in several parts of Southwestern United States. Its occurrence in human populations in this country is of increasing public health importance; more cases (40) were reported in 1983 than in any previous year since 1920 (CDC, 1984k). The control of epizootic plague and control measures directed against the vector (Oriental rat flea, *Xenopsylla cheopis*) represent the most important prevention program against human plague,

but active immunization is of additional protective value in select high-risk persons.

A formaldehyde-inactivated *Yersinia pestis* vaccine is licensed for use in the United States (CDC, 1982h). Adequate serologic responses have been demonstrated in 83%, 90%, and 90% of adult volunteers after one, two, and three doses (1 ml each) of vaccine, respectively (Bartelloni et al., 1973). Immunization is associated with a reduced incidence and severity of clinical plague following exposure. Vaccine administration is recommended for:

- Laboratory and field personnel working with *Y. pestis* organisms resistant to antimicrobial agents
- Persons engaged in aerosol experiments with *Y. pestis*
- Persons engaged in field operations in areas where plague is enzootic and where prevention of exposure is not possible (e.g., disaster areas)

Plague vaccination should also be considered for:

- Laboratory personnel regularly working with *Y. pestis* or plague-infected rodents
- Persons whose vocations bring them into regular contact with wild rodents or rabbits in areas with enzootic plague
- Persons traveling to plague endemic areas, especially if travel is not limited to urban areas (CDC, 1982h, 1984j)

Primary immunization consists of three intramuscular doses of vaccine for both adults and children. Generally, a second dose is given 4 weeks after the initial dose, and the third dose is given 4 to 12 weeks after the second dose. If an accelerated schedule is required, three doses can be administered at least 1 week apart. Three booster doses should be given at approximately 6-month intervals under circumstances of continuing plague exposure. Subsequently, booster doses at 1- to 2-year intervals should provide good protection under most circumstances. Persons exposed to patients with known plague pneumonia or to *Y. pestis* aerosol in the laboratory should be given a 7- to 10-day course of antimicrobial therapy (tetracycline, chloramphenicol, or streptomycin) regardless of their previous immunization history.

Primary immunization may result in mild systemic symptoms, such as general malaise, headache, fever, and mild lymphadenopathy, or local erythema and induration at the injection site in approximately 10% of recipients, especially with repeated injections. Sterile abscesses or hypersensitivity reactions (urticaria or reactive airway symptoms) have been reported rarely. Severe local or systemic reactions to plague vaccine contraindicate revaccination. Plague vaccine should not be administered to individuals with a known hypersensitivity to any of the vaccine constituents, such as beef protein, soy, casein, or phenol. Because safety of plague vaccine administered during pregnancy has not been established, it should not be used unless there is a substantial risk of infection (CDC, 1982h).

Pneumococcal Vaccine

Pneumococcal infections are common and account for considerable morbidity in healthy children. Although there are 83 types of pneumococci, only a few types account for more than 80% of pneumococcal infections, which include otitis media, pneumonia, bacteremia, and meningitis. Diagnosis is usually easy and therapy successful. One exception is pneumococcal meningitis, which is often complicated and occasionally fatal. Further, penicillin resistance has been described, including strains resistant to multiple antibiotics. These events give emphasis to an immunologic approach for the control of pneumococcal infections. Some children are particularly susceptible to severe or even fatal pneumococcal infection, including those with functional or anatomic asplenia (e.g., congenital absence, surgical removal, or sickle cell anemia with autosplenectomy), those with nephrotic syndrome, and those with congenital or acquired immunodeficiencies (CDC, 1984u; American Academy of Pediatrics, 1994).

A polyvalent pneumococcal vaccine containing a purified polysaccharide antigen derived from the capsules of 14 of the 83 individual strains of pneumococci was licensed for use in the United States in 1977. In 1983, it was replaced by a 23-valent vaccine, each dose of which contains 25 µg of each polysaccharide antigen (as compared with its predecessor, which contained a 50-µg dose of each antigen). This new vaccine confers protective levels of antibodies to a larger number of serotypes while providing less total polysaccharide and, possibly, fewer irritants and pyrogens (Robbins et al., 1983). The 23 serotypes contained in the vaccine are responsible for over 88% of cases of pneumococcal bacteremia in the United States.

Clinical trials in healthy adults in South Africa (Austrian et al., 1976; Smit et al., 1977) and in New Guinea (Riley et al., 1977) have demonstrated the vaccine's high efficacy (serologic response and prevention of disease secondary to vaccine serotypes). Although the duration of protection afforded by the vaccine is unknown, persistence of antibodies has been demonstrated 5 years after immunization. Persons who have received the 14-valent pneumococcal vaccine should not be revaccinated with the 23-valent vaccine, since the maximum increase in protection does not warrant an increased risk of adverse reactions from revaccination (Lawrence et al., 1983). Adverse reactions associated with initial vaccination include (CDC, 1984u):

- Erythema and pain at the injection site in half of the recipients
- Fever, myalgia, and severe local reactions in less than 1% of recipients
- Severe systemic reactions in approximately 5 per 1 million doses administered

In children over 2 years old with sickle cell disease, an octavalent pneumococcal vaccine has demonstrated adequate immunogenicity and some protective efficacy against systemic pneumococcal infections (Ammann et al., 1977). However, vaccine failures have been reported in individuals with this disease and in other children (Sumaya et al., 1981). Unfortunately, children under 2 years old respond poorly to pneumococcal vaccine, and healthy children up to 5 years old may respond suboptimally to some vaccine serotypes, including those most often associated with clinical disease (Klein, 1981; Douglas et al., 1983). Children with steroid-resistant nephrotic syndrome may not respond as well to the vaccine as others (Spika et al., 1982). Although pneumococcal vaccine can decrease the incidence of recurrent otitis media in certain infants and children (Howie et al., 1984), it is not recommended for this purpose.

Pneumococcal vaccine currently is recommended for children over 2 years of age with:

- Sickle cell disease or other causes of functional or anatomic asplenia (including splenectomy)
- Nephrotic syndrome
- Cerebrospinal fluid leaks
- Conditions associated with immunosuppression (including HIV infection)

A single (0.5-ml) dose given subcutaneously or intramuscularly is recommended. Vaccine should be administered at least 2 weeks before elective splenectomy and as long as possible before planned immunosuppressive therapy. Vaccine is also recommended for adults who are at increased risk of pneumococcal disease and its complications, including those with chronic cardiopulmonary, hepatic, or renal disease, as well as healthy individuals 65 years and older (CDC, 1984u).

Revaccination with pneumococcal vaccine should be considered after 3 to 5 years for children under age 10 years (at revaccination), children at risk for severe pneumococcal infection (e.g., patients with asplenia), and groups of patients that have rapid disappearance of antipneumococcal antibody after vaccination (e.g., patients with sickle cell anemia, nephrotic syndrome, or renal failure, and transplant recipients). Revaccination also should be considered for older children and adults at high risk for pneumococcal infection who were vaccinated previously at age 6 or younger (American Academy of Pediatrics, 1994).

Rabies Vaccine

Although human rabies occurs infrequently in the United States, some 25,000 individuals each year require prophylaxis after known or potential exposure to rabies. Carnivorous wild animals (skunks, foxes, coyotes, raccoons, and bats) account for about 85% of proven cases of animal rabies in this country; the prevalence of rabies among these animal populations has increased in recent years. Domestic animals (dogs and cats) represent only a small proportion of proven rabid animals, but they account for most postexposure courses of rabies prophylaxis given annually (Helmick, 1983). Rodents (squirrels, hamsters, gerbils, rats, and mice) and lagomorphs (rabbits and hares) are rarely infected and have not been associated with rabies in the United States (Mann, 1983).

Only six cases of human rabies were reported in the United States during 1980 to 1984, two of which were acquired from dog bites received outside the country (CDC, 1981b, 1981c, 1983d, 1983e, 1984f, 1984x, 1985b). This exceedingly low incidence attests to the efficacy of postexposure prophylaxis using the recommended vaccine and immunoglobulin preparations. In fact, rabies has not been reported in any patient who has received currently recommended postexposure prophylaxis (Bernard et al., 1982; CDC, 1984n). Although rabies is associated with an almost universally fatal outcome, the need for prophylaxis should be evaluated carefully, since available prophylactic methods are rarely complicated by severe adverse reactions. However, the longer that treatment is postponed, the less likely it is to be effective.

Human Diploid Cell Vaccines

Human diploid cell vaccines (HDCVs) were licensed for use in the United States in 1980. HDCV is supplied as 1.0-ml single-dose vials of lyophilized vaccine with accompanying diluent. It is administered intramuscularly, generally in the deltoid area. These preparations represent a significant advantage over previous vaccines (inactivated duck embryo and nervous tissue–derived vaccines no longer available in the United States) with respect to immunogenicity, reaction rates, and convenience. Essentially all recipients develop protective antibody titers that persist for at least 2 years. Local reactions (pain, erythema, or swelling) occur in 25% of recipients, and mild systemic reactions (nausea, abdominal pain, headache, or myalgia) have been noted in about 20%. Systemic and occasionally severe allergic reactions have been reported to occur at a rate of 1 per 1000 HDCV doses administered to more than 400,000 individuals (CDC, 1984s). Transient neuroparalytic reactions have been observed even less commonly, at 1 per 170,000 vaccinees worldwide (Bernard et al., 1982).

Rabies Immune Globulin and Antiserum

Antirabies human immune serum globulin (RIG) concentrated by cold ethanol fractionation from plasma of hyperimmunized human donors is available from Cutter Laboratories (Hyperrab) and Merieux Institute (Imogam). The content of rabies-neutralizing antibody is standardized to contain 150 IU/ml. It is supplied in 2-ml (300-IU) and 10-ml (1500-IU) vials for pediatric and adult use, respectively. Antirabies serum (ARS), available from Selavo, is a concentrated serum obtained from hyperimmunized horses. Neutralizing antibody content is standardized to contain 1000 IU per vial.

RIG is well tolerated in most recipients, although local pain and low-grade fever may result. Anaphylaxis, angioneurotic edema, or other systemic reactions have not been reported. However, ARS produces serum sickness in approximately 40% of adult recipients, and in a small number of children, anaphylactic reactions occur. Therefore, although RIG and ARS are both effective, RIG is the product of choice and is recommended unless unavailable. When ARS must be used, the patient must be tested for sensitivity to equine serum (Hattwick et al., 1974; Bahmanyar et al., 1976; CDC, 1984n).

Vaccine and Rabies Immune Globulin Usage

Postexposure Prophylaxis. Recommendations for the management of individuals following possible exposure to rabies include meticulous attention to flushing and cleaning of the wound with soap and water in addition to active immunization and passive immune globulin administration. The need for preventive measures must be individualized. This decision depends on circumstances precipitating the exposure; the species, clinical state, and availability of the animal inflicting the wound; and the local prevalence of rabies in animal populations. Bites or nonbite exposures (scratches, abrasions, open wounds, or mucous membranes contaminated with saliva) must be considered significant.

A combination of active (HDCV) and passive immunization (RIG) almost always is indicated for the treatment of bites and nonbite exposures inflicted by rabid animals as well as by those suspected of being rabid (Table 29–5). When possible, the brains of wild animals (skunks, foxes, coyotes, raccoons, and bats) or symptomatic dogs or cats implicated in an exposure should be examined for evidence of rabies at the CDC. Active and passive immunization always should be initiated promptly and vaccine administration should be discontinued only if laboratory results are negative. Individuals exposed to healthy dogs or cats that are available for observation do not require immediate prophylactic treatment. Implicated healthy domestic dogs or cats should be quarantined and observed by a veterinarian for at least 10 days; if suggestive symptoms develop, the exposed individuals should begin postexposure prophylaxis promptly, and the brain of the animal should be examined. An unknown (escaped) animal must be regarded as rabid (see Table 29–5).

HDCV therapy must be provided as early as possible but should be used regardless of the time interval after exposure. After initial vaccine administration, four additional 1.0-ml intramuscular doses are given at 3, 7, 14, and 28 days. Routine serologic testing is not indicated after postexposure prophylaxis and is reserved only for those whose immune response may be impaired by primary disease or by immunosuppressive therapy. Pregnancy is not a contraindication to rabies prophylaxis.

RIG is administered only once, at the beginning of antirabies prophylaxis, to provide immediate passive protection until adequate antibody titers are achieved from active HDCV immunization. If not administered initially together with the vaccine, RIG can be given up to 8 days afterwards; it is not indicated after that, since antibody responses to the vaccine have likely occurred. The recommended dose of RIG is 20 IU/kg. About half the dose of RIG should be infiltrated into the area surrounding the wound and the remainder administered intramuscularly.

Pre-exposure Prophylaxis. Active immunization for pre-exposure prophylaxis in high-risk groups (vet-

Table 29–5. Rabies Postexposure Prophylaxis Guide, United States, 1991

Animal Type	Evaluation and Disposition of Animal	Postexposure Prophylaxis Recommendations
Dogs and cats	Healthy and available for 10 days observation	Do not begin prophylaxis unless animal develops symptoms of rabies*
	Rabid or suspected rabid†	Immediate vaccination and RIG
	Unknown (escaped)	Consult public health officials for advice
Skunks, raccoons, bats, foxes, and most other carnivores; woodchucks	Regarded as rabid unless geographic area is known to be free of rabies or until animal proven negative by laboratory tests†	Immediate vaccination and RIG
Livestock, ferrets, rodents, and lagomorphs (rabbits and hares)	Consider individually	Consult public health officials. Bites of squirrels, hamsters, guinea pigs, gerbils, chipmunks, rats, mice, other rodents, rabbits, and hares almost never require antirabies treatment.

*During the 10 day holding period, treatment with RIG and vaccine should be initiated at the first sign of rabies in the biting dog or cat. The symptomatic animal should be killed immediately.

†The animal should be killed and tested as soon as possible. Holding for observation is not recommended. Vaccination is discontinued if immunofluorescent test of the animal is negative.

RIG = human rabies immune globulin vaccine.

Adapted from American Academy of Pediatrics. In Peter G, ed. 1994 Red Book: Report of the Committee on Infectious Diseases, 23rd ed. Elk Grove Village, Ill., American Academy of Pediatrics, 1994.

erinarians, animal handlers, selected laboratory workers, persons visiting countries where rabies is endemic, and persons whose pursuits may involve frequent contact with rabid animals) should be considered. For this purpose, an initial 1.0-ml intramuscular injection of HDCV is given followed by a second dose 7 days later and a third injection 3 weeks after the second. Under conditions of continued exposure, booster doses should be given or serologic testing performed as recommended (CDC, 1984n). Pre-exposure prophylaxis also can be given using the Merieux Institute HDCV preparation packaged for intradermal use; a series of 0.1-ml doses is administered in the lateral aspect of the upper arm, following a schedule similar to that recommended for intramuscular administration (CDC, 1983c). Routine postvaccination serology after pre-exposure prophylaxis is necessary only for those suspected of being immunosuppressed. In individuals who have received adequate pre-exposure prophylaxis, postexposure prophylaxis consists of two 1.0-ml intramuscular doses of HDCV, the first dose administered at the time of the exposure and a second dose 3 days later. RIG is not required under these circumstances.

Typhoid Vaccine

The overall prevalence of typhoid fever is significantly lower in the United States than in highly endemic countries, but the potential for importation into this country from Central and South America is well recognized. Most of the 350 to 600 cases reported annually in the United States since 1963 have been acquired during foreign travel (CDC, 1982a; Taylor et al., 1983). The gradual elimination of typhoid fever in the United States during the past half century reflects improved public health measures, including optimal sanitation methods and identification and reporting of affected individuals. Active immunization with typhoid vaccine represents only an ancillary preventive public health measure to be used in selected settings to prevent transmission from known infected individuals.

Immunizing Antigens

Two typhoid vaccines are available in the United States for civilian use. The older of the two is a heat-phenol–inactivated preparation for parenteral administration. A live, attenuated vaccine prepared from the Ty21a strain of *Salmonella typhi* recently has become available. This vaccine can be administered orally. Unfortunately, data concerning its efficacy and safety for children under 6 years of age are limited and it is not yet recommended for use in this age group.

In field trials, the parenteral vaccine and the Ty21a vaccine have had similar efficacy. Unfortunately, protection depends somewhat on the challenge inoculum. Demonstrated protection to small inocula of *S. typhi* can be overcome with a high-inoculum challenge.

Vaccine Usage

Specific indications for typhoid vaccination in the United States include household or other intimate exposure to a known typhoid carrier and foreign travel to areas where typhoid fever is endemic.

Yellow Fever Vaccine

Because yellow fever does not occur in the United States, prevention is considered only for purposes of international travel. As is true for other arboviral diseases, urban disease can be prevented best by suppressing or eradicating mosquito vectors. Another effective preventive measure is to immunize persons living in or traveling to areas where yellow fever is endemic (CDC, 1984w).

Immunizing Antigen

The yellow fever vaccine (YFV) licensed in the United States is a live, attenuated preparation derived from the 17D viral strain prepared in chick embryos (CDC, 1984w). In contrast to the previously used Dakar strain preparation, the 17D strain has been associated only rarely with significant neurologic complications (two cases of encephalitis following administration of 34 million doses of vaccine). Mild side effects, including low-grade fever, headache, and myalgia, have been observed in 2% to 5% of recipients. Immediate hypersensitivity reactions, including rash, urticaria, and reactive airway symptoms, are extremely uncommon (less than 1 per 1 million doses) and occur primarily in individuals with histories of egg allergy (CDC, 1984w). Immunity after vaccination with the 17D strain virus has been demonstrated to persist for more than 10 years (Wisseman and Sweet, 1962; Rosenzweig et al., 1963).

Vaccine Usage

Yellow fever vaccine is recommended for individuals over 9 months of age traveling to or residing in areas of yellow fever endemicity (parts of Africa and South America). Vaccination for international travel is required by local health regulations in individual countries. To obtain an international certificate of vaccination, a YFV approved by the World Health Organization and administered at a designated YFV center is required. Such centers in the United States can be located by contacting state and local health departments.

Primary immunization consists of a single, subcutaneous injection of 0.5 ml reconstituted, freeze-dried vaccine for both adults and children. Revaccination is required no more frequently than every 10 years. In preparation for imminent travel, other live virus vaccines can be given at a different site simultaneously with YFV; if not given on the same day, the administration of multiple live virus vaccines should be separated by at least 4 weeks. Cholera vaccine and YFV administration should be separated by at least 3 weeks; if time constraints preclude this, they can be given simultaneously (Felsenfeld et al., 1973). A prospective study of individuals given YFV and commercially available immune globulin indicated no attenuation of the immune response to YFV compared with controls (CDC, 1984w).

Precautions and Contraindications

Although no adverse effects of YFV on the developing fetus have been demonstrated, vaccine administration to pregnant women should be avoided. Pregnant women and infants under 9 months of age should be considered for vaccination only when travel to high-risk areas is required and high-level protection against mosquito exposure is not feasible. As is true of other live viral vaccines, YFV should not be administered to patients with altered immune states as a result of underlying disease or immunosuppressive therapy. Documented hypersensitivity to eggs is a contraindication to vaccination. However, experience in the armed forces suggests that allergy sufficiently severe to preclude vaccination is uncommon and occurs only in those individuals who are unable to eat eggs. If international quarantine regulations represent the only reason to immunize a patient known to be hypersensitive to eggs, attempts should be made to obtain a waiver. If immunization of an individual with a questionable history of egg hypersensitivity is considered essential because of a high-risk of exposure, an intradermal skin test may be given as directed in the YFV package insert (CDC, 1984w).

INVESTIGATIONAL ACTIVE IMMUNIZING AGENTS

Human Immunodeficiency Virus Vaccines

Several candidate HIV vaccines are undergoing clinical trials. Most of these vaccines are genetically engineered products based on the HIV envelope proteins gp120 and gp160. HIV vaccine development has focused not only on prevention of infection but also on slowing of immune attrition in individuals already infected with the virus. In one study (Redfield et al., 1991), candidate vaccine rgp160 (MicroGeneSys, Inc.) was administered in a dose-escalating manner to HIV-infected adults. There was no evidence of systemic or immune toxicity. New humoral immune responses were noted to some epitopes of gp160, and almost all subjects developed new lymphoproliferative responses that were sustained with sequential boosting. It is speculated that novel vaccine-induced immune responses directed against recombinant envelope antigens may result in delayed HIV disease progression.

Studies are beginning of HIV envelope vaccines for active immunization of pregnant HIV-infected women and prevention of vertical HIV transmission. The rationale for these studies is based on preliminary findings indicating that pregnant HIV-infected women may be less likely to transmit infection if they have high titers of anti-HIV neutralizing antibody. Vaccine studies in HIV-exposed newborn infants also have commenced.

Cytomegalovirus Vaccine

About 1% of newborns in the United States are infected congenitally with cytomegalovirus (CMV), and 10% to 20% of these manifest significant neurologic defects. Certain allograft recipients are also at high risk for severe CMV disease; at least 90% of renal transplant patients excrete CMV postoperatively. The development of CMV vaccines has been targeted at diminishing morbidity associated with CMV disease in these and other high-risk patient groups.

Live, attenuated vaccines, passaged in human tissue culture, have been developed and tested in Britain (AD 169 strain) (Stern, 1984) and the United States (Towne strain) (Plotkin et al., 1984). Following subcutaneous administration to normal volunteers, both humoral and cell-mediated immune responses are observed. However, the duration of the immune response or protection afforded is not known. Controlled trials have demonstrated that the use of CMV vaccine in seronegative renal transplant candidates may not diminish the rate of CMV infection after transplantation but may decrease the severity of acquired CMV disease. Viremia or shedding of vaccine-type CMV has not been demonstrated after immunization, and adverse reactions to the vaccine are limited to minor local reactions.

Before CMV vaccine can be used on a large scale, studies are required to evaluate if vaccine-induced antibody in pregnant women reduces the risk of disease in offspring. Further, the protective efficacy of the vaccines against multiple strains of CMV and the possible risks of latent infection or oncogenesis associated with vaccination need to be defined.

Group B Streptococcal Vaccine

Group B *Streptococcus* (GBS) is the leading cause of neonatal sepsis and meningitis. Morbidity and mortality rates remain high despite the use of antimicrobials and intensive supportive care. Serotype III is responsible for about two thirds of all GBS infections in infants. Although less information is available about other serotypes, high titers of transplacental antibody to type III GBS capsular polysaccharide prevents the development of disease in exposed neonates. Because high levels of maternal type-specific anti-GBS antibody should protect full-term newborns, immunization of pregnant women with purified type-specific vaccine has been considered as an approach to control of GBS infections. In general, the immunogenicity of purified GBS capsular polysaccharide has been disappointing, with response rates of 40% to 80% in nonimmune adults (Baker and Kasper, 1985). However, one study (Baker et al., 1988) reported that type III vaccine was tolerated well by pregnant women and that opsonically active antibody could be demonstrated in their infants.

Tularemia Vaccine

Human tularemia occurs primarily in the south central United States, where the disease is enzootic in both domestic and wild animals. Prevention of human disease depends on the prevention of transmission either (1) directly from infected animals (rabbits, squirrels, skunks, muskrats, woodchucks, coyotes, and others) or animal products; or (2) indirectly from infected vector insects (e.g., ticks or deer flies). Active immunization rarely is indicated except in high-risk settings, such as persons engaged in laboratory work involving *Francisella tularensis* (American Academy of Pediatrics, 1994).

A live, attenuated tularemia vaccine for intradermal use is available in the United States as an investigational product from the CDC. In laboratory workers, vaccine administration has reduced the incidence of typhoidal tularemia and the severity of ulceroglandular disease (Burke, 1977), but its efficacy in the prevention of naturally occurring disease is unknown.

PASSIVE IMMUNIZATION AGENTS

Varicella-Zoster Immune Globulin (VZIG)

Early studies demonstrated the efficacy of zoster immune globulin (ZIG), prepared from patients convalescing from herpes zoster, in preventing chickenpox among exposed, susceptible, normal or high-risk children when administered within 72 hours after exposure. The scarcity of plasma from patients convalescing from zoster used to prepare ZIG resulted in a limited supply of this material. Thus, techniques were developed to prepare a globulin of similar potency from plasma of normal donors with high varicella-zoster antibody. This VZIG is available in ample supply in the United States.

Since VZIG became available for use in 1978, both serologic and clinical evaluations have demonstrated that the product is equivalent to ZIG in preventing or modifying clinical disease in susceptible immunocompromised patients exposed to varicella. VZIG (human) is a sterile, 10% to 18% solution of the globulin fraction of human plasma (primarily IgG) in 0.3 molar glycine stabilizer and 1:10,000 thimerosol preservative. It is prepared by Cohn ethanol precipitation. This product is available through regional distribution centers in conjunction with the American Red Cross as well as from hospital pharmacies.

VZIG Usage

The appropriateness of VZIG administration after a known or suspected exposure to varicella depends on the susceptibility of the exposed individual, whether the exposure is likely to result in infection, and whether the exposed individual is at high risk for complications of varicella.

Both normal and immunocompromised adults and children who have had clinical varicella based on a carefully obtained history can be considered immune. Bone marrow transplant recipients, however, represent an exception to this rule. Because subclinical primary infections rarely occur (estimated to be less than 5% of infections among normal children), children under 15 years old without histories of clinical varicella should be considered to be susceptible unless serologic studies demonstrate adequate immunity. Most normal adults with negative or unknown histories of clinical varicella are probably immune, based on very low attack rates of varicella in adult populations after household or hospital exposure.

Multiple serologic techniques have been developed to determine susceptibility to varicella. The complement-fixating test is the most commonly available serologic assay, but its overall usefulness is limited by its lack of sensitivity and specificity as well as the fact that about two thirds of patients lack detectible complement-fixing antibody to varicella within a year after clinical infection. Other more sensitive assays—including fluorescent antibody membrane antigen (FAMA), immune adherence hemagglutination assay (IAHA), enzyme-linked immunosorbent assay (ELISA), and neutralization antibody assay—are not generally available and have not been fully evaluated, especially in immunocompromised populations. Furthermore, even sensitive antibody assays may not be useful in assessing the likelihood that neonates and young infants exposed to varicella will develop clinical disease.

Exposure criteria for which VZIG is indicated among susceptible individuals at risk for severe varicella infection include one of the following types of exposure to persons with chickenpox or zoster:

- Continuous household contact
- Playmate contact (generally more than 1 hour of play indoors)
- Hospital contact (in same two- to four-bed room or adjacent beds in a large ward or prolonged face-to-face contact with an infectious staff member or patient)
- Newborn contact (newborn of mother who had onset of chickenpox 5 days or less before delivery or within 48 hours after delivery)

Each of these criteria is contingent on the possibility that VZIG can be administered within 96 hours (preferably sooner) after the earliest known exposure.

Specific recommendations for use of VZIG among persons meeting appropriate exposure criteria are outlined in Table 29–6. In general, patients receiving monthly doses of intravenous immunoglobulin should be protected and do not require VZIG. However, VZIG should be considered if exposure occurs more than 3 weeks after the most recent dose of immunoglobulin or if the patient has advanced HIV disease with a markedly depressed CD4+ lymphocyte count.

Infants and Children

Immunocompromised Children. Passive immunization of susceptible immunocompromised children following significant exposure to chickenpox or zoster represents the most important use of VZIG. This includes children with primary immunodeficiency disorders or neoplastic diseases and children whose treatment is considered immunosuppressive.

Newborns of Mothers With Varicella. VZIG is indicated for newborns of mothers who develop chickenpox within 5 days before or 48 hours after delivery. Infants of mothers who develop clinical varicella more than 5 days before delivery are thought to be protected from varicella complications by transplacentally acquired maternal antibody. No evidence exists to suggest that infants born to mothers who develop varicella more than 48 hours after delivery are at increased risk for serious complications.

Table 29–6. Recommendations for Use of Varicella-Zoster Immune Globulin (VZIG)

Exposure Criteria*
1. One of the following types of exposure to persons with chickenpox or zoster:
   a. Continuous household contact
   b. Playmate contact (generally >1 hour of play indoors)
   c. Hospital contact (in same two- to four-bed room or adjacent beds in a large ward or prolonged face-to-face contact with an infectious staff member or patient)
   and
2. Time elapsed after exposure is such that VZIG can be administered within 96 hours but preferably sooner

Candidates for VZIG†
1. Susceptible to varicella-zoster (see text)
2. Significant exposure, as listed above
3. Age <15 years; administration to immunocompromised adolescents and adults and to other older patients on an individual basis (see text)
4. One of the following underlying illnesses or conditions:
   a. Leukemia or lymphoma
   b. Congenital or acquired immunodeficiency, including the acquired immunodeficiency syndrome
   c. Immunosuppressive treatment
   d. Newborn of mother who had onset of chickenpox within 5 days before delivery or 48 hours after delivery
   e. Premature infant (≥28 weeks' gestation) whose mother has no history of chickenpox
   f. Premature infants (<28 weeks' gestation or ≤1000 g) regardless of maternal history

*Patients must meet both criteria.
†Patients must meet both exposure criteria above.
Adapted from Centers for Disease Control. MMWR 33(7):84–100, 1984, and American Academy of Pediatrics. In Peter G, ed. 1994 Red Book: Report of the Committee on Infectious Diseases, 23rd ed. Elk Grove Village, Ill., American Academy of Pediatrics,1994, pp. 510–517.

Postnatal Exposure of Newborn Infants. Premature infants exposed to varicella postnatally should be evaluated on an individual basis. Because the risk of complications from postnatally acquired varicella in the premature infant is unknown, it is reasonable to administer VZIG to exposed premature infants whose mothers have negative or uncertain histories of varicella exposure; these infants should be considered at risk as long as they are hospitalized. All exposed infants under 28 weeks' gestation or with birth weight of 1000 g or less should receive VZIG regardless of maternal history because of the uncertainty of acquiring transplacental maternal antibody. Full-term infants who develop varicella after postnatal exposure are not known to be at increased risk for complications of chickenpox as compared with older children, so VZIG is not recommended for full-term infants regardless of the mother's immune status.

VZIG in Adults

Immunocompromised Adults. Complications of varicella in immunocompromised adults are substantially greater than in normal individuals. Most (85% to 95%) immunocompromised adults with negative or unknown histories of previous varicella are immune. Nonetheless, adults who are believed to be susceptible and who have had significant exposures should receive VZIG.

Normal Adults. Varicella can be severe in normal, healthy adults. Epidemiologic and clinical studies indicate that normal adults who develop varicella have a 9- to 25-fold greater risk of complications, including death, than normal children. Most adults with negative or uncertain histories of varicella are immune, so a decision to administer VZIG to an adult must be individualized. If sensitive laboratory screening tests for varicella are available, they might be used to determine susceptibility if time permits.

Pregnant Women. Some investigators have recommended VZIG administration for pregnant women with negative or uncertain histories of varicella who were exposed significantly in the first or second trimester to try to prevent congenital varicella syndrome or in the third trimester to prevent neonatal varicella. However, no evidence exists that administering VZIG to a susceptible pregnant woman prevents viremia, fetal infection, or congenital varicella syndrome. Thus, the primary (perhaps only) indication for VZIG in pregnant women is to prevent varicella complications in a susceptible adult rather than to prevent intrauterine infection.

VZIG in Hospital Settings

Health care personnel with negative or uncertain histories of chickenpox should be evaluated in a manner similar to that for other adults. If possible, sensitive laboratory tests for determining susceptibility can be used to assess candidacy for VZIG and to determine possible work restrictions that may be necessary during the incubation period, especially when large numbers of individuals have been exposed.

Ideally, all health care personnel caring for patients with varicella or zoster should be immune. Other control measures to prevent or control nosocomial varicella outbreaks include (1) strict isolation precautions, (2) isolation of exposed patients, and (3) early discharge, when possible. Potentially susceptible hospital personnel with significant exposure should not have direct patient contact from approximately the 10th through the 21st day after exposure, the period during which chickenpox may occur. These control measures should apply regardless of whether potentially susceptible exposed personnel or patients receive VZIG. Data on clinical attack rates and incubation periods of varicella following VZIG administration in this setting are lacking. However, studies of immunocompromised children with negative histories of varicella treated with VZIG who have had intense exposures, such as in a household setting, demonstrate that about one third to one half develop clinical varicella and might be infectious. Further, VZIG may prolong the average incubation period in immunocompromised patients from 14 to 18 days, but the vast number of cases occur within 28 days of exposure in immunocompromised, VZIG-treated patients. Thus, personnel who receive VZIG should probably not work in patient areas for 10 to 28 days after exposure if no illness occurs, and patients who receive VZIG should be isolated during this interval if early discharge is not possible.

VZIG Administration

VZIG is of maximum benefit when administered as soon as possible after a presumed exposure but may be effective when given as late as 96 hours after exposure. No evidence exists documenting the usefulness or efficacy of VZIG in treating clinical varicella or zoster or in preventing disseminated zoster. The duration of protection afforded by VZIG administration is uncertain, but, based on the known half-life of immune globulin (approximately 3 weeks), high-risk patients who are re-exposed more than 3 weeks after a previous dose of VZIG should receive another full dose.

VZIG is supplied in vials containing 125 units per vial (1.25 ml). The generally recommended dose is 125 units per 10 kg (22 lb) of body weight up to a maximum of 625 units (5 vials). However, the minimum dose recommended is 125 units, and fractional doses are not advised. Some investigators recommend exceeding a total dose of 625 units in some immunocompromised adults. VZIG should be administered intramuscularly, as directed. It should never be administered intravenously.

Adverse reactions to VZIG administration are rare; local discomfort, pain, redness, or swelling occurs at the injection site in about 1% of recipients. Less frequent systemic reactions, such as gastrointestinal symptoms, malaise, headaches, rash, or respiratory symptoms, occur in approximately 0.2% of recipients. Severe reactions, such as angioneurotic edema and anaphylactic shock, have been reported rarely (<0.1%). When VZIG is indicated for patients with severe thrombocytopenia or any other coagulation disorder that would generally contraindicate intramuscular injections, the expected benefits should outweigh the risks.

Human Immune Serum Globulin

There are only a few well accepted indications for ISG (e.g., immunodeficiency, hepatitis A prophylaxis, and measles prophylaxis). In most situations for which its use is considered, either ISG or IVIG can be used. However, ISG has advantages in terms of cost and ease of administration.

Hepatitis A Virus Prophylaxis

The value of ISG in the prevention or attenuation of hepatitis A virus (HAV) infection is well established (Krugman and Ward, 1961–1962). Individuals exposed to HAV are afforded protection against symptomatic disease by the prompt administration of ISG by the intramuscular route. It is recommended for all household contacts as soon as possible after exposure. The use of ISG more than 2 weeks after exposure or after onset of illness is not recommended. Serologic testing is not generally indicated because it may delay the administration of ISG. ISG is also recommended for contacts of HAV cases occurring in day care centers. If a case is identified in a child, a staff member, or the household of two or more families of attendees, ISG, 0.02 ml/kg, should be given to all children and staff. In custodial institutions, such as those for the mentally retarded, HAV infection is highly transmissible; when outbreaks occur, residents and staff having close personal contact with identified patients should receive 0.02 ml/kg of ISG (American Academy of Pediatrics, 1994).

Exposures to HAV in classrooms or other places in schools generally do not represent significant risk for infection. ISG is not generally indicated except in the unusual instance of a school-centered epidemic, for which ISG is recommended for close contacts of identified patients. Similarly, routine administration of ISG to hospital personnel caring for patients with HAV is not indicated. Rather, emphasis should be placed on hand washing and proper isolation procedures in the management of patients. In most cases, the source of food- or water-borne HAV epidemics is usually recognized too late for ISG to be effective. However, if administered within 2 weeks after ingestion of identified HAV-contaminated water or food, it may be effective.

ISG is generally not indicated in newborn infants whose mothers had HAV during pregnancy, unless the mother is jaundiced and otherwise actively symptomatic at the time of delivery. While administration of 0.02 ml/kg ISG is recommended in this setting, adequate documentation of its value is lacking.

In most cases, tourist travel does not require the prophylactic administration of ISG. However, individuals traveling to underdeveloped areas, such as tropical rural villages, should receive ISG, 0.02 ml/kg, if they anticipate staying less than 3 months. Those who require long-term protection should receive 0.06 ml/kg ISG and should receive additional booster doses every 4 to 5 months or receive the hepatitis A vaccine. ISG can be given with hepatitis A vaccine if the traveler will be exposed before the 1 month needed to ensure immunity from the vaccine (American Academy of Pediatrics, 1994).

Measles Prophylaxis

Human immune serum globulin has been shown to prevent or modify clinical measles in susceptible individuals when given within 6 days of exposure. The recommended dose of ISG is 0.25 ml/kg (or a maximum dose of 15 ml). It may be especially indicated for susceptible household contacts of measles patients, particularly contacts under 1 year old, for whom the risk of complications is highest. Live measles vaccine should then be given about 3 months later when measles antibody titers have diminished, and if the child is then at least 15 months old. Immunocompromised children should receive 0.5 ml/kg of ISG after measles exposure (or a maximum dose of 15 ml). Although ISG usually prevents measles in susceptible normal children following exposure, it may not be effective in certain children with acute leukemia or other conditions associated with altered immunity. A child regularly receiving intramuscular or intravenous ISG

preparations for the treatment of antibody immunodeficiency need not receive additional prophylaxis if exposed to measles.

Other Considerations Regarding Human Immune Serum Globulin

Human immune serum globulin is sometimes used in circumstances in which only questionable or no proof of efficacy exists. For example, massive doses of ISG have been used in an attempt to prevent rubella in recently exposed pregnant women. However, there is little evidence that even 20 to 40 ml of ISG offers any protection. Similarly, there is no evidence for efficacy of ISG in the management or treatment of asthma or severe allergic diathesis, burn patients, or most acute infections, including severe, even life-threatening bacterial or viral diseases. Of particular importance is the lack of efficacy of ISG in the management of undifferentiated recurrent upper respiratory tract infections (see Chapter 9).

Adverse reactions to ISG are largely limited to the discomfort or pain experienced on administration. Severe systemic reactions are uncommon, but anaphylaxis and collapse have been reported. A higher risk of systemic reactions is associated with inadvertent intravenous administration, so ISG should always be given intramuscularly in a large muscle mass and not by any other route. Mild systemic symptoms (fever, chills, sweating) are sometimes observed in individuals receiving repeated doses. Because ISG preparations contain trace amounts of IgA, persons who are selectively IgA deficient may develop IgA antibodies and have systemic symptoms (chills, fever, and shock-like symptoms) in response to subsequent doses of ISG, plasma, or whole blood transfusions (American Academy of Pediatrics, 1994).

Special Human Immune Serum Globulins

These preparations differ from ISG only with respect to the selection of donors. Individuals known to have high titers of a specific desired antibody are selected for preparation of these products as compared with random selections of adults for ISG. Available special ISGs include (1) hepatitis B immune globulin (see hepatitis B vaccine), (2) rabies immune globulin (see rabies vaccine), (3) tetanus immune globulin (see tetanus vaccine), (4) varicella-zoster immune globulin, (5) cytomegalovirus intravenous immune globulin, and (6) Rh immune globulin (Rho-Gam). Several others, including HIV hyperimmune intravenous immunoglobulin (HIVIG), respiratory syncytial virus intravenous immunoglobulin (RSV-IVIG), and bacterial polysaccharide immune globulin, are being evaluated in clinical trials.

Intravenous Immune Globulin (IVIG)

A complete discussion of the use of IVIG in immunodeficiency and autoimmune and inflammatory diseases is given in Chapter 9.

References

American Academy of Pediatrics. Revision of recommendation for use of rifampin prophylaxis of contacts of patients with *Haemophilus influenzae* infections. Pediatrics 74:301–302, 1984.

American Academy of Pediatrics. *Haemophilus* type B polysaccharide vaccine. Pediatrics 76:322–324, 1985a.

American Academy of Pediatrics: Recommendations for using pneumococcal vaccine in children. Pediatrics 75:1153–1158, 1985b.

American Academy of Pediatrics. Acellular pertussis vaccines: recommendations for use as the fourth and fifth doses. Pediatrics 90:121–123, 1992a.

American Academy of Pediatrics. Universal hepatitis B immunization. Pediatrics 89:795–800, 1992b.

American Academy of Pediatrics. Report of Committee on Infectious Diseases. The Red Book. Evanston, Ill., American Academy of Pediatrics, 1994.

American Academy of Pediatrics. Recommendations for the use of live attenuated varicella vaccine. Pediatrics 95:791–796, 1995.

Ammann AJ, Addiego J, Wara DW, Lubin B, Smith WB, Mentzer WC. Polyvalent pneumococcal-polysaccharide immunization of patients with sickle-cell anemia and patients with splenectomy. N Engl J Med 297:897–900, 1977.

Asano Y, Nagai T, Miyata T. Long-term protective immunity of recipients of the Oka strain of live varicella vaccine. Pediatrics 75:667–671,1985.

Austrian R, Douglas RM, Schiffman G, Coetzee AM, Koornhot HJ, Hayden-Smith S, Reid RDW. Prevention of pneumococcal pneumonia by vaccination. Trans Assoc Am Phys 89:184–192, 1976.

Avery ME, Wofsdorf J. Diagnosis and treatment: approaches to newborn infants of tuberculous mothers. Pediatrics 42:519–522, 1968.

Bahmanyar M, Fayaz A, Nour-Salchi S. Successful protection of humans exposed to rabies infections: postexposure treatment with the new human diploid cell rabies vaccine. JAMA 248:3136–3138, 1982.

Baker CJ, Kasper DL. Group B streptococcal vaccines. Rev Infect Dis 7:458–467, 1985.

Baker CJ, Rench MA, Edwards MS, Carpenter RJ, Hays BM, Kasper DL. Immunization of pregnant women with a polysaccharide vaccine of group B streptococcus. N Engl J Med 319:1180–1185, 1988.

Band JD, Chamberland ME, Platt T, Weaver RE, Thornsberry C, Fraser DW. Trends in meningococcal disease in the United States, 1975–1980. J Infect Dis 148:754–758, 1983.

Barin R, Goudeau A, Denis F, Yvonnet B, Chiron JP, Coursaget P, DiapMar I. Immune response in neonates to hepatitis B vaccine. Lancet 1:251–253, 1982.

Barkin RM, Samuelson JS, Gotlin LP. DTP reactions and serologic response with a reduced dose schedule. J Pediatr 105:189–194, 1984.

Bartelloni PJ, Marshall JD Jr, Cavanaugh DC. Clinical and serological responses to plague vaccine U.S.P. Milit Med 138:720–722, 1973.

Beasley RP, Hwang L-Y, Lee GC-Y, Lan C-C, Roan C-H, Huang F-Y, Chen E-L. Prevention of perinatally transmitted hepatitis B virus infections with hepatitis B immune globulin and hepatitis B vaccine. Lancet 2:1099–1102, 1983.

Beasley RP, Hwang L-Y, Lin CC, Chien C-S. Hepatocellular carcinoma and hepatitis B virus: a prospective study of 22,707 men in Taiwan. Lancet 2:1129–1132, 1981.

Berger R, Just M. Vaccination against hepatitis A: control 3 years after the first vaccination. Vaccine 10:295, 1992.

Berkowitz CD, Ward JI, Meier K, Hendley JC, Brunnell PA, Barkin RA, Zahradnik J, Samuelson J, Gorden L. Safety and immunogenicity of *Haemophilus influenzae* type b polysaccharide and polysaccharide diphtheria toxoid conjugate vaccines in children 15–24 months. J Pediatr 110:509–514, 1987.

Bernard KW, Smith PW, Kader FJ, Moran MJ. Neuroparalytic illness and human diploid cell rabies vaccine. JAMA 248:3136–3138, 1982.

Bernier FH. Improved inactivated poliovirus vaccine: an update. Pediatr Infect Dis 5:289–292, 1986.

Bijkerk H. Surveillance and control of poliomyelitis in The Netherlands. Rev Infect Dis 6(Suppl.):S451–S456, 1984.

Black SB, Shinefield HR. Northern California Permanente Medical Care Program, Departments of Pediatrics Vaccine Study Group. b-Capsa I. *Haemophilus influenzae*, type b, capsular polysaccharide vaccine safety. Pediatrics 79:321–325, 1987.

Black SB, Shinefield HR, Fireman B, Hiatt R, Polen M, Vittinghoff E. Efficacy in infancy of oligosaccharide conjugate *Haemophilus influenzae* type b (HbOC) vaccine in a United States population of 61,080 children. Pediatr Infect Dis J 10:97–104, 1991.

Bottiger M. Long-term immunity following vaccination with killed poliovirus vaccine in Sweden, a country with no circulating poliovirus. Rev Infect Dis 6(Suppl.):S548–S551, 1984.

Brachman PS, Gold H, Plotkin SA, Fekety FR, Werrin M, Ingraham NR. Field evaluation of a human anthrax vaccine. Am J Public Health 52:632–645, 1962.

Broome CV, Fraser DW. Pertussis in the United States, 1979: a look at vaccine efficacy. J Infect Dis 144:187–190, 1981.

Burke DS. Immunization against tularemia: analysis of the effectiveness of live *Francisella tularensis* vaccine in prevention of laboratory-acquired tularemia. J Infect Dis 135:55–60, 1977.

Candel S. Epididymitis in mumps, including orchitis: further clinical studies and comments. Ann Intern Med 34:20–24, 1951.

[CDC] Centers for Disease Control. Cholera vaccine. MMWR 27(20):173–174, 1978a.

[CDC] Centers for Disease Control. SHEW, USPHS, Diphtheria surveillance, Report no. 12, July 1978b.

[CDC] Centers for Disease Control. Goal to eliminate measles from the United States. MMWR 27(41):391, 1978c.

[CDC] Centers for Disease Control. Meningococcal polysaccharide vaccines. MMWR 27(35):327–329, 1978d.

[CDC] Centers for Disease Control. Bacterial meningitis and meningococcemia—United States, 1978. MMWR 28(24):277–279, 1979a.

[CDC] Centers for Disease Control. BCG vaccines. MMWR 28(21):241–244, 1979b.

[CDC] Centers for Disease Control. Diphtheria, tetanus and pertussis: guidelines for vaccine prophylaxis and other preventive measures. MMWR 30(32):392–407, 1981a.

[CDC] Centers for Disease Control. Human rabies acquired outside the United States from a dog bite. MMWR 30(43):537–540, 1981b.

[CDC] Centers for Disease Control. Human rabies—Oklahoma. MMWR 30(28):343–349, 1981c.

[CDC] Centers for Disease Control. Annual summary. MMWR 31(54):142–144, 1982a.

[CDC] Centers for Disease Control. Childhood immunization initiative, United States—5-year follow-up. MMWR 31(17):231–232, 1982b.

[CDC] Centers for Disease Control. Measles prevention. MMWR 31(17):217–231, 1982e.

[CDC] Centers for Disease Control. Mumps vaccine. MMWR 31(46):617–625, 1982f.

[CDC] Centers for Disease Control. Pertussis surveillance. MMWR 31(25):333–336, 1982g.

[CDC] Centers for Disease Control. Plague vaccine. MMWR 31(22):301–304, 1982h.

[CDC] Centers for Disease Control. Poliomyelitis prevention. MMWR 31(3):22–34, 1982i.

[CDC] Centers for Disease Control. Rubella—United States, 1979–1982. MMWR 31(42):568–575, 1982j.

[CDC] Centers for Disease Control. Efficacy of mumps vaccine—Ohio. MMWR 32(30):391–398, 1983b.

[CDC] Centers for Disease Control. Field evaluations of pre-exposure use of human diploid cell rabies vaccine. MMWR 32(46):601–603, 1983c.

[CDC] Centers for Disease Control. Human rabies—Michigan. MMWR 32(12):159–160, 1983d.

[CDC] Centers for Disease Control. Imported human rabies. MMWR 32(6):78–86, 1983e.

[CDC] Centers for Disease Control. Influenza vaccines, 1983–1984. MMWR 32(26):333–337, 1983f.

[CDC] Centers for Disease Control. General recommendations on immunization. MMWR 32(1):1–17, 1983g.

[CDC] Centers for Disease Control. The safety of hepatitis B virus vaccine. MMWR 32(10):134–136, 1983h.

[CDC] Centers for Disease Control. Anthrax and anthrax vaccine—adult immunization. MMWR 33(1S):33S–34S, 1984a.

[CDC] Centers for Disease Control. Practices Advisory Board—adult immunization. MMWR 33(1S):28S–29S, 1984b.

[CDC] Centers for Disease Control. Cholera—healthy information for international travel 1984. MMWR 33:70–71, 1984c.

[CDC] Centers for Disease Control. Hepatitis B vaccine: Evidence confirming lack of AIDS transmission. MMWR 33(49):685–687, 1984e.

[CDC] Centers for Disease Control. Human rabies—Texas. MMWR 33(33):469–470, 1984f.

[CDC] Centers for Disease Control. Measles—United States, 1983. MMWR 33(8):105–108, 1984g.

[CDC] Centers for Disease Control. Mumps outbreak—New Jersey. MMWR 33(29):421–430, 1984h.

[CDC] Centers for Disease Control. Mumps—United States, 1983–1984. MMWR 33(38):533–535, 1984i.

[CDC] Centers for Disease Control. Plague—adult immunization. MMWR 33(1S):29S–30S, 1984j.

[CDC] Centers for Disease Control. Plague in the United States, 1983. MMWR 33(1S):15S–21S, 1984k.

[CDC] Centers for Disease Control. Rabies prevention—United States, 1984. MMWR 33(28):393–408, 1984n.

[CDC] Centers for Disease Control. Rubella prevention. MMWR 33(22):301–318, 1984p.

[CDC] Centers for Disease Control. Rubella vaccination during pregnancy—United States, 1971–1983. MMWR 33(26):365–373, 1984q.

[CDC] Centers for Disease Control. Supplementary statement of contraindications to receipt of pertussis vaccine. MMWR 33(13):169–171, 1984r.

[CDC] Centers for Disease Control. Systemic allergic reactions following immunization with human diploid cell rabies vaccine. MMWR 33(14):185–187, 1984s.

[CDC] Centers for Disease Control. Tuberculosis—United States, 1983. MMWR 33(28):412–415, 1984t.

[CDC] Centers for Disease Control. Update: Pneumococcal polysaccharide vaccine usage—United States. MMWR 33(20):273–281, 1984u.

[CDC] Centers for Disease Control. Yellow fever vaccine. MMWR 32(52):679–688, 1984w.

[CDC] Centers for Disease Control. Human rabies—Pennsylvania. MMWR 33(45):633–635, 1984x.

[CDC] Centers for Disease Control. Diphtheria, tetanus, and pertussis: guidelines for vaccine prophylaxis and other preventive measures. MMWR 34(27):405–426, 1985a.

[CDC] Centers for Disease Control. Human rabies acquired outside the United States. MMWR 34(17):235–236, 1985b.

[CDC] Centers for Disease Control. Meningococcal vaccines. MMWR 34(18):255–259, 1985c.

[CDC] Centers for Disease Control. Polysaccharide vaccine for prevention of *Haemophilus influenzae* type b disease. MMWR 34(15):201–205, 1985d.

[CDC] Centers for Disease Control. Suboptimal response to hepatitis B vaccine given by injection into the buttock. MMWR 34(8):105–113, 1985f.

[CDC] Centers for Disease Control. Poliomyelitis prevention: enhanced-potency inactivated poliomyelitis vaccine. MMWR 36(22):139–140, 1987.

[CDC] Centers for Disease Control. Update prevention of *Haemophilus influenzae* type b disease. MMWR 37(2):13–16, 1988.

[CDC] Centers for Disease Control. Measles prevention: recommendations of the Immunization Practices Advisory Committee (ACIP). MMWR 38(S-9):1–18, 1989.

[CDC] Centers for Disease Control. Summary of notifiable diseases—United States, 1990. MMWR 39:1–61, 1990.

[CDC] Centers for Disease Control. Hepatitis B virus: a comprehensive strategy for eliminating transmission in the United States through universal childhood vaccination. MMWR 40(RR-13):1–25, 1991.

[CDC] Centers for Disease Control. Retrospective assessment of vaccination coverage among school-aged children—selected U.S. cities, 1991. MMWR 41:103–107, 1992a.

[CDC] Centers for Disease Control. Pertussis vaccination: acellular pertussis vaccine for reinforcing and booster use. MMWR 41(RR-1):1–10, 1992b.

[CDC] Centers for Disease Control. Standards for pediatric immunization practices. MMWR 42(RR-5):1–13, 1993a.

[CDC] Centers for Disease Control. Prevention and control of influenza. Part I. Vaccines. MMWR 42(RR-6):1–14, 1993b.

[CDC] Centers for Disease Control. Laboratory-based surveillance for meningococcal disease in selected areas—United States, 1989–1991. MMWR 42(SS-2):21–30, 1993c.

[CDC] Centers for Disease Control. Hepatitis surveillance report no. 55. Atlanta, Centers for Disease Control and Prevention, 1994.

Chen ST, Edsall G, Peel MM, Sinnathvray TA. Timing of antenatal tetanus immunization for effective protection of the neonate. Bull WHO 61:159–165, 1983.

Cherry J, Feigin RD, Lobes LA, Hinthorn DR, Shackelford PG, Shirley RH, Lins RD, Choi CS. Urban measles in the vaccine era: a clinical epidemiologic and serologic study. J Pediatr 81:217–230, 1972.

Cherry J, Feigin RD, Shackelford PG, Hinthorn DR, Schmidt RR. A clinical and serologic study of 103 children with measles vaccine failure. J Pediatr 82:802–808, 1973.

Christensen PE, Schmidt H, Bang HO, et al. An epidemic of measles in Southern Greenland in 1951. Acta Med Scand 144:430–450, 1953.

Clemens JD, Chuong JJH, Feinstein AR. The BCG controversy: a methodological and statistical reappraisal. JAMA 249:2362–2369, 1983.

Cochi SL, Broome CV, Hightower AW. Immunization of U.S. children with *Haemophilus influenzae* type B polysaccharide vaccine: a cost-effectiveness model of strategy assessment. JAMA 253:521–529, 1985.

Cody CL, Baraff LJ, Cherry JD, March SM, Manclark CR. Nature and rates of adverse reactions associated with DTP and DT immunizations in infants and children. Pediatrics 68:650–660, 1981.

Coulehan JL, Hallowell C, Michaels RH, Welty TK, Lui N, Kvo JSC. Immunogenicity of a *Haemophilus influenzae* type B vaccine in combination with diphtheria-pertussis-tetanus vaccine in infants. J Infect Dis 148:530–534, 1983.

Crossley K, Irvine P, Warren JB, Lee BK, Mead K. Tetanus and diphthera immunity in urban Minnesota adults. JAMA 242:2298–2300, 1979.

Daum RS, Granoff DM. A vaccine against *Haemophilus influenzae* type b. Pediatr Infect Dis 4:355–357, 1985.

Dixon CW. Smallpox. London, JA Churchill, 1962.

Douglas RM, Paton JC, Duncan SJ, Hansman DJ. Antibody response to pneumococcal vaccination in children younger than five years of age. J Infect Dis 148:131–137, 1983.

Edsall G, Elliott MW, Peebles TC, Levine L, Eldred MC. Excessive use of tetanus toxoid boosters. JAMA 202:17019, 1967.

Ellison RT III, Kohler PF, Curd JG, Judson FN, Keller LB. Prevalence of congenital or acquired complement deficiency in patients with sporadic meningococcal disease. N Engl J Med 308:913–916, 1983.

Enders JF, Katz SL, Milovanovic MW, Holloway A. Studies on an attenuated measles virus vaccine. I. Development and preparation of the vaccine. N Engl J Med 263:153–159, 1960.

Feigin RD, Baker CJ, Herwaldt LA, Lampe RM, Mason EO, Whitney SE. Epidemic meningococcal disease in an elementary school classroom. N Engl J Med 307:1255–1257, 1982.

Felsenfeld O, Wolf RH, Gyr K, Grant LS, Dutta NK, Zarifi AZ, Zafari Y. Simultaneous vaccination against cholera and yellow fever. Lancet 1:457–458, 1973.

Fenner F. Global eradication of smallpox. Rev Infect Dis 4:916–922, 1982.

Fleming DW, Leibenhaut MH, Albanes D, Cochi SL, Hightower AW, Makintuber S, Helgerson SD, Broome CV. Contributing Group: Secondary *Haemophilus influenzae* type B in day care facilities: risk factor and prevention. JAMA 254:509–514, 1985.

Fox AS, Lepow ML: Tuberculin skin testing in Vietnamese refugees with a history of BCG vaccination. Am J Dis Child 137:1093–1094, 1983.

Fox JP. Eradication of poliomyelitis in the United States: a commentary on the Salk reviews. Rev Infect Dis 2:277–281, 1980.

Fulginiti VA. Simultaneous measles exposure and immunization. Arch Ges Virusforsch 16:300–304, 1964.

Fulginiti VA, Arthur JH, Pearlman S, Kempe CH. Altered reactivity to measles virus: skin test reactivity and antibody response to measles virus antigens in recipients of killed measles virus vaccine. J Pediatr 75:609–616, 1969.

Fulginiti VA, Leland OS, Kempe CH. Evaluation of measles immunization methods. Am J Dis Child 105:509, 1963.

Fulginiti VA, Eller JJ, Downie AW. Altered reactivity to measles virus: atypical measles in children previously immunized with inactivated measles virus vaccines. JAMA 202:1075–1078, 1967.

Fulginiti VA, Arthur JH, Pearlman DS. Altered reactivity to measles virus: local reactions following attenuated measles virus immunization in children who previously received a combination of inactivated and attenuated vaccines. Am J Dis Child 115:671–675, 1968.

Fulginiti VA, Eller JJ, Sieber OF, Joyner JW, Minamitani M, Meiklejohn G. Respiratory virus immunization. I. A field trial of two inactivated respiratory virus vaccines: an aqueous trivalent parainfluenza virus vaccine and an alum-precipitated respiratory syncytial virus vaccine. Am J Epidemiol 89:435–448, 1969.

Glezen WP. Consideration of the risk of influenza in children and indications for prophylaxis. Rev Infect Dis 2:408–420, 1980.

Glezen WP, Frank AL, Taber LH, Tristan MP, Vallbona C, Paredes A, Allison JE. Influenza in childhood. Pediatr Res 17:1029–1032, 1983.

Gold R, Lepow ML, Goldschneider I, Draper TF, Gotschlich EC. Kinetics in antibody production of group A and group C meningococcal polysaccharide vaccines and administered during the first six years of life: prospects for routine immunization of infants and children. J Infect Dis 140:690–697, 1979.

Goldsmith S, Rosenberg E, Pollaczek EH. A study of the antibody response to a dose of tetanus toxoid. N Engl J Med 267:485–487, 1962.

Good RA, Kelly WD, Rotstein J, Varco RL. Immunologic deficiency diseases. Progr Allergy 6:187–319, 1962.

Greenwood BM, Hassan-King M, Whittle HC. Prevention of secondary cases of meningococcal disease in household contacts by vaccination. Br Med J 1:1317–1319, 1978.

Grenier B, Hamza B, Biron G, Xueref C, Viarme F, Roumiantzeff M. Seriommunity following vaccination in infants by an inactivated poliovirus vaccine prepared on Vero cells. Rev Infect Dis 6(Suppl):S545–S547, 1984.

Gross PA, Lee H, Wolff JA, Hall CB, Minnefore AB, Lazicki ME. Influenza immunization in immunosuppressed children. J Pediatr 92:30–35, 1978.

Hankins WA, Gwaltney JM Jr, Hendley JO, Farquhar JD, Samuelson JS. Clinical and serological evaluation of a meningococcal polysaccharide vaccine: groups A, C, Y and W 135(41306). Proc Soc Exp Biol Med 169:54–57, 1982.

Hattwick MAW, Rubin RH, Music S, Sikes RK, Smith JS, Gregg MB. Postexposure rabies prophylaxis with human rabies immune globulin. JAMA 227:407–410, 1974.

Helmick CG. The epidemiology of human rabies postexposure prophylaxis, 1980–1981. JAMA 250:1990–1996, 1983.

Herman JJ, Radin R, Schneiderman R. Allergic reaction to measles (rubeola) vaccine in patients hypersensitive to egg protein. J Pediatr 102:196–199, 1983.

Herrman KL, Halstead SB, Wiebenga NH. Rubella antibody persistence after immunization. JAMA 247:193–196, 1982.

Hilleman M, Buynak EB, Weibel RE. Development and evaluation of the Moraten measles virus vaccine. JAMA 206:487–491, 1968a.

Hinman AR, Orenstein WA, Bloch AB, Bart KJ, Eddins, DL, Amler RW, Kirby CD. Impact of measles in the United States. Rev Infect Dis 5:439–444, 1983.

Hirtz DG, Nelson KB, Ellenberg JH. Seizures following childhood immunizations. J Pediatr 102:14–18, 1983.

Howie VW, Ploussard J, Sloyer JL, Hill JC. Use of pneumococcal polysaccharide vaccine in preventing otitis media in infants: different results between racial groups. Pediatrics 73:79–81, 1984.

Hurwitz ES, Schonberger LB, Nelson DB, Holman RC. Guillain-Barré syndrome and the 1978–1979 influenza vaccine. N Engl J Med 304:1557–1561, 1981.

Innis BL, Snitbhan R, Kunasol P. Protection against hepatitis A by inactivated vaccine. JAMA 271:1328–1334, 1994.

Jacobs RL, Lowe RS, Lanier BQ. Adverse reactions to tetanus toxoid. JAMA 247:40–42, 1982.

Jacobson JA, Filice GA, Holloway JT. Meningococcal disease in day-care centers. Pediatrics 59:299–300, 1977.

Jereb JA, Kelly GD, Porterfield DS. The epidemiology of tuberculosis in children. Semin Pediatr Infect Dis 4:220–231, 1993.

Kanai K: Japan's experience in pertussis epidemiology and vaccination in the past thirty years. Jpn J Med Sci Biol 33:107–143, 1980.

Katz SL, Enders JF, Holloway A. Studies on attenuated measles virus vaccine. VIII. General summary and results of vaccination. N Engl J Med 263:180, 1960.

Kaythy H, Karanko V, Peltola H, Sarno S, Makela PH. Serum antibodies to capsular polysaccharide vaccine in group A *Neisseria meningitidis* followed for three years in infants and children. J Infect Dis 142:861–868, 1980.

Kaythy H, Peltola H, Karanko V. The protective level of serum antibodies to the capsular polysaccharide of *Haemophilus influenzae* type b. J Infect Dis 147:1100, 1983.

Kaythy H, Karanko V, Peltola H. Serum antibodies after vaccination with *Haemophilus influenzae* type b capsular polysaccharide and responses to reimmunization: no evidence of immunologic tolerance or memory. Pediatrics 74:857–865, 1984.

Kempe CH, Fulginiti VA. The pathogenesis of measles virus infection. Arch Ges Viruforsch 16:103–128, 1964.

Kendrick P. A field study of alum-precipitated combined pertussis vaccine and diphtheria toxoid for active immunization. Am J Hyg 38:193–202, 1943.

Klein JO. The epidemiology of pneumococcal disease in infants and children. Rev Infect Dis 3:246–253, 1981.

Krugman S. Further-attenuated measles vaccine: characteristics and use. Rev Infect Dis 5:477–481, 1983.

Krugman S. Present status of measles and rubella immunization in the United States: a medical progress report. J Pediatr 90:1–5, 1977.

Krugman S, Ward R. Infectious hepatitis: current status of prevention with gamma globulin. Yale J Biol Med 34:329–333, 1961–1962.

Lange B, Shapiro SA, Waldman MTG, Proctor E, Arbeter A. Antibody responses to influenzae immunization of children with acute lymphoblastic leukemia. J Infect Dis 140:402–406, 1979.

Lapinleimu K. Elimination of poliomyelitis in Finland. Rev Infect Dis 6(Suppl):S457–S460, 1984.

Lawrence EM, Edwards KM, Schiffman G, Thompson JM, Vaughn WK, Wright RF. Pneumococcal vaccine in normal children: primary and secondary vaccination. Am J Dis Child 137:846–850, 1983.

Leads from the MMWR. JAMA 259:2527–2528, 1988.

Lepow ML, Peter G, Glode MP, Daum RS, Calnen G, Knight KM, Mayer D, Kuo JSC, Lui NST. Response of infants to *Haemophilus influenzae* type B polysaccharide and diphtheria-tetanus-pertussis vaccines in combination. J Infect Dis 149:950–955, 1984.

Lerman SJ, Bollinger M, Brunken JM. Clinical and serologic evaluation of measles, mumps, and rubella (HPV-77: DE-5 and RA 27/3) virus vaccines, singly and in combination. Pediatrics 68:18–22, 1981.

Lewis FA, Gust ID, Bennett MM. On the etiology of whooping cough. J Hyg 71:139, 1973.

Lieu T, Cochi SL, Black SB. Cost-effectiveness of a routine varicella vaccination program for U.S. children. JAMA 271:375–381, 1994.

Luelmo F. BCG vaccination. Am Rev Resp Dis 125(Suppl):70–73, 1982.

Mann JM. Systematic decision-making in rabies prophylaxis. Pediatr Infect Dis 2:162–167, 1983.

Meningococcal Disease Surveillance Group. Meningococcal disease: secondary attack rate and chemoprophylaxis in the United States, 1974. JAMA 235:261–265, 1976.

Merigan TC, Petralli JK, Wilbur J. Circulating human interferon induced by measles vaccination and its *in vitro* antiviral efficacy (abstract). Clin Res 13:197, 1965.

Miller DL, Alderslade R, Ross EM. Whooping cough and whooping cough vaccine: the risks and benefits debate. Epidemiol Rev 41:1–24, 1982.

Miller DL, Ross EM, Alderslade R, Bellman MH, Rawson NSB. Pertussis immunization and serious acute neurological illness in children. Br Med J 282:1595–1599, 1981.

Miller LW, Older JJ, Drake J, Zimmerman S. Diphtheria immunization: effect upon carriers and the control of outbreaks. Am J Dis Child 123:197–199, 1972.

Moore M, Katona P, Kaplan JE, Schonberger LB, Hatch MH. Poliomyelitis in the United States 1969–1981. J Infect Dis 146:558–563, 1982.

Mortimer EA Jr, Jones PK. An evaluation of pertussis vaccine. Rev Infect Dis 1:927–932, 1979.

Munford RS, Taunay A deE, de Morais JS, Fraser DW, Feldman RA. Spread of meningococcal infection within households. Lancet 1:1275–1278, 1974.

Nathanson N, Bodian D. Experimental poliomyelitis following intramuscular virus infection. III. The effect of passive antibody on paralysis and viremia. Bull Johns Hopkins Hosp 111:198–220, 1962.

National Vaccine Advisory Committee. The measles epidemic: the problems, barriers, and recommendations. JAMA 266:1547–1552, 1991.

Nightingale E. Recommendations for a national policy on poliomyelitis vaccination. N Engl J Med 297:249–253, 1977.

Ogra PL, Karzon DT, Righthand F. Immunoglobulin response in serum and secretions after immunization with live and inactivated poliovaccine and natural infection. N Engl J Med 279:893–900, 1968.

Orenstein WA, Bart KJ, Hinman HR, et al. The opportunity and obligation to eliminate rubella from the United States. JAMA 251:1988–1994, 1984.

Osterholm MT, Rambeck JH, White KE. Lack of protective efficacy and increased risk of disease within 7 days after vaccination associated with *Haemophilus influenzae* type b (Hib) polysaccharide (PS) vaccine use in Minnesota (abstract). Abstracts of the 27th ICAAC, New York, 1987.

Pacheco SE. The risks of intravenous immunoglobulin. Semin Pediatr Infect Dis 3:147–149, 1992.

Paisley JW, Bruhn FW, Lauer BA, McIntosh K. Type A2 influenza viral infections in children. Am J Dis Child 132:34–36, 1978.

Peebles TC, Levine L, Eldred MC, Edsall G. Tetanus-toxoid emergency boosters: a reappraisal. N Engl J Med 280:575–581, 1969.

Peltola H, Kaythy H, Sivonen A, Makela PH. *Haemophilus influenzae* type b capsular polysaccharide vaccine in children: A double-blind field study of 100,000 vaccines 3 months to 5 years of age in Finland. Pediatrics 60:730–737, 1977a.

Peltola H, Makela PH, Kaythy H, Jousimies H, Herva E, Hallstrom K, Sivonen A, Renkonen O-V, Pettay A, Karanko V, Ahvanen P, Sarna S. Clinical efficacy of meningococcus group A capsular polysaccharide vaccine in children three months to five years of age. N Engl J Med 297:686–691, 1977b.

Peltola H, Kaythy H, Virtanen M, Markela PH. Prevention of *Haemophilus influenzae* type b bacteremic infections with the capsular polysaccharide vaccine. N Engl J Med 310:1561–1566, 1984.

Peter G. Childhood immunizations. N Engl J Med 327:1794–1800, 1992.

Pincus DJ, Morrison D, Andrews C, Lawrence E, Sell SH, Wright PF. Age-related response to two *Haemophilus influenzae* type b vaccines. J Pediatr 100:197–201, 1982.

Plotkin SA, Smiley ML, Friedman HM, Starr SE, Fleischer GR, Wlodaver G, Dafoe DC, Friedman AD, Grossman RA, Bahker CF. Prevention of cytomegalovirus disease by Towne strain live attenuated vaccine. In Plotkin SA, Michelson S, Pagano JS, Rapp F, eds. CMV: Pathogenesis and Prevention of Human Infection. New York, Alan R Liss, 1984, pp. 271–284.

Preblud SR, Serdula MK, Frank JA Jr, Brandling-Bennett AD, Hinman AR. Rubella vaccination in the United States: a ten year review. Epidemiol Rev 2:171–194, 1980.

Preblud SR, Orenstein WA, Koplan JP, Bart KJ, Hinman AR. A benefit-cost analysis of a childhood vaccination program. Postgrad Med J 61:17–22, 1985.

Puziss M, Wright GG. Studies on immunity in anthrax. X. Gel-Absorbed protective antigen for immunization of man. J Bacteriol 85:230–236, 1963.

Rauh LW, Schmidt R. Measles immunization with killed virus vaccine. Am J Dis Child 109:232–234, 1965.

Redfield RR, Birx DL, Ketter N, Tramont E, Polonis V, Davis C, Brundage JF, Smith G, Johnson S, Fowler A, Wierzba T, Shafferman A, Volvovitz F, Oster C, Burke DS. A phase I evaluation of the safety and immunogenicity of vaccination with recombinant gp160 in patients with early human immunodeficiency virus infection. N Engl J Med 324:1677–1684, 1991.

Redmond SR, Pichichero ME. *Haemophilus influenzae* type b disease: an epidemiologic study with special reference to day-care centers. JAMA 252:2581–2584, 1984.

Riley ID, Tarr PI, Andrews M, Pfeiffer M, Howard R, Challands P, Jennison G, Douglas RM. Immunization with a polyvalent pneumococcal vaccine: reduction of adult respiratory mortality in a New Guinea highlands community. Lancet 1:1338–1341, 1977.

Robbins JB, Austrian R, Lee C-J, Rastogi SC, Schiffman G, Henrichsen J, Makela PH, Broome CV, Facklam RR, Tiesjema RH, Parke JC Jr. Consideration for formulating the second-generation pneumococcal capsular polysaccharide vaccine with emphasis on the cross-reactive types within groups. J Infect Dis 148:1136–1159, 1983.

Rosenzweig EC, Babione RW, Wisseman CL Jr. Immunological studies with group B arthropod-borne viruses. IV. Persistence of yellow fever antibodies following vaccination with 17D strain yellow fever vaccine. Am J Trop Med Hyg 12:230–235, 1963.

Sabin AB. Strategies for elimination of poliomyelitis in different parts of the world with use of oral poliovirus vaccine. Rev Infect Dis 6(Suppl.):S391–S396, 1984.

Sako W. Studies on pertussis immunization. J Pediatr 30:29–40, 1947.

Salk D. Eradication of poliomyelitis in the United States. II. Experience with killed poliovirus vaccine. Rev Infect 2:243–257, 1980a.

Salk D. Eradication of poliomyelitis in the United States. III. Polio vaccines—practical considerations. Rev Infect Dis 2:258–273, 1980b.

Salk J, Salk D. Control of influenza and poliomyelitis with inactivated vaccines. Science 195:834–847, 1977.

Sandberg ET. Intravenous immunoglobulin preparations. Semin Pediatr Infect Dis 3:144–146, 1992.

Santosham M, Wolff M, Reid R, Hohenboken M, Bateman M, Goepp J, Cortese M, Sack D, Hill J, Newcomer W, Capriotti L, Smith J, Owen M, Gahagan S, Hu D, Kling R, Lukacs L, Ellis RW, Vella PP, Calandra G, Matthews H, Ahonkhai V. The efficacy in Navaho infants of a conjugate vaccine consisting of *Haemophilus influenzae* type b polysaccharide and *Neisseria meningitidis* outer-membrane protein complex. N Engl J Med 324:1767–1772, 1991.

Sato Y, Kimura M, Fukumi H. Development of a pertussis component vaccine in Japan. Lancet 1:122–126, 1984.

Schlech WF III, Ward JI, Band JD, Hightower A, Fraser DN, Broome CV. Bacterial meningitis in the United States, 1978–1981. The national bacterial meningitis surveillance study. JAMA 253:1749–1754, 1985.

Schneerson R, Barrera O, Sutton A, Robbins JB. Preparation, characterization and immunogenicity of *Haemophilus influenzae* type b polysaccharide protein conjugates. J Exp Med 152:361–376, 1980.

Schonberger LB, Kaplan J, Kim-Farley R, Moore M, Eddins DL, Hatch M. Control of paralytic poliomyelitis in the United States. Rev Infect Dis 6(Suppl.):S424–S426, 1984.

Schwarz AJ. Immunization against measles: development and evaluation of a highly attenuated live measles vaccine. Ann Pediatr (Stockh) 202:241–252, 1964.

Scolnick EM, McLean AA, West DJ, McAleer WJ, Miller WJ, Buynak EB. Clinical evaluation in healthy adults of a hepatitis B vaccine made with recombinant DNA. JAMA 251:2812–2815, 1984.

Siber GR, Werner BG, Halsey NA, Reid R, Almeido-Hill J, Garrett SC, Thompson C, Santosham M. Interference of immune globulin with measles and rubella immunization. J Pediatr 122:204–211, 1993.

Smit P, Oberholzer D, Hayden-Smith S, Koornhof HJ, Hilleman MR. Protective efficacy of pneumococcal polysaccharide vaccines. JAMA 238:2613–2616, 1977.

Smith MH. National Childhood Vaccine Injury Compensation Act. Pediatrics 82:264–269, 1988.

Spika JS, Halsey NA, Fish AJ, Lum GM, Laver BA, Schiffman G, Giebink GS. Serum antibody response to pneumococcal vaccine in children with nephrotic syndrome. Pediatrics 69:219–223, 1982.

Stern H. Live cytomegalovirus vaccination of healthy volunteers: Eight-year follow-up studies. In Plotkin SA, Michelson S, Pagano JS, Rapp F, eds. CMV: Pathogenesis and Prevention of Human Infections. New York, Alan R Liss, 1984, pp. 263–269.

Stewart GT. Vaccination against whooping cough: efficacy versus risks. Lancet 1:234–239, 1977.

Sultz HA, Hart BA, Zielezny M. Is mumps virus an etiologic factor in juvenile diabetes mellitus? J Pediatr 86:654–656, 1975.

Sumaya CV, Harbison RW, Britton HA. Pneumococcal vaccine failures: two case reports and review. Am J Dis Child 135:155–158, 1981.

Tada H, Yanagida M, Mishina J, Fuji T, Baba K, Ishikowa S, Aihara S, Tsuda F, Miyakawa Y, Makota M. Combined passive and active immunization for preventing perinatal transmission of hepatitis B virus carrier state. Pediatrics 70:613–619, 1982.

Taunay A deE, Galvao PA, de Morais JS, Gotschlich EC, Feldman RA. Disease prevention by meningococcal serogroup C polysaccharide vaccine in preschool children: results after eleven months in São Paulo, Brazil. Pediatr Res 8:429, 1974.

Taylor DN, Pollard RA, Blake PA. Typhoid in the United States and the risk to the international traveler. J Infect Dis 148:599–602, 1983.

Thompson NJ, Glassroth JL, Snider DE Jr, Farer LS. The booster phenomenon in serial tuberculin testing. Am Rev Respir Dis 119:587–597, 1979.

Townsend JT, Baringer JR, Wolinsky JS. Progressive rubella panencephalitis: late onset after congenital rubella. N Engl J Med 292:990–993, 1975.

Tsolia M, Gershon A, Steinberg S, Gelb L. Live attenuated varicella vaccine: evidence that the virus is attenuated and the importance of skin lesions in transmission of varicella-zoster virus. J Pediatr 116:184–189, 1990.

van Wezel AL, van Steenis G, van der Marel P, Osterhaus ADME. Inactivated poliovirus vaccine: current production methods and new developments. Rev Infect Dis 6(Suppl.):S335–S340, 1984.

von Seefried A, Chun JH, Grant JA, Letvenuk L, Pearson EW. Inactivated poliovirus vaccine and test development at Connaught Laboratories Ltd. Rev Infect Dis 6(Suppl. 2):S345–S349, 1984.

Wahdan MH, Rizk F, El-Akkad AM, El Ghoroury AA, Hablas R, Girgis NI, Amer A, Boctar W, Sippel JE, Gotschlich EC, Triav R, Sanborn WR, Cvjetanovic B. A controlled field trial of a serogroup A meningococcal polysaccharide vaccine. Bull WHO 48:667–673, 1973.

Ward JI, Fraser DW, Baraff LJ, Plikaytis BD. *Haemophilus influenzae* meningitis: a national study of secondary spread in household contacts. N Engl J Med 301:122–126, 1979.

Watson BM, Piercy SA, Plotkin SA, Starr SE. Modified chickenpox in children immunized with the Oka/Merck varicella vaccine. Pediatrics 91:17–22, 1993.

Werzberger A, Mensch B, Kuter B. A controlled trial of a formalin-inactivated hepatitis A vaccine in healthy children. N Engl J Med 327:453–457, 1992.

Wilfert CM. Mumps meningoencephalitis with low cerebrospinal fluid glucose, prolonged pleocytosis and elevation of protein. N Engl J Med 280:850, 1960.

Wilkins J, Wehrle PF. Additional evidence against measles vaccine administration to infants less than 12 months of age: altered immune response following active/passive immunization. J Pediatr 94:865–869, 1979.

Wilkins J, Wehrle PFA. Evidence for reinstatement of infants 12–14 months of age into routine measles immunization programs. Am J Dis Child 132:164–166, 1978.

Wilkins J, Wehrle PF. Further characterization of responses of infants and children to meningococcal A polysaccharide vaccine. J Pediatr 94:828–832, 1979.

Wisseman CL Jr, Sweet BH. Immunological studies with group B arthropod-borne viruses. III. Response of human subjects to revaccination with 17D strain yellow fever vaccine. Am J Trop Med Hyg 11:570–575, 1962.

Wood WB Jr. Studies of the mechanism of recovery in pneumococcal pneumonia. J Exp Med 73:201–222, 1941.

Yeager AS, Davis JH, Ross LA. Measles immunization: successes and failures. JAMA 237:347–351, 1977.

Chapter 30

Immunologic Mechanisms in Infectious Diseases

Gerald T. Keusch

Beginning at birth, and sometimes in utero, the human encounters an enormous array of microorganisms with vastly different structure and biochemistry, diverse properties, and an enormous variance in their ability to colonize the host and cause infectious disease. Although the immune system may be thought of as a means to protect us from the pathogenic microorganisms, this is undoubtedly a reflection of only one of the specialized functions of a general mechanism that developed to distinguish self from non-self. The immune system is highly complex and interactive, utilizing both soluble and cell-to-cell communication to activate and regulate immune responses, and it is essential for survival.

Because immune mechanisms and microorganisms have evolved in close association, it is no surprise that the interaction of host and pathogen represents a balance of reactions of the two organisms, sometimes favoring the microbe and sometimes favoring the host. Even disease may represent a balance in which the organism initially causes pathology, but the otherwise healthy host mounts an immune response that ultimately controls the infection. We may envision this interaction as a constant war in which slight tactical advantages to one or the other participant shift the balance in its favor. This view is supported by the fact that only a minor population of microorganisms are virulent for humans, indicating that specialized properties are required for virulence. Acquisition of these traits may have occurred over millennia of evolution,

or they may be rapidly transferred from one genus to another by sudden insertion of genes, as with plasmid transfer from one bacterium to a recipient strain.

Epidemiologic changes may also account for virulence, and it is possible that the occurrence of acquired immunodeficiency syndrome (AIDS) is an example of this, in which a virus, human immunodeficiency virus (HIV), with the property of inactivating normal immune mechanisms, has gained a new route of access to the human because of behavioral factors.

It is important to recognize that the interaction of microbe and host is not a static one and that the immune system is not a monolithic structure. The balance is also reflected in the dose-response relationship of infectious disease: a small inoculum of organisms may be contained by the host; however, a larger inoculum may cause disease. Even the immunity induced by vaccines is not absolute. Immunization with imperfect killed typhoid vaccine is effective, but the protection afforded can be overcome by increasing the infecting dose of typhoid bacilli. In many instances, the time factor becomes paramount; a host capable of responding within hours may eradicate a pathogen before symptoms result, whereas another individual with a slower response time may not.

To these general principles, we must add the concepts of commensalism and symbiosis, which describe interactions between microorganisms and a host that benefit one or both, respectively, while doing no harm to either. Undoubtedly, both types of relationships exist with our "normal flora," the vast microbial mass that is present on the mucous membranes and skin. These organisms ordinarily cause no disease and may be helpful by their metabolic activities and secreted products; however, if they gain access to the tissues of the host, the consequences can be disastrous. Systemic spread can occur because of (1) compromised immune function, (2) traumatic breaches of the mucosal and skin barriers by accident, or (3) medical procedures such as instrumentation and surgery.

Earlier chapters have described the specific components of the immune system in great detail. This chapter examines the function of the immune system from the perspective of a pathogenic microorganism and defines the conditions and adaptations in both host and organism that determine the ultimate balance in the host-pathogen interaction. To accomplish this, pathogenic mechanisms are described in order to understand how successful pathogens overcome host defenses. Then the host response to specific organisms is presented in order to define how the immune system prevents or controls an infection once initiated.

THE NORMAL FLORA

It is reasonable to begin with a discussion of normal flora, a confined microbial population containing many potential pathogens that ordinarily cause no harm (Keusch and Gorbach, 1995). To provide an idea of the enormity of this microbial mass, if we were to disaggregate an adult human into individual cells, we would find the number of bacterial cells alone that are present in the flora to exceed the number of mammalian cells by 1000-fold. This vast population is not randomly distributed on skin and mucous membranes. Rather, specific organisms populate specific niches, determined by ecologic factors, including anaerobiosis, the presence of required nutrients, resistance to host factors such as gastric acid, and the presence of specific attachment sites for cell surface constituents. The overwhelming majority of organisms in the mouth and the colon, for example, are strict anaerobes, favored in the reduced oxygen tension present in the gingival crevice and in the colonic lumen. Facultative anaerobes, able to survive in the presence or absence of oxygen, may be found as well, but in lower numbers. Such bacteria are present on the skin surface, hair follicles, and glands, where they may use oxygen and lower oxygen tension, permitting more strict anaerobes to grow as well. The breast-fed newborn acquires a specific intestinal flora with a predominance of *Bifidobacterium bifidus,* which restricts the implantation of Enterobacteriaceae, and only later do these organisms colonize. In contrast, the formula-fed infant rapidly develops a more "adult" type flora. Administration of antibiotics can also perturb the specific components of the flora, eliminating antibiotic-sensitive organisms and allowing others to implant or to increase in number (Lidbeck and Nord, 1993).

Microbial properties undoubtedly play a role in the selection of normal flora. Certain strains are capable of

long-term residence, whereas others of the same genus are not. The normal inhabitants appear to be ecologically regulated and to occupy specific and distinctive habitats. This flora tends to be stable in individuals, and under normal conditions all niches are occupied and resistant to displacement. A pathogen must have specific properties to colonize, multiply, and invade tissues under these circumstances.

However, the host must restrict the growth of the flora as well. If the rate of multiplication of an *Escherichia coli* grown under optimal in vitro conditions (doubling time of 20 minutes) were duplicated in the gut lumen, a single organism would multiply to more than 10^{14} in just over 14 hours. This obviously does not occur, and in vivo doubling times are much longer owing to a variety of control mechanisms, including shedding, competition for available nutrients, enteric secretions, peristalsis, and intestinal immune mechanisms. That these mechanisms indeed are effective is attested to by the dramatic increase in microbial number after death, indicating that nutrition is not the limiting factor.

MICROBIAL PATHOGENICITY

In all but a few examples, pathogenic microorganisms must establish themselves in or on the host; multiply in particular cells, organs, or sites; and possibly produce physiologically active metabolites such as toxins (Table 30–1). All of this must be accomplished while avoiding the mobilization of host defenses. The exceptions are toxin-producing organisms such as food poisoning strains of *Staphylococcus,* which multiply outside of the host in food and produce enterotoxins, which are ingested and cause disease.

Colonization of the Host

The initial contact between organism and host is the superficial epithelium of the skin or mucous membranes. When these barriers are intact, they represent a significant impediment to microbial invasion. However, if the barrier is broken, penetration can occur and infection is initiated. The examples may be as different as *Staphylococcus aureus* entering the subcutaneous tissues through a damaged cuticle, causing paronychia, and the deposition on the skin of the protozoan *Trypanosoma cruzi* during the feeding of the insect vector with subsequent systemic invasion of the host, resulting in Chagas' disease. Many organisms do not require a mechanical break in the epithelial barrier, as they have evolved ways to overcome these barriers.

Table 30–1. Determinants of Microbial Pathogenicity

1. Colonization
2. Tissue invasion
3. Multiplication within the host
4. Dissemination
5. Resistance to host defenses
6. Production of specific virulence factors

Specific mechanisms may vary in the conjunctiva and in the respiratory, intestinal, and genitourinary tracts; however, the principles are similar (Finlay and Falkow, 1989). The infecting inoculum may be deposited, ingested, or inhaled, migrating along ostia such as the urethra, or it may be introduced by a foreign body; these are different for different organisms, depending on their properties in the environment and the methods employed for transmission (Sparling, 1983). Indeed, these differences account for the varied sites of infection and nature of the resulting disease.

Examples of colonization mechanisms have been well studied in both the gastrointestinal and genitourinary tracts. To illustrate these, we can discuss one genus of bacteria, *E. coli.* Although all *E. coli* look alike under the microscope and share a vast number of biochemical properties, they may be separated by serologic analysis of the antigenic polysaccharides of their lipopolysaccharide exterior (O or somatic antigens), capsular polysaccharides (K antigens) if present, and flagellar proteins (H antigens), found in most *E. coli,* which are motile by means of these appendages. The most useful serologic classification uses O and H antigens together, and it is of interest that of the more than 9000 combinations possible, only a limited handful are potential pathogens (Levine, 1987). One such group is termed enterotoxigenic *E. coli* or ETEC, which causes watery diarrhea by means of toxins that induce isotonic secretion by the intestinal epithelial cells (see below). Because the genetic information for toxin synthesis is contained in plasmids in ETEC, theoretically any *E. coli* can be toxigenic. However, a very restricted number of serotypes are regularly recovered from patients, and these organisms are found to possess surface structures containing antigenic determinants that mediate attachment of the organism to the intestinal epithelial cell brush border.

Attachment of a bacterial cell to a mammalian cell involves two large surfaces, both of which are negatively charged owing to the presence of ionizable surface constituents, including the carboxyl groups of teichoic, glucuronic, and hyaluronic acids on the former and the sialic acid groups on the latter. This presents a mutually repellent charge on the two cells that must be overcome for adherence to occur. Indeed, attractant forces exist, including various weak interactions such as focal ionic attractions, van der Waals forces, hydrogen bonding, and hydrophobic interactions. The strength of these forces is altered by the distance between the cells, the temperature, the ionic strength of the environment, and the radius of curvature of the two surfaces in apposition to one another (van Oss, 1990). As the radius decreases, repellent forces decrease much more steeply than do attractant forces, resulting in a net increase in the attraction of the two cells. As this tends to bring the cells closer together, interactions between hydrophobic regions on the two surfaces can develop, for example, between stretches of apolar amino acids, hydrogen atoms, or methyl or methoxy groups on lipids. Displacement of water then results in a favorable change in free energy and strong adherence. On the basis of these physicochemical prin-

ciples, we might predict that adhesive factors on bacteria would likely be placed on long, thin appendages with a small radius of curvature at the tip relative to the organism itself and that the surface might be less negatively charged or highly hydrophobic and carry a determinant capable of recognizing complementary groups on the epithelial cell surface to be colonized.

In fact, in many instances this is precisely what nature has evolved. Most ETECs have long, thin filaments, termed *pili* or *fimbriae,* radiating out from the surface, giving them a hairy appearance when appropriately visualized under the electron microscope. These structures express attachment antigens that are characteristically localized at the fimbrial tip (Buhler et al., 1991; Hultgren et al., 1991, 1993) where they may bind to cell surface receptors (Stromberg et al., 1991).

These ETEC products are called colonization factor antigens (CFAs) (Krogfelt, 1991), and many antigenically distinctive CFAs have been described, including CFA/I, CFA/II (a complex of three *coli* surface (CS) antigens, CS1, CS2, and CS3), CFA/III, CFA/IV (a complex of CS4, CS5, and CS6), CS7, PcFO9, PcFO159, PcFO166, H4, and CS17. Geographic variation in CFA expression is well known; CFA/I is common in Asia, CFA/II is common in the Middle East, and CFA/IV is common in Latin America (McConnell et al., 1991; Wolf et al., 1993).

Expression of these factors correlates with production of *E. coli* heat-stable enterotoxin (ST) but not heat-labile enterotoxin (LT). Most CFA-positive organisms agglutinate erythrocytes from certain species of animals in the presence of mannose (mannose-resistant hemagglutination, or MRHA), which is considered by some to be a model of the specific receptor-ligand interactions occurring at the intestinal epithelial cell surface (Darfeuille-Michaud et al., 1990). CS2 is the only non-fimbriate and non-hemagglutinating member of the CFA I–IV group; however, all are highly hydrophobic, (van Loosdrecht et al., 1990). Selective deletion of the CFA genes results in a noncolonizing avirulent strain, demonstrating the clinical importance of the colonization factor.

The identification of cell surface carbohydrate structures as the receptors for adhesins is particularly well illustrated by the uropathogenic *E. coli,* many of which possess a mannose-resistant hemagglutinin that has specificity for carbohydrate determinants of the human P blood group system (Vaisanen et al., 1981). These bacteria recognize neutral glycolipids on the cell surface that express a terminal disaccharide consisting of galactose linked $\alpha 1 \rightarrow 4$ to galactose (Leffler and Svanborg-Eden, 1980) by means of a fibrillar adhesin encoded by the *papE* gene (Kuehn et al., 1992). The pilus is therefore known as the *P-pilus* (for P blood group) or *Pap-pilus* (for pyelonephritis-associated pilus).

The same glycolipid receptor is present on human kidney and bladder uroepithelial cells, to which the organisms avidly attach (Roche and Moxon, 1992). Using a mouse pyelonephritis model, which simulates many of the features of ascending human urinary tract infection (UTI), and using genetically manipulated bacterial strains expressing either the mannose-sensitive common type 1 pilus or the P-pilus, only the latter mediates the in vivo attachment necessary for infection to occur (O'Hanley et al., 1985). Moreover, immunization with P-pili, but not type 1 pili, prevents colonization and infection, which provides further evidence of the importance of the adherence lectin in pathogenesis.

As might be anticipated in nature, urinary tract pathogens are also endowed with other adherence mechanisms, and a simple vaccine consisting of P-pilus antigens will not eradicate urinary tract infection as a human disease problem. In fact, strong focal adherence of bacteria to individual bladder cells might facilitate the elimination of the organisms as the host cells are sloughed and passed in the urine (McLean and Nickel, 1991). Rapid clearance of P-pilus or type 1 pilus expressing transformants of an adhesin-negative *E. coli* strain isolated from a patient with stable bacteriuria has been demonstrated (Andersson et al., 1991). The phenomenon of protein-carbohydrate interactions in cell-cell adherence mechanisms (Hultgren et al., 1993) also suggests the potential of therapeutic detachment of pathogens through the use of synthetic receptors or carbohydrate haptens (Karlsson et al., 1992).

Other groups of microorganisms are also endowed with attachment mechanisms. For example, *Mycoplasma pneumoniae* has a specialized terminal structure consisting of a central core with a dense central filament surrounded by an envelope formed by an extension of the plasma membrane. This structure, called the *attachment organelle,* contains adherence proteins that have been localized to the terminal knob of the rod-like extensions observed on detergent-treated organisms (Stevens and Krause, 1992). These rods are trypsin-sensitive and are involved in attachment to cells via neuraminidase-sensitive, long-chain, surface sialo-oligosaccharides of I (branched) or i (linear) type cold agglutinins (Loveless et al., 1992). In addition, the organisms make a number of glycosidases capable of modifying host cell glycoconjugates (Kahane et al., 1990).

These mechanisms are at least superficially similar to the attachment of another respiratory pathogen, influenza virus, via its membrane hemagglutinin, which binds to neuraminidase-sensitive receptors. Indeed, the virus expresses both hemagglutinin and neuraminidase on its surface and uses these factors to attach to and detach from the host target cell.

Invasion of Host Tissues

Systemic pathogens must gain entrance to the host tissues, often through intact barriers (Finlay, 1990). A particularly well-studied example is the invasive mechanism employed by *Shigella* sp., the cause of bacillary dysentery. The capacity to invade host cells has been clearly associated with clinical virulence, since either natural noninvasive variants or genetically altered noninvasive mutants of invasive strains are avirulent in animal models and in human experimental infections (Sansonetti, 1992). The process must be very efficient in *Shigella,* for fewer than 100 organisms constitutes a human infectious dose resulting in clinical disease.

Genetic studies of invasion have shown that multiple chromosomal and plasmid genes, both structural and regulatory, play a role (Hale, 1991).

Shigella invasion is, in essence, the process of phagocytosis, except that it is epithelial cells that, albeit not designed to be professional phagocytes, have somehow been induced to ingest the organism. This results in formation of phagocytic vacuoles by a process analogous to that of neutrophils, involving polymerization of actin and reorganization of the host cell cytoskeleton (Goldberg and Sansonetti, 1993). The signal for this is transmitted by plasmid-mediated outer membrane proteins, known as *invasion plasmid antigens* or *(Ipa)* (Buysse et al., 1987), by an as yet uncertain biochemical mechanism. Deletion of the large (120 to 140 megadaltons) plasmid that encodes these antigens renders the organism noninvasive and avirulent. Certain *E. coli* share the ability of *Shigella* to invade host cells and use the identical or highly conserved molecules to accomplish the task, encoded on large plasmids like those in *Shigella* (Sansonetti, 1992). The evidence suggests a common ancestor for the invasion gene in enteroinvasive *E. coli,* which later moved into *Shigella.*

Recent but already classic work on *Yersinia* invasion of mammalian host cells has identified a single gene product, *invasin,* that mediates the invasive process (Isberg et al., 1993) and host cell structures of the β_1 integrin class that serve as the relevant receptor for *invasin* (Isberg and Leong, 1990). The use of cinemicroscopy has allowed Falkow and colleagues to describe a kinetic ruffling of the host cell membrane as a characteristic response to invasive *Salmonella,* resembling but distinct from the ruffling induced by growth factors and mediated by small GTPases, such as rac or rho (Jones et al., 1993). Ruffles, known to be induced by mitogens or oncogenes as well, are sites of extensive filamentous actin rearrangement associated with active pinocytosis. It is of interest that the ruffles induced by an invasive *Salmonella* results in the ingestion of a noninvasive isolate added to the culture, a process termed *passive entry* (Francis et al., 1993).

Multiplication Within the Host

Invasion alone would not necessarily be a problem if multiplication of the organisms did not occur as well (Finlay and Falkow, 1989). In fact, construction of *Shigella–E. coli* hybrids capable of invading but not multiplying within the host intestinal epithelial cell have verified this concept, as the organism is incapable of causing illness (Formal et al., 1983). Similarly, a galactose epimerase–deficient mutant of *Salmonella typhi* has been found to invade but not survive within cells because the enzyme defect renders the organism susceptible to toxic metabolites that build up in concentration during initial growth. In fact, this strain, Ty 21a, appears to be a most effective live oral vaccine strain because of these properties, for it invades and activates an immune response but then dies off before causing disease.

Microorganisms that multiply within cells are protected from immune mechanisms of host defense. The viruses, of course, must replicate intracellularly, for they are metabolically incapable of surviving outside of cells. Other organisms capable of independent extracellular life may also multiply intracellularly, including bacteria (*Legionella pneumophila* and *Mycobacterium tuberculosis,* for example) and protozoa (e.g., *Toxoplasma gondii* and *Leishmania* sp.). Studies of the mechanisms of intracellular survival of *L. pneumophila* suggest a single genetic locus that is responsible for inhibiting phagosome-lysosome fusion and recruitment of host cell organelles with the bacteria-containing phagosome (Berger and Isberg, 1993). This locus, designated *dot* for defect in organelle trafficking, complements the defect in two classes of mutant *L. pneumophila* that fail to grow intracellularly, one defective for fusion and recruitment of organelles, and the second defective for the latter alone. This suggests the possibility that organelle recruitment is in some way necessary for intracellular growth.

Some genetic studies have revealed two distinct loci on a cloned DNA segment from *M. tuberculosis* that mediate invasion and survival of the resulting *E. coli* recombinant in mammalian host cells (Arruda et al., 1993). *M. tuberculosis* therefore appears to have evolved a strategy in which the organism is transferred to phagosome vesicles that are not fused with lysosomes wherein preferential bacterial multiplication occurs (McDonough et al., 1993). The failure of such unfused vesicles to acidify may be the critical mechanism by which the organism is able to multiply (Crowle et al., 1991). Other data suggest that microbial lipoarabinomannan may contribute as well, by inhibiting interferon-γ–mediated macrophage activation (Chan et al., 1991).

T. gondii is not particular in cell preference, and in essence any mammalian cell will do. One reason suggested for this is the ability of the parasite to bind host-derived laminin and the ability of laminin to bind to β_1 integrin receptors common to virtually all nucleated cell types (Furtado et al., 1992). The parasite then enters the cell within a parasitophorous vacuole that is unable to fuse with other endocytic or biosynthetic organelles, a block that cannot be overcome by killing the parasite after its initial entry into the cell (Joiner et al., 1990). However, by altering the parasite's route of entry by coating the organism with antibody and infecting a CHO cell line that bears the Fc receptor, fusion will occur. This suggests that fusion blockade is a function of the route of entry and not secretion of a soluble factor by the parasite itself.

Multiplication is also obviously important to extracellular organisms, which must have sufficient resistance to host microbicidal mechanisms to survive. In some instances, for example, *S. pneumoniae,* it has been well demonstrated that the polysaccharide capsule of the organism endows it with the ability to resist phagocytosis (Avery and Dubos, 1931). In fact, it is difficult to find other properties of the pneumococcus to account for its ability to cause disease, except that it induces an inflammatory response while avoiding ingestion by neutrophils in sufficient numbers to greatly multiply. In the lung, this inflammation fills up the alveoli with fluid, interfering with gas exchange, resulting in the symptoms of pneumonia; if the organism reaches the meninges, the resulting inflammation causes the clinical manifestations of acute meningitis. A special case is the long-term survival of certain systemic metazoan pathogens, for example, adult stage schistosomes or filarial worms, which survive for many years within the venous or lymphatic systems, constantly resisting cells and circulating factors of the immune system with impunity.

Although it is of importance for the organisms to survive and multiply, it is equally important in most instances not to rapidly overwhelm and kill the host, for this may limit the transmission of the organism to new susceptibles to the detriment of the species. This is especially true of highly human-adapted microorganisms, for there is no other reservoir of transmission. Principles of ecologic balance thus dictate that organisms capable of causing rapidly lethal infection should not do this in all infected individuals. In cases such as anthrax, in which transmission may be from contact with dead infected tissue, these principles are not applicable.

Dissemination of Microorganisms

With some exceptions, such as diphtheria, in which organisms localized to the pharyngeal epithelial surface produce a lethal toxin that is systemically spread, most organisms causing systemic disease must disseminate throughout the host to reach target cells or tissues, of which there may be more than one. One novel mechanism postulated for the gonococcus is to "hitchhike" by attachment to sperm and ride upstream against the movement of cilia into the fallopian tube, where it causes acute salpingitis (Sparling, 1983). Organisms that penetrate epithelial or mucosal surfaces often reach the blood stream and circulate throughout the body. This may not produce any symptoms, as, for example, the initial bacteremia in *S. typhi* infection resulting in sequestration within hepatic mononuclear phagocytes, or it may cause potentially fatal clinical septicemia. Since the complement and antibody present in plasma can rapidly kill many organisms without the participation of phagocytic cells, circulating microorganisms are usually found to be resistant to this bactericidal mechanism. It is presumably for the same reason that the complement-sensitive epimastigote stage of *T. cruzi* is not present in the circulation, although both epimastigotes and trypomastigotes may be released from infected cells, for only the complement-resistant trypomastigote survives.

Staphylococcus aureus bacteremia often causes disseminated microabscesses throughout the body (Sheagren, 1984). One mechanism of spread is within phagocytic cells that ingest but do not kill the organism and instead are themselves killed in the process. These circulating microcolonies of *S. aureus* are then widely deposited in different tissues, producing the characteristic multiple small abscesses of this infection. Viremia is also common in systemic viral infection; however, the blood stream can best be considered a pathway to reach the right target cell that permits attachment and penetration of the virus, which must reach the intracellular milieu to replicate. The same is true of some helminth larvae with a systemic phase in their life cycle. For example, *Trichinella spiralis* larvae are born live from the female worm in the gut epithelium. They invade the circulation and are widely distributed; using their sharp stylus-like anterior end, they indiscriminantly burrow into diverse types of cells. For all but skeletal muscle, this is a lethal event for the larva. However, in myocytes, the larva survives and continues its development into an infectious cyst that is the transmission stage of the parasite.

MECHANISMS OF DISEASE

The foregoing discussion deals primarily with mechanisms of infection, and it should be re-emphasized that individual pathogens may utilize several of the mechanisms described to encounter and infect the host. These processes may be entirely asymptomatic and constitute the incubation period of an infectious illness. Once established in their preferred site, pathogenic organisms can then produce cellular and organ dysfunction or destruction, resulting in the clinical manifestations of disease. A number of distinct mechanisms are involved in this phase of the host-pathogen interaction (Table 30–2).

The Inflammatory Response

One important cause of disease manifestations is the inflammatory response induced by the invading pathogen (Sparling, 1983). Although this is clearly an important component of host defense, adventitious tissue damage may also result from an exuberant response with detrimental clinical effects. Inflammation begins with a chemotactic signal or leukocyte migration. One well-defined class of microbial signals is a series of N-formylated low-molecular-weight peptides produced by bacteria. The best studied of these is N-formyl-methionyl-leucyl-phenylalanine (f-met-leu-phe), which brings about the directed migration (chemotaxis) of both polymorphonuclear leukocytes (PMNs) and monocytes/macrophages, when injected into tissue or in vitro. Other mediators can also cause chemotaxis. For example, neutral proteases of microorganisms can directly cleave the third (C3)) and fifth (C5) components of the complement system, generating active fragments with chemotactic function and anaphylatoxin activity, which increase vascular permeability and assist in the diapedesis or movement of leukocytes from the intravascular compartment to the tissues.

Table 30–2. Mechanisms of Disease or Tissue Damage in Infections

1. Inflammatory response
2. Endotoxin
3. Peptidoglycan
4. Capsular polysaccharides
5. Toxins

Whether or not this mechanism is biologically significant is not clear; however, activation of complement by the organism's surface constituents or antigens results in the generation of the same complement activation products. This is biologically important, as demonstrated by the abnormal host response in patients with genetic defects of the complement system (see Complement and Host Defense). Release of leukocyte enzymes with proteolytic activity, or activation of the clotting or kinin systems, can directly damage tissue. The accumulation of leukocytes may protect the host (the laudable pus mentioned in historical medical writings), but can also result in abscess formation with adverse clinical implications.

Some organisms induce an organized inflammatory reaction known as a *granuloma*, containing macrophages and T lymphocytes and often eosinophils or PMNs. This is characteristic of mycobacterial infection, in which the granuloma both functions to contain the spread of the organism and causes tissue pathology. In *Schistosoma mansoni* infection, the granuloma forms around the eggs produced by adult worm pairs, which are swept into the liver from the portal vein. There is an antigen-specific induction of the host inflammatory response that ultimately destroys the eggs (Weinstock, 1992). However, once formed, other antigens stimulate granuloma cells to produce fibrogenic factors, resulting in the characteristic fibrosis of schistosomiasis (Wyler, 1992). It is the latter that has clinical importance, for the presence of the adult worms and the eggs by themselves does no harm. Rather, the host fibrosis response is the mechanism for clinical symptoms. For this reason, schistosomiasis is a classic example of immunopathogenesis of disease.

Endotoxin

The lipopolysaccharide (LPS) constituents (endotoxin) of the outer membrane of gram-negative bacteria are highly active molecules that play an important role in many infections (Martich et al., 1993). The LPS from different organisms has a common structure, including a toxic lipid (lipid A), a core oligosaccharide containing ketodeoxyoctanoic acid (KDO), and a richly variable outer O polysaccharide that expresses the distinctive antigens of the different organisms. Most, if not all, of the biologic effects of LPS, including induction of fever (pyrogenicity), direct activation of the alternative complement pathway as well as Hageman's factor and the kinin-forming system, are caused by the lipid A component, a hydrophobic domain of LPS situated in the outer monolayer of the outer membrane of the organism (Raetz, 1993). This is now known to act by regulating a number of protein mediators of host responses collectively known as *cytokines*, many of which are produced by macrophages activated by LPS (Watson et al., 1994). This requires the interaction of LPS via the lipid A moiety with a hepatocyte-derived acute-phase plasma glycoprotein called *LPS-binding protein* (LBP) and the subsequent binding of the LPS-LBP complex to cellular receptors mediating lipid A–dependent responses (Ulevitch, 1993). In the presence of LBP, lipid A cytokine responses occur at lower concentrations by at least 1000-fold and the rate of cytokine release is dramatically enhanced (Hailman et al., 1994).

To make matters more complex, LBP is related to another lipid A–binding protein present in neutrophil granules, *bactericidal/permeability increasing protein* (BPI), which exerts a profound bactericidal effect on gram-negative bacilli. A membrane protein or proteins of 70 to 80 kD, and possibly a second protein or proteins of 30 to 40 kD, that interact with lipid A have been identified by photochemical cross-linking with labeled LPS derivatives and are proposed to represent the LPS cellular receptors (Morrison et al., 1993). Less ambiguous is the involvement of the glycosyl-phosphatidyl-inositol (GPI)–anchored macrophage membrane differentiation antigen, CD14, in transduction of the LPS activation signals in macrophages (Ziegler-Heitbrock and Ulevitch, 1993), which appears to occur through a protein tyrosine phosphorylation mechanism (Weinstein et al., 1993) and activation of transcription factor NF-κB (Read et al., 1993).

LPS-induced changes are associated with mobilizing host defense mechanisms to inflammatory challenge, and these are essential for host survival. At the same time, these responses represent double-edged swords, capable of causing major clinical problems if present in excess. Thus, clinical diseases associated with LPS activation of host responses include sepsis syndrome and septic shock, thermal injury, and possibly liver failure, and ischemic and inflammatory bowel disease (Manthous et al., 1993a). Specific organ effects on myocardium, lungs, kidney, brain, and the gastrointestinal tract that result in physiologic deterioration have also been described (Manthous et al., 1993b). Given this intimate relationship between the beneficial and harmful clinical effects of endotoxin, it is not surprising that mice deficient for either the interferon-γ receptor (Car et al., 1994) or tumor necrosis factor (TNF) 55-kD receptor (Pfeffer et al., 1993) have been shown to resist endotoxic shock. In the latter case, the TNF receptor–deficient animals became much more susceptible to live bacterial challenge (Schwab, 1993), perhaps because of shared binding sites with LPS on peripheral blood monocytes (Rabin et al., 1993).

Peptidoglycan

The bacterial cell wall is not there simply to maintain the structure of the microorganism; it also has the capacity to induce host injury responses (Bone, 1994). The major constituent of the cell wall is peptidoglycan (PG), which is a polymer of N-acetyl-D-glucosamine linked β 1→4 to N-acetyl-muramic acid with attached short peptide side chains that are cross-linked by peptide bridges to form a rigid structure. Species specificity resides in the different primary structure of the amino acids used to form the interchain peptide bridges. Peptidoglycan exhibits certain endotoxin-like properties, including pyrogenicity, complement activation (both classical and alternative pathways), and adjuvanticity (Schwab, 1993), perhaps because of shared binding

sites with LPS on peripheral blood monocytes (Rabin et al., 1993). Staphylococcal PG has also been shown to inhibit phagocytosis of *S. aureus* by human PMNs and induces leukopenia when injected into experimental animals (Spika et al., 1982). These effects are abrogated by anti-PG antibody.

Experimental injection of PG from group A β-hemolytic *Streptococcus pyogenes* into mice can induce a chronic inflammatory response in heart muscle that superficially resembles the lesions of rheumatic fever (Schwab, 1993). When it is administered to rats, a migratory polyarthritis develops, including synovitis, pannus formation, and joint destruction. It is reported that PG is several times more potent than LPS in the activation of the alternative pathway of complement. The adjuvant action of PG is contained primarily in a muramyl-alanyl-isoglutamine dipeptide (MDP), and the question has been raised whether this property might not account for the induction of autoimmune tissue responses in appropriate hosts. Since the metabolism of PG within phagocytic cells is slow and the material persists, PG can chronically activate macrophages to become cytotoxic for target cells, which suggests a possible mechanism for PG-induced tissue damage (Smialowicz and Schwab, 1977).

Metabolism of pneumococcal PG by N-acetylmuramyl-L-alanine amidase, the autolytic enzyme of *S. pneumoniae*, results in a product that induces purpura when injected into experimental animals (Chetty and Kreger, 1981). With the use of a model organ culture of human fallopian tubes, soluble PG products produced during growth of *Neisseria gonorrhoeae* (a unique characteristic of this organism) by the action of gonococcal PG:PG-6-muramyl transferase (transglycosylase), including non-reducing disaccharide tetrapeptide and tripeptide monomers designated "anhydro-monomers," have been shown to damage the tissue in vitro, with a loss of ciliated cells (Melly et al., 1984). Neither muramyl dipeptide nor N-acetylglucosamine in high concentration reproduced the abnormalities. These few examples are enough to indicate the potential relevance of this structural component of bacterial cell walls to virulence of the organisms.

Capsular Polysaccharides

Mention has been made of antiphagocytic capsular polysaccharides that aid certain microorganisms to evade host defenses and establish infection. Additional roles for capsular polysaccharides clearly exist. One such role is in the production of disease manifestations caused by *Bacteroides fragilis*. Many studies in the past decade have established this organism as a major anaerobic pathogen of humans. One of the now classic diseases due to *B. fragilis* is intra-abdominal sepsis and abscess formation. The establishment of experimental animal models for this process has helped to clarify the role of the surface oligosaccharide structures of the organism as a major virulence factor. Other *Bacteroides* species do not possess this cellular component. It was found that substitution of killed *B. fragilis* or of purified capsular material for the live inoculum in these experimental models resulted in intra-abdominal abscess just as if the live organism had been introduced (Onderdonk et al., 1990). Although the LPS from the bacterium was also able to promote abscess formation, the capsular material was much more active on a stoichiometric basis.

Recently, the capsule has been purified and its chemical structure determined. It is a complex of two distinct polysaccharides, each with repeating units of negatively charged carboxyl or phosphate groups and positively charged amino groups, both of which are required for induction of abscesses (Tzianabos et al., 1993). These studies confirm that the capsule is the critical factor in the model disease. The *Bacteroides* LPS is structurally different from that of Enterobacteriaceae, lacking two carbohydrates unique to the latter (KDO and L-glycero-D-mannoheptose), and it does not exhibit the biologic properties of endotoxin either. The mechanism of abscess promotion by the capsular material is unclear, and no direct toxic effect on PMN function has been demonstrated in vitro.

Toxins

Manifestations of a number of infectious diseases are due to the action of microbial toxins. Early in the microbiologic era, clinical diphtheria and tetanus were shown to be due to protein toxins and the preparation of toxoid vaccines resulted in successful prophylactic immunization. Many other organisms are also toxigenic, and there is renewed interest in these molecules as agents of disease (Alouf and Freer, 1991).

Diphtheria toxin is relatively well understood. Its structure is fully defined, and the biologically active portion is well characterized as an adenosine diphosphate (ADP)–ribosylating enzyme for its target substrate, elongation factor 2 (EF-2), which is used for cellular protein synthesis (Pappenheimer, 1993). Susceptible cells have a toxin receptor, recently cloned and identified as a heparin-binding epidermal growth factor–like precursor (Naglich et al., 1992), A translocation domain of the toxin allows the enzymatically active portion to cross the host cell membrane to reach its cytoplasmic target (London, 1992), where it catalytically inhibits protein synthesis and kills the cell. The most important target is the myocardial muscle cell, and cell death results in an inflammatory myocarditis.

Cholera toxin is also an ADP-ribosylating enzyme, acting on the guanosine triphosphate (GTP)–binding protein of the regulatory subunit of cellular adenylate cyclase (Spangler, 1992). Toxin binds to cell surface GM_1 ganglioside and is translocated to the cell interior where ADP ribosylates the regulatory subunit and activates the cyclase, resulting in marked elevation of cellular cyclic adenosine monophosphate (cAMP). If the target cell is in the intestinal epithelium, this causes the secretion of isotonic fluid, which is the diarrheal stool of the disease. In contrast to diphtheria toxin, cholera toxin does not cause structural damage.

Pseudomonas exotoxin A is a third ADP-ribosylating protein, very similar in action to diphtheria toxin on the same substrate, EF-2, but with distinct tissue tro-

pism. However, in contrast to the two toxins mentioned, the role of the *Pseudomonas* toxin in infection due to *Pseudomonas aeruginosa* remains uncertain (Wick et al., 1990). Membrane-damaging cytolytic toxins are also produced by a number of other organisms, at least in vitro, for example, streptolysins from *S. pyogenes* (Wannamaker, 1983). Their role in disease causation is also not certain.

IMMUNE RESPONSES TO INFECTIOUS AGENTS

Just as microbial virulence is polygenic and complex, so is the host immune response to these diverse agents. Although we generally (and arbitrarily) divide the immune response into component parts for convenience, it is clear that the entire system functions as an interactive network with often overlapping functions. Indeed, there clearly is redundancy in mechanisms to contain and control infection. Nevertheless, specialization is evident in the workings of immune mechanisms, for hosts with genetic or acquired defects of specific limbs of the system are not universally susceptible to all classes of infectious agents (Table 30–3) (Stiehm et al., 1986). In general, defects of cell-mediated immunity are associated with severe intracellular infections as a result of viruses, protozoa, fungi, and certain facultative intracellular bacteria. In contrast, defects of neutrophil function, or of antibody or complement production, are associated with invasive pyogenic infections caused primarily by bacteria and, to a lesser extent, by certain viral or fungal infections.

These clinical observations make it clear that no one immune mechanism is responsible for defense against a single class of infectious agents; rather, specific biologic features of the infectious agent determine which immune mechanism(s) is (are) most important for protection (Table 30–4). This suggests that host immune responses are geared to the pathogenic potential of the

Table 30–3. Specific Infections Complicating Genetically Determined Immunodeficiencies

| Pathogen | Immune System Affected | | | |
	Phagocytic	T-Cell	Complement	Antibody
Bacteria				
Staphylococci	+ + +		+ +	+ + +
Coliforms	+ + +		+ +	+
Haemophilus influenzae	+		+	+ + +
Mycobacterium tuberculosis		+ + +		
Fungi				
Candida	+ +	+ +		
Aspergillus	+ + +			
Cryptococcus		+ + +		
Viruses				
Herpesviruses		+ + +		
Enteroviruses		+		+ +
Protozoa				
Pneumocystis carinii		+ + +		

Table 30–4. Antimicrobial Immune Mechanisms

1. Complement-mediated lysis
2. Complement- or antibody-mediated opsonization
3. Phagocytosis and intracellular killing
4. Antibody-dependent cellular cytotoxicity of viruses or bacteria
5. Antibody-dependent (eosinophil) cellular cytotoxicity of helminths
6. Antibody neutralization (viruses, toxins, colonization factors)
7. T cell–dependent macrophage activation (interferon-γ)
8. Cytotoxic T lymphocytes
9. Natural killer cells
10. Interferon

infecting organism; therefore, it is essential to think about host-pathogen interactions in order to understand the immune response. It should also be emphasized that the mere mounting of a particular immune response does not necessarily result in a protective host defense but may be an associated epiphenomenon or even a mechanism for the microorganism to evade the immune system, as, for example, the polyclonal B-cell activation observed in malaria or leishmaniasis.

Complement and Host Defense

Activation of the complement system results in the appearance of a number of mediators of the immune system and the inflammatory response (Frank, 1992) (see Chapter 7). As such, complement is centrally located in the immunologic network for efficient mobilization of these responses. The soluble factors C3a, C5a, and C4a (in high concentration) induce histamine secretion by mast cells and basophils, which promotes vasodilatation. C3a and C5a increase vascular permeability and can enhance the diapedesis of leukocytes from the intravascular to extravascular compartments where the invading microorganism is localizing. C5a is the most potent chemoattractant produced by the host, and it both increases PMN adhesiveness and stimulates the respiratory burst of these cells to activate microbicidal mechanisms. In addition, C5a mediates the release of leukotrienes, another class of activators of the inflammatory response. C3d and C3e, secondary cleavage products of C3b, can modulate some B-lymphocyte functions and can mobilize PMNs from bone marrow to induce leukocytosis, respectively.

At the same time, cell-bound products of the cascade play important roles. C3b is a major opsonic factor, allowing recognition of the C3b coated organism by phagocytic cells through their C3b receptor. C4b can function in the neutralization of viruses. Deposition of C5a on the surface of the organism initiates the assembly of the membrane attack complex, which results in the death and lysis of cells susceptible to this action. Some organisms are resistant to this effect of the complement cascade by forming factors that destroy complement components, failing to bind activated complement components, or shedding complement proteins deposited on the cell surface (Frank, 1992). It is not

surprising that such bacteria preferentially cause systemic sepsis.

The essential role of the complement system is revealed by the study of patients with genetic defects at specific loci of the cascade. (See Chapter 17.) These may separately affect the initiating factors of the classical or alternative pathways, may be located at the bridge point of the two pathways, C3, or may be specifically localized to the terminal components common to both pathways, but after the formation of the activated fragments of C3. A review of the infections associated with these defects is revealing (Ross and Densen, 1984). Deficiency of the initiating components of classical pathway activation is accompanied by apparent susceptibility to *S. aureus* or *S. pneumoniae, Haemophilus influenzae, Neisseria,* gram-negative rods, and herpesviruses. Genetic defects in the alternative pathway are much less frequent. Two families with a sex-linked defect in properdin have been described in which severe meningococcal infections have affected males. C3-deficient patients have suffered from problems with encapsulated bacteria, primarily the pneumococcus, but also *H. influenzae* and neisserial infection. Defects of components C5 to C9 are associated with recurrent infections due to the meningococcus or gonococcus.

Review of all reported patients with genetic complement deficiencies reveals that 25% (61/242) have experienced frequently recurrent (90 episodes in the 61 patients) systemic infections with either *Neisseria meningitidis* or *N. gonorrhoeae* (see Chapter 17). The highest incidence has been in the C5-deficient patients. An additional observation of relevance is that the incidence of group Y *N. meningitidis* infection in patients with defects in the late complement components is increased fourfold over that observed in normal patients. This suggests that the direct bactericidal effect of the late components is of particular importance for defense against this organism. Immunization with capsular antigens to induce early complement component–dependent opsonizing antibody should reduce the risk of such individuals to meningococcal disease (Figueroa et al., 1993).

In contrast, an experimental model of pneumococcal bacteremia in the guinea pig has demonstrated that complement is critically involved in the clearance of the organism from the blood stream and survival from the experimental infection (Brown et al., 1983). Whereas specific antibody greatly enhanced the host response, complement activation by either pathway was essential. These findings are consistent with the preponderance of *S. pneumoniae* infections in C3-deficient patients, and it suggests that the role of complement in pneumococcal infection is as an opsonin to promote the efficient uptake and killing of the organism by phagocytic cells (Bruyn et al., 1992).

Phagocytosis and Microbicidal Activity

The principal effector phagocytic cells are the PMNs and the mononuclear phagocytes (monocytes and macrophages). Because of the role of T lymphocytes in the activation of macrophage microbicidal activity, this is discussed later in the context of cell-mediated immunity. Eosinophils may play a role in the host response to helminthic infections, in which the cells attach to and damage the worm, even though ingestion of the parasite is impossible because of its size (Gleich et al., 1993).

Neutrophil phagocytosis and intracellular microbicidal activity constitute a complex process, dependent upon humoral factors supplied by activation of complement and by the production of specific antibodies. PMNs are required to migrate to the site of infection, to recognize and ingest the organism in a phagocytic vesicle, and to form phagolysosomes by fusing with primary and secondary lysosomes that degranulate into the fused vesicle, depositing antimicrobial factors and metabolizing oxygen products to form highly toxic oxygen radicals (Baggiolini et al., 1993). When all of this is accomplished, a variety of ingested microorganisms can be killed.

The accumulation of leukocytes in injured, inflamed, or infected tissues is a critical host response. The mechanisms involved are complex and are regulated by the coordinated expression and/or activation of leukocyte and endothelial cell adhesion molecules (Nourshargh, 1993). These molecules, termed *selectins,* control the cell-cell interactions that permit diapedesis to and trapping of phagocytic cells at the site of inflammation (Bevilacqua and Nelson, 1993). The release of cytokines and other metabolic products of activated leukocytes, for example, nitric oxide and various free radicals (Moncada and Higgs, 1993), either may serve the host in a protective manner or may aggravate the organ pathology of the systemic inflammatory response syndrome (Dinarello et al., 1993).

Considerable insight into the function and role of phagocytic antimicrobial cells in infectious disease is gained by examination of the clinical problems faced by patients with genetically determined defects in cell function who have normal numbers of poorly functioning cells and of patients with neutropenia who have low numbers of cells that may or may not be functionally intact (see Chapters 15 and 16). One interesting problem is presented by patients with defects in chemotaxis of neutrophils. At least 25 genetic or acquired conditions are associated with defective chemotaxis, sometimes in conjunction with other functional abnormalities (see Chapters 13 and 15).

A more restricted chemotactic abnormality, albeit variable in extent, is present in patients with the hyperimmunoglobulin E syndrome (see Chapters 13 and 15). This has been attributed to suppressive factors released from mononuclear cells. Beginning in the first few weeks or months of life, these individuals suffer from repeated staphylococcal infections of skin that become chronic and from persistent pulmonary infections with *S. aureus* that often progress to tissue destruction and pneumatoceles. Although PMNs do accumulate in the lesions, their migration is delayed and subnormal. It appears that the delay in response to bacterial invasion allows infection in skin or lung to become established but is nevertheless sufficient to prevent systemic spread. The elevation in IgE levels, often with specificity for staphylococcal cell walls, is not helpful and may

be a defect in lymphocyte function that regulates IgE production. Aberrations in anti-staphylococcal antibody in other Ig classes have been described, including an excess of IgM but not IgG antibody and a deficit of anti–*S. aureus* IgA in serum, which correlated with the incidence of infection at mucosal surfaces and adjacent lymph nodes (Dreskin et al., 1985). It is likely that immunoregulatory abnormalities underlie these findings, which may contribute to the infection problems in the afflicted subjects.

There are a number of genetic disorders of PMN microbicidal function (see Chapter 15). In chronic granulomatous disease (CGD), for example, phagocyte chemotaxis, ingestion of organisms, and degranulation of lysosomes proceed normally; however, the cells fail to produce microbicidal products such as H_2O_2 via the oxidative burst (Curnutte, 1993). Intracellular organisms, therefore, are not killed, and the result is severe and prolonged infections, often progressing to granuloma formation consisting of mononuclear cells. A limited number of organisms are consistently isolated, principally *S. aureus,* and, less commonly, *Aspergillus* and *Candida* sp., *Chromobacterium violaceum, Pseudomonas cepacia,* and a variety of gram-negative rod Enterobacteriaceae. These problem organisms have been noted to share one apparently important characteristic—they produce the enzyme catalase, which breaks down H_2O_2 produced during their metabolism. In contrast, catalase-negative organisms such as *S. pneumoniae, S. pyogenes,* and viruses do not seem to be problems for the individual with CGD. It is believed that this is due to utilization by the CGD leukocyte of H_2O_2 produced by the microorganism in the phagolysosome to generate toxic oxygen radicals.

The same pattern of infection seen in CGD also occurs in patients with Chédiak-Higashi syndrome (CHS) (see Chapters 15 and 16). In this disorder, degranulation of lysosomes is abnormal, although other aspects of phagocytosis and respiratory burst are intact. In vitro studies demonstrate abnormal early kinetics of killing of *S. aureus* as well as streptococci, but after 20 minutes of incubation the rate of killing parallels normal leukocytes (Root et al., 1972). This suggests that initial intracellular killing is dependent on lysosomal factors, whereas the later microbicidal activity is due to the respiratory burst and production of oxygen radicals. In addition to this defect, there is a peripheral neutropenia in patients with CHS, which undoubtedly contributes to the functional abnormalities (Blume and Wolff, 1972). This disease also illustrates that a rapid and full response of phagocytic cells is important to host defense mechanisms against pyogenic organisms.

Patients with severe neutropenia but intact cell-mediated immunity suffer from frequent skin, mucosal, and systemic infections, generally initiated by bacteria that are normally resident at these sites (Lee and Pizzo, 1993) (see Chapters 15 and 31). The predominant organisms are *S. aureus* and facultative gram-negative rods, including *E. coli, Klebsiella pneumoniae, P. aeruginosa,* and *Enterobacter* sp. This strongly suggests that phagocytic cells present in mucosal linings and exiting the body through these surfaces play an important role in restricting mucosal flora to the surface and the lumen. In addition, particularly when the normal flora has been deranged by the use of antimicrobial drugs, fungal infections due to *Candida, Aspergillus,* and *Mucor* species are observed. This implies that even in the presence of severe neutropenia, an intact normal flora can inhibit the growth and invasiveness of fungi. The risk of infection is also increased when normal barriers such as skin are breached by intravenous lines and when the respiratory or urinary tract is damaged by instrumentation, indwelling airways, or catheters, as discussed in Chapter 31.

Humoral Immunity

The production of antibodies is a highly specific immune response to individual antigenic determinants. Antibodies can distinguish proteins differing in one amino acid or polysaccharides that vary only in the spatial organization of the same sequence of sugars. The generation of the repertoire of antibodies of such exquisite specificity is complex, genetically determined, and under the control and regulation of T lymphocytes for most antigens (Berek and Ziegner, 1993). During an antibody response, both the isotype (immunoglobulin type) and idiotype (antigenic specificity) change from IgM to IgG predominance and from low affinity to high affinity, respectively. It seems reasonable to suggest that the early IgM response is not of high affinity in order to permit rapid production of antibodies that can still recognize the antigen and thus function in the early antimicrobial host defenses (Brunham and Holmes, 1983). IgM is a potent activator of complement, which functions as an opsonin when C3b is deposited on the microbial surface and is recognized by the C3b receptor on PMNs and macrophages. However, because of its size, IgM is restricted to the intravascular compartment. Later production of IgG to microbial surface determinants enhances the opsonic activity because the phagocytes can engage the free Fc portion of the antibody by means of their Fc receptors, and the antibody can be readily delivered to extravascular sites of infection. Defects in IgG subclasses may contribute to selective susceptibility to pathogens (Kuijpers et al., 1992). For example, deficiency in IgG2 subclass antibody, often accompanied by reduced IgG4 and/or IgA antibody, results in reduced antibody responses to bacterial capsular antigens and recurrent or chronic infections with encapsulated organisms (see Chapter 11).

Much of our understanding of the importance of humoral immunity as a host defense has come from clinical studies of patients with congenital immunoglobulin deficiency states. Recent studies have focused on another way to examine this, that is, the perceived improvement in health status attributable to immunoglobulin replacement therapy (Gardulf et al., 1993). This study showed that prior to initiation of treatment, these patients reported more episodes of infection and perceived greater dysfunction, measured as emotional state, mobility, social interactions, sleep, rest, work, and recreation, than a non-immunocompromised but otherwise similar reference group. After 18 months of replacement therapy, however, health-related func-

tions and behaviors and self-rated state of health both improved and were associated with higher IgG levels prior to scheduled immunoglobulin infusions. Increasingly, such "quality of life" indicators are going to be evaluated as critical outcome measures of therapy.

Opsonization

The importance of antibody opsonins for host defense is amply documented by the clinical problems experienced by patients with congenital Bruton-type agammaglobulinemia (Stiehm et al., 1986). Beginning in the first few months of life when maternal antibody disappears, these patients experience recurrent bacterial infections of the respiratory mucosal lining, including sinuses, middle ear, bronchi, and lungs. Bacteremia with secondary meningitis or septic arthritis is common (see Chapter 11). The organisms commonly involved in these infections are encapsulated, such as the pneumococcus, *H. influenzae,* or *N. meningitidis,* which become resident on respiratory mucosal surfaces, as well as *S. aureus,* all of which resist phagocytosis until opsonized. In the case of *S. aureus,* antibody may also play a role following phagocytosis, for phagosome-lysosome fusion is potentiated by antibody coating of the organism, without which the bacterium may survive in the unfused vesicle (Leijh et al., 1979). Repeated administration of pooled IgG from normal donors repletes the antibody pool in these patients and reduces the frequency and severity of infection.

Clinical observations in the pre-antibiotic era in patients with pneumococcal pneumonia and bacteremia are also revealing. Patients rapidly became ill and often died in the first few days of infection (Finland, 1979). If they survived, they remained gravely ill until quite suddenly, about 1 week after infection, rapid improvement would occur. This dramatic change, called the "crisis," can be attributed to the development of increasing titers of high-affinity IgG antibody and to the sudden increase in opsonizing capacity of the plasma, leading to ingestion of extracellular organisms by PMNs and microbial death. Administration of type-specific antiserum, usually produced in horses, was a significant advance in therapy (serotherapy) before chemotherapy was available (Finland, 1979). Although patient survival was improved, serum sickness was a frequent complication, as antibodies to the foreign protein developed, resulting in immune complex deposition.

Secretory Antibodies

Antibodies serve multiple other functions in addition to opsonization. A good example is the antibody secreted onto mucosal surfaces, generally dimeric secretory immunoglobulin A (sIgA), which may function to prevent microbial colonization (see Chapter 8). Good experimental evidence exists that mucosal anticolonization immunity protects against infection with toxigenic *E. coli* bearing the colonization factors to which immunity has been induced (Svennerholm et al., 1990). Indeed, secretion of sIgA antibodies that recognize a single epitope on enteric pathogens can protect against colonization or invasion of the gut mucosa

(Neutra and Kraehenbuhl, 1993). Humans also respond to a prototype oral vaccine against these organisms, consisting of formalin-inactivated bacteria bearing CFA/I and CFA/II plus the β-subunit of cholera toxin, with a specific intestinal sIgA response to the colonization antigens (Ahren et al., 1993). Such antibodies may be present in breast milk and serve to protect suckling infants, or they may develop in the course of infection and play an important part in recovery. In part, because of a lack of mucosal antibodies, chronic giardiasis may occur in patients with Bruton's syndrome as well as in those with selective IgA deficiency (Roberts-Thomson, 1993).

Antitoxins

Neutralization of the biologic effects of microbial toxins is a distinctive role of antibody, for it affects microbial products rather than the organism itself. Whether the antibody recognizes the biologically active α-subunit and prevents its function or is specific for the β-subunit and inhibits toxin binding to target tissues, the result is neutralization of toxin activity. Because many toxin-mediated diseases develop rapidly after infection, and because the toxin may become tightly bound to or internalized in the target cell, the optimal time for antibody production is before the toxin is introduced, for this can be completely protective. This is precisely the aim of immunization with toxoid vaccines to prevent such diseases as tetanus or diphtheria.

The normal delay in production of antibodies in either of these diseases, unfortunately, can be fatal, for the pathophysiologic events are already in motion and the damage is done by the time the antibody can be produced in natural infection. In diphtheria infection, recovery is associated with the formation of specific antitoxin, which protects the host from toxin produced during the late stages of the infection and confers long-lasting immunity to subsequent encounters with the organism. In contrast, the dose of tetanus toxin resulting in disease symptoms is significantly less than the immunizing dose, and if the subject survives, a second infection may result. Patients with tetanus must therefore be immunized with toxoid in order to prevent repeat attacks.

Virus Neutralization

Virus neutralization is another function of antibodies. While neutralizing antibodies are generally directed to surface antigens of the virus (Greenspan et al., 1983), certain internal sequences (e.g., epitopes of VP1 and VP4 of poliovirus) may be targets for neutralizing antibodies because internal peptides of these antigens induce virus-neutralizing antibody. The mechanism for this may involve the ability of such ''internal'' antigens to display reversible temperature-dependent conformational flexibility by means of which they become reversibly surface exposed at 37°C (Li et al., 1994). Antibody binding to viruses can result in several effects, including alterations in viral charge or shape, and blockade of attachment sites on the surface of the virus. Antibody binding can also result in viral aggregation, thus preventing uptake into susceptible cells, or cause viral lysis in the circulation during viremia, often in conjunction with complement. Viral replication is prevented within cells invaded by the antibody-coated virus particle.

Paralytic poliomyelitis, chronic echovirus infection of the gut or meninges (Misbah et al., 1992) and chronic antigenemia in hepatitis B infection are a few examples of problems in the agammaglobulinemic subject, whereas other agents, such as measles and rubella, present no particular problem (Hermaszewski and Webster, 1993). This is undoubtedly a reflection of the importance of cell-mediated immunity and T-cell–mediated mechanisms in the response to the latter viruses.

IgA Antibody-Dependent Cellular Cytotoxicity

Recurrent enteritis is also a problem for the agammaglobulinemic patient (Stiehm et al., 1986). Although some of this may be due to the lack of anti-colonization factor secretory IgA, studies in experimental animals have begun to define an antibody-dependent, cell-mediated cytotoxicity (ADCC) of lymphocytes against enteric pathogens (Tagliabue et al., 1984). The antibody isotype involved appears to be IgA when lymphocytes are obtained from the intestine. The importance of ADCC is not yet clear for host defense in the gut, but the possibility is intriguing, for the anti-complementary environment of the intestinal lumen obviates complement-mediated mechanisms from playing a significant role in microbicidal activity in this locale.

IgG Antibody-Dependent Cellular Cytotoxicity

Another mechanism of as yet uncertain in vivo importance is the complement-independent ADCC reaction involving IgG. ADCC responses to bacteria are mediated by small lymphocytes termed *K* or *killer cells,* which lack surface markers of either B or T lymphocytes but possess high-affinity receptors for the Fc portion of immunoglobulin. Antigenic specificity is provided by the antibody, rather than being a property of the lymphocyte itself, and is not restricted by the major histocompatibility antigens (Sissons and Oldstone, 1980). This activity is more efficient in vitro at lower concentrations of antibody than is granulocyte-mediated cytotoxicity, suggesting that it could play a physiologic role at complement- and antibody-poor sites, such as mucosal surfaces, or in isolated body compartments, such as the central nervous system.

Another form of ADCC involving eosinophils as effector cells has been proposed in the host response to helminths (Elsas et al., 1990). Whereas eosinopenia is usually observed in acute bacterial or protozoal infections, eosinophilia is a characteristic of many helminthic infections in humans, including trichinosis, schistosomiasis, filariasis, and larva migrans syndromes due to helminths, for which the human is not a definitive host and in whom the worm cannot mature to the adult stage. In vitro studies have demonstrated that eosinophils adhere to and eventually damage antibody-coated helminth larvae, including schistosomes, newborn *Trichinella spiralis,* and microfilaria of *Wuchereria bancrofti* and *Onchocerca volvulus.* The mechanism of adherence and larvicidal activity is not certain but is associated with IgG antibody, and complement is not required.

Cell-Mediated Immunity

Many immune responses to infectious agents directly involve mononuclear cells, including T lymphocytes and macrophages, rather than humoral immunity, although soluble molecules serve as mediators for communication and activation of the effector cells of the response (Schrader, 1991). The multiplicity of the cell-to-cell interactions that occur in this complex immunologic network, along with the secreted mediators of lymphocytes and macrophages, lymphokines, and monokines, have already been discussed in previous chapters.

Cell-mediated antimicrobial responses may be characterized by granuloma formation. In addition to the well-known granulomatous response to *M. tuberculosis,* similar histologic reactions occur in other infections, such as *Chlamydia trachomatis,* lymphogranuloma venereum strains infecting rectal mucosa (Quinn et al., 1981), or following the deposition of *Schistosoma* eggs in liver or bladder, depending on the species of worm and its preferred locale (Weinstock, 1992). In these examples, the granuloma serves to contain the organism, which is not necessarily killed. In schistosomiasis, in addition to isolating the egg and ultimately killing the larva inside, the granuloma is the proximate cause of the pathology of the infection, as egg antigens induce release of fibrogenic granuloma products that induce fibrosis and scarring of tissue with significant physiologic consequences (Wyler, 1992). In a number of intracellular infections, e.g., *S. typhi, Toxoplasma gondii,* or *Leishmania* sp., the macrophage is a critical target cell in which the organism multiplies, defying its microbicidal mechanisms (Hall and Joiner, 1991). However, later in infection, when sensitized T lymphocytes develop, the interaction of these cells with the infected macrophage activates its intracellular microbicidal systems through the mediation of interferon-γ (Flynn et al., 1993) and other cytokines, such as TNF (Kaufmann, 1993), and modulated by other soluble host-derived factors, prominent among which is interleukin-10 (IL-10) (Oswald et al., 1992).

The induction of T-cell reactivity requires processing of protein antigens and transport to the surface of antigen-presenting cells (APCs) (Knight and Stagg, 1993) for presentation to T cells in association with molecules of the major histocompatibility complex (MHC) (Yewdell and Bennink, 1993). This leads to a clonal expansion of reactive T cells following complex inductive and regulatory events that control this process (Rothenberg, 1992). This, in turn, results in the release of lymphocyte products that lead to the attraction, immobilization, and activation of mononu-

clear phagocytes for microbial killing. Microbicidal activity is multifactorial, including increased secretion of neutral serine proteases (Hudig et al., 1993), production of reactive oxygen radicals and nitric oxide (Nathan and Hibbs, 1991), and enhanced phagocytosis and intracellular processing of microorganisms (Dunlap and Briles, 1993).

The development of antimicrobial capacity correlates well with the appearance of delayed-type skin hypersensitivity (DTH) to antigens from the organism eliciting the response (Rosenstreich, 1993); however, experimental examples exist in which an effective protective macrophage microbicidal response can be separated from defective DTH responses (Hernandez-Frontera and McMurray, 1993).

As studied in animals, transfer of acquired resistance to naive animals is possible with transfer of activated T lymphocytes but not with serum. Although the induction of the cell-mediated response is antigen (organism)-specific, it has long been known that primed cells activated by the same antigen responsible for the original sensitization demonstrate antimicrobial responses to other intracellular pathogens and, in this sense, are "nonspecific" (Mackaness, 1969). For as yet uncertain reasons, such cell-mediated responses are best elicited by living organisms, although recent insights into the molecular and physiologic changes induced in both living microorganisms and host cells during cell-cell interactions suggest that the repertoire of stimulating and reactive molecules may differ when live organisms are used.

HOST DEFENSES IN CELL-MEDIATED IMMUNITY

Cytotoxic T Lymphocytes

Cell-mediated responses to viruses also occur, often involving direct cell lysis of virus-infected cells bearing virus antigens at their surface by a class of cytotoxic T lymphocytes (CTLs). Recognition of the virus antigen in this response is genetically restricted and occurs in conjunction with HLA determinants. Defects in cell-mediated immunity result in frequent and severe viral infections, such as varicella, herpesviruses, and cytomegalovirus, and with other intracellular pathogens, including *Pneumocystis carinii* and *Mycobacterium tuberculosis* (Dunlap and Briles, 1993) (see Chapters 12 and 31). In such patients, even immunization with the live attenuated bacille Calmette-Guérin (BCG) vaccine strain of *Mycobacterium bovis* or its use as a therapeutic agent for cancer can result in disseminated progressive mycobacterial infections of the lungs and other organs (Abramowsky et al., 1993; Kristjansson et al., 1993).

An interesting example is the role of CTLs in defense against influenza A virus infection, in which humoral antibody responses to the hemagglutinin (H) and neuraminidase (NA) antigens of the virus are correlated with disease prevention, for example, following influenza immunization (Bender and Small, 1992). Passive immunization of previously unexposed mice prevents pneumonia due to virus challenge but, interestingly, does not affect the localized rhinotracheitis except when anti-influenza IgA is administered. In contrast, recovery from infection is best correlated with the CTL response. This is most clearly demonstrated in studies of athymic nude mice infected with the virus, in which adoptive transfer of specific CTLs allows clearance of virus from the lungs and the administration of antibody blocks shedding but only for the duration of the therapy. A partial explanation for the increased severity of influenza in the elderly may relate to an age-dependent decrease in CTL activity, resulting in increased spread of the virus throughout the respiratory tract as well as prolonged shedding.

It is likely that the relative roles of antibody and cellular immunity will vary for different viruses or for the same virus in hosts with different immune capacities or degree of virus exposure. Two brief examples will suffice. First, recurrent varicella may occur in individuals with high titer circulating antibody when cell-mediated immunity is suppressed. Second, varicella infection may be prevented or illness modified following exposure in such T-cell–deficient patients by the use of varicella-zoster immune globulin (Zaia et al., 1983).

Natural Killer Cells

Another class of cytotoxic lymphocytes is the natural killer (NK) cells. NK cells are large, low-density, granular, T-cell receptor and surface immunoglobulin–negative lymphocytes that do not require immunologically specific activation to function (Lanier and Phillips, 1992). They were originally described as natural tumoricidal cells; however, increasingly a role in response to infection, particularly viral infection, has been described (Bancroft, 1993). These cells are modulated by interactions with MHC class I molecules, including an influence of both the MHC class I groove and the peptides that bind in this site (Karre, 1993). A variety of NK-associated (NKa) cell surface markers defined by monoclonal antibodies have also been reported to be present on these cells, overlapping with those found on cells of other lineages, including T cells, macrophages, and granulocytes (see Chapters 2, 10, and 12). There is some evidence that NK cells respond to activation stimuli, including interleukin-2 and interferon-γ and that some distinctive subpopulations may differ in activation signal specificity and clinical function (Ciccone et al., 1992).

The best evidence for a role of NK cells in antiviral defense comes from experimental animal infections. Depletion and adoptive transfer of purified cell populations are employed to identify those cells involved in the host response, and most often several cell populations exert an impact. For example, in herpes simplex virus infections, a role for CD4$^+$ and CD8$^+$ lymphocytes and macrophages in addition to NK cells is suggested, along with evidence that interferon-α and -γ and interleukin-2 modify these responses (Rinaldo and Torpey, 1993).

Similar data have been obtained for a role of NK cells in host defense to a coxsackievirus B4 infection of the pancreas (Vella and Festenstein, 1992). Studies of murine cytomegalovirus (MCMV) provide strong genetic evidence for the particular importance of NK cells in antiviral defense. Innate resistance among inbred mouse strains to MCMV has long been associated with NK cell activity, and adaptive transfer of these cells restores the antiviral response (Bukowski et al., 1985). Genetic resistance to MCMV is a result of the presence of an autosomal, non-MHC encoded gene, *Cmv-1*, which, in mice, controls MCMV replication in the spleen (Scalzo et al., 1992). The gene is closely linked to the NK complex region on murine chromosome 6, and specific in vivo depletion of NK cells by a monoclonal antibody abolished restricted splenic replication of MCMV. In contrast, neither a relationship to interferon production nor an effect of depleting mature CD4$^+$ or CD8$^+$ cells on virus growth is found. That this mechanism is specific for some, but not all, viruses is indicated by the lack of correlation between NK activity and response to lymphocytic choriomeningitis virus in the same animals. The relevance of NK-mediated antiviral activity in human infection remains to be determined.

Interferons

Interferon, originally described in 1957 as an antiviral protein, is now known to be a family of molecules with diverse immunoregulatory properties (such as induction of NK activity) as well as antiviral and antitumor effects (Itri, 1992). Three distinct classes of interferons are produced:

- α or leukocyte interferon
- β or fibroblast interferon
- γ or immune interferon

Interferon-α, an acid-stable nonglycosylated protein, and interferon-β, an acid-stable glycoprotein, are produced when cells are exposed to viruses or to double-stranded RNAs or related polyanions. Interferon-γ, an acid-labile glycoprotein, is produced during antigen or mitogen stimulation of lymphocytes and has relatively more immunoregulatory effect than direct antiviral properties. IFN-α and IFN-β have significant antiviral activity. See Chapter 2 for an additional discussion of the interferons.

In experimental settings, interferons exhibit a broad range of antimicrobial action, extending to bacteria, *Chlamydia*, protozoa, and rickettsia (Stiehm et al., 1982). This may be a consequence of interferon's effects on cellular immunity, including enhancement of macrophage phagocytosis, increased expression of surface MHC antigens and Fc receptors, augmented T cell–mediated cytotoxicity, and induction of NK cells (Koziel and Walker, 1992). Interferon-γ is thought to be the major cytokine activator of macrophages (Flynn et al., 1993).

As a consequence of considerable animal experimentation and early human clinical trials, interferons are now approved by the U.S. Food and Drug Administration (FDA) for five clinical applications, including interferon-α for treatment of hairy cell leukemia, condyloma acuminatum, Kaposi sarcoma, and hepatitis C virus (HCV); and interferon-γ for chronic granulomatous disease, with other promising indications (including tumors, HIV, and other viral infections) still under study (Baron et al., 1991).

HCV infection is illustrative of the problems with interferon therapy as a single modality. This is a progressive, relentless chronic hepatitis, which appears to have the additional problem of infection of the graft when liver transplantation is carried out (Sherlock, 1994). The efficacy of interferon-α was originally hailed as a breakthrough; however, longer experience suggests that the effect is primarily on the cytopathic effects of HCV rather than primarily antiviral. Moreover, further experience shows that approximately 50% of patients do not respond with a reduction in virus titers, and at least half of those who do respond experience relapse. Thus, the overall response rate is a disappointing 25%, and current efforts are directed toward identifying patients likely to respond, determining the side effects of the treatment, and exploring the possibility of combined therapy (Davis, 1994).

The role of interferons in HIV other than for treatment of Kaposi sarcoma is also problematic; some evidence links enhanced interferon responses with the progression of viral replication and disease, and other data suggest that interferons can maintain the virus in a latent state (Francis et al., 1992). In addition, in vitro studies demonstrate that HIV, in contrast to other viruses, does not induce monocyte interferon production and, in fact, blocks the interferon response to poly(I):poly(C) (Laurence, 1990). Thus, interferons may play different roles at different stages of HIV infection in combination with other cytokines and cytokine antagonists (Poli and Fauci, 1993).

SUPPRESSION OF IMMUNE FUNCTION BY INFECTIOUS AGENTS

There is little need to reiterate here how microorganisms activate the immune system. This is covered in detail in Part I of this textbook and is the same whether the antigen involved is living or dead. In some instances, this immune activation results in pathology, producing characteristic signs and symptoms of the disease associated with the involved organism. By contrast, some infectious agents have the ability to interact with and suppress the immune system and therefore cause immunodeficiency. Some data suggest that rubella virus infection may underlie certain acquired dysgammaglobulinemias or hypogammaglobulinemias (Schimke et al., 1969), and an association between cytomegalovirus and combined immunodeficiency has been postulated (Groshang et al., 1984). The most striking example is also the most recently described, the effect of the HIV virus on T cells in the causation of the profound immunodeficiency known as AIDS.

This important virus is discussed in detail in Chapter 18.

HIV Infection

Understanding of the pathogenesis of AIDS and the progressive destruction of immunologically active cells

leading to a profound immunodeficiency (Fauci, 1993), susceptibility to a variety of infectious diseases, both opportunistic and nonopportunistic, and severe lymphoproliferative disorders (Schnittman and Fauci, 1994) has increased dramatically over the past decade. It is now clear that although HIV infection ultimately causes immunosuppression, it also leads to a vigorous early immune response to the virus itself, including both neutralizing antibody and cellular responses that lyse infected cells in vitro (Fauci et al., 1991).

Unfortunately, there is no evidence that these responses eliminate the virus (Bolognesi, 1993); indeed, there is extensive evidence that the virus continuously replicates in lymphoid tissues over the entire course of the infection, even during the ''latent phase,'' when it is difficult to find virus in the periphery (Fauci, 1993). Important interactions with inflammatory stimuli, agents potentially able to act as superantigens (Posnett, 1992) (e.g., cytomegalovirus) and cytokines (Vicenzi and Poli, 1994) serve to regulate HIV replication in a complex manner, in part mediated by activation of nuclear transcription factors (Duh et al., 1989).

Ultimately, progression of HIV to AIDS and its associated immunodeficiency is the result of ineffective immune control and unrestricted proliferation of the virus. Although the long-term hope is that pre-exposure vaccine-induced neutralizing antibody, ADCC, or cell-mediated immunity will protect the host, in general, effective viral vaccines are most likely to be developed when the virus itself naturally induces immunity, and there is no convincing evidence that this occurs in HIV. Attempts at postexposure immunization to boost the host protective response have also been promoted, but there is no convincing evidence that this approach will be clinically effective (Schnittman and Fauci, 1994).

Epstein-Barr Virus Infection

It is interesting to compare effects on the host of HIV infection of the CD4$^+$ T lymphocyte with Epstein-Barr virus (EBV), which has a striking tropism for B lymphocytes. This virus is the cause of heterophile antibody-positive infectious mononucleosis (IM), in which EBV initially infects the epithelium of the upper respiratory tract and salivary glands (Tosato and Blaese, 1985) (see Chapter 27). B lymphocytes also become infected in the oropharynx and disseminate the virus to distant lymphoid organs and the peripheral blood. Although EBV-infected B cells can grow indefinitely in vitro and the virus has the property of similarly immortalizing normal B cells in culture, the lymphocytosis associated with the appearance of atypical cells is predominantly the CD8$^+$ suppressor-cytotoxic phenotype. Even after full recovery from IM, small numbers of EBV-positive peripheral B cells can be isolated that spontaneously outgrow in culture and the virus can still be recovered from oral secretions. This is true even though antibodies develop to EBV specific glycoproteins that appear on the surface of the infected B cell and preclude subsequent viremia.

Cell-mediated immunity can be demonstrated as well in patients with infectious mononucleosis. T lymphocytes capable of mediating cytotoxic reactions to EBV-infected cells are present, independent of major histocompatibility complex (MHC) restriction (Tosato and Blaese, 1985). In addition, suppressor T cells are activated that profoundly inhibit normal lymphocyte proliferation and immunoglobulin production in vitro in response to antigens or mitogens. However, isolated B cells from patients with IM can be stimulated by EBV to immunoglobulin production, indicating that the B cells are normally responsive when separated from T-suppressor cells, which act as a control mechanism for B-cell activation by the virus. This suppression is expressed primarily during the early stages of B-cell activation in vitro.

It is believed that the suppressor and cytotoxic functions of T cells may represent different mechanisms of host defense in patients with acute IM. EBV-infected cells are susceptible to cytotoxic T-cell elimination early in infection; later on, the small proportion of EBV-positive B cells remaining are under suppressor T-cell influences that inhibit their proliferation as well as their maturation into suitable targets for the cytotoxic T lymphocyte to act upon. Hence, small numbers of virus-positive B cells persist, amounting to approximately 3 per million B cells when all suppressor T cells are removed, and in effect there is an effective control mechanism for EBV-infected cells without eliminating all such cells.

The complex immunologic response to EBV-infected B cells resulting in T-cell control and clinical cure of IM is followed by ultimate disappearance of the suppressor T cells from the circulation. In a few patients, however, exaggerated, persistent T-cell suppression can lead to acquired common variable hypogammaglobulinemia. Well-documented cases of acquired hypogammaglobulinemia have occurred directly after IM, involving all classes of immunoglobulin in the X-linked lymphoproliferative syndrome (Provisor et al., 1975) (see Chapter 12).

Studies of similar cases demonstrate a normal number of circulating B cells that, however, fail to generate immunoglobulins following in vitro stimulation with pokeweed mitogen, and the presence of suppressor T cells, which inhibit immunoglobulin production by normal B cells (Tosato and Blaese, 1985). An intermediate situation has also been observed with persistent, chronic, symptomatic IM with normal immunoglobulin levels and circulating suppressor cells that, in coculture experiments, inhibit immunoglobulin synthesis by normal cells.

The immune response induced by EBV may also lead to the development of B-cell malignancies. In a few patients receiving bone marrow transplants (see Chapters 19, 27, and 32), fatal lymphoproliferation of latent EBV-infected host or donor cells has developed following treatment with an anti–T-cell monoclonal antibody (anti-P 19) to suppress graft-versus-host reactions. Ablation of the T-suppressor control mechanism for EBV-positive B cells is the likely cause of this complication. In addition, some patients receiving kidney transplants and who have been immunosuppressed with cyclosporine, have also developed B-cell lymphoproliferative syndromes involving EBV-infected cells (Craw-ford et al., 1980). Genetically determined inability to induce EBV suppressor cells may also be associated with EBV infection in certain patients with the X-linked lymphoproliferative syndrome (Purtilo, 1981).

References

Abramowsky C, Gonzalez B, Sorensen RU. Disseminated bacillus Calmette-Guerin infections in patients with primary immunodeficiencies. Am J Clin Pathol 100:52–56, 1993.

Ahren C, Wenneras C, Holmgren J, Svennerholm, AM. Intestinal antibody response after oral immunization with a prototype cholera B subunit–colonization factor antigen enterotoxigenic Escherichia coli vaccine. Vaccine 11:929–934, 1993.

Alouf JE, Freer JH. Sourcebook of Bacterial Protein Toxins. London, Academic Press, 1991.

Andersson P, Engberg I, Lidin-Janson G, Lincoln K, Hull R, Hull S, Svanborg C. Persistence of Escherichia coli bacteriuria is not determined by bacterial adherence. Infect Immun 59:2915–2921, 1991.

Arruda S, Bomfim G, Knights R, Huima-Byron T, Riley LW. Cloning of an M. tuberculosis DNA fragment associated with entry and survival within cells. Science 261:1454–1457, 1993.

Avery OT, Dubos R. The protective action of a specific enzyme against type III pneumococcus infections in mice. J Exp Med 54:73–89, 1931.

Baggiolini M, Boulay F, Badwey JA, Curnutte JT. Activation of neutrophil leukocytes: chemoattractant receptors and respiratory burst. FASEB J 7:1004–1020, 1993.

Bancroft GJ. The role of natural killer cells in innate resistance to infection. Curr Opin Immunol 5:503–510, 1993.

Baron S, Tyring SK, Fleishman WR Jr, Coppenhaver DH, Niesel DW, Klimpel GR, Stanton GJ, Hughes TK. The interferons. Mechanisms of action and clinical applications. JAMA 266:1375–1383, 1991.

Bender BS, Small PA Jr. Influenza: pathogenesis and host defense. Semin Respir Infect 7:38–45, 1992.

Berek C, Ziegner M. The maturation of the immune response. Immunol Today 14:400–404, 1993.

Berger KH, Isberg RR. Two distinct defects in intracellular growth complemented by a single genetic locus in Legionella pneumophila. Mol Microbiol 7:7–19, 1993.

Bevilacqua MP, Nelson RM. Selectins. J Clin Invest 91:379–387, 1993.

Blume RS, Wolff SM. The Chédiak-Higashi syndrome: studies in four patients and a review of the literature. Medicine 51:247–280, 1972.

Bolognesi DP. The immune response to HIV: implications for vaccine development. Semin Immunol 5:203–214, 1993.

Bone RC. Gram-positive organisms and sepsis. Arch Intern Med 154:26–34, 1994.

Brown EJ, Hosea SW, Frank MM. The role of antibody and complement in the reticuloendothelial clearance of pneumococci from the bloodstream. Rev Infect Dis 5:S797–S805, 1983.

Brunham RC, Holmes KK. Immune mechanisms involved in bacterial infections. In Gallin JR, Fauci AS, eds. Advances in Host Defense Mechanisms: Lymphoid Cells, Vol. 2. New York, Raven Press, 1983, pp. 69–100.

Bruyn GA, Zegers BJ, van Furth R. Mechanisms of host defense against infection with Streptococcus pneumoniae. Clin Infect Dis 14:251–262, 1992.

Buhler T, Hoschutzky H, Jann K. Analysis of colonization factor antigen I, an adhesin of enterotoxigenic Escherichia coli O78:H11: fimbrial morphology and location of the receptor-binding site. Infect Immun 59:3876–3882, 1991.

Bukowski JF, Warner JF, Dennert G, Welsh RM. Adoptive transfer studies demonstrating the antiviral effect of natural killer cells in vivo. J Exp Med 161:40–52, 1985.

Buysse JM, Stover CK, Oaks EV, Venkatesan M, Kopecko DJ. Molecular cloning of invasion plasmid antigen (ipa) genes from Shigella flexneri: analysis of ipa gene products and genetic mapping. J Bacteriol 169:2561–2569, 1987.

Car BD, Eng VM, Schnyder B, Ozmen L, Huang S, Gallay P, Heumann D, Aguet M, Ryffel B. Interferon gamma receptor deficient mice are resistant to endotoxic shock. J Exp Med 170:1437–1444, 1994.

Chan J, Fan XD, Hunter SW, Brennan PJ, Bloom BR. Lipoarabinomannan, a possible virulence factor involved in persistent *Mycobacterium tuberculosis* within macrophages. Infect Immun 59:1755–1761, 1991.

Chetty C, Kreger A. Role of autolysin in generating the pneumococcal purpura-producing principle. Infect Immun 31:339–344, 1981.

Ciccone E, Moretta A, Moretta L. Specific functions of human NK cells. Immunol Lett 31:99–103, 1992.

Crawford DH, Thomas JA, Janossy G, Sweny P, Fernando ON, Morehead JF, Thompson JH. Epstein-Barr virus nuclear antigen positive lymphoma after cyclosporin A treatment in patients with renal allograft. Lancet I:1355–1366, 1980.

Crowle AJ, Dahl R, Ross E, May MH. Evidence that vesicles containing living, virulent *Mycobacterium tuberculosis* or *Mycobacterium avium* in cultured human macrophages are not acidic. Infect Immun 59:1823–1831, 1991.

Curnutte JT. Chronic granulomatous disease: the solving of a clinical riddle at the molecular level. Clin Immunol Immunopathol 67:S2–S15, 1993.

Darfeuille-Michaud A, Aubel D, Chauviere G, Rich C, Bourges M, Servin A, Joly B. Adhesion of enterotoxigenic *Escherichia coli* to the human colon carcinoma cell line Caco-2 in culture. Infect Immun 58:893–902, 1990.

Davis GL. Interferon treatment of chronic hepatitis C. Am J Med 96:41S–46S, 1994.

Dinarello CA, Gelfand JA, Wolff SM. Anticytokine strategies in the treatment of the systemic inflammatory response syndrome. JAMA 269:1829–1835, 1993.

Dreskin SC, Goldsmith PK, Gallin JI. Immunoglobulins in the hyperimmunoglobulin E and recurrent infection (Job's) syndrome. Deficiency of anti–*Staphylococcus aureus* immunoglobulin. Am J Clin Invest 75:26–34, 1985.

Duh RJ, Maury WJ, Folks TM, Fauci AS, Rabson AB. Tumor necrosis factor α activates human immunodeficiency virus type 1 through induction of nuclear factor binding to the NF-κB sites in the long terminal repeat. Proc Natl Acad Sci U S A 86:2336–2340, 1989.

Dunlap NE, Briles DE. Immunology of tuberculosis. Med Clin North Am 77:1235–1251, 1993.

Elsas PX, Elsas MI, Dessein AJ. Eosinophil cytotoxicity enhancing factor: purification, characterization and immunocytochemical localization on the monocyte surface. Eur J Immunol 20:1143–1151, 1990.

Fauci AS. Multifactorial nature of human immunodeficiency virus disease: implications for therapy. Science 262:1011–1018, 1993.

Fauci AS, Schnittman SM, Poli G, Koenig S, Pantaleo G. Immunopathogenic mechanisms in human immunodeficiency virus (HIV) infection. Ann Intern Med 114:678–693, 1991.

Figueroa J, Andreoni J, Densen P. Complement deficiency states and meningococcal disease. Immun Res 12:295–311, 1993.

Finland MM. Pneumonia and pneumococcal infections with special reference to pneumococcal pneumonia. Am Rev Respir Dis 120:481–502, 1979.

Finlay BB. Cell adhesion and invasion mechanisms in microbial pathogenesis. Curr Opin Cell Biol 2:815–820, 1990.

Finlay BB, Falkow S. Common themes in microbial pathogenicity. Microbiol Rev 53:210–230, 1989.

Flynn JL, Chan J, Triebold KJ, Dalton DK, Steward TA, Bloom BR. An essential role for interferon gamma in resistance to *Mycobacterium tuberculosis* infection. J Exp Med 178:2249–2254, 1993.

Formal SB, Hale TL, Sansonetti PJ. Invasive enteric pathogens. Rev Infect Dis S702–S707, 1983.

Francis ML, Meltzer MS, Gendelman HE. Interferons in the persistence, pathogenesis, and treatment of HIV infection. AIDS Res Human Retrovir 8:199–207, 1992.

Francis CL, Ryan TA, Jones BD, Smith SJ, Falkow S. Ruffles induced by *Salmonella* and other stimuli direct macropinocytosis of bacteria. Nature 364:639–642, 1993.

Frank MM. The mechanism by which microorganisms avoid complement attack. Curr Opin Immunol 4:14–19, 1992.

Furtado GC, Cao Y, Joiner KA. Laminin on *Toxoplasma gondii* mediates parasite binding to the beta 1 integrin receptor alpha 6 beta 1 on human foreskin fibroblasts and Chinese hamster ovary cells. Infect Immun 60:4925–4931, 1992.

Gardulf A, Bjorvell H, Gustafson R, Hammarstrom L, Smith CI. The life situations of patients with primary antibody deficiency untreated or treated with subcutaneous gammaglobulin infusions. Clin Exp Immunol 92:200–204, 1993.

Gleich GJ, Adolphson CR, Leiferman KM. The biology of the eosinophilic leukocyte. Ann Rev Med 44:85–101, 1993.

Goldberg MB, Sansonetti PJ. *Shigella* subversion of the cellular cytoskeleton: a strategy for epithelial colonization. Infect Immun 61:4941–4946, 1993.

Greenspan NS, Schwartz DH, Doherty PC. Role of lymphoid cells in immune surveillance against viral infection. In Gallin JL, Fauci AS, eds. Advances in Host Defense Mechanisms. Lymphoid Cells, Vol. 2. New York, Raven Press, 1983, pp. 101–142.

Groshang T, Horowitz S, Lovchik J, Davis A, Hong R. Chronic cytomegalovirus infection, immunodeficiency and monoclonal gammopathy antigen driven malignancy? J Pediatr 88:217–223, 1984.

Hailman E, Lichenstein HS, Wurfel MM, Miller DS, Johnson DA, Kelley M, Busse LA, Zukowski MM, Wright SD. Lipopolysaccharide (LPS)–binding protein accelerates the binding of LPS to CD14. J Exp Med 179:269–277, 1994.

Hale TL. Genetic basis of virulence in *Shigella* species. Microbiol Rev 55:206–224, 1991.

Hall BF, Joiner KA. Strategies of obligate intracellular parasites for evading host defenses. Immunol Today 12:A22–A27, 1991.

Hermaszewski RA, Webster AD. Primary hypogammaglobulinemia: a survey of clinical manifestations and complications. Q J Med 86:31–42, 1993.

Hernandez-Frontera E, McMurray DN. Dietary vitamin D affects cell-mediated hypersensitivity but not resistance to experimental pulmonary tuberculosis in guinea pigs. Infect Immun 61:2116–2121, 1993.

Hudig D, Ewoldt GR, Woodard SL. Proteases and lymphocyte cytotoxic killing mechanisms. Curr Opin Immunol 5:90–96, 1993.

Hultgren SJ, Normark S, Abraham SN. Chaperone-assisted assembly and molecular architecture of adhesive pili. Ann Rev Microbiol 45:383–415, 1991.

Hultgren SJ, Abraham S, Caparon M, Falk P, St. Geme JW 3d, Normark S. Pilus and nonpilus bacterial adhesins: assembly and function in cell recognition. Cell 73:887–901, 1993.

Isberg RR, Leong JM. Multiple beta 1 chain integrins are receptors for invasin, a protein that promotes bacterial penetration into mammalian cells. Cell 60:861–871, 1990.

Isberg RR, Yang Y, Voorhis DL. Residues added to the carboxyl terminus of the Yersinia pseudotuberculosis invasin protein interfere with recognition by integrin receptors. J Biol Chem 268:15840–15846, 1993.

Itri LM. The interferons. Cancer 70:940–945, 1992.

James SP. The gastrointestinal mucosal immune system. Dig Dis 11:146–156, 1993.

Joiner KA, Furhman SA, Miettinen HM, Kasper LH, Mellman I. *Toxoplasma gondii:* fusion competence of parasitophorous vacuoles in Fc receptor–transfected fibroblasts. Science 249:641–646, 1990.

Jones BD, Paterson HF, Hall A, Falkow S. *Salmonella typhimurium* induces membrane ruffling by a growth factor-receptor-independent mechanism. Proc Natl Acad Sci U S A 90:10390–10394, 1993.

Kahane I, Reisch-Saada A, Almagor M, Albeliuck P, Yatziv S. Glycosidase activities of mycoplasmas. Int J Med Microbiol 273:300–305, 1990.

Karlsson KA, Angstrom J, Bergstrom J, Lanne B. Microbial interaction with animal cell surface carbohydrates. Acta Pathol Microbiol Immunol Scand Suppl 27:71–83, 1992.

Karre K. Natural killer cells and the MHC class I pathway of peptide presentation. Semin Immunol 5:127–145, 1993.

Kaufmann SH. Immunity to intracellular bacteria. Ann Rev Immunol 11:129–163, 1993.

Keusch GT, Gorbach SL. Enteric microbial ecology and infection. Bacteria. In Haubrick WS, Schaffner F, Berk JE, et al., eds. Bockus Gastroenterology, 5th ed., Vol 2. Philadelphia, WB Saunders, 1995, pp. 1115–1130.

Knight SC, Stagg AJ. Antigen-presenting cell types. Curr Opin Immunol 5:374–382, 1993.

Koziel MJ, Walker BD. Viruses, chemotherapy and immunity. Parasitology 105:S85–S92, 1992.

Kristjansson M, Green P, Manning HL, Slutsky AM, Brecher SM, von Reyn CF, Arbeit RD, Maslow LN. Molecular confirmation of bacillus Calmette-Guérin as the cause of pulmonary infection following urinary tract instillation. Clin Infect Dis 17:228–230, 1993.

Krogfelt KA. Bacterial adhesion: genetics, biogenesis, and role in pathogenesis of fimbrial adhesins of *Escherichia coli*. Rev Infect Dis 13:721–735, 1991.

Kuehn MJ, Heuser J, Normark S, Hultgren SJ. P pili in uropathogenic *E. coli* are composite fibres with distinct fibrillar adhesive tips. Nature 356:252–255, 1992.

Kuijpers TW, Weening RS, Out TA. IgG subclass deficiencies and recurrent pyogenic infections, unresponsiveness against bacterial polysaccharide antigens. Allergy Immunopathol 20:28–34, 1992.

Lanier LL, Phillips JH. Natural killer cells. Curr Opin Immunol 4:38–42, 1992.

Laurence J. Immunology of HIV-1 infection. I: Biology of the interferons. AIDS Res Hum Retroviruses 6:1149–1156, 1990.

Lee JM, Pizzo PA. Management of the cancer patient with fever and prolonged neutropenia. Hematol Oncol Clin North Am 7:937–960, 1993.

Leffler H, Svanborg-Eden C. Chemical identification of a glycosphingolipid receptor for *Escherichia coli* attaching to human urinary tract epithelial cells and agglutinating human erythrocytes. FEMS Microbiol Lett 8:127–134, 1980.

Leijh PCJ, van den Barselaar MT, van Zwet TL, Daha MR, van Furth R. Requirement of extracellular complement and immunoglobulin for intracellular killing of micro-organisms by human monocytes. J Clin Invest 63:772–784, 1979.

Levine MM. *Escherichia coli* that cause diarrhea: enterotoxigenic, enteropathogenic, enteroinvasive, enterohemorrhagic, and enteroadherent. J Infect Dis 155:377–389, 1987.

Li Q, Yafal AG, Lee YM, Hogle J, Chow M. Poliovirus neutralization by antibodies to internal epitopes of VP4 and VP1 results from reversible exposure of these sequences at physiological temperature. J Virol 68:3965–3970, 1994.

Lidbeck A, Nord CE. Lactobacilli and the normal human anaerobic microflora. Clin Infect Dis 16(Suppl. 4):S181–S187, 1993.

London E. Diphtheria toxin: membrane interaction and membrane translocation. Biochim Biophys Acta 1113:25–51, 1992.

Loveless RW, Griffiths S, Fryer PR, Blauth C, Feizi T. Immunoelectron microscopic studies reveal differences in distribution of sialo-oligosaccharide receptors for *Mycoplasma pneumoniae* on the epithelium of human and hamster bronchi. Infect Immun 60:4015–4023, 1992.

Mackaness GB. The influence of immunologically committed lymphoid cells on macrophage activity in vivo. J Exp Med 129:973–992, 1969.

Manthous CA, Hall JB, Samsel RW. Endotoxin in human disease. Part 1: Biochemistry, assay, and possible role in diverse disease states. Chest 104:1572–1581, 1993a.

Manthous CA, Hall JB, Samsel RW. Endotoxin in human disease. Part 2: Biologic effects and clinical evaluations of anti-endotoxin therapies. Chest 104:1872–1881, 1993b.

Martich GD, Boujoukos AJ, Suffredini AF. Response of man to endotoxin. Immunobiology 187:403–416, 1993.

McConnell MM, Hibberd ML, Penny ME, Scotland SM, Cheasty T, Rowe B. Surveys of human enterotoxigenic *Escherichia coli* from three different geographical areas for possible colonization factors. Epidemiol Infect 106:477–484, 1991.

McDonough KA, Kress Y, Bloom BR. Pathogenesis of tuberculosis: interaction of *Mycobacterium tuberculosis* with macrophages. Infect Immun 61:2763–2773, 1993.

McLean RJ, Nickel JC. Bacterial colonization behaviour: a new virulence strategy in urinary infections? Med Hypoth 36:269–272, 1991.

Melly MA, McGee ZA, Rosenthal RS. Ability of monomeric peptidoglycan fragments from *Neisseria gonorrhoeae* to damage human fallopian-tube mucosa. J Infect Dis 149:378–386, 1984.

Misbah SA, Spickett GP, Ryba PC, Hockaday JM, Kroll JS, Sherwood C, Kurtz JB, Moxon ER, Chapel HM. Chronic enteroviral meningoencephalitis in agammaglobulinemia: case report and literature review. J Clin Immunol 12:266–270, 1992.

Moncada S, Higgs A. The L-arginine-nitric oxide pathway. N Engl J Med 329:2002–2012, 1993.

Morrison DC, Lei MG, Kirikae T, Chen TY. Endotoxin receptors on mammalian cells. Immunobiology 187:212–226, 1993.

Naglich JC, Metherall JE, Ressell DW, Eidels L. Expression cloning of a diphtheria toxin receptor: identity with a heparin binding EGF-like growth factor precursor. Cell 69:1051–1066, 1992.

Nathan CF, Hibbs JB Jr. Role of nitric oxide synthesis in macrophage antimicrobial activity. Curr Opin Immunol 3:65–70, 1991.

Neutra MR, Kraehenbuhl JP. The role of transepithelial transport by M cells in microbial invasion and host defense. J Cell Sci 17:209–215, 1993.

Nourshargh S. Mechanisms of neutrophil and eosinophil accumulation in vivo. Am Rev Resp Dis 148:S60–S64, 1993.

O'Hanley P, Lark D, Falkow S, Schoolnik G. Molecular basis of *Escherichia coli* colonization of the upper urinary tract in BALB/c mice. Gal-gal pili immunization prevents *Escherchia coli* pyelonephritis in the BALB/c mouse model of human pyelonephritis. J Exp Med 75:347–360, 1985.

Onderdonk AB, Cisneros RL, Finberg R, Crabb JH, Kasper DL. Animal model system for studying virulence of and host response to *Bacteroides fragilis*. Rev Infect Dis 12(Suppl. 2):S169–S177, 1990.

Oswald IP, Wynn TA, Sher A, James SL. Interleukin-10 inhibits macrophage microbicidal activity by blocking the endogenous production of tumor necrosis factor alpha required as a costimulatory factor for interferon gamma–induced activation. Proc Natl Acad Sci U S A 89:8676–8680, 1992.

Pappenheimer AM Jr. The story of a toxic protein, 1888–1992. Protein Sci 2:292–298, 1993.

Pfeffer K, Matsuyama T, Kundig TM, Wakeham A, Kishihara K, Shahinian A, Wiegmann K, Ohashi PS, Kronke M, Mak TW. Mice deficient for the 55 kd tumor necrosis factor receptor are resistant to endotoxic shock, yet succumb to *L. monocytogenes* infection. Cell 73:457–467, 1993.

Poli G, Fauci AS. Cytokine modulation of HIV expression. Semin Immunol 5:165–173, 1993.

Posnett DN. Superantigen implicated in dependence of HIV-1 replication in T cells on TCR V beta expression. Nature 358:255–259, 1992.

Provisor AJ, Iacuone JJ, Chilcote RR, Neiburger RG, Crussi FG, Baehner RL. Acquired agammaglobulinemia after a life-threatening illness with clinical and laboratory features of infectious mononucleosis in three related male children. N Engl J Med 293:62–65, 1975.

Purtilo D. Immune deficiency predisposing to Epstein-Barr virus–induced lymphoproliferative diseases: the X-linked lymphoproliferative syndrome as a model. Adv Cancer Res 34:279–312, 1981.

Quinn TC, Corey L, Chaffee RG, Schuffler MD, Brancato FP, Holmes KK. The etiology of anorectal infections in homosexual men. Am J Med 71:395–406, 1981.

Rabin RL, Bieber MM, Teng NN. Lipopolysaccharide and peptidoglycan share binding sites on human peripheral blood monocytes. J Infect Dis 168:135–142, 1993.

Raetz CRH. Bacterial endotoxins: Extraordinary lipids that activate eucaryotic signal transduction. J Bacteriol 175:5745–5753, 1993.

Read MA, Cordle SR, Veach RA, Carlisle CD, Hawiger J. Cell-free pool of CD14 mediates activation of transcription factor NF-kappa B by lipopolysaccharide in human endothelial cells. Proc Natl Acad Sci U S A 90:9887–9891, 1993.

Rinaldo CR Jr, Torpey DJ 3d. Cell-mediated immunity and immunosuppression in herpes simplex virus infections. Immunodeficiency 5:33–90, 1993.

Roberts-Thomson IC. Genetic studies of human and murine giardiasis. Clin Infect Dis 16(Suppl. 2):S98–S104, 1993.

Roche RJ, Moxon ER. The molecular study of bacterial virulence: a review of current approaches, illustrated by the study of adhesion in uropathogenic *Escherichia coli*. Pediatr Nephrol 6:587–596, 1992.

Root RK, Rosenthal AS, Balestra DJ. Abnormal bactericidal, metabolic, and lysosomal functions of Chédiak-Higashi syndrome leukocytes. J Clin Invest 51:649–665, 1972.

Rosenstreich DL. Evaluation of delayed hypersensitivity: from PPD to poison ivy. Allerg Proc 14:395–400, 1993.

Ross SC, Densen P. Complement deficiency states and infection: epidemiology, pathogenesis, and consequences of neisserial and other infections in an immune deficiency. Medicine 63:243–273, 1984.

Rothenberg EV. The development of functionally responsive T cells. Adv Immunol 51:85–214, 1992.

Sansonetti PJ. Molecular and cellular biology of *Shigella flexneri* invasiveness: from cell assay systems to shigellosis. In Sansonetti PJ, ed. Pathogenesis of Shigellosis. Current Topics in Microbiology and Immunology. Berlin; Springer-Verlag, 1992, pp. 1–19.

Scalzo AA, Fitzgerald NA, Wallace CR, Gibbons AE, Smart YC, Burton RC, Shellam GR. The effect of the *Cmv-1* resistance gene, which is linked to the natural killer cell gene complex, is mediated by natural killer cells. J Immunol 149:581–589, 1992.

Schimke RN, Bolano C, Kirkpatrick CH. Immunologic deficiency in the congenital rubella syndrome. Am J Dis Child 118:626–633, 1969.

Schnittman SM, Fauci AS. Human immunodeficiency virus and acquired immunodeficiency syndrome: an update. Adv Intern Med 39:305–355, 1994.

Schrader JW. Peptide regulatory factors and optimization of vaccines. Molec Immunol 28:295–299, 1991.

Schwab JH. Phlogistic properties of peptidoglycan-polysaccharide polymers from cell walls of pathogenic and normal-flora bacteria which colonize humans. Infect Immun 61:4535–4539, 1993.

Sheagren JN. *Staphylococcus aureus.* The persistent pathogen. N Eng J Med 310:1368–1373, 1984.

Sherlock DS. Chronic hepatitis C. Disease-a-Month 40:117–196, 1994.

Sissons JGP, Oldstone MBA. Antibody-mediated destruction of virus-infected cells. Adv Immunol 29:209–260, 1980.

Smialowicz R, Schwab JH. Cytotoxicity of rat macrophages activated by persistent or biodegradable bacterial cell walls. Infect Immun 17:599–606, 1977.

Spangler BD. Structure and function of cholera toxin and the related *Escherichia coli* heat-labile enterotoxin. Microbiol Rev 56:622–647, 1992.

Sparling PF. Bacterial virulence and pathogenesis: an overview. Rev Infect Dis 5:S637–S646, 1983.

Spika JS, Peterson PK, Wilkinson BJ, Hammerschmidt DE, Verbrugh HA, Verhoef J, Quie PG. Role of peptidoglycan from *Staphylococcus aureus* in leukopenia, thrombocytopenia, and complement activation associated with bacteremia. J Infect Dis 146:227–234, 1982.

Stevens MK, Krause DC. *Mycoplasma pneumoniae* cytadherence phase-variable protein HMW3 is a component of the attachment organelle. J Bacteriol 174:4265–4274, 1992.

Stiehm ER, Kronenberg LH, Rosenblatt HM, Bryson Y, Merigan TC. Interferon: immunobiology and clinical significance. Ann Intern Med 96:80–93, 1982.

Stiehm ER, Chin TW, Haas A, Peerless AG. Infectious complications of the primary immunodeficiencies. Clin Immunol Immunopathol 40:69–86, 1986.

Stromberg N, Nyholm PG, Pascher I, Normark S. Saccharide orientation at the cell surface affects glycolipid receptor function. Proc Natl Acad Sci U S A 88:9340–9344, 1991.

Svennerholm AM, Wnneras C, Holmgren J, McConnell MM, Rowe B. Roles of different coli surface antigens of colonization factor II in colonization by and protective immunogenicity of enterotoxigenic *Escherichia coli* in rabbits. Infect Immun 58:341–346, 1990.

Tagliabue A, Boraschi D, Villa L, Keren DF, Lowell GH, Rappuoli R, Nencioni L. IgA-dependent cell-mediated activity against entero-

pathogenic bacteria: distribution, specificity, and characterization of the effector cells. J Immunol 133:988–992, 1984.

Tosato G, Blaese RM. Epstein-Barr virus infection and immunoregulation in man. Adv Immunol 37:99–149, 1985.

Tzianabos AO, Onderdonk AB, Rosner B, Cisneros RL, Kasper DL. Structural features of polysaccharides that induce intra-abdominal abscesses. Science 262:416–419, 1993.

Ulevitch RJ. Recognition of bacterial endotoxins by receptor-dependent mechanisms. Adv Immunol 53:267–289, 1993.

Vaisanen V, Elo J, Tallgren L, Siitonen A, Makela P, Svanborg-Eden C, Kallenius G, Svenson SB, Hultberg H, Korhonen T. Mannose-resistant hemagglutination and P antigen recognition characteristics of *E. coli* causing pyelonephritis. Lancet 2:1366–1369, 1981.

van Loosdrecht MC, Norde W, Zehnder AJ. Physical chemical description of bacterial adhesion. J Biomater Appl 5:91–106, 1990.

van Oss CJ. Aspecific and specific intermolecular interactions in aqueous media. J Mol Recognit 3:128–136, 1990.

Vella C, Festenstein H. Coxsackievirus B4 infection of the mouse pancreas: the role of natural killer cells in the control of virus replication and resistance to infection. J Gen Virol 73:1379–1386, 1992.

Vicenzi E, Poli G. Regulation of HIV expression by viral genes and cytokines. J Leuk Biol 56:328–334, 1994.

Wannamaker LW. Streptococcal toxins. Rev Infect Dis 6:S723–S732, 1983.

Watson RWG, Redmond HP, Bouchier-Hayes D. Role of endotoxin in mononuclear phagocyte-mediated inflammatory responses. J Leuk Biol 56:95–103, 1994.

Weinstein SL, June CH, DeFranco AL. Lipopolysaccharide induced protein tyrosine phosphorylation in human macrophages is mediated by CD14. J Immunol 151:3829–3838, 1993.

Weinstock JV. The pathogenesis of granulomatous inflammation and organ injury in schistosomiasis: interactions between the schistosome ova and the host. Immunol Invest 21:455–475, 1992.

Wick MJ, Hamood AN, Iglewski BH. Analysis of the structure-function relationship of *Pseudomonas aeruginosa* exotoxin A. Molec Microbiol 4:527–535, 1990.

Wolf MK, Taylor DN, Boedeker EC, Hyams KC, Maneval DR, Levine MM, Tamura K, Wilson RA, Echeverria P. Characterization of enterotoxigenic *Escherichia coli* isolated from U.S. troops deployed to the Middle East. J Clin Microbiol 31:851–856, 1993.

Wyler DJ. Why does liver fibrosis occur in schistosomiasis? Parasitol Today 8:277–279, 1992.

Yewdell JW, Bennink JR. Antigen processing: a critical factor in rational vaccine design. Semin Hematol 30(Suppl. 4):26–30, 1993.

Zaia JA, Levin MJ, Preblud SR, Leszcynski J, Wright GG, Ellis RJ, Curtis AC, Valerio MA, LeGore J. Evaulation of varicella-zoster immune globulin: protection of immunosuppressed children after household exposure to varicella. J Infect Dis 147:737–743, 1983.

Ziegler-Heitbrock HWL, Ulevitch RJ. CD14: Cell surface receptor and differentiation marker. Immunol Today 14:121–125, 1993.

Chapter 31

Infection in the Compromised Host

James D. Cherry and Ralph D. Feigin

Certain inherited and acquired disorders are associated frequently with infections by organisms that produce no significant disease in most normal individuals. The infections in compromised hosts are due to organisms indigenous to the host or found commonly in the environment and are frequently referred to as opportunistic infections (Hart et al., 1969; Klainer and Beisel, 1969; Bode et al., 1974; Young et al., 1974; Hewitt and Sanford, 1974; Feigin and Shearer, 1975; Feigin and Matson, 1992). The clinical evaluation and treatment of immunologically compromised children with possible opportunistic infection are now frequent occurrences.

It is important to emphasize that the relationship between the host and the exogenous and endogenous microbial surroundings is a dynamic one. Specific microbial virulence can be expressed only in comparative terms because of daily variations in the total spectrum and concentration of microorganisms to which the host is exposed and the changes in host defense mechanisms. *Pathogenicity*, which is the capacity of a microorganism to cause disease, is not an absolute term. Frequently, highly "pathogenic" microorganisms do not cause disease in exposed "susceptible" individuals, and on other occasions "nonpathogens" cause disease in "normal healthy" persons. In addition to the risks of opportunistic infection, the compromised child is susceptible to all microorganisms to which normal children are susceptible, and the illnesses in the compromised children are frequently more severe and protracted.

Although infections in compromised children always have occurred, their relative importance has increased steadily over the last 40 years. The major change over time has been in the specific microorganisms causing fatalities and the fact that in the past compromised children frequently died as the result of their first systemic infections. Today, compromised children have a history of survival from repeated serious infections. A major problem of the present era is the large number of infections in the compromised host that are hospital-acquired. These nosocomial infections tend to be more difficult to manage because they are due to microorganisms from the hospital environment that frequently are resistant to conventional antimicrobial therapy (Eickhoff, 1972, 1975; Hewitt and Sanford, 1974; Moore, 1974; Westwood et al., 1974; Neu, 1984; Gardner and Goldmann, 1992).

INFECTION IN CHILDREN COMPROMISED BY ANATOMIC DEFECTS

Opportunistic infections frequently are associated with the following anatomic defects: (1) dermal sinus tracts, (2) congenital and acquired cardiac defects, (3) urinary tract abnormalities, and (4) cleft palate. The microorganisms responsible for infections in children with anatomic defects and an approach to treatment and prevention are presented in Table 31–1.

Dermal Abnormalities of the Craniospinal Axis

Congenital dermal abnormalities of the craniospinal axis are more common than generally appreciated (Powell et al., 1975; Givner and Kaplan, 1993). About 1% of children have midline defects; fortunately, only a small fraction of these defects communicate with the central nervous system and become infected. Powell and colleagues (1975) reviewed the literature and found 110 infections of dermal sinuses. The most common infectious agents were those of normal bowel or skin flora (Table 31–1). Some infections were nosocomial.

Because the morbidity and mortality from dermal sinus tract infections are great, prevention by surgical correction is indicated whenever defects are noted. An approach to therapy is listed in Table 31–1.

Table 31–1. Infection in the Host Compromised by Anatomic Defects

Predisposing Causes	Opportunistic Organisms Isolated Most Frequently	Approach to Treatment of Infections	Prevention of Infections
Dermal abnormalities of the craniospinal axis	*Corynebacterium* sp., *Proteus* sp., *Escherichia coli*, *Staphylococcus epidermidis*, *S. aureus*, diphtheroids, *Pseudomonas aeruginosa*, *Alcaligenes faecalis*, *Bacteroides* sp., *Haemophilus aphrophilus*, *Streptococcus* sp.	1. Gram-stained smear and culture of lesion drainage and cerebrospinal fluid. 2. Incision and drainage if abscess present. 3. Prior to identification of an organism, immediate therapy with systemic antibiotics (choice made on basis of Gram stain). If the etiologic agent is in doubt, antibiotic therapy should include coverage for *S. aureus*, *S. epidermidis*, *Corynebacterium* sp., and Enterobacteriaceae. 4. Repair of defect.	1. Careful evaluation of all skin defects. 2. Surgical repair of all defects that might communicate with the central nervous system.
Cardiac defects	*Streptococcus* viridans group, *S. pneumoniae*, other streptococci, enterococci, *S. aureus*, *S. epidermidis*, *Neisseria* sp., many gram-negative bacilli, *Candida* sp., *Aspergillus* sp., *H. aphrophilus*, *Corynebacterium* sp., *Neisseria* sp., *Pseudomonas cepacia*, *Aerococcus viridans*, *Aspergillus fumigatus*	1. Multiple blood specimens for culture prior to therapy 2. Penicillin therapy for susceptible (MIC ≤0.2 μg/ml penicillin G) *Streptococcus* viridans group; penicillin or vancomycin and an aminoglycoside for enterococci and resistant viridans group *Streptococcus*; penicillinase-resistant penicillin or vancomycin for *Staphylococcus* sp.	1. Prophylactic administration of recommended antibiotics during dental and other procedures resulting in extensive bacteremia*
Obstructive lesions of the urinary tract	*E. coli*, other gram-negative bacilli; enterococci, *S. epidermidis*	1. Smear and quantitative culture of urine. 2. Urologic evaluation and corrective surgery. 3. Antibiotic therapy based on results of culture.	1. Corrective surgery. 2. Prophylactic antibiotics.
Cleft palate	*E. coli*, other gram-negative bacilli; *H. influenzae*, *Streptococcus* sp., *S. aureus*	1. Culture of ear drainage. 2. Antibiotic therapy based on culture data. 3. Tympanostomy tube insertion.	1. Tympanostomy tube insertion. 2. Prophylactic antibiotics. 3. Surgical repair of cleft palate.

*Data from Dajani AS, Bisno AL, Chung KJ, et al. JAMA 264:2919–2922, 1990.
Abbreviation: MIC = minimal inhibitory concentration.

Cardiac Defects

Children with congenital and acquired heart disease may develop acute or subacute bacterial endocarditis. The most common etiologic agents include viridans group streptococci, *Streptococcus pneumoniae*, other non–beta-hemolytic streptococci, enterococci, *Staphylococcus aureus*, and *Staphylococcus epidermidis* (Caldwell et al., 1971; Mendelsohn and Hutchins, 1979; Johnson and Rhodes, 1982; Kramer et al., 1983; Stanton et al., 1984; Van Hare et al., 1984; Noel et al., 1988; Elward et al., 1990; Starke, 1992; Saiman et al., 1993). Subacute bacterial endocarditis in children with congenital cardiac defects has also been reported in association with other opportunistic organisms, including *Haemophilus aphrophilus* (Johnson and Rhodes, 1982), *Neisseria* sp. (Brodie et al., 1971; Scott 1971), diphtheroids (Merzbach et al., 1965; Van Hare et al., 1984), *Moraxella* (Christensen and Emmanouilides, 1967), *Enterobacter* sp. (Caldwell et al., 1971; Stanton et al., 1984), *Pseudomonas* sp. (Johnson and Rhodes, 1982; Kramer et al., 1983), *Escherichia coli* (Johnson and Rhodes, 1982), *Klebsiella pneumoniae* (Stanton et al., 1984), *Candida* sp. (Mendelsohn and Hutchins, 1979; Saiman et al., 1993), *Serratia* sp. (Stanton et al., 1984), *Haemophilus* sp. (Blair and Weiner, 1979; Stanton et al., 1984), *Kingella kingae* (Odum et al., 1984), beta-hemolytic streptococci groups B, C, and G (Goldberg et al., 1985; Saiman et al., 1993), *Aspergillus* sp. (Barst et al., 1981; Saiman et al., 1993), and *Actinobacillus actinomycetemcomitans* (Van Hare et al., 1984).

In addition to microbial infections within the heart, infants with congenital heart disease have an increased risk of severe illness when infected with respiratory syncytial virus (Hall, 1992; MacDonald et al., 1982). An approach to prevention and treatment is presented in Table 31–1.

Urinary Tract Abnormalities

Obstructive lesions of the urinary tract increase the risk of infection significantly. In addition to the usual gram-negative enteric microorganisms that cause urinary tract infections in children without demonstrable structural malformations, organisms of low virulence such as *S. epidermidis* are noted in infections in children with obstructive defects (Deinard and Libit, 1972).

Cleft Palate

Otitis media is an almost universal complication of cleft palate (Paradise et al., 1969; Paradise and Bluestone, 1974; Paradise, 1976). The increased susceptibility in children with cleft palate is thought to be due to a functional impairment of the opening mechanisms of the eustachian tube. There has been little microbiologic study of otitis media in children with cleft palates. Because otitis media occurs in early infancy in these children, *E. coli* and other gram-negative bacilli are frequent pathogens as well as *Haemophilus influenzae*, *S. pneumoniae*, and *S. aureus*.

INFECTION IN CHILDREN COMPROMISED BY CHANGES IN OR PROCEDURES THAT BYPASS THE SKIN OR MUCOUS MEMBRANE BARRIERS

The skin and mucous membranes represent important barriers to infection. The intact skin generally resists infection by organisms that may contaminate it, and few microorganisms are able to penetrate it (Burtenshaw, 1948; Aly et al., 1972, 1975; Cooperstock, 1992). Situations in which the skin or mucous membrane barriers to infection have been compromised and thereby predispose the host to opportunistic infection are presented in Table 31–2.

Catheters

Intravascular Catheters

In the present era, the care of the majority of hospitalized children involves the use of one or more intravascular catheters, and these catheters are the most common cause of nosocomial bacteremias (Maki and Band, 1981). Catheter types include peripheral intravenous catheters, short-term arterial and central venous lines, long-term cuffed silicone central lines such as Broviac and Hickman catheters, and implanted venous access systems. Opportunistic infections occur with all intravascular access lines (Band and Maki, 1979, 1980; Buxton et al., 1979; Rhame et al., 1979; Adams et al., 1980; Begala et al., 1982; Jarvis et al., 1983; Moyer et al., 1983; Shinozaki et al., 1983; Palmer, 1984; Press et al., 1984; Tomford et al., 1984; Wang et al., 1984; Flynn et al., 1987a, 1988; Jarvis, 1987; Decker and Edwards, 1988; Wurzel et al., 1988; Freeman et al., 1990; Richet et al., 1990; Rupar et al., 1990; Dawson et al., 1991; Furfaro et al., 1991; Gorelick et al., 1991; Ingram et al., 1991; Severien and Nelson, 1991; Riikonen et al., 1993).

In simple (noncuffed) catheters, infections are classified as exit site infections (local infection at the point where the catheter exits the skin), septic infections, or combination infections. Cuffed catheters also are associated with exit site and septic infections; in addition, they also may have tunnel infections (infections of the subcutaneous track that extends proximally from the skin exit site to the point where the catheter enters the vein) (Decker and Edwards, 1988).

Bacteremia or fungemia with organisms commonly found on the skin has been reported in 0.4% to 5% of patients with simple intravenous catheters (Harbin and Schaffner, 1973; Maki et al., 1973). The rate of septicemia associated with prolonged intravenous catheterization as used for providing total nutrition parenterally has been even higher (Goldman and Maki, 1973; Begala et al., 1982; Press et al., 1984; Decker and Edwards, 1988; Wurzel et al., 1988; Riikonen et al., 1993). *S. epidermidis*, *S. aureus*, *Streptococcus* group D and *Streptococcus* viridans group, *Bacillus* sp., *Pseudomonas* sp., *Bacteroides* sp., *Serratia*, *Citrobacter*, *Enterobacter* sp., *Acinetobacter* sp., and other organisms have been recovered from patients receiving total parenteral alimentation

Table 31–2. Infection in the Child Compromised by Procedures That Bypass the Skin or Mucous Membrane Barriers

Predisposing Causes	Opportunistic Organisms Isolated Most Frequently	Approach to Treatment of Infections	Prevention of Infections
Intravenous catheters	*Staphylococcus epidermidis, Staphylococcus aureus, Enterococcus* sp., *Streptococcus* sp., *Bacteroides* sp., *Escherichia coli, Acinetobacter* sp., *Pseudomonas* sp., *Citrobacter* sp., *Klebsiella* sp., *Enterobacter* sp., *Bacillus* sp., *Serratia* sp., *Cryptococcus* sp., *Candida* sp., *Torulopsis glabrata, Malassezia furfur, Corynebacterium* sp., *Mycobacterium* sp.	1. Removal of catheter, if possible, especially with persistently positive blood culture or clinical signs suggesting persistent infection. 2. Aspiration of blood through the line, and obtain peripheral blood for culture. 3. Culture of tip of removed catheter. 4. Culture of infusing solution. 5. Culture of skin at site of insertion. 6. If patient febrile, start therapy with a penicillinase-resistant penicillin or vancomycin and an aminoglycoside. Consider addition of a third-generation cephalosporin. 7. Examination of catheter tip for a thrombus by ultrasonography. 8. If thrombus is present, prolonged antimicrobial therapy will be necessary; line will need to be removed frequently.	1. When possible, use of scalp vein needles rather than plastic catheters. 2. Frequent change of intravenous site and administration set. 3. Use of surgical preparation prior to placing catheter. 4. Fewer infections occur with subcutaneous ports than with external catheters. 5. Intravenous antibiotic prophylaxis preoperatively. 6. Adequate staff training in the care of indwelling catheters. 7. Line placed preferably in upper body.
Urinary catheters	Gram-negative enteric bacilli, *Pseudomonas* sp., *Serratia* sp., *Acinetobacter* sp., *Staphylococcus epidermidis, Candida* sp., *Alcaligenes* sp., *Enterococcus* sp., *Proteus mirabilis*	1. Gram-stained smear, culture of urine, and culture of blood. 2. Removal of catheter, if possible. 3. If patient is febrile, immediate therapy with systemic antibiotics (choice made on basis of Gram stain). Frequently, therapy includes an aminoglycoside. 4. Treat *Proteus* sp., even if patient is asymptomatic, to prevent calculi. 5. If removal of catheter is not possible, local therapy with either continuous antibiotic or acetic acid bladder irrigation.	1. Careful attention to sterile technique during catheter insertion. 2. Use of a closed drainage system or continuous bladder irrigation with acetic acid or antibiotic solution.
Inhalation therapy equipment	*S. aureus, Streptococcus pneumoniae*, other streptococci, *Haemophilus influenzae, Pseudomonas* sp., *Serratia* sp., *Klebsiella pneumoniae, Acinetobacter* sp., *Flavobacterium* sp., *Alcaligenes* sp., other gram-negative bacilli	1. Culture from patient's respiratory tract. 2. Initial therapy usually includes an aminoglycoside and a third-generation cephalosporin.	1. Use of a specific regimen for cleaning inhalation therapy equipment. 2. Infection control protocols to monitor associated infections.

(Dudrick et al., 1968; Groff, 1969; Boeckman and Krill, 1970; Curry and Quie, 1971; Rodrigues et al., 1971; Dillon et al., 1973; Saleh and Schorin, 1987; Decker and Edwards, 1988). Tissue invasion by fungi has been documented; *Candida albicans* and *Torulopsis glabrata* appear to be the principal offenders (Freeman and Litton, 1974). Broviac catheter–related outbreaks of sepsis due to *Malassezia furfur* in infants receiving intravenous

fat emulsions have been described (Powell et al., 1984; Azimi et al., 1988).

Bacteremia related to intravenous therapy may occur even if local signs of inflammation are absent. Frequently, however, signs of inflammation, thrombosis, or purulent material are observed at the site of catheterization. When positive cultures or clinical signs suggest infection due to intravenous therapy with short-term catheters (noncuffed), the therapy should be discontinued immediately. Therapy may be re-established at another site, if necessary. After the removal of a contaminated intravenous catheter, bacteremia or fungal septicemia may resolve spontaneously without specific antimicrobial therapy. When positive cultures or clinical signs suggest persistent infection, appropriate antimicrobial drugs should be administered.

Central venous lines with Broviac and Hickman catheters are usually left in place for considerable periods of time. Infection rates in different studies have varied from 0.47 to 7.59 per 1000 catheter use days (Begala et al., 1982; Press et al., 1984; Decker and Edwards, 1988; Wurzel et al., 1988). Press and associates (1984) have shown that exit site infections in patients with Hickman catheters usually can be cured with antibiotics alone without removal of the catheter. They also noted that tunnel infections usually necessitate catheter removal. They suggest that exit site and tunnel infections be treated with antibiotics. Removal of the catheter should be considered if clinical improvement (no persistence of fever, bacteremia, and local inflammation) has occurred after 48 hours of treatment. Our experience in patients on total parenteral nutrition who are immunocompetent with bacteremia is that they frequently can be cured with appropriate antimicrobial treatment without removal of the line.

Routine replacement of all apparatus used for intravenous administration every 72 hours can decrease significantly the hazard of extrinsic contamination (Maki et al., 1987; Snydman et al., 1987). All bottles containing fluids for intravenous administration should be inspected immediately prior to use for cracks and turbidity. When peripheral intravenous administration is required, a small needle rather than a plastic catheter should be used; use of needles has been associated with a lower incidence of septicemia and phlebitis than that of catheters (Crossley and Matsen, 1972; Peter et al., 1972). Topical antibiotic preparations applied repeatedly to the site of catheter insertion have been widely used to prevent infections. Although some studies have suggested benefit from this procedure, there is the added risk of infection with more resistant bacterial strains (Maki et al., 1973).

Guidelines for the prevention of infections of arterial lines have been described in detail by Mermel and Maki (1989) and Shinozaki and associates (1983).

Intravenous catheter–associated sepsis may be caused by the infusion of contaminated intravenous fluids. Infection related to contaminated intravenous fluids has been caused by *Enterobacter cloacae, Enterobacter agglomerans, Pseudomonas* sp., *Citrobacter freundii, Klebsiella* sp., *Serratia* sp., and yeasts (Maki et al., 1973a, 1976; Jarvis et al., 1983). Nosocomial infection outbreaks with *E. agglomerans* and *E. cloacae* have been related to fluid contamination during the manufacturing process.

Urinary Catheters

The use of indwelling urinary catheters is a common cause of opportunistic infection (Kunin and McCor-

mack, 1966; Stamm, 1975; Wong and Hooton, 1981; Lohr et al., 1989; Meanes, 1991). In addition to common gram-negative enteric bacteria, many highly resistant organisms such as *Pseudomonas* sp., *Acinetobacter, Achromobacter, Candida,* and *Serratia* have been incriminated frequently (Ederer and Matsen, 1972; Schonebeck, 1972; Maki et al., 1973b). The approach to prevention and treatment of catheter-associated urinary tract infections is presented in Table 31–2.

Inhalation Therapy

Nosocomial pneumonias are common in immunocompromised patients, and the most common associated factor is mechanical ventilation. The incidence, risk factors, and etiologic agents of these pneumonias have been well studied in adults, but few recent studies have been conducted in pediatric intensive care units (Barzilay et al., 1988; Leu et al., 1989; Rello et al., 1991; Nielsen et al., 1992; George, 1993; Kollef, 1993). Etiologic diagnosis of pulmonary infections in patients on ventilators is difficult because of contamination by oropharyngeal flora. In a study in baboons, Johanson and colleagues (1988) found that tracheal aspirates revealed 78% of the organisms found in lung tissue, but false-positive cultures occurred frequently. *S. aureus, S. pneumoniae,* other streptococci, *H. influenzae, Pseudomonas aeruginosa, Serratia marcescens, Acinetobacter* sp., *Flavobacterium* sp., *Achromobacter* sp., *Klebsiella pneumoniae,* and other gram-negative bacilli have been the organisms implicated most commonly (Edmondson et al., 1966; Mertz et al., 1967; Pierce et al., 1970; Sanders et al., 1970; Reinhardt et al., 1980; Rello et al., 1991; Nielsen et al., 1992).

In the past, contaminated reservoir nebulizers were a problem, but with present-day cleaning and maintenance programs, this source of infection is uncommon. However, when an outbreak occurs in an intensive care unit, specimens for culture should be obtained from the equipment (e.g., reservoirs). Specific regimens for the cleaning and maintenance of inhalation therapy equipment (particularly nebulizers and tubing) should be adopted and continuously employed.

Surgery

Opportunistic infections are common in surgical patients (Riley, 1969; Cruse and Foord, 1980; Cruse, 1981; CDC, 1981; Davis et al., 1984; Sleigh and Peutherer, 1988; Olson and O'Conner-Allen, 1989; Horan et al., 1993). Although the surgical patient is compromised primarily because of the disruption of the skin and mucous membrane protective barriers, other aspects of therapy such as the use of intravenous and urinary catheters and inhalation therapy devices also contribute to the overall infection risk. A complete discussion of infection in surgical patients is beyond the scope of this chapter.

General Surgery

Wound infection is the most common opportunistic problem in surgical patients. The incidence of wound infection varies greatly among different centers and in the type of surgery performed. In "clean" surgical cases, an incidence rate of wound infection can be expected to be between 2% and 5%. The most common etiologic agents and an approach to prevention are presented in Table 31–3.

When a fever develops in a child postoperatively, infection by opportunistic microorganisms must be considered. Appropriate cultures and serologic tests are mandatory to establish an etiologic diagnosis. The many types and varied nature of the opportunistic organisms that produce disease postoperatively prevent the suggestion of a single specific antibiotic regimen as appropriate for all patients.

Table 31–3. Infection in the Child Compromised by Surgical Procedures

Type of Surgery	Opportunistic Organisms Isolated Most Frequently	Approach to Treatment of Infections	Prevention of Infections
General surgery	*Staphylococcus aureus, S. epidermidis, Streptococcus* sp., *Escherichia coli, Clostridia* sp., *Klebsiella pneumoniae, Enterobacter* sp., *Pseudomonas* sp., *Proteus* sp., other gram-negative bacilli, *Bacteroides* sp., and other anaerobes, *Candida* sp., and other fungi, *Pasteurella multocida, Bacillus subtilis, Alcaligenes faecalis, Aeromonas hydrophila*	1. Gram-stained smear, and culture from wound; blood specimens for culture. 2. Withhold antibiotic therapy until specimens for culture have been obtained.	1. Discourage use of prophylactic antibiotics unless they have been demonstrated to be useful in controlled trials in the particular surgical condition. 2. Discourage unnecessary use of urinary and intravenous catheters and respirators. 3. Careful attention to aseptic techniques. 4. Routine hospital surveillance of surgical infections.
Cerebrospinal fluid shunts	*S. epidermidis, S. aureus, Bacillus* sp., diphtheroids, gram-negative enteric bacilli	1. Gram-stained smear and cultures of CSF, blood, and shunt. 2. In patients with a ventriculo-atrial shunt, obtain multiple blood specimens for culture. 3. Immediate therapy with vancomycin and an aminoglycoside. Possible change of antibiotic therapy following culture results. 4. Direct aspiration of shunt reservoir or valve. 5. Removal of infected shunt.	1. Prophylactic administration of a penicillinase-resistant penicillin during the perioperative period.
Burns	*Streptococcus* sp., *Staphylococcus* sp., *Pseudomonas* sp., *Serratia* sp., *Aeromonas hydrophila, Klebsiella* sp., *Flavobacterium* sp., *Enterobacter* sp., *Escherichia coli, Proteus* sp., *Providencia* sp., *Enterococcus* sp., *Candida* sp., *Mucor* sp., *Aspergillus* sp., *Geotrichum, Helminthosporum, Alternaria, Fusarium, Cryptococcus,* herpes simplex virus, varicella-zoster virus	1. Burn wound biopsy specimen and blood specimens for culture. 2. If patient febrile or toxic, immediate therapy with a penicillinase-resistant penicillin or vancomycin and an aminoglycoside. 3. Use of IVIG in selected cases.	1. Low-dose prophylaxis with penicillin. 2. Careful cleaning of the burned skin and meticulous protective care. 3. Anticipatory treatment for invading and translocating organisms. 4. Early wound closure.
Cardiac surgery	*Staphylococcus aureus, S. epidermidis,* diphtheroids, *Acinetobacter* sp., *Serratia* sp., *Pseudomonas* sp., *Candida* sp., *Aspergillus* sp., *Salmonella* sp., Enterobacteriaceae	1. Multiple blood specimens for culture prior to therapy.	1. Prophylactic administration of a penicillinase-resistant penicillin or cefazolin during the perioperative period. 2. Prophylaxis is started immediately before the operative procedure, repeated during prolonged procedures, and continued for no more than 24 hours postoperatively to minimize occurrence of microbial resistance.

Abbreviations: CSF = cerebrospinal fluid; IVIG = intravenous immunoglobulin.

Cerebrospinal Fluid Shunts

Odio and associates (1984) reviewed the records of 516 cerebrospinal fluid (CSF) shunt procedures in 297 patients from 1975 through 1981. There were three ventriculoatrial (VA) and 513 ventriculoperitoneal (VP) shunt procedures. Fifty-nine shunt infections (11%) occurred in 50 (17%) of the children. Staphylococci accounted for 75% of the infections, with *S. epidermidis* being more common than *S. aureus*. There were 11 (19%) infections with gram-negative bacilli, and two or more pathogens were isolated in 15% of the infections. In a more recent study involving 273 VP and 75 VA shunts in children, the infection rate was 8% (Kontny et al., 1993). The rate of infection was 13.6% for operations lasting more than 90 minutes and 5.2% for those with a duration of less than 30 minutes.

Most shunt infections are caused by microorganisms considered to be normal flora of the skin. Recovery of such organisms from the CSF, the shunt, or blood of patients with shunts should be regarded as presumptive evidence of infection. Hypocomplementemic glomerulonephritis is a well-recognized complication of shunt infection (Black et al., 1965; Stickler et al., 1968; McKenzie and Hayden, 1974). Most commonly, *S. epidermidis* has been implicated as the organism associated with this syndrome.

Fever is an almost universal manifestation of shunt infection. Erythema of the skin overlying the tubing used for diversion of the CSF is virtually diagnostic of infection. Children with infection of VA shunts generally have bacteremia, whereas patients with infection of VP shunts rarely have positive blood cultures and may have negative CSF cultures. Thus, when fever is observed in a child with a VA shunt, multiple blood cultures should be obtained, because generally they will permit an etiologic diagnosis. Direct aspiration of the shunt reservoir or valve is a helpful procedure for establishing the diagnosis of an infection of the shunt in patients who are not receiving antibiotics.

Patients with infected shunts should be treated with antibiotics directed specifically toward the offending organisms. Prior to the isolation and identification of the etiologic agent, treatment should include coverage for *Staphylococcus* sp., diphtheroids, and *Bacillus* sp. (Nydahl and Hall, 1965; Shurtleff et al., 1974; Schoenbaum et al., 1975; Odio et al., 1984; Walters et al., 1984; Yogev, 1985).

Because many strains of *S. epidermidis* are resistant to methicillin, an initial treatment regimen of vancomycin and an aminoglycoside is suggested. Although it is occasionally possible to successfully treat shunt infections with antibiotics alone, it is usually safer and necessary to remove the infected shunt (Walters et al., 1984; Odio et al., 1984; Yogev, 1985).

The temporal association of surgery to infection of VA and VP shunts with *S. epidermidis* and *S. aureus* (Schoenbaum et al., 1975; Odio et al., 1984) suggests that administration of antistaphylococcal antibiotics prophylactically in the perioperative period may be warranted. In one uncontrolled study of 80 adult patients, shunt infection was reduced from 19% to 3% when a regimen of parenteral methicillin, followed by oral dicloxacillin, was employed (Salmon, 1972). Odio and associates (1984) noted infections in 38% of 89 procedures in which prophylaxis was not used but in only 6% of 427 procedures when prophylaxis was given. Schoenbaum and colleagues (1975) and Yogev (1985) also noted lower infection rates when prophylactic antistaphylococcal antibiotics were administered. By contrast, others (Tsingoglou and Forrest, 1971; Naito et al., 1973) have not noted benefits when prophylactic antibiotics have been employed. Langley and associates (1993) performed a meta-analysis on the efficacy of antimicrobial prophylaxis, and they concluded that perioperative use of antimicrobial agents significantly reduces the risk of infection.

Burns

Thermal injury is unfortunately commonplace and is associated with significant morbidity and mortality in children. Opportunistic infection accounts for about half of all burn-associated fatalities (Feller and Crane, 1970; MacMillan, 1980). The damage resulting from a burn destroys the normal skin barrier to infection, allowing normal skin bacteria as well as environmental contaminants a portal of entry (Pruitt et al., 1984). In addition, Alexander and Meakins (1972) noted abnormalities in neutrophil function in patients with burns. Killing of *Staphylococcus* and *Pseudomonas* organisms by neutrophils was less efficient than was the killing of *Serratia* and streptococci. Alexander (1971a) also noted a circadian periodicity of neutrophil function; the time of day at which activity was minimal could be associated with an increased risk of sepsis in the burned patient.

In addition to neutrophil dysfunction, burn injury may be associated with abnormal vascular responses, diminished uptake of particles by the reticuloendothelial system, abnormal responses to antigens, and delayed rejection of homografts (Alexander, 1971a; Pruitt et al., 1984) (see Chapter 19).

Prior to the antibiotic era, infections with *Streptococcus pyogenes* were of most importance in patients with burns (Alexander, 1971b). Associated with the frequent use of penicillin therapy in patients with burns, streptococcal complications were controlled, but penicillin-resistant strains of *S. aureus* became a problem.

After the introduction and widespread use of penicillinase-resistant penicillins and cephalosporins, staphylococcal infections decreased in prominence in patients with burns, and gram-negative organisms became the predominant pathogens. Septicemia with *P. aeruginosa* was frequent. During the last 15 years, however, methicillin-resistant strains of staphylococci have developed, and because of this, sepsis caused by staphylococcal infection is again a major problem.

Septicemia in children with burns also has been related to *S. epidermidis*, *Serratia* sp., *Aeromonas hydrophila*, *Klebsiella* sp., *Enterobacter* sp., *Flavobacterium* sp., *Pseudomonas* sp., *E. coli*, *Proteus* sp., *Providencia* sp., *Candida* sp., *Mucor*, *Aspergillus* sp., *Geotrichum*, *Helminthosporium*,

Alternaria, Fusarium, and *Cryptococcus* (Peterson and Baker, 1959; Rabin et al., 1961; Foley, 1969; Benjamin et al., 1970; Alexander and Meakins, 1972; Abramovsky et al., 1974; Phillips et al., 1974; Spebar and Lindberg, 1979; Pruitt et al., 1984; MacMillan, 1980; Tredget et al., 1992; Sheridan et al., 1993). Viral invasion of the burned area also may occur: children with burns are particularly susceptible to herpes simplex infection. In addition, Linnemann and MacMillan (1981) noted that 22% of pediatric burn patients had serologic evidence of cytomegalovirus infections.

An approach to the treatment and prevention of opportunistic infections in children with burns is presented in Table 31–3 (Alexander, 1971b; Shuck, 1972; MacMillan, 1980; Pruitt et al., 1984).

Cardiac Surgery

Cardiac surgery has been associated with a significant risk of postoperative infection due to opportunistic microorganisms. *S. aureus* and *S. epidermidis, Salmonella, Serratia,* diphtheroids, *Acinetobacter lwoffi, Enterobacter* sp., *Pseudomonas* sp., *C. albicans,* and *Aspergillus* are the opportunists that have been implicated most frequently (Pike et al., 1951; Koiwai and Nahas, 1956, Brandt and Swahn, 1960; Watanakunakorn et al., 1968; Shafer and Hall, 1970; Griffin et al., 1973; Kammer and Utz, 1974; Wilson et al., 1975; Bernhard, 1975; Fisher et al., 1981; Flynn et al., 1987b; Wilhelmi et al., 1987; Boyce et al., 1990). An approach to prevention and treatment of infections in cardiac surgery patients is presented in Table 31–3.

INFECTION IN CHILDREN COMPROMISED BY INHERITED DISORDERS OF IMMUNITY

Disorders of Polymorphonuclear Leukocyte Function or Number

The development of the polymorphonuclear phagocytic system is presented in Chapter 5, and the pathophysiology and clinical aspects of these disorders are presented in Chapter 15.

Chronic Granulomatous Disease of Children

The clinical manifestations of chronic granulomatous disease (CGD) include marked lymphadenopathy, pneumonitis, suppuration of nodes, hepatomegaly, dermatitis, splenomegaly, liver and perianal abscesses, diarrhea, genitourinary granulomata, and osteomyelitis, particularly of the small bones of the hands and feet (Johnston and Baehner, 1971; Mills and Quie, 1980; Tauber et al., 1983; Quie and Hetherington, 1984). This condition is due to an inherited defect of leukocyte bactericidal function in which there is impaired intracellular killing of catalase-producing microorganisms (see Chapter 15). Bacteria such as *S. pneumoniae* and *S. pyogenes* do not cause unusual difficulty in patients with CGD because they generate hydrogen peroxide but not catalase. On the other hand, catalase-

positive organisms such as *S. aureus* and gram-negative enteric bacteria are troublesome. *S. aureus* has been isolated frequently from patients with this disease.

Systemic abscesses and other infections with organisms of low virulence such as *Enterobacter* sp., *E. coli, S. epidermidis, Serratia* sp., *Pseudomonas* sp., *Proteus* sp., *Salmonella* sp., *Candida* sp., and *Aspergillus* sp. are common (Johnston and Baehner, 1971; Lazarus and Neu, 1975). Infections with *Torulopsis* sp., *Hansenula polymorpha, Pneumocystis carinii, Streptococcus intermedius, Nocardia* sp., *Actinomyces israelii, Alcaligenes faecalis, Chromobacterium* sp., *Acinetobacter* sp., and *Mycobacterium fortuitum* have also been reported (Johnston and Baehner, 1971; Lazarus and Neu, 1975; Chusid et al., 1975; McGinnis et al., 1980; Mills and Quie, 1980; Gallin et al., 1983; Tauber et al., 1983; Quie and Hetherington, 1984). Disseminated infection with bacille Calmette-Guérin (BCG) has been noted in three immunized children with CGD (Esterly et al., 1971; Verronen, 1974).

Treatment of infection in patients with CGD must be dictated by the organisms producing the infections and their sensitivity patterns. In patients with suspected sepsis, treatment parenterally with a semisynthetic penicillinase-resistant penicillin and with an aminoglycoside antibiotic such as gentamicin is recommended until results of cultures are available. Drainage of abscesses is imperative. Antibiotic therapy must be continued for extended periods of time as dictated by the course of infection. Rifampin may be particularly effective in some patients because it may exert a bactericidal effect intracellularly (Ezer and Soothill, 1974; Jacobs and Wilson, 1983). Isoniazid, fosfomycin, clindamycin, trimethoprim-sulfamethoxazole, and chloramphenicol also readily cross cellular membranes and inhibit intracellular bacteria, so that they also could be useful when infecting organisms are sensitive (Quie, 1973; Gmünder and Seger, 1981; Jacobs and Wilson, 1983; Hoger et al., 1985). In this regard, Thompson and Soothill (1970) noted clinical improvement in two children with CGD who were treated with isoniazid and para-aminosalicylic acid, in spite of the fact that neither was affected by known mycobacterial infections. Granulocyte infusions have been suggested as an adjunct of therapy in life-threatening infections (Raubitschek et al., 1973; Tauber et al., 1983; Gallin et al., 1983). Corticosteroids in conjunction with antimicrobial therapy have been used to reduce obstruction caused by inflammation in three patients with CGD (Chin et al., 1987; Quie and Belani, 1987).

Attempts at prevention of infection in children with CGD have been disappointing. Continuous antibiotic therapy prophylactically has been advocated (Phillapart et al., 1972; Ammann and Wara, 1975; Johnston et al., 1975). In nine patients with CGD, nafcillin therapy appeared to reduce the number of infectious episodes (Phillapart et al., 1972). In contrast to these findings, Lazarus and Neu (1975) point out that the majority of fatalities that occur in children with CGD are due to gram-negative bacillary bacteria; they suggest that some of these deaths may be due to changes in the flora of children treated prophylactically with penicillinase-resistant penicillins.

In another study, the number of infectious episodes and the severity of bacterial infections were reduced in four or five children with CGD who were placed on long-term sulfisoxazole treatment (Johnston et al., 1975). The decrease in the number of infections was out of proportion to the demonstrable direct antibacterial effect of the drug. There was a modest enhancement of bactericidal activity of leukocytes in all five patients in the presence of sulfisoxazole, but studies of phagocytosis-associated oxidative metabolism in patients' cells have not revealed a metabolic basis for improved killing. Two children with CGD who we have followed also appeared to benefit from continuous sulfisoxazole prophylactic administration. More recently, there have been several reports of prophylactic success with trimethoprim-sulfamethoxazole (Kobayashi et al., 1978; Mendelsohn and Berant, 1982; Gallin et al., 1983; Tauber et al., 1983; Frayha and Biggar, 1983; Margolis et al., 1990). In contrast, McCrae and Raeburn (1972) noted no benefit from either clofazimine or cotrimoxazole treatment in one child with CGD.

Anderson (1981) noted that the administration of oral ascorbate in three children resulted in slight increases in neutrophil hexose monophosphate shunt and staphylocidal activity and reduction in the occurrence of obvious infections. In contrast with Anderson's findings, Foroozanfar and associates (1983) treated three patients with ascorbate for 8 months and were unable to document any improvement in the intracellular killing of microorganisms.

Recently, in vitro and in vivo studies have shown that interferon-γ can partially correct the metabolic defect in phagocytes of patients with CGD (Sechler et al., 1988; Mühlebach et al., 1992; Curnutte, 1993). In a controlled trial involving 128 patients with CGD, it was found that interferon-γ therapy was effective in reducing the frequency of serious infections (International Chronic Granulomatous Disease Cooperative Study Group, 1991). Patients were treated with interferon-γ (50 μg/M^2 of body surface area) three times a week.

Bone marrow transplantation has been tried in three cases, and in one case improvement persisted for 3 years (Gallin et al., 1983; Tauber et al., 1983).

Job's/Hyper IgE Syndrome

Job's syndrome (hyperimmunoglobulin E recurrent-infection syndrome) is a condition in which fair, red-headed girls experience repeated episodes of "cold" staphylococcal abscesses of the skin, subcutaneous tissue, or lymph nodes (Davis et al., 1966; Donabedian and Gallin, 1983; Quie and Hetherington, 1984) (see Chapters 13 and 15). Infections are also caused by *C. albicans*, *H. influenzae*, *S. pyogenes*, gram-negative pathogens, and other fungi (Shyur and Hill, 1991). When patients known to be afflicted with Job's syndrome are infected, appropriate cultures should be obtained and initial treatment with a semisynthetic penicillinase-resistant penicillin should ensue. Continuous antibiotic

therapy prophylactically with a penicillinase-resistant penicillin is a worthwhile approach in the severely affected child. Hattori and colleagues (1993) reported on a 13-year-old boy who had marked clinical improvement with trimethoprim-sulfamethoxazole therapy; associated with this clinical improvement was improvement in neutrophil function and a decrease in serum IgE concentration.

Glucose-6-Phosphate Dehydrogenase Deficiency

Leukocytes of patients with glucose-6-phosphate dehydrogenase (G-6-PDH) deficiency are unable to kill *S. aureus*, *E. coli*, or *Serratia* normally (Cooper et al.,1972) (see Chapter 15). The treatment and prevention of clinical infections should be similar to that employed in CGD.

Chédiak-Higashi Syndrome

This inherited autosomal recessive disorder is associated with recurrent pyogenic infection. Patients with this syndrome suffer infections similar to those in CGD (*S. aureus*, *Serratia*); in addition, they suffer excessively from infections with catalase-negative organisms (Ammann and Wara, 1975).

Treatment must be based on the recovery of the etiologic agents and the determination of their sensitivity patterns. In the septic child, initial therapy with a penicillinase-resistant penicillin and an aminoglycoside antibiotic such as gentamicin is recommended. The use of low-dose penicillin or trimethoprim-sulfamethoxazole prophylaxis should be considered in patients with recurrent infections with sensitive organisms. Affected children may also benefit from pneumococcal vaccine. Bone marrow transplantation may be lifesaving (Feigin and Matson, 1992).

Neutropenia

Congenital neutropenia may occur as an isolated deficit, with aplastic anemia, or in some patients with agammaglobulinemia or other immunodeficiency diseases (Kauder and Mauer, 1966; Baehner, 1972; Feigin and Shearer, 1975) (see Chapter 15). Neutropenia associated with pancreatic insufficiency and malabsorption also is a well-defined clinical syndrome (Shmerling et al., 1969). Cyclic neutropenia is another syndrome in which circulating white blood cells are depressed at intervals of about 3 weeks, and this is associated with aphthous stomatitis and fever (Wright et al., 1981).

Acquired neutropenias are a more common clinical problem than those of congenital disease. They most frequently are associated with drug administration. Acquired neutropenia also may be associated with overwhelming infection, collagen disease, allergic disorders, neoplasms, myelophthisic disorders, hypersplenism, and radiation.

In all neutropenic syndromes except cyclic neutropenia, severe pyogenic infections are the rule. Although infection with common pathogens is the usual occurrence, sepsis due to opportunistic organisms such as *Acinetobacter* sp., *Serratia* sp., *Pseudomonas* sp., *S. epidermidis*, and fungi is also frequent.

Prevention of infections in the neutropenic patient is a formidable challenge. As in the Chédiak-Higashi syndrome, prophylaxis with low-dose penicillin or trimethoprim-sulfamethoxazole may be useful in children with congenital neutropenia who have recurrent infections with sensitive organisms.

The treatment of infections in children with neutropenia is dependent on data derived from cultures taken prior to therapy. In treating infections with *Pseudomonas* sp. and other gram-negative bacilli, it is important to use two synergistic antimicrobial agents, such as ceftazidime and gentamicin. The clinical manifestations of infection in neutropenic patients are different from those in non-neutropenic patients. Sickles and colleagues (1975) noted that exudation, fluctuation, ulceration or fissure, local heat, swelling, and regional adenopathy were less commonly found in patients with malignancies who were profoundly granulocytopenic than in similar patients without granulocytopenia. Only erythema and local pain or tenderness were common findings in both granulocytopenic and non-granulocytopenic patients. The response to therapy in children with neutropenia generally is slower than in normal children.

Patients with both congenital or acquired neutropenia may respond to granulocyte-macrophage or granulocyte colony-stimulating factors (GM-CSF, G-CSF) (Welte et al., 1990; Dale, 1994). Patients have been treated with G-CSF for more than 3 years without adverse effects.

Splenic Deficiency

The pathophysiology of splenic deficiency is discussed in Chapters 11 and 19. The major cause of splenic deficiency is surgical removal, but congenital asplenia and splenosis also occur (Pedersen, 1983). In splenic deficiency disorders, there is an increased susceptibility to overwhelming infection with *S. pneumoniae*, *Neisseria meningitidis*, and *H. influenzae*. Rarely, other streptococci, *Staphylococcus* sp., *E. coli, Klebsiella, Salmonella*, and *P. aeruginosa* cause septicemia (Chilcote et al., 1976; Walker, 1976). In endemic areas, persons with splenic deficiency are also at increased risk of severe and often fatal infections with *Plasmodium* and *Babesia* spp. protozoan diseases (Editorial, *Lancet*, 1976; Katz, 1982). The pneumococcus is the major risk in asplenic children. The experience to date suggests that, although splenectomy increases the risk of infection in all persons, susceptibility is in large part influenced by the underlying disease state for which splenectomy was performed. Until recently, the pneumococcus has been highly susceptible to penicillin, and therefore penicillin prophylaxis has been recommended. Most authorities agree that asplenic children with malignancies, thalassemia, histiocytosis, and other debilitating diseases should be placed on prophylactic penicillin. In children in whom splenectomy was performed because of

trauma, there is less agreement in regard to prophylaxis.

It is our belief that children under the age of 3 years should receive prophylaxis and that in older children the parents should be offered an option. If prophylaxis is undertaken, it must be emphasized to the parents that haphazard compliance is probably worse than no antibiotic administration. If a continuous prophylactic regimen is not employed, the parents should have a supply of amoxicillin/clavulanate potassium (Augmentin) readily available. At the first sign of respiratory illness, the patient's physician should be contacted and Augmentin therapy (40 mg/kg/day, based on the amoxicillin component, in divided doses every 8 hours) immediately instituted. It must be emphasized that all febrile illnesses must be considered potentially serious and immediate medical attention sought. For prophylaxis, oral penicillin G two times a day should be employed. Children under 5 years of age should receive 200,000 U/dose; those over 5 years of age, 400,000 U/dose. Alternatively, oral penicillin V can be used (125 mg twice daily for children under 5 years of age and 250 mg twice daily for older children).

In recent years there has been a worldwide increase in pneumococci that are resistant to penicillin (Klugman et al., 1990; Rauch et al., 1990; Friedland et al., 1992; Jacobs, 1992; Tan et al., 1993). The majority of so-called resistant strains are intermediately resistant (MICs of 0.1 to 1 µg/ml), but some are highly resistant (>1 µg/ml); some of these latter strains are also resistant to third-generation cephalosporins. Whether this resistance will make present penicillin prophylaxis ineffective is not known at this time. When sepsis is a possibility, immediate therapy with a third-generation cephalosporin has been recommended in the past. At present, because of the possibility of highly resistant organisms, we would recommend the use of vancomycin intravenously (40 mg/kg/day every 6 hours) as well as the third-generation cephalosporin (cefotaxime, 200 mg/kg/day every 6 hours).

Asplenic children 2 years of age and older should receive polyvalent pneumococcal polysaccharide vaccine and quadrivalent meningococcal polysaccharide vaccine. These children should also receive their regularly scheduled *H. influenzae* type b immunization series.

Sickle Cell Disease and Other Hemoglobinopathies

An increased incidence of pneumonia, osteomyelitis, meningitis, and genitourinary infections due to *S. pneumoniae, H. influenzae, Salmonella* sp., *Edwardsiella tarda*, and *Mycoplasma* sp. has been described in children with hemoglobinopathies (Rubin et al., 1968; Barrett-Connor, 1971; Shulman et al., 1972; Sachs et al., 1974; Wong et al., 1992). Aspects of pathophysiology are discussed in Chapter 19.

All children at appropriate ages should be given pneumococcal, meningococcal, and *H. influenzae* type b vaccines. Therapy of bacterial infections in children with sickle cell disease requires an aggressive approach.

Prior to therapy, cultures of blood, stool, and throat as well as bone and joint lesions, if present, should be obtained. In the toxic child, initial therapy with cefotaxime and vancomycin is indicated. In the older child with pneumonia, therapy with erythromycin or tetracycline for *M. pneumoniae* should also be started.

B-Cell Immunodeficiencies

The prototype B-cell deficit is X-linked agammaglobulinemia (Bruton, 1952); other B-cell immunodeficiencies are itemized in Table 9–2 and are discussed in Chapter 11. Opportunistic infections occur because the lack of secretory antibody allows infection of mucosal surfaces, and this infection can spread systemically because of the absence of serum cytotoxic or neutralizing antibody or an antibody that participates in antibody-dependent cellular cytotoxicity (Stiehm et al., 1986). The lack of antibody-antigen interaction may lead to impaired complement activation, decreased chemotaxis, and a deficiency of opsonization and phagocytosis of microorganisms.

The following clinical illness categories are manifestations of B-cell immunodeficiencies: recurrent pneumonia and otitis media, pharyngitis-tonsillitis, sinusitis, bronchiectasis, conjunctivitis, rhinitis, meningitis, septicemia, persistent infectious diarrhea and viral encephalitis, viral hepatitis, cholangitis, paralytic poliomyelitis, mycoplasma arthritis, and chronic cystitis and urethritis (Hausser et al., 1983; Stiehm et al., 1986). Classically, recurrent infections are due to encapsulated bacteria such as *S. pneumoniae, S. aureus, H. influenzae, N. meningitidis,* and *P. aeruginosa* (Gitlin et al., 1959). More recently, severe, recurrent, or chronic infections have been noted with other bacteria, viruses, protozoa, and mycoplasmas (Wilfert et al., 1977; Saulsbury et al., 1980; Sloper et al., 1982; Ponka et al., 1983; Erlendsson et al., 1985; Stiehm et al., 1986). In Table 31–4, a list of opportunistic infectious agents in B-cell deficiency states is presented. Particularly troublesome have been

Table 31–4. Infection in the Host Compromised by B-Cell and T-Cell Immunodeficiency Syndromes

Immunodeficiency Syndrome	Opportunistic Organisms Isolated Most Frequently	Approach to Treatment of Infections	Prevention of Infections
B-cell immunodeficiences	Encapsulated bacteria (*Streptococcus pneumoniae, Staphylococcus aureus, Haemophilus influenzae,* and *Neisseria meningitidis*), *Pseudomonas aeruginosa, Campylobacter* sp., enteroviruses, rotaviruses, *Giardia lamblia, Cryptosporidium* sp., *Pneumocystis carinii, Ureaplasma urealyticum,* and *Mycoplasma pneumoniae*	1. Intravenous immune globulin (IVIG), 200 to 800 mg/kg. 2. Vigorous attempt to obtain specimens for culture prior to antimicrobial therapy. 3. Incision and drainage if abscess present. 4. Antibiotic selection based on sensitivity reports.	1. Maintenance IVIG for patients with quantitative and qualitative defects in immunoglobulin (IgG) metabolism (200 to 800 mg/kg every 3–5 weeks). 2. In chronic recurrent respiratory disease, vigorous attention to postural drainage. 3. In selected cases (recurrent or chronic pulmonary or middle ear), prophylactic administration of ampicillin, penicillin, or trimethoprim/sulfamethoxazole.
T-cell immunodeficiencies	Encapsulated bacteria (*S. pneumoniae, H. influenzae, S. aureus*), facultative intracellular bacteria (*M. tuberculosis,* other *Mycobacterium* sp., *Listeria monocytogenes*), *Escherichia coli, Pseudomonas aeruginosa, Enterobacter* sp., *Klebsiella* sp., *Serratia marcescens, Salmonella* sp., *Nocardia* sp., viruses (cytomegalovirus, herpes simplex virus, varicella-zoster virus, Epstein-Barr virus, rotaviruses, adenoviruses, enteroviruses, respiratory syncytial virus, measles virus, vaccinia virus, parainfluenzae viruses), protozoa (*P. carinii, Toxoplasma gondii, Cryptosporidium* sp.), and fungi (*Candida* sp., *Cryptococcus neoformans, Histoplasma capsulatum*)	1. Vigorous attempt to obtain specimens for culture prior to antimicrobial therapy. 2. Incision and drainage if abscess present. 3. Antibiotic selection based on sensitivity reports. 4. Early antiviral treatment for herpes simplex and varicella-zoster viral infections. 5. Topical and nonadsorbable antimicrobial agents frequently useful.	1. Prophylactic administration of trimethoprim-sulfamethoxazole for prevention of *P. carinii* pneumonia. 2. Oral nonadsorbable antimicrobial agents to lower concentration of gut flora. 3. No live virus vaccines, or bacille Calmette-Guérin vaccine. 4. Careful tuberculosis screening.

enteroviral syndromes such as chronic encephalitis, dermatomyositis, and vaccine-induced paralytic poliomyelitis. In Table 31–4, a general approach to the treatment and prevention of infections in B-cell immunodeficiencies is presented. The availability of intravenous immunoglobulin (IVIG) has had a major impact on the treatment and prevention of infections in children with B-cell deficiencies (Liese et al., 1992).

T-Cell Immunodeficiencies

There are many T-cell immunodeficiencies; these are itemized in Table 9–2 and are described in Chapter 12. The prototype T-cell deficiency is thymic aplasia (DiGeorge's syndrome), in which there is failure of development of the third and fourth pharyngeal pouches (DiGeorge, 1968); although patients with this syndrome have a marked T-cell defect, immunoglobulins are not depressed. In contrast, children with the severe combined immunodeficiency syndrome (SCID) have marked defects of both B-cell and T-cell systems (Buckley, 1983; Rosen et al., 1984).

Severe infections in children with T-cell immunodeficiencies can be caused by organisms that cause common illnesses in normal children. In addition, children with T-cell defects may suffer severe disease from opportunistic infections with organisms that rarely cause disease in normal hosts. Infectious agents that frequently cause disease in children with T-cell immunodeficiencies are presented in Table 31–4.

There are several unique infections in T-cell deficiency states (Stiehm et al., 1986; Hughes, 1993). Chronic diarrhea is caused by Cryptosporidium sp., Giardia lamblia, and rotaviruses, and chronic pulmonary infection is caused by respiratory syncytial virus, parainfluenza viruses, cytomegalovirus, and adenoviruses. Persistent C. albicans infections involving the mucous membranes, scalp, skin, and nails occur in chronic mucocutaneous candidiasis. Males with X-linked lymphoproliferative syndrome have a specific immune defect to Epstein-Barr virus. When a person is infected with this virus, a severe or fatal infection occurs because of a killer cell response directed against both infected and noninfected cells (Sullivan et al., 1983). Children with cartilage-hair hypoplasia, a rare autosomal recessive disorder with short-limbed dwarfism, are particularly susceptible to severe varicella-zoster and vaccinia infections (Hong et al., 1972). In children with combined immunodeficiency, death has followed immunization with live viral vaccines or with BCG (Rosen and Janeway, 1964; Hitzig et al., 1968).

An approach to treatment and prevention of infections in patients with T-cell immunodeficiencies is presented in Table 31–4.

Selective IgA Deficiency

Selective IgA deficiency (see Chapter 14) occurs in about one in 700 persons. Many afflicted persons are healthy; others have recurrent respiratory or gastrointestinal infections, or both (Burgio et al., 1980; Shyur and Hill, 1991). Infections in children with selective IgA deficiency should be treated vigorously with specific antimicrobial agents indicated by appropriate cultures. Immune serum globulin treatment is contraindicated in selective IgA deficiency because the product contains insufficient amounts of IgA for adequate replacement but sufficient amounts to sensitize the patient so that anti-IgA antibodies develop.

Complement Immunodeficiencies

Complement immunodeficiencies are listed in Table 9–2 and described in detail in Chapter 17. The following complement deficiencies—C2, C3, C5, C6, C7, and C8—have been associated with disseminated infections with encapsulated and other bacterial organisms (Hyatt et al., 1981; Goldstein and Marder, 1983; Stiehm et al., 1986; Shyur and Hill et al., 1991). Specific organisms include S. pneumoniae, S. pyogenes, H. influenzae, N. meningitidis, N. gonorrhoeae, S. aureus, Salmonella typhi, E. coli, other gram-negative enteric bacteria, Proteus sp., Pseudomonas sp., and Klebsiella sp. Illnesses have included septicemia, meningitis, pneumonia, sinusitis, and arthritis. Patients with known infection-associated complement defects should be treated vigorously with an appropriate antibiotic such as cefotaxime at the onset of febrile illnesses. Appropriate cultures prior to therapy will dictate further therapy. In life-threatening instances, the administration of complement-containing plasma may be beneficial. Children of appropriate age will benefit from pneumococcal, H. influenzae type b, and meningococcal vaccines.

Cystic Fibrosis

Children with cystic fibrosis experience premature death owing to pulmonary insufficiency, which results from chronic pulmonary infection (see Chapter 22). In these children, infections due to S. aureus, P. aeruginosa, coliform bacteria, and Haemophilus sp. are common. The management of infection in children with cystic fibrosis is a major and continuous challenge. In the antibiotic era, the longevity of children with cystic fibrosis has increased substantially. However, the exact role of antibiotics in this increased survival period is not clear. Several different methods of antibiotic administration are employed at different cystic fibrosis centers, and there are few differences in outcome among these centers. At some centers, continuous prophylaxis with oral or aerosolized antibiotics is used. At other centers, antibiotics are employed only at times of exacerbation of pulmonary symptoms.

There is little evidence to support the concept that continuous aerosolized and oral antibiotic prophylaxis diminishes the presence of pulmonary infection more than could be achieved by meticulous attention to pulmonary toilet without continuous antibiotic administration. Continuous administration of antibiotics (orally or by the aerosol route) may predispose the patient to colonization and infection with saprophytic strains of bacteria, which are resistant to multiple antibiotics.

In our opinion, it is best to use antibiotics in children with cystic fibrosis at times when respiratory-related changes occur (e.g., fever, increased sputum, increased breathing difficulty). Therapy should be guided by sputum cultures, but in many instances of minor respiratory worsening, patients often will improve somewhat on antibiotics that would not be expected to be effective on the basis of sensitivity data. Oral cephalosporins, penicillinase-resistant penicillins, sulfonamides, ampicillin, chloramphenicol, and tetracycline all enjoy frequent use. In children with greater clinical deterioration, parenteral antibiotics are indicated. If culture reveals a predominant growth of coagulase-positive staphylococci, a penicillin such as oxacillin is indicated. In the usual situation in which *P. aeruginosa* is the major organism in the sputum, therapy should include an aminoglycoside antibiotic to which the pathogen is sensitive. At the present time, gentamicin with mezlocillin or piperacillin is a satisfactory regimen. Sensitivities always should be performed so that when resistance to gentamicin is noted, another aminoglycoside (e.g., tobramycin, amikacin) can be employed.

Diabetes Mellitus

Children and adults with diabetes mellitus have a decreased resistance to bacterial and fungal infections. Pyelonephritis and perinephric abscesses due to *S. aureus* and *S. epidermidis*, *E. coli*, *Proteus*, *Clostridium* sp., and *Actinomyces* sp. have been reported frequently (McCabe, 1972; Vejlsgaard, 1973). The increased incidence of bacteremia and pyelonephritis in diabetic patients may be attributable, in part, to a greater frequency of hospitalization and catheterization (see Chapter 19).

Infection by *Mucor*, *T. glabrata*, and *Candida* sp. has been noted with greater frequency in children with diabetes mellitus than in the normal host. It is of interest that *Mucor* (Baker and Severance, 1948; Martin et al., 1954; Marks et al., 1970) was not reported in the United States until 1943, shortly after the introduction of antibiotic therapy, although diabetes mellitus and other diseases associated with an increased risk of *Mucor* infection have been present for centuries (Gregory et al., 1943). This suggests that the increased frequency of fungal disease is related to the repeated use of antibiotics. The management of infection in diabetic children depends on careful attention to even trivial infections. Cultures should be done and appropriate antibiotic therapy instituted.

INFECTION IN CHILDREN COMPROMISED BY ACQUIRED DISORDERS OF IMMUNITY

Malignancy

In children with cancer, infection is a major problem and also may be a terminal event (Kosmidis, 1980; Miser and Miser, 1980; Nachman and Honig, 1980; Siegel et al., 1980; Jackson et al., 1982; Wong and Ogra, 1983; Brown, 1984; Hughes, 1984; Friedman et al., 1984; Saarinen, 1984; Lewis et al., 1985; Steele, 1985; Pizzo et al., 1991a, 1991b; Katz and Mustafa,

1993; Koll and Brown, 1993). In general, children with solid tumors have less frequent and severe infections than do children with lymphoproliferative diseases (Levine et al., 1974; Hughes, 1974; Nachman and Honig, 1980). Hughes (1974), in a study of 482 children with malignancies, noted that infection was most common in children with leukemia and least common in those with Wilms' tumor. Disseminated infections were more likely in lymphoproliferative diseases, whereas localized infections were more frequent with solid tumors. In an analysis of fever and neutropenia in children with neoplastic disease, Nachman and Honig (1980) noted an infection rate of 36.7% in children with leukemia, whereas the rate was only 15% in children with solid tumors. Septicemia occurred in 58.3% of the leukemic children and in 35.7% of those children with solid tumors. In contrast, 42.8% of infections in children with solid tumors were pulmonary, whereas lung infections accounted for only 25% of the infections in children with leukemia.

Therapeutic maneuvers that are associated with a minimal risk of infection in the normal host become significant hazards to children with cancer. Intravenous fluids, scalp vein needles, indwelling intravenous and urinary catheters, transfusions, and use of respirators all have been associated with opportunistic infection in children with cancer. Bronchial or urinary tract obstruction by tumor growth also may predispose to infection. Chemotherapy may be complicated by gangrenous stomatitis and necrotizing enteropathy, which may be associated with septicemia due to gram-negative organisms. Rectal fissures and perirectal abscesses may serve as sources of infection in children with cancer, and fatal infections have developed in patients with Hodgkin's disease after splenectomy performed for staging of the disease.

The single most important factor that predisposes patients with cancer to infection is granulocytopenia (Bodey et al., 1966; Hughes, 1971; Katz and Mustafa, 1993). In an extensive study, Bodey (1984) noted that the incidence of infectious episodes in persons with leukemia increased with decreasing blood granulocyte levels. An absolute neutrophil count of 500/mm^3 is a critical value. Below this value, the risk of infection is high. In addition, the duration of granulocytopenia is directly related to risk of developing infection.

Granulocytopenia in patients with cancer may be related to their primary disease or may be the result of therapy provided. In some cases, neutrophil function may be impaired in children with leukemia both in relapse and in remission, even though the number of circulating leukocytes is normal (Strauss et al., 1970; Skeel et al., 1971). Decreased chemotaxis and digestive capacity of neutrophils have been reported in patients with Hodgkin's disease and myelocytic leukemia (Rosner et al., 1970; Holland et al., 1971).

Lymphopenia or a deficiency in T-lymphocyte function or both may contribute to the development of viral or fungal disease in cancer patients (Bodey et al., 1966; Levy and Kaplan, 1974). Patients with lymphoma are particularly susceptible to infection produced by facultative intracellular organisms, and in these individuals macrophage function may be altered (Sinkovics and Smith, 1970).

No reduction in the concentration of serum immunoglobulins or complement components has been noted in most patients with leukemia or lymphoma other than that induced by chemotherapy (Ragab et al., 1970; Gooch and Fernbach, 1971). The concentration of specific antibodies, however, may be altered. In children with acute leukemia who were receiving combination chemotherapy, heat-stable opsonins specific for *P. aeruginosa* fell precipitously, whereas those specific for *S. epidermidis* remained unchanged (Wollman et al., 1975).

Because of the extensive immunologic defects in children with malignancies, the spectrum of agents associated with opportunistic infections is great and involves both gram-positive and gram-negative bacteria, fungi, viruses, and protozoa. The incidence of infections caused by specific microbial agents varies among geographic areas and hospital centers and during different time periods in the same location. A listing of the more usual causative agents in serious infections as well as an approach to infection prevention and treatment is presented in Table 31–5. In an analysis of fatal infections in children with leukemia, Hughes (1971) noted that gram-negative bacillary organisms were the etiologic agents in over one half of the study group. *P. aeruginosa* was the most common etiologic agent noted. Surprisingly, one fifth of the infections were due to *C. albicans*, and only 17 of the 199 infections were due to *S. aureus*. There were 11 terminal viral infections, and eight fatalities were due to protozoa.

In contrast with the findings of Hughes (1971), Saarinen (1984) in Helsinki surveyed infections in 100 children with acute lymphoblastic leukemia and noted a total absence of disseminated candidiasis, a relative infrequency of gram-negative septicemia, and a predominance of septicemias due to gram-positive organisms. In 165 septic episodes in pediatric patients with leukemia and lymphoma at Memorial Sloan-Kettering Cancer Center, the most common etiologic agents were the following: *S. viridans*, 16.3%; *E. coli*, 15.2%; *Serratia* sp., 12.1%; *S. epidermidis*, 11.5%; *P. aeruginosa*, 9.1%; fungi, 7.3%; *Klebsiella* sp., 5.5%; and *S. aureus*, 4.9% (Brown, 1984).

Recent changes in the patterns of infections in patients with malignancies are (1) an increase in infections caused by gram-positive cocci (coagulase-negative staphylococci, *Streptococcus* sp., and *Enterococcus* sp.), (2) a decrease in infections caused by *E. coli* and an increase in infections by other Enterobacteriaceae (e.g., *Klebsiella* sp., *Enterobacter* sp., *Serratia* sp.) and non–enterobacteriaceae-fermentatitive and nonfermentative bacilli, and (3) emergence of multiple-resistant infectious organisms (Koll and Brown, 1993).

In leukemia, the cause of fever and presumed infection is associated with the stage of disease (Kosmidis et al., 1980). At the time of diagnosis of leukemia, the cause of fever is found in only about one third of cases. Of the infections documented, about one third are bacterial and two thirds are viral. During induction therapy, fever is usually due to bacterial infection. During remission, most fevers are due to viral infections; during relapse, febrile episodes are most commonly due to viruses, bacteria, and fungi. Documented bacterial and fungal septic episodes virtually always are associated with severe neutropenia. Pneumonia due to *P. carinii* usually does not occur early in the course of childhood malignant disease but is noted during remission and relapse (Siegel et al., 1980).

Immunosuppression

Immunosuppressive therapy is employed in a large number of human diseases, such as rheumatoid arthritis and other connective tissue diseases, inflammatory bowel disease, chronic active hepatitis, several hematologic diseases, nephrotic syndrome and nephritis, many allergic conditions, and a large number of other poorly understood illnesses (Skinner and Schwartz, 1972). Immunosuppressive therapy is also employed in organ transplantation, and drugs that cause immunosuppression are an integral part of cancer chemotherapy. Opportunistic infection in malignancies has been presented earlier, and infection problems related to organ transplantation are covered in a subsequent section.

Infections are responsible for significant morbidity and mortality in children receiving immunosuppressive therapy. The incidence of infections and their etiology and severity are dependent on both the basic underlying disease process and the immunosuppressive agents employed (see Chapters 19 and 27).

Experimental evidence suggests that predisposition to infection in patients who have been immunosuppressed with steroids is a reflection of a multifaceted derangement of the normal mechanisms of host resistance. This may include depression of leukocyte chemotaxis and local inflammatory responses, interference with the acquisition or expression of cell-mediated functions, impairment of phagocytosis and killing of bacteria, and depression of interferon synthesis (Ward, 1966; Claman, 1972; Dale and Petersdorf, 1973; Zurier and Weissman, 1973). Nitrogen mustard, cyclophosphamide, busulfan, and chlorambucil (biologic alkylating agents); cytosine arabinoside, 5-fluorouracil, azathioprine, 6-mercaptopurine, and 6-thioguanine (antimetabolites); methotrexate (folic acid antagonist); and cyclosporine all interfere with replication of cells. These drugs may suppress primary and secondary antibody responses and delayed hypersensitivity in some individuals (Schwartz, 1965; Steinberg et al., 1972).

Although it is clear that immunosuppressive therapy increases the general risk of opportunistic infection, it is difficult to quantitate this risk and to separate it from the risk associated with the disease for which immunosuppression was undertaken. For example, a short course of corticosteroid therapy in asthma is of little increased risk to the patient. On the other hand, the risk is considerably greater in the child receiving long-term therapy for an illness such as systemic lupus erythematosus. The spectrum of possible opportunistic infection associated with immunosuppression includes all the microorganisms listed in Table 31–5. The possibilities in any specific patient depend on his or her

Table 31–5. Infection in the Host Compromised by Malignancy, Immunosuppression, or Transplantation

Category	Opportunistic Organisms Isolated Most Frequently	Approach to Treatment of Infections	Prevention of Infections
Malignancy	Bacteria—*Pseudomonas aeruginosa* and other sp., *Escherichia coli*, *Enterobacter* sp., *Klebsiella* sp., *Acinetobacter* sp., *Proteus* sp., *Serratia* sp., other gram-negative bacilli, *Bacteroides* sp., and other anaerobes, *Staphylococcus aureus, S. epidermidis*, *Streptococcus* sp., enterococci, diphtheroids, *Listeria* sp., *Haemophilus influenzae*, *Salmonella* sp., *Mycobacterium tuberculosis* and other *Mycobacterium* sp. Fungi—*Candida albicans* and other *Candida* sp., *Aspergillus* sp., *Cryptococcus neoformans*, *Histoplasma capsulatum*, *Fusarium* sp., *Trichosporon beigelii, Torulopsis glabrata*, *Curvularia* sp., *Mucor* sp. Viruses—varicella-zoster virus, cytomegalovirus, herpes simplex, hepatitis B and C, Epstein-Barr, adenoviruses, measles, papovavirus Parasites—*Pneumocystis carinii*, *Toxoplasma gondii*, *Cryptosporidium* sp., *Strongyloides stercoralis*	1. Obtain appropriate Gram-stained smears and specimens for culture (blood, urine, CSF, intravenous sites, and wounds), even of minor lesions prior to onset of therapy. 2. When possible, choose antibiotic combinations for specific etiologic agents (employ bactericidal rather than bacteriostatic antibiotics). 3. With occurrence of fever (three oral temperature readings of 38°C in a 24-hour period or a single temperature of ≥38.5°C), initiate empiric antimicrobial therapy. Several regimens have been successful; a cost-effective approach is monotherapy with ceftazidime. 4. Once therapy has been started, allow ample time for effect; therapy should rarely be less than 7 days. In neutropenic patients, continue therapy until the absolute neutrophil count is >500 cells/mm³. 5. Institute empiric therapy with antifungal agents in patients who are neutropenic with fever that is unresponsive to antibiotics.	1. Prophylactic administration of trimethoprim-sulfamethoxazole to prevent *Pneumocystis carinii* pneumonia. 2. Avoidance of unnecessary hospitalization. 3. Avoidance of antibiotics and catheters unless specifically indicated. 4. Routine surveillance culture specimens (throat, stool, and axilla) at regular intervals may be useful. 5. Use of VZIG, ISG, or IVIG (measles), and HBIG, if exposed. 6. Use of pneumococcal, *H. influenzae* type b, and influenza vaccines. 7. Use of acyclovir (250 mg/M² every 8 hours) in herpes simplex–seropositive patients during intensive therapy for acute leukemia. 8. Administration of varicella vaccine in children with acute lymphocytic leukemia in remission who have not had varicella.
Immunosuppression	Same as Malignancy, above.	Same as Malignancy, above.	1. Avoidance of unnecessary hospitalization. 2. Avoidance of antibiotics and catheters unless specifically indicated. 3. Use of VZIG, ISG or IVIG (measles), and HBIG if exposed.
Transplantation	Same as Malignancy, above, plus: Bacteria—*Listeria monocytogenes*, Viruses—parainfluenzae, respiratory syncytial, parvovirus B19 Fungi—*Coccidioides immitis*, *Blastomyces dermatitidis*	Same as Malignancy, above, plus: Use of ganciclovir and IVIG to treat cytomegalovirus infections.	Same as Malignancy, above, plus: 1. Reduction of total bowel flora of microorganisms with nonadsorbable antibiotics. 2. Removal of dietary items that may contain significant microbial contamination. 3. When blood products are necessary, use (if possible) of cytomegalovirus-seronegative products in patients who are cytomegalovirus-seronegative. 4. Consideration of prophylactic ganciclovir in cytomegalovirus-seropositive transplant recipients or when the donor was seropositive and the recipient was seronegative.

Abbreviations: IV = intravenous; CSF = cerebrospinal fluid; VZIG = varicella-zoster immune globulin; ISG = human immune serum globulin; IVIG = human intravenous immune serum globulin; HBIG = hepatitis B immune globulin.

endogenous and exogenous surroundings at the time of suppressive therapy. The nonhospitalized child is particularly at extra risk to common viral and bacterial contagious diseases as well as factors associated with the home environment (i.e., bacteria and viruses from household pets, fungi in the soil). In contrast, the frequently hospitalized child has a much greater risk of systemic infection with nosocomial, highly resistant bacteria. It should be remembered that all live viral vaccines are contraindicated in immunosuppressed children. An approach to prevention and treatment of infections is presented in Table 31–5.

Transplantation

Organ and tissue transplantation in children is presented in detail in Chapter 32. Opportunistic infections are common in transplant recipients and are a threat to both the patient's life and the survival of the transplanted tissue. Immunosuppressive therapy is an integral part of the process of transplantation; predictably, infections following transplantation are similar to those associated with immunosuppression. In addition, the transplantation process *per se* and the rejection process predispose the host to infection, particularly with viruses. Infection risks and the microorganisms involved are also related to the organ or tissue being transplanted (renal, liver, heart, or bone marrow). A general listing of causes of infection and an approach to prevention and treatment are presented in Table 31–5.

Kidney Transplantation

Renal transplantation in children presently is very successful, with 1-year survival rates of 97% for living-related kidney transplants and 93% for cadaver kidney transplants (So and Simmons, 1992). However, infections are common and are a major cause of morbidity and mortality (Najarian et al., 1986; Potter et al., 1986; Brayman et al., 1992; Harmon, 1991).

Early infections after transplantation are most often bacterial and involve the urinary tract, the graft and wound site, vascular catheters, and the lungs (So and Simmons, 1992; Deen and Blumberg, 1993). Urinary tract infections are most common and are due to *E. coli* and other gram-negative bacilli, enterococci, and coagulase-negative staphylococci.

Late-onset infections involve a multitude of opportunistic agents. Predisposing factors include immunosuppression, graft rejection, and antibiotics. Etiologic agents of most importance are cytomegalovirus, Epstein-Barr virus, herpes simplex virus, varicella virus, *Candida* sp., *Aspergillus* sp., *Mycobacterium* sp., *Toxoplasma gondii*, and *P. carinii*. Deaths are often due to polymicrobial infections involving cytomegalovirus and bacterial, fungal, or parasitic agents.

Cytomegalovirus infection can be a primary infection when a seronegative recipient receives a kidney from a seropositive donor, or it can be reinfection in seropositive recipients. Several approaches have been used to prevent cytomegalovirus infections. These include IVIG, cytomegalovirus immune globulin (CMVIG), high-dose oral acyclovir, and ganciclovir (Pakkala et al., 1992; So and Simmons, 1992; Conti et al., 1993; Prokurat et al., 1993; Snydman, 1993; Werner et al., 1993). Results among studies have varied. No regimen prevented primary infection, but the use of either of the antivirals or immune globulins reduced the severity and frequency of clinical manifestations of infection.

Liver Transplantation

Today, liver transplantation offers hope to children with acute fulminant hepatic failure and end-stage chronic liver disease (Kuhls and Leach, 1992). Of children receiving transplants, 70% to 90% survive for 1 year, and long-term survivals are common. However, serious infections following transplantation occur in 40% to 70% of pediatric patients, and infection is the leading cause of death (Andrews et al., 1987; Hiatt et al., 1987; Vacanti et al., 1987; Zitelli et al., 1987).

Children with liver transplants have similar risks of infection as other solid organ transplant recipients. In addition, they have an added risk from the gastrointestinal flora, which is in direct contact with the biliary drainage system and the frequent occurrence of postoperative biliary stasis or vascular insufficiency, or both, resulting in ischemia in a segment of the liver.

Common locations of infection in children with liver transplants are the wound, the central venous catheter, the liver, the extrahepatic intra-abdominal region, the urinary tract, and the lung. The major causes of liver and extrahepatic intra-abdominal infections are bacteria and include gram-negative enteric bacilli, *P. aeruginosa*, streptococci, enterococci, and enteric anaerobes. Although anaerobes are the most prevalent organisms in the flora of the large bowel, they are a relatively infrequent cause of post-transplantation infection. Infections caused by *Candida* sp. and *T. glabrata* also are common. Cytomegalovirus and adenoviruses also may cause hepatitis.

Infections relating to immunosuppression are similar to those in other transplant recipients and include viruses (cytomegalovirus, varicella-zoster, Epstein-Barr, herpes simplex, adenoviruses, parvovirus B19, respiratory viruses, hepatitis viruses), protozoa (*P. carinii*, *T. gondii*, and *Cryptosporidium parvum*), and endogenous fungi and bacteria (*Histoplasma capsulatum*, *Mycobacterium tuberculosis*, and other *Mycobacterium* sp.) (Kuhls and Leach, 1992; Nour et al., 1993).

The rate of infections after liver transplantation can be reduced by using perioperative antibiotics intravenously, nonabsorbable antibiotics orally, and perhaps high-dose acyclovir (Bailey et al., 1993; Mollison et al., 1993; Saliba et al., 1993; Smith et al., 1993).

Heart Transplantation

Compared with renal, liver, and bone marrow transplantation, the experience in children with heart transplantation is relatively limited (Fricker et al., 1987; Green et al., 1989; Kaplan, 1992). Children with heart transplants have similar risks of infections resulting from immunosuppression as do liver transplant recipients. The most important early postoperative infections are similar to those that are associated with other major thoracic surgeries, including pneumonia, mediastinitis, lung abscess, and wound infections. Common causative organisms include *Pseudomonas* sp. and other gram-negative bacilli, *Staphylococcus* sp., streptococci, and other organisms of the upper respiratory tract flora.

Respiratory viruses (respiratory syncytial virus, influenza viruses, and adenoviruses) are also an important cause of morbidity and mortality during the early postoperative period. Late infections in heart transplant patients are similar to those that occur in liver transplant recipients.

Bone Marrow Transplantation

Infection and graft-versus-host disease and the interaction between these two factors are the major source of morbidity and mortality in bone marrow transplant recipients (Wasserman et al., 1988; Zaia, 1992; Hiemenz and Greene, 1993; Sable and Donowitz, 1994). The major difference between bone marrow transplantation and solid organ transplantations is the occurrence of neutropenia in all bone marrow transplant recipients. There is an extensive literature relating to the prevention and treatment of infections in bone marrow transplantation; however, there are few studies that deal exclusively with children. This is an important omission because, in general, children tolerate many antimicrobial agents, such as aminoglycosides and amphotericin B, better than do adults and also accept certain unpleasant regimens, such as the oral use of nonabsorbable antibiotics, with better compliance.

Infection risks in bone marrow transplantation can be separated into four time periods:

1. Pretransplantation.
2. Pre-engraftment.
3. Early post-engraftment.
4. Late post-engraftment.

The occurrence of infection during the *pretransplantation* period depends on the underlying condition and its stage of treatment. Neutropenia is the main defect. The most common infections are bacteremias and septicemias due to aerobic gram-negative bacilli and local infections (skin, soft tissue, intraoral, and urinary) due to cutaneous local flora.

The *pre-engraftment* period begins with the onset of neutropenia, lasts 4 to 6 weeks, and is always associated with mucositis. Bacterial infections predominate during this period. In the past, the most common systemic infections were due to gram-negative bacilli, either from the patient's enteric flora or from the hospital environment. Infection with these organisms is still common, but in recent years, there has been an increase in aerobic gram-positive coccal infections due to *S. aureus, S. epidermidis,* streptococci, and enterococci. Opportunistic fungal infections also occur, with those due to *Candida* sp. being most common. Severe hemorrhagic mucositis due to reactivation of latent herpes simplex virus is also common.

The *early post-engraftment* period, which lasts for about 1 to 3 months after transplantation, is indicated by absolute neutrophil count values increasing to higher than 500 cells/mm³. With the recovery from neutropenia, the risk of gram-negative and gram-positive bacterial sepsis is reduced. During this period, there is severe combined immunodeficiency, and this problem may be complicated by graft-versus-host disease and its treatment. A major problem in this period is reactivation of latent cytomegalovirus or primary infection in a previously cytomegalovirus-seronegative pa-

tient. Manifestations of cytomegalovirus infection include asymptomatic virus shedding, fever, hepatitis, leukopenia, thrombocytopenia, gastrointestinal disease, and pneumonia.

Other infectious risks during this period are due to adenoviruses, Epstein-Barr virus, influenza viruses, parainfluenza viruses, respiratory syncytial virus, papovaviruses (JC and BK), *Candida* sp., *Aspergillus* sp., and other environment fungi, *Pneumocystis carinii,* and *Toxoplasma gondii.*

The *late post-engraftment* period is complicated by chronic graft-versus-host disease and its treatment. A major problem in this period is reactivation of latent varicella-zoster virus and frequent dissemination of disease. Another risk factor that must be considered during this period is infection due to encapsulated organisms such as *S. pneumoniae, H. influenzae,* and *N. meningitidis.*

The approach to prevention and treatment of infections in bone marrow transplant recipients is outlined in Table 31–5. Hemorrhagic mucositis can be prevented by the prophylactic use of acyclovir, and *P. carinii* pneumonia can be prevented by the prophylactic use of trimethoprim-sulfamethoxazole. The use of clotrimazole troches or nystatin has reduced the frequency and severity of oropharyngeal candidiasis, and the use of oral nonabsorbable antimicrobials has reduced the occurrence of sepsis due to gram-negative bacilli.

Empiric treatment of febrile episodes with broad-spectrum antibiotics and persistent fevers with amphotericin B have decreased the rates of morbidity and mortality during the period of neutropenia.

Acquired Immunodeficiency Syndrome

The acquired immunodeficiency syndrome (AIDS) is an illness caused by persistent infection with the human immunodeficiency virus (HIV). By definition, AIDS occurs when an HIV-infected person has an opportunistic infection or evidence of severe immunosuppression (<200 CD4⁺ T-lymphocytes/μl or a CD4⁺ T-lymphocyte percentage of total lymphocytes of less than 14) (CDC, 1987, 1992). In Chapter 18, the historical, epidemiologic, and immunologic aspects of HIV infections in children are presented. In this chapter, specific infections and their diagnosis and treatment in HIV-infected children are discussed.

Patients with AIDS have a broad-based immunodeficiency that involves the following cells: T cells, macrophages, monocytes, B cells, and natural killer cells (Flynn and Shenep, 1992; Hanson and Shearer, 1992). Combined effects include depletion of CD4 lymphocytes, diminished or absence of delayed-type hypersensitivity, decreased production of interleukin-2 and interferon-γ, depletion of T cells, impaired chemotaxis and phagocytosis, decreased specific antibody response to specific antigen challenge, hypergammaglobulinemia, and impaired cytotoxicity (see Chapters 11, 15, 16, and 18).

The classification system for HIV infection in children under 13 years of age is presented in Table 31–6. Criteria for Class P-2 symptomatic infection subclasses are

Table 31–6. Summary of the Initial Classification System of HIV Infection in Children Under 13 Years of Age*

Class P-0: Indeterminate Infection

Class P-1: Asymptomatic Infection
  Subclass A. Normal immune function
  Subclass B. Abnormal immune function
  Subclass C. Immune function not tested

Class P-2: Symptomatic Infection
  Subclass A. Nonspecific findings
  Subclass B. Progressive neurologic disease
  Subclass C. Lymphoid interstitial pneumonitis
  Subclass D. Secondary infectious diseases
    Category D-1. Specified secondary infectious diseases listed in the CDC surveillance definition for AIDS
    Category D-2. Recurrent serious bacterial infections
    Category D-3. Other specified secondary infectious diseases
  Subclass E. Secondary cancers
    Category E-1. Specified secondary cancers listed in the CDC surveillance definition for AIDS
    Category E-2. Other cancers possibly secondary to HIV infection
  Subclass F. Other diseases possibly due to HIV infection

*For new classification, see Chapter 18.
  From Centers for Disease Control. 1987 classification system for HIV infection in children under 13 years of age. MMWR 36:225–236, 1987.
  Abbreviations: AIDS = acquired immunodeficiency syndrome; CDC = Centers for Disease Control; HIV = human immunodeficiency virus.

presented in Table 31–7, and conditions included in the 1993 AIDS surveillance case definition for adolescents and adults are presented in Table 31–8.

Today almost all new HIV infections in young children are a result of the congenital or perinatal transmission of the virus from an infected mother.

Clinical manifestations of illness in children infected with HIV can be due to the primary HIV infection, the exaggerated and persistent effects of a congenital infection (e.g., cytomegalovirus, *Toxoplasma gondii*), the exaggerated and often persistent effects of a regular human pathogen (e.g., respiratory syncytial virus), exaggerated anatomically localized infections (e.g., otitis media), and true opportunistic infections with organisms that do not cause disease in normal hosts (Oleske et al., 1983; Scott et al., 1984; Shannon and Ammann, 1985; Krasinski, 1988; Rubinstein, 1983; Vernon et al., 1988; Falloon et al., 1989; Chandwani et al., 1990; Frenkel et al., 1990; Leibowitz et al., 1990, 1991, 1993; Mitchell et al., 1990; Leggiadro et al., 1991; Principi et al., 1991; Scott, 1991; Barnett et al., 1992; Flynn and Shenep, 1992; Hanson and Shearer, 1992; Hoyt et al., 1992; Lewis et al., 1992; Vandersteenhoven, 1992; Hanson, 1993; Rutstein et al., 1993).

Eighty percent of HIV-infected newborns have clinical manifestations of disease during the first 24 months of life (Scott, 1991). Initial manifestations may be nonspecific and include hepatomegaly or splenomegaly or both, generalized lymphadenopathy, failure to thrive, and developmental delay.

Recurrent bacterial infections with common pediatric pathogens (*H. influenzae* type b, *S. pneumoniae*, *S. aureus*, and *Salmonella* sp.) are common. Septicemia is most common; other illnesses include pneumonia, meningi-

tis, urinary tract infection, osteomyelitis, septic arthritis, and deep-seated abscesses. Also common are otitis media, sinusitis, and skin infections that do not respond as well to conventional antimicrobial therapy as do similar infections in children without HIV infections.

Case reports of new opportunistic infections and unusual clinical manifestations of known pathogens are being reported every day (Kline and Dunkle, 1988; Lacroix et al., 1988; Markowitz et al., 1988; Wong and Ross, 1988; Di John et al., 1990; Hughes and Parham, 1991; Friedland et al., 1992; Gradon et al., 1992; Silliman et al., 1993; Glaser et al., 1994). For example, fatal cases of both measles pneumonia and varicella encephalitis without rash have been reported (Markowitz et al., 1988; Silliman et al., 1993). Farm animals and pets may be a source of unusual infections in AIDS patients (Glaser et al., 1994). Of particular risk is bacillary angiomatosis due to *Rochalimaea henselae* and *Rochalimaea quintaum*, which can be acquired from cats, and cutaneous granulomas due to *Mycobacterium marinum*, which can be acquired from fish tanks.

Other illnesses in AIDS patients may include toxic shock syndrome, supraglottitis, very late onset group B streptococcal infection, severe molluscum contagiosum, disseminated *Acanthamoeba* infection and septicemia due to *Moraxella catarrhalis* (Kline and Dunkle, 1988; Lacroix et al., 1988; Wong and Ross, 1988; Di John et al., 1990; Hughes and Parham, 1991; Friedland et al., 1992). Recently, Gradon and associates (1992) have presented a review of unusual opportunistic pathogens in patients with AIDS by anatomic location of the infections.

Prevention of Infection

The approach to prevention and treatment of infections in HIV-infected children is continually changing (the therapy of the primary HIV infection is presented in Chapter 18). Children with HIV infections should receive all regularly scheduled immunizations, except that inactivated polio vaccine rather than oral polio vaccine should be given (American Academy of Pediatrics, 1994a). In addition, family members who are to be immunized should also receive inactivated polio vaccine rather than oral polio vaccine. Children with HIV infections should also receive yearly influenza immunization, and those 2 years of age and older should receive pneumococcal vaccine.

Because inadequate immune responses following measles immunization in HIV-infected children are common, children exposed to measles should be given immune serum globulin prophylaxis (0.5 ml/kg, maximum 15 ml) unless they are routinely receiving IVIG and have received a dose within 3 weeks of exposure. If HIV-infected children experience an injury with a wound classified as tetanus prone, they should receive tetanus immune globulin (human), regardless of their vaccination status.

Pneumocystis carinii pneumonia is the most important HIV-associated opportunistic infection in children. Infection with this agent is often fatal, and the median survival time following successful treatment of a first

Table 31–7. Summary of Subclasses of Symptomatic (P-2) HIV Infections in Children Younger Than 13 Years of Age

Subclass A—Nonspecific Findings
Includes children with two or more unexplained nonspecific findings persisting for more than 2 months, including fever, failure-to-thrive, or weight loss of more than 10% of baseline, hepatomegaly, splenomegaly, generalized lymphadenopathy (lymph nodes measuring at least 0.5 cm present in two or more sites, with bilateral lymph nodes counting as one site), parotitis, and diarrhea (three or more loose stools per day) that is either persistent or recurrent (defined as two or more episodes of diarrhea accompanied by dehydration within a 2-month period).

Subclass B—Progressive Neurologic Disease
Includes children with one or more of the following progressive findings: (1) loss of developmental milestones or intellectual ability, (2) impaired brain growth (acquired microcephaly and/or brain atrophy demonstrated on computerized tomographic scan or magnetic resonance imaging scan), (3) progressive symmetrical motor deficits manifested by two or more of these findings: paresis, abnormal tone, pathologic reflexes, ataxia, or gait disturbance.

Subclass C—Lymphoid Interstitial Pneumonitis
Includes children with a histologically confirmed pneumonitis characterized by diffuse interstitial and peribronchiolar infiltration of lymphocytes and plasma cells and without identifiable pathogens, or, in the absence of a histologic diagnosis, a chronic pneumonitis—characterized by bilateral reticulonodular interstitial infiltrates with or without hilar lymphadenopathy—present on chest x-ray for a period of at least 2 months and unresponsive to appropriate antimicrobial therapy. Other causes of interstitial infiltrates should be excluded, such as tuberculosis, *Pneumocystis carinii* pneumonia, cytomegalovirus infection, or other viral or parasitic infections.

Subclass D—Secondary Infectious Diseases
Includes children with a diagnosis of an infectious disease that occurs as a result of immune deficiency caused by infection with HIV.
   Category D-1. Includes patients with secondary infectious disease due to one of the specified infectious diseases listed in the CDC surveillance definition for AIDS: *Pneumocystis carinii* pneumonia, chronic cryptosporidiosis, disseminated toxoplasmosis with onset after 1 month of age, extraintestinal strongyloidiasis, chronic isosporiasis, candidiasis (esophageal, bronchial, or pulmonary), extrapulmonary cryptococcosis, disseminated histoplasmosis, noncutaneous extrapulmonary or disseminated mycobacterial infection (any species other than leprae), cytomegalovirus infection with onset after 1 month of age, chronic mucocutaneous or disseminated herpes simplex virus infection with onset after 1 month of age, extrapulmonary or disseminated coccidioidomycosis, nocardiosis, and progressive multifocal leukoencephalopathy.
   Category D-2. Includes patients with unexplained, recurrent, serious bacterial infections (two or more within a 2-year period), including sepsis, meningitis, pneumonia, abscess of an internal organ, and bone/joint infections.
   Category D-3. Includes patients with other infectious diseases, including oral candidiasis persisting for 2 months or more, two or more episodes of herpes stomatitis within a year, or multidermatomal or disseminated herpes zoster infection.

Subclass E—Secondary Cancers
Includes children with any cancer described below in categories E-1 and E-2.
   Category E-1. Includes patients with the diagnosis of one or more kinds of cancer known to be associated with HIV infection, as listed in the surveillance definition of AIDS and indicative of a defect in cell-mediated immunity: Kaposi's sarcoma, B-cell non-Hodgkin's lymphoma, or primary lymphoma of the brain.
   Category E-2. Includes patients with the diagnosis of other malignancies possibly associated with HIV infection.

Subclass F—Other Diseases
Includes children with other conditions possibly due to HIV infection not listed in the above-mentioned subclasses, such as hepatitis, cardiomyopathy, nephropathy, hematologic disorders (anemia, thrombocytopenia), and dermatologic diseases.

From Centers for Disease Control. 1987 classification system for HIV infection in children under 13 years of age. MMWR 36:225–236, 1987.

episode is less than 4 months in infants and children. Therefore, prophylaxis is a high priority (CDC, 1995). Because *P. carinii* pneumonia occurs early in life and because HIV infection is often difficult to diagnose during early infancy, prophylaxis must be initiated in the first few months of life and often before HIV infection has been definitively diagnosed. Recommendations for initiation of *P. carinii* pneumonia prophylaxis are presented in Table 31–9. Drug regimens for prophylaxis are presented in Table 31–10. The mainstay of prophylaxis is trimethoprim-sulfamethoxazole, but aerosolized pentamidine in older children, dapsone, and intravenous pentamidine are also effective (Kletzel et al., 1991; Orcutt et al., 1992; Carr et al., 1993; Stavola and Noel, 1993; Hand et al., 1994).

IVIG Prophylaxis

Because children with AIDS have defective humoral as well as cellular immunity, IVIG has been used prophylactically and is recommended by the Working Group on Antiretroviral Therapy: National Pediatric HIV Resource Center (1993). IVIG is recommended for children with hypogammaglobulinemia (immunoglobulin G [IgG] <250 mg/ml) and recurrent serious bacterial infections, and for children who fail to form antibodies to common antigens such as measles. The dose of IVIG is 400 mg/kg every 4 weeks (American Academy of Pediatrics, 1994a).

Other Prophylactic Measures

Prophylaxis or maintenance therapy should also be used in the following instances (CDC, 1993b):

1. Household or day care contact with active tuberculosis. Treat with isoniazid for 9 to 12 months (if there is a known exposure to a drug-resistant strain, a multiple-drug regimen is necessary).
2. Varicella-zoster immune globulin should be administered to those exposed to varicella or herpes zoster.

Table 31–8. Conditions Included in the 1993 AIDS Surveillance Case Definition

Candidiasis of bronchi, trachea, or lungs
Candidiasis, esophageal
Cervical cancer, invasive*
Coccidioidomycosis, disseminated or extrapulmonary
Cryptococcosis, extrapulmonary
Cryptosporidiosis, chronic intestinal (>1 month's duration)
Cytomegalovirus disease (other than liver, spleen, or nodes)
Cytomegalovirus retinitis (with loss of vision)
Encephalopathy, HIV-related
Herpes simplex: chronic ulcer(s) (>1 month's duration); or bronchitis, pneumonitis, or esophagitis
Histoplasmosis, disseminated or extrapulmonary
Isosporiasis, chronic intestinal (>1 month's duration)
Kaposi sarcoma
Lymphoma, Burkitt's (or equivalent term)
Lymphoma, immunoblastic (or equivalent term)
Lymphoma, primary, of brain
Mycobacterium avium complex or *M. kansasii*, disseminated or extrapulmonary
Mycobacterium tuberculosis, any site (pulmonary* or extrapulmonary)
Mycobacterium, other species or unidentified species, disseminated or extrapulmonary
Pneumocystis carinii pneumonia
Pneumonia, recurrent*
Progressive multifocal leukoencephalopathy
Salmonella septicemia, recurrent
Toxoplasmosis of brain
Wasting syndrome due to HIV

*Added in the 1993 expansion of the AIDS surveillance case definition.
From Centers for Disease Control and Prevention. 1993 revised classification system for HIV infection and expanded surveillance case definition for AIDS among adolescents and adults. MMWR 41(No. RR-17):15, 1992.

3. Those treated for cytomegalovirus infection should be placed on a maintenance regimen with ganciclovir or foscarnet.

4. Patients treated for cryptococcal meningitis should be placed on maintenance therapy with oral fluconazole.

5. Patients with persistent or recurrent mucocutaneous candidiasis should be placed on maintenance therapy with topical clotrimazole; if this measure fails, use ketoconazole or fluconazole.

6. Patients treated for ocular or central nervous system toxoplasmosis should be placed on maintenance therapy with daily pyrimethamine-sulfadiazine and folinic acid.

7. Patients with frequently recurring severe herpes simplex infections should be given oral acyclovir daily.

8. Children treated for disseminated *Mycobacterium avium* infections should be considered for prophylaxis with rifabutin.

Malnutrition

Children with chronic severe malnutrition are immunologically compromised and suffer frequently from opportunistic infections (see Chapters 15, 17, and 19). In children with protein-calorie malnutrition, the following immunologic defects have been noted: decreased concentrations of C1q, C1s, C3, C5, C6, C8, C9, and C3 proactivator, depression in T-cell function, defective intracellular bacterial killing by leukocytes, and significant reductions in the migration of polymorphonuclear leukocytes to sites of inflammation (Yoshida et al., 1967; Geefhuysen et al., 1971; Smythe et al., 1971; Chandra, 1972; Sellmeyer et al., 1972; Seth and Chandra, 1972; Freyre et al., 1973; Neumann et al., 1975; Ferguson et al., 1974; Neumann, 1981). These deficits, acting alone or in concert, undoubtedly predispose these children to infection with opportunistic microorganisms. In addition, infections with normal pathogens can frequently be expected to be more severe than in the immunologically competent host.

Serum immunoglobulin deficiencies have not been

Table 31–9. Recommendations for *Pneumocystis carinii* Pneumonia (PCP) Prophylaxis and CD4+ Monitoring for Human Immunodeficiency Virus (HIV)–Exposed Infants and HIV-Infected Children by Age and HIV Infection Status

Age/HIV Infection Status	PCP Prophylaxis	CD4+ Monitoring
Birth to 4–6 wk, HIV exposed	No prophylaxis	1 mo
4–6 wk to 4 mo, HIV exposed	Prophylaxis	3 mo
4–12 mo		
HIV infected or indeterminate	Prophylaxis	6, 9, and 12 mo
HIV infection reasonably excluded	No prophylaxis	None

1–5 yr, HIV infected†	Prophylaxis if:
	  CD4+ count is <500 cells/μl or
	  CD4+ percentage is <15%‡
		Every 3–4 mo*

6–12 yr, HIV infected	Prophylaxis if:
	  CD4+ count is <200 cells/μl or
	  CD4+ percentage is <15%‡
		Every 3–4 mo*

*More frequent monitoring (e.g., monthly) is recommended for children whose CD4+ counts or percentages are approaching the threshold at which prophylaxis is recommended.
†Children 1–2 years of age who were receiving PCP prophylaxis and had a CD4+ count of <750 cells/μl or percentage of <15% at <12 months of age should continue prophylaxis.
‡Prophylaxis should be considered on a case-by-case basis for children who might otherwise be at risk for PCP, such as children with rapidly declining CD4+ counts or percentages, or children with category C conditions (see Chapter 18 and Table 18–3). Children who have had PCP should receive lifelong PCP prophylaxis.
Adapted from Centers for Disease Control and Prevention. Revised guidelines for prophylaxis against *Pneumocystis carinii* pneumonia for children. MMWR 44(RR-4):1–11, 1995.

Table 31–10. Drug Regimens for the Prophylaxis of *Pneumocystis carinii* Pneumonia in Children

I. Recommended regimen (children ≥1 month of age):

Trimethoprim/sulfamethoxazole (TMP-SMX) 150 mg TMP/M²/day with 750 mg SMX/M²/day given orally in divided doses twice a day (b.i.d.) 3 times per week on consecutive days (e.g., Monday,Tuesday, and Wednesday).
Acceptable alternative TMP-SMX dosage schedules:

   A. 150 mg TMP/M²/day with 750 mg SMX/M²/day given orally *as a single daily dose*, three times per week on consecutive days (e.g., Monday, Tuesday, and Wednesday)
   B. 150 mg TMP/M²/day with 750 mg SMX/M²/day orally divided b.i.d. and *given 7 days/week*
   C. 150 mg TMP/M²/day with 750 mg SMX/M²/day given orally divided b.i.d. and given three times per week on alternate days (e.g., Monday, Wednesday, and Friday)

II. Alternative regimens, if TMP-SMX is not tolerated:

Aerosolized pentamidine *(≥5 years of age)* 300 mg given via Respirgard II inhaler monthly. **Dapsone** *(≥1 month of age)* 1 mg/kg (not to exceed 100 mg) given orally once daily. If neither aerosolized pentamidine nor dapsone is tolerated, some clinicians use **intravenous pentamidine** (4 mg/kg) given every 2 or 4 weeks.

Adapted from Centers for Disease Control. Guidelines for prophylaxis against *Pneumocystis carinii* pneumonia for children infected with human immunodeficiency virus. MMWR 40(RR-2):9, 1991.

found consistently, but deficits in specific antibody responses despite normal or elevated total serum immunoglobulins have been observed (Cannon, 1945; Work et al., 1973). Transient deficiency of nasal secretory IgA has been reported in malnourished children in Thailand (Sirisinha et al., 1975). With nutritional repletion, cellular immunity, serum complement activity, and polymorphonuclear leukocyte function return toward normal.

Children with protein-calorie malnutrition are particularly susceptible to severe and progressive measles virus infection and disseminated herpes simplex virus infection. Severe and protracted bacterial urinary tract, pulmonary, and gastrointestinal infections are common, as are chronic diarrheas due to parasites. Particularly troublesome are infections with gram-negative enteric bacilli and *M. tuberculosis* infections (Faber, 1938; Becker et al., 1963; Phillips and Wharton, 1968; Morley, 1969; James, 1972).

Nephrotic Syndrome

Prior to the use of antibiotics and corticosteroids, peritonitis due to *S. pneumoniae*, group A streptococci, staphylococci, and *H. influenzae* type b was a relatively common and often fatal complication of nephrotic syndrome. Although peritonitis due to these microorganisms still occurs, systemic infection due to gram-negative bacilli has been observed with increasing frequency (Wilfert and Katz, 1968). Patients with nephrotic syndrome have been found to have cellular and humoral immune defects and a decreased bacterial killing by neutrophils (Yetgin et al., 1980). Pneumococcal vaccine should be administered to those 2 years of age or older (Fikrig, 1978). This disorder is discussed in Chapters 17, 19, and 25.

Uremia

Renal failure is associated with an increased risk of infection with opportunistic organisms (Welt et al., 1970; Haag-Weber and Hörl, 1993). Common offending microorganisms include *Enterobacter, Staphylo-*coccus, Serratia, Bacteroides, Candida, Mucor, herpesviruses, and *Pneumocystis.*

Reasons for the increased propensity for infection have been sought (see Chapter 19). Lymphopenia has been observed frequently; a depressed and delayed response to tuberculin, coccidioidin, histoplasmin, *Candida*, trichophytin, and mumps as well as impaired allograft rejection have been reported in patients who were uremic (Dammin et al., 1957; Riis and Stougaard, 1959; Kirkpatrick et al., 1964; Lang et al., 1966). Inability of lymphocytes to proliferate in response to antigens has been well documented and has been related in part to a plasma factor in uremic patients (Elves et al., 1966; Silk, 1967; Ming et al., 1968). The increased risk of infection with saprophytic fungi, herpesviruses, and *Pneumocystis* in uremic patients may be related to the depression of T-cell function.

Immunoglobulin concentrations generally have been normal. Polymorphonuclear leukocyte production is apparently normal, but a defect in the early phase of the acute inflammatory response has been suggested (Wilson et al., 1965; Haag-Weber and Hörl, 1993).

Exudative Enteropathy

When an excessive loss of protein occurs into the gastrointestinal tract, significant reduction in albumin and gamma globulin, particularly IgG, may be noted (see Chapters 12, 19, and 23). Disorders in which exudative enteropathy has been noted include acute gastrointestinal infection, Ménétrier's disease (protein loss with giant hypertrophy of the gastric mucosa), gluten-induced enteropathy, intestinal lymphangiectasia, kwashiorkor, Hirschsprung's disease, gastrointestinal neoplasms, allergic gastroenteritis, regional enteritis, ulcerative colitis, jejunal malformations, gastrocolic fistula, angioneurotic edema, postgastrectomy syndrome, congestive heart failure, constrictive pericarditis, and aminopterin administration (Waldmann and Schwab, 1965; Waldmann, 1966; Feigin and Shearer, 1975). Infection related specifically to the IgG deficiency is rare.

In patients with intestinal lymphangiectasia, however, hypogammaglobulinemia may be accompanied by lymphopenia and skin anergy, and impaired homograft rejection has been documented in these individuals (Strober et al., 1967; Weiden et al., 1972). The increased susceptibility of some of these children to infection is related to the loss of immunoglobulins and lymphocytes with disruption of the normal circulation of small lymphocytes from the blood into lymphoid tissues and back to the blood (Gatti et al., 1970). Persistent giardiasis in children with this disease has resolved when there was improvement in the clinical and immunologic status of the patient (Feigin and Shearer, 1975).

Inflammatory Bowel Disease

Granulomatous colitis and ulcerative colitis (see Chapter 23) *per se* do not appear to predispose the host to opportunistic infection. When those disorders are treated with corticosteroids, however, opportunistic infection with bacteria, viruses, fungi, and parasites may occur. Infection is usually systemic, but *Candida* endophthalmitis (localized infection) has been noted in a child who was receiving corticosteroids for ulcerative colitis (Haning et al., 1973).

Inflammatory Disease of Connective Tissue

Abnormalities in immunoglobulins and antibodies that react with body tissue constituents or with other immunoglobulins, e.g., rheumatoid factors, have been noted in patients with collagen diseases (see Chapter 24). When opportunistic infections with *Candida, Aspergillus, Mucor*, and *Pneumocystis* occur in patients with connective tissue disorders, they are most likely related to the administration of corticosteroids and other immunosuppressive agents (Klainer and Beisel, 1969). Infection with *Pseudomonas, Listeria, Staphylococcus, Serratia*, diphtheroids, *Nocardia, Candida, Aspergillus, Cryptococcus, Mucor*, cytomegalovirus, varicella-zoster virus, and *Pneumocystis* may be seen in patients with significant involvement of the reticuloendothelial system (Feigin and Shearer, 1975).

INFECTION IN THE NEWBORN INFANT

From an immunologic point of view, all newborn infants (full-term as well as premature) can be considered to be compromised. Most neonatal infections are opportunistic in that the principal offending microorganisms are those that are readily cultured from the exogenous and endogenous environments of normal individuals. Specific immunodeficiencies of newborns are presented in Chapter 10.

The greatest infection risk for the newborn infant is the surrounding environment, and an important defect that the infant at birth has is the total lack of a microbial flora. Natural antibiosis and competitive inhibition among organisms are important host defense mechanisms that are not available to the newborn. The events leading to the acquisition of a flora are critical in the

determination of which infants will become infected. In general, the infant who receives a balanced dose of organisms from the mother runs a lower risk of infection than the infant heavily colonized with a single organism from the environment.

In recent years, IVIG has been used in several controlled and uncontrolled studies to treat and prevent infections in low-birth-weight infants (NIH Consensus Conference, 1990; Magny et al., 1991; Baker et al., 1992; Kinney et al., 1991; Weisman et al., 1992; Hill, 1993). These studies were reviewed at an National Institutes of Health (NIH) Consensus Conference in 1989 and more recently by Hill (1993). Of six prophylaxis studies, two showed marginal benefit and four of five treatment studies showed benefit. One treatment study in animals indicated that the IVIG impaired the antibacterial activity of antibiotics in animals infected with group B streptococci (Kim, 1989).

From the available data, it is our opinion that evidence for prophylaxis is insufficient to recommend its use. Similarly, the data regarding therapy are such that it should not be used routinely but perhaps should be reserved for specific individual cases.

GENERAL APPROACH TO TREATMENT OF INFECTION IN THE COMPROMISED HOST

The general principles of diagnosis and treatment of opportunistic infections are the same as those applied when infections are caused by organisms normally considered to be pathogenic. The possibility of opportunistic infections can be anticipated in association with certain clinical situations, and the physician can frequently predict the types of organisms that may be responsible for specific infections that are suspected or observed. The physician must alert the laboratory to the possibility of opportunistic infection, and, in turn, the microbiologist must not regard the isolation of a normally saprophytic microorganism as a contaminant, particularly if it is recovered repeatedly from specimens obtained from the same patient.

It is important to emphasize that the relationship between a microorganism and the host is a dynamic one. Virulence can be expressed only in comparative terms because of daily variations in the mechanisms of host defense and the microorganisms to which the host is exposed. Any microorganism can produce disease in an appropriate host.

Opportunistic microorganisms do not produce disease in a haphazard manner. Thus, diagnosis and treatment need not be initiated haphazardly. For example, in the compromised host with an indwelling venous catheter, periodic blood specimens should be obtained for culture and the site of insertion of the catheter should be examined carefully. The tip of the catheter should be cultured routinely on removal. Similarly, cultures of sputum or tracheal aspirates should be obtained repeatedly in children who have a tracheostomy and who are receiving inhalation therapy. In this manner, the physician can detect sequential changes in the microbial flora of the patient. Cultures of this type assume special importance in children who are immunosuppressed, because in these individuals, the usual clinical signs of infection may be absent.

Once appropriate cultures and serologic tests designed to establish an etiologic diagnosis have been obtained from the immunologically compromised child, therapy should be initiated immediately in most instances. Prior to the identification of a specific infectious agent, initial treatment must be guided by the underlying disease process with which the patient is afflicted and the types of organisms that most commonly are responsible for infection in these individuals (see Tables 31–1 through 31–8). When a specific organism is recovered and specific sensitivities are obtained, therapy may be changed accordingly.

Approach to Diagnosis

Serious infections in compromised children usually have only a limited number of clinical manifestations (fever, respiratory distress, abdominal distress, neurologic complaints, skin and soft tissue lesions, and bone or joint complaints) and sites of infection (septicemia, pneumonia, peritonitis or abdominal abscess, meningitis or brain abscess, skin cellulitis and ulcers, soft tissue abscess, arthritis, and osteomyelitis). However, each clinical category of infection can be due to a multitude of different microorganisms, including common bacteria, mycobacteria, fungi, parasites, and viruses. In preceding sections and tables of this chapter, the various microorganisms most frequently associated with opportunistic infections in children with specific immunologic defects are presented.

Septicemia

In hospitalized children with severe combined immunodeficiencies, malignancies, and immunosuppression, fever is a frequent occurrence, and in most instances this fever is due to septicemia. The approach to diagnosis should be easy, but all too frequently undue delay occurs because of failure to collect appropriate cultures. Multiple blood cultures should be obtained.

In addition to blood cultures, cultures from all other possible sites of infection should be obtained. Cutdown sites, intravenous catheters, and the urine should be cultured.

Pneumonia

Pneumonia is the second most common problem in compromised patients, and all too frequently antibiotics are started prior to appropriate cultures. Because many children with pneumonia due to opportunistic microorganisms also have septicemia, multiple blood cultures should be obtained. In addition, sputum smears and cultures should be obtained. In virtually all instances in which pleural fluid is visible by radiograph, a thoracentesis should be performed. In many instances when only "pleural thickening" is observed, a thoracentesis reveals 1 or 2 ml of diagnostically useful fluid. In many instances, more invasive diagnostic study is

indicated (Prober et al., 1984; Commers et al., 1984; Johanson et al., 1988; Dichter et al., 1993). The nature of subsequent studies depends on the skill of the physician's consulting services. Diagnostic bronchoscopy with bronchoalveolar lavage or direct lung tap frequently is rewarding. Open lung biopsy is often necessary.

Other Infections

Arthritis, osteomyelitis, cellulitis, and abscess areas should be needled for culture prior to therapy. Frequently, these culture attempts are facilitated by having a small amount of saline in the syringe. If the tap is dry, the saline can be pushed into and withdrawn from the site of suspected infection. Cerebrospinal fluid should be obtained for culture whenever there is the slightest suspicion of central nervous system infection.

Handling of Cultures

Positive cultures are the hallmark of therapeutic success. Frequently, extensive and invasive surgical procedures are performed for diagnosis and the specimens are then handled improperly. All cultures obtained from deep sites should be inoculated into aerobic and anaerobic bacterial media as well as into fungal and mycobacterial media. Multiple smears should be made and treated with Gram's stain, methenamine silver stain, hematoxylin-eosin, or other appropriate tissue stains. From specimens obtained from the lung and urine, cerebrospinal fluid, and, frequently, blood, viral cultures also are indicated.

Approach to Therapy

Empiric Treatment for the Neutropenic Febrile Cancer or Bone Marrow Transplant Patient

Following the initial collection of appropriate cultures, all neutropenic cancer and bone marrow transplant patients with fever of unknown origin should be started immediately on empiric antimicrobial therapy (Cherry, 1983; Bodey, 1984; Frazier et al., 1984; Winston et al., 1984; Pizzo et al., 1991a; Zaia, 1992; Katz and Mustafa, 1993; Pizzo, 1993; Sable and Donowitz, 1994). Empiric therapy must consist of broad-spectrum agents because the variation of types of organisms and their susceptibility patterns are legion (see Table 31–5). There are many possible empiric antimicrobial regimens. In the past, we suggested using an aminoglycoside (amikacin, gentamicin, netilmicin, or tobramycin) in combination with either an anti-*Pseudomonas* penicillin (azlocillin, carbenicillin, ticarcillin, mezlocillin, or piperacillin) or a third-generation cephalosporin and a penicillinase-resistant penicillin (nafcillin or oxacillin). More recent experience indicates that empiric therapy can be simplified and made less costly by the use of ceftazidime monotherapy (Pizzo et al., 1991a; Pizzo, 1993). Following the results of cultures and sensitivities, the antimicrobial regimen can be altered. Combination treatment (an anti-*Pseudomonas* penicillin and an aminoglycoside) should be employed for all infections with gram-negative bacillary infections. For infections with gram-positive cocci, a narrow-spectrum penicillin, penicillinase-resistant penicillin (depending on sensitivity of the organism), or vancomycin is adequate for the treatment of the infection. However, it has been noted on occasion that in patients treated initially with single narrow-spectrum drugs, secondary gram-negative bacterial infections develop. Because of this problem, it may be important to administer an aminoglycoside or ceftazidime along with the specific treatment for the gram-positive organism.

When cultures do not reveal a bacterial etiology for the fever and a patient remains febrile on ceftazidime monotherapy, further empiric treatment must be considered. After additional cultures we would suggest adding an aminoglycoside and perhaps vancomycin to the regimen. With continued fever, empiric antifungal treatment must be considered. We would suggest the routine empiric administration of amphotericin B if fever has persisted for more than 7 days; amphotericin B should be added to the regimen at an earlier time if the patient's clinical condition is deteriorating.

The duration of antimicrobial treatment in the neutropenic cancer or bone marrow transplantation patient is not well established. If the patient remains neutropenic, therapy should be continued for at least 7 days after the child's temperature has returned to normal. However, because relapse or re-infection is common, it is frequently recommended that once treatment is started, it be continued until the child is no longer neutropenic (i.e., absolute granulocyte count ≥500/mm³) (Pizzo et al., 1984).

Bacterial Infections

Selected antimicrobial agents useful for the treatment of severe bacterial infections in children who are compromised immunologically are presented in Table 31–11. Both the dosage and usual susceptible organisms are listed. Frequently, in seriously ill children, antibiotic therapy must be started before culture results are available. Because gram-negative bacillary infections are most common in compromised children and because many are hospital-acquired, the likelihood of multiple drug resistance is great. Thus, initial therapy should provide broad bactericidal coverage (see previous discussion). At some centers where gentamicin has been used extensively, many infections due to gentamicin-resistant organisms have been observed. In these instances, another aminoglycoside antibiotic (based on hospital laboratory sensitivity patterns), such as amikacin, netilmicin, or tobramycin, should be used.

In Table 31–11, antimicrobial dosage is listed by square meter as well as by kilogram. This is of little importance with penicillins and cephalosporins but can be very important with aminoglycoside antibiotics. Children who are underweight for their age tend to have relatively greater blood volumes and extracellular fluid spaces than their weights would indicate. Therefore, dosages calculated by kilogram nearly always will be too low. Underdosage is a common occurrence with aminoglycoside therapy in children with cystic fibrosis. In addition, because the gap between effective therapeutic and toxic levels of aminoglycoside antibiotics is small, it is imperative to determine peak and trough blood levels when these drugs are administered. The specific in vitro sensitivity of the infectious agent for which treatment is provided also must be determined.

Pseudomonas infections should always be treated with both an aminoglycoside and an anti-*Pseudomonas* penicillin or ceftazidime because significant synergism has been described. Anti-*Pseudomonas* penicillins should not be used as single drugs in the treatment of *Pseudomonas* infections because therapeutic results have been disappointing and resistance rapidly develops. Trimethoprim-sulfamethoxazole on occasion can be lifesaving in illnesses that are due to multiresistant gram-negative bacillary infections.

When anaerobic infections are suspected, chloramphenicol, clindamycin, or metronidazole should be added to the therapeutic regimen. The exception to this statement occurs in pulmonary disease, in which large doses of penicillin G or carbenicillin will be satisfactory.

Vancomycin is a useful drug that should be administered to patients with multiresistant staphylococcal, enterococcal, and streptococcal infections and in serious streptococcal and staphylococcal infections in allergic individuals. *M. pneumoniae* infections are frequently of greater severity in compromised patients and should be treated vigorously with erythromycin.

Tuberculosis in compromised patients frequently is far advanced before it is recognized by the physician. In addition, the recent emergence of tuberculosis due to drug-resistant *M. tuberculosis* is a major problem (CDC, 1993a). At present, a four-drug regimen with isoniazid, rifampin, pyrazinamide, and streptomycin or ethambutol is recommended for initial empiric treatment.

Viral Infections

Viral infections are responsible for considerable morbidity and mortality in compromised children. Although specific antiviral therapy is still at a rudimentary stage of development in contrast to antibacterial therapy, there is much that can be offered to the patient. Useful therapeutic agents are listed in Table 31–12. Topical ophthalmic preparations of acyclovir, idoxuridine, trifluridine, and vidarabine have all been shown to be effective in treating acute keratoconjunctivitis and recurrent epithelial keratitis caused by herpes simplex virus. No topical antiviral agent is presently useful for treating recurrent skin herpes simplex viral infections.

The use of amantadine in early influenza A infection would appear to be supported by adequate scientific data, and in the clinical situation in which influenza A infection is suspected, this therapy is recommended. Ribavirin, administered by aerosol generator, appears to be therapeutically effective in respiratory syncytial and influenza viral infections in immunocompetent

Table 31–11. Selected Agents Useful in Treating Severe Bacterial Infections in Immunologically Compromised Children*

Agent	Dose	Usual Susceptible Organisms	Comments
Amikacin	15–40 mg/kg/day (420–1100 mg/M^2/day) q8h IM or IV (30 min infusion)	*Enterobacter* sp., *Escherichia coli*, *Klebsiella pneumoniae*, *Proteus* sp., *Providencia* sp., *Serratia* sp., *Acinetobacter* sp., *Pseudomonas* sp., nontuberculous mycobacteria	Blood levels 1 hr and 8 hr (peak and trough) after administration frequently necessary to ensure adequate concentration without toxicity.
Ampicillin	100–300 mg/kg/day (2.8–8.4 g/M^2/day) q4h IM or IV (5 min infusion)	Enterococci, streptococci, *Listeria monocytogenes*, *E. coli*, *Proteus mirabilis*, *Salmonella* sp., *Shigella* sp., *Haemophilus influenzae*	When administered in conjunction with an aminoglycoside, synergism frequently occurs.
Aztreonam	90–120 mg/kg/day (2.6–3.4 g/M^2/day) q6–8h IM or IV	Most aerobic gram-negative bacteria; virtually devoid of activity against aerobic gram-positive and anaerobic organisms	Useful when gram-negative aerobic bacteria are resistant to cephalosporins, penicillins, and aminoglycosides; superinfection with gram-positive organisms is a problem.
Carbenicillin	200–500 mg/kg/day (5.6–14.0 g/M^2/day) q4h IV (5 min infusion)	Many *Bacteroides* sp. and other anaerobes; with gentamicin, amikacin, or tobramycin for *Pseudomonas aeruginosa* and other gram-negative bacilli	Should always be used in conjunction with an aminoglycoside antibiotic.
Cefazolin	25–50 mg/kg/day (0.7–1.4 g/M^2/day) q6h IM or IV (5 min infusion)	*Staphylococcus aureus*, *Staphylococcus epidermidis*, group A beta-hemolytic streptococci, *Streptococcus pneumoniae*	When administered in conjunction with an aminoglycoside, synergism frequently occurs.
Cefoperazone	100–150 mg/kg/day (2.8–4.2 g/M^2/day) q6–8h IV (10–20 min infusion)	Most gram-positive and gram-negative aerobes except *L. monocytogenes*, enterococci (many anaerobes sensitive)	Particularly useful in biliary tract infections.
Cefotaxime	100–200 mg/kg/day (2.8–5.6 g/M^2/day) q6–8h IV (10–20 min infusion)	Most gram-positive and gram-negative aerobes except *L. monocytogenes* and enterococci	
Ceftriaxone	50–100 mg/kg/day (1.4–2.8 g/M^2/day) q12h IV (10–20 min infusion)	Similar to cefotaxime	
Cefuroxime	100–200 mg/kg/day (2.8–6.7 g/M^2/day) q6–8h IV (10–20 min infusion)	Most gram-positive cocci (except enterococci), *H. influenzae*, *Neisseria meningitidis*	
Chloramphenicol	50–100 mg/kg/day (1.4–2.8 g/M^2/day) q6h PO or IV (30 min infusion)	*Salmonella* sp., *Shigella* sp., *H. influenzae*, anaerobes, gram-negative bacilli	
Ciprofloxacin	20–30 mg/kg/day q12h IV or PO	*Enterococcus faecalis*, *Staphylococcus* sp., *Citrobacter* sp., *Enterobacter cloacae*, *E. coli*, *H. influenzae*, *Haemophilus parainfluenzae*, *Klebsiella pneumoniae*, *Morganella morganii*, *Proteus* sp., *Providencia* sp., *P. aeruginosa*, *Serratia marcescens*	Not approved for patients <18 yr of age; causes arthropathy in juvenile animals.
Clarithromycin	15 mg/kg/day in 2 divided doses. 10–30 mg/kg/day in 2 divided doses for *Mycobacterium avium–intracellulare*	*Legionella* sp., *Chlamydia trachomatis*, *S. aureus* (methicillin sensitive), *Streptococcus* sp., *Enterococcus* sp., *Neisseria gonorrhoeae*, anaerobic cocci, *Campylobacter jejuni*, *H. influenzae*, *Bacteroides* sp., *Mycobacterium leprae*, *Mycobacterium kansasii*, *M. avium–intracellulare*, *Corynebacterium* sp., *L. monocytogenes*, *Clostridium perfringens*, *Peptococcus*, *Peptostreptococcus*, *Bordetella pertussis*, *Moraxella catarrhalis*, *Pasteurella multocida*	Safety not established for patients <12 yr of age.
Clindamycin	10–40 mg/kg/day (280–1120 mg/M^2/day) q6h IM or IV (30 min infusion)	Anaerobes	
Erythromycin	30–50 mg/kg/day (840–1400 mg/M^2/day) q6h PO or IV (1 h infusion)	*Mycoplasma pneumoniae*, *Chlamydia* sp., *Legionella* sp., *S. aureus*, *Streptococcus* sp., *B. pertussis*	
Ethambutol	25 mg/kg/day (700 mg/M^2/day) for 2 mo then 15 mg/kg/day (420 mg/M^2/day) PO	*Mycobacterium tuberculosis*, atypical mycobacteria	Used in conjunction with isoniazid, rifampin, and pyrazinamide.
Gentamicin	5–7.5 mg/kg/day (140–210 mg/M^2/day) q8h IM or IV (30 min infusion)	*Enterobacter* sp., *E. coli*, *K. pneumoniae*, *Proteus* sp., *Providencia* sp., *P. aeruginosa*, *Citrobacter* sp., *Serratia* sp.	Blood levels 1 hr and 8 hr (peak and trough) after administration frequently necessary to ensure adequate concentration without toxicity.
Imipenem-cilastatin	40–60 mg/kg/day (1.1–1.7 g/M^2/day)	Active against most gram-positive cocci and gram-negative bacilli	Not approved for children. Useful for organisms resistant to cephalosporins, penicillins, and aminoglycosides; usually used in conjunction with an aminoglycoside; has propensity to induce seizures.
Isoniazid	10–20 mg/kg/day (280–560 mg/M^2/day) (maximum 500 mg/day) PO or IM	*M. tuberculosis*, atypical mycobacteria	Used in conjunction with ethambutol, streptomycin, rifampin, and pyrazinamide.

Table continued on following page

Table 31–11. Selected Agents Useful in Treating Severe Bacterial Infections in Immunologically Compromised Children* *Continued*

Agent	Dose	Usual Susceptible Organisms	Comments
Kanamycin	15–20 mg/kg/day (420–560 mg/M²/day) q8h IM or IV (30 min infusion)	*Enterobacter* sp., *E. coli, K. pneumoniae, Proteus* sp., *Providencia* sp., *Serratia* sp., *Acinetobacter* sp.	
Metronidazole	15–50 mg/kg/day (420–1400 mg/M²/day) q6h IV or PO	Most anaerobes	
Mezlocillin	300 mg/kg/day (8.4 g/M²/day) q4–6h IV (10–20 min infusion)	Similar to carbenicillin but, in general, is more active	Should always be used with an aminoglycoside antibiotic.
Nafcillin	100–200 mg/kg/day (2.8–5.6 g/M²/day) q4–6h IM or IV (5 min infusion)	*S. aureus*	
Norfloxacin	400 mg q12h PO	Similar to ciprofloxacin	Not approved for patients <21 yr of age; causes arthropathy in juvenile animals.
Ofloxacin	400–800 mg/day q12h PO	*Chlamydia trachomatis*; otherwise similar to ciprofloxacin	Not approved for children; causes arthropathy and osteochrondrosis of juvenile animals.
Oxacillin	100–200 mg/kg/day (2.8–5.6 g/M²/day) q4–6h IM or IV (5 min infusion)	*S. aureus*	
Penicillin	50,000–300,000 U/kg/day (1.4–8.4 million U/M²/day) q4h IM or IV (5 min infusion)	*Streptococcus* sp., *Neisseria* sp., *Clostridium* sp., *Pasteurella multocida*, oropharyngeal anaerobes, *Streptococcus moniliformis*.	
Piperacillin	200–300 mg/kg/day (5.6–8.4 g/M²/day) q4h IV or IM (30 min infusion)	Similar to carbenicillin but, in general, is more active	Should always be used in combination with aminoglycoside.
Pyrazinamide	20–30 mg/kg/day (560–840 mg/M²/day) or 20 mg/kg (560 mg/M²) twice weekly PO	*M. tuberculosis*, atypical mycobacteria	Use in mycobacteria infections with resistant organisms in conjunction with other agents.
Rifampin	10–20 mg/kg/day (280–560 mg/M²/day) (maximum 600 mg/day) PO	*M. tuberculosis*, atypical mycobacteria	For tuberculosis, use in conjunction with isoniazid, pyrazinamide, streptomycin, and ethambutol.
Streptomycin	15–30 mg/kg/day (420–840 mg/M²/day) IM	*M. tuberculosis*, atypical mycobacteria	Used in three-drug or four-drug therapy with isoniazid, rifampin, pyrazinamide, and ethambutol; has synergistic role in therapy of bacterial endocarditis.
Tetracycline	20–40 mg/kg/day (560–1120 mg/M²/day) q6h PO or IV (2 hr infusion)	*M. pneumoniae, Chlamydia* sp.	
Ticarcillin	200–300 mg/kg/day (5.6–8.4 g/M²/day) q4–6h IV (10–20 min infusion)	Similar to carbenicillin	Should always be used with an aminoglycoside antibiotic.
Tobramycin	3–5 mg/kg/day (84–140 mg/M²/day) q8h IM or IV (30 min infusion)	*Enterobacter* sp., *E. coli, K. pneumoniae, Proteus* sp., *Providencia* sp., *Serratia* sp., *Acinetobacter* sp., *Pseudomonas* sp., *Citrobacter* sp.	Blood levels 1 hr and 8 hr (peak and trough) after administration frequently necessary to ensure adequate concentration without toxicity.
Trimethoprim-sulfamethoxazole	Trimethoprim 10–20 mg/kg/day (280–560 mg/M²/day) Sulfamethoxazole 50–100 mg/kg/day (1.4–2.8 g/M²/day) q12h PO or IV	*Providencia* sp., *Salmonella* sp., *Serratia* sp., *Shigella* sp., *E. coli, Klebsiella* sp., *Enterobacter* sp., *M. morganii, Proteus* sp., *H. influenzae, Shigella flexneri, Shigella sonnei*	Useful when organisms resistant to aminoglycosides.
Trisulfapyrimidines	120 mg/kg/day (3.4 g/M²/day) q6h PO for 4 wk	*Nocardia*	
Vancomycin	40–60 mg/kg/day (1200–1800 mg/M²/day) q6h IV (30 min infusion)	*S. aureus, S. epidermidis, Streptococcus* sp., enterococci, *Clostridium difficile*	For treatment of an enterococcal infection, used with an aminoglycoside antibiotic; for *Clostridium difficile* enteritis, administered 50 mg/kg/day PO.

*Consult drug product information sheets (package inserts) and other sources for more complete administration and toxicity data. Some doses and administration suggestions in this table may be different from those recommended by the manufacturer.

Data from Nelson JD. Pocketbook of Pediatric Antimicrobial Therapy, 10th ed. Baltimore, Williams & Wilkins, 1993; Feigin RD, Cherry JD. Texbook of Pediatric Infectious Diseases, 3rd ed. Philadelphia, WB Saunders, 1992.

children and adults. Gelfand and colleagues (1983) and McIntosh and associates (1984) reported encouraging results in three children with severe combined immunodeficiency syndromes infected with respiratory syncytial virus or parainfluenza virus type 3.

Mucocutaneous herpes simplex viral infections are common in immunocompromised children; they are frequently severe and chronic, being the cause of significant morbidity (Wong and Hirsch, 1984; Bryson, 1984). These infections can be treated successfully with acyclovir. Similarly, both exogenous (varicella) or endogenous (zoster or disseminated zoster) infections with varicella-zoster virus can be treated effectively with acyclovir. In addition to treatment, recurrences of illness due to herpes simplex virus can be prevented by the prophylactic use of acyclovir. Similar, but less effective, is the use of maintenance therapy with ganciclovir to prevent recurrence of the clinical manifestations of cytomegalovirus infection in immunosuppressed patients.

Fungal Infections

Fungal infections are a major cause of death in compromised children. In many instances, vigorous antibiotic therapy has been carried out, but extensive fungal infection is found at autopsy. In particular, *Candida* overgrowth is common in compromised patients receiving antibiotic therapy. This overgrowth should be

Table 31–12. Selected Agents Useful in Treating Viral Infections in Immunologically Compromised Children*

Type	Agent	Dose and Method of Administration	Susceptible Viruses	Comments
Topical	Acyclovir	Eye—5% ointment q3–4h	Herpes simplex, varicella-zoster	
	Idoxuridine	Eye—0.1% solution q1h; 0.5% ointment q4h	Herpes simplex	
	Trifluridine	Eye—1% solution q2h (max., 9 drops/eye/24h)	Herpes simplex	
	Vidarabine	Eye—3% ointment, 1/2″, 5 times/day	Herpes simplex, varicella-zoster	
Systemic	Acyclovir	15–45 mg/kg/day (420–1350 mg/M²/day) q8h IV (1-h infusion)	Herpes simplex and varicella-zoster	
	Amantadine	1–9 yr: 4.4–8.8 mg/kg/day (125–250 mg/M²/day) q12h PO (Max., 150 mg/day) 9–12 yr: 100 mg PO q12h	Influenza A	
	Didanosine	7–10 mg/kg/day (200–300 mg/M²/day) PO q8–12h	Human immunodeficiency virus (HIV)	Should be used if zidovudine intolerance or failure.
	Foscarnet	180 mg/kg/day (5 g/M²/day) IV q8h for 14–21 days, then 60–120 mg/kg/day (1.7–2.4 g/M²/day) q24h for maintenance	Cytomegalovirus	
	Ganciclovir	10 mg/kg/day (300 mg/M²/day) IV q12h for 14–21 days 5 mg/kg/day (150 mg/M²/day) IV q24h for long-term suppression 10 mg/kg/day (300 mg/M²/day) IV q12h for 1 wk, then 5 mg/kg/day (150 mg/M²/day) IV q24h for prophylaxis	Cytomegalovirus	
	Ribavirin	Administered by aerosol generator (6 g in 300 ml sterile USP water) 12–18h exposure per day	Respiratory syncytial virus	In vitro studies have shown efficacy against influenza, parainfluenza, and measles virus. Clinical studies of this agent for treatment of influenza and parainfluenza virus are in progress.
	Ramantidine	5 mg/kg/day (150 mg/M²/day) q12h Maximum dose <10 yr 150 mg/day, ≥10 yr 200 mg/day	Influenza A	Approved for prophylactic use.
	Vidarabine	15–30 mg/kg/day (420–840 mg/M²/day) (12-h infusion) for 10–14 days	Herpes simplex, varicella-zoster	
	Zidovudine	<12 yr: 24 mg/kg/day (720 mg/M²/day) PO q6h (maximum 800 mg/day) ≥12 yr: 500–600 mg/day in 3–6 divided doses	HIV	

*Consult drug product information sheets (package inserts) and other sources for more complete administration and toxicity data. Some doses and administration suggestions in this table may be different from those recommended by the manufacturer.

Data from Nelson JD. Pocketbook of Pediatric Antimicrobial Therapy, 10th ed. Baltimore, Williams & Wilkins, 1993; Feigin RD, Cherry JD. Textbook of Pediatric Infectious Diseases, 3rd ed. Philadelphia, WB Saunders, 1992; American Academy of Pediatrics. Antiviral drugs. In Peter G, ed. 1994 Red Book: Report of the Committee on Infectious Diseases, 23rd ed. Elk Grove Village, Ill., American Academy of Pediatrics, 1994, pp. 568–569.

treated vigorously with topical agents because it is quite probable that dissemination can be reduced. Useful antifungal agents are listed in Table 31–13.

For systemic fungal disease, the most effective agent is amphotericin B. This is a drug with considerable toxicity, but with judicious use, it can be highly effective. In children, in whom renal functional abnormalities are usually less of a problem, dosage can frequently be pushed higher and treatment continued longer than in adult patients. When amphotericin B is used, it is important to determine blood concentrations of amphotericin B and the sensitivity of the fungus. These tests are not performed in many hospital laboratories, but they are available in reference laboratories. After institution of therapy with amphotericin B, it should be continued for at least 3 weeks and usually for at least 6 weeks. Flucytosine is also a potent antifungal agent. However, in our experience, it has proved disappointing when used as the single therapeutic agent. In therapy of *Candida* infections, we frequently use both amphotericin B and flucytosine together. Fluconazole, itraconazole, and ketoconazole are three relatively new antifungal agents that, when used on the basis of sensitivity studies, can occasionally be used in place of amphotericin B. Itraconazole has been used successfully in invasive *Aspergillus* sp. infections and fluconazole and ketoconazole in disseminated *Coccidioides immitis* infections. Fluconazole is also effective in cryptococcal meningitis.

Parasitic Infections

The major parasitic infections causing opportunistic infection in immunologically compromised children are due to *P. carinii*, *T. gondii*, and *Cryptosporidium* sp. Occasionally, *Entamoeba histolytica*, *Isospora belli*, and *Giardia* are also problems. Selected agents useful in treating parasitic infections in immunologically compromised children are presented in Table 31–14.

PREVENTION OF INFECTION IN THE COMPROMISED CHILD

Prevention of infection in the compromised child varies with the nature and degree of the individual defect (see Tables 31–1 through 31–5). For example, children with splenic deficiency syndromes need only pneumococcal vaccine and specific antibiotic prophylaxis against selected bacteria, and patients with simple

Table 31–13. Selected Agents Useful in Treating Fungal Infections in Immunologically Compromised Children*

Type	Agent	Dose and Method of Administration	Susceptible Fungi	Comments
Topical	Nystatin	Cream, ointment, powder, oral suspension, oral tablets, vaginal tablets 100,000 to 1 million U/day q.i.d.	*Candida* sp.	
	Clotrimazole	1% ointment or solution b.i.d. to q.i.d.	*Candida* sp., dermatophytes	
	Miconazole	Cream b.i.d. to q.i.d.	*Candida* sp., dermatophytes	
Systemic	Amphotericin B	0.8–1.5 mg/kg/day (22–42 mg/M²/day) q.d. or q.o.d. IV (3–4h infusion)	*Aspergillus* sp., *Blastomyces, Candida* sp., *Coccidioides immitis, Cryptococcus neoformans, Histoplasma capsulatum, Mucor, Paracoccidioidomycosis, Phaeohyphomycosis, Zycomycosis*	In children, an initial dose of 0.25 mg/kg is usually well tolerated, increasing by 0.25 mg/kg daily until 1.0 mg/kg is reached; in severely ill patients, the first 4 doses can be given 6 hr apart, then adjusted to q.d. or q.o.d.
	Fluconazole	3–6 mg/kg (84–168 mg/M²/day) IV or PO once daily	Mucosal candidiasis, cryptococcal meningitis, *Candida* urinary tract infection	
	Flucytosine	50–150 mg/kg/day (1.4–4.2 g/M²/day) q6h PO	*Candida* sp., *Cryptococcus neoformans*	Used in conjunction with amphotericin B.
	Itraconazole	200 mg PO once or twice daily for adults; dose for children not established	*Aspergillus* sp., *Blastomyces dermatitidis, C. immitis, Cryptococcus neoformans*	
	Ketoconazole	3.3–6.6 mg/kg/day (100–200 mg/M²/day) q.d. PO	*Blastomyces dermatitidis, Candida* sp., *C. immitis, H. capsulatum, Paracoccidioides brasiliensis, C. neoformans, Pseudallescheria boydii*	*Drug of choice for chronic mucocutaneous candidiasis.*
	Miconazole	20–40 mg/kg/day (600–1200 mg/M²/day) IV q8h (30–60 min infusion)	*Candida* sp.	

*Consult drug product information sheets (package inserts) and other sources for more complete administration and toxicity data.
Data from Nelson JD. Pocketbook of Pediatric Antimicrobial Therapy, 10th ed. Baltimore, Williams & Wilkins, 1993; Feigin RD, Cherry JD. Textbook of Pediatric Infectious Diseases, 3rd ed., Philadelphia, WB Saunders, 1992; American Academy of Pediatrics. Antimicrobials and related therapy. In Peter G, ed. 1994 Red Book: Report of the Committee on Infectious Diseases, 23rd ed. Elk Grove Village, Ill., American Academy of Pediatrics, 1994, pp. 560–562.

Table 31–14. Agents Useful in Treating Selected Parasitic Infections in Immunologically
Compromised Children*

Parasitic Agent	Therapy of Choice and Dose	Comments
Entamoeba histolytica (severe infection)	Metronidazole 35–50 mg/kg/day (1–1.4 g/M²/day) q8h PO for 10 days or Dehydroemetine 1.0–1.5 mg/kg/day (29–41 mg/M²/day) (maximum 90 mg) q12h IM for 5 days either drug followed by Iodoquinol 40 mg/kg/day (1.1 g/M²/day) q8h PO for 20 days or if hepatic abscess Chloroquine phosphate 10 mg base/kg (maximum 300 mg base) (290 mg/M²/day) q24h PO for 2–3 wk	Dehydroemetine available from Centers for Disease Control and Prevention.
Giardia lamblia	Quinacrine HCl 6 mg/kg/day (170 mg/M²/day) q8h PO (maximum dose 300 mg/day) for 7 days	Alternative therapies: metronidazole, furazolidine.
Isospora belli	Trimethoprim-sulfamethoxazole (TMP/SMX) 10 mg TMP—50 mg SMX/kg/day (280 mg TMP—1.4 g SMX/M²/day) q6h PO for 10 days then 5 mg TMP—25 mg SMX/kg/day q12h for 3 wk	
Pneumocystis carinii	See Table 31–10	
Strongyloides stercoralis	Thiabendazole 50 mg/kg/day (1.4 g/M²/day) q12h PO, maximum dose 3 g/day for 2 days (5 days or longer for disseminated disease)	Clarithromycin proven effective in adults.
Toxoplasma gondii	Pyrimethamine 2 mg/kg/day (60 mg/M²/day) q12h PO for 3 days then 1 mg/kg/day (maximum 25 mg/day) × 4 wk plus Sulfadiazine 100–200 mg/kg/day (2.8–5.4 g/M²/day) q6h PO × 4 wk	
Cryptosporidium sp.	Spiramycin 100 mg/kg/day (2.4 g/M²/day) q6h PO	Spiramycin is an investigational drug; no data are available relating to children; octreotide may control diarrhea; paromomycin and azithromycin also possibly effective.

*Consult drug product information sheets (package inserts) and other sources for more complete administration and toxicity data.
Data from Nelson JD. Pocketbook of Pediatric Antimicrobial Therapy, 10th ed. Baltimore, Williams & Wilkins, 1993; Feigin RD, Cherry JD. Textbook of Pediatric Infectious Diseases, 3rd ed. Philadelphia, WB Saunders, 1992; American Academy of Pediatrics. Drugs for parasitic infections. In Peter G, ed. 1994 Red Book: Report of the Committee on Infectious Diseases, 23rd ed. Elk Grove Village, Ill., American Academy of Pediatrics, 1994, pp. 576–599.

immunoglobulin deficiency need only replacement therapy. However, prevention of infection in the more severely compromised child (immunosuppressed, transplant recipient, combined immunodeficiency) requires considerable organization and expense. Frequently, ill-advised preventive measures can lead to greater opportunistic infection rather than protection.

Baseline Studies

In newly acquired immunologic defects as well as hereditary defects, it is important to determine the past microorganism experience of the patient as well as that of close family contacts. A generous amount of serum should be obtained for routine serologic baseline value determinations at the time and the majority of the specimen saved for future comparative study. The following baseline antibody studies should be performed: *Toxoplasma*, cytomegalovirus, herpes simplex, varicella-zoster virus, and measles. A tuberculin and *Candida* skin test should be placed, and tuberculin testing of family members also should be carried out frequently.

Surveillance Cultures

When patients with severe immunodeficiencies with neutropenia are seen initially, baseline cultures of throat and stool should be obtained to determine bacterial and fungal flora. The throat and urine specimens should be cultured for viruses in patients with B-cell and T-cell immunodeficiencies.

Stool examination for ova and parasites also is indicated. In severely compromised children, routine culture monitoring should frequently be continued, as changes in flora can be used to predict forthcoming disease.

Immunization

Following historic and serologic data, many active and passive immunologic procedures can be useful. Inactivated polio and influenza vaccines should be administered to all patients. Passive immunization with varicella-zoster immune globulin or other gamma globulins should be used following known exposures. Tetanus and diphtheria immunizations should be kept up to date.

General Care of Severely Compromised Patients

Patients with immunologic defects should not have undue exposure when being treated at home. Patients should be discouraged from having contact with pets and should avoid crowds and other situations that may involve heavy exposure to potentially infectious microorganisms. In the hospital, protective care should be practiced. Some protective care practices place considerable restrictions on the patient, visitors, and the medical staff. Poorly carried out protective care procedures are frequently worse than no protective care procedures at all.

In general, immunocompromised children should be cared for with infection precautions that are not different from routine good patient care techniques (Garner and Simmons, 1983). For these children, routine techniques must be emphasized and enforced. All personnel and others having contact with the child must wash their hands before, during, and after patient care. Immunocompromised children should be separated from patients who are infected or who have conditions that result in infection transmission. Private rooms should be used whenever possible.

The hallmark of good protective care is handwashing. Unfortunately, in many elaborate settings this is overlooked or is performed improperly. There are two types of handwashing. The first is the surgical scrub; the second is a quick wash designed only to remove surface bacteria likely to have been picked up from recent contact. Except when certain procedures (e.g., catheter insertion) are to be carried out, the single quick wash is all that should be done (Sprunt et al., 1973; Steere and Mallison, 1975). This is particularly important for persons spending a considerable amount of time with the child in protective care. If their hands contain normal flora, they are less likely to become heavily colonized with more resistant gram-negative bacillary organisms from the hospital environment.

Although frequently employed, masks offer little in the way of protective care. The mask that remains on for a prolonged period of time concentrates organisms, so that if it is touched (e.g., rubbing the nose), it creates a greater hazard than no mask at all.

Because opportunistic infections with hospital organisms are the major problem in the severely compromised individual, protective practices should be directed against these agents. Hospital equipment involved in multiple patient use must be carefully monitored. This equipment includes respirators, ophthalmoscopes, pumps, stands, thermometers, and so on. Other environmental sources of gram-negative organisms, including flower vases, improperly maintained soap dispensers, water-surrounded bar soap, and raw fruits and vegetables, should be monitored carefully.

Second only to handwashing in the success of protective care is the exclusion of personnel and visitors who are disseminators of microorganisms. All persons with respiratory illnesses or cutaneous lesions of any sort should not be allowed in the room of an immunocompromised patient.

Prophylactic Antimicrobial Agents

Although there is considerable controversy relating to the role of prophylactic antimicrobial agents in the prevention of opportunistic infections, it is clear that in some instances they have a place. In patients with urinary catheters, serious systemic infections can be prevented by using a continuous bladder rinse with either a neomycin-polymyxin or a 0.25% acetic acid solution.

Silver and sulfa compounds locally can be useful in reducing systemic infections in burn patients. Nonadsorbable antibiotics can be used to reduce the total number of organisms in the gastrointestinal tract; this would appear to be useful in transplantation patients.

The systemic use of antibiotics can be expected to be successful prophylactically when a particular drug is used to prevent infections with one or two specific organisms. Penicillin administration can be used to prevent pneumococcal infections in asplenic individuals and streptococcal infection at the time of dental surgery in persons with cardiac defects. Prevention of staphylococcal infection of prostheses (heart valves, CNS shunts) with oxacillin or nafcillin administration may be possible. Prophylactic administration of trimethoprim-sulfamethoxazole is useful for the prevention of *Pneumocystis* infections in children on immunosuppressive therapy.

The administration of acyclovir orally to adults with leukemia and following bone marrow transplantation has been successful in preventing troublesome cutaneous herpes simplex virus lesions (Anderson et al., 1984; Wade et al., 1984).

Prophylactic Intravenous Immunoglobulin (IVIG)

IVIG is highly effective in patients with agammaglobulinemia. Recent studies indicate its usefulness in selected children with HIV infections (see Chapter 18).

References

Abramovsky CR, Quinn D, Bradford WD, Conant NF. Systemic infection by *Fusarium* in a burned child. J Pediatr 84:561–564, 1974.

Adams JM, Speer ME, Rudolph AJ. Bacterial colonization of radial artery catheters. Pediatrics 65:94–97, 1980.

Alexander JW. Immunological considerations in burn injury and the role of vaccination. In Stone H, Polk HC, eds. Contemporary Burn Management. Boston, Little, Brown & Co, 1971a, pp 265–280.

Alexander JW. Control of infection following burn injury. Arch Surg 103:435–441, 1971b.

Alexander JW, Dionigi R, Meakins JL. Periodic variation in the antibacterial function of human neutrophils and its relationship to sepsis. Ann Surg 173:206–213, 1971.

Alexander JW, Meakins JL. A physiologic basis for the development of opportunistic infection in man. Ann Surg 176:273–287, 1972.

Aly R, Maibach HI, Shinefield HR, Strauss WG. Survival of pathogenic microorganisms on human skin. J Invest Dermatol 58:205–210, 1972.

Aly R, Maibach HI, Rahman R, Shinefield HR, Mandel AD. Correlation of human in vivo and in vitro cutaneous antimicrobial factors. J Infect Dis 131:579–583, 1975.

American Academy of Pediatrics. HIV Infection and AIDS. In Peter G, ed. 1994 Red Book: Report of the Committee on Infectious Diseases, 23rd ed. Elk Grove Village, Ill., American Academy of Pediatrics, 1994a, pp 254–270.

American Academy of Pediatrics. Antiviral drugs. In Peter G, ed. 1994 Red Book: Report of the Committee on Infectious Diseases, 23rd ed. Elk Grove Village, Ill., American Academy of Pediatrics, 1994b, pp 568–569.

American Academy of Pediatrics. Drugs of choice for invasive and other serious fungal infections. In Peter G, ed. 1994 Red Book: Report of the Committee on Infectious Diseases, 23rd ed. Elk Grove Village, Ill., American Academy of Pediatrics, 1994c, pp 560–561.

American Academy of Pediatrics. Drugs for parasitic infections. In Peter G, ed. 1994 Red Book: Report of the Committee on Infectious Diseases, 23rd ed. Elk Grove Village, Ill., American Academy of Pediatrics, 1994d, pp 576–599.

Ammann AJ, Wara DW. Evaluation of infants and children with recurrent infection. Curr Probl Pediatr 4:1–47, 1975.

Anderson H, Scarffe JH, Sutton RNP, Hickmott E, Brigden D, Burke C. Oral acyclovir prophylaxis against herpes simplex virus in non-Hodgkin lymphoma and acute lymphoblastic leukaemia patients receiving remission induction chemotherapy: a randomised double blind, placebo controlled trial. Br J Cancer 50:45–49, 1984.

Anderson R. Assessment of oral ascorbate in three children with chronic granulomatous disease and defective neutrophil motility over a 2-year period. Clin Exp Immunol 43:180–188, 1981.

Andrews W, Fyock B, Gray S, Coln D, Hendrickse W, Siegel J, Belknap R, Hogge A, Benser M, Kennard B, Stewart S, Albertson N. Pediatric liver transplantation: the Dallas experience. Transplant Proc 19:3267–3276, 1987.

Azimi PH, Levernier K, Lefrak LM, Petru AM, Barrett T, Schenck H, Sandhu AS, Duritz G, Valesco M. *Malassezia furfur*: a cause of occlusion of percutaneous central venous catheters in infants in the intensive care nursery. Pediatr Infect Dis J 7:100–103, 1988.

Baehner RL. Disorders of leukocytes leading to recurrent infection. Pediatr Clin North Am 19:935–956, 1972.

Bailey TC, Ettinger NA, Storch GA, Trulock EP, Hanto DW, Dunagan WC, Jendrisak MD, McCullough CS, Kenzora JL, Powderly WG. Failure of high-dose oral acyclovir with or without immune globulin to prevent primary cytomegalovirus disease in recipients of solid organ transplants. Am J Med 95:273–278, 1993.

Baker CJ, Melish ME, Hall RT, Casto DT, Vasan U, Givner LB, the Multicenter Group for the Study of Immune Globulin in Neonates. Intravenous immune globulin for the prevention of nosocomial infection in low-birth-weight neonates. N Engl J Med 327:213–219, 1992.

Baker RD, Severance AO. Mucormycosis with report of acute mycotic pneumonia (abstract). Am J Pathol 24:716–717, 1948.

Band JD, Maki DG. Infections caused by arterial catheters used for hemodynamic monitoring. Am J Med 67:735–741, 1979.

Band JD, Maki DG. Steel needles used for intravenous therapy. Morbidity in patients with hematologic malignancy. Arch Intern Med 140:31–34, 1980.

Barnett ED, Klein JO, Pelton SI, Luginbuhl LM. Otitis media in children born to human immunodeficiency virus–infected mothers. Pediatr Infect Dis J 11:360–364, 1992.

Barrett-Connor E. Bacterial infection and sickle cell anemia: An analysis of 250 infections in 166 patients and a review of the literature. Medicine 50:97–112, 1971.

Barst RJ, Prince AS, Neu HC. Aspergillus endocarditis in children: case report and review of the literature. Pediatrics 68:73–78, 1981.

Barzilay Z, Mandel M, Keren G, Davidson S. Nosocomial bacterial pneumonia in ventilated children: clinical significance of culture-positive peripheral bronchial aspirates. J Pediatr 112:421–424, 1988.

Becker W, Naude DT, Kipps A, McKensie D. Virus studies in disseminated herpes simplex infections associated with malnutrition in children. S Afr Med J 37:74–76, 1963.

Begala JE, Maher K, Cherry JD. Risk of infection associated with the use of Broviac and Hickman catheters. Am J Infect Control 10:17–23, 1982.

Benjamin RP, Callaway L, Conant NF. Facial granuloma associated with Fusarium infection. Arch Dermatol 101:598–600, 1970.

Bernhard VM. Management of infected vascular prostheses. Surg Clin North Am 55:1411–1417, 1975.

Black JA, Challacombe DN, Ockenden BG. Nephrotic syndrome associated with bacteremia after shunt operations for hydrocephalus. Lancet 2:921–924, 1965.

Blair DC, Weiner LB. Prosthetic valve endocarditis due to *Haemophilus parainfluenzae* biotype II. Am J Dis Child 133:617–618, 1979.

Bode FR, Pare JAP, Fraser RG. Pulmonary diseases in the compromised host. Medicine 53:255–293, 1974.

Bodey GP. Antibiotics in patients with neutropenia. Arch Intern Med 144:1845–1851, 1984.

Bodey GP, Buckley M, Sathe YS, Freireich EJ. Quantitative relationships between circulating leukocytes and infection in patients with acute leukemia. Ann Intern Med 64:328–340, 1966.

Boeckman CR, Krill CE, Jr. Bacterial and fungal infections complicating parenteral alimentation in infants and children. J Pediatr Surg 5:117–126, 1970.

Boyce JM, Potter-Bynoe G, Opal SM, Dziobek L, Medeiros AA. A common-source outbreak of *Staphylococcus epidermidis* infections among patients undergoing cardiac surgery. J Infect Dis 161:493–499, 1990.

Brandt L, Swahn G. Subacute bacterial endocarditis due to coagulase negative *Staphylococcus albus*. Acta Med Scand 166:125–132, 1960.

Brayman KL, Stephanian E, Matas AJ, Schmidt W, Payne WD, Sutherland DER, Gores PF, Najarian JS, Dunn DL. Analysis of infectious complications occurring after solid-organ transplantation. Arch Surg 127:38–48, 1992.

Brodie E, Adler JL, Daly AK. Bacterial endocarditis due to an unusual species of encapsulated *Neisseria; Neisseria* mucosa endocarditis. Am J Dis Child 122:433–437, 1971.

Brown AE. Neutropenia, fever, and infection. Am J Med 76:421–428, 1984.

Bruton OC. Agammaglobulinemia. Pediatrics 9:722–727, 1952.

Bryson YJ. The use of acyclovir in children. Pediatr Infect Dis 3:345–348, 1984.

Buckley RH. Immunodeficiency. J Allergy Clin Immunol 72:627–643, 1983.

Burgio GR, Duse M, Monafo V, Ascione A, Nespoli L. Selective IgA deficiency: clinical and immunological evaluation of 50 pediatric patients. Eur J Pediatr 133:101–106, 1980.

Burtenshaw JML. The autogenous disinfection of the skin. Dermatology 158–185, 1948.

Buxton AE, Highsmith AK, Garner JS, West M, Stamm WE, Dixon RE, McGowan JE, Jr. Contamination of intravenous infusion fluid: effects of changing administration sets. Ann Intern Med 90:764–768, 1979.

Caldwell RL, Hurwitz RA, Girod DA. Subacute bacterial endocarditis in children. Am J Dis Child 122:312–315, 1971.

Cannon PR. The relationship of protein metabolism to antibody production and resistance to infection. Advances in Protein Chemistry 135–154, 1945.

Carr A, Penny R, Cooper DA. Efficacy and safety of rechallenge with low-dose trimethoprim-sulphamethoxazole in previously hypersensitive HIV-infected patients. AIDS 7:65–71, 1993.

[CDC] Centers for Disease Control. National nosocomial infections study report: annual summary, 1978, issued March 1981.

[CDC] Centers for Disease Control. Update: Acquired Immunodeficiency Syndrome—United States. MMWR 34:245–248, 1985.

[CDC] Centers for Disease Control. Classification system for human immunodeficiency virus (HIV) infection in children under 13 years of age. MMWR 36:225–236, 1987.

[CDC] Centers for Disease Control. 1993 revised classification system for HIV infection and expanded surveillance case definition for AIDS among adolescents and adults. MMWR 41(RR-17):1–19, 1992.

[CDC] Centers for Disease Control and Prevention. Initial therapy for tuberculosis in the era of multidrug resistance: recommendations of the advisory council for the elimination of tuberculosis. MMWR 42(RR-7):1–8, 1993a.

[CDC] Centers for Disease Control and Prevention. Recommendations on prophylaxis and therapy for disseminated *Mycobacterium avium* complex for adults and adolescents infected with human immunodeficiency virus. MMWR 42(RR-9):17–20, 1993b.

[CDC] Centers for Disease Control and Prevention. 1995 revised guidelines for prophylaxis against *Pneumocystis carinii* pneumonia for children infected with or perinatally exposed to human immunodeficiency virus. MMWR 44(RR-4):1–11, 1995.

Chandra RK. Immunocompetence in undernutrition. J Pediatr 81:1194–1200, 1972.

Chandwani S, Borkowsky W, Krasinski K, Lawrence R, Welliver R. Respiratory syncytial virus infection in human immunodeficiency virus–infected children. J Pediatr 117:251–254, 1990.

Cherry JD. Selection of antimicrobial agents for initial treatment of suspected septicemia in infants and children. Rev Infect Dis 5:S32–S39, 1983.

Chilcote RR, Baehner RL, Hammond D, and the investigators and Special Studies Committee of the Children's Cancer Study Group. Septicemia and meningitis in children splenectomized for Hodgkin's disease. N Engl J Med 295:798–800, 1976.

Chin TW, Stiehm ER, Falloon J, Gallin JI. Corticosteroids in treatment of obstructive lesions of chronic granulomatous disease. J Pediatr 111:349–352, 1987.

Christensen CE, Emmanouilides GC. Bacterial endocarditis due to *Moraxella* new species I. N Engl J Med 277:803–804, 1967.

Chusid MJ, Parrillo JE, Fauci AS. Chronic granulomatous disease: diagnosis in a 27-year-old man with *Mycobacterium fortuitum*. JAMA 233:1295–1296, 1975.

Claman HN. Corticosteroids and lymphoid cells. N Engl J Med 287:388–397, 1972.

Commers JR, Robichaud KJ, Pizzo PA. New pulmonary infiltrates in granulocytopenic cancer patients being treated with antibiotics. Pediatr Infect Dis 3:423–428, 1984.

Conti DJ, Freed BM, Lempert N. Prophylactic immunoglobulin therapy improves the outcome of renal transplantation in recipients at risk for primary cytomegalovirus disease. Transplant Proc 25:1421–1422, 1993.

Cooper MR, DeChatelet LR, McCall CE, LaVia MF, Spurr CL, Baehner RL. Complete deficiency of leukocyte glucose-6-phosphate dehydrogenase with defective bactericidal activity. J Clin Invest 51:769–778, 1972.

Cooperstock MS. Indigenous flora in host economy and pathogenesis. In Feigin RD, Cherry JD, eds. Textbook of Pediatric Infectious Diseases, 3rd ed. Philadelphia, WB Saunders, 1992, pp 91–119.

Crossley K, Matsen JM. The scalp-vein needle: a prospective study of complications. JAMA 220:985–987, 1972.

Cruse P. Wound infection surveillance. Rev Infect Dis 3:734–737, 1981.

Cruse PJE, Foord R. The epidemiology of wound infection: a 10-year prospective study of 62,939 wounds. Symp Surg Infect 60:27–40, 1980.

Curnutte JT. Conventional versus interferon-γ therapy in chronic granulomatous disease. J Infect Dis 167:S8–S12, 1993.

Curry ER, Quie PG. Fungal septicemia in patients receiving parenteral hyperalimentation. N Engl J Med 285:1221–1225, 1971.

Dajani AS, Bisno AL, Chung KJ, Durack DT, Freed M, Gerber MA, Karchmer AW, Millard D, Rahimtoola S, Shulman ST, Watanakunakorn C, Taubert KA. Prevention of bacterial endocarditis: recommendations by the American Heart Association. JAMA 264:2919–2922, 1990.

Dale DC. Potential role of colony-stimulating factors in the prevention and treatment of infectious diseases. Clin Infect Dis 18:S180–S188, 1994.

Dale CD, Petersdorf RG. Corticosteroids and infectious diseases. Med Clin North Am 57:1277–1287, 1973.

Dammin GJ, Cough NP, Murray JE. Prolonged survival of skin homografts in uremic patients. Ann NY Acad Sci 64:967–976, 1957.

Davis SD, Schaller J, Wedgwood RJ. Job's syndrome: recurrent "cold" staphylococcal abscesses. Lancet 1:1013–1015, 1966.

Davis SD, Sobocinski K, Hoffman RG, Mohr B, Nelson DB. Postoperative wound infections in a children's hospital. Pediatr Infect Dis 3:114–116, 1984.

Dawson S, Pai M, Smith S, Rothney M, Ahmed K, Barr R. Right atrial catheters in children with cancer: a decade of experience in the use of tunnelled, exteriorized devices at a single institution. Am J Pediatr Hematol Oncol 13:126–129, 1991.

Decker MD, Edwards KM. Central venous catheter infections. Pediatr Clin 35:579–612, 1988.

Deen JL, Blumberg DA. Infectious disease considerations in pediatric organ transplantation. Semin Pediatr Surg 2:218–234, 1993.

Deinard AS, Libit SA. Coagulase negative staphylococci bacteria in a child. Pediatrics 49:300–302, 1972.

Dichter JR, Levine SJ, Shelhamer JH. Approach to the immunocompromised host with pulmonary symptoms. Hematol/Oncol Clin North Am 7:887–912, 1993.

DiGeorge AM. Congenital absence of the thymus and its immunologic consequences: concurrence with congenital hypoparathyroidism. In Bergsma D, Good RA, eds. Immunologic Deficiency Diseases in Man. New York, The National Foundation, 1968, pp 116–123.

Di John D, Krasinski K, Lawrence R, Borkowsky W, Johnson JP, Schieken LS, Rennels MB. Very late onset of group B streptococcal disease in infants infected with the human immunodeficiency virus. Pediatr Infect Dis J 9:925–928, 1990.

Dillon JD, Jr, Schaffner W, Van Way CW III, Meng HL. Septicemia and total parenteral nutrition: distinguishing catheter-related from other septic episodes. JAMA 223:1341–1344, 1973.

Donabedian H, Gallin JI. The hyperimmunoglobulin E–recurrent infection (Job's) syndrome: a review of the NIH experience and the literature. Medicine 62:195–208, 1983.

Dudrick SJ, Wilmore DW, Vars HM. Long-term total parenteral nutrition with growth, development and positive nitrogen balance. Surgery 64:134–142, 1968.

Ederer GM, Matsen JM. Colonization and infection with *Pseudomonas cepacia*. J Infect Dis 125:613–618, 1972.

Editorial: Infective hazards of splenectomy. Lancet 1:1167–1168, 1976.

Edmondson EB, Reinarz JA, Pierce AK, Sanford JP. Nebulization equipment: a potential source of infection in gram-negative pneumonias. Am J Dis Child 111:357–360, 1966.

Eickhoff TC. Hospital infections. Disease of the Month. Chicago, Year Book Medical Publishers, 1972.

Eickhoff TC. Nosocomial infections. Am J Epidemiol 101:93–97, 1975.

Elves MW, Israels MCG, Collinge M. An assessment of the mixed leukocyte reaction in renal failure. Lancet 1:682–685, 1966.

Elward K, Hruby N, Christy C. Pneumococcal endocarditis in infants and children: report of a case and review of the literature. Pediatr Infect Dis J 9:652–657, 1990.

Erlendsson K, Swartz T, Dwyer JM. Successful reversal of echovirus encephalitis in X-linked hypogammaglobulinemia by intraventricular administration of immunoglobulin. N Engl J Med 312:351–353, 1985.

Esterly JR, Sturner WQ, Esterly NB, Windhorst DB. Disseminated BCG in twin boys with presumed chronic granulomatous disease of childhood. Pediatrics 48:141–144, 1971.

Ezer G, Soothill JR. Intracellular bactericidal effects of rifampicin in both normal and chronic granulomatous disease polymorphs. Arch Dis Child 49:463–466, 1974.

Faber K. Tuberculosis and nutrition. Acta Tuberc Scand 12:287–335, 1938.

Falloon J, Eddy J, Wiener L, Pizzo PA. Human immunodeficiency virus infection in children. J Pediatr 114:1–30, 1989.

Feigin RD, Matson DO. Opportunistic infections: the compromised host. In Feigin RD, Cherry JD, eds. Textbook of Pediatric Infectious Diseases, 3rd ed. Philadelphia, WB Saunders, 1992, pp 960–989.

Feigin RD, Shearer WT. Opportunistic infection in children. I and II. In the compromised host. J Pediatr 87:507–514, 677–694, 1975.

Feller I, Crane KH. National burn information exchange. Surg Clin North Am 50:1425–1436, 1970.

Ferguson AC, Lawlor GJ, Neumann CG, Oh W, Stiehm ER. Decreased rosette-forming lymphocytes in malnutrition and intrauterine growth retardation. J Pediatr 85:717–723, 1974.

Fikrig SM, Schiffman G, Philipp JC, Moel DI. Antibody response to capsular polysaccharide vaccine of *Streptococcus pneumoniae* in patients with nephrotic syndrome. J Infect Dis 137:818–821, 1978.

Fisher MC, Long SS, Roberts EM, Dunn JM, Balsara RK. *Pseudomonas maltophilia* bacteremia in children undergoing open heart surgery. JAMA 246:1571–1574, 1981.

Flynn PM, Shenep JL. Acquired immunodeficiency syndrome. In Patrick CC, ed. Infections in Immunocompromised Infants and Children. New York, Churchill Livingstone, 1992, pp 161–177.

Flynn PM, Shenep JL, Stokes DC, Barrett FF. *In situ* management of confirmed central venous catheter–related bacteremia. Pediatr Infect Dis J 6:729–734, 1987b.

Flynn PM, Van Hooser B, Gigliotti F. Atypical mycobacterial infections of Hickman catheter exit sites. Pediatr Infect Dis J 7:510–513, 1988.

Flynn PM, Weinstein RA, Nathan C, Gaston MA, Kabins SA. Patients' endogenous flora as the source of "nosocomial" *Enterobacter* in cardiac surgery. J Infect Dis 156:363–368, 1987a.

Foley FD. The burn autopsy: fatal complications of burns. Am J Clin Pathol 52:1–13, 1969.

Foroozanfar N, Lucas CF, Joss DV, Hugh-Jones K, Hobbs JR. Ascorbate (1 gm/day) does not help the phagocytic killing defect of X-linked chronic granulomatous disease. Clin Exp Immunol 41:99–102, 1983.

Frayha HH, Biggar WD. Chronic granulomatous disease of childhood: a changing pattern? J Clin Immunol 3:287–291, 1983.

Frazier JP, Kramer WG, Pickering LK, Culbert S, Brandt K, Frankel LS. Antimicrobial therapy of febrile children with malignancies and possible sepsis. Pediatr Infect Dis 3:40–45, 1984.

Freeman J, Goldmann DA, Smith NE, Sidebottom DG, Epstein MF, Platt R. Association of intravenous lipid emulsion and coagulase-negative staphylococcal bacteremia in neonatal intensive care units. N Engl J Med 323:301–308, 1990.

Freeman JB, Litton AA. Preponderance of gram-positive infections during parenteral alimentation. Surg Gynecol Obstet 139:905–908, 1974.

Frenkel LD, Gaur S, Tsolia M, Scudder R, Howell R, Kesarwala H. Cytomegalovirus infection in children with AIDS. Rev Infect Dis 12:S820–S826, 1990.

Freyre EA, Chabes A, Poémape O, Chabes A. Abnormal Rebuck skin window response in kwashiorkor. J Pediatr 82:523–526, 1973.

Fricker FJ, Griffith BP, Hardesty RL, Trento A, Gold LM, Schmeltz K, Beerman LB, Fischer DR, Mathews RA, Neches WH, Park SC, Zuberbuhler JR, Lenox CC, Bahnson HT. Experience with heart transplantation in children. Pediatrics 79:138–146, 1987.

Friedland LR, Raphael SA, Deutsch ES, Johal J, Martyn LJ, Visvesvara GS, Lischner HW. Disseminated *Acanthamoeba* infection in a child with symptomatic human immunodeficiency virus infection. Pediatr Infect Dis J 11:404–407, 1992.

Friedland LR, Shelton S, Paris M, Rinderknecht S, Ehrett S, Krisher K, McCracken GH Jr. Dilemmas in diagnosis and management of cephalosporin-resistant *Streptococcus pneumoniae* meningitis. Pediatr Infect Dis J 12:196–200, 1993.

Friedman LE, Brown AE, Miller DR, Armstrong D. *Staphylococcus epidermidis* septicemia in children with leukemia and lymphoma. Am J Dis Child 41:715–719, 1984.

Furfaro S, Gauthier M, Lacroix J, Nadeau D, Lafleur L, Mathews S. Arterial catheter–related infections in children: a 1-year cohort analysis. Am J Dis Child 145:1037–1043, 1991.

Gallin JI, Buescher ES, Seligmann BE, Nath J, Gaither T, Katz P. Recent advances in chronic granulomatous disease. Ann Intern Med 99:657–674, 1983.

Gardner P, Goldmann DA. Hospital control of infections: nosocomial infections. In Feigin RD, Cherry JD, eds. Textbook of Pediatric Infectious Diseases, 3rd ed. Philadelphia, WB Saunders, 1992, pp. 2145–2157.

Garner JS, Simmons BP. CDC guideline for isolation precautions in hospitals and CDC guideline for infection control in hospital personnel. Infect Control 4:245–325, 1983.

Gatti RA, Stutman O, Good RA. The lymphoid system. Ann Rev Physiol 32:529–546, 1970.

Geefhuysen J, Rosen EU, Katz J, Ipp T, Metz J. Impaired cellular immunity in kwashiorkor with improvement after therapy. Br Med J 4:527–529, 1971.

Gelfand EW, McCurdy D, Rao CP, Middleton PJ. Ribavirin treatment of viral pneumonitis in severe combined immunodeficiency disease (letter). Lancet 2:732–733, 1983.

George DL. Epidemiology of nosocomial ventilator-associated pneumonia. Infect Control Hosp Epidemiol 14:163–169, 1993.

Gitlin D, Janeway CA, Apt L, Craig JM. Agammaglobulinemia. In Lawrence HS, ed. Cellular and Humoral Aspects of the Hypersensitive States. New York, Hoeber Medical Division, Harper & Row, 1959, pp 375–441.

Givner LB, Kaplan SL. Meningitis due to *Staphylococcus aureus* in children. Clin Infect Dis 16:766–771, 1993.

Glaser CA, Angulo FJ, Rooney JA. Animal-associated opportunistic infections among persons infected with the human immunodeficiency virus. Clin Infect Dis 18:14–24, 1994.

Gmünder FK, Seger RA. Chronic granulomatous disease: mode of action of sulfamethoxazole/trimethoprim. Pediatr Res 15:1533–1537, 1981.

Goldberg P, Shulman ST, Yogev R. Group C streptococcal endocarditis. Pediatrics 75:114–116, 1985.

Goldman DA, Maki DG. Infection control in total parenteral nutrition. JAMA 223:1360–1364, 1973.

Goldstein IM, Marder SR. Infections and hypocomplementemia. Ann Rev Med 34:47–53, 1983.

Gooch WM III, Fernbach DJ. Immunoglobulins during the course of acute leukemia in children: effects of various clinical factors. Cancer 28:984–989, 1971.

Gorelick MH, Owen WC, Seibel NL, Reaman GH. Lack of association between neutropenia and the incidence of bacteremia associated with indwelling central venous catheters in febrile pediatric cancer patients. Pediatr Infect Dis J 10:506–510, 1991.

Gradon JD, Timpone JG, Schnittman SM. Emergence of unusual opportunistic pathogens in AIDS: a review. Clin Infect Dis 15:134–157, 1992.

Green M, Wald ER, Fricker FJ, Griffith BP, Trento A. Infections in pediatric orthotopic heart transplant recipients. Pediatr Infect Dis J 8:87–93, 1989.

Gregory JE, Golden A, Haymaker W. Mucormycosis of the central nervous system: a report of 3 cases. Bull Johns Hopkins Hosp 73:405–419, 1943.

Griffin JR, Pettit TH, Fishman LS, Foos RY. Blood-borne *Candida* endophthalmitis: a clinical and pathologic study of 21 cases. Arch Ophthalmol 89:450–456, 1973.

Groff DB. Complication of intravenous hyperalimentation in new-borns and infants. J Pediatr Surg 4:460–464, 1969.

Haag-Weber M, Hörl WH. Uremia and infection: mechanisms of impaired cellular host defense. Nephron 63:125–131, 1993.

Hall CB. Respiratory syncytial virus. In Feigin RD, Cherry JD, eds. Textbook of Pediatric Infectious Diseases, 3rd ed. Philadelphia, WB Saunders, 1992, pp 1633–1656.

Hand IL, Wiznia AA, Porricolo M, Lambert G, Caspe WB. Aerosolized pentamidine for prophylaxis of *Pneumocystis carinii* pneumonia in infants with human immunodeficiency virus infection. Pediatr Infect Dis J 13:100–104, 1994.

Haning HAL, Johnston R, Touloukian R, Margolis CZ. Successfully treated *Candida* endophthalmitis in a child. Pediatrics 51:1027–1031, 1973.

Hanson CG, Shearer WT. Pediatric HIV infection and AIDS. In Feigin RD, Cherry JD, eds. Textbook of Pediatric Infectious Diseases, 3rd ed. Philadelphia, WB Saunders, 1992, pp 990–1011.

Hanson IC. Respiratory infections in HIV-infected children. Immunol Allergy Clin North Am 13:205–217, 1993.

Harbin RL, Schaffner W. Septicemia associated with scalp-vein needles. South Med J 66:638–640, 1973.

Harmon WE. Opportunistic infections in children following renal transplantation. J Pediatr Nephrol 5:118, 1991.

Hart PD, Russell E Jr, Remington JS. The compromised host and infection: II. Deep fungal infection. J Infect Dis 120:169–191, 1969.

Hattori K, Hasui M, Masuda K, Masuda M, Ogino H, Kobayashi Y. Successful trimethoprim-sulfamethoxazole therapy in a patient with hyperimmunoglobulin E syndrome. Acta Paediatr 82:324–326, 1993.

Hausser C, Virelizier JL, Buriot D, Griscelli C. Common variable hypogammaglobulinemia in children: clinical and immunologic observations in 30 patients. Am J Dis Child 137:833–837, 1983.

Hewitt WL, Sanford JP. Workshop on hospital-associated infections. J Infect Dis 130:680–686, 1974.

Hiatt JR, Ament ME, Berquist WJ, Brems JF, Brill JE, Colonna JD II, El Khoury G, Quinones WJ, Ramming KP, Vargas JH, Busuttil RW. Pediatric liver transplantation at UCLA. Transplant Proc 19:3282–3288, 1987.

Hiemenz JW, Greene JN. Special considerations for the patient undergoing allogeneic or autologous bone marrow transplantation. Hematol Oncol Clin North Am 7:961–1002, 1993.

Hill HR. Intravenous immunoglobulin use in the neonate: role in prophylaxis and therapy of infection. Pediatr Infect Dis J 12:549–559, 1993.

Hitzig WH, Barandun S, Cottier H. Die schweizerische form der agammaglobulinamie. Ergeb Inn Med Kinderheilkd 27:79–154, 1968.

Hoger PH, Seger RA, Schaad B, Hitzig WH. Chronic granulomatous disease: uptake and intracellular activity of Fosfomycin in granulocytes. Pediatr Res 19:38–44, 1985.

Holland JF, Senn H, Banerjee T. Quantitative studies of localized leukocyte mobilization in acute leukemia. Blood 37:499–511, 1971.

Hong R, Ammann AJ, Huang S, Levy RL, Davenport G, Bach ML, Bach FH, Bortin MM, Kay HEM. Cartilage-hair hypoplasia: effect of thymus transplants. Clin Immunol Immunopathol 1:15–26, 1972.

Horan TC, Culver DH, Gaynes RP, Jarvis WR, Edwards JR, Reid CR, and the National Nosocomial Infectious Surveillance (NNIS) System. Nosocomial infections in surgical patients in the United States, January 1986–June 1992. Infect Control Hosp Epidemiol 14:73–80, 1993.

Hoyt L, Oleske J, Holland B, Connor E. Nontuberculous mycobacteria in children with acquired immunodeficiency syndrome. Pediatr Infect Dis J 11:354–360, 1992.

Hughes WT. Fatal infections in childhood leukemia. Am J Dis Child 122:283–287, 1971.

Hughes WT, Feldman S, Cox F. Infectious diseases in children with cancer. Pediatr Clin North Am 21:583–615, 1974.

Hughes WT. Hematogenous histoplasmosis in the immunocompromised child. J Pediatr 105:569–575, 1984.

Hughes WT, Parham DM. Molluscum contagiosum in children with cancer or acquired immunodeficiency syndrome. Pediatr Infect Dis J 10:152–156, 1991.

Hughes WT. Prevention of infections in patients with T cell defects. Clin Infect Dis 17:S368–S371, 1993.

Hyatt AC, Altenburger KM, Johnston RB Jr, Winkelstein JA. Increased susceptibility to severe pyogenic infections in patients with an inherited deficiency of the second component of complement. J Pediatr 98:417–419, 1981.

Ingram J, Weitzman S, Greenberg M, Parkin P, Filler R. Complication of indwelling venous access lines in the pediatric hematology patient: a prospective comparison of external venous catheters and subcutaneous ports. Am J Pediatr Hematol Oncol 13:130–136, 1991.

International Chronic Granulomatous Disease Cooperative Study Group. A controlled trial of interferon gamma to prevent infection in chronic granulomatous disease. N Engl J Med 324:509–516, 1991.

Jackson ME, Wong KY, Lampkin B. *Pseudomonas aeruginosa* septicemia in childhood cancer patients. Pediatr Infect Dis 1:239–241, 1982.

Jacobs MR. Treatment and diagnosis of infections caused by drug-resistant *Streptococcus pneumoniae*. Clin Infect Dis 15:119–127, 1992.

Jacobs RF, Wilson CB. Activity of antibiotics in chronic granulomatous disease leukocytes. Pediatr Res 17:916–919, 1983.

James JW. Longitudinal study of the morbidity of diarrheal and respiratory infections in malnourished children. Am J Clin Nutr 25:690–694, 1972.

Jarvis WR. Epidemiology of nosocomial infections in pediatric patients. Pediatr Infect Dis J 6:344–351, 1987.

Jarvis WR, Highsmith AK, Allen JR, Haley RW. Polymicrobial bacteremia associated with lipid emulsion in a neonatal intensive care unit. Pediatr Infect Dis 2:203–208, 1983.

Johanson WG, Jr, Seidenfeld JJ, Gomez P, De Los Santos R, Coalson JJ. Bacteriologic diagnosis of nosocomial pneumonia following prolonged mechanical ventilation. Am Rev Respir Dis 137:259–264, 1988.

Johnson CM, Rhodes KH. Pediatric endocarditis. Mayo Clin Proc 57:86–94, 1982.

Johnston RB Jr, Baehner RI. Chronic granulomatous disease: correlation between pathogenesis and clinical findings. Pediatrics 48:730–739, 1971.

Johnston RB Jr, Wilfert CM, Buckley RH, Webb LS, DeChatelet LR, McCall CE. Enhanced bactericidal activity of phagocytes from patients with chronic granulomatous disease in the presence of sulphisoxazole. Lancet 1:824–827, 1975.

Kammer RB, Utz JP. *Aspergillus* species endocarditis: the new face of a not so rare disease. Am J Med 56:506–521, 1974.

Kaplan SL. Heart transplants: infections in immunocompromised infants and children. In Patrick CC, ed. Infections in Immunocompromised Infants and Children. New York, Churchill Livingstone, 1992, pp 251–260.

Katz JA, Mustafa MM. Management of fever in granulocytopenic children with cancer. Pediatr Infect Dis J 12:330–339, 1993.

Katz M. Parasitic infections. J Pediatr 87:165–178, 1975.

Katz M. Babesiosis. Pediatr Infect Dis 1:219–221, 1982.

Kauder E, Mauer AM. Neutropenias of childhood. J Pediatr 69:147–157, 1966.

Kim KS. High-dose intravenous immune globulin impairs antibacterial activity of antibiotics. J Allergy Clin Immunol 84:579–588, 1989.

Kinney J, Mundorf L, Gleason C, Lee C, Townsend T, Thibault R, Nussbaum A, Abby H, Yolken R. Efficacy and pharmacokinetics of intravenous immune globulin administration to high-risk neonates. Am J Dis Child 145:1233–1238, 1991.

Kirkpatrick CH, Wilson WEC, Talmadge DW. Immunologic studies in human organ transplantation. I. Observation and characterization of suppressed cutaneous reactivity in uremia. J Exp Med 119:727–742, 1964.

Klainer AS, Beisel WR. Opportunistic infection: a review. Am J Med Sci 258:431–455, 1969.

Kletzel M, Beck S, Elser J, Shock N, Burks W. Trimethoprim-sulfamethoxazole oral desensitization in hemophiliacs infected with human immunodeficiency virus with a history of hypersensitivity reactions. Am J Dis Child 145:1428–1429, 1991.

Kline MW, Dunkle LM. Toxic shock syndrome and the acquired immunodeficiency syndrome. Pediatr Infect Dis J 7:736–738, 1988.

Klugman KP. Pneumococcal resistance to antibiotics. Clin Microbiol Rev 3:171–196, 1990.

Kobayashi Y, Amano D, Ueda K, Kagosaki Y, Usui T. Treatment of seven cases of chronic granulomatous disease with sulfamethoxazole-trimethoprim (SMX-TMP). Eur J Pediatr 127:247–254, 1978.

Koiwai EK, Nahas HC. Subacute bacterial endocarditis following cardiac surgery. AMA Arch Surg 73:272–278, 1956.

Koll BS, Brown AE. Changing patterns of infections in the immunocompromised patient with cancer. Hematol Oncol Clin North Am 7:753–769, 1993.

Kollef MH. Ventilator-associated pneumonia: a multivariate analysis. JAMA 270:1965–1970, 1993.

Kontny U, Höfling B, Gutjahr P, Voth D, Schwarz M, Schmitt HJ. CSF shunt infections in children. Infection 21:89–92, 1993.

Kosmidis HV, Lusher JM, Shope TC, Ravindranath Y, Dajani AS. Infections in leukemic children: a prospective analysis. J Pediatr 96:814–819, 1980.

Kramer HH, Bourgeois M, Liersch R, Kuhn H, Nebler L, Meyer H, Sievers G. Current clinical aspects of bacterial endocarditis in infancy, childhood and adolescence. Eur J Pediatr 140:253–259, 1983.

Krasinski K, Borkowsky W, Bonk S, Lawrence R, Chandwani S. Bacterial infections in human immunodeficiency virus–infected children. Pediatr Infect Dis J 7:323–328, 1988.

Kuhls TL, Leach CT. Infections in pediatric liver transplant recipients. In Patrick CC, ed. Infections in Immunocompromised Infants and Children. New York, Churchill Livingstone, 1992, pp 231–250.

Kunin CM. Detection, Prevention and Management of Urinary Tract Infections: A Manual for the Physician Nurse and Allied Health Worker. Philadelphia, Lea & Febiger, 1972.

Kunin CM, McCormack RC. Prevention of catheter-induced urinary-tract infections by sterile closed drainage. N Engl J Med 274:1155–1161, 1966.

Lacroix J, Ahronheim G, Girouard G. *Pseudomonas aeruginosa* supraglottitis in a six-month-old child with severe combined immunodeficiency syndrome. Pediatr Infect Dis J 7:739–741, 1988.

Lang PA, Ritzmann SE, Merian FL, Lawrence MC, Levin WC, Gregory R. Cellular evolution in induced inflammation in uremic patients. Tex Rep Biol Med 24:107–111, 1966.

Langley JM, LeBlanc JC, Drake J, Milner R. Efficacy of antimicrobial prophylaxis in placement of cerebrospinal fluid shunts: meta-analysis. Clin Infect Dis 7:98–103, 1993.

Lazarus GM, Neu HC. Agents responsible for infection in chronic granulomatous disease in childhood. J Pediatr 86:415–417, 1975.

Leggiadro RJ, Kline MW, Hughes WT. Extrapulmonary cryptococcosis in children with acquired immunodeficiency syndrome. Pediatr Infect Dis J 10:658–662, 1991.

Leibovitz E, Cooper D, Giurgiutiu D, Coman G, Straus I, Orlow SJ, Lawrence R. Varicella-zoster virus infection in Romanian children infected with the human immunodeficiency virus. Pediatrics 92:838–842, 1993.

Leibovitz E, Rigaud M, Chandwani S, Kaul A, Greco MA, Pollack H, Lawrence R, Di John D, Hanna B, Krasinski K, Borkowsky W. Disseminated fungal infections in children infected with human immunodeficiency virus. Pediatr Infect Dis J 10:888–894, 1991.

Leibovitz E, Rigaud M, Pollack H, Lawrence R, Chandwani S, Krasinski K, Borkowsky W. *Pneumocystis carinii* pneumonia in infants infected with the human immunodeficiency virus with more than 450 CD4 T lymphocytes per cubic millimeter. N Engl J Med 323:531–533, 1990.

Leu H-S, Kaiser DL, Mori M, Woolson RF, Wenzel RP. Hospital-acquired pneumonia: attributable mortality and morbidity. Am J Epidemiol 129:1258–1267, 1989.

Levy R, Kaplan HS. Impaired lymphocyte function in untreated Hodgkin's disease. N Engl J Med 290:181–186, 1974.

Lewis IJ, Hart CA, Baxby D. Diarrhoea due to Cryptosporidium in acute lymphoblastic leukaemia. Arch Dis Child 60:60–62, 1985.

Lewis LL, Butler KM, Husson RN, Mueller BU, Fowler CL, Steinberg SM, Pizzo PA. Defining the population of human immunodeficiency virus–infected children at risk for *Mycobacterium avium–intracellulare* infection. J Pediatr 121:677–683, 1992.

Liese JG, Wintergerst U, Tympner KD, Belohradsky BH. High- vs. low-dose immunoglobulin therapy in the long-term treatment of X-linked agammaglobulinemia. Am J Dis Child 146:335–339, 1992.

Linnemann CC Jr, MacMillan BG. Viral infections in pediatric burn patients. Am J Dis Child 135:750–753, 1981.

Lohr JA, Donowitz LG, Sadler JE III. Hospital-acquired urinary tract infection. Pediatrics 83:193–199, 1989.

MacDonald NE, Hall CB, Suffin SC, Alexson C, Harris PJ, Manning JA. Respiratory syncytial viral infection in infants with congenital heart disease. N Engl J Med 307:397–400, 1982.

MacMillan BG. Infections following burn injury. Surg Clin North Am 60:185–196, 1980.

Magny J-F, Bremard-Oury C, Brault D, Menguy C, Voyer M, Landais P, Dehan M, Gabilan J-C. Intravenous immunoglobulin therapy for prevention of infection in high-risk premature infants: report of a multicenter double-blind study. Pediatrics 88:437–443, 1991.

Maki DG, Goldman DA, Rhame FS. Infection control in intravenous therapy. Ann Intern Med 79:867–887, 1973a.

Maki DG, Hennekens CG, Phillips CW, Shaw WV, Bennett JV. Nosocomial urinary tract infection with *Serratia marcescens*: an epidemiologic study. J Infect Dis 128:579–587, 1973b.

Maki DG, Band JD. A comparative study of polyantibiotic and iodophor ointments in prevention of vascular catheter–related infection. Am J Med 70:739–744, 1981.

Maki DG, Rhame FS, Mackel DC, Bennett JV. Nationwide epidemic of septicemia caused by contaminated intravenous products. I. epidemiologic and clinical features. Am J Med 60:471–485, 1976.

Maki DG, Botticelli JT, LeRoy ML, Thielke TS. Prospective study of replacing administration sets for intravenous therapy at 48- vs. 72-hour intervals: 72 hours is safe and cost-effective. JAMA 258:1777–1781, 1987.

Margolis DM, Melnick DA, Alling DW, Gallin JI. Trimethoprim-sulfamethoxazole prophylaxis in the management of chronic granulomatous disease. J Infect Dis 162:723–726, 1990.

Markowitz LE, Chandler FW, Roldan EO, Saldana MJ, Roach KC, Hutchins SS, Preblud SR, Mitchell CD, Scott GB. Fatal measles pneumonia without rash in a child with AIDS. J Infect Dis 158:480–483, 1988.

Marks MI, Langston C, Eickhoff TC. *Torulopsis glabrata*: an opportunistic pathogen in man. N Engl J Med 283:1131–1135, 1970.

Martin FP, Lukeman JM, Ranson RF, Geppert LJ. Mucormycosis of central nervous system associated with thrombosis of the internal carotid artery. J Pediatr 44:437–516, 1954.

McCabe WR: Pyelonephritis. In Hoeprich PD, ed. Infectious Diseases. New York, Harper & Row, 1972, pp. 507–521.

McCrae WM, Raeburn JA. Chronic granulomatous disease: an attempt to stimulate phagocytic activity. Lancet 1:1370–1371, 1972.

McGinnis MR, Walker DH, Folds JD. Hansenula polymorpha infection in a child with chronic granulomatous disease. Arch Pathol Lab Med 104:290–292, 1980.

McIntosh K, Kurachek SC, Cairns LM, Burns JC, Goodspeed B. Treatment of respiratory viral infection in an immunodeficient infant with ribavirin aerosol. Am J Dis Child 138:305–308, 1984.

McKenzie SA, Hayden K. Two cases of "shunt nephritis." Pediatrics 54:806–808, 1974.

Meanes E. Current patterns in nosocomial urinary tract infections. Urology 37:9–12, 1991.

Mendelsohn G, Hutchins GM. Infective endocarditis during the first decade of life: an autopsy review of 33 cases. Am J Dis Child 133:619–622, 1979.

Mendelsohn HB, Berant M. Chronic granulomatous disease: a new clinical variant. Acta Paediatr Scand 71:869–872, 1982.

Mermel LA, Maki DG. Epidemic bloodstream infections from hemodynamic pressure monitoring: signs of the times. Infect Control Hosp Epidemiol 10:47–53, 1989.

Mertz JJ, Scharer L, McClement JH. A hospital outbreak of *Klebsiella* pneumonia from inhalation therapy with contaminated aerosol solutions. Am Rev Respir Dis 95:454–460, 1967.

Merzbach D, Freundlich E, Metzker A, Falk W. Bacterial endocarditis due to corynebacterium. J Pediatr 67:792–796, 1965.

Mills EL, Quie PG. Congenital disorders of the functions of polymorphonuclear neutrophils. Rev Infect Dis 2:505–517, 1980.

Ming PL, Ming SC, Dammin GJ: Effect of uremia and azathioprine on lymphocyte response to phytohemagglutinin. Pediatr Proc 27:432, 1968.

Miser JS, Miser AW. Staphylococcus aureus sepsis in childhood malignancy. Am J Dis Child 134:831–833, 1980.

Mitchell CD, Erlich SS, Mastrucci MT, Hutto SC, Parks WP, Scott GB. Congenital toxoplasmosis occurring in infants perinatally infected with human immunodeficiency virus 1. Pediatr Infect Dis J 9:512–518, 1990.

Mollison LC, Richards MJ, Johnson PDR, Hayes K, Munckhof WJ, Jones R, Dabkowski PD, Angus PW. High-dose oral acyclovir reduces the incidence of cytomegalovirus infection in liver transplant recipients. J Infect Dis 168:721–724, 1993.

Moore WL Jr. Nosocomial infections: an overview. Am J Hosp Pharm 31:832–838, 1974.

Morley D. Severe measles in the tropics. I. Br Med J 1:297–300, 1969.

Moyer MA, Edwards LD, Farley L. Comparative culture methods on 101 intravenous catheters: routine, semiquantitative, and blood cultures. Arch Intern Med 143:66–69, 1983.

Mühlebach TJ, Gabay J, Nathan CF, Erny C, Dopfer G, Schroten H, Wahn V, Seger RA. Treatment of patients with chronic granulomatous disease with recombinant human interferon-gamma does not improve neutrophil oxidative metabolism, cytochrome b558 content or levels of four antimicrobial proteins. Clin Exp Immunol 88:203–206, 1992.

Nachman JB, Honig GR. Fever and neutropenia in children with neoplastic disease: an analysis of 158 episodes. Cancer 45:407–412, 1980.

Naito H, Toya S, Schizawa H, Iizaka Y, Tsukumo D. High incidence of acute postoperative meningitis and septicemia in patients undergoing craniotomy with ventriculoatrial shunt. Surg Gynecol Obstet 137:810–812, 1973.

Najarian JS, So SKS, Simmons RL, Fryd DS, Nevins TE, Ascher NL, Sutherland DER, Payne WD, Chavers BM, Mauer SM. The outcome of 304 primary renal transplants in children (1968–1985). Ann Surg 204:246–258, 1986.

Neu HD. Unusual nosocomial infections. Disease a Month, 30:1–68, 1984.

Neumann CG. Malnutrition and infection. In Powands MC, Canonico PG, eds. Infection: The Physiologic and Metabolic Responses of the Host. New York, Elsevier, North Holland Biomed Press, 1981, pp. 320–357.

Neumann CG, Lawlor GJ Jr, Stiehm ER, Swendseid ME, Newton C, Herbert J, Ammann AJ, Jacob M. Immunologic responses in malnourished children. Am J Clin Nutr 28:89–104, 1975.

Nielsen SL, Røder B, Magnussen P, Engquist A, Frimodt-Møller N. Nosocomial pneumonia in an intensive care unit in a Danish university hospital: incidence, mortality and etiology. Scand J Infect Dis 24:65–70, 1992.

NIH Consensus Conference. Intravenous immunoglobulin: prevention and treatment of disease. JAMA 264:3189–3193, 1990.

Noel GJ, O'Loughlin JE, Edelson PJ. Neonatal *Staphylococcus epidermidis* right-sided endocarditis: description of five catheterized infants. Pediatrics 82:234–239, 1988.

Nour B, Green M, Michaels M, Reyes J, Tzakis A, Carlton Gartner J, McLoughlin L, Starzl TE. Parvovirus B19 infection in pediatric transplant patients. Transplantation 56:835–838, 1993.

Nydahl BC, Hall WH. The treatment of staphylococcal infection with nafcillin with a discussion of staphylococcal nephritis. Ann Intern Med 63:27–43, 1965.

Odio C, McCracken GH, Jr, Nelson JD. CSF shunt infections in pediatrics: a seven-year experience. Am J Dis Child 138:1103–1108, 1984.

Odum L, Jensen KT, Slotsbjerg TD. Endocarditis due to *Kingella kingae*. Eur J Clin Microbiol 3:263–266, 1984.

Oleske J, Minnefor A, Cooper R Jr, Thomas K, de la Cruz A, Ahdieh H, Guerrero I, Joshi VV, Desposito F. Immune deficiency syndrome in children. JAMA 249:2345–2349, 1983.

Olson MM, O'Connor-Allen M. Nosocomial abscess. Arch Surg 124:356–361, 1989.

Orcutt TA, Godwin CR, Pizzo PA, Ognibene FP. Aerosolized pentamidine: a well-tolerated mode of prophylaxis against *Pneumocystis carinii* pneumonia in older children with human immunodeficiency virus infection. Pediatr Infect Dis J 11:290–294, 1992.

Pakkala S, Salmela K, Lautenschlager I, Ahonen J, Häyry P. Anti-CMV hyperimmune globulin prophylaxis does not prevent CMV disease in CMV-negative renal transplant patients. Transplant Proc 24:283–284, 1992.

Paradise JL, Bluestone CD, Felder H. The universality of otitis media in 50 infants with cleft palate. Pediatrics 44:35–42, 1969.

Paradise JL, Bluestone CD. Early treatment of the universal otitis media in infants with cleft palate. Pediatrics 53:48–54, 1974.

Paradise JL. Management of middle ear effusions in infants with cleft palate. Ann Otol Rhinol Laryngol 85:285–288, 1976.

Pedersen FK. Postsplenectomy infections in Danish children splenectomized 1969–1978. Acta Paediatr Scand 72:589–595, 1983.

Peter G, Lloyd-Still JD, Lovejoy FH Jr. Local infection and bacteremia from scalp vein needles and polyethylene catheters in children. J Pediatr 80:78–83, 1972.

Peterson JE, Baker TJ. An isolate of *Fusarium roseum* from human burns. Mycologia 51:453–456, 1959.

Phillapart AI, Colodney AH, Baehner RL. Continuous antibiotic therapy in chronic granulomatous disease: preliminary communication. Pediatrics 50:923–925, 1972.

Phillips I, Wharton B. Acute bacterial infections in kwashiorkor and marasmus. Br Med J 1:407–409, 1968.

Phillips JA, Bernhardt HE, Rosenthal SG. *Aeromonas hydrophila* infections. Pediatrics 53:110–112, 1974.

Pierce AK, Sanford JP, Thomas GD, Leonard JS. Long-term evaluation of decontamination of inhalation-therapy equipment and the occurrence of necrotizing pneumonia. N Engl J Med 282:528–531, 1970.

Pike RM, Schulze ML, McCullough M. Isolation of *Mima polymorpha* from a patient with subacute bacterial endocarditis. Am J Clin Pathol 21:1094–1096, 1951.

Pizzo PA. Management of fever in patients with cancer and treatment-induced neutropenia. Drug Ther 18:1323–1332, 1993.

Pizzo PA, Commers J, Cotton D, Gress J, Hathorn J, Hiemenz J, Longo D, Marshall D, Robichaud KJ. Approaching the controversies in antibacterial management of cancer patients. Am J Med 76:436–449, 1984.

Pizzo PA, Rubin M, Freifeld A, Walsh TJ. The child with cancer and infection: I. Empiric therapy for fever and neutropenia, and preventive strategies. J Pediatr 119:679–694, 1991a.

Pizzo PA, Rubin M, Freifeld A, Walsh TJ. The child with cancer and infection: II. Nonbacterial infections. J Pediatr 119:845–857, 1991b.

Ponka A, Tilvis R, Kosunen TU. Prolonged campylobacter gastroenteritis in a patient with hypogammaglobulinemia. Acta Med Scand 213:159–160, 1983.

Potter D, Feduska N, Melzer J, Garovoy M, Hopper S, Duca R, Salvatierra O. Twenty years of renal transplantation in children. Pediatrics 77:465–470, 1986.

Powell DA, Aungst J, Snedden S, Hansen N, Brady M. Broviac catheter–related *Malassezia furfur* sepsis in five infants receiving intravenous fat emulsions. J Pediatr 105:987–990, 1984.

Powell KR, Cherry JD, Hougen TJ, Blinderman EE, Dunn MC. A prospective search for congenital dermal abnormalities of the craniospinal axis. J Pediatr 87:744–750, 1975.

Press OW, Ramsey PG, Larson EB, Fefer A, Hickman RO. Hickman catheter infections in patients with malignancies. Medicine 63:189–200, 1984.

Principi N, Marchisio P, Tornaghi R, Onorato J, Massironi E, Picco P.

Acute otitis media in human immunodeficiency virus–infected children. Pediatrics 88:566–571, 1991.

Prober CG, Whyte H, Smith CR. Open lung biopsy in immunocompromised children with pulmonary infiltrates. Am J Dis Child 138:60–63, 1984.

Prokurat S, Drabik E, Grenda R, Vogt E. Ganciclovir in cytomegalovirus prophylaxis in high-risk pediatric renal transplant recipients. Transplant Proc 25:2577, 1993.

Pruitt BA, Jr, McManus AT. Opportunistic infections in severely burned patients. Am J Med 76:146–154, 1984.

Quie PG. Infections due to neutrophil malfunction. Medicine 52:411–417, 1973.

Quie PG, Hetherington SV. Patients with disorders of phagocytic cell function. Pediatr Infect Dis 3:272–280, 1984.

Quie PG, Belani KK. Corticosteroids for chronic granulomatous disease. J Pediatr 111:393–394, 1987.

Rabin ER, Lundberg GD, Mitchell ET. Mucormycosis in severely burned patients: report of two cases with extensive destruction of the face and nasal cavity. N Engl J Med 264:1286–1289, 1961.

Ragab AH, Lindqvist KJ, Vietti TJ, Choi SC, Osterland CK. Immunoglobulin pattern in childhood leukemia. Cancer 26:890–894, 1970.

Raubitschek AA, Levin AS, Stites DP, Shaw EB, Fudenberg HH. Normal granulocyte infusion therapy for aspergillosis in chronic granulomatous disease. Pediatrics 51:230–233, 1973.

Rauch AM, O'Ryan M, Van R, Pickering LK. Invasive disease due to multiply resistant *Streptococcus pneumoniae* in a Houston, Texas, day-care center. Am J Dis Child 144:923–927, 1990.

Reinhardt DJ, Kennedy C, Malecka-Griggs B. Selective nonroutine microbial surveillance of in-use hospital nebulizers by aerosol entrapment and direct sampling analyses of solutions in reservoirs. J Clin Microbiol 12:199–204, 1980.

Rello J, Quintana E, Ausina V, Castella J, Luquin M, Net A, Prats G. Incidence, etiology, and outcome of nosocomial pneumonia in mechanically ventilated patients. Chest 100:439–444, 1991.

Rhame FS, Maki DG, Bennett JV. Intravenous cannula-associated infections. In Bennett JV, Brachman PS, eds. Hospital Infections. Boston, Little, Brown & Co., 1979, pp. 433–442.

Richet H, Hubert B, Nitemberg G, Andremont A, Buu-Hoi A, Ourbak P, Galicier C, Veron M, Boisivon A, Bouvier AM, Ricome JC, Wolff MA, Pean Y, Berardi-Grassias L, Bourdain JL, Hautefort B, Laaban JP, Tillant D. Prospective multicenter study of vascular-catheter–related complications and risk factors for positive central-catheter cultures in intensive care unit patients. J Clin Microbiol 28:2520–2525, 1990.

Riikonen P, Saarinen UM, Lähteenoja K-M, Jalanko H. Management of indwelling central venous catheters in pediatric cancer patients with fever and neutropenia. Scand J Infect Dis 25:357–364, 1993.

Riis P, Stougaard J. The peripheral blood leukocytes in chronic renal insufficiency. Dan Med Bull 6:85–90, 1959.

Riley HD, Jr. Hospital-associated infections. Pediatr Clin North Am 16:701–734, 1969.

Rodrigues RJ, Shinya H, Wolff WI, Puttlitz D. *Torulopsis glabrata* fungemia during prolonged intravenous alimentation therapy. N Engl J Med 284:540–541, 1971.

Rosen FS, Janeway CA. Dangers of vaccination in lymphopenic infants. Pediatrics 33:310–311, 1964.

Rosen FS, Cooper MD, Wedgwood RJP. The primary immunodeficiencies. N Engl J Med 311:235–242, 300–310, 1984.

Rosner F, Valmont I, Kozinn PJ, Caroline L. Leukocyte function in patients with leukemia. Cancer 25:835–842, 1970.

Rubin HM, Eardley W, Nichols BL. *Shigella sonnei* osteomyelitis and sickle cell anemia. Am J Dis Child 116:83–87, 1968.

Rubinstein A. Acquired immunodeficiency syndrome in infants. Am J Dis Child 137:825–827, 1983.

Rupar DG, Herzog KD, Fisher MC, Long SS. Prolonged bacteremia with catheter-related central venous thrombosis. Am J Dis Child 144:879–882, 1990.

Rutstein RM, Cobb P, McGowan KL, Pinto-Martin J, Starr SE. *Mycobacterium avium–intracellulare* complex infection in HIV-infected children. AIDS 7:507–512, 1993.

Saarinen UM. Severe infections in childhood leukemia: a followup study of 100 consecutive ALL patients. Acta Paediatr Scand 73:515–522, 1984.

Sable CA, Donowitz GR. Infections in bone marrow transplant recipients. Clin Infect Dis 18:273–284, 1994.

Sachs JM, Pacin M, Counts GW. Sickle hemoglobinopathy and *Edwardsiella* tarda meningitis. Am J Dis Child 128:387–388, 1974.

Saiman L, Prince A, Gersony WM. Pediatric infective endocarditis in the modern era. J Pediatr 122:847–853, 1993.

Saleh RA, Schorin MA. *Bacillus* sp. sepsis associated with Hickman catheters in patients with neoplastic disease. Pediatr Infect Dis J 6:851–856, 1987.

Saliba F, Eyraud D, Samuel D, David MF, Arulnaden JL, Dussaix E, Mathieu D, Bismuth H. Randomized controlled trial of acyclovir for the prevention of cytomegalovirus infection and disease in liver transplant recipients. Transplant Proc 25:1444–1445, 1993.

Salmon JH. Adult hydrocephalus: evaluation of shunt therapy in 80 patients. J Neurosurg 37:423–428, 1972.

Sanders CV, Jr, Luby JP, Johanson WG, Jr, Barnett JA, Sanford JP. *Serratia marcescens* infection from inhalation therapy medications: nosocomial outbreak. Ann Intern Med 73:15–21, 1970.

Saulsbury FT, Winkelstein JA, Yolken RH. Chronic rotavirus infection in immunodeficiency. J Pediatr 97:61–65, 1980.

Schoenbaum SC, Gardner P, Shillito J. Infections of cerebrospinal fluid shunts: epidemiology, clinical manifestations and therapy. J Infect Dis 131:543–552, 1975.

Schonebeck J. Asymptomatic candiduria: prognosis, complications and some other clinical considerations. Scand J Urol Nephrol 6:136–146, 1972.

Schwartz RS. Immunosuppressive drugs. Prog Allergy 9:246–303, 1965.

Scott GB. HIV infection in children: clinical features and management. J AIDS 4:109–115, 1991.

Scott GB, Buck BE, Leterman JG, Bloom FL, Parks WP. Acquired immunodeficiency syndrome in infants. N Engl J Med 310:76–81, 1984.

Scott RM. Bacterial endocarditis due to *Neisseria flava*. J Pediatr 78:673–675, 1971.

Sechler JMG, Malech HL, White CJ, Gallin JI. Recombinant human interferon-γ reconstitutes defective phagocyte function in patients with chronic granulomatous disease of childhood. Proc Natl Acad Sci U S A 85:4874–4878, 1988.

Sellmeyer E, Bhettay E, Truswell AS, Meyers OL, Hansen JDL. Lymphocyte transformation in malnourished children. Arch Dis Child 47:429–435, 1972.

Seth V, Chandra RK. Opsonic activity, phagocytosis and bactericidal capacity of polymorphs in undernutrition. Arch Dis Child 47:282–284, 1972.

Severien C, Nelson JD. Frequency of infections associated with implanted systems vs. cuffed, tunneled Silastic venous catheters in patients with acute leukemia. Am J Dis Child 145:1433–1438, 1991.

Shafer RB, Hall WH. Bacterial endocarditis following open heart surgery. Am J Cardiol 25:602–607, 1970.

Shannon KM, Ammann AJ. Acquired immune deficiency syndrome in childhood. J Pediatr 106:332–342, 1985.

Sheridan RL, Ryan CM, Pasternack MS, Weber JM, Tompkins RG. Flavobacterial sepsis in massively burned pediatric patients. Clin Infect Dis 17:185–187, 1993.

Shinozaki T, Deane RS, Mazuzan JE, Hamel AJ, Hazelton D. Bacterial contamination of arterial lines. A prospective study. JAMA 249:223–225, 1983.

Shmerling DH, Prader A, Hitzig WH, Giedion A, Hadorn B, Kuhni M. The syndrome of exocrine pancreatic insufficiency, neutropenia, metaphyseal dysostosis and dwarfism. Helv Paediatr Acta 24:547–575, 1969.

Shuck JM. Infection control in burns—topical and systemic. Surg Clin North Am 52:1425–1438, 1972.

Shulman ST, Bartlett J, Clyde WA Jr, Ayoub EM. The unusual severity of mycoplasmal pneumonia in children with sickle cell disease. N Engl J Med 287:164–167, 1972.

Shurtleff DB, Foltz EL, Weeks RD, Loeser J. Therapy of *Staphylococcus epidermidis*: infections associated with cerebrospinal fluid shunts. Pediatrics 53:55–62, 1974.

Shyur S-D, Hill HR. Immunodeficiency in the 1990s. Pediatr Infect Dis J 10:595–611, 1991.

Sickles EA, Green WH, Wiernik PH. Clinical presentation of infection in granulocytopenic patients. Arch Intern Med 135:715–719, 1975.

Siegel SE, Nesbit ME, Baehner R, Sather H, Hammond GD. Pneumonia during therapy for childhood acute lymphoblastic leukemia. Am J Dis Child 134:28–34, 1980.

Silk MR. The effect of uremic plasma on lymphocyte transformation. Invest Urol 5:195–199, 1967.

Silliman CC, Tedder D, Ogle JW, Simon J, Kleinschmidt-DeMasters BK, Manco-Johnson M, Levin MJ. Unsuspected varicella zoster virus encephalitis in a child with acquired immunodeficiency syndrome. J Pediatr 123:418–422, 1993.

Sinkovics JG, Smith JP. Septicemia with *Bacteroides* in patients with malignant disease. Cancer 25:663–671, 1970.

Sirisinha S, Suskind R, Edelman R, Asvapaka C, Olson RE. Secretory and serum IgA in children with protein-calorie malnutrition. Pediatrics 55:166–170, 1975.

Skeel RT, Yankee RA, Henderson ES. Hexose monophosphate shunt activity of circulating phagocytes in acute leukemia. J Lab Clin Med 77:975–984, 1971.

Skinner MD, Schwartz RS. Immunosuppressive therapy. N Engl J Med 287:221–227, 281–286, 1972.

Sleigh JD, Peutherer JF. Changing patterns of bacterial and viral infections in surgery. Br Med Bull 44:403–422, 1988.

Sloper KS, Dourmashkin RR, Bird RB, Slavin G, Webster ADB. Chronic malabsorption due to cryptosporidiosis in a child with immunoglobulin deficiency. Gut 23:80–82, 1982.

Smith SD, Jackson RJ, Hannakan CJ, Wadowsky RM, Tzakis AG, Rowe MI. Selective decontamination in pediatric liver transplants: a randomized prospective study. Transplantation 55:1306–1309, 1993.

Smythe PM, Brereton-Stiles GG, Grace HJ, Mafoyane A, Schonland M, Coovadia HM, Loening WEK, Parent MA, Vos GH. Thymolymphatic deficiency and depression of cell mediated immunity in protein-calorie malnutrition. Lancet 2:939–944, 1971.

Snydman DR. Review of the efficacy of cytomegalovirus immune globulin in the prophylaxis of CMV disease in renal transplant recipients. Transplant Proc 25:25–26, 1993.

Snydman DR, Donnelly-Reidy M, Perry LK, Martin WJ. Intravenous tubing containing burettes can be safely changed at 72-hour intervals. Infect Control 8:113–116, 1987.

So SKS, Simmons RL. Infections following kidney transplantation in children. In Patrick CC, ed. Infections in Immunocompromised Infants and Children. New York, Churchill Livingstone, 1992, pp. 215–230.

Spebar MJ, Lindberg RB. Fungal infection of the burn wound. Am J Surg 138:879–882, 1979.

Sprunt K, Redman W, Leidy G. Antibacterial effectiveness of routine hand washing. Pediatrics 52:264–271, 1973.

Stamm WE. Guidelines for prevention of catheter-associated urinary tract infections. Ann Intern Med 82:386–390, 1975.

Stanton BF, Baltimore RS, Clemens JD. Changing spectrum of infective endocarditis in children: analysis of 26 cases, 1970–1979. Am J Dis Child 138:720–725, 1984.

Starke JR. Infections of the heart: infective endocarditis. In Feigin RD, Cherry JD, eds. Textbook of Pediatric Infectious Diseases, 3rd ed. Philadelphia, WB Saunders, 1992, pp 326–343.

Stavola JJ, Noel GJ. Efficacy and safety of dapsone prophylaxis against *Pneumocystis carinii* pneumonia in human immunodeficiency-virus–infected children. Pediatr Infect Dis J 12:644–647, 1993.

Steele RW. Infection in the immunocompromised host. Pediatr Infect Dis 4:309–314, 1985.

Steere AC, Mallison GF. Handwashing practices for the prevention of nosocomial infections. Ann Intern Med 83:683–690, 1975.

Steinberg AD, Plotz PH, Wolff SM, Wong VG, Agus SG, Decker JL. Cytotoxic drugs in treatment of nonmalignant diseases. Ann Intern Med 76:619–642, 1972.

Stickler GB, Shin MH, Burke EC, Holley KE, Miller RH, Segar WE. Diffuse glomerulonephritis associated with infected ventriculoatrial shunt. N Engl J Med 279:1077–1082, 1968.

Stiehm ER, Chin TW, Haas A, Peerless AG. Infectious complications of the primary immunodeficiencies. Clin Immunol Immunopathol 40:69–86, 1986.

Strauss RR, Paul BB, Jacobs AA, Simmons C, Sbarra AJ. The metabolic and phagocytic activities of leukocytes from children with acute leukemia. Cancer Res 30:80–88, 1970.

Strober W, Wochner RD, Carbone PP, Waldmann TA. Intestinal lymphangiectasia: a protein losing enteropathy with hypogammaglobulinemia, lymphocytopenia and impaired homograft rejection. J Clin Invest 46:1643–1656, 1967.

Sullivan JL, Byron KS, Brewster FE, Baker SM, Ochs HD. X-linked lymphoproliferative syndrome. J Clin Invest 71:1765–1778, 1983.

Tan TQ, Mason EO Jr, Kaplan SL. Penicillin-resistant systemic pneumococcal infections in children: a retrospective case-control study. Pediatrics 92:761–767, 1993.

Tauber AI, Borregaard N, Simons E, Wright J. Chronic granulomatous disease: a syndrome of phagocyte oxidase deficiencies. Medicine 62:286–309, 1983.

Thompson EN, Soothill JF. Chronic granulomatous disease: quantitative clincopathological relationships. Arch Dis Child 45:24–32, 1970.

Tomford JW, Hershey CO, McLaren CE, Porter DK, Cohen DI. Intravenous therapy team and peripheral venous catheter–associated complications: a prospective controlled study. Arch Intern Med 144:1191–1194, 1984.

Tredget EE, Shankowsky HA, Joffe AM, Inkson TI, Volpel K, Paranchych W, Kibsey PC, Alton JD, Burke JF. Epidemiology of infections with *Pseudomonas aeruginosa* in burn patients: the role of hydrotherapy. Clin Infect Dis 15:941–949, 1992.

Tsingoglou S, Forrest DM. A technique for the insertion of Holter ventriculo-atrial shunt for infantile hydrocephalus. Br J Surg 58:367–372, 1971.

Vacanti JP, Lillehei CW, Jenkins RL, Donahoe PK, Cosimi AB, Kleinman R, Grand RJ, Cho SI. Liver transplantation in children: the Boston Center experience in the first 30 months. Transplant Proc 19:3261–3266, 1987.

Vandersteenhoven JJ, Dbaibo G, Boyko OB, Hulette CM, Anthony DC, Kenny JF, Wilfert CM. Progressive multifocal leukoencephalopathy in pediatric acquired immunodeficiency syndrome. Pediatr Infect Dis J 11:232–237, 1992.

Van Hare GF, Ben-Shachar G, Liebman J, Boxerbaum B, Riemenschneider TA. Infective endocarditis in infants and children during the past 10 years: a decade of change. Am Heart J 107:1235–1240, 1984.

Vejlsgaard R. Studies on urinary tract infections in diabetics: III. significant bacteriuria in pregnant diabetics and in matched controls. Acta Med Scand 193:337–341, 1973.

Vernon DD, Holzman BH, Lewis P, Scott GB, Birriel JA, Scott MB. Respiratory failure in children with acquired immunodeficiency syndrome and acquired immunodeficiency syndrome–related complex. Pediatrics 82:223–228, 1988.

Verronen P. Presumed disseminated BCG in a boy with chronic granulomatous disease of childhood. Acta Paediatr Scand 63:627–630, 1974.

Wade JC, Newton B, Flournoy N, Meyers JD. Oral acyclovir for prevention of herpes simplex virus reactivation after marrow transplantation. Ann Intern Med 100:823–828, 1984.

Waldmann TA. Protein-losing enteropathy. Gastroenterology 50:422–443, 1966.

Waldmann TA, Schwab PJ. IgG (7S gamma globulin) metabolism in hypogammaglobulinemia: studies in patients with defective gamma globulin synthesis, gastrointestinal protein loss, or both. J Clin Invest 44:1523–1533, 1965.

Walker W. Splenectomy in childhood: a review in England and Wales, 1960–64. Br J Surg 63:36–43, 1976.

Walters BC, Hoffman HJ, Hendrick EB, Humphreys RP. Cerebrospinal fluid shunt infection: influences on initial management and subsequent outcome. J Neurosurg 60:1014–1021, 1984.

Walzer PD, Schultz MG, Western KA, Robbins JB. *Pneumocystis carinii* pneumonia and primary immune deficiency diseases of infancy and childhood. J Pediatr 82:416–422, 1973.

Wang EEL, Prober CG, Ford-Jones L, Gold R. The management of central intravenous catheter infections. Pediatr Infect Dis 3:110–113, 1984.

Ward PA. The chemosuppression of chemotaxis. J Exp Med 124:209–226, 1966.

Wasserman R, August CS, Plotkin SA. Viral infections in pediatric bone marrow transplant patients. Pediatr Infect Dis J 7:109–115, 1988.

Watanakunakorn C, Carleton J, Goldberg LM, Hamburger M. *Candida* endocarditis surrounding a Starr-Edwards prosthetic valve: recovery of *Candida* in hypertonic medium during treatment. Arch Intern Med 121:243–245, 1968.

Weiden PL, Blaese RM, Strober W, Block JB, Waldmann TA. Impaired lymphocyte transformation in intestinal lymphangiectasia: evidence for at least two functionally distinct lymphocyte populations in man. J Clin Invest 51:1319–1325, 1972.

Weisman LE, Stoll BJ, Kueser TJ, Rubio TT, Frank CG, Heiman HS, Subramanian KNS, Hankins CT, Anthony BF, Cruess DF, Hemming VG, Fischer GW. Intravenous immune globulin therapy for early-onset sepsis in premature neonates. J Pediatr 121:434–443, 1992.

Welt LG, Black HR, Krueger KK. Symposium on uremic toxins. Arch Intern Med 126:773–780, 1970.

Welte K, Zeidler C, Reiter A, Müller W, Odenwald E, Souza L, Riehm H. Differential effects of granulocyte-macrophage colony-stimulating factor and granulocyte colony-stimulating factor in children with severe congenital neutropenia. Blood 75:1056–1063, 1990.

Werner BG, Snydman DR, Freeman R, Rohrer R, Tilney NL, Kirkman RL, the Treatment IND Study Group. Cytomegalovirus immune globulin for the prevention of primary CMV disease in renal transplant patients: analysis of usage under treatment IND status. Transplant Proc 25:1441–1443, 1993.

Westwood JCN, Legacé S, Mitchell MA. Hospital-acquired infection: present and future impact and need for positive action. Can Med Assoc J 110:769–774, 1974.

Wilfert CM, Katz SL. Etiology of bacterial sepsis in nephrotic children, 1963–1967. Pediatrics 42:840–843, 1968.

Wilfert CM, Buckley RH, Mohanakumar T, Griffith JF, Katz SL, Whisnant JK, Eggleston PA, Moore M, Treadwell E, Oxman MN, Rosen FS. Persistent and fatal central nervous system echovirus infections in patients with agammaglobulinemia. N Engl J Med 296:1485–1489, 1977.

Wilhelmi I, Bernaldo de Quirós JCL, Romero-Vivas J, Duarte J, Rojo E, Bouza E. Epidemic outbreak of *Serratia marcescens* infection in a cardiac surgery unit. J Clin Microbiol 25:1298–1300, 1987.

Wilson WEC, Kirkpatrick CH, Talmage DW. Suppression of immunologic-responsiveness in uremia. Ann Intern Med 62:1–14, 1965.

Wilson WR, Jaumin PM, Danielson GK, Giuliani ER, Washington JA, Geraci JE. Prosthetic valve endocarditis. Ann Intern Med 82:751–756, 1975.

Winston DJ, Gale RP, Meyer DV, Young LS, the UCLA Bone Marrow Transplantation Group. Infectious complications of human bone marrow transplantation. Medicine 58:1–31, 1979.

Winston DJ, Ho WG, Champlin RE, Gale RP. Infectious complications of bone marrow transplantation. Exp Hematol 12:205–215, 1984.

Winston DJ. Use in viral infections. In Stiehm ER (moderator). Intravenous immunoglobulins as therapeutic agents. Ann Intern Med 107:367–382, 1987.

Wollman MR, Young LS, Armstrong D, Haghbin M. Anti-*Pseudomonas* heat-stable opsonins in acute lymphoblastic leukemia of childhood. J Pediatr 86:376–381, 1975.

Wong DT, Ogra PL. Viral infections in immunocompromised patients. Med Clin North Am 67:1075–1092, 1983.

Wong ES, Hooton TM. Guideline for prevention of catheter-associated urinary tract infections. In Guidelines for the Prevention and Control of Nosocomial Infections. U.S. Department of Health and Human Services, Centers for Disease Control, 1981, pp. 1–5.

Wong KK, Hirsch MS. Herpes virus infections in patients with neoplastic disease: diagnosis and therapy. Am J Med 76:464–478, 1984.

Wong VK, Ross LA. *Branhamella catarrhalis* septicemia in an infant with AIDS. Scand J Infect Dis 20:559–560, 1988.

Wong W-Y, Overturf GD, Powars DR. Infection caused by *Streptococcus pneumoniae* in children with sickle cell disease: epidemiology, immunologic mechanisms, prophylaxis, and vaccination. Clin Infect Dis 14:1124–1136, 1992.

Work TH, Ifekwunigwe A, Jelliffe DB, Jelliffe P, Neumann CG. Tropical problems in nutrition. Ann Intern Med 79:701–711, 1973.

Working Group on Antiretroviral Therapy. National Pediatric HIV Resource Center. Antiretroviral therapy and medical management of the human immunodeficiency virus–infected child. Pediatr Infect Dis J 12:513–522, 1993.

Wright DG, Dale DC, Fauci AS, Wolff SM. Human cyclic neutropenia: clinical review and long-term followup of patients. Medicine 60:1–13, 1981.

Wurzel CL, Halom K, Feldman JG, Rubin LG. Infection rates of Broviac-Hickman catheters and implantable venous devices. Am J Dis Child 142:536–540, 1988.

Yetgin S, Gur A, Saatci U. Non-specific immunity in nephrotic syndrome. Acta Paediatr Scand 69:21–24, 1980.

Yogev R. Cerebrospinal fluid shunt infections: a personal view. Pediatr Infect Dis 4:113–118, 1985.

Yoshida T, Metcoff J, Frenk S, DeLaPena C. Intermediary metabolites and adenine nucleotides in leukocytes of children with protein-calorie malnutrition. Nature 214:525–526, 1967.

Young RC, Bennett JE, Geelhoed GW, Levine AS. Fungemia with compromised host resistance: a study of 70 cases. Ann Intern Med 80:605–612, 1974.

Zaia JA. Infections associated with bone marrow transplantation. In Patrick CC, ed. Infections in Immunocompromised Infants and Children. New York, Churchill Livingstone, 1992, pp. 261–276.

Zitelli GJ, Gartner JC, Malatack JJ, Urbach AH, Miller JW, Williams L, Kirdpatrick B, Breinig MK, Ho M. Pediatric liver transplantation: patient evaluation and selection, infectious complications, and lifestyle after transplantation. Transplant Proc 19:3309–3316, 1987.

Zurier RB, Weissman G. Anti-immunologic and anti-inflammatory effects of steroid therapy. Med Clin North Am 57:1295–1307, 1973.

Chapter 32

Transplantation

Rebecca H. Buckley

Although replacement of injured or diseased parts of the body with those of others has been an aspiration of many for centuries, this feat was accomplished only within the past 40 years. This achievement followed recognition of the immunologic nature of graft re-jection, first demonstrated by the skin grafting experiments of Medawar (1944). He showed that the first skin graft from an unrelated donor was rejected more rapidly, and that autologous grafts were never rejected. Medawar (1946) later demonstrated that injections of leukocytes sensitized the recipient to subsequent skin grafts from the leukocyte donor and inferred from this that leukocytes carried transplantation antigens.

Prior to 1955, only isolated reports of attempted (largely unsuccessful) organ transplants had appeared in the scientific literature. Since then, the explosive growth of transplantation is attested by the fact that, by 1993, 315,737 kidney transplants had been reported from 507 transplant centers worldwide along with 48,965 bone marrow transplants from 261 centers, 29,395 heart transplants from 232 centers, 34,307 liver transplants from 170 centers, 5516 pancreas or pancreas-kidney transplants from 193 centers, and 2817 lung transplants from 89 centers (Terasaki and Cecka, 1994).

Organ and tissue transplantation have the greatest potential application to pediatrics, because fatal or debilitating disease of single organs is more common in young patients. In addition to the proven usefulness of renal transplantation for renal failure; bone marrow transplantation for immunodeficiency, aplastic anemia, leukemia, and inborn errors of metabolism; liver transplantation for biliary atresia; and skin transplantation for burns, other organs and tissues have also been transplanted successfully in children, including the lungs and the heart, the parathyroids, and the pancreas. The future holds the possibility that re-infusions of autologous marrow cells that have been transfected with normal genes to successfully correct defective ones will likely be another major therapeutic advance.

Despite progress in the technical aspects of organ transplantation and in the development of immunosuppressive agents capable of preventing graft rejection, the histocompatibility barrier still limits success in bone marrow transplantation for certain types of diseases. This chapter presents current knowledge of the major transplantation antigens, cells, antibodies, and types of reactions responsible for graft rejection; the methods available for identifying such antigens and for matching donor and recipient; the means by which the immune response can be manipulated to control graft rejection; and the clinical experience with various organ and tissue grafting in pediatrics.

HISTOCOMPATIBILITY ANTIGENS AND DONOR-RECIPIENT PAIRING

The Major Histocompatibility Complex

Transplantation or histocompatibility antigens are those antigens present on tissue cells that are capable of inducing an immune response in a genetically dissimilar (allogeneic) recipient, resulting in their rejection. Much of the information on histocompatibility antigens came initially from studies in inbred strains of mice, in which at least 30 independently segregating genetic loci encoding for such antigens were identified (Klein, 1975). Their gene products are called *alloantigens,* since they occur as genetically dissimilar forms within the species. Early on, it was noted that although genetic disparity between donor and recipient mice

for any of these loci led to eventual graft rejection, differences in the H-2 genetic complex resulted in the most rapid and vigorous rejection. Thus, the H-2 complex was identified as the major histocompatibility complex (MHC) of mice; loci coding for antigens evoking weaker responses were termed *minor* loci.

In every mammalian species that has been studied subsequently, a single genetic complex has been found to encode histocompatibility antigens with rejection-inducing potency similar to those of H-2. Examples of MHCs in other species include the B complex in chickens, the AgB complex in rats, the DLA complex in dogs, the SLA locus in swine, the RhL-A complex in monkeys, and the H-1 complex in rabbits. Each MHC is genetically complex because it includes many different loci, each encoding separate cell surface proteins, and because of the extreme polymorphism of those loci.

The Human Major Histocompatibility Complex: HLA

Recognition of this genetic region in 1967 (Bach and Amos, 1967) was the result of a 15-year effort by many investigators throughout the world and was a major breakthrough for clinical organ and tissue transplantation. Similarities between histocompatibility antigens of animals and humans began to be appreciated when Amos (1953) identified transplantation antigens on mouse leukocytes by leukoagglutination and Dausset (1954) found that 90% of 60 multitransfused subjects had leukocyte agglutinins in their sera. Dausset then correctly deduced that leukocyte alloantigens present in transfused blood were frequently responsible for alloimmunization against human histocompatibility antigens. A far more common cause of such alloimmunization was appreciated in 1958, however, when Payne and Rolfs and van Rood and colleagues independently demonstrated alloantibodies to human leukocyte antigens (HLAs) in sera from multiparous women. It was later recognized that such antibodies are also found in the sera of recipients of tissue or organ grafts.

Beginning in 1964, a series of International Histocompatibility Workshops were held in which sera and cells were exchanged by participants throughout the world. Analyses of data from these Workshops resulted in the identification of multiallelic genetic loci and the definition of their gene products. Convincing evidence for the existence of a single chromosomal region controlling the inheritance of the major human histocompatibility antigens was presented in 1967 by Bach and Amos; they showed that compatibility by leukocyte typing correlated with compatibility in mixed leukocyte culture (MLC) in pairs of siblings from seven large families (Amos and Bach, 1968).

The World Health Organization (WHO) Nomenclature Committee in 1968 proposed that the leukocyte antigens controlled by the closely linked genes of the human MHC be designated by the letters HLA. This Committee has convened every 2 to 3 years since; the most recent meeting was held in March of 1994 (Bodmer et al., 1995). At each meeting, new genes,

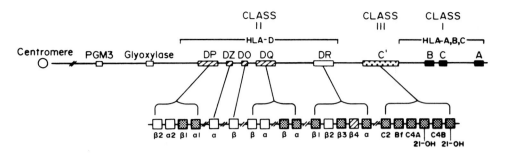

Figure 32–1. Schematic representation of the human leukocyte antigen (HLA) region on the short arm of human chromosome 6. Open squares in the HLA-D region represent genes that may not be expressed.

alleles, and antigens were identified. Thus, a very large number of genes have been found within the HLA region over the past 25 years, and enormous strides have been made in understanding the serology, biochemistry, and biologic functions of their gene products (Bodmer et al., 1995). Certain conditions are required for acceptance of new HLA allele DNA sequences by the WHO Committee, including sequencing performed in both directions and a preference for full-length DNA sequences (Bodmer et al., 1995).

Nomenclature, Location, and Structure

The multiple genetic loci of the human MHC reside on the short arm of chromosome 6 (Fig. 32–1). They and their cell surface and soluble protein products are divided into three classes (I, II, and III) on the basis of their tissue distribution, structure, and function (Bodmer, 1986; Bach and Sachs, 1987). Class I and II genes encode for HLA cell surface antigens which are codominantly expressed and class III for several components of the complement system; all share important roles in immune function.

Class I MHC antigens are present on all nucleated cells and are each composed of a 45-kD α heavy chain encoded by genes of the HLA-A, -B, or -C loci on chromosome 6 and associated noncovalently with a 12-kD protein, β_2 microglobulin (β_{2m}) encoded by a gene on chromosome 15 (Thorsby, 1987). The α chains are composed of approximately 340 amino acid residues that form three extracellular domains, a transmembrane part and an intracytoplasmic tail (Fig. 32–2). The β chain (β_{2m}) is nonpolymorphic and consists entirely of a single extracellular domain of 100 amino acids. The alloantigenic activity of class I antigens is determined exclusively by hypervariable regions of the N-terminal domains of the 45-kD α heavy chain (Lopez de Castro et al., 1985). These proteins, similar to products of the K and D loci in the mouse, are now recognized as the principal targets for CD8$^+$ cytotoxic T cells (Bach and Sachs, 1987).

By contrast, MHC class II antigens have a more limited tissue distribution and are expressed only on B lymphocytes, monocytes-macrophages, Langerhans cells, dendritic cells, endothelium, activated T lymphocytes, and epithelial cells. Each is a heterodimer composed of noncovalently associated α and β chains of approximately 230 amino acid encoded by genes of the HLA-D region. The α chains have a molecular mass between 29 and 34 kD; the β chains, between 25 and 28 kD.

Both chains form two extracellular domains, a transmembrane part, and an intracytoplasmic tail (see Fig. 32–2). Class II antigens, also known as *B-cell alloantigens* and immune-associated or "Ia" antigens, are the primary targets for CD4$^+$ T-helper lymphocytes.

The genetic organization of the HLA loci is depicted schematically in Figure 32–1. In addition to the well-known HLA class I A, B, and C genes shown, there are seven more class I genes: HLA-E, HLA-F, HLA-G, HLA-H, HLA-J, HLA-K, and HLA-L and three well-known class II "families" of genes, referred to as HLA-DR, -DQ, and -DP (Table 32–1) (Bodmer et al., 1995). Each of the latter families includes at least one α gene and one or more β genes. Thus, since genes of two separate MHC loci encode the α and β chains of each family's heterodimer, one cannot refer simply to "the" DR, DQ, or DP gene but must also specify the α or β chain gene. Only the DP and DQ α chains are polymorphic; the DR α chain shows no variation. One nonpolymorphic α gene and nine β genes have been identified in the DR family.

In most DR haplotypes (see below), the product of the α gene associates on the cell surface with the product of the DRβ 1 gene to form the DR $\alpha\beta$1 heterodimer. The DRβ 1 gene is highly polymorphic; it has more than 100 alleles encoding for variations on the 14 classic DR antigens (Bodmer et al., 1995). The DRβ 3 allele encodes additional "supertypic" DR molecules, variations on DR52, and the DRβ 4 allele for variations

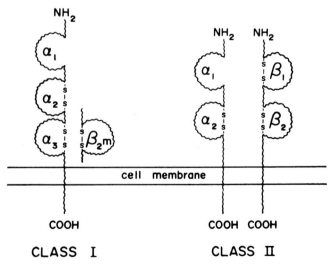

Figure 32–2. Schematic of the molecular composition of HLA class I and II antigens.

Table 32–1. Names for Genes in the Major Histocompatibility Complex (HLA System)

Name*	Previous Equivalents	Molecular Characteristics
HLA-A	—	Class I α-chain
HLA-B	—	Class I α-chain
HLA-C	—	Class I α-chain
HLA-E	E, 'pr6.2'	Associated with class 16.2-kB Hind III fragment
HLA-F	F, '5.4'	Associated with class 15.4-kB Hind III fragment
HLA-G	G, '6.0'	Associated with class 16.0-kB Hind III fragment
HLA-H	H, AR, '12.4'	Class I pseudogene associated with 5.4-kB Hind III fragment
HLA-J	cda 12	Class I pseudogene associated with 5.9-kB Hind III fragment
HLA-K	HLA-70	Class I pseudogene associated with 7.0-kB Hind III fragment
HLA-L	HLA-92	Class I pseudogene associated with 9.2-kB Hind III fragment
HLA-DRA	DRα	DR α chain
HLA-DRB1	DRβI, DR1B	DR β1 chain determining specificities DR1, DR2, DR3, DR4, DR5, etc
HLA-DRB2	DRβII	Pseudogene with DR β-like sequences
HLA-DRB3	DRβIII, DR3B	DR β3 chain determining DR52 and Dw24, Dw25, Dw6 specificities
HLA-DRB4	DRβIV, DR4B	DR β4 chain determining DR53
HLA-DRB5	DRβIII	DR β5 chain determining DR51
HLA-DRB6	DRBX, DRBσ	DRB pseudogene found on DR1, DR2, and DR10 haplotypes
HLA-DRB7	DRBψ1	DRB pseudogene found on DR4, DR7, and DR9 haplotypes
HLA-DRB8	DRBψ2	DRB pseudogene found on DR4, DR7, and DR9 haplotypes
HLA-DRB9	M4.2 β exon	DRB pseudogene, isolated fragment
HLA-DQA1	DQχ1, DQ1A	DQ α chain as expressed
HLA-DQB1	DQβ1, DQ1B	DQ β chain as expressed
HLA-DQA2	DXχ, DQ2A	DQ α-chain–related sequence, not known to be expressed
HLA-DQB2	DXβ, DQ2B	DQ β-chain–related sequence, not known to be expressed
HLA-DQB3	DVβ, DQB3	DQ β-chain–related sequence, not known to be expressed
HLA-DOB	DOβ	DO β chain
HLA-DMA	RING6	DM α chain
HLA-DMB	RING7	DM β chain
HLA-DNA	DZα, DOα	DN α chain
HLA-DPA1	DPα1, DP1A	DP α chain as expressed
HLA-DPB1	DPβ1, DP1B	DP β chain as expressed
HLA-DPA2	DPα2, DP2A	DP α-chain–related pseudogene
HLA-DPB2	DPβ2, DP2B	DP β-chain–related pseudogene
TAP1	RING4, Y3, PSF1	ABC (ATP Binding Cassette) transporter
TAP2	RING11, Y1, PSF2	ABC (ATP Binding Cassette) transporter
LMP2	RING12	Proteasome-related sequence
LMP7	RING10	Proteasome-related sequence

*Gene names given in bold type have been assigned since the 1991 Nomenclature report.
Abbreviations: ATP = adenosine triphosphate.
From Bodmer JG, Marsh SGE, Albert ED, et al: Nomenclature for factors of the HLA system, 1994. Tissue Antigens 44:1–18, 1994. © 1994, Munksgaard International Publishers Ltd, Copenhagen, Denmark.

on DR53. DR52 occurs with DR3, DR5, DR6, and DR8 and DR53 with DR4, DR7, and DR9. DRβ 2 and DRβ 6–9 genes are not expressed and are referred to as *pseudogenes* (see Table 32–1) (Bodmer et al., 1995).

The DQ gene family contains two α chain genes, of which one is very polymorphic, and three β chain genes, one of which encodes the presently recognized DQ antigens. It has not been clearly established whether the other α and β chain genes of the DQ family are expressed. DQ antigens are referred to as being *supertypic* to DR antigens. This means that whenever a particular DQ specificity is present, any one of several DR specificities may be present. For example, all Caucasians who are DR1+, DR2+, or DRw6+ are also DQ1+. It is generally considered that DQ is the homolog of murine I-A and DR the homolog of murine I-E.

The DP family has two α and two β genes; only one of each has an expressed gene product. Finally, there are other genes within the HLA region, including DOB, DMA, DMB, DNA, TAP1 and TAP2, and LMP2 and LMP7 (see Table 32–1) (Bodmer et al., 1995).

Thus, on cells expressing both class I and class II HLA

antigens, there are three class I antigens and three or more (usually four) class II heterodimers. Table 32–1 lists the names of the genes in the HLA region given official recognition by the WHO Nomenclature Committee in 1994. Of the known genetic systems in humans, HLA is the most polymorphic. There are 50 currently recognized HLA A alleles, 97 B alleles, 34 C alleles, more than 100 DR alleles, more than 60 DQ alleles, and more than 65 DP alleles. These alleles occur with different frequencies in various ethnic and racial groups.

Prior to DNA typing, HLA antigens were defined largely by their reactions with antibodies. However, T lymphocytes recognize antigenic specificities different from those recognized by antibodies, referred to as lymphocyte-defined subtype *polymorphisms* (Gregersen et al., 1986). For example, a person typed as DR4 can have five different lymphocyte-defined subtypes (e.g., Dw4, Dw10) that are differentially recognized by T cells. Each subtype is characterized by a different allele of the DR β 1 locus. One of three hypervariable (H) regions of the N-terminal domain of DR β appears to be the most important in T cell recognition of these

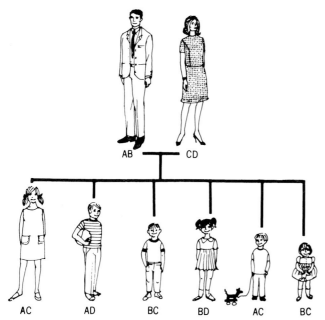

Figure 32–3. Schematic representation of the inheritance of human leukocyte antigens (HLAs). The letters A, B, C, and D are arbitrary symbols for the four parental chromosome 6s bearing the major histocompatibility complex (MHC). The four (or five) closely linked genes in this chromosomal region are usually transmitted to the offspring *en bloc*, and the fixed combination of one each A, B, C, D (and DR) antigens is referred to as a haplotype (see Table 32–3). There are two pairs of HLA-identical siblings among the offspring in this family, two with haplotypes A and C and two with B and C. (Reproduced from Amos DB. Immunologic and genetic aspects of kidney transplantation. In Strauss MB, Welt LG [eds]. Diseases of the Kidney, 2nd ed. Boston, Little, Brown, 1971.)

different antigenic specificities (Bell et al., 1985; Wu et al., 1986).

Class III genes are located between the HLA B and D loci and determine the structure of three components of the complement system: C2, C4, and factor B (Arnett, 1986). C2 and factor B are each encoded by single loci. The C4 protein is encoded by two genetic loci (C4A and C4B), which appear to be separated by the gene for 21-hydroxylase. Class III loci are also highly polymorphic, particularly C4A and C4B, yielding multiple electrophoretically distinct allotypic gene products or no gene product at all (*null alleles*). Of all normal individuals, 19% carry the null allele at C4A (designated C4A*QO) and 28% carry the null allele at C4B (C4B*QO). For total C4 deficiency (which is extremely rare), null genes must be present on both chromosome 6s at both the C4A and C4B loci. Heterozygous C2 deficiency (C2*QO) occurs in approximately one in 300 individuals and homozygous C2 deficiency in one in 10,000.

Because the recombination fraction between the HLA loci has been shown by family studies to be just under 1% (~1/3000th of the total genome), this region has been predicted to include several hundred genes (Bodmer, 1986). In addition to the loci depicted in Figure 32–1, there is evidence for close linkage of the MHC to the loci regulating the Rodgers and Chido erythrocyte antigens, phosphoglucomutase isoenzymes,

and the gene controlling the 21-hydroxylase–deficient form of congenital adrenal hyperplasia (Bach and Sachs, 1987).

Inheritance

HLA antigens are inherited in a mendelian dominant manner. However, because of the closeness of the different loci of the MHC and the resultant low crossover frequency, HLA genes are also always inherited *en bloc*. This fixed combination of genetic determinants is referred to as a *haplotype*. Because chromosome 6 is an autosome, all individuals have two HLA haplotypes (one for each chromosome) and there will be only four possible combinations of these haplotypes among the offspring of any two parents.

A schematic representation of the inheritance of HLA antigens in a hypothetical family is shown in Figure 32–3. Within a given family, 25% of siblings will be HLA identical, 50% will be haploidentical, and 25% will differ by both haplotypes. Since each locus is multiallelic, the number of possible combinations among unrelated individuals is enormous. The actual number, however, is less than the theoretical number, because certain combinations of antigens occur more frequently than expected on the basis of chance. Three such pairs of HLA-A and -B loci antigens are A1 and B8, A3 and B7, and A29 and B12. This phenomenon is referred to as linkage disequilibrium; further examples are given in Table 32–2. It has been postulated that linkage disequilibrium may have arisen because of selective advantage provided by certain combinations of alleles. The most important combination in the United States Caucasian population is A1,B8,C7,DR3, DR52,DQ2, and a C4A null gene. This haplotype, interestingly, is associated with multiple autoimmune diseases.

Natural HLA Antibodies

Because of the occasional hyperacute rejection of kidney or heart transplants by recipients not known to have been previously sensitized with HLA antigens, Rapaport and Chase (1964) have suggested that "natural" antibodies, analogous to antibodies to A and B blood group substances, may exist for HLA antigens. These investigators immunized guinea pigs, mice, rabbits, and rats with heat-killed group A streptococci and observed accelerated rejection of skin allografts indistinguishable from rejection caused by presensitization with donor tissue antigens (Rapaport, 1970). Heterologous serum from animals preimmunized with streptococcal antigens has also been effective in accelerating graft rejection when administered to skin graft

Table 32–2. Two Common Extended Haplotypes Exemplifying Linkage Disequilibrium*

A1, B8, Cw7, DR3, DRw52, DQw2, C4A.QO
A3, B7, DR2, DRw10, DQw1

*Based on white populations.

recipients (Rapaport et al., 1969). These observations suggest that antigens in nature resemble HLA antigens and may account for some unexplained cases of hyperacute rejection.

The ABO System

The importance of ABO erythrocyte antigens in transplantation was demonstrated by Dausset and Rapaport (1966), who showed that the survival of skin grafts from type AB donors in type O recipients was shortened if the recipients were preimmunized with AB erythrocytes. Ceppellini and associates (1969) found that skin from type A1 or B donors grafted onto unrelated type O recipients underwent a significantly accelerated rejection. By contrast, no decrease in survival was observed if the donor had either type A2 or O blood; this suggested that A2 may be less important as a transplantation antigen. It is of note, however, that ABO incompatibility does not lead to a shortened skin graft survival time in two thirds of HLA identical sibling donor-recipient combinations. This, together with the fact that ABO incompatibility does not cause stimulation in mixed leukocyte cultures, indicates that ABO compatibility is of much less importance than HLA compatibility in graft survival, except for primarily vascularized grafts, such as kidney and heart.

The importance of ABO compatibility for graft acceptance has been most clearly demonstrated in kidney transplantation, where hyperacute rejection caused by cytotoxic antibodies to A1 or B blood group substances is seen when kidneys from type A1, B, or AB donors are transplanted into type B, A, or O recipients (Kissmeyer-Nielsen et al., 1966). This is due to the fact that ABO blood group antigens are present on kidney grafts, particularly those from A or B secretors, and preformed naturally occurring antibodies to blood group substances are present in mismatched recipients. The blood group antigen A2 appears to be less immunogenic because of a lack of the blood group A type 4 chain glycolipid (Breimer et al., 1987). Results of blood group A2 kidney transplants into type O recipients have been comparable with those into ABO-compatible recipients (Brynger et al., 1984; Breimer et al., 1985).

In contrast to the kidney, the liver is immunologically privileged, in the sense that it has increased resistance to antibody-mediated hyperacute rejection. This has allowed successful liver transplantation despite a positive cross-match and ABO-incompatible combinations (Hitzig and Willi, 1961).

The donor and recipient, if possible, should be ABO-compatible, as defined by the laws of transfusion (Breimer et al., 1985). The donor of an organ graft should not possess A or B blood group antigen if that antigen is absent in the recipient. Conversely, the donor of bone marrow or other immunocompetent tissue grafts for an immunologically incompetent recipient should possess A or B blood group antigen if that antigen is present in the recipient. Finally, in bone marrow transplantation, if both donor and recipient are immunologically competent, ABO compatibility should be present in both directions.

Other Systems

There are undoubtedly other antigens that determine histocompatibility in humans, since even HLA-identical sibling allografts are eventually rejected unless immunosuppressive agents are used (Amos et al., 1969). These antigens may be organ-specific or tissue-specific antigens or, more likely, minor locus histocompatibility antigens similar to those identified in the mouse (Graff and Bailey, 1973).

Donor Selection

Two general methods are used to pair donors and recipients for transplantation. The first involves the detection of HLA antigens on donor and recipient leukocytes by either serologic or DNA typing methods; the second method involves the measurement of the response of immunocompetent cells from the recipient to antigens present on donor cells (and *vice versa* for bone marrow transplantation).

Serotyping

Many serologic methods have been used to detect histocompatibility antigens; these include leukocyte agglutination, cytotoxicity, complement-fixation, and mixed agglutination. Lymphocyte cytotoxicity has the greatest reproducibility and practicality: a micromethod is now in widespread use (Terasaki and McClelland, 1964). Polyclonal antisera used in these assays are obtained from multiparous women or from volunteers who have undergone leukocyte alloimmunization. In addition, monoclonal antibodies are now available for a large number of specificities.

A two-stage method is used in which lymphocytes are first incubated with the antisera and then incubated with rabbit complement (Sullivan and Amos, 1986). Dead cells appear larger and darker, and there is a clear distinction between the nucleus and cytoplasm under phase-contrast microscopy. Because considerable skill is required to detect cytotoxicity by this method, however, the cells are usually preincubated with a vital dye (such as trypan blue, eosin, nigrosin, or ethidium bromide) and cell death is indicated by uptake of the dye. Cytofluorography can also be used to detect HLA antigens if monoclonal antibodies are available for the informative antigens.

In routine typing for HLA-A, -B or -C antigens, peripheral blood mononuclear cells (MNCs) from the potential donor and recipient are tested against a panel of antisera having known HLA specificities. In typing for HLA class II antigens, it is necessary to first obtain a B-lymphocyte-enriched cell population. This is done by passing the MNCs over nylon wool or anti-F(ab)'2 columns or incubating them in anti-F(ab)'2 dishes, then eluting the SIg⁺ B cells with human immunoglobulin (IgG) (Sullivan and Amos, 1986).

If the potential donor and recipient are first-degree relatives, the parents and siblings should be tested so that genotyping as well as phenotyping can be accomplished. By comparing the reaction patterns of the parents with those of their children, one can identify the two paternal and two maternal haplotypes. In such an analysis, an attempt is made to determine the HLA antigens that are inherited *en bloc* (i.e., the haplotype for each of the four parental chromosomes bearing HLA genes). Siblings can be identified who have identical haplotypes (i.e., who are HLA-identical) and who have no haplotypes in common (i.e., are haplo-distinct) (see Fig. 32–3).

An example of such a genotypic analysis is present in Table 32–3. The data presented from this hypothetical family represent a great oversimplification of what takes place in actual practice, since usually several different antisera are used to test for the presence of one HLA antigen. Some of these have broader specificities than others, therefore possibly containing cross-reactive antibodies or more than one anti-HLA antibody. It is occasionally not possible to detect all parental HLA antigens with this technique. Nonetheless, observations on the intrafamilial reaction patterns usually permit genotyping even when all antigens are not identified.

Sequence-Specific Oligonucleotide Genotyping of HLA Polymorphism

Sequence-specific oligonucleotide (SSO) genotyping permits far more precise and detailed HLA typing than can ever be achieved by serologic or lymphocyte functional typing methods. It is carried out on polymerase chain reaction (PCR)–amplified DNA by oligonucleotide hybridization and is most useful for accurate matching of HLA class II specificities, a feat difficult to do reliably by conventional serologic HLA typing because of the extensive polymorphism of class II antigens. A number of variations on this technique have been developed, but a particularly useful semiautomated method was developed by Cros and colleagues (1992). This consists of an oligonucleotide hybridization assay done on microtiter plates, followed by automatic colorimetric reading. The entire typing assay can be completed in less than 4 hours and has been validated on more than a thousand haplotypes in prospective DR typing of patients and their potential donors (Cros et al., 1992). It is simple enough for routine laboratory use.

Another DNA-based matching technique is that of universal heteroduplex generator (UHG) cross-matching (Clay et al., 1994). This is a rapid and simple method of screening prospective bone marrow donors for HLA-DPB1 compatibility with the recipient. The method relies on the visual comparison of PCR heteroduplex banding patterns on nondenaturing polyacrylamide minigels. It determines whether pairs or groups of samples are HLA-DPB1 matched or mismatched but does not permit direct assignment of HLA-DPB1 alleles. In a comparative study with SSO typing, 52 of 56 (93%) pairs showed concordant findings in UHG cross-matching (Clay et al., 1994).

Lymphocyte Defined Antigen Typing

Lymphocyte-defined HLA class II antigens are detected through their stimulatory capacity in the mixed leukocyte reaction (MLR). This test is performed by mixing blood leukocytes from donor and recipient in tissue culture for 5 to 6 days and noting, through ^{3}H-thymidine incorporation, the amount of DNA synthesis; the latter indicates the degree of reactivity of the two cell populations against alloantigens of each other (Bach and Hirschhorn, 1964; Bain et al., 1964).

One-Way Mixed Leukocyte Reaction. In actual practice, the bidirectional response in a mixed leukocyte reaction is usually prevented so that the reactivity of each cell population can be measured separately. This is accomplished by pretreating one population of cells with either x-irradiation or mitomycin C to arrest DNA synthesis and cell division, the so-called "one-way" MLR (Amos and Bach, 1968). The treated cells are still alive, with HLA class II membrane antigens intact, and hence are able to stimulate the untreated lymphoid cell population. The responding cell population is composed entirely of T lymphocytes, whereas the stimulating cells consist of B lymphocytes and monocytes, both of which bear HLA class II antigens.

The one-way MLR is used in intrafamilial typing to confirm that siblings who appear HLA-identical by serotyping are also identical for T-lymphocyte–defined antigens. Unless extensive DNA typing is done, the one-way MLR using homozygous typing cells as stimulators is the only means of defining some HLA class II antigens (Mempel et al., 1973). If the responder cell shares the HLA-D locus specificity with the homozygous typing cell, it does not react in MLR, whereas lack of identity between the two cell populations results in a positive MLR. The results of HLA-D typing correlate primarily with DRB compatibility, but the precision in donor matching with SSO typing is far greater than with either HLA-D typing or direct MLR testing (Mickelson et al., 1994).

Primed Lymphocyte Typing. A modification of the MLR, the primed lymphocyte typing (PLT) test, avoids the 5- to 6-day lag period necessary for peak MLR responsiveness (Sheehy and Bach, 1976). In PLT, "known" homozygous typing stimulator cells are cultured for 9 to 14 days with responder cells known to lack that specificity. The responder cells are now primed and can be cloned (Bach et al., 1979) or are kept in a frozen state ready to use. "Unknown" stimulator cells are then added; a specific and rapid (within 24 hours) proliferation by the primed responder cells indicates that the unknown stimulator cells bear the same D region specificity as the known homozygous stimulator cells.

Prior to the development of DNA typing, PLT was the principal test used to define HLA-DP specificities. This test also has the advantage of not necessarily requiring homozygous typing cells (which are often difficult to obtain); in intrafamilial typing, any known stimulator cell population sharing one haplotype with the responder cells can be used to prime for detection of the antigens of the non-shared haplotype of the stimulator cells (Mempel et al., 1973).

Cell-Mediated Lympholysis. Another matching technique involving an initial MLR is cell-mediated lympholysis (CML); CML is useful in demonstrating

Table 32–3. Genotypic Analysis for Human Leukocyte Antigens (HLAs) in a Hypothetical Family*

Reactions with Antisera Detecting Official HLAs

Family Member	Arbitrary Symbols for HLA Chromosomes	HLA-A Locus				HLA-B Locus					HLA-C Locus			HLA-DR Locus			
		1	2	3	10	7	8	13	15	w3	w4	w5	w6	1	2	3	4
Father	A / B	+	+				+	+			+		+	+	+		
Mother	C / D			+	+				+	+		+	+			+	+
Sibling I	A / C	+		+				+		+		+	+	+		+	
Sibling II	A / D	+			+			+	+				+	+			+
Sibling III	B / C		+	+			+			+	+	+			+	+	
Sibling IV	B / D		+		+		+		+		+		+		+		+
Sibling V	A / C	+		+				+		+		+	+	+		+	
Sibling VI	B / D		+		+		+		+		+		+		+		+

Haplotypes

HLA Chromosomes	HLA-A Locus				HLA-B Locus					HLA-C Locus			HLA-DR Locus			
	1	2	3	10	7	8	13	15	w3	w4	w5	w6	1	2	3	4
Father A	+						+					+	+			
Father B		+				+				+				+		
Mother C			+						+		+				+	
Mother D				+				+				+				+

*By observing the reaction pattern similarities and differences between the offspring and the parents and by determining the reactions which always occur together in a single individual, one can deduce the two HLAs controlled by each parental chromosome (i.e., the haplotype). Each haplotype consists of one each of HLA-A, -B, -C, and -DR antigens (see Table 32–1). All patterns found in the children represent various combinations of one paternal and one maternal haplotype. Siblings I and V are HLA-identical, as are Siblings IV and VI.

HLA class I antigen identity or differences between donor and recipient. In this assay, a MLR is established for 5 days; during this time, the stimulator cells gradually die, leaving only the responding cells. The responding cells are then tested for their cytolytic specificity using ^{51}Cr-labeled target cells from the donors of both the responding and stimulator cells and from other subjects. The target cells are preincubated with phytohemagglutinin (PHA) for 3 days and mixed with the responder (effector) cells from the MLR. After 3 to 4 hours, the supernatant is analyzed for its ^{51}Cr content, which reflects the amount of target cell lysis. If the chromium release is equivalent for pairs of target cells, they share HLA class I antigens. Extensive studies have shown that class II antigens are responsible for the stimulation of CD4$^+$ helper/inducer T cells in CML, and HLA class I antigens are the targets for CD8$^+$ cytotoxic T cells. Thus, although class II antigenic differences lead indirectly to the formation of cytotoxic effector cells, the targets of the latter are cells bearing disparate class I antigens (Bach and Sachs, 1987).

Cross-Matching

Serologic Cross-Matching. Serologic cross-matching is a form of matching of donor and recipient and is of particular importance to the success of primarily vascularized grafts, such as kidney and heart. Serum from the prospective recipient is tested against cells from the potential donor for the presence of antibodies to red blood cell and/or HLA antigens. The two-stage microlymphocytotoxicity test is usually used to detect the latter. In most transplant centers, patients awaiting kidney or heart transplants are screened monthly for serum anti-HLA antibodies to a reference cell panel. This cross-match should also be performed near the time of the actual transplant, since these antibodies can form within a short period, particularly if the recipient is receiving blood transfusions. On the other hand, the reactivity of sera from such patients can diminish despite once having a high titer (Sanfilippo et al., 1984).

The presence of such antibodies correlates with hyperacute renal graft rejection (Kissmeyer-Nielsen et al., 1966). For this reason, a positive serologic cross-match in the past has been considered an absolute contraindication to renal transplantation. However, not all lymphotoxic antibodies in patients with positive cross-matches are directed against class I HLA antigens. Some appear to have specificities for only class II antigens on B lymphocytes, and a number of renal allografts have been successfully carried out in their presence (Carpenter and Morris, 1978). Reed and coworkers (1987) demonstrated that the presence of anti–anti-HLA (i.e., anti-idiotypic) antibodies (shown by blocking of lymphocytotoxic activity of anti-donor HLA antibody) correlated well with graft acceptance, whereas the presence of anti-anti–anti-HLA antibodies that potentiated the cytotoxic activity of anti-donor HLA antibodies correlated with graft rejection.

Cellular Cross-Matching. Cellular cross-matching procedures have been mentioned, and the MLR is the most crucial of these. However, the CML test can provide evidence of prior sensitization to class I antigens of the donor.

Value of HLA Typing in Clinical Organ Transplantation

Most of the information about HLA typing has been derived from renal, bone marrow, and corneal transplantation. Although typing for intrafamilial transplants of all types is of great value, the usefulness of HLA typing in cadaveric kidney grafting has been a point of much controversy since cyclosporine became available (Terasaki and Cecka, 1994). Renal grafts from HLA-identical sibling donors have a 3-year survival of about 90%, those from family members sharing one haplotype have a 3-year survival of about 80%, and those from siblings with two different haplotypes have a 3-year survival of about 70%, the same rate as those with cadaveric grafts (Terasaki and Cecka, 1994).

Analyses from several centers have indicated that survival of kidneys well matched for class I antigens (i.e., sharing three or four antigens) is improved by 10% to 30% over those of less well-matched grafts (van Rood, 1987). Data from the London Transplant Group indicate that matching for B locus antigens is more important than matching for A locus antigens (Festenstein et al., 1986). Transplants that could not be matched for both B locus antigens but were completely matched for Bw4/Bw6 also did very well. In addition, the London group reported that since 1978 excellent results were obtained with HLA-DR but not with DQ matching (Festenstein et al., 1986). The advantage of matching for HLA-B and DR in cadaveric renal transplantation was also supported in a worldwide survey by Opelz and coworkers (1987) and in a similar analysis by the Eurotransplant group (van Rood, 1987). HLA matching is particularly important in patients who have become presensitized to MHC antigens prior to renal transplantation or in patients undergoing a second transplant, because 45% of patients with early rejection of primary grafts become sensitized to HLA antigens and reject most subsequent transplants (Barber et al., 1985; Perdue, 1985).

In regard to corneal grafts, HLA matching usually does not influence the rate of rejection; the exception is high-risk patients whose corneas are severely vascularized or who have had two or more previous grafts (Sanfilippo et al., 1986).

Until the past 15 years, strict HLA matching was crucial for success in bone marrow transplantation, as both graft rejection and lethal graft-versus-host (GVH) reactions are common complications. Until 1980, usually only HLA-identical siblings could be used as bone marrow donors; rarely, other relatives (e.g., parents or cousins) were found to be identical for class II HLA antigens when there had been consanguineous marriages (Mickelson et al., 1976). The development of techniques to deplete post-thymic T cells from donor marrow has permitted numerous successful half-matched marrow transplants with no or minimal GVH disease over the past two decades (Buckley et al., 1993).

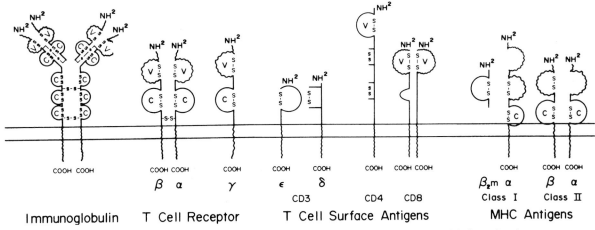

Figure 32–4. Cell surface receptors sharing structural homologies with immunoglobulin molecules. Other candidates include intracellular adhesion molecules (ICAMs), such as I-CAM and N-CAM.

HLA and the Immune Response

Class I and II chains of HLA molecules are closely related structurally to each other and to many other recognition structures of the immune system. The domains closest to the cell membrane (Iα_3, β_2m, IIα_2, and IIβ_2) show strong sequence homologies (see Fig. 32–2). They also have sequences similar to those found in immunoglobulin heavy and light chains, in α, β and γ chains of the T-cell receptor, and in CD3, CD4 and CD8 T-cell surface antigens. Because of their shared sequence homologies, these molecules have been designated as members of the *immunoglobulin gene superfamily* (Fig. 32–4) (Hunkapiller and Hood, 1986). These closely related molecules may have evolved from a common ancestral gene (Kronenberg et al., 1986).

Evidence that products of MHC genes are involved in immune responsiveness was first presented in 1969 by McDevitt and Chinitz; they described linkage of so-called MHC immune response (Ir) genes in mice to defects in responsiveness to certain antigens. Numerous subsequent studies have confirmed and expanded those observations (Tiwari and Terasaki, 1985).

Currently, it is believed that MHC gene products are involved in most, if not all, responses to T-dependent antigens. Thus, soluble antigens must first be processed and degraded by antigen-presenting cells (APCs: [macrophages, dendritic cells, or B cells]) and a resulting peptide presented in the groove of an HLA class II antigen to a T-lymphocyte capable of recognizing that peptide before a proliferative response is elicited. Thus, the HLA molecule serves as a crucial component of recognition units responsible for immune cell interaction and T-lymphocyte activation. Although self-HLA molecules do not normally stimulate a response by autologous T cells, when a foreign antigenic peptide is associated with self–class I or II antigens on target cells or APCs, an autologous T cell receptor capable of recognizing that peptide in the context of self-MHC interacts with the APC and a signal is sent to the nucleus of that T cell to become activated (Fig. 32–5). Foreign antigens associated on the cell surface with autologous class I molecules are recognized by CD8[+]

cytotoxic T cells; antigens associated with class II molecules are recognized by CD4[+] helper/inducer T cells.

Thus, these self-HLA antigens serve as both restricting and regulating molecules, since the T cells do not recognize soluble foreign antigens on cells that do not bear self-HLA antigens, and the HLA antigen class with which the foreign antigen is associated determines which type of T-cell function is activated. By contrast, foreign HLA antigens alone appear to be sufficient to activate receptors on CD4[+] T cells to cause them to proliferate and on CD8[+] T cells to make them become cytolytic for cells bearing those foreign antigens (Krensky, 1985).

Further restrictions imposed by the MHC are conferred on pre–T cells while they are differentiating in the thymus (Zinkernagel, 1978). Studies using irradiated parental or F_1 hybrid mice reconstituted with bone marrow cells from the F_1 hybrid indicate that MHC antigens of the recipient (probably those on recipient epithelial or dendritic cells within the thymus) influence the differentiating T cells to have restricted cytotoxic T-cell activity against virus-infected tissues. Indeed, the genetic environment in which T cells develop is very important. Haploidentical stem cells that enter the thymus of a human recipient with severe combined immunodeficiency (SCID) develop into thymocytes that are positively selected by HLA antigens on thymic

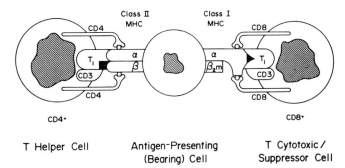

Figure 32–5. Schematic of cell-cell interactions involving the T-cell receptor (Ti), HLA class I and II molecules, and T-cell surface antigens CD4 and CD8.

epithelial cells and on resident dendritic cells, so that they learn to recognize recipient B and antigen-presenting cells as self; those not selected die by apoptosis (Roberts et al., 1989). The positively selected cells are then negatively selected by the infant's self-peptides in the clefts of the HLA antigens so that cells with the potential to react against the recipient are deleted (Schiff and Buckley, 1987).

HLA and Disease Associations

Since the relationships between H-2 phenotypes and susceptibility of mice to virus-induced tumors were established (Lilly et al., 1964), there has been considerable interest in the association of HLA phenotypes and disease susceptibility in humans. These associations may provide information relevant to the pathogenesis, diagnosis, and genetics of the disease. The first evidence that MHC genes might be associated with a specific disease was reported by Amiel (1967), who noted an increased frequency of the HLA antigen "4c" in patients with Hodgkin's disease. This antigen was later shown to include HLA-B5, HLA-B15, and HLA-B18.

Since 1967, a large number of diverse diseases have been been found to be associated with increased or decreased frequencies of various HLA antigens (Table 32–4) (Tiwari and Terasaki, 1985). These include autoimmune, suspected autoimmune and infectious diseases, primary immunodeficiencies and various forms of malignancy, all of which are considered immunologic diseases. However, similar associations have been reported for HLA and conditions, such as narcolepsy, that have no conceivable immunologic basis. Although the associations listed are all statistically significant and some are particularly striking, in only one case is the association absolute—that of narcolepsy with DR2. Beyond that, the magnitudes of the effect on risk varies greatly (Adams, 1987):

- Very strong for ankylosing spondylitis and B27 (risk increased 69-fold, i.e., ×69)
- Moderate for Goodpasture's syndrome and DR2 (×13.8)
- Slight for many diseases (e.g., systemic lupus erythematosus) and B8 (×2.7)

Reasons for the lack of complete correlation include the possibility that the MHC antigens reflect genes that are not themselves responsible for the disease susceptibility but are closely linked to the as yet unidentified disease-causing genes (Coppin and McDevitt, 1986). Such an association would reflect linkage disequilibrium between the two loci. Another likely possibility is that the disease under question, while phenotypically homogeneous, may be genetically heterogeneous. Further, the disease may also be affected by genes outside the MHC and by environmental factors.

This has been illustrated best by studies of the molecular basis of HLA DR4 associations with rheumatoid arthritis (Nepom et al., 1986, 1987). Although this association has been reported in numerous studies and multiple ethnic groups, one fourth to one third of individuals affected with rheumatoid arthritis do not

have the HLA-DR4 antigen and among those who do, there is evidence for an effect of specific combinations of other MHC alleles with DR4 (Arnett, 1986; Nepom et al., 1986; Winchester, 1986; Nepom et al., 1987). However, it is now apparent that the HLA-DR4 allospecificity is expressed on a family of at least six different related but distinct haplotypes (Nepom et al., 1986, 1987). In other words, the different haplotypes all react with DR4-specific alloantisera yet stimulate each other in a MLR; that is, they have different lymphocyte-defined (Dw/LD) DR4 antigens (Nepom et al., 1986, 1987). Dw4 (DR4) and Dw14 (DR4) DR1 genes appear to be alleles that confer disease risk in rheumatoid arthritis, whereas Dw10 (DR4) does not.

Similarly, although type I insulin-dependent diabetes mellitus (IDD) is closely associated with HLA DR3 and/or DR4 positivity, this is not absolute (Platz et al., 1982; Wolf et al., 1983). Some molecular and genomic studies of this association resulted in the cloning of a polymorphic DNA endonuclease fragment that associates IDD with HLA-DQ, specifically HLA-DQ 3.2 (DQw3) much more closely than with any DR specificity (Michelsen and Lernmark, 1987; Nepom et al., 1987). Likewise, another DQ beta gene complementary DNA (cDNA) probe has demonstrated a close linkage of HLA-DQ beta chain polymorphism to myasthenia gravis (Bell et al., 1986). Finally, the allele DRβ1* 1302 was recently associated with protection against persistent hepatitis B virus infection among both children and adults in The Gambia (Thursz et al., 1995). Further studies of this type should clarify some of the currently weak associations of MHC antigens with other diseases.

In the search for mechanisms whereby certain diseases are associated with abnormal frequencies of particular MHC antigens, an early hypothesis suggested that they are a result of abnormal or defective immune response genes closely linked to loci controlling MHC antigens (McDevitt and Bodmer, 1974). However, DNA sequence analysis of the MHC has revealed only genes for cell surface antigens and complement proteins (Hood et al., 1983). Moreover, defective immune response genes would not explain MHC-associated nonimmunologic diseases.

Another hypothesis suggests antigenic cross-reactivity between HLA antigens and certain microorganisms, with failure to recognize antigenic determinants on invading microorganisms, thereby allowing infection to occur. In support of this postulate, Ebringer and Ghudoom (1986) found evidence that cross-reactivity between HLA-B27 and microbial antigens is implicated in the pathogenesis of B27-associated conditions. Lopez et al., (1993) reported finding two CTL T-cell clones with the same T-cell receptor that had cross-reactivity between HLA-B27 and HLA-DR2 as a result of a shared structural motif between HLA-B27 and the DR2 B5*0101 chain. The authors postulated that HLA-B27 spondyloarthropathies may be the product of an autoimmune T-cell response against a tissue-specific peptide specifically presented by HLA-B27 in joint tissues.

A final hypothesis suggests that the HLA antigens themselves may serve as cell membrane receptors for

Table 32–4. Summary of Most Significant Human Leukocyte Antigens (HLAs) and Disease Association

Disease	Race	Studies N	Patients No.	Patients % +	Controls % +	RR	Disease	Race	Studies N	Patients No.	Patients % +	Controls % +	RR
Rheumatoid Arthritis							*Psoriasis Vulgaris*						
B27	C	17	861	16	9	2.0	B13	C	36	2579	19	5	4.1
DR4	C	17	1127	68	25	3.8	B17	C	35	2515	19	7	5.3
Bw54	O	3	221	24	11	2.5	B37	C	15	804	7	2	3.9
DR4	O	5	348	66	39	2.8	Cw6	C	7	353	56	15	7.5
DR4	N	3	109	40	10	5.4	DR7	C	5	296	48	23	3.2
							B13	O	5	336	24	8	3.3
Juvenile Rheumatoid Arthritis													
B27	C	15	1146	25	9	3.9	B17	O	4	224	12	9	1.9
DR5	C	5	422	34	15	3.3	B37	O	3	206	20	2	8.4
							Cw6	O	4	262	27	4	8.5
							DR7	O	2	148	10	1	7.6
Ankylosing Spondylitis													
B27	C	40	2130	89	9	69.1	*Pemphigus Vulgaris*						
B27	O	7	211	85	15	207.9	A26	CJ	5	117	60	20	4.8
B27	N	2	33	58	4	54.4	B38	CJ	5	117	59	21	4.6
							DR4	CJ	3	62	91	32	14.6
Acute Anterior Uveitis													
B27	C	10	520	47	10	8.2	*Dermatitis Herpetiformis*						
							B8	C	14	498	75	22	9.8
Reiter's Disease							DR3	C	4	126	82	20	17.3
B27	C	25	906	80	9	37.1	*Behçet's Disease*						
Juvenile Diabetes Mellitus							B5	C	6	150	31	12	3.8
B8	C	39	4322	40	21	2.5	B5	O	6	199	68	33	4.5
B15	C	36	4052	22	14	2.1	*Idiopathic Hemochromatosis*						
DR3	C	13	1174	46	22	3.3	A3	C	11	493	72	28	6.7
DR4	C	12	1051	51	25	3.6	B7	C	11	493	48	26	2.9
Bw54	O	8	453	39	11	5.6	B14	C	10	481	19	6	2.7
DR3	O	4	139	38	14	4.8	*Sjögren's Syndrome*						
DR4	O	4	139	49	25	2.6	B8	C	6	184	50	24	3.3
B8	N	6	337	19	11	2.4	Dw3	C	4	105	64	24	5.7
B15	N	5	299	6	5	2.2							
DR3	N	3	135	57	28	3.2	*Systemic Lupus Erythematosus*						
DR4	N	3	135	46	11	6.7	B8	C	17	855	40	20	2.7
							DR3	C	9	316	42	21	2.6
Graves Disease													
B8	C	18	1445	4	23	2.5	*Goodpasture's Syndrome*						
DR3	C	4	333	56	25	3.7	DR2	C	2	25	88	27	13.8
B35	O	3	162	42	14	4.4							
Celiac Disease							*Multiple Sclerosis*						
B8	C	16	696	68	22	7.6	B7	C	38	4964	37	24	1.8
DR3	C	5	194	79	22	11.6	DR2	C	13	1051	51	27	2.7
DR7	C	4	137	60	15	7.7	*Myasthenia Gravis*						
Narcolepsy							B8	C	12	747	44	19	3.3
DR2	C	2	45	100	22	129.8							
DR2	O	1	92	100	34	358.1							

Abbreviations: N = number of studies; No. = number of patients; C = Caucasian; O = Oriental; N = Negro; J = Jewish; % + = percent positive; RR = relative risk.
From Tiwari JL, Terasaki PI. HLA and Disease Associations. New York, Springer-Verlag, 1985, p. 33.

certain viruses (van Rood, 1986). Viral modification of transplantation antigens may cause autologous T cells to proliferate and react against the cells bearing the modified determinants (Dougherty and Zinkernagel, 1975). Relevant to this hypothesis are the findings of a significant excess of HLA-DR7 and a significant deficiency of HLA-DR2 in patients with chronic persistent infection with hepatitis B virus (Almarri and Batchelor, 1994).

GRAFT REJECTION

Mechanisms of Graft Rejection

Role of Lymphatics

Adequate lymphatic drainage of the graft site is necessary for graft sensitization. This was illustrated by the experiment of Barker and Billingham (1967), who raised skin flaps connected by narrow pedicles containing arteries and veins alone or arteries, veins, and lymphatics. Skin allografts placed on the flaps connected by all three vessels were destroyed in the usual length of time, whereas those placed on flaps without a lymphatic supply persisted as long as the flaps were viable. When another graft from the same donor was placed elsewhere on that host, the graft on the skin flap was promptly rejected, showing that lymphatics are not needed for graft rejection once sensitization occurs. Although blood vessels transport the effectors of rejection and vascular destruction is a prominent feature of rejection, vascular alterations are not essential for rejection because cytolysis can occur within Millipore chambers containing only immunocytes and target cells.

Events of Rejection

Histologic studies of skin grafts have provided most of the knowledge of the events of graft rejection. Within a few days after a histoincompatible skin graft is made, vascularization of the graft bed occurs and the site appears to be healing. A few days later, however, the grafted tissue appears darker; by the sixth day, there is vascular dilatation and tortuosity, with perivascular accumulation of mononuclear cells. These processes continue until thrombosis of the vascular supply occurs, the cellular infiltrate extends throughout the graft, and complete rejection occurs, usually after 10 to 11 days.

The rejection process begins much earlier for a second graft from the same donor. Rejection begins just at the time vascular connections are established and is usually complete in 7 days or less. In an even more rapid form of rejection, the *white graft phenomenon,* vascularization does not occur at all.

Although mononuclear cell infiltration is a prominent feature of rejection, the extent of damage does not always correlate with the degree of infiltration; indeed, the more rapid the rejection, the less the infiltrate. Conversely, slowly rejecting grafts may have intense accumulations of mononuclear cells (and even plasma cells) (the *blue graft phenomenon*) (Eichwald et al., 1966). Kidney graft rejection is accomplished by subendothelial depositions on the capillary basement membrane and infiltration of lymphoid cells, plasma cells, and macrophages. The extent of rejection is best correlated with the proportion of nonviable cells in the grafted tissue.

The Role of Antibody

Because the cellular infiltrates in most rejected grafts resemble those of delayed hypersensitivity reactions, and since graft rejection can be passively transferred with lymphoid cells but not with serum antibody even in high doses, most investigators have believed that graft rejection was mediated solely through the action of the small lymphocyte. The relatively intact capacity of patients with congenital X-linked agammaglobulinemia to reject allografts also attests to the major role of thymus-dependent immunity.

This view was modified when cytotoxic antibodies were found in recipients of allogeneic grafts and when less than perfect correlation was found between the mononuclear cell infiltration and the degree of rejection. The strongest evidence for a role for antibody in graft rejection is the hyperacute rejection of primarily vascularized organs, such as the kidney and heart. Humoral antibodies can be demonstrated in recipients undergoing these reactions (Kissmeyer-Nielsen et al., 1966). These antibodies combine with HLA antigens on endothelial cells with subsequent complement fixation and accumulation of polymorphonuclear cells. Endothelial damage then occurs, probably as a result of enzymes released from polymorphonuclear leukocytes; platelets then accumulate, thrombi develop, and the result is renal cortical necrosis or myocardial infarction.

The Cellular Basis of Graft Rejection

Results from both in vitro studies in humans and in vivo investigations in animals of cellular responses to MHC-encoded alloantigens support roles for both $CD4^+$ T-helper and $CD8^+$ cytotoxic T lymphocytes as well as macrophages in the rejection process (Schneider et al., 1986; Bach and Sachs, 1987). When different combinations of class I and class II antigen-bearing cells in MLR and CML experiments were used, it was learned that both helper and cytotoxic lymphocytes collaborate in the generation of cytotoxic responses.

Over the past decade, considerably more information has accrued about the nature of this collaboration and the rejection response in general (Suthanthiran and Strom, 1994). It is known that allograft rejection results from the coordinated activation of alloreactive T cells and antigen-presenting cells (APCs). Although acute rejection is a T cell–dependent process, the destruction of the allograft results from a broad array of effector mechanisms. Cell-cell interactions and the release of multiple types of cytokines lead to the recruitment of $CD4^+$ T cells, $CD8^+$ cytotoxic T cells, antibody-forming B cells, and other proinflammatory leukocytes.

The initial event is antigenic stimulation of recipient T cells capable of recognizing intracellularly processed fragments of foreign proteins embedded in the grooves of the MHC proteins expressed on the surface of APCs. Some of the recipient's T cells may recognize donor antigenic peptides presented on the surface of donor APCs; other T cells may recognize donor antigen after it is processed and presented by the recipient's APCs. On stimulation with antigens, the T-cell receptor/CD3/CD4 or CD8 complex physically associates with several intracellular protein tyrosine kinases.

Tyrosine phosphorylation activates the coenzyme phospholipase Cγ1 to hydrolyze phosphatidylinositol 4,5-biphosphate and the generation of inositol 1,4,5-triphosphate and diacylglycerol. Diacylglycerol, in the presence of intracellular calcium mobilized by inositol triphosphate, binds to and activates protein kinase C, which promotes the expression of several nuclear regulatory proteins and causes transcriptional activation and expression of genes central to T-cell division (such as the genes encoding interleukin-2 [IL-2] and its receptor) (Suthanthiran and Strom, 1994).

One of the participants in the signal transduction process is *calcineurin*, a calcium- and calmodulin-dependent serine-threonine phosphatase. Inhibition of calcineurin's phosphatase activity appears to be the fundamental mechanism of action of cyclosporine and tacrolimus, two potent immunosuppressive agents that have played major roles in the success of allografting over the past decade.

Stimulation of T cells through their antigen receptor is not sufficient to initiate T-cell activation, unless costimulation is provided by interaction of other ligand-receptor pairs present on the surfaces of T cells and APCs during their encounter. Some of these interactive pairs include the T-cell surface molecule, CD2, and its ligand, CD58 on APCs; CD11a/CD18:CD54; CD5:CD72; CD40 ligand:CD40; and CD28:CD80. Unless signals are provided through one or more of these receptor-ligand interactions or by cytokines (such as IL-1 and IL-6 from the APC), T-cell anergy or tolerance induction occurs when the T-cell receptor interacts with the APC. Thus, T-cell accessory proteins and their ligands on APCs are target molecules for anti-rejection therapy. If costimulation does occur, the T cell becomes activated, and this leads to stable transcription of the IL-2 gene and other genes important in T cell activation.

As noted earlier, cyclosporine and tacrolimus interfere significantly with the activation process initiated by interaction of APCs with the T-cell receptor and many of the costimulatory molecules. An exception, however, is the CD28:CD80 costimulatory pathway, which is independent of protein kinase C and calcium but can also lead to stable transcription of the IL-2 gene and other activation genes. That pathway is resistant to inhibition by cyclosporine and tacrolimus. Stimulation of the B cell by antigen occurs through its antigen receptor (i.e., surface immunoglobulin), but costimulation is also required for B-cell activation. This costimulation can be provided by cytokines released by T cells or through many of the same T-cell protein–ligand pairs important in T-cell–APC costimulation, as these ligands are also present on B cells.

Once T-cell activation has occurred, autocrine T-cell proliferation continues as a consequence of the expression of the IL-2 receptor. Interaction of IL-2 with its receptor triggers the activation of protein-tyrosine-kinases and phosphatidylinositol-3-kinase, resulting in translocation into the cytosol of an IL-2 receptor–bound serine-threonine kinase, Raf-1. This in turn leads to the expression of several DNA-binding proteins, such as c-jun, c-fos, and c-myc, and to progression of the cell cycle (Suthanthiran and Strom, 1994). The consequence of all of these events is the development of graft-specific, infiltrating cytotoxic T cells. Cytokines from the T cells also activate macrophages and other inflammatory leukocytes and cause up-regulation of HLA molecules on graft cells. The activated T cells also stimulate B cells to produce anti-graft antibodies. Ultimately, all of these cellular and humoral factors destroy the graft.

Nonspecific Immunosuppression

Because there is no method to suppress the host's immune response to antigens of the graft and at the same time maintain other immune responses, rejection must be prevented with nonspecific immunosuppressive agents. These include radiation, corticosteroids, cytotoxic agents, antilymphocyte antibodies, and cyclosporine and tacrolimus (see Chapter 19). The success of transplantation between unrelated donor and recipient can be attributed to the use of these agents. Because these agents depress both specific and nonspecific immunity, they render the recipient more susceptible to both infection and malignancy (Strom, 1987). Indeed, infection is the most important cause of transplant recipient mortality. Thus, all patients must have their immunosuppressive regimen fine-tuned to prevent rejection, yet minimize the risk of infection; too high a dose and infection supervenes, and too small a dose and the graft is rejected.

Corticosteroids

On entering the cell, steroids bind to a specific intracellular receptor. The steroid-receptor complex then enters the nucleus, leading to alterations in DNA transcription, messenger ribonucleic acid (mRNA) translation, and modification of enzyme synthesis. Steroids prevent transcription of macrophage IL-1-encoding RNA and thereby block the synthesis of IL-1. This in turn results in decreased stimulation of IL-2 and other lymphokine production by antigen-activated T-helper cells. Thus, essential growth factors are not produced, and the overall effect is decreased DNA, RNA, and protein synthesis and slowing of the rejection process. Steroids also stabilize cellular and lysosomal membranes and, in so doing, inhibit phagocytosis, retard the release of proteolytic enzymes, and prevent destruction of the grafted cells.

Prednisone is used prophylactically in most renal transplantations, beginning with a dose of 2 mg/kg/day; this is usually continued indefinitely but at a progressively lower dose. It has been successfully discontinued in some recipients of HLA-identical kidney grafts who then receive azathioprine alone (Siegler et al., 1977). Intravenous injection of prednisolone in a high dose (20 to 30 mg/kg) is particularly valuable in reversing acute organ rejection crises (Bell et al., 1971); the steroid is usually given for three doses on consecutive or alternate days.

Cytotoxic Agents

The cytoxic agents are a complex and heterogeneous group of chemicals, each having different biochemical effects at various points in the cell cycle. Nevertheless, all of these agents affect the structure or properties of DNA. The most common cytotoxic agents are:

- The purine antagonists, 6-mercaptopurine (6-MP) and azathioprine (Imuran)
- Methotrexate, a folic acid antagonist

• Cyclophosphamide (Cytoxan), an alkylating agent similar to nitrogen mustard

Purine Antagonists

Azathioprine has been the most widely used immunosuppressive agent in transplantation, although its therapeutic index is no higher than that of 6-MP, from which it differs by an imidazole ring. It damages cells because its metabolites are incorporated into purine nucleotides, and this inhibits the synthesis of DNA, thereby blocking proliferation of immunocompetent lymphoid cells. Its major effect is on T cells, and there is a lesser effect on B cells (Bach and Strom, 1985). Until the availability of cyclosporine, azathioprine was used by almost all renal transplant centers as the principal immunosuppressive agent, usually in combination with prednisone. In some centers, a high dose (5 mg/kg/day) of azathioprine is used for 2 preoperative and the first 2 postoperative days, tapering to a maintenance dose of 2 to 3 mg/kg/day by 1 week. In other centers, the latter dose is begun initially to avoid fluctuation in the immunosuppressive effect. The intravenous dose is one-half the oral dose.

Because bone marrow toxicity is a major side effect of azathioprine administration, hemoglobin levels, white blood cell (WBC) count, and platelet counts must be followed closely (daily during the first 2 weeks, several times a week for the next 2 to 3 months, and at lesser intervals thereafter). WBC counts in the range of 3000 to 5000/mm³ or less are an indication for reducing the dose, but a rapidly falling count at a higher level can also signify this need.

During renal failure, the oral dose of azathioprine should not exceed 1.5 mg/kg/day, and the actual dose is dictated by the WBC count. The drug can also lead to hepatotoxicity, usually manifested by mild to marked jaundice, but occasionally manifested only by elevated liver enzymes (Bach and Strom, 1985).

Methotrexate

Because methotrexate is excreted by the kidney, there has been reluctance to use it in kidney transplantation. Methotrexate has been employed most successfully in the prevention of graft-versus-host disease in aplastic anemia or in leukemia patients undergoing bone marrow transplantation (Thomas et al., 1975).

Cyclophosphamide

Cyclophosphamide is an effective substitute for azathioprine in renal and liver transplantation, offering the advantage of lessened liver toxicity (Bach and Strom, 1985). The dose is usually one-half that of azathioprine. The same precautions should be followed with regard to monitoring blood counts because leukopenia is common. Cyclophosphamide in high doses has been especially useful in conditioning patients for acceptance of bone marrow transplants (Santos, 1974).

Antilymphocyte and Antithymocyte Globulins

Antibodies from animals immunized with human lymphoid cells are effective immunosuppressive agents (Russell and Cosimi, 1979). These consist of the IgG fraction of sera from horses or rabbits immunized with either lymphoid cells (antilymphocyte globulin, ALG) or thymocytes (antithymocyte globulin, ATG), or of rat or murine monoclonal antibodies to T-cell surface antigens (CD3, CD2) (Cosimi et al., 1981) or IL-2 receptors (Soulillou et al., 1987). The advantage of the use of a monoclonal antibody to IL-2 receptors is that such receptors are present only on activated T lymphocytes; thus, the main effect is on T cells possibly activated by graft antigens. Administration of these foreign antibody molecules has, however, been followed by the development of serum sickness, chills, fever, and/or anaphylaxis. These reactions are more common if treatment is interrupted and reinstituted or continued for long periods of time.

The immunosuppressive potency of these antibodies can be assayed by their ability to prevent skin graft rejection in subhuman primates or by their ability to reduce the number of circulating CD2+ or CD3+ cells (Cosimi et al., 1981; Bach and Strom, 1985). The development of certain treatment regimens, including intravenous administration regimens, has reduced the incidence of allergic reactions (Bach and Strom, 1985). ALG is usually begun at the time of renal transplantation and continued on a daily or alternate-day schedule for 4 to 6 weeks.

In general, ALG or ATG decreases the onset, severity, and number of rejection episodes. The steroid-sparing effects of ALG and ATG are less consistent, but there is some evidence for this effect. Several studies have reported improved transplant survival with their use (Cosimi et al., 1981; Bach and Strom, 1985; Leone et al., 1987). Such antibodies are particularly useful in reversing acute graft rejection occurring in the first 2 weeks. However, antibodies eventually develop in the recipient to the foreign epitopes on these molecules, including anti-idiotypic antibodies, thereby causing their immune elimination and reducing their efficacy as immunosuppressive agents (Jeffers et al., 1986).

Radiation

The extreme lethality of total body irradiation has precluded its wide use in clinical organ transplantation. The present use of radiation is limited to local irradiation of the renal graft bed, total body irradiation for preparation of leukemic patients for bone marrow transplantation, and total lymphoid irradiation (Slavin et al., 1978; Strober, 1984). In the latter procedure, the skull, lungs, long bones, and pelvis are shielded and all major lymphoid organs, including the thymus and spleen, are exposed to 200 rad/day, five times a week, until a total dose of 3400 rad is reached. Studies in this model suggest that the state of tolerance is maintained by antigen-specific T cells.

Cyclosporine

A fungal metabolite of *Tolyplocadium inflatum*, cyclosporine is a neutral, hydrophobic, cyclical peptide containing 11 amino acids (White, 1983). It was recognized as a potentially valuable immunosuppressive agent in the late 1970s and has been used extensively in human organ transplantation for the past decade. Because of its extreme hydrophobicity, the drug must be dissolved in oil for administration; it is noncytotoxic and nonmyelosuppressive.

Cyclosporine gains access to the cell cytoplasm by binding to the isomerase protein, cyclophilin; the complex then acts on an intracellular enzyme to prevent the translocation of signals evoked by antigenic stimuli from the surface to the nucleus of the T cell. In this manner, it blocks transcription of the IL-2 gene. Thus, its predominant immunosuppressive effect is produced by blocking IL-2 synthesis and IL-2 receptor expression, thereby interfering with activated CD4$^+$ helper T-lymphocyte function (Bach and Strom, 1985; Shevach, 1985; Strom, 1987). The release of other lymphokines, including interferon-gamma (IFN-γ), B-cell stimulation factors, and cytotoxic differentiation factor, is also inhibited. Thus, T-cell proliferation and differentiation of precursor cytotoxic lymphocytes are blocked.

Cyclosporine has little capacity to interfere with the responsiveness of activated T lymphocytes (already expressing growth factor receptors) to cytokines. In summary, the cumulative effect of cyclosporine is the prevention of full activation of CD8$^+$ cytotoxic T cells, CD4$^+$ helper T cells, B cells, and macrophages by depriving them of the necessary CD4$^+$ helper cell stimulants. An improved oral formulation of cyclosporine (Neoral), soon to be available, has more uniform absorption and is less dependent on bile (Calne, 1994).

Tacrolimus (FK 506)

Tacrolimus (FK 506) is a macrolide compound isolated from *Streptomyces tsukubaensis* with potent immunosuppressive properties (Kino et al., 1987). To gain entry to the cell cytoplasm, tacrolimus binds to an isomerase protein in the some way as cyclosporine does, but the protein is a different one—the tacrolimus, or FK-binding, protein. The complex acts on the same enzyme system as does cyclosporine/cyclophilin to prevent T-cell receptor signal transduction to the nucleus. Tacrolimus inhibits formation of IL-2, IL-3, interferon (IFN-γ), and other cytokines by T cells in vitro. In this manner, it inhibits the MLR and was approximately 100 times more potent than cyclosporine as an immunosuppressive agent in animal organ transplantation (Kino et al., 1987; U.S. Multicenter FK 506 Liver Study Group, 1994).

In one study comparing tacrolimus and cyclosporine immunosuppressive regimens for liver transplantation, 1-year patient survival rates were similar (88%) and graft survival rates were not significantly different (82% and 79%, respectively) (U.S. Multicenter FK 506 Liver Study Group, 1994). Tacrolimus was associated with significantly fewer episodes of acute corticosteroid-resistant, or refractory rejection, but there were many more side effects that necessitated discontinuation of the drug. The most serious side effects were nephrotoxicity and neurotoxicity. More recently, hypertrophic cardiomyopathy has been associated with the use of tacrolimus in pediatric transplant patients; the condition resolved after reducing the dose, discontinuing the drug, or changing to cyclosporine (Atkison et al., 1995).

Combination Therapy

From the preceding text, it can be appreciated that no agent is the perfect immunosuppressive drug. Cytotoxic agents, steroids, and cyclosporine (or tacrolimus) all affect antigen-driven T-cell proliferation at different points in the T-cell activation process. Thus, the combined use of all three types of agents should provide a synergistic rather than mere additive effect (Bach and Strom, 1985; Strom, 1987).

Specific Immunosuppression

Specific immunosuppression is defined as suppression of the host's (and/or donor's, in the case of bone marrow transplantation) immune response against donor (and/or host in marrow transplantation) alloantigens without suppression of responses to other antigens.

Tolerance

Tolerance (specific immunologic unresponsiveness) is an induced state occurring as a consequence of specific deletion or suppression of a clone of cells that react with a specific antigen (Dresser and Mitchison, 1968). Most attempts to achieve specific immunosuppression have been directed toward manipulation of either graft antigens or the specific antigen receptors on cells capable of mediating rejection. The antigen receptors include both T-cell and B-cell (e.g., antibody) receptors.

The first example of specific immunosuppression was the ''neonatal tolerance'' observed by Billingham and colleagues (1953). They injected adult bone marrow cells intravenously into neonatal mice and found that such animals, even as adults, would accept donor type skin grafts indefinitely. Although this is not feasible in humans, other approaches designed to induce specific immunosuppression show promise.

Modification of the antigenicity of endocrine tissues (thyroid, pancreatic islet cells) by culturing the tissues for a period of time prior to transplantation has resulted in indefinite graft survival across the MHC or even across species in experimental animals (Lafferty et al., 1976; Sollinger et al., 1976; Lacy et al., 1979; Bowen et al., 1980). The mechanism of this modification is not completely clear, but it appears to be due to loss of cells rich in class II MHC antigens (dendritic and other APCs). This possibility is supported further by the studies of Faustman and associates (1981), who obtained extended survival of pancreatic islets treated with anti-Ia antibodies. Thus, it may be possible to avoid an effective immune response against a tissue if class II antigens are absent.

Other studies in experimental animals have shown that avoidance of class II antigens is sufficient for acceptance of grafts of only certain tissues, namely primarily vascularized organs, such as the kidney (Pescovitz et al., 1984), and not others, namely skin, where class I differences led to rejection (Kortz and Sachs, 1987). The liver also appears to be capable of long-term acceptance, even in the face of disparities of antigens of both MHC classes.

Another means of inducing specific immunosuppression in animals has been to administer antigen after a nonspecific immunosuppressive agent, such as anti-lymphocyte globulin (ALG) (Monaco and Wood, 1970) or azathioprine (Tyler et al., 1987). The fact that reduced doses or, in some cases, actual discontinuation of immunosuppressive agents still allows for successful maintenance of renal or hepatic allografts suggests that some degree of specific tolerance may be induced in human organ transplantation (Nagao et al., 1982).

In attempts to modify the receptors for antigens on T and B cells, Binz and Wigzell (1975) first reported successful abrogation of graft rejection in animals through the administration of anti-idiotypic antibodies produced by immunizing with antisera or alloreactive T cells. These findings could not be duplicated by others. Monoclonal anti-MHC antibodies have also been used as immunogens for such anti-idiotypic antibodies (Devaux et al., 1982; Sachs et al., 1985). Although the anti-idiotypic antibodies were potent inhibitors of humoral immune responses against the MHC antigens involved, they did not modify T-cell responses to those antigens or prolong skin graft survival (Bluestone et al., 1986). This fits with the knowledge that B- and T-cell antigen receptors differ in the epitopes recognized. Thus, administration of anti-idiotypic agents is not currently useful as the sole means of inducing specific immunosuppression for graft acceptance; however, anti-idiotypic T cells may be the mechanism for otherwise induced MHC tolerance in rats (Lancaster et al., 1985).

Enhancement

Enhancement is a form of antibody-mediated specific immunosuppression first appreciated when it was noted that administration of an antibody to a tumor prevented its rejection (Kaliss, 1958). Enhancement now has been extended to grafts of incompatible normal tissues (Stuart et al., 1970; French and Batchelor, 1972).

In this phenomenon, antiserum to the graft blocks the response of host lymphoid cells to the grafted tissues; in bone marrow transplantation, donor serum blocks the attack of grafted immunocompetent cells against host tissues. This is thought to be the mechanism underlying the beneficial effect of donor-specific blood transfusions employed in some centers to improve outcomes in haploidentical renal transplantation (Salvatierra et al., 1987; Tyler et al., 1987).

The mechanism of enhancement is unknown. The antibody may interfere with recognition of antigenic determinants by nonimmune lymphocytes *(afferent inhibition)*, may have a direct effect on the immunocyte *(central inhibition)*, or may mask the antigen *(efferent inhibition)*. The existence of *active enhancement* tends to preclude afferent inhibition, since both sensitized lymphocytes and blocking factors coexist. Moreover, *tolerance* following enhancement can be transferred by cells and not serum from enhanced animals (French and Batchelor, 1972). An idiotype–anti-idiotype mechanism may be one explanation for this phenomenon (Sachs, 1987). Unfortunately, enhancement has not been successful for prolonging survival of grafts other than kidney or in species other than the rat.

Prior Bone Marrow Transplantation

A final possible means of specifically modifying the host's immune response for organ grafting is that of first performing bone marrow transplantation from the prospective donor to the host. Thus far, this has been done primarily in experimental animals for obvious reasons (e.g., danger to the host of immunosuppression for marrow acceptance and the risk of a GVH reaction). Nevertheless, if rigorous T-cell depletion of donor marrow is used, a GVH reaction can be prevented, as already demonstrated for animals (Muller-Ruchholtz et al., 1976) and humans (Buckley et al., 1986, 1993). Depletion of donor marrow T cells and ablation of host immune cells by conditioning regimens lead to incomplete immunoreconstitution because the T cells that arise have matured in a thymus that is histoincompatible with donor marrow B and APCs (Singer et al., 1981). This problem has been circumvented experimentally by using total lymphoid irradiation (i.e., the long bones are shielded from irradiation) (Slavin et al., 1978) or by reconstituting total-body irradiated animals with a mixture of T-cell–depleted syngeneic and allogeneic bone marrow cells (Ildstad and Sachs, 1984). Both techniques have led to mixed chimeras. In the latter case, the animals were tolerant to donor grafts, lacked GVH disease, and were completely immunologically reconstituted. The first method was not successful in sensitized hosts, but the second method was (Sachs, 1987).

Regardless of the mechanism of specific immunosuppression, the development of a predictable means of inducing unresponsiveness only to the foreign histocompatibility antigens of the grafted tissue cells would represent a major breakthrough for the field of organ and tissue transplantation.

Differences in Tissue Acceptability

As already alluded to earlier, certain allogeneic tissues are accepted better than others. These differences may be due to (Russell and Cosimi, 1979):

- Variation in the degree of expression of HLA antigens on certain tissues
- The presence of unique or special antigens on certain tissues
- Differences in the resistance to immune attack of various tissues
- Differences in the anatomic site to which the tissue is transplanted

Because lymphocytes are particularly rich in HLA antigens, several approaches have been used to reduce their number in grafted organs or tissues. These include radiation or perfusion of kidneys, and culturing endocrine tissues (e.g., pancreas, thyroid) (Lafferty et al., 1976).

Differentiation antigens or other unique antigens may exist on cells from certain tissues (e.g., liver, lung) that evoke a strong immune reaction; their importance in clinical organ transplantation is not yet known. Certain cells (e.g., chondrocytes) are less susceptible to rejection than others. By contrast, some organs (e.g., the heart) are rejected more readily (Russell and Cosimi, 1979). Finally, the site of grafting is important because allografts survive longer in "privileged" sites, such as the anterior chamber of the eye, the interior of the brain, and probably the interior of the testis. The liver is also considered to be a "protected" organ to some extent. Grafts in these sites may be protected by a diminished blood supply or a lessened traffic of lymphoid cells.

PEDIATRIC RENAL TRANSPLANTATION

At one time, children were considered poor candidates for renal transplantation because of (1) the surgical technical problems of small vessels and donor organ–recipient size disparities and (2) growth impairment, orthopedic complications, and psychosocial problems resulting from the high-dose steroids required to prevent rejection. That kidney transplantation can be carried out successfully in children, however, has been repeatedly established at many centers over the past three decades; survival and graft function have been comparable with those in adults (McEnery et al., 1992; Broyer et al., 1993; Najarian et al., 1993; Tejani et al., 1993; Cecka and Terasaki, 1994; Batisky et al., 1994).

At present there are more than 10,000 functioning renal allografts in children worldwide (Ettenger et al., 1990; McEnery et al., 1992; Broyer et al., 1993; Tejani et al., 1993; Batisky et al., 1994; Cecka and Terasaki, 1994). The increased number of kidney transplants performed in children over the past three decades has paralleled the dramatic increase in renal transplantation in adults worldwide during that period. Moreover, since 1980, 1-year survival of cadaveric kidney grafts at most centers has increased from 50% to 80% and 1-year patient survival rates from more than 80% to more than 90% (Lundgren, 1987; Ettenger et al., 1990; McEnery et al., 1992; Broyer et al., 1993; Najarian et al., 1993; Tejani et al., 1993; Batisky et al., 1994; Cecka and Terasaki, 1994).

Many factors have contributed to these improvements, including improved surgical techniques and better approaches to prevent graft rejection. In particular, the use of donor-specific (Salvatierra et al., 1987) or random donor (So et al., 1986) blood transfusions, and the introduction of cyclosporine as a basic immunosuppressive agent have been of great benefit (Lundgren et al., 1987; Ettenger et al., 1990).

Despite spectacular improvement in dialysis techniques and the availability of this form of therapy to very young infants (Nevins and Kjellstrand, 1983), renal transplantation remains the treatment of choice for end-stage renal disease (ESRD) in patients of nearly all ages (Rivat et al., 1977; Ettenger et al., 1990; Broyer et al., 1993; Najarian et al., 1993; Tejani et al., 1993; Batisky et al., 1994). A successful kidney transplant brings about improvements in overall body function and in the quality of life that cannot be achieved with even the most advanced dialysis techniques.

There is no lack of patients for such transplants. Estimates of new cases of end-stage renal disease range from 1.5 to 3 per million people annually. In the United States, between 360 and 720 infants and children are newly diagnosed as having end-stage renal disease each year (Ettenger and Fine, 1986). It is important, however, that all the advances of the past three decades be brought to bear on pediatric renal transplants of the future. In this regard, many advocate that such transplants be performed only at centers where there are teams of experienced personnel and adequate resources (Ettenger et al., 1990; McEnery et al., 1992; Najarian et al., 1993; Tejani et al., 1993).

Indications

The three main causes of end-stage renal disease in infants and children are, in descending order of frequency, glomerulopathies of various types, congenital hypoplasia-dysplasia, and obstructive uropathy (Ettenger et al., 1990; McEnery et al., 1992; Cecka and Terasaki, 1994). In contrast to adult patients, a much higher percentage (49%) of pediatric renal transplant recipients have underlying congenital urinary tract disease (Ettenger and Fine, 1986; So et al., 1986; Ettenger et al., 1990; McEnery et al., 1992). Chronic glomerulonephritis is the most frequent underlying disorder in children age 6 years or older. Below age 6, congenital nonobstructive and obstructive renal disease are the most common conditions leading to the need for kidney transplantation. Wilms' tumor is the principal malignancy seen in the pediatric age group, but this indication for transplantation accounts for fewer than 5% of those performed (Ettenger et al., 1990; Najarian et al., 1993).

The only patients with end-stage renal disease who should be excluded from consideration for kidney transplantation are those with malignancy that cannot be brought under control or those with debilitating irreversible brain injury (So et al., 1986; Ettenger et al., 1990; Najarian et al., 1993). Thus, neither age nor pre-existing illness, such as diabetes or collagen-vascular disease, is an absolute contraindication to transplantation (Ettenger et al., 1990; McEnery et al., 1992; Broyer et al., 1993; Najarian et al., 1993; Cecka and Terasaki, 1994).

Donor Selection

Rates of Success

As discussed previously, renal transplant procedures are the most successful when related donors are involved. Best results are obtained when the donor is an identical twin; 2-year survival with a functioning kidney occurs in 87% to 100% of identical twin recipients and 30-year patient and graft survival are 70% and 55%, respectively (Cecka and Terasaki, 1994). A failure in this situation is usually secondary to development of the primary disease in the grafted kidney. The next best results are achieved when related donors are used. The 1-year graft survival rate in pediatric recipients of cadaver kidneys from 1988 to 1992 ranged from 70% to 84% and the 3-year rate was 58% to 67%. The latter rates were significantly poorer than in the related groups (Cecka and Terasaki, 1994).

Clearly, HLA matching improves the outcome of renal grafts not only when related donors are available but also when cadaver kidneys are used (Opelz, 1987; van Rood, 1987; Ettenger et al., 1990; McEnery et al., 1992). The loci statistically most important for matching appear to be HLA-B and -DR (Festenstein et al., 1986). Because of the ethical problems surrounding the use of minors as donors, HLA-identical sibling transplant procedures are not performed as often as in adults. As mentioned, the donor of the organ graft should not possess either A or B blood group antigens if that antigen is absent in the recipient (Breimer et al., 1987). In addition, living donors with hypertension should not be used. Finally, the serologic cross-match between the recipient's current serum and the donor's lymphocytes must be negative to minimize the chance of hyperacute rejection from preformed antileukocyte antibodies (Cicciarelli and Terasaki, 1983).

The fact that kidney grafts are tolerated by about 50% of the recipients who had had antibodies to donor HLA antigens in the past but not at the time of transplantation (Sanfilippo et al., 1984) indicates that "sensitization" is a changeable state. Anti–anti-HLA (i.e., anti-idiotype) antibodies were found in the sera of patients who tolerated their grafts, as opposed to antibodies (possibly anti-anti–anti-HLA antibodies) in the sera of those who experienced acute rejections, which potentiated the cytotoxic activity of a previously positive serum (Reed et al., 1987). This observation led to the recommendation that in the future cross-matches be done to detect these two different types of anti-idiotypic bodies (Reed et al., 1987).

Transplantation in Infants Under Age 1

Prior to 1985, renal transplantation in infants younger than 1 year of age had generally met with dismal success, with only 2 of 13 reported cases surviving with functioning grafts (Ettenger and Fine, 1986). Most of those had received cadaver kidneys, and many were from anencephalic donors. However, the experience with 13 such transplants (12 from living-related donors) at the University of Minnesota between 1978 and 1985 was good, and 12 of the 13 were alive with functioning grafts from 2.0 to 7.5 years after transplantations (So et al., 1986). Because of the adverse effects of end-stage renal disease on growth and development, the tendency in recent years has been to transplant as early as possible, particularly if a living-

related donor is available (So et al., 1987; Najarian et al., 1993). At major centers, such as those at the University of California at Los Angeles and the University of Minnesota, up to 50% of the pediatric renal transplantations are performed by the time the child is 5 years of age (Ettenger et al., 1990; Najarian et al., 1993). Because of the adverse experience to date, however, some say that cadaveric transplantations should not be performed in the first year of life and that anencephalic donors should not be used routinely because of their high percentage of renal malformations and generally poor renal function (Broyer et al., 1985; Fine, 1987).

Preparation of the Recipient

The development within the last two decades of improved dialysis techniques has been of major importance to successful renal transplantation in children (Nevins and Kjellstrand, 1983). The objective of dialysis is to correct electrolyte imbalances and reduce the blood urea nitrogen (BUN) to 50 to 70 mg/dl, thus avoiding a marked diuresis in the immediate post-transplantation period. Hemodialysis should be performed within 24 to 36 hours of transplantation of a kidney from a related donor. Although this is usually not possible when cadaver donors are used, the technique of continuous ambulatory peritoneal dialysis (CAPD) developed over the past several years has yielded results comparable with those for hemodialysis (Ettenger and Fine, 1986).

Surgical Procedures

For adults and most children, the renal transplant operation has become standardized (Simmons and Najarian, 1984). The earlier practice of removing the patient's diseased kidneys 2 to 3 weeks before transplantation has not been carried out routinely in recent years, except in patients with hypertension or infection, and nephrectomy is now performed at the time of transplantation.

For children weighing 15 kg or more, an extraperitoneal surgical approach is made. The donor renal vein and artery are anastomosed end-to-end to the recipient's distal inferior vena cava and distal aorta or common iliac artery, respectively. One of the major advances has been in overcoming the technical problems of transplanting adult kidneys into small children (So et al., 1986).

For infants and children weighing less than 15 kg, the kidney is transplanted intraperitoneally. The donor renal vein and artery are anastomosed end-to-side to the recipient inferior vena cava and aorta or common iliac vessels, respectively (Miller et al., 1983).

Immunosuppressive Regimens

Until cyclosporine became available in the early 1980s, most centers used a combination of azathioprine (Imuran), in initial doses of 3 to 5 mg/kg/day and maintenance doses of 2 to 3 mg/kg/day, and prednisone, in initial doses of 1 to 3 mg/kg/day (or 70 to 100 mg/M²/day) and maintenance doses of 0.2 to 0.3 mg/kg/day, to prevent graft rejection. Both drugs were begun 2 to 3 days prior to transplantation when a living donor was available or as soon as knowledge of a potential cadaver kidney was obtained. The maintenance dose of azathioprine was adjusted downward, if necessary, to maintain a WBC count of greater than 4000/mm³.

Beginning in 1983 and 1984, many centers began to use cyclosporine (in lieu of azathioprine) and lower doses of prednisone for immunosuppression (Tejani et al., 1986; Ettenger et al., 1990; McEnery et al., 1992). Cyclosporine has been given in varying doses at different centers but is generally given intravenously over 2 to 3 hours in doses of 3 to 10 mg/kg during or just after transplantation and of 7.5 to 10 mg/kg on the day after. It is subsequently administered orally at doses of 15 to 17.5 mg/kg/day as a single dose or in two divided doses for 1 to 2 weeks, then gradually tapered to 6 to 12.5 mg/kg/day by 9 weeks, depending on signs of toxicity or rejection and blood levels. Alternately, it is given on the basis of body surface area (500 mg/M² daily, reducing by 50 mg/M² weekly to 300 mg/M²). Trough blood levels are monitored by a radioimmunoassay and doses are adjusted to maintain them above 200 ng/ml. Prednisone is given at a dose of 0.5 mg/kg on the day of transplantation and gradually reduced to 0.1 to 0.2 mg/kg/day by 12 weeks. In some centers, prednisone is discontinued after 4 or 5 months following transplantation; in others, a maintainance dose is given on an alternate-day schedule (Ettenger et al., 1990).

The North American Pediatric Renal Transplant Cooperative Study (Tejani et al., 1993b) evaluated 568 cadaver kidney and 492 live-donor recipients. Patients receiving only prednisone and azathioprine showed a greater incidence of rejection prior to 30 days, a greater incidence of hospitalization for rejection and for hypertension over the next 6 months, and a greater loss of allograft in the first 6 months compared with patients receiving prednisone and cyclosporine or those receiving all three drugs. Serum creatinine levels were lower in the cadaver kidney recipients receiving all three drugs than in those receiving just cyclosporine and prednisone, but there was no difference in the live-donor recipients' creatinine levels when those two treatment regimens were compared. However, antibiotic requirements were higher in the three-drug group (Tejani et al., 1993b).

Although cyclosporine has shown clear superiority over azathioprine as an initial immunosuppressive agent, its major side effect in children as well as adults has been nephrotoxicity (Ettenger et al., 1990). Neurotoxicity has also occurred (Atkinson et al., 1984). A number of groups have recommended that cyclosporine be used only for the first 90 days, as they were successfully switched to azathioprine at a dose of 2.5 to 3 mg/kg/day (Hoitsma et al., 1987; Morris et al., 1987; Ettenger et al., 1990; McEnery et al., 1992; Hollander et al., 1995) and a temporarily higher dose of prednisone.

Thus, combinations of various immunosuppressive agents permit much lower doses of prednisone than used in the past and, therefore, obviate the many deleterious effects of steroids on growth and other parameters. Moreover, the nephrotoxicity of cyclosporine can be minimized by discontinuing it after the first 3 to 6 months, since acute rejection episodes are unlikely to occur after this time. Even in centers where conventional regimens (i.e., azathioprine and prednisone) are used, lower doses of prednisone (and alternate-day regimens) can be used without increasing the incidence of rejection or graft loss (Ettenger et al., 1990). In this schedule, prednisone is given at 0.5 mg/kg/day initially and tapered to 0.25 mg/kg by 12 weeks, then switched to alternate-day dosages ranging from 2 to 3 mg/kg.

In the past, acute rejection episodes have been treated with intravenous pulses of methylprednisolone as high as 30 mg/kg daily for 3 days (Bell et al., 1971). However, Kauffman et al. (1979) found pulses of 3 mg/kg to be equally effective, so that most centers now use lower steroid doses. The major reason is the recognition of the deleterious effects of high cumulative doses of corticosteroids (Ettenger and Fine, 1986). Other modalities of therapy, therefore, have been sought to control acute rejection. Among the most useful has been either equine ATG for 5 days or the murine monoclonal anti–T-cell antibody OKT3 (2.5 to 10 mg/day for 1 to 14 days). ATG is usually effective only for reversing rejection episodes in low-risk patients (i.e., those with living-related donor kidneys or two DR antigen-matched cadaveric kidneys [Ettenger and Fine, 1986]), but OKT3 may reverse rejection crises in high-risk patients who are resistant to high-dose methylprednisolone and/or ATG (Leone et al., 1987).

Post-transplantation Problems

Rejection

Rejection is the most common problem during the 3 months immediately after transplantation (Ettenger and Fine, 1986; So et al., 1986; Ettenger et al., 1990; McEnery et al., 1992; Tejani et al., 1993). Most such episodes, however, can be partially or completely reversed by one of the earlier-mentioned immunosuppressive agents. Rejection episodes are classified as follows:

1. *Hyperacute rejection* occurs within minutes or hours after the anastomosis takes place, mainly in recipients with preformed antileukocyte antibodies. It is thought to be either an Arthus or a Schwartzman type of reaction.

2. *Accelerated rejection* occurs on the second to the fifth day after transplantation. It is thought to represent a secondary cell-mediated and/or antibody response to antigens present in the donor kidney.

3. *Acute rejection*, the most common form, is due to a primary allogeneic response occurring within the first 7 to 21 days after transplantation and may be of varying severity: (a) *mild* (functional abnormalities easily reversed by prednisone or ATG); (b) *moderate* (clinical symptoms of fever, anorexia, arthralgia, hypertension, enlargement and tenderness of the kidney, and func-

tional changes reversible after 1 to 2 weeks with either large doses of steroids, ATG or OKT3); or (c) *severe* (marked deterioration, often necessitating resumption of hemodialysis).

4. *Chronic rejection* occurs when the tenuous graft tolerance is disturbed, 3 or more months after transplantation. It is characterized by marked proteinuria, hypertension, and the nephrotic syndrome. A kidney biopsy is usually necessary to distinguish rejection from cyclosporine nephrotoxicity.

Hyperacute, accelerated, and chronic rejection almost always lead to transplant failure, although occasionally the accelerated form can be reversed by high-dose methylprednisolone or anti–T-cell antibody therapy. Graft loss accounts for most prolonged hospital stays for renal transplant patients (Arbus et al., 1993). Most of these patients receive a second kidney. Subsequent grafts from living donors have an improved survival, but those from cadavers do not (Barber et al., 1985; Tejani et al., 1993; Cecka and Terasaki, 1994).

Other problems of the immediate post-transplantation period include acute tubular necrosis (particularly if cadaver kidneys are used and the ischemic time is prolonged), ureteral leaks (Ehrlich, 1984), and recurrence of the hemolytic-uremic syndrome, especially in patients who are treated with cyclosporine (Leithner et al., 1985). Hypertension, if present before transplantation, is eventually ameliorated, although it usually persists for the first 6 months and may persist in a mild form indefinitely.

Primary Disease Recurrence

Recurrence of the primary renal disease in the grafted kidney does occur, but the overall frequency is low (Cameron, 1982; Laine et al., 1993; Touraine et al., 1994). The diseases most likely to recur fall into three categories:

- Primary glomerulonephritis (particularly focal glomerulosclerosis with the nephrotic syndrome)
- Systemic diseases that involve the kidney (mainly insulin-dependent diabetes mellitus, systemic lupus erythematosus, and Henoch-Schönlein purpura)
- Metabolic diseases (e.g., cystinosis and oxalosis)

Because of the low frequency of recurrence of these primary diseases, however, none is a contraindication for renal transplantation (Iwatsuki et al., 1984; McEnery et al., 1992; Cecka and Terasaki, 1994).

Growth Retardation

Growth retardation is a major problem in pediatric renal transplantation (Ettenger et al., 1990; McEnery et al., 1992; Tejani et al., 1993a; Hokken-Koelega et al., 1994b). Initially, this is a result of the end-stage renal disease itself. Despite successful renal transplantation, growth failure is perpetuated by conventional immunosuppressive regimens that employ high-dose steroids.

Another contributing factor is the age of the recipient. When transplantation is performed shortly before puberty, growth spurts fostered by normally functioning grafts have usually led to epiphyseal closure, so that true "catch-up" growth and normal adult stature rarely occur. The lower-dose and/or alternate-day steroid regimens that have been used more recently have improved growth rates and prevented other unwanted steroid side effects (Ettenger et al., 1990; McEnery et al., 1992). In addition, significant amelioration of this problem is accomplished by early transplantation, particularly during the first year of life (Najarian et al., 1993). Some say, however, that unless a living-related donor is available, transplantation is best postponed until after age 1 year (Fine, 1987). With combination immunosuppressive regimens using low-dose or alternate-day steroids, lessened growth failure can be expected without compromised graft survival (Fine, 1987).

Finally, one study showed a sustained improvement in height when growth hormone therapy was administered to a group of severely growth-retarded post–renal transplant adolescents for 2 years (Hokken-Koelega et al., 1994a).

Orthopedic Problems

Orthopedic problems in renal transplantation include slipped femoral epiphyses, spontaneous fractures, and aseptic necrosis, all of which may lead to crippling deformities. Osteoporosis may result in axial compression fractures and osteonecrosis of the lower extremities (Ruderman et al., 1979). The cause of osteoporosis is uncertain, but it may be related to steroid therapy, antecedent uremia, inactivity, and renal osteodystrophy. Secondary hyperparathyroidism does not usually necessitate parathyroidectomy at the time of transplantation, as it can be managed with a low-calcium, high-phosphate diet and eventually subsides spontaneously.

Psychiatric Problems

Psychiatric problems are common in pediatric renal transplantation, particularly in adolescents, in large part due to their obesity, cushingoid changes, and loss of physical attractiveness. The latter problems have not been completely obviated by cyclosporine and steroid reduction, since hirsutism and a disproportionate cushingoid appearance have been observed in patients receiving cyclosporine. Suicide is not uncommon. Other nonimmunologic causes of death include electrolytic imbalance, infection, pulmonary embolism, cerebral hemorrhage, recurrence of Wilms' tumor, and reticulum cell sarcoma of the brain. However, infection is the most frequent cause of death, in large part a result of the immunosuppression.

Prognosis

Despite the sequelae of rejection, recurrence of disease, growth retardation, and orthopedic and psychiatric problems, renal transplantation is clearly as successful in children as in adults, and there is strong support for its continued and expanded use in pediatric end-stage renal disease (So et al., 1986; Ettenger et al., 1990; McEnery et al., 1992; Broyer et al., 1993; Najarian et al., 1993; Batisky et al., 1994; Cecka and Terasaki, 1994).

PEDIATRIC LIVER TRANSPLANTATION

Liver transplantation had its inception in 1963 when Starzl and coworkers (1986, 1987) replaced the diseased liver of a 3-year old child who had extrahepatic biliary atresia. Although that patient died, subsequent successes have established liver transplantation as standard therapy for a variety of advanced chronic liver diseases in both children and adults (Flye and Hendrisak, 1986; Starzl et al., 1986, 1987).

Prior to a consensus meeting at the National Institutes of Health in 1983, most liver transplant procedures were carried out in only five centers (Denver and Pittsburgh in the United States, Cambridge in England, Hannover in Germany, and Groninger in the Netherlands), and fewer than a thousand hepatic graft procedures had been performed. At present, at least 170 centers worldwide are performing liver transplantation regularly, and 34,307 such procedures had been reported by 1993 (Starzl et al., 1986; Bismuth et al., 1987; Belle et al., 1994). Infants and children account for approximately 15% of all recipients (Starzl et al., 1986, 1987; Belle et al., 1994).

High mortality was common before the 1980s because of surgical technical and organ preservation problems, choice of recipients with hopelessly advanced disease, overwhelming infection, and graft rejection. Since 1983, however, 1-year survival rates have increased from 25% to 40% to 61% to 78%, depending on the age and health of the recipient, the underlying condition, and various clinical considerations. This improvement has resulted from better surgical techniques but, most importantly, from the use of cyclosporine (Starzl et al., 1987).

Indications

Liver transplantation is indicated in the following cases (Mowat, 1987):

- Chronic end-stage liver disease
- Fulminant acute liver failure
- Cancer limited to the liver

The most common causes of chronic end-stage liver disease in children include the biliary atresia syndromes (accounting for nearly 50% of all transplant operations); metabolic diseases (representing roughly 25%), such as alpha$_1$-antitrypsin deficiency, Wilson's disease, Crigler-Najjar syndrome, tyrosinemia, glycogen storage disease types I and IV, protoporphyria, sea-blue histiocyte syndrome and others; bile duct hypoplasia; Byler's familial cholestasis; and chronic active hepatitis (Flye and Hendrisak, 1986; Starzl et al., 1986; Belle et al., 1994). Three infants with newborn liver

failure underwent successful surgery, receiving allogeneic livers, but one infant succumbed to overwhelming fungal sepsis (Lund et al., 1993).

Fulminant hepatitis and primary hepatic tumors (hepatoblastomas, hepatocellular tumors, and cholangiocarcinomas) are rare indications for liver transplantation in children. Hepatocellular carcinoma is often a result of maternal transmission of hepatitis B; for two such infants, the procedure was successful and there was no tumor recurrence; however, there was a recurrence of hepatitis B infection (Yandza et al., 1993).

The difficult clinical problem is to select patients who are not too ill to survive the procedure but who are sufficiently ill to warrant a high-risk procedure. Practically, patients who meet two of the following four criteria are considered candidates (van Thiel, 1985):

- A total bilirubin of 15 mg/dl or greater
- A prothrombin time greater than the control by 5 seconds and uncorrectable with vitamin K
- A serum albumin level of 2.5 g/dl or lower
- Hepatic encephalopathy that prevents normal function despite optimal medical therapy

Preoperative Evaluation

The potential recipient should be evaluated carefully to make certain that the underlying cause of the liver failure has been diagnosed accurately, to ascertain that hydration is adequate, to assess renal status, to determine whether or not encephalopathy is present, and to identify any potential source of infection. Angiography, ultrasound, Doppler CT, and magnetic resonance imaging (MRI) can be used to evaluate whether vascular or biliary abnormalities are present. Of particular importance is the determination of patency of the portal vein. If the portal vein is thrombosed, perfusion of the graft can be accomplished by means of a vascular graft; however, this markedly increases the surgical complexity and failure rate of the transplant procedure.

Donor Operation

Current organ preservation and surgical techniques limit the time possible for donor organ storage to 6 to 12 hours at most, with best results in those held for less than 6 hours (Flye and Hendrisak, 1986; Starzl et al., 1986). Especially in the pediatric age group, good matching of donor and recipient size is mandatory for surgical implantation of the orthotopic graft. Donor weight limits are usually set at 30% below to 10% above the recipient's weight. This narrow range markedly reduces the number of potential appropriate organ donors for children. Because of these considerations, decisions regarding suitability of the organ are based only on the potential donor's ABO blood type, HIV antibody status, organ size, liver function tests, and stability of the heart-bearing cadaver. Usually, neither HLA matching nor serologic cross-matching is considered.

Proper harvest of the donor liver is crucial, since the

liver cannot tolerate either warm or cold ischemia as well as a donor kidney. Multiple organs are usually harvested from a single heart-bearing cadaver. The liver is dissected first, followed by the kidneys and the heart. After the initial dissection of all organs, the abdominal viscera are perfused through the aorta with cold intracellular electrolyte (Collins') solution while the heart is perfused to induce cardioplegia. Rapid core cooling of the liver and kidneys is accomplished in this fashion, which practically eliminates any period of warm ischemia. Livers harvested in this manner will function if reimplanted within 8 to 12 hours.

Recipient and Transplant Operations

Removal of the diseased liver is often the most difficult aspect of orthotopic liver transplantation, which in its totality is one of the most technically demanding of all surgical procedures. Because of problems such as portal hypertension, coagulation defects, and metabolic imbalances, the major intraoperative problems are hemodynamic and metabolic, with hyperkalemic cardiac arrest remaining a major risk. During donor hepatectomy, the entire venous return from the abdominal viscera and from the lower half of the body is clamped off. This technique produces two deleterious effects; it markedly reduces overall cardiac output and produces marked venous hypertension in the splanchnic and renal circulations. In adults and larger children, this problem is diminished by constructing a veno-venous bypass wherein the blood in the portal vein and inferior vena cava is shunted through a centrifugal pump similar to those used in cardiopulmonary bypass and returned to the superior vena cava via the axillary vein. Although this procedure increases the technical complexity of the operation, it markedly diminishes the fluid accumulation in the splanchnic bed and diminishes the incidence of renal failure postoperatively. In smaller children with vessels that are too small to cannulate and bypass effectively, reliance is placed on the natural collateral venous circulation. Younger infants naturally tolerate this type of clamping better. Unlike the situation in adults, prior abdominal surgery has little overall impact on the prognosis in pediatric liver transplantation.

Although all of the operative steps, up to actual removal of the liver, can be performed in the recipient while the donor organ is in transit, the actual native hepatectomy is not done until the donor organ arrives in the operative suite. Suprahepatic vena caval and portal venous donor-recipient anastomoses are performed first in order to re-establish portal blood flow and end the cold ischemia time. End-to-end hepatic artery and infrahepatic vena caval anastomoses are done next, then end-to-end choledochostomy is performed. Assessment of allograft function begins during the operation with assessment of bile output and correction of coagulation factor deficiencies.

Immunosuppression and Postoperative Care

Methylprednisolone is given intravenously at a dose of 4 mg/kg preoperatively and is reduced by a rapidly tapering schedule postoperatively. After surgical recovery, azathioprine is given at a dose of 2 mg/kg for about 15 days, then gradually tapered. Cyclosporine, 6 mg/kg, is given intravenously and blood levels are monitored. Tacrolimus is also available at some centers; the dose is usually 0.05 mg/kg every 12 hours intravenously initially, then orally at 0.12 mg/kg every 12 hours thereafter (U.S. Multicenter FK 506 Liver Study Group, 1994). If acute tubular necrosis is present, tacrolimus may be withheld and OKT3 given instead. In one randomized trial of OKT3-based (for the 14 initial days) versus cyclosporine-based prophylaxis after liver transplantation, there was a lower incidence of acute rejection, renal function was better, and the incidence of severe infections was lower in the OKT3 group at 1 year after transplantation (Farges et al., 1994). Four-year patient and graft survival rates in the OKT3 group (69% and 61%, respectively) were not statistically different from those in the cyclosporine group (62% and 54%, respectively).

Major postoperative problems may occur (1) immediately (0 to 24 hours), (2) early (24 to 48 hours), (3) subacutely (2 to 12 days), or (4) later (13 days and beyond) (van Thiel, 1985). Fluid overload is the most common immediate problem, and hepatic arterial or portal vein thrombosis is the major early complication (usually signaling graft failure). Biliary leaks are the next most frequent early or subacute problem. Infection and renal dysfunction may also occur subacutely. Graft rejection or viral hepatitis is a late complication.

A form of chronic rejection, the "vanishing bile duct syndrome" has been correlated with a complete mismatch for class I antigens (Donaldson et al., 1987). Patients without serious complications are ordinarily hospitalized for 3 weeks, are then followed closely as outpatients, and can return home by 6 weeks. Most patients have excellent graft function, with serum bilirubin and transaminase values in the normal or moderately elevated range.

Prognosis

As already noted, 1-year survival rates following liver transplantation have improved dramatically since 1983. Rejection episodes occur in approximately two thirds in the first 6 months; these usually subside after 3 days of high-dose methylprednisolone (Solu-Medrol), but some patients require OKT3 or ATG therapy for reversal. In general, most programs achieve 75% to 80% 1-year survival rates in children, and some centers report a rate as high as 90%. Across all indications, the estimated probability of a pediatric recipient surviving for 5 years is 70%, and the estimated probability of surviving without retransplantation is 58% (Belle et al., 1994).

Causes of death include acute and chronic rejection, infection, vascular surgical complications, liver infarction, and cerebrovascular accidents. Patients with cholestatic chronic liver disease or end-stage liver disease caused by metabolic disorders, such as alpha$_1$-antitrypsin deficiency, survive longer than those with fulminant liver failure or postnecrotic cirrhosis (e.g., postneonatal hepatitis or chronic active hepatitis) (Belle et al., 1994).

There is considerable controversy over whether to operate on patients with chronic hepatitis B infections. In a retrospective study of European patients who were hepatitis B surface antigen (HbsAg)–positive at the time of transplantation, survival was 75% at 1 year and 63% at 3 years; most patients were given long-term immunoprophylaxis with anti-Hbs immune globulin, but the risk of recurrent infection at 3 years was 50% (Samuel et al., 1993).

Patients with malignancy fare least well, with less than a 50% 2-year survival.

In one French study, patients who received liver transplants before age 2 had poor growth velocity by the third year after transplantation (Codoner-Franch et al., 1994); however, the authors found that long-term improvement in height usually occurred in most patients when surgery took place after age 2 years, particularly if the patients were kept on an alternate-day steroid regimen.

Chimerism

Chimerism, the presence of genetically different components within an animal or person, is an interesting phenomenon that has been reported more and more frequently after liver transplantation (Starzl et al., 1992a, 1992b, 1994; Collins et al., 1993). Graft-versus-host reactions (GVH) have long been known to occur in some liver transplant recipients. One such patient was investigated after recovery from GVH-mediated myelosuppression and found to have donor-type stem cells (Collins et al., 1993). This phenomenon was also extensively investigated by PCR analysis of tissues from two patients with type IV glycogen storage disease and from one with type I Gaucher's disease 26 to 91 months after surgery (Starzl et al., 1994). Donor-type HLA-DR DNA was found in the heart of both patients with glycogen storage disease; in the skin of one; and in the skin, intestine, blood, and bone marrow of the patient with Gaucher's disease. The cardiac deposits of amylopectin in the patients with type IV glycogen storage disease and the lymph node deposits of glucocerebroside in the patient with Gaucher's disease were reportedly dramatically reduced. The authors concluded that systemic microchimerism occurs after allogeneic liver transplantation and that this can ameliorate pancellular enzyme deficiencies.

In addition to stem cells, however, the liver is also a source of many other hematopoietic cell lineages; thus it is not clear that all of the chimeric cells arose from hepatic stem cells. The authors also speculate that the chimerism, which they think may occur almost uniformly in liver transplant recipients, also accounts for tolerance of the recipient to the liver and resultant graft acceptance (Starzl et al., 1992a, 1992b). They point out that a number of liver transplant recipients have discontinued their immunosuppressive drugs altogether without graft rejection (Starzl et al., 1992b).

Liver Transplantation from Living-Related Donors

As is the case for all solid organ transplantation, lack of suitable donors is a major problem for liver transplantation. Xenotransplantation is being explored as an alternative, but there have been no successes yet (Starzl et al., 1993). Since 1988, this problem has been approached at several centers by partial hepatectomies of living-related donors (Yamaoka et al., 1994). In a report from Japan (Yamaoka et al., 1994), 73 living-related transplants had been given to 72 patients, and 59 recipients were alive and well with the original graft and normal liver function at follow-ups 3 to 47 months afterward. The left lateral segment was used in 46 cases, the left lobe in 25 cases, and the right lobe in one case. Donor safety is much greater with use of the left lateral segment; the recipients undergo total hepatectomies.

PEDIATRIC HEART TRANSPLANTATION

The first human heart transplant was performed in December 1967. By February 1992, 22,650 heart transplantations had been reported to the International Heart Transplantation Registry (Kaye, 1993). More than 1000 patients have been pediatric recipients (Fricker et al., 1987), and most of these operations have been performed since 1983.

Indications

The various forms of cardiomyopathy are the most common pediatric indications for heart transplantation, followed by congenital heart disease. Congenital heart disease includes hypoplastic left heart syndrome and other forms of complex congenital heart defects. Absolute contraindications include the presence of active uncontrolled infection in the recipient, insulin-dependent diabetes mellitus, active or recent malignancy, gastroduodenal ulcer, a positive serologic HLA cross-match, ABO incompatibility, elevated pulmonary arterial resistance, HIV antibodies, and significant chronic end-organ dysfunction (Ardehali et al., 1994; Breen et al., 1994; Michler et al., 1994). Patients with increased pulmonary vascular resistance are referred for heart-lung transplantation.

As with other forms of organ transplantation, a paucity of available organs is a major limitation, particularly in the pediatric age group. The cardiac allografts are selected by matching ABO blood group and approximate body weight and heart size. Contraindications for donation include the presence of severe cardiac disease and unresolved systemic infection. A history of resuscitation or the receipt of inotropic agents is not necessarily an exclusion.

Immunosuppression

Immunosuppressive regimens for heart transplantation are similar in many respects to those already described for renal and hepatic grafts. Usually a combination of high-dose (10 mg/kg) intravenous methylprednisolone is given intraoperatively after a loading dose of 4 mg/kg azathioprine preoperatively (Fricker et al., 1987; Brown et al., 1993). Prednisone is given postoperatively at 3 mg/kg/day but tapered rapidly to 0.2 mg/kg by day 10; azathioprine is continued at 1 to 2 mg/kg/day; and cyclosporine is begun immediately postoperatively at 2.5 mg/kg, with doses adjusted to maintain blood levels at around 200 ng/ml. OKT3 induction therapy has also been used with great success (Brown et al., 1993). High-dose methylprednisolone, ALS/ATG, or OKT3 monoclonal antibody has been used to treat acute rejection episodes, and methotrexate or total lymphoid irradiation has been used for chronic rejection (Chinnock et al., 1993).

In November 1989, the Pittsburgh group (Armitage et al., 1993) began a prospective study using FK 506 as the primary immunosuppressive agent. High-dose methylprednisolone was given intraoperatively and on the first postoperative day; afterward, the patient was maintained on prednisone 0.1 mg/kg/day orally, until it was discontinued after the first normal findings from an endomyocardial biopsy. No azathioprine was given. Survival in that group of patients has been 82% at 1 and 3 years, and the actuarial freedom from grade 3A rejection in the FK 506 group was 60% at 3 and 6 months after transplantation compared with 20% and 12%, respectively, in the group treated with cyclosporine-based, triple-drug therapy. Of 24 children, 20 (83%) in the FK 506 group were receiving no steroids (Armitage et al., 1993). The prevalence of hypertension was 4% in the FK 506 group versus 70% in the cyclosporine group, and renal toxicity of FK 506 was mild. FK 506 did not produce hirsutism, gingival hyperplasia, or abnormal facial bone growth. These apparent advantages of FK 506 bode well for the pediatric age patient facing cardiac transplantation and life-long immunosuppression.

Complications

Post-transplantation complications include (1) hemodynamic problems during the first few days, (2) rejection episodes, and (3) side effects of immunosuppression. Hemodynamic problems are more likely to occur if there is increased pulmonary arterial resistance or if the donor heart is in less than optimal condition.

Rejection episodes are more difficult to detect when cyclosporine is the principal immunosuppressive agent, but they can be diagnosed by endomyocardial biopsy (Caves et al., 1973). The frequency of rejection is greatest within the first 6 months after transplantation. Although the frequency of rejection episodes may not be diminished by cyclosporine, their severity has been. The result is that many fewer hearts have been lost to this complication; as noted above, FK 506 has had an even greater beneficial impact on this problem (Armitage et al., 1993).

A retrospective analysis by Opelz and Wujciak (1994) revealed that graft survival in heart transplantation was significantly influenced by the extent of HLA compatibility. In addition, use of a male donor heart into a female recipient has also been associated with a higher incidence of rejection (Kawauchi et al., 1993).

Postoperative pulmonary hypertension can be a major cause of early death after heart transplantation, particularly in older children, especially those with congenital heart disease who received a graft that had been preserved more than 6 hours (Fukushima et al., 1994).

Because a much lower dose of steroids is required with either cyclosporine-based or FK 506 immunosuppression than with azathioprine plus steroids alone, the frequency of infectious complications is lower. This is particularly true because steroids have been discontinued altogether in a number of patients (Armitage et al., 1993; Canter et al., 1994). Nevertheless, bacterial, fungal, and viral infections still occur with significant frequency (Miller et al., 1994).

Viral infections, such as cytomegalovirus (CMV) and hepatitis, represent the major cause of morbidity in pediatric transplant patients and account for 19% of all deaths (Bernstein, 1993; Elkins et al., 1993; Miller et al., 1994). CMV accounts for 25% of serious infections and occurs either as a primary infection or as a reactivation. Encouragingly, however, acyclovir prophylaxis was associated with a lower than expected frequency of CMV infection after heart transplantation (Elkins et al., 1993).

Lymphomas have developed in a number of patients (93 of 7634) receiving cyclosporine and azathioprine plus antilymphocyte antibodies for rejection episodes (Opelz and Henderson, 1993). The tumors have often regressed following reduction or discontinuation of these agents. The nephrotoxic effects of cyclosporine have led some groups to switch from cyclosporine to conventional therapy after 2 or 3 years in order to avoid renal toxicity after the risk of rejection has diminished.

Prognosis

Since the introduction of cyclosporine more than 12 years ago, the results of cardiac transplantation have improved greatly. The International Heart Transplantation Registry has shown a 71% 4-year survival rate for patients receiving cyclosporine-based, triple-immunosuppression therapy compared with a 41% survival rate for those given immunosuppression with only azathioprine and prednisone (Kaye, 1993). Survival, however, is influenced by the age of the recipient; patients younger than age 40 have a better survival rate. Especially impressive have been results of cardiac transplantation procedures performed in newborn infants or in infants in the first year of life (Assaad, 1993; Bailey et al., 1993; Zales and Stapleton, 1993).

The largest experience with infant transplant surgery has been at Loma Linda, California (Assaad, 1993; Bailey et al., 1993), where 140 transplants were performed in 139 infants from 1985 until 1993. These patients ranged in age from 3 hours to 12 months. Overall survival was 83%, with 5-year actuarial survival at 80%; 5-year survival of 60 newborn recipients was

84%. Of 66 children aged 7 hours to 18 years who received heart transplants at Pittsburgh from 1982 to 1992, 67% were surviving at 4 months to 8 years after transplantation; all had returned to age-appropriate activities (Mempel et al., 1973). Since mid-1988, 1- and 3-year survival rates were 82% in children with congenital heart disease and 90% in children with cardiomyopathy. Somewhat lower survival rates were achieved at other institutions (LeBidois et al., 1992; Turrentine et al., 1994). The longest-surviving recipient was leading a normal life 18 years after the procedure (Kaye, 1993). These results, coupled with the excellent rehabilitation achieved, offer great promise for the future.

HEART-LUNG AND LUNG TRANSPLANTATION

Since 1984, combined heart and lung transplants have been performed successfully at 27 institutions in 186 patients of all ages who had both end-stage heart and lung disease (Kaye, 1993). The indications were congenital heart disease, primary pulmonary hypertension, cystic fibrosis, and other end-stage lung diseases.

Heart-lung transplantation has been used most successfully in the treatment of cystic fibrosis (Hodson, 1992; Dennis et al., 1993; Madden et al., 1993; Maynard, 1994), and has become an established form of treatment over the last few years. Actuarial survival at 1 and 3 years after transplantation was 78% and 65%, respectively, in 28 patients with cystic fibrosis, compared with 77% and 65% in patients without cystic fibrosis undergoing heart-lung transplantation. The pharmacokinetics of oral cyclosporine are altered by poor enteral absorption in patients with cystic fibrosis, however, such that they usually require much higher oral doses to achieve the desired plasma level (Tsang et al., 1994). Patients with immunodeficiency disorders who have end-stage lung disease and cor pulmonale may also be candidates for a transplant.

The 5-year actuarial survival for recipients to 18 years of age is approximately 40% (Kaye, 1993). These are less favorable than comparable figures for cardiac transplantation alone primarily as a result of a higher perioperative mortality of 29% in the heart-lung procedure, and a higher incidence of infection (Starnes and Jamieson, 1986; Kaye, 1993). Obliterative bronchiolitis remains the most serious late complication after heart-lung or lung transplantation (Hodson, 1992; Maynard, 1994).

As of 1993, 109 lung transplantations were reported to the Registry and 30 of these were in pediatric-age patients (Kaye, 1993). Ten patients underwent lung transplantation for primary pulmonary hypertension; 3, for congenital heart disease; and 17, for a variety of congenital and acquired pulmonary disorders, with cystic fibrosis leading the list. The 1-year actuarial survival in these patients was approximately 70%, but little information is available for times beyond 1 year.

Donor organ availability is an even greater problem for heart-lung and lung transplantation than for other organs and tissues, since both heart and lungs must be normal. If the recipient's heart is normal, it can be used as a donor heart for a second patient. There is an extreme scarcity of healthy donor lungs because pulmonary edema, aspiration, and pneumonia commonly occur in brain-dead patients.

As a potential means of providing organs for more patients, single-lung transplantation has been advocated by some (Toronto Lung Transplant Group, 1986). Single-lung transplantation has been advocated for adult patients with end-stage emphysema or pulmonary fibrosis. Four of five patients with the latter condition were long-term survivors after a unilateral lung transplant, with improved lung function, normal PaO_2 values, and a good quality of life (Toronto Lung Transplant Group, 1986). A combined liver, heart, and lung transplantation was performed successfully in a patient who had primary biliary cirrhosis and primary pulmonary hypertension (Wallwork et al., 1987).

TRANSPLANTATION OF PANCREATIC TISSUE

Indications

Even though endocrine deficiencies can be treated with hormone administration, permanent cure can theoretically be achieved through organ or tissue transplantation. This is particularly attractive in diabetes, since, despite insulin administration, it is a leading cause of uremia and blindness and remains the third leading cause of death in the United States (Tyden et al., 1986).

Human pancreatic transplantation has been limited primarily to transplantation of the intact gland or segments thereof (Calne, 1986; Sutherland and Moudry, 1987a, 1987b; Robertson, 1992; Sutherland et al., 1994). Prior to 1977, only 57 segmental or whole pancreatic transplants had been performed in 55 patients (Sutherland and Moudry, 1987a). As with other forms of organ transplantation, the past 27 years have witnessed a tremendous increase in transplantation of the pancreas. From 1966 to 1994, more than 5000 pancreatic transplants were reported to the International Pancreas Transplant Registry (Sutherland et al., 1994). Most of these were simultaneous pancreas-kidney transplants, but some were simultaneous pancreas-liver, some simultaneous pancreas-kidney-liver, and some simultaneous pancreas-heart.

There appears to be a beneficial effect from combining pancreas and kidney transplantation, since most such diabetic recipients have irreversible renal disease. In those dually grafted, cadaver renal graft functional rates at 1 year were comparable to those in diabetics given only renal grafts. Moreover, the dually transplanted patients were found to have no further deterioration in retinopathy or neuropathy.

The various immunosuppressive regimens used have included combinations of cyclosporine, azathioprine, and prednisone (yielding the best results) or prednisone with either one of the other two agents (Sutherland and Moudry, 1987a; Robertson, 1992; Sutherland et al., 1994).

Prognosis

Clearly, the results of pancreatic transplantation have improved with time, with 1-year graft survival rates rising from 42% prior to 1978 to 75% from 1987 to 1993. Graft survival rates were lower (48%) for those who received the pancreas after the kidney or for those who received a pancreas alone. Five-year graft function averaged between 50% and 60%. The improvement is largely due to the introduction of cyclosporine. However, the major technical problem of what to do with the exocrine ducts appears to have been successfully overcome by anastomosing them to the bladder; the earlier practice of enteric drainage resulted in lower graft survival rates (Sutherland et al., 1994). Although pancreatic islet cell transplantation has been successful in reversing the diabetic state of pancreatectomized or streptozocin- or alloxan-treated rats (Ballenger and Lacy, 1972), it has been helpful thus far in only a few humans with diabetes (Robertson, 1992).

TRANSPLANTATION OF PARATHYROID TISSUE

Autotransplantation of parathyroid tissue is useful in the treatment of primary (Ross et al., 1986) and secondary hyperparathyroidism (Wells et al., 1978; Sitges-Serra and Caralps-Riera, 1987). In this procedure, a total parathyroidectomy is performed and the extirpated glands are sliced into small (1 × 2 mm) pieces and placed in culture medium. Some 20 to 25 such pieces are then implanted into a site on the volar surface of the nondominant forearm. The remaining pieces are frozen for future use. The incidence of hypoparathyroidism after total parathyroidectomy plus autotransplantation has ranged from 13% to 40%, however, and there have been several cases of late graft failure (Sitges-Serra and Caralps-Riera, 1987).

SKIN TRANSPLANTATION

The principal indication for a skin allograft is a burn affecting more than 80% of the body surface, an invariably fatal injury. In these patients, the burn sites are covered with cultured allogeneic epidermal cells grown from cadaveric skin (Madden et al., 1986) and whatever autologous skin is available. Culturing the epidermal cells eventually results in loss of DR antigen expression (Hefton et al., 1984). Wound healing is significantly hastened for first-degree and second-degree burns but not for third-degree burns (Madden et al., 1986). It is possible that the allografted cells survive only temporarily and that they are gradually replaced by autologous epidermal cells (Madden et al., 1986).

BONE TRANSPLANTATION

Bone transplantation has been used primarily to replace large segments of the long bones or the pelvis with nonviable allogeneic bone in patients with bone tumors. In several series, success rates as high as 89% have been reported (Friedlander et al., 1983; Czitrom et al., 1986). No immunosuppression or HLA donor typing is used.

BONE MARROW TRANSPLANTATION

Historical Aspects

The observation by Lorenz et al. (1952) that lethally irradiated animals could be reconstituted by bone marrow cells stimulated attempts to apply this therapy to patients with bone marrow failure. However, such transplants were unsuccessful except in identical twins (Pillow et al., 1966) until the late 1960s after the human major histocompatibility complex (MHC) was discovered (Amos and Bach, 1968).

Since 1955, more than 50,000 bone marrow transplantations have been performed worldwide in the treatment of nearly 50 different fatal diseases (O'Reilly et al., 1984; Good, 1987; Martin et al., 1987; Thomas, 1987; Armitage, 1994; Rowlings et al., 1994). A large number of them have been in children, where they have been more successful than in adults (Thomas, 1987; Armitage, 1994; Rowlings et al., 1994).

The objective of marrow transplantation is to replace defective, absent, or malignant cells of the recipient with normal replicating hematopoietic and immunocompetent cells. Normal bone marrow contains self-replicating cells that can give rise to erythrocytes, granulocytes, cells of the monocyte-macrophage lineage, megakaryocytes, and immunocompetent T and B cells (Wu et al., 1967, 1968; Brenner et al., 1993).

Problems Unique to Bone Marrow Transplantation

Certain unique problems distinguish bone marrow transplantation from grafting of solid organs, such as the kidney, liver, and heart. The first problem is that immunocompetent cells in both recipient and donor marrow have the potential of rejecting each other, resulting in marrow graft rejection on the one hand and graft-versus-host disease (GVHD) on the other (Martin et al., 1987). The second concern is that successful unfractionated marrow grafting usually requires strict donor and recipient MHC class II antigen compatibility to avoid such reactions (O'Reilly et al., 1984; Good, 1987; Martin et al., 1987).

Finally, except for patients with severe combined immunodeficiency (SCID), complete DiGeorge anomaly, or identical twin donors, even HLA-identical recipients have to be pretreated with lethal doses of irradiation or cytotoxic agents to prevent graft rejection (Martin et al., 1987; O'Reilly, 1987). Immunosuppressive agents commonly used to ensure the acceptance of solid organ grafts have deleterious effects on the very cells one is trying to engraft in patients with genetically determined immunodeficiency. Therefore, immunosuppressive and myeloablative agents must be given *before* infusion of the marrow to avoid injury to the donor cells.

Indications

Diseases treated successfully by bone marrow transplantation include the following (O'Reilly et al., 1984; Good, 1987; Martin et al., 1987; Thomas, 1987):

- Radiation injury
- Several primary immunodeficiency disorders
- Congenital hematologic abnormalities, including hemoglobinopathies, aplastic anemia, acute leukemia, and chronic myeloid leukemia
- Solid tumors, such as neuroblastoma and lymphoma
- A number of inborn errors of metabolism

In addition, autologous marrow transplantation has been used in conjunction with lethal irradiation or chemotherapy in the treatment of patients with some hematologic malignancies, solid tumors, or breast cancer (Rowlings et al., 1994).

The rationale for bone marrow transplantation in leukemia is the hope that the leukemic cells can be reduced or eliminated by irradiation or chemotherapy and the grafted allogeneic normal cells can then reject any remaining leukemic cells (Weiden et al., 1979). This concept of adoptive immunotherapy for leukemia, although supported by higher recurrence rates in identical twin transplants (Fefer et al., 1977; Gale and Champlin, 1984), is challenged by reports of patients in whom allogeneic engraftment was achieved but who had recurrences of their leukemia and of patients in whom the leukemia recurred in cells of donor type (Thomas et al., 1975; Thomas, 1987). Nevertheless, transplants into leukemic recipients using T-cell–depleted marrow have been associated with a higher degree of leukemia recurrence (Maraninchi et al., 1987).

Prevention of Rejection

Factors influencing the likelihood of engraftment include:

1. The immunocompetence of the recipient.
2. The degree of MHC disparity of donor and recipient.
3. The degree of presensitization of the recipient to the histocompatibility antigens of the donor.
4. The number of marrow cells administered.
5. The pretransplant immunosuppression given the recipient.
6. Whether or not T-cell depletion techniques are used.

As already noted, unfractionated bone marrow transplantation is unique in its requirement for MHC class II antigen compatibility. However, even MHC-compatible donor marrow will be rejected unless the recipient is immunosuppressed or profoundly immunodeficient. Such rejection probably occurs on the basis of non-MHC minor locus histocompatibility antigen differences. Unfractionated marrow cells can become engrafted in HLA-disparate recipients if they lack cellular immunity, but fatal graft-versus-host disease can be anticipated.

Presensitization of dogs to donor antigens by blood transfusion increases the likelihood of rejection of DLA-identical marrow (Martin et al., 1987). Thus, prospective marrow recipients should not receive blood transfusions from potential sibling donors or from other family members because these will increase the risk of sensitization to minor locus antigens not controlled by the MHC.

Between 3 and 10.9×10^8/kg of nucleated marrow cells are required to achieve engraftment in aplasia and leukemia (Martin et al., 1987). By contrast, patients with SCID have required far fewer cells; as few as 4×10^6 unfractionated nucleated marrow cells per kilogram recipient body weight have resulted in immunologic reconstitution (O'Reilly et al., 1984). The difference is undoubtedly due to the presence of ample hematopoietic cells other than lymphocytes in the immunodeficient recipients, whereas the conditioning regimens in leukemia and aplasia leave the marrow devoid of cellular elements. However, despite receiving much higher numbers of T cell–depleted marrow cells, some patients with severe T-cell deficiency have not achieved engraftment (O'Reilly et al., 1986).

Except for recipients of syngeneic (identical twin) marrow or those with SCID, all bone marrow transplant recipients need preconditioning to achieve engraftment. Immunosuppressive and myeloablative agents must be given prior to infusion of the marrow to avoid injury to the donor cells. The agents used most widely have been x-irradiation, procarbazine, cyclophosphamide, busulfan, and ATG. In nonmalignant conditions, such as aplasia or immunodeficiency, preparation of the recipient need only be directed at immunosuppression and "spacing" (i.e., making room in the marrow for donor cells. Thus total body irradiation (TBI) required to eradicate malignant cells is not necessary.

Preparation of patients with acute leukemia or other malignancies for marrow transplantation is more complex because 1000 to 1200 rad of TBI is usually used to eradicate the tumor cells (Martin et al., 1987). A combination of 2 to 4 mg/kg of busulfan daily for 4 days, followed by 50 mg/kg cyclophosphamide daily for 2 days, has been commonly employed for nonmalignant conditions (Blazar et al., 1985). A similar regimen has also been used by Tutschka (1986) for leukemia patients as an alternative to TBI and cyclophosphamide, resulting in considerably less morbidity in the early post-transplant period, no increase in leukemia recurrence, and better survival rates.

Marrow Transplant Procedure

Unfractionated bone marrow transplantation is the simplest of all transplantation procedures, offering little risk to the donor, because it involves removal of a tissue that is readily regenerated. The bone marrow cells are usually obtained by aspiration with a 14- or 16-gauge needle from multiple sites along both iliac crests, over the length of the sternum, or (in children) from the upper one third of the tibia, while the donor is under general anesthesia (Thomas et al., 1975; Martin et al., 1987). The aspirate is placed in heparinized tissue culture medium, then passed through metal screens with diminishing apertures to remove bone spicules. Nucleated marrow cells are then enumerated and given intravenously in a manner similar to that of a blood transfusion.

Graft-Versus-Host Reactions

GVH reactions are the major barrier to widespread successful application of bone marrow transplantation to the correction of many different diseases (Glucksberg et al., 1974; O'Reilly et al., 1984; Martin et al., 1987; O'Reilly, 1987; Deeg and Henslee-Downey, 1990; Ferrara and Deeg, 1991; Parkman, 1991). The principal reason for this is that the recipient with a lethal T-cell defect (or one made equally T cell–deficient by irradiation or chemotherapy) cannot reject bone marrow, matched or mismatched (Ferrara and Deeg, 1991). By contrast, engrafted genetically different immunocompetent donor T cells recognize foreign HLA antigens on the recipient's cells and respond to them (Glucksberg et al., 1974; Deeg and Henslee-Downey, 1990; Ferrara and Deeg, 1991; Parkman, 1991). In the case of unfractionated marrow transplants from HLA-D mismatched donors, this reaction of the donor T lymphocytes against the recipient is almost invariably fatal.

GVH reactions are usually mild and self-limited in infants with SCID not given pretransplant immunosuppression who receive unfractionated HLA-identical marrow (O'Reilly et al., 1984; Good, 1987; O'Reilly, 1987; Parkman, 1991). However, in 60% of recipients given pretransplant irradiation or immunosuppressive drugs, GVH reactions are moderate to severe and they are fatal in 15% to 20% despite HLA identity (Glucksberg et al., 1974; Martin et al., 1987; Deeg and Henslee-Downey, 1990). This is likely a result of recognition by donor T cells of recipient minor locus histocompatibility or Y chromosome–associated transplantation antigens, since a significantly higher incidence of GVH disease occurs in male aplasia and immunodeficient patients given MHC-matched unfractionated female marrows than in patients receiving MHC and sex-matched marrows (Bortin and Rimm, 1977; Martin et al., 1987).

The severity of GVH reactions increases with the recipient's age (Storb et al., 1986; Parkman, 1991); the use of HLA-matched unrelated donors; and, if a related donor is not HLA-identical, with the degree of genetic disparity.

Clinical Features of GVH Reactions

Graft-versus-host reactions begin 6 or more days after transplantation (or after transfusion, in the case of nonirradiated blood products) (Anderson and Weinstein, 1990). Reactions include fever, a morbilliform maculopapular erythematous rash, and severe diarrhea (Glucksberg et al., 1974). The rash becomes progressively confluent and may involve the entire body surface; it is both pruritic and painful and eventually leads to marked exfoliation. Eosinophilia and lymphocytosis develop, followed shortly by hepatosplenomegaly, exfoliative dermatitis, protein-losing enteropathy, bone marrow aplasia, generalized edema, marked susceptibility to infection, and death (Skinner et al., 1986; Gratama et al., 1987; Parkman, 1991). Skin biopsy specimens reveal basal vacuolar degeneration or necrosis, spongiosis, single-cell dyskeratosis, eosinophilic necrosis of epidermal cells, and a dermal perivascular round cell infiltration (Woodruff et al., 1976; Deeg and Henslee-Downey, 1990). Similar necrotic changes occur in the liver and intestinal tract and eventually in most other tissues.

Grading of the severity of GVH disease is based on the severity and number of organ systems involved (Glucksberg et al., 1974; Thomas et al., 1975). The four categories generally defined are:

Grade 1. 1+ to 2+ skin rash without gut involvement and with no more than 1+ liver involvement.

Grade 2. 1+ to 3+ skin rash with either 1+ to 2+ gastrointestinal involvement or 1+ to 2+ liver involvement or both.

Grade 3. 2+ to 4+ skin rash with 2+ to 4+ gastrointestinal involvement with or without 2+ to 4+ liver involvement. Decrease in performance status and fever also characterize grades 2 and 3, with increasing severity per stage.

Grade 4. The pattern and severity of GVHD is similar to those in grade 3 with extreme constitutional symptoms.

If the patient does not die and if the acute GVH reaction persists, the reaction is termed "chronic" after 100 days. Chronic GVH disease may evolve from acute GVH reactions or may develop in the absence of or after resolution of acute GVH disease. It occurs in approximately 45% to 75% of conditioned patients receiving matched bone marrow transplants (Martin et al., 1987; Weisdorf et al., 1990; Parkman, 1991). Skin lesions of chronic GVH disease resemble scleroderma, with hyperkeratosis, reticular hyperpigmentation, atrophy with ulceration, and fibrosis and limitation of joint movement. Other manifestations include the sicca syndrome, disordered immunoregulation—as evidenced by autoantibody and immune complex formation and polyclonal and monoclonal hyperimmunoglobulinemia (Noel et al., 1978; Graze and Gale, 1979), idiopathic interstitial pneumonitis, and frequent infections (Skinner et al., 1986; Parkman, 1991).

Treatment of GVH Reactions

Many regimens have been employed to mitigate GVH reactions in both MHC-incompatible and -compatible bone marrow transplants. In MHC-compatible bone marrow transplants into patients with SCID or complete DiGeorge anomaly, it is not usually necessary to give immunosuppressive agents to prevent or mitigate GVH disease, although occasionally steroids are used to treat more severe forms of the condition. However, for unfractionated HLA-identical marrow transplants into all patients for whom pretransplant chemotherapy is given to prevent rejection, it is necessary to use prophylaxis against GVH disease. Patients are usually given cyclosporine daily for 6 months or methotrexate (15 mg/M² on the first day after transplantation and 10 mg/M² on the third, sixth, and eleventh days and weekly thereafter until day 100) or both (in which case a shorter course of methotrexate is used (Storb et al., 1986; Martin et al., 1987; Parkman, 1991).

Once GVH disease has become established, it is extremely difficult to treat. Antithymocyte serum, steroids, and murine monoclonal antibodies to human T-cell surface antigens have ameliorated some, but the course has been inexorably fatal in others similarly treated (Martin et al., 1987; O'Reilly, 1987; Deeg and Henslee-Downey, 1990; Parkman, 1991). Currently, anticytokine and anticytokine receptor antibodies are being evaluated for their potential efficacy in mitigating GVH disease (Deeg and Henslee-Downey, 1990). Recently, determining the frequency of recipient-specific T-cell precursors in donor blood by limiting dilution analysis and identification of IL-2–producing cells after in vitro stimulation with recipient mononuclear cells has been found to correlate with the severity of subsequent GVH disease in HLA-identical sibling bone marrow transplants (Theobald et al., 1992; Schwarer et al., 1993). This approach could be used prospectively to intensify GVH disease prophylaxis when the only available HLA-identical sibling donor has a high frequency of such recipient-specific T-cell precursors (Theobald et al., 1992; Schwarer et al., 1993).

The best approach to GVH reactions is a preventive one. The agents already mentioned have not prevented GVH reactions entirely; moreover, in children with genetically determined severe T-cell deficiency, they adversely affect the very cell one is trying to engraft. By far, the best preventive approach is the removal of all post-thymic T cells from the donor marrow (see below).

Post-transplantation Problems

Multiple problems occur during the post-transplantation period, particularly in conditioned patients. Thus, marrow transplantation should be carried out only by experienced teams.

Anemia and Thrombocytopenia

Multiple red blood cell and platelet transfusions are usually necessary for conditioned patients during the 7 to 20 days before engraftment occurs. All transfusions that contain immunocompetent cells should be irradiated with from 1500 to 3000 rad to prevent GVH reactions (Martin et al., 1987), and, if the recipient is CMV-seronegative, the transfusion should be from CMV-seronegative donors (Tutschka, 1986). Family members can be used as blood donors during this period; they are preferred, so as to minimize the risk of hepatitis and HIV infections. Platelets from an HLA-matched sibling are preferred, inasmuch as they are not as subject to immune elimination as are randomly selected platelets.

Infection

The immunodeficiency (Noel et al., 1978; Graze and Gale, 1979) that occurs in the post-transplantation period for patients who have had conditioning regimens, regardless of whether GVH disease is present, is responsible for the high incidence of infections in those patients during the first 100 days after marrow cell infusion (Skinner et al., 1986; Martin et al., 1987). Another contributing factor is the profound granulocytopenia that occurs in conditioned patients for 11 to 18 days after transplantation. However, the use of recombinant granulocyte colony-stimulating factor (G-CSF) has reduced the severity of this problem. The advent of GVH disease prolongs the impaired immunity (Noel et al., 1978; Graze and Gale, 1979) and further heightens the susceptibility to infection. Protective isolation is necessary, and most transplant groups use laminar flow isolation units (Martin et al., 1987). Because such hosts are highly susceptible to opportunistic viral, fungal, and facultative intracellular microorganisms, untreatable infections develop frequently (Skinner et al., 1986).

The most problematic agents include *Candida albicans, Pneumocystis carinii,* cytomegalovirus, herpes simplex, varicella zoster virus, Epstein-Barr virus (EBV), parainfluenza, enteroviruses, and adenoviruses (Skinner et al., 1986). Bacterial infections with high-grade pathogens also occur but, if identified in time, can usually be treated effectively with antibiotics. Intravenous and oral immune globulin therapies have also helped to reduce the frequency and severity of infections caused by common bacterial and viral agents. Trimethoprim-sulfamethoxazole has vastly reduced the mortality from *P. carinii* pneumonia and is an effective prophylactic agent for this infection. Long-term therapy with ribavirin has provided some amelioration of parainfluenza infections. Acyclovir is highly effective in treating varicella zoster and herpes simplex infections and may have some prophylactic effect for EBV infections. Nevertheless, little other than the development of normal host T-cell function will abrogate ongoing infections with CMV, EBV, enteroviruses, and adenoviruses (DeVoe et al., 1985). Infections frequently lead to death before successful engraftment can occur; this is particularly true if severe GVH reactions occur.

Veno-occlusive Disease

Veno-occlusive disease (VOD) is a major cause of mortality following conditioning regimens employing cytoreductive agents that damage hepatic vascular endothelium (McDonald et al., 1985; Eltumi et al., 1993). Distinguishing VOD from other causes of liver damage can be difficult after bone marrow transplantation, particularly when thrombocytopenia poses an unacceptable risk for diagnostic percutaneous liver biopsy in the early post-transplant period. Until recently, the diagnosis was made on clinical criteria; however, serum concentrations of the aminopropeptide of type III procollagen (PIIINP) above a standard deviation score of 8 were found to be 100% predictive of VOD and to be similarly useful in the diagnosis and monitoring of this condition (Eltumi et al., 1993).

Identification of Engraftment

Four types of markers are used to identify donor cells in marrow recipients:

- Chromosomal differences (Korver et al., 1987; Vossen et al., 1993; Van Den Berg et al., 1994)
- Erythrocyte and leukocyte antigens
- Serum allotypes (Korver et al., 1987)
- DNA sequence polymorphisms (Ginsburg et al., 1985; Blazar and Filipovich, 1990)

If the donor and recipient are of the opposite sex, karyotypic markers can be detected as early as 2 weeks after grafting. Serum immunoglobulin allotypic markers are particularly useful in documenting chimerism of B cells. The advantage of DNA sequence polymorphisms is that they do not require cell division, so that the origin of even nondividing cells, such as monocytes or natural killer cells, can be determined (Ginsburg et al., 1985; Blazar and Filipovich, 1990).

Time to Immune Reconstitution

The time course of immune reconstitution varies, depending on (Buckley et al., 1986; Martin et al., 1987):

1. Whether or not the donor marrow is T cell–depleted.
2. Whether or not agents are administered after transplantation to prevent GVH reactions.
3. Whether or not GVH disease develops.

Normal T-cell and B-cell function can be seen as early as 12 days following administration of unfractionated HLA-identical marrow cells to infants with SCID (Sindel et al., 1984; DeVoe et al., 1985). On the other hand, T-cell function does not develop until 90 to 120 days following administration of T cell–depleted haploidentical marrow cells, and B-cell function may require 2 or 3 years or longer to develop (Buckley et al., 1986).

In matched marrow transplants into leukemia or aplasia patients or into any patient requiring conditioning and GVH disease prophylaxis, the period of immunodeficiency can be prolonged well beyond 100 days (Noel et al., 1978; Graze and Gale, 1979). Natural killer cell function appears earlier than T-cell function, at around 4 to 8 weeks (Rooney et al., 1986). When T cells do appear, they may present with normal subset populations (Buckley et al., 1986) or with a profound CD4 deficiency and CD8 predominance if there is GVH disease (Janossy et al., 1986). Earlier development of

antibody production has been achieved by immunizing the donor and the recipient with an antigen or vaccine shortly before transplantation; the antibody is produced by donor B cells (Lum et al., 1986).

HLA-Identical Bone Marrow Transplantation for Severe T-Cell Deficiency

The only adequate therapy for patients with severe forms of cellular immunodeficiency is immunologic reconstitution by transplantation of immunocompetent tissue. Although fetal liver and thymus appeared ideal for this because they have very low GVH potential (Uphoff, 1958) and are rich in precursors of immune cells, their success in conferring immune function on such patients has been, at best, only 10% to 15% (O'Reilly et al., 1985). Moreover, the immune function that developed was incomplete and unsustained.

Shortly after discovery of HLA in 1967 (Bach and Amos, 1967), immune function was conferred in two patients with invariably fatal genetically determined immunodeficiency diseases by transplanting into them HLA-identical allogeneic bone marrow cells (Bach et al., 1968; Gatti et al., 1968). One patient had SCID (Gatti et al., 1968), and the other had Wiskott-Aldrich syndrome (Bach et al., 1968). The correction of those two very different defects, as well as the subsequent correction of many other types of primary immunodeficiency by bone marrow transplantation, has taught us that the defects in most such conditions are intrinsic to cells of one or more hematopoietic lineages. Thus, bone marrow has been and remains the tissue of choice for immunoreconstitution (Good, 1987; O'Reilly, 1987).

Until 1980, only HLA-identical unfractionated bone marrow could be used for this purpose because of lethal GVH disease that ensued if mismatched donors were used (Bortin and Rimm, 1977). In most cases, both T-cell and B-cell immunity have been reconstituted by such fully matched transplants, with evidence of function detected as early as 2 weeks after transplantation (O'Reilly et al., 1984; Sindel et al., 1984; DeVoe et al., 1985; Good, 1987).

Analysis of the genetic origins of the immune cells in the engrafted patients has revealed that although the T cells are all of donor origin, the B cells in approximately half are those of the recipient (O'Reilly et al., 1984). Initially, it was considered that bone marrow was effective in conferring immunity on patients with SCID because it provided normal stem cells, but it is apparent from the later experience with T cell–depleted marrow (Buckley et al., 1986) that the early restoration of immune function in unfractionated HLA-identical marrow transplants is by adoptive transfer of mature T and B cells with the donor marrow (Sindel et al., 1984; DeVoe et al., 1985). As noted above, however, unfractionated bone marrow transplantation has not been possible for more than 75% of the immunodeficient patients who could have benefited, as they had no HLA-identical donors. As a consequence, most of these patients died (Bortin and Rimm, 1977).

HLA-Haploidentical Bone Marrow Transplantation for Severe T-Cell Deficiency

Historical Aspects

Because of the low availability of HLA-matched sibling donors for patients with lethal T-cell defects, many approaches were tried to avoid lethal GVHD when mismatched donors were used. From 1968 to 1980, all of these methods were unsuccessful except for fetal tissue transplants, which gave only marginal and unsustained immunologic improvement (Bortin and Rimm, 1977). However, the fact that totally HLA-disparate fetal liver cells could correct the immune defect in a few such patients without causing GVH reactions gave hope that HLA-disparate marrow stem cells could do the same if all T cells could be removed. Early success in T-cell depletion was achieved in experimental animals by treating donor marrow or spleen cells with anti–T cell antisera or agglutinating the unwanted cells with plant lectins (Muller-Ruchholtz et al., 1976; Reisner et al., 1978). The remaining immature marrow or splenic non–T cells restored lymphohematopoietic function to lethally irradiated MHC-disparate recipients without lethal GVH reactions.

Methods of T-Cell Depletion

Soybean Lectin and Sheep Erythrocyte Agglutination. Following these leads, methods were developed to deplete post-thymic T cells from human marrow. The most widely used and successful method for accomplishing this involves agglutination of most mature marrow cells with soybean lectin and subsequent removal of T cells from the unagglutinated marrow by sheep erythrocyte rosetting and density-gradient centrifugation (Reisner et al., 1983; Schiff et al., 1987). Patients treated with haploidentical (i.e., half-matched) parental stem cells prepared by this method have had minimal or no GVH reactions (Buckley et al., 1986; Fischer et al., 1986b; O'Reilly et al., 1986; Buckley, 1987).

Monoclonal Antibody and Complement Lysis. A second method of depleting post-thymic T cells from donor marrow involves incubating it with monoclonal antibodies to human T cells plus a source of complement (Filipovich et al., 1984; Waldmann et al., 1984; Reinherz et al., 1982). Antibodies employed for this purpose have included T12, Leu 1, CT-2, and Cam-PATH-1. T-cell depletion may not be as effective with this approach, possibly because of modulation of T-cell antigens from the surface of the T cells without destroying them. As a consequence, somewhat more frequent and severe GVH disease has been observed.

Sheep Erythrocyte Agglutination. A final approach has been to use sheep erythrocyte rosette depletion alone to remove T cells from haploidentical donor marrow (Fischer et al., 1986a, 1986b). Because different centers have used different numbers of rosette depletions and different methods of modifying the sheep red blood cells (i.e., no modification, neuraminidase or AET*-treatment), it has been difficult to evalu-

ate whether this approach is as effective as the others in removing post-thymic T cells. In one center, only a single rosetting step is done, with the intent to leave a few post-thymic T cells (Fischer et al., 1986a). GVH reactions are then modulated by giving the recipient cyclosporine continuously for various time periods following the transplantation.

Time Course and Nature of Engraftment

The time to development of immune function following haploidentical stem cell grafts is quite different from that after unfractionated HLA-identical marrow. Lymphocytes with mature T-cell phenotypes and functions fail to rise significantly until 3 to 4 months after transplantation (Fig. 32–6); normal T-cell function is reached between 4 and 7 months (Buckley et al., 1986). B-cell function develops much more slowly, averaging 2 to 2.5 years for normalization in some; others do not develop B-cell function altogether, despite normal T-cell function (Buckley et al., 1986; O'Reilly et al., 1986). Genetic analyses of the cells from such chimeric patients have revealed all T cells to be genetically donor, whereas the B and antigen-pre-

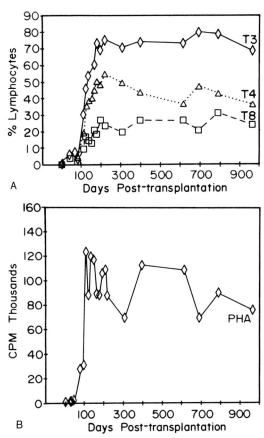

Figure 32–6. Development of lymphocytes with mature T-cell phenotypes *(A)* and function *(B)* in a male infant with severe combined immunodeficiency following a maternal bone marrow stem cell transplant. All cells dividing in response to phytohemagglutinin (PHA) had a female karyotype. The 90- to 100-day lag before the maternal stem cells are matured completely by the infant's thymus is reminiscent of the time it takes for mature T cells to appear in the human embryo. CPM = counts per minute.

---

*Aminoethylisothiuronium bromide.

senting cells almost always remain those of the recipient (Buckley et al., 1986; O'Reilly et al., 1984, 1986).

These observations indicate that the thymic microenvironment of most infants with SCID is capable of differentiating half-matched normal stem cells to mature and functioning T lymphocytes that can cooperate effectively with host B cells for antibody production (Buckley et al., 1986). Thus, the genetic defect in most does not involve the thymus.

Studies of these chimeric children reveal that the genetically donor cells that matured from stem cells to functioning mature T cells in the patient are tolerant of host class I and II HLA antigens and become autoreactive against the original donor's mononuclear cells (Schiff and Buckley, 1987). In addition, studies by the author and her associates (Roberts et al., 1989) found that some cloned tetanus toxoid–specific T cells from these chimeras prefer host APCs, i.e., are "educated" to recognize host as self, as has been noted in murine models (Singer et al., 1981). The finding that functioning B cells are those of the host indicates that the genetic defect does not affect the B cells in some of these patients (Buckley et al., 1986).

Efficacy of Bone Marrow Transplantation in Immunodeficiency Diseases

Although precise figures are not available, more than 900 patients worldwide with different forms of genetically determined immunodeficiency have been given bone marrow transplants over the past 27 years in attempts to correct their underlying immune defects (Table 32–5). From 1968 to 1977, only 14 (or 29%) of 48 infants with SCID worldwide were long-term survivors of successful HLA class II compatible bone marrow transplants (Bortin and Rimm, 1977). Possibly because of earlier diagnosis before untreatable opportunistic infections develop, the results have improved considerably over the last decade (Fischer et al., 1986b, 1990, 1994; Buckley, 1987; Buckley et al., 1993). A worldwide survey by the author revealed that 210 of 265 (79%) patients with primary immunodeficiency transplanted with HLA-identical marrow over the past 27 years survive with good immune function (see Table 32–5).

Most encouraging, however, are the results of half-matched stem cell transplants in patients with severe T-cell deficiency (Buckley et al., 1993). From the same formal and informal survey, the author ascertained that 554 such transplantations had been performed over the past 15 years and, of those, 297 (or 54%) of the patients were surviving with functioning grafts. The significance is even more impressive when it is realized that most of the 554 recipients would have died had not the new T-cell depletion techniques been developed.

Other types of immunodeficiency corrected by HLA-identical bone marrow transplants since 1968 include the Wiskott-Aldrich syndrome (55 patients) (Bach et al., 1968; Parkman et al., 1978; O'Reilly et al., 1984; Fischer et al., 1986a), the bare lymphocyte syndrome (4), the Chédiak-Higashi syndrome (7) (Fischer et al.,

1986b), DiGeorge anomaly (2) (Goldsobel et al., 1987), chronic granulomatous disease (14) (Foroozanfar et al., 1977), and leukocyte adhesion defect type 1(LAD-1) (6) (O'Reilly et al., 1984; Fischer et al., 1986b).

As shown in Table 32–5, however, haploidentical transplants have not been nearly as successful in the latter types of immune defects as in patients with SCID, possibly because pretransplant immunosuppression of these patients has been uniformly necessary to prevent graft rejection. This makes the patient much more susceptible to opportunistic infections because of ablation of phagocytic cells and the longer time course to engraftment of T cell–depleted marrow. Only 19 of 56 patients with Wiskott-Aldrich syndrome and 7 of 24 with Omenn syndrome have had successful haploidentical stem cell transplants. By contrast, 12 of 16 patients with LAD-1 have had successful haploidentical marrow transplants.

Efficacy of Bone Marrow Transplantation in Malignancy

The success of marrow transplantation in curing malignancy depends on a number of factors, the most important of which include the type of malignant disease, the stage of that disease, and the age of the recipient (Thomas, 1987). Although autologous and syngeneic (identical twin) marrow have been used successfully in the treatment of various forms of malignancy, by far the greatest experience and success has been with allogeneic (genetically different) marrow (Martin et al., 1987; O'Reilly, 1987; Thomas, 1987; Rowlings et al., 1994).

In contrast to the success noted above with T cell–depleted haploidentical marrow in treating infants with lethal genetic defects of T-cell function, this approach has been confounded by resistance to engraftment and leukemia recurrence when applied to the treatment of malignancies (Maraninchi et al., 1987; O'Reilly, 1987). Thus, most successful allogeneic bone marrow transplants for malignant diseases have been with unfractionated HLA-identical marrow. However, since only 25% to 30% of patients have HLA-identical siblings, alternative donor types have been sought (Beatty et al., 1985). Surprisingly, unfractionated marrow from family donors who share one genetically identical HLA haplotype but whose other haplotype differs from the patient's other haplotype by only one HLA locus has achieved results similar to those with marrow from HLA-matched sibling donors in the treatment of patients with malignancy (Beatty et al., 1985).

A possible breakthrough was reported in solving the graft failure repeatedly seen with T cell–depleted haploidentical marrow infusions for leukemia. Aversa and his colleagues (1994) from Italy found that by (1) increasing the size of the graft inoculum 7-fold to 10-fold by adding G-CSF-mobilized haploidentical donor peripheral blood stem cells (depleted of T cells by soy lectin/sheep erythrocyte rosetting) to similarly T–cell–depleted donor marrow cells, and (2) using a highly immunosuppressive and myeloablative conditioning

Table 32–5. Survey of Bone Marrow Transplantation for Immunodeficiency Diseases, 1968–1995

Type of Immune Defect	Total No. of Patients		No. of Patients with HLA-Identical Donor		No. of Patients with Haplo-Identical Donor		No. of Patients with Unrelated Donor	
	No. Transplanted	No. Surviving	No. Transplanted	No. Surviving	No. Transplanted	No. Surviving	No. Transplanted	No. Surviving
Severe combined immunodeficiency*	517	341	119	100	382	230	16	11
Wiskott-Aldrich syndrome	143	91	61	55	56	19	26	17
Nezelof syndrome	49	23	13	10	34	13	2	0
Omenn syndrome	39	18	9	8	24	7	6	3
Major histocompatibility complex antigen deficiency	30	13	8	4	20	7	2	2
Leukocyte adhesion defect, type 1	26	21	7	6	16	12	3	3
Chédiak-Higashi syndrome	18	13	9	7	4	0	5	5
Chronic granulomatous disease	10	6	7	4	0	0	3	2
Purine nucleoside phosphorylase deficiency	8	4	5	2	2	2	1	0
DiGeorge anomaly	7	2	3	2	4	0	0	0
Cartilage-hair hypoplasia	6	3	2	2	3	1	1	0
Hyper-IgM immunodeficiency	6	3	2	1	3	1	1	1
X-linked lymphoproliferative syndrome	5	2	5	2	0	0	0	0
Other illnesses	21	12	15	7	6	5	0	0
TOTAL patients (% survival)	889	551 (62%)	265	210 (79%)	554	297 (54%)	66	44 (67%)

*Including adenosine deaminase deficiency.

Data provided during 1994–1995 by the following physicians listed alphabetically, plus the author Rebecca Buckley (Durham): Douglas Barrett (Gainesville); Mary Ellen Conley (Memphis); Morton J. Cowan (San Francisco); A. Fasth (Goteborg); A. Filopovich (Minneapolis); Alain Fischer (Paris); William Friedrich (Ulm); Harv Harfi (Ryad, Saudi Arabia); Richard Hong (Wisconsin); Nina Kapoor (Oklahoma and Columbus); Hans Ochs (Seattle); F. Porta (Brescia, Italy); Reinhard Seger (Zurich); William Shearer (Houston); Trudy Small (Sloan-Kettering); E. Richard Stiehm (UCLA); Kenneth Weinberg (Los Angeles); Howard Weinstein (Boston Children's); and John Zieglar (Australia).

regimen (single fraction fast total body irradiation, ATG, cyclophosphamide, and thiotepa), they achieved engraftment in 16 of 17 patients with end-stage chemoresistant leukemia. Nine patients died from transplant-related toxicity and two relapsed, but six are alive and event-free after a median follow-up of 230 days. Higher probabilities of relapse (60% to 70%) account for lower survival rates for patients with end-stage leukemia (10% to 20%) and advanced Hodgkin's disease or lymphomas (15% to 20%) (Thomas, 1987).

A summary of the results of HLA-identical sibling bone marrow transplants for various stages and types of leukemia and lymphoma over a 15-year period was published by Thomas in 1987. Table 32–6 (from that review) provides Thomas' estimate from the published literature and his group's experience of the probability of survival and of relapse according to the type and stage of malignant disease. The best survival rates (50% to 70%) with the lowest probability of relapse (20%) occurred in patients younger than 20 years of age who had acute nonlymphocytic leukemia (ANL) transplanted in first remission and in patients with chronic myelogenous leukemia (CML) transplanted in chronic phase (Goldman et al., 1986).

Clearly, HLA-identical bone marrow transplantation is the treatment of choice for those two categories of patients. These statistics were upheld by those from analyses by European Leukemia Cooperative Groups (Zittoun et al., 1995) on transplants in acute myelogenous leukemia and by the International Bone Marrow Transplant Registry on 16,905 allogeneic marrow transplants for any disease reported over a 20-year period (Rowlings et al., 1994).

For patients with acute myelogenous leukemia during first complete remission the projected rate of disease-free survival at 4 years was 55% for allogeneic transplantation, 48% for autologous transplantation, and 30% for intensive chemotherapy (Zittoun et al., 1995). For the autologous transplants (done when there is no HLA-identical donor), autologous remission marrow is purged with 4-hydroperoxycyclophosphamide, cryopreserved, and then reinfused after the pa-

tient has been given intensive cytoreductive therapy (Yeager et al., 1987). For patients with CML, the 3-year leukemia-free survival rate was 57% for transplantations done in the first chronic phase, 41% in accelerated or second chronic phase, and 18% in more advanced disease (Rowlings et al., 1994).

Because approximately 45% of patients with acute lymphoblastic leukemia (ALL) have been cured by combination chemotherapy (Rivera et al., 1993) and the probability of event-free survival has steadily increased with advances in this therapy (to a recent high of 71%), most of these patients do not undergo bone marrow transplantation. However, many such patients have received transplants in second remission when they were in good condition and the prognosis was known to be poor with chemotherapy alone (Barrett et al., 1994).

In an analysis comparing data in the International Bone Marrow Transplant Registry on such transplants with results of continued chemotherapy in children with ALL treated by the Pediatric Oncology Group, Barrett and colleagues (1994) found that the mean probability of a relapse at 5 years was significantly lower among the transplant recipients than among the chemotherapy recipients (45% versus 80%). At 5 years, the probability of leukemia-free survival was higher after transplantation than after chemotherapy (40% versus 17%). This survival rate was somewhat higher than the 29% reported by Weisdorf et al., (1994) at a median of 7.8 years.

Changing Indications for Autologous Marrow Transplantation

The data from the International Bone Marrow Transplant Registry suggest that the use of autologous marrow infusions is increasing at a rate greater than 20% per year and now exceeds use of allogeneic bone marrow transplants (Rowlings et al., 1994). In addition, the most common indication for autologous marrow infusion changed from non-Hodgkin's lymphoma in

Table 32–6. Summary of Reported Results of Marrow Transplantation for Malignant Disease

	Probability of Survival*	Probability of Relapse†	Longest Time Since Transplant (Years)
End-stage acute leukemia	0.10–0.20	0.70	15
ALL in second remission	0.33–0.50	0.60	10
ANLL in first remission			
Age <20 yr	0.50–0.70	0.20	10
Age >20 yr	0.35–0.50	0.20	10
CML: Blastic phase	0.10–0.15	0.80	10
Accelerated phase	0.20–0.40	0.60	7
Chronic phase	0.50–0.70	0.20	10
Advanced Hodgkin's and lymphomas	0.15–0.20	0.60	14

*A Kaplan-Meier analysis of the probability that a patient will be on a plateau for long-term survival.
†A Kaplan-Meier analysis of the probability of relapse if death does not occur from other causes.
Abbreviations: ALL = Acute lymphoblastic leukemia; CML = chronic myelogenous leukemia; ANLL = acute nonlymphocytic leukemia.
From Thomas ED. Marrow transplantation for malignant disease. Am J Med Sci 294(2):75–79, 1987. Based on data from Kaplan EL, Meier PJ. Am Statistical Assoc 53:457–481, 1958.

1989 to 1990 to breast cancer in 1991 to 1992 (Treasure, 1994). Approximately 35% of all autologous infusions in 1992 were for breast cancer, primarily in women with advanced disease.

Efficacy of Bone Marrow Transplantation in Aplastic Anemia

Both identical twin and unfractionated HLA-identical marrow have effected cures of severe marrow aplasia (Storb et al., 1984; Bortin and Gale, 1986; Pillow et al., 1966; Casper et al., 1990). The fact that approximately 50% of adult patients with this condition improve dramatically after immunosuppressive therapy (ATG/ALG, cyclosporine, and/or androgens) suggests that immunologic mechanisms have an etiologic role in some forms of aplasia. In children, however, a majority of cases appear to be due to stem cell abnormalities, since HLA-identical bone marrow transplantation is far more successful than immunosuppressive therapy (Casper et al., 1990).

During the past decade, many transplant centers have reported favorable outcomes of matched marrow transplants in children; long-term, disease-free survival increased from 47% in 1978 to 1980 to between 70% and 80% in the more recent larger series (Casper et al., 1990). Therefore, bone marrow transplantation should be considered the treatment of choice for children with severe aplastic anemia (especially those under 6 years of age), if an HLA-identical sibling donor is available.

For patients without an HLA-identical sibling or who are over age 40 years, immunosuppressive therapy is the treatment of choice, as non–HLA-identical grafts have had very poor outcomes (Storb et al., 1984; Casper et al., 1990). However, even if a favorable response occurs after immunosuppressive therapy, the actuarial incidence of relapse is 35% (Schrezenmeier et al., 1993). Multiple transfusions prior to marrow transplantation should be avoided if marrow transplantation is a possibility, as transfusions can sensitize the recipient. Use of more intense conditioning regimens, including radiation, as well as large numbers of marrow cells ($>4 \times 10^8$ cells/kg) has helped to overcome this problem (Casper et al., 1990).

Efficacy of Bone Marrow Transplantation in Hemoglobinopathies, Osteopetrosis, and Metabolic Storage Diseases

Lucarelli and associates (1987) reported on 40 Italian patients with homozygous β thalassemia who underwent transplantation with HLA-identical marrow following conditioning with busulfan and cyclophosphamide; 30 were surviving and 28 were without thalassemia, giving actuarial probabilities of survival and disease-free survival at 2 years of 75% and 69%, respectively. Altogether, more than 537 patients with homozygous β thalassemia received transplants from 1982 to 1992, and the probabilities of survival, disease-free survival, and rejection were 0.85, 0.80, and 0.05, respectively (Lucarelli et al., 1993). Sixty-four patients

with the mildest disease classification (class 1) had even better probabilities of 0.92, 0.85, and 0.04, respectively. Because of the high efficacy of marrow transplantation, the authors recommended that all such patients who have healthy HLA-identical siblings undergo this treatment. Transplantation has also been carried out in more than 50 patients with sickle cell disease, and 41 were surviving at between 1 and 75 months after transplantation (Beutler, 1994).

The European Bone Marrow Transplantation Group reported on 69 patients with autosomal recessive osteopetrosis who were given HLA-identical or haploidentical bone marrow transplants between 1976 and 1994 (Gerritsen et al., 1994). Recipients of genotypically HLA-identical marrow had an actuarial probability for 5-year survival, with osteoclast function, of 79%. Recipients of phenotypically HLA-identical marrow from a related or unrelated donor had an actuarial probability for 5-year survival, with osteoclast function, of 38%, and those who received HLA-haploidentical marrow from a related donor had an actuarial probability for 5-year survival, with osteoclast function, of only 13%.

Of approximately 12 patients with metabolic diseases who underwent transplantation with matched bone marrow, 8 were surviving with durable engraftment (O'Reilly et al., 1984).

Other diseases treated successfully with bone marrow transplantation include: histiocytosis X (Ringden et al., 1987), paroxysmal nocturnal hemoglobinuria (Antin et al., 1985), Fanconi's anemia, congenital aregenerative anemias, acute myelofibrosis, four types of polysaccharidoses, Gaucher's disease (Chan et al., 1994), metachromatic leukodystrophy, thrombocytopenia–absent radii syndrome (Brochstein et al., 1992), and other mucolipidoses (O'Reilly et al., 1984; Krivit and Whitley, 1987).

Remaining Problems with Haploidentical T Cell–Depleted Transplants

In addition to the longer period of susceptibility to infection caused by the longer time course to development of immune function following haploidentical stem cell transplants, four principal problems have been encountered in mismatched transplants which occur much less frequently in matched transplants:

- Resistance to engraftment
- Inadequate B-cell function
- Development of B-cell lymphomas
- Leukemia recurrence

Resistance to Engraftment

Resistance to engraftment (Cudkowicz, 1975; O'Reilly et al., 1986) has been particularly difficult to overcome in patients with some pre-existing T-cell function given haploidentical stem cell transplants, even though they have received lethal conditioning regimens (Fischer et al., 1986b, 1986c). Though the reasons for this are not clear, some success in circumventing this problem has been reported by Fischer and colleagues (1986c). Following their observations that conditioned LAD-1 patients readily accepted half-matched stem cell transplants, those authors employed in vivo pretreatment of the recipient with a monoclonal antibody to the alpha-chain of leukocyte function–associated antigen (LFA-1) and achieved rapid engraftment of haploidentical marrow in seven of seven conditioned patients who had had some pretreatment T-cell function (Fischer et al., 1986c). Because LFA-1 is an adhesion protein important in immune cell interaction, the authors speculated that the antibody interfered with host recognition of the graft. Subsequent experience with this approach has been less promising, however, and this has not been employed in patients with leukemia, where resistance to engraftment of haploidentical T-cell–depleted marrow has been a major problem (O'Reilly, 1987).

Inadequate Development of B-Cell Function

Donor B-cell engraftment is rarely achieved in patients with SCID who have undergone transplantation with haploidentical stem cells and who do not receive conditioning regimens (O'Reilly et al., 1986). This is also true in a majority of those who receive unfractionated HLA-identical marrow without conditioning (Buckley et al., 1993). Nevertheless, a majority of these patients who receive matched marrow eventually have normal B-cell function, whereas this is not the case for many who receive half-matched marrow. Lack of B-cell function may be due to intrinsic defects in the patient's own B cells or to the fact that the latter must be "helped" by half-matched rather than fully HLA-matched T cells. Recent evidence that B cells of boys with X-linked SCID do not isotype-switch, even with normal T cells, suggests that the problem may be intrinsic to the B cells in that type of SCID (Buckley, unpublished data). Because of this problem, some centers condition patients with SCID prior to half-matched marrow transplants, with the hope of enhancing donor B-cell engraftment. However, when this is done, there are many more infection-related deaths (Fischer et al., 1986a) and the agents used may have long-term undesirable effects on other body tissues.

Most centers, therefore, opt for no pretransplant conditioning, and they administer immune globulin to recipients who remain deficient in B-cell function following haploidentical stem cell transplants despite normal T-cell function. The author has been encouraged by her own experience to date with nonconditioned T cell–depleted haploidentical marrow transplants in which more than 50% of the patients with SCID successfully engrafted have developed some B-cell function, with antibody responses to bacteriophage ϕX174 being comparable in some to those of recipients of unfractionated HLA-identical marrow—despite the fact that the B cells remain those of the host (Buckley et al., 1993). The development of B-cell function also indicates that patients with some forms of SCID do have intrinsically normal B cells.

B-Cell Lymphomas

The development of B-cell lymphomas has also been a problem in recipients of half-matched stem cell transplants (Trigg et al., 1985), whereas they are almost never seen in HLA-identical transplants (Good, 1987). Most of these have been EBV-positive, and most have been in recipients of monoclonal antibody T cell–depleted marrow. Garcia and colleagues (1987), however, reported the development of a B-cell lymphoma not associated with EBV in a patient with SCID who had received T cell–depleted haploidentical marrow. The long period before development of normal T-cell function is thought to be related to the propensity for such tumors to develop.

Leukemia Recurrence

Finally, the higher leukemia recurrence rate in recipients of T cell–depleted marrow already referred to (Maraninchi et al., 1987) has led a number of transplant groups to abandon the use of T-cell depletion in bone marrow transplantation for leukemia.

FETAL TISSUE TRANSPLANTATION

Although transplantation of fetal liver and/or thymus has been attempted many times over the past three decades in the correction of SCID, DiGeorge anomaly, or other severe T-cell deficiency, it has rarely been permanently successful, except possibly in patients with DiGeorge anomaly (August et al., 1968; Cleveland et al., 1968). However, the improved immune function observed in DiGeorge patients following fetal thymus transplantation may have been due to growth of autologous thymic tissue, since a majority of these patients have tiny nests of autologous thymic tissue and some parathyroid glands in the mediastinum. Chimerism has rarely, if ever, been proved in any DiGeorge patient after a fetal thymus implant. Moreover, as already noted, because the complete DiGeorge anomaly has been corrected by HLA-identical bone marrow transplantation (Goldsobel et al., 1987), that should be the treatment of choice if an HLA-identical sibling donor is available (see Chapter 12).

Between 1975 and 1981 (before T cell–depleted haploidentical marrow transplantation became feasible), numerous attempts were made to correct SCID with fetal liver or fetal liver plus thymus. Some degree of success was achieved, as evidenced by chimerism and improved immune function, but the immunoreconstitution observed was slow to develop, only partial at best and lost with time (Buckley et al., 1976; O'Reilly et al., 1985). Another approach attempted was that of using cultured (mature) thymic epithelium. However, only marginal and unsustained improvement was observed and a high incidence of B-cell lymphomas was reported in recipients of such cultured thymuses (Borzy et al., 1979). These procedures are also described in Chapter 12.

References

Adams DD. Protection from autoimmune disease as the third function of the major histocompatibility gene complex. Lancet 2:245–250, 1987.

Almarri A, Batchelor JR. HLA and hepatitis B infection. Lancet 344:1194–1195, 1994.

Amiel JL. Study of the leukocyte phenotypes in Hodgkin's disease. In Curtoni ES, Mattiuz PL, Tosi RM, eds. Histocompatibility Testing. Copenhagen, Munksgaard, 1967, pp. 79–81.

Amos DB. The agglutination of mouse leukocytes by iso-immune sera. Br J Exp Pathol 34:464–470, 1953.

Amos DB, Bach FH. Phenotypic expressions of the major histocompatibility locus in man (HL-A): leukocyte antigens and mixed leukocyte culture reactivity. J Exp Med 128:623–637, 1968.

Amos DB, Seigler HF, Southworth JG, Ward FE. Skin graft rejection between subjects genotyped for HLA. Transplant Proc 1:342–346, 1969.

Anderson KC, Weinstein JH. Transfusion-associated graft-versus-host disease. N Engl J Med 323:315–321, 1990.

Antin JH, Ginsburg D, Smith BR, Nathan DG, Orkin SH, Rappeport JM. Bone marrow transplantation for paroxysmal nocturnal hemoglobinuria: eradication of the PNH clone and documentation of complete lymphohematopoietic engraftment. Blood 66:1247–1250, 1985.

Arbus GS, Sullivan EK, Tejani A. Hospitalization in children during the first year after kidney transplantation. Kidney Int 44:83–86, 1993.

Ardehali A, Laks H, Drinkwater DC, Ziv ET, Sorensen TJ, Hamilton MA, Warner-Stevenson L, Moriguchi JB, Kobashigawa JA. Cardiac transplantation at UCLA. In Terasaki PI, Cecka JM, eds. Clinical Transplants 1993. Los Angeles, UCLA Tissue Typing Laboratory, 1994, pp. 119–128.

Armitage JM, Fricker FJ, del Nido P, Starzl TE, Hardesty RL, Griffith BP. A decade (1982 to 1992) of pediatric cardiac transplantation and the impact of FK 506 immunosuppression. J Thoracic Cardiovasc Surg 105:464–473, 1993.

Armitage JO. Bone marrow transplantation. N Engl J Med 330:827–838, 1994.

Arnett FC. HLA genes and predisposition to rheumatic diseases. Hosp Pract, 1986, pp. 89–100.

Assaad A. Post-transplantation management of the newborn and the immunosuppressive role of prostaglandin E1. J Heart Lung Transplant 12:191–194, 1993.

Atkinson K, Biggs J, Darveniza P, Boland J, Concannon A, Dodds A. Cyclosporine associated central nervous system toxicity after allogeneic bone marrow transplantation. Transplantation 38:34–37, 1984.

Atkison P, Joubert G, Barron A, Grant D, Paradis K, Seldman E, Wall W, Rosenberg H, Howard J, Williams S, Stiller C. Hypertrophic cardiomyopathy associated with tacrolimus in paediatric transplant patients. Lancet 345:894–896, 1995.

August CS, Rosen FS, Filler RM, Janeway CA, Markowski B, Kay HEM. Implantation of a fetal thymus: restoring immunological competence in a patient with thymic aplasia (DiGeorge's syndrome). Lancet 2:1210–1211, 1968.

Aversa F, Tabilio A, Terenzi A, Velardi A, Falzetti F, Giannoni C, Iacucci R, Zei T, Martelli MP, Gambelunghs C, Rossetti M, Caputo P, Latini P, Aristei C, Raymondi C, Reisner Y, Martelli MF. Successful engraftment of T cell depleted haploidentical "three-loci" incompatible transplants in leukemia patients by addition of recombinant human granulocyte colony-stimulating factor-mobilized peripheral blood progenitor cells to bone marrow inoculum. Blood 84:3948–3956, 1994.

Bach FH, Albertini RJ, Joo P, Anderson JL, Bortin MD. Bone marrow transplantation in a patient with Wiskott-Aldrich syndrome. Lancet 2:1364–1366, 1968.

Bach FH, Amos DB. Hu-1: major histocompatibility locus in man. Science 156:1506–1508, 1967.

Bach FH, Hirschhorn K. Lymphocyte interaction, a potential histocompatibility test in vitro. Science 143:813–814, 1964.

Bach FH, Inouye H, Hank JA, Alter BJ. Human T lymphocyte clones reactive in primed lymphocyte typing and cytotoxicity. Nature 281:397–409, 1979.

Bach FH, Sachs DH. Transplantation immunology. N Engl J Med 317:489–492, 1987.

Bach JF, Strom TB. The Mode of Action of Immunosuppressive Drugs. New York, Elsevier, 1985.

Bailey LL, Gundry SR, Razzouk AJ, Wang N, Sciolaro CM, Chiavarelli M. Bless the babies: one hundred fifteen late survivors of heart transplantation during the first year of life. J Thoracic Cardiovasc Surg 105:805–815, 1993.

Bain B, Magdalene RV, Lowenstein L. The development of large immature mononuclear cells in mixed leukocyte cultures. Blood 23:108–116, 1964.

Ballenger WF, Lacy PE. Transplantation of intact pancreatic islets in rats. Surgery 72:175–186, 1972.

Barber WH, Curtis JJ, Whelchel JD, Luck RG, Diethelm AG. Outcome of second kidney allografts following failure of transplants from living-related donors. Transplantation 40:225–228, 1985.

Barker CF, Billingham RE. The role of regional lymphatics in the skin homograft response. Transplantation 5:962–966, 1967.

Barrett AJ, Horowitz MM, Pollock BH, Zhang M, Bortin MM, Buchanan GR, Camitta BM, Ochs J, Graham-Pole J, Rowlings PA, Rimm AA, Klein JP, Shuster JJ, Sobocinski KA, Gale RP. Bone marrow transplants from HLA-identical siblings as compared with chemotherapy for children with acute lymphoblastic leukemia in a second remission. N Engl J Med 331:1253–1258, 1994.

Batisky DL, Wyatt RJ, Fitzwater DS, Gaber AO, Roy S. Pediatric renal transplant experience in Memphis, Tennessee. Transplant Proc 26:54–56, 1994.

Beatty PG, Clift RA, Mickelson EM, Nisperos B, Flournoy N, Martin PJ, Sanders JE, Stewart P, Buckner CD, Storb R, Thomas ED, Hansen JA. Marrow transplantation from related donors other than HLA-identical siblings. N Engl J Med 313:765–771, 1985.

Bell J, Smoot S, Newby C, Toyka K, Rassenti L, Smith K, Hohlfeld R, McDevitt H, Steinman L. HLA-DQ beta chain polymorphism linked to myasthenia gravis. Lancet 1:1058–1060, 1986.

Bell JI, Denny D, McDevitt HO. Structure and polymorphism of murine and human class II major histocompatibility antigens. Immunol Rev 84:51–71, 1985.

Bell PRF, Calman KC, Wood RFM, Briggs JC, Paton AM, MacPherson SG. Reversal of acute clinical and experimental organ rejection using large doses of intravenous prednisolone. Lancet 1:876–888, 1971.

Belle SH, Beringer KC, Detre KM. Trends in liver transplantation in the United States. In Terasaki PI, Cecka JM, eds. Clinical Transplants 1993. Los Angeles, UCLA Tissue Typing Laboratory, 1994, pp. 19–36.

Bernstein D. Update on cardiac transplantation in infants and children. Crit Care Med 21:354–355, 1993.

Beutler E. Bone marrow transplantation beyond treatment of aplasia and neoplasia. West J Med 160:129–132, 1994.

Billingham RE, Brent L, Medawar PB. Actively acquired tolerance of foreign cells. Nature 172:603–606, 1953.

Binz H, Wigzell H. Shared idiotypic determinants on B and T lymphocytes reactive against the same antigenic determinants: I. Demonstration of similar or identical idiotypes on IgG molecules and T cell receptors with specificity for the same alloantigen. J Exp Med 142:197–211, 1975.

Bismuth H, Ericzon BG, Rolles K, Castaing D, Otte JB, Ringe B, Sloof M. Hepatic transplantation in Europe: first report of the European Liver Transplant Registry. Lancet 2:674–767, 1987.

Blazar BR, Filipovich AH. Identification of transfused blood cells in children with SCID by analysis of multiple cell lineages using restriction fragment length polymorphisms. Bone Marrow Transplant 5:327–333, 1990.

Blazar BR, Ramsay NKC, Kersey JH. Pretransplant conditioning with busulfan and cyclophosphamide for nonmalignant diseases. Transplantation 39:597, 1985.

Bluestone JA, Leo O, Epstein SL, Sachs DH. Idiotypic manipulation of the immune response to transplantation antigens. Immunol Rev 90:5–27, 1986.

Bodmer JG, Marsh SGE, Albert ED, Bodmer WF, Dupont B, Erlich HA, Mach B, Mayr WR, Parham P, Sasazuki T, Schreuder GMT, Strominger JL, Svejgaard A, Terasaki PI. Nomenclature for factors of the HLA system, 1994. Tissue Antigens 44:1–18, 1995.

Bodmer WF. HLA today. Hum Immunol 17:490–503, 1986.

Bortin MM, Gale RP. Current status of allogeneic bone marrow transplantation: a report from the International Bone Marrow Transplant Registry. In Terasaki PI, ed. Clinical Transplants 1986. Los Angeles, UCLA Tissue Typing Laboratory, 1986, pp. 17–28.

Bortin MM, Rimm AA. Severe combined immunodeficiency disease: characterization of the disease and results of transplantation. JAMA 238:591–600, 1977.

Borzy MS, Hong R, Horowitz SD, Gilbert E, Kaufman D, DeMendonca W, Oxelius VA, Dictor M, Pachman L. Fatal lymphoma after transplantation of cultured thymus in children with combined immunodeficiency disease. N Engl J Med 301:565–568, 1979.

Bowen KM, Andrus L, Lafferty KJ. Successful allotransplantation of mouse pancreatic islets to non-immunosuppressed recipients. Diabetes 29S:98–104, 1980.

Breen TJ, Keck B, Hosenpud JD, White R, Daily OP. Thoracic organ transplants in the United States from October 1987 through December 1992: a report from the UNOS Scientific Registry for Organ Transplants. In Terasaki PI, Cecka JM, eds. Clinical Transplants 1993. Los Angeles, UCLA Tissue Typing Laboratory, 1994, pp. 37–46.

Breimer ME, Brynger H, Le Pendu J, Oriol R, Rydberg L, Samuelsson BE, Vinas J. Blood group ABO incompatible kidney transplantation: biochemical and immunochemical studies of blood group A glycolipid antigens in human kidney and characterization of the antibody response (antigen specificity and antibody class) in O recipients receiving A2 grafts. Transplant Proc 19:226–230, 1987.

Breimer ME, Brynger H, Rydberg L, Samuelsson BF. Transplantation of blood group A2 kidneys to O recipients: biochemical and immunological studies of blood group A antigens in human kidneys. Transplant Proc 17:2640–2643, 1985.

Brenner MK, Rill DR, Holladay MS, Heslop HE, Moen RC, Buschle M, Krance RA, Santana VM, Anderson WF, Ihle JN. Gene marking to determine whether autologous marrow infusion restores long-term haemopoiesis in cancer patients. Lancet 342:1134–1137, 1993.

Brochstein JA, Shank B, Kernan NA, Terwilliger JW, O'Reilly RJ. Marrow transplantation for thrombocytopenia-absent radii syndrome. J Pediatr 121:587–589, 1992.

Brown JW, Turrentine MW, Kesler KA, Mahomed Y, Darragh R, Evans K, Thompson L, Caldwell R. Triple drug immunosuppression for heart transplantation in infants and children. J Heart Lung Transplant 12:265–274, 1993.

Broyer M, Donckerwoicke R, Brunner F, Brynger H, Jacobs C, Kramer P, Selwood N, Wing A. The European experience with treatment of end-stage renal disease in young children. In Cummings NB, Klahr S, eds. Chronic Renal Disease: Causes, Complications and Treatment. New York, Plenum Publishing, 1985, pp. 347–354.

Broyer M, Ehrich J, Jones E, Selwood N. Five year survival of kidney transplantation in children: data from the European (EDTA-ERA) Registry. Kidney Int 44:22–25, 1993.

Brynger H, Rydberg L, Samuelsson BE, Sandberg L. Experience with 14 renal transplants with kidneys from blood group A (subgroup A2) to O recipients. Transplant Proc 16:1175–1176, 1984.

Buckley RH. Bone marrow transplantation in treatment of severe primary T cell immunodeficiency: recent advances. Pediatr Ann 16:412–421, 1987.

Buckley RH, Schiff SE, Sampson HA, Schiff RI, Markert ML, Knutsen AP, Hershfield MS, Huang AT, Mickey GH, Ward FE. Development of immunity in human severe primary T cell deficiency following haploidentical bone marrow stem cell transplantation. J Immunol 136:2398–2407, 1986.

Buckley RH, Schiff SE, Schiff RI, Roberts JL, Markert ML, Peters W, Williams LW, Ward FE. Haploidentical bone marrow stem cell transplantation in human severe combined immunodeficiency. Semin Hematol 30:92–104, 1993.

Buckley RH, Whisnant JK, Schiff RI, Gilbertsen RB, Platt MS. Correction of severe combined immunodeficiency by fetal liver cells. N Engl J Med 294:1076–1081, 1976.

Buckner CD. Bone marrow transplantation. N Engl J Med 292:823–843, 1975.

Calne RY. Pancreas transplantation. Progr Allergy 38:395–403, 1986.

Calne RY. Immunosuppression in liver transplantation. N Engl J Med 331:1154–1155, 1994.

Cameron JS. Glomerulonephritis in renal transplants. Transplantation 34:237–245, 1982.

Canter CE, Moorhead S, Saffitz JE, Huddleston CB, Spray TL. Steroid withdrawal in the pediatric heart transplant recipient initially treated with triple immunosuppression. J Heart Lung Transplant 13:74–80, 1994.

Carpenter CB, Morris PJ. The detection and measurement of pre-transplant sensitization. Transplant Proc 10:509–513, 1978.

Casper JT, Truitt RR, Baxter-Lowe LA, Ash RC. Bone marrow transplantation for severe aplastic anemia in children. Am J Pediatr Hematol-Oncol 12:434–448, 1990.

Caves PK, Stinson EB, Billingham ME, Rider AK, Shumway NE. Diagnosis of human cardiac allograft rejection by serial cardiac biopsy. J Thorac Cardiovasc Surg 66:461–466, 1973.

Cecka JM, Terasaki PI. The UNOS Scientific Renal Transplant Registry. In Terasaki PI, Cecka JM, eds. Clinical Transplants 1993. Los Angeles, UCLA Tissue Typing Laboratory, 1994, pp. 1–18.

Ceppellini R, Bigliani S, Curtoni ES, Leigheb G. Experimental allotransplantation in man: II. The role of A1, A2 and B antigens: III. Enhancement by circulating antibody. Transplant Proc 1:390–394, 1969.

Chan KW, Wong LTK, Applegarth D, Davidson AGF. Bone marrow transplantation in Gaucher's disease: effect of mixed chimeric state. Bone Marrow Transplantation 14:327–330, 1994.

Chinnock RE, Baum MF, Larsen R, Bailey L. Rejection management and long term surveillance of the pediatric heart transplant recipient: the Loma Linda experience. J Heart Lung Transplant 12:255–264, 1993.

Cicciarelli J, Terasaki P. Sensitization patterns in transfused kidney transplant patients and their possible role in kidney graft survival. Transplant Proc 15:1208–1211, 1983.

Clay TM, Culpan D, Howell WM, Sage DA, Bradley BA, Bidwell JL. UHG crossmatching: a comparison with PCR-SSO typing in the selection of HLA-DPB1–compatible bone marrow donors. Transplantation 58:200–207, 1994.

Cleveland WW, Fogel BJ, Brown WR, Kay HEM. Fetal thymus transplant in a case of DiGeorge's syndrome. Lancet 2:1211–1214, 1968.

Codoner-Franch P, Bernard O, Alvarez F. Long term follow-up of growth in height after successful liver transplantation. J Pediatr 124:368–373, 1994.

Collins RH, Anastasi J, Terstappen LWM, Nikaein A, Feng J, Fay JW, Klintmalm G, Stone MJ. Brief report: donor-derived long term multilineage hematopoiesis in a liver transplant recipient. N Engl J Med 328:762–770, 1993.

Coppin HL, McDevitt HO. Absence of polymorphism between HLA-B27 genomic exon sequences isolated from normal donors and ankylosing spondylitis patients. J Immunol 137:2168–2172, 1986.

Cosimi AB, Colvin RB, Burton RC, Rubin RH, Goldstein G, Kung PC, Hansen WP, Delmonico FL, Russell PS. Use of monoclonal antibodies to T cell subsets for immunologic monitoring and treatment in recipients of renal allografts. N Engl J Med 305:308–314, 1981.

Cros P, Allibert P, Mandrand B, Tiercy J, Mach B. Oligonucleotide genotyping of HLA polymorphism on microtitre plates. Lancet 340:870–873, 1992.

Cudkowicz G. Genetic control of resistance to allogeneic and xenogeneic bone marrow grafts in mice. Transplant Proc 7:155–159, 1975.

Czitrom AA, Langer F, McKee N, Gross AE. Bone and cartilage allotransplantation: a review of 14 years of research and clinical studies. Clin Orthop 208:141–145, 1986.

Dausset J. Leuco-agglutinins: IV. Leuco-agglutinins and blood transfusion. Vox Sang 4:190–198, 1954.

Dausset J, Rapaport FT. The role of ABO erythrocyte groups in human histocompatibility reactions. Nature 209:209–211, 1966.

Deeg HJ, Henslee-Downey PJ. Management of acute graft-versus-host disease. Bone Marrow Transplant 6:1–8, 1990.

Dennis C, Caine N, Shkarples L, Smyth R, Higenbottam T, Stewart S, Wreghitt T, Large S, Wells FC, Wallwork J. Heart-lung transplantation for end-stage respiratory disease in patients with cystic fibrosis at Papworth Hospital. J Heart Lung Transplant 12:893–902, 1993.

Devaux D, Epstein SL, Sachs DH, Pierres M. Cross-reactive idiotypes of monoclonal anti-Ia antibodies: characterization with xenogeneic anti-idiotypic reagents and expression in anti-H2 humoral responses. J Immunol 129:2074–2081, 1982.

DeVoe PW, Buckley RH, Shirley LR, Darby CP, Ward FE, Mickey GH, Raab-Traub N, Vandenbark GH. Successful immune reconstitution in severe combined immunodeficiency despite Epstein-Barr virus and cytomegalovirus infections. Clin Immunol Immunopathol 34:48–59, 1985.

Donaldson PT, O'Grady J, Portmann B, Davis H, Alexander GJM,

Neuberger J, Thick M, Calne RY, Williams L. Evidence for an immune response to HLA class I antigens in the vanishing bile duct syndrome after liver transplantation. Lancet 1:945–948, 1987.

Dougherty PC, Zinkernagel RM. A biologic role for the major histocompatibility antigens. Lancet 1:1406–1409, 1975.

Dresser DW, Mitchison NA. The mechanism of immunological paralysis. Adv Immunol 8:120–181, 1968.

Ebringer A, Ghudoom M. Ankylosing spondylitis, HLA-B27, and *Klebsiella*: cross-reactivity and antibody studies. Ann Rheum Dis 45:703–704, 1986.

Ehrlich RM. Surgical complications of renal transplantation. Ann Intern Med 100:246–257, 1984.

Eichwald EJ, Wetzel B, Lustgraaf EC. Genetic aspects of second-set skin grafts in mice. Transplantation 4:260–273, 1966.

Elkins CC, Frist WH, Dummer JS, Stewart JR, Merrill WH, Carden KA, Bender HW. Cytomegalovirus disease after heart transplantation: is acyclovir prophylaxis indicated? Ann Thoracic Surg 56:1267–1273, 1993.

Eltumi M, Trivedi P, Hobbs JR, Portmann B, Cheeseman P, Downie C, Risteli J, Risteli L, Mowat AP. Monitoring of veno-occlusive disease after bone marrow transplantation by serum aminopropeptide of type III procollagen. Lancet 342:518–521, 1993.

Ettenger RB, Fine RN. Pediatric renal transplantation. In Garovoy MR, Guttmann RD, eds. Renal Transplantation. New York, Churchill Livingstone, 1986, pp. 339–435.

Ettenger RB, Rosenthal JT, Marik J. Cadaver renal transplantation in children: results with long-term cyclosporine immunosuppression. Clin Transplant 4:329–336, 1990.

Farges O, Ericzon B, Bresson-Hadni S, Lynch SV, Hockerstedt K, Houssin D, Galmarini D, Faure J, Baldauf C, Bismuth H. A randomized trial of OKT3-based versus cyclosporin-based immunoprophylaxis after liver transplantation. Transplantation 58:891–898, 1994.

Faustman D, Hauptfeld V, Lacy P, Davie J. Prolongation of murine islet allograft survival by pretreatment of islets with antibody directed to determinants. Proc Natl Acad Sci U S A 78:5156–5159, 1981.

Fefer A, Buckner CD, Thomas ED, Cheever MA, Clift RA, Glucksberg H, Neiman PE, Storb R. Cure of hematologic neoplasia with transplantation of marrow from identical twins. N Engl J Med 297:146–148, 1977.

Ferrara JLM, Deeg HJ. Graft-versus-host disease. N Engl J Med 324:667–674, 1991.

Festenstein H, Doyle P, Holmes J. Long-term follow-up in London transplant group recipients of cadaver renal allografts. N Engl J Med 314:7–14, 1986.

Filipovich AH, Youle RJ, Neville DM, Vallera DA, Quinones R, Kersey JH. Ex vivo treatment of donor bone marrow with anti–T cell immunotoxins for prevention of graft-versus-host disease. Lancet 1:469–472, 1984.

Fine RN. Growth after renal transplantation in children. J Pediatr 110:414–416, 1987.

Fischer A, Durandy A, de Villartay J-P, Vilmer E, Le Deist F, Gerota I, Griscelli C. HLA-haploidentical bone marrow transplantation for severe combined immunodeficiency using E rosette fractionation and cyclosporine. Blood 67:444–449, 1986a.

Fischer A, Friedrich W, Levinsky R, Vossen J, Griscelli C, Kubanek B, Morgan G, Wagemaker G, Landais P. Bone marrow transplantation for immunodeficiencies and osteopetrosis: European survey, 1968–1985. Lancet 1:1080–1083, 1986b.

Fischer A, Griscelli C, Blanche S. Prevention of graft failure by an anti-LFA-1 monoclonal antibody in HLA-mismatched bone marrow transplantation. Lancet 2:1058–1061, 1986c.

Fischer A, Landais P, Friedrich W. European experience of bone marrow transplantation for severe combined immunodeficiency. Lancet 336:850–854, 1990.

Fischer A, Landais P, Friedrich W, Gerritsen B, Fasth A, Porta F, Vellodi A, Benkerrou M, Jais JP, Cavazzana-Calvo M, Souillet G, Bordigoni P, Morgan G, Van Dijken P, Vossen J, Locatelli F, di Bartolomeo P. Bone marrow transplantation (BMT) in Europe for primary immunodeficiencies other than severe combined immunodeficiency: a report from the European Group for BMT and the European Group for Immunodeficiency. Blood 83:1149–1154, 1994.

Flye MW, Hendrisak MD. Liver transplantation in the child. World J Surg 10:432–441, 1986.

Foroozanfar N, Hobbs JR, Hugh-Jones K, Humble JG, James DCO, Selwyn S, Watson JG, Yamamura M. Bone marrow transplantation from an unrelated donor for chronic granulomatous disease. Lancet 1:210–213, 1977.

French ME, Batchelor JR. Enhancement of renal allografts in rats and man. Transplant Rev 13:115–141, 1972.

Fricker FJ, Griffith BP, Hardesty RL, Trento A, Gold LM, Schmeltz K, Beerman LB, Fischer DR, Mathews RA, Neches WH, Park SC, Zuberbuhler JR, Lenox CC, Bahnson HT. Experience with heart transplantation in children. Pediatrics 79:138–146, 1987.

Friedlander GE, Mankin HJ, Sell KW. Osteochondral Allografts. Biology, Banking and Clinical Applications. Boston, Little, Brown & Co, 1983.

Fukushima N, Gundry SR, Razzouk AJ, Bailey LL. Risk factors for graft failure associated with pulmonary hypertension after pediatric heart transplantation. J Thoracic Cardiovasc Surg 107:985–989, 1994.

Gale RP, Champlin RE. How does bone marrow transplantation cure leukaemia? Lancet 2:28–30, 1984.

Garcia CR, Brown NA, Schreck R, Stiehm ER, Hudnall SD. B cell lymphoma in severe combined immunodeficiency not associated with the Epstein-Barr virus. Cancer 60:2941–2947, 1987.

Gatti RA, Meuwissen HJ, Allen HD, Hong R, Good RA. Immunological reconstitution of sex-linked lymphopenic immunological deficiency. Lancet 2:1366–1369, 1968.

Gerritsen EJA, Vossen JM, Fasth A, Friedrich W, Morgan G, Padmos A, Vellodi A, Porras O, O'Meara A, Porta F, Bordigoni P, Cant A, Hermans J, Griscelli C, Fischer A. Bone marrow transplantation for autosomal recessive osteopetrosis. J Pediatr 125:896–902, 1994.

Ginsburg D, Antin JH, Smith BR, Orkin SH, Rappeport JM. Origin of cell populations after bone marrow transplantation: analysis using DNA sequence polymorphisms. J Clin Invest 75:596–603, 1985.

Glucksberg H, Storb R, Fefer A, Buckner CD, Neiman PE, Clift RA, Lerner KG, Thomas ED. Clinical manifestations of graft-versus-host disease in human recipients of marrow from HL-A-matched sibling donors. Transplantation 18:295–304, 1974.

Goldman JM, Apperley JF, Jones L, Marcus R, Goolden AWG, Batchelor R, Hale G, Waldmann H, Reid CD, Hows J, Gordon-Smith E, Catovsky D, Galton DAG. Bone marrow transplantation for patients with chronic myeloid leukemia. N Engl J Med 314:202–207, 1986.

Goldsobel AB, Haas A, Stiehm ER. Bone marrow transplantation in DiGeorge syndrome. J Pediatr 111:40–44, 1987.

Good RA. Bone marrow transplantation symposium: bone marrow transplantation for immunodeficiency diseases. Am J Med Sci 294:68–74, 1987.

Graff R, Bailey DW. The non-H2 histocompatibility loci and their antigens. Transplant Rev 15:26–49, 1973.

Gratama JW, Stijnen T, Weiland HT, Hekker AC, de Gast GC, Zwaan FE, Weijers TF, D'Amaro J, The TH, Vossen JMJJ. Herpes virus immunity and acute graft-versus-host disease. Lancet 1:471–474, 1987.

Graze PR, Gale RP. Chronic graft-versus-host disease: a syndrome of disordered immunity. Am J Med 66:611–620, 1979.

Gregersen PK, Shen M, Song QL, Merryman P, Degar S, Seki T, Maccari J, Goldberg D, Murphy H, Schwenzer J, Wang, CY, Winchester RJ, Nepom GT, Silver J. Molecular diversity of HLA-DR4 haplotypes. Proc Natl Acad Sci U S A 83:2642–2646, 1986.

Hefton JM, Amberson JB, Biozes DG, Weksler ME. Loss of HLA expression by human epidermal cells after growth in culture. J Invest Dermatol 83:48–50, 1984.

Hitzig WH, Willi H. Hereditare lymphoplasmocytase dysginesie. Schweiz Med Wochenschr 91:1625–1633, 1961.

Hodson ME. Heart-lung transplantation for cystic fibrosis. Eur J Pediatr 151:55–58, 1992.

Hoitsma JA, van Lier HJJ, Wetzels JFM, Berden JHM, Koene RAP. Cyclosporine treatment with conversion after three months versus conventional immunosuppression in renal allograft recipients. Lancet 1:584–586, 1987.

Hokken-Koelega ACS, Stijnen T, de Ridder MAJ, de Muinck Keizer-Schrama MPF, Wolff ED, de Jong MCJW, Donckerwolcke RA, Groothoff JW, Blum WF, Drop SLS. Growth hormone treatment in growth-retarded adolescents after renal transplant. Lancet 343:1313–1317, 1994a.

Hokken-Koelega ACS, van Zaal MAE, de Ridder MAJ, Wolff ED, de Jong MCJW, Donckerwolcke RA, de Muinck Keizer-Schrama MPF, Drop SLS. Growth after renal transplantation in prepubertal children: impact of various treatment modalities. Pediatr Res 35:367–371, 1994b.

Hollander AAMJ, van Saase JLCM, Kootte AMM, van Dorp WT, van Bockel HJ, van Es LA, van der Woude FJ. Beneficial effects of conversion from cyclosporin to azathioprine after kidney transplantation. Lancet 345:610–614, 1995.

Hood L, Steinmetz M, Malissen B. Genes of the major histocompatibility complex of the mouse. Annu Rev Immunol 1:529–568, 1983.

Hunkapiller T, Hood L. The growing immunoglobulin gene superfamily. Nature 323:15–16, 1986.

Ildstad ST, Sachs DH. Reconstitution with syngeneic plus allogeneic or xenogeneic bone marrow leads to specific acceptance of allografts or xenografts. Nature 307:168–170, 1984.

Iwatsuki S, Rabin BS, Shaw BW, Starzl TE. Liver transplantation against T cell positive warm crossmatches. Transplant Proc 16:1427–1429, 1984.

Janossy G, Prentice HG, Grob JP, Ivory K, Tidman N, Grundy J, Favrot M, Brenner MK, Campana D, Blacklock HA, Gilmore MJML, Patterson J, Griffiths PD, Hoffbrand AV. T lymphocyte regeneration after transplantation of T cell depleted allogeneic bone marrow. Clin Exp Immunol 63:577–586, 1986.

Jeffers GJ, Fuller TC, Cosimi AB, Russell PS, Winn HJ, Colvin RB. Monoclonal antibody therapy: anti-idiotypic and non-antiidiotypic antibodies to OKT3 arising despite intense immunosuppression. Transplantation 41:572–578, 1986.

Kaliss N. Immunological enhancement of tumor homografts in mice: mice. a review. Cancer Res 18:992–1003, 1958.

Kauffman HP, Stormstad AS, Sampson D, Stawicki AT. Randomized steroid therapy of human kidney transplant rejection. Transplant Proc 11:36–38, 1979.

Kawauchi M, Gundry SR, Alonso de Begona J, Fullerton DA, Razzouk AJ, Boucek MM, Nehlsen-Cannarella S, Bailey LL. Male donor into female recipient increases the risk of pediatric heart allograft rejection. Ann Thoracic Surg 55:716–718, 1993.

Kaye MP. Pediatric thoracic transplantation: the world experience. J Heart Lung Transplant 12:344–350, 1993.

Kino T, Hatanaka H, Miyata S. FK-506, a novel immunosuppressant isolated from a *Streptomyces*. II. Immunosuppressive effect of FK-506 in vitro. J Antibiot (Tokyo) 40:1256–1265, 1987.

Kissmeyer-Nielsen F, Olsen S, Petersen VP, Fjeldborg O. Hyperacute rejection of kidney allografts associated with pre-existing humoral antibodies against donor cells. Lancet 2:662–665, 1966.

Klein J. Biology of the Mouse Histocompatibility Complex: Principles of Immunogenetics Applied to a Single System. Berlin: Springer, 1975.

Kortz EO, Sachs DH. Mechanisms of specific transplantation tolerance induction by vascular allografts across a class I difference in miniature swine. Transplant Proc 19:861–863, 1987.

Korver K, De Lange GG, Langloid van den Bergh R, Schellekens PTA, Van Loghem E, van Leeuwen F, Vossen JM. Lymphoid chimerism after allogeneic bone marrow transplantation. Transplantation 44:643–650, 1987.

Krensky AM. The human cytolytic T lymphocyte response to transplantation antigens. Pediatr Res 19:1231–1234, 1985.

Krivit W, Whitley CB. Bone marrow transplantation for genetic diseases. N Engl J Med 316:1085–1087, 1987.

Kronenberg M, Siu G, Hood L, Shastri N. The molecular genetics of the T cell antigen receptor and T cell antigen recognition. Ann Rev Immunol 4:529–591, 1986.

Lacy PE, Davie JM, Finke EH. Prolongation of islet allograft survival following in vitro culture (24°C) and a single injection of ALS. Science 204:312–313, 1979.

Lafferty KJ, Bootes A, Dart G, Talmage DW. Effect of organ culture on the survival of thyroid allografts in mice. Transplantation 22:138–149, 1976.

Laine J, Jalanko H, Holthofer H, Krogerus L, Rapola J, von Willebrand E, Lautenschlager I, Salmela K, Holmberg C. Post-transplantation nephrosis in congenital nephrotic syndrome of the Finnish type. Kidney Int 44:867–874, 1993.

Lancaster F, Chui YL, Batchelor JR. Anti-idiotypic T cells suppress rejection of renal allografts in rats. Nature 315:336–337, 1985.

LeBidois J, Kachaner J, Vouhe P, Sidi D, Tamisier D. Heart transplantation in children: mid-term results and quality of life. Eur J Pediatr 151:59–64, 1992.

Leithner C, Sinzinger H, Pohanka E, Schwarz M, Kretschmer G, Syre G. Occurrence of hemolytic uremic syndrome under cyclosporine treatment: accident or possible side effect mediated by a lack of prostacyclin-stimulating plasma factor. Transplant Proc 15:2787–2789, 1985.

Leone MR, Alexander SR, Barry JM, Henell K, Funnell MB, Goldstein G, Norman DJ. OKT3 monoclonal antibody in pediatric kidney transplant recipients with recurrent and resistant allograft rejection. J Pediatr 111:45–50, 1987.

Lilly F, Boyse EA, Old LI. Genetic basis of susceptibility to viral leukaemogenesis. Lancet 2:1207–1209, 1964.

Lopez de Castro JA, Barbosa JA, Krangel MS, Biro PA, Strominger JL. Structural analysis of the functional sites of Class I HLA antigens. Immunol Rev 85:149–168, 1985.

Lopez D, Barber DF, Villadangos JA, Lopez de Castro JA. Cross-reactive T cell clones from unrelated individuals reveal similarities in peptide presentation between HLA-B27 and HLA-DR2. J Immunol 150:2675–2686, 1993.

Lorenz E, Cogdon C, Uphoff D. Modification of acute radiation injury in mice and guinea pigs by bone marrow injection. Radiology 58:863–877, 1952.

Lucarelli G, Galimberti M, Polchi P, Giardini C, Politi P, Baronciani D, Angelucci E, Manenti F, Delfini C, Aureli G, Muretto P. Marrow transplantation in patients with advanced thalassemia. N Engl J Med 316:1050–1055, 1987.

Lucarelli G, Galimberti M, Polchi P, Angelucci E, Baronciani D, Giardini C, Andreani M, Agostinelli F, Albertini F, Clift RA. Marrow transplantation in patients with thalassemia responsive to iron chelation therapy. N Engl J Med 329:840–844, 1993.

Lum LG, Seigneuret MC, Storb R. The transfer of antigen-specific humoral immunity from marrow donors to marrow recipients. J Clin Immunol 6:389–396, 1986.

Lund DP, Lillehei CW, Kevy S, Perez-Atayde A, Maller E, Treacy S, Vacanti JP. Liver transplantation in newborn liver failure: treatment for neonatal hemochromatosis. Transplant Proc 25:1068–1071, 1993.

Lundgren G. Widening indication of kidney transplantation—are there limits? Transplant Proc 19:63–66, 1987.

Lundgren G, Albrechtsen D, Flatmark A, Gabel H, Klintmalm G, Persson H, Groth CG, Brynger H, Frodin L, Husberg B, Maurer W. Thorsby E. HLA matching and pretransplant blood transfusions in cadaveric renal transplantation: a changing picture with cyclosporin. Lancet 2:66–69, 1987.

Madden BP, Kamalvand K, Chan CM, Khaghani A, Hodson ME, Yacoub M. The medical management of patients with cystic fibrosis following heart-lung transplantation. Eur Respir J 6:965–970, 1993.

Madden MR, Finkelstein JL, Staiano-Coico L, Goodwin LW, Shires GT, Nolan EE, Hefton JM. Grafting of cultured allogeneic epidermis on second and third degree burn wounds on 16 patients. J Trauma 26:955–962, 1986.

Maraninchi D, Blaise D, Rio B, Leblond V, Dreyfus F, Gluckman E, Guyotat D, Pico JL, Michallet M, Ifrah N, Bordigoni A. Impact of T cell depletion on outcome of allogeneic bone marrow transplantation for standard risk leukaemias. Lancet 2:175–178, 1987.

Martin PJ, Hansen JA, Storb R, Thomas ED. Human marrow transplantation in immunological perspective. Adv Immunol 40:379–438, 1987.

Maynard LC. Pediatric heart-lung transplantation for cystic fibrosis. Heart Lung 23:279–284, 1994.

McDevitt HO, Bodmer WF. HLA immune response genes, and disease. Lancet 1:1269–1275, 1974.

McDevitt HO, Chinitz A. Genetic control of the antibody response: relationship between immune response and histocompatibility (H-2) type. Science 163:1207–1208, 1969.

McDonald GB, Sharma P, Matthews DE, Shulman HM, Thomas ED. The clinical course of 53 patients with venocclusive disease of the liver after marrow transplantation. Transplantation 39:603–608, 1985.

McEnery P, Stablein D, Arbus G, Tejani A. Renal transplantation in children. N Engl J Med 326:1727–1732, 1992.

Medawar PB The behaviour and fate of skin autografts and skin homografts in rabbits. J Anat 78:176–199, 1944.

Medawar PB. Immunity to homologous grafted skin: II. The relationship between antigens of blood and skin. Br J Exp Pathol 27:15–24, 1946.

Mempel W, Gross-Wilde H, Baumann P, Netzel B, Steinbauer-Rosenthal I, Scholz S, Bertrams J, Albert ED. Population genetics of the MLC response: typing for MLC determinants using homozygous and heterozygous reference cells. Transplant Proc 5:1529–1534, 1973.

Michelsen B, Lernmark A. Molecular cloning of a polymorphic DNA endonuclease fragment associates insulin dependent diabetes mellitus with HLA-DQ. J Clin Invest 79:1144–1152, 1987.

Michler RE, Chen JM, Mancini DM, Reemtsma K, Rose EA. Sixteen years of cardiac transplantation: The Columbia-Presbyterian Medical Center Experience. In Terasaki PI, Cecka JM, eds. Clinical Transplants 1993. Los Angeles, UCLA Tissue Typing Laboratory, 1994, pp. 109–118.

Mickelson EM, Fefer A, Storb R, Thomas ED. Correlation of the relative response index with marrow graft rejection in patients with aplastic anemia. Transplantation 22:294–330, 1976.

Mickelson EM, Guthrie LA, Etzioni R, Anasetti C, Martin PJ, Hansen JA. Role of the mixed lymphocyte culture (MLC) reaction in marrow donor selection: matching for transplants from related haploidentical donors. Tissue Antigens 44:83–92, 1994.

Miller LC, Lum CT, Bock GH, Simmons RL, Najarian JS, Mauer SM. Transplantation of the adult kidney into the very small child: technical considerations. Am J Surg 145:243–247, 1983.

Miller LW, Naftel DC, Bourge RC, Kirklin JK, Brozena SC, Jarcho J, Hobbs RE, Mills RM. Infection after heart transplantation: a multiinstitutional study. J Heart Lung Transplant 13:381–393, 1994.

Monaco AP, Wood ML. Studies on heterologous antilymphocyte serum in mice: VII. Optimal cellular antigen for induction of immunologic tolerance with antilymphocyte serum. Transplant Proc 2:489–496, 1970.

Morris PJ, Allen RD, Thompson JF, Chapman JR, Ting A, Dunnill MS, Wood RFM. Cyclosporin conversion versus conventional immunosuppression: long term follow-up and histological evaluation. Lancet 1:586–592, 1987.

Mowat AP. Liver disorders in children: the indications for liver replacement in parenchymal and metabolic diseases. Transplant Proc 19:3236–3241, 1987.

Muller-Ruchholtz W, Wottge HU, Muller-Hermerlink HK. Bone marrow transplantation in rats across strong histocompatibility barriers by selective elimination of lymphoid cells in donor marrow. Transplant Proc 8:537–541, 1976.

Nagao T, White JW, Calne RY. Kinetics of unresponsiveness induced by a short course of cyclosporine A. Transplantation 33:31–35, 1982.

Najarian JS, Almond S, Gillingham KJ, Mauer SM, Chavers BM, Nevins TE, Kashtan CE, Matas AJ. Renal transplantation in the first five years of life. Kidney Int 44:40–44, 1993.

Nepom GT, Hansen JA, Nepom BS. The molecular basis for HLA class II associations with rheumatoid arthritis. J Clin Immunol 7:1–7, 1987.

Nepom GT, Seyfried CA, Nepom BS. Immunogenetics of disease susceptibility: new perspectives in HLA. Pathol Immunopathol Res 5:37–46, 1986.

Nevins TE, Kjellstrand CM. Hemodialysis for children—a review. Int J Pediatr Nephrol 4:155–169, 1983.

Noel DR, Witherspoon RP, Storb R, Atkinson K, Doney K, Mickelson EM, Ochs HD, Warren RP, Weiden PL, Thomas ED. Does graft-versus-host disease influence the tempo of immunologic recovery after allogeneic human marrow transplantation? An observation on 56 long term survivors. Blood 51:1087–1105, 1978.

O'Reilly RJ, Kirkpatrick D, Kapoor N, Collins N, Brochstein J, Kernan N, Flomenberg N, Pollack M, Dupont B, Lopez C, Reisner Y. A comparative review of the results of transplants of fully allogeneic fetal liver and HLA-haplotype mismatched, T cell depleted marrow in the treatment of severe combined immunodeficiency. In Gale RP, Touraine J, Lucarelli G, eds. Fetal Liver Transplantation. New York, Alan R. Liss, 1985, pp. 327–342.

O'Reilly RJ, Brochstein J, Collins N, Keever C, Kapoor N, Kirkpatrick D, Kernan N, Dupont B, Burns J, Reisner Y. Evaluation of HLA-haplotype disparate parental marrow grafts depleted of T lymphocytes by differential agglutination with a soybean lectin and E rosette depletion for the treatment of severe combined immunodeficiency. Vox Sang 51:81–86, 1986.

O'Reilly RJ. Current developments in marrow transplantation. Transplant Proc 19:92–102, 1987.

O'Reilly RJ, Brochstein J, Dinsmore R, Kirkpatrick D. Marrow transplantation for congenital disorders. Semin Hematol 21:188–221, 1984.

Opelz G. HLA matching and transplant survival: effect of HLA matching in 10,000 cyclosporin-treated cadaver kidney transplants. Transplant Proc 19:92–102, 1987.

Opelz G, Henderson R. Incidence of non-Hodgkin lymphoma in kidney and heart transplant recipients. Lancet 342:1514–1516, 1993.

Opelz G, Wujciak T. The influence of HLA compatibility on graft survival after heart transplantation. N Engl J Med 330:816–819, 1994.

Parkman R. Human graft-versus-host disease. Immunodefic Rev 2:253–264, 1991.

Parkman R, Rappeport J, Geha R, Belli J, Cassadya R, Levey R, Nathan DG, Rosen RS. Complete correction of the Wiskott-Aldrich syndrome by allogeneic bone marrow transplantation. N Engl J Med 298:921–927, 1978.

Payne R, Rolfs MR. Fetomaternal leukocyte incompatibility. J Clin Invest 37:1756–1763, 1958.

Perdue ST. Risk factors for second transplants 1985. In Terasaki PI, ed. Clinical Kidney Transplants. Los Angeles, UCLA Tissue Typing Laboratory, 1985, pp. 191–203.

Pescovitz MD, Thistlethwaite JR, Auchincloss H, Ildstad ST, Sharp TG, Terrill R, Sachs DH. Effect of class II antigen matching on renal allograft survival in miniature swine. J Exp Med 160:1495–1508, 1984.

Pillow RP, Epstein RB, Buckner CD, Giblett ER, Thomas E. Treatment of bone marrow failure by isogeneic marrow infusion. N Engl J Med 275:94–97, 1966.

Platz P, Jakobsen BK, Morling M, Ryder LP, Svejgaard A, Thomsen M, Christy M, Kromann H, Been J, Nerup J, Green A. A genetic analysis of insulin-dependent diabetes mellitus. Diabetologia 21:108–115, 1982.

Rapaport FT. Role of streptococcal and other heterologous antigens in transplantation. Transplant Proc 2:447–453, 1970.

Rapaport FT, Chase RM. Homograft sensitivity induction by Group A streptococci. Science 145:407–408, 1964.

Rapaport FT, Markowitz AS, McCluskey RT. The bacterial induction of homograft sensitivity: III. Effects of Group A streptococcal membrane antisera. J Exp Med 129:623–645, 1969.

Reed E, Hardy M, Benvenisty A, Lattes C, Brensilver J, McCabe R, Reemtsma K, King DW, Suciu-Foca N. Effect of antiidiotypic antibodies to HLA on graft survival in renal allograft recipients. N Engl J Med 316:1450–1455, 1987.

Reinherz EL, Geha R, Rappeport JM, Wilson M, Penta AC, Hussey RE, Fitzgerald KA, Daley JF, Levine H, Rosen FS, Schlossman SF. Reconstitution after transplantation with T lymphocyte-depleted HLA haplotype-mismatched bone marrow for severe combined immunodeficiency. Proc Natl Acad Sci U S A 79:6047–6051, 1982.

Reisner Y, Kapoor N, Kirkpatrick D, Pollack MS, Cunningham-Rundles C, Dupont B, Hodes RJ, Good RA. Transplantation for severe combined immunodeficiency with HLA-A, B, D, DR incompatible parental marrow cells fractionated by soybean agglutinin and sheep red blood cells. Blood 61:341–348, 1983.

Reisner Y, Itzicovitch L, Meshorer A, Sharon, N. Hematopoietic stem cell transplantation using mouse bone marrow and spleen cells fractionated by lectins. Proc Natl Acad Sci U S A 75:2933–2936, 1978.

Ringden O, Ahstrom L, Lonnqvist B, Baryd I, Svedmyr E, Gahrton G. Allogeneic bone marrow transplantation in a patient with chemotherapy-resistant progressive histiocytosis X. N Engl J Med 316:733–735, 1987.

Rivat L, Rivat C, Daveau M, Ropartz C. Comparative frequencies of anti-IgA antibodies among patients with anaphylactic transfusion reactions and among normal blood donors. Clin Immunol Immunopath 7:340–348, 1977.

Rivera GK, Pinkel D, Simone JV, Hancock ML, Crist WM. Treatment of acute lymphoblastic leukemia—30 years' experience at St. Jude Children's Research Hospital. N Engl J Med 329:1289–1295, 1993.

Roberts JL, Volkman DJ, Buckley RH. Modified MHC restriction of donor-origin T cells in humans with severe combined immunodeficiency transplanted with haploidentical bone marrow stem cells. J Immunol 143:1575–1579, 1989.

Robertson RP. Pancreatic and islet transplantation for diabetes—cures or curiosities? N Engl J Med 327:1861–1868, 1992.

Rooney CM, Wimperis JZ, Brenner MK, Patterson J, Hoffbrand AV, Prentice HG. Natural killer cell activity following T cell depleted allogeneic bone marrow transplantation. Br J Haematol 62:413–420, 1986.

Ross AJ, Cooper A, Attie MF, Bishop HC. Primary hyperparathyroidism in infancy. J Pediatr Surg 21:493–499, 1986.

Rowlings PA, Horowitz MM, Armitage JO, Gale RP, Sobocinski KA, Zhang M, Bortin MM. Report from the International Bone Marrow Transplant Registry and the North American Autologous Bone Marrow Transplant Registry. In Terasaki PI, Cecka JM, eds. Clinical Transplants 1993. Los Angeles, UCLA Tissue Typing Laboratory, 1994, pp. 101–108.

Ruderman RJ, Poehling GG, Gray R, Nardone M, Goodman W, Seigler HF. Orthopedic complications of renal transplantation in children. Transplant Proc 11:104–106, 1979.

Russell PS, Cosimi AB. Transplantation. N Engl J Med 301:470–479, 1979.

Sachs DH. Specific immunosuppression. Transplant Proc 19:123–127, 1987.

Sachs DH, Bluestone JA, Epstein SL. Anti-idiotype responses in transplantation immunology. Transplant Proc 17:549–552, 1985.

Salvatierra O, Melzer J, Vincenti F, Amend WJC, Tomianovich S, Potter D, Husing R, Garovoy M, Feduska NJ. Donor-specific blood transfusions versus cyclosporine—the DST story. Transplant Proc 19:160–166, 1987.

Samuel D, Muller R, Alexander G, Fassati L, Ducot B, Benhamou J, Bismuth H. Liver transplantation in European patients with the hepatitis B surface antigen. N Engl J Med 329:1842–1847, 1993.

Sanfilippo F, MacQueen JM, Vaughn WK, Foulks GN. Reduced graft rejection with good HLA-A and B matching in high risk corneal transplantation. N Engl J Med 315:29–35, 1986.

Sanfilippo F, Vaughn WK, Spees EK, Bollinger RR. Cadaver renal transplantation ignoring peak reactive sera in patients with markedly decreasing pre-transplant sensitization. Transplantation 38:119–124, 1984.

Santos GW. Immunosuppression for clinical marrow transplantation. Semin Hematol 11:341–351, 1974.

Schiff SE, Buckley RH. Modified responses to recipient and donor B cells by genetically donor T cells from human haploidentical bone marrow chimeras. J Immunol 138:2088–2094, 1987.

Schiff SE, Kurtzberg J, Buckley RH. Studies of human bone marrow treated with soybean lectin and sheep erythrocytes: stepwise analysis of cell morphology, phenotype and function. Clin Exp Immunol 68:685–693, 1987.

Schneider TM, Kupiec-Weglinski JW, Towpik E, Strom TB, Tilney NL. Studies on mechanisms of acute rejection of vascularized organ allografts. Hum Immunol 15:320–329, 1986.

Schrezenmeier H, Marin P, Raghavachar A, McCann S, Hows J, Gluckman E, Nissen C, van't Veer-Korthof ET, Hinterberger LW, van Lint MT, Frickhofen N, Bacigalupo A. Relapse of aplastic anaemia after immunosuppressive treatment: a report from the European Bone Marrow Transplantation Group SAA Working Party. Br J Haematol 85:371–377, 1993.

Schwarer AP, Jiang YZ, Brookes PA, Barrett AJ, Batchelor JR, Goldman JM, Lechler RI. Frequency of anti-recipient alloreactive helper T cell precursors in donor blood and graft-versus-host disease after HLA-identical sibling bone marrow transplantation. Lancet 341:203–205, 1993.

Sheehy MJ, Bach FH. Primed LD typing (PLT)—technical considerations. Tissue Antigens 8:157–171, 1976.

Shevach EM. The effects of cyclosporin A on the immune system. Annu Rev Immunol 3:397–423, 1985.

Siegler HF, Ward FE, McCoy RE, Weinreth JL, Gunnells JC, Stickel DL. Long term results with forty-five living related renal allograft recipients genotypically identical for HLA. Surgery 81:274–283, 1977.

Simmons RL, Najarian JS. Kidney transplantation. In Simmons RL, Finch ME, Ascher NL, Najarian JS, eds. Manual of Vascular Access, Organ Donation, and Transplantation. New York, Springer-Verlag, 1984, pp. 292–328.

Sindel LJ, Buckley RH, Schiff SE, Ward FE, Mickey GH, Huang AT, Naspitz C, Koren H. Severe combined immunodeficiency with natural killer cell predominance: abrogation of graft-versus-host disease and immunologic reconstitution with HLA-identical bone marrow cells. J Allergy Clin Immunol 73:829–836, 1984.

Singer A, Hathcock KS, Hodes RJ. Self-recognition in allogeneic radiation bone marrow chimeras: a radiation-resistant host element dictates the self specificity and immune response gene phenotype of T helper cells. J Exp Med 153:1286–1301, 1981.

Sitges-Serra A, Caralps-Riera A. Hyperparathyroidism associated with renal disease. Surg Clin North Am 67:359–377, 1987.

Skinner J, Finlay JL, Sondel PM, Trigg ME. Infectious complications in pediatric patients undergoing transplantation with T lymphocyte depleted bone marrow. Pediatr Infect Dis 5:319–324, 1986.

Slavin S, Reitz B, Bieber CP, Kaplan HS, Strober S. Transplantation tolerance in adult rats using total lymphoid irradiation: permanent survival of skin, heart, and marrow allografts. J Exp Med 147:700–707, 1978.

So SKS, Mauer SM, Nevins TE, Fryd DS, Sutherland DER, Ascher NL, Simmons RL, Najarian JS. Current results in pediatric renal transplantation at the University of Minnesota. Kidney Int 30:25–30, 1986.

So SKS, Chang PN, Najarian JS, Mauer SM, Simmons RL, Nevins TE. Growth and development in infants after renal transplantation. J Pediatr 110:343–350, 1987.

Sollinger HW, Burkholder PM, Rasmus WR, Bach FH. Prolonged survival of xenografts after organ culture. Surgery 81:74–79, 1976.

Soulillou JP, Le Mauff B, Olive D, Delaage M, Peyronnet P, Hourmant M, Mawas C, Hirn M, Jacques Y. Prevention of rejection of kidney transplants by monoclonal antibody directed against interleukin 2. Lancet 1:1339–1342, 1987.

Starnes VA, Jamieson SW. Current status of heart and lung transplantation. World J Surg 10:442–449, 1986.

Starzl TE, Iwatsuki S, Shaw BWJ, Gordon RD, Esquivel C. Liver transplantation in the cyclosporin era. Prog Allergy 38:366–394, 1986.

Starzl TE, Esquivel C, Gordon R, Todo S. Pediatric liver transplantation. Transplant Proc 19:3230–3235, 1987.

Starzl TE, Demetris AJ, Trucco M, Ramos H, Zeevi A, Rudert WA, Kocova M, Ricordi C, Ildstad S, Murase N. Systemic chimerism in human female recipients of male livers. Lancet 340:876–877, 1992a.

Starzl TE, Demetris AJ, Murase N, Ildstad S, Ricordi C, Trucco M. Cell migration, chimerism and graft acceptance. Lancet 339:1579–1582, 1992b.

Starzl TE, Fung J, Tzakis A, Todo S, Demetris AJ, Marino IR, Doyle H, Zeevi A, Warty V, Michaels M, Kusne S, Rudert WA, Trucco M. Baboon to human liver transplantation. Lancet 341:65–71, 1993.

Starzl TE, Demetris AJ, Trucco M, Ricordi C, Ildstad S, Terasaki PI, Murase N, Kendall RS, Kocova J, Rudert WA, Zeevi A, van Thiel D. Chimerism after liver transplantation for type IV glycogen storage disease and type I Gaucher's disease. N Engl J Med 328:745–749, 1994.

Storb R, Thomas ED, Buckner CD, Appelbaum FR, Clift RA, Deeg HJ, Doney K, Hanson JA, Prentice RL, Sanders JE, Stewart P, Sullivan KM, Witherspoon RP. Marrow transplantation for aplastic anemia. Semin Hematol 21:27–35, 1984.

Storb R, Deeg HJ, Whitehead J, Appelbaum F, Beatty P, Bensinger W, Buckner CD, Clift R, Doney K, Farewell V, Hansen J, Hill R, Lum L, Martin P, McGuffin R, Sanders J, Stewart P, Sullivan K, Witherspoon R, Yee G, Thomas ED. Methotrexate and cyclosporine compared with cyclosporine alone for prophylaxis of acute graft-versus-host disease after marrow transplantation of leukemia. N Engl J Med 314:729–735, 1986.

Strober S. Natural suppressor (NS) cells, neonatal tolerance, and total lymphoid irradiation: exploring obscure relationships. Ann Rev Immunol 2:219–237, 1984.

Strom TB. The immunopharmacology of graft rejection. Transplant Proc 19:128–129, 1987.

Stuart FP, Fitch FW, Rowley DA. Specific suppression of renal allograft rejection by treatment with antigen and antibody. Transplant Proc 483:488, 1970.

Sullivan KA, Amos DB. The HLA system and its detection. In Rose NR, Friedman H, Fahey JL, eds. Manual of Clinical Laboratory Immunology. Washington, DC, American Society for Microbiology, 1986, pp. 835–846.

Suthanthiran M, Strom TB. Renal transplantation. N Engl J Med 331:365–394, 1994.

Sutherland DER, Moudry KC. Pancreas Transplant Registry report. Transplant Proc 4:5–7, 1987a.

Sutherland DER, Moudry KC. Clinical pancreas and islet transplantation. Transplant Proc 19:113–120, 1987b.

Sutherland DER, Moudry-Munns K, Gruessner A. Pancreas Transplant Results in United Network for Organ Sharing (UNOS) United States of American (USA) Registry with a comparison to non-USA data in the International Registry. In Terasaki PI, Cecka JM, eds. Clinical Transplants 1993. Los Angeles, UCLA Tissue Typing Laboratory, 1994, pp. 47–70.

Tejani A, Butt MH, Khawar MR, Phadke K, Adamson O, Hong J, Fusi M, Trachtman H. Cyclosporine experience in renal transplantation in children. Kidney Int 30:35–43, 1986.

Tejani A, Fine R, Alexander S, Harmon W, Stablein D. Factors predictive of sustained growth in children after renal transplantation. J Pediatr 122:397–402, 1993a.

Tejani A, Stablein D, Fine R, Alexander S. Maintenance immunosuppression therapy and outcome of renal transplantation in North American children: a report of the North American Pediatric Renal Transplant Cooperative Study. Pediatr Nephrol 7:132–137, 1993b.

Terasaki PI, Cecka JM. Clinical Transplants, 1993. Los Angeles, UCLA Tissue Typing Laboratory, 1994.

Terasaki PI, McClelland JD. Microdroplet assay of human serum cytotoxins. Nature 206:998–1000, 1964.

Theobald M, Nierle T, Bunjes D, Arnold R, Heimpel H. Host-specific interleukin-2-secreting donor T cell precursors as predictors of acute graft-versus-host disease in bone marrow transplantation between HLA-identical siblings. N Engl J Med 327:1613–1617, 1992.

Thomas ED. Marrow transplantation for malignant disease. Am J Med Sci 294:75–79, 1987.

Thomas ED, Storb R, Clift RA, Fefer A, Johnson FL, Neiman PE, Lerner KG, Glucksberg H, Buckner CD. Bone marrow transplantation. N Engl J Med 292:823–843, 1975.

Thorsby E. Structure and function of HLA molecules. Transplant Proc 19:29–35, 1987.

Thursz MR, Kwiatkowski D, Allsopp CEM, Greenwood BM, Thomas HC, Hill AVS. Association between an MHC Class II allele and clearance of hepatitis B virus in The Gambia. N Engl J Med 332:1065–1069, 1995.

Tiwari JL, Terasaki PI. HLA and Disease Associations. New York; Springer-Verlag, 1985.

Toronto Lung Transplant Group. Unilateral lung transplantation for pulmonary fibrosis. N Engl J Med 314:1140–1145, 1986.

Touraine J, Roncarolo M, Plotnicky H, Bachetta R, Spits H. T lymphocytes from human chimeras do recognize antigen in the context of allogeneic determinants of the major histocompatibility complex. Immunol Lett 39:9–12, 1994.

Treasure T. Autologous bone marrow and peripheral blood progenitor transplant for breast cancer. Lancet 344:418–419, 1994.

Trigg ME, Billing R, Sondel PM, Exten R, Hong R, Bozdech MJ, Horowitz SD, Finley JL, Moen R, Longo W, Erickson C, Peterson A. Clinical trial depleting T lymphocytes from donor marrow for matched and mismatched allogeneic bone marrow transplants. Cancer Treat Rep 69:377–386, 1985.

Tsang VT, Johnston A, Heritier F, Leaver N, Hodson ME, Yacoub M. Cyclosporin pharmacokinetics in heart-lung transplant recipients with cystic fibrosis. Eur J Clin Pharmacol 46:261–265, 1994.

Turrentine MW, Kesler KA, Caldwell R, Darragh R, Means L, Mahomed Y, Brown JW. Cardiac transplantation in infants and children. Ann Thoracic Surg 57:546–554, 1994.

Tutschka PJ. Diminishing morbidity and mortality of bone marrow transplantation. Vox Sang 51:87–94, 1986.

Tyden G, Lundgren G, Ost L, Kojima Y, Gunnarsson R, Ostman J, Groth CG. Progress in segmental pancreatic transplantation. World J Surg 10:404–409, 1986.

Tyler JD, Anderson CB, Sicard GA. Interleukin 2 response inhibition following donor specific transfusions given with azathioprine. Transplant Proc 19:258–261, 1987.

Uphoff DE. Preclusion of secondary phase of irradiation syndrome by inoculation of fetal hematopoietic tissue following lethal total body X irradiation. J Natl Cancer Inst 20:625–632, 1958.

U.S. Multicenter FK 506 Liver Study Group. A comparison of tacrolimus (FK 506) and cyclosporine for immunosuppression in liver transplantation. N Engl J Med 331:1110–1115, 1994.

Van Den Berg H, Vossen JM, van den Bergh RL, Bayer J, van Tol MJD. Detection of Y chromosome by in situ hybridization in combination with membrane antigens by two-color immunofluorescence. Lab Invest 64:623–628, 1994.

van Rood JJ. HLA antigens as carrier molecules. Hum Immunol 17:237–247, 1986.

van Rood JJ. Prospective HLA typing is helpful in cadaveric renal transplantation. Transplant Proc 19:139–143, 1987.

van Rood JJ, Eernisse JG, van Leewen A. Leukocyte antibodies in sera from pregnant women. Nature 181:1735–1736, 1958.

van Thiel DH. Liver transplantation. Pediatr Ann 14:474–480, 1985.

Vossen JM, van Leeuwen JEM, van Tol MJD, Joosten AM, Van Den Berg H, Gerritsen EJA, Haraldsson A, Meera Khan P. Chimerism and immune reconstitution following allogeneic bone marrow transplantation for severe combined immunodeficiency disease. Immunodeficiency 4:311–313, 1993.

Waldmann H, Hale G, Cicidalli G, Weshler Z, Manor D, Rachmilewitz EA, Polliak A, Or R, Weiss L, Samuel S, Brautbar C, Slavin S. Elimination of graft-versus-host disease by in vitro depletion of alloreactive lymphocytes with a monoclonal rat anti-human lymphocyte antibody (Campath-1). Lancet 2:483–486, 1984.

Wallwork J, Williams R, Calne RY. Transplantation of liver, heart and lungs for primary biliary cirrhosis and primary pulmonary hypertension. Lancet 2:182–184, 1987.

Weiden PL, Flournoy N, Thomas ED, Prentice R, Fefer A, Buckner CD, Storb R. Antileukemic effect of graft-versus-host disease in human recipients of allogeneic marrow grafts. N Engl J Med 300:1068–1073, 1979.

Weisdorf D, Haake R, Blazar B, Miller W, McGlave P, Ramsay N, Kersey J, Filipovich A. Treatment of moderate/severe acute graft-versus-host disease after allogeneic bone marrow transplantation: an analysis of clinical risk features and outcome. Blood 75:1024–1030, 1990.

Weisdorf DJ, Woods WG, Nesbit ME, Uckun F, Dusenbery K, Kim T, Haake R, Thomas W, Kersey JH, Ramsay NKC. Allogeneic bone marrow transplantation for acute lymphoblastic leukaemia: risk factors and clinical outcome. Br J Haematol 86:62–69, 1994.

Wells SA, Stirman JA, Bolman RM, Gunnells JC. Transplantation of the parathyroid glands: clinical and experimental results. Surg Clin North Am 58:391–402, 1978.

White DJG. Cyclosporin A: clinical applications and immunology. Clin Immunol Allergy 3:287–304, 1983.

Winchester RJ. The HLA system and susceptibility to diseases: an interpretation. Clin Aspects Autoimmunity 1:9–26, 1986.

Wolf E, Spencer KM, Cudworth AG. The genetic susceptibility to type I (insulin-dependent) diabetes: analysis of the HLA-DR association. Diabetologia 24:224–230, 1983.

Woodruff JM, Hansen JA, Good RA, Santos GW, Slavin RE. The pathology of the graft-versus-host reaction (GVHR) in adults receiving bone marrow transplants. Transplant Proc 8:675–684, 1976.

Wu AM, Till JE, Siminovitch L, McCulloch EA. A cytological study of the capacity for differentiation of normal hemopoietic colony-forming cells. J Cell Physiol 69:177–184, 1967.

Wu AM, Till JE, Simonovitch L, McCulloch EA. Cytological evidence for a relationship between normal hemopoietic colony-forming cells and cells of the lymphoid system. J Exp Med 127:455–463, 1968.

Wu S, Saunders TL, Bach FH. Polymorphism of human Ia antigens generated by reciprocal intergenic exchange between two DR loci. Nature 324:676–679, 1986.

Yamaoka Y, Tanaka K, Ozawa K. Liver Transplantation from Living-Related Donors. In Terasaki PI, Cecka JM, eds. Clinical Transplants 1993. Los Angeles, UCLA Tissue Typing Laboratory, 1994, pp. 179–184.

Yandza T, Alvarez F, Laurent J, Gauthier F, Dubousset A, Valayer J. Pediatric liver transplantation for primary hepatocellular carcinoma associated with hepatitis virus infection. Transplant Int 6:95–98, 1993.

Yeager AM, Kaizer H, Santos GW, Saral R, Colvin OM, Stuart RK, Braine HG, Burke PJ, Ambinder RF, Burns WH, Fuller DJ, Davis JM, Karp JE, May WS, Rowley SD, Sensenbrenner LL, Vogelsang GB, Wingard JR. Autologous bone marrow transplantation in patients with acute non-lymphocytic leukemia, using ex vivo marrow treatment with 4-hydroperoxycyclophosphamide. N Engl J Med 315:141–147, 1987.

Zales VR, Stapleton PL. Neonatal and infant heart transplantation. Pediatr Clin North Am 40:1023–1046, 1993.

Zinkernagel RM. Thymus function and reconstitution of immunodeficiency. N Engl J Med 298:222, 1978.

Zittoun RA, Maandelli F, Roel-Willemze R, de Witte T, Labar B, Resegotti L, Leoni F, Damasio E, Visani G, Papa G, Caronia F, Hayat M, Stryckmans P, Rotoli B, Leoni P, Peetermans ME, Dardenne M, Vegna ML, Petti MC, Solbu G, Suciu S. Autologous or allogeneic bone marrow transplantation compared with intensive chemotherapy in acute myelogenous leukemia. N Engl J Med 332:217–223, 1995.

APPENDIX 1

CLUSTER DESIGNATION NOMENCLATURE FOR HUMAN LEUKOCYTE DIFFERENTIATION ANTIGENS

Janis V. Giorgi

Leukocytes, also known as white blood cells, are responsible for immune responses, inflammation, and protection of the host against foreign pathogens. The membranes of leukocytes display an array of molecules that allow the various types of white blood cells to carry out their functions, interact with one another, and home to sites of immunologic activity (Lanier and Jackson, 1992; Barclay et al., 1993; Schlossman et al., 1995). Hundreds of different molecules have been identified on leukocytes. The function, structure, and leukocyte distribution of some of these molecules, known as leukocyte differentiation antigens (LDAs), have been defined (Table 1).

Much of our knowledge of the function, structure, and distribution of LDAs comes from studies using monoclonal antibodies (MAbs). Monoclonal antibodies against human LDAs have usually been produced in mice by injecting them with different types of leukocytes (e.g., thymocytes, tonsil cells, bone marrow, lymphocytes, and platelets). In order to pool knowledge so that faster progress can be made in understanding the immune system, scientists working on MAbs against LDAs often share reagents. In addition to informal exchanges, comprehensive formal exchanges, known as workshops, are held every few years. For these workshops, scientists prepare collaborative protocols, exchange thousands of reagents, and meet to share and interpret their results. These workshops lead not only to new knowledge, but also to an organized, internationally recognized system for keeping track of available MAbs.

Often, multiple MAbs are found that react with the same molecule on the surface of leukocytes. These molecules are considered to be discrete by the workshops when all investigators performing the tests agree that at least two MAbs react with a given molecule. For example, the two MAbs must reliably immunoprecipitate the same molecule and have identical reactivity with a broad panel of cell types. Monoclonal antibodies that react similarly are said to belong to the same "cluster designation" or "cluster of differentiation" (CD). MAb CDs are numbered consecutively. Since the first workshop, when CD1 to CD15 were defined, the current number of assigned CDs has grown to 130. Most of these are listed in Table 1. The naming system for human LDAs is referred to as the *CD nomenclature.*

The CD names refer to the monoclonal antibodies, not the LDAs. Thus, a MAb that reacts with the low-affinity immunoglobulin E (IgE) Fc receptor is called a CD23 MAb. Accordingly, it is proper to state that "staining was done with a CD23 MAb." Each individual MAb also has its own clone name. For example, Leu3a, OKT4, and T4 are all CD4 MAbs. Notably, MAbs that belong to the same CD may have different biologic activities. For example, Leu3a but not OKT4 blocks human immunodeficiency virus (HIV) binding to CD4$^+$ cells. Often, especially if the exact structure and function of the antigen with which the MAbs react is unknown or is complex, the antigen itself may be referred to by the CD number followed by the word "antigen" or "molecule." The literature can sometimes be confusing because these conventions are not always followed. One of the most common mistakes is to refer to an MAb as "anti-CDx" (e.g., "anti-CD3"; the proper phrase is "a CD3 MAb"). A second common mistake is to use the term "CDx" to signify the antigen itself (e.g., "soluble CD4" instead of "soluble CD4 molecule").

Table 1 lists the names of the defined clusters of MAbs as of November 1993 (Schlossman et al., 1995). No new clusters will be granted international recognition until the results of the next workshop are available, scheduled for November 1996. Information in the column indicating "leukocyte distribution" underscores the fact that only a few antigens are restricted to a particular cell lineage; for example, CD3 MAbs react only with T cells. The next workshop will investigate nine major categories of molecules or cell types. These categories of molecules are adhesion structures, cytokine receptors, and non-lineage antigens; the categories of cell types are B cells, endothelial cells, myeloid cells, natural killer cells, platelets, and T cells. Immature, mature, and activated cells often have distinct arrays of LDAs compared with one another, and there are large differences between cells that belong to differ-

Table 1. Human Leukocyte Differentiation Antigens

Monoclonal Antibody Cluster Designation	Leukocyte Distribution	Function of Antigen	Molecular Weight (10^3)*
CD1a	Thymocytes; Langerhans cells		49, 12
CD1b	Thymocytes; Langerhans cells		45, 12
CD1c	Thymocytes; Langerhans cells		43, 12
CD2	T; NK subset	LFA-2; CD58 receptor; E-rosette receptor	50
CD2R	Activated T	Activation-related epitope	50
CD3	T	TCR complex; γ, δ, ϵ, ζ chains	16, 20, 25–28
CD4	T subset; monocytes	MHC class II; HIV receptor	56
CD5	T;B subset	CD72 receptor	67
CD6	T		100
CD7	T;NK; platelets		40
CD8	T and NK subsets	MHC class receptor	68; 32–34
CD8β			68; 32–34
CD9	Platelets; pre-B; monocytes		24
CD10	Pre-B; PMN	Neutral endopeptidase; CALLA	100
CD11a	Leukocytes	α_1 integrin; CD54 receptor; LFA-1α	180
CD11b	Monocyte/myeloid; NK; T subset	α_M integrin; complement receptor type 3	165
CD11c	Monocyte/myeloid; NK; T subset	α_x integrin; complement receptor type 4	150
CDw12	Monocytes; PMN		90–120
CD13	Monocytes; PMN	Aminopeptidase N	150
CD14	Monocytes	Receptor for LPS-LPS binding protein complex	55
CD15	PMN; activated T	Lewis x Ag (X hapten)	CHO
CD15s	PMN; monocytes, eosin; lymph; epithelial	Sialylated Lewis x Ag	CHO
CD16	NK;PMN; T subset	IgG Fc receptor type III A and B	50–65
CD16b	NK;PMN; T subset	IgG Fc receptor type III B	48–60
CDw17	PMN; monocytes; platelets	Lactosylceramide	
CD18	Leukocytes	β_2 integrin	95
CD19	B; follicular dendritic		90
CD20	B		95; 33, 35, 37
CD21	B; follicular dendritic	Complement receptor type 2; EBV receptor	145
CD22	B	Adhesion receptor	130; 140
CD23	B	Low affinity IgE Fc receptor	45–50
CD24	B; PMN; follicular dendritic		38/41
CD25	T and B subsets; activated T	IL-2 receptor α	55
CD26	T	Dipeptidylpeptidase IV	110
CD27	T; plasma cells		110; 55
CD28	T subset	B7/BB1 antigen receptor	80; 44
CD29	Leukocytes; platelets	β_1 integrin	110; 130
CD30	Activated B; T		120; 105
CD31	Platelets; monocytes; PMN; NK; T subsets	gpIIa', endocam	140
CD32	Monocytes; PMN; B; platelets	IgG Fc receptor type II	40
CD33	Monocytes		67
CD34	Progenitor cells	L-selectin (CD62L) ligand	105–120
CD35	B; monocytes; PMN; erythrocytes	Complement receptor type 1; C3bR	160–250
CD36	Platelets; monocytes	gpIV; malaria receptor	88
CD37	B	Signal transduction	40–52
CD38	NK; thymocytes; activated T; plasma cells	ADP-ribosyl cyclase	45
CD39	B; macrophages; alloactivated T		78; 70–100
CD40	B	Costimulatory molecule for B; survival R	48/44
CD41	Platelets	α IIb integrin, gpIIB/IIIa	135; 120, 23
CD42a	Platelets	Clotting factor receptor, gpIX	22
CD42b	Platelets	Clotting factor receptor, gpIbα	160; 135, 23
CD42c	Platelets	Clotting factor receptor, gpIbβ	22
CD42d	Platelets	Clotting factor receptor, gpV	85
CD43	Leukocytes	Leucosialin (sialophorin)	95
CD44	Leukocytes	Hyaluronic acid receptor (H-CAM)	80–90
CD44R	Leukocytes	Specific for exon V9	
CD45	Leukocytes	Phosphatase (common leukocyte antigen)	180, 190, 205, 220
CD45RA	Most T; B; NK	Phosphatase	220, 205
CD45RB	Most T; B; NK	Phosphatase	190-205, 220
CD45RO	Activated/memory T	Phosphatase	180
CD46	Leukocytes; platelets	Membrane cofactor protein; measles virus R	66/56
CD47	Leukocytes; platelets	Integrin-associated protein, neurophilin	47–52
CD48	Leukocytes		43
CD49a-f	Leukocytes; platelets	Six variants, α_{1-6} integrins (VLA-1-6)	120-210
CD50	Leukocytes	ICAM-3; ligand of LFA-1	120; 124
CD51	Leukocytes; platelets	α integrin; vibronectin receptor	125, 25
CD52	Leukocytes	Signaling; defined by Campath-1 MAb	21–28
CD53	Leukocytes	Signal transduction	32–40
CD54	Activated lymphocytes; macrophages	ICAM-1, CD11a/18 ligand	90
CD55	Leukocytes	Decay accelerating factor	70; 75
CD56	NK; T subset	N-CAM	220/140
CD57	NK and T subset		CHO
CD58	Leukocytes	LFA-3; CD2 ligand	65–70
CD59	Leukocytes; platelets		18–20
CDw60	T subset; platelets	GD3 ganglioside	CHO
CD61	Platelets	β_3 integrin	95; 110
CD62E	Cytokine-activated endo; some leukocytes	E-selectin	115
CD62L	HEV; activated endo; lymph subset; monocytes; PMN; eosin	L-selectin; CD34 receptor	75–80

Table 1. Human Leukocyte Differentiation Antigens *Continued*

Monoclonal Antibody Cluster Designation	Leukocyte Distribution	Function of Antigen	Molecular Weight (10^3)*
CD62P	Endo; platelets; PMN; monocytes; lymph subset, NK	P-selectin	130; 150
CD63	Activated platelets	gp53	53
CD64	Monocytes	IgG Fc receptor type I	75
CDw65	PMN; monocytes	Fucoganglioside; ceramide-dodecasaccharide	CHO
CD66a	PMN	Biliary glycoprotein	160–180
CD66b	PMN	CEa gene member 6 (formerly CD67)	95–100
CD66c	PMN	Non–cross-reactive Ag	90
CD66d	PMN	CEA gene member 1	30
Cd66e	PMN	CEA	180–200
CD68	Monocytes; macrophages		110
CD69	Activated lymphocytes; platelets		34/28
CD70	Activated B and T	CD27 ligand	70, 90, 160; 75, 95, 170
CD71	Proliferating cells	Transferrin receptor	180; 95
CD72	B	CD5 ligand	86; 43/39
CD73	B; T subset	Ecto 5′-nucleotidase	69
CD74	B; monocytes	MHC class II associated invariant chain	41, 35, 33
CDw75	B; T subset		CHO
CDw76	B; T subset		CHO
CD77	Activated B	Globotriaosylceramide	CHO
CDw78	B		
CD79a-b	B	sIg receptor complex Igα and Igβ	33–40
CD80	Activated B and T; monocytes	CD28 ligand; B7/BB1	60
CD81	B; neuroblastoma	TAPA-1	26
CD82	Epithelial; endo	Signaling	50–53
CD83	Circulating dendritic; Langerhans	Defined by HB15 MAb	43
CDw84	Leukocytes		73
CD85	B and plasma cells; monocytes		120
CD86	B and plasma cells		80
CD87	PMN; monocytes; activated T lines	Urokinase plasminogen activator receptor	50–65
CD88		C5a receptor	40
CD89	PMN; monocytes; macrophages	IgA Fc receptor	55–70
CDw90	T; CD34+ bone marrow subset	Thy-1	25–35
CD91	Phagocytes	α₂-macroglobulin receptor	600; 515/85
CDw92	PMN; monocytes		70
CD93	PMN; monocytes		110; 120
CD94	NK; T subset	KP43	70; 43 dimer
CD95		Fas	42
CD96		Tactile (T-cell activation increased late expression)	240, 180, 160; 160
CD97		Activation Ag	74, 80, 89
CD98	Leukocytes (except myeloid); endo; stromal	4F2	120; 80, 40
CD99	T subset, broad	coded by autosomal X	32
CD99R			
CD100	Lymphocytes		300; 150
CDw101	T subset; PMN; monocytes	On T subset that proliferates to CD28 MAb	240 dimer; 140
CD102	Endo; platelets; leukocyte subset	ICAM-2	60
CD103	Intraepithelial lymphocytes	αᴱ integrin; human mucosal lymphocyte–1 Ag	175; 150, 25
CD104	Epithelial; thymocytes	β₄ integrin	200; 220
CD105		Endoglin, T-cell growth factor β₁ and β₃ receptor	180; <105
CD106		VCAM-1	90, 95; 100, 110
CD107a	Platelets	LAMP-1 activation	110
CD107b		LAMP-2	120
CDw108	Activated T; stromal		80
CDw109	Activated T; activated platelets, endo	? Signal transduction	170/150
CD115	Myeloid	Colony-stimulating factor–1 receptor	150
CDw116		Granulocyte macrophage colony-stimulating factor receptor	75, 85
CD117	Early hematopoietic	Stem cell factor receptor, c-Kit	145
CDw119	Broad	Interferon-γ receptor	90
CD120a		Tumor necrosis factor receptor type 1	55
CD120b		Tumor necrosis factor receptor type 2	75
CDw121aB		IL-1 receptor I	80
CD121b		IL-1 receptor II	68
CD122		IL-2 receptor β	75
CDw124		IL-4 receptor	140
CD126		IL-6 receptor	80
CDw127		IL-7 receptor	75
CDw128		IL-8 receptor	58–67
CDw130		gp130 (cytokine receptors)	130

*Molecular weight values are according to information provided at the Fifth Leukocyte Differentiation Antigen Workshop, Boston, March 3–7, 1993. The values separated by a semicolon represent unreduced versus reduced forms.

Data from Lanier et al., 1992, and Shaw et al., 1995.

Abbreviations: ADP = adenosine diphosphate; Ag = antigen; B = B cell; CALLA = common acute lymphoblastic leukemia antigen; CEA = carcinoembryonic antigen; EBV = Epstein-Barr virus; endo = endothelium; eosin = eosinophil; HCAM = homing cell adhesion molecule; HEV = high endothelial venules; HIV = human immunodeficiency virus; ICAM = intracellular Ig, immunoglobulin adhesion molecule; IL = interleukin; LAMP = lysosome-associated membrane protein; LFA = leukocyte function associated; LPS = lipopolysaccharide; lymph = lymphocytes; MAb = monoclonal antibody; MHC = major histocompatibility complex; N-CAM = neural cell adhesion molecule; NK = natural killer cell; PMN = polymorphonuclear cells; T = T cell; TAPA = target of antiproliferative antibody; TCR = T-cell receptor; V-CAM = vascular cell adhesion molecule; VLA = very late activation.

ent lineages. When known, one or more functions for the molecule defined by the MAb CDs is provided in Table 1 along with the molecular weight.

Not all the functionally important molecules on leukocytes belong to the class of antigens under consideration by the LDA workshops. For example, those molecules involved in antigen recognition by T cells (i.e., the α, β, γ, and δ chains of the T-cell receptor) are not included. Likewise, the molecules involved in antigen recognition by B cells (i.e., the immunoglobulin molecules) are excluded. The major histocompatibility complex (MHC) molecules, such as HLA-DR, are important in leukocyte function but are excluded because they are considered in the separate nomenclature scheme of human histocompatibility antigens known by a rather similar name (i.e., human leukocyte antigens [HLA]). These antigens are involved in transplant rejection.

The hundreds of different molecules on leukocytes and the thousands of available MAbs against them are overwhelming, even for cellular immunologists. The CD nomenclature is a system to keep track of this information. CD nomenclature may become outdated as knowledge of the functions of LDAs matures. However, MAbs against LDAs will remain important tools for probing lymphocyte biology, and the use of the CD nomenclature will probably persist as a shorthand for exchanging ideas and knowledge even if the functions and structure of all the LDAs became known.

A point that may be of special interest is that, in addition to their use in basic studies of human biology and disease, the MAbs that are designated by the CD nomenclature have applications in clinical care. Several MAbs, including those designated CD3, CD25, and CD11a, have been administered therapeutically as immunosuppressive agents in solid organ or bone marrow transplantation. Other MAbs are used for ex vivo selection or deletion of cells for transplant (e.g., CD34 to select stem cells). Second, MAbs are used to classify primary and secondary immunodeficiencies, including low numbers of T and B cells in severe combined immunodeficiency disorder (SCID) or SCID accompanied by natural killer cell defects (Giorgi et al., 1992). HIV disease management uses CD4$^+$ cell number and CD38 antigen expression as major markers of disease stage and for prognosis. Finally, MAbs are used extensively to classify leukemias and lymphomas in a valuable adjunct to the management of these malignancies (Landay and Duque, 1992).

References

1. Barclay AN, Birkeland ML, Brown MH, Beyers AD, Davis SJ, Somoza C, Williams AF: The Leucocyte Antigen Facts Book. London, Academic Press, 1993.
2. Giorgi JV, Kesson AM, Chou CC: Immunodeficiency and infectious disease. In Rose NR, DeMacario EC, Fahey JL, Friedman H, Penn GM, eds: Manual of Clinical Laboratory Immunology, 4th ed. Washington, DC, American Society for Microbiology, 1992, pp. 174–181.
3. Landay AL, Duque RE: Hematopoietic neoplasms. In Rose NR, DeMacario EC, Fahey JL, Friedman H, Penn GM, eds: Manual of Clinical Laboratory Immunology, 4th ed. Washington, DC, American Society for Microbiology, 1992, pp. 191–200.
4. Lanier LL, Jackson AL: Monoclonal antibodies: Differentiation antigens expressed on leukocytes. In Rose NR, DeMacario EC, Fahey JL, Friedman H, Penn GM, eds: Manual of Clinical Laboratory Immunology, 4th ed. Washington, DC, American Society for Microbiology, 1992, pp. 157–163.
5. Schlossman SF, Boumsell L, Gilks W, Harlan JM, Kishimoto T, Morimoto C, Ritz J, Shaw S, Silverstein R, Springer T, Tedder TF, Todd RF, eds: Oxford, Oxford University Press, 1995.

APPENDIX 2

PRINCIPAL HUMAN CYTOKINES

Susan F. Plaeger

	Molecular Weight (kD)	Immune Cells That Secrete	Immune Target Cells	General Function in Immune system	Association with Pathology/Therapeutic Potential	Comments
IL-1	17	MO, T, B lymphs, NK, PMN	T, B lymphs, MO, PMN	Cell activation and induction of effector function in inflammation and immunity	Increased in chronic inflammation, autoimmune disease; inhibitors or antagonists as potential therapeutics	2 proteins (α, β) with same receptors; IL-1 receptor antagonist competes for binding
IL-2	15–18	T, B lymphs	T, B lymphs, NK, MO, PMN	T and B cell activation and expansion; cytolytic enhancement	Increased in serum in allograft rejection; therapeutic potential in cancer, infectious disease (HIV) and transplantation	T_H1-associated cytokine
IL-3	28	T lymphs, thymic epithelium	Hematopoietic stem and progenitor cells	Synergizes for cell proliferation and differentiation	Therapeutic potential in pancytopenia, bone marrow failure	Also known as multi-CSF; member of hematopoietic cytokine family
IL-4	19	T lymphs	B, T lymphs, NK, MO, progenitor cells	Cell growth and differentiation, Ig isotype selection	Increase associated with lack of protective immunity in some parasitic infections (e.g., leishmaniasis); therapeutic potential in cancer, nematode infestations, HIV infection	T_H2-associated cytokine
IL-5	45	T lymphs	Eosinophils, basophils (B lymphs)	Cell growth, differentiation, and activation, chemotaxis	Increased levels in eosinophilia; therapeutic potential in atopic diseases	B-cell effects in humans may be limited; T_H2-associated cytokine
IL-6	21	T, B lymphs, MO	B, T lymphs, NK, thymocytes	Broad effects on cell growth, differentiation, and activation	Increased levels in diseases with immune activation (e.g., autoimmune, HIV, immune malignancy)	Growth factor for certain malignant cells
IL-7	20	Bone marrow, thymic stroma	B, T lymphs, NK, MO, thymocytes	Cell growth and differentiation, cytolytic potentiator	Therapeutic potential in immune deficiency, HIV infection, malignancies	Originally known as lymphopoietin-1
IL-8	8	T lymphs, MO, PMN	PMN	Cell activation, chemotaxis, adhesion	Increased in inflammatory diseases	Member of chemokine family of pro-inflammatory cytokines
IL-9	40	T lymphs	T, B lymphs, mast cells, thymocytes	Growth of activated T cells; mast cell growth differentiation (synergizes with IL-3 and/or IL-4)	May have tumorigenic potential; inhibitors as potential therapy in atopic diseases for suppression of IgE	Autocrine growth factor
IL-10	19	T lymphs, mast cells	T, B lymphs, MO thymocytes	Suppression of MO function; cell growth and differentiation	Potential association with chronic parasitemia; therapeutic potential as anti-inflammatory inhibitors as potential antiviral therapy	Homologous to open reading frame of EBV genome; T_H2-associated cytokine
IL-11	19	Stromal cells	Bone marrow progenitors	Synergizes for cell growth and differentiation	Therapeutic potential in thrombocytopenia	Shares biologic activities with IL-6
IL-12	75 hetero-dimer	B lymphs, MO, PMN	T lymphs, NK	Cytotoxic protentiator; cell growth and differentiation (T_H1 development)	Therapeutic potential in toxic shock, some parasitic infections, HIV infection	Mediator between adaptive and natural immunity; originally called NK cell stimulating factor

Table continued on following page

Appendix 2

	Molecular Weight (kD)	Immune Cells That Secrete	Immune Target Cells	General Function in Immune system	Association with Pathology/Therapeutic Potential	Comments
IL-13	10	T lymphs	MO, B lymphs	Cell adhesion, differentiation and activation; proliferation and isotype switching	Therapeutic potential as anti-inflammatory	Overlapping function with IL-4
IL-14	53	T cells; malignant B cells	B cells	Induction of B cell proliferation; inhibition of Ig secretion; selective expansion of B cell subpopulations	Not known	Shares activities with IL-4; formerly called high-molecular-weight B-cell growth factor
IL-15	14–15	Human stromal cells, MO	T, B lymphs, monocytes, NK cells, endothelial cells	Shared bioactivities with IL-2	Not known	Utilizes IL-2 receptor β and γ components; may require a unique receptor subunit as well
IFN-α, β	18–20	Leukocytes; fibroblasts	T, B lymphs, MO, NK	Antiproliferative effects; stimulates MO differentiations, APC activity, MHC expression; augments CTL generation and function; augments NK function; immune regulation	Potent antiviral activity, but may enhance viral pathology in certain infections; antitumor activity; IFN-α widely used to treat malignancies	>20 variants in IFN-α family
IFN-γ	20	T lymphs (T$_H$1) NK	T, B lymphs, MO, NK	Cell activation differentiation; up-regulation of MHC; cytolytic potentiator, antibody isotype selection	Therapeutic potential as antiviral (<IFN-α or β), antiprotozoal; effective in treatment of certain malignancies, chronic granulomatous disease	T$_H$1-associated cytokine
TNF-α	17	MO/MAC	T, B lymphs, MO, PMN	Mediation of inflammatory response; tumor cell killing; cell activation and cytokine secretion	Increased levels in cachexia, autoimmune disease, septic shock, HIV; therapeutic potential of inhibitors in these conditions; therapeutic potential in cancer, infections	Also called cachectin; shares receptors with TNF-β
TNF-β	25	T lymphs	T, B lymphs, MO, PMN	See TNF-α above, although generally less potent than TNF-α	See TNF-α above	Also called lymphotoxin; approximately 30% homology with TNF-α
GM-CSF	22	T, B lymphs, MO, mast cells, PMN	PMN, MO	Stimulation of proliferation, maturation, and function of hematopoietic cells; induction of cytokines from MO	Treatment of neutropenia/pancytopenia, post-bone marrow transplantation; augmentation of cell yield from transplant donors	
G-CSF	18–22	MO, PMN	PMN	Stimulation of PMN proliferation, differentiation, and activation	Treatment of neutropenia (fewer adverse effects than GM-CSF)	Shares sequence homology with IL-6
M-CSF	45–70	MO, B, T lymphs	MO/MAC	Stimulation of MO and other mononuclear phagocyte proliferation, differentiation, and survival; induction of cytokine release from MO and MO cytotoxic function	May have a role in autoimmune disease, osteoporosis, some malignancies; therapeutic potential in cancer and fungal disease; may lower plasma cholesterol	
TGF-β	25 Homo-dimer	Platelets, MO	T, B lymphs, NK, thymocytes, MO	Suppression of proliferation and inflammation; chemoattractant; suppression of cytotoxic function; down-regulation of antibody secretion (IgG, IgM); up-regulation of IgA	Therapeutic potential in wound healing, autoimmune disease, transplant rejection; inhibitors for glomerulonephritis	5 Isoforms

Note: Many cytokines have multiple effects on a wide variety of cell types. This table is not all-inclusive but is directed primarily toward immunologic effects in humans.

Abbreviations: APC = antigen-presenting cell; CSF = colony-stimulating factor; CTL = cytotoxic T lymphocyte; EBV = Epstein-Barr virus; G-CSF = granulocyte colony stimulating factor; GM-CSF = granulocyte-macrophage colony-stimualting factor; HIV = human immunodeficiency virus; IFN = interferon; Ig = immunoglobulin; IL = interleukin; lymphs = lymphocytes; MAC = macrophage; MHC = major histocompatibility complex; MO = monocyte; M-CSF = macrophage colony-stimulating factor; PMN = polymorphonuclear neutrophil; NK = natural killer; TGF = transforming growth factor; T$_H$1, T$_H$2 = T cell of heavy-chain phenotype, TNF = tumor necrosis factor.

References

Ambrus JL, Pippin J, Joseph A, Xu C, Blumenthal D, Tamayo A, Claypool K, McCourt D, Srikiatchatochorn A, Ford RJ. Identification of a cDNA for a human high-molecular-weight B-cell growth factor. Proc Natl Acad Sci U S A, 90:6330–6334, 1993.

Appasamy PM. Interleukin-7: biology and potential of clinical applications. Cancer Invest 11:487–499, 1993.

Armitage RJ, Macduff BM, Eisenman J, Paxton R, Grabstein KH. Il-1 has stimulatory activity for the induction of B cell proliferation and differentiation. J Immunol 154:483–490, 1995.

Davies DR, Wlodawer A, Cytokines and their receptor complexes. FASEB J 9:50–56, 1995.

Gately MK. Interleukin-12: a recently discovered cytokine with potential for enhancing cell-mediated immune responses to tumors. Cancer Invest 11:500–506, 1993.

Giri JG, Ahdieh M, Eisenman J, Shanebeck K, Grabstein K, Kumaki S, Namen A, Park LS, Cosman D, Anderson D. Utilization of the β and γ chains of the IL-2 receptor by the novel cytokine IL-15. EMBO J 13:2822–2830, 1994.

Herbert CA, Baker JB. Interleukin-8: a review. Cancer Invest 11:743–750, 1993.

Holland G, Zlotnik, A. Interleukin-10 and cancer. Cancer Invest 11:751–758, 1993.

Johnson CS. Interleukin-1: therapeutic potential for solid tumors. Cancer Invest 11:600–608, 1993.

Johnson HM, Bazer FW, Szente BE, Jarpe MA. How interferons fight disease. Sci Am 28 May 1994, pp 68–75.

Klein B. Cytokine, cytokine receptors, transduction signals, and oncogenes in human multiple myeloma. Semin Hematol 32:4–19, 1995.

Lindeman A, Mertelsmann R. Interleukin-3: structure and function. Cancer Invest 1:609–623, 1993.

Lotz M. Interleukin-6. Cancer Invest 1:732–742, 1993.

Mahanty S, Nutman TB. The biology of interleukin-5 and its receptor. Cancer Invest 11:624–634, 1993.

Neben S, Turner K. The biology of interleukin 11. Stem Cells Dayton 11:156–162, 1993.

Puri RK, Siegel JP. Interleukin-4 and cancer therapy. Cancer Invest 11:473–486, 1993.

Renauld JC, Houssiau F, Louahed J, Vink A, Van Snick J, Uyttenhove C. Interleukin-9. Adv Immunol 54:79–97, 1993.

Rubin JT. Interleukin-2: its biology and clinical application in patients with cancer. Cancer Invest 11:460–469, 1993.

Index

Note: Page numbers in *italics* refer to illustrations;
page numbers followed by t refer to tables.